The Clinical Practice of Medical-Surgical Nursing

The Clinical Practice of Medical-Surgical Nursing

Marjorie Beyers, R.N., M.S.N.
Director, Evanston Hospital School of Nursing
Evanston, Illinois

Susan Dudas, R.N., M.S.N.
Nurse Consultant, Department of Health, Education, and Welfare,
Public Health Service, Division of Resource Development,
Nursing Section, Chicago, Illinois; Independent Nurse Practitioner
and Ostomy Care Specialist, Whiting, Indiana

Little, Brown and Company
Boston

Copyright © 1977 by Little, Brown and Company (Inc.)

First Edition

All rights reserved. No part of this book may be reproduced in any form or by any electronic or mechanical means, including information storage and retrieval systems, without permission in writing from the publisher, except by a reviewer who may quote brief passages in a review.

Library of Congress catalog card no. 76-56022

ISBN 0-316-09262-2 (C)
ISBN 0-316-09263-0 (P)

Printed in the United States of America

This book is dedicated to our families

Contributing Authors

Cornelia van der staay Kenner, M.S.N.
Instructor in Surgical Nursing, Department of Surgery, Southwestern Medical School, University of Texas Health Science Center at Dallas; Assistant Professor, University of Texas College of Nursing

Mary Ann Krol, M.S.N.
Assistant Professor, Medical-Surgical Nursing, Loyola University School of Nursing, Chicago

Mary Marrs, B.S.N.
County Health Nurse, Boone County, Indiana

Virginia Myers Mermel, M.S.N.
Doctoral Candidate (D.N.Sc.); Instructor, Georgetown University School of Nursing, Washington, D.C.

Eileen Mulqueeny, M.S.N.
Assistant Specialist, University of Hawaii School of Medicine, Honolulu; formerly Assistant Professor, University of Hawaii School of Nursing

Irene Schreck, M.S.N.
Assistant Professor, Marquette University College of Nursing, Milwaukee, Wisconsin

Contents

Contributing Authors vi

Preface viii

Acknowledgments ix

part I		Concepts Basic to Clinical Practice in Nursing	
chapter 1		Health and Disease States	3
		Basic Concepts 5 Communicable Diseases and Infections 64 The Patient Requiring Surgery 80 The Patient with Cancer 105	
chapter 2		Fluid and Electrolyte Balance Virginia Mermel	149
part II		Clinical Nursing Care	
chapter 3		Patients with Respiratory System Dysfunction	195
chapter 4		Patients with Cardiovascular System Dysfunction Eileen Mulqueeny	311
chapter 5		Patients with Hematopoietic and Lymphatic System Dysfunction	413
chapter 6		Patients with Kidney and Urinary Tract Dysfunction	467
chapter 7		Patients with Gastrointestinal System Dysfunction	523
chapter 8		Patients with Selected Endocrine Disorders	621
chapter 9		Patients with Reproductive System Dysfunction	733
chapter 10		Patients with Musculoskeletal System Dysfunction Irene Schreck	805
chapter 11		Patients with Nervous System Dysfunction	889
chapter 12		Patients with Eye Dysfunction	991
chapter 13		Patients with Ear, Nose, and Throat Dysfunction	1033
chapter 14		Patients with Integumentary System Dysfunction	1093
chapter 15		Patients with Thermal Injuries Cornelia Kenner	1135
chapter 16		Patients in Shock Mary Ann Krol	1177
		Index	1207

Preface

This book is a representation of the knowledge of nursing practice in the evolving field of medical-surgical nursing. From their varied experiences, the authors have confirmed that the proper basis for nursing practice is a sound knowledge of health and disease in the broadest sense—how one stays healthy, the physiologic and psychological changes in illness or dysfunction, and the adaptations people make to changes in their health status—and have developed this book accordingly. Peripheral to this basis for nursing practice are the myriad nursing specialties such as acute care, chronic care, gerontologic care, public health care, and advisor or consultant to other care givers. Another determinant is the organizational structure within which nurses function; these structures are of necessity and purpose different in many respects, and the differences influence nursing practice.

The scope of the book is the nursing care of adults with medical-surgical illnesses. The book is primarily intended for undergraduate nursing students who have a beginning competence in the knowledge and skills fundamental to nursing and who have completed basic social and physiologic science courses. It is expected that the student is able to integrate this previously acquired knowledge with new knowledge in this book. The practicing nurse will find this book a useful reference. Assessment of the patient's condition, care and treatment methods, decisions about care, and evaluation of the patient's response and progress from acute illness to rehabilitation are considered in relation to the basic disease processes most frequently encountered in the adult population.

In Part I, the reader is drawn into the health-illness arena with its many variables. Discussed are the health care practices commonly encountered in medical-surgical nursing: medical therapy, surgery, fluid and electrolyte balance, oncology. In Part II the systems approach is used for autonomous chapters that may be studied in sequence or at random. The straightforward presentation of the content enables the faculty to have greater flexibility in using the book in a given curriculum. Trauma and emergency care are integrated with the content along with the major problems created by dysfunction within a system. Care of the patient in shock or with thermal injuries is included in separate chapters because the patients who undergo these complex problems may have one or many conditions representative of the interaction among body systems.

The authors have deliberately selected a narrative presentation to encourage students to learn through understanding relationships among events. Too often nurses have been taught to learn long lists of events without connection with the implications of these events to a basic physiologic process or to the alternative outcomes. Human beings are different; they react individually to illness and they cannot be fully cared for on the basis of a common list of events or actions. The nurse who learns relationships and who integrates information can become increasingly sensitive to these individual differences among people and can better adapt to changes in the patient's condition and in the approaches to giving care.

It is the authors' opinion that the core of nursing practice remains the one-to-one nurse-patient relationship. This relationship is often directed by imperatives of the patient's major illness or disease. The imperatives influence the nurse's immediate actions, decisions, and care planning tailored to the individual patient.

Nursing is an ideologic yet scientific profession. While this view may seem dichotomous, it is the underlying message of this book. The authors have attempted to subtly define the role of the nurse in explaining the nursing implications in the content presented. Not all nurses will agree with the stated implications, but the authors assume that all nurses in practice do accept responsibility for their personal practice of medical-surgical nursing. It is the authors' hope that this book will serve as a useful reference for them.

M. B. and S. D.

Acknowledgments

The authors are grateful for the encouragement and support of their colleagues in this endeavor, particularly Margaret Brown, Elizabeth Federer, and Janet Weeks. Special mention is given to June Werner, Chairperson, Clinical Department of Nursing at Evanston Hospital, whose continuous support was invaluable, as well as to the many head nurses and clinical instructors at Evanston Hospital who provided clinical information and resources, including Selma Arp, Verneal Frank, Rita Garber, Marie Falls, Jessica McNamara, Judy Swanson, and Wendy Law.

Special recognition is given to illustrators Lana Lewandowski and Jim Chiros, and to photographer Ron Hurst, whose illustrations and photography have substantially clarified many of the aspects of nursing care depicted in this book. We thank all the patients who cooperated in this photography, particularly Jim Hathaway and Bob Copeland, and would like to acknowledge the efforts of the many persons who assisted in preparation of the manuscript: Pauline Augustian; Mary Ellen Bach; Lori Ann Beyers; Caryl Ericsson; Rose Dudas; Leona Manata; Michael, Michelle and Susan Manata; Lee Paige; Nancy Sergel; Irene Taylor; and Nancy Zimmerman and those who provided library resources: Barbara Kuntze, Susan Schoenbeck, Rose Slowinski, and Caryl Rubin.

We are appreciative of the guidance and expertise provided by the staff at Little, Brown and Company, particularly Marty White and Christopher Campbell and especially Anne Merian, our mentor extraordinaire. In addition, we express our appreciation to the many persons who reviewed specific chapters in the book or who contributed valuable clinical information, advice, suggestions, and corrections. Among them are:

Charles R. Baxter, M.D., F.A.C.S.
Professor, Department of Surgery, Southwestern Medical School, University of Texas Health Science Center at Dallas

Fred Bozett, M.S.N.
Assistant Professor, University of San Francisco, San Francisco, California

Alice Bradee, M.S.N.
Assistant to the Director of Staff Education, Madison General Hospital, Madison, Wisconsin

Sue Driscoll, M.S.N.
Clinical Specialist, University of Wisconsin, Madison, Wisconsin

Cynthia Dunsmore, B.S.N.
Faculty, Evanston Hospital School of Nursing, Evanston, Illinois

Mary Gordon, R.N., M.S.
Clinical Specialist, Parkland Memorial Hospital, Dallas, Texas

Evelyn Greathouse, R.N.
Staff Nurse, Operating Room, St. Anthony's Hospital, Crown Point, Indiana

Maureen Groër, Ph.D.
Associate Professor, School of Nursing, Lewis University, Lockport, Illinois

John L. Hunt, M.D.
Assistant Professor, Department of Surgery, Parkland Memorial Hospital, Dallas, Texas

Anita Kedas, M.S.N.
Clinical Nurse Specialist in Rehabilitation, Veterans Administration Hospital, Danville, Illinois

Margaret (Peggy) Keeler, M.S.N.
Clinical Specialist in Nursing Education, Veterans Administration Hospital, Palo Alto, California

Maralyn Keyes, M.S.N.
Director of Staff Development, Lutheran General Hospital, Park Ridge, Illinois

Nancy Laatsch, M.S.N.
Nursing Coordinator, Evanston Hospital, Evanston, Illinois

Ellen McDonald, B.S.N.
Coordinator, Gastrointestinal Clinic, Mt. Sinai Hospital, Milwaukee, Wisconsin

Ralph Meyer, Jr., M.D.
Head, Division of Physiology, Department of Basic Science, Marquette University, Milwaukee, Wisconsin

Bonnie Myers, B.S.N.
Faculty, Evanston Hospital School of Nursing, Evanston, Illinois

Peter H. Nennhaus, M.D.
Cardiovascular Surgeon, Evanston, Illinois

Elizabeth O'Connor, R.N., E.T.
Holy Cross Hospital, Silver Springs, Maryland

Andrew A. Pandazi, M.D., S.C.
Urologist, Milwaukee, Wisconsin

Phyllis Patterson, M.S.N.
Clinical Specialist in Hematology, University of Michigan, Ann Arbor

Anne Porter, M.S.N.
Faculty, Evanston Hospital School of Nursing, Evanston, Illinois

John E. Read, M.D.
Ophthalmologist, Chesterton, Indiana

Barbara Rolling, M.S.N.
Clinical Nurse Expert, Outpatient Nursing Service, National Institutes of Health, Bethesda, Maryland

Francis Rotter, M.D.
Orthopedic Surgeon, St. Michael's Hospital, Milwaukee, Wisconsin

Gloria Smokvina, M.S.N.
Doctoral Candidate, Wayne State University, Detroit, Michigan

Thora Vervoren, B.S., R.Ph.
Director of Pharmacy Services, Columbia Hospital, Milwaukee, Wisconsin

Vivian Weatherby, R.N., E.T.
Suburban Hospital, Bethesda, Maryland

Judy Zoellner, M.S.N.
Director, Continuing Education, Evanston Hospital, Evanston, Illinois

part I Concepts Basic to Clinical Practice in Nursing

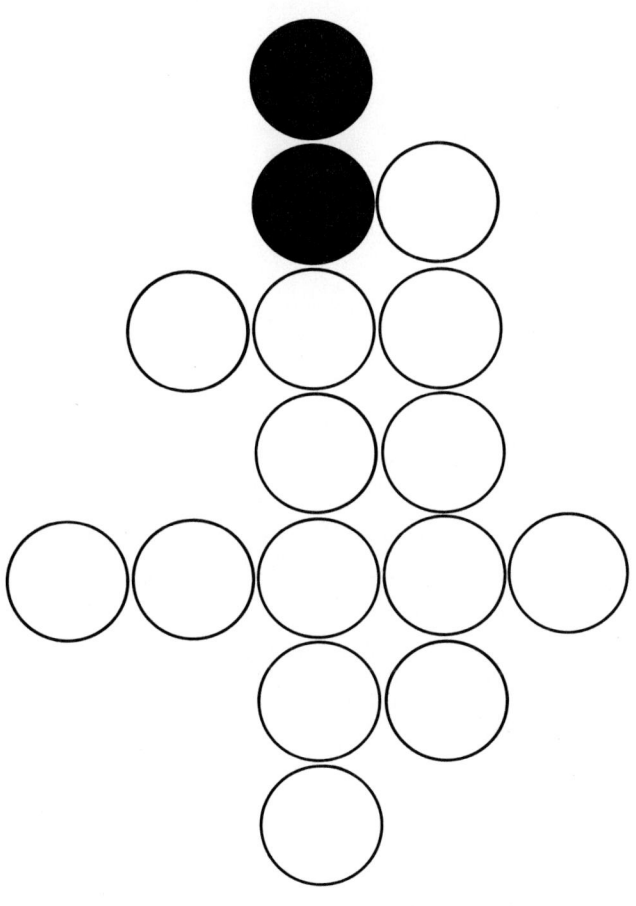

NOTICE

The indications and dosages of all drugs in this book have been recommended in the medical literature and conform to the practices of the general medical community. The medications described do not necessarily have specific approval by the Food and Drug Administration for use in the diseases and dosages for which they are recommended. The package insert for each drug should be consulted for use and dosage as approved by the FDA. Because standards for usage change, it is advisable to keep abreast of revised recommendations, particularly those concerning new drugs.

chapter 1

Health and Disease States

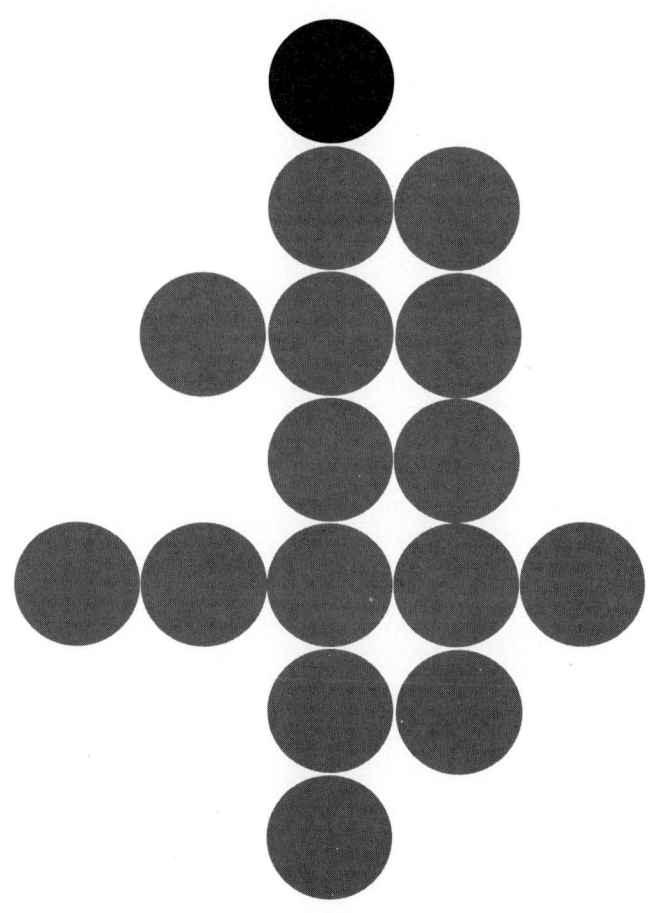

Basic Concepts

Nursing is a universal profession; nursing care is a legitimate and authorized function of the nurse. The Council of National Representatives of the International Council of Nurses adopted a new definition of *nurse* in August 1975. This definition is as follows:

A nurse is a person who has completed a programme of basic nursing education and is qualified and authorized in her/his country to practice nursing. Basic nursing education is a formally recognized programme of study which provides a broad and sound foundation for the practice of nursing and for post-basic education which develops specific competency. At the first level, the educational programme prepares the nurse, through study of behavioural, life and nursing sciences and clinical experience, for effective practice and direction of nursing care, and for the leadership role. The first level nurse is responsible for planning, providing and evaluating nursing care in all settings for the promotion of health, prevention of illness, care of the sick and rehabilitation; and functions as a member of the health team. In countries with more than one level of nursing personnel, the second level programme prepares a nurse, through study of nursing theory and clinical practice, to give nursing care in cooperation with and under the supervision of a first level nurse [36].

The focus of nursing, as defined in this statement, is ". . . the promotion of health, prevention of illness, care of the sick and rehabilitation" and has broad and complex implications for the nurse. Because health and illness are very personal and private matters for any person, the recipient of nursing care must be a participant in the operational aspects of nursing care. In medical care one does not deal with absolutes of cause and effect, but rather with processes. These include processes of physiologic, psychological, and societal natures. There is no one best way to deal with a person's health problems; even outcomes of good quality care cannot be determined in advance or be assured because of factors no one can explain. We do not know why, given the correct and appropriate care and treatment, some people recover and others do not. Nurses therefore can achieve their goals only through working within these processes. While certain facts and principles are generally accepted in the scientific arena, these facts and principles must be applied to the processes that are operational in the care situation and must be viewed as guidelines or signposts in the selection of specific activities to meet the requisites of any given situation.

Facts, principles, and concepts change in importance and in perspective within a situation. Knowledge of contingencies, individual differences, situational variances, and environmental influences must be learned along with the facts, principles, and concepts of illness and disease if the nursing student is to be successful.

No one textbook can include all the aspects of nursing care that must be learned by a nursing student. The scope of this book is defined as the care of adults who have medical-surgical illnesses or the potential for developing health problems. It is expected that the student who is to study the content in this book will have a basic knowledge of anatomy, physiology, chemistry, nutrition, microbiology, social sciences, and introductory nursing care. It is also expected that the student will correlate the content herein with that found in medical and other nursing texts, current journals, and other sources of behavioral and physiologic science information.

The content for this book was selected and developed with the following in mind:

1. There are no absolutes or definite answers or solutions to all health care problems.
2. Because each person presents a unique set of needs, individualized nursing care must be determined from a generalized background of knowledge and experience.
3. Even though each person has a unique health status or set of illness problems, certain criteria can be evaluated to define a person's unique needs within a broad scope of knowledge.
4. The human body functions as an integrated unit with multiple interacting systems and subsystems.
5. In order to understand the functioning of the integrated human being, it is helpful to dissect the broader entity to learn about and to understand the systems and subsystems that contribute to the whole.
6. Integration of content related to nursing care depends on internalizing knowledge and experience from many different sources. A sense of wholeness is achieved by the nursing student through synthesis of the knowledge and experience.

7. A person who becomes a nurse continues to be a student throughout life, since the nurse and the recipient of health care continually evolve in attaining maturity in a continually changing environment.
8. In the process of evolution, each nurse and patient develops concepts of role, function, and purpose based on a continually developing philosophy and framework of supporting concepts, principles, and facts.

Stated in another way, this text has been developed from the viewpoint that there are emerging sets of knowledge about health and illness and alternative avenues for care. The information presented herein focuses on processes that can be applied to many different but somewhat similar situations.

The content has been organized so as to facilitate the student's understanding of the processes of illness, treatment modalities, identifiable expected outcomes of care, and preventive measures. The chapters provide a body systems approach to these processes. By studying the body systems as divisions of human function related to physiologic systems, it is possible to study each system for its own properties, characteristics, and dysfunction. This does not negate the importance of viewing an illness in the broader sense of a person's total body functioning. Any system can be divided into component parts. For adults with medical-surgical illnesses, the functioning of the cell systems and subsystems provides a reasonable and practical basis for the study of expected outcomes of defined illnesses.

Nursing knowledge as currently studied provides a baseline for the student's entry to the profession. Within this context, the professional nurse must continue to develop health care knowledge and skills as information is revealed or discovered so that there is a continual building of an operational and ever-current repertoire of competencies.

As the environment, society, and culture evolve, so do the role and function perceptions of the individual who participates in this broader environment. Each nursing student must initially define a personal concept of nursing that is true to his or her self-concept and must relate positively to the concept of the professional nurse within the profession and in keeping with the broader concept of the system of health care provided by all health professionals.

Nursing care is based on knowledge of man as an integrated being who lives in and is dependent on an environment. The concept of environment may be applied also to the singular unit of a cell, as every cell exists in a unique environment within the body. Environment is also important to the integrity of internal body processes and to behavior within the organism. A person functions in relation to his immediate environment: room temperature, humidity, stressors, and stimuli. Even the space a person occupies is surrounded by the broader environment of family and community, and communities relate to broader determinations of space, which may include the world in its orbital environment. The total functioning of the individual therefore is complexly integrated within the body, as man relates to his environment and participates in situations and events in his own personal orbit.

Each aspect of human functioning, from the singular cell to the broad concept of the world in space, is complex. The amount of knowledge man has about the cell and about the events that happen between the singular unit of the cell and the multiple components of space is overwhelming. The amount of knowledge that is unknown must be equally overwhelming. In order to develop a perspective for the scope of nursing care, the nurse must first examine the functioning of the human body in relation to the space it occupies.

Human beings and the space they occupy are interdependent. Their perceived relationships with others and with the environment often determine their concepts and attitudes toward functioning. **Illness** may be defined as acute or chronic maladaptation, and **health** may be considered a relative state in which a person functions in an interdependent way to perform work. (Work refers to any activity.) Throughout life a person seeks to define health and illness in terms of their impact on his functioning.

The concept of what is a state of health may change as the person matures. For example, a person who has developed chronic constipation may, at the time of the onset, consider himself "sick" or ill. As the condition persists and no pathologic cause is found, the condition becomes part of that person's usual daily situation. If the person adjusts to the condition and deals with the constipation as a characteristic of his daily functioning he is said to have adapted. On the other hand, if he continues to perceive constipation as an illness he is never really healthy or well as long as the particular condition persists.

Certain changes in human functioning are accepted as components of the normal aging process. Examples are the physiologic changes of arteriosclerosis and osteoporosis. Consequently, for many people the concept of a state of health is directly related to age; arterial dysfunction in a young adult is abnormal and constitutes a state of disease. The same condition in a 60-year-old person is expected and therefore normal and congruent with a concept of health for this person. Gradually declining perceptual abilities in vision and hearing are also expected, as are many of the psychological changes associated with aging. It should be pointed out, however, that chronologic age and physiologic age are not necessarily directly related.

What is considered to be maximal functioning for a given person may also vary with the degree or amount of stresses that person experiences. These stresses may arise from internal physiologic processes, from interaction with others, and from environmental stressors such as an influenza epidemic. In most instances, the stresses one experiences are a product of the total set of life events in a given time and are difficult to categorize with specificity.

Much has been written about human adaptation. It is known that a person has certain innate capabilities for adaptation and the ability or potential to learn new patterns and skills. It is also known that a person has some degree of control over his life events but is also subject to unknowns—events that occur without forewarning and often with no explainable cause—events which, despite their uncertainty and uncontrollability, can be adapted to or which may be so stressful that adaptive resources may become immobilized.

Humanity works continually to achieve order and a sense of control over the events that influence human life. For example, research on major health problems such as diabetes, heart disease, blood dyscrasias, and nervous system diseases is ongoing. Breakthroughs in research enable us to better understand and treat disease. Identification of a new vaccine may be important in controlling a communicable disease; the ability to provide for exogenous hormones is necessary in the treatment of endocrine imbalances. Knowledge about the risk factors that cause heart disease can help a person learn to avert the disease. As humanity strives to discover more about diseases and their causation, the very diseases being studied are evolving, changing in nature and effect. Even as scientists discover how to prevent or treat existing diseases, new pathologic processes become evident, further challenging human creativity and ingenuity.

All these considerations lead one to understand that nursing care, focused on prevention of disease and care of the sick, is of necessity based on an inexact science that contains threads of specific knowledge, general application, and generalized sets of premises throughout. How does a nurse cope with this complex and elusive description of nursing care and content? In order to be effective, each nurse must define a role, support that role with knowledge, and practice the skills necessary to achieve the objectives of the role.

Just as the cell is the singular autonomous unit of the human body, a person is a singular autonomous unit of a broader system. The person, whether a nurse or a recipient of care, interacts in the broader system just as the cell interacts in tissue. Physiologically, tissues form organs that may be considered equivalent to families in a community. Further, systems comprise an integrated functioning unit of the body, which can be equated to the society in which communities of people exist. The role of the nurse in this society is an interactive role in which the nurse relates to singular units, individual patients whose behavior is integrated in the broader systems of family, community, and society.

In the following pages, these ideas will be discussed in detail. The cell and its relation to body processes, functions of the body, and disease processes along with modes of intervention will be discussed in a general way.

The Cell

Cellular activity is regulated and controlled by numerous processes, such as water and electrolyte balance and hormonal and nervous system activity. Within the body there are many different types of cells, each with specific functions and of varying sizes and shapes. The fine differentiation of cells accommodates the many ongoing processes in the body.

Osmotic equilibrium is common to all cells as water and charged and uncharged molecules are exchanged among cells and their intracellular spaces. The electrolytes (charged) are important in enabling the cells to maintain membrane potential differences. A negative potential difference exists between the inside of the cell and its surrounding extracellular space. This difference is the **membrane potential,** which regulates the entry or exit of electrolytes to and from the cell. The cell membrane prevents passage of large molecules and permits passage of water, small molecules, and lipid soluble substances.

Movement of molecules to and from cells occurs through simple diffusion, diffusion assisted by carriers, electrical potentials, and solvent drag. Each of these processes is operational in providing the cell with the materials it requires for maintaining life and function.

The cell membrane has diverse functions and serves as an insulator for electric energy, as a barrier for movement of certain molecules and water, and as a means of containment for intracellular structures. Within the confines of the cell membrane, cellular organelles are present in the cytoplasm, which is a semifluid gel-like material. The primary composition of the cell is protein made up of amino acid chains connected by peptide bonds. The possibilities for different structural arrangements are great because there are more than twenty different amino acids that can be connected in pairs. The particular structural arrangement of any given cell is determined by the genetic code, which is found in chromosomes in the nucleus of each cell.

The **nucleus** of the cell is an organelle that controls the replication, regulation, and maintenance of the cell. Survival of the cell is a function of the nucleus. When cells divide (mitosis), the nucleus divides to pass on the hereditary message of that cell's structure, growth, and developmental requisites so that a given type of cell can be replicated exactly and maintained. Chromosomes, which contain these messages, are deoxyribonucleic acid (DNA) and ribonucleic acid (RNA) and protein. DNA contains the code for the cell and is necessary for protein synthesis. Nucleotides comprised of base, sugar, and phosphate make up the DNA and RNA molecules.

The arrangement of the different available bases forms a genetic code for the DNA. The codon of an amino acid is its three-base sequence, which is particular for a given gene. Bases of nucleotides are of two types: **pyrimidine bases,** which are cytosine and thymine, and **purine bases,** which are named adenine and guanine. These two types of bases are joined, so that one of the pyrimidine bases is joined with one of the purine bases in variable sequences. DNA molecules are then formed by pairing of the purine and pyrimidine bases in sequence as determined by the codon.

The DNA molecule provides the framework that specifies how the protein molecule is arranged. The gene carries this information and is considered the hereditary unit of the cell. Attached to chromosomes, genes are capable of exactly reproducing with the cell's division and controlling the synthesis of protein as carried to the ribosomes with messenger RNA (mRNA).

Messenger RNA is formed in the nucleus and enters the cell cytoplasm where it is gathered by ribosomes, another cellular organelle. RNA strands form the basis of synthesis for other protein molecules. The RNA carries the cellular message or code and attracts another type of RNA (transfer RNA), which occurs in different specificities, each type being attracted to its match-specific code of RNA. Enzymes in the ribosomes catalyze the binding of the mRNA and the tRNA. When the protein molecule is completed, it is released to the cytoplasm.

Enzymes are protein substances formed from amino acids in the cell. Present in minute amounts, enzymes are potent catalysts of cellular activity. Some enzymes are retained within the cell whereas others are released from the cells for function in organs or in systems. Digestive enzymes are good examples of the latter.

Synthesis of DNA and RNA requires not only enzymes but also an energy source. This energy source is adenosine triphosphate (ATP), which is formed in the **mitochondria,** the organelles that are the cell's powerhouse. The mitochondria take in nutrients and convert them to ATP. Energy is stored in

ATP until needed. Release of energy from ATP takes place by its conversion to adenosine diphosphate (ADP).

Another component of cells are the threadlike structures called endoplasmic reticulum. Endoplasmic reticulum connects the nucleolar membrane to the outer cell membrane. It increases the surface for chemical reactions and serves as a transport pathway. The threads of endoplasmic reticulum are constantly being broken and re-formed by the action of the cytoplasm. Ribosomes collect on the granular type of endoplasmic reticulum, which serves to promote protein synthesis. The other type of endoplasmic reticulum is agranular and is found predominantly in cells that have high levels of lipid synthesis. Some cells contain both granular and agranular endoplasmic reticulum; however, more often, one or the other type is found.

The **Golgi apparatus** is also a functioning organelle that synthesizes and secretes various materials, usually in the form of granules. **Lysosomes,** another type of organelle, contain hydrolytic enzymes and are concerned with the digestion and degradation of large molecules. Lysosomes also store potentially harmful enzymes to protect the cellular structure from their action. If the lysosomes rupture, releasing these destructive enzymes, death of the cell (necrosis) may occur.

Other cellular structures include centrioles and centrisomes, which function in cell division and are replicated prior to the cell's division. They are also associated with subcellular movement, being the basal structure for cilia and flagella formation. Vacuoles are enclosed by membranes and are found in the cytoplasm. They contain fluid and they function to maintain internal cellular pressure. It is thought that the vacuoles assist movement of the cytoplasm toward the cell membrane for gas exchange from the cytoplasm across the membrane. Finally, the nucleolus, formed by chromosomes, is a compact body within the nucleus and contains protein and RNA. Ribosomes are thought to be formed in the nucleolus, and these ribosomes are transported to the nucleus and then to the cellular cytoplasm.

Cells are held together by **intracellular ground substance,** including hyaluronic acid and chondroitin sulfate. **Hyaluronic acid,** a polysaccharide, retains water and has a high molecular weight. Its viscosity provides for flexibility, and it serves as a lubricant and buffer for cellular movement. **Chondroitin sulfate** is a firmer structure than hyaluronic acid and is comprised of polysaccharides and protein. It serves as the matrix for fibrous elements of cellular connections including elastin, collagen, and reticulin. The function of chondroitin sulfate is to support and glue the cells together.

In the following chapters, much information is included about the specific function of particular types of cells as they relate to body systems. The fantastic capability of the cell to function autonomously is protective of total body functioning. In certain disease states, there is unusual destruction or interference with cellular function, and the cell's ability to replicate and to conduct internal metabolic activities is important in the rebuilding or replacement processes that are encouraged by treatment and therapies.

The cells of the body are significant in total body functioning. For the body to function as an integrated whole, its singular units, the cells, must be functioning so that the tissues and organs they form can function appropriately. In a sense the capability of the human body to live and the effectiveness of the individual's ability to relate to society can be considered as an aggregate of single cellular function in concert with other cells. As with the Gestalt psychology the end result, human behavior, is greater and different from merely the total of all of the cell's functioning, but all are necessary for the effectiveness of the product of human behavior.

Metabolism

The human body both uses and produces energy. The source of this energy is in the environment, and there is an interdependency between a person and his or her environment in the utilization of energy. When a person gains energy, there is a loss of energy in the immediate environment. Similarly, when a person loses energy, there is a gain of energy in the immediate environment. The first law of thermodynamics (the law of energy conservation) explains this exchange: In this law, there is a definite quantity of energy in a given system; a gain or loss of energy causes an equal gain or loss of energy in surrounding systems [50, 65].

The basic unit of energy is the kilogram-calorie (kcal or kilocalorie), which is the standard unit for the amount of heat required to increase the temperature of one kilogram of water by 1° centigrade. The environmental production of foodstuffs provides for human energy, and food is necessary for the production and use of energy. The principle of conservation of energy is important in energy exchange, as human waste materials such as urine, feces, perspiration, and carbon dioxide are used in the environment just as fuel produced in the environment is used by man. The processes of energy production and use are known as metabolism.

Metabolic needs vary in different environmental conditions and in response to internal body changes. The processes for production and use of energy are complicated. Not all fuel is always used to perform physical work or to maintain body function; the excess energy is stored for later use. Some energy is eliminated in the form of the various body excrements. Expenditure of chemical energy (equivalent to the amount of heat expended by the body in a given period of time) is the metabolic rate. Measurement of the body's production of energy in the basal state (expenditure of energy for a given period of time when a person is in a resting state) is a diagnostic test, known as BMR, the basal metabolic rate. It is calculated by oxygen consumption during the period when the temperature and metabolic and muscular work are decreased to a basal level. Certain variables in the BMR include increases in normal periods of growth such as during childhood and pregnancy. Men generally have higher BMRs than do women.

People expend different amounts of energy in their daily lives. This is usually discussed in terms of work. Work is defined as activity, including rest, exercise, and cognitive human functions. The least amount of energy expended by any individual occurs during sleep. At rest, either sitting or lying down, the body's energy expenditure increases slightly over that expended during rest. With increasing performance of work, there are upward gradations in the expenditure of energy.

Light activity (work) includes writing or office work. Standing while performing light activity slightly increases the energy expenditure. Getting dressed, walking, and performing housekeeping activities are classified as moderate activity and require about double the energy expenditure of light activity. Skiing and running are examples of heavy activity and require expenditures of about ten times the expenditure of energy for light activity [65].

Moderate work requires about 3800 kcal in a 24-hour period, which is approximately three times the resting metabolic rate [50]. Hard work, in comparison, requires four to eight times the resting metabolic requirements. A person engaged in manual labor (hard work) requires about 6200 kcal in 24 hours [50]. The kilocalories a person requires for expenditure of energy are derived from the oxidation of fuel, mainly carbohydrates and fats. Energy exchange in man is basically derived from the bonding of both molecular and potential energy. Ingested food is processed in the body via a number of important metabolic pathways. (Digestion and absorption of food is discussed in Chapter 7.)

Carbohydrates are transformed into glucose in the body, as most of the carbohydrate metabolic pathways utilize glucose. Upon entry to the cell, glucose is phosphorylated to form glucose 6-phosphate, which enters one of the major pathways for glucose metabolism. These include the pentose phosphate pathway, the Embden-Meyerhof pathway (an anaerobic glycolysis pathway), and the Krebs or citric acid cycle, which is an aerobic pathway. The Krebs cycle is the major energy-producing cycle in which glucose, through several intermediary steps, is converted to 3-carbon pyruvate, which is converted to water and carbon dioxide for energy. Acetyl CoA is the important pivotal product in the Krebs cycle, which is produced by aerobic oxidation of pyruvic acid. Acetyl CoA is pivotal because it serves as an intermediate between the metabolic conversions of glucose and fatty acid. Energy produced or liberated through the Krebs cycle is stored in high energy phosphate bonds called ATP (adenosine triphosphate).

The Embden-Meyerhof pathway provides for the conversion of glucose to pyruvic to lactic acid. The pentose phosphate pathway provides for storage of glycogen or for the formation of pentose sugars.

Fats (lipids) produce energy through interconversions of lipid and glucose pathways, through the central metabolic intermediate, acetyl CoA. Fats and excess carbohydrates can be stored as an energy source through the lipid metabolic pathways. Lipogenesis is the process through which lipids are transformed into long chain fatty acids, which in turn are combined with alphaglycerol phosphate to form triglycerides. As these energy stores are required by the body, the process is reversed so that fatty acids and glycerol are formed, glycerol entering the metabolic pathway for glucose, and fatty acids being broken down to form acetyl CoA to enter the Krebs cycle.

Proteins are generally not used as energy sources and are conserved for body building processes. In times of need, however, proteins can be converted through hydrolysis to constituent amino acids, which are deaminized or transaminized to form keto acids and can enter the Krebs cycle to produce energy.

The two major classifications of metabolic activity are catabolism and anabolism. **Catabolism** is the degradation of complex molecules into simple molecules [65]. Most of the processes of catabolism involve oxidation and hydrolysis; it is important to recall that the binding of hydrogen and carbon are important in production of chemical energy. Catabolic processes provide energy.

The opposite process, **anabolism,** stores energy through synthesis of nutrients. Anabolism is dependent on catabolic processes because the storage processes require energy produced by catabolism. A common metabolic necessity for both anabolism and catabolism is the phosphate radical, through which high energy bonds of ATP provide a major source of chemical energy.

The three major sources of fuel for the body's energy, then, are carbohydrates, fats, and proteins, in the order of preferential use. This fuel as provided by foods is chemical in nature, and metabolism is basically a chemical process. Vitamins and minerals are essential to cell growth and function and are also important in metabolism.

The nutrients that are ingested, processed, and used for energy through metabolism are mobile within the body. Together they are pooled molecules and atoms that are readily exchanged in the storage and production of energy.

The ability of the human body to store chemical fuel for energy is seemingly unlimited. The major storage nutrient is fat; the body converts excess carbohydrate and protein to fat for storage, primarily in adipose tissue. Certain regulatory processes take place to enable the body to respond to both internal and external energy requirements. One process, the metabolic interchange of nutrients—carbohydrates and proteins and fat—provides a constant supply of energy through maximum utilization of the fuel available at any given time. Fuel in the body in excess of body needs is stored to be used when the intake of fuel may be reduced or lacking.

Primary regulatory controls of metabolism include neuroendocrine functions. The hypothalamus is a central control site of metabolism, and its function in this regard is multiple. One function of the ventromedial region of the hypothalamus is its mechanism for recognition of hunger and satiety. The hunger-satiety mechanism is not well understood. Several factors are known however: People tend to eat more in cold temperatures and less in warmer environments, so that environmental temperature probably affects hunger by influencing internal body temperature. It has also been noted that physiologic hunger is related to fat stores, with ingestion of food being less when the fat stores are higher. Signs of hunger include both decreased blood sugar and increased gastric contractions. The hypothalamus seems to have a coordinating function in hunger, relating hormonal stimulation to the information provided by sensors for endocrine levels, body temperature, blood glucose levels, and other indications of the status of the fuel supply and utilization.

An example of this is the relationship between internal body temperature and hunger. As heat is produced following ingestion of food, neural sensors in the hypothalamus detect the increased temperature and hunger is decreased [50, 65]. This is a very individualized function, as heat production from metabolism varies considerably with individuals. As discussed in Chapter 8, the hypothalamus is also important in regulation of the release of tropic hormones from the anterior pituitary gland. The tropic hormones influence hormonal activity of the adrenal and thyroid glands, both of which figure in metabolic processes. Cortisol, synthesized by the adrenal gland, increases gluconeogenesis (production of glucose from glucogenic amino acids, lactate, and glycerol) while thyroid hormone stimulates the metabolic rate of the body. Growth hormone release, stimulated by the hypothalamus directly, increases protein synthesis. Other hormones, such as glucagon and insulin from the pancreas, influence glucose metabolism. Calcium, a major body electrolyte involved in bone formation and in many body functions, is influenced by parathyroid hormone.

Water and electrolytes are also regulated partly by hormones. These substances are very important to the metabolic processes and in the digestion of nutrients. All these hormones are synthesized and released through feedback loops, which form complicated interaction systems designed to achieve a state of balance in body function. Many of the hormonal systems are regulated by direct or indirect neural control, so that the body functions are integrated in response to energy requisites for physiologic and psychological activity. In summary, maintenance of the balance among fuel needs, fuel storage, and energy utilization requires complexly integrated processes. Some aspects of the resultant body behavior can be evaluated.

In providing nursing care, it is important to use validated methods and measurements to assess body functions. Some methods or observations are used to assess the effectiveness of variable body functions that are difficult to attribute to any given or specific process. Others are pertinent to specific body functions and lend themselves more easily to direct or indirect measurement.

Some body functions are variable because of individual differences; there are large, small, wide, and thin people, all with different square meter surface areas of the body. Within these size and shape variables, there are also differences in normal rates and levels among individuals in a size classification. What is considered normal or baseline for one person may be different from another person's normal baseline. Examples are the different normal levels of metabolic rates and blood pressure rates among individuals.

Age is an important variable in body function. In general, metabolic and other body function processes increase during growth and decrease gradually as aging progresses. Even age, however, is not directly related to the body's function, because some healthy people at age 80 are capable of producing more work than other healthy people can produce at age 50.

Assessment of body function can be approached from the point of view of the effectiveness of human interaction. Basically social creatures, humans interact with people and their environment. Certain characteristics may be evaluated on the basis of the capability of humans to interact. Of these, the ability to perceive and to integrate information is characteristic of an effectively functioning person. Visual, auditory, tactile, and olfactory stimulation along with proprioception are important routes for sensory input, and all are dependent on having sufficient energy. The ability to think, to problem solve, and to communicate also are dependent on energy processes. These functions can be generally evaluated by assessing a person's level of consciousness, alertness, ability to learn, ability to communicate, and ability to perform work in a thoughtful and purposeful way. Even these characteristics are variable among individuals, despite the state of health. Everyone has a highly individual capacity for mental processes, for interacting, and for experiencing. The capacity for self-awareness may be basic to all these interactive and thoughtful processes.

The development of self-awareness is a function of highly integrative processes that depend on interaction with other people in the environment. People tend to know themselves in relation to other people and to conditions and things in their environment. Each person has innate emotional responses and the capacity for self-expression. There are also genetically inherited tendencies for aptitudes and capabilities that influence the development of self—musical ability, creativity, and artistic ability are examples. Other people, particularly family members and those who have an impact on a person's life (significant others such as friends, teachers, and clergy) are greatly influential in a person's development of self-awareness. The sensitivities one develops for awareness are often a product of interaction processes as the person's self evolves in the growth and maturation phases of life. While self-awareness is difficult to assess, it influences interaction and consequently is predominant in any nursing assessment. The person's degree of self-awareness influences that person's ability to communicate health status or to participate in measurement or observation activities in assessment.

A person's total functioning as an integrated unit is evaluated through interaction processes. Nurses can augment this interaction through development of constructive, supportive, and therapeutic interactions. Interviewing, teaching, and counseling skills are essential for nurses in this interaction as is competence in specific nursing therapies and diagnostic measures. In addition, knowledge of human functioning is an integral part of the interactive skills used in nursing care. An analogy can be drawn between the integrative functioning of mind and body to achieve total human functioning and the integration of knowledge, interactive skills, and competence in giving nursing care.

On a physiologic level, assessments may be made and documented precisely so that definite levels or measurements may be obtained. Yet the interpretation of these measurements depends on consideration of the unknown quantity of interaction between mind and body. Physiologic measurements such as respiratory quotient, muscular strength, and blood pressure give specific readings. These readings must be interpreted in view of the influential internal and external factors of emotional tension, anxiety, or even anger. Only in controlled laboratory experiments are these events measured with a minimum of outside influences. Many standardized physiologic measurements are obtained through controlled experiments, and these standardized measurements are helpful in assessing a given person's function on a comparative basis. Knowledge of body processes derived from experimentation is helpful in assessment and provides the background information necessary for the nurse's decision-making processes.

When considering the energy expenditure of a given individual, mechanical efficiency of approximately 20 to 30 percent is possible [50]. Energy from carbohydrates is the best source of fuel in terms of efficiency, as compared to that derived from fats, because more energy is expended in fat oxidation than in carbohydrate oxidation. Emotional and physiologic factors influence the efficiency of human activity. The quality of nutrients ingested, the level of fatigue, the physiologic condition, and the nature of the work itself determine the degree of efficiency.

As discussed in Chapter 10, the ability to exercise, the effects of rest and exercise, and the effects of long-term immobilization all depend on reciprocal and integrated functions of the respiratory, circulatory, and metabolic systems. Exercise involves various forms of energy; thermal energy is produced but not utilized by the body; chemical, mechanical, and electrical energy are all utilized and produced by the body.

Oxygen consumption is an essential component of energy production and use. One measure of oxygen utilization is the respiratory quotient (RQ), which is defined as the volume of oxygen consumed in relation to the volume of carbon dioxide expired in a given period. Because food is oxidized in metabolism, the RQ is a measure of the breakdown of chemicals in food through oxidation to produce energy. The breakdown of chemicals is influenced by respiratory rates and exercise levels as well. Oxygen consumption is also directly related to the expenditure of energy.

The phrase **maximal oxygen consumption** refers to the maximum amount of energy derived from aerobic metabolism through which energy is released and therefore available for expenditure. The maximal oxygen consumption tends to be greater in youth than in old age. Although there are physiologic variations among individuals in the rate of maximal oxygen consumption, there is a fairly constant level of capability for a given person. This constant rate is attained by the second or third minute of exhausting work. Maximum oxygen consumption can be increased. For example, athletes who undergo training can develop greater maximal oxygen consumption rates. Long-term inactivity results in decreased oxygen consumption. Since oxygen consumption is a product of respiratory, circulatory, and metabolic activities as augmented or controlled by the neuroendocrine systems, genetic variations in these systems capabilities influence the rate of maximum oxygen consumption.

When a person has worked at capacity for energy production he becomes exhausted. Following work resulting in exhaustion, a person is said to have oxygen debt. **Oxygen debt** is the amount of energy required to restore the high-energy phosphate bonds that have been released, especially from muscles. Restoration of high-energy systems is necessary following exhausting work [50].

The body, in its inimitable ability to provide checks, balances, and alternative modes of functioning, is also capable of subsidizing aerobic metabolism with anaerobic metabolism. Anaerobic energy production predominates when the expenditure of energy exceeds that capable of being produced by oxidative or aerobic metabolism. When oxygen utilization increases, anaerobic metabolism provides the extra energy requirements. In anaerobic metabolism, muscular breakdown of glycogen results in the formation of lactic acid. The resulting increase in lactate production builds up in the muscles and is diffused into the blood. This alternative pathway of anaerobic metabolism can produce energy until the accumulation of lactic acid is sufficient to cause a state of acidosis. Acidosis impedes the ability to work and may, in debilitated persons, lead to the development of numerous ill effects including shock. The mechanisms of shock resulting from lactic acid acidosis are given in greater detail in Chapter 16.

Oxygen consumption therefore is required for energy production and is a measure of energy expenditure. The ability of a person to be active depends not only on metabolic production of energy, but also on circulation and respiration. The limits of the pulmonary capability for ventilation directly influence the ability to work (see Chap. 3). Impaired circulation or disturbances in the capability of the blood to carry oxygen to the cells also decreases the ability to work, just as the capability of the cardiac musculature influences work.

The effects of exercise on the circulatory system are significant. Because oxygen use is increased during exercise, there is a concomitant requirement for increased cardiac output. There is also dilatation of capillaries and arterioles in the muscles being used in the exercise. The body pushes its circulatory resources to the areas of greatest need by shunting blood to these areas from other more inactive body parts such as the viscera and skin. Through vasoconstriction, circulation to these areas is decreased during exercise.

Another measurement of energy expenditure is the production of body heat as thermal energy is released by the body. As with other aspects of body function, there are specific mechanisms for maintenance of optimal body heat. During work, heat production increases and the heat regulatory center in the hypothalamus is "set" at a level higher than that for resting or less active states. When energy is released by the muscular activity, the circulatory system conducts the heat to the peripheral blood vessels. The circulation also delivers water to the sweat glands, and the peripheral blood vessels dilate so that heat may be lost through evaporation of water and through convection and radiation.

Periods of rest usually follow periods of extreme activity. During periods of rest, the body replenishes its supplies to accommodate future exercise. Rest is an essential need of the body, even when a person does not engage in strenuous activity. The body has built-in mechanisms or cycles for regulation of, or for achieving, a balance between exercise and rest. Both are related to and important for basic body functions. Exhausting work causes maximum oxygen consumption and increased metabolism, circulation, and ventilation. Its opposite, sleep, causes decreased oxygen consumption, metabolism, circulation, and ventilation. Body temperature changes in relation to these factors. During sleep the body's major supply of heat is from the viscera, trunk, and brain. Heat is conserved through vasoconstriction of the periphery. As may be recalled, during periods of work the muscles supply most of the body heat.

While body processes produce thermal energy, the body does not use this form of energy. Body heat is important, however, for supporting body processes. The optimum temperature for cellular enzymatic function is about 37°C (99°F) [50]. Heat is a product of chemical energy, just as work is a product of chemical energy utilization. Much experimentation has been done to discover the relation among various aspects of body function and the rhythms of the body. It has been found that there is normally an increase in body temperature prior to awakening. People who awaken quickly tend to have this increase prior to awakening whereas those who awaken with difficulty have less of an increase in body temperature prior to awakening. During sleep the lowest body temperature in a 24-hour cycle is reached. Deep body temperature can fluctuate ± 5°C from the normal mean in the diurnal rhythm [65]. Each person has a 24-hour temperature cycle, with the highest point occurring in late afternoon or evening for those who sleep during the night. The natural temperature cycle occurs with constancy and is not influenced by food intake or by exercise [5, 44, 50].

Body Rhythms

Numerous other body processes are also cyclic. Pulse rate is cyclic and tends to rise and fall at times corresponding to body temperature increases or decreases. In fact, the subject of rhythms nicely demonstrates how a single individual functions in relation to his environment. There are cyclic rhythms in many areas: the changing of seasons, the phases of the moon and tide, and night and day are some of the easily recognized rhythms. **Circadian rhythms** (diurnal rhythms) or sleep-waking cycles are synchronized with rhythms in adrenal function and influence the metabolism of food and cardiac and respiratory functions. Body circadian rhythms are thought to be in phase with the rhythms in the environment. Cycles of light and darkness in the environment are more visible than cycles in body function, many of which are thought to be self-regulated. In addition to circadian rhythms, there are also ultradian rhythms, with cycles shorter than 24 hours, and infradian cycles of longer than 24 hours.

Eating, brain wave rhythms, and hormonal release are some of the functions related to ultradian rhythms within the circadian rhythms. It is considered that the integration of body functioning and the sense of harmony with the environment are dependent on the phasing of rhythms found throughout nature. Discordance in rhythms can lead to a number of abnormal conditions. It has been theorized that some behavioral illnesses, tumor growth, and many other forms of illness may be related to interrupted rhythms or to stressful events at times in the circadian rhythm when the person can least effectively deal with the stress. Desynchronization of body rhythms may produce dysfunction in body processes and cause some of these illnesses [5, 44, 76].

As more is discovered about body rhythms, nursing care can be more specifically planned to incorporate this knowledge of body function in care and treatment to enhance the effectiveness of nursing care. Peaks and troughs of circadian rhythms influence body functions. Foods may be metabolized differently in different phases of the cycle, which has implications for timing the intake of food for the greatest nutritional and metabolic effectiveness. Cell division is speeded up in certain phases of the cycle so that the giving of medications may be planned for the time of maximum effectiveness. Behavior is also related to circadian rhythms, having implications for optimum times for learning and for counseling. Performance of work, alertness, and visual, olfactory, auditory, and other sources of sensory stimuli perception have been shown to change during the phases of the circadian rhythms. All of these circadian effects have implications for the timing of nursing activities. Another example of planning care according to rhythms is the provision for rest and exercise.

Rest and exercise are basic needs. There are circadian rhythmic variations in sleep patterns. The circadian pattern of sleep is thought to stem from hypothalamic function and is established usually by the age of 2 years. Studies of sleep states [44, 50] indicate that there is a phase of **slow wave sleep** (SWS), which is associated with reduced and constant rates of respiration and cardiovascular functions. Muscle tone is reduced during slow wave sleep, and the person in this state is aroused with difficulty. In the second sleep state, **desynchronized sleep** (DS), the respiratory, cardiovascular, and autonomic nervous system functions are paradoxical. Rapid eye movements (REM) are also noted. A person cycles back and forth from slow wave sleep to desynchronized sleep. There are more REM periods as the waking time draws near and as the body temperature begins to rise. Both slow wave sleep and desynchronized sleep are necessary for health. Children have longer periods of SWS than adults.

When deprived of REM periods in sleep, the individual makes up for the loss by experiencing more REM periods in the next sleep period. Slow wave sleep periods increase when a person has exercised more than usual or has experienced the loss of a sleep period [76]. Several behavioral effects result from loss of sleep. Lethargy and depression follow deprivation of slow wave sleep, and anxiety and irritability are experienced following loss of REM sleep. The type of activity determines to some extent the type of sleep pattern [44, 50, 65]. For example, new experiences or learning tend to require greater needs for REM sleep.

Variations in sleep patterns are significant

in the hospital setting, particularly when hospital routines, treatment patterns, and the patient's adjustment interfere with the normal sleep patterns. Certain drugs, for example, antihypertensives, interfere with the REM phase of sleep. Nurses should be aware of the impact these factors have on the hospitalized person's behavior. Care should be given to minimize the factors that interfere with sleep and to promote rest by accommodating the timing of care to the patient's normal sleep pattern [5].

Another interesting observation is the finding that there is interference with the consolidation of learned responses in people who are deprived of REM sleep. DeWied [21] reports an experimental theory that this interference may be caused by chemicals that act directly on the cells of the central nervous system. This theory stems from animal research to determine the influence of hormones on motivation, learning, and memory. It was found that the amino acid sequence 4 through 10 of ACTH and vasopressin directly influenced the learning and motivation of the animals studied. Because ACTH is released as part of the normal stress response in humans, it has been postulated that the same sequence may stimulate the human central nervous system when an important event is experienced. Learning in the presence of vasopressin is retained longer, even if vasopressin is withdrawn. ACTH seems to augment motivation only if it is present *during* the learning behavior. There is impaired learning with ACTH deficiency, and memory impairment occurs with vasopressin deficiency in the animals studied. The components of the amino acid sequence that cause these changes do not influence the activity in the target organ, the adrenal glands, for ACTH.

Genetic Influences

The evolutionary implications of the effect of chemicals on the brain lead one to contemplate the importance of heredity as a factor in behavior. As mentioned in the discussion of the cell, genes carry messages for the traits and characteristics of an individual. While the environment influences the development of the individual's behavior, the genetic inheritance and environmental effects are difficult to differentiate. The genetic makeup of an individual is termed **genotype**.

Phenotype is the expression of the interaction of the environment on the genotype. The genetic makeup of any individual occurs through random pairing of chromosomes from the parents.

There are two genes present for every trait in a given individual, and his or her phenotype is the expression of the dominant gene traits. If **homozygous,** the pair of genes correspond and can be a pair of either dominant or recessive genes. The trait then expressed is either dominant or recessive accordingly. If, however, the trait genes are present in combination of one dominant and one recessive, the genes are **heterozygous** and the dominant allele is expressed in the phenotype. The alternate forms of genes are **alleles.**

Genetic constitution determines characteristics of appearance and behavior: size, shape, coloring, aptitudes, strength, chemical makeup, and propensities for health and disease. Because of the influence of genetic makeup, it can be said that the occurrence of all illness is influenced by a person's genetic constitution. Certain diseases are recognized to be definitely inherited.

Penetrance describes the frequency of the disease expressed by the phenotype. Penetrance is considered to be a relative term because the gene may cause the effects of the disease in such a mild form that it is not detected in the affected individual. In other persons the effects of the disease are readily observable. This phenomenon is termed **expressivity** and defines the degree of severity of the effects of the disease in the affected individual. The concepts of penetrance and expressivity describe individual variations in the effects of genes. Reasons for the variations are at this time poorly defined, although the importance of the interaction of genes and the total internal and external environment are recognized.

Some diseases are genetically inherited as autosomal dominant; others are autosomal recessive, and some are sex-linked. In **autosomal dominant diseases,** if heterozygous, the dominant gene expresses the disease and the recessive gene is not expressed, but may have some effect on the expression of the trait. If homozygous, the corresponding dominant genes may produce a stronger effect.

Autosomal recessive genes must be homozygous to express the abnormality. Both genes in the pair are corresponding and recessive. In some instances neither gene in the pair is dominant or recessive; this pairing is called codominance. The ABO blood groups described in Chapter 5 are an example of codominance. Intermediate inheritance in which the dominant expression is modified by the recessive gene is similar to codominance. In general, autosomal dominant and recessive diseases affect both males and females. Autosomal dominant traits are transmitted to half of the children of parents with heterozygous traits and one of the parents expresses the disorder. Because of the latter, autosomal dominant diseases demonstrate a positive family history in which the disease is expressed in succeeding generations.

Autosomal recessive traits must be homozygous to be expressed, and parents with autosomal recessive trait expression are not affected with the disease if the gene is heterozygous in each parent. Their children, however, will inherit the gene. These diseases cannot be traced then, as they are not expressed in succeeding generations. The normal dominant trait is expressed in the heterozygous individuals. Recessive diseases are expressed by the homozygous genes and are generally of greater severity than autosomal dominant diseases because both genes, being recessive, complement one another.

When a trait for a disease is carried by a sex chromosome, the expression of the disease is sex-linked and can be either dominant or recessive. If the gene is carried on the X chromosome and is recessive or dominant, the affected father will pass the trait on to his daughters. His sons will not be affected, but his daughter's children may carry the gene if female, or express the disease if male. The male is hemizygous for the abnormal gene, which means that his single X chromosome (the other being Y) carries the gene. The female child expresses the disease if homozygous for the recessive trait. Sex-linked diseases are usually recessive.

The genetic constitution of an individual then may contribute to the expression of a disorder or disease, or it may lead to the propensity for the development of diseases throughout life. At the same time, the genetic constitution of an individual may be such that the individual has a "strong constitution" and is able to resist disease and to remain healthy, with a great capacity for productivity. The entire subject of genetics is developmental, and the reader is advised to seek other references for more information about the subject. Let it suffice to say that individual variations among people make each nursing care situation unique and challenging as the nurse assesses needs and plans the care appropriate for a given individual.

Adaptive Responses

The question still remains: How does the environment affect the individual in either increasing or decreasing his or her risks for development of illness? A report of a June 1973 conference, *Stressful Life Events: Their Nature and Effects* [22], contains the results of studies conducted primarily at Cornell University Medical College [22]. The following conclusions derived from these studies are pertinent to nursing:

1. Exposure to culture change, social change, and change in interpersonal relations may lead to a significant change in health if (a) a person has preexisting illness or susceptibility to illness, and he perceives the change as important to him, or (b) there is a significant change in his activities, habits, ingestants, exposure to disease-causing agents, or in the physical characteristics of his employment.

2. Exposure to culture change, social change and change in interpersonal relations may lead to no significant change in health if (a) the person has no significant preexisting illness or susceptibility to illness, or if he does not perceive the change as important to him, and (b) there is no significant change in his activities, habits, ingestants, exposure to disease-causing agents, or in the physical characteristics of his environment.

3. If a culture change, social change, or change in interpersonal relations is not associated with a significant change in the activities, habits, ingestants, exposure to disease-causing agents, or in the physical characteristics of the environment of a person, then its effect upon his health cannot be defined solely by its nature, its magnitude, its acuteness or chronicity, or its apparent importance in the eyes of others.

In addition, the conference report [22] contained much interesting information and many theories about the nature of an individual's response to the life events he encounters in relation to his development of illness. In general, researchers found stressors to include both positive and negative life events. In some of the reported studies, it was demonstrated that people tend to be affected by similar types or classifications of stress, despite their geographic or economic status.

As would be expected, illness behaviors were more predominant in people who tended to be less flexible, in those with fewer supporting systems in the community (friends and neighbors), and in those who tended to be less settled and less well satisfied with themselves in relation to their family, social, and work roles. For some of these people, the development of illness as perceived by them provided a coping mechanism through which they dealt with their frustrations [22].

Humans have several normal responses to disease-producing agents in their environment. These protective and automatic responses do not require thought on the part of the individual to initiate the protection they afford. Three of these responses will be discussed in detail, as they are basic to many illness processes and in the resolution of a variety of diseases or illnesses. These three processes are the inflammatory response, the immune response, and the pain response.

THE INFLAMMATORY RESPONSE

The **inflammatory response,** in its broadest definition, is an adaptive response essential to life. It involves recognition of and dealing with potentially harmful events that are capable of causing injury to body cells. As such, the inflammatory response is the body's defense reaction to trauma or injury or to invasion by microorganisms. Sources of trauma abound in the environment and may include any of the forms of energy that are productive in performing the work of the body. These energy sources are potentially harmful if they are excessive and thus are able to overcome the body's defenses, or if the person is in a weakened condition rendering him unable to withstand their effects, thereby causing a pathologic condition. Trauma may result from mechanical, thermal, chemical, or electrical sources. The trauma may occur quickly, and the traumatic incident may end abruptly, or it may occur through continued exposure. A gunshot wound is an example of acute trauma. A tight-fitting shoe may produce continued mechanical pressure, causing irritation and the formation of a blister, an example of a more slowly occurring trauma. When trauma of any type occurs and the body surfaces have been penetrated, the inflammatory response is initiated.

Another source of injury to body cells is invasion by bacteria, viruses, and parasites. The inflammatory response is important in defending the body from this invasion by microorganisms. Yet other sources of injury are the products of the immune response and changes in tissue or body cells resulting from other diseases. Necrosis of tissue is an example, as are toxic products of the immune response that extend the process of the disease to surrounding tissues.

The body actually has many protective mechanisms. They all function to keep potentially harmful agents from coming into contact with the internal cells of the body. The skin, with its antibacterial secretions; mucous membranes, with the ability to produce mucus, which has an antimicrobial action; the action of cilia, which trap and help remove particles before they are able to reach the lower respiratory tract; and many body secretions such as tears, which contain lysozyme, also having an antimicrobial action, are all examples of body defenses.

Once the body surface has been penetrated, however, the inflammatory response becomes operational. The condition that ensues is **inflammation** of the part affected, specifically implied by the suffix **-itis,** as in appendicitis, cellulitis, or cystitis. Any factor that causes inflammation—temperature extremes, mechanical pressure, electrical stimuli, radiation, invasion by pathogenic microorganisms or foreign bodies, or the accumulation of cellular and metabolic products—may initiate the inflammatory response. The inflammation may be referred to as acute, subacute, or chronic. The last may begin as acute and become chronic, or it may begin as an insidious process. In each case, the inflammatory response involves a sequence of processes for localization and interference with the advancement of the inflammation. The period of the inflammatory response is accompanied by and followed by repair of the injury.

Assessment of the phases of the inflammatory response is dependent on understanding the processes that take place when the body responds to potentially injurious substances. For purposes of integrating the assessment factors with physiologic events, the two will be discussed together. Initially, vascular changes take place with temporary constriction, then dilatation of arteries, veins, and capillaries. The blood flow to the area of inflammation increases and causes the involved area to become reddened and to feel warm. The acceleration of the blood flow to the inflamed area is followed by a slowing of blood flow, sludging of the red blood cells, and enlargement of the lining cells of the vessel walls. A **flare,** which is an area of redness, is noted at the site of the inflammation.

As the vessels undergo changes, the leukocytes tend to leave their normal flow path in the vessel and adhere to the vessel wall. The vessel walls become increasingly permeable and fluid from the microcirculation, which is high in protein materials, leaks into the surrounding areas, and forms a **wheal,** a rounded area of edema at a *localized* site of inflammation. Edema indicates that lymph flow has increased to the site of the inflammation, and that the osmotic pressure has increased. The edema associated with inflammation is caused by accumulation of exudate in the tissues. The extent of the edema (or swelling) is variable, increasing as the area of inflammation extends. Edema may be localized to a specific site of injury, or it may include an entire organ or body part, as a swollen arm. The increased pressure in the small vessels comprising the microcirculation and the decreased colloid osmotic pressure within the vessels cause proteins, blood plasma, leukocytes, and fluid to be lost into the surrounding extravascular spaces through **diapedesis,** the migration of blood cells from the vessels into the extracellular space.

Histamine, which is released early following injury to cells, augments vasodilatation and increases vessel permeability. While many of the factors that influence the inflammatory response are not well understood, such as the role of histamine, it is thought that certain mediators may increase the emigration of the leukocytes. It is also thought that some of these mediators may be a cause of pain associated with inflammation. In addition to histamine, bradykinin and kallidin, polypeptides that form through partial hydrolysis of proteins, also cause vasodilatation in the inflamed area. These kinins are destroyed by kininases. Other mediators, such as the globulin permeability factor, are also present, but their functions in inflammation are not well defined.

A number of different types of blood cells are drawn to the inflamed area. These include erythrocytes, platelets, and leukocytes that collect on the endothelium and adhere to the vessel walls. These cells are rolled along the surfaces of the vessel wall, creating a margin around the inflamed area. This process is called margination and outlines the area of inflammation. Of the cells that collect, polymorphonuclear neutrophilic leukocytes are the primary cells in the phagocytic action of the blood cells directly on foreign particles such as chemicals, bacteria, or cellular debris (phagocytosis). The polymorphs, as they are often named, arise from the bone marrow and are released to circulating blood, from which they become available for diapedesis. The process of chemotaxis (chemical attraction) assists in attraction of polymorphs to the foreign substances.

Foreign substances are incorporated into the cytoplasm of the polymorph cells. The cytoplasm contains digestive enzymes in the granular substance and the digestive enzymes act on the foreign substances, forming vacuoles in the process. These vacuoles are **phagosomes. Opsonins** (IgG) are antibody substances that also promote the ingestion of bacterial products by coating the bacteria or foreign body, encouraging phagocytosis. Eventually, a pus cell is formed. This is simply a polymorphonuclear leukocyte that has become necrotic.

Once the bacteria are located within the vacuoles or phagosomes, they come into contact with the cellular lysosomes. The contact between the vacuole and lysosome causes a phagolysosome to form. The lysosomes release hydrolytic and proteolytic enzymes to inactivate or kill the invading bacteria. It should be noted that bacteria may kill the leukocytes, causing the proteolytic enzymes to be released and thereby dissolving dead tissue.

Other cells, eosinophils and monocytes, also migrate to the inflamed area and are also capable of phagocytosis. Eosinophils are formed in the bone marrow and are attracted to the site of inflammation by increased histamine. Monocytes in tissues are called macrophages and are sometimes referred to as histocytes. These cells are present in many tissues, such as in the Kupffer cells of the liver. Monocytes also originate in the stem cells of the bone marrow. (Cells that travel in the blood are **monocytes** and those located in the tissues are **macrophages.**) Macrophages are scavenger cells. Both types of cells have phagocytic action, being capable of engulfing bacteria and cellular debris.

The inflammatory response can spread and involve surrounding tissues, or it may be localized with a defined and circumscribed area in which a wall is formed about a collection of pus. Pus contains living and dead polymorphs, macrophages, and necrotic tissue. Pus is formed by suppuration, and is a yellow alkaline substance. The suppurative stage of the inflammatory process may be summarized as follows. As the polymorphs reach the end of their short life span, they liberate enzymes that digest the cellular debris. Macrophages have a longer life span and are important in the process of "cleaning up" the products of inflammation. The resulting action of enzymes is the formation of yellow pus, which eventually drains or is absorbed through the lymphatic system. The method for drainage depends on the type and site of injury. In abscess formation, there is usually localized suppuration and limited inflammation in which the liquified cavity is contained by a wall of living tissue. The liquified material extends or directs itself to the direction of least resistance, forming a head from which the drainage occurs. In some instances a sinus is formed as a route of discharge for the pus. This is often the case when a hair follicle or sebaceous gland is involved in an infection. In other instances fistulas may occur. A **fistula** is a tract or route of exit that forms between mucous membranes or between an organ and the surface of the skin. An ulcer is another type of formation from which sloughing occurs. In other instances, suppurative material is absorbed by surrounding tissues and lymphatics. Exudate differs according to the areas involved in inflammation. When the exudate is low in protein, it is **serous** and is usually clear and watery. **Fibrinous** exudate contains fibrinogen molecules and is thicker than serous exudate. **Purulent** exudate results from large numbers of white cells (leukocytes). **Hemorrhagic** exudate results from rupture of vessels.

The process of phagocytosis requires metabolic energy and is associated with increased oxygen consumption, increased utilization of glucose, and increased synthesis of RNA. If anaerobic conditions exist, lactic acid production increases. For this reason, the person with an inflammatory response is expected to have increased respirations, increased pulse rate, and increased temperature. When the inflammatory response is related to bacterial infection, increased temperature is related to endogenous pyrogens (fever-producing substances) which reach the temperature regulating centers via the circulation. Pain, another symptom, is caused by a number of factors. One factor is increased pressure on surrounding tissue because of edema. The nerve endings are affected in this response. It should be noted that bone pain is more severe because there is no space for edema to extend. As mentioned previously, mediators may cause pain, e.g., serotonin has been thought to cause pain.

If the process of phagocytosis is effective, the acute inflammation will be resolved and the irritating substances will have been dealt with. In many instances, the immune response, which is described later, is important in the inactivation of the microorganisms or in dealing with the foreign substances.

When an acute inflammation is not resolved, the person may develop a chronic inflammation. An inflammation may also be chronic from the outset as in granulomatous responses. There is usually an increase in eosinophils, which are often found to accompany allergic responses. The macrophages become more differentiated, becoming either lipophages, which appear when fat necrosis occurs; siderophages, which appear when there is destruction of blood cells as in hemorrhage; and multinucleate cells, which are many macrophages fused together. The last are called giant cells. In addition to these differences, the cellular exudate is different in chronic inflammation. The cells appearing in the exudate are mainly mononuclear cells (plasma cells, lymphocytes, and macrophages) rather than the polymorphs seen in acute inflammation. There is also an increased growth of connective tissue in the area of chronic inflammation.

The system or organ basic to the processes of inflammation and important to maintenance of the fluidity of the blood is the reticuloendothelial system. The cells of this system are found throughout the body, being the most highly concentrated in the spleen and lymph nodes. The monocytes and macrophages, already mentioned, are very important cells in this system. Other aspects of the reticuloendothelial system are described more fully in Chapter 5.

In summary, the inflammatory process includes three main phenomena: the vascular response, the production of inflammatory exudate, and tissue changes that take place as a result of inflammation. The end result of tissue changes must be described in relation to the cause of the inflammation. For example, wounds heal differently, depending on the causative factors. The wound resulting from surgery is quite different from one that results from trauma.

A discussion of the types of wounds that may occur facilitates understanding of this point. Among the types of traumatic wounds that may occur are lacerations, abrasions, and stab wounds. **Lacerations** are cuts that may be clean or ragged; they may involve either subcutaneous tissues or extend deeper, involving internal organs. An **abrasion** is caused by friction and results in shearing of the skin. **Stab wounds** are punctures of the skin that may be superficial or deep.

Wounds may also be caused by extremes of temperature; heat causes destruction of cells and if sufficient, the heat may cause protein to coagulate. Lesser heat injuries are characterized by erythema. Care of the thermally injured patient is the topic of Chapter 15. Extreme cold may cause injury because of vasoconstriction, which leads to tissue ischemia (as in frostbite). Radiation may damage cells, as discussed later in this chapter. Electricity causes wounds typified as burns at the point of entry and exit. In some instances electric currents may be sufficient to cause death, as with contacting a high voltage line. Chemicals, either acids or alkalis, cause injury by burning and corroding the tissues. A **contusion** is a blow that ruptures the small blood vessels so that blood leaks into the intracellular tissues, causing a hematoma.

All these wounds may initiate the inflammatory process. It is important to note that the emergency care given may directly influence the healing time of the wound. Infection delays the healing time and must be avoided if possible. Wounds with foreign material imbedded in the area are particularly subject to infection. First aid should be given carefully to prevent further damage. The wound is covered with a sterile (if possible) or clean dressing, the wounded part is immobilized, and the patient is quickly transported to a hospital for further care. When it is not possible to take the patient to an emergency room immediately, the wound should be cleaned, the edges approximated by using a clean bandage, and the part immobilized until treatment can be obtained. If care must be delayed for days, attempts should be made to remove foreign material, being careful not to extend the wound. Wounds that are properly repaired early tend to heal more quickly and with less residual damage such as infection or scarring.

Wound repair constitutes return of the wounded area to its former condition or as nearly so as possible. This process involves both healing and regeneration. Healing refers to wound closure, while regeneration refers to renewed tissue. Factors important in repair include removal of debris and any irritants from the wound and replacement of the tissue or structuring of the part so that further reconstruction may be accomplished. The process of healing begins with the enzymatic action of removal of debris and dead tissue and continues with the absorption of the exudate. Finally, formation of fibrous tissue in a process called organization occurs. Traumatic wounds heal more slowly than surgical wounds. Surgical wounds usually heal by first intention, as is described later in this chapter. Traumatic wounds, in contrast, usually heal by secondary union, healing by granulation.

Emergency care of the wound includes cleaning it with an antiseptic for removal of foreign material and bacteria. If the wound is not treated within 12 hours, the physician provides for a wound covering, but does not close the wound because of the danger of bacterial infection. In this instance the wound heals by granulation with gradual regeneration of tissue to fill in the gaps of the wound. If the wound is large, surgical intervention may be required to explore and repair the wound. It is necessary to provide for drainage of exudate so that formation of exudate does not create pressure and thus interfere with the blood supply to the wound during the healing. As with any inflammatory response, the rapidity of healing is influenced by the person's age, decreasing as the person becomes older, by hormonal balance, and by the general physical condition. A well-nourished person tends to heal more quickly than one who is undernourished for any reason. In many instances the inflammatory response is related to internal disease processes, which influence resolution or healing.

Internal disease processes influence repair of wounds. A person with systemic vascular disease, for example, may have extreme difficulty in coping with a traumatic wound because of impaired circulation. In some instances, the disease has led to initiation of the inflammatory response so that the condition is continuous. Rheumatoid arthritis is typical of this type of condition and is also indicative of the complementary relationship between inflammatory and immune responses.

The complementary relationship between immune and inflammatory responses is complex. The action of macrophages, for example, supports the immune response through engulfment of the invasive foreign materials. In some instances the products of the immune response cause an inflammatory response. This relationship between the two responses makes it difficult to separate them when describing the processes. The inflammatory response has several broad functions in ridding the body of particles of cells and metabolic products not needed, as well as in removing microorganisms. Similarly, the immune response has many applications for protection of the body. The relationships between the inflammatory response and the immune response are discussed more fully in the following pages.

THE IMMUNE RESPONSE

Adaptation is a fascinating and complex set of processes involving specific psychological and physiologic functions as well as general body integrative functions. The **immune response** is one of these adaptive processes and exemplifies the complexity of adaptation. Unique to vertebrates and variable among species, the immune response is influenced by environment, genetic inheritance, embryonic life, age, and hormonal balance.

The environment in which humans live greatly influences variations in the immune response among species and races. Through living in different environments, people are thought to have developed different sensitivities and tolerances for substances as required for protection in particular environments. Differences in the immune responses are genetically inherited also, and differences in immune sensitivities and tolerances are developed during embryonic life. The exposure of a people to an environment, the exposure of an embryo to an environment, and the continuous life exposure of an individual to different environments all influence the immune response.

The effectiveness of an immune response varies according to the stage and condition in the life cycle as well as to the types of substances encountered in the environment. The ability to resist infection is decreased in childhood and in old age; the state of health influences the effectiveness of the immune system. It is known that hormonal imbalances and debilitation cause a decreased ability to resist infection.

As an adaptive process, immunity serves several purposes. By definition, **immunity** is a protective adaptive response, specific to harmful substances. (Microorganisms are included in the category **harmful substances** to which an individual has had prior exposure.) The immune response provides the body with a means of eliminating harmful substances or rendering them harmless. In addition to providing protection from potentially harmful substances from the environment, the immune response also aids in the control of abnormal cell growth within the body and for removal of worn-out cells through cellular metabolism.

The immune response may be disease-producing as well as protective. Allergy and hypersensitivity are examples of altered responses to the immune process and cause tissue damage or destruction or interference with normal body function. Some people develop diseases related to the immune response, either because of abnormal immunity to self-substances (autoimmune diseases) or because of a deficiency in the immune response (immunodeficiency disease).

Immunity can be divided into two major types: humoral and cellular. **Humoral immunity** is a function of serum antibody formation in response to antigens. **Cellular immunity** is a cell-mediated process in which cells sensitized by antigens react directly with the antigen. Both humoral and cellular immunity are thought to be interdependent, although the processes of each are different.

There is a balance between humoral and cellular immunity in the body.

Antigens are substances that are capable of initiating the immune response. This response is called immunogenicity. Another name for antigen is immunogen. Antibodies are products of the immune response that react specifically with antigens. **Antigenicity** is the ability of antigens to react with antibodies. Antigens are complex macromolecules containing protein, often in combination with carbohydrate or lipid. In order to be antigenic, a substance must have a molecular weight of at least 5,000 [89] and a firm molecular structure. **Haptens** are incomplete antigens, substances that are capable of acting as antigens only when they are bound to a carrier molecule. Haptens have a lower molecular weight than antigens and are not capable of eliciting an immune response unless they are bound to a carrier substance.

Antibodies are protein substances synthesized by the body in response to antigens. For a reaction to antigens to occur, antibodies must be combined with antigens. Although there is much to be discovered about antigen-antibody responses, it is known that there is a relation between the specificity of the antibody responses and the antigen that has stimulated the antibody formation. Antibodies belong to the classes of immunoglobulins. There are five different classes of antibodies, each class being an **isotype** and each having a pair of light and heavy chains. The abbreviation Ig is used to signify immunoglobulin, and the classes or isotypes are designated by the Greek letters for G, A, M, D, and E (γ, α, μ, δ, and ϵ). Each Greek letter signifies a different isotype with an identifying different heavy chain. Each class of immunoglobulin, IgG, IgA, IgM, IgD, and IgE, is further subdivided into subclasses (Fig. 1-1). These subclasses, referred to by number, such as IgG_1, IgG_2, and so on, are **allotypes.** They represent further differences in heavy chain formation in each class. The differences in heavy chain formation are attributed to genetic variations. IgG isotypes, for example, have four different subclasses of allotypes, numbered 1 to 4, which are distinct, genetically transmitted allotypes.

The IgG isotypes are the most predominant and frequently found, occurring primarily in the blood and extravascular spaces. Most of the immunity for blood-borne agents is provided by the IgG isotypes; in fact about 80 percent or more of the immunoglobulins in the serum are IgG. Infants have high IgG levels at birth. IgG levels begin to decrease at about 6 to 8 months of age. The levels present at about 4 to 5 years of age are maintained into adulthood. It is important to note that IgG antibodies are the only class with the capability of crossing the placenta and therefore are the only ones that can be transmitted from the mother to the baby, providing protection from viruses and from gram-positive organisms.

IgM immunoglobulins make up 5 to 10 percent of those found in the serum. The IgM isotypes are the largest of the immunoglobulin molecules and are similar to the IgG isotypes in function. The newborn begins synthesizing IgM antibodies at birth, reaching adult levels in about one year. Because the IgM antibodies do not cross the placenta, the newborn infant initially has low levels of IgM antibodies and therefore is more susceptible to gram-negative organisms.

IgA immunoglobulins are next in order of prevalence in the body after the IgG. Adult levels are attained at about the age of 7. These immunoglobulins are found in saliva, tears, respiratory and gastric mucin, lymphoid tissues of the gastrointestinal tract, genitourinary and respiratory passages, mammary secretions, and bile. The IgA isotypes protect mucous membranes and are usually excreted by the body so that their levels in the serum are usually low. Bound IgA releases histamine at the site of the immune reaction. The exact manner in which IgA functions for antimicrobial activity is not understood. It is known that IgA isotypes protect against proteolytic enzymes and form nonabsorbable complexes in the external secretory systems of the body. IgA are predominant in respiratory, gastrointestinal, and genitourinary infections and may confer passive immunity.

IgD immunoglobulins and IgE immunoglobulins are found in the mucosa of the respiratory and gastrointestinal tracts. It is thought that both are involved in many allergic reactions. IgE levels, like IgA levels, are fairly constant throughout life. No specific role has been identified in IgD reactions, whereas IgE has been found to mediate hypersensitivity reactions and atopic diseases. Dermatitis and asthma are two examples of the atopic diseases.

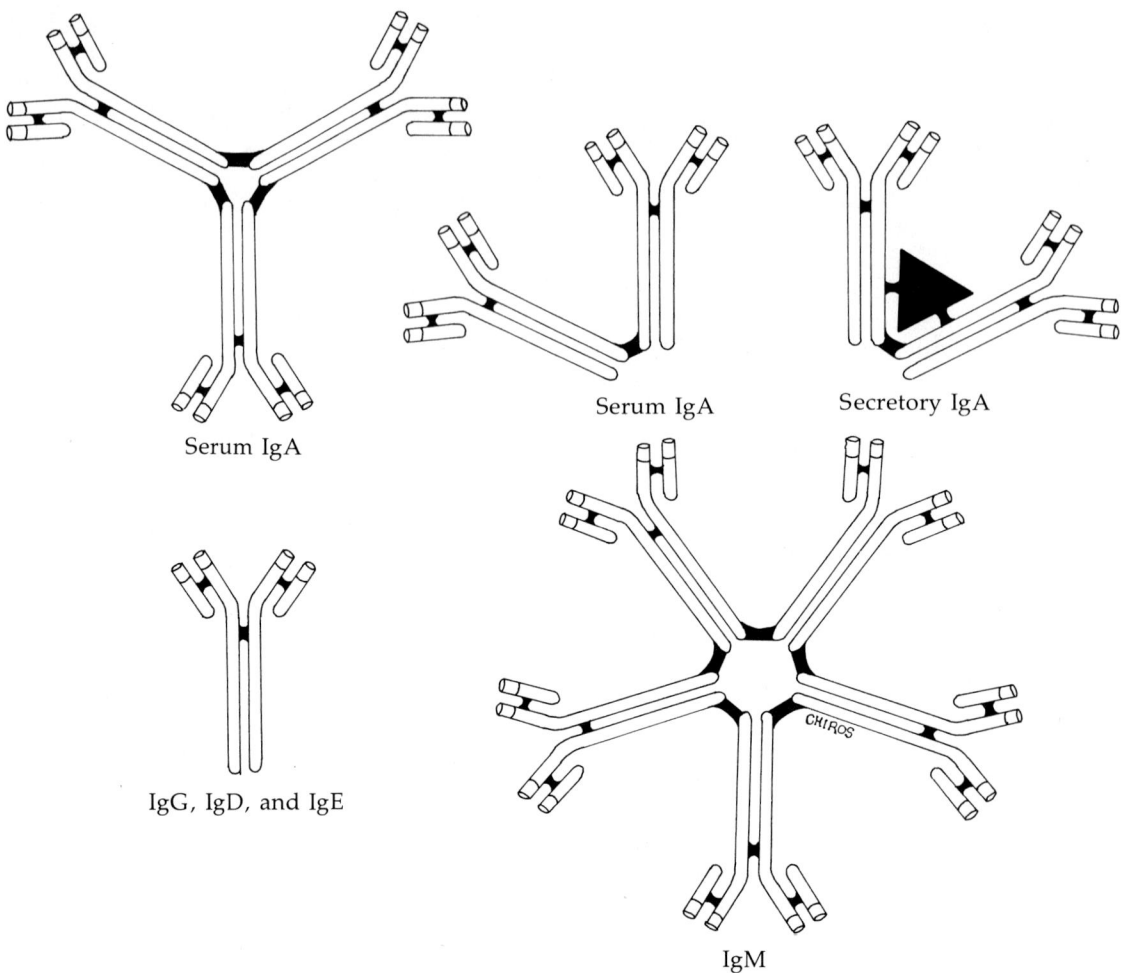

Figure 1-1
Diagram of antibodies.

The humoral or serologic component of the immune system, in which antigens stimulate production of antibodies, is called B-cell division. In this component, antibodies that are immunoglobulins are produced principally by the plasma cells. Precursors of B cells that produce antibodies probably arise from the bone marrow. In addition to the plasma cells, certain lymphoblasts may also produce antibodies. Generally, a cell that is capable of producing antibodies or immunoglobins is a **lymphocyte.**

The basis for the development of B cells in man is not known. Lymphoid tissue, which is a broad designation for the body tissues that synthesize antibodies, includes the central lymphoid structures, the thymus and lymphoid tissues in the gastrointestinal tract, and the peripheral lymphoid tissues or organs; the spleen; and lymph nodes. Tonsils forming Waldeyer's ring, Peyer's patches in the ileum, the vermiform appendix, and bone marrow cells are sites of specific lymphoid tissues. The central lymphoid structures mature at about one year of age, with peripheral lymphoid tissue attaining adult size at approximately 6 years (Fig. 1-2).

The second component of the immune system, cellular immunity, is the **T cell,** which is responsible for cellular-mediated immunity. T cells are formed during embryogenesis, and their formation is dependent on the thymus gland, which attains its greatest mass just prior to puberty and thereafter decreases in size. In contrast, the spleen achieves its full weight in adulthood.

Health and Disease States 25

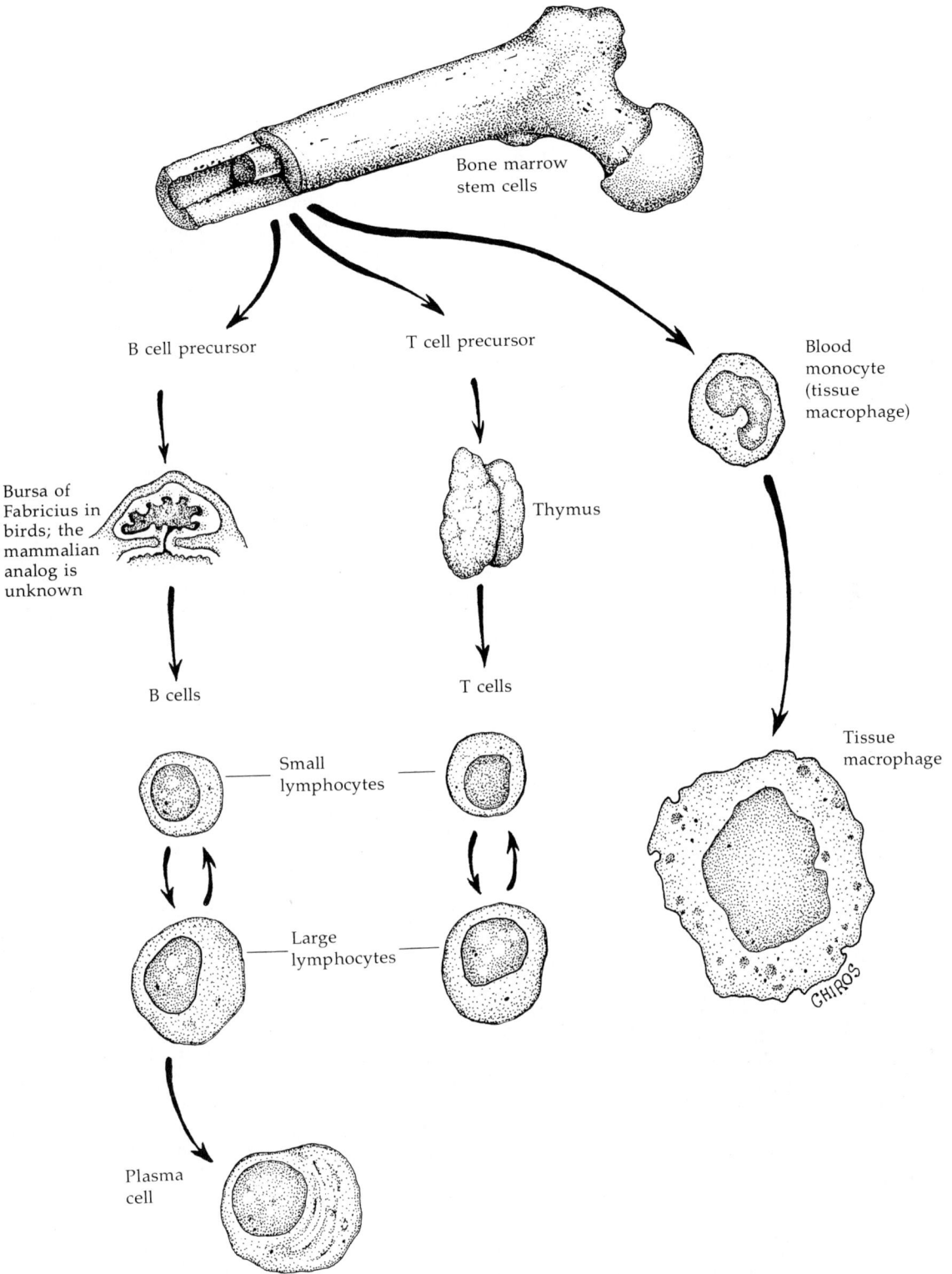

Figure 1-2
Development of cells in immune response.

In cell-mediated immunity, sensitized lymphoid cells recognize the antigen. This component of immunity is a defense mechanism against substances including parasites, fungi, and cancer growth, and it functions in transplant rejections. The lymphocytes of the T-cell component are sensitized to antigens through exposure. The resulting immune responses are highly specific.

There are differences in the degree of antibody-antigen responses in the immune system. The term **specificity** indicates that antibodies are specific for certain antigens. This concept is applicable to both serologic or humoral immunity and cell-mediated immunity. A portion of each antigen molecule reacts with the antibody; this portion is the **antigenic determinant. Affinity** is the strength of the attraction between the antigen and the antibody. **Avidity** is the strength of the bond formed after the antigen and antibody have made contact. The antigens that stimulate antibody formation initially have antigenic determinants for that antibody. Other antigens may contain some but not all determinants of the initiating antigen and are capable of forming a cross reaction with the antibody produced by the initial antigen. Antibodies react most strongly with the antigens that initially trigger their formation and less strongly with antigens that contain fewer of the antigenic determinants for the antibody as in a cross reaction.

The concept of specificity also applies to cellular immune responses. There is a stronger reaction with antigens that have initiated the initial response than with antigens that are related but not precisely the same. The process through which antibodies react with antigens in a specific relationship is **recognition.** It is thought that the surface of the cells in both components of the immune system, the humoral antibody system and the cell-mediated system, has receptors capable of recognizing and reacting with antigens. Exactly how recognition occurs is not known. It has been postulated that the mechanisms of recognition are the same or similar for both components.

When an antigen is introduced into the body for the first time, this initial contact causes a primary response. The antigen is taken up by macrophages, which process the antigen and help it become recognized by the lymphoid tissue. It is necessary that the antigen comes into direct contact with lymphoid tissue for antibody to be produced. A few days following introduction of the antigen into the body, precursors of antibody-forming cells are released into the circulation and distributed throughout the body, to the lymph nodes, and to the spleen. These precursors arise from stem cells in the bone marrow. Within the bone marrow the cells are not differentiated; these cells are **lymphocytes.** These lymphocytes may differentiate to become one of three types of cells: plasma cells, sensitized lymphocytes, or macrophages, all of which are important in the immune response. Once the precursor cells have differentiated and have left the bone marrow, they no longer are capable of differentiation. According to the clonal selection theory, the body has capability for recognition of any foreign material that might be encountered throughout life.

The precursor lymphocytes from the bone marrow may become either B cells or T cells. The B cells are developed in gastrointestinal tract lymphoid tissue and the T cells are developed in the lymphoid tissue of the thymus. It is thought that the precursors of the antibody-forming cells may have receptors for recognition of specific antigens. How this takes place is a matter of speculation. It may be that the macrophages process the antigen so that recognition may occur. Another theory is that an interaction between T cells and B cells is necessary for recognition. Yet another theory postulates that T cells are responsible for recognition and that these cells react first, transmitting the information to the B cells. Following production of the precursor cells, which are thought to have receptors for recognition of specific antigens, however this takes place, 5 to 7 days are required for plasma cells to produce antibodies. Once the primary response has been established, there is an ability within the immune system to remember the antigen that stimulated the response.

The concept of memory is important in the secondary response of the immune system. Further stimulation of the immune response by the same antigen, that is, an antigen with the same structure as the initiating antigen, causes a second reaction, which is more rapid and stronger than the first, or primary, reaction. This secondary response is also called the anamnastic response. In the secondary response a burst of antibody production peaks after a few days and then diminishes so that the serum antibody titers are gradually reduced. A little understood control mechanism functions to prevent unchecked formation of antibodies. It is speculated that T cells may suppress antibody formation to control the response.

Two types of antibodies, antiantibodies and antireceptor antibodies, also function to control the antibody responses. Antiantibodies are common to a species and are called idiotypes. The **antiantibody** reacts with another antibody and thereby prevents the ability of the second antibody to become bound to an antigen. The **antireceptor antibody** reacts with the reactor (recognition) site on the surface of the antibody molecules so that the receptor site is not available for binding with antigens. Antireceptor antibodies block or limit the ability of the antibody to be bound to an antigen.

Another concept important in the control of the immune response is that of **tolerance.** In this process, antibodies are not produced to react to a known antigen. Tolerance may occur naturally or it may be induced. Natural tolerance is thought to occur during embryonic life. Because the fetus is isolated in the mother's womb, it comes into contact only with its own antigens, or self-antigens. Consequently the embryo develops tolerance for its self-antigens. If, however, foreign antigens are introduced during embryonic life, the fetus develops tolerance for these foreign antigens and does not have the ability to recognize them as foreign later in life.

Acquired tolerance is induced, usually by such methods as irradiation or by administration of antimetabolic drugs. An antigen that induces tolerance is a **tolerogen,** which may be administered to develop tolerance. Generally, tolerance is established most easily when the antigens serving as tolerogens are most closely related to those of the host. It is important to note that the dosage of antigen administered influences the reaction. In many instances high or low doses of antigen may induce tolerance, whereas an intermediate dosage induces an antibody response [82]. Once tolerance has been established, it must be supported to continue. This support is usually accomplished by periodic administration of the tolerogen.

Tolerance can be reversed by many methods. One is by introducing cross-related antigens which have some antigenic determinants in common with the antigens that induced tolerance.

The concept of immune tolerance is very important in several areas of practical application: in preparing and administering immunizations and in treating people who require organ transplants or those who have abnormal immune responses. The mechanisms of tolerance are not yet well understood. Some authorities believe that everyone has tolerance for certain continuously present antigens and that the immune system is able to maintain a state of balance through some sort of feedback mechanisms to keep the immune response in check. This balance is important for preventing tissue destruction as a result of immune response products while also maintaining sufficient protection for the body against harmful substances. For these reasons it is thought that the mechanism of tolerance is probably an ongoing and active process.

Immunity occurs naturally in the normally functioning immune system, and antibodies are constantly present in the body, usually in low titers. Artificial or acquired immunity may be produced to establish a response to antigens that are known to produce disease. This process is called immunization and it requires isolation of antigenic substances that must be appropriately prepared and administered to induce the specific immune response desired. Innate or natural immunity and acquired immunity may be classified as active or passive. **Passive immunity** occurs when antibodies are introduced into the body, such as occurs naturally in the fetus in utero, by maternal antibodies or by introduction of antibodies or pooled human immunoglobulin with specific antibodies. **Active immunity** is produced innately by contact with antigens in the environment, or artificially by contact with antigens purposefully introduced into the body, as in immunizations. Passive immunity is usually short-term immunity. Active immunity lasts longer and may extend for years or for the person's lifetime.

Antigens enter the body through various routes, via skin and the mucous membranes of the respiratory and gastrointestinal tracts. Artificially introduced antigens may be administered via these routes as well as via intradermal, intramuscular, and intravenous routes. Artificial antigens are most often combined with an adjuvant to "hold" the antigen so that it is released slowly and thereby creates a stronger reaction. The protocols established for administration of antigens are designed to establish immunity for as long as possible. Knowledge of primary and secondary reactions is used to determine the number of doses required to maintain the longest lasting immunity possible and to prevent development of tolerance.

A number of different substances are used as immunogens. These substances include killed bacteria, toxoids of bacteria, inactivated live or attenuated viruses, and killed organisms. The route selected for administration of the immunogen is determined to accomplish the most effective immunity possible. For example, oral polio vaccine reaches the lymphoid tissues of the gastrointestinal tract. The polio virus is contracted by swallowing infected material [87]. It is thought that local application or administration of the vaccine augments the action of the antibodies, because the isotype most often present in the local area is increased. For example, IgA antibodies increase most when the immunogen is applied to the mucous membranes of the respiratory tract, where IgA antibodies are found in the greatest number.

Even though a great degree of purification has been achieved in the preparation of vaccines to produce a specific immunity, it is not yet possible to establish purely specific immunity with vaccines. Differences in the antigen-antibody structures in both the vaccine and the receptor cells of the person being immunized may contribute to differences in reactions to the immunizations. Despite these differences, the effectiveness of immunization for prevention of widespread disease from infectious agents is important for positive health practices involving immunization programs. Unfortunately, immunizations are not available for every type of potentially harmful microorganism. There are, however, immunizations for many of the major communicable diseases including typhoid, polio, *viral* diseases such as influenza, smallpox, measles, mumps, and rubella, pertussis, cholera, and plague.

It is possible to measure the effectiveness of the immune response in laboratories by replicating the several different processes through which antigen-antibody responses produce immunity in the body. Some antigen-antibody complexes are capable of more than one type of process to render the foreign agent harmless. Because of the known responses of the antigen-antibody complexes, however, it is possible to establish controlled conditions in which the type of antibody, the antigen, and the levels of antigen and antibody can be distinguished or determined. Classification of these processes includes precipitation, agglutination, opsonization, lysis, and complement fixation. All these processes are determined by the amount of antigen, the available antibody, and the presence of enzymes, complement, and other factors that support the processes.

These reactions are replicated in laboratory tests including the Coombs test, the Paul Bunnel test, the Widal test, and the rheumatoid factor test, all of which depend on agglutination (clumping of cells). Each cell has a number of antigenic determinants, and agglutination reactions occur in both specific antigen-antibody reactions and cross-reacting antigen-antibody contacts. Complement fixation tests replicate the activity of antigen-antibody complexes upon complement to render it fixed.

The ability of antibodies to become attached to the receptor sites of the virus cell prevents its attachment to host cells, thereby neutralizing the virus. Radioimmunoassay is commonly used in laboratories to measure antibody levels and to detect the levels of substances such as hormones that enter into antigen-antibody reactions. Another measurement method is immunofluorescence, which utilizes a reagent or dye to establish fluorescent groups in proteins to measure the antigen-antibody activity. Dye-labeled antibodies reacting with specific antigens can be studied with an ultraviolet light in immunofluorescence techniques. Opsonization utilizes the process of phagocytosis of immunogenic particles through the reaction of the antibodies in the presence of complement.

As more is discovered about the specific aspects of the immune response, the ability to provide for artificial immunity, to intervene in immune diseases, and to promote growth of transplants will be improved.

Altered Immune Responses

Many diseases are associated with the immune response. Some of these diseases have been known as immune diseases for many years while others are diseases more recently associated with immune responses. There are many different ways to describe these disorders. For purposes of introduction to the subject, a discussion of the pathology of immune-related diseases follows.

There are several kinds of altered immune responses. Those mediated by antibodies include toxic complex responses, atopic reactions, neutralization, and cytotoxic reactions. All these responses require prior exposure of the antigen and a period of 1 to 2 weeks from the time the antigen is again introduced into the body until the secondary response occurs. The antibody reactions are most specific for antigens that stimulated their production and less specific for cross-reactive antigens. Each response is influenced by the nature and location of the antigen or the antibody tissue specificity or both, or by sensitization to the antigen. Usually the degree of hypersensitivity to the antigen diminishes with time. Reexposure of the antigen, however, involves an increasingly rapid and more intense reappearance of the hypersensitivity reaction. This reaction was explained earlier as the anamnestic response. Hypersensitivity mediated by antibodies can be transferred with serum antibody, and it is possible to accomplish temporary desensitization by administration of the antigen in repeated doses so that the antibodies present are bound or taken up by the doses of antigen. In this way the antibodies are not available for antigen-antibody reactions.

Cell-mediated immune responses include delayed and granulomatous hypersensitivity reactions. These responses occur between the antigen and lymphocytes. Cell-mediated reactions are localized and are not transferred by circulating antibody. It is thought that the granulomatous reactions may involve insoluble antigens as opposed to the soluble antigens common to humoral-mediated reactions.

While immune reactions will be discussed separately according to the classifications of the type of reaction, it should be noted that immune reactions usually do not occur as a single entity. Usually the immune reactions occur in combination; the primary response may be an atopic reaction, but a toxic complex response may come into play. It is thought that some reactions may stimulate other types of reactions and that the toxic complex reaction may be involved in all the immune reactions in which tissues are injured or destroyed. In some instances the reactions are variations of one another; neutralization reactions, for example, are actually variations of the toxic complex reactions. The granulomatous reaction may be a variation of the delayed hypersensitivity reaction.

In many instances a primary reaction may be associated with the causation or manifestation of any given disease. For this reason, disease processes most commonly associated with a particular type of immunologic response are included as the response is being discussed.

The immune response may be induced by any number of natural or artificial antigenic substances. It should be noted that the chemicals of drugs often act as haptens and can be combined in the body to become complete antigens, capable of inducing the immune response. The various immune responses associated with drug administration are not emphasized in this text, and the reader is referred to a pharmacology text for this information.

While the immune response is normally protective, it also can destroy tissue or interfere with tissue function. **Atopy,** also called allergic reactions, and **anaphylactic reactions** are perhaps the most commonly known of the altered immune responses that can produce tissue damage. These reactions occur when antigens react with previously sensitized cells. In tissues the most commonly affected cell is the **mast cell;** in the blood, **basophils** are the most commonly affected cells. As antigens react with these sensitized cells, pharmacologically active substances are released, causing changes in the tissues. The pharmacologically active substances are chemical mediators, among the most predominant being histamine and slow-reacting substance (SRS) in man. Others include serotonin, bradykinin, acetycholine, and heparin.

Chemical Mediators

In order to understand the abnormal reaction that ensues when antigens stimulate the sensitized antibodies, causing the release of chemical mediators, it is helpful to review the pharmacologic action of the mediators. Histamine, the most predominant in man, causes dilatation of capillaries and arterioles and increased tissue permeability, contraction of smooth muscles, and increased gastric secretion. The pharmacologic blocking of these actions is achieved by antihistamines. Serotonin is found in platelets, the spleen, the gastrointestinal tract, in mast cells, lung tissue, and the brainstem. Serotonin acts to contract smooth muscle, to decrease central nervous system activity, and to increase intestinal peristalsis and the respiratory rate. Serotonin also provokes histamine release.

The release of SRS is coincidental with the release of histamine but its action is slower than that of histamine [87]. The release of SRS is not blocked by antihistamines, an important point in the treatment of symptoms. Acetylcholine is mostly localized at the neural synaptic connections and causes peripheral vasodilatation. Cholinesterase inactivates acetylcholine.

Heparin is found in mast cells. It decreases coagulation of the blood and changes the surface of the blood cell and blood vessel walls. The release of heparin accounts for the prolonged clotting time that occurs in anaphylaxis.

Signs and symptoms resulting from the action of the chemical mediators depend on the location of the immune response. If, for example, histamine is released in the respiratory airways, the contraction of smooth muscle and mucus production both contribute to narrowing or blocking the airways, interfering with ventilation. The action of histamine in the gastrointestinal tract does not cause blocking in the same way as in the airways, because the products can be eliminated more easily from the gastrointestinal tract through increased peristalsis. The route of entry then sometimes determines the signs and symptoms resulting from the antigen-antibody response. In anaphylactic shock, the sensitized cells of the shock organs are activated, usually through intravenous administration of an antigen. Anaphylactic shock, however, can occur as a result of oral, subcutaneous, or intramuscular injection of antigens. In other instances the route of entry elicits specific symptoms. Antigens causing extrinsic asthma are inhaled and stimulate the bronchial mucosa. Urticaria may result from orally ingested antigens, and atopic dermatitis results from antigenic contact with the skin.

Allergic Reactions

Allergic reactions are stimulated by antibodies termed **reaginic antibodies,** which are found in all the immunoglobulin groups of antibodies. IgE predominates in allergic reactions and is a skin-fixing antibody that binds to the mast cells or basophils. Anaphylaxis may be mediated by both IgE and IgG. Diagnostic tests for determination of the presence of reaginic antibodies of the IgE class are limited because the serum levels of IgE are very minimal and cannot be measured easily. Skin tests using application of allergens to the skin evoke a response in sensitive individuals. The radioallergosorbent test (RAST) is done by binding radiolabeled anti-IgE to IgE bound to the antigen to determine the amount of bound IgE. Some centers also use the radioimmunosorbent test (RIST) to measure the IgE concentrations. This test is very useful in differentiating between intrinsic and extrinsic asthma.

Other tests include the Schultz-Dale test and the Prausnitz-Küstner (P-K) reaction. The Schultz-Dale test is done with animal organs that are sensitized to react with specific antigens. The degree of the reaction is measured by the organ contraction. The P-K reaction uses human IgE fixed to the skin, which causes a cytophilic affinity for the mast cells in the dermal plasma membrane.

The signs and symptoms of allergic and anaphylactic reactions may be variable. Anaphylactic reactions may be either localized or systemic. Localized reactions include formation of wheals or hives and flare, itching, and sometimes urticaria. Systemic reactions include contraction of smooth muscles, increased permeability of the small blood vessels, bronchospasm, wheezing, dyspnea, bradycardia, and faintness; circulatory shock and death may occur within 2 hours.

Conditions such as asthma, hay fever, hives, and eczema are examples of atopic, or allergic, responses. The signs and symptoms depend on the route of entry of the antigen into the body or to the area of contact, the dose of the antigen, and the sensitivity of the given organs to the antigen. It is postulated that sensitivity may be genetically controlled and that familial tendencies exist. There may then be a hereditary predisposition to allergic reactions. It is also possible that susceptible people have higher IgE levels than normal or that their IgE is of a variant type. Another possibility in causation of allergic reactions is that sensitive people may be more sensitive to the pharmacologic action of cell mediators.

Treatment of allergic reactions is not specific because so many aspects of the processes of the allergic response are not understood. Included in these processes are the elicitation of the immune response by the antigens and the antigen-antibody reaction, the release of chemical mediators, and the activity of the autonomic nervous system. The antigen-antibody response has been discussed previously, but some points about the enzyme system and the autonomic nervous system should be discussed for clarity.

At the cellular level, the enzyme system that is activated to release mediators may be a function of both alpha and beta adrenergic receptors. Cyclic AMP, controlled by the stimulation of alpha and beta receptors, determines the amount of mediators available. It should be noted that there is provision for cellular regulation of the enzymes as the beta receptors activate adenyl cyclase, which increases cyclic AMP, while alpha receptors decrease cyclic AMP. Drugs may be used to intervene in this balance of receptor activity. For example, norepinephrine stimulates the alpha receptors to increase enzymes and sensitization to allergens. Isoproterenol stimulates beta receptors and decreases allergic sensitivity. Theophylline prevents cyclic AMP breakdown and decreases sensitivity to antigens.

It is possible that allergic reactions may in part be caused by loss of balance between alpha and beta receptors in the end organs. These organs include the muscles of the bronchial and the gastrointestinal tract. Decreases in cyclic AMP, from stimulation of alpha receptors, may cause end-organ cells to become activated. For some reason, the beta cell receptors are not able to respond by increasing cyclic AMP, which would relax smooth muscle cells and counterbalance the alpha effect. If this theory is correct, some allergic responses may not be caused by alterations of immune system responses, but rather by the imbalance between alpha and beta receptors.

On a broader level, there is also a balance in the autonomic nervous system between the parasympathetic (cholinergic) and sympathetic (adrenergic) systems. If there is imbalance, for example, if the sympathetic system effects override those of the parasympathetic system, bronchial constriction, gastrointestinal peristalsis, dilatation of the bladder sphincter and arteries, and pupil constriction predominate. It is possible that some of the allergic reactions may be primarily due to autonomic nervous system imbalances. More likely, the allergic reactions are complex interactions among many factors.

Because of the inability to detail all the processes of the allergic response, treatment cannot be truly specific to the cause. Intervention can take place at any level, however. The person who is sensitive to allergens might first prevent the response by avoiding the allergen. If this is not possible, hyposensitization, desensitization, or tolerance can be achieved so that the IgE receptor is reduced to diminish the response that occurs when the person does come into contact with the allergen. This therapy is not always successful, however. Other treatment modalities include those of controlling the level of cyclic AMP with drugs or decreasing sympathetic stimulation, or blocking of parasympathetic symptoms. As is discussed in later chapters in relation to specific disease processes, the role of the person's emotional state is also important in the incidence of allergic reactions. It is not known how the emotional state affects the allergic response, but it is known that this response is a complex one, stimulated by multiple factors.

Delayed Hypersensitivity Reaction

Another classification of altered immune responses is the **delayed hypersensitivity reaction**. In this reaction, specifically modified lymphocytes react to antigens when they come into contact with the receptor sites. At the site of localization of the antigen, the cells become infiltrated with monocytes and lymphocytes. This infiltration, through a little understood mechanism, causes tissue destruction. Cell mediators are released from damaged cells and can affect cells surrounding those involved in the antigen response. The cell mediators can cause injury or destruction to these surrounding tissues.

As the name implies, delayed hypersensitivity may occur days or weeks following the contact with the allergen. Because many of the studies of this type of reaction were first done with tuberculin, delayed hypersensitivity is sometimes also called the tuberculin-type reaction. This type of reaction is a cellular reaction as opposed to the humoral antibody reaction of allergic reactions. The altered cell–mediated immunity response involves destruction of cells or an inability of cells to function and is the delayed hypersensitivity reaction.

The tuberculin test demonstrates the events occurring in delayed hypersensitivity reactions. When tuberculin antigens are injected into the skin, no reaction occurs for 4 to 6 hours. The induration and swelling then occur, reaching a peak between 24 and 48 hours. Mononuclear cells accumulate, particularly around the small veins, and the dermis eventually becomes invaded (see color insert Figure 1 on page 1078A).

Allergens causing contact allergy, such as poison ivy, cosmetics, clothing, and adhesive tape, are highly reactive chemical compounds. They are also lipid-soluble and therefore can penetrate the epidermis. In the epidermis the chemicals, which are incomplete antigens or haptens, combine with some factor, yet unknown, to form a complete antigen. This reaction may be evoked in nonsensitive as well as sensitive people. A greater amount of the antigen is required to stimulate a response in nonsensitized people than in sensitized individuals. The visible response to the contact allergen is redness, induration, and vesiculation. Because the epidermis must be penetrated by the antigen, contact dermatitis reactions may take longer than dermal reactions initiated by injection of antigen (tuberculin testing) into the dermis. It is important to note that the reaction to chemical haptens is dependent on a vascular supply, indicating that hematogenous cells do carry the sensitivity [87].

Cell-mediated delayed hypersensitivity reactions are important in a number of viral diseases such as influenza, herpes simplex, variola, and mumps; in mycotic infections such as dermatophytes and *Candida*; and in protozoal infections, insect bites (see color insert Figure 2 on page 1078A), and infestations by parasites. The parasitic organisms are not directly toxic, but it is thought that the inflammatory reactions they produce may cause the hypersensitivity reaction. When these antigens first come into contact with the body, there is no reaction. Later, cell-mediated hypersensitivity develops to help the host to limit the infection or to destroy the organism. Cellular destruction may occur as a byproduct of the hypersensitivity reaction.

In addition to the infectious diseases related to delayed hypersensitivity, many other diseases are associated with delayed hypersensitivity responses. For example, certain genetic phenotypes of the HL-A system (which will be discussed later) have been found in some people with immunopathologic diseases such as lupus erythematosis, active hepatitis, myasthenia gravis, ankylosing spondylitis, and psoriasis. There is much ongoing research in this area, and it may be that these diseases can be better treated when and if specific alterations in immune response are identified.

Donor Grafts and Organ Transplants

Much related research has been ongoing in the field of organ transplants and grafting. Grafts refer to placement of skin or tissue from a donor to an individual to replace missing or damaged skin or tissue or to improve function or appearance. Donor graft rejections are cell-mediated delayed hypersensitivity reactions. The rejection of donor tissue occurs when the recipient reacts to donor tissue antigens that are foreign to him. These antigens are called transplantation antigens. The names of grafts indicate the relation of the donor graft to the recipient: **homografts,** or **allografts,** are transplants between individuals in the same species. An **isograft** is a tissue transplant between two persons with identical genetic strains. **Xenograft** is a graft from a donor of a species different from that of the recipient, such as an animal graft applied to a recipient human [87].

Other terms used in transplants are **autograft,** which is a graft from one part of the body to another in the same person; **orthotopic graft,** which means that an organ or tissue is transplanted into its anatomically designated position; and **heterotopic graft,** which is tissue transplanted to an abnormal position. When tissue antigens are the same for both the donor and the recipient they are said to be **histocompatible.** When tissue antigens between the donor and the recipient are different, a state of **histoincompatibility** exists [83].

Allograft rejections occur when tissue is transplanted from one individual to an immunocompetent person of the same species. When tissue is transplanted from the self, or from a genetically identical person, such as a monozygotic twin, the allograft rejection does not occur. Grafts between different species (xenografts) cause rapid and severe rejection reactions.

When grafts are placed, revascularization (development of blood supply to the graft) occurs on about the second or third day and is completed by about the sixth to seventh day. After the first week, the signs of rejection begin in the deep layers of the graft. This response is similar to the tuberculin reaction, with infiltration and edema. In 9 to 10 days, thrombosis occurs, and necrosis of tissue with sloughing of the graft occurs in 11 to 14 days. The entire process is called the first-set rejection.

The second graft causes a more rapid and intense rejection because preformed antibody is now present against the antigens in the donor graft. The second-set rejection takes only 4 to 5 days for necrosis and tissue ischemia to occur.

Rejections are mediated by the cellular type of allergic reaction, and humoral antibodies may also be involved in rejection. This is related to the histocompatibility of the donor graft and the recipient. The ABO erythrocyte and leukocyte systems and the HL-A system are important in determining compatibility. Some antigens are specific to a species; others are specific to a given organ of the body. In allograft rejection, it is the antigenic differences between the donor and the recipient of the same species that determine the rejection. These antigens are **isoantigens**. The HL-A system of antigens is shared by most of the nucleated body cells. The name human leukocyte locus A (HL-A) was originally given to the system because early research concentrated on leukocytes. The system now includes antigens of a much broader scope; however, the name still is used.

The HL-A system comprises more than forty different specificities controlled by an allelic pair of autosomal cistrons. (A **cistron** is a linear array of codons required for synthesis of a single polypeptide chain.) Each cistron has information for two HL-A antigens, each HL-A with a maximum of two specificities in each of its two subdivisions: segregant series or the first and second sublocus. Because of the many possible variables, the chances of achieving histocompatibility by exactly matching two unrelated individuals are about one in a million.

In addition to the HL-A system, the blood-group antigens of the ABO system are important in matching grafts. These blood groups are particularly important in matching blood transfusions with the recipient and are discussed more fully in Chapter 5.

Determining histocompatibility between the graft donor and the recipient or host is important in preparations for transplantation. As mentioned earlier, grafts from identical twins are histocompatible and therefore more likely to "take." When grafts are taken from donors who are relatives, better histocompatibility can be achieved than when the grafts are taken from nonrelated individuals or from nonrelated cadavers. A number of pregraft activities are important to augment growth of the graft in the recipient. Tissue typing is done to match the ABO and Rh antigens and antigens of the HL-A system. Tests are also done to determine the presence of cytotoxic antibodies in the recipient to the donor cells.

Measures can also be taken to repress or suppress the rejection of allografts. Antimetabolites and alkylating agents that act on the lymphoid cells have particular affinity for the cells of the T-cell division, and this activity reduces the immune competence of the individual. Corticosteroids are also used to decrease the activity of lymphocytes that are sensitized for donor antigens. Corticosteroids suppress T-cell lymphocytes associated with cell-mediated activity more than humoral activity, and they interfere with antibody synthesis when given in large enough doses. The side effects of corticosteroids may inhibit their use for immunosuppression in some patients.

Antilymphocytic serum has also been prepared for administration prior to grafting. This serum is prepared by immunizing horses with human lymphoid tissues to develop human antiserum. It contains a globulin fraction that is effective in suppressing the immune response, although its mechanism of action is not understood. Humoral immunity is not affected; it is postulated that the serum blocks recognition of antigens in some way. There is much experimentation with different methods to establish tolerance or enhancement to antigens in an effort to induce immune suppression prior to grafting. With present practice, there is always the possibility that a graft may take for several years and then be rejected. Persons treated with immunosuppressive drugs have a tendency to develop infections and there is a higher incidence of malignancy following immunosuppression in these people. Both of these problems are major ones.

In addition to histocompatibility, there are many other important considerations in determining the feasibility of organ transplants. In general, transplantation of the kidney is most successful because the kidney is easiest to replace anatomically. In addition, the kidney has considerable reserve function so that even if some tissue destruction occurs, the transplanted kidney can still maintain some function. There are also artificial means for supplying kidney function through dialysis, if necessary. Other solid organs are not as easy to transplant, and the rejection affects functioning of the whole organ. Transplants of hearts and livers have been done, but survival rates for these transplants are lower than those for kidney transplants.

Another advantage of kidney transplants is that a kidney may be donated by a relative or by an identical twin, increasing the probability of success. The kidney, however, is one of the few solid organs that are duplicated in the body. There is only one heart and only one liver. Thus, most solid organs cannot be donated by live persons, and for transplantation of these organs cadavers must be used. Some transplanted organs are able to grow because the body has some *immune privileged* sites where grafts can take; these sites include the meninges of the brain and the anterior chamber of the eye. Because these areas have no lymph drainage, there is less stimulation of the graft by immune cells of the host's lymph tissue [82].

Granulomatous Reaction

Yet another type of immune response is the granulomatous reaction, which may be stimulated by foreign bodies or through hypersensitivity reactions to insoluble antigens. These reactions are similar to delayed hypersensitivity reactions, but are even more delayed. In granulomatous reaction, there is formation of an insoluble colloid, leading to epithelial cell growth which, together with other reticuloendothelial cells such as giant cells and histocytes, forms a granuloma. Examples of these reactions include diseases such as sarcoidosis and leprosy. One form of tuberculosis may be caused by the granulomatous hypersensitivity reaction.

The Arthus Reaction

One of the types of immune response that are considered to be central to other types is the Arthus reaction, or the toxic complex reaction. **Arthus reaction** refers to an experimental model in which antigen was demonstrated to produce a secondary response of increased antibody titers, agglutination of platelets, mast cell degranulation, and release of pharmacologically active substances. The transudation of molecules and activation of the complement system cause considerable vasculitis with hemorrhage, thrombosis, and acute inflammation. It is thought that reactions of the Arthus type are the result of antibody reactions with antigens in the tissue or by formation of complexes of soluble antigen and antibody. IgG antibodies are the predominant isotypes that cause precipitation.

The soluble antigen-antibody complexes are formed by the precipitation antibody to create microprecipitates in and around small vessels or in the bloodstream. When lodged in the blood vessels, the circulating complexes can cause inflammation. When they are activated by chemotaxic factor, the complexes fix complement so that the leukocytes release lysosomal enzymes, which cause destruction of the tissues.

Serum sickness is an example of an Arthus reaction and results when the elastic portion of the lamina of the arteries is destroyed. In serum sickness the antibody titers first increase, then complexes form between antigen and antibody and are deposited on vascular walls. The immune complexes cause an inflammatory response. Another example of a disease related to the Arthus reaction is glomerulonephritis. One cause is alteration of the basement membrane of glomeruli from the destruction of small vessels. There are also other causes of glomerulonephritis.

Collagen diseases are other examples of the Arthus or toxic complex reaction. These diseases may affect multiple organs and tissues throughout the body. There is evidence that immunopathology may be a major causative factor in collagen diseases. Among the collagen diseases are systemic lupus erythematosus, polyarteritis nodosa, scleroderma, dermatomyositis, and rheumatoid arthritis. In both rheumatoid arthritis and systemic lupus erythematosus, there is formation of autoantibodies to the person's own tissue. There seems to be a relation between collagen diseases and other autoimmune and granulomatous diseases. Many people who are affected with one of these altered immune responses also are affected by others.

The specific cause of systemic lupus erythematosus (SLE) is not known. It is postulated that an antigen, perhaps a virus, causes the immune response of this collagen disease. It is possible that, having developed autoimmunity, the toxic complex reaction destroys the small vessels and leads to the fragmentation and destruction of collagen fibers that occur in the collagen diseases. The signs and symptoms of the disease are variable and are related to destruction of tissue and formation of fibrinous areas.

Previously the LE cell (a polymorphonuclear neutrophil, formed by an antibody capable of reacting with deoxyribonucleic acid [DNA]) was diagnostic of SLE. Currently, identification of antinuclear antibodies usually of the IgG type, but also IgM or IgD, is considered diagnostic of SLE. These antinuclear antibodies act against the nucleus of damaged cells. The antinuclear antibodies cannot act against healthy cells, but require some factor that causes cell damage to gain entry. Once the antinuclear antibodies have reacted with nuclear antigens, complement is formed and the cell structure is damaged, causing interference with function or destruction of the cells. It is thought that these reactions may be the cause of the multiple lesions that occur in the spleen, in the basement membranes of the skin, and in the choroid plexus of the brain in people with systemic lupus erythematosus.

No one knows why there are so many degrees of severity of lupus erythematosus or why the spontaneous remissions and exacerbations occur during the course of the disease. There is also no explanation for the myriad of disease patterns found among people with lupus. Lesions may be found in a combination of many organs: skin, heart, vessels, central nervous system, and kidneys may all be involved either totally or in combinations. Because of this lack of knowledge about the cause, treatment is usually geared to decreasing the inflammatory reaction by use of corticosteroids and immunosuppressive drugs. Renal or nervous system involvement is the most common cause of death in SLE.

Rheumatoid arthritis is another collagen disease that evades diagnosis and classification. The symptoms begin with inflammation of the synovia, followed by formation of a granulomatous inflammation called pannus. The synovia is filled with lymphocytes and plasma cells, which cause the hyperplasia. Nodules may form in the subcutaneous tissue, and in some persons there is also inflammation of the vessel walls and of the myocardium.

As with SLE, a rheumatoid factor has been isolated. This factor is usually an IgM antibody, which specifically acts with the person's self-IgG. Increased levels of this rheumatoid factor have been found in people experiencing exacerbations of the disease, along with increases in IgG in the cytoplasm of the complexes. It is thought that there may be a cyclic effect in which antigens, yet to be identified, stimulate the production of anti-IgG antibody. The antigen-antibody complexes may lead to the formation of the rheumatoid factor, which in turn may perpetuate formation of antibody complexes to activate complement. The complement activation may result in proliferation of lymphocytes and plasma cells in the synovium, and these cells may assume lymphoid tissue function to further produce the rheumatoid factor.

Whatever the process that takes place, people with rheumatoid arthritis have pain and scarring as a result of the granulomatous inflammation. The scars lead to decreased joint mobility, so that both the pain and the immobility must be treated to provide comfort and to prevent contractures. Experimentation continues to uncover more information about the causation of these evasive collagen diseases.

Cytotoxic or Cytolytic Reactions

Another type of allergic reaction is the cytotoxic or cytolytic reaction, in which circulating antibody reacts with antigenic cell components or with antigens attached to the cells. Erythrocytes, leukocytes, platelets, and vascular endothelium have antigens on the cell membranes, and the complement system may be activated by antigen-antibody reactions, thereby destroying the integrity of the cell membrane.

Complement, made up of the components of the enzyme system of the cell, causes lysis or death. The complement system is an accessory system that immunologically supports the suppurative inflammatory process. Complement includes more than ten serum proteins, interacting in sequence. Each component is identified by a number: C1, C2, and so on. The major complements make up 7 to 10 percent of the total serum globulin, and the reaction sequence is moderated by inhibitors and inactivators so that balance is maintained. The proteins in the complement system react with antigen-antibody complexes, causing the cellular trauma and inflammation that are basic to the cytotoxic and cytolytic reactions. It may be that these reactions are also important in precipitating the toxic complex reactions. Specific complement proteins have been found to be decreased in lupus erythematosus and glomerulonephritis. While the cytolysis that follows fixation eliminates the antigen, it can also destroy the cells. Therefore, complement has a positive and a negative action. Transfusion reactions, erythroblastosis fetalis, agranulocytosis, and thrombocytopenic purpura are some of the disorders that can be classified as complement-related cytotoxic reactions. Many bleeding disorders and abnormal bleeding tendencies are exaggerated by the complement system. The cycle of events that occur in these disorders can be triggered by many events; for example, inflammation, trauma, responses to certain endotoxins, and antibody-antigen reactions.

Erythrocytes from donor blood may stimulate circulating antibody of the host when a blood transfusion is given. Blood typing prior to transfusion is important as more than sixty different blood group factors are *currently recognized* as leading to antibody reactions with donor blood. The Rh system and the ABO system are the most predominant in blood reactions and can be detected by crossmatching the donor and recipient blood prior to transfusion. Blood groups have different antigenic specificities on the surfaces of the erythrocytes, and these individual blood group characteristics are inherited.

In transfusion reactions, the patient's antibody reacts with the donor's antigen. A reverse transfusion reaction, in which the patient's antigen reacts with the donor's antibody, may occur. In erythroblastosis, the donor's antigen reacts with the host's antibody. The woman carrying an Rh-positive fetus is sensitized in the first pregnancy, becoming immunized by the Rh-positive erythrocytes that pass into her blood from the fetus during delivery. During the second pregnancy, the antibody response to antigen has been established. Because maternal IgG crosses the placenta, the antibodies can cause death of the fetal erythrocytes. Another condition, autoallergic hemolytic anemia, results when the antibody and antigen complexes form within the body as the antibodies to antigens in self-erythrocytes.

Acute granulocytosis is an allergic reaction to drugs that adhere to the leukocytes. The drugs act as haptens and become bound to become complete antigens. Sulfapyridine is an example of a drug that can cause acute agranulocytosis. There are also drugs that can induce hemolytic reactions because they are capable of adhering to red cells. Penicillin is an example of a drug that can act as a hapten, becoming a complete antigen and binding to the erythrocytes. Allergic reactions may also occur to platelets, and the result is hemorrhage and purpura.

It is interesting to note that cytotoxic reactions may contribute to many autoallergic diseases, occurring as secondary mechanisms to the primary mechanism of delayed hypersensitivity, and demonstrating the overlapping of the various types of immune responses.

Classification of Hypersensitivity Reactions
These reactions may be classified in types from I to IV as follows:

Type I reactions Anaphylactic reactions include both systemic and local anaphylaxis, cytolytic and cytotoxic reactions, transfusion reactions, toxic-complex reactions, and delayed cellular hypersensitivity reactions.

In these reactions, a foreign antigen reacts with antibodies in the tissues that have been formed through previous sensitization by contact with the antigen. The effects of tissue damage are partly explained by release of histamine or other pharmacologically active substances from the mast and basophilic cells. The reaginic antibody has a particular affinity for the cell membrane and can remain fixed to it for many weeks, explaining the delayed reactions.

Local anaphylaxis is caused when the antigen gains contact to a body surface such as the mucous membranes of the respiratory airways. Systemic anaphylaxis indicates that there is increased sensitivity to a foreign substance.

Desensitization may be accomplished by raising the level of the circulating antibody to take up the antigen, thereby preventing the antigen from reaching the tissue cells covered with reaginic antibody.

Type II reactions The antigenic component is part of a tissue cell, or is closely associated to the tissue cell. IgG and IgM antibodies cause cytotoxic or cytolytic effects, usually involving activation of complement (transfusion reactions).

Type III reactions Complexes between the antigen and the antibody form in the blood or tissues in conditions in which there is a high level of circulating antibody. The complexes form mechanical blockages, particularly in the small vessels (serum sickness).

Type IV reactions Delayed cellular hypersensitivity reactions involve a mixed cellular reaction that involves lymphocytes and macrophages. The antigen may be introduced by skin contact or by intracellular infectious agents, which become antigenic by binding with proteins in the skin. The results are localized signs of redness, swelling, formation of vesicles, and scaling and exudation of fluid. Local anaphylaxis occurs more frequently than systemic anaphylaxis. Systemic anaphylaxis may be drug-induced or may result from bee stings in hypersensitive people. Desensitization is accomplished by giving small doses of subcutaneously injected antigen to which the patient is hypersensitive. The doses are repeated and slowly increased to develop antibodies that block the antigen from contact with the reaginic antibody that coats the tissue cells. To determine which substances a person may be hypersensitive to, intradermal injection of antigens is done. This test does not give conclusive evidence of specific hypersensitivities, however, as cross reactions may occur in the tests. It is also difficult to isolate every antigen to which a person may be sensitive.

The IgG antibodies in the serum have a high degree of organ specificity. Immune-related diseases such as thyroiditis (see Chap. 8) may occur. IgG or IgM antibodies are usually involved in cytolytic or cytotoxic mechanisms. They combine with the antigens of microorganisms to immobilize them. Kidney disease may occur because antibodies capable of reacting with the glomerular capillary basement membrane (GBM antigen) or antibodies reacting with circulating antigen-antibody complexes have been produced.

The study of immunopathology is continuing, and in the future there may be valid evidence that many diseases are caused or influenced by specific immune mechanisms. Study of the immune response in cancer is currently of vital interest. Cancer, the abnormal and continued growth of cells of a given tissue, is a subject of much concern. It is postulated that the body has defense mechanisms that operate to prevent or limit tumor growth. One of these mechanisms may be the immune response to tissue antigens.

There are many types of tumor antigenic responses. Some of these responses are loss of normal antigenic specificity, development of new antigenic specificities that are not normally present in tissue, and embryonic reversion in which there are embryonic or fetal antigens. Organ-specific and histocompatible tumor-specific transplantation antigens (TSTA) have been demonstrated in experimental animals. These TSTAs are either specific for a given tumor or they can be shared by many tumors. **Autochthonous** is the word used to indicate the relation between the tumor and the host.

A carcinoembryonic antigen has been found to be present normally in low levels. People who have malignant tumors often have higher levels of this antigen. While not diagnostic for cancer, the levels of this antigen may be useful in evaluating the success of therapy for cancer. If, for example, the levels decrease following therapy, the person's prognosis can be considered to be more favorable than if the levels remain the same or increase. Another substance, alpha fetoprotein, has been identified. This substance is a serum protein secreted from cells and is found in high concentrations in adults with hepatic tumors. It is also found in pregnant women, and in very low levels in normal adults.

There is increased incidence of carcinoma

in persons who have received immunosuppressive therapy for any reason. It is postulated that immunosuppressive therapy may affect the T-cell component, leading to a decreased control of lymphoid-cell proliferation.

Although there is little conclusive evidence, it can be speculated that malignancy may occur as a result of a breakdown of the immune surveillance system. This breakdown may occur because of lack of specific tumor antigen, development of immune tolerance or decreased immune enhancement, or antigenic modulation of the tumor/host. There may be an imbalance in the host response, with decreased antigen stimulation or decreased antibody response. Another theory is that immunosuppressive cells may develop or that tumor growth occurs in immunologically privileged sites.

Primary Immunodeficiency Disorders

In addition to the types of immune responses discussed thus far, there are also primary immunodeficiency disorders. There are many of these disorders and, in an effort to bring some order to the diffuse naming of them, the World Health Organization has developed a Classification of Primary Immunodeficiency Disorders [87]. Some of these diseases are briefly described in the following paragraphs as they illustrate the effects of immunosuppression.

Agammaglobulinemia was one of the first described immunodeficiency states, having been discovered in 1952. It is a congenital sex-linked disorder that becomes evident at about the sixth to the ninth month of age, as the maternally transmitted immunoglobulin levels decrease. The infant has deficiencies in all five classes of immunoglobulins, with absence of plasma cells in the connective tissue, lymph nodes, and the spleen. There is also absence of germinal follicles in the lymph nodes and in the spleen, so that the infant has impaired antibody-formation capabilities. The infant is given prophylactic antibody therapy or gamma globulin injections to protect him from infection. Cell-mediated immunity is intact so that the infant is able to recover from viral infections, with the exception of viral hepatitis. Agammaglobulinemia is associated with the occurrence of rheumatoid arthritis, dermatomyositis, and vasculitis, or with malignancy of the lymphoreticular system.

Selective immunoglobulin deficiency is an isolated IgA deficiency. **Dysgammaglobulinemia** is a deficiency of one or more of the immunoglobulin classes, with IgA deficiency being the most frequently occurring. These infants have recurrent gastrointestinal infections with sprue-like symptoms and many allergic respiratory problems. It is thought that the disease may be autosomal, either recessive or dominant.

In **transient hypogammaglobulinemia of infancy** there is a delay in the onset of the synthesis of immunoglobulins. The disease is self-limiting, lasting to the age of from 15 to 18 months. These infants are susceptible to pyogenic-organism–induced infections, with IgG or IgA levels being either absent or diminished. IgM levels are often elevated or normal. Many of these infants are found to have hypertrophic tonsils and adenoids.

Deficiencies in cellular immunity include the Di George syndrome. In this condition there is absence of the parathyroid and thymus glands, and the newborn infant often manifests hypocalcemic tetany. The T-cell component may be totally deficient, whereas the B-cell division is normal and functioning. Often, the infant has associated anomalies of the trachea, the esophagus, the heart, or the great vessels. Because cell-mediated immunity is deficient, the infant is susceptible to fungal infections, to viruses, and to gram-negative infections. The affected infants usually die in infancy.

Episodic lymphopenia and lymphocytotoxin are associated with immunologic amnesia in which there is suppression of T-cell mediated immunity. These infants have recurrent bacterial and viral infections, and there is evidence of low IgM levels. Eczema is often found. The basic problem is that the infant's immunologic memory is impaired. These infants usually do not survive childhood.

Another condition that is associated with depressed cellular immunity is immunodeficiency with normal or hyperimmunoglobulinemia. This condition is similar to the Di George syndrome, but is usually less severe as the child usually has no parathyroid or thymus abnormalities. The infant is susceptible to severe infections since the ability to form antibodies is impaired because of the depletion of T-cell dependent lymphoid tissues.

Madame Louis Bar syndrome is an immunodeficiency disease with progressive cerebellar ataxia and recurrent sinus and pulmonary infections. Telangiectasia is also present. Wiskott-Aldrich syndrome is a sex-linked recessive, genetically transmitted disease in which the affected child has low IgA levels. The major problem in this condition is a defect in the processing of antigens by macrophages, which affects both the humoral and cellular immunity. The T-cell and B-cell divisions of the immune system are blocked. The result is that the infant is susceptible to infections, develops thrombocytopenic purpura and atopic eczema, but can respond normally to certain antigens.

Adults can acquire immunodeficiency as a result of the formation of thymomas. The defects in cellular immunity may influence all types of immunoglobulins, and antibody formation is generally impaired. There is increased incidence of arthritis and other collagen diseases in these persons. Hypogammaglobulinemia is a central finding in this disease.

Severe combined immunodeficiency, in which both humoral and cell-mediated immunity are impaired, occurs in two types. The Swiss type is autosomal recessive and becomes manifest in the first few weeks of infancy. The United States type may be less severe than the Swiss type and is sex-linked recessive. People with the United States type (thymic alymphoplasia) are unable to reject allografts, have a susceptibility for infection, and often die during childhood.

Variable immunodeficiencies occur, probably because of genetic factors, although environmental factors have been implicated in their causation. These patients tend to have many different syndromes including sprue-like syndrome, formation of granulomas in organs, an increased incidence of malignancy, and a high frequency of collagen diseases. They also tend to have hemolytic anemia, pernicious anemia, and gastric atrophy. The deficiencies in the immune system are variable, but cell-mediated immunity is usually normal. The only treatment available currently is the administration of gammaglobulin.

Immunodeficiency diseases occur in many different forms, and all represent some problem in the immune system. Some are specific for one type of immunoglobulin, others are variable in immunoglobulin deficiencies, still others are specific for cell-mediated immunity or involve only the humoral antibody-mediated immunity. The types of signs and symptoms found in infants and adults are similar to those found in diseases thought to be associated with alterations in the normal immune response, such as pernicious anemia, collagen diseases, and purpura. Study of the progress and the etiology of the immunodeficiency diseases is very helpful therefore in adding to one's knowledge of the immune response. It is well established that the immune response is very important in many disease processes. One develops great respect for the complexity of the normal adaptive capabilities of the body when discussing the types of disorders that may occur, the types of processes that are as yet elusive, and the potential for future treatment modalities that may prove beneficial in treating or curing many diseases.

THE PAIN RESPONSE

Another of the protective mechanisms of the body is the pain sensation. Pain may be the first symptom of the presence of an abnormal condition in the body and is often the stimulus for the affected individual to seek medical assistance. Thus, pain sensations may be viewed as a warning signal of the body to prevent damage, injury, or malfunction. An obvious example of how pain sensations are a protective mechanism is the body's quick response to a painful stimulus, such as touching a hot stove. The absence of pain sensations in this situation would cause injury and damage were the hand not removed immediately. The absence of pain sensations in an area of the body, as in spinal cord injury, may lead to extensive tissue damage.

Pain is also a protective influence on the outcome of a disease process. Observation of the patient's expressions of pain assists the physician in the diagnosis of a pathologic condition and in the selection of appropriate therapy. This diagnostic factor is important for the nurse to consider when caring for the patient with pain, but in whom a diagnosis has not been made. Early administration of analgesics may mask the pain symptom to such a degree that an accurate diagnosis may be prevented or delayed, and the nurse must explain to the patient the reasons for withholding medications temporarily and provide other nursing comfort measures. Thus, continual pain or changes in its location, intensity, and characteristics may be significant in helping the physician determine the diagnosis and thus define the appropriate intervention.

Regardless of the protective component of pain, it is a distressing sensation and in cases such as the pain associated with advanced cancer it serves no biologic purpose. Pain may be damaging psychologically and physiologically when it is excessive and chronic as well as when it is uncontrolled. In fact, severe pain may be a major factor in the development of shock and thus may cause a life-threatening situation.

An important element of pain is the patient's expression of pain (verbal and nonverbal behavior) and the nurse's response to the type of expression observed. Endurance of pain is valued by many persons, and intolerance for a specific type of pain expression may seriously impair the patient's ability to obtain pain relief.

The prevention and/or control of pain is also an important aspect in giving nursing care. Certain procedures may increase the patient's pain, and the nurse's efforts must be directed toward minimizing the pain. The administration of injections, for example, may create pain for certain patients. Therefore, pain associated with the technique must be minimized by the nurse's skill in administering the injection as well as by the intellectual preparation of the patient for the injection. Judicious use of analgesics prior to painful treatments is also an important aspect of the nurse's role in preventing pain, especially in the use of analgesics prior to dressing changes for the severely burned patient. Another example is the use of analgesics for the postoperative patient in order to obtain cooperation and effectiveness in coughing and ambulation. In order to understand the cause of pain and the appropriate measures to control or relieve pain, a review of the pain mechanism is necessary.

The Mechanism of Pain

Although the pain experience is complex and many aspects of the experience or its control are still not understood, three essential components for the pain sensation to occur are clearly identified. These three types of structures include (1) receptors that are sensitive to pain stimuli, (2) the impulse pathway for the transmission of pain, and (3) cortical centers for the perception, interpretation, and initiation of responses. The sensory nerve fibers, whose free nerve endings in the skin and other organs form the pain receptors, are the peripheral sites for the transmission of pain. It is felt that some chemical substance(s)—possibly bradykinin or histamine—released from the cells or formed in damaged tissues excites the pain nerve endings. The primary pathway for pain transmission is the lateral spinothalamic tract, which ascends in the anterior spinal column to the brainstem and the thalamus. The sensory nerve fibers are of two types, namely, myelinated and nonmyelinated. **Myelinated nerve fibers** are large fibers that transmit impulses rapidly and are responsible for the sharp pain felt the instant injury occurs. **Nonmyelinated fibers** are smaller and conduct sensations more slowly. The nonmyelinated fibers are responsible for the diffuse or aching pain that follows the initial sensation of sharp pain. The different types of receptors are thought to be the basis for the varying types of sensation that occur with a single stimulus. In addition, tissue ischemia and muscle spasms are related to pain stimulation.

Some pain impulses that enter the spinal cord produce a reflex response, passing immediately to motor neurons. This reaction is observed when a pinprick to the body causes immediate withdrawal of the extremity. Other pain impulses enter the spinal cord and ascend the anterolateral spinothalamic tract to the thalamus and to the appropriate sensory area of the cerebral cortex, causing the person to cry out in response to the pain. At this point, interpretation occurs in relation to the site of the pain, its quality, and intensity. Figure 1-3 illustrates the pathway of pain impulses. The impulses received at the cortical level result in the initiation of impulses that activate the physical and psychological responses to the pain stimulus.

A recently proposed theory, the gate control theory, has been developed by Melzack and Wall [113]. These researchers claim that impulses carried to the dorsal spinal gray matter by the myelinated fibers activate cells in the substantia gelatinosa (functional units of densely packed cells that extend the length of the spinal cord) which depress synaptic transmission and thus close the "gate" to transmission of other impulses. If the stimulus is increased in intensity or prolonged, there is greater relative activity of the non-

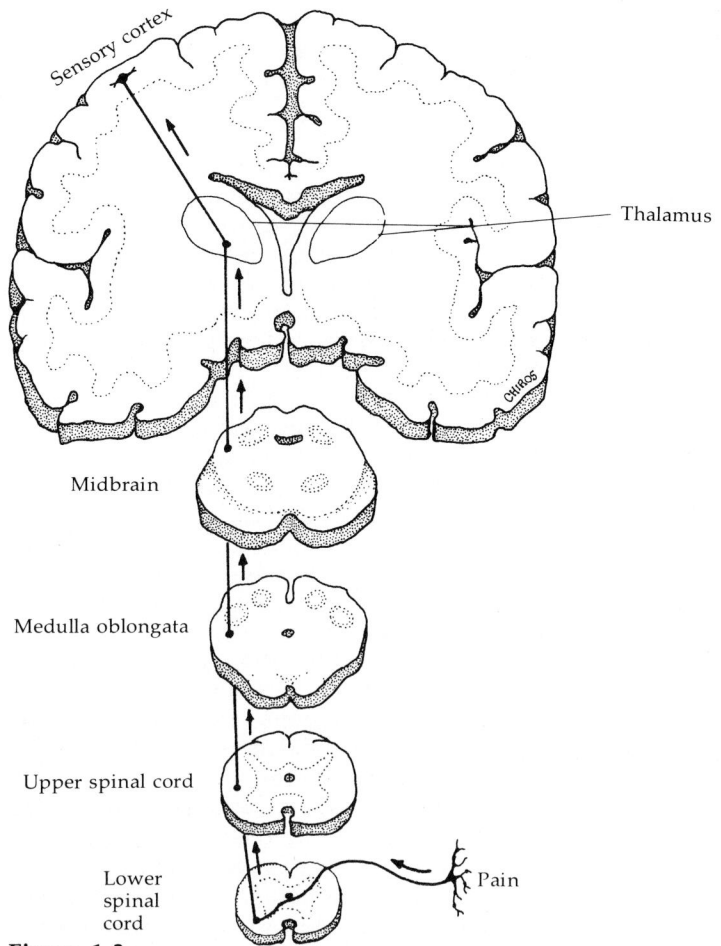

Figure 1-3
The sensory pathway for pain; temperature sensations are transmitted by the same pathway. Pain sensations are transmitted via the anterolateral tract and lateral lemniscus to the thalamus and then via the internal capsule to the cortex. The sensory pathway may be interrupted at various sites to control intractable pain by neurosurgical techniques.

myelinated fibers that mediate pain and the gate then opens, allowing transmission of pain signals. In the gate theory it is postulated that fibers from the reticular formation and the cortex carry signals that modulate pain and color its perception with the individual's mental state, emotions, and past experience. The gate theory thus proposes that pain is a complex perceptual experience that alters sensory input. This theory is the basis for the initiation of various pain therapies that will be discussed later in this chapter. The gate theory, however, is still considered controversial and is criticized by some authorities as lacking experimental support.

Pain Perception and Reactions

Pain is primarily a subjective experience that increases awareness of the body and limits awareness of the surroundings. The pain itself cannot be seen, but rather the effects of pain or the reaction to the pain stimulus are observable. Pain is an individualized experience, influenced by the meaning of the pain to the patient. Perception of the pain depends upon the intensity and frequency of the pain impulses, but the reaction to pain is also influenced by learned experiences. For example, the experience of pain may tend to cause the patient to anticipate more painful experiences.

Pain threshold is that point or level at which a stimulus first causes an awareness of pain or, in other terms, the intensity of stimulation that can be perceived as pain. Although some authorities feel that pain threshold is fairly constant and uniform and that differences reflect the responses to the pain stimuli, other authorities feel that pain threshold may vary from one person to another and at different times and under different conditions in any given individual. Inflammation or injury of tissues near the nerve endings may increase sensitivity to pain (as with sunburn). This state of increased sensitivity to pain is known as hyperalgesia. It has been noted that a second pain stimulus may actually raise the pain threshold of other parts of the body. Certain drugs, including alcohol, may depress the cerebral cortex and thus raise the pain threshold. Environmental distractions may raise the pain threshold, while the lack of environmental stimuli may lower the pain threshold. Nurses have frequently noted that patients have increased pain during the night, when ordinary stimuli from the environment are at a minimum.

When pain is experienced, the reaction to the pain is reflected physiologically and psychologically in autonomic, psychic, and skeletal muscle reactions in differing degrees, depending on the intensity and duration of the pain. Autonomic responses to intense or prolonged pain include alterations in blood pressure, constriction of blood vessels resulting in skin that is cool to touch, gastrointestinal distress, increased respiratory rate, nausea and vomiting, pallor, dilated pupils, increased perspiration, and tachycardia.

Involuntary and voluntary responses of skeletal muscle are readily recognized in actions of the patient. Grimacing or clenching of the fists and restlessness may be observed. Muscle tone is increased in an attempt to immobilize the affected part, as observed in patients with abdominal pain who present with rigidity of the abdomen.

Psychic reactions include anxiety, apprehension, verbalization of the pain and suffering, restlessness, fear, and anger. Some persons, however, withdraw and suffer in silence. Anxiety increases the perception of pain and tends to intensify the pain. Stimulation of ascending fibers of autonomic areas of the brainstem causes nausea and diaphoresis.

Some of the factors that influence the perception of and reaction to pain, in addition to those already cited, include attitudes toward pain and values placed on the endurance of pain; social, cultural, and economic factors; the environment and the type of situation in which the pain is experienced; and the psychological and physiologic state of the individual. The latter situation can be illustrated by the decreased response to pain in persons who are unconscious.

Types of Pain

Superficial pain occurs when surface structures are affected by painful stimuli. Superficial pain is sometimes referred to as direct pain because the pain localizes where the point of stimulus occurs. This type of pain is usually felt as a sharp localized sensation at the site of stimulation.

Deep pain arises from structures in deeper tissues, such as the muscle, periosteum, and viscera. It may also be localized, arising directly from the site of stimulus or more often, it is poorly localized and dull and aching. Pain experienced at a site other than the area of stimulus is **referred pain,** for example, the pain of a visceral structure perceived as occurring in an area on the body surface. The pain of angina pectoris is a classic example of referred pain; it arises in the heart, but is projected to various regions of the body, including the jaw, midsternal region, the left arm, or the epigastrium. Therefore the symptom of pain must be considered in conjunction with other signs and symptoms, and it must be described accurately to be of diagnostic value.

Although the mechanism of referred pain is not clearly understood, it is generally known that the area of stimulation and the area where pain is felt are both innervated by nerve fibers that arise from the same segment of the spinal cord. The pain impulses from sensory fibers in certain viscera, skeletal muscles, and superficial tissues are delivered to the same segment of the spinal cord from which they ascend via a common spinothalamic tract to the thalamus and the cerebral cortex. Faulty localization in the brain may be due to the infrequency of visceral pain impulses as compared to the frequency of cutaneous impulses. Previous experiences (i.e., learned pain pathways) contribute to the referral of the pain to other superficial sites rather than to the viscera.

Other types of pain are classified as acute, chronic, psychogenic, projected, and intractable. **Acute pain** usually has a sudden onset and is either sharp or violent and unrelenting. The term acute also implies pain of a shorter duration. Appropriate analgesics and treatment of the cause are the means of controlling this type of pain. If acute pain is psychogenic in nature the same principle applies, that is, the psychological needs or basis for the pain must be determined, and psychotherapy or psychological techniques are utilized in treating the underlying cause.

Chronic pain is continual and persists or recurs for an indefinite period of time. Its onset is generally a gradual one, and the pain tends to be refractory to treatment. Pain associated with rheumatoid arthritis and peripheral vascular insufficiency are examples of chronic pain. This type of pain is exhausting and generally debilitating. Depression and frustration are associated with its long-term presence. In addition, the patient may develop adaptive or defensive patterns of behavior when the pain lasts for weeks or years.

Intractable pain is chronic pain that is resistant to usual treatment and persists for a long duration in spite of treatment. The causes of intractable pain involve individual nerve trunks, the ganglion, the spinal cord, or thalamic structures of the cerebrum. A classic example of intractable pain is that associated with certain types of advanced cancer. The severe and persistent pain interferes with the patient's ability to carry on a normal life pattern and even interferes with the maintenance of nutrition and personal hygiene habits. Thus the patient with intractable pain often presents in a debilitated state and often with distinct personality changes.

Psychogenic pain is generally defined as pain that is independent of peripheral stimulation and is due to emotional factors. No anatomic or physiologic cause can be detected, but the pain is actually felt by the patient due to complex psychological factors. **Projected pain** is perceived as arising at the site of the pain receptors served by the pathway in which such pain would originate. The impulses, however, actually originate at a point along the pain pathway beyond the peripheral pain receptors. An example of this type of pain is **phantom limb pain.** Although a limb has been removed, the patient has pain and other sensations, as though the limb is still there. In other words, previously established pain pathways localize the pain arising from stimuli within the stump, and the pain is thus projected to the portion of the limb that was removed.

Specific types of pain are discussed in those chapters related to the clinical abnormalities associated with the pain. For example, the pain of tic douloureux and headache as well as of central pain syndromes is discussed in Chapter 11. Pain associated with cancer is discussed later in this chapter.

PAIN ASSESSMENT

Accurate assessment of pain depends on close attention to the patient's verbal description of the pain as well as observation of other physical and psychological signs present. Because pain is a subjective symptom, information on the nature, intensity, and location of pain must be obtained from the patient. The patient should be encouraged to describe the pain in his own words, but if he is unable to describe it, a range of words may be offered by the nurse. A variety of terms are used, such as pricking, burning, aching, throbbing, sharp, cramping, dull, stabbing, and excruciating. In addition, the onset of pain, its duration, predisposing factors, the measures used to combat the pain, and what the pain means to the person are other considerations. In evaluating the significance of the pain and its effect on the patient, the nurse must assess the patient's vital signs, other existing physical problems, and the absence of any complicating factors. For example, the patient who describes substernal pain is evaluated for potential cardiovascular problems, and his circulatory status is evaluated. If the pain is of cardiac origin, immediate intervention is necessary, depending on the severity of the symptom.

The general appearance and facial expressions and bodily movements should be observed. The presence of diaphoresis, tachycardia, and tachypnea are noted. The emotional response of the patient and the ability to be distracted from the pain are also assessed. The site of the pain is examined. For example, specific localization of pain in an operative wound, beyond the time of usual incisional pain, should alert the nurse to examine the surgical incision for tenderness, swelling, discoloration, firmness or rigidity, and warmth. The patient's position may be significant in assessing the pain syndrome. He or she may be lying with knees drawn up, or clasping a body part. The patient may be stiff and rigid, refusing to move in order to immobilize himself to prevent pain. All observations and interventions must be accurately recorded.

Thus, pain is assessed in its total context, taking into account all factors that affect the patient physiologically and psychologically. A patient who is completely involved with the pain cannot be distracted from awareness of the pain, is extremely tense, irritable, restless, and usually is breathing rapidly and perspiring excessively. The patient's diagnosis and vital signs determine the need for immediate intervention in such a situation. The nurse must also learn to differentiate between situations when psychological comfort measures are most important and those in which immediate physiologic measures are required.

In both of the above situations, however, the nurse's role in reducing the patient's anxiety cannot be overemphasized. Listening to the patient, acknowledging his discomfort, and demonstrating a willingness to try to relieve the pain contributes to the reduction of anxiety. Often, talking about the pain and describing the discomfort is helpful in relieving some of the patient's distress. If, however, the nurse implies doubt or denial that the pain exists or that the patient is not acting in an acceptable manner for expressing pain, the patient's pain and discomfort are likely to increase.

If the pain is not a symptom of an acute emergency situation, various methods may be utilized to relieve the pain. The patient's position is evaluated to determine if it is a contributing factor. For example, the patient who is lying on a catheter drainage tube and causing bladder distention may be immediately relieved when the tube is freed and patency is reestablished. The patient suffering from gas pains postoperatively may obtain more relief and comfort from an enema and increased ambulation than from administration of a narcotic. A painful limb may be relieved by elevating it. If the pain in the limb is related to a tight cast, additional steps such as bivalving the cast may be necessary in order to prevent permanent damage. Again, the importance of looking at the total situation, rather than at the expression of pain alone, is essential in determining the significance of the pain and the appropriate type of nursing or other intervention.

Providing for adequate rest and quiet is also important in reducing the patient's irritability and awareness of pain. Efficient and purposeful actions of the nurse also are important factors in making the patient physically and psychologically comfortable. Noisy and excessive stimulation may increase the patient's irritation so that the patient is able to express these feelngs of irritation only by complaining of painful discomfort. Massaging the areas of pressure for the patient who has remained immobilized for prolonged periods may be another aspect of providing for patient comfort and relief of pain.

Accurate assessment of pain can be difficult. This assessment is affected not only by the individual's response to the pain but also by the nurse's own attitude toward pain and the appropriate ways that pain is expressed. Thus the intensity and the importance of the pain may be viewed differently by the patient and the nurse. These differences in the perception of pain often result in conflict between the patient and the nurse concerning how the pain is to be treated.

Strauss and associates [120] have studied pain from a perspective other than the traditional one of the pain itself or the one-to-one interaction between the patient and nurse or physician. This "organization-work-interactional" perspective is concerned with the setting in which the pain and the management of pain occur and the interaction between the staff and patient as well as among the different staff members. They investigated the management of pain in various settings, the intensive care unit, emergency room, recovery room, cancer unit, and a burn unit. In the intensive care unit they found that the primary work was related to therapeutics and recovery care in contrast to comfort care. Emergency room staff were primarily concerned with diagnosis or immediate treatment despite the patient's pain; the recovery room staff was primarily concerned with close monitoring for potential complications. These findings were contrasted to a unit with cancer patients where appropriate relief of pain and comfort were the primary focus. Strauss and associates also found that patient socialization was an important factor in influencing pain expression by patients in a burn unit, and they determined that staff expectations regarding appropriate types of pain or pain expression are an important factor in the way pain is managed and in the nurse-patient relationship. These investigators concluded that "staff is not genuinely accountable for much of its interaction with or behavior toward the patient in pain." In addition they felt that improvement in the care of patients in pain will not occur until "it becomes a matter of collective concern and organizational accountability."

Weiner [125] applied this perspective in describing pain assessment on an orthopedic unit where she found that problems arose when there was a discrepancy in how staff assessed pain and how patients assessed their own pain. She also placed importance on the absence of accountability for failure to listen, understand, or provide comfort care of the patient. She found that perceptions of causes, signs, or visibility of pain (difficulty in objectively validating the pain), relief procedures, and endurance of pain were the sources of discrepancy. She also found that staff tended to force patients into enduring pain by placing a high value on stoicism. Staff often viewed pain as being of psychogenic origin and even supported this belief by their interpretations of some relief procedures. For example, ultrasound techniques were not viewed as effective measures by some of the staff. Thus, when patients obtained relief from pain by these methods, the staff were convinced that the pain was psychogenic in origin. Weiner recommended the establishment of a pain profile on admission to determine the patient's special routine or pattern of handling pain, previous effective methods in other hospitalizations, and any specific information about dealing with the pain. This determination can be threatening, however, to nurses who are made uncomfortable when patients with chronic pain try to advise them on what is effective or ineffective intervention. The patient's knowledge of drugs and their actions may be the result of long experience with various prescriptions and may be threatening to the nurse; thus a negative or antagonistic relationship may be established [125].

Management of Pain

Interest in the appropriate management of pain is increasing as various pain centers across the country investigate the mechanisms of pain and appropriate therapy. The Multidisciplinary Pain Clinic at the University Hospital in Seattle, Washington, is a demonstration center for pain management. Techniques at this center are varied and are based on an assessment of the patient's pain. A patient diary in which activities, medications, and episodes of pain are described is used as a basis for the patient's and the staff's definitions of pain. A high incidence of back pain is found among the patients coming to the clinic. Clinic personnel include anesthesiologists, neurosurgeons, psychiatrists, psychologists, nurses, physical therapists, occupational therapists, and internists, among others. Prior to treatment a personality inventory is also established by means of various psychological tests, most often the Minnesota Multiphasic Personality Inventory (MMPI). Drug-dependent patients are detoxified after an initial assessment of the patient's drug pattern. In some settings, for example, the patient gets any drug asked for in the first 48 hours to develop a drug profile. Then pain cocktails of combinations of various drugs with reduced narcotic content are administered at specific intervals. The nurse has an important role at this time in providing psychological support and in observing the patient closely for withdrawal symptoms.

Operant conditioning may be used as a technique to "unlearn" the pain the patients have learned to feel. Behavior modification techniques are developed, depending on the personality and drug profile of the individual patient. Basically the goal of this therapy is to reinforce the pain-free status by rewarding the patient whenever he or she functions actively and does not utilize his pain as a means for obtaining relief. Patient contracts are often utilized in order to obtain the patient's cooperation in this treatment approach [98]. The importance of the multidisciplinary approach cannot be overemphasized, because all health professionals are needed to provide effective management of pain. The various types of interventions used in the management of pain will now be discussed. The reader is also encouraged to obtain references and resources, including pharmacology textbooks devoted entirely to pain management, for a more extensive background in current pain research.

Analgesic drug therapy The use of various medications is probably the most common approach to the management and control of pain. Analgesics are used to alter pain perception by interfering with the transmission of painful stimuli from peripheral sites or by altering perceptive and subjective responses to pain at cerebral levels. Medications utilized include strong, addictive narcotics (morphine sulfate and substitutes such as meperidine hydrochloride), various oral nonaddictive analgesic drugs (salicylates), and ointments and topical agents. The danger of addiction and drug dependency on strong medications requires judicious prescriptions and administration. The use of strong medications in the control of chronic pain is to be discouraged, because of their tendency to induce addiction. Withholding narcotics when the patient is in need of relief from exquisite pain is inappropriate also. Administration of analgesics requires an accurate evaluation of the patient's physical and emotional state and need for the medication, as well as knowledge about the action of the drug, the anticipated therapeutic effects, the potential side or toxic effects, and alternatives for pain control. Usually a prescription for the analgesic dictates the limitations of dosage and the frequency of administration, both of which must be adhered to. The nurse, however, is responsible for evaluating the effectiveness of the medication and notifying the physician if the relief obtained is inadequate. Administration of medications should not be a substitute for nursing care measures, and the nurse should evaluate alternative means for pain relief. The nurse should also keep in mind that the therapeutic effects of an analgesic may be inhibited by anxiety, poor positioning, worry, and other factors. The presence of anxiety may indicate the need for a medication with a mood-ameliorating effect. The promptness in administering the analgesic is also an important factor because the longer the patient suffers, the more apprehensive he becomes, making it difficult to achieve adequate relief. Also, the medication prescribed may specifically relieve mild or moderate pain but be ineffective in relieving intense pain.

The drugs used to relieve pain include those that depress pain perception, reduce the patient's response to pain, or relax muscle spasm. Mild, aching pain is generally treated with mild analgesics such as acetylsalicylic acid (aspirin), combinations with phenacetin and caffeine, propoxyphene (Darvon), and other drugs. These mild drugs even in large doses are not useful in severe pain.

Drugs that reduce pain perception include the strong analgesics such as morphine, codeine, and meperidine hydrochloride (Demerol), which are opiates and potentially are addicting drugs. Of these, codeine has the least potential for addiction. Other opiate preparations are the semisynthetic compounds hydromorphone (Dilaudid) and oxymorphone (Numorphan), and the synthetic drugs fentanyl (Sublimaze), anileridine (Leritine), methadone (Dolophine), levorphanol (Levo-Dromoran), and phenazocine (Prinadol) [4]. All these strong analgesics, however, produce one or more adverse reactions, including central nervous system depression, oversedation, mood alteration, respiratory and circulatory depression, bowel and urinary tract dysfunction, and nausea and vomiting.

A major aspect of the use of these drugs is the danger of physical and psychological dependence on the analgesics. Patients whose pain has a considerable psychogenic component are particularly likely to develop drug dependency. Such a patient asks frequently for the drug and increasingly wants larger doses in order to obtain the physical and psychological effects derived from the drug. The original need for the drug to alleviate pain becomes replaced by the patient's dependence on the drug to distort reality and promote both physical and psychological comfort. In certain patients, however, as in the patient with advanced cancer, the importance of pain relief is primary, and the danger of drug addiction in terminal stages as a rationale for withholding of the drug is totally unrealistic.

If the patient is apprehensive and anxious, administration of hypnotics or sedatives (sodium amytal or phenobarbital) or a tranquilizer (prochlorperazine [Compazine] or diazepam [Valium]) may be prescribed as an adjunct to an analgesic. Sedatives and hypnotics alter the psychic components of pain. When muscle spasm is a factor in the cause of the pain, muscle relaxants (diazepam or carisoprodol [Rela, Soma]) may be indicated.

In addition to analgesics, other measures may assist in relieving pain. For example, moist or dry heat may be applied to relieve muscle tension or spasm and promote pain relief. This relief is also facilitated by the increased rate of blood flow through the area of muscle tension. Cold applications may be indicated to reduce the accumulation of tissue fluid and to produce a local anesthetic effect. The reduction in inflammatory swelling in some situations may promote pain relief. Again, the physician or the nurse or both must carefully assess the dynamics of the specific pain situation to determine whether hot or cold applications are appropriate.

The supportive aspects of nursing care serve as substitutes in some situations for analgesic drug administration or as an adjunct to the use of the drugs. Acknowledgment of the patient's suffering, attention to proper body alignment and positioning, spending more time with the patient, and general comfort measures such as mouth care, fluid intake, back massage, and splinting of the incision of a postoperative patient during movement and coughing are examples of some of these supportive measures. Controlling environmental factors that are disturbing to the patient and providing diversional activities are also important nursing measures in promoting pain relief.

Placebos Placebos are inactive substances intended to have no pharmacologic effects but which may be used in selected situations to evaluate or treat pain or both. Their use is primarily in patients whose pain has overtones of psychogenic origin. The suggestibility factor is a major aspect in the use of these substances, which include sodium bicarbonate, vitamins, distilled water, lactose capsules, or physiologic saline solution. In other words, the patient thinks he is being given a pain medication to relieve his discomfort. In evaluating the effects of placebos, two groups of persons have been identified. Placebo reactors are individuals who frequently are relieved of discomfort with the use of placebos, and negative or nonreactors are those who are psychologically predisposed to resist relief from the drugs or placebos. In studying the effect of placebos on reactors and nonreactors, Walike [122] found that placebo reactors tended to exhibit higher dependency and lower ego strength and self-sufficiency than nonreactors. The use of placebos in pain management is a controversial one and must be done judiciously and only under the physician's order. The danger of the patient learning that he has been given placebos for pain relief can be detrimental to his ability to trust any person in the medical profession. Therefore the use of placebos should be evaluated in terms of its purpose, duration, and appropriateness.

Because placebos can be effective in some situations emphasizes the importance of the suggestibility factor in obtaining relief with a variety of nursing measures. Billars [90] verified the importance of the suggestibility factor in a small study done to determine the effect of suggestions that a specific action would relieve pain. She proposed that suggestions coupled with a reasonable action and explanation might make any nursing measure more effective. (In other words, the nurse should convey that the medication or nursing measure will relieve the pain.)

Hypnosis Hypnosis is a type of therapy that is based on the power of suggestion via the process of focusing attention as a means of altering an individual's reactions, in this case pain. The technique should be used only by trained persons because there are dangers associated with the technique, and untoward effects have occurred.

The patient is placed in a trance-like state that is either light, medium, or deep. Once the trance-like state is achieved, a variety of procedures may be employed to relieve pain. Direct suggestions that the patient will lose his pain or will change his response to the pain may be utilized. (The latter technique is called a psychological lobotomy by some authorities.) Psychiatric therapy may be given during the trance-like state. Anesthesia and analgesia may be used in addition to hypnosis. Hilgard [104] proposes that hypnosis can be helpful for many patients and can be supplemental to chemical analgesics when their use is ill-advised or when relief through smaller drug doses is desirable. It is generally felt that about 20 percent of the population can be placed into the deep stages of hypnosis.

Again it should be emphasized that the technique of hypnosis should be used only by trained persons who are also able to cope with potential complications related to posthypnotic stages and the psychological disturbances that may arise following placement in the hypnotic stage.

Acupuncture Although acupuncture is often thought of as a type of hypnosis, proponents of the technique emphasize the distinct difference that the patient undergoing acupuncture knows what is being done, in contrast to the patient under hypnosis, who is unaware of what is being done. It has been shown that hypnosis is a factor in the success of acupuncture technique because it has been determined that poor candidates for hypnosis are poor candidates for acupuncture. The importance of acupuncture in the treatment of chronic pain has gained considerable interest in this country since the use of the technique in China was evaluated by various American physicians. Its potential for relief of pain problems of psychological and physiologic origin is being evaluated currently, and its effect is thought to be related to the gate control theory. It is being used currently, for example, in the treatment of tension headaches, migraine, peptic ulcer, and low back pain. Acupuncture therapy is not readily available in the United States. Controversy continues about its acceptability as a form of scientific medical therapy.

Acupuncture involves the insertion of needles through the skin up to a few inches at selected points in the body, determined by the type of pain relief desired. The needles are either twirled or electrical currents are passed through them. Analgesia may be produced to the point that major surgery may be accomplished. The advantages and potential of acupuncture are related to the relative simpleness of the technique, since body functions are not affected by it. Thus the patient remains awake and is able to ambulate freely after undergoing acupuncture. Postanesthetic morbidity and residual depression are not present. The disadvantage is that the technique does not work successfully on all patients and may cause emotional distress when no relief is attained. Controlled studies to determine the effectiveness of the technique are required to determine its true value and its appropriate application.

Peripheral nerve stimulation Peripheral nerve or dorsal column stimulation involves the surgical implantation of electrodes along the spine, either around the peripheral nerve or against the dorsal column of the spinal cord. The technique requires a laminectomy and is based on the gate control theory, which suggests that electrical stimulation relieves pain by blocking or closing the gate to transmission of pain impulses from the spinal cord to the brain. A subcutaneous receiver of the electrode is powered by a compact external system that is similar in design to a cardiac pacemaker. The patient carries the battery-operated device to generate the electrical impulse as prescribed for relief of pain. The technique has proved to be effective in patients with pain syndromes related to low back pain, as well as in patients with cancer and rheumatoid arthritis.

Previously, transcutaneous electrical stimulation was done as a screening or evaluation technique to determine the potential benefits of electrode implantation in the relief of pain. Thus, another modification of the original method has now come into use in the treatment of pain. In transcutaneous electrical stimulation, small electrical currents are passed through the skin to create impulse transmission within the large fibers to stimulate enough positive excitation and subsequently inhibit pain impulses. The electrodes are placed in the region of the patient's pain (or over the peripheral nerve pathway) and are connected by cables to a small, lightweight and battery-operated pulse generator. The stimulator does not pose an electrical hazard, but the technique is not recommended for patients with cardiac pacemakers because of potential interference with and inhibition of the output of some demand cardiac pacemakers. The electrical stimulation is felt as a tingling or buzzing sensation; some patients find the stimulation extremely unpleasant and are unable to tolerate it. It has proved to be effective, however, in pain relief for some patients with chronic low back pain, peripheral neuropathies, and phantom limb pain.

The location for the placement of the electrodes, the voltage, and the frequency and duration of application are determined on an individual basis by the physician. The nurse and patient observe the effects of stimulation in relieving pain. The electrical stimulators can be obtained only via a physician's prescription. There is a potential hazard if these stimulators are used in the case of new persistent pain that is symptomatic of underlying disease different from that for which the stimulator is prescribed.

There is also a possibility that physical or psychological dependence on the stimulator may occur, but this dependence has not been proved or demonstrated. The patient must be taught to use precautions in the use of the stimulator. For example, skin irritation may occur if excessive stimulation is used or if an inadequate amount of electrode jelly is used in applying the electrodes. The patient must also be instructed in care of the generator and to avoid submerging it in water or cleaning agents or dropping it and causing damage.

The use of the transcutaneous stimulator is undergoing considerable evaluation presently. Its use has expanded to postoperative thoracic surgery. One report [97] indicated that the transcutaneous stimulator was used postoperatively in the care of patients with thoracic surgery in conjunction with routine analgesic medications. The study showed that patients treated with the external stimulator developed fewer postoperative complications [97]. It was felt that the stimulator relieved pain and facilitated better coughing and deep breathing by the patient and thus resulted in fewer complications.

Neurosurgical pain relief When intractable pain cannot be controlled effectively by analgesics or other techniques, surgical interruption of the pain pathway may be indicated. Usually neurosurgical pain relief procedures are done in patients with advanced stages of cancer or with excessive pain associated with tic douloureux (trigeminal neuralgia). When pain intractability is so severe that the patient's total life pattern is disrupted, neurosurgical procedures may be done in other disease states as well. The surgical procedure must be precise so that unnecessary loss of sensations other than pain does not occur. There are several approaches to surgical treatment of pain, depending on the location and severity of the pain.

When the source of pain is localized to a relatively small area of the body, neurectomy is done. This interruption of peripheral nerves is accomplished by severing or crushing peripheral sensory nerve fibers from the affected area or by means of injection. Peripheral nerve blocks may be accomplished with local anesthetics such as lidocaine, or neurolytic drugs such as absolute alcohol or phenol, for temporary relief of pain. Lidocaine provides pain relief for 1½ to 6 hours. Although absolute alcohol and phenol produce neurolysis with interruption of pain impulses for up to 6 months, they are used infrequently due to their severe toxic effects. They may produce necrosis, sloughing of superficial tissues, and occasionally peripheral neuritis of the blocked nerve [95].

A rhizotomy procedure involves interruption of the sensory pathway that carries impulses from the affected area just before the nerve enters the spinal cord. Thus the fibers are severed or crushed in the area between the associated dorsal ganglion and the cord, creating a permanent sensory deficit; a laminectomy is necessary to accomplish this procedure. The procedure is used primarily to relieve pain in the upper part of the trunk. It also causes loss of the sense of touch and position in the area.

A laminectomy is usually necessary to accomplish a cordotomy. This procedure involves the division of bilateral or unilateral spinothalamic tracts in the spinal cord. A unilateral cordotomy involves an incision in the anterolateral pathway opposite the side on which the pain is located. This procedure also results in loss of the temperature sense, but leaves other sensations and motor function intact.

Patients who are unable to tolerate the surgical procedure and those who have terminal cancer are usually treated by percutaneous cervical cordotomy. This procedure requires a short convalescence and is generally well tolerated. A needle is inserted into the neck below and behind the mastoid process in order to cause stereotaxic destruction of the anterolateral spinothalamic tracts. A local anesthetic is used. Occasionally edema from the cordotomy produces pressure on the pyramidal tract, resulting in transient weakness of the same side of the body. Ordinarily the patient is ambulated within 24 hours if there is no paresis. A problem may occur with bladder dysfunction (either incontinence or distention), particularly when bilateral cordotomy is done.

Other neurosurgical procedures include tractotomy, which is the surgical division of the anterolateral pathway in the brainstem by craniotomy, and frontal lobotomy, which is the destruction of cerebral tissue in the frontal lobes of the brain. Both of these procedures may be accomplished for intractable pain, but are rarely done, because of the associated neurologic deficits.

When these procedures are accomplished, the nurse must be aware that the denervated tissues are no longer supplied with sensory innervation and are highly vulnerable to injury. Sensations of pain and temperature are no longer present and injury can occur without the patient being aware of it. The patient and family must be thoroughly instructed in measures to prevent such injury from occurring. Otherwise, burn injuries, decubiti, or trauma may occur. In addition, these patients should be checked for bladder dysfunction, constipation, and for diminished strength of extremities to detect any motor dysfunctions resulting from the surgery.

Stereotaxic brain surgery may be done to treat intractable pain. The use of radiation for this purpose is an example of a closed approach to this technique. In the open stereotaxic procedure, a probe or needle is inserted into one or more sites in the brain via a burr hole in the skull. A heating current is then applied via the probe to cause coagulation of adjacent tissue. A neurolytic agent is injected when the needle technique is used.

Additional aspects of stereotaxic techniques are presented in Chapter 11. More information on postoperative aspects related to neurosurgery are found in that chapter also.

The management of intractable pain is a complex problem and requires the use of a variety of treatment methods, some of which have been discussed in this section. Throughout the management of pain, the importance of an understanding and concerned nurse who assesses pain accurately within its total context and follows through with appropriate intervention cannot be overestimated.

In some patients who have derived some psychological gains by the presence of intractable pain, successful treatment of the intractable pain may require a difficult readjustment in their lives. Neurotic features have often been associated with chronic pain. Sternbach and Timmermans [119], however, in their study of 113 patients over a 2-year period, demonstrated that neuroticism associated with chronic pain is the result of pain and may be reversible when the pain is reduced or abolished.

Implications of Adaptation for Nursing Processes

The preceding discussion of the inflammatory, immune, and pain responses elucidates the complexity of the body functions. These responses have been presented as protective of body function while also having the capability of causing disease. The latter may occur for several reasons. The response may be inadequate in dealing with the potentially harmful agent, alterations in response may reverse the expected protective effect, and changes in the environment may render the responses ineffective. In each instance the concept of adaptation is related to the maintenance of health; ineffective adaptation or failure to adapt is related to the occurrence of disease. The processes through which the body adapts can be described from both physiologic and psychological bases. Understanding of these processes is important in determining how to support or facilitate the patient's optimum body function.

The phrase **optimum body function** implies a relative condition since definition of optimum is difficult. We know, for example, that people have both psychological and physiologic reserves that allow for wide variations in capabilities. The stress response described by Seyle [66] is an example of body responses that provide for use of reserves to meet crises. Compensatory cardiovascular function allows for maintenance of cellular oxygenation; in fact, most body systems contain subsystems that have checks, balances, and alternate and overlapping functions to protect and preserve functioning. Individual capabilities for psychological functioning also elude attempts to define limits. It is not known how to determine or predict behavioral capabilities. Personally, most of us wonder or speculate how we would react in times of crises. We are often surprised at the capabilities of people to adapt to and master seemingly impossible situations. In general, humans have abilities to maintain life and functions that are automatic, learned, and developed as well as capabilities that may never be tested in a lifetime.

A basic concept in the maintenance of body function is that of homeostasis. Originally described by Claude Bernard in relation to physiologic maintenance of the body's internal milieu, the concept of homeostasis has been expanded to describe interactive body functions as we know them today. Many aspects of Bernard's original thesis still apply while some of his explanations for how the dynamic but steady state is maintained have been changed.

An excellent example of homeostasis is the fluid and electrolyte balance in the body. Despite the constant flux of water and electrolytes within the body, with ever-changing environmental influences and variable intake of fluids and electrolytes, the body is able to maintain constancy in fluid and electrolyte balance. How the body maintains constancy (the steady state) in temperature ranges despite variations in environmental temperatures, the internal production of thermal energy, and exercise levels is another example of homeostasis. The ability to maintain cellular oxygenation despite changes in posture, exercise levels, and intake of nutrients affecting cellular metabolism is yet another example.

While homeostasis refers to physiologic function, the concept of adaptation is more easily applied to total body function. Earlier, biologic adaptation to changing environments through genetic mutations was discussed. This form of adaptation provides for reproduction of the species and for maintenance of life through long-term evolutionary processes. Adaptation also takes place within the body in response to highly integrated and interdependent processes. Synthesis and release of thyroid hormone is an example of the body's ability to adapt to a wide variety of physiologic and psychological stimuli. The integration of behavior of psychological and physiologic origins is demonstrated by the simple act of blushing. Blushing is an emotional response that also involves changes in circulation. Anxiety, which causes increased gastric motility, may lead to diarrhea in some persons, indicating the integration of body responses.

For purposes of analysis, one often studies theories of physiologic and psychological adaptation as separate entities. In practice, the nurse must synthesize these theories through perspectives of the total situation: the environment and the patient's emotions and physiologic capabilities, coping patterns, and stage in life. Physiologic adaptation is difficult to separate from psychological adaptation. Often the question of whether physiologic illness results from or causes psychological problems has no answer. It may be that the basic mechanism of many disease processes will be found to be caused by a basic central process. For example, people with irritable bowel syndrome often have behavioral changes. The question is, which set of symptoms comes first, the emotional or the physical symptoms? Or, are both caused by the same disease process with varying patterns of onset and demonstration of symptoms in different individuals?

The integration of the functions of the mind and body is also important in nursing care because a patient's ability to adapt to an illness may directly influence whether the illness becomes chronic or whether the patient can master the learning and changes necessary to overcome the effects of the illness state so that it is resolved or made compatible with health. Coping mechanisms have been defined to explain behaviors used to adapt to life situations. These coping mechanisms include events such as problem-solving and learning, and adjustment mechanisms, such as the defense mechanisms a person integrates into his patterns of behavior. The individual's genetic makeup is important in describing his propensities for development of an individual coping pattern.

Even coping mechanisms or resulting patterns are integrated. For example, certain individuals tend to have propensities for the development of symptoms or illnesses. Often the individual can identify this tendency in himself. Some people tend to develop diarrhea when fatigued or under stress. Others may develop respiratory distress or musculoskeletal symptoms when experiencing similar stresses. It has been speculated that the basis for these propensities may be genetically transmitted. It is possible that they are learned behaviors produced by interaction with others and with the environment, being also influenced by the types of stresses a person undergoes throughout life. In some instances the risks for developing specific types of illnesses are directly related to the environmental hazards. Coal miners, for example, are particularly susceptible to black lung disease; people who live in unsanitary or crowded conditions are especially susceptible to communicable diseases such as tuberculosis. From an individual point of view, there is no certainty about how a person will react to a specific set of circumstances. Some people with low back pain are able to participate in active sports, whereas others with a similar condition are unable to be active.

It becomes obvious that any illness event must be evaluated by the nurse in terms of the patient's past, present, and future situation. The effects of the pre-illness experiences must be understood if the present illness is to be diagnosed with accuracy. This information may be important in efforts to bring about necessary changes so that when the present illness is resolved the patient does not return to a situation that will cause recurrence of the illness. If, for example, a person is admitted to the hospital for treatment of anginal pain, the pain can be relieved through treatment. If the events that led to anginal pain are not understood and dealt with, the patient may remain subject to similar or the same stresses that precipitated the angina, and may again experience symptoms. Eventually, the patient may be admitted with a myocardial infarction that might have been prevented with thorough evaluation and appropriate care, including changes in his way of life at the time of the initial hospitalization. This situation brings to the fore two very important questions that must be dealt with by the nurse. The first is: What is the nurse's right, role, and responsibility for becoming this involved with another person's life? The second is: What is the right of the person with the illness to maintain his own freedom to select or to accept care? Both of these questions must be considered in a broad context of the health care system.

The role of the nurse is evolving in accord with the roles of others within the health care system. The right to health care for everyone is a central theme in explorations and the development of health care systems. Health care is generally spoken of as a right of people in the United States. Yet there are those who question the availability, accessibility, and equality of health care, as well as the capabilities of health care workers to provide this right within the present health care system. There are admittedly wide variations in the quality, availability, and accessibility of health care throughout the country. Further complicating the definition of health care as a right is the lack of clarity about the level of health care included in this right. Does it include immunizations, health assessment, dental care, and eye examinations? Does it also include therapies, medications, x-ray, supportive measures, teaching, and counseling? What is the right of a person with a long-term or chronic illness for continued care? Finally, what is the person's right for maintaining life? When is a person really dead? Formerly, ordinary and extraordinary treatment modalities were defined as the capability for effective intervention in crises situations. In current practice the delineation between the two is less clear, and assisting or supporting life through technologic measures has become more ordinary in certain situations.

As nursing care roles evolve, they must evolve in concert with the development of standards of "rights for health care." If, for example, it is determined that every citizen has a right to certain health care measures, delivery of these measures must be assured in the health care system. This thesis has all sorts of implications such as who will pay, who will give the services, and how will the citizen learn of his rights, accept these rights, and be assured access to the designated level of health care.

The right to health care is much more difficult to manage than such systems as the sanitary system, which assures clean water, disposal of waste, and a healthy environment. For the most part, citizens who have the right for sanitation generally enjoy this right in an automatic way. One turns on the tap and water is delivered through a public works process that has identifiable managers, mechanisms, and legislative backing. It is unlikely that one would fail to use the tap water or would select water from an unpure alternative source. While this is an oversimplification, it does demonstrate the differences between the rights to sanitation and to health care. For the latter a person must go somewhere or perform some interactive activity involving relationships with other people, installation of equipment in central locations, and involved recordkeeping and follow-through processes.

Health care defies being placed "on tap." As health and illness are very personal matters, the choices for seeking and using health care systems are personal. Even if a person does seek care, there are problems associated with appropriate use of the care and treatment given. Drugs can be misused, or the advice or learning necessary to achieve health may be rejected. Having the right, if services are available, does not imply appropriate utilization.

The basic rights of health care issue is a subject of research, philosophy, value systems, legislation, economic feasibility, and, particularly, professional standards. A study entitled *Social Networks and Health Care Consumership; Applications of Models of Health Service Utilization* deals with social network variables in the use of health services [63]. This study explores the decision-making process in deciding whether health care is needed and where to seek it. The major steps outlined are readiness as related to the level of concern, definition of the problem, investigation and evaluation of health services available, and, finally, selection. The study indicates that in making decisions about health care the decision maker operates within his or her social network: family, employers, fellow employees, friends, and community members.

While the sample investigated is small, an interesting finding was that 67.5 percent of the respondents sought health care information from their physician first. Of all the respondents, 35.8 percent reported that they depended on their own intuition about their health, using information from books, magazines, and television, whereas 20 percent sought information from friends and relatives. Thus, even though these respondents sought health information from physicians first, the physician was not the exclusive or final source for health care information. It was found that concern about health increased with increasing age, the presence of known illness, and decreased income.

Another important measurement in this study was the time element in seeking health services. The results indicated that 44 percent of the respondents sought advice from a nuclear family member. This finding implies that the knowledge and attitudes of the nuclear family members are an important factor in whether health care will be sought and where to go for this care. Interestingly enough, the respondents with highly developed extended friendship systems tended to delay less in seeking treatment while those with highly developed extended family relationships delayed longer in attaining health care. The latter has implications from the point of view of health counseling. If a person is supported by family members and has a high interactive level with them, he may not be motivated to seek health care unless the extended family system encourages him to do so. Again, knowledge and attitudes greatly influence the use of health services. Finally, individuals with no well-developed social networks, termed **isolates** in this study, delayed the longest in seeking health care for their problems. This finding implies that "private persons" do not interact much with others and will probably not seek outside help unless a problem becomes very grave.

While this study is inclusive of only a small sample, it does centralize the problems in seeking, using, and selecting health care that must be dealt with by nurses. The basic constructs of the study are invaluable to nurses who are concerned with improving the health care in a community. Some of the most salient constructs are that a person must first identify a non-normal state and must decide that the problem is medical. Once these conclusions have been reached, the person must have faith in the health services, be uncomfortable enough to seek care, and have sufficient money and time to undergo the care and treatment. This study emphasizes the importance of perceptions about health care in utilization of the care. These perceptions are generally highly influenced by persons with whom there is interaction in life.

A person who seeks care enters into another interactive process. The nurse continually interacts with patients in the caregiving process. To be effective, the nurse must make every interaction meaningful by following a logical and orderly pattern in this interaction. The concept of accountability permeates the nurse's interactions, and to be accountable, the nurse has to delineate the services offered and given so that results or outcomes can be measured. The nurse has to communicate these matters clearly to the patient so that he or she will understand what can be expected and feel satisfied that seeking care is a worthwhile endeavor. During this time the nurse establishes both the nurse's role and the nature of the services offered by the particular agency. Protocols for assessment vary from one setting to another, and the nurse's role may also vary. For example, assessment in some settings may be limited to interview but may include physical examination in others.

ASSESSMENT

The starting point or initiation of the nurse-patient relationship is a phase of assessment. A person seeks health care for multitudinous reasons, and the purpose of his or her presence in the health care setting must be determined prior to taking any action.

How does the patient perceive his situation? Usually this can be ascertained by establishing the reason for the visit. If the problem is easily definable, the process of discovery is facilitated. If the problem is vague and ill-defined, the nurse must help clarify the patient's situation through interview and other assessment techniques.

Assessment is an ongoing part of the nursing process that begins with the establishment of baseline data and continues with data collection to determine the patient's status at any given point in time as care is progressing. It is important to view assessment in the perspective of its relation to both time and place. An individual grows, develops, and changes throughout life. His status on any given day, at any hour during the day, will never be replicated because he is moving forward in time. Documentation therefore applies to the time the data were collected. Similarly, reactions are influenced by many factors. If the person is uncomfortable in the setting or with the people he may not be able to clearly express his thoughts.

Assessment tools or methods include observation, interviewing, listening, and measuring. The stimuli presented by the patient elicit a reaction in the nurse. Experience and a positive role concept enable the nurse to react in a way that is beneficial to the interaction. An open mind is basic to assessment because many cues or clues to concerns or problems are so subtle that they are easily missed by a nurse who is preoccupied or reacting to the patient's behavior.

Among the determinants of the approach the nurse uses in assessment is, first of all, the reason the patient seeks care. In some instances the nurse may initiate care, which will make a difference in approach because it now is the nurse who must establish a common understanding about the purpose of care. The most successful approach to assessment is usually one that deals directly with the predominant or most distressing complaint. This complaint may be so stressful that a person who normally would not seek care has become motivated to accept help. Some people do not seek care readily, and numerous inhibitions prevent them from obtaining care unless they perceive their problem to be life-threatening. By dealing directly with the predominant concern, the nurse not only conveys acceptance and understanding but also facilitates development of a trusting relationship. Once this type of relationship is established, the nurse can more effectively broaden the scope of the assessment.

Of import in the communication and the relationship established by the nurse are several components of assessment. These components include discovery of barriers that may impede communication, such as language barriers, speech difficulties, intellectual capability, attention span, and physical limitations or constraints. Barriers may also stem from experiences or relationships; previous health care experiences, if not positive, may interfere with acceptance of the present situation. Family relationships may present barriers also if there is nonacceptance of health care within the family unit, if there are cultural or religious impediments to acceptance of health care, or if the patient is presenting problems directly related to or involving another family member.

Just as many factors indigenous to a person, including his or her physical and emotional condition, influence approaches to assessment, so do those factors unique to the nurse. Interviewing skills and clinical expertise are necessary for a successful assessment. These skills determine the nurse's ability to understand the patient's problem, to perceive the motivation for seeking care, and to evaluate the circumstances that may have bearing on the nurse-patient relationship. The ability to follow through with data collected in the assessment requires the nurse to have knowledge of the implications of the assessment and the ability to problem solve, to set limits, and to intervene effectively in assisting the patient. The nurse also must be able to validate certain assessment factors by means of background medical and nursing histories. It is sometimes difficult to maintain objectivity in an assessment if the nurse has had prior experience in caring for a given patient. Knowledge of previous health care and problems may be extremely beneficial in determining the current status of the person, but it can be detrimental if the previous information masks or obscures the present data related to a newly developing condition. Even determining the approach to use in assessment is a form of assessment. The nurse carefully estimates the patient's ability to participate in the assessment procedure by first evaluating his or her sensory perceptions. The nurse quickly ascertains whether the person can see, hear, or respond to touch. Another "instant" observation is that of determining emotional status, estimated by nonverbal cues and how the patient communicates the purpose of his visit. An alert nurse quickly estimates the level of trust presented by the patient, and his ability to concentrate and to express feelings and attitudes. The nurse also must be astute in picking up indications of pain or discomfort and of the patient's dependence on those who may accompany him. The role of significant others in assessment may be important in either impeding or facilitating the assessment. Because subsequent care planning and implementation are based on the assessment, all aspects of the nursing process can be carried out successfully only if the basic assessment is accomplished with preciseness.

Physical Examination

The physical examination is done to detect abnormalities that can be found through observation, palpation, percussion, or auscultation. The examination usually begins with the patient's head and neck and proceeds in an orderly sequence to include the chest, arms and hands, and the abdomen, back, trunk, legs, and feet. Percussion, auscultation, and palpation are done systematically as the nurse examines each body part. Observation of the condition of the skin overlying each body part is also done systematically. Methods used for this examination are explained in each chapter of this book and will not be repeated in this section.

Throughout the examination the nurse makes observations of the patient's general status. These observations include estimation of the patient's self-concept, perception of his health status, and acceptance of his limitations and, in general, level of satisfaction with his personal status. An alert nurse who has determined a general overview of the patient's problems—if there are problems—also determines the patient's motivation to change or to accept treatment, his self-determination and ability to set and meet goals, possible sources of conflict, and unfulfilled expectations. All these are estimated in the initial assessment and thereafter are validated through nurse-patient interactions during subsequent contacts.

A standard form for documenting information and observations during the assessment phase is helpful in the interpretation and consolidation of data. Care planning is augmented in this manner. The form usually includes assessment findings, history obtained through interviewing and from other sources, assessment of the functioning of each system or type of disease process, information about the person's life patterns, nutritional status, housing and family or significant other relationships, accessibility and availability of resources, social relationships including employment, diversional, and recreational activities, stage in life and coping patterns, and concept of illness or wellness as perceived by the patient. The data required for completion of this form can be obtained during an interview and developed in ongoing contacts with the patient.

Physical examination provides an opportunity to further explore data obtained in the patient's history. Many nurses are accustomed to obtaining this information from the physician's examination data. Some nurses have developed physical examination skills and conduct the examination themselves to ascertain the person's current status. Important data are also obtained from laboratory tests such as complete blood count, urinalysis, other tests, and x-rays. The laboratory data are necessary to complete a basic examination and are often obtained routinely when an examination is done to establish baseline data.

PLANNING NURSING CARE

Having completed an initial assessment, the nurse proceeds to develop a plan for care that outlines the goals and procedures to be implemented in managing the patient's care needs. Many different types of care can be initiated, depending on the needs and problems found. In the hospital setting, the nurse's care plan is developed in collaboration with the physician's plan so that the two support common goals. The specific role for each is frequently dependent on institutional protocols, and the level of communication frequently depends on the expertise and role perception of the nurse and the physician.

When the nurse is functioning in a clinic or in the home, the physician may or may not be actively involved in care at the initial assessment. In this instance the physician becomes an important resource person, the nurse referring patients with specific identified problems or those who have significant medical care needs requiring the physician's attention. In many instances the nurse functions in giving ongoing care to people who have chronic or long-term problems and often sees people who have been referred by the physician to a care agency such as the visiting nurse association. A basic medical plan of care accompanies the referral, and the nurse establishes a baseline evaluation through assessment on initial contact with the patient. The interdependence of the nurse and physician roles is ongoing in this type of situation as the nurse informs the physician of problems that may develop, maintains contacts with the physician to jointly determine the patient's progress, and seeks counsel and support in solving difficult problems that do not respond to nursing management.

In general the nurse performs an important coordinating function through care contacts. Because of the nurse's involvement and knowledge of the patient's use of health resources, effectiveness of treatment, and evaluation of emerging needs and problems, the nurse is in a position to refer the patient to appropriate resources and to ascertain whether the patient actually sought and received care.

The broadness of the nurse's role in caring for people makes categorization of components of the role difficult. Care given varies with the setting: Acute care situations require emphasis on technology, complicated procedures, and care measures. Chronic care situations require emphasis on teaching, counseling, retraining, or readjusting the patient's self-concept in accordance with his capabilities and limitations. Clinic and outpatient settings emphasize assessment, evaluation, teaching, and counseling. Home care situations emphasize family relationships, resolution of conflicts, counseling, and assistance in helping the family become self-sufficient. All these situations have different innate care emphases; however, all require that the nurse have a good repertoire of information about human behavior, human needs, and anticipated or expected needs associated with identified care needs. Every person has a unique and individual set of problems. Many of these problems can be related to anticipated outcomes of specific types of situations, disease processes, or personal needs related to age, sexuality, and social roles.

All these aspects of situations are taken into account when planning for care. The goals for care are relevant only if they are compatible with the patient's life. Consider a person who is found to have cardiovascular disease. The knowlege of the presence of the disease may have a different impact on this person than on another person with the same disease. The nurse knows the expected and potential outcomes that directly relate to the disease process and then must apply or transfer this knowledge of probable outcomes to the individual's responses.

A diagnosis may be accepted differently by different patients. If a patient has suspected that he has a problem and this problem is verified by a medical authority, he may experience a feeling of relief. This feeling may stem from the support the medical diagnosis gives to his own feelings about himself. The issue for this patient may be that of proving that he or she has not imagined the health problem. There is also something comforting about knowing that a condition is treatable. Another person with the same diagnosis may respond to the news with pessimism. This pessimism may represent the attitude of a person who has delayed seeking diagnosis and who has built up many fears and anxieties. Confirmation of the diagnosis reinforces the fears and anxieties. Other responses include nonacceptance, disbelief, or, in general, denial of the problem. Yet another person may respond with a myriad of ill-defined worries and fears about his ability to maintain life styles within the diagnosis.

These examples of individual responses to diagnosis are pertinent to care planning. The consequences of these responses in the outcomes of the patient's total adjustment and acceptance of treatment must be dealt with in the plan of care. The nurse must develop subgoals that support attainment of the central goal so that the patient's adaptation to the diagnosis and treatment will be effective.

A treatment and care plan may be similar for each of these patients in respect to medications, diet, activity, and other measures. Nonetheless, this plan may not be equally effective for each patient because of individual attitudes about prognosis. The negative responses must be resolved. Denial must be resolved if the patient is to participate in treatment. Ill-defined worries and fears must be dealt with as they may produce considerable stress and intensify the physiologic disturbance.

Patient Variables

A number of variables are cogent to the problems of care and treatment. The meaning of the diagnosis is sometimes the broadest consideration as it is inclusive of all the components of the patient's life. His age, sexuality, social and employment roles, personal concept and attitudes, and family unit are some of the most obvious components. A person is born with innate biologic propensities for the way he manages his life; these are nurtured and developed through life experiences, with the family being the dominant influence in early life.

During growth and maturation, humans are continually influenced by social norms and roles that help them to define themselves and form relationships with others. Adolescence is considered a culturally imposed phase of life requiring adjustment and conformation with role expectations. Young adults are faced with socially prescribed roles of selecting a mate or a single life, of choosing occupations or careers, and of selecting a place in the social milieu. Selections made at this time often define subsequent roles and relationships. As a consequence they are of import in determination of personal identity.

In the middle years, the individual is part of a social unit that usually binds him in a strong sense of belonging. This may be a career, a family, or a geographic location. During these years the person is generative, that is, he or she is producing through building roles in an occupation or career, raising a family, or contributing to the development or maintenance of other productive enterprises. Personal identity is closely aligned with social groups, family, employment groups, or career-oriented or community groups.

Life patterns begin to change as old age begins. Some of the groups a person has been closely aligned with also change. Children are grown and leave home so that the family situation requires adjustment. The demands previously made from the building or generative activities change in character and the individual becomes less active.

Later a person becomes one of the aged population. Retirement from active work, loss of close relationships with social groups that have held important personal meanings, and loss of the marital partner are sources of conflict for the aged. At the same time, energy levels decline and physiologic adaptation slows with aging. The aged person tends to review past life events and may spend time in the resolution of his feelings about important life events.

Knowledge about life patterns gives the nurse a frame of reference for evaluating factors that either have caused the illness or on which the illness will have an impact. Knowledge of the general demands of the phases of life enables the nurse to anticipate these conflicts and direct the interaction to discovery and validation of the patient's actual or perceived concerns. The nurse can focus on these concerns in terms of general knowledge of life's social roles and may assist the patient in recognizing and dealing with conflicts.

Life events are associated with stress or conflict resolution, particularly as a person moves from one stage of life to another. While social roles are extremely important, the nurse must discover how that person relates to the social role. A person who considers physical attractiveness necessary in establishing relationships with others may be in conflict with the appearance of gray hair, aging skin, and decreased energy. Another conflict may arise from changing relationships in marriage. Still other conflicts arise from expectations concerning children or the failure of children to meet these expectations. Loss of employment or income is another conflict for some elderly persons.

The actual disease process or illness may result from or have an impact on the patient's behavior in all his roles. The illness becomes an integral part of his life responses, representing a coping pattern for some or influencing the coping patterns of others. The illness may directly influence the basic concept of identity. For example, a woman may become very concerned about her ability to have a close relationship with a man following a mastectomy. This basic worry influences her concept of herself as a woman, which may in turn diminish her ability to participate in or contribute to a wide variety of social activities, cutting off outlets for both emotional support and satisfying activity. Another woman may not perceive a mastectomy in this manner, but instead may logically accept the diagnosis and treatment, and pursue her usual social roles with minimum interference.

Disease generates a response. The response is a highly individual matter that includes all the forces that have been integrated with personality and behavior patterns. Sexuality is a major force that has an influence on physiologic and psychological coping mechanisms. Studies have shown that the behavior of female infants is different from that of male infants. Learned patterns of behavior are inevitably different for each sex because the behavior of the infant creates a reciprocal response that continues to influence interactions throughout life. Individual responses in social roles are affected by and influence learned behavior patterns. In this regard sexuality is a dominant force in behavior.

Culture is another dominant force that influences behavior patterns. Differences in culturally influenced behaviors are more visible when one lives in a foreign country. These differences are less visible in geographic locations in which the majority of the inhabitants have assimilated the culture of that geographic area, and have in fact influenced the development of the culture. The nurse must develop a sensitivity to cultural differences among people, particularly as they reflect potential responses to illness and acceptance of care. This sensitivity is pertinent to the visible demography of the area in which one is actively giving care. Cultural variations are more obvious in some locations than in others. The nurse who grows up and continues to reside and work in a given geographic location may never be exposed to extremes in cultural variations because the nurse's perceptions are similar to those of the population in the nurse's care spheres.

An awareness of differences in life patterns influenced by socioeconomic norms is essential in planning relevant care and treatment. In many instances the socioeconomic levels are closely tied to social roles. Not only does socioeconomic status influence self-concept and role conceptualization, but it also determines the resources available for care and treatment.

Many responses are general to human nature; physiologic responses tend to be similar whether the person is rich, poor, married, single, employed, or not. The physiologic changes that are expected following a hysterectomy are an example. These changes occur in the human species with consistency. However, they appear in varying degrees and in varying extremes according to total behavior. Certain anticipated responses, then, are associated with most of the identified disease processes that are influenced by learned behavior. The nurse who knows about these anticipated responses can assist the patient's adjustment by validating these responses in any given individual and by dealing with them in the care plan. Many individual variations in behavior are not explained by culture, socioeconomic status, or sexuality. These individual responses reflect different personality characteristics or traits and highly individualized coping patterns. These coping patterns are essential components of adaptation to illness. The nurse can be effective in helping a patient discover and develop appropriate coping patterns for adjusting or adapting to disease. Some of the techniques used are counseling, behavior modification, and primarily teaching the patient how to cope in a direct and effective manner.

Not infrequently the nurse is confronted with problems that arise from the family unit and that contribute to the conflicts the patient is experiencing. A broad view of the interactive and interdependent coping patterns that are part of a family system is necessary if the patient is to develop effective coping patterns, not only for adjusting to the disease but also for relating effectively within the family unit. The dependency and interaction within the family unit is pertinent to any family member's care. The nurse must ascertain probable sources of conflict such as failure to support a special diet or to purchase medications. This effort, however, is complicated by the limited contact some nurses have with family members, particularly in hospital situations. More often than not, the nurse learns about and views family members from the hospitalized person's perspective or from the family member who most frequently visits the patient in the hospital.

Nurses who practice in home care situations have the advantage of working with the patient in his own environment. Contact with family members may also be limited in this situation because the nurse often visits while family members are at work or school. However, the patient may relate the concerns and problems of family relationships more directly in the home than in the hospital because hospitalization tends to somewhat isolate the patient from these concerns. They are more evident and immediate in the home.

The effects of hospitalization are cogent to behavior during hospitalization. Isolation from the family unit or disruption of usual patterns for any person, whether living alone or in a family group, may disrupt self-concept and feelings of security. The number of hospital events, many unfamiliar, which the patient is expected to participate in, expends much of his energy for adaptation. New and unusual routines, in fact an entirely new social structure is imposed on the patient and may negate his reliance on his normal coping patterns. The patient cannot take a walk or raid the refrigerator, or get angry with a "safe" person. These coping mechanisms are activities that are normal outlets in the home situation. Removal from home coupled with fears and anxieties about the outcomes of hospitalization adds to a patient's stress level. If the patient also has a disease process that diminishes his energy, he may have great difficulty while in the hospital. Older people, who have greater difficulty than younger people in adjusting to change, may be in extreme duress during hospitalization.

Discharge Planning
Even discharge from the hospital may be stress-producing because the patient must reenter the home or family unit. Absence and return of a family member requires adjustment for each person in the family. The interactions during this adjustment phase may help or hinder recovery, depending on the strength and health of the family unit. The nurse should be aware of the stresses experienced with discharge and act to smooth the process as much as possible. Some people, particularly the aged, are moved to a temporary convalescent center or nursing home following hospital discharge. In some instances the change may prove too great for the person's diminished adjustment capabilities.

The nurse must plan care for the duration of the patient's hospitalization and for the phase of adjustment following hospitalization. Discharge planning is essential in this part of the nursing process. The resources and facilities in a given community vary but should be known to the nurse so that appropriate referrals for follow-up care can be made. Teaching family members or significant others is an important aspect in discharge planning. Teaching prior to an event, however, may not be effective in the long run.

Often, while the patients are still in the hospital, nurses teach them about self-care measures required following hospitalization. Although the patient may fully understand these measures at the time of discharge, newly developing problems or conflicts may interfere with the ability to carry out self-care measures at home. Without reinforcement of previous learning and with the occurrence of new problems, patients may not remember important measures. Anxiety levels may also interfere with carrying out measures independently in the home. Home care requirements for patients with short-term illnesses are different from those of patients with long-term or chronic illnesses. Therefore discharge planning must take into account the needs for continued care and reinforcement of learning following hospitalization. Posthospitalization home visits should be made early so that patients can be assisted in their adaptation to prevent frustration, to decrease stress, and to prevent complications. Counsel and support are two central needs during the posthospitalization phase.

In subsequent chapters attention is given to the needs of people who have certain types of diseases. This information is basic not only to care planning but also to implementation of care plans. While each type of problem has unique implications for care measures, the process of giving care is universal. While the process factors in giving care are related to disease or illness, the same factors are applicable to health teaching and measures for prevention of disease. Basically, interactions follow the same or similar patterns whether the nurse is working with the well, potentially ill, or ill population.

In some respects nurses deal directly in either one-to-one situations or in units such as the family. The composite picture of the health status of a community may seem obscure to the nurse who concentrates on these small units of the community. This composite, however, influences human behavior and helps the nurse anticipate and relate to commonly occurring problems within the community whether they are related to disease or to maintenance of wellness.

Wellness is an elusive and subjective concept and at best is considered a relative state. A person may have many physiologic imbalances yet consider himself to be well. Another person may consider himself ill yet have no visible or demonstrable imbalances. **Wellness** may be defined as ability to adapt, to relate effectively, and to function at a nearly maximum level according to capability. Wellness can be related to productivity; if a person is able to produce and consume energy he is active in and contributes to his environment at some level.

A relative view of wellness is pertinent to the nurse's role in the rehabilitation and care of chronically ill patients. In some disease processes, the patient experiences long-term effects of diminished function. The effects may be diminished abilities to problem solve because of cerebral anoxia, loss of ability to walk as with spinal cord injury, or many other forms of functional disruption. The rehabilitative process is a component of all care and may be utilized in convalescence from acute and temporary illness as well as in long-term or chronic and debilitating diseases. Rehabilitation measures are also inclusive of specific techniques important for retraining, for adapting to loss of function such as learning to use a prosthesis, and for supplementing or substituting for lost function as with use of records for the blind or learning laryngeal speech by those with laryngectomies.

In many instances rehabilitation requires specialized nursing skills according to the patient's particular illness. These skills are discussed more fully in subsequent chapters. Teaching and counseling, however, are two prominent roles of nurses in all aspects of rehabilitation. Patients' needs evolve as their conditions change so that teaching and counseling are ongoing matters.

Patient Teaching in Patient Care

Teaching is one of the most satisfying yet difficult roles in nursing. It may be conducted in a large-scale public information program, in a series of individual or group sessions, over the long term with people who have long-term health problems, or in a brief and single contact. The nurse does not always have feedback to determine whether teaching has been effective. In some instances, teaching cannot be documented as it is an integral part of a general conversation. As accountability for the nurse's teaching role evolves, however, there is increasing need to document and evaluate teaching from the aspect of actual learning that has taken place.

Much of the nurse's teaching is conducted in relation to illness processes, their prevention or treatment. The readiness and learning abilities of patients are consistent issues in developing effective teaching techniques. Learning abilities are also concerns in teaching people how to stay well when they have no perceived problems. When people are seeking health care, they may have high anxiety levels that interfere with learning. The patient who has just been told that he requires an operation is usually not ready to learn about postoperative measures. He is probably preoccupied with the general implications of surgery rather than with specific aspects of care. Sometimes, humans have limited perspectives of their problems. For example, if a person is convinced that his primary problem is a skin lesion when he is also found to have anemia, the skin lesion must be treated before he can accept dealing with the anemia.

Some generalizations about teaching can be made. People who are able to learn, who problem solve well, and who are motivated to learn can learn content from individualized methods such as pamphlets, movies, or slide-tape programs. Those who have impaired vision or hearing may require different learning formats. Nonetheless, everyone who learns basic content must apply or translate that content to his own needs. This type of learning has emotional overtones and thus implies that interaction is necessary in dealing with feelings and attitudes. The nurse can discuss the content of the patient's needs and develop a plan realistic and pertinent to his or her life, personal concerns, worries, and anxieties.

To be useful, teaching must be relevant. It should be realistic in terms of the materials and resources available to the learner and applicable to his life situation. If the goal of teaching is to help a person become independent in caring for himself, lists of do's and don't's may not be sufficient. Rather, general information along with examples of how it probably applies to the events the learner will experience is required. The nurse should explore "what if" types of situations with the patient in an effort to prepare him for adjusting to his changing life situations. In many instances care systems, particularly in hospitals, are geared to making the patient dependent on the health personnel. Teaching should enable a person to become as independent as possible.

Evaluation of learning is difficult because changes in behavior may or may not be visible. To evaluate learning outcomes, the nurse is limited to measurement of outcomes that can be realistically observed as feedback for evaluation of both the learning and the teaching. The outcomes should be cooperatively defined by the nurse and the patient so that the goals are commonly understood. In so doing much valuable information can be obtained from the patient about how he learns and what he needs to know and do to achieve the desired outcomes. Teaching a single person how to prepare a diabetic diet may not be relevant if that person eats out consistently. If the goal is to provide a correct diet, the means used to attain this goal might better be focused on the selection of appropriate foods from restaurant menus.

Teaching on the basis of a person's needs and previous knowledge augments transferral of new information or skills to his knowledge and life style. It is best accomplished within the person's own milieu. If this is not possible, then teaching is carried out in the patient's own context. The patient should set the tone for the way information is communicated; words and phrases should be used in keeping with his perceptions and usual modes of communication to facilitate understanding.

Significant others, family members or persons involved in the patient's care, must also be included in the teaching to ensure that it will be used. The nurse should ascertain who will be affected by this teaching. Who will support and reinforce the teaching? Who will carry out the care measures? Who needs to know what changes are significant? The persons identified in these questions benefit from being included in the teaching programs.

Teaching is never complete because a person's needs are continually changing. Therefore, resources for continued evaluation and for teaching needs must be defined for that person. Who does he or she see or call when problems arise? How do they contact and utilize resources? The nurse should provide information and contacts to answer these types of questions.

The type of teaching done by the nurse depends on the nature of the patient's needs, the extent and duration of the problem, and the potential for changes in the patient's condition. These factors have implications for continued use of health resources and, to be effective, the nurse must be familiar with appropriate places and channels for referral in the community.

Counseling the Patient

Counseling is a role that nurses have assumed naturally as part of the process of giving care. Documentation of counseling, which is so much a part of nursing interactions, requires analysis of the content of the interactions. Teaching and counseling techniques have much in common; in both, the nurse must begin with information or cues the patient presents. The initial nurse-patient contact often determines the effectiveness of subsequent contacts. The nurse's technique is important. By listening attentively, the nurse can discern what is uppermost in the patient's mind. Initiating counseling with these data provides the link of understanding necessary in counseling and teaching. Failure to relate to the patient's foremost concerns may "turn him off" because it conveys either a lack of acceptance or an inability to understand the problems as perceived by the patient.

Patience in exploration of a person's perceived needs and status is the keynote to effective counseling. The nurse may fulfill the counseling role simply by helping the patient clarify his own situation through an exploratory conversation. The definition of problems is a positive outcome of counseling. Many times, a person is able to act independently in solving his own problems, once they are voiced and accepted. In other instances, the nurse refers the patient to appropriate resources for resolution of the problems. It may be best to recommend several alternative resources so that the patient can make his own selection. When the nurse senses that the patient will not follow through in selection, he or she can assist the patient by arranging the first visit to the referral agency. The patient then has the option of deciding whether to continue using that agency. The nurse can also facilitate a positive interaction with the referral agency by giving them a resume of the reason for the referral.

Counseling is most effective if the assistance given corresponds to the patient's own motivation for seeking assistance. The patient must feel a need for counseling and must believe that the time spent in counseling is worth the effort. It is also necessary that the patient make a commitment to the activities associated with counseling and that the counselor is open and honest about what services or assistance can actually be offered. The scope of counseling is broad. In general the nurse can offer realistic support through listening and problem solving and through delineation of helpful activities. The wise nurse limits the scope of counseling and freely uses referrals when the patient's problems are beyond the scope of the nurse's expertise. Referrals may be made to other nurses or to other health professionals, to persons in community agencies, or to other community organizations offering the required services.

The overall goal of counseling is similar to that for teaching, that is, to help a patient become as independent as possible. Independence is derived from a multiplicity of factors: a feeling of competence, security in having correct information, and a sense of assurance in being able to act appropriately in situations. In nursing, counseling may be direct or indirect. **Direct counseling** is working with the individual involved. **Indirect counseling** is working with others to solve problems or conflicts related to another person's care. The latter is applicable when another person is caring for someone who is unable to care for himself. Direct counseling is also effective in working with units of people; a family that is working to resolve care problems may benefit from direct counseling in which all the affected members are present. A group of people with similar health problems may benefit from group counseling in which the members can offer each other support. Group process is particularly useful when there is conflict or misunderstanding, or lack of knowledge among members of the group.

Nurses also benefit from counseling. This counseling is pertinent to nurses who work in stressful environments such as intensive care units. It is important that nurses know how to use consultation as well as how to function effectively as counselors. Consultation is a supportive interaction based on sharing. To effectively use consultation, the nurse must deal with perceived needs for problem solving, for additional knowledge and information, and for resolving conflicts within the care situation. Growth is facilitated by consultation geared to gaining new perspectives and devising new or different approaches to care. This type of growth-oriented consultation is beneficial in the continual development of nursing knowledge and expertise.

EVALUATION OF NURSING CARE

Nursing is evolving and changing, which means that nurses must continually develop new approaches and new knowledge through evaluation of care. Current emphasis on quality assurance, in which the nurse thoughtfully acts in an accountable manner and documents the nursing care given, requires skills in planning, evaluating, and recording. There is controversy about how nursing care can best be evaluated. Should it be evaluated in terms of process or in terms of outcome?

Process evaluation includes analysis of the rationale for nursing activities and evaluation of the performance of these activities. This is a type of formative evaluation because it takes place during the developing phases of an activity or set of activities. Outcome evaluation is concerned with developing criteria for desirable effects of the actions and measuring the end product, or the results of the actions. When one examines nursing care, many activities are constructed as essentials in the process. These constructs or critical events can be defined in many instances. For example, in catheterization, some of the constructs include opening the sterile pack correctly, using sterile technique to preserve the sterility of the catheter, correctly preparing the patient for catheterization by explaining the procedure—to name a few. The performance of these constructs and the thought processes of the nurse who plans and carries them out in a process evaluation can be measured. Using the same example, an outcome criterion might be to relieve pressure in the bladder, to measure output from the bladder, or to prevent bladder infection. These criteria or expected outcomes are standards to be achieved. The measurement of outcome is simpler than that of process, particularly in the interactive components of any performance.

An article written by Doris Block [9] emphasizes correlation between process and outcome evaluation. This correlation seems reasonable, but it requires careful consideration of the crucial constructs of care. The relation between process and outcome is, in some instances, direct and measurable, but it may be a matter of chance in others. For example, not every person who has developed a bladder infection has been catheterized with incorrect technique, and technique may be violated without a resultant bladder infection. This point is made to exemplify the problems inherent in assuring quality care. These care problems necessitate thorough evaluation of process and outcomes via research to determine cause and effect of actions and outcomes in controlled situations. In actuality, there are always reasons why the results obtained in controlled situations cannot be replicated in actual care situations. Knowledge of the probability and variables in relationships between cause and effect can, however, contribute validity to the evaluation of either process or outcome or both.

One of the major impediments to outcome or process evaluation in medical and nursing care is the vast body of knowledge and information that is theoretical. Many times diagnosis is determined according to theories or "educated guesses." Even when a diagnosis is clear cut, the underlying disease process may be ill-defined because the basic causes of many diseases are as yet unknown. The wide variation not only in disease processes but also in individual responses to disease processes further complicates outcome or process evaluation. Care, treatment modalities, and expected outcomes are continually being reevaluated according to new insights, newly developing theories, and specific findings in health and disease oriented research.

DISEASE PROCESSES

The causes of disease have been a subject of medical study for centuries. Numerous classifications have been devised in an attempt to clarify the nature of disease processes. For many diseases there is no known cause, even though much of the process is understood. In some diseases, the effects are known, but the processes that cause these effects are obscure. Frequently, diseases are classified in more than one way. A disease may bring about changes in cellular structure, or in the shape of an organ or its function. Some of these changes are grossly visible; others are detectable only through laboratory techniques. Some diseases are best known by their symptoms and signs. Others are known by the type of pathology involved, such as infection and cancer. Sometimes the names or classifications given to diseases give no clue to the pathologic processes, particularly when they are named for the people who discovered them. Currently the trend is to avoid use of eponyms in describing diseases.

Another way of classifying disease is according to onset and duration. **Acute illness** or disease has a sudden onset and may be of short duration. An acute illness may be resolved and is then called short-term. It may, however, become prolonged or cause complications of longer duration and then becomes a long-term or **chronic illness.** Sometimes chronic illness can be resolved over a long period, lasting months or years. Often chronic illness lasts a lifetime and the basic condition does not change. **Exacerbation** of a disease is the recurrence of acute signs and symptoms. **Remission** is a temporary withdrawal of the signs and symptoms.

Many studies of disease are concerned with the **epidemiology** of disease. Epidemiologic methods for study of disease, which are considered to be the diagnostic process of public health, include collection of data about the occurrence, frequency, and distribution of both health and disease. The cause of diseases can be inferred indirectly from epidemiologic data. Studies indicate at what age, in which sex and race, and in what geographic locations certain diseases occur. Culture, habits, customs, and attitudes toward health care are all included in epidemiologic studies. The outbreak of disease is referred to as its **incidence,** which means the number of new cases that occur in a given period of time. **Prevalence** is another term used in epidemiology and refers to the total number of cases present in a given period. Both the incidence of new cases and the presence of disease of longer duration are included in prevalence. **Mortality rates** are derived according to causes of death; these rates are calculated as the total number of deaths for any given cause divided by the total number of people in the population being studied. **Morbidity rates** give information about the ratio of disease to health in a given population.

Epidemiology is important in the study of disease for evaluation of environmental and other factors that contribute to health or disease, as evidenced in the population studied. If the population in a given community or a specific geographic location has a high incidence of a particular disease, research can be focused on discovery of the contributory factors in that location. These factors include the presence of natural or man-made agents such as toxic substances, nutrition patterns, and the temperature and vegetation in the given area.

Many of the studies to discover the level of

health or disease in a community are **retrospective.** They involve accumulation of data that summarize past events through surveys and questionnaires. Some of the studies are **random samples** obtained by interviews or surveys. Other studies are compiled continuously, such as those concerned with the reported causes of death and the age at death. If the incidence of a certain disease process is high in a specific age group in a particular area, this population is said to be **at risk.**

Nurses are concerned not only with the care of sick people but also with the factors that contribute to health. For this reason, much of the nurse's health teaching and counseling is based on knowledge about the known risk factors in diseases. Nurses are also involved in giving care that provides the greatest benefit for the patient. Treatment of diseases such as cancer involves choices in treatment modalities. Some of the effects of radiation therapy for cancer, for example, may be harmful to the body cells. The decision to be made is whether the negative effects of radiation therapy outweigh the results that would occur if this type of therapy is not given. When disease results from treatment or therapy, it is **iatrogenic.** Dental caries resulting from radiation therapy to the head and neck is an example of an iatrogenic disease.

Application of Basic Concepts in Selected Clinical Situations

Certain treatment modalities are used in the treatment of many diseases, just as certain types of pathologic processes occur in any system of the body. Surgical intervention is an example of a treatment modality that has widespread application. Communicable diseases, infection, and neoplastic growths are examples of pathologic processes that also affect any system of the body. Each is described separately in this chapter so that the knowledge gained can be applied as the subsequent chapters are studied.

Communicable Diseases and Infections*

In the following pages, communicable and infectious diseases will be discussed. **Communicable diseases** are diseases that spread among people and are caused by pathogenic microorganisms. These diseases are usually named according to the symptoms or the causative organism.

Each communicable (or contagious) disease has a typical pattern of transmission from reservoir to host, period of incubation, of communicability, generalized signs and symptoms, and treatment.

Infection is different from an infectious (communicable) disease. An infection may result when microorganisms normally present in the body and within the environment multiply and grow beyond normal limits. Conditions that favor the growth of the organism beyond normal limits include a disruption of the body's protective mechanisms, such as a break in the skin surface, and lowered resistance for any reason, such as a debilitating disease. Microorganisms may also cause disease when they increase in number or virulence, thus being able to overcome the person's resistance.

Infection is defined as "the entry and development or multiplication of an infectious agent in the body of man or animals" [128]. Several commonly used terms help to describe the process through which infections occur. A **carrier** is a person (or animal or bird) who is otherwise apparently well, but who harbors pathogenic microorganisms that live and multiply in his body without overtly causing disease. The carrier is able to transmit the infectious agent to others, who may then become infected. **Contamination** is the presence of viable organisms capable of causing infections, and **susceptibility** is the tendency to become ill if and when there has been exposure to a pathogenic organism. The person who becomes ill as a result of infection with a pathogenic organism has insufficient or poor resistance to the disease. The inflammatory and immune responses previously discussed explain how resistance is developed. A **contact** is a person or animal who has associated with another person or animal who is contaminated or infected with pathogenic organisms. The person who is in contact with an infected person may contract the disease if his resistance is insufficient [128].

Other terms used frequently in communicable disease control include the words endemic, epidemic, and pandemic. **Endemic** is the continual presence of a disease or infec-

*By Mary Marrs.

tious agent in a community at normal or usual levels. **Epidemic** refers to a temporary and significant increase in the incidence of disease, above the normal expected levels. **Pandemic** refers to a worldwide epidemic. **Sporadic** diseases occur occasionally and are present in a small number of people.

Nurses who practice actively in the control of communicable diseases in a community deal with the multiple factors that influence the spread of these diseases. Basically the most central factors that operate in the chain of infection are the following. In the chain of communicable diseases there must be a causative agent, a **host** (humans, animals, or birds that harbor the infectious agent), the proper environment for growth of the agent, and transmission to the susceptible host. The **causative agent** is a pathogenic microorganism that is classified as bacterial, viral, rickettsial, protozoal, fungal, or helminthic. **Reservoir** is the term used for the human, animal, or substance that provides an environment conducive to the life of the organism. The usual channels of escape of the microorganism from humans include the respiratory tract, the gastrointestinal tract, the genitourinary tract, or any open lesion, or in the case of infestations it may be mechanical escape such as with lice or scabies [173].

TRANSMISSION OF COMMUNICABLE DISEASES

The **transmission** or escape of the microorganism from one place to another occurs in one of several different ways. In some instances transmission occurs through **direct contact** of a noninfected person with an infected person or source. **Indirect contact** refers to infection of a noninfected person who comes into contact with substances that have been contaminated by an infected person. Impetigo is a communicable disease that may be spread through indirect contact. Use of contaminated drinking glasses or water fountains, or touching articles that have been contaminated are examples of indirect contact.

Infectious agents are spread from one place to another through vehicles, through the air, or by vectors. A **vehicle** is an inanimate substance that is contaminated and which can support growth of the organism. Food, water, drugs, or blood are such vehicles. Microorganisms are spread through the air in the form of droplet nuclei or in dust particles. The common cold is an infection caused by an agent that spreads through droplet nuclei; staphylococci spread through dust particles. A vector may be an insect, which has six legs; or an arachnid, which has eight legs. Both insects and arachnids are termed **arthropods.** Mosquitos, fleas, and lice are insects that may spread disease; ticks and mites are arachnids that may spread disease.

Nurses must be aware of the means through which infectious agents spread diseases. There are many instances in which nurses can prevent contact with microorganisms through use of good aseptic technique, such as correct hand washing, using only *uncontaminated* equipment (disposable syringes) and isolating patients who have infectious diseases. Control of droplet spread of infections through sneezing, coughing, or from sputum is also important for the nurse. Droplet nuclei are small residues of droplets that have evaporated. Dust is ever present and can become contaminated through agents found on clothing or linens, or in soil.

Any person who is exposed to microorganisms has the potential for becoming a host (or reservoir). The portals of entry of microorganisms are the same as the escape portals in transmission of the microorganism; the respiratory tract, ingestion of food via the gastrointestinal tract, or mucous membranes or breaks in the skin.

In determining whether the exposed person will develop the disease a microorganism causes, it is important to review some of the factors that influence susceptibility or resistance to disease. First, the virulence or strength of the organism is important. Highly virulent organisms are more powerful than those with low virulence, and the highly virulent ones are more difficult to resist, even by "healthy" persons. The number of organisms is also important in determining the disease-producing potential of the organism. A person may be able to resist a few microorganisms, but may not be able to resist them in large numbers. A number of other important considerations in resistance to infection include genetic makeup and acquired resistance. Finally, the individual state in terms of physical condition, nutritional state, emotional state, and the total number of stresses at any given time influence a person's ability to resist infection.

Nurses who work in the community or in the hospital setting should be aware that environmental and other factors influence a person's status at any given time. Certain people, especially the very young and the aged, are highly susceptible to infection, as are those who have debilitating illnesses. Crowded or unsanitary conditions, malnutrition for any reason, or alterations in the immune system also influence susceptibility to infections. In general, immunization programs take into account the special needs of people in these categories. This is particularly true of immunization programs geared to prevent viral influenza, in which the most highly susceptible persons are immunized first when possible and appropriate. Other immunization programs, such as those for measles, mumps, rubella, and diphtheria are developed for target populations such as young children. Some immunization programs are developed for everyone in the community. Immunization for poliomyelitis is an example of a preventive measure designed for every person.

COMMUNICABLE DISEASE CONTROL METHODS

We have at our disposal today the reality of controlling many communicable diseases through immunization. These immunizations, however, are helpful for disease control only if they are used properly. One of the problems of the population, particularly very young parents, is their lack of knowledge of the need for immunizations for their infants and children. Often, the nurse may encounter complete ignorance of the dangers and side effects of the many once feared childhood diseases because the young parents have never seen or heard of them. Other people reject immunizations because of cultural or religious beliefs. Looking through old death records from the turn of the century gives one a chilling reminder of these fearsome diseases; one can see that whole families were wiped out within weeks by communicable diseases such as diphtheria or measles.

Knowledge about available immunizations, about how they should be given, and the time intervals for boosters is another responsibility of nurses. It is also important for nurses to know about the kind of protection and immunity these immunizations provide and the conditions under which they should not be given. Unless the ground rules are observed, the population served by nurses may not be served well. Nurses should also maintain immunizations for protection of their own health.

Records of family immunizations are important. It is necessary to establish an orderly method for tabulating immunizations along with strong education and follow-up programs to ensure that the required immunizations are given. The programs should provide for correct spacing to ensure effective primary responses and booster effects (as described under The Immune Response). It has been found, for example, that administration of booster doses prior to a child's entrance to nursery school or the primary grades is particularly important.

At times, some people develop a disease for which they have been given immunization. In these cases, it can be found that specific contraindications were not observed when administering the vaccine or that the immunizing materials were improperly stored or, in some instances, were administered after exposure to the disease so that there was not sufficient time for the recipient to develop antibodies. Some people develop hypersensitivity responses to materials used in the preparation of vaccines or immunizations.

Although no vaccine in use has ever been 100 percent effective, research is ongoing to determine vaccine effectiveness and to reappraise the vaccine administration methods used to block the transmission of the causative organisms. A classic example of the results of these evaluative processes is the withdrawal of smallpox vaccine from the list of required childhood immunizations. Several factors influenced the decision, the greatest of these being a tremendous decrease in the risk of actual disease resulting from worldwide protection of susceptible individuals. With decreased incidence of outbreaks, the complications experienced from the vaccination itself exceeded the number of cases of the disease. Therefore, containment and blockage of transmission of the causative agent are utilized to control any outbreaks. In the present policy, administration of the vaccine is confined to susceptible people in areas in which the disease has occurred in order to contain the disease within this area.

When considering a method of control for

communicable diseases, all known facts should first be gathered and then considered with particular attention to the method of transmission and the virulence of the organism involved. The book *Control of Communicable Diseases in Man* [128] is the basic reference used by health workers who are involved in the control of communicable diseases. This book is the official report of the American Public Health Association (APHA) and is a readily available and handy reference. In this reference aspects of communicable diseases are discussed according to their identification, occurrence, infectious agents, the reservoir, mode of transmission, incubation period, period of communicability, susceptibility and resistance, and methods of control. The last includes preventive measures for control in limited contacts and in epidemics and internationally applicable measures. The control procedures and measures given for each communicable disease in the APHA reference are specific. They are intended to control the patient's contacts in his immediate environment to prevent the spread of his disease.

In general these control measures include reporting the disease to the local health authority by the doctor, nurse, or other designated person; isolation or quarantine to minimize contacts with noninfected persons; and the use of concurrent disinfection measures to prevent transmission according to the mode of transmission of the specific infectious agent (respiratory secretions, sputum, and contaminated substances used by the infected person, or handling of feces). In addition, location of contacts so that immunization measures or treatment can be given is necessary to contain the infectious agent and control the spread of the disease.

While the APHA book is extremely useful in determining control or preventive measures, the nurse should also be aware of local and state regulations concerning communicable diseases. Regulations about reporting and control measures vary from one area of the country to another. It is necessary for the nurse to realize that the national statistics about communicable diseases are only as good as the local data collection in every area of the country. The information collected at the local level is the basis for the state statistics and for corresponding surveillance programs for control. Therefore care and attention should be given to the collection and tabulation of information about the incidence of communicable diseases.

Some diseases are internationally quarantinable. These include cholera, plague, smallpox, yellow fever, and other diseases under surveillance by the World Health Organization. In the latter category are louse-borne relapsing fever, typhus fever, poliomyelitis, malaria, and influenza. Local reporting is determined according to the need for and the ability to control specific diseases, for the development of programs for controlling specific diseases, and for data collection for specific epidemiologic study. Weekly bulletins* are sent to state and local health departments to provide information to local health workers about current outbreaks throughout the world and to issue corresponding immunization requirements necessary for traveling from one area to another. It is important that the traveler be informed of the booster requirements for international travel and that he carry along with his passport a listing of all current and accountable immunizations and vaccinations to be checked and verified when entering other countries.

Surveillance, outbreak control or search, and containment are public health strategies. They are important for widespread control of communicable diseases extending from the world to a given person's home. These strategies also are useful tools for nurses to implement in situations in which the spread of infection must be controlled: in hospitals, homes, institutions, clinics, or any situation in which people congregate.

Surveillance

A comprehensive surveillance program consists in four basic functions: (1) collection of data relevant to the extent of the infection and to the potential for its transmission to others, (2) consolidation of the data in terms of the important variables such as time, place, and persons infected or exposed, (3) epidemiologic and statistical analysis, and (4) dissemination and interpretation of the basic data to persons involved in surveillance and control programs [138].

---

*Morbidity and mortality weekly reports are provided by the National Center for Disease Control, Atlanta, Georgia, an agency of the United States Public Health Service.

Surveillance data can be obtained in an active or passive manner. Passive surveillance data include reports from physicians, laboratories, or health agencies. The actual reporting by these persons and agencies is dependent on the attitudes of and assistance sought by infected persons. It is important for the nurse to remember that the concept of illness varies with groups and individuals, and often this concept is related to environmental, cultural, or economic factors. Age, degree of the illness, and complications influence the decision to seek treatment or report a communicable disease. For example, a family in the low income group may seek medical treatment only for the principal wage earner in the family because the basic income is absolutely essential to the family's livelihood. The cost of medical treatment may cause many persons to refrain from seeking assistance for seemingly "normal" illness. An example is the common cold, which may be a precursor to many different illnesses. The infected person may not seek medical attention because it is well known that the remedy for the common cold consists in rest, taking fluids, aspirin, and proper nutrition. One may consider that the lack of a known or specific cure makes the effort of being told about these common remedies by a physician or nurse not worth the expense involved. In other instances, such as illness in a young infant or child, transient illness is considered normal if it is mild. Care of the infant might create no need for changes in routines. If the family is oriented to the concept that transient illness is normal, no family member is likely to seek treatment. Therefore many illnesses are never diagnosed by a physician and are never reported.

Because the incidence of unreported illness in the community is considerable, active surveillance may be employed to provide supplementary information. This type of surveillance requires activities that search for feedback from study populations through surveys, phone calls, and home visitation. The communication methods known to be effective in a given area should be used in active surveillance. If newspaper and radio advertisements about the surveillance program are means of reaching large groups of people, they should be utilized. If there is sufficient staff available, and if the interest of the community is aroused, much valuable information can be obtained through active surveillance programs. Television, radio, or newspapers may be used to disseminate information about the typical symptoms of rubella, for example. A phone number can be given so that people can call if rubella symptoms are present in their household or neighborhood. Personal contact through follow-up visits can then be made to determine the actual situation, to establish the diagnosis, to investigate the source of the infection and the mode of transmission, to identify susceptible persons, and to gather information on their immune status. When a given area is studied in this manner, information can be gathered, data can be consolidated and summarized, and programs can be established to determine priorities and operational containment measures to control the disease.

Public Education
Public health is a broad and encompassing field that is often associated with immunizations and control of communicable diseases. While disease control is only one aspect of public health activity, it is a very important one. The fact that the present generation of people growing up has minimal knowledge of childhood diseases and consequently no fear of them or of their consequences is a tribute to the effective work of public health agencies. It is also proving to be a hazard, however, because immunization rates are gradually declining and the incidence of some diseases is increasing as inadequate numbers of susceptible persons take advantage of immunization programs. In some states, this problem is being rectified by passage of laws requiring immunizations. In some communities, officials require immunization programs as part of the community services. Most school systems have established immunization requirements to protect their populations.

The same category of contagious or communicable disease in the adult population can also be discussed in terms of decreasing incidence. In many instances, diseases that once ravaged the adult population have diminished through improved procedures for handling, packaging, and transporting food, through improved sanitation systems, and through improved housing conditions. All these efforts are part of the function of the Public Health Department in a community, county, or state as well as the National Center for Disease Control in Atlanta, Georgia, which conducts ongoing research and program development for protection of the public.

One of the concerns for those who work in public health is the proliferation of varying types of health centers (storefront clinics) and the mobility of the population. It has become difficult to bring a semblance of order to the efforts to control communicable diseases because there is often no local control of health care and treatment for given individuals. The fragmentation of health care in the current delivery system, with people seeking their treatment from a number of unrelated health services, negates orderly collection of health information and use of services. This fragmentation of health care services not only produces real problems for case finding and follow-up for the health agencies, but also interferes with the important roles of health counseling and teaching that health workers can perform if they have the opportunity to develop ongoing relationships with the people who use health services. The declining rates of immunizations could well be a product of this type of fragmentation of health services. People ought to have a comprehensive health record with a reliable provider of care. This factor has important implications for the need to develop strong and effective health departments and to coordinate services in the health care system.

Many states have attempted to protect individuals by passing laws requiring immunizations. Most of these programs are related to attending school or taking part in other formalized activities within the community. These programs do not reach every segment of the population because large numbers of children of preschool age and aged persons in the highly susceptible groups are not actively involved in congregate functions as at school or employment. There is continual need for study and the development of programs to reach every segment of the population and to coordinate health services. In many instances, local health departments are endeavoring to achieve the latter by developing central control record systems for immunizations and for other types of care under their jurisdiction.

Many health departments are also engaged in active public education programs. These programs are designed to inform the public of positive health practices important in the prevention of disease. Communications media are used in these programs, as people tend to get information most easily through accustomed sources. Newspapers and local radio stations are utilized in these programs. Other sources of communication include a coloring book developed to explain the important immunizations for children. This book, when given to school-age children, is also a means of reaching parents who may read the "coloring book" information when the child brings it home from school. Maternity packets developed for target populations explain immunization programs necessary for preschool children. This particular program is designed to increase the number of immunizations obtained by preschool children in addition to giving new parents information about positive health pratices for themselves and their children. Informing people of the care needed to remain healthy is recognized as an important aspect of public health. Nurses should be aware of these public health programs and should be prepared to reinforce them when appropriate in any contact with people.

The importance of community education programs in an age in which people have had minimal personal experiences with communicable diseases is recognized by health workers. A discussion based on a communicable disease may help explain control of communicable disease among identified risk groups. Rubella, for example, usually occurs in children in the 5- to 9-year age group and is most prevalent in the spring and winter. Also at risk are pregnant women who have not in their early years had rubella and who are in their first trimester of pregnancy. If they now develop rubella, the virus can cross the placental barrier and damage the fetus. Infants with congenital rubella syndrome carry the virus for an undetermined period and can be the source of infection for unprotected women of childbearing age who are at risk, particularly those who work in newborn nurseries.

People at risk are protected by use of a live virus vaccine developed in 1969. Previous to this development, collected figures showed a high incidence of rubella every 6 to 9 years, and the next outbreak was then expected to occur in 1970. Not only was the 1970 (or 1971) predicted outbreak averted through the use of immunization, but also a general reduction in the incidence of rubella was achieved.

The target populations for rubella immunization are children more than 1 year of age, school-age children in the primary grades, and adolescent girls prior to the childbearing age. If young women are immunized later, it must be ascertained that they are not pregnant at the time of vaccination or that they have no probability of becoming pregnant within 3 months of the vaccination. It is difficult to immunize when there is the possibility of pregnancy in a population group designated for a mass immunization program because of the individual variations in status. Some states try to control rubella in this age group by requiring a rubella titer (HI) along with the other necessary premarital tests as a method of ensuring control, to prevent the transmission of maternal rubella infection and resultant damage to the fetus. This example demonstrates the intertwining of data collection, interpretation of data, definition and implementation of programs, and resultant control of a specific disease [178].

Another area of emphasis in recent times is the improvement of record keeping for tabulation of immunizations. Many records are brief to the point of excluding data important for conducting an ongoing immunization program. Because immunizing agents are continually being developed and improved, differences in their effects should be noted. It is also helpful to know how long the particular type of vaccine has been in use. Many immunizing agents were originally killed viruses, to be given in multiple doses, and sometimes requiring follow-up booster administration. These agents have been replaced with one-time administration of live virus vaccine with the capability of providing lifetime immunity. For this reason the immunizations given should be fully documented so that future evaluation of the recipient's needs can be carefully evaluated. Thus the records should specify the manufacturer's name for the vaccine used and the dosage and other pertinent information.

Nurses should also be aware of the priorities established in immunization programs. When, for example, there is a shortage of the immunizing agent, populations at risk (those with the greatest susceptibility) are given preference in the immunization program. Priorities for determining immunization programs are also based on identification of the most harmful disease prevailing, especially when the administration of more than one immunizing agent at any given time will not produce the desired immunity in a given individual.

Some of the newer immunizing agents are still undergoing research to determine their long-term effects. Mumps vaccine was introduced in 1968. Studies [178] concerning the duration of protection indicate that the antibodies developed in immunized individuals have persisted since their first immunization. Mumps occurs most frequently in school-age children, with only 15 percent of the reported cases occurring after puberty.

Combination vaccines are presently available. An example is the measles-rubella (MR) vaccine given via a single injection. Measles, mumps, and rubella (MMR) also can be given in a single injection. Yet, another example is a combination of diphtheria, pertussis, and tetanus vaccines (DPT). It has been shown that MMR or MR given with trivalent oral polio vaccine (TOPV) is effective. Antibody responses obtained in the combination administration are comparable to the responses obtained when each component vaccine is given at different times. There has been no increase in either the frequency or the severity of the clinical reactions of persons given the combination vaccines. This research is essential in the development of immunization programs. It is advisable to give as much protection as possible to the person being immunized since that person may not return for follow-up immunization programs.

It is necessary to develop effective follow-up programs for people who have been immunized. The Sabin oral poliomyelitis immunization programs conducted in the early 1960s were very effective. By 1964, 88 percent of the children in the 1- to 4-year age group had received the polio vaccine. By 1973, however, only 63 percent of the children in the same age group were adequately immunized [178]. This statistic implies that the delivery system for polio vaccination has become less adequate and that an epidemic of poliomyelitis could result if the trend toward decreasing immunization is not reversed. Nurses who are aware of these trends can be instrumental in helping community agencies see the need for immunization programs and they may be able to provide positive stimulus to initiation of programs.

The Nurse's Role

Nurses also have an important role in assisting with surveillance activities. There is need for continuous scrutiny of agents that cause communicable disease so that control measures can be taken. This type of surveillance is the function of the city, county, and state public health departments, and it includes many types of activities. Systematic collection of morbidity and mortality reports, data from field investigations about epidemics and individual cases, studies of immunity levels in the population, laboratory reports identifying infectious agents, and the availability and use of protective measures such as vaccines and insecticides are important sources of information for the interpretation and evaluation of epidemiologic data in active surveillance.

Because many families tend to be less concerned with communicable diseases than previously, when the incidence was high and threatening to family life, the nurse must actively engage in public information programs and in counseling individuals. These activities are particularly applicable components of health teaching and counseling of families with members who have chronic illnesses, elderly members, or persons who are in particular populations at risk. The same need for teaching applies to individuals who are in a position to influence the health status of other people, such as those in day care centers, in homes for the aged, or in other types of community based programs providing human services.

Each nurse has an important role in investigating epidemiologic data and in breaking the chain of infectious diseases. The activities are integral to the other care roles the nurse assumes. Principles of epidemiologic investigation are similar to other forms of nursing assessment. Recognition and validation of the presence of communicable illnesses *(time, place,* and *number of cases)* give information about what might be expected so that control measures can be taken early. If there is a possibility that an epidemic exists, information should be gathered and action to control the disease should be taken as early as possible.

The major difference between assessment of a person's health status and needs and an epidemiologic survey is that the survey is oriented to groups. Programs to control communicable diseases must also be oriented to the total environment, the larger group.

Nurses are in a position to observe human behavior in relation to health and disease. This role is often not given the attention it should be given as a key element in the progress toward solving problems related to prevention of disease. In many instances, advances in the control and treatment of diseases have come about because an astute and knowledgeable observer noted the implications of the relationships among the events taking place. Often the events are overlooked because they tend to be common, everyday occurrences. A well-known historic example is the initial observation and awareness during the Spanish-American War of the importance of the mosquito in disease causation. Mosquitos are common and could go unnoticed; in this historic discovery, Walter Reed, an army surgeon, noted the relation between the mosquito and the occurrence of disease (yellow fever). Nurses are in a position to note analogous events and to determine the relationships among these events and their effects.

As more is learned about diseases, one of the important tasks is that of disseminating what has been discovered so that the new information can be integrated into the lifestyles of people. Conveying the implications of what has been discovered is often difficult as attitudes and feelings about diseases are cultural as well as individual. Teaching people to understand and to deal with communicable diseases, infections, and illness in general often involves dealing with misinformation, superstitions, and family traditions.

Health teaching is complex because of multitudinous factors. The following anecdote illustrates this point. Several years ago, a nurse was trying to deal with a persistent problem of head lice (pediculosis capitus) in an ethnic neighborhood. The problem occurred within a school situation, and control measures were undertaken by a public health nurse in cooperation with the school nurse and with community nurses. The nurses used printed instructions with diagrams and pictures—they developed every type of teaching aid they could think of and had available. Still, the problem kept recurring and spreading throughout the school. Finally, one nurse sat down and talked about the discouraging situation with one of the families, only to discover in this conversation that head lice were a sign of health to these people.

On the basis of this information, the nurse realized why the one-to-one surveillance was not effective. The families had indeed been following the nurse's instructions to the letter, even to removing the last nit from the head. But then they would place the live specimen back on the head of the child because it was their guarantee that the child was healthy. They had been brought up with the belief that the child who has head lice is healthy. If the louse had not stayed on the child's body, the child would be considered ill. (In the case of body lice, this is true, because body lice will attempt to leave the body of the person whose temperature exceeds a tolerable temperature for the lice.) The families had learned to associate the presence of lice with health from observations made by watchful mothers years and years ago. The information had been passed from generation to generation, and the present families had believed it from childhood. While they were in fact completely cooperative in the health measures advised by the nurses, they also remained faithful to the teachings of their predecessors.

Since early times, human beings have been aware that unidentified elements or forces can cause illness in varying degrees. Lacking specific knowledge about the causes of illness, human beings have sought to protect themselves from the unknown by using various charms and rituals to cure or control illnesses. These practices have been handed down from generation to generation and become ingrained from early infancy. It is difficult to replace the traditions, beliefs, and folklore of different cultures with current, proved knowledge about the means to prevent and treat disease.

The nurse must thus remain cognizant of the varying cultural beliefs, traditions, and folklore when giving care. Because today's society is highly mobile, there is an intertwining of longstanding cultural beliefs and practices and the nurse may come across people who use an admixture of different cultural practices. Beliefs and feelings must be respected as a part of individuality; the nurse must be able to help a person learn the acceptable methods and correct approaches for disease prevention, control, and treatment. In order to do this, the nurse must use adaptable teaching methods and a great deal of ingenuity.

The information that needs to be taught about communicable diseases and their control includes information about methods for control, prevention, and care. The control methods are continually changing as new rules, regulations, and policies are developed according to the needs at any given period of time. These are designated by national and state health departments and are communicated to local health personnel for implementation. Measures for prevention include the policies that have been developed for specific situations as well as universal measures that are used in protecting people from infectious agents. Care and treatment measures are designated according to the problems presented by an individual with the disease. Each of these areas will be discussed more fully in the following pages.

Public Safety

When the health of a community (or of a state or nation) is at risk because of a high incidence of communicable disease at a given time, control of that disease becomes a matter of public safety. To ensure public safety, regulations and policies are developed by national, state, and local health departments for implementation in the appropriate places. These places usually include public institutions, places of employment, and any area where people tend to congregate in large numbers, such as train stations and airports. When the preventive measures require ongoing implementation, legislation may be passed to ensure protection of the public.

It is interesting to note that public health legislation did not originate within the medical profession, but that it was often dictated by esthetic and olfactory considerations. For example, the recently revised sanitary code of New York City has relieved the Commissioner of Health of his obligation to look for dead horses in the street [171]. It has become necessary to continually revise and update public health legislation to meet the current needs of people. Many factors are constantly changing and are influencing the type of protection needed. One of these factors is that environmental changes bring about concomitant changes in the balance between the host and the disease-producing agent.

A number of natural disasters may bring about changes in this balance. Floods produce enteric infections, because the uncontrolled waters mix with sewage and drinking water. The safety of the drinking water becomes questionable, and specific temporary measures must be undertaken to protect the public. This situation requires that information be disseminated publicly so that the area population will know how to protect itself from disease. Other changes in the environment include increases in the mosquito population during rainy seasons. This increase may raise the incidence of mosquito-borne diseases such as encephalitis. In order to prevent an epidemic of encephalitis, public health measures include efforts to reduce the mosquito population via spraying with appropriate agents and the dissemination of information about protective measures so that people can protect themselves from contact with the mosquitos. Information about the recognizable signs and symptoms of the disease and specific information about the required care and treatment of the affected population are also stated publicly so that people will know what is happening and will be encouraged to seek care if needed.

Sometimes, efforts to restore the balance between host and agent result in the appearance of a new problem. In a mouse extermination program in a New York City apartment house, a new disease, **rickettsialpox**, appeared when parasitic mites left the cold bodies of the mice to find new homes on the warm bodies of the tenants [171]. Some of the main elements in disease control that can contribute to this upset in the balance between host and agent are food supplies, the use of pesticides, the removal of wastes including body excrement, and climates that foster the growth of bacteria or other microorganisms. The water supply is a major element that also requires constant attention to ensure public safety.

For each of these elements there is public legislation. Sanitation systems provide for public safety through the proper elimination of wastes; laws concerning food packaging, preservation, and transport ensure safe supplies of food; public works departments ensure safety of the water supply; and community controls in the use of pesticides ensure that pesticides with known detrimental effects on the balance of nature are banned. There are also provisions for assisting communities during natural catastrophes such as floods, earthquakes, and droughts.

In addition to public legislation, there are regulations and measures taken by health departments at every level to provide the public with information on self-protection. These measures are concerned with the preparation and handling of food in the home or in restaurants, procedures to ensure cleanliness in handling laundry, ventilation systems, and the use of disinfectants or pesticides as well as general housekeeping. In general, removal of sources of bacterial growth is translated into methods that can be used by every person in self-protection. The nurse must be aware of these measures and must be able to explain them to people who require this teaching.

Because these protective methods are basic to a normal state, nurses sometimes forget that many people do not know these basics and must be taught. The simple act of removing crumbs and dust to eliminate insects and mice may need to be taught along with some of the basic principles for precluding bacterial growth. The latter include use of both heat and refrigeration. Bacteria and their products are readily destroyed by heat given that the temperature and duration of the heat are sufficient. Coldness prevents the growth of bacteria. Another basic method for preventing disease is that of washing food products before use to reduce microorganisms to an acceptable level and remove residues of pesticides that may have been used in the growing or storing procedures. In some geographic areas, the need to create a dry place for storage of food is important, as moisture promotes bacterial growth. Warm humid climates make such measures for initiating dry storage spaces necessary. The cooking methods used are also important in the preservation of health. Microorganisms may thrive in improperly cooked foods, making the correct preparation of foods an important area for teaching people how to protect themselves from such microorganisms.

Another area that deserves attention when discussing the balance between the host and the infectious agent is that of the use of antibiotics, which has led to the creation of drug-resistant strains of bacteria. Some patients who undergo antibiotic therapy do not demonstrate overt signs and symptoms of infections, but continue to be carriers. This is particularly a problem in hospitals and in institutions where many people gather together, so that the possibility of transmission is increased. In some instances the effects of trauma and treatment have resulted in the development of more virulent strains of bacteria so that ordinary resistance is insufficient in developing immunity to the virulent strains [156]. Using antibiotics indiscriminately can also sensitize the patient to these medications.

The nurse's activities toward public protection therefore must take into account the effects of the protective measures that are being used. It is important to remain informed about public health practices within communities and to make thoughtful decisions about control procedures. Often, a solution to an immediate problem creates other far-reaching problems that may be more difficult to solve. The cost of public and private programs, their potential effectiveness, the accessibility of the materials and supplies needed for these programs, and their long-term effects influence the decision about initiating specific programs.

Infection Control

Because much of the public health literature deals with national and community based programs that have far-reaching effects, one sometimes loses sight of some of the basic procedures that can be carried out easily and inexpensively in the home. One of the most fundamental means of protection from infectious agents is hand washing. This simple act can be taught and reinforced in the nurse's dealings with people. Thorough hand washing is taught in most fundamental nursing courses. This measure should become second nature to nurses, wherever they practice: in the home, in hospitals, or in other health agencies.

Hand washing can also be taught to children in schools and in home situations. Some teachers in elementary schools are able to teach the importance of hand washing by setting aside a specific time for children to wash their hands. This is especially educative immediately preceding lunch and after using the bathroom.

Hand washing is an important aspect of all isolation procedures in hospitals and in homes, but it is often neglected by nurses. One study of hand washing [150] used Feldman's hand washing criteria and ranked activities enumerated by Fulkerson of the Center for Disease Control in Atlanta, Georgia. The CDC ranks activities from cleanest to the most contaminated. The study indicated that among the group investigated, hand washing procedures were lax in some or many aspects of these criteria. This finding is surprising because hand washing is an elemental and essential aspect of care.

Many people with communicable diseases and infections are being cared for in general hospitals. To care for these people correctly, infection control committees have been established to develop guidelines and policies for protective care of hospital populations. This protection is geared to prevention of cross-infection and to protection of noninfected people. An epidemiologically oriented manual has been developed by the CDC [133]. This manual offers current guidelines and procedures for the care of patients with diseases that might be seen in hospitals in the United States. It spells out the types of isolation recommended and the precautions necessary to prevent transmission of disease to patients or personnel. It is hoped that the data collected concerning the need for private rooms, the use of masks, gowns, and gloves, and precautions necessary for removal of excreta, secretions, soiled articles, and personal belongings will be referred to in the development of uniform, practical systems of dealing with these diseases in the hospital setting. Because such programs are costly, care should be taken to develop practical programs based on facts. When there is question or doubt, studies can be conducted within an organization to develop appropriate procedures for the particular situation in that hospital.

As with many other aspects of medical care and treatment, there often is controversy about the infection control procedures that are developed. Often, the nurse will find variability in programs among hospitals. One of the reasons for this variability is that the control of infections is constantly being studied and that the findings may have institutional implications. Often a specific institution develops and uses procedures that have been successful in controlling infections in that institution. It is considered sensible for them to maintain these programs, rather than to experiment with new or different procedures, only to find that the control is not satisfactory. The nurse should be aware of this perspective when evaluating a given institution's policies and procedures as they are often as much a matter of the institution's total organizational structure and physical facility as they are a matter of protection of a person or persons with a disease or of protection of personnel.

Nosocomial infections All nurses must be continuously aware of the potential for the development of infections in the hospital setting. Hospital-acquired infections are termed **nosocomial infections.** These infections develop during hospitalization and are not present or incubating at the time of admission to the hospital. Nosocomial infections are distinguished from community-acquired infections, that is, infections present when the patient is admitted to the hospital. It is essential however to consider patients with community-acquired infections as potential sources of nosocomial infections by the spread of these infections to susceptible persons within the hospital setting.

Approximately 5 percent of all patients admitted to general hospitals in the United States will develop a nosocomial infection. Diagnosis and therapy add at least a third of a billion dollars annually to the cost of hospitalization for the patients who acquire nosocomial infections. More importantly, these infections have resulted in the death of some patients and certainly in prolonged hospitalization and delayed recovery for others [135, 155, 156].

Several factors have been implicated in the increasing occurrence of nosocomial infections: negligence in aseptic technique, particularly in the basic principles of hand washing; overdependence on antibiotics; longer and more complicated operations; various types of therapy and instrumentation; and lowered resistance due to age or chronic illness, drug therapy such as with steroids, cancer chemotherapy, and irradiation. Complicated treatment modalities, while life-saving in many situations, have also introduced other means for pathogenic invasion. Some life-saving procedures require instrumentation and thus are potential iatrogenic causes of infection: respiratory therapy, catheterization, dialysis, intravenous therapy, and total parenteral nutrition.

The Joint Commission for Accreditation of Hospitals requires that all hospitals have an infection control committee. New criteria on measures to evaluate the effectiveness of such committees are being developed. Infection committees are generally composed of the hospital epidemiologist, physician representatives of the major clinical departments, the pathologist or a representative from the bacteriology department, an infection control nurse, the director of nursing or nursing supervisor or both, and administrative representatives. Other persons may be temporary or permanent members of the committee. These persons include the head of housekeeping, inhalation therapists, and dietary and other personnel.

The functions of an infection control committee are to determine hospital policies related to infection control and to provide for implementation of those policies. These functions include the development of mechanisms for effective surveillance of nosocomial infections, the promotion of control measures, assuring the adequate and appropriate use of the microbiology laboratory, and the distribution of information on infection control to medical and hospital staff. A hospital epidemiologist familiar with fundamental biostatistics is essential for an effective infection control program. Depending on the size of the hospital, this staff position may be a full-time or part-time one.

The infection control nurse is responsible for detecting and recording nosocomial infections on a systematic and current basis and for analyzing the data with the hospital epidemiologist. Thus a background in epidemiology, microbiology, and basic statistics, as well as a good clinical background, is an essential qualification for the infection control nurse. The infection control nurse and the epidemiologist are responsible for the initial epidemiologic investigations of all significant clusters of infection above the endemic (or usual) level. Specific tasks include daily review of bacteriology laboratory reports to note positive cultures (and follow-up chart reviews to determine clinical significance) and daily ward rounds to review patients on isolation, patients with fever, patients receiving antibiotics, and high-risk patients such as those undergoing catheterization or other types of instrumentation. An effective relationship with hospital staff will facilitate this investigation, because nurses and other staff who are cognizant of the importance of preventing nosocomial infections will communicate readily with the infection control nurse.

Not only must attention be given to hospitalized patients, but outpatient departments and the employee health service program must be assessed. Potential sources for nosocomial infections and contacts with infected persons must be ascertained among hospital employees and patients.

The infection control nurse determines attack rates and rates of infection according to the total hospital population. These rates are also determined in particular units or services and are compared with endemic situations (the usual incidence at the particular institutions) in order to determine areas in which potential epidemics are developing or clusters of infections are occurring. The number of nosocomial infections divided by the population at risk (usually determined as the number of discharges during the month) gives the rate of infection [138, 173].

The responsibility for infection control lies not only in the hands of the infection control committee, but in every employee of the hospital. The nurse, particularly, is in a strategic position to be a role model in infection control by practicing rigid aseptic techniques, by being aware of potential hazards in the development of nosocomial infection, and by identifying high-risk patients. The nurse should also be alert to symptoms that indicate potential infection, such as fever, cellulitis, purulent drainage from a surgical wound, and increased coughing and sputum expectoration.

Nurses with a keen awareness of the hazards of nosocomial infections know that the host factor is a major factor in who becomes infected. They should recognize their responsibility for identifying high-risk persons. Three categories of susceptible patients have been identified: (1) patients with exogenously impaired defense mechanisms, including those on corticosteroid therapy, antineoplastic agents, immunosuppressive therapy, or systemic antimicrobial drugs; (2) patients undergoing instrumentation procedures, such as with intravenous or indwelling urinary catheters, and diagnostic examinations of the gastrointestinal, respiratory, or urinary tracts; (3) patients with certain medical conditions, including malignancies, diabetes, chronic lung disease, collagen disease, and certain cardiovascular disorders (e.g., rheumatic heart disease). Precautions in nursing care are indicated with these patients, and assessment and observation for impending infections are essential elements of any plan of care for them [155].

In addition to knowing which patients are most susceptible to nosocomial infections, the nurse should be aware of the most frequent sites of these infections so that special efforts can be made to combat them. The three most frequent sites of nosocomial infections are (1) the urinary tract, (2) surgical wounds, and (3) the respiratory tract. A discussion of urinary tract infection (UTI) follows, as an example of a prevalent nosocomial infection that can in most cases be prevented.

When one considers that an estimated 400,000 patients in this country acquire a UTI during hospitalization, one should be concerned with efforts to control this problem [135, 160]. Junin [160] further states that the leading cause of gram-negative bacteremia and death due to sepsis in hospitals is associated with instrumentation of the urinary tract, particularly with the indwelling urinary catheter. Thus, measures to insure safety in urologic instrumentation must be adhered to.

Bacteria acquired from several sources have been implicated in catheter-associated infections of the urinary tract. Urinary catheter insertion may introduce microorganisms that inhabit the distal urethra; cross-contamination of urinary catheters (via hospital personnel) is another important mode of transmission. The risk of developing a UTI increases with duration of catheterization. Consequently, the Hospital Infections Branch of the Center for Disease Control has made several recommendations for urinary catheter care in order to reduce the number of nosocomial infections from this source [139]. These recommendations include (1) restriction of indwelling catheters to only absolutely necessary situations and not for the convenience of personnel; (2) strict aseptic technique in the insertion of catheters, and insertion of catheters by only those persons adequately trained in the technique; (3) daily or twice daily perineal care to clean the meatal-catheter junction with an antiseptic soap; (4) application of an antimicrobial ointment when needed; (5) use of a sterile closed drainage system that is not opened unless absolutely necessary for irrigation of an obstructed catheter and only under strict aseptic technique; (6) aspiration techniques (for sterile specimen collections) from the distal catheter using a sterile syringe and a small gauge needle after preparing the site with tincture of iodine or alcohol, or both; (7) maintenance of collecting bags *always below* the level of the bladder; (8) separation of catheterized patients whenever possible to avoid the potential for cross-contamination; and (9) elimination of the procedure of routine catheter change, unless indicated by malfunction or accumulation of concretions in the catheter [139]. Adherence to these recommendations should reduce the incidence of nosocomial UTI. Measures to control the second most common site of nosocomial infections, the surgical wound, are discussed later in this chapter.

Attention should be focused on the increasing incidence of hospital-acquired respiratory infections associated with the use of inhalation therapy equipment. Ironically, patients who require inhalation therapy are often in weakened physical states and are thus susceptible to nosocomial infections. Many of the parts of the inhalation equipment are made of materials that prohibit autoclaving; thus inadequate decontamination has been a major factor in the incidence of nosocomial infections. Some manufacturers have recognized these inherent problems and are now marketing autoclavable breathing circuits, including nebulizers and humidifiers. Complicated machines for administering anesthetics may also be sources of gram-negative organisms when inhaler hoses, rebreathing bags, suction tubes, and face masks are improperly or inadequately decontaminated. The increased incidence of respiratory tract infections therefore warrants close monitoring of measures to prevent cross-contamination of patients via inhalation therapy equipment. When equipment cannot be autoclaved, it is most effectively cleaned in activated gluteraldehyde [158]. *Pseudomonas* organisms grow very well in nebulizer solutions at room temperature; therefore these solutions should be freshly prepared, and hoses and bottles should be changed and sterilized daily [158].

Another type of nosocomial infection in patients and personnel is that of hepatitis. Specific information on the care of patients with hepatitis is found in Chapter 7. Here, however, it is important to emphasize that the increased use of blood and blood components, particularly in patients undergoing renal dialysis or immunosuppression therapy, is a major factor in the increased incidence of viral hepatitis, particularly hepatitis B. Renal dialysis patients are particularly susceptible because of additional hazards associated with the procedure. Certain types of gram-negative "water" bacteria, among them *Pseudomonas, Xanthomonas, Aeromonas,* and *Flavobacterium* species, grow rapidly in dialysate, especially when it contains carbonaceous and nitrogenous waste products from the patient's blood [148, 149]. Thus, bacterial contamination may become excessive. Although neither the water used to prepare dialysis fluids nor the dialysis fluids need be sterile (completely free from viable microorganisms), microbial contamination should be maintained at a low level, thus requiring close attention to the water treating system, the dialysate distribution systems and, in some cases, the type of dialyzer [148, 149].

In the past there has been a great deal of emphasis on the importance of routine environmental sampling as a means of detecting highly contaminated reservoirs of infection. Currently the accepted view is that environmental sampling is important as part of an epidemiologic investigation, as a means of determining the cost-effectiveness of housekeeping practices, or as a staff education project. Serious objections to routine environmental monitoring have been raised by the American Hospital Association and others, particularly since there is a singular lack of correlation between environmental data and nosocomial infection rates [136, 147]. Thus, more attention must be given to other ways of monitoring control measures to prevent nosocomial infections. As has been emphasized, cross-contamination and the lack of stringent hand washing have been the major factors in the increased incidence of nosocomial infections.

Isolation measures When it has been determined that a patient harbors an infection, isolation techniques are established to protect other patients and personnel. In this case isolation is actually the separation of the infected person for the period of communicability of the infecting organisms. The organism is isolated by isolating the person, in order to control contact with excreta or objects contaminated by the person. Knowledge of the type of organism involved, its mode of transmission, and its entry and exit modes is an essential factor for determining the specific type of isolation indicated. An important concept to remember is that the *organism*, not the patient, is isolated. The emotional trauma of human isolation can be detrimental to the complete recovery of the patient. Isolation may also be established for the purpose of protecting the patient from contamination when resistance to infection is impaired. This concept is termed **reverse isolation.** It is most frequently used for patients undergoing immunosuppression in cancer chemotherapy or in organ transplants.

The Center for Disease Control guidelines for hospitals [131, 133] divide isolation into five types: (1) respiratory, (2) enteric, (3) wound and skin, (4) strict, and (5) reverse, or protective. Basic to all these types is meticulous hand washing before and after contact with the patient.

Respiratory isolation is used when the organism is transmissible by the airborne route. The patient should be in a private room. The wearing of a mask is indicated, and patient instruction regarding the handling of disposable contaminated tissues must be emphasized. Enteric isolation is used when the causative organism is transmitted by fecal contamination. Even before a stool culture confirms the presence of an enteric infection, precautions should be taken. The patient is provided with private bathroom facilities when possible and is taught the importance of personal hygiene and proper hand washing. Gloves may be necessary when hands are likely to become grossly contaminated. Because linens might contain fecal contamination, they should be double bagged for transfer to the laundry. When viral hepatitis (hepatitis A or B) is suspected, enteric precautions and needle precautions are instituted.

Wound and skin isolation is designed to prevent direct contact with the organism. Gowning and gloving by personnel and double bagging of linens and other articles in direct contact with the organism are essential.

Strict isolation is carried out for controlling highly communicable organisms with multiple routes of transmission. Methods for preventing airborne, enteric, and contact transmission are necessary. Protective or reverse isolation is accomplished to prevent susceptible patients with lowered resistance from acquiring an infection.

Basic to all these procedures is the nurse's knowledge of the causative organism and its mode of transmission, and adherence to correct hand washing techniques. The risk of personnel acquiring transient hand carriage of organisms is usually greatest after contact with excretions, secretions, or blood. Although hand washing with an antiseptic agent between patient contacts is theoretically desirable, hand washing with soap, water, and mechanical friction is considered sufficient to remove most transiently acquired organisms. The CDC recommends antiseptics for hand washing before surgery and other high-risk invasive procedures, but recommends soap and water for other hand washing [133, 135, 174]. Steere and Mallison [174] found that antiseptic agents may produce excessively dry skin if used frequently and lead to dermatitis, thereby negating the purpose of hand washing.

Thus the nurse must examine the individual situation and evaluate bacteriology reports as well as the patient's physiologic and psychological state and level of understanding in order to determine the specific isolation regimen to carry out.

The concept of isolating the organism and not the patient can be illustrated in the management of a patient admitted to a general hospital with a suspected diagnosis of pulmonary tuberculosis. In the past, this patient would have been placed in segregated areas, under strict isolation, and caps, gowns, and masks were worn by all involved personnel. A great deal of insecurity and fear prevailed among the personnel when caring for this patient and frequently this insecurity and fear was conveyed to the patient. Today the characteristics of the causative organism and its mode of transmission determine the specific approach to isolation measures rather than completely isolating the patient.

The tubercle bacillus is transmitted by airborne contamination, primarily by means of droplet nuclei from the moisture produced during coughing, sneezing, or laughing by the patient whose sputum contains the organism. Inhalation and implantation on lung tissue of these bacillus-laden droplet nuclei are necessary for transmission to be completed [134, 165, 166]. Larger particles are unable to penetrate the lungs due to the protective mechanisms in the upper respiratory tract. Tubercle bacilli are nonmotile organisms and are readily killed by heat, drying, sunshine, and ultraviolet light [134]. Thus tubercle bacilli on fomites such as linen, furniture, books, and floors do not constitute a significant infection hazard and do not require special handling [134, 165]. Hand washing is an efficient method of removing organisms picked up from fomites or by direct contact with infected sputum.

The primary method for preventing secretions from becoming airborne and contaminating the environment is isolation of the organism. The patient is taught how to cover his nose and mouth with disposable tissues when coughing, raising sputum, sneezing, or laughing. All contaminated tissues are placed in bags for subsequent burning. (Some settings use special containers, and the contents are later flushed in the sewage system.)

Initiation of appropriate chemotherapy, generally with two or three antituberculosis agents, readily eliminates the tubercle bacilli from the sputum and reduces the cough and the amount of sputum expectorated. This process usually requires several days to two weeks in most patients, unless they prove to be drug-resistant.

When patient instruction for proper handling of sputum and administration of chemotherapy have been initiated, other isolation measures are not indicated. This recommendation assumes that the patient is in a well-ventilated room *without* recirculation of air, which is vital if air contamination is to be prevented. Gowning and masking of personnel are therefore not necessary. If the patient is unwilling or is unable to cooperate in isolating the organisms, masking the patient or isolation procedures with masking by personnel may be necessary.

The major hazard from tuberculosis (TB) actually occurs when patients not suspected of having TB are later diagnosed with the condition. Thus, the nurse who readily teaches all patients to properly handle sputum and disposable tissues when the patient has a symptom of coughing is practicing good preventive care. When a patient is first diagnosed as having TB after being hospitalized for some time, all personnel who might have become infected must be identified. The success of this procedure and subsequent management is facilitated by an active TB surveillance program in the employee health program. Individuals with negative skin reactions to TB tests are evaluated, and therapy is initiated for those who have become infected. Usually a Mantoux test (intradermal tuberculin hypersensitivity test) is preferred because it is a reliable test. Personnel are usually tested immediately (unless they already have a positive reaction as determined on preemployment testing) and again 10 weeks after exposure.

Once chemotherapy is started, the patient is soon discharged from the hospital. In fact, many patients with TB diagnosed in a physician's office or in an outpatient clinic are not hospitalized at all. Emphasis in the care of the TB patient centers on ensuring that the patient will continue to take prescribed medications on an outpatient basis. The disease must be reported to the local health department. Follow-up care requires communication with the public health department and the visiting nurse association.

Thus the isolation techniques of the past have been modified as the result of increased knowledge about TB, the tubercle bacillus, and its mode of transmission; bacteriologic testing to determine the number and virulence of tubercle bacilli in the sputum; and effective and appropriate chemotherapy. Additional information on TB is found in Chapter 3.

COMMUNITY IMPLICATIONS

In the management of TB it is necessary to inform the health department in the patient's community of events that influence infection control in the community so that follow-up can be maintained. Many events are instrumental in creating problems of infection control in communities. Central among them is that many patients are discharged prior to obtaining laboratory results, a consequence in part of the emphasis on monitoring hospital days. When laboratory results confirming the diagnosis are received following the patient's discharge, care may become fragmented, and there is usually a delay in communicating the information from one agency to another. Another problem frequently encountered is the lack of discharge planning or failure to follow up on discharge planning.

The patient may leave the hospital armed with information, medications, and materials necessary for continued treatment at home. Without positive reinforcement in the home situation the patient's motivation may wane or his lack of understanding may become evident. His condition may worsen, spread to others, or become complicated.

Another problem is the fragmentation of health services within a community. With the myriad of health agencies springing up in some communities, communication between new and established agencies about specific patients is very difficult. The community health nurse, when being referred to a problem or when finding a problem, often has to initiate an investigation to validate the care and treatment given. In most communities the health department is the central coordinating agency with the knowledge and resources to develop operational programs for the control and prevention of diseases in the community. Health department personnel perceive the community impact of communicable diseases whereas personnel in independent health agencies tend to be most concerned with the immediate problems of a specific individual. Unless these specific incidences of disease are reported to the central coordination agency, however, an explosive outbreak may occur.

Personnel who staff the emergency rooms of hospitals should be alert to the potential for community outbreaks when they see a patient with a communicable disease. The emergency room staff should have good relationships with the health department for reporting and observing potential problems. Often an alert observer in the emergency room can first detect signs of a developing problem that can be handled to protect other people from developing diseases.

While the roles of people who work in hospitals are different from the roles of those who work in health departments, it is necessary that each group understand the function of the other. Cooperation is essential for the care of individual patients and the protection of the community. Through cooperation it is possible to reduce the effects of communicable diseases. Someone in the hospital setting, by informing the health department of a communicable disease, may be the key in averting a **point epidemic,** an epidemic in which a common source of contaminant or infectious agent causes disease in an explosive manner, with several cases of the disease breaking out at one time. **Contact epidemics,** those that spread from person to person, with the incidence of the disease developing over a longer period of time, can also be allayed if the chain of infection is broken early.

The health department staff has a central role in the protection of community members. This role is based on knowledge of the community's resources, socioeconomic groups, living patterns, housing, sanitation, education system, available human resources, health care patterns, age groups, gaps in health services, disease pockets, and areas of low resistance. All these factors are data that are available over a long period of time. Maintenance of good records, retrospective active surveillance studies, and other means of collecting data are utilized in obtaining this information.

Program planning is done on the basis of this carefully acquired information. Depending on staffing and available resources, program planning will be tedious and time-consuming as well as challenging and rewarding. Prevention and control of communicable diseases are the hallmarks of sound public health activities.

The discussion of infection control is pertinent to the following discussion of the patient requiring surgery. Infection, however, is only one of the many factors that must be controlled for the patient's safety throughout the surgical experience.

The Patient Requiring Surgery

Surgical procedures are done for several reasons: (1) to obtain tissue for examination, (2) to visualize internal structures as a means of diagnosis, (3) to cure disease by removing the diseased tissue or organs, (4) to repair or remove traumatized tissue and structures, (5) to relieve symptoms by means of palliative procedures, (6) to improve appearance by cosmetic procedures, and (7) to perform prophylactic procedures.

Biopsy procedures for examination of tissue with a microscope may be done in a variety of ways. The specimen is used to confirm a diagnosis, estimate prognosis, or to determine the course of a disease and appropriate treatment. Use of the frozen-section technique for diagnosis assists in determining which therapeutic approach to follow. The **frozen-section** technique is a rapid method of examination of a specimen during an operation when immediate information is needed on whether a piece of tissue is malignant. A specimen of tissue is quick-frozen, cut by a microtome, and stained immediately. Although this technique does not permit detailed study of the cells, rapid diagnosis of possible malignant lesions can be made. The most frequent use of the technique is in the case of breast biopsy, when tissue is examined as a basis for performing a radical mastectomy vs. removal only of a cyst. The skill of the pathologist is of paramount importance in this technique.

Other types of biopsies are the **punch biopsy,** in which a hollow instrument similar to a large needle is introduced into a cavity and a piece of tissue is removed, and **excisional biopsy,** in which a lesion or mass is removed and is later examined for diagnosis of the disease. Tissue for examination via microscope may also be obtained by scraping the surface of a lesion, as in the case of dilation and curettage, when tissue is obtained from the cervix or uterus. Some biopsies do not have to be done in an operating room, although they require aseptic approaches. Histologic examination of cells obtained from sputum or other secretions (e.g., the Papanicolaou technique, which is described later) and needle aspiration in which fluid is removed from a lesion or cavity for examination with microscope and diagnosis are two examples.

Exploratory surgery is done in order to establish a diagnosis by visualizing internal structures. In some cases no further excision (other than removal of some lymph nodes) may be indicated. For example, on finding extensive cancer involvement, the surgeon may have no choice other than to close the incision. Exploratory laporotomy may be done to determine the staging (the extent) of malignant disease as a basis for prescribing therapy. Staging operations are used in Hodgkin's disease and lymphoma (see Chap. 5).

Curative surgery is the removal of diseased tissue or a diseased organ, as in an appendectomy, in which the diseased appendix is removed. When a portion of an organ or the total organ is removed, surgical reconstruction is necessary. When a portion of the stomach or duodenum is diseased and removed, for example, the continuity of the gastrointestinal tract must be restored by anastomosis. Curative surgery does not always require removal of a diseased organ, however. A classic example of curative surgery is that of reconstruction and repair of cardiac congenital defects. Incision and drainage of an abscess is a curative measure. Specific types of curative surgery are discussed in subsequent chapters. It is important to remember that although a surgical procedure may be curative, it may also result in altered function and appearance. An illustration is the amputation of a gangrenous leg; although the basic disease that caused the gangrene to develop is not cured, the gangrenous process in that specific anatomic location is cured and in some cases does not recur in any other part of the body. Curative surgery and its implications in relation to cancer is discussed later in this chapter.

Surgery often is done to **repair or remove traumatized tissue.** The increasing numbers of automobile accidents and violent crimes have resulted in multiple injuries that require complex surgical techniques for repair and reconstruction. Skin graft procedures for the treatment of burn injuries is only one example of surgery to restore damaged tissue to its normal appearance. Splenectomy, the removal of the spleen, is often done when the organ is damaged in traumatic events.

Palliative surgery is done to relieve symptoms even when there is no hope for cure. For example, obstructive lesions due to cancer may be removed, although metastasis has already occurred to other parts of the body. A colostomy to relieve intestinal obstructions, and urinary diversions to remove a diseased bladder, are examples of palliative surgery. These same operations, however, may be considered curative if the extent of the disease is localized. There is considerable overlap between some curative and palliative procedures because some of the same methods are used in both. A distinct example of palliative surgery is that of neurosurgery for pain relief, as described earlier in this chapter.

Another type of surgery is that of **reconstruction.** Although reconstruction may be included as a stage in the category of surgical intervention to repair congenitally deformed or traumatized tissue, some types of reconstructive surgery are done specifically for cosmetic purposes only. Examples are face-lifting procedures and breast reconstruction. These latter surgeries are **elective** types of surgery, but the patient still is vulnerable and is at the risk of complications related to infection, anesthesia, and inadvertent trauma or injury during the procedure. Perhaps these types of surgery may be categorized under **prophylactic surgery,** in that a disease—specifically, emotional illness—may in some cases be averted by reconstruction of parts of the body the patient views as defective. Other types of prophylactic surgery are those in which precancerous lesions, such as polyps in the gastrointestinal tract, are removed. Prophylactic operations are also done in certain types of cancer; an example is oophorectomy (removal of ovaries) to prevent recurrence of cancer of the breast, which is considered to be hormone-dependent.

Surgery may be classified according to the urgency of the operation. In this classification, surgery may be an emergency, urgent, scheduled, required, elective, or optional. **Emergency** surgery is indicated in life-threatening situations such as hemorrhage from a bleeding vessel, perforation of an organ, or repair of a gunshot wound.

Urgent surgery includes operations that require correction to prevent further injury or damage to tissues, such as removal of kidney stones or obstructive tumors. Hysterectomy (removal of the uterus) and cholecystectomy (removal of the gallbladder) are examples of surgery that can be either urgent or elective. **Elective** surgery is not absolutely necessary but is performed for the patient's well-being, such as removal of scars, or hysterectomy for asymptomatic fibroids. A subgroup of elective surgery (**optional** surgery) is that which the patient requests, such as a sterilization procedure.

Surgical procedures may also be classified as major or minor types of operations, depending on their complexity, anticipated blood loss and trauma, and length and depth or type of anesthesia required. It is important for the nurse to remember that no type of surgery is viewed as being minor in the eyes of the patient or his family, and all operations have potential for unforeseen complications.

Regardless of the type of operation required by a patient, the event itself imposes psychological and physiologic stresses on the patient and his family or other significant persons in his or her life. The safe and therapeutic care of a patient prior to surgery, during surgery, and postoperatively requires understanding of the factors essential to satisfactory physical and psychological preparation of the patient and of factors that affect the body's defense against the trauma of surgical intervention as well as of anesthesia and the medications used. The science of surgery has been refined to such a degree that an increasing number of surgical procedures are now performed with reasonable safety and considerable benefit to the patient. Improvements in surgical techniques, anesthesia, management, physiologic monitoring, supportive measures, and treatments have made possible a variety of surgical procedures, including complex cardiac, liver, and pancreatic operations.

Various personnel come in contact with the surgical patient. This patient must adjust to the stress of hospitalization, which requires admission to a particular unit and staff and transfer to the operating room, recovery room, and in some cases to an intensive care unit. The patient necessarily experiences several strange and bewildering environments and equipment and various stressful and sometimes embarrassing procedures. All these events make the patient feel vulnerable, insecure, frightened, and cause a temporary loss of identity. Efforts to allay these feelings must be made at all stages of the surgical event by open communication between the patient and the involved hospital staff.

Pertinent information about the patient must be recorded and transmitted to the various departments to assure continuity of care. Not only must the surgical procedure be safe and precise, but asepsis must be assured. The patient must also be protected from complications or injury while the anesthetic is being administered. Preoperatively, intraoperatively, and postoperatively, care must be planned to assure the physical and psychological comfort of the patient. Aspects of these three stages of the surgical experience will now be discussed.

PREOPERATIVE CARE

The goal of preoperative preparation is to promote the best possible physical and psychological state of the patient. This goal is facilitated by an accurate determination of the strengths and limitations of the patient that are likely to affect the outcome of the operation. A trusting relationship should be established so that the patient will feel free to express his fears about the operation and to ask any questions about the operation and hospitalization. The fear of the unknown, anesthesia, pain, disability, and the operative findings all affect the patient's psychological state. The patient's understanding about the state of his health and the planned surgery should be determined so that needs for teaching can be ascertained. The patient's previous experiences in surgery, depending on the type of surgery, and previous experiences with anesthesia, will also affect his or her attitude toward the current procedure and will indicate the approach to use in teaching the patient.

Vital signs and body weight are taken to obtain a baseline for operative and postoperative evaluation. The nurse also determines the presence of allergies or other possibly complicating factors, the patient's use of any medications, and any dietary restrictions. Habits such as smoking or alcoholic intake are assessed in relation to their effect on the patient's tolerance of anesthesia and surgery. The patient's nutritional state and fluid and electrolyte balance are also determined by means of physical assessment, history taking, and laboratory methods. The presence of associated conditions that increase surgical risk are determined, and appropriate treatment is provided. Anemia, fluid and electrolyte imbalance, pulmonary, cardiac, and renal disease, obesity, diabetes, and psychic and emotional disturbances are disorders that increase the risk in surgery. Obesity is a risk factor in that obese patients are highly susceptible to infection. In addition, obesity may interfere with postoperative pulmonary function by reducing vital capacity due to excessive pressure on the diaphragm. Elderly patients, often presenting with chronic diseases, also have difficulty in adapting to the prolonged stresses associated with surgery.

The surgical patient is also assessed for the presence of infection, such as upper respiratory tract infection or a skin infection such as boils or pimples. The danger of bacterial contamination of the surgical wound may necessitate postponement of surgery until the infection is controlled. Infection of the upper respiratory tract, for example, can predispose to pulmonary complications and also may require postponement of surgery.

Laboratory studies are indicated to determine the presence of other conditions that increase surgical risks. A white blood cell count, red blood cell count, hemoglobin, hematocrit, and urinalysis are done routinely. An elevated white blood count may be a factor in the disease process for which surgery is planned. In many cases, however, surgery may be contraindicated if there is an elevated white blood count, suggesting an infection of an unknown source. Surgery is also contraindicated in the presence of an abnormally low white blood count, which would inhibit essential defense mechanisms. Previously undetected anemia may be determined by an abnormal hemoglobin. If the hemoglobin level is below 9 to 10 gm per 100 ml blood, elective surgery is delayed until the source of the anemia is determined; in other cases, transfusions of packed blood cells are administered prior to surgery. Blood glucose levels and the blood urea nitrogen are usually determined preoperatively.

A chest x-ray is usually obtained. The x-ray is particularly important for detecting the presence of emphysema or bronchitis, which generally requires preoperative treatment. Abnormal pulmonary findings should alert the staff and anesthesiologist to the potential for postoperative pulmonary complications unless special precautions are taken. An electrocardiogram is also taken to determine the cardiac status of the patient if the operation is to be complex, prolonged, or likely to be associated with complications, or if the patient is over the age of 40.

A complete history and physical examination of the pulmonary, cardiovascular, neurologic, endocrine, renal, hepatic, and gastrointestinal systems are necessary. These examinations are important in determining the capacity of the patient to tolerate the administration of an anesthetic and the stress of surgery and in estimating his potential for recovery. Other diagnostic procedures are indicated by the specific type of surgery anticipated. Chronic medical conditions must be controlled prior to subjecting the patient to the additional stress of a surgical procedure. For example, the diabetic patient must be well controlled, and the patient with hypertension must be treated appropriately.

Prevention of anxiety, or at least recognition of its presence, is one of the primary responsibilities of the nurse. The unique meaning of the surgery to the patient should be determined. Often, hospital personnel categorize certain operations as minor or usual procedures. It is important to realize, however, that *any* surgery is unique in the view of the person who is to undergo it. When the operation involves the loss of a body part and necessitates changes in life patterns, the threat to body image is a devastating experience. Extreme anxiety or depression or both may be assessed as being detrimental to the patient and, in some cases, the operation may be postponed for psychotherapeutic intervention.

Preparation for surgery requires adequate time for teaching the patient about the surgical procedure and how he will be expected to participate in postoperative care. Adequate preparation helps to relieve the patient's anxiety, obtain his cooperation and participation, and hasten the recovery process. Preoperative teaching may be done by the nurse on the surgical unit; in some settings the operating room staff is responsible for the preoperative teaching. Either group or individual teaching methods may be used, depending on the institutional procedure and on the specific needs of the individual patient. Some institutions use a particular nurse or team for preoperative teaching with the aid of written and audiovisual materials. Although there may be procedural variations, the fact remains that preoperative teaching is an essential component in the care of surgical patients. Lindeman and Van Aerman [204] showed that structured preoperative teaching improved the ability of patients to deep breathe and cough postoperatively and also significantly reduced the mean length of hospitalization. Dumas [189] found that a lower incidence of postoperative vomiting occurred as the result of specific nursing actions during the preoperative period. Preoperative visits by operating room staff also appear to increase the efficiency of nursing care in the operating and recovery rooms. The staff learn pertinent information about the patient prior to surgery, and the patient is able to recognize a familiar face in the operating room. A preoperative visit by the anesthesiologist is also routinely made to orient the patient about anesthesia and to determine the appropriate agent.

The content of the preoperative teaching should include information on hospital policies, procedures (including premedication) for surgical preparation, the anticipated type of incision, expectations of the patient, functions of various hospital personnel, and the purpose of various types of fairly routine postoperative procedures such as the administration of intravenous fluids and oxygen, and gastrointestinal intubation. The content should, of course, be adapted to the needs of the particular patient. Proper coughing and deep-breathing exercises should be demonstrated, and patients should be given an opportunity to practice them. Demonstrations on turning and proper positioning also should be given, and explanations of the purpose of early ambulation and leg exercises should be emphasized. Patients should also be oriented to the purposes of the recovery room and the intensive care unit if such care is anticipated.

The patient must be oriented to the type of surgery anticipated. Informed consent implies that the patient understands what is being done and the risks involved. The consent form also includes signing for a particular type of anesthetic (general, spinal, or local). The nurse is generally the person responsible for having the patient sign the consent permit and must confirm that the permit indicates precisely the type of procedure anticipated. The nurse must also determine whether the patient understands the content of the form. If there are any problems with interpretations, the surgeon is contacted. Under no circumstances is the patient coerced into signing, nor is the patient to be under the effects of any medication that would impair his understanding. The legal implications of the operative permit must be respected. Although informed consent implies understanding of the procedures, the nurse must also assess when the patient's anxiety may be intensified by excessive information. There should be continued assessment of the patient's ability to handle and interpret information.

Depending on the type of surgery, the patient is often given an enema the evening before surgery. Results of the enema are carefully recorded. Surgery of the colon requires particular preparation, as described in Chapter 7. The enema is given to lessen the likelihood of fecal spillage into the peritoneal cavity if intestinal trauma should occur, and exposure of the operative site in pelvic surgery is facilitated by an empty bowel. Also, the possibility of incontinence and contamination is reduced, when relaxation of sphincter muscles occurs during anesthesia. In hemorrhoidectomies and gynecologic repairs, it is desirable to delay the first postoperative bowel movement to avoid strain on the sutures.

A healthy and intact skin is the first line of defense against injury, including mechanical and biologic injury associated with the incision. Preoperative preparation of the skin therefore is directed toward restricting biologic injury and preventing infection. The surgical site and surrounding area are shaved to decrease the number of microorganisms entering the wound. Shaving may be done the evening before surgery or it may be delayed until the patient enters the operating room suite. It has been found that a prolonged interval between shaving and the actual surgery increases the incidence of the infections. Regardless of when it is done, care must be taken to avoid cuts and nicks in the skin. If cuts or abrasions occur, they should be reported. In some cases, the operation may even be postponed until healing occurs. Wet shaving is preferred to a dry procedure. Some institutions use depilatory creams for hair removal. Although the technique is effective in avoiding abrasions, there is the danger of sensitivity to some of the chemicals. Other protocols use clippers rather than razors to remove gross hair. If not contraindicated, a daily bath with a bacteriostatic soap for several days prior to surgery may be prescribed as a means of reducing potential skin sources of infection. General cleanliness and proper hygiene are necessary to ensure skin integrity and cleanliness.

The patient is restricted from fluids and food for 8 to 10 hours preoperatively to assure an empty stomach and to prevent vomiting and potential aspiration as well as distention of the gastrointestinal tract. The patient, however, is well hydrated prior to the fluid restriction period. If necessary, intravenous fluids are given to provide adequate hydration. For patients undergoing major abdominal surgery, a nasogastric tube is usually inserted to empty the stomach and prevent postoperative vomiting and gastrointestinal distention. The nurse must consider the patient's total health status and other therapies. Essential medications, such as insulin and antiarrhythmic drugs are administered. Dosages, however, may be changed prior to surgery. The patient who has been on anticoagulants will require antidotes during the preoperative period. The nurse must therefore consider the implications of all medications the patient has been receiving and should contact the surgeon about any questions regarding their restriction or administration. A sedative is usually prescribed to ensure that the patient attains a good night's rest before undergoing surgery. The patient is awakened in the morning in time for last-minute details in preparation before being given preoperative medication about 1 hour prior to surgery. All procedures essential during the immediate preoperative period must be accomplished before the patient is given the preanesthetic medication. The medication is prescribed to have its effect on the patient at the initiation of anesthesia and thus must be administered specifically and accurately. If there are problems and delays, the anesthetist or the surgeon or both should be notified. The precise timing of the preoperative medication for the patient receiving local anesthesia is important in having the patient relaxed and sedated prior to initiation of the local anesthetic and the operation itself.

Prior to receiving the injection, the patient is asked to empty his bladder in order to prevent distention and possible injury to the bladder as well as to facilitate exposure of pelvic organs. In some surgical procedures a retention catheter is inserted prior to surgery. A fresh operative gown is worn to surgery. Any nail polish the patient is wearing is removed in order to facilitate observation of impaired tissue perfusion. Jewelry, wigs, breast forms, ocular prostheses, and hearing aids are removed from patients and placed in safekeeping in order to prevent loss or damage. If a prosthesis is implanted and cannot be removed, that fact should be recorded. Dentures or bridge plates are removed because of the danger of aspiration, loss, or breakage. However, procedures such as facial reconstruction may require that the patient retain his dentures during the procedure. Also, some patients are so sensitive about being seen without dentures that special permission is given to allow them to retain the dentures until the anesthesia is started. The anesthetist should be informed about this change from the usual procedure. Hairpins are removed and the hair braided (if long) and covered with a cap, either on the unit or when the operative suite is reached. Special precaution is taken in regard to the care of contact lenses; often, patients or their nurses forget to remove these lenses prior to surgery. There is a danger of loss of the lenses as well as of corneal injury while the patient is unconscious.

A preoperative checklist is completed to ensure that the patient has been properly prepared prior to administration of the preoperative medication. Laboratory values are evaluated and the surgeon and the anesthesiologist are notified of pertinent abnormalities. Vital signs are again taken and abnormal deviations (not previously present) are reported prior to the administration of preoperative medication. The patient's chart is marked for any special precautions, such as drawing attention to pertinent medications the patient is receiving or any other significant and unusual factors. It is important that the patient's identification, his chart, and other pertinent details are precisely checked at each point in preoperative care and prior to moving the patient from his room.

Once all these details have been attended to, the patient is ready to receive the preoperative medication at the prescribed time. The medication usually includes a sedative or a tranquilizer to allay anxiety and to facilitate smooth induction of anesthesia. An analgesic such as morphine or meperidine hydrochloride (Demerol) is given to provide additional sedation and relaxation. A vagolytic agent, such as atropine sulfate or scopolamine, is given to decrease pulmonary and oropharyngeal secretions and to obliterate vagal reflexes. The patient soon complains of mouth dryness after the latter medication and should be advised that this effect is an expected sensation.

The side rails are raised once the medication is given, and the patient is instructed to stay in bed. A call light should be available so the patient can readily call for assistance.

The nurse should note whether any family members are present. Once the patient has been moved from the unit, the family is directed to the waiting room where they will be able to confer with the surgeon after the operation. The family should be advised as to the anticipated length of the operation and as to the recovery room procedures during the immediate postoperative period.

After the patient is transported to surgery, his room is cleaned and prepared for his return. A postoperative bed is prepared and essential equipment such as an intravenous pole, an emesis basin, and tissues is made available.

INTRAOPERATIVE CARE

The patient being transferred to the operating room suite needs protection from both physical and psychological trauma. Although the patient may be drowsy from the preoperative medications, he is aware of the sounds and sights around him. It is important that events be explained to him as they happen and that he not be left unattended for prolonged periods while waiting for the surgical procedure to be initiated. During the operation, the patient is cared for directly as well as indirectly by a number of persons. These members of the surgical team and their functions and responsibilities are discussed in the following section.

The Surgical Team

All members of the surgical staff are concerned with the safety and welfare of the patient. The surgeon is the leader of the surgical team. His or her prime concern is to perform the operation in an effective and safe manner. The knowledge and skill of the surgeon is paramount in the recovery of the patient, and skill in handling organs and tissue gently but efficiently is vital to the prevention of complications. The surgeon's primary concern is with decisions related to the surgical approach necessitated by the findings, effective hemostasis and prevention of injury to tissues, and the patient's physiologic response to the surgery. The surgeon is dependent on others in the operating suite for physiologic monitoring.

The anesthesiologist, who is a physician trained in the administration of anesthetics, is responsible for providing a smooth induction of the anesthesia in order to prevent pain and to maintain satisfactory degrees of relaxation of the patient for the duration of the surgical procedure. The anesthesiologist has the primary responsibility for monitoring the physiologic status of the patient and continually monitors oxygen exchange, circulatory functions, systemic circulation, and the patient's vital signs. An anesthesiologist advises the surgeon of impending complications, but is expected to intervene independently. For many operations, an anesthetist, that is, a nurse who has been trained to administer anesthetics, is responsible for the induction of anesthesia. In these situations the nurse-anesthetist requires medical direction in complicated situations that are beyond the limits of protocols.

Within the operating suite, nurses may have one of two roles, either that of circulating nurse or of scrub nurse. Although nurses function as scrub nurses in many settings, operating room technicians also may function in the scrub nurse role.

The role of the scrub nurse (or technician) is to help provide an aseptic environment and to anticipate the needs of the surgeon during the operation. The name **scrub nurse** is derived from the requirement that this person scrub his or her hands and forearms before participating as a member of the surgical team. A surgical scrub involves the use of methodical and timed scrubbing with a bacteriostatic agent to reduce the number of transient, resident, and deep flora of the hands and arms, making them surgically clean [201]. (The reader is referred to the bibliography and other sources for detailed information on scrubbing techniques.)

Subsequent to the scrubbing procedure, the scrub nurse dons sterile gown and gloves and proceeds to assemble sterile equipment and instruments in readiness for the surgical procedure. Instruments are handed to the surgeon or his assistant according to requirements at different stages in the procedure. The scrub nurse is also responsible for preparing needles and sutures prior to initiation of the suturing phases. In addition, the scrub nurse is responsible for maintaining a neat and orderly sterile field to facilitate prompt availability of specific instruments and for monitoring sponge counts (also needles and instruments) to make certain that none is lost or accidentally retained in the patient. This latter function is done with the cooperation of other scrubbed personnel and the circulating nurse. Sponge counts are done prior to the surgery, before closure of the peritoneum (or other cavity covering), and again prior to closure of the skin.

The circulating nurse also is responsible for maintenance of aseptic technique of all personnel but does not scrub or wear sterile gloves or gown. Management of the environment and the safety of the patient are the primary concerns of the circulating nurse. This responsibility includes providing for psychological comfort prior to and during induction of anesthesia. Initial assessment of the patient and continued monitoring are major responsibilities of the circulating nurse. The circulating nurse is the *liaison* between scrubbed personnel, the rest of the surgical department, and the rest of the hospital. She or he saves all discarded sponges and participates in the sponge count. The circulating nurse observes the surgical procedure and also anticipates needs for equipment, instruments, medications, and blood units, and prepares labels for the specimens for the laboratories. The role is a broader one than that of the scrub nurse. Thus the circulating nurse should be a registered nurse.

Depending on the type of surgery being done, the surgeon may have one or two assistants who are either physicians, surgeons, or medical students. (All these persons must also scrub and wear sterile attire and gloves.) These individuals assist in retracting the operative site so that exposure is assured. They also assist in maintaining hemostasis and other functions as needed.

Theoretically, the team described is the extent of essential personnel in a specific surgical suite. In practice, both medical and nursing students may be in the area for an observation learning experience, as may be other staff members who are learning new responsibilities. The number of persons in the operating room should be restricted because increased numbers of persons only increases the likelihood of contamination and subsequent infection.

In addition to the personnel mentioned, other persons also are concerned with the welfare of the patient and are responsible for the environment and the maintenance of a safe and aseptic surgical area. Housekeeping personnel, orderlies, cleaning aides who wash and clean instruments and equipment, and staff members who sterilize instruments and supplies all have a vital role in maintaining a safe and aseptic environment for the surgical patient. Maintenance personnel and engineers also have an important role in maintaining a safe and aseptic environment. Providing for air conditioning that delivers air under pressure with a complete change and filtering of air every 5 to 10 minutes is an example of a responsibility of the engineering department.

Surgical Asepsis

Aseptic technique must be followed rigidly in order to prevent the transmission of microorganisms from the environment to the surgical wound and sterile field of the patient. Contamination may occur from instruments or supplies that have not been properly sterilized as well as from personnel who are carriers of or are infected by pathogenic organisms. For example, the noses and throats of hospital personnel are a major source of virulent organisms, especially staphylococci. The use of properly fitting high-efficiency masks is absolutely essential to the maintenance of an aseptic environment. The masks should fit snugly over the bridge of the nose, along the side of the face, and under the chin. In addition, laughing and excessive talking is prohibited in the operating room to prevent forced expiration and excessive moisture and contamination of the mask. Moist masks are replaced with dry ones, because filtration effectiveness decreases as the moisture becomes excessive.

The health of personnel in the operating suite is routinely monitored so that carriers or infected persons (e.g., persons with boils or sore throats) are not allowed in operative areas. By design, the operating room usually is isolated from all other hospital traffic, and the number of persons within the area should be limited to essential staff only. The correlation between the number of bacteria in the air or indirectly in the surgical wound and the activity and number of personnel in the operating room has been frequently noted [182, 187, 201]. Legitimate observers are accommodated best in separate viewing rooms, but unfortunately, the majority of operating rooms do not have this type of facility.

In the operating room suite, staff wear designated clothing instead of clothing worn in other areas of the hospital or outside the hospital. (**Antistatic** clothing is also indicated as a safety factor in the operating room.) In addition, a cap or turban is used to completely cover the hair. Special coverings are provided for persons with beards while they are within the operating room area.

All materials and instruments coming in contact with the wound are sterilized before they are used in the operative procedure.

Sterilization is defined as the complete destruction of all forms of microbial life, including spores. The most effective type of sterilization is that of steam under pressure, or autoclaving. Some instruments and articles, however, are injured or made defective by autoclaving, so that other techniques are necessary. Dry heat, for example, is used for sterilizing oils and powders.

Ethylene oxide is useful in the sterilization of intricate and delicate instruments and articles made of heat-labile materials. The effectiveness of ethylene oxide sterilization is determined by proper gas concentration, adequate duration of the sterilization cycle, proper temperature, relative humidity, and the gaseous mixture. In addition, precautions are taken to provide for aeration in a well-ventilated chamber for removal of toxic residual gas. If adequate aeration time is not provided for diffusion of the gas from the package before the articles are used, serious chemical burns or skin and mucous membrane irritation may result on contact with the residual gas.

Immersion in sporacidal chemical solutions is another type of sterilization and is used for articles for which the previously mentioned methods are contraindicated. Two substances that are used for chemical sterilization are formaldehyde-alcohol solutions and activated glutaraldehyde. The latter solution must be fresh (not more than 2 weeks old) to be effective. These agents necessitate time-consuming sterilization methods, taking 10 to 12 hours or longer. The nurse must be knowledgeable about the proper application of these agents. Inadequate immersion may only disinfect articles rather than sterilize them. **Disinfection** destroys pathogenic organisms, but not various spore-forming bacteria. The nurse must also be knowledgeable about substances whose effectiveness is controversial or documented as unsafe. For example, benzalkonium chloride (Zephiran) has been used extensively as a disinfectant and antiseptic. The limitations of this product have been documented in the literature [212, 220]. Microbial contamination of Zephiran solutions has also been reported.

Various products are used in the operating room area (as well as in other areas of the hospital) for the purpose of creating aseptic conditions. The use of these products should be limited to their specific purpose. The nurse therefore must clearly understand the terms that describe the actions of specific agents and should not substitute these agents for other purposes.

In contrast to a **germicidal agent,** which destroys pathogenic organisms, a **bacteriostatic agent** only inhibits the activity of the microorganisms and does not destroy them. An **antiseptic** is an agent that combats microorganisms, but is limited to use on tissue. An antiseptic therefore cannot be used for disinfecting surfaces or instruments. A **disinfectant** is a chemical agent applied to inanimate objects. Alcohol or alcohol-iodine combinations are considered appropriate antiseptics, except for use on mucous membranes; diluted solutions of iodophors are generally used for treating mucous membranes. In addition to knowing the appropriate use of specific agents, the nurse must follow the correct instructions for appropriate concentrations of the various agents. The reader is referred to the reference list at the end of this chapter for specific resources related to this information.

The importance of preventing infection in surgical wounds has already been emphasized. Of paramount importance is the proper cleaning of the patient's skin to remove bacteria in the area of the incision. Various solutions are used, and skin preparation procedures vary in different institutions. Iodine, alcohol, or iodophors are the solutions currently used most often in surgical scrubs. Regardless of the solution used, the operative site is thoroughly cleaned mechanically prior to surgery. If shaving has not already been done, the circulating nurse also shaves (or clips) the area and checks it for cuts, abrasions, infections, or skin lesions. The circulating nurse prepares the skin after the patient is under an appropriate level of anesthesia. Cleaning consists in a mechanical scrub that begins at the incision site and is continued outward toward the periphery. Usually the scrub is timed as a 5-minute scrub. The extent of the preparation should always be considerably wider than the anticipated site of the incision. In the case of an abdominal preparation, the umbilicus is initially cleaned with cotton-tipped swabs to remove dirt that may be embedded.

After the mechanical cleaning of the site, sterile draping is applied by the scrubbed personnel to create a sterile field. Many surgeons drape an adherent plastic sheet over the operative area and make the incision through it. This technique provides a tight seal between the open wound and resident bacteria on the adjacent intact skin.

In a typical abdominal operation, the incision is made with a sterile blade cutting through the skin and subcutaneous tissue. This blade is not used again during the procedure. Immediately, subcutaneous bleeders are clamped with curved hemostats and subsequently are ligated with catgut, silk, or cotton ligatures. The assistant sponges the area to aid in visualizing other sources of bleeding. The edges of the incision are isolated by means of towel clips prior to incising the fascia and peritoneum. Another knife or curved cutting scissor is used to incise the muscle, deep fascia, and the peritoneum. The abdomen is then explored (unless an acute inflammation is present, when such a procedure is contraindicated) prior to definitive surgery. When the definitive surgery is accomplished, when the patient's organs are in proper position, and after an initial sponge count has been confirmed, the procedure for closure is initiated. The incision is then closed by layers in the reverse of the cutting procedure. Prior to final skin closure, another sponge count is taken.

During the operation, various types of sutures are used. **Ligatures** are free pieces of suture (i.e., not threaded with a needle) for tying blood vessels. **Sutures** are threads, wires, or other material used to stitch tissues together. There are two general types of suture: absorbable and nonabsorbable. **Absorbable** sutures are digested or absorbed by the body tissues after a certain period of time. These sutures include plain catgut, chromic catgut (which is coated with chromic acid to cause a slower absorption), and polyglycolic synthetics. **Nonabsorbable** sutures remain permanently in body tissues, unless they are used for skin suturing, in which case they are removed. Nonabsorbable sutures include those of silk, cotton, nylon, wire, and mersilene. In order to minimize tissue reaction, the least amount of suture material safely possible is used in relation to the type of tissue involved and the type of holding power required. Meticulous hemostasis and precise approximation of wound edges are essential to assure proper wound healing. Skin closure is accomplished with either a continuous or an interrupted suture line. Although the continuous suture line is done rapidly and is strong because of its even distribution of tension, the entire line is disrupted if the suture should break. In an interrupted or alternate suture technique each suture is tied and cut separately and thus takes longer to accomplish. If one suture should break, however, the others are able to hold the wound together.

Other modifications of suturing technique include the vertical mattress suture for concave surfaces, where edges are prone to inversion; the Gillies horizontal dermal suture for anchoring a point of the skin; and a running subcuticular suture [209]. In most wounds or incisions a single layer of closely placed skin sutures is used, but two layers of sutures may be used on facial wounds, where minimal scarring is a primary goal [209].

For selected patients with abdominal surgery, and particularly for the obese patient, retention sutures may be used in addition to usual suturing. **Retention** sutures are heavy sutures made of nylon and are used to encompass the abdominal wall, that is, the skin, fat, fascia, muscle, and peritoneum, from inside the peritoneal cavity through to the skin. These sutures provide a strong means of holding the wound together, but the method tends to cause more postoperative pain than do closures done by layers. Some surgeons modify their use of retention sutures by placing them after the peritoneum is closed, thus penetrating only the layers from the fascia to the skin. Retention sutures are usually left in place for 2 to 3 weeks [190, 209].

Skin clips, staples, or adhesive strips may be used in lieu of suturing. Although skin clips prevent inversion of skin edges and generally result in optimum healing, they may appear unsightly to the patient and they tend to snag on bedclothes. Adhesive strips do not bring deeper tissues together nor do they control bleeding from wound edges. Some surgeons use a combination of suturing and adhesive strips by removing the sutures within several days postoperatively and applying tape as a replacement.

Wound healing is facilitated by skillful handling of tissues, minimal foreign bodies (sutures) in the wound, adequate hemostasis and prevention of hematoma formation, eradication of dead space, and appropriate use of drains. Other factors related to wound healing are discussed later in this chapter. After closure of the wound, a sterile dressing is applied.

Anesthesia

A surgical procedure is made possible by the safe and appropriate administration of anesthetics to induce anesthesia. **Anesthesia** is the loss of sensation due to interference with normal neural function. Anesthesia prevents pain, relaxes muscles, and allays anxiety. There are two major classifications of anesthesia: general and regional. **General** anesthesia produces loss of consciousness and thus affects the total person. **Regional** anesthesia blocks pain receptors and conduction fibers in a specific area, which is predetermined by the site selected for instillation of the anesthetic agent.

General anesthesia may be administered by inhalation, intravenous injection, or rectal induction. The ideal general anesthetic produces analgesia, complete loss of consciousness, complete muscle relaxation, and hyporeflexia, and yet is safe and has minimal side effects. No single anesthetic meets all these criteria, so a combination of several agents is used to obtain the optimal effects of each, and to decrease likelihood of toxicity.

The type of anesthesia selected for a specific patient depends on the type of surgery, the depth of anesthesia required, the anticipated length of the procedure, the patient's condition, previous experiences with anesthesia, and preferences, and the available equipment and skill of the anesthesiologist. Before selecting the anesthetic to use in a given patient, the anesthesiologist considers the smoking and drinking habits of the patient as well as the presence of pulmonary, hepatic, renal, or cardiovascular disease. Histories of allergies are also an important consideration. If a nonsurgical problem that constitutes a risk is detected in the preoperative examination, the risks of delaying the surgery until the problem is corrected is weighed against the risks of the problem not being treated. For example, even if pulmonary disease creates a risk for a given patient, in emergency situations an anesthetic is given in spite of this problem.

General anesthesia is used for major head and neck surgery, intracranial surgery, thoracic surgery, and upper abdominal surgery. **Inhalation** anesthesia requires the administration of gases or liquid agents in volatile form combined with oxygen by inhalation via mask-breathing, through an endotracheal tube, or by open drop. The last technique, which is used infrequently, involves dropping the liquid directly onto layers of gauze or onto an absorbant face mask held over the patient's mouth and nose while protecting the eyes from any contact with the solution. The anesthetic agent enters the circulatory system at the alveolar-capillary site.

The advantages of the inhalation anesthetics are related to their effectiveness as analgesics and as muscle relaxants, and in allaying anxiety. Their disadvantages are related to their depressive effects on the cardiovascular and respiratory systems. Inhalation agents are associated with cardiac arrest, vomiting and aspiration, respiratory obstruction (due to increased mucus production and tongue relaxation), shock, hypotension, bronchospasm, and laryngospasm. Bronchospasm and laryngospasm may be controlled by the use of endotracheal intubation. Inhalation agents also cause peripheral dilatation, so that shivering is often observed postoperatively. Protection against chills and prevention of shivering are nursing concerns postoperatively, because shivering increases oxygen demands, an important factor in the cardiac or debilitated patient.

Certain of the gases and liquids used in inhalation anesthesia are highly flammable, and when they are mixed with air or oxygen, they are explosive. When these agents are used, precautions are necessary to elimination sources of ignition. Conductive floors and the use of conductive shoes or shoe covers by personnel are necessary to ensure proper conductivity of static electricity into the floor. To avoid starting static sparks, operating room personnel must not wear nylon or rayon slips or uniforms. Smoking in the vicinity of the operating room is not allowed, nor is the use of electrocautery permitted. (If cautery is needed, a noninflammable anesthetic agent is used.) Some of the characteristics of selected anesthetic agents used for general anesthesia are presented in Table 1-1.

Induction of inhalation anesthesia takes place in four stages, which vary according to the agents and premedications used. **Stage I** ranges from the beginning of the administration of the gas or drug to the loss of consciousness. During this stage the patient appears drowsy, dizzy, and inebriated. It is important that a nurse or someone stay close by to assist the patient if any complications should arise. The room is kept quiet and talking is kept at a minimum. It is also important to remember that hearing is the last sense to be lost during induction of anesthesia so that conversation should be limited to essential and appropriate communication. The patient's condition, for example, should not be discussed at this time.

Stage II is the period from the loss of consciousness until relaxation is achieved. The patient remains susceptible to external stimuli and should not be touched suddenly. This stage is a potentially excitable period; the patient breathes irregularly and may move his arms and legs or body. The nurse should quietly remain at the patient's side and be ready to restrain the patient if needed.

Stage III is the surgical anesthesia stage and follows from the period of relaxation to the loss of reflexes and the depression of vital functions. During this period the patient's respirations are regular, the pupils are contracted, the eyes stop oscillating, the eyelid reflexes disappear, the jaw relaxes, and the swallowing, gag, and laryngeal reflexes are abolished. The auditory sensation is not lost until this stage. When the anesthesiologist indicates that stage III has been reached, the circulating nurse proceeds with the surgical preparation of the skin. Stage III may be further divided into four planes, according to the degree at which reflexes are repressed or paralyzed. Plane 1 is the lightest phase; plane 4 is the deepest, with paralysis of intercostal muscles. Plane 2 of stage III is considered the appropriate one for surgical procedures.

Stage IV is the danger stage, when there is excessive depression of vital functions. Cardiac arrest and respiratory failure may occur. If stage IV occurs, the circulating nurse must be ready to assist the anesthesiologist in preventing cardiac arrest. Resuscitative equipment is always available in the immediate vicinity of any operating room suite.

The circulating nurse should also assist the anesthesiologist during the insertion of the endotracheal tube, if it is to be used. Endotracheal intubation is used during general anesthesia to facilitate control over respiration, to maintain a patent airway, and to facilitate removal of secretions. Intubation, however, may result in vocal cord trauma, throat soreness, and tracheolaryngeal edema.

Table 1-1
Selected agents used for general and local anesthesia

Agent	Route of administration	Characteristics
General anesthetics		
Gases		
Nitrous oxide (N₂O)	Inhalation	Nonexplosive gas, but supports combustion. Must always be administered with at least 20% oxygen. Useful for brief anesthesia (dentistry, labor). Combined with volatile liquid, barbiturate, strong analgesic, and muscle relaxant for surgical anesthesia
Ethylene	Inhalation	Highly flammable and explosive. Unpleasant odor. Rapid induction and recovery. Provides good analgesia but poor muscle relaxation. Used with 20% oxygen. Less used than nitrous oxide because it is explosive. Causes unpleasant aftertaste
Cyclopropane	Inhalation	Explosive; produces rapid induction, good analgesia, and adequate muscle relaxation. Often used for patients in shock who require surgery. Frequently causes nausea, vomiting, headache, postoperative hypotension, and respiratory depression
Volatile liquids		
Ether (ethyl ether; diethyl ether)	Inhalation; open drop	Flammable; explosive. Potent anesthetic with pungent, irritating odor. Slow induction, prolonged recovery. Minimal cardiovascular effects; therefore useful in poor-risk patients. High incidence of nausea and vomiting. Causes increased secretions
Enflurane (Ethrane)	Inhalation	Nonflammable. Similar properties to halothane, but is thought to provide better analgesia and muscle relaxation. Central nervous stimulation is seen in anesthesia
Halothane (Fluothane)	Inhalation	Nonexplosive. Rapid induction with little excitement. Degree of muscle relaxation inadequate; requires supplemental agents. Circulatory depressant in high concentrations, causing hypotension. Generally given with nitrous oxide. Associated with liver damage; not used in patients with history of jaundice or suspected liver disease
Methoxyflurane (Penthrane)	Inhalation	Nonflammable, nonexplosive. Slow induction compared to halothane. Good muscle relaxation and good analgesia. Associated with impaired renal function (renal insufficiency with increased output) and hepatic necrosis. Prolonged postoperative depressant action
Trichloroethylene (Trilene)	Inhalation	Nonflammable. Slow induction, slow recovery, and inadequate muscle relaxation for surgical anesthesia. Used widely in obstetrics. Relatively safe as analgesic. May cause rapid, shallow respirations and arrhythmias
Vinyl ether (Vinethene)	Inhalation	Explosive. Effects similar to those of ethyl ether, but more potent. Rapid induction, but incomplete muscle relaxation. Contraindicated for long operations due to potential hepatic and renal toxicity. May cause convulsions; not used in patients with history of seizures. Used in brief operations
Ethyl chloride	Inhalation	Flammable. Rapid induction, but incomplete muscle relaxation. Depresses myocardium, reduces cardiac output
Thiopental sodium (Pentothal sodium)	Intravenous	Commonly used agent. Used for initial induction prior to inhalation agent. May be used alone for brief procedures. Short-acting barbiturate. Rapid, smooth induction, generally pleasant sensation. May cause laryngospasm, respiratory depression, muscle twitching. Asthmatics or patients with allergies may not tolerate drug. Problems with use in patients with long history of barbiturate use

Table 1-1 (Continued)

Agent	Route of administration	Characteristics
Ketamine hydrochloride (Ketaject, Ketalar)	Intravenous (also intramuscularly)	May be used alone in brief procedures. Rapid induction agent. A "dissociative anesthetic (may cause confusion, hallucinations, disorientation). Patient must be protected from excessive stimuli (including sudden touching) during recovery. May cause increased CSF pressure and transient rise in blood pressure
Fentanyl and droperidol (Innovar)	Intravenous	Combination synthetic narcotic analgesic and tranquilizer. May be habit-forming. Used with nitrous oxide for neuroleptic effect. Danger of circulatory collapse. Requires close monitoring of blood pressure and respiration due to depressant effect. Narcotic analgesics should be used sparingly in the early postoperative period
Local anesthetics		
Lidocaine (Xylocaine)	Topical, intravenous, subcutaneous, spinal	Rapid action and of longer duration than procaine. Has excellent powers of diffusion; used also in managing cardiac arrhythmias
Dibucaine hydrochloride (Nupercaine hydrochloride)	Spinal, topical	Slow onset of action, but one of the most toxic and long-acting local anesthetics
Procaine (Novocain)	Subcutaneous, intramuscular, intravenous, spinal	Low toxicity and lack of local irritation. Slow action. Danger of idiosyncratic and severe reactions. Slow absorption and prolonged effect. Usually given with epinephrine
Tetracaine hydrochloride (Pontocaine)	Topical, spinal	Much more potent than procaine. Longer duration of action than procaine or lidocaine, and more toxic than either

When the patient has reached the proper stage of anesthesia, the circulating nurse and anesthesiologist place him or her in the correct position for the surgical procedure. Abdominal surgery, for example, is likely to require a dorsal recumbent position. The lithotomy position is used for vaginal repairs and some perineal surgeries. Regardless of the type of surgery or particular position used, the patient is carefully and securely strapped into position. He is not strapped too tightly or his arms restrained so tightly that circulation is impaired. The arm with the intravenous site is carefully supported and positioned so that abduction will not be excessive. Lengthy and excessive abduction of the arm can result in paralysis of the brachial plexus (nerve network that supplies the arm, forearm, and hand). Bony prominences are generally padded to prevent nerve and tissue damage. The nurse must consider all these precautions because the patient must be protected from injury while under anesthesia.

As stated previously, the anesthesiologist is responsible for the physiologic monitoring of the patient during the operation. The period of induction is probably the most critical period. Subsequently, recovery from anesthesia is another critical period in the operative experience.

Neuromuscular-blocking agents are used with general anesthesia to provide sustained skeletal muscle relaxation during surgical procedures, particularly in abdominal surgery. They may also be used to facilitate endotracheal intubation. These agents must be carefully controlled because of their effect on the respiratory muscles. Improper use could lead to respiratory failure. Neuromuscular-blocking agents are associated with hypotension, bradycardia, arrhythmias, and inadequate postoperative ventilation. Patients receiving digitalis are particularly vulnerable to ventricular arryhythmias because the neuromuscular-blocking agents potentiate the action of digitalis.

These agents are classified as either nondepolarizing (competitive) or depolarizing. Nondepolarizing drugs compete with acetylcholine at the neuromuscular junction of the skeletal muscle and block the transmission of impulses. Thus paralysis of the muscle fibers results. Gallamine triethiodide (Flaxedil) and tubocurarine (curare) are examples of nondepolarizing agents. Depolarizing agents produce a sustained depolarization at the motor end plate, making the end-plate receptors refractory to acetylcholine. These agents are rapid acting. The most common drug used for this purpose is succinylcholine chloride (Anectine).

Intravenous anesthetics provide a simple, pleasant, and rapid loss of consciousness, but they have a weak analgesic action. They have no muscle-relaxing properties and they are used primarily to produce unconsciousness prior to the administration of inhalation anesthesia. The intravenous agents, however, may be used as single agents during brief procedures such as oral surgery or pelvic examinations.

The dangers of the intravenous agents are laryngospasm, bronchospasm, hypotension, and respiratory arrest. Thiopental sodium (Pentothal) is the most commonly used intravenous anesthetic.

Rectal anesthesia is infrequently used, but may be given for rapid induction and reduction of preoperative anxiety prior to the administration of an inhalation anesthetic. One of the agents used for rectal anesthesia is tribromoethanol (Avertin), which may cause respiratory depression, hypotension, and liver and kidney damage. Thiopental sodium may also be used for rectal anesthesia, but it may cause respiratory depression and hypotension.

As previously stated, regional or local anesthesia is used to anesthetize specific regions of the body without causing loss of consciousness. The anesthetic is placed upon the surface to be anesthetized or is injected into a nerve or nerve pathway that controls pain sensation to a particular area, thereby blocking the transmission of painful stimuli to the brain. Regional anesthesia includes the following types: topical, local infiltration, nerve block, spinal anesthesia, saddle block, epidural block, and caudal block. The patient is awake during the operation, although narcotics or barbiturates may be used as adjunct medications. Vasoconstrictors may be added to solutions for infiltration, nerve block, epidural, and spinal anesthesia to prolong the effect of the anesthetic and reduce risk of toxic reactions. The patient is able to cough and breathe normally, so that respiratory complications are not likely to occur. The use of regional anesthesia is limited to short procedures, as patients are generally anxious and fearful at being awake during the procedure. In addition, some regional anesthetic agents may cause systemic depression. Spinal anesthesia, in particular, may result in hypotension. Prior sensitization to the agents used in regional anesthesia may result in anaphylactic reactions.

Topical anesthetics are sprayed or dropped on mucous membranes in the nasopharynx, the mouth, the vagina, or the rectum, primarily to facilitate diagnostic procedures. Some topical agents are sold "over the counter," such as Nupercainal and Solarcaine. Topical anesthetics used for ocular surgery are discussed in Chapter 12.

Local injection and infiltration of anesthetic drugs directly into the tissues at the incision site may be used for superficial or minor procedures such as biopsies or simple suturing. Only the peripheral nerves around the area of the incision are blocked. Therefore it is not practical to use this method of anesthesia for extensive or deep tissue surgery. The most frequently used drug for this technique is lidocaine (Xylocaine). Care is taken that the agent is not injected into a vein, because of the danger of anaphylactic reactions. Local anesthetics such as procaine hydrochloride (Novocain) are used widely in dentistry.

Regional **nerve blocks** require the injection of anesthetic agents into the nerve plexus that controls pain sensation to a particular area. The same drugs that are used for local anesthesia are also used in this type of anesthesia, but the area affected is greater in regional nerve block. The technique may be used to anesthetize an entire finger (digital nerve block) or the entire upper arm (axillary block), for example. Allergic reactions may occur with regional blocks. In addition, ischemic necrosis due to decreased circulation may result. The potential for this latter complication, though rare, requires that the nurse carefully observe the circulation of the affected body part when this technique is used.

For certain operations performed below the

level of the diaphragm, nerve blockage is attained by intrathecal injection of appropriate drugs. Depending on the level and site of injection, the anesthesia produced is referred to as spinal, saddle block (also called low spinal), or caudal. **Spinal** anesthesia is used in certain abdominal, pelvic, or lower extremity operations. The anesthetic agent, in these cases, is injected into the subarachnoid space to block the nerve roots leading to the operative site. Close monitoring of the patient is necessary to ascertain that the level of the anesthesia is not above the level of the T4 spinal cord segment, which could result in respiratory paralysis.

When spinal anesthesia is used, the circulating nurse assists the anesthesiologist by maintaining the patient in the proper position. The anesthetic is administered while the patient is either in a sitting position with his arms resting over a stand, or more commonly in a side-lying position with the back arched outward. The latter position facilitates insertion of the needle between the lumbar vertebrae into the spinal canal. Postural preventive measures are taken to avoid a rise in the anesthesia level or a toxic reaction, which would threaten respiratory function. The patient is observed for effects on the autonomic nervous system, particularly hypotension and bradycardia. Motor nerve functions are the last to be affected and the first to be restored. Thus, during recovery, the patient may first be able to wiggle his toes, but may not be able to distinguish touch or sensation in the extremity. The nurse who feels secure that the patient is satisfactorily recovered from spinal anesthesia once he is able to wiggle his toes is functioning mistakenly, however. The ability to wiggle toes indicates that the motor blockade is wearing off, but the patient still is affected by autonomic blockade and is still vulnerable to hypotension.

Spinal anesthesia is relatively safe in the hands of a skilled anesthesiologist. The technique does not require extensive equipment and drugs, and it can be used when surgery is required and pulmonary disease in the patient contraindicates the use of general anesthesia. Excellent muscle relaxation is provided. Many patients, however, are fearful of spinal anesthesia. The bizarre and unpleasant feeling of numbness and paralysis in the extremities and the tingling and vibratory sensations may create anxiety and apprehension. The patient should be warned that these sensations are to be expected, and these aspects should be discussed with the patient preoperatively.

Complications of spinal anesthesia include hypotension and respiratory depression, as has been cited. Headaches from spinal anesthesia are thought to be due to the reduction of cerebrospinal fluid pressure caused by seepage of the fluid through the dural puncture site. Hypersensitivity of the patient, poor hydration, and the use of a large spinal needle are often considered as predisposing factors. Therefore, use of a small spinal needle (22 to 25 gauge), administration of adequate fluids, and the maintenance of a flat position for approximately 4 to 12 hours postoperatively are measures used to combat this complication. While the patient is under spinal anesthesia, the nurse should be particularly concerned about his position and avoidance of pressure on the affected portions of the body. Circulatory problems and nerve damage may result if the patient is allowed to lie in awkward positions. The patient is unaware of the position of his extremities while under the influence of spinal anesthesia.

Neurologic complications such as arachnoiditis may result from the use of unsterile medications or equipment or improper technique. In the case of preexisting central nervous system disease, muscle weakness and other complications (such as paraplegia) may occur.

Saddle block anesthesia is accomplished by the injection of an anesthetic into the dural sac at the third and fourth lumbar space. It is used commonly in obstetrics because it produces anesthesia of the perineal area mainly. The effects are like those of spinal anesthesia.

Caudal anesthesia is used in obstetrics also. The anesthetic is injected through the lower end of the sacrum into the caudal area of the spinal canal. It affects the caudal nerve roots, rendering the cervix, vagina, and perineum insensitive to pain.

Several nonanesthetic agents and measures may be used to supplement general and regional anesthetics. These ancillary agents reduce preoperative apprehension, counteract undesirable reflexes, facilitate induction, provide smooth maintenance and recovery, reduce the amount of general anesthetic required, and fortify anesthetics of low potency [179]. As indicated previously, sedatives, hypnotics, and antianxiety agents may be used preoperatively. Narcotics are used to produce analgesia and sedation before and after surgery. Phenothiazines are often administered to produce drowsiness and to control nausea and vomiting. Anticholinergic drugs such as atropine and scopolamine are given to reduce the excessive secretions that some inhalation anesthetics cause. Neuromuscular-blocking agents have been discussed in relation to their use in obtaining sustained skeletal muscle relaxation during surgical anesthesia. They are necessary in abdominal surgery as well as in facilitating endotracheal intubation. In thoracic surgery they are used to produce apnea so that respiration can be controlled.

Hypothermia is the induced reduction of the temperature of all or part of the body and is sometimes used as an adjunct to anesthesia to control bleeding and reduce metabolism. In amputations, local hypothermia is used to alter local circulation and to lower cell metabolism. The involved area is packed in ice or wrapped in a special refrigeration apparatus. In addition, tourniquets are applied to inhibit circulation. This procedure is generally started about 3 to 5 hours prior to surgery.

To obtain generalized hypothermia by surface cooling, the patient's entire body is immersed in an ice water bath, or more commonly, wrapped in a cooling blanket through which iced water and alcohol are circulated in its coils. For cardiac and neurologic surgical procedures, extracorporeal cooling devices are used to cool the blood outside the body before reinfusing the cooled blood into the patient. The body temperature may be reduced to between 28 and 30°C (82.4 to 86°F). When hypothermia is accomplished and during rewarming, the patient is closely observed for impending respiratory depression and cardiac arrest, as well as for skin irritations (and potential frostbite), and labile temperatures. Skin care, with application of body oils or lotion, and frequent position changes are necessary when surface cooling methods are used. Monitoring of vital signs and of intake and output is essential. Postoperatively the patient is rewarmed slowly with application of blankets. The shivering factor, often encountered in the use of hypothermia, is controlled by use of sedatives, ataractics, and muscle relaxants.

When a narcotic is used during anesthesia it may cause **hypoventilation.** Narcotic antagonists may be necessary and include naloxone (Narcan), doxapram (Dopram), and levallorphan tartrate (Lorfan). These drugs may cause nausea and vomiting. If patients undergoing anesthesia are known to be narcotic addicts, narcotic antagonists are contraindicated and are given only if absolutely necessary. Otherwise, withdrawal symptoms may be initiated.

As the surgeon is beginning to conclude the operation, the anesthesiologist has already begun to lighten the anesthesia to facilitate as rapid a recovery as possible postoperatively. The patient, however, is still susceptible to complications due to the anesthetic agent used. These complications include cardiac arrest, respiratory depression, airway obstruction due to excessive mucus formation and depression of the medullary center, bronchospasm, laryngospasm, circulatory impairment, hypotension and shock, vomiting, and aspiration. An infrequent but usually fatal complication is that of **malignant hyperthermia,** or malignant hyperpyrexia. This sudden and life-threatening rise in body temperature occurs during the administration of the anesthetic. The temperature may rise as high as 43 to 44°C (110 to 112°F). If the temperature is not controlled immediately, respiratory and metabolic acidosis, intravascular coagulation, tissue hypoxia, and hypovolemia result. The fatality rate is high, generally between 70 and 80 percent. Although the specific cause of the condition is not known, combinations of certain drugs and anesthetic agents such as halothane and succinylcholine have been implicated. A major component of the syndrome appears to be genetic susceptibility. Often there is a history of previous occurrences of the syndrome either in a member of the family or in the patient. Here again is another example of how an accurate patient history may have an important impact on the surgical outcome.

Malignant hyperthermia tends to occur in children or young adults. Its onset, while the patient is under the influence of the anesthetic, is insidious. When malignant hyperthermia occurs the anesthesia is discontinued, the patient is cooled by one of the previously described methods, and immediate correction of hypoxia, acidosis, hypovolemia, and fluid imbalance is undertaken. Even in patients who survive this crisis there may be brain damage as a result of severe cerebral hypoxia. Postoperatively the patient is observed for fluid and electrolyte imbalances, symptoms of cerebral hypoxia, and respiratory depression.

As the patient is being transferred from the operating room to the recovery room, care is taken that the patient is handled gently to avoid injury and vasomotor effects resulting in hypotension. The anesthesiologist accompanies the patient to the recovery room to assure that the respiratory and circulatory systems are functioning properly.

POSTOPERATIVE CARE

The patient remains in the recovery room until he has recovered from anesthesia and his vital signs are stable. The recovery room is staffed so that close observation is possible. Emergency equipment as well as suctioning and other essential equipment are readily available in this setting. Recovery from anesthesia generally takes between 1 and 2 hours, but is varied, depending on the physiologic state of the patient, on the length and type of surgery, and on the anesthetic agents used.

Immediately, the patient's respiratory status is checked to determine the adequacy of the airway. If the patient is still unconscious an oral airway or an endotracheal tube is used to maintain the airway. The oral airway, a rubber or plastic hollow tube, is inserted into the oropharyngeal cavity to prevent the tongue from slipping back into the throat and occluding the airway. Suctioning through the airway is essential to maintaining patency of the airway.

The endotracheal tube is inserted into the trachea, via either the nose or the mouth, and a ventilator may be attached to the tube to provide for alveolar exchange. The anesthesiologist determines the regulation of the ventilator, as required by the patient's condition and specific needs.

Vital signs are checked and the patient's color, skin condition, peripheral pulses, wound dressing, and essential monitoring equipment are checked and regulated. After the patient has been settled, the nurse receives a report from the anesthesiologist. The report should include information on the type of surgery done, any complications or potential complications, the findings, blood and fluid replacement, urine output, type of anesthetic used and the patient's tolerance to it, and any drains or special equipment utilized during surgery.

The recovery room admission note should indicate the time the patient was received, his level of consciousness, and information on the assessment of the vital signs, wound status, and types of equipment.

Close observation of the patient is absolutely essential because the patient at this stage is vulnerable to a variety of complications, most important of which are those related to his respiratory and cardiovascular status. The two most significant early pulmonary complications are those of **acute respiratory obstruction** and **atelectasis**. The patient should be placed on his side, unless contraindicated by the type of surgical procedure. If the patient must remain supine, his head is turned to the side and his chin is extended. This positioning prevents aspiration of mucus or vomitus, which can occur as the result of diminished swallowing and gag reflexes. As stated previously, the patient's tongue may fall back and obstruct the airway unless an oral airway or endotracheal tube is in place.

On awakening, the patient is immediately encouraged to deep breathe and to repeat this activity at regular intervals during the recovery period (unless assisted ventilation is being used).

The patient is also observed closely for any signs of hypoxia, as demonstrated by rapid shallow breathing; noisy snoring or gasping respirations; a thready pulse; increased restlessness; and confusion. Laryngeal spasm may occur as a side effect of anesthesia and requires immediate intervention. The most significant sign of laryngeal spasm is an audible "crowing" sound accompanied by stridor, restlessness, and subsequent cyanosis. Oxygen must be administered immediately and suctioning of saliva, blood or mucus is necessary. The anesthesiologist should be called while the nurse is initiating manual respiration via an Ambu bag until other resuscitative methods are started. An endotracheal tube is necessary in laryngeal spasm in order to assure a patent airway and controlled respiration. (Administration of a muscle relaxant is usually necessary to facilitate intubation.)

Patient restlessness and disorientation

to some degree during recovery from anesthesia generally disappear as consciousness is again attained. Usually oxygen is administered via nasal cannula during recovery if an endotracheal tube and controlled ventilation are not provided. The nurse must carefully assess whether the patient's restlessness is due to pain or to hypoxia. Administration of a narcotic to a hypoxic patient will further depress the respiratory system.

Most inhalation anesthetics wear off fairly rapidly because of their low solubility in blood and the body tissues. Therefore pain sensation returns quickly and administration of an analgesic may be indicated. Either morphine or meperidine hydrochloride (Demerol) is given slowly intravenously, assuming that the vital signs are satisfactory. Such an injection takes effect within 3 to 5 minutes, but subsides within 45 minutes. During this time the patient may waken and complain of pain, but soon return to sleep. The nurse, in evaluating the patient's need for pain medication, always weighs the importance of minimizing the pain (to avoid complications related to increased stress caused by pain) against the dangers of overmedication and potential respiratory depression.

When an endotracheal tube is to be left in place, additional care and monitoring are required. A detailed discussion of care of the patient with an endotracheal tube and controlled ventilation is provided in Chapter 3. When the endotracheal tube is removed, the patient must be observed for adequate spontaneous respiration and adequate ventilation. Arterial blood gas measurements and spirometry are used to determine the appropriate time for extubation. These aspects of maintenance of pulmonary function are also discussed in detail in Chapter 3.

In addition to the complications already mentioned, the patient recovering from anesthesia is susceptible to the development of cardiac arrhythmias and cardiac arrest. Emergency resuscitation equipment must be available for immediate use in the recovery room. Aspects of care in cardiac resuscitation are discussed in Chapter 4.

Accurate assessment of the cardiovascular and respiratory status of the patient is a vital precaution. Even in the absence of specialized monitoring equipment, the nurse is able to make accurate assessments by observing vital signs closely, using chest auscultation methods, observing chest expansion, and assessing the patient's color, level of consciousness, and skin condition.

Postoperatively the patient is also vulnerable to hemorrhage and shock. Hemorrhage may be either external or internal. The wound dressing is observed frequently for any incidence of fresh bleeding. Tubes or drainage equipment are observed for bloody drainage. The symptoms of hemorrhage are increased pallor, diaphoresis, cool skin, oliguria, thirst, rapid and shallow respirations, decreased blood pressure and temperature, and restlessness. Early detection of signs and symptoms of internal hemorrhage is imperative in the prevention of hypovolemic shock, an abnormal state of inadequate cellular metabolism. Care of the patient in shock is discussed in Chapter 16.

Although the recovery room setting is an intensive care setting and there is considerable activity related to the care of patients recovering from anesthesia, as quiet an environment as possible should be maintained. It is important to remember that just as hearing is the last sense to be lost during induction of anesthesia, it is also the first sense to be regained during recovery. The sounds of other patients moaning and groaning, retching and vomiting, and of suctioning and other equipment can be extremely frightening to a patient as he awakens from anesthesia. The patient needs quiet assurance, an orientation to his location, and prompt attention to his needs in order to allay his anxiety.

When the patient has recovered sufficiently from the anesthesia and his vital signs are again stabilized, he is transferred either to his own room or to the intensive care unit for continued care. Patients who have undergone extensive and complicated surgery, who are poor surgical risks, or who have experienced cardiac arrest or respiratory insufficiency during or after surgery usually require continued intensive care and specialized monitoring.

When the patient is to be moved to either the intensive care unit or his own room, the routine precautions for transferring a patient are taken. Again, a thorough report is given to the personnel who will now be responsible for his care so that continuity of care will be provided.

Important ongoing aspects of postoperative care are related to assessment of vital signs, encouraging the patient to cough and deep breathe every hour, changing his position at regular intervals, and using narcotics judiciously to relieve pain. If the patient does not receive adequate relief from his pain, he is not likely to cough and deep breathe effectively, but will instead splint his side and tend to breathe rapidly and shallowly to protect himself from further pain. Patients with high abdominal or thoracotomy incisions are less likely to breathe well or cough effectively because the proximity of the wound to the diaphragm causes pain on coughing and results in poor ventilation. Therefore the nurse must be particularly diligent in assessing the effectiveness of deep breathing and coughing in these patients. Splinting the incision with the hands or with a pillow will often be helpful in encouraging the patient to cough. Often the patient is fearful of injuring the incision by coughing deeply, and splinting of the incision will enable him to feel secure. The color and consistency of the mucus should be noted. Thick, foul-smelling and yellowish or greenish sputum indicates the presence of an infection.

The earliest sign of atelectasis and pneumonia, the most common postoperative complications, is that of bronchial breathing, which can be detected with a stethoscope during auscultation. This sign often occurs before fever or other signs of pneumonia are evident. Alelectasis and pneumonia result from stasis of secretions and mucus, due to ineffective coughing.

Maintenance of fluid and electrolyte balance is extremely important during the postoperative period. Inadequate replacement of fluid losses may result in dehydration and electrolyte deficits. Intake and output must be recorded accurately. Infusions must be administered correctly and at the appropriate rate. Antiemetics should be administered for nausea and vomiting before excessive amounts of fluids are lost. Nasogastric intubation may be necessary if vomiting continues. Electrolyte values on laboratory reports should be examined carefully and the surgeon notified of significant abnormalities. Renal function should be monitored carefully, as inadequate renal function in the presence of extensive fluid administration may result in fluid overload and threaten cardiac and pulmonary function.

The patient who has undergone extensive surgery generally has a retention catheter in place, so that renal output can easily be monitored. If inadequate renal outflow occurs in the presence of hypotension, renal failure should be suspected. Details of renal failure are discussed in Chapter 6.

Within 8 to 10 hours postoperatively, patients should void, particularly after abdominal or gynecologic surgery. Anesthesia effects, pain, fear, and tension, however, may contribute to the patient's inability to void. The bladder is checked for distention by palpating for fullness above the symphysis pubis. Bladder distention is suspected if the patient voids only small amounts frequently. The patient may be assisted to the bathroom to promote bladder function in a natural atmosphere and natural pattern, assuming his or her physiologic status can tolerate the activity. The male patient often may be able to void once he is allowed to stand at the bedside. Other measures to encourage voiding are discussed in Chapter 6. Only as a last resort is catheterization attempted. Nonetheless, the patient who has a distended bladder but is unable to void even with ambulation and other inducements requires catheterization. A distended bladder also causes pressure on the operative site and can lead to other complications.

Adequate rest and comfort are important for the patient to be able to withstand the stress of the surgical procedure and to facilitate his recovery from anesthesia. Usually narcotics such as morphine, meperidine hydrochloride (Demerol), or codeine are administered by injection for analgesia during the first 24 hours after surgery. These medications may be required beyond that period in patients who have had extensive surgery. Although it is important for the patient to be comfortable, the nurse must use good judgment in administering the prescribed narcotics. Respiratory depression must be avoided, and the patient must not be so sedated that he is unable to cooperate in coughing and deep breathing and in exercises to improve circulation. Vital signs are checked prior to narcotic administration for assurance that the patient is not hypotensive and in danger of further depression due to additional medication. Frequent changes in position, oral hygiene, and other comfort measures may relieve the patient of distress and the narcotic may not be needed.

After the first 24 to 48 hours, new orders are

usually written for pain management. A less potent narcotic or a smaller dosage of the same narcotic may be ordered. Depending on the status of the patient, an oral medication may be preferred. If the patient continues to ask for narcotics after several days postoperatively, the nurse should report the problem. The patient may be developing a complication or is becoming dependent on the medication. Other reasons for increasing discomfort should be determined. For example, the patient with gas pains and a distended abdomen may request narcotics frequently to relieve his distress. A rectal tube (if not contraindicated by the type of surgery) may promote much relief and negate the need for a narcotic. Releasing a too tight bandage or assisting the patient to ambulate may also help to relieve pain and discomfort.

Movement and early ambulation are encouraged postoperatively to prevent complications related to circulatory stasis and weakness as well as respiratory complications such as hypostatic pneumonia. Early in his recovery period the patient is encouraged to move, turn, flex his ankles and legs, cough, and deep breathe. Either the night following surgery or on the following day the patient is usually assisted in ambulation. This does not mean moving only from the bed to the chair, but in the room and in the hall. Ambulation to this extent should be done at least twice on the first postoperative day and increasingly thereafter in both time and distance as the patient increases in independence and ability. Early ambulation not only promotes adequate circulation and prevents pulmonary embolism or thrombophlebitis, but it also promotes psychological well-being. The patient is often surprised at how well he is able to tolerate ambulation and is encouraged in his recovery ability. Depending on his tolerance, the patient is also allowed to gradually assume responsibility for his own personal hygiene.

When the patient is first started with ambulation, he is assisted slowly and smoothly in adjusting to the vertical position and in avoiding strain on the incision. For the patient who is moved too quickly and is also somewhat dehydrated, the change in position may be too great and his adaptive mechanisms may not be adequate. Fainting may occur and the patient will become hesitant about attempting ambulation later. Patients should be encouraged to walk in an upright position and should not be allowed to bend in an attempt to protect the incision. For patients with circulatory problems or those who have had vascular surgery, support hose (elastic stockings) may be used to promote venous return and prevent venous stasis. The stockings should be removed daily and reapplied as often as necessary to prevent wrinkling, which could cause constriction. Patients should also be advised of the importance of not crossing their legs or having the knee gatch of the bed elevated, both of which increase venous stasis.

The nutritional status of the patient is closely monitored. Depending on the type of surgical procedure that was done, the patient may be restricted from fluids for 24 to 48 hours and may have a nasogastric tube in place. Ordinarily the patient is allowed to drink fluids when he has recovered from anesthesia as long as he has no nausea and is not vomiting. Broth, tea, fruit juices, soups, and Jell-O are often well tolerated by some patients, even on the night of surgery. These patients progress within a day or so to soft foods. About 2 or 3 days postoperatively, they are able to tolerate a full, nutritious diet. If the patient does not have a natural bowel movement, an enema may be ordered 3 or 4 days postoperatively. Proper nitrogen balance is essential for wound healing and postoperative recovery. The importance of an adequate nutritional intake cannot be overemphasized.

When the patient's surgery requires prolonged fluid and food restriction, other means of nutrition must be provided, either by total parenteral nutrition or by nasogastric tube feedings. These measures are described in detail in Chapters 2 and 7.

Several additional postoperative complications may occur. These include paralytic ileus and gastric dilatation, particularly in patients with gastric surgery or those who have had spinal anesthesia. These complications are discussed in Chapter 7. The patient is checked for abdominal distention postoperatively to detect these complications, which are suspected in the presence of frequent vomiting and continued absence of gastric motility (neither gas nor feces is passed by rectum). Another complication resulting from either fluid or food restriction or inadequate oral intake of nutrition is that of acute parotitis. The condition, however, is associated primarily with poor oral hygiene and extreme debilitation. **Acute parotitis,** which is an inflammation of the parotid gland, produces swelling, pain, and redness at the site of the gland. Surgical incision, drainage, and the administration of antibiotics may be necessary. The importance of oral hygiene and adequate fluid and food intake cannot be overemphasized in the prevention of acute parotitis.

Singultus (hiccoughs) is a transient condition that may persist and lead to complications. Hiccoughs are most likely to occur with abdominal surgery, and they generally result from irritation of the phrenic nerve due to a distended abdomen, gastric dilatation, paralytic ileus, peritonitis, or subdiaphragmatic abscess. Anxiety may also be a precipitating factor. Although hiccoughs may be regarded lightly and may be considered more an annoyance or a nuisance, they can cause exhaustion, vomiting, and fluid and electrolyte imbalance. In addition, they may interfere with nutritional intake. They also may be a predisposing factor in wound dehiscence, which will be discussed shortly.

Hiccoughs are treated by gastric lavage or suction, administration of carbon dioxide, having the patient rebreathe his own air from a paper bag, or by administration of antispasmodics (e.g., atropine), sedatives, or tranquilizers. When the hiccoughs are uncontrollable, a phrenic nerve block or phrenic nerve crushing procedure may be necessary.

Fever is a common symptom that occurs as a slight elevation during the first day or so following surgery. In this case, dehydration and tissue damage may be an important factor. A marked elevation of temperature (above 38°C; 100.4°F) or a persistent fever is a serious symptom and requires further investigation. A pulmonary complication, a wound infection, a urinary tract infection, or thrombophlebitis should be suspected. The wound should be checked for swelling or drainage. A culture of wound drainage is indicated. Urinary tract infections, as mentioned earlier in this chapter, are the most frequent cause of nosocomial infections and should be suspected when the patient has had a retention catheter in place. Fluid intake is encouraged. A urine specimen is collected for culture and sensitivity, and appropriate antibiotic therapy is initiated. UTI should be suspected when the patient complains of dysuria or frequency of urination.

Thrombophlebitis is suspected when the patient complains of pain in the calf of his leg or if swelling, warmth, or tenderness is noted at the site. Venous stasis and increased blood coagulability may occur postoperatively because of dehydration and hypovolemia related to hemorrhage. It is a frequent complication after gynecologic surgery and may be related to prolonged immobilization in a lithotomy position with tight leg straps. Obesity and prolonged immobilization are predisposing factors. The care of patients with thrombophlebitis is discussed in detail in Chapter 4.

Wound infection is another important cause of fever and is a serious complication that usually causes prolonged hospitalization and prolonged recovery. Wound care and the prevention of wound infections will now be discussed in the context of wound healing.

Surgical Wound Healing

Uncomplicated surgical wounds heal by the process of primary union, also known as first intention. **Primary union** is a form of connective tissue repair that involves the proliferation of fibroblasts and capillary buds and the subsequent laying down of collagen to produce a scar. Primary union is the usual consequence of most tissue damage [190, 217]. Connective tissue repair may also occur by secondary union, a process that takes place when excessive loss of tissue prevents primary union.

Robbins describes the process of primary union as consisting in several stages [217]. Initially the line of the incision, after the wound is closed with sutures, is filled with a blood clot. As the surface of the clot dries it retracts and draws the edges of the wound together as a means of superficial healing. A crust or scab forms and seals the wound. Within 24 hours an inflammatory reaction results in the margins of the wound, and a polymorphonuclear infiltrate becomes visible. At this time, reepithelialization of the surface and fibrous bridging of the subepithelial defect begin. The fibrin meshwork in the blood clot provides a structural scaffold along which the epithelial cells, fibroblasts, and capillary buds migrate [190, 217]. Within a few days fibroblasts and capillary beds in the deeper levels invade the fibrin clot and bridge the defect. Initially the surface epithelium is thin, but proliferation soon results in the multilayered differentiated squamous epithelium characteristic of normal epidermis. In this area of the wound, however, the hair follicles, sweat glands, and sebaceous glands that have been destroyed cannot be replaced. New vessels are compressed by the continued proliferation of the fibroblasts and eventually are obliterated so that the scar becomes devascularized and pale. Collagen is detectable in about 4 to 5 days and builds up during the next 2 or 3 weeks, resulting in increased strength of the wound. It is generally felt that tensile strength is achieved within 3 to 4 weeks and may be at normal levels by the end of the second postoperative month [190, 217].

In an open wound or where there has been a significant loss of tissue and a large amount of exudate or necrotic debris has been removed, the defect must be filled by a slow buildup of newly formed, highly vascularized connective tissue. This type of healing is **secondary union,** or secondary intention, and involves the development of granulation tissue comprised of young fibroblasts and capillaries. Secondary union is a slow process and is not completed until all the debris has been removed and the defect is reepithelialized. In this process, large areas of scar tissue are produced.

The phases of wound healing are divided into the lag phase, the healing phase, and the maturation phase. The **lag phase** is the first 4 to 7 days postoperatively when fluid containing plasma, blood cells, and fibrin travels from the tissues into the wound and fuses the cut surfaces. The **healing phase** occurs during the next 7 days when fibroblasts multiply rapidly, bridging the wound edges and restoring continuity. This phase begins rapidly, diminishes progressively, and terminates at about the fourteenth day. The next 7 days (fourteenth to twenty-first day postoperatively) are the **maturation phase,** when there is solid healing of the wound by deposition of fibrous connective tissue (scar formation) [190, 217].

On the basis of this information, the nurse can appreciate that severe stress and strain on the wound should be avoided during the first 2 or 3 weeks postoperatively. Following this period, gradual increase in activity is necessary in order to reestablish normal or near-normal tensile strength. Sutures are generally left in place for 5 to 7 days, but they are removed earlier for certain incisions, such as in thyroidectomy or in plastic surgery in order to decrease scarring.

The criterion for the removal of sutures is that there is sufficient collagen across the defect so that the unsupported wound can withstand stress without being disrupted. Therefore the nature of the stresses imposed on the wound site determine the length of time sutures are needed. As discussed previously, retention sutures may be needed for 2 or 3 weeks after certain abdominal surgical procedures. Tendon wounds also require extra suture support for 2 to 3 weeks. The soles of the feet, the palms of the hands, and the extensor surfaces of the elbows or knees require sutures for 10 to 12 days because of slow healing at these sites and constant exposure to extensive stress.

When there is extensive drainage or an infected wound, healing is delayed. Other techniques using drains, tubes, and catheters at the wound site are necessary to promote healing. The purpose of these techniques is to facilitate the escape of body fluids when it would be detrimental to allow these fluids (blood, lymph, pancreatic juices, intestinal juices, bile, and pus) to accumulate within body cavities. These techniques are most often used to drain abscesses and intestinal contents when leakage of an anastamosis may occur, and to decompress the gastrointestinal tract or other body sites. An example of the latter purpose is the decompression of the common bile duct by means of a T tube after common bile duct surgery. This procedure is described in Chapter 7.

Various types of drains may be used. The most common is the **Penrose drain,** which is made of soft rubber and which causes little tissue reaction. It is sutured to the skin and a safety pin is placed externally in order to maintain its position. The Penrose drain acts primarily by capillary action, drawing any pus or fluid along its surfaces through a stab wound made adjacent to the main incision. A cigarette drain may be placed inside a Penrose drain to assist in absorbing the drainage. A Foley catheter may be inserted to provide for drainage or, in the case of gastrostomy, it may be used as a means of postoperative feeding into the stomach.

A **sump tube** is a double-lumen device that prevents adjacent tissue from clogging the opening in the suction tube by means of an outer screen of perforated tubing. It is usually used when large volumes of fluid output are expected and it is usually attached to either continuous or intermittent low suction.

The nurse should always know when a drain or tube has been placed in a wound and must check for malfunction as well as make certain that the tubes are not kinked. The nurse must attach the proper type of drainage apparatus, depending on whether the tube or catheter is to be attached to intermittent or continuous suction or is to drain by gravity. The drainage is measured and the amount is noted in the output record. The color, consistency, volume, and any change in the quality of the discharge are described in the nursing notes. Significant odors are also described.

There may be bleeding from the drains, and there is danger of sepsis. The drain may also be lost accidentally if there is undue tension on it. The nurse must take precautions to prevent undue tension on drains or tubes and should take care not to accidentally pull on them when changing dressings.

If a wound is clean and has no drains, the dressings are often removed within 24 hours and the wound is exposed. **Wound exposure** (open technique) minimizes wound infection by eliminating the warm, moist environment of drainage-soaked sealed dressings. Some patients, however, are disturbed by the exposure and request that the wound be covered. Usually the first dressing change is done by the surgeon so that he can examine the incision. Subsequent dressings are changed by the nurse. The nurse should record the appearance of the wound, any discoloration, tenderness, or pain, whether the incision is intact or whether there is any drainage. The type and amount of drainage should be described specifically. The frequency of dressing change is determined by the amount of drainage present. The objective is to keep the wound dry.

In certain operations, such as radical mastectomy, closed wound suction may be used. The primary purpose of closed wound drainage is to establish external pressure with equal distribution to facilitate fixing of the opposing planes of tissue, thereby obliterating any space between them. Closed wound suction is indicated when a large volume of debris and serosanguinous fluid is anticipated. An apparatus frequently used in such cases is the Hemovac system, which involves the use of wound tubes connected to an evacuator system. This system removes serosanguinous fluids that could retard tissue granulation. Gentle, even pressure is exerted by means of negative pressure created by compression of the evacuator system. The directions provided on the evacuator system must be followed precisely. Precautions are taken to prevent the tubes from becoming kinked or disconnected, and the evacuator is emptied of drainage as it accumulates. An excellent pictorial demonstration of the use of these tubes is available in the recent literature [224].

Wound healing is facilitated by good nutrition, particularly adequate amounts of protein; vitamin C, which is essential for collagen formation; fluid and electrolyte balance; and an adequate blood supply. Wound healing takes place more readily in the young healthy person than in the aged person.

Delayed or impaired wound healing may be the result of inadequate nutrition, hypoproteinemia and vitamin C deficiency, anemia, and a diminished blood supply to the area, as in arteriosclerosis. Wound healing is also delayed by steroid administration; cortisone inhibits the initial inflammatory response and thus inhibits subsequent fibroplasia and collagen formation. Ionizing radiation interferes with wound healing, as do obesity, diabetes, or debilitating diseases like cancer. Increased abdominal pressure due to distention strains the sutures and predisposes to delayed healing. Local factors that contribute to poor wound healing include infection, hematoma formation, excessive foreign body in the wound (e.g., sutures), and local ischemia. Excessive retraction of tissue during the surgical procedure may also predispose to poor wound healing. Inadvertent tissue strangulation due to excessive tension of the sutures during closure also alters the healing process. Hematomas may interfere with adequate circulation to the wound and thus interfere with healing. Most often, hematoma formation occurs as the result of difficult or incomplete hemostasis or in extensive resection.

Cruse [187] classifies surgical wounds as clean, clean-contaminated, contaminated, or dirty. A **clean wound** is one in which the gastrointestinal tract or respiratory tract was not entered during the operation. In addition, no apparent inflammation was encountered during the procedure and there was no break in aseptic technique. A thyroidectomy wound is an example of a clean wound.

A **clean-contaminated wound** is one in which the gastrointestinal or respiratory tract was entered, but no significant spillage occured during the procedure.

A **contaminated wound** is one in which inflammation and pus formation were found during surgery, and spillage from the hollow viscus occurred. This category includes fresh, or early, traumatic wounds and procedures in which a break in aseptic technique occurred.

A **dirty wound** is one in which pus is encountered or a perforated viscus is discovered during the operation. Long-standing traumatic wounds are included in this category.

The wound healing process is evaluated by regularly observing the status of the wound. The nurse should observe for any type of drainage from the wound as well as for signs of local inflammatory reactions. Defective wound healing is detected when the wound edges fail to seal within 2 to 3 days or if serosanguinous fluid appears between the skin sutures. Restlessness, fever, warmth, redness, swelling, and abnormal pain at the wound site are signs and symptoms associated with the onset of wound infection.

Purulent drainage from a wound is cultured for the causative organism and sensitivity studies are done to determine the appropriate type of antibiotic to use. The wound is often opened in order to achieve proper drainage. Wound irrigations may also be prescribed to facilitate removal of purulent drainage and debris. Isolation procedures oriented to skin and wound precautions are also instituted. The importance of aseptic technique in dressing changes, and the importance of thorough hand washing before and after dressing changes, cannot be overemphasized.

An infected wound complicates the postoperative course and results in prolonged hospitalization and delayed recovery.

In addition to wound infection, other complications are dehiscence and evisceration.

Wound **dehiscence** is the partial or total separation of layers of the wound enclosure. (see color insert Figure 11 on page 1078C). A small area of separation may be treated by the application of adhesive "butterfly" strips to approximate the wound edges. In other cases, however, large amounts of serosanguinous fluid may suddenly gush from a previously satisfactory-appearing wound as a result of the separation of the fascial edges. Wound dehiscence most often occurs between the seventh and tenth postoperative days and is associated with distention, excessive coughing, and hiccoughing. A heavy dressing is applied and the patient is instructed to stay in bed and to avoid coughing. The surgeon is notified, and the insertion of drains and resuturing are necessary. Wound dehiscence may proceed to evisceration if these protective measures are not taken immediately. Nonetheless, evisceration may occur suddenly, even without warning or dehiscence.

Wound **evisceration** is the protrusion of viscera through the separated edges of an abdominal wound closure (all layers of tissue are disrupted and the peritoneal cavity is exposed). The patient often describes the sensation that "the stitches gave away." This situation is an emergency and the surgeon is notified immediately. The nurse should cover the protruding coils of intestine with sterile towels or sterile dressings moistened with normal saline and check the patient's vital signs. The patient is observed for signs of impending shock. Reassurance and a calm, efficient atmosphere are provided to allay the anxiety and apprehension of the patient. The patient is advised to lie still and limit his movements while waiting for the surgeon. The surgical department is notified of the impending surgery. Gastric suction may be prescribed to relieve distention is order to avoid retching and further trauma to the wound.

The patient who has experienced wound dehiscence or wound evisceration or both is generally frightened and apprehensive. Even after the wound has been resutured, the patient may hesitate to move or to cough because he fears recurrence of the event. The nurse must provide reassurance and psychological comfort measures during this period. Otherwise the patient may suffer other complications related to inadequate ambulation and inadequate pulmonary ventilation subsequent to the second surgical procedure. Again, wound dehiscence is a source of discouragement and insecurity as the patient's progress is handicapped and hospitalization is prolonged.

Discharge Planning

The length of time a patient needs in order to recuperate from his operation depends on his preoperative physical and mental condition, the magnitude of the operation, and whether any postoperative complications develop. Preparation of the patient and his family for the patient's discharge is begun early in the postoperative period. Uncomplicated postoperative recovery usually requires a fairly short period of hospitalization. Patients are often discharged within 7 days, even after major surgery, thereby placing a greater responsibility on the nurse for early discharge planning.

The patient is instructed in all aspects of his postoperative management, including wound care, personal hygiene, proper nutrition, and appropriate types of activity, and he or she is advised that heavy lifting is generally to be avoided for a period of 6 weeks. The homemaker is given specific instructions about restrictions related to household management. For example, a female patient may assume that vacuuming and other light housekeeping may be appropriate fairly early in her recovery period, when these activities are actually contraindicated early in her convalescent period.

Patients who have had extensive surgery and altered physiologic functioning (colostomy, radical mastectomy) require specific and detailed instructions in management. These requirements are described in subsequent chapters.

At discharge, the patient is given specific instructions about when to see the surgeon after hospitalization. Patients who are unable to manage their recuperation adequately are referred to a home health care agency for continued supervision and follow-up care.

Cancer

The word **cancer** has various meanings; it is derived from the Latin word for crab. Its use in medical terminology is based on the similarity between the characteristics of a crab and the manner in which cancer invades adjacent tissue. Clinically, cancer is defined as a neoplastic process in which there is an uncontrolled proliferation of abnormal cells that interfere with normal functions and can spread into normal tissues throughout the body [287]. The malignant (uncontrolled) process may lead to a fatal outcome unless adequate therapy halts the process.

The term cancer has several conceptual meanings as well, including death, pain, mutilation, debilitation, and dependency. It is therefore important for the nurse to understand what the diagnosis of cancer means to the patient and his or her family in order to work effectively with them. In addition, the nurse must examine his or her own definition of cancer because the care given the patient is directly affected by the nurse's own attitude toward the disease.

Although cancer is the second leading cause of death in the United States and continues to affect 1 in 4 persons, a sense of hopelessness should not be a universal reaction to the diagnosis. Cancer is not a single disease, but rather many entities, most of which can be cured or controlled if detected in an early, localized stage. Advances in cancer prevention, early detection, and improved treatment modalities have made an impact on the survival status of many cancer patients.

In order to have a realistic approach to the care of patients with cancer, the nurse must understand (1) the nature of cancer, (2) the terminology of cancer, (3) the mechanisms of metastasis, (4) preventive and diagnostic methods, (5) carcinogenesis [those factors producing cancer], (6) the treatment modalities used to control cancer, and (7) the palliative measures available when cure is not feasible. In addition, the nurse must realize that successful treatment of the patient with cancer requires a team approach and open communication among the team members, the patient, and the patient's family. The following discussions are concerned with all these factors.

Terminology of Cancer

Oncology literally means "the study of tumors." In practice, however, the term has a broader meaning and includes all aspects relating to tumors, including the prevention, diagnosis, and treatment of patients with tumors (or neoplastic disease). Oncologic nursing has become a specialty field for nurses and encompasses the areas of detection, prevention, diagnosis, direct nursing care, and research.

Neoplasia means "new tissue" and thus in-includes benign and malignant growths. A **neoplasm** is a mass of new and abnormal tissue and it is a term that is generally used interchangeably with the term **tumor**. Tumor, however, is a more inclusive term and technically is not synonymous with neoplasm. A tumor, for example, is an abnormal swelling due to an increased number of cells, but it also may be an accumulation of blood or fluid in a localized area, as in injuries or inflammatory processes. In practice tumor is frequently used to mean both benign and malignant neoplasms.

The term **benign neoplasm** implies that the neoplasm is relatively harmless as compared to a malignant neoplasm because benign neoplasms are not recurrent and do not progress to other sites. All benign neoplasms cannot be considered relatively harmless, however. Depending on the location of the benign neoplasm, this space-occupying lesion may press on vital structures (e.g., a vital artery) and interfere with essential functions. Thus a benign neoplasm may precipitate a fatal outcome.

A **malignant neoplasm** is a potentially life-threatening condition. Yet some malignant neoplasms are characteristically slow growing and less likely to metastasize, so that their threat may not be as great as that of the type of benign neoplasm discussed above. Table 1-2 indicates the primary differences that distinguish benign neoplasms from malignant ones. The reader is reminded, however, that the differentiation between these two categories is not always clear-cut. It is therefore important to remember that there are exceptions to general categories and that some benign neoplasms may even become malignant. An example is the relatively high incidence of malignant transformations of benign epithelial papillomas of the colon, specifically the villous pattern. In addition, for unknown reasons, individuals also show a great variance in their response to specific neoplasms.

Neoplasms are named according to the site of origin or the type of tissue involved. There are at least 100 different types of cancer, and they are classified by their microscopic appearance and by site of origin. Table 1-3 classifies selected examples of common types of tumors. The suffix *-oma*, which denotes a tumor, is attached to the root word that iden-

Table 1-2
Selected characteristics of benign and malignant neoplasms

Benign neoplasm	Malignant neoplasm
Cells in tumor are fairly well differentiated; appear typical with well-organized, orderly growth pattern	Cells are atypical and vary in abnormality from well-differentiated to anaplastic stages; disorderly patterns of growth with many mitotic figures*
Generally encapsulated. If not encapsulated, there usually is a well-defined area around the lesion with sharply circumscribed margins	Rarely encapsulated
Remains localized at site of origin; does not have the ability to metastasize	Frequently metastasizes
Tends to grow slowly but steadily. Growth is usually limited, although some benign ovarian cysts grow to large size	Tends to grow rapidly but erratically; rate of growth varies with type of lesion, and some grow slowly
Tends to grow by expansion and causes pressure effects	Tends to infiltrate normal tissue* and to grow by expansion
Rarely recurs after removal; cured by total excision	Frequently recurs
Slowly progressive and may remain stationary or regress	Usually fatal if untreated

*Anaplasia (primitive, embryonic-type and poorly differentiated cells) and evidence of invasion of normal tissues are the major criteria by which a diagnosis of cancer is made in a primary lesion. Sometimes it is extremely difficult, if not impossible, to determine whether a tumor is malignant or benign.

Table 1-3
Classification of selected neoplasms

Type of tissue	Benign	Malignant
Connective tissue		*Sarcomas*
Fibrous tissue	Fibroma	Fibrosarcoma
Cartilage	Chondroma	Chondrosarcoma
Bone	Osteoma	Osteogenic sarcoma
Fatty tissue	Lipoma	Liposarcoma
Muscle tissue		
Smooth muscle	Leiomyoma	Leiomyosarcoma
Striated muscle	Rhabdomyoma	Rhabdomyosarcoma
Endothelial tissue		
Blood vessels	Hemangioma	Angiosarcoma (or hemangiosarcoma)
Blood cells; lymphoid tissue		
Hematopoietic cells		Leukemia
Lymphoid tissue		Malignant lymphoma
		Lymphocytic leukemia
		Hodgkin's disease
		Reticulum cell sarcoma
Plasma cell		Multiple myeloma
Nervous tissue		
Nerve tissue	Neuroma	Neurofibrosarcoma
Glia		Glioma
Meninges	Meningioma	Malignant meningioma
Epithelial tissue		*Carcinomas*
Squamous cells	Squamous cell papilloma	Squamous cell carcinoma
Basal cells		Basal cell carcinoma
Gland cells	Adenoma	Adenocarcinoma
Liver cells	Liver cell adenoma	Hepatocellular carcinoma (commonly termed hepatoma)
Lung		Bronchiogenic carcinoma
Placental epithelium	Hydatidiform mole	Choriocarcinoma
Mixed tumors; compound tumors (tumors derived from one type of neoplastic cell, from one or more germ layer)	Teratoma	Malignant teratoma

tifies the cell type of tumor origin. For example, a tumor arising in fibrous tissue is a **fibroma** and one in a gland is an **adenoma**. This rather simplified explanation is not universally applicable, however. As illustrated in the classification of benign tumors of epithelial origin, some tumors are classified on the basis of their microscopic patterns, others on their macroscopic patterns, and still others by the cells of origin [286].

Malignant neoplasms are either carcinomas or sarcomas, and these terms are incorporated into the nomenclature along with the term denoting cell type. A **carcinoma** is a cancer of epithelial cells, which comprise the skin and linings of organs. A **sarcoma** is a cancer of connective tissue such as muscle, bone, and cartilage. Thus, an **adenocarcinoma** is a lesion in which neoplastic epithelial cells grow in glandular patterns. These guides to the nomenclature are not consistently followed in practice however. For example, **malignant melanoma** is commonly used in lieu of the term melanocarcinoma, and **hepatoma** is commonly used to denote carcinoma of hepatic cell origin in preference to the term hepatocellular carcinoma. **Lymphomas** are malignant tumors of lymphoid tissue. Malignant tumors of the lymphoid and hematopoietic system are classified as sarcomas.

Nature of Cancer

As described earlier, all cells have the inherent ability to divide and multiply. In normal cellular proliferation, the process is controlled and is initiated by an appropriate stimulus, as in injury with the normal cellular response for wound healing. In addition, normal cellular proliferation ceases when the need for new tissue has been met. These cells are typical of the tissue from which they arise and are capable of carrying out the specialized function of the normal functioning tissue. These characteristics are defined as differentiated cells.

Cellular proliferation is abnormal when it occurs without an appropriate stimulus and when it is not needed by the body. In fact, neoplasms grow without regard for the needs of the body and often interfere with the normal functioning of specific body organs. Besides serving no useful purpose, malignant neoplasms frequently grow at the expense of normal tissues by utilizing essential nutrients and depriving normal cells of these nutrients. A person with a malignant neoplasm is frequently malnourished and debilitated in appearance.

Theoretically, cancer arises when a single normal cell changes into a malignant neoplastic cell, either by natural mutation (genetic alterations) or following chemical, viral, or radiation induction. Although it is not known exactly how the change occurs, it is felt that disturbances in the regulatory functions of the nucleic acids DNA and RNA are involved in the malignant process. In the normal development of various organs and body parts, cells undergo differentiation in size, appearance, and arrangement. Under morphologic examination such cells can be readily identified as originating from a specific organ or body part and are thus classified as well differentiated. Although the cells in some malignant neoplasms are fairly typical in appearance, others may be so abnormal and immature that they lack any resemblance to healthy or normal cells. This loss of differentiation is termed **anaplasia.** The extent of the loss of differentiation is a factor used in determining the degree of malignancy of the tumor. A neoplasm with poorly differentiated (or undifferentiated) cells carries a poorer prognosis than a neoplasm composed of well-differentiated cells having infrequent mitoses and a slow growth rate.

In addition to the **parenchyma** (proliferating neoplastic cells), neoplasms are composed of a supporting structure known as the stroma. The **stroma** is composed of connective tissue, blood vessels, and lymphatics. Neoplasms with stromal proliferation of connective tissue create firm, hard **scirrhus** masses. In some cases the stroma of the tumor contains an infiltrate of lymphocytes, plasma cells, and histiocytes which is thought to be an immunologic reaction against the tumor.

Mechanisms of Metastasis

Malignant neoplasms have the ability to **metastasize** (grow in separate and distinct sites from the primary lesion). Metastasis may occur via any one of four processes: (1) direct extension or infiltration into adjacent tissues, (2) lymphatic spread to distant organs, (3) hematologic dissemination, and (4) implantation. Of these processes, lymphatic spread is the most commonly occurring type of metastasis.

Cancer cells invade the lymphatic vessels and spread to local lymph nodes by embolization. Lymphatic spread tends to follow the natural drainage pathways, as demonstrable by axillary node involvement from a primary cancer of the breast. Cancer cells may bypass regional nodes or pass through without entrapment [287].

Cancer cells may penetrate the wall of an organ and invade local contiguous organs, generally following the path of least resistance. Thus, tumors of the bone are unlikely to penetrate beyond the confines of the periosteum but rather grow within the marrow cavity.

During a surgical diagnostic or therapeutic procedure, fragments of cancer cells may be carried from the original site and be transplanted to another site. This outcome may occur via the surgical instruments or via the surgeon's gloved hands. Several measures are necessary to prevent such iatrogenic spread of the cancer. Tumors must be manipulated or palpated gently. Care is taken to prevent the release of cancer cells into the bloodstream. For example, arteries and veins of a tumor are ligated before the tumor is manipulated. In some settings, precautions are taken during the surgical procedure itself by removing all instruments contaminated with cancer cells prior to closure, following radical surgery, in order to prevent implantation in another area, including the incision. The surgical wound may also be irrigated with distilled sterile water or antineoplastic agents prior to closure. Judicious handling of the primary cancer site can decrease the likelihood of metastasis by minimizing the shedding of tumor cells. The potential for shedding tumor cells is also the basis for the use of preoperative radiation to inactivate tumor cell activity and facilitate removal of the involved organ without transplanting tumor cells to other sites.

Veins and capillaries may be penetrated by the cancer cells and transmit the cancer to other organs, depending on the venous drainage patterns. For example, cancer of the digestive tract is carried by the portal vein to the liver. Hematologic dissemination appears to be an important factor in metastasis to the five most common sites; the lung, the liver, the lymph nodes, bone, and the brain. Lung tumors may metastasize via the arterial system and frequently spread to the brain because of the high rate of blood flow to the cerebrum. Some types of cancer, such as cancer of the breast, may metastasize to various organs, including the bone, the lung, the brain, or the liver. The spleen is infrequently involved in metastasis, although it is often involved in lymphomas.

Certain types of cancer are less likely to metastasize than are other types. This fact is important to consider in determining the implications of a diagnosis of cancer. For example, basal cell carcinoma of the skin grows very slowly and does not invade the blood and lymph vessels, nor does it metastasize to other parts of the body. Thus, basal cell carcinoma has a high cure rate. Breast and lung cancer and adenocarcinoma of the stomach and colon, however, are unpredictable and may invade and metastasize early.

Malignant neoplasms are generally classified according to a staging procedure. The purpose in staging cancer is to obtain a concise description of the apparent extent of the disease as a basis for facilitating communication, in determining the prognosis, in planning appropriate treatment protocols, and in evaluating the effect of treatment. **Clinical staging** is done by using various tests and examinations of accessible sites. **Surgical staging** requires surgical procedures such as biopsies and exploratory surgery for cancer at inaccessible sites to determine whether the cancer has spread and to which sites. These techniques are followed by pathologic or histologic staging for confirmation of the clinical diagnosis.

Staging is a uniform international classification system and should not be confused with the grading of a tumor. The grading procedure is a histologic designation and is dependent on the examining pathologist's judgment and skill. Staging classifications may vary according to the type of organ involved. For example, classification of cancer of the bladder by the Jewett method is done according to the involvement of bladder layers and lymph nodes. Staging in Hodgkin's disease and lymphomatosis is discussed in Chapter 5.

The use of staging can be illustrated by the usual method for staging cancer of the cervix. The stages are as follows:

Stage 0 Preinvasive carcinoma, located on the surface of the cervix; termed carcinoma in situ.
Stage I Invasive carcinoma, but confined to the cervix.
Stage II Cancer extends beyond the cervix, but not to the pelvic wall.
Stage III Carcinoma extends to the pelvic wall and/or involves the lower third of the vagina.
Stage IV Carcinoma has invaded the rectum and/or bladder beyond previously described limits; metastatic sites are present outside the true pelvis.

A new approach to the classification of tumors is the TNM staging system, which has evolved from collaboration of the International Union Against Cancer (UICC) and the American Joint Committee for Cancer Staging and End Stage Reporting (AJCCS). This system has three components: **T** for the primary tumor; **N** for regional nodes; and **M** for metastasis. These components may be further divided into subscripts to describe the progression of the disease (increases in tumor size) and the presence or absence of metastasis. Supplementary information utilizes symbols to designate specific radiologic study. Treatment is prescribed once the tumors have been staged clinically, surgically, and pathologically, using protocols as guidelines for tested treatment modalities.

Carcinogenesis

Although the specific cause of cancer is not known, considerable knowledge is available about **carcinogenesis,** the production of cancer. Carcinogens are agents that are capable of inducing cancer in man and animals and include viruses, chemicals, physical agents, and hormones. These agents require exposure over a sufficient period of time and usually in large enough doses. Environmental factors play a part in carcinogenesis, as verified by epidemiologic studies of the incidence of different types of cancer in various parts of the world. For example, there is a high incidence of cancer of the stomach in Japan, Iceland, and Finland and it is considered to be related to the high intake of smoked fish. Cancer of the colon is increasingly found in the United States and has recently been linked to the high fat content (particularly beef) in the diet. In addition, there is evidence that some cancers appear to have a familial tendency, as noted by the increased incidence of cancer of the breast in families and retinoblastoma in several members of one family. Thus there is increasing evidence that susceptibility to different types of cancer is to some extent under genetic control. Susceptibility to certain types of cancer is also related to age and sex.

The origin of various animal tumors has been linked to infection by RNA tumor viruses, as demonstrated by the onset of sarcomas and leukemias in chickens injected with viruses of cancerous tissues. Studies are being carried out to determine viral causes of human cancers, particularly in leukemia, breast cancer, and sarcomas. The Epstein-Barr virus, a type of herpesvirus, has been implicated in Burkitt's lymphoma and also in nasopharyngeal cancer. Cancer of the cervix is another type of cancer currently being studied for possible viral etiology. It is thought that viruses disturb metabolic processes of the cells, destroying the cells or adversely affecting the genetic code of the cells, thereby leading to the development of cancer.

Chemical carcinogens include a variety of substances, such as tar, soot, aniline dyes, the hydrocarbons in cigarette smoke, air pollutants, nickel, asbestos, and arsenicals. Industrial exposure to aniline dye has been implicated in the development of bladder cancer among aniline dye workers. Lung cancer has developed in persons inhaling asbestos and in workers in nickel mines. Vinyl chloride, which is used in making polyvinyl chloride plastic materials, has been linked to the development of hemangiosarcoma of the liver.

Smoking has long been implicated as a major causal factor in the development of lung cancer. Statistics have shown that habitual cigarette smokers have a higher incidence of lung cancer than do nonsmokers. Smoking has also been implicated in the development of cancer of the mouth, esophagus, and larynx. Air pollution caused by industrial wastes, automobile exhausts, and other sources have also played a part in the increased incidence of lung cancer.

Physical agents that have been identified as carcinogenic are ionizing radiation, ultraviolet rays, and sunlight. Ionizing radiation from x-rays or radioactive isotopes have been implicated in the development of leukemia as well as of other types of cancer. An increased incidence of skin cancer is found in persons whose skins are exposed to strong sunlight for extended periods. Skin cancer, for example, is more prevalent among rural inhabitants than among urban dwellers and is also more common in fair-skinned persons than in dark-skinned persons. Physical trauma has been implicated in carcinogenesis when long-term irritation and inflammation have contributed to neoplastic formation. An example of this is the onset of cancer of the oral cavity associated with long-term irritation from ill-fitting dentures. Often, patients will relate the incidence of a neoplasm to an injury. In reality, the injury causes the person to examine the site more closely, at which time a previously unnoticed growth is then detected.

Hormones have been implicated in the development of certain types of cancer. For example, substantial evidence has recently shown that administration of diethylstilbestrol (DES) during pregnancy may produce adenocarcinoma of the vagina in female offspring.

The nurse has a major role in educating the public about the dangers of carcinogenic agents. The nurse should also practice habits that prevent unnecessary exposure to these agents. Educational programs to reduce the number of smokers should be supported. Warning labels on cigarette packages about the tar and nicotine content have helped to discourage the use of cigarettes with higher tar content and have also encouraged persons to change to filtered cigarettes when unable to stop smoking.

Continued research on chemical carcinogenesis is one means of attacking the incidence of cancer by preventive methods. Adequate screening of chemicals should be done before new chemicals are used. Discovery of carcinogenic agents and subsequent control or elimination of these agents are important to reducing exposure and subsequent development of cancer. The Food and Drug

Administration (FDA) of the United States Department of Health, Education and Welfare conducts tests and evaluates the carcinogenic activity of chemical compounds including drugs, food additives, cosmetics, and insecticides. Legislation then follows to control or eliminate the use of agents identified as carcinogenic.

Cancer Detection and Diagnosis

The basic principle in any cancer control program is to find the patient with cancer in the early stage of the disease, before any metastasis occurs. Early detection of cancer as a method to attack the morbidity and mortality in cancer is facilitated by regular medical physical examinations, including various screening and diagnostic tests.

The nurse is in a unique case-finding position because of frequent contacts with many persons and increased opportunities to observe for signs of cancer. Utilizing knowledge of the most frequent sites of cancer and of carcinogenic factors, the nurse can identify high-risk persons. All nurses, not only those in cancer detection centers, should be oriented to educating the public in cancer prevention and detection. Increased awareness and skill in physical assessment should also contribute to the nurse's role in cancer detection. In addition to physical assessment skills, the nurse must combine skills of psychological comfort to provide emotional support to the person who is suspected of having cancer.

In screening patients for cancer, a thorough history will help to determine whether there is a strong family history of cancer. Questions should also disclose information on a family history of precancerous diseases such as familial polyposis and Gardner's syndrome, two types of colonic disease that predispose to cancer. A history of pernicious anemia or gastric atrophy or both, for example, is an important factor in the detection of stomach cancer. Social habits and environmental and occupational factors related to the individual's life should be investigated to determine patients with high risk for certain cancers. For example, the status of the respiratory system, including cytology of the sputum, of an individual who has been a heavy smoker for 20 years requires particular assessment. Women who start sexual activity early and have multiple partners and pregnancies are at risk for cancer of the cervix. Occupational exposure to carcinogenic chemicals such as asbestos, petroleum, and aniline dyes requires particular monitoring of the urinary and respiratory systems. Thus the history will give the examiner a high index of suspicion of cancer in certain situations. The history should include data on all the body systems, because a patient may forget to mention slight differences or changes until specifically asked about them. For example, a patient may not consider a slight change in bowel patterns an important factor to discuss until specifically asked about such a change.

The physical examination includes inspection and palpation of all accessible sites and orifices. Inspection and palpation of the skin surface emphasizes particularly those surfaces exposed to the sun or to frequent trauma or irritation, such as the lower lip in pipe smokers of long standing. The face is the most frequent site of skin cancers, and therefore these cancers are amenable to early detection. Skin cancer generally begins with a small painless sore that does not heal. The patient should be asked about the duration of any observable lesion.

About 90 percent of all cancers of the mouth are amenable to early detection because these are usually squamous cell carcinomas originating from surface epithelium and thus are accessible to visualization. A systematic examination of the mouth, combining visualization and digital palpation of the oral cavity, can be effective in detecting early, asymptomatic lesions. Clues from the history should alert the nurse to look for specific susceptible sites.

The fact that about 50 percent of all intraoral malignant lesions arise in the tongue mandates careful examination of the tongue. The finding of leukoplakia in the oral cavity is important, since this is considered a precancerous lesion. Small innocuous, macular, plaque-like, red velvety or keratotic lesions should arouse the examiner's suspicion. The larynx and surrounding areas are examined, and the node-bearing areas of the neck and the thyroid gland are palpated. Specific information on the assessment of the oral cavity, the head and neck, and the thyroid gland is given in subsequent chapters on the specific body systems.

The importance of an annual physical examination cannot be overemphasized in detecting asymptomatic or early cancer. Its value can be further illustrated in the early detection of breast cancer, cervical cancer, and colonic cancer.

Various methods are used to detect cancer of the breast at an early asymptomatic stage. The importance of monthly breast self-examination must be stressed, especially since most breast tumors are first discovered by the woman herself. The technique for self-examination of the breasts is described in Chapter 9. The nurse should assess the patient's knowledge and practice of self-examination and should use the examination as a time for reinforcing the proper technique. The breast should be examined in both a sitting and supine position. Although emphasis is placed on examination of the breast in female patients, the reader is reminded that men also have breast tissue and that palpation of the male breast is also indicated. If a lump or any breast abnormality such as asymmetry, nipple discharge, nipple retraction, skin retraction, or thickening or ulceration is detected, further diagnostic measures are indicated to determine what type of lesion is present. Any mass should be regarded as potentially cancerous until proved otherwise. Excisional biopsy or, in some cases, needle aspiration, is used to determine the type of lesion. Specific therapy is indicated by the biopsy results. Other screening techniques, which are adjuncts to the physical examination and breast self-examination, are mammography, xerography, and thermography. Even though there is controversy over the use of these procedures currently, a discussion is warranted.

Mammography is the radiographic examination of the soft tissue of the breast without the use of contrast medium. A low energy x-ray beam is used to outline the structure of the breast, to demonstrate the absence or presence of a breast lesion, and to determine whether the lesion is benign or malignant. The patient scheduled for a mammography should be advised that the procedure is essentially a painless one and does not require injection of a radiopaque substance. Films will be taken with the patient in a sitting position with the breast positioned on a small wooden block. Other films are taken while the patient is in a side-lying position and in a slightly rotated supine position. Some females have complained of discomfort in the breast during lengthy or repeated repositioning of the breast, which may be necessary in some situations. Otherwise there is no physical discomfort, although psychologically the patient may feel threatened and fearful of the results of the examination.

Mammography is most useful in detecting cancer in certain susceptible females with any of the following characteristics: familial history of breast cancer, previous breast biopsy or breast surgery, signs and symptoms of breast disease, previous mastectomy of the opposite breast, and large pendulous breasts that are difficult to examine by palpation. In addition, women who have never married or who have not lactated are more likely than other women to develop cancer of the breast and are candidates for mammography. Currently, the use of mammography is being challenged by some authorities who feel that the examination causes undue exposure to radiation and may actually cause breast cancer. The examination is not a routine screening test, however, and should be limited primarily to females over 35 years of age.

Thermography involves the use of heat-sensitive devices and an infrared camera to record areas of elevated skin temperature. Elevated skin temperature may be associated with cancer of the breast. The test requires complex interpretation, and there has been controversy over its usefulness.

Xerography, according to some authorities, gives a more detailed picture of a breast than mammography does. It is a xeroradiographic process, but a low dose of radiation is required.

The annual physical examination (or more often when indicated in selected susceptible females) should always include a pelvic examination and a cervical smear for cytologic examination. The smear must be fixed with either alcohol or a commercial fixing agent to assure an adequate specimen. The patient is asked about the presence of any vaginal discharge as well as about her menstrual pattern. Even a small amount of bleeding in the postmenopausal patient is an important and significant sign.

The **Papanicolaou smear** test involves aspiration of the vaginal pool that collects in the posterior fornix or upper third of the vagina and the swab or scraping technique of the cervix to obtain tissue specimens and aspirations from the external os. In some protocols a Schiller's test is done; an aqueous solution of iodine is used to stain the mucous membrane of the cervix. The Schiller test is used to identify specific abnormal sites for biopsy techniques, because abnormal tissue will not take the Schiller's stain. The Schiller's staining technique, however, is not specific for neoplastic epithelium. In addition to the specimen collection, the examination includes careful inspection of the external genitalia, examination of the cervix and vagina with a speculum (after a vaginal pool specimen has been taken), and bimanual palpation of the uterus and adnexa. The patient with abnormal cells requires a biopsy and other appropriate diagnostic procedures to determine a definite diagnosis and appropriate therapy. Other diagnostic methods such as colposcopy, laparoscopy, and exploratory laparotomy are discussed in Chapter 9.

The patient is thoroughly instructed in the purpose of these tests as well as in the procedures. Certain instructions are essential for accuracy of the smear collections. For example, the female scheduled for a Pap smear is instructed to eliminate douching for at least 24 hours prior to having the test. In addition, the nurse who shows awareness of the patient's anxiety about a possible diagnosis of cancer in relation to diagnostic tests consistently provides psychological support and comfort. Opportunities for patient teaching regarding personal hygiene and cancer detection methods should be utilized.

Exfoliative cytology, as accomplished in cervical smear diagnostic methods, is based on the examination of cells shed from the surface of certain tissues into body cavities. The technique is also used in examining the cells of other orifices, such as sputum, mouth smear, gastric washings, and nipple discharge or ulceration.

A combined rectovaginal examination of the pelvis in the female will provide an opportunity to inspect the perianal area via digital examination and to palpate for a retroflexed uterus; the uterus is otherwise nonpalpable. Digital examination of the rectum is also essential in male patients to determine the status of the prostate gland (irregularities or unusually firm areas) and also to evaluate the presacral and perirectal tissues. A rectal examination and proctosigmoidoscopy is generally recommended in both males and females over the age of 40 as a part of the annual physical examination. These procedures are an essential part of any cancer detection program since 70 to 75 percent of colon and rectal cancers can be detected by these methods. The finding of abnormalities should be followed by a barium enema and biopsy of any lesions.

Certain basic laboratory tests are an essential part of a cancer detection examination. These tests include such laboratory examinations as hemoglobin level and hematocrit determination, white blood cell count and differential, urinalysis, and chest x-ray when indicated. The annual vaginal and cervical smear is essential for all females over the age of 20. A stool guaiac test for occult blood is also a screening test for the detection of colon and rectal cancer. Other diagnostic tests are done as indicated by specific findings during the screening examination. These tests include scans of specific organs, specific x-rays, and endoscopic examinations. Computerized tomography is another important diagnostic tool.

Although emphasis on detecting asymptomatic cancer has increased, public education regarding the seven danger signals of cancer is very important. The nurse should emphasize, however, that the seven danger signals may be indicative of diseases other than cancer and that only physical examination and specific diagnostic tests can validate the specific cause of the symptoms. Too often the fear of cancer prohibits a person from seeking further investigation of these early signs of cancer. It has been suggested that delay in seeking help on the recognition of symptoms of cancer appears to be a conscious and deliberate act rather than a failure to perceive the symptom or to comprehend its consequences [257]. The importance of the annual physical examination, even in the absence of symptoms, cannot be overemphasized. The seven danger signals are identified by the American Cancer Society as follows:

Change in bowel or bladder habits
A sore that does not heal (especially a painless one)
Unusual bleeding or discharge
Thickening or lump in breast or elsewhere
Indigestion or difficulty in swallowing
Obvious change in wart or mole
Nagging cough or hoarseness

The public must be educated more effectively toward reducing the fear of cancer and emphasizing the importance of seeking medical assistance immediately on detection of one of these signs. The threat of cancer causes various reactions. Some people fear the radical types of treatment often required for cancer and seek unproved cancer remedies for a "miracle cure." Cancer quackery may promise such cures and may receive considerable publicity and support even from influential citizens. An example of such an unproved method of cancer remedy can be illustrated by the lengthy controversy over the use of the drug Krebiozen (Carcalon). Extensive federal investigation of this drug has cited it as having no anticancer activity, although it has been widely supported and used. The tragedy of cancer quackery is that the patient who uses these unproved methods delays seeking appropriate therapy until the cancer has progressed beyond control and spends considerable money in the process. In addition, some of these remedies may be dangerous. An example is Laetrile (amygdalin), which has been promoted as an anticancer agent even though it has been shown that amygdalin, which is obtained from apricot seeds, may break down into a toxic agent, cyanide.

The nurse has an important role in educating the public about the dangers of using unproved remedies and in publicizing the characteristics of quacks in order to help patients avoid seeking their help. Secrecy about the treatment and guarantees that a cure in all or at least a vast majority of cases treated has been achieved are major characteristics that should lead one to suspect the remedy. The nurse should also be supportive of patients during the long and uncomfortable phases of conventional treatment in order to prevent their becoming discouraged and susceptible to quackery.

The National Cancer Institute of the National Institutes of Health is the central focus of government-supported research in cancer and coordinates both federal and nonfederal research programs, and the national program against cancer. The National Cancer Act of 1971 further expanded the National Cancer Program to establish better connections between cancer research and its clinical application. The program is designed to reduce the incidence, morbidity, and mortality in human cancer. Two types of cancer centers have been developed at selected sites across the country. These types are the **comprehensive center** to conduct long-term multidisciplinary programs in cancer biomedical research, cancer clinical services and investigations, cancer training and education and community programs of cancer diagnosis, epidemiology, and preventive medicine, and the **specialized center** with programs in one or more but not all of the aspects listed for the comprehensive center [253].

The American Cancer Society is a nongovernmental agency which finances research, produces educational materials for both professionals and the public, and offers certain patient services. It also offers supportive services to patients through its volunteer visitor programs, and some chapters of the society provide equipment and supplies needed by individual patients.

Treatment of Cancer

The four modes of therapy used in cancer management are (1) surgical intervention, (2) radiation therapy, (3) chemotherapy, and (4) immunotherapy. It seems appropriate to add supportive therapy as a fifth mode. Supportive therapy includes pain relief and blood transfusions. The type of tumor, the site of origin, and the anatomic extent of the disease are the factors that determine the treatment approach and whether a combination of treatment modalities is indicated.

SURGICAL INTERVENTION

Surgical intervention is the most frequently used primary treatment of cancer and it may be curative, palliative (or supportive), or preventive. Surgical techniques are also used in diagnosing the condition. Surgical excision is used for biopsy techniques. Biopsy may also be done by needle aspiration in some cases. Exploratory laparotomies are also done in diagnostic staging of lymphomas, Hodgkin's disease, and other cancers. Surgery is also an important aspect of cancer prevention as illustrated in the surgical removal of conditions that predispose to cancer, such as polyps in the colon, ulcerations, and moles.

Improved surgical techniques and postoperative management have facilitated the use of aggressive surgery to eradicate cancer cells or to provide palliation. Extensive operations, often viewed as mutilating procedures, such as resection of multiple organs, hemipelvectomy, and pelvic exenteration, are being accomplished. The potential effects of these extensive operations are evaluated in light of unacceptable complications, functional morbidity, and mortality. Radical surgery should not be such that the patient's recovery is jeopardized, either physiologically or psychologically. At the same time, surgery should not be so limited that recurrence occurs because inadequate but expendable tissue was not removed. The patient must be informed of the risks of aggressive surgery, as well as of the meaning of expected physiologic alterations, in addition to being informed of the risks associated with less aggressive treatment. For example, the patient for whom pelvic exenteration is indicated is advised that both a fecal stoma and a stoma for urinary diversion are created in this operation.

Total rehabilitation after extensive surgery for cancer requires the specialized resources of various professional personnel working together in a team approach. This approach also utilizes volunteers and nonprofessional persons from programs such as the Reach to Recovery of the American Cancer Society. This team approach is exemplified in the patient who requires extensive head and neck surgery and subsequent reconstructive surgery. The expertise and emotional support from various professional staff, including the specialist in prosthesis construction, are essential components of a therapeutic and rehabilitative approach to this type of curative surgery. The skills and expertise of the surgeon and the nurse are inadequate if cosmetically and functionally acceptable prostheses are not available to the patient with extensive facial and oral surgery. Total rehabilitation is also inhibited unless the patient and family are included in all phases of the treatment period.

The surgical technique is dependent on the findings at the time of surgery as well as on the preferred approach of the individual surgeon. Cancer of the breast, for example, may be treated by lumpectomy (removal of only visible tumor), by simple mastectomy (amputation of the breast), or by radical mastectomy (removal of the breast, pectoral muscles, and the axillary lymph nodes). Studies are being done currently to compare the effectiveness of each of these approaches in preventing recurrences. Controversy still surrounds the use of lumpectomy procedures. In addition to the previously mentioned approaches to surgical treatment of cancer of the breast, either prophylactic oophorectomy (removal of the ovaries) or irradiation of the ovaries may be the treatment of choice in the premenopausal patient with cancer of the breast. These procedures eliminate hormonal stimulation and inhibit the growth of cancer cells that may have already spread to other areas of the body. Additional surgery may include bilateral adrenalectomy or hypophysectomy (removal of the pituitary gland). The pituitary hormone causes the adrenal glands to secrete estrogen as a compensatory mechanism after the ovaries have been removed. The pituitary gland also seems to direct hormonally dependent cancers to distant sites in the body. Thus, hypophysectomy may be indicated to retard metastasis and to provide relief of pain for the patient with advanced cancer of the breast.

Surgical excision of malignant neoplasms in their early stages has the greatest potential as a curative measure. Curative surgery assumes the elimination of all cancer cells and the absence of recurrence of the disease for over 5 years after the initial treatment. Generally, a margin of healthy tissue is also removed in these surgical resections in order to assure prevention of metastasis. The lymph nodes that drain the area of the primary site as well as the tumor itself are removed when metastasis through the lymphatic system is questionable or likely. Surgical intervention is the primary form of treatment for cancer of the colon and rectum, the breast, the stomach, the uterus, and other organs. Specific surgical procedures are discussed in subsequent chapters in relation to the specific body systems.

In addition to surgical resection, **cryosurgery** is being utilized in the treatment of certain types of cancer. This technique, which destroys tumors by freezing them with liquid nitrogen, is being used to treat cancer of the skin and mouth and other superficial cancers.

Even if a cure is not attainable, prolonged survival has been achieved with the use of aggressive surgical techniques. **Palliative surgery** attempts to treat the complications of cancer even when total removal of cancer cells is not possible. An example of palliative surgery is the surgical treatment of bowel obstruction by formation of a colostomy, or surgical correction of fistula formation associated with colonic cancer. Ostomy procedures have prolonged the lives of patients with cancer of the colon even when a cure is not possible. Palliative surgery also may be done to relieve pain caused by extension of a tumor pressing on surrounding nerves.

RADIATION THERAPY

The goal of radiation therapy is to destroy or inhibit the growth of cancer cells without causing irreparable damage to adjacent normal tissue. All radiation occurs in the form of waves of electromagnetic energy, which causes ionization on application to body tissues. Absorption of radiation energy results in suppression or cessation of cell mitosis, and disruption of oxygen and nutrients. The treatment is based on the principle that tissues with large numbers of dividing cells are more susceptible to ionizing radiation than are normal cells. Tumors are classified as being radiosensitive, moderately radiosensitive, and radioresistant. The type and extent of the tumor therefore determine the type of radiation therapy selected or if it is to be used at all. For example, the leukemias and lymphomas are radiosensitive. The lymphomas may be cured by radiation therapy as may certain local leukemias. Total body radiation therapy can bring about a remission in leukemia.

The patient may receive radiation therapy by one of three modes: (1) **external beam** therapy delivered by the conventional orthovoltage machine, which is used in treating superficial lesions as deep as 4 to 5 cm, or the supervoltage machines such as the betatrons, cobalt 60, cyclotrons, or linear accelerators (these latter machines have an energy greater than 1 million electron volts, also known as 1 mev), (2) **sealed internal radiation** in the form of either temporary or permanent implantations, or (3) **unsealed** internal or systemic radiation therapy by means of one of several radionuclides (radioisotopes).

The term **radiation** usually incites fear in the patient and his family. The destructive effects of radiation are well known, and many patients find it difficult to comprehend its potential therapeutic effect. In addition, patients often fear that they will become radioactive and thus will endanger others.

Some patients also view radiation therapy as a measure of last resort in terminal cancer. The patient's understanding and perception of radiation therapy should be discussed in order to prepare him adequately for the type of therapy he is to undergo.

The nurse should understand the principles of self-protection from radiation exposure. The maximum permissible dose for radiation workers is 5 rem (roentgen equivalent man) for persons over the age of 18 as established by the International Committee on Radiation Protection. The measurement **rem** refers to a unit of radiation dose equivalent to biologic effectiveness. Nurses and other personnel who frequently care for patients receiving radiation therapy wear film badges or docimeters to record their exposure to radiation. Time, distance, and shielding measures to prevent excessive exposure to radiation include the limiting of time in contact with the radiation source, increasing the distance from the source, and storing radioactive materials in lead containers.

Radiation therapy may be used as a single treatment with a goal of cure, as in patients with early Hodgkin's disease, cancer of the cervix, or certain head and neck cancers. Radiation therapy has proved to be successful in extending survival for 5 years or more in at least 90 percent of men with seminoma of the testes, 80 percent of children with retinoblastoma, 75 percent of patients with Hodgkin's disease, and about 50 percent of patients with squamous cancer of the cervix or cancer of the nasopharynx, if the disease is detected early [246]. Radiation therapy may be the preferred treatment in cases in which surgical excision of the tumor may result in loss of function of an organ. Such a situation occurs in cancer of the larynx detected at an early stage. The voice function is preserved when radiation is used, whereas surgical treatment may also be successful but results in loss of the voice function. Radiation therapy may also be the preferred treatment when certain brain lesions are not accessible by surgical techniques.

Radiation therapy may also be used in combination with surgery, preferably preoperatively. At this stage the goal is to inhibit metastasis by destroying peripheral cells of the involved organ and to shrink the tumor to facilitate surgical removal. Postoperatively, radiation may be used when a primary lesion is removed but lymph nodes cannot be resected. Preoperative radiation is preferred because metastasis may increase as a result of tumor manipulation during surgery. Radiation may also be used as palliative therapy to produce symptomatic relief of pain in skeletal metastasis, as in advanced cancer of the breast.

Toxic effects, known as radiation sickness, are characterized by anorexia, nausea, vomiting, diarrhea, general malaise, lethargy, and weakness. The symptoms are generally related to the dose of radiation administered, as well as the type and volume of tissue being treated. Discontinuance of the therapy, or at least reduction in dosage, may be required. Nursing care involves protecting the patient from the toxic effects of radiation therapy by providing adequate nutritional intake via high caloric and high protein diets, drug therapy (antiemetics) to counteract nausea and vomiting, meals at preferred times, and adequate rest. Conservation of energy is a major aspect of the patient's tolerance for radiation therapy and the nurse must assist the patient in finding ways to do this appropriately. Intake of adequate fluids is encouraged to facilitate the elimination of uric acid, which increases from tumor breakdown, and pain medication is provided for alleviation of discomfort. People vary in their response to therapy, and some patients become discouraged when weakness and lethargy increase after therapy is started. Emotional support during this period is of paramount importance.

External Radiation Therapy

External radiation is applied via x-ray machines varying from conventional machines to those of megavoltage or supervoltage capability. The latter machines include the linear accelerator, the Van de Graaff generators, the betatron, and the cobalt 60 or cesium 127 bombs. Dosages are prescribed in **rads,** units of absorbed dose of ionizing radiation. The machines are large and complex pieces of equipment that are frightening to the patient who has to lie beneath them in a room all by himself. The major role of the nurse in working with the patient who is to undergo external radiation treatment is to orient the patient to the purpose of the therapy and to the procedure. Prior to the first treatment, it is especially helpful if personnel spend time in the treatment room with the patient before the initiation of therapy. This time will enable the patient to examine the surroundings, ask questions, and become familiar with the machine before being left alone. He is instructed to remain in the exact position he is placed to ensure that the proper site for the therapy is reached, and shielding is provided for nontreated sites. The patient is also advised that the intercommunication system will enable him to communicate with the technicians outside the room.

Patients are usually tired after the treatment and should be provided with rest. Usually radiation therapy is prescribed four to five times weekly; the actual treatment period takes only a few minutes.

While the machine is functioning, no personnel are allowed in the therapy room. A viewing screen or television monitoring system permits observation of the patient during treatment. Once the treatment is over, there is no danger to the personnel. The patient receiving external radiation is not a source of radioactivity. A major advantage of the megavoltage or supervoltage machines is that they are more penetrating and less likely to injure the surface skin layer than in conventional x-ray therapy. Megavoltage radiation also has better-defined, sharper beam edges and is thus less injurious to bone tissue. In order to reach the specific organ involved, however, external radiation techniques also affect other normal tissues exposed to the field of treatment. These tissues primarily include the skin, mucous membrane, fat, connective tissue, muscle, bone, and cartilage. Bone marrow depression is a complication of radiation therapy, requiring consistent monitoring of blood counts and platelet levels. The nurse must protect the patient from infection and teach the patient these protective measures. If thrombocytopenia occurs, the patient must be protected from injury and bleeding. Blood transfusions are given for severe anemia.

An adequate nutritional intake may be difficult to achieve if radiation is being administered to the abdominal area, with resultant nausea and vomiting or diarrhea. Monitoring of the patient's weight is important in evaluating the adequacy of nutritional intake. If the oral cavity is being treated, oral hygiene is essential to counteract the dry mouth, the difficulty in swallowing, the sore throat, and the metallic taste or loss of taste associated with the therapy. Mild mouthwashes and local analgesics such as anesthetic sprays may be useful. A high pressure dental-type of spray utilizing one-half strength hydrogen peroxide and water is particularly effective in cleaning the mouth of patients with malignant oral tumors and those receiving radiation to the oral cavity. The treated mucous membrane is particularly sensitive to irritants such as alcohol, cigarettes, and hot or spicy foods. All these products should be eliminated from the diet of these patients. A soft bland diet, with nutritious liquid supplements, is most palatable at this time. Dental caries may occur with oral radiation; often, teeth that are in poor condition are removed prior to initiation of oral radiation therapy.

In addition to these reactions to external radiation therapy, skin reactions occur. Local skin reactions, which are characterized by redness, burning, itching, and dryness, are usual and expected. These reactions should not be referred to as burns, because this description implies overradiation, which is not the case. Several precautions related to skin care are necessary. The area to be treated is marked with indelible ink by the radiologist to serve as a guide for treatment. The patient is cautioned not to wash the marks off. Mild soap and water may be used to clean the area, but massaging, rubbing, or scrubbing should be avoided to prevent skin irritation and breakdown. In some institutional protocols, even water is not allowed on this area.

Medications, lotions, or ointments are not applied to the skin being irradiated because they interfere with the effects of the radiation therapy and irritate the skin. If the skin is not broken and is not moist and weeping, cornstarch may be applied lightly to the area several times a day to control the itching sensation but should be discontinued immediately if the skin becomes broken. If the skin should blister, peel, or crack the radiologist should be consulted for specific treatment.

If the head and neck area is being treated, the use of cosmetic creams is restricted. If the scalp is being exposed to radiation, the use of dyes, color shampoos, and permanents is prohibited. If the axillary area is being treated, deodorants should not be used.

The patient is advised to protect the radiated skin from irritation due to exposure to the sun or to extreme cold. Heat therapies, such as sunlamps, hot water bottles, heating pads, or electric blankets should not be used on these areas. The patient is warned that skin exposed to x-ray therapy is sensitive and susceptible to skin reactions, and is cautioned about avoiding injury, friction, or infection. No adhesive or cellophane tape should be used on the area being treated. Loose-fitting clothing should be used; tight girdles, for example, are contraindicated when the abdomen is being irradiated.

In addition to skin reactions, fatigue and other effects may occur, depending on the site being treated. For example, pelvic radiation may cause cystitis with bleeding and burning sensations. Radiation to the scalp will cause alopecia if the hair roots are destroyed. Pneumonitis often occurs when the chest area is treated. The nurse should specifically observe for anticipated skin reactions as well as for untoward reactions related to the specific sites being irradiated.

Internal Sealed Radiation Therapy

Radium is a radioactive material that emits gamma rays (as well as alpha and beta rays) and is used primarily for internal implantation for a specified period of time. Other sealed sources of radionuclides used for temporary implants include cobalt 60 and cesium 137. Radium, in the form of sealed sources such as wires, seeds, needles, plaques, tubes, or applicators, is inserted into body cavities such as the vagina or the nasopharynx. Radium needles are implanted to treat some cancers of the upper lip, oral cavity, and the tongue.

One of the most frequent uses of radium therapy is the temporary implantation of radium in cancer of the cervix. The dosage is prescribed in milligram hours, which refers to the effect produced on a specific area by 1 mg of radium for 1 hour (e.g., 100 mg radium left in place for 48 hours results in a total dosage of 4,800 mg hours of radium). Radium implantation creates a hazard for nursing personnel, because of gamma ray emission, until the source is removed from the patient and from the room. This hazard requires that personnel adhere to the principles of time, distance, and shielding when caring for the patient with a radium implant. A film badge or dosimeter is worn by persons who frequently work with cancer patients receiving internal radiation therapy. Pregnant nurses should not be assigned to patients receiving radium therapy, and nurses caring for these patients should rotate their assignments regularly.

Patients with radium implants frequently fear that they are a hazard to others. Visitors should be instructed to limit their time at the patient's bedside while the implant is in place. Pregnant women and children are not permitted to visit. The patient should be forewarned that nursing care will be minimal but that all essential care will be given while the implant is in place, and also that efforts will be made to spend appropriate time with him or her to prevent excessive isolation. Backrubs are omitted. Linen is changed only if necessary; perineal care is omitted in patients with a vaginal implant, unless absolutely necessary. The patient should understand that nurses or personnel who work frequently with patients receiving radiation therapy are required to protect themselves from excessive exposure by adhering to the principles of time, distance, and shielding. The patient with a radium implant is generally placed in a private room or in a room with patients who are past the childbearing age and require minimal care or other patients with radium implants.

Many patients feel that radiation is the last resort for extensive disease and will need to be informed that frequently it is the preferred treatment. The physician should thoroughly orient the patient to the expectations for the treatment. If the therapy is in reality a palliative one, this information should be given to the patient.

In the case of cervical radium implantation, the patient is advised of the need for bed rest and restricted movement in order to prevent displacement of the implant. The head of the bed is generally kept flat or limited to an elevation of 15 degrees. Turning is done in a log-rolling fashion.

An enema and a douche are given preoperatively. Perineal skin shaving and the usual preoperative routines such as restriction of oral intake and preoperative sedation are followed. A Foley catheter is inserted to prevent bladder distention and possible displacement of the radium applicator. The patient is taught not to touch, displace, or remove the applicator once it is in place.

Various types of radium applicators are used. Afterloading applicators permit more convenient radium insertion and limit radiation exposure in the operating room, recovery room, and x-ray room. In this technique the applicator (ovoid or tandem) is inserted in the operating room, an x-ray is then taken to determine its position, and the radium is later inserted into the applicator either in a treatment room or in the patient's room.

An appropriately tagged and identified radium carrier and long forceps are kept in the patient's room in case of accidental displacement and for subsequent removal of the implant. The room and the bed of the patient are clearly marked with specific instructions and information about the length of time the implant is to be retained. When the patient returns from the operating room, the position of the applicator is checked, vital signs are taken, and the patient is made comfortable. Precautions and instructions about activity are repeated. The number of applicators and the prescribed time for therapy should be noted. The position of the applicators should be checked at least every 4 hours. The functioning of the retention catheter should be monitored.

The patient is observed for symptoms of elevated temperature, nausea, vomiting, and malaise, which indicate radiation reactions or infection. If these symptoms occur, the physician is notified for directions for treatment of the symptom or early removal of the implant or both. The physician should be notified also of any suspicious vaginal drainage that may indicate the formation of vesicovaginal fistulas.

Although linens, bandages, and forceps are not contaminated by contact with the applicators, tubes, seeds, or wires, they are checked for the presence of applicators that may have become dislodged or accidentally removed. Frequently, linens and all other materials are kept in the patient's room until all the radium has been removed and accounted for. No special waste precautions are necessary since no secretions or discharges from patients being treated with sealed sources of radiation are contaminated. Urine and feces are removed in the usual manner, but the bedpan is checked for any sign of an applicator.

When the radium is removed (or when it has been accidentally removed), it should be immediately placed into the lead container. (The Radiation Safety Officer should be notified in case of accidental removal.) The radium should not be handled directly with the hands, but always with long-handled forceps, picking up the applicators by the string. All applicators should be accounted for. In some settings, x-rays are routinely ordered to verify that all applicators have been removed. If the patient with a vaginal implant should inadvertently get out of bed, there is a danger of loss or dislodgement with potential damage to normal structures. An x-ray should be taken immediately to determine if any of the applicators has changed position; the radium should be removed in this case.

After removal of the radium, the patient usually is given an enema, a douche, and a bath. If all the radium is accounted for, the patient is usually discharged from the hospital after several hours, assuming there is no excessive vaginal discharge or that the patient does not have difficulty in voiding after the catheter is removed.

As mentioned previously, other types of vehicles are used for radium implants in the treatment of cancer at various sites. The care will vary according to the site involved, but the nurse will still follow the principles of giving essential care and of time, distance, and shielding for protection against excessive radiation.

Internal Unsealed Radiation Therapy

Nurses are more familiar with the term **radioisotope** than with **radionuclide;** however, the latter term is preferred by nuclear medicine specialists and will be used in this chapter. A radionuclide is the nucleus of a chemical element plus its orbiting electrons that has become unstable and emits radiant energy. The action of a radionuclide in the body is the same as that of its stable form, the nuclide, in terms of absorption, distribution, biochemical effects, metabolism, and secretion, except that in the unstable form energy is emitted.

Institutions practicing nuclear medicine must be licensed by the Atomic Energy Commission and must have a Radiation Protection Supervisor who has the responsibility for establishing procedures for the safe use of all radioactive materials, including the storage, handling, and disposal of these agents. Nuclear medicine areas are identified with a three-bladed purple or magenta symbol on a yellow background.

Radionuclides are used for both diagnostic and therapeutic purposes. For diagnostic purposes, tracer doses are used. Tracer doses are administered either orally or by injection and then are located and traced by sensitive machines as the substance circulates and concentrates in particular organs and tissues. Extremely small doses of radionuclides are used for diagnostic purposes, so that patients who have received tracer doses are not in danger of cellular destruction. Nor are personnel caring for the patient in danger of exposure to the radionuclide.

A **scintillation scanner** is an instrument that records radioactivity for diagnostic purposes by measuring the uptake of a radioisotope by a specific organ. The technique is useful for identifying malignant growths and other lesions. The scanner is passed back and forth over the area of the body being studied and it records "hot" and "cold" areas on a graphic type of picture or recording. **Hot spots** are concentrations of the radionuclide at the site of a malignant growth; **cold spots** indicate a lack of concentration of the radionuclide in a specific area, as distinguished from the surrounding tissue, which does concentrate the substance. Thus scanning is based on the theory that radioactive substances are distributed uniformly throughout normal tissue of specific organs.

The greatest contribution of radionuclides is their ability to detect lesions in radiologically "nonaccessible" organs such as the pancreas and the spleen, as well as in the evaluation of parenchymal disease by means of scans of the kidney, liver, bone, and lung. The success of the scanning technique is dependent on visualizing differences in relative concentrations of gamma-emitting isotopes in specific tissues. The choice of radionuclide depends on the organ or system under study, the method of biologic transport of the radionuclide, and its degree of concentration within the organ [283]. In addition, the radionuclide chosen should have the least potential for damage to the target organ and the shortest possible half-life. Thus radionuclides are diagnostic when they are concentrated in a specific organ, such as radioactive iodine for the diagnosis of thyroid tumors, or if they are excreted by an organ. In addition, compounds may be tagged with the radionuclide to trace its path through a specific metabolic pathway, as in the use of vitamin B_{12} tagged with cobalt 60 in the diagnosis of pernicious anemia.

The scanning techniques are generally safe and pain-free procedures and cause limited discomfort, except for the prolonged length of time required to remain in a specific position during the procedure and the intravenous injection of the radionuclide.

The patient being oriented to the scanning technique, is advised as to how the isotope will be administered (either orally by capsule or liquid or intravenously, depending on the specific nuclide) and the time interval before the scan is actually done. (The time required for assimilation of the radionuclide varies according to the organ being examined, as well as the nuclide being used.) The patient is also advised about the scanner machine itself; it can be described as being similar to x-ray machines, with which most persons are familiar. Patients should be assured that the scanner will not touch them, which is a frequently expressed fear of many patients, and that the scanner simply receives the signals of the radionuclide and a picture or diagram is formed to indicate the distribution of the agent in the specific organ. Patients are also advised that no special precautions are required after the test, because only tracer doses of the specific radionuclide are used.

Two types of detectors are used for radionuclidic imaging. One is the rectilinear scanner, which moves back and forth across the specific area and records the concentration of radioactivity within or around the lesion by means of parallel lines. This picture takes approximately 5 to 45 minutes to be completed. In contrast to this technique, the stationary scanner or camera produces a rapid complete image of the entire organ or system at one time.

When therapeutic dosages of radionuclides are given, specific precautions are required, because the patient himself literally is a source of radioactivity as long as the injected radionuclide remains within his body and emanates rays of radiant energy. The nurse caring for this patient must therefore know the specific radionuclide that has been used; its half-life (the time it takes for one-half of the atoms in the radionuclide to decay, that is, to lose one-half its original energy); the mode of administration; the date of administration; the type of radiation emitted (gamma rays or beta particles); and the manner in which it is metabolized and excreted.

The patient who has received therapeutic doses of a radionuclide is isolated and his room is tagged with the radioactivity symbol. Specific precautions in the total care of this patient should be outlined and readily available on the patient's chart and in the hallway by the door of the patient's room. The nurse should quickly contact the specific radiation officer in the hospital in the event of contamination of the room or other articles by spillage of contaminated secretions.

The nurse should remember to abide by the principles of distance, time, and shielding in the care of these patients and should limit the length of time in close contact with the patient (i.e., within three feet of the patient). Patient care is given as rapidly as possible, but not at the sacrifice of quality as needed by the given patient. Rotation of personnel is adhered to, to avoid overexposure of individual staff members. The nurse should provide psychological support to the patient by explaining carefully the rationale for the radiation precautions and stress that the treatment and the precautions are a temporary measure. Telephone contacts, conversations over the intercom, and watching television or participating in other diversional activities are important factors in helping the patient to tolerate lengthy isolation. Plans for diversional activities should actually be made prior to treatment, so that the nurse and patient together can decide on significant and important activities.

Some of the commonly used radionuclides include but are not limited to the following: cobalt (^{60}Co), gold (^{198}Au), iodine (^{131}I), and phosphorus (^{32}P). Each one of these elements, or any others used, requires special precautions. It is the responsibility of the nurse working with the patient to follow institutional protocols for management of patients with specific radionuclide therapy. Therapeutic ^{131}I has a half-life of 8.1 days. About 50 percent of this substance will be excreted from the body within 24 hours, most of it in the urine and the rest in saliva and perspiration. It can also be excreted in vomitus and feces. Thus, the nurse must take precautions with urine, linens, and feeding utensils and plates when caring for a patient who has undergone ^{131}I therapy. (Rubber gloves should be worn when handling contaminated materials and isolation gowns should be worn as protective covering.) Usually, urine is collected into a shielded container to monitor radionuclide excretion and the patient is taught to collect the specimen. The patient is encouraged to drink at least 2,000 ml of water during the first 24 hours to aid the excretion of ^{131}I. Paper utensils are usually used for a specified time. The utensils and linens are collected in impermeable bags so that they can be checked for contamination prior to disposal or incineration. If gloves become contaminated, they are washed in soap and water before being removed.

Phosphorus 32 (^{32}P) produces only beta radiation. It is most frequently used to control effusions in body cavities, being instilled in a colloidal suspension form directly into the specific cavity. When this suspension has been instilled, the nurse should turn the patient every 10 to 15 minutes for the first two hours to ensure proper distribution of the fluid [238]. The patient does not create a radiation hazard to anyone working with him because of the limited range of beta radiation. However, if there is seepage or drainage from a wound at the site of instillation, the drainage will be contaminated. Evan's blue dye is usually added to ^{32}P so that it can be easily visualized by its blue stain on dressings and linen in case of seepage and subsequent contamination. The nurse should wear gloves whenever handling any material suspected of being contaminated and should contact the radiation officer about the contamination. Contaminated dressings, bedclothes, and other items are kept in impermeable bags (waxed, lined paper, or plastic) until monitored by the radiation safety officer prior to disposal.

Radioactive gold (^{198}Au) may be injected into either the pleural or the abdominal cavity although it is used less often because it may cause fibrosis. Spills of contaminated drainage may occur from the injection site or from drainage tubes in the cavity. The nurse should wear rubber or plastic gloves when wiping up small spills with disposable absorbing materials. Usually ^{198}Au is prepared so that it causes a purple stain, which can readily be identified on contaminated clothing or articles. The half-life of ^{198}Au is less than 3 days, so that the precaution period is relatively short.

Some patients may receive radionuclide therapy and be discharged shortly after the dose is administered. Such patients must be instructed carefully about measures to protect other members of their family while they still contain radioactive substances. The patient is advised to avoid holding children and to sleep alone, but is encouraged to participate in other usual family activities. Special precautions associated with specific types of radionucludes are also discussed with the patient. For example, if ^{131}I has been used, the patient should flush the toilet several times after use in order to dilute the potentially contaminated urine. The patient is also advised of the half-life of the specific radionuclide (which usually are those with short half-lives for patients being treated on an outpatient basis) so that he will know when precautions can be discontinued.

Regardless of the type of radionuclide utilized, the nurse must always recognize the importance of obtaining essential information about the specific precautions in individual patient situations. Precautions should be followed explicitly to ensure that therapeutic results are obtained from the use of these agents without creating hazards for the personnel caring for the patient.

CHEMOTHERAPY

Another mode of therapy in the management of the patient with cancer is **chemotherapy,** the use of specific drugs. More than 40 drugs have been developed and have proved useful in some types of cancer in controlling the disease, in providing palliation by relieving pain, and in prolonging survival. Chemotherapy may be used as a single treatment modality in some situations or it may be combined with one or more of the other modalities.

Traditionally, chemotherapy has been used only in patients with disseminated or advanced disease, but its use is no longer limited. Currently, chemotherapy is being used as an early treatment method combined with surgery or radiation therapy or both, before symptoms of recurrence occur. This approach was initiated when evidence was accumulated that at the time of initial therapy with surgery or radiation, a large number of patients with solid tumors already had microscopic sites of metastatic cancer beyond the scope of the primary therapy. Relapses have occurred in patients who have been considered as having localized disease and have apparently been due to undetected metastasis at initial diagnosis and therapy. Chemotherapy in the early stages of the disease is indicated to destroy undetectable cancer cells throughout the patient's body. Some drugs are being utilized about 2 to 3 weeks postoperatively.

It is also felt that aggressive chemotherapy is better tolerated with less toxicity while the patient is asymptomatic and especially when the patient is able to tolerate a good oral intake. Disseminated disease results in anorexia and loss of adequate nutritional intake, which contributes to poor tolerance of chemotherapy.

Chemotherapy is making an impact in the management of patients with cancer by prolonging survival rates associated with certain types of cancer. For example, the use of chemotherapy is considered potentially curative in choriocarcinoma, with the use of high doses of methotrexate or actinomycin D or both. Remissions have also occurred with chemotherapy in the treatment of lymphomas, leukemias, and testicular tumors.

Chemotherapy may produce regression of primary tumors and may retard the development of secondary growths. Pain and other secondary effects of cancer may be relieved by these agents, improving the patient's wellbeing and the quality of his life.

Chemotherapeutic drugs used in the treatment of cancer include alkylating agents, antimetabolites, antibiotics, plant alkaloids, and hormones. Selected agents are listed in Table 1-4, including indications, precautions, and toxic effects.

The **alkylating** agents have a cytoxic effect and act on DNA in the cell nucleus to hinder cell growth and mitosis. **Antimetabolites** are synthetic substances such as purine or pyrimidine analogs or folic acid antagonists. These drugs are similar to the substances that nourish normal cells during growth and development. When antimetabolites are administered, they are taken up by cancer cells and interfere with the metabolic processes and the manufacture of protein in the malignant cells.

Antibiotics used in antineoplastic therapy interfere with RNA synthesis. **Plant alkaloids** act by interfering with mitosis during a specific stage (metaphase). L-Asparaginase is a unique cancer drug; it is an enzyme that depletes the supply of an essential amino acid, asparagine, in malignant cells. The natural and synthetic hormones tend to alter the hormonal imbalance that supports certain hormone-dependent cancers.

The major factor that limits chemotherapy is that agents used lack specificity and act on both normal and neoplastic cells, causing toxic effects that often require discontinuance of the drug. The ideal chemotherapeutic agent is not available. Such an agent would interfere with cancer cell viability by inhibiting growth and reproduction without causing untoward effects on normal cells. Antineoplastic drugs are most effective on rapidly growing tumors (large portions of the tumor cells are in the miotic cycle). Consequently, normal cells that reproduce rapidly are also affected by these agents, particularly the bone marrow, epithelial cells of the gastrointestinal tract, hair follicles, and skin. Thus bone marrow depression (with leukopenia, thrombocytopenia, and anemia), stomatitis, nausea and vomiting, gastrointestinal ulcerations, diarrhea, and alopecia are common toxic effects of many of the chemotherapeutic agents. These toxic effects, as well as others applicable to specific drugs, require frequent assessment of the patient. Medical and nursing intervention is required to combat these side effects, as will be discussed shortly.

In addition to drug toxicity, other limiting factors related to cancer chemotherapy are those of drug resistance and tumor growth fractions. The increased use of combination therapy, in lieu of single agent therapy, is directed at all three of these limitations. **Tumor growth fraction** is the term used to indicate that only a fraction of cells within a tumor move through the replication cycle at any one point in time. The other cells are in a resting phase and are generally unaffected by anticancer drugs. Thus, proliferating cells demonstrate certain phases in the cell cycle of growth and division. Mitosis has four phases: prophase, metaphase, anaphase, and telephase. Some of the chemotherapeutic drugs affect the cell only during one or more of these phases (phase-specific agents) whereas others of these drugs affect the cell at various stages of the entire cycle (noncyclic-specific). Combination therapy provides the maximal therapeutic effects of several drugs, including effects at different stages of the cell cycle. Careful dosage calculation and cycling schedules are carried out to prevent cumula-

Table 1-4
Selected drugs used in cancer chemotherapy

Drug	Route of administration	Major indications	Toxic effects and precautions
Alkylating agents*			
Mechlorethamine hydrochloride (Mustargen, nitrogen mustard)	Intravenous, intracavity, peritoneal, pleural	Chronic leukemia, Hodgkin's disease, lymphomas, cancer of lung, ovaries, breast	Nausea, vomiting, anorexia, bone marrow depression. A vesicant agent; causes blisters on skin contact; nurse should wear gloves in preparing drug. Avoid extravasation
Cyclophosphamide (Cytoxan, Endoxan)	Oral, intravenous	Acute leukemia, chronic lymphocytic leukemia, Hodgkin's disease; cancer of lung (especially oat cell), cancer of breast, multiple myeloma, Wilms' tumor, neuroblastoma, Burkitt's lymphoma	Nausea, vomiting, anorexia, stomatitis, hemorrhagic cystitis, skin reactions, alopecia, bone marrow depression. Force fluids to combat hemorrhagic cystitis
Triethylene thiophosphoramide (Thio-tepa)	Intravenous, intracavity	Carcinoma of breast, lung, ovaries. Chronic lymphatic leukemia, Hodgkin's disease, lymphomas	Bone marrow depression, nausea, vomiting
Phenylalanine mustard (Mephalan, Alkeran, L-Sarcolysine)	Oral	Multiple myeloma, malignant melanoma, cancer of ovaries or testes	Bone marrow depression, moderate nausea
Chlorambucil (Leukeran)	Oral	Chronic lymphocytic leukemia, Hodgkin's disease, lymphoma, trophoblastic neoplasms (carcinoma of testes, e.g.)	Bone marrow depression. Large doses cause dermatitis and hepatotoxicity
Busulfan (Myleran)	Oral	Chronic myelocytic leukemia, polycythemia vera	Bone marrow depression
Antimetabolites			
Methotrexate (Amethopterin, MTX)	Oral, intravenous infusion, or intrathecally	Acute lymphocytic leukemia, choriocarcinoma, cancer of testes, lymphosarcoma, cancer of cervix	Anorexia, nausea, vomiting, stomatitis, gastrointestinal ulceration, bone marrow depression, hepatotoxicity, nephrotoxic, alopecia, (Citrovorum factor administered with methotrexate in some protocols to prevent toxicity)
5-Fluorouracil (5-FU)	Intravenous infusion, intra-arterial infusion, also orally	Cancer of colon, pancreas, ovary, breast	Nausea, vomiting, stomatitis, bone marrow depression, diarrhea, alopecia, skin eruptions
Fluorodeoxyuridine (Floxuridine, FUDR)	Regional arterial infusion only	Cancer of breast, colon, stomach, bile duct, ovaries, cervix, liver	Anorexia, nausea, vomiting, stomatitis, diarrhea, bone marrow depression
6-Mercaptopurine (Purinethol, 6-MP)	Oral	Leukemia	Nausea, vomiting, bone marrow depression
Thioguanine (6-TG)	Oral, (investigational IV)	Acute leukemia	Nausea, vomiting, bone marrow depression, photosensitivity

*Alkylating agent; maximum toxicity may occur 2 to 3 weeks after the last dose is given.

Table 1-4 (Continued)

Drug	Route of administration	Major indications	Toxic effects and precautions
Cytosine arabinoside (Cytosar, Ara-C)	Intravenous (or subcutaneous), or intrathecally	Acute granulocytic and lymphocytic leukemia, lymphomas	Bone marrow depression, nausea, vomiting, diarrhea, stomatitis, hepatic toxicity. Leukopenia may be very severe
Antibiotics			
Doxorubicin (Adriamycin)	Intravenous	Hodgkin's disease, acute leukemia, lymphomas, breast cancer, ovarian cancer, cancer of bladder, lung, thyroid, Wilms' tumor, neuroblastoma, osteogenic sarcoma	Bone marrow depression, cardiotoxicity with heart failure, nausea, stomatitis, alopecia
Daunorubicin (Daunomycin)	Intravenous	Acute granulocytic and lymphocytic leukemia	Same as above
Bleomycin (Blenoxane)	Intravenous, intramuscular, subcutaneous	Hodgkin's disease, non-Hodgkin's lymphoma, testicular carcinoma	Nausea, vomiting, fever, dermatitis, stomatitis, alopecia, pulmonary fibrosis (periodic chest x-rays indicated), pneumonitis, anaphylactic shock in susceptible persons, bone marrow depression, nail and skin pigment changes
Dactinomycin (Actinomycin D, Cosmegen)	Intravenous	Osteogenic sarcoma, Wilms' tumor, testicular carcinoma, choriocarcinoma	Nausea, vomiting, alopecia, acne, stomatitis, diarrhea, bone marrow depression. Local irritant; tissue damage with extravasation
Streptozotocin (investigational)		Selectively destroys insulin-producing islet cells of pancreas, malignant insulinoma, carcinoid tumors	Nausea, vomiting, renal tubular defects
Mithramycin (Mithracin)	Intravenous		Elevated BUN, CNS effects, confusion, delirium, anorexia, dermatitis, hypocalcemia
Mitomycin (Mutamycin, Bristol)	Intravenous	Gastrointestinal, adenocarcinoma, breast cancer, hepatic cell carcinoma	Bone marrow depression, skin reactions, alopecia, nausea, vomiting, fever, necrosis and sloughing at injection site
Plant alkaloids			
Vinblastine sulfate (Velban)	Intravenous	Hodgkin's disease, lymphomas	Nausea, vomiting, neuropathy, paresthesia, bone marrow depression, alopecia, stomatitis. Local irritant; causes tissue sloughing if extravasated
Vincristine sulfate (Oncovin)	Intravenous	Acute lymphocytic leukemia, Hodgkin's disease, lymphomas, neuroblastoma	Bone marrow depression, neurotoxicity, alopecia, peripheral neuritis, paralytic ileus

Table 1-4 (Continued)

Drug	Route of administration	Major indications	Toxic effects and precautions
Hormones			
Estrogens:			
Diethylstilbesterol (DES)	Oral	Metastatic cancer of breast (postmenopausal), prostate carcinomas	Fluid and salt retention, hypercalcemia, feminization in male patients
Ethinyl estradiol (Estinyl)	Oral	Breast carcinoma (postmenopausal)	Implicated in vaginal carcinoma of offspring. Sexual impotence in males
Progestins:			
Hydroxyprogesterone caproate (Delalutin)	Intramuscularly	Endometrial carcinoma, prostatic carcinoma	Edema, changes in menstrual flow
Megestrol (Megace)	Oral	Endometrial carcinoma	
6-Methylhydroxyprogesterone (Provera)	Oral	Endometrial, renal cell, and breast carcinoma	
Androgens:			
Testosterone propionate	Intramuscularly	Breast cancer (especially for premenopausal patients)	Hair growth, fluid and salt retention, hypercalcemia, masculinization
Fluoxymesterone (Halotestin, Ultandren)	Oral	Breast cancer	Same as above
Adrenocorticosteroids:			
Prednisone (Meticorten)	Oral	Hodgkin's disease, lymphomas, multiple myeloma, lymphocytic leukemia, breast cancer	Increased susceptibility to infection, peptic ulcer, emotional changes, fluid retention, electrolyte imbalance, steroid diabetes
Dexamethasone (Decadron)	Oral	Same as above	Same as above
Miscellaneous cytotoxic agents			
BCNU (investigational) (bis-chloroethyl-nitrosourea) (Carmustine)	Intravenous	Hodgkin's disease, metastatic and primary brain tumors, lymphomas, multiple myeloma, malignant melanoma	Bone marrow depression, nausea, vomiting, local inflammation, renal and hepatic toxicity
Procarbazine (methylhydrazine, Matulane)	Oral (investigational IV)	Hodgkin's disease, lymphomas, bronchogenic carcinoma	Nausea, bone marrow depression, CNS depression. Possesses monoamine oxidase inhibitory effect; therefore cheese, bananas, tea, coffee, wine, and sympathomimetic tricyclic antidepressants are to be avoided
Hydroxyurea (Hydrea)	Oral	Chronic granulocytic leukemia, malignant melanoma	Nausea, bone marrow depression, alopecia
L-Asparaginase	Intravenous	Acute lymphoblastic leukemia	Nausea, vomiting, hepatic dysfunction, hyperglycemia, hypoalbuminemia, bone marrow depression, hyperlipidemia, hypersensitivity reactions

Table 1-4 (Continued)

Drug	Route of administration	Major indications	Toxic effects and precautions
Dacarbazine (DTIC-Dome, DIC)	Intravenous	Malignant melanoma, Hodgkin's disease	Bone marrow depression, nausea and vomiting. Local tissue irritation if extravasation occurs
Quinacrine (Atabrine)	Intrapleural	Bronchogenic carcinoma	Local pain, fever

tive toxicities of the drugs. In addition, drug-free intervals are provided to allow the patient's normal tissues to be repaired before therapy is again initiated. In some settings, anticoagulants are used as an adjunct to chemotherapy. The rationale for this approach is to prevent the fibrin substratum needed for capillaries to move into a growing tumor and thus decrease oxygenation of tumor cells and increase their susceptibility to cytotoxic agents [251].

The cancer chemotherapeutic agents are administered systemically (orally or intravenously), regionally by isolation-perfusion or intra-arterial infusion, or locally by instillation into a body cavity such as the pleural or peritoneal cavities. In addition, a drug such as methotrexate may be instilled intrathecally. This latter approach, for example, is used in the treatment of meningeal leukemia.

The selection of specific drugs is determined by the primary tumor site, the presence of overt metastasis, the extent of metastasis, the physical status of the patient, and other existing diseases that might have an affect on the cancer therapy. Prior to the initiation of chemotherapy, the patient's hematologic status is determined. The nutritional status of the patient is also determined, because patients in negative nitrogen balance are not appropriate candidates for chemotherapy. Evaluation of the patient, considering the advantages and potential benefits of the drug as weighed against the risks involved, may result in a decision not to use specific chemotherapeutic agents.

The patient and the family should be thoroughly oriented to the purpose of the proposed drug regimen and to its anticipated therapeutic and toxic effects. The patient is also advised about how untoward effects will be treated. The level of information and the detail of the explanations depends on the patient's level of understanding and ability to tolerate extensive and complicated information. The patient is advised that frequent monitoring of his hematologic status will require frequent venipunctures for blood analysis. The importance of adequate nutritional intake during therapy must be emphasized.

Prior to initiation of chemotherapy, the patient's body systems are assessed to obtain baseline data for evaluating anticipated changes. In addition to the evaluation of the hematologic and nutritional status, the patient's weight is determined. Oral and anal orifices are examined for the presence of any lesions, and the integrity of the skin is assessed.

Toxic Effects and Side Effects

Toxicity and side effects of chemotherapeutic agents require appropriate nursing intervention. Nausea and vomiting are treated by the judicious use of antiemetic drugs. Small frequent feedings are helpful, and carbonated drinks are often well tolerated. If the fluid and nutritional status is threatened, intravenous fluid therapy and nutritional nasogastric tube feedings or total parenteral nutrition may be necessary. Diarrhea is treated with drugs such as Lomotil or Kaopectate as well as by modification of the diet to eliminate irritating foods.

Stomatitis, which refers to inflamed and painful mouth ulcerations, requires frequent and proper oral hygiene. To prevent further trauma, pain, or infection, soft toothbrushes (or the commercial Toothette products) are used in mild stomatitis; even these soft toothbrushes may be painful in severe stomatitis. Mouth care is essential before each meal to improve appetite and to stimulate salivary flow, even when stomatitis is not present. Mouth care is indicated every 4 hours for mild stomatitis and every 2 hours for severe stomatitis [240]. Mouthwashes consisting of saline-diluted hydrogen peroxide (one part hydrogen peroxide to four parts of saline) are beneficial germicidal oxidizing measures. If the patient is unable to expectorate, a spray of the solution may be instilled, followed by gentle suctioning. If the patient has dentures, these should be removed in the presence of stomatitis in order to prevent further mechanical injury; they are not replaced until the stomatitis improves. Regular assessment of the mouth is indicated to determine the presence of stomatitis and the effectiveness of oral hygiene measures. Painful lesions may be treated with viscous xylocaine applied to the mucus membrane [240].

The symptoms of nausea, anorexia, and vomiting also interfere with oral intake. Bland, nonirritating foods are prescribed; the patient is advised to avoid highly seasoned foods and hot foods. These patients generally tolerate cold fluids better. Small, frequent feedings of high caloric and high protein foods are encouraged. Dietary supplements are also fairly well tolerated when flavored with commercial extracts. Cold drinks, ice cream, and popsicles are soothing and generally tolerated, and they also provide necessary calories and fluid intake. Fluid intake is important in maintaining fluid and electrolyte balance and in promoting elimination of the end products of the various chemotherapeutic agents in the drug regimen.

Alopecia is another frequently encountered toxic effect associated with cancer chemotherapy. Although the technique is controversial, some practitioners advise the use of a tourniquet around the forehead for 10 to 15 minutes during and after intravenous administration of drugs that cause alopecia [270] in order to reduce blood flow to the scalp and reduce the damage to the hair follicles. In addition, the patient is cautioned to avoid hair brushing, and to use gentle combing instead. The use of wigs, turbans, scarves, or night caps is a helpful measure. Alopecia is particularly distressing for patients. Encouragement that the hair will regrow after therapy is discontinued is generally reassuring.

In addition to oral ulcerations associated with certain drugs, rectal and anal lesions are frequently encountered. These body areas should be examined carefully and regularly. Rectal temperatures are contraindicated for patients receiving drugs such as methotrexate that are likely to cause rectal lesions.

Some of these effects are tolerable, with the judicious use of nursing measures and various medications as previously mentioned. Certain toxic reactions, however, require reduction in dosages and even discontinuance of certain drugs. One of the most dangerous toxic reactions is that of bone marrow depression, associated with the majority of the agents used. This toxic reaction leads to host susceptibility to infections and impaired antibody production. The onset of leukopenia makes the patient vulnerable to infections. Thrombocytopenia precipitates bleeding, and anemia precipitates lethargy, lack of energy, and susceptibility to skin breakdown and poor healing. Early in the treatment process, the patient is instructed about reducing exposure to other infected persons and is observed for signs of respiratory infection, the most common infection in cancer patients. Viral and fungal infections also frequently occur. When the white blood count falls to below 2,000 per cubic millimeter, **reverse isolation** techniques are indicated. Bone marrow transplants may be needed. However, the use of reverse isolation is controversial because these immunosuppressed patients develop infections due to endogenous flora, for which reverse isolation has proved ineffective. In certain settings, a protective environment is facilitated by the use of the life island or the laminar air flow unit.

The **life island** is a patient isolation system in which the patient's hospital bed is enclosed in a plastic canopy. Air inside the canopy is filtered to remove all airborne microorganisms, and only sterilized materials are placed in the unit. Arm-length gloves built into the side of the unit are used for any contact with the patient. The close and abnormal environment is generally so distressful for the patient that its use on a long-term basis is limited.

The **laminar air flow unit** consists of a self-cleaning unit that is installed in a private room. A constant stream of purified air passes through the unit's microfilters, which screen out organisms smaller than any pathogenic particle. All equipment is sterilized prior to its entry and use in the patient's unit. Sterile gowns, caps, masks, gloves, and shoe covers are used by personnel when in contact with the patient. Although this arrangement is generally preferable to the life island, the need for psychological support to prevent sensory deprivation in such a setting cannot be overemphasized.

In addition to those precautions taken to prevent the introduction of pathogenic organisms into the environment of the patient with severe bone marrow depression, the patient requires protection against his own endogenous organisms. Oral antibiotics or oral antifungal agents or both are usually administered to suppress potentially pathogenic organisms.

In addition to the frequently encountered toxic effects of chemotherapy, there are specific and potentially dangerous effects associated with some of the agents. These effects are listed in Table 1-4. When patients are on various agents, the nurse must be familiar with toxic effects of all the agents as well as with those nursing measures indicated to assess the presence of impending toxicity. For example, doxorubicin (Adriamycin), which is a commonly used agent, has the potential for causing toxic cardiac effects leading to myocardial damage and cardiac failure. Assessment of the cardiac status, including periodic electrocardiograms, is absolutely essential when this drug is used.

Administration of bleomycin makes the patient susceptible to pneumonitis and pulmonary fibrosis. Thus, assessment of the patient's respiratory status and observation for symptoms of dyspnea and wheezing should be accomplished regularly; chest x-rays should also be taken at periodic intervals.

When the patient is receiving cyclophosphamide (Cytoxan) he is encouraged to drink at least two quarts of water daily to prevent the onset of hemorrhagic cystitis, one of the potential toxic effects associated with the use of Cytoxan. Certain drugs (methotrexate) are nephrotoxic and others (L-asparaginase) are hepatotoxic, requiring serum evaluation of various blood elements to monitor the effects of these drugs. The neurotoxic effects of vincristine (Oncovin) must be prevented by routine assessment of the peripheral nerves and tendon reflexes and subsequent reduction of dosage or discontinuance of the drug. The reader is referred to Table 1-4 for other details on the chemotherapeutic agents and is advised to become thoroughly oriented to the characteristics of these drugs.

In many settings the nurse is responsible for administering the parenteral chemotherapeutic agents. Extreme care in the preparation of the drug and careful administration are absolutely essential. The patient receives frequent venipunctures for blood analysis and for administration of the drugs. The frequent venipunctures result in fragile or sclerosed veins, limiting the sites available for puncture. Skill in intravenous techniques is essential in the prevention of further damage or pain for the patient. Drugs should be properly diluted and administered slowly. When possible, compatible drugs for combined therapy are mixed in a single syringe to facilitate administration. Infiltration of the drug should be avoided, since tissue sloughing may occur, especially with nitrogen mustard, 5-fluorouracil, vincristine, vinblastine, dactinomycin, and streptozotocin [250].

Even when the patient is intellectually prepared for the development of toxic side effects of chemotherapy, depression and discouragement often occur when the toxic effects occur. Discouragement is often expressed as doubt about the value of the therapy and the desire to discontinue the regimen. Psychological support is particularly important as the patient attempts to resolve his feelings about the therapy and as interventions are planned to counteract the side effects.

Among the protocols for combination chemotherapy given in repeated cycles are COAP (Cytoxan, Oncovin, Ara-C, and prednisone); MOPP (nitrogen mustard, Oncovin, procarbazine, and prednisone), which is used in the treatment of Hodgkin's disease; and Adriamycin and Cytoxan in combination for advanced breast cancer. Another protocol for breast cancer is the addition of 5-fluorouracil to the latter regimen. High doses of methotrexate with Adriamycin for the treatment of osteogenic sarcoma is still another example of an effective combination therapy regimen.

Other Methods of Administration

Besides the oral and intravenous administration of chemotherapeutic agents for the systemic treatment of cancer, drugs may be administered by regional perfusion and arterial infusion methods. **Isolation-perfusion** is the administration of concentrated doses of chemotherapeutic agents through a closed system with isolated arteriovenous recirculation via catheters inserted into the major artery and vein of an extremity. For example the iliac, femoral, or popliteal arteries and veins are used to treat melanomas and sarcomas of the lower extremity. A totally occlusive tourniquet is applied to the extremity to isolate the area from the systemic circulation. Using a pump oxygenator, the extremity is perfused with oxygenated blood containing the chemotherapeutic agent. The length of the treatment varies according to the drug being used and the site being treated. After the cannulas are removed, the patient is observed for local tissue reactions such as erythema and blistering and for pain in the extremity. Pain following the perfusion is an ominous sign and almost always indicates severe injury to normal tissue. Normally there is no pain except that associated with the trauma of the injection site. Regional perfusion techniques are also used in treating abdominal or lower pelvic tumors. A laparotomy is done in order to block the blood supply to the tumor area by clamping of the mesenteric artery and vein and using the pump oxygenator and medication. Catheters are introduced into the femoral artery and vein.

Intra-arterial infusion is the percutaneous insertion of a catheter into a major artery under fluoroscopic control or under direct visualization in a surgical procedure to administer a high concentration of a chemotherapeutic agent directly to a cancerous organ. When the correct location is confirmed by injection of radiopaque dye, and arteriograms confirm a satisfactory perfusion, continuous infusion of the chemotherapeutic drug is started. This technique is used, for example, in the treatment of liver metastasis with intrahepatic arterial infusion of 5-fluorouracil. Battery operated tubing pumps with disposable plastic reservoirs of the appropriately diluted agent are now available as portable infusion equiment for long-term use. Such an apparatus is the Sigmamotor ML-6 infusion package,* which administers an uninterrupted flow of the medication for 7 days without changing the apparatus. The infuser has a clock mechanism for controlling the administration of the drug. This technique facilitates outpatient treatment of infusion therapy over a period of several months if necessary. Patient teaching related to the care of the apparatus requires caution in maintaining the proper position of the arterial catheter. Hemorrhage, sepsis, tissue irritation, and the onset of toxic drug effects are potential problems associated with the treatment.

A modification of the infusion technique is the use of central nervous system intrathecal chemotherapy by means of a cerebrospinal fluid reservoir such as the Ommaya reservoir (Fig. 1-4). This procedure involves a burr hole incision and catheter insertion into a ventricle of the nondominant side of the patient's brain. A polyethylene reservoir of a chemotherapeutic agent provides even distribution of the agent. Complications associated with this technique include infections, seizures, bacterial meningitis, and cellulitis.

Investigational Therapy

Different approaches to chemotherapy administration are always under study, just as new drugs continue to be investigated. In selected settings nurses may thus be involved with investigational therapy, which places increased responsibility on the nurse in the observation of therapeutic and unexpected toxic effects. When patients are selected for investigational therapy, *informed consent is*

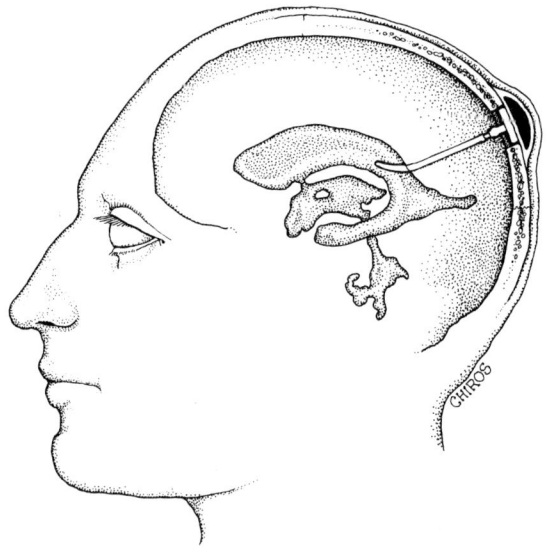

Figure 1-4
Ommaya reservoir connected to the lateral ventricle.

---

*Sigmamotor Corporation, Middleport, New York.

absolutely essential, so that the patient is knowledgeable about the potential therapeutic and toxic effects. Before drugs are approved for general use, they are evaluated according to a three-phase process. The use of investigational drugs is governed by federal regulations, which require that only qualified oncologists prescribe the medications. Phase I involves the use of the drug only in patients with advanced disease, for whom conventional therapy is not adequate. This phase establishes clinically acceptable doses and schedules in terms of toxic and therapeutic effects, since previous doses have been determined only in animal studies.

Phase II continues with the administration of the drug to patients with advanced disease, but now the patients must meet measurable disease criteria for drug evaluation to identify antitumor activity of the agent against specific types of cancer. The antitumor activity of the drug is evaluated by changes determined in tumor size measurement and x-ray studies.

Phase III is the evaluation of the drug in testing on a large scale, using patients with a specific type of cancer, as determined by previous phases of the investigation. Randomized trials are carried out to compare the new drug against standard forms of therapy in terms of effectiveness, side effects, and consistency in response. The toxic effects of the drug are evaluated according to the potential benefit of the drug.

Throughout the procedures for investigational therapy, the patient is kept informed of his progress and is protected from developing severe toxic effects during the efforts to evaluate the drug's effectiveness. Psychological support is essential as the patient becomes discouraged when initial hope is tempered by the reality of minimal therapeutic effects.

Regardless of the setting in which the nurse practices his or her profession, the nurse must have thorough knowledge of the chemotherapeutic agents being administered to assure safe and therapeutic care for the patient. Consistent and accurate assessment of the patient is imperative in the detection of impending toxic effects and in the provision of appropriate nursing interventions. The importance of psychological support during the tedious and often uncomfortable chemotherapeutic procedures cannot be overemphasized.

IMMUNOTHERAPY

The fourth treatment modality used in cancer therapy is that of immunotherapy. Although it is still in the developmental stage, immunotherapy is thought by some authorities to be a potentially unique and effective resource in treating both localized and disseminated cancer.

The increased incidence of cancer among patients who have had organ transplants and who have received immunosuppressive drugs has drawn attention to the immunity aspects of cancer. As discussed earlier in this chapter, an immune response is the body's production of specific antibodies or sensitized cells to neutralize or attack antigens, which may be foreign protein, a chemical, a bacterium, or a virus. Examples given were those related to stimulation of T cells (lymphocytes that mature in the thymus) resulting in sensitized lymphocytes and the production of immunoglobulins in response to stimulation of B cells (lymphocytes derived from bone marrow to become plasma cells).

Many cancer cells have protein structures on their membranes and thus possess specific tumor antigens which should initiate an immune response to this foreign protein. However, cancer cells appear to be protected in some way from the immune response [246]. Studies are under way to determine what these cancer protective mechanisms are, as are continued studies of the immune system itself.

The goal of immunotherapy is to stimulate the body's defense mechanisms for biochemically attacking foreign cells and substances and to reject the cancer cells. The fact that immune responses occur in tumor growth is considered as a basis for diagnostic measures in cancer, such as the use of radioimmunoassay methods for identifying patients with otherwise undetected cancer cells. For example, carcinoembryonic antigen (CEA) has been found to be elevated in the serum of a significant number of patients with colon cancer. Similar biochemical markers are determined as elevated in breast cancer, such as human chorionic gonadotropin and a compound identified as N^2N^2-dimethylguanosine [246]. It is hoped that immunodiagnostic tests can be developed to facilitate early diagnosis of many cancers and detection of recurrences.

Several survey techniques are used to assess the patient's immune status as a basis for administering agents to stimulate the host's immune mechanism. These survey techniques include measurement of serum-blocking antibody titer (antibodies elicited by tumor antigen and blocking lymphocyte-mediated interaction and destruction of tumor cells) [280]. Other immune system surveys include delayed hypersensitivity skin testing to assess the patient's capacity to respond to treatment by non-specific immunotherapeutic stimulants and testing of sensitization to a chemical antigen, dinitrochlorobenzene (DNCB) [280].

Because tumor antigens have not been isolated, specific immunization techniques to increase specific antitumor activity are not available, although possible immunospecific effects have been reported [246, 280]. Immunotherapy currently is centered on stimulating a patient's immune defenses generally with chemical or microbial agents to which the patient has been previously sensitized. The general response in some cases has been tumor regression; the technique has been used primarily with small tumor masses and cancer cells. The effectiveness of immunotherapy combined with one or more of the other modes of treatment is under extensive study [252].

Immunotherapy has been used in the treatment of malignant melanoma. Bacillus Calmette-Guérin (BCG) vaccine is administered to patients with multiple melanoma either by intravenous, or more commonly by intralesional or scarification, techniques. Scarification requires breaking but not deeply lacerating the patient's skin five times. The BCG vaccine is then dropped onto the broken skin and covered with plastic film. The patient is instructed to keep the area dry and the dressing on for 24 hours, after which the skin may be washed gently. The patient may develop symptoms of influenza with aching, fever, swollen regional lymph nodes, and malaise, but this reaction is temporary and lasts only 24 to 48 hours. As the patient's lymphocytes attack the BCG, it is hoped that they will also attack tumor cells and produce antibodies against the tumor. Intralesional therapy is accomplished by injecting the BCG vaccine directly into the melanoma. The regression or disappearance of injected and noninjected lesions has resulted with this technique. Immunotherapy has also been used in the treatment of human leukemia and sarcomas, but there is controversy over its effectiveness in these cases. BCG treatment must be handled judiciously; some deaths have been recorded as a result of anaphylactic reactions.

Terminal Illness

The stage of terminal illness and impending death brings another crisis in the life of the cancer patient and his family. Although terminal illness and death are included in this discussion of cancer, this discussion applies to terminal illness and the process of dying and death from any cause.

Terminal illness is that stage of illness when all treatment measures have failed in the control of the disease process and symptoms of deterioration increase in severity. Nursing care of the terminally ill patient is directed toward making the patient physically and psychologically comfortable. Depending on the individual situation, the patient may be hospitalized or at home. In either case, the nurse is responsible for assessing the general appearance of the patient, his strength, color, mobility, skin integrity, pain status, and psychological status to determine the changes needed in the plan of care. In the hospital this assessment is done on a daily (or more frequent) basis; in the home, it is done by the visiting nurse or by telephone using the family's assessment data; in the clinic, it is done at every visit. Assessment of all body systems is essential. Impending problems must be detected to prevent untoward discomfort from preventable complications.

Fatigue and weakness are predominant symptoms of the patient in the terminal stages of cancer. Various factors contribute to increased fatigue, including associated anemia, anorexia, decreased caloric intake, weight loss, pain, loss of muscle mass, and inadequate assimilation of nutritive elements. The term **cachexia** is used to describe this progressive weakness, wasting, and weight loss. It is felt that neoplasms increase their demand for normal metabolites at the expense of normal tissue, leading to muscle wasting and loss of body fat. Anorexia, gastrointestinal disturbances and obstruction, malabsorption syndromes, and excess losses of protein all contribute to the state of cachexia. The nurse should therefore initiate activities toward conservation of the patient's energy, increased caloric intake, and prevention of infections to which the patient is susceptible.

Attention to specific details of dietary management is essential. DeWys and associates [247] have found that among many cancer patients there is both a decreased taste sensation and an increased taste threshold for sweets. Another substantial finding is that an aversion to meat is correlated with a lowered taste threshold for butter. Observing the patient's intake and eating patterns and discussing the diet with the patient may indicate the need for modifications in the diet plan. For example, the patient who has a meat aversion should obtain protein from eggs, cheese, and other sources. Increased seasoning and sweetening of food may be helpful in efforts to increase intake in persons with elevated sucrose thresholds.

A high protein intake is necessary. Usually smaller and more frequent meals with high protein snacks in between are better tolerated than are three large meals. For patients having difficulty in chewing or swallowing, blenderized meals or strained baby foods may be taken. High protein eggnogs may appeal to some patients. Commercial dietary supplements such as Sustargen, Nutriment, Suscatel, and Vivonex are often used. Vivonex is particularly useful because it is an easily absorbed low residue diet. When these foods cannot be taken orally, nasal gastric tubes are inserted to provide nourishment, or total parenteral nutrition is used. In some cases, particularly when there is an obstruction of the esophagus, a gastrostomy is performed.

Personal hygiene is accomplished by the patient to the extent that he is able; in some cases, the nurse or the family must provide total hygienic care. If the patient is extremely weak and has only minimal energy for very few independent activities, the patient should decide what these activities will be and the staff should make every effort to abide by his decision. For example, the male patient may decide that shaving himself is the most important activity he can do independently and should be allowed to do so as long as is possible. Although he may be able to shave, he may then be unable to bathe or feed himself and will require assistance in these activities. The nurse must constantly assess how much tolerance of activity the patient has and then adjust activity plans with his participation in any decisions that are made.

The bedridden patient is susceptible to tissue breakdown. Turning the patient at regular intervals and providing regular back massage will stimulate the skin and promote relaxation. Wrinkle-free and dry bedding is of paramount importance in preventing skin breakdown. Air pressure mattresses and other devices may be necessary. The patient with cancer has enough problems in maintaining a semblance of comfort and should not be allowed to develop decubiti or other complications, which only add to his discomfort and further complicate his care. Vascular thrombosis is another potential complication and is related to dehydration and inactivity. Thrombosis is prevented by active and passive exercises of both of the extremities. As long as the patient is able, ambulation is encouraged.

The patient is assessed as to his elimination capabilities. Symptoms of incontinence or urine retention are evaluated and appropriate interventions initiated either by bladder programs or, if necessary, by the use of a retention catheter. Often dehydration, pain medications, and inactivity contribute to constipation, which should be combated with suppositories, increased fluid intake, stool softeners, or enemas. When patients are able to take only minimal nutrients and fluids, daily weights and intake and output are recorded to determine the need for fluid and electrolyte replacement. Depending on the type of intake the patient has, and the presence of draining wounds and the types of medications the patient is taking, the nurse should observe for symptoms of fluid and electrolyte imbalance. This aspect of care is discussed in detail in Chapter 2.

It has been estimated that hypercalcemia complicates the course of malignant disease in about 10 to 30 percent of cancer patients [242]. Serious central nervous system, renal, and cardiac dysfunction may result from this potentially fatal problem. Hypercalcemia is most often associated with mixed osteolytic and osteoblastic metastasis, particularly from breast cancer and bone destruction by tumor. The large amounts of calcium resorbed surpass the renal clearance capabilities of the patient. The nurse should therefore carefully observe susceptible patients for this complication, noting symptoms such as anorexia, nausea, thirst, weakness, and lethargy as well as changes in central nervous system functioning that may lead the nurse to suspect brain metastasis rather than electrolyte disturbances.

In addition to observing for the toxic signs discussed, the nurse should observe for diarrhea, which may result from chemotherapy or radiation therapy, particularly when the pelvic or abdominal area has been irradiated. Diarrhea is treated with medications and appropriate low residue or bland foods. Bone marrow depression may be present as a result of the various therapies, and the patient must be protected from both infections and trauma resulting in bleeding, as discussed in earlier sections of this chapter.

For the terminally ill, adequate relief of pain is absolutely essential. It should be noted, however, that not all cancer patients suffer great pain. Sometimes the pain of cancer is not related to the disease itself but rather to the secondary effects of the illness. For example, a decubitus results from prolonged bed rest and decreased nutrition; painful joints are due to improper positioning or lack of exercise; a dry unkempt mouth is due to decreased intake and inadequate mouth care. Therefore, pain relief also includes the prevention of complications that cause secondary pain. The patient is allowed to participate in the plan for pain relief. When the pain has been controlled, the patient becomes able to concentrate on other aspects of his life as long as is possible. The effect of pain medication is assessed regularly to determine when the patient's need for relief necessitates a larger dose of medication or a different medication. Often, patients may hesitate to ask for pain medication even though they are suffering, because the social stigma associated with requesting medication and the social approval of stoicism inhibit this request. Again the terminally ill patient should not have to waste his limited energy in trying to please others but rather should be allowed to feel free and open about requesting medication as needed.

There has probably been more interest recently in adequate pain relief and a lessening of the fear of addiction in relation to the management of pain in cancer. The management of pain in the terminally ill should be directed toward making the patient comfortable without making him so unaware of his environment that he is unable to react with others. Rather than placing a patient on PRN doses, medications are often given around the clock.

Initially the mildest analgesic, such as aspirin, is used. Later, codeine and stronger narcotics may be used in the control of increasing pain. These narcotics or other agents are supplemented with antiemetic drugs or tranquilizers to assist in potentiating the action of the analgesic drugs. It is interesting that at the St. Christopher Hospice in Great Britain, which is an institution for the terminally ill, combinations of drugs are used, but diamorphine (heroin) is a major drug used. Medications are given every 4 hours. The patients are not allowed to suffer but are relieved of pain on an individually prescribed dosage and schedule to support a pain-free and alert patient. Thorazine and its derivatives are also used. The personnel at the Hospice have found that when the patient is secure in the knowledge that medication will be given routinely every 4 hours, he or she does not anticipate pain and is thus more relaxed and less anxious [306, 318]. The effects of the drug therapy, however, are evaluated closely and continuously, and adjustments are made as needed.

Another enlightened approach to pain management used in some settings in the United States is the Brompton mixture for relief of pain in terminal disease. This approach also prescribes medication every 4 hours around the clock rather than PRN to prevent pain and to erase the memory of pain. The drug mixture is changed to meet the individual patient's needs. A Brompton elixir that is often used includes: 10 mg morphine, 10 mg cocaine, 5 ml ethyl alcohol (vodka), 5 ml syrup, and 20 ml chloroform water. The elixir totals 30 ml and is given orally. Thorazine or another phenothiazine syrup may be added to this mixture. In some settings, heroin is substituted.

The drug that is used in pain management is probably not as important as the assessment of the individual patient and the security that pain relief provides. As mentioned earlier, it is important to begin pain management with the milder medications, leaving the more potent drugs to the later stages of the terminal illness.

At St. Christopher's Hospice, pain medications are not the only methods used to provide pain relief. There is an emphasis on the use of touch and listening to the patient. The patient's identity is emphasized in order to allow the patient to die in dignity. When admitted to this hospital, the patient brings his own belongings and treasures; he is not made anonymous by hospital gowns and impersonalized surroundings. The family is involved as much as desired by the patient and the family members. When the family elects to care for the patient at home, home care services are provided. The philosophy of the hospital is the conscious acceptance of dying and death as a part of the process of living. Unique to this institution is the continued contact and assistance to family members after the patient's death for varying lengths of time [306].

There is much to learn from considering the approaches used at this prototype institution for the terminally ill. McCorkle [319] investigated the effects of touch as nonverbal communication on seriously ill patients. Her study demonstrated that the use of touch indicated that the nurse cared about the patient and that this gesture facilitated rapport between patient and nurse within a short period of time. The patient with cancer or any other terminal illness may or may not directly express the various fears that generally underlie such a state. The fear of death and the fear of pain associated with terminal illness are the major concerns of the patient. The fear of rejection and abandonment is a theme often associated with a terminal illness. Patients with a diagnosis of cancer therefore are predisposed to depression due to the changes in the pattern of living associated with the dissease or with the various treatment methods. What the terminal illness and impending death mean to the patient can be determined only by developing a trusting relationship and open communication with the patient. Only through listening to the patient and observing nonverbal behavior can the nurse make a judgment about what the patient feels about the total situation. The importance of open communication cannot be overemphasized.

Pienschke [280a] studied four approaches to revealing diagnosis and prognosis to cancer patients and found that the initial manner in which a patient was told his diagnosis and prognosis influenced his response to his illness and the methods of treatment. The four approaches are (1) **open-open:** disclosure by direct confrontation of the exact nature of the diagnosis and the realistic appraisal of the prognosis; (2) **open-guarded:** disclosure of the diagnosis but avoiding the fact of the high probability of death as the outcome; (3) **guarded-open:** guarded information about the diagnosis, but open discussion of the seriousness of the illness; and (4) **guarded-guarded:** both the diagnosis and prognosis are kept from the patient. Pienschke studied the effect of these approaches on the patient's confidence in his doctors and nurses, the patient's satisfaction with the information received about his illness, the patient's satisfaction with nursing care, and the adequacy of the care given. The study found that the open approach to diagnosis was predominantly used but that the guarded approach was predominantly used for revealing prognosis. The study also showed that the patients had greater confidence in the professional staff when the open-open approach was used, and that the guarded-guarded approach tended to place a strain on both the patient and the professional staff. The study also supports the importance of providing an open line of communication between the medical and nursing staff and the patient, so that the patient can participate in decisions about his care management during the terminal stages. Openness is a vital element in care, as the patient tends to feel hopeless as the disease obviously progresses beyond the means of control available. Hopelessness and helplessness, which often go hand in hand in the presence of cancer and other terminal diseases, are increased when the patient loses his self-esteem and identity. Measures to increase the patient's self-esteem and identity will serve to make the patient more secure and comfortable. Again, the patient should be asked about his ideas and feelings about aspects of his care; the nurse can learn about the patient's own beliefs and concerns only by providing opportunities for such discussions and free expression. If the nurse or other personnel are unwilling to spend time with the patient, the patient may interpret the staff's behavior as rejection when in reality the staff may simply be uncomfortable in talking with him during the last stages of his illness.

Glaser and Strauss, Kubler-Ross, and

others [302, 311] have found that patients usually know that they are dying even when they have not been told directly. Facial expressions, demeanor, tone of voice, and evasive or vague replies are some of the obvious ways in which doctors and nurses transmit information to a patient, even without being aware of doing so. When this behavior reflects a change from the previous ways of handling information and communication with the patient, the patient quickly grasps the meaning of the changed behavior.

The fact that professional staff experience pain and emotional stress when talking with patients about dying has long been recognized. Interest in gaining skill in communicating with dying patients has increased as professionals seek assistance in coping with terminal patients. Weekly discussions and conferences for staff working with dying patients are helpful if experienced resource people are available to assist the staff in coping. These types of conferences have been shown to improve staff and patient behavior and to enhance staff morale. Professional staff also need opportunities to express their own feelings about death and caring for the dying to objectively evaluate the care given to the terminally ill patients.

The nurse who is aware of the patient's need for help in resolving the issue of his terminal illness and impending death can assist the patient by identifying the person most effective in giving him help and support in this crisis. Patients who are dying often identify a single person who would be most effective in helping them. They usually identify a favorite person, one who has conveyed caring and concern for them. Thus, the person who is most helpful to individual patients changes, depending on the individual patient as well as on the rapport attained with specific staff members.

In addition to providing the patient with opportunities to discuss his fears, feelings, and desires about his care and illness, the nurse should provide time to talk with the family. The family should be allowed a role in the care of the terminally ill patient, even in the institutional setting. The nurse should observe and listen for cues that indicate the family's desire to participate in the care of the patient. At times, the nurse must intervene when it becomes obvious that the family members are participating too extensively and at the expense of their own health. The family may then be relieved of guilt feelings by the nurse's approach to them for reducing their participation or at least modifying their time and involvement.

Often the family members are concerned over the financial aspects of the illness and may overextend themselves in trying to meet work obligations, home responsibilities, and time at the hospital. When finances are a problem, the nurse should obtain the assistance of the hospital social worker to determine potential resources for assistance. Financial concerns are a realistic consideration, especially in light of the expensive treatments that are often associated with cancer management. (For example, Adriamycin, a drug that is used fairly often in chemotherapy, may cost from $800 to $2,000 alone for one course of therapy; yet it may be only one of several drugs and modes of therapy used [246].)

Death and Dying

There has been an increased interest in the process of dying and death during the last decade. The increased numbers of persons living to older ages, and the changes in family structure and functions, have made an impact on the process of dying in our society. Whereas in previous years the dying person was within a tight family and community structure during terminal stages, persons now often die alone or at least with minimal family support. From home care of the dying, the care has shifted into specialized institutions for an estimated 75 percent of those who die. Thus the process of dying tends to take place in unfamiliar settings and is managed by institutional personnel rather than by the family. This fact places responsibility on the health professions to personalize the institutional methods of caring for patients during their terminal stages of illness. The field of thanatology (study of death) has developed during the last decade, and increasingly the terminal stages of patients' illnesses have been studied.

Glaser and Strauss [302] studied the process of dying, particularly in relation to awareness of the patient's oncoming death. Dying patients were studied in the context of their hospital environments, in six different hospital settings. These investigators identified four types of awareness in relation to the patient's awareness of oncoming death. These four types are: (1) **closed awareness,** in which the staff knew the diagnosis but the patient did not, (2) **suspected awareness,** in which the staff continued to act as though recovery was expected, but the patient suspected the truth, (3) **mutual pretense awareness,** in which both patient and staff were aware of impending death but acted as though the patient would get well, and (4) **open awareness,** in which both the patient and staff were aware of impending death and discussed it openly. Needless to say, the last type of awareness was least often encountered. The first three were found to put the patient into isolation without adequate resources. These investigators also found that the burden of dealing with the patient in relation to awareness of terminal illness rested primarily on the nursing staff because physicians chose not to tell patients about their status. Glaser and Strauss also cited the nonaccountability for the psychosocial aspects of care as a major factor in the manner in which care was given to patients during terminal stages of illness.

Although the practice of not telling patients of the terminal nature of their illness has decreased, the problem now relates to *how* to tell the patient and his family. When advised of the terminal nature of the illness, patients and families react in various ways. Some react by attempting a full life before death and use the time to settle affairs and plan the future of family members. They do this fully realizing the implications of the diagnosis and impending death. Others react by declining any treatment and then seek other resources, including quackery, for a quick and miracle cure. Others deny the illness and its terminal verdict by not acknowledging the facts as they are given to them. This reaction generally is a temporary protective and defense mechanism to handle intolerable information. Although denial is generally temporary, nurses may encounter some patients who even to the last days of life deny that they are dying. This type of situation is distressful for both the patient and the staff. When denial no longer can be utilized adequately, the patient begins to search for reasons for the illness and impending death, which is the first step in the process of understanding and accepting the illness and impending death.

Terminal care generally relates to the final weeks, days, or hours of life, but Weisman [330] considers it to begin at that unspecified point when the aim of treatment is no longer to cure but to preserve life and to relieve distress, to palliate, and to maintain comfortable existence as long as possible. He identifies three stages of fatal illness: (1) the period from the onset of symptoms until the diagnosis is made; the period includes delay, denial, and postponement as methods of coping; (2) the interval between diagnosis and onset of the terminal decline, a period characterized by changes in the equilibrium of denial and acceptance with the use of defenses of mitigation and displacement; and (3) the terminal stage, or the period when active treatment is found to have diminishing value and emphasis shifts to symptomatic relief. During these stages various psychological reactions are observed. Weisman stresses that fear of abandonment is one of the major concerns at this time.

Kubler-Ross [311] identifies five stages in the dying process, with shock being the initial reaction and leading to **denial,** the first distinct stage. **Anger** is the second stage, a time when the nurse and other personnel should recognize that the patient's anger may be randomly directed at anyone in his environment. The third and generally the shortest stage is that of **bargaining,** in which the patient offers something (such as good behavior) in exchange for a postponement of death. **Depression,** which usually results from evidence of increased symptomology, is the fourth stage, before the fifth and final stage of **acceptance.** (The reader is referred to the bibliography for other references by this well-recognized authority in the dying process.)

Kubler-Ross has qualified stages of dying with the admonition that not all patients go through these stages, nor do they go through them in a specific order [313]. It has also been recognized that patients may pass through a stage and return to it at a later time. Nurses can help document this process by more accurate recording of comments, attitudes, and behavior of the patient and the family during the process of dying.

Kubler-Ross's theory has been criticized as being subjective and inadequate in its lack of explicitly specifying a procedure for determining the specific stage of the patient's coping mechanisms. These critics feel that misperceiving a stage could result in negative consequences for the patient [327].

Hinton [305] has studied the dying process and has assessed mood, physical distress, level of consciousness, and awareness of dying. He found depression to be frequently present during the 8 weeks prior to death, but also acknowledged that drugs may have influenced this finding. Weisman and Kastenbaum [330] used a technique known as psychological autopsy in studying terminal illness. Through interdisciplinary conferences, they tried to reconstruct the final phases of life of a recently deceased patient. They identified two different groups of these persons on the basis of their response to impending death. These two groups were (1) those persons who appeared aware of and accepting of impending death and withdrew from daily activities and (2) those who were aware of imminent death but engaged in daily life activities and even initiated new ones. In contrast to Kubler-Ross, these two investigators did not observe stages of dying but rather a pattern of behavior that was adopted and persisted until death.

Similar to the stages of dying or reactions to a terminal prognosis, the process of anticipatory grief is thought to involve specific stages of reaction to the dying patient. **Anticipatory grief** may be demonstrated by both the patient and his family. In fact, the patient with terminal illness must be allowed to grieve in anticipation of his death. This aspect of behavior is a natural part of the dying and grieving process, and the patient will require support during this process. The inability of family members or staff to face the terminal aspect of the patient's illness, or the patient's need to grieve for his losses (his loved ones, his life), may contribute to an isolated and impersonal way of dying unless efforts are made to facilitate communication with the patient rather than denying or preventing this need. Professionals, according to Glaser and Strauss [302] and others, have an obligation to help people die gracefully and to live even while they are dying. The trajectory of death (the course of dying) should be based on how the patient wishes it to be carried out.

Interest in the study of the process of dying continues. Currently it appears in nursing circles that Kubler-Ross's approach to understanding the process is the most accepted approach. Her writings have influenced many persons in nursing to observe dying patients more closely and to become less fearful of working with them. Death and dying have become important concerns for the nursing profession, and nurses are attempting to find appropriate ways to assist patients and their families to adjust to and to facilitate a dignified and peaceful death. Nurses, who work more closely with dying patients than do most other professionals, have unique opportunities to become more involved in the care of the dying, and also to document more accurately the observations and feelings of patients and their families. Through self-examination of the nurse's own feelings about death, denial, and psychological comfort, the nurse will be better able to cope with caring for the terminally ill. Certainly the nurse's attitude in caring for the terminally ill patient will affect the comfort of the patient and the family. When nurses practice the current approaches toward care of the terminally ill, they closely observe the degree of denial and acceptance of death, the conversations about dying, and the patient's feelings about dying, just as they observe vital signs and signs of physical complications in monitoring the physiologic changes in their patients. To observe the psychological factors carefully and accurately, the nurse listens to the patient and provides time for discussing the patient's feelings and concerns about terminal illness, how he is changing, and how the dying process should be handled. Emphasis is placed on helping the patient live one day at a time while coping with problems as they arise. If a trusting and meaningful relationship has been established, the nurse will then know what persons, possessions, and events have meant the most to the patient during his healthy life and will also know what is most important to him at this time. This knowledge should then guide the nurse in providing for those most significant persons and possessions at the time of impending death. Thus the patient will have the support of still other significant persons, the nurse and other staff, through the process and will not have to feel abandoned, as so many dying patients have feared.

Caring for the dying patient can be threatening and taxing for the nurse. But the assurance that all that is possible has been done to make the patient comfortable is also very satisfying, to both the nurse and the family. Helping the patient to have a dignified death is a primary nursing goal in the care of the terminally ill patient and thus requires specific nursing interventions.

Life-sustaining Techniques

The development of resuscitative techniques and the various mechanical devices to maintain life functions and the development of human transplant procedures have necessitated a redefinition of death. The conventional definition of **death** has been the cessation of all vital functions, but the modern definition requires adjustment of this definition in terms of irreversible brain damage. (The brain is more sensitive than any other organ to the lack of oxygen and nutrients. Destroyed brain cells cannot be regenerated.) However, this latter issue presents more controversy in relation to an appropriate definition of irreversible brain damage.

Criteria that have been used by one study group [304a] to define irreversible brain damage include: (1) total unresponsiveness, that is, complete absence of all central nervous system activity, (2) complete lack of spontaneous movements or spontaneous ventilation, (3) absence of cephalic reflexes, and (4) electrocerebral silence. The last two criteria are generally reflected by an isoelectric or zero-line electroencephalogram. However, the EEG records only the activity of the cerebral cortex and allows no conclusions about the function of subcortical brain structure. Universal acceptance of these criteria therefore is not currently present. In addition, there is no agreement on the need for a repeated evaluation of these criteria 24 hours after the initial evaluation. The definition of death, therefore, is not only a medical one, but also a legal one. The controversy over the legality of this definition continues throughout the country.

The answers to questions related to the prolonging or not prolonging of life are not clearly defined legally or morally. Two types of euthanasia have been identified. **Negative euthanasia** occurs when ordinary treatment is given (nutrition, comfort measures, pain relief) but nothing is done to hasten the death of a person. **Positive euthanasia** is that which occurs when specific measures are taken to hasten death. Recent legal actions related to abortion cases and situations of euthanasia indicate that varying conflicts about these aspects still require resolution.

The controversy over what constitutes a dignified death also continues. The Euthanasia Educational Council has instituted a Living Will Program. The documents provided under this program state that in the event of no reasonable expectation of recovery, the signer requests to die and not be kept alive by artificial means or heroic measures. The document is seen as a means to relieve families of guilt relative to not prolonging life in the absence of potential for recovery.

Although the document is not legally binding, it does serve as a guide for family members and medical personnel in handling the terminal stages. In fact, bills are being introduced in some state legislatures to make the document legally binding.

This entire scope of dying, in relation to the definition and the legal aspects of euthanasia, appears to be in transition. The reader is advised to keep updated on developments in this area.

References

GENERAL

1. Aitken, J. *Coordinated Health Services for the Aged* (League Exchange #10). New York: National League for Nursing, 1976.
2. Seventy-fifth anniversary issue. *Am. J. Nurs.* 75 (10), 1975.
3. Allport, F. H. *Theories of Perception and the Concept of Structure*. New York: Wiley, 1955.
4. AMA Department of Drugs. *AMA Drug Evaluations* (2nd ed.). Acton, Mass.: Publishing Sciences Group, 1973. Pp. 205–281.
5. Aschoff, J. Circadian systems in man and their implications. *Hosp. Pract.* 11:51, 1976.
6. Bates, B. *A Guide to Physical Examination*. Philadelphia: Lippincott, 1974.
7. Battistella, R. M. The right to adequate health care. *Nurs. Digest* 4:12, 1976.
8. Bickley, H. C. *Practical Concepts in Human Disease*. Baltimore: Williams & Wilkins, 1974.
9. Bloch, D. Evaluation of nursing care in terms of process and outcome: Issues in research and quality assurance. *Nurs. Res.* 24:256, 1975.
10. Bonner, C. D. *Homburger and Bonner's Medical Care and Rehabilitation of the Aged and Chronically Ill* (3rd ed.). Boston: Little, Brown, 1974.

11. Brammer, L. *The Helping Relationship: Process and Skills.* Englewood Cliffs, N. J.: Prentice-Hall, 1973.
12. Brink, P. J. (ed.). *Transcultural Nursing.* Englewood Cliffs, N. J.: Prentice-Hall, 1976.
13. Bristow, O. *Discharge Planning for Continuity of Care* (League Exchange #112). New York: National League for Nursing, 1976.
14. Browning, M., and Minehan, P. *The Nursing Process in Practice.* New York: American Journal of Nursing Co., 1974.
15. Buckingham, W., Sparberg, M., and Brandfonbrener, M. *A Primer of Clinical Diagnosis.* New York: Harper & Row, 1971.
16. Carkhuff, R. R. *The Art of Helping.* Englewood Cliffs, N. J.: Prentice-Hall, 1973.
17. Clute, K. F. Law and Health—Some Current Challenges. In *Politics and Law in Health Care Policy.* New York: Milbank Memorial Foundation, 1973. Pp. 139–200.
18. Coelho, G. V. *Coping and Adaptation.* New York: Basic Books, 1975.
19. Corso, J. F. Sensory progress and age effects in normal adults. *J. Gerontol.* 26:98, 1971.
20. *Current Estimates from the Health Interview Survey. United States—1974.* Washington D. C.: U. S. Department of Health, Education, and Welfare, Public Health Service, Health Resources Administration, 1975.
21. De Wied, D. Hormonal influence on motivation, learning, and memory processes. *Hosp. Pract.* 11:123, 1976.
22. Dohrenwend, B. S., and Dohrenwend, B. P. *Stressful Life Events: Their Nature and Effect.* New York: Wiley, 1974.
23. Dubos, R. *Man, Medicine and Environment.* New York: Praeger, 1968.
24. Epstein, C. *Nursing the Dying Patient.* Englewood Cliffs, N. J.: Prentice-Hall, 1975.
25. Eshleman, J. R. *The Family: An Introduction.* Boston: Allyn & Bacon, 1974.
26. Fawcett, J. The family as a living open system: An emerging conceptual framework for nursing. *Int. Nurs. Rev.* 22:113, 1975.
27. Fowkes, W., and Hunn, V. *Clinical Assessment for the Nurse Practitioner.* St. Louis: Mosby, 1973.
28. Fried, C. An analysis of "equality" and "rights" in medical care. *Hosp. Prog.* 57:44, 1976.
29. Friedman, G. *Primer of Epidemiology.* New York: McGraw-Hill, 1974.
30. Gibson, J. J. *The Senses Considered as Perceptual Systems.* Boston: Houghton Mifflin, 1966.
31. Gasfield, A. J. D. *PSROs: The Law and the Health Consumer.* Cambridge, Mass.: Ballinger, 1975.
32. Gubrium, J. *Time Roles and Self in Old Age.* New York: Behavioral Publications, 1976.
33. Hansell, N. *The Person-In-Distress.* New York: Behavioral Publications, 1976.
34. U. S. Department of Health, Education, and Welfare, Public Health Service, Health Resources Administration. *Health: United States–1975.* Rockville, Md.: National Center for Health Statistics, 1975.
35. Helson, H. *Adaptation Level Theory.* New York: Harper & Row, 1964.
36. ICN adopts definition of "nurse." *Int. Nurs. Rev.* 22 (204):184, 1975.
37. Johnson, W., and Moeller, D. *Living with Change.* New York: Harper & Row, 1972.
38. Kane, R. L., and Kane, R. A. *Federal Health Care (with Reservations).* New York: Springer, 1976.
39. Kane, R. L. *The Health Gap: Medical Services and the Poor.* New York: Springer, 1976.
40. Kübler-Ross, E. *Death, The Final Stage of Growth.* Englewood Cliffs, N. J.: Prentice-Hall, 1975.
41. LaBele, B. Health care and the aged. *J. Gerontol. Nurs.* 1:20, 1975.
42. LeBow, M. D. *Behavior Modification: A Significant Method in Nursing Practice.* Englewood Cliffs, N. J.: Prentice-Hall, 1973.
43. Leeser, I. R. *Community Health Nursing* (Nursing Outline Series). Flushing, N. Y.: Medical Examination Publishing, 1975.
44. Luce, G. C. *Biological Rhythms in Human and Animal Physiology.* New York: Dover, 1971.
45. Marram, G. D., Schlegel, M. W., and Bevis, Em. O. *Primary Nursing.* St. Louis: Mosby, 1974.
46. McKay, R. *Practitioner Preparations in Nursing Education Programs: A Workshop Report.* Washington D. C.: U.S. Department of Health, Education, and Welfare, Health Manpower Branch, Region VIII, 1975.
47. Milio, N. *The Care of Health in Communities.* New York: Macmillan, 1975.
48. Mims, F. H. (ed.). Symposium on human sexuality. *Nurs. Clin. North Am.* 10:3, 1975.
49. Moses, D. V. Assessing behavior in the elderly. *Nurs. Clin. North Am.* 7:225, 1972.
50. Mountcastle, V. B. (ed.). *Medical Physiology* (13th ed.). St. Louis: Mosby, 1974.
51. Muhlenkamp, A. F. Perception of life change events by the elderly. *Nurs. Res.* 24:109, 1975.
52. Murray, R. L. E. (ed.). Symposium on the concept of body image. *Nurs. Clin. North Am.* 7:593, 1974.
53. Murray, R., and Zentner, J. *Nursing Assessment and Health Promotion throughout the Life Span.* Englewood Cliffs, N. J.: Prentice-Hall, 1975.
54. Patient assessment: Taking a patient's history (Programmed Instruction). *Am. J. Nurs.* 74:293, 1974.

55. Patrick, D. Toward an operational definition of health. *J. Health Soc. Behav.* 14:6, 1973.
56. Patterson, G. *Families: Application of Social Learning to Family Life.* Champaign, Ill. Research Press, 1971.
57. Peery, T. M., and Miller, F. N., Jr. *Pathology: A Dynamic Introduction to Medicine and Surgery* (2nd ed.). Boston: Little, Brown, 1971.
58. Phaneuf, M. *The Nursing Audit.* New York: Appleton-Century-Crofts, 1972.
59. Porter, I. *Heredity and Disease.* New York: McGraw-Hill, 1968.
60. Race, A. R., Leecraft, J. F., and Crist, T. *The Sex Scene: Understanding Sexuality.* New York: Harper & Row, 1975.
61. Redman, B. *The Process of Patient Teaching in Nursing* (2nd ed.). St. Louis: Mosby, 1972.
62. Roberts, S. L. *Behavioral Concepts and the Critically Ill Patient.* Englewood Cliffs, N. J.: Prentice-Hall, 1976.
63. Salloway, J. C. *Social Networks and Health Care Consumership: Applications of Models of Health Service Utilization.* Springfield, Va.: National Technical Information Service, 1974.
64. Sana, J. M., and Judge, R. D. *Physical Appraisal Methods in Nursing Practice.* Boston: Little, Brown, 1975.
65. Selkurt, E. E. *Basic Physiology for the Health Sciences.* Boston: Little, Brown, 1975.
66. Selye, H. *The Stress of Life.* New York: McGraw-Hill, 1956.
67. Sherman, J., and Fields, S. *Guide to Patient Evaluation.* Flushing, N. Y.: Medical Examination Publishing, 1974.
68. Smyth, K. (ed.). Symposium on teaching patients. *Nurs. Clin. North Am.* 6:571, 1971.
69. Spradley, B. W. *Contemporary Community Nursing.* Boston: Little, Brown, 1975.
70. Starr, B. D., and Goldstein, H. S. *Human Development and Behavior.* New York: Springer, 1975.
71. Sutterly, D. C. *Perspectives in Human Development.* Philadelphia: Lippincott, 1973.
72. Taylor, D., and Johnson, O. *Systematic Nursing Assessment.* Bethesda, Md.: U. S. Department of Health, Education, and Welfare, Publ. No. (HRA) 74–17, 1974.
73. Timiras, P. *Developmental Physiology and Aging.* New York: Macmillan, 1972.
74. Wandelt, M., and Ager, J. *Quality Patient Care Scale.* New York: Appleton-Century-Crofts, 1974.
75. Wandelt, M., and Stewart, D. *Slater Nursing Competencies Rating.* New York: Appleton-Century-Crofts, 1974.
75a. Washington University Department of Medicine. E. C. Boedeker and J. H. Dauber (eds.), *Manual of Medical Therapeutics* (21st ed.). Boston: Little, Brown, 1974.
76. Weitzman, E. D. Biologic rhythms and hormone secretion patterns. *Hosp. Pract.* 11:79, 1976.
77. Whaley, L. F. *Understanding Inherited Disorders.* St. Louis: Mosby, 1974.
78. Woods, N. F. *Human Sexuality in Health and Illness.* St. Louis: Mosby, 1975.
79. Wooley, F. R., Warnick, M. W., Kane, R. L., and Dyer, E. D. *Problem-Oriented Nursing.* New York: Springer, 1974.
80. Wu, R. *Behavior and Illness.* Englewood Cliffs, N. J.: Prentice-Hall, 1973.
81. Zimmer, M. J. Symposium on quality assurance. *Nurs. Clin. North Am.* 9:303, 1974.

INFLAMMATION AND THE IMMUNE RESPONSE

82. Eisen, H. *Immunology.* New York: Harper & Row, 1974.
83. Gordon, B. L. *Essentials of Immunology* (2nd ed.). Philadelphia: Davis, 1974.
84. Harvey, A. M., and Johns, R. J. *The Principles and Practice of Medicine* (18th ed.). New York: Appleton-Century-Crofts, 1972.
85. Jolik, W. K., and Smith, D. *Zinsser Microbiology* (15th ed.). New York: Appleton-Century-Crofts, 1972.
86. National Institute of Allergy and Infectious Disease. *Immunology Research: An Introduction.* Bethesda, Md.: U.S. Department of Health, Education, and Welfare, Publ. No. (NIH) 73–529, 1973.
87. Sell, S. *Immunology, Immunopathology and Immunity* (2nd ed.). New York: Harper & Row, 1975.
88. Smith, A. L. *Principles of Microbiology* (7th ed.). St. Louis: Mosby, 1973.
89. Sodeman, W., and Sodeman, W. *Pathologic Physiology: Mechanisms of Disease* (5th ed.). Philadelphia: Saunders, 1974.

PAIN

90. Billars, K. S. You have pain? I think this will help. *Am. J. Nurs.* 70:2143, 1970.
91. Bobey, M. J. Psychological factors affecting pain tolerance. *J. Psychosom. Res.* 14:371, 1970.
92. Bumpus, J. F. Effective pain control with electroacupuncture. *Am. J. Acupuncture* 3:140, 1975.
93. Copp, L. A. The spectrum of suffering. *Am. J. Nurs.* 74:491, 1974.
94. Crowley, D. M. *Pain and Its Alleviation.* Los Angeles: University of California Press, 1962.
95. Derrick, W. S. The management of chronic pain. *Cancer* 23:269, 1973.

96. Drakontides, A. B. Drugs to treat pain. *Am. J. Nurs.* 74:508, 1974.
97. Electrical stimulation reduces complications after surgery. *J.A.M.A.* 230:1623, 1974.
98. Fordyce, W. An application of behavior modification technique to a problem of chronic pain. *Behav. Res. Ther.* 6:105, 1968.
99. Gaumer, W. R. Electrical stimulation in chronic pain. *Am. J. Nurs.* 74:505, 1974.
100. Goloskov, J., and LeRoy, P. Use of the dorsal column stimulator. *Am. J. Nurs.* 74:506, 1976.
101. Gutterman, P., and Shenkin, H. A. Saline frontal lobotomy in the treatment of intractable pain. *J.A.M.A.* 199:123, 1967.
102. Guyton, A. C. *Textbook of Medical Physiology.* Philadelphia: Saunders, 1971. Pp. 577–591.
103. Guzman, F., and Lim, R. K. The mechanism of action of the non-narcotic analgesics. *Med. Clin. North Am.* 52:3, 1968.
104. Hilgard, E. R. The alleviation of pain by hypnosis. *Pain* 1:213, 1975.
105. Indeck, W., and Printy, A. Skin application of electrical impulses for relief of pain. *Minn. Med.* 58:305, 1975.
106. Johnson, J. E., and Rice, V. H. Sensory and distress components of pain: Implications for the study of chronic pain. *Nurs. Res.* 23:203, 1974.
107. Loeser, J. D., Black, R. G., and Christman, A. Relief of pain by transcutaneous stimulation. *J. Neurosurg.* 42:308, 1975.
108. Mastrovito, R. C. Psychogenic pain. *Am. J. Nurs.* 74:514, 1974.
109. McCaffery, M. *Nursing Management of the Patient with Pain.* Philadelphia: Lippincott, 1972.
110. McLachlan, E. Recognizing pain. *Am. J. Nurs.* 74:496, 1974.
111. Melzack, R. How acupuncture works: A sophisticated western theory takes the mystery out. *Psychol. Today* 6:28, 1973.
112. Melzack, R. Prolonged relief of pain by brief intense transcutaneous somatic stimulation. *Pain* 1:357, 1975.
113. Pain mechanisms: A new theory. *Science* 150:971, 1965.
114. Pain. I. Basic concepts and assessment (Programmed Instruction). *Am. J. Nurs.* 66:1085, 1966.
115. Melzack, R., and Wall, P. Pain. II. Rationale for intervention (Programmed Instruction). *Am. J. Nurs.* 66:1345, 1966.
116. Pawl, R. P. Percutaneous radio frequency electrocoagulation in the control of chronic pain. *Surg. Clin. North Am.* 55:167, 1975.
117. Shealy, C. N., and Maurer, D. Transcutaneous nurse stimulation for control of pain. *Surg. Neurol.* 2:45, 1974.
118. Siegele, D. The gate control theory. *Am. J. Nurs.* 74:498, 1974.
119. Sternback, R., and Timmermans, G. Personality changes associated with reduction of pain. *Pain* 1:177, 1975.
120. Strauss, A., Fagerhaugh, S. Y., and Glaser, B. Pain: An organizational-work-interactional perspective. *Nurs. Outlook* 22:560, 1974.
121. Therrien, B., and Salmon, J. H. Precutaneous cordotomy for relief of intractable pain. *Am. J. Nurs.* 68:2594, 1968.
122. Walike, B., and Meyer, B. Relation between placebo reactivity and selected personality factors. *Nurs. Res.* 15:119, 1966.
123. Way, E. L. (ed.). *New Concepts in Pain and Its Clinical Management.* Philadelphia: Davis, 1967.
124. Weisenberg, M., Kriendler, M. L., Schachat, R., and Werboff, J. Pain: Anxiety and attitudes in Black, White and Puerto Rican Patients. *Psychosom. Med.* 37:123, 1975.
125. Wiener, C. L. Pain assessment on an orthopedic ward. *Nurs. Outlook* 23:508, 1975.

COMMUNICABLE DISEASE AND INFECTIONS

126. Bartlett, R. C. Control of Hospital-Associated Infection. In *Manual of Clinical Microbiology* (2nd ed.). Atlanta, Ga.: Center for Disease Control, 1974. Chap. 91.
127. Beland, I., and Passos, J. *Clinical Nursing* (3rd ed.). New York: Macmillan, 1975.
128. Benenson, A. S. (ed.). *Control of Communicable Diseases in Man* (12th ed.). Washington, D.C.: American Public Health Association, 1975.
129. Braxton, M. Epidemiology—What It's All About. In *Infection Control* (Publ. No. 20–1582). New York: National League for Nursing, 1975.
130. Brown, M. S. What you should know about communicable diseases and their immunizations. Part I, *Nursing 75* 5:9; Part II, *Nursing 75* 5:10, 1975.
131. Castle, M. Isolation. Precise procedures for better protection. *Nursing 75* 5:50, 1975.
132. Castle, M., and Osterhout, S. Urinary tract catheterization and associated infection. *Nurs. Res.* 23:170, 1974.
133. Center for Disease Control. *Isolation Techniques for Use in Hospitals* (rev.). Atlanta, Ga.: U.S. Department of Health, Education, and Welfare, Public Health Service, Publ. No. 017-023-00094-2, 1976.
134. Center for Disease Control. *Guidelines for Prevention of TB Transmission in Hospitals.* Atlanta, Ga.: U. S. Department of Health, Education and Welfare, Public Health Service, 1975.

135. Center for Disease Control. III. Methods of Prevention and Control of Nosocomial Infections. In *National Nosocomial Infections Study Quarterly Report* (4th quarter 1972). Atlanta, Ga.: Center for Disease Control, 1972.
136. Center for Disease Control. *Microbial Environmental Surveillance in the Hospital* (Training Document). Bureau of Epidemiology, Atlanta, Ga.: Center for Disease Control, 1970 (reprint. 1976).
137. Center for Disease Control. *Morbid. Mortal. Wkly Rep.* 25 (2), 1976.
138. Center for Disease Control. *Outline for Surveillance and Control of Nosocomial Infections,* Atlanta, Ga.: U.S. Department of Health, Education, and Welfare, Public Health Service, 1974.
139. Center for Disease Control. Recommendations for Prevention and Control of Catheter-Related Urinary Tract Infections and Statement on Microbiologic Sampling in the Hospital by Committee on Infections within Hospitals, American Hospital Association. In *National Nosocomial Infections Study Quarterly Report* (1st, 2nd quarters 1973). Atlanta, Ga.: Center for Disease Control, 1974.
140. Center for Disease Control. *Recommendations for the Prevention of IV-Associated Infections.* Atlanta, Ga.: U.S. Public Health Service, Publ. No. 00-2185, 1973.
141. Center for Disease Control. Recommendation of the Public Health Service Advisory Committee on Immunization Practices. *Morbid. Mortal. Wkly Rep.* 24 (23), 1975.
142. Center for Disease Control. Recommendations for health department supervision of tuberculosis patients. *Morbid. Mortal. Wkly Rep.* 23:75, 1974.
143. Center for Disease Control. Collected recommendations of the Public Health Service Advisory Committee on Immunization Practices. ACIP Recommendations (Supplement). *Morbid. Mortal. Wkly Rep.* 21 (25), 1972.
144. Center for Disease Control. Statement on Microbiologic Sampling in the Hospital by Committee on Infections within Hospitals, American Hospital Association. In *National Nosocomial Infections Study Quarterly Report* (1st, 2nd quarters 1973). Atlanta, Ga.: Center for Disease Control, 1974.
145. Chavigny, K. H. Nurse epidemiologist in the hospital. *Am. J. Nurs.* 75:4, 1975.
146. Conrad, J. L. (ed.). *Immunization Against Disease* (U.S. Department of Health, Education, and Welfare, Public Health Service, Health Services and Mental Health Administration). Atlanta, Ga.: Center for Disease Control, 1972.
147. Eickhoff, T. Role of Environmental Sampling. In *Proceedings of the International Conference on Nosocomial Infections.* Atlanta, Ga.: Center for Disease Control, 1970.
148. Favero, M. S. Microbiological hazards associated with artificial kidney machines. *APIC Newslett.* 2:9, Oct. 1974.
149. Favero, M. S. et al. Gram-negative water bacteria in hemodialysis systems. *Health Lab. Sci.* 12:321, 1975.
150. Fox, M. K., Langner, S. B., and Wells, R. How good are handwashing techniques? *Am. J. Nurs.* 74:9, 1974.
151. Garner, J. Nurse epidemiologist. Instrumental in infection control. *AORN J.* 20:261, 1974.
152. Garner, J. S., Bennett, J. V., Scheckler, W. E., Maki, D. G., and Brachman, P. S. Surveillance of Nosocomial Infections. In *Proceedings of the International Conference on Nosocomial Infections.* Atlanta, Ga.: Center for Disease Control, 1970.
153. Hoeprich, P. D. *Infectious Disease: A Guide to the Understanding and Management of the Infectious Process.* Hagerstown, Md.: Harper & Row, 1972.
154. Hymovich, D. P., and Barnard, M. U. *Family Health Care.* New York: McGraw-Hill, 1973.
155. Council of Hospital and Related Institutional Nursing Services. *Infection Control* (Publ. No. 20-1582). New York: National League for Nursing, 1975.
156. *Infection Control in the Hospital.* Chicago: American Hospital Association, 1970.
157. Irelan, L. M. *Low-Income Life Styles.* U.S. Department of Health, Education, and Welfare, Social and Rehabilitation Service, Office of Research and Demonstration, 1971.
158. Knight, V. Instruments and infection. *Hosp. Pract.* 2:82, 1967.
159. Kovarovic, S. Infection Control in a Governmental Hospital. In *Infection Control* (Publ. No. 20-1582). National League for Nursing, New York: 1975.
160. Kunin, C. M. *Detection, Prevention, and Management of Urinary Tract Infections* (2nd ed.). Philadelphia: Lea & Febiger, 1974.
161. McInnes, M. E. *Essentials of Communicable Disease.* St. Louis: Mosby, 1975.
162. Mikat, D. M., and Mikat, K. W. *A Clinician's Dictionary Guide to Bacteria* (2nd ed.). Indianapolis: Lilly Co., 1975.
163. Mulholland, S. G. Analysis and significance of nosocomial infection rates. *Ann. Surg.* 180:827, 1974.
164. Murray, R., and Zentner, J. Guidelines for more effective health teaching. *Nursing 76* 6:2, 1976.
165. National Tuberculosis and Respiratory Dis-

ease Association. Guidelines for the general hospital in the admission and care of tuberculosis patients (Prepared by the Ad Hoc Committee on the Treatment of Tuberculosis Patients in General Hospital). *Am. Rev. Respir. Dis.* 99:631, 1969.
166. National Tuberculosis Association. Infectiousness of tuberculosis (A Report of the NTA Ad Hoc Committee on Treatment of Tuberculosis Patients in General Hospitals). *Am. Rev. Respir. Dis.* 96:836, 1967.
167. National Tuberculosis and Respiratory Disease Association. Standards for tuberculosis treatment in the 1970's (A Statement by the Ad Hoc Committee on Quality Care for Tuberculosis). *Am. Rev. Respir. Dis.* 102:992, 1970.
168. Rycroft, P. Infection Control in the Community. In *Infection Control*. New York: National League for Nursing, Department of Hospital and Related Institutional Nursing Services, 1975.
169. *Salmonella Surveillance* (Rep. No. 124, 4th quarter 1974). Center for Disease Control, U.S. Department of Health, Education, and Welfare, Public Health Service, Publ. No. CDC 76-8219, Atlanta, Ga.: Center for Disease Control, 1975.
170. Sanford, J. P. The Hospital Reservoir (Speech presented before American College of Surgeons Symposium on the Control of Surgical Infections, Fort Lauderdale, Florida, March 6, 1970). Atlanta, Ga.: Center for Disease Control, 1970.
171. Smillie, W. G., and Kilbourne, E. D. *Preventive Medicine and Public Health* (3rd ed.). New York: Macmillan, 1963.
172. Spaulding, E. H. Role of Chemical Disinfection in the Prevention of Nosocomial Infections. In *Proceedings of the International Conference on Nosocomial Infections*. Atlanta, Ga.: Center for Disease Control, 1970.
173. Spencer, F. J. *Principles of Epidemiology*. Atlanta, Ga.: U.S. Department of Health, Education, and Welfare, Public Health Service Center for Disease Control, 1975.
174. Steere, A. C., and Mallison, G. F. Handwashing practices for the prevention of nosocomial infections. *Ann. Int. Med.* 83:683, 1975.
175. Taplin, D., and Mertz, P. M. Flower vases in hospitals as reservoirs of pathogens. *Lancet* 2:1279, 1973.
176. Terris, M. Approaches to an epidemiology of health. *Am. J. Public Health* 65:1037, 1975.
177. Wenzel, K. The role of the infection control nurse. In P. J. Brachman (ed.), Symposium on infection and the nurse. *Nurs. Clin. North Am.* 5:89, 1970.
178. Witte, J. J. Recent advances in public health immunization. *Am. J. Public Health* 64:939, 1974.

THE PATIENT REQUIRING SURGERY

179. AMA Department of Drugs. Agents Applied Locally—Antiseptics and Disinfectants (chap. XI, pp. 645–657). Drugs Used in Anesthesia (chap. IV, pp. 205–249). In *AMA Drug Evaluations* (2nd ed.). Acton, Mass.: Publishing Sciences Group, 1973.
180. Auld, M., et al. Wound healing. *Nursing 72* 2:36, 1972.
181. Bakutis, A. Anesthesia reactions. *Nursing 72* 2:16, 1972.
182. Ballinger, W. F., Treybal, J. C., and Vose, A. B. *Alexander's Care of the Patient in Surgery* (5th ed.). St. Louis: Mosby, 1972.
183. Beaumont, E. Hypo/hyperthermia equipment. Product survey. *Nursing 74* 4:34, 1974.
184. Bruegel, M. A. Relationship of preoperative anxiety to perception of postoperative pain. *Nurs. Res.* 20:26, 1971.
185. Castle, M. Wound care. Clear-cut ways to speed healing. *Nursing 75* 5:40, 1975.
186. Center for Disease Control. Food and Drug Administration warning—Contaminated detergent solution. *Morbid. Mortal. Wkly Rep.* 18:366, 1969.
187. Cruse, P. J. E., and Foord, R. A five year prospective study of 23,649 surgical wounds. *Arch. Surg.* 107:206, 1973.
188. Devney, A. M., and Kingsbury, B. A. Hypothermia in fact and fantasy. *Am. J. Nurs.* 71:1725, 1971.
189. Dumas, R. G. Psychological preparation for surgery. *Am. J. Nurs.* 63:52, 1963.
190. Dunphy, J. E. (ed.). *Wound Healing. A Medcom Update for the 70s*. Pearl River: Davis & Geck, 1974.
191. Dushoff, I. M. A stitch in time. *Emer. Med.* 5:21, 1973.
192. Fehlau, M. T. Applying the nursing process to patient care in the operating room. *Nurs. Clin. North Am.* 10:617, 1975.
193. Garfield, J. M. Psychological problems in anesthesia. *Am. Fam. Physician* 10:60, 1974.
194. Grahm, L. E., and Myers, E. Evaluation of anxiety and fear in adult surgical patients. *Nurs. Res.* 20:113, 1971.
195. Harrington, J. D. Symposium on intensive care of the surgical patient. *Nurs. Clin. North Am.* 10:1, 1975.
196. Heydman, A., and Stegman, M. R. One in a thousand. *Am. J. Nurs.* 71:1944, 1971.
197. Houghton, C. et al. The effect of anemia on wound healing. *Ann. Surg.* 179:163, 1974.
198. Johnson, J. E. Effects of structuring patient's expectations on their reactions to threatening events. *Nurs. Res.* 21:499, 1972.

199. Johnson, J. E. et al. Psychosocial factors in the welfare of surgical patients. *Nurs. Res.* 19:24, 1970.
200. Laufman, H. What's wrong with our operating rooms. *Am. J. Surg.* 122:332, 1971.
201. LeMaitre, G., and Finnegan, J. *The Patient in Surgery: A Guide for Nurses* (3rd ed.). Philadelphia: Saunders, 1975.
202. Libman, R. H., and Keithley, J. Relieving airway obstruction in the recovery room. *Am. J. Nurs.* 75:603, 1975.
203. Lindeman, C. A., and Stetzer, S. L. Effect of preoperative visits by operating room nurses. *Nurs. Res.* 22:4, 1973.
204. Lindeman, C. A., and Van Aerman, B. Nursing intervention with the presurgical patient. The effects of structured and unstructured preoperative teaching. *Nurs. Res.* 20:319, 1971.
205. Mallison, G. F. Housekeeping in operating suites. *AORN J.* 21:213, 1975.
206. Maykowski, K., and Fabre, D. Nursing assessment of the surgical intensive care patient. *Nurs. Clin. North Am.* 10:83, 1975.
207. Mehaffy, N. L. Assessment and communication for continuity of care for the surgical patient. *Nurs. Clin. North Am.* 10:625, 1974.
208. Minckley, B. B. Physiologic and psychologic responses of elective surgical patients. *Nurs. Res.* 23:392, 1974.
209. Myers, M. B. Sutures and wound healing. *Am. J. Nurs.* 71:1725, 1971.
210. Nardi, G. L., and Zuidema, G. D. *Surgery: A Concise Guide to Clinical Practice* (3rd ed.). Boston: Little, Brown, 1972.
211. Nolan, M. G. (ed.). Symposium on perspectives in operating room nursing. *Nurs. Clin. North Am.* 10:613, 1975.
212. Ogden, A. E., and Rathnell, T. K. Infections and benzalkonium solutions. *J.A.M.A.* 193:978, 1965.
213. Parsons, M. C., and Stephens, G. J. Postoperative complications: Assessment and intervention. *Am J. Nurs.* 74:240, 1974.
214. Peacock, E. E., and Van Winkle, W., Jr. *Surgery and Biology of Wound Repair*. Philadelphia: Saunders, 1970.
215. Postlethwaitt, R. W. Principles of Operative Surgery: Antisepsis, Techniques, Sutures and Drains. In Sabiston, D. C., *Davis-Christopher Textbook of Surgery* (10th ed.). Philadelphia: Saunders, 1972.
216. Powell, M. An environment for wound healing. *Am. J. Nurs.* 72:1862, 1972.
217. Robbins, S., and Angell, M. *Basic Physiology*. Philadelphia: Saunders, 1971.
218. Seropian, K., and Reynolds, G. M. Wound infections after preoperative depilatory versus razor preparation. *Am. J. Surg.* 121:251, 1971.
219. Smith, R. B. et al. In a recovery room. *Am. J. Nurs.* 73:70, 1973.
220. Spaulding, E. H. Role of Chemical Disinfection in the Prevention of Nosocomial Infections. In *Proceedings of the International Conference on Nosocomial Infections*. Atlanta, Ga.: Center for Disease Control, 1970. Pp. 247–254.
221. Williams, S. R. Care of the Surgery Patient. In *Nutrition and Diet Therapy* (2nd ed.). St. Louis: Mosby, 1973.
222. Winslow, E. H., and Fuhs, M. F. Preoperative assessment for postoperative evaluation. *Am. J. Nurs.* 73:1372, 1973.
223. Wolfer, J. A., and Davis, C. E. Assessment of surgical patients' preoperative emotional condition and postoperative welfare. *Nurs. Res.* 19:402, 1970.
224. Wound suction. Better drainage with fewer problems. *Nursing 75* 5:52, 1975.

THE PATIENT WITH CANCER

225. Achte, K. A., and Vauhkonen, M. L. Cancer and the psyche. *Omega* 2:46, 1971.
226. AMA Department of Drugs. Antineoplastic Agents. In *AMA Drug Evaluations* (2nd ed.). Acton, Mass.: Publishing Sciences Group, 1973. Chap. 88, pp. 835-861.
227. American Cancer Society. *A Cancer Source Book for Nurses*. New York: American Cancer Society, 1975.
228. American Cancer Society. *'76 Cancer Facts and Figures*. New York: American Cancer Society, 1975.
229. American Cancer Society. *Nutrition for Patients Receiving Chemotherapy and Radiation Treatment*. New York: American Cancer Society, 1974.
230. American Cancer Society. *Unproven Methods of Cancer Management*. New York: American Cancer Society, 1971.
231. Ansfield, F. J. *Cancer Chemotherapy: When Should It Be Instituted?* (Tape #476). Madison, Wisc.: Nursing Dial Access, 1975.
232. Ansfield, F. J. *Indications for Use of 5 FU in Advanced Cancer* (Tape #95). Madison, Wisc.: Nursing Dial Access, 1974.
233. Ansfield, F. J. *Selection of Patients for Cancer Chemotherapy* (Tape #75). Madison, Wisc.: Nursing Dial Access, 1975.
234. Armstrong, D., and Tedder, E. Care of patients with the carcinoid syndrome. *Nurs. Clin. North Am.* 4:171, 1969.
235. Axtell, L. M. et al. *End Results in Cancer* (Rep. No. 4). Bethesda, Md.: U.S. Department of Health, Education, and Welfare, Publ. No. (NIH) 73-272, 1972.

236. Bast, R. C., Jr. et al. BCG and cancer. Part 1. *N. Engl. J. Med.* 290:1413, 1974.
237. Bates, B. *A Guide to Physical Examination.* Philadelphia: Lippincott, 1974.
238. Behnke, H. D. (ed.). *Guidelines for Comprehensive Nursing Care in Cancer.* New York: Springer, 1973.
239. Bouchard, R., and Owens, N. *Nursing Care of the Cancer Patient* (2nd ed.). St. Louis: Mosby, 1972.
240. Bruya, M. A., and Madrira, N. P. Stomatitis after chemotherapy. *Am. J. Nurs.* 75:1349, 1975.
241. Buehler, J. A. What contributes to hope in the cancer patient? *Am. J. Nurs.* 75:1353, 1975.
242. Buescu, A. et al. Cancer hypercalcemia—A pragmatic approach. *Clin. Bull.* 5:91, 1975.
243. Buschke, F., and Parker R. G. *Radiation Therapy in Cancer Management.* New York: Grune & Stratton, 1972.
244. Davies, R. K. et al. Organic factors and psychological adjustments in advanced cancer patients. *Psychosom. Med.* 35:469, 1973.
245. Delmonte, L., and Oettgen, H. F. BCG in the therapy of cancer. *Clin. Bull.* 5:69, 1975.
246. DeVita, V. T., and Rauscher, F. J. *Fact Sheet: Advances in Cancer Treatment–1974.* Bethesda, Md.: National Cancer Institute, 1975.
247. DeWys, W. D., and Wazlters, K. Abnormalities of taste sensation in cancer patients. *Cancer* 36:1888, 1975.
248. Dietz, J. H. Rehabilitation of the cancer patient: Its role in the scheme of comprehensive care. *Clin. Bull.* 5:104, 1975.
249. DiPalma, J. Drug therapy today. Radiopharmaceuticals: Nuclear-age drugs for diagnosis and treatment. *R.N.* 38:59, 1975.
250. DuPriest, R. W. et al. Streptozotocin therapy in 22 cancer patients. *Cancer* 35:358, 1975.
251. Elias, G. et al. Heparin and chemotherapy in the management of inoperable lung carcinoma. *Cancer* 36:129, 1975.
252. Faraci, R. P. et al. BCG-induced protection against malignant melanoma: Possible immunospecific effect in a murine system. *Cancer* 35:372, 1975.
253. Fink, D. J. The cancer control program. *Cancer* 35:72, 1975.
254. Fortner, J. G., and Shiu, M. H. Organ transplantation and cancer. *Surg. Clin. North Am.* 54:871, 1974.
255. George, M. M. Long-term care of the patient with cancer. *Nurs. Clin. North Am.* 8:623, 1973.
256. Godwin, J. D. Carcinoid tumors. An analysis of 2837 cases. *Cancer* 36:569, 1975.
257. Hackett, T. P. et al. Patient delay in cancer. *N. Engl. J. Med.* 289:14, 1973.
258. Hadden, J. W. Thymopoietin, ubiquitin and the differentiation of lymphocytes. *Clin. Bull.* 5:66, 1975.
259. Hedrick, J. L. *Smoking, Tobacco and Health.* Bethesda, Md.: U.S. Department of Health, Education, and Welfare, 1969.
260. Hicks, S. *Cancer Diagnosis. Crisis for Patient and Family* (Tape #436). Madison, Wisc.: Nursing Dial Access, 1970.
261. Hilkemeyer, R. Nursing care in radium therapy. *Nurs. Clin. North Am.* 2:83, 1967.
262. Hoover, R., and Fraumeni, J. F., Jr. Risk of cancer in renal transplant recipients. *Lancet* 2:55, 1973.
263. Hoover, H. C., and Ketcham, A. S. Techniques for inhibiting tumor metastasis. *Cancer* 35:5, 1975.
264. Islet, C. (ed.). Newest treatment for cancer: Immunotherapy. *R.N.* 39:35, 1976.
265. Jackson, B. S., and Armenaki, D. W. A tumor classification system. *Am. J. Nurs.* 76:1320, 1976.
266. Jones, S. et al. Combination chemotherapy with Adriamycin and cyclophosphamide for advanced breast cancer. *Cancer* 36:90, 1975.
267. Jewett, H. Cancer of the bladder—Diagnosis and staging. *Cancer* 32:1072, 1973.
268. Keough, G., and Niebel. Oral cancer detection—A nursing responsibility. *Am. J. Nurs.* 73:684, 1973.
269. Levin, D. L. et al. *Cancer Rates and Risks* (2nd ed.). Bethesda, Md.: U.S. Department of Health, Education, and Welfare, National Cancer Institute, Publ. No. (NIH) 76-691, 1974.
270. Marino, E. B., and LeBlanc, D. H. Cancer chemotherapy. *Nursing 75* 5:22, 1975.
271. Mastrovito, R. C. Cancer: Awareness and denial. *Clin. Bull.* 4:142, 1974.
272. Milligan, C. et al. Screening for cervical cancer. *Am. J. Nurs.* 75:1343, 1975.
273. Muto, T. et al. The evolution of cancer of the colon and rectum. *Cancer* 36:2251, 1975.
274. *National Cancer Institute. Fact Book 1975.* Bethesda, Md.: U.S.Department of Health, Education, and Welfare, Publ. No. (NIH) 75-512, 1975.
275. *National Cancer Program Planning Conference* (Summary Report for Cancer Control). Bethesda, Md.: U.S. Department of Health, Education, and Welfare, Publ. No. (NIH) 76-965, 1975.
276. National Institutes of Health. *Research Advances 1975.* Bethesda, Md.: U.S. Department of Health, Education, and Welfare, Publ. No. (NIH) 75-3, 1975.
277. Nutrition, diet and cancer. *Dairy Counc. Dig.* 46:25, 1975.

278. Peck, A. Emotional reactions to having cancer. *Cancer* 22:284, 1972.
279. Peery, T. M., and Miller, F. N., Jr. *Pathology: A Dynamic Introduction to Medicine and Surgery* (2nd ed.). Boston: Little, Brown, 1971.
280. Peterson, B. H., and Kellogg, C. J. *Current Practices in Oncologic Nursing.* St. Louis: Mosby, 1976.
280a. Pienschke, S. D. Guardedness or openness on the cancer unit. *Nurs. Res.* 22:484, 1973.
281. *Precautions in the Management of Patients Who Have Received Therapeutic Amounts of Radionuclides.* Washington, D.C.: National Council on Radiation Protection and Measurements, 1970.
282. Prehn, R. T. Cancer and the immune response. *Proc. Inst. Med. Chic.* 29:339, 1973.
283. Quinn, J. L. *Radionuclides in the Diagnosis of Cancer.* New York: American Cancer Society, 1971.
284. Rauscher, F. J. *Fact Sheet: Adriamycin.* Bethesda, Md.: U.S. Department of Health, Education, and Welfare, National Institutes of Health, 1975.
285. Rhoads, J. E. The control of large bowel cancer. *Cancer* 36:2314, 1975.
286. Robbins, S., and Angell, M. *Basic Pathology.* Philadelphia: Saunders, 1971.
287. Rubin, P. (ed.). *Clinical Oncology for Medical Students and Physicians* (4th ed.). New York: American Cancer Society, 1974.
288. Schabel, F. M., Jr. Concepts for systematic treatment of micrometastasis. *Cancer* 35:15, 1975.
289. Schmidt. B. C. et al. *National Cancer Program* (Report of President's Cancer Panel). Bethesda, Md.: U.S. Department of Health, Education, and Welfare, Publ. No. (NIH) 75-354, 1974.
290. Seifurt, P. et al. Comparison of continuously infused 5-Fluorouracil with bolus injection in treatment of patients with colorectal adenocarcinoma. *Cancer* 36:123, 1975.
291. Shimkun, M. *Science and Cancer* (2nd rev.). Bethesda, Md.: U.S. Department of Health, Education and Welfare, Publ. No. (NIH) 75-568, 1973.
292. Silverstein, M. J., and Morton, D. L. Cancer immunotherapy. *Am. J. Nurs.* 73:1178, 1973.
292a. Smart, C. et al. Phase I. Study of Ftorafur, an analog of 5-Fluorouracil. *Cancer* 36:103, 1975.
293. Van Roosenbeek, E., and Delclos, L. *The Radioactive Patient. Care, Precautions and Procedures in Diagnosis and Therapy.* Flushing, N.Y.: Medical Examination Publishing, 1975.
294. Watson, R. C. The whole body scan. Computed tomography (CT)—A major advance in the diagnosis of cancer. *Clin. Bull.* 6:47, 1976.
295. Weisburger, J. H. Large bowel cancer. Metabolic epidemiology and carcinogenesis. *Cancer* 36:2385, 1975.
296. Weston, J. *Nurse's Role in Cancer Detection* (Tape #547). Madison, Wisc.: Nursing Dial Access, 1975.
297. Zamcheck, N. The present status of CEA in diagnosis, prognosis and evaluation of therapy. *Cancer* 36:2460, 1975.

TERMINAL ILLNESS; DEATH AND DYING

298. Becker, E. *The Denial of Death.* New York: Free Press, 1973.
299. Caughill, R. E. *The Dying Patient: A Supportive Approach.* Boston: Little, Brown, 1976.
300. Epstein, C. *Nursing the Dying Patient: Learning Processes for Interaction.* Reston, Md.: Reston Publishing, 1975.
301. Feifel, H. (ed.). *The Meaning of Death.* New York: McGraw-Hill, 1959.
302. Glaser, B. G., and Strauss, A. L. *Awareness of Dying.* Chicago: Aldine, 1965.
303. Gonda, T. Pain relief, addiction and the dying patient. *J. Thanatol.* 1:146, 1970.
304. Greinacher, N., and Muller, A. *The Experience of Dying.* New York: Herder & Herder, 1974.
304a. Harvard Medical School, Ad Hoc Committee to Examine the Definition of Brain Death. A definition of irreversible coma. *J.A.M.A.* 205:387, 1968.
305. Hinton, J. M. The physical and mental distress of dying. *Q. J. Med.* 32:1, 1963.
306. Ingles, T. St. Christopher's Hospice. *Nurs. Outlook* 22:759, 1974.
307. Janis, K. M. Determination of Death in the Terminally Ill Patient. In M. B. Ravin and J. H. Modell (eds.), *Introduction to Life Support.* Boston: Little, Brown, 1973. Pp. 166-175.
308. Kahana, E. Attitudes of young men and women toward awareness of death. *Omega* 3:37, 1974.
309. Kastenbaum, R., and Weisman, A. D. The Psychological Autopsy as a Research Procedure in Gerontology. In D. P. Kent, R. Kastenbaum, and S. Sherwood (eds.), *Research Planning and Action for the Elderly.* New York: Behavioral Publications, 1972.
310. Kaüffer, C. A Medical View of the Process of Death. In ref. 304, pp. 33–53.
311. Kübler-Ross, E. Dying as a Human-Psychological Event. In ref. 304, pp. 48–54.
312. Kübler-Ross, E. *On Death and Dying.* New York: Macmillan, 1969.
313. Kübler-Ross, E. *Death: The Final Stage of*

314. Kutscher, A. H. Anticipatory Grief, Death and Bereavement: A Continuum. In E. Wyschogrod (ed.), *The Phenomenon of Death: Faces of Mortality*. New York: Harper & Row, 1973. Pp. 40–53.
315. Kutscher, A. H., Jr. *Death and Bereavement*. Springfield, Ill.: Thomas, 1969.
316. Langone, J. *Death Is a Noun: A View of the End of Life*. Boston: Little, Brown, 1972.
317. Lester, D., Getty, C., and Kneisl, C. R. Attitudes of nursing students and nursing faculty toward death. *Nurs. Res.* 23:50, 1974.
318. Liegner, L. M. St. Christopher's Hospice, 1974. Care of the dying patient. *J.A.M.A.* 234:1047, 1975.
319. McCorkle, R. Effects of touch on seriously ill patients. *Nurs. Res.* 23:125, 1974.
320. Quint, J. C. Personalizing institutional care of the dying. *J. Thanatol.* 2:60, 1970.
321. Quint, J. C. The dying patient: A difficult nursing problem. *Nurs. Clin. North Am.* 2:763, 1967.
322. Quint, J. C. *The Nurse and the Dying Patient*. New York: Macmillan, 1967.
323. Quint, J. C. The threat of death: Some consequences for patients and nurses. *Nurs. Forum* 8:286, 1969.
324. Schoenberg, B. et al. *Loss and Grief: Psychological Management in Medical Practice*. New York: Columbia University Press, 1970.
325. Schoenberg, B. et al. *Psychosocial Aspects of Terminal Care*. New York: Columbia University Press, 1972.
326. Schoenberg, B. et al. *Anticipatory Grief*. New York: Columbia University Press, 1974.
327. Schulz, R., and Aderman, D. Clinical research and the stages of dying. *Omega* 5:137, 1974.
328. Sudnow, D. *Passing On: The Social Organization of Dying*. Englewood Cliffs, N.J.: Prentice-Hall, 1967.
329. Troup, S. B., and Greene, W. A. (eds.). *The Patient, Death and the Family*. New York: Scribner, 1974.
330. Weisman, A. D. Care and Comfort for the Dying. In S. B. Troup and W. A. Greene (eds.), *The Patient, Death and the Family*. New York: Scribner, 1974. Pp. 97-111.
331. Wyschogrod, E. (ed.). *The Phenomenon of Death: Faces of Mortality*. New York: Harper & Row, 1973.

Note: Entry preceding 314 continues from previous page: *Growth*. Englewood Cliffs, N.J.: Prentice-Hall, 1975.

chapter 2

Fluid and Electrolyte Balance

Virginia Mermel

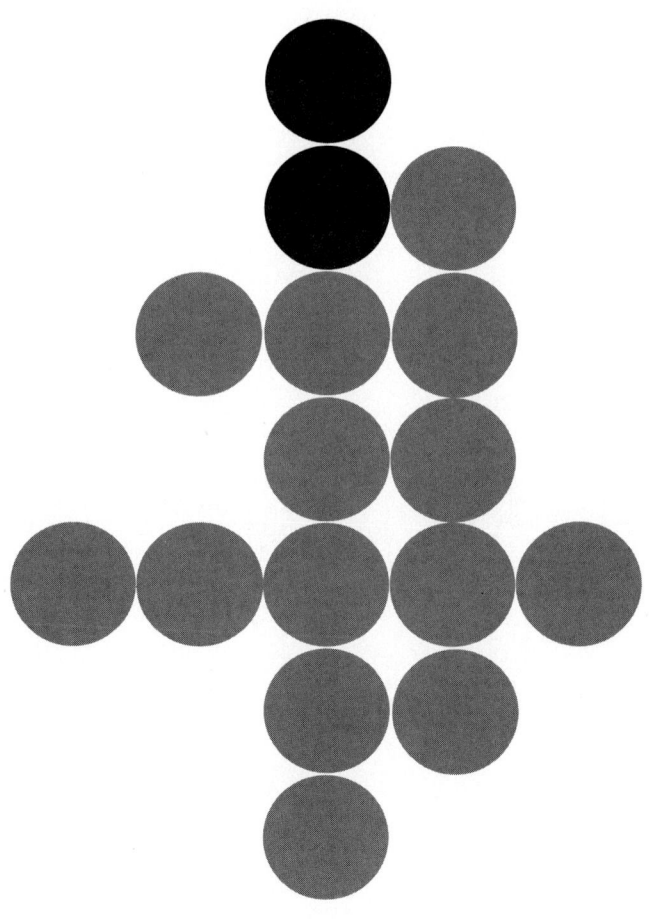

The nurse does not approach a person in order to assess his or her needs for nursing without knowledge of normal physiology and the alterations that can occur in the structure and function of the human body. This chapter is designed with this logical progression in mind.

The normal state of fluids and electrolytes in the body will be presented and will be followed by discussions of the regulating mechanisms that maintain the normal state in the face of variable external and internal environments. Evidence that the control or regulating mechanisms of the body are not adequate to the task of maintaining normal balance will be presented as clinical disease or as a symptom complex. Both the normal and the disease states have implications for nursing. The **normal state** is a baseline of data to guide the nurse in maintaining positive health in any adult for whom he or she cares. The normal state also is the goal to be attained by nursing intervention in situations of altered balance. The **disease state** describes the internal changes that occur with an alteration in the body's ability to function and the symptoms that arise when the body's psychological and physiologic coping mechanisms fail. These situations will indicate the specific nursing needs of a patient and will be discussed in relation to the process of nursing.

Common Concepts

There are several concepts basic to an understanding of fluids and electrolytes in the body. A central one is the idea of **polarities**, the opposite effects at the two extremes of a continuum. This concept is discussed in terms of increase-decrease, positive-negative, and hyper- and hypo-states. Examples of this concept abound in nature and are based on the principle of interdependency of essential parts. A simple example is provided by a tablespoon of salt in a glass of water. Increasing the amount of water decreases the previous ratio of salt to water. Another example is that of nitrogen: When the amount of nitrogen ingested is greater than the amount excreted, the body is said to be in positive nitrogen balance. When the amount excreted is greater than that ingested, the body is in negative nitrogen balance.

Homeostasis is a second concept essential to the comprehension of body fluids. The renowned physiologist Walter Cannon coined the term and described its meaning so well that it bears repeating verbatim.

The coordinated physiological processes which maintain most of the steady states in the organism are so complex and so peculiar to living beings—involving, as they may, the brain and nerves, the heart, lungs, kidneys, and spleen, all working cooperatively—that I have suggested a special designation for these states, homeostasis. The word does not imply something set and immobile, a stagnation. It means a condition—a condition which may vary but which is relatively constant [1].

As Cannon pointed out, homeostasis is a dynamic state in which the body is continually regulating itself. Homeostasis is sometimes referred to as the steady state, and absence of homeostasis as imbalance. The healthy body is a homeostatic organism. An example of this dynamic mechanism occurs when a person who has ingested a greater amount of fluid than is needed by the body experiences an increased output of dilute urine.

A third concept, closely allied to homeostasis, is that of adapting. **Adapting** is the act of striving toward a positive, viable condition, and **adaptation** is the state that is evidenced when that result is achieved. Adaptation always refers to accomplished change, and when we say that an organism is adapting to its environment, we are saying that it is changing in order to cope with the demands made by that environment. **Maladaptation** is the opposite concept and indicates that the organism has not moved in a positive direction. Helson considers adaptation to be a learning state and views it as always having two aspects: Whenever one mode of adaptation becomes prominent, a corresponding mode recedes in importance [3]. For example, if retention of sodium is adaptive for an organism, the forces that normally promote sodium excretion will diminish.

It must be remembered that, in adaptation, although the body is seeking a functional state and can adjust to a variety of unusual stimuli, there is a limit beyond which it can no longer cope and external intervention and support are necessary to sustain life. Helson believes that homeostasis is a class of adaptation that refers to steady states [3]. If any distinction can be made between adaptation and homeostasis, it is that in adaptation the organism seeks to contend with threatening stimuli in almost any way possible in order to survive, whereas in homeostasis the organism is committed to returning to a previous, well-defined state. The person who has respiratory insufficiency, for example, and is unable to eliminate excess carbon dioxide from his circulating blood, learns to live with higher than normal levels of this metabolic waste product. He is said to have adapted, but he is not in homeostasis.

Feedback and equilibrium are two terms that also describe the body's maintenance processes. **Equilibrium** is a state in which opposing forces counteract each other. In the body this equilibrium is evidenced when the amount of fluid intake precisely balances the amount of fluid output. **Dynamic equilibrium** is the balance between shifting and opposing forces characteristic of living processes. **Disequilibrium** exists when one of two opposing forces is for some reason more powerful than the other and dominates the relationship; it is illustrated in the loss of large amounts of fluids through vomiting and the corresponding inability to ingest enough liquid to keep the body fluids in balance.

Feedback is a term derived from systems theory and is the return of part of the output of a process to its source in order to modify or reinforce that process. A good example of feedback is provided by the respiratory system. An increase in the amount of carbon dioxide in the blood leads to an increased rate of respirations, with the result that more carbon dioxide is excreted from the lungs and the carbon dioxide level in the blood falls.

Normal State of Fluids and Electrolytes

The normal state of fluids and electrolytes in the body provides a picture of the healthy person. It is basic to understanding the deviations that occur in response to external and internal stimuli.

One of the difficulties in understanding fluid balance has been the extensive use of chemical terms to describe this phenomenon. The following relevant terms are defined as they are used in this chapter:

body water Simple, pure water contained in the body.
body fluid Body water plus the electrolytes and nonelectrolytes dissolved in that water; the intracellular and extracellular fluid.
electrolytes Chemical substances that form electrically charged particles when they are in a solution. For example: sodium$^+$, potassium$^+$, and chloride$^-$.
nonelectrolytes Chemical substances that do not form electrically charged particles when they are in a solution. For example: urea, glucose, and creatine.
ion An atom or group of atoms having either a positive charge (a cation) or a negative charge (an anion) of electricity. Sodium$^+$ and chloride$^-$ are ions; sodium$^+$ is a cation, chloride$^-$ an anion.
molecule A chemical combination of two or more atoms that form a specific chemical substance; the smallest unit of a substance that retains the characteristics of that substance.
solute A substance that is dissolved in a solvent.
solution A liquid mixture of two or more substances molecularly dispersed throughout one another in a homogenous manner; a solute and a solvent.
solvent A liquid that is capable of dissolving a solute.
osmosis The passage of water molecules from an area of greater concentration to an area of lesser concentration when they are separated by a membrane that selectively prevents the passage of solute molecules, but is permeable to the solvent.
osmotic pressure The pressure needed to reverse the forces of osmosis.

In addition to these descriptive terms, several different units of measure are used in referring to body fluids when measuring the number of molecules, electrical charges, or particles of a solute per unit volume as well as the volume of the solution.

cubic centimeter or milliliter (cc or ml) One cubic centimeter is the volume contained in an area 1 cm long by 1 cm wide by 1 cm high. A **milliliter** is the volume contained in 1/1,000 of a liter. These two measurements are equal.
equivalent (eq) A measurement of electrical charges. One equivalent is 1 mole of an ionized substance divided by its valence and can be expressed in grams. For example: 1 mole of sodium chloride with a gram molecular weight of 58.5 and a valence of 2 is equal to 29.2 grams (58.5 ÷ 2 = 29.2). A **milliequivalent (mEq)** is 1/1,000 of an equivalent; 2 eq of sodium chloride = 2,000 mEq of sodium chloride.

liter (L) The volume contained in an area 10 cm long by 10 cm wide by 10 cm high.

milligrams percent (mg%) One thousandth of a gram per 100 milliliters of a solution, preferably expressed as mg/100 ml.

mole (M) The amount of a substance or of a chemical equivalent to its mass and expressed in grams (gram molecular weight) as, 1 mole of sodium chloride is equal to 23 + 35.5 = 58.5 grams. A **millimole (mM)** is 1/1,000 of a mole; 1 mM of sodium chloride = 58.5 milligrams.

osmol (Osm) The particles of a substance. One osmol equals the molecular weight of a substance in grams divided by the number of freely moving particles each molecule liberates in solution; 1 Osm of sodium chloride = 58.5 grams ÷ 2 = 29.7 grams. Therefore 1 mole of sodium chloride = 2 Osm. A **milliosmol (mOsm)** is 1/1,000 of an osmol; 1 mOsm of sodium chloride = 29.7 mg.

The four significant variables that are descriptive of body fluids are volume, distribution, composition, and function.

VOLUME

The greater part of the human body is composed of body fluid. A 70-kilogram person (approximately 150 pounds) has 40 liters of body fluid, which accounts for approximately 60 percent of the body weight. Age, sex, and amount of adipose tissue all affect the relative amount of body fluid to body weight. A newborn infant's total body weight is composed of 75 percent fluid; this percentage progressively decreases until old age. The obese person has a decreased percentage of body fluid because fat cells do not hold fluid to the same extent as do other cells. The average female also has a lower content of body fluid than the average male has due to the greater number of fat cells in the structure of the female body.

DISTRIBUTION

A second important variable is the distribution of body fluid. The body fluid is contained within two large, chemically different compartments: the extracellular fluid (ECF) and the intracellular fluid (ICF) compartment. The term compartment is usually dropped in speaking of them, and body fluids are referred to as either intracellular or extracellular fluids.

Intracellular fluid comprises 25 of the 40 liters of total body fluid (Table 2-1) and is collectively contained within the trillions of minute cells in the body. **Extracellular fluid** is referred to as either interstitial fluid or plasma. This is a practical and useful designation but it is not physiologically accurate. The ECF actually exists in numerous different spaces, all of which are meaningful in the study of total body fluid, although some of the amounts are very small. The total amount of ECF in the human body is 15 liters. It is primarily distributed in the following manner: plasma or intravascular fluid, about 3 liters; interstitial fluid, which surrounds the cells, accounts for approximately 12 liters; and small amounts of cerebrospinal fluid, which bathes the spinal cord and brain; intraocular fluid, the fluid within the eyes; secretions of the gastrointestinal tract; inaccessible bone water; and the "potential spaces." Although the potential spaces usually do not contain large amounts of fluids, they can expand to contain significant amounts. These spaces are sometimes called the third space and exist in the peritoneal cavity, pericardial cavity, joint spaces, the bursae, and between the visceral and parietal pleurae of the lungs. The fluid of the potential spaces communicates freely with the interstitial spaces.

COMPOSITION

The body fluid is composed of water, electrolytes, and nonelectrolytes. Intracellular and extracellular fluid compartments contain the same kinds of electrolytes and nonelectrolytes, but the concentrations of each differ significantly. Table 2-2 lists the concentrations of the various ions and molecules in the body fluid compartments.

Table 2-1
Distribution of body fluids in a person weighing 70 kilograms

Extracellular Fluid (L)		Intracellular fluid (L)
Interstitial*	Plasma	
12	3	25

*Interstitial fluid includes the fluids found in the cerebrospinal spaces, intraocular spaces, gastrointestinal tract, bones, and potential spaces.

Table 2-2
Concentrations of ions and molecules in the two fluid compartments of the body

Intracellular fluid	Ions and molecules	Extracellular fluid
2–10 mEq/L	Sodium (Na^+)	138–142 mEq/L
135–155 mEq/L	Potassium (K^+)	3.8–5.0 mEq/L
<1 mEq/L	Calcium (Ca^{++})	<5 mEq/L
58 mEq/L	Magnesium (Mg^{++})	1–2 mEq/L
4–10 mEq/L	Chloride (Cl^-)	92–105 mEq/L
8–10 mEq/L	Bicarbonate (HCO_3^-)	24–28 mEq/L
30–45 mEq/L	Phosphate (HPO_4^{--})	1 mEq/L
2 mEq/L	Sulfate (SO_4^{--})	0.5 mEq/L
0–20 mg/100 ml	Glucose	90 mg/100 ml
200 mg/100 ml	Amino Acids	30 mg/100 ml
2–95 gm/100 ml	Cholesterol / Phospholipids / Neutral fat	0.5 gm/100 ml
	Proteinate:	6–8 gm/100 ml
	Plasma proteins	14.6–19.4 mEq/L

The most significant electrolyte in the ECF is sodium, which accounts for 90 percent of all ECF solutes. The ECF also contains large quantities of chloride and bicarbonate and small concentrations of potassium, magnesium, and phosphate. In contrast, the ICF contains large amounts of potassium, phosphate, and magnesium and only small quantities of sodium, chloride, and bicarbonate.

FUNCTION

The importance of body water cannot be overstressed. In addition to the role it plays as a vital component of the fluid compartments, it serves the body as a solvent in which the many solutes available for cell function are dissolved. Body water transports to and from the cells the gases, nutrients, waste products, and products of cellular metabolism. It assists the body in heat regulation by the evaporation of perspiration and it is important in maintaining the delicate hydrogen ion balance in the body. Body water provides the water of hydrolysis so that foods may be digested. And, finally, body water provides a medium for the excretion of waste from the body.

Sodium is the most significant cation in the extracellular fluid and it contributes greatly to the osmolality of that compartment. The primary role of sodium is in controlling the distribution of water throughout the body. It is able to function in this capacity partly because of its dominance in quantity and partly because it does not easily cross the cell membrane. A decrease in the serum sodium concentration will promote water excretion by inhibiting antidiuretic hormone. This water loss is directed toward establishing a normal concentration of sodium. Conversely, an increase in serum sodium concentration stimulates the release of antidiuretic hormone, causing the retention of water and the subsequent dilution of sodium to its normal level. Sodium also facilitates the transport of carbon dioxide by bicarbonate and is a major alkali, or base, in the maintenance of hydrogen ion balance. The irritability of nerve and muscle tissue is promoted by sodium, as is the conduction of nerve impulses.

Potassium is the principal cation of cellular fluid. It assists in the transport of oxygen as potassium oxyhemoglobin and promotes the transport of carbon dioxide as bicarbonate in the erythrocyte. Potassium in the body activates a number of enzymatic reactions and it aids in the regulation of hydrogen ion balance. The structure and function of the kidneys are dependent on the normal physiologic values of potassium. Adequate function of the heart, skeletal, and smooth muscles and the conduction of nerve impulses require adequate concentrations of potassium.

Calcium is an extremely versatile cation. The primary role of calcium is as the major component of teeth and bones, both in their initial development and in maintaining their viability. Calcium functions as an enzyme activator in facilitating skeletal muscle contraction. Normal values of calcium are necessary for proper heart muscle contraction. Calcium facilitates the transmission of nerve impulses and is an important component of all cell membranes. Calcium ions influence the conversion of prothrombin to thrombin in the blood clotting process.

Magnesium is primarily a cation of the intracellular fluid. Its concentration is approximately one-sixth that of potassium and it is believed to function in much the same manner. It serves the body as a catalyst for many intracellular enzymatic reactions, especially those having to do with carbohydrate metabolism. Magnesium facilitates the normal functioning of the nervous system, skeletal muscle contraction, and normal cardiac rhythm and it promotes regulation of the blood phosphorus level.

Proteins are the only dissolved substances in the plasma that do not diffuse easily into the interstitial fluid from the capillaries. As such they play an important role in the pressure that exists at the capillary membrane. This pressure is called colloid osmotic or oncotic pressure, to distinguish it from osmotic pressure, which exists at the cell membrane. Not only do most of the proteins remain in the plasma, but their negative charge requires large amounts of cations to remain with them in order to maintain electroneutrality. Proteins comprise about three-fourths of the body's solids and are the **building blocks** of the body. Proteins break down into the amino acids that are essential for body growth and maintenance of the life of the cell. Transportation of oxygen, muscle contraction, repair of tissue, and the structure of enzymes and genes are all dependent on protein.

Normal Balance of Body Fluids

In the healthy person, **body fluid homeostasis** is maintained by balancing the amount of intake and utilization of fluids, electrolytes, and nonelectrolytes with the amount excreted. Body water is balanced as follows:

Sources of body water	Range per day (ml)
Ingested water	500–1,700
Water contained in solid foods	800–1,000
Water from oxidation of food and body tissues	200– 300
Total	1,500–3,000

Losses of body water	Range per day (ml)
Insensible	
Water vapor loss through lungs and skin	850–1,200
Sensible	
Water loss through urine	600–1,600
Water loss through feces	50– 200
Total	1,500–3,000

The insensible, or imperceptible, loss of body water goes on continuously even when water intake is reduced to zero. Water is available for urinary excretion only after the needs of insensible loss have been met. No electrolytes are lost in moderate perspiration; only during profuse sweating is sodium excreted.

Electrolytes and nonelectrolytes are obtained by the body from the food and beverages ingested in a normal diet. Excess electrolytes and nonelectrolytes are excreted primarily in the urine and feces. The more important fluid constituents and their dietary sources are as follows:

Fluid constituent	Recommended daily allowances [5]	Dietary sources
Sodium	6 gm	Table salt
Potassium	60–100 mEq	Concentrated meat broth, skim milk, bananas, orange juice, tomato juice, peaches
Calcium	0.8 gm	Milk, milk products, cheese, butter, vegetables, fruit
Magnesium	0.3 gm	Nuts, seafood, whole grains, cocoa
Chloride	Not established	Table salt
Protein	0.8 gm per kilogram of body weight	Eggs, milk, meat

Movement of Body Fluids

The body fluid compartments are separated from each other by the membranes of the cells and capillaries. These membranes are **selectively permeable,** which means that they allow the passage of some ions and molecules but not of others. The selective permeability of these membranes performs an important regulatory function for the fluid compartments by maintaining a specific internal environment, different from that of the surrounding external environment. Although fluids and electrolytes are in constant motion in their various compartments, their relative concentrations (see Table 2-2) remain constant in the healthy person.

There is still much to be learned concerning the structure and function of cell and capillary membranes. One model of the structure of cell membrane that has received wide acceptance is the fluid mosaic model of Singer [6]. This model describes the cell membrane as being composed primarily of lipids and proteins in various fluid states and arranged in a mosaic pattern. In this pattern the areas of lipids that extend across the width of the membrane are interrupted at various intervals by protein molecules that may either extend across the membrane or be partially embedded in the lipid matrix.

Lipid-soluble fluids and substances pass easily through the lipid portion of the cell by becoming dissolved in it or by going through openings (pores) on its surface. Oxygen is an example of a gas that is soluble in lipids and passes through the cell membrane with ease. If a substance is water-soluble, it enters the cell along the side of the protein molecule. Movement of fluids and solutes through the pores of the lipid layer depends on the size of the molecule or ion, its electrical charge, and the effect of certain substances on the diameter of the pore. For example, mannitol, sucrose, and lactose all have greater diameters than does the average pore and cannot pass directly through it. If a positive ion such as calcium is lining a pore wall, it will repel other positive ions that attempt to pass through. Antidiuretic hormones can act on the pore wall to increase its diameter and allow greater movement of fluids and solutes.

DIFFUSION

Fluids and electrolytes move across cell and capillary membranes by several processes, but the primary ones are diffusion and active transport. The process of diffusion can be further categorized as simple diffusion, facilitated diffusion, and osmosis.

Simple diffusion, the random movement of molecules and ions in liquids and gases, occurs as a normal kinetic motion of matter. Each molecule has motion of its own and in addition bounces off other molecules, which helps to propel it. In simple diffusion, molecules and ions always move from areas of high concentration to areas of low concentration until they are distributed equally. Diffusion occurs within a compartment or between compartments if the membrane separating the compartments is permeable to the ion or molecule.

In **facilitated diffusion,** a substance that does not easily cross the cell membrane is assisted in doing so. For example, glucose does not easily dissolve in lipids, but it can combine with a second substance that renders it lipid-soluble and as such it crosses the membrane. This facilitated diffusion of glucose can occur only if its concentration is greater outside the cell than inside.

OSMOSIS

Osmosis is a special case of diffusion of water and it occurs when the concentration of water becomes greater in one compartment than in another. Therefore the water molecules move from the area of greater concentration to the area of lesser concentration. The classic example of osmosis is that of an equal volume of pure water and a solution of sodium chloride existing on opposite sides of a selectively permeable membrane. The presence of the sodium chloride molecules has reduced the number of water molecules on the sodium chloride side to below the number of water molecules on the pure water side. The membrane, due to its selective permeability, will not permit the sodium chloride molecules to move to the area of the pure water. Water thus moves from the pure water side to the side of the sodium chloride solution. If the pure water and the sodium chloride solution are conceptualized as existing in a U-shaped tube separated by a selectively permeable membrane, osmotic pressure can be envisioned. The water will pass from the pure water side across the membrane until the level of the sodium chloride solution becomes much higher than that of the pure water. Eventually the pressure of the sodium chloride solution at the membrane becomes great enough to *oppose* the pure water osmosis. This pressure is the **osmotic pressure** of the sodium chloride solution.

Osmotic pressure is an important concept in the understanding of fluids and electrolytes. The osmotic pressure exerted by nondiffusible ions and molecules in a solution is determined by the number of particles per unit volume of that fluid and not by their size or activity. The large, slow particles are averaged with the small, fast ones and an equal amount of energy (ability to exert pressure) is assigned to each particle. The *osmol* unit is used to express the number of particles in a solution that are capable of exerting pressure against a membrane. Osmolality and osmolarity characterize the concentration of osmols. **Osmolarity** refers to the number of osmols per liter of **solution** and **osmolality** represents the number of osmols per liter of **solvent**. The numerical difference between the two is small, and osmolality is the more useful term because this factor is the quantity most often measured.

Because the osmolality of plasma is approximately the same as the osmolality of ECF and ICF, the body is generally considered to be **iso-osmolar:** having the same osmolality. In the healthy person serum osmolality is about 285 to 305 milliosmols (mOsm) per liter. Iso-osmolar intravenous fluids contain approximately the same number of osmotically active particles as does normal serum, 285 to 305 mOsm per liter. When the osmolarity of one solution is compared with that of another, it is spoken of in terms of tonicity. A solution such as isotonic saline contains 310 mOsm per liter and is isotonic to plasma. A solution of 10% invert sugar in water, which has 555 mOsm per liter, is hypertonic to plasma; a solution of 0.45% sodium chloride with 154 mOsm per liter is hypotonic to plasma.

When osmotic pressure is the result of the presence of protein molecules it is termed **colloidal osmotic pressure,** or **oncotic pressure.** Although the amount of pressure exerted by proteins at the capillary membrane is not great, proteins are an important factor in plasma pressure because they do not diffuse across the membrane.

ACTIVE TRANSPORT

Active transport is the second major process whereby fluids and solutes move from one compartment to another. As just discussed under diffusion, the movement of solutes and fluid always occurs from an area of greater concentration to an area where these factors are less prominent. **Active transport** is the means whereby solutes and solvents move "up hill" against gradients and go from areas where they have had low concentration to areas where they are already highly concentrated. The mechanism of active transport is similar to that of facilitated diffusion in that substances are moved through membranes by means of carriers. Carriers have not actually been identified for any cell types. The term **carrier** is given to a process that seems to operate as a carrier would. The carrier attaches itself to a substance, moves it through the membrane, and finally returns to its original position to pick up more substance. Since active transport is movement against a gradient, however, it requires energy in the course of movement, which is the difference between active transport and facilitated diffusion. Active transport occurs not only across cell membranes but also across membranes within the cell and entire cellular layers such as the intestinal epithelium, epithelium of the renal tubules, and many other layers.

A special case of active transport dealing with sodium and potassium is the **sodium pump.** It was noted in the distribution of electrolytes that large quantities of sodium exist extracellularly and large quantities of potassium exist intracellularly. Sodium and potassium can diffuse through the cell wall, and if this diffusion is not counteracted, the concentrations of each would eventually equilibrate. In such a situation the amounts of sodium and potassium available to the compartments where they are critically needed would be inadequate. The sodium pump acts by means of a carrier substance that attaches itself to sodium inside the cell and transports it to the exterior. Once out of the cell the carrier substance changes somewhat, attaches itself to potassium, and moves across the membrane to the interior of the cell. The pump transports about three sodium ions for every two potassium ions and is especially important in preventing continual swelling of the cells. The cells contain many nondiffusible substances that tend to cause osmosis of water to their interior. The sodium pump opposes this tendency and prevents cellular distention.

A mechanism of specific relevance for water and solute movement in relation to the capillary walls is that of hydrostatic pressure. **Hydrostatic pressure** is the result of the weight of water. In a large container of water, the pressure at the water's surface is equal to the atmospheric pressure, but the pressure rises 1 mm Hg for each 13.6 mm distance below the water. In the human vascular system, hydrostatic pressure is maintained by an adequate fluid volume. When a person stands still, the pressure in his right atrium is approximately 0 mm of mercury and in the veins of his feet it is 90 mm of mercury. At the arteriole end of the capillaries, the hydrostatic pressure is greater than the colloid osmotic pressure and fluid moves outward. Fluid returns to the vascular system at the venule end of the capillary bed because the colloid osmotic pressure is greater than the hydrostatic pressure and reabsorption is favored. This concept that a balance of hydrostatic pressure and colloid osmotic pressure is responsible for fluid balance was originally proposed by E. H. Starling in the late nineteenth century. Modifications of his proposal have been made in the intervening years, but the basic model remains valid.

Regulation of Body Fluids

Numerous factors and body systems are involved in the conservation and excretion of body water, electrolytes, and nonelectrolytes. As was noted in the discussion of normal balance, the body has a limited number of avenues whereby it can obtain necessary fluids and nutrients and dispose of excesses. Yet the body fluids play a significant role in every biochemical reaction in the body. The opportunities for gross irregularities to occur are almost endless. The ability of the body to correct some of its own problems without outside help and most of its problems with a little help is a tribute to its beautifully integrated regulatory systems.

The body signals its need for a greater ingestion of water by means of thirst. The thirst mechanism plays an important role in regulating the volume and tonicity of the body fluids. The major physiologic stimulus for thirst is a 1 to 2 percent decrease in total body water. Such a decrease causes a rise in the osmolarity of the ECF (hypertonic) and a resultant mild cellular dehydration. The neurons of the hypothalamic nuclei, known as the thirst center, respond to this dehydration and transmit stimulatory impulses to the cerebral cortex and into consciousness. The need for water then becomes translated into the behavior of drinking. The opposite situation occurs when the ECF becomes hypotonic and the volume of fluid within the neurons expands. Inhibitory impulses are transmitted to the cerebral cortex and the need to ingest fluid is not felt.

Thirst may also be stimulated by a contracted vascular or extracellular volume. When volume is decreased, water moves from the cells into the extracellular spaces to reestablish transcellular osmotic equilibrium and all the body fluids become hypotonic. The exact mechanism by which a reduced extracellular volume stimulates the thirst center is not clearly known. It may be related to decreased arterial pressure in the carotid and aortic baroreceptors, which accompanies a fall in cardiac output. Also a decrease in intrathoracic blood volume, as in blood loss, quiet standing, the upright position, and positive pressure breathing, decreases the tension in the left atrial wall and great pulmonary veins and stimulates thirst.

Other stimuli to the thirst center have been identified as emotional stress and pain; increased temperature of the blood perfusing the hypothalamus; drugs such as isoproterenol hydrochloride (Isuprel), morphine, and barbiturates; and possibly stimulation of carotid body chemoreceptors by low oxygen tension.

The sensation of thirst may also occur in the presence of expansion of total body water of interstitial volume when the "effective" circulating blood volume, blood pressure, and cardiac output are reduced. These conditions may arise secondarily to such pathologic conditions as congestive heart failure, cirrhosis of the liver with ascites or edema, and the nephrotic syndrome.

Thirst is inhibited by conditions opposite those that are stimulatory; for example, **expansion** of the intravascular volume of the neurons of the hypothalamic nuclei, expanded vascular and extracellular volume, and **increased** intrathoracic blood volume. Occasionally emotional stress will inhibit thirst; and drugs such as alcohol, phenytoin sodium (Dilantin), atropine, and possibly epinephrine are also inhibitory. Acute cold exposure with peripheral vasoconstriction that shifts the blood volume centrally leads to inhibition of thirst.

The excretion of excess body fluids from the renal system is influenced by two potent hormones: **antidiuretic hormone** (ADH) and **aldosterone.** ADH promotes increased water reabsorption from both the distal tubules and the collecting ducts of the kidney; it increases the size of the pores in the lipid layer of these kidney cells until water is absorbed with ease. In the absence of ADH, the pores of the epithelial cells in the distal tubules and collecting ducts become very small, that is, too small for the water molecule to pass through. As a result tubular fluid is excreted as urine.

The overall effect of ADH is to decrease the volume of urine and increase the concentration of urine with a resulting conservation of body water.

Antidiuretic hormone is formed in the hypothalamic nuclei and stored in the posterior lobe of the pituitary gland. The production site of ADH is anatomically near the thirst center and is carefully integrated physiologically. The stimuli for thirst also stimulate the release of ADH, and the thirst inhibitors inhibit ADH release. Two stimuli for the release of ADH must be emphasized: acute hemorrhagic hypotension and major surgical procedures. Acute hemorrhage is a situation not only of decreased vascular volume but also of decreased pressure, and it is one of the most powerful stimuli for the immediate release of ADH. Major surgical procedures present numerous instances of stimuli for the release of ADH both during an operation and postoperatively. These include premedications, anesthesia, traction on the viscera, decreased cardiac output, pain, and emotional stress.

The second hormone of major significance in regulating body fluids is aldosterone. Aldosterone promotes the reabsorption of sodium and chloride and the excretion of potassium and hydrogen ions in the distal tubules of the kidney. It acts on specific protein receptors in renal cells to enhance sodium transport back into the kidney cells. The absorption of sodium and chloride increases the osmolality of extracellular fluid which, as indicated above, stimulates the secretion of ADH and leads to conservation of water. Simply stated, aldosterone conserves sodium.

Aldosterone is a potent mineralocorticoid secreted by the adrenal glands. The secretion of aldosterone is primarily dependent on the renal enzyme **renin**. The sequence of events leading to aldosterone secretion has been theorized as follows: A reduction in ECF volume or vascular volume is reflected in the arterial bed in the distal tubules and stimulates renal secretion of renin. Renin acts upon angiotensinogen, which is present in the circulating blood, and converts it to angiotensin I, which has an extremely weak vasoconstrictive action. A converting enzyme changes angiotensin I to angiotensin II, which has a powerful vasoconstrictive action and counteracts the reduced vascular volume. Angiotensin II and probably I stimulate the adrenal cortex to secrete aldosterone. As aldosterone promotes sodium retention, it contributes to the expansion of the ECF compartment and finally to an increase in the vascular volume.

The renin-angiotensin mechanism is the primary stimulator of aldosterone secretion, but it is not the only one. ACTH has an effect when first administered pharmacologically, but this effect does not seem to last. Potassium depletion diminishes the secretion of aldosterone, and potassium excess increases it.

Other hormones affect the regulation of fluids and electrolytes, but not to the same extent as do ADH and aldosterone. Cortisol can increase sodium reabsorption in the distal tubules of the kidney, similarly to aldosterone. Cortisol also increases the glomerular filtration rate, which increases the volume of glomerular filtrate. Thyroid hormones increase renal blood flow and tubular reabsorption of sodium and lead to either increased or decreased excretion of water and electrolytes. Phosphate, bicarbonate, sodium, and potassium are increased in the urine by the action of parathyroid hormone on the proximal tubules. Parathyroid hormone decreases calcium in the urine, except in hypercalcemia, when calcium is excreted.

The renal system is one of the most complex biochemical mechanisms in the body. Its role in regulating the composition and volume of body fluids is central to the body's ability to function as a homeostatic organism.

The function of the kidneys is to excrete excesses of ingestion and metabolic waste products and to retain the solutes and water that are vital to life. The nephron is the operative anatomic unit in the kidney that carries out homeostatic regulation and does so by concentration or dilution of the urine.

The nephron, of which there are about one million in the kidneys, is composed of an afferent arteriole, a glomerulus which is encased in Bowman's capsule, an efferent arteriole, the proximal convoluted tubule, collecting tubules, and peritubular capillaries. Each of these structures plays a specific part in water and electrolyte balance.

Blood enters the nephron through the arcuate artery and proceeds through the afferent arteriole to the glomerulus. The glomerulus is an arrangement of about fifty parallel capillaries that filter out plasma much as do any other capillaries in the body. It is, however, highly permeable and allows passage of almost all substances with molecular sizes less than that of plasma proteins. After filtration, the blood leaves the glomerulus by the efferent arteriole and enters the vascular bed of the kidney. The glomerular filtrate that has collected in Bowman's capsule continues to the proximal tubule. The quantity of glomerular filtrate formed each minute in all nephrons is the **glomerular filtration rate (GFR),** and in a normal person it averages approximately 125 ml per minute. About 98 to 99 percent of the filtrate is reabsorbed by the epithelial cells of the tubules, and only 1 to 2 percent becomes urine.

As the glomerular filtrate moves through the tubules and the loop of Henle, substances are either secreted or absorbed by the tubular epithelium. The substances move from the peritubular fluid (ECF) to the tubular lumen (glomerular filtrate) and back across the tubular membrane either by diffusion or by active transport, just as occurs with other membranes in the body. The substances that are absorbed by active transport include glucose, sodium ions, amino acids, calcium ions, potassium ions, phosphate ions, and urate ions. Substances such as hydrogen ions are actively secreted or moved from the epithelial cells to the lumen of the tubules. Water diffuses by means of osmosis from the tubular lumen to the ECF, or vice versa, depending on the compartment with the greatest concentration of solute. Urea also diffuses into the ECF due to a concentration difference; the ECF is positive in relation to the tubular fluid and as a result negative ions such as chloride, phosphate, and bicarbonate diffuse into the tubules according to differences in electrical and chemical concentrations. Potassium is secreted by diffusion from the epithelial cells to the tubular lumen after sodium is actively absorbed; because the electrical potential in the lumen is so negative, the positive ion potassium is needed for balance. Table 2-3 is a graphic representation of the movement of these solutes and fluid.

The eventual concentration of a given substance in the urine is dependent on the amount that has been reabsorbed from the glomerular filtrate and the relative reabsorption of water. If a greater percentage of **water** is reabsorbed the substance becomes concentrated in the urine; if a greater percentage of the **substance** is reabsorbed the urine will become dilute (see Table 2-4 for common constituents of normal urine).

Table 2-3
Movement of solutes and fluids across membranes of the kidney tubules

Tubular membrane	Tubular lumen		Tubular membrane	Renal blood capillaries
	Glomerular filtrate			Extracellular fluid
Epithelial cells	Glucose, Amino acids, Sodium ions, Calcium ions, Potassium ions, Phosphate ions, Urate ions	Active transport	Epithelial cells	
	←		Active transport	Hydrogen ions
	Water	Osmosis ———		
	←		Osmosis	Water
	Urea, Chloride ions, Phosphate ions, Bicarbonate ions	Diffusion ———		
	←		Diffusion	Potassium

Table 2-4
Normal values for 24-hour urine excretion

	Normal Values
Calcium (usual diet)	100–250 mg
Chloride	100–250 mEq/24 hr (dependent on sodium reabsorption)
Hemoglobin and myoglobin	None
Osmolality	290 mOsm/kg water
pH	4.6–8.0 (average 6.0) (depends on diet)
Potassium	25–100 mEq/24 hr (dependent on sodium reabsorption)
Protein	
Qualitative	0
Quantitative	10–150 mg/24 hr
Sodium	80–180 mEq (varies with dietary ingestion of salt)
Glucose	0

Hydrogen Ion Balance

The discussion thus far has been directed toward the balance of water and some of the more abundant electrolytes, and little mention has been made of the important concept of hydrogen ion balance. The separation of the two has been purely for reasons of clarity, for in reality they are highly interdependent mechanisms in the body.

Hydrogen ions are produced in the body in two ways. The normal metabolism of fats and carbohydrates yields carbon dioxide and water, which combine to form carbonic acid. Carbonic acid then dissociates into hydrogen and bicarbonate.

$$CO_2 + H_2O \rightarrow H_2CO_3 \rightarrow H^+ + HCO_3^-$$

Carbon dioxide / Water / Carbonic acid / Hydrogen / Bicarbonate

The second source of free hydrogen is by metabolic oxidation of some proteins. Body homeostasis operates to prevent the accumulation of excess hydrogen in the body by excreting CO_2 via the respiratory system and the metabolically derived hydrogen through the kidney tubules. Certain amounts of hydrogen are essential to the body for proper cellular metabolism, adequate functioning of the enzyme systems, and attachment of oxygen to hemoglobin.

The amount of hydrogen in the body is the **hydrogen ion concentration.** In the past, this concentration was referred to as acid base balance. An **acid** is a substance that is capable of giving up a proton when in solution; a **base** is a substance capable of receiving a proton. As the hydrogen ion is frequently the proton that attaches to or dissociates from substances, therefore making the difference in the amount of acids or bases, hydrogen ion concentration came into use as the more accurate term.

The term **pH** is derived from the German language and can be translated as the "power of hydrogen." It is the index used to quantify the free hydrogen ion concentration in the body. In other words, the pH of a solution is a measure of its hydrogen ion concentration and indicates the degree of acidity of alkalinity of that solution. The range of pH for any solution is from 0 to 14, with neutrality or an exact balance of acids with bases occurring at 7. Solutions that have a pH of 0 are completely acid, those with a pH of 14 are completely alkaline. In the healthy person, the pH of plasma is 7.4, a situation of slight base excess.

The pH of a solution is determined by computing the value of the negative logarithm of the hydrogen ion concentration of that solution. In many solutions this concentration can be measured directly. In serum, however, this concentration is difficult to measure and as a result an equation, the **Henderson-Hasselbalch equation,** has been developed to determine serum pH. The equation is complex, but essentially it employs the values of the serum concentrations of carbon dioxide and bicarbonate ions expressed as a ratio of bicarbonate ions to carbon dioxide* (HCO_3^-/CO_2). A ratio of 20 mEq of bicarbonate to 1 mEq of carbon dioxide in the equation will yield a pH of 7.4, the normal value of serum.

The pH value is used to indicate quantities of hydrogen in the body rather than the usual electrolyte measure, mEq, because of the ex-

---

*Carbon dioxide is used in the equation instead of carbonic acid because of the difficulty in determining carbonic acid values. The equation takes into account the different concentrations of these substances in normal serum.

Table 2-5
Normal concentrations of arterial blood gases* and hydrogen ion in the intravascular compartment

Partial pressure of oxygen (P_{O_2})	80–100 mm Hg
Partial pressure of carbon dioxide (P_{CO_2})	38–45 mm Hg
Hydrogen ion concentration (pH)	7.34–7.4

*Gases are measured in terms of partial pressure since the sum of the pressure of all gases is the total gas pressure and therefore an individual gas exerts only a partial pressure.

tremely small numbers involved. For example, the normal serum pH value of 7.4 converts to 0.00004 mEq per liter. The pH is a discrete measurement and it is helpful to remember that a fall in serum pH from 7.4 to 7.1 indicates that the amount of hydrogen in the body has doubled (see Table 2-5 for normal values of arterial blood gases and hydrogen ion concentration).

Hydrogen and potential hydrogen, CO_2, are not produced in the body in steady amounts, and as a result the body must regulate their available quantities until excretion can rid the body of excesses. There are three primary means of regulation: the chemical buffering system, the respiratory system, and the renal system. Each of these systems operates to maintain the pH of the body within normal limits in order to facilitate optimal functioning of chemical reactions. These systems also operate in a time sequence, with the chemical system responding to increased hydrogen ions within a fraction of a second, the respiratory system responding in a matter of minutes, and the renal system within a few hours to a day or more.

Chemical Buffering System

The common definition of a **buffer** is an object that acts to lessen or absorb shock. This role is precisely that of the chemical buffers in the body fluids. They operate to lessen the effect of excess quantities of acid or base by absorbing them. Buffers are associated pairs of chemicals. One member of the pair is a weak acid that reacts with a strong base to form water and a salt of the acid, thereby neutralizing the effect of the base. The other member is the salt of the acid that reacts with a strong acid to form a weak acid and a salt. The terms **strong** and **weak** characterize the abilities of acids and bases to dissociate into their component ions. Therefore when a strong acid that can easily release its hydrogen is converted into a weak acid that will not easily give up its hydrogen, the addition of hydrogen ions to the extracellular fluid has been prevented. In the same way, conversion of a strong base to a weak base limits the release of excessive hydroxyl ions into the solution. In both instances, compounds that have a great potential for altering the body pH are prevented from doing so.

The bicarbonate-carbonic acid system is the primary buffer of extracellular fluids. When a strong acid such as hydrochloric acid is added to extracellular fluid, a bicarbonate salt such as sodium or potassium bicarbonate will react with it, yielding weak carbonic acid and the salt, sodium chloride. For example:

HCL	+	$NAHCO_3$	→	H_2CO_3	+	NACL
Strong acid		Salt		Weak acid		Salt
(Hydrochloric acid)		(Sodium bicarbonate)		(Carbonic acid)		(Sodium chloride)

The other member of this buffering pair, carbonic acid, will react with a strong base such as sodium hydroxide to yield sodium bicarbonate and water. The chemical reaction is as follows:

NAOH	+	H_2CO_3	→	$NAHCO_3$	+	H_2O
Strong base		Weak acid		Salt		
(Sodium hydroxide)		(Carbonic acid)		(Sodium bicarbonate)		(Water)

The phosphate buffering system acts in much the same manner as the bicarbonate-carbonic acid system but utilizes different chemical buffers, the acid salts sodium dihydrogen phosphate and disodium hydrogen phosphate. The phosphate buffer acts primarily within the cells, especially within red blood cells and cells of the kidney tubules.

Protein acts in the tissue cells and plasma and is the most plentiful buffer in the body. It also functions in the same way as the bicarbonate-carbonic acid buffer: converting strong acids and bases to weak ones. A protein buffer that acts solely within the erythrocyte and is the most important buffer of carbonic acid is **hemoglobin.**

Respiratory Regulation of Hydrogen Ions

Respiratory control of hydrogen ion concentration is accomplished via control of the carbon dioxide content of the plasma. Carbon dioxide is continually being formed as a waste product of metabolism. It diffuses into the interstitial fluids and then into the blood where it is transported to the alveoli and enters into the normal oxygen–carbon dioxide exchange process of the lungs.

If the rate of carbon dioxide production remains constant, the primary factor affecting the amount of carbon dioxide in the blood is the **rate of alveolar ventilation.** Increasing the respiratory rate times two (from 20 to 40 respirations per minute) can raise the pH from 7.4 to 7.63. Decreasing the rate by three-fourths (from 20 to 5 respirations per minute) reduces the pH from 7.4 to 7.0. In typical feedback fashion, the hydrogen ion concentration acts directly on the respiratory center in the medulla, increasing the respiratory rate when the hydrogen ion concentration is high and decreasing the rate when the hydrogen ion concentration is low. In summary, excess carbon dioxide in the blood stimulates the respiratory center to increase alveolar ventilation and promote carbon dioxide removal; decreased carbon dioxide stimulates the respiratory center to decrease the respiratory rate, thereby conserving carbon dioxide.

Renal Regulation of Hydrogen Ions

The kidneys regulate hydrogen ion concentration mainly by increasing or decreasing bicarbonate ion concentration in the blood. They do so by a series of complex actions that take place in the kidney tubules.

In the epithelial cells of the renal tubules, carbon dioxide, under the influence of the enzyme carbonic anhydrase, combines with water to form carbonic acid, which dissociates into the hydrogen ion and the bicarbonate ion. The hydrogen ion is then secreted through the membrane into the glomerular filtrate.

Renal blood capillaries extracellular fluid	Tubular membrane epithelial cell	Glomerular filtrate
$CO_2 \longrightarrow$	$CO_2 + H_2O$ H_2CO_3 $\begin{bmatrix}\text{Carbonic}\\ \text{anhydrase}\end{bmatrix}$	$H^+ + HCO_3^-$ H^+ $\longleftarrow$ Na^+

Each time a hydrogen ion is secreted into the tubule, a sodium ion is reabsorbed into the epithelial cell. The carbon dioxide concentration in the extracellular fluid is the stimulus for this process: The greater the carbon dioxide concentration in the extracellular fluid the more rapidly the reaction occurs and the more rapidly hydrogen ions are secreted. Therefore any of the factors that influence carbon dioxide concentration, such as metabolic production or respiratory rate, will also influence tubular membrane secretion of hydrogen.

The reabsorption of bicarbonate ions from the glomerular filtrate proceeds in relation to the hydrogen ions that have been secreted into the tubules. The bicarbonate ions combine with the hydrogen ions in the tubules to form carbonic acid, which dissociates into carbon dioxide and water. The carbon dioxide diffuses back through the epithelial cells to the extracellular fluid, and the water is excreted as urine.

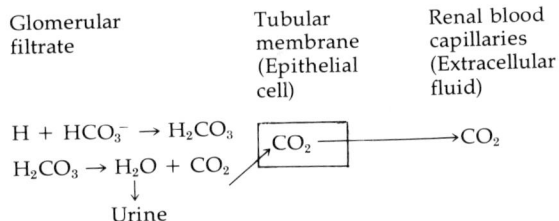

The effect of these actions has been the removal of all the bicarbonate ions from the glomerular filtrate and thus the possibility that they will be excreted in urine. The bicarbonate ion that was originally formed in the epithelial cells combines with the sodium and diffuses back into the extracellular fluid as sodium bicarbonate.

Epithelial cell	Extracellular fluid
$HCO_3^- + NA \rightarrow NAHCO_3$	$\longrightarrow NAHCO_3$

To summarize, the presence of carbon dioxide in the extracellular fluid, a potential source of hydrogen ions (acid) to the body, initiates a chain of events across the epithelial cells of the renal tubules that leads to the formation of sodium bicarbonate and its release into the extracellular fluid. The net effect is that a greater amount of base becomes available to the body.

Alterations in Body Fluids

Alterations in the volume, distribution, composition, and thus ultimately the function of body fluids lead to imbalances with which the body cannot cope, even when fully using its powers of regulation. These changes may be primary, such as those related to inadequate intake of essential nutrients, or secondary as the result of changes in body organ structure due to disease or trauma.

Imbalances in body fluids rarely involve simply the water or one specific electrolyte or nonelectrolyte. Because of their complex interdependency, a change in one soon leads to a change in another. Also, the physical laws that govern the body processes—isoosmolality, electroneutrality, pressure—do not regard all the characteristics of a given molecule or ion when reaching for a state of equilibrium. If a positive ion is needed and sodium is not available, the body will substitute potassium. If tonicity is required and cellular potassium is inadequate, the cell will substitute sodium.

Problems of Water Balance

DEHYDRATION

Dehydration is a deficit in the amount of body water necessary for the body to carry out its normal functioning. It is the result of decreased intake with normal or increased output, normal intake with increased losses, or possibly an increased intake that cannot compensate for losses that are extreme. In some instances there may not be a deficit in total body water; a person may have the normal 40 liters of fluid, but a quantity of it may be sequestered in the third spaces and thus be unavailable for use.

Having said that simple losses of water are rare, it is now necessary to state that they do occur. A simple water deficit may result from an intake of fluids that has not kept pace with losses of fluid. In such a situation, the extracellular fluid becomes hypertonic in relation to the cellular fluid. As water is the most freely moving substance in the body, the first response of the body is to equilibrate the hypertonic and hypotonic fluids by osmosis from the interior of the cells to the extracellular space. As a result, the cells become shrunken and cellular dehydration exists. Cellular dehydration stimulates the release of antidiuretic hormone by the pituitary gland, which acts on the kidney tubules to conserve the available water by reabsorbing it from the tubule lumen.

Nursing Assessment

Certain conditions are more likely than others to lead to dehydration. In the assessment of any adult, the nurse must be aware of which persons are at risk in order to plan and institute measures that will prevent potential problems from becoming real ones. The population at risk also identifies those persons who may already be suffering from the problem of dehydration.

Population at risk AGED PERSONS Aged persons have a tendency to become dehydrated. With the process of aging more and more whole nephrons deteriorate, and the renal function of reabsorption diminishes. When older people ingest enough fluids, their bodies are quite capable of maintaining normal balance; but they often do not do so. Among the reasons elderly persons may not drink sufficient fluids are (1) they have developed habits of drinking minimal amounts of fluids, (2) elderly persons, especially females who suffer from incontinence, may restrict fluid intake to prevent the occurrence of incontinence, (3) physical diseases may prohibit the elderly from obtaining fluids readily. If incontinence is present and fluids are restricted, an undesirable side effect is the limitation of bladder distensibility and the increased incidence of infection. If an older person lives alone and is ill without adequate fluids being made available, he may come to the nurse's attention in a severely dehydrated state. Nurses should be particularly aware therefore of the fluid intake of older persons, especially those who live alone or are physically disabled.

DISEASE OR TRAUMATIC STATES Almost any disease has the potential for altering the normal balance of body fluids; however, the following conditions have the greatest probability of doing so:

kidney diseases lead to impaired concentration of water with resulting diuresis.
ulcerative colitis accompanied by diarrhea leads to large losses of fluid from the gastrointestinal tract.
undiagnosed or uncontrolled diabetes mellitus with polyuria causes excretion of large amounts of glucose into the kidneys and produces the physiologic need of the kidneys to dilute this concentration.
burns not only disrupt the integrity of the skin, allowing frank exudation of fluid, but also increase the permeability of the capillaries, leading to fluid loss from the circulation.
salicylate poisoning with fluid loss due to associated hyperventilation.
cirrhosis of the liver and **abdominal cancer** may cause a shifting of fluid from the extracellular spaces to the peritoneal cavity (ascites).
cerebral injuries with damage to the thirst center or to the respiratory center or both, with resultant hyperventilation.
diabetes insipidus, in which damage to the hypothalamic nuclei results in the absence of antidiuretic hormone and a resultant profuse diuresis of dilute urine.
hormonal imbalances in which a decrease in the normal functioning of antidiuretic hormone and aldosterone leads to a decreased ability of the kidneys to conserve water.

SITUATIONAL OR THERAPEUTIC FACTORS
mechanical devices such as laryngectomy tubes and tracheostomy tubes create trauma and discomfort in the initial phases of insertion and inhibit the patient's ability and willingness to ingest fluids.
extreme debilitation or critical illness makes swallowing difficult or impossible.
drainage from wounds or suction apparatuses can lead to large losses of fluid.
the unavailability of water, which may occur when people are lost and unable to find a source of water, or during catastrophic floods and tornados when the water supply becomes contaminated or the water supply routes are damaged.

GENERALIZED SYMPTOMS
the symptoms that arise as a consequence of other illness states can either decrease fluid intake or accelerate its loss.
fever increases loss of body fluid by increasing the metabolic rate and results in increased utilization of water.
fluid shifts such as ascites, pulmonary edema, and peripheral edema limit the amount of fluid available for normal functioning by rendering it unavailable for use.
a decreased level of consciousness limits a person's ability to ingest adequate amounts of fluid.
vomiting can account for major fluid losses via the gastrointestinal tract.
hemorrhage leads to rapid losses of extracellular fluid.
excessive ventilation, as is seen in severe acidosis, leads to large losses of fluid from the lungs.

Subjective and objective assessment data The dehydrated patient will exhibit certain symptoms and signs that the nurse will be able to observe during the assessment. A given patient is not likely to exhibit all the symptoms and signs detailed below. The presence, however, of symptoms that represent two or more body systems should alert the nurse to consider dehydration as a diagnosis and to search for further data to support this conclusion.

Subjective and objective assessment data are descriptive of the basic problem of a less than adequate amount of body fluids.

general systemic involvement. Weight loss, general fatigue; appears weak and ill.
integumentary system. Flushed appearance of skin, especially the face; warm feeling of the skin; loss of skin elasticity; decreased perspiration; decreased salivation with dry "cottony" feeling in mouth; dry, cracked lips; decreased tearing.
cardiovascular system. Tachycardia and lowered blood pressure.
central nervous system. Personality changes, decreased level of consciousness, fever.
urinary system. Anuria or oliguria, dark color of urine, increased specific gravity of urine. Severe dehydration can result in renal failure.
gastrointestinal system. Extreme thirst,

nausea and vomiting, decreased fluid intake, diarrhea. If a patient is unable to eat, hypoproteinemia will develop with an accompanying low plasma colloidal osmotic pressure and an increase in the movement of fluids from the circulating volume to the interstitial spaces.

hematologic system. Serum sodium greater than 150 mEq per liter, elevated hematocrit, elevated blood urea nitrogen levels.

It is important to remember that one of the gravest consequences of dehydration is hypovolemic shock. Dehydration may exist in varying degrees; hypovolemic shock may be considered an extreme form of dehydration. Although the most usual cause of hypovolemic shock is hemorrhage, any complex of factors that significantly reduces the circulating blood volume can lead to hypovolemic shock. The reader is referred to Chapter 16 for a detailed description of hypovolemic shock and its management.

Methods of assessment The usual methods of assessment, such as interviewing the patient and family relative to the patient's health history, physical examination, observation, analysis of medical and laboratory records, and measurement of vital signs are all used to gather data to provide adequate information for a diagnosis of dehydration. In taking the history, specific attention is given to such factors as the amount of food and fluid intake and the amount of fluid losses by normal or abnormal routes the patient has experienced in the past few days.

Nursing Diagnosis
The nursing diagnosis includes not only the conclusions drawn from analysis of the assessment data but also a phrase concerning the possible cause of the patient's condition. The nursing diagnosis should be specific to a given patient. It emphasizes either the condition of the patient and the cause, or the significant presenting problem and the pathologic condition that precipitated it.

Some possible diagnostic statements emphasizing the pathologic condition and causation are

Dehydration related to hemorrhage.
Dehydration related to inability to swallow.
Dehydration related to ascites [4].

Statements emphasizing the presenting problem might be

Decreased level of consciousness related to dehydration.
Weight loss related to dehydration.
Dry skin and mucous membranes related to dehydration.

An alternative diagnostic statement as proposed by the National Conference on Classification of Nursing Diagnosis [2] is

Depletion of body fluids.

Nursing Plan
The nursing objectives are directed toward alleviation of the patient's symptoms and reversal of the underlying pathophysiologic mechanism. Nursing objectives are always stated in terms of the specific patient's needs and problems. The following objectives, however, would apply to most patients experiencing dehydration:

Replacement of fluid losses that exceed fluid intake.
Prevention of physical, social, and psychological deterioration occurring as a consequence of pathologic condition.
Promotion of patient's self-care activities to preillness state.
Facilitate medical regimen.

Nursing Intervention
Nursing interventions are activities carried out by the nurse in order to meet the objectives of the nursing plan. They are directed toward specific results or outcomes for the patient.

Offer oral fluids Explain to the patient the need to increase oral intake if not contraindicated by his condition or symptoms. Discuss with him why his intake is inadequate, the normal needs of his body, and the ways he or she feels the deficit could be corrected. Determine his fluid likes and dislikes and desired times for ingestion. Any plan that is developed should be done *with* the patient and not *for* him, unless his condition is such that he is unable to participate.

Teach the patient to promote his own fluid intake by scheduling his times of ingestion and setting goals for himself. If a patient is physically and emotionally able to do so, he can manage his intake adequately, requiring only support of his efforts and provision of the fluids. At times an interested family member will be willing to participate in helping the patient to increase his fluid intake.

Position the patient comfortably to facilitate drinking. Do not hesitate to ask the family to provide favorite fluids that may not be available in the institution, and present fluids aesthetically and in quantities that are not overwhelming. The use of a small glass can give the patient the satisfaction of completing a task by being able to empty it.

Common fluids to offer are milk, juice, and water. Variety can be provided by including soups, bouillons, and foods that have a high fluid content (ice cream, sherbet, and puddings).

Many solid foods have a high fluid content. These foods are not usually counted in a fluid record, but the patient can be encouraged to select them for his menu. Some examples are:

Food	Amount	Water content (ml)
Cottage cheese	5½ tablespoons	65
Cantaloupe	average slice	230
Fresh peach	one medium	110
Fresh pineapple	2-inch slice	210
Watermelon	large slice	315

All foods and fluids offered must meet any dietary restrictions the patient has, such as a low-sodium or measured diabetic diet.

Administer intravenous fluids Intravenous fluids are part of the medical regimen. The nurse does not order the quantity nor the constituents of the intravenous fluids but has several responsibilities relative to their administration.

Explain to the patient and his family the reason intravenous fluids are being given, the procedure of administration, any limitations that will be imposed on the patient, and the proposed duration of this type of therapy. Intravenous fluids are so commonplace to nurses that nurses tend to forget how frightening this intrusive procedure can be to patients who are experiencing it for the first time, or to those who have had discomfort or distress during previous experiences. Establish or monitor, or both, the flow rate of the fluids. The amount of fluids to be administered per minute is converted to drops according to the flow meter on the administration set. Do not increase the rate of fluids without consulting the physician; fluids that are infused at too great a speed overload the extracellular fluid compartment and lead to circulatory overload.

Monitor the infusion site for signs of infiltration into the soft tissues or for inflammation of the vein. Infiltration occurs when the needle becomes dislodged from the vein and fluid accumulates in the tissues. The infusion site will be edematous, hard, and painful and usually the fluids will have slowed or stopped running. If they have not stopped, the nurse should discontinue them immediately. Application of warm compresses to the edematous area will help reduce the edema. Inflammation is evidenced by redness along the vein, swelling, and pain. The infusion should be stopped and the physician notified.

Prevent limitations in mobility due to the infusion. Although the patient's position is often very important to the proper functioning of the infusion, patients should be encouraged to move. The use of an arm board can provide stability to the infusion site and lessen the patient's fears of dislodging the needle.

CALCULATIONS OF INTRAVENOUS FLOW RATES
The drop factor varies with different commercial parenteral administration sets. The specific set will indicate its drop factor on the label (that is, the number of drops delivering 1 ml of solution). The desired number of drops per minute to administer a specific amount of fluid can be determined by using the following formula:

Drip rate

$$= \frac{\text{volume ordered} \times \text{drops/milliliter}}{\text{time expressed in minutes}}$$

$$= \text{drops per minute}$$

For example:
The drip rate is as follows for an order of 1,000 ml of 5% dextrose in water to be infused in 4 hours (using a Baxter/Travenol administration set with a drop factor of 10).

$$\frac{1,000 \text{ ml} \times 10}{240 \text{ minutes}} = 42 \text{ gtt per minute}$$

Some manufacturers have devised calculators to determine desired flow rates when employing their administration sets.

Maintain an accurate record of intake and output Measure and record all oral and intravenous intake. Measure and record all output (urine, suction, liquid stools, bleeding, wound exudates or drainage, vomitus), and estimate incontinence losses. Sheets and dressings can be weighed to determine the amount of fluid they may contain. Teach the patient to measure and record his own intake and output as much as possible. Involve an interested family member in helping the patient or assisting the nurses to maintain an accurate record. Support the patient and family in their efforts, and do not let them become overanxious when their efforts fail.

Communicate the oral and intravenous fluid replacement plan to all persons who are caring for the patient

Maintain the integrity of the skin and mucous membranes The dehydrated patient usually experiences a decrease in all body secretions (refer to the section on assessment). Therefore certain nursing measures are indicated, including the following:

Bathe patient only every other day; liberally apply lotion to skin at least twice a day.
Give specific care to nose, mouth, and lips every 4 hours, or more often if necessary.
Encourage or assist patient to change his position in bed frequently.
If the patient is unresponsive, administer moisturizing drops to the eyes every 4 hours.

Maintain adequate nutrition Provide diet with adequate amounts of protein, fats, carbohydrates, minerals, and vitamins.

Measure and record significant signs Pulse, respirations, blood pressure, temperature, central venous pressure, and weight.

Support medical therapy The goal of medical therapy in the treatment of dehydration is to replace the fluid and electrolyte losses that have been incurred. Replacement is not only calculated on the amount of obvious losses but also requires an additional 1,500 ml to cover insensible loss. The therapy will be specific to the individual patient but in general, the physician will order fluids that are isotonic to the normal serum, such as isotonic sodium chloride or 5% dextrose in distilled water.

Nursing Evaluation
The success of nursing interventions in making a positive difference in the health of the dehydrated patient can be measured by evaluating the status of the patient in terms of outcome criteria.

If at assessment it was determined that the patient was ingesting 1,000 ml of fluid less than his output or less than his physiologic need of 2,500 ml, one of the specific objectives of the nursing care plan would be that of increasing oral fluid intake by 1,000 ml per day. The nursing intervention is directed toward this goal. The outcome criterion would be: Oral fluid intake of 2,500 ml every 24 hours during hospitalization. Simple comparison of the intake record with the criterion will indicate the success or failure of the nursing intervention.

The nursing process may be conceptualized as occurring in a circular fashion. Information about the patient is acquired by **assessment**. A summary statement of the assessment data ia made in the nursing **diagnosis**. The nursing **plan** details objective judgments that can alter the patient's present illness state or maintain positive aspects of his health. Nursing **interventions** are actions designed to accomplish these objectives, and **outcome criteria** are explicit statements by which achievement of the objectives can be measured. If the outcome criteria are not met, each step of the process must be reexamined to determine why they were not. Assessment data may have been inadequate, the nursing plan may not have been specific enough for the patient, the nursing intervention may have been well designed but insufficiently administered, or the outcome criteria may have been unrealistic. Conversely, if the outcome criteria are achieved, the nursing process is reviewed in order to determine whether any one of the assessment data, objectives, or interventions was more significant than others in achieving positive results. This final analysis of the total nursing process is **evaluation**.

WATER INTOXICATION

Water intoxication, or overhydration, is a condition of fluid in the body compartments in excess of the normal 60 percent of body weight. It is a situation of an increased or normal intake with a decreased output. The excess fluid in the extracellular compartment causes it to be hypotonic in relation to the intracellular fluid and leads to movement of fluid into the cells and a resulting cellular swelling or distention. Normally, cellular distention causes the pituitary gland to stop secreting antidiuretic hormone and diuresis occurs. If, however, the functioning of antidiuretic hormone has in some way been interrupted, diuresis will not occur. The extracellular fluid compartment continues to expand and develops an increased pressure. As a result, aldosterone secretion ceases and the kidneys excrete sodium with a minimum amount of water. The extracellular fluid becomes more hypotonic and a vicious cycle develops.

Nursing Assessment

Population at risk DISEASE STATES

congestive heart failure with a resulting low renal blood flow and low urinary output.
acute renal insufficiency when urinary output is decreased or absent.
cerebral lesions that lead to excessive secretion of antidiuretic hormone.
psychogenic polydipsia wherein a person voluntarily ingests extremely large amounts of fluids. The behavior is psychologically motivated.
adrenal insufficiency and a resulting decrease in aldosterone secretion that leads to excessive sodium losses and the sequence of events described under water intoxication.

SITUATIONAL FACTORS

fear, pain, acute infections, anesthetics, analgesics, and **acute stress** all stimulate the secretion of antidiuretic hormone, which in some cases may be excessive and lead to water retention.
overadministration of therapeutic fluids by nonoral routes: intravenous, rectal.

Subjective and objective data A distinct difference in observable symptoms occurs relative to the rapid or gradual onset of water intoxication. In **rapid onset** the symptoms start suddenly, are primarily neurologic in origin, and may be strange behavior, loss of attention, confusion, staring, aphasia, lack of coordination, sleeplessness interspersed with violent behavior, shouting, delirium, extreme muscle weakness, convulsions, and coma. In water intoxication of **gradual onset** the symptoms occur slowly and are also primarily neurologic in origin: weakness, apathy, sleepiness, anorexia, nausea, vomiting, personality changes, disorientation or psychosis, convulsions, or coma may occur.

In addition, various subjective and objective symptoms may be observed in either sudden or gradual onset.

integumentary system. Warm, moist feeling and flushed appearance of skin; marked salivation, marked tearing.
central nervous system. Gross muscle weakness, isolated muscle twitching, diminished or absent tendon reflexes.
urinary system. Volume is usually low but may be high; low specific gravity of urine; however, there may be greater than normal amounts of sodium and chloride.
general systemic involvement. Total body weight gain in excess of 5 percent of previous weight; edema of the ankles, sacrum, eyelids; generalized body edema (anasarca).
hematologic system. Decreased hemoglobin concentration; decreased hematocrit; decreased mean corpuscular hemoglobin concentration; blood urea nitrogen is normal or low unless previously high; potassium is normal or low; serum sodium concentration is decreased below 130 mEq per liter and may fall to 115 mEq per liter. The critical factor is the rapidity of sodium dilution with a rapid fall leading to convulsions.

Nursing Diagnosis

Some possible nursing diagnoses according to the previously explained concepts would be

Water intoxication related to congestive heart failure.
Water intoxication related to renal insufficiency.

Water intoxication related to overadministration of intravenous fluids.

Or, alternatively,

Ankle edema related to water intoxication.
Confusion related to acute water intoxication.
Vomiting related to water intoxication.

The diagnosis suggested by the National Conference on Classification of Nursing Diagnosis is

Excess of body fluids.

Nursing Plan

Nursing objectives that would apply to most patients experiencing water intoxication are

Promote reversal of excess fluid state.
Maintain integrity of the skin and mucous membranes.
Promote physical mobility.
Prevent physical, social, and psychological deterioration, which can occur as a consequence of the pathologic condition.

If the neurologic symptoms predominate, the following objectives are indicated:

Limit environmental stimuli.
Provide for safety of the patient.

Nursing Intervention

Withhold oral fluid for 24 hours Explain to the patient the reasons for limiting his fluid intake in order to avoid adding fluid to an already overloaded state. In addition, within a 24-hour period, the body will lose approximately 1,000 ml of fluid via the lungs and skin plus any that may be excreted by the kidneys. The insensible loss can make a considerable difference in a patient with a moderate excess of body fluids.

Provide safety devices when patient is in bed or ambulatory If the patient has an altered level of consciousness, siderails must be used to prevent him from falling out of bed. He must also be prevented from using hazardous objects such as a razor, an oral thermometer, or any glass equipment. Similar precautions must be observed if the patient is lucid but is experiencing muscle weakness. The care of the person who has convulsions or is comatose is detailed in Chapter 11.

Care for the skin The edematous areas of the overhydrated patient's skin are exceptionally susceptible to decubitus ulcer formation. The excess amount of fluid in these tissue spaces limits the blood flow to the cells and as a result limits their nutrition, placing them in a highly vulnerable position. If, in addition, the patient is not fully mobile, all the hazards of pressure are added to the already susceptible tissue. The following nursing interventions are directed toward *prevention* of decubitus ulcers:

Turn the patient frequently, using as many different positions as possible in order to reduce pressure.
Massage the skin of edematous areas to promote circulation.
Eliminate extra bedding and plastic pillows or sheets to reduce heat formation.
Keep bedding and clothing dry to prevent excoriation.

Care for mucous membranes Excessive tearing and salivation increase the possibility of infection; therefore the eyes and mouth must be cleaned and maintained in as nearly a normal state of hydration as possible.

Maintain accurate record of all output Measure and record all instances of fluid output. If the patient is capable of doing so, he can be taught to maintain his own output record. The family may also be taught to participate in this aspect of care.

Weigh patient daily Accurate daily weights provide a measure of fluid loss. The patient should be weighed at the same time every day, wearing the same clothing, and on the same scale.

Maintain quiet, nonstressful environment The high probability of neurologic symptoms occurring indicates the need to limit further stimulation of the central nervous system. Quiet movements, no radio or television, reduction of noise outside the patient's room, and elimination of unnecessary conversation all promote a more peaceful environment.

Support medical regimen Medical therapy is directed toward correcting the underlying disorder and the resulting symptoms. Fluid intake is always monitored and usually is restricted. Some authors suggest administration of hypertonic saline if the serum sodium falls to very low levels, but they caution against the dangers inherent in this therapy and recommend its use only in rare cases.

Evaluation

Evaluation of the effectiveness of nursing intervention is accomplished by use of outcome criteria (see the evaluation section on dehydration). The criteria would be written in relation to the objectives of the nursing care plan and the individual patient. For example, if prevention of skin breakdown is one of the nursing objectives, the outcome criterion could be written as: No evidence of redness or excoriation on any skin surfaces. Simple inspection of the patient's skin would attest to whether or not the goal has been accomplished.

Problems of Electrolyte Balance

HYPONATREMIA

Hyponatremia literally means less sodium in the blood. Clinically the serum sodium level falls below the normal range of 135 to 142 mEq per liter. The serum sodium value is not an indication of the total body stores of sodium but of the ratio of sodium to water in the extracellular fluid. The *total* body stores of sodium may be high, normal, or low. A low serum sodium concentration is the result of increased amounts of body fluids due to increased ingestion or retention of water or of losses of sodium greater than losses of water. As was indicated earlier, sodium is the most abundant electrolyte in the extracellular fluid and as such makes a great contribution to the osmotic pressure of the extracellular fluid compartment. With sodium loss, the extracellular fluid becomes hypotonic in relation to the cells, water moves *into* the cells, and there is a resulting drop in extracellular volume, including plasma or blood volume, as the body endeavors to correct the diminished sodium concentration. For reasons that are not clearly understood, albumin, a plasma protein, also drops with a drop in serum sodium. The decreased protein in the intravascular spaces lowers its osmotic pressure and renders it hypotonic in relation to the extravascular spaces. As a result, fluid leaves the plasma and enters the interstitial spaces, leading to a further decrease in circulating volume and an increase in tissue fluid.

The decreased osmolality of the extracellular fluid causes the hypothalamic nuclei to cease the secretion of antidiuretic hormone; water is excreted freely from the kidneys in an effort to restore the normal concentration of extracellular sodium. The diminished extracellular volume initiates the chain of events that leads to aldosterone secretion and results in kidney reabsorption of sodium, another effort directed toward helping expand the extracellular fluid compartment.

To summarize, a decrease in the ratio of sodium to water in the extracellular fluid compartment leads to efforts by the body to correct the low ratio of sodium by moving water out of the extracellular compartment into the cells, tissue spaces, and urine and by retrieving sodium from possible excretion in the urine.

Nursing Assessment

Population at risk DISEASE STATES

chronic congestive heart failure with excessive extracellular fluid because of diminished cardiac output or excessive sodium loss due to administration of diuretics, or severely reduced dietary sodium intake.

starvation or malnutrition states for reasons not clearly known but thought to be related to incapacity of the sodium pump and the accumulation of intracellular sodium.

peritonitis with collection of fluid in the peritoneal cavity due to the inflammatory process.

intestinal obstruction with collection of fluid in the intestines.

acute pancreatitis where fluid moves into the diseased area in response to the inflammatory process.

severe burns, which lead to collection of fluid in the blisters or interstitial spaces. Such a shift of fluid, which contains large quantities of sodium, will usually occur within the first 48 to 72 hours following a burn.

GENERALIZED SYMPTOMS

vomiting causes a loss of the normal sodium content of the gastric juices.

- **diarrhea** leads to a loss of sodium with the water of liquid stool.
- **diaphoresis** results in loss of sodium through the skin.
- **ascites** represents a shift of fluid from the extracellular spaces to the tissue spaces but not a shift of sodium.
- **fistulas of the gastrointestinal or biliary tract** with loss of fluid into body cavities or through the skin.
- **hemorrhage** with a resulting large loss of extracellular fluid.

SITUATIONAL OR THERAPEUTIC FACTORS

- **postoperatively or following accidental injuries** in which trauma to the tissues leads to a shift of sodium and potassium across the cell membrane; sodium enters the cells and potassium leaves it.
- **excessive use of diuretics,** which leads to renal excretion of sodium.
- **gastrointestinal suction** mechanically removes the gastric contents, which are rich in sodium.

Subjective and objective data When sodium loss occurs rapidly, as in severe hemorrhage or burns, the patient will present the symptoms of shock (see Chap. 16). With a less rapid onset of hyponatremia, the following symptoms will be exhibited:

- **cardiovascular system.** Orthostatic hypotension, tachycardia, headache, giddiness, low blood pressure, and collapsing pulse all result from the decreased circulating blood volume.
- **musculoskeletal system.** General weakness and/or specific muscle weakness.
- **neurologic system.** In severe loss of sodium, mental confusion, delirium, stupor, or coma may develop.
- **gastrointestinal system.** Anorexia, nausea, vomiting.
- **urinary system.** Specific gravity usually normal; low urinary output, possibly anuric; low sodium and chloride concentrations.
- **hematologic system.** Serum sodium values of less than 135 mEq per liter, elevated hematocrit, mean corpuscular volume of red blood cells elevated, low chloride or bicarbonate, depending on which of these ions is lost with the sodium; high serum potassium; elevated blood urea nitrogen.
- **integumentary system.** Loss of skin turgor and elasticity; soft, sunken eyeballs.

Nursing Diagnosis

The diagnosis of hyponatremia is usually made explicit by the physician. For the purposes of nursing, this diagnostic label can be accepted and expanded to include information more contributory to the care of the patient. For example, some possible diagnoses might be

Hyponatremia related to severe burns.
Hyponatremia related to prolonged vomiting.
Hyponatremia related to trauma.

Or, alternatively,

Muscle weakness related to hyponatremia.
Orthostatic hypotension related to hyponatremia.
Mental confusion related to hyponatremia.

Nursing Plan

The objectives of the nursing plan would be to promote correction of the underlying cause of decreased serum sodium concentration, maintain a safe environment for the patient, and prevent secondary disabilities that might arise as a consequence of the pathologic condition.

Nursing Intervention

Maintain accurate records of intake and output

Assist patient when he or she is ambulatory and provide for protection from falls or injury when left alone The problems of muscle weakness and neurologic alterations jeopardize the patient's ability in self-care. If the problem is that of muscle weakness, self-injury is prevented by physical assistance when moving, support when left alone in a chair, and protection when in bed. Explain to the patient the reasons he is unable to ambulate as freely as when he was not ill and caution him against attempting to ambulate alone. If mental confusion is the problem, explain to the patient and his family the reasons for protective devices and assist the patient to be as autonomous as his condition permits. In more severe states of altered levels of consciousness, the patient must be closely observed and completely cared for by the nurse.

Maintain quiet, tension-free environment
Because of the possibility of neurologic complications, stimulation of the central nervous system should be kept to a minimum. Not only a quiet environment but clear and explicit explanations to the patient about his care and his progress are helpful in reducing stress.

Irrigate gastric suction apparatuses with normal saline The use of an isotonic irrigating solution will minimize the loss of gastrointestinal electrolytes. Specific interventions will differ, based on whether the hyponatremia is due to a decreased intake of sodium, a loss of sodium greater than water, or an increase in extracellular fluid.

Encourage the ingestion of foods and fluids high in sodium when there is a decreased intake or loss of sodium Examples of such items are common table salt, milk, meat, eggs, carrots, beets, celery, and asparagus. When there is an increase in extracellular fluid, the situation is very similar to that of water intoxication. The similarity is that both are situations of increased fluid volume; the difference is that in hyponatremia the ratio of sodium to water is decreased and in water intoxication this ratio usually remains unchanged. The nursing interventions for hyponatremia due to increased extracellular fluid are primarily directed toward the problems of extracellular fluid excess. As the interventions have been described in the water intoxication section, those interventions that are applicable will be repeated, but the reader is asked to review the water intoxication section for a full description (see page 169).

Care for the skin
Care for the mucous membranes
Weigh patient daily

Administer prescribed medical therapy Medical therapy is directed toward treating the sodium loss and decreasing the excess fluid.

Nursing Evaluation
Evaluation of the efficacy of the nursing intervention can be accomplished only by use of outcome criteria. If one of the nursing objectives has been to prevent disabilities related to the underlying pathologic condition and the patient is experiencing a great deal of muscle weakness with concomitant immobility, an appropriate nursing intervention would be passive exercises to maintain muscle tone. The outcome criterion could be stated as: Muscle tone adequate to support normal movement when the patient is able to ambulate. If this statement is true at the time the muscle weakness has subsided, the nursing objective would be met.

HYPERNATREMIA

Hypernatremia is the situation in which the ratio of sodium to extracellular fluid is elevated. The patient's level of serum sodium will be greater than 145 mEq per liter. High levels of serum sodium may result from greater than normal ingestion or administration of saline solutions or inadequate fluid intake. The extracellular fluid is hypertonic in relation to the cells, and cellular dehydration occurs.

Nursing Assessment

Population at risk DISEASE STATES

severe burns in which large amounts of fluids are lost from the skin.
diabetes mellitus when prolonged glucose diuresis has resulted in water losses exceeding those of sodium.
diabetes insipidus with large urinary losses of water that may occur postoperatively in patients with neurologic disease or in persons with intracranial injury.
certain liver diseases in which the normal inactivation of aldosterone does not occur and sodium reabsorption in the renal tubule becomes excessive.
cerebral tumors in which the neurons of the thirst center have been destroyed and sensations of thirst are absent.

SITUATIONAL OR THERAPEUTIC FACTORS

steroid therapy wherein cortisone, although a glucocorticoid, may increase sodium retention.
weak, elderly, disabled, or comatose persons who are unable to ingest adequate amounts of fluids.
patients receiving high protein feedings dissolved in minimal amounts of water. The breakdown of protein leads to urea formation, which requires large amounts of fluid for its excretion.

administrations of excessive amounts of sodium solutions.

Subjective and objective data Most persons with hypernatremia are seriously ill due to the underlying disease. Specific signs and symptoms are difficult to isolate, but may include the following:

central nervous system. Depression of the central nervous system produces lethargy that may progress to coma; reflexes may be hyperactive; muscle rigidity and tremor may be present; spasticity, epileptiform seizures, and possibly convulsions.
musculoskeletal system. Generalized muscle weakness.
general systemic involvement. Low grade fever.
renal system. Blood urea nitrogen may be three or four times normal; concentration of urine occurs.

Nursing Diagnosis
The diagnosis of hypernatremia is usually made by the physician. The nursing diagnosis would include significant information relative to the clinical condition. Some examples might be

Hypernatremia related to severe burns.
Hypernatremia related to steroid therapy.
Hypernatremia related to cerebral tumor.

Or, alternatively,

Epileptic seizures related to hypernatremia.
Muscular weakness related to hypernatremia.
Lethargy related to hypernatremia.

Nursing Plan
The objectives of the nursing plan and, consequently, the nursing intervention for a patient with **hypernatremia** are similar to those for a patient with **hyponatremia** due to the altered sodium concentrations and changes in fluid volume in both cases. In instances for which the nursing care has already been described, only a statement will be made to indicate its inclusion.

Facilitate the medical regimen toward reversal of hypernatremic state.
Prevent physical and psychological deterioration related to the disorder.
Maintain safe environment for the patient.

Nursing Intervention
Maintain accurate records of intake and output
Assist when ambulatory and protect from injury when left alone
Maintain quiet, tension-free environment
Measure and record significant signs Temperature, pulse, respirations, and blood pressure should be measured every 2 to 4 hours.

Discontinue any hypertonic or saline intravenous solutions if the hypernatremia is due to an excess intake of sodium without an increase in extracellular fluid Hypernatremia due to a decrease in fluid volume primarily presents the same problems as those of dehydration. Those interventions that have been discussed in the section on dehydration are listed below.

Offer and encourage oral fluids.
Administer intravenous fluids.
Maintain accurate record of intake and output.
Communicate fluid replacement plan to all persons who are caring for the patient.
Maintain the integrity of the skin and mucous membranes.
Maintain adequate nutrition.
Measure and record significant signs. Temperature, pulse, respirations, and blood pressure are monitored frequently. Daily weights provide a measure of the reversal of the dehydrated state.
Support prescribed medical therapy.

Nursing Evaluation
An outcome criterion for a patient with hypernatremia might be based on an assessment finding of lethargy. A specific nursing intervention designed to prevent disabilities due to this state might be: Assist with ambulation and protect from falling. The outcome criterion would be stated as ambulation accomplished safely at all times. If the patient has no slips or falls, the nursing objective has been met.

HYPOKALEMIA

Hypokalemia, or hypopotassemia, is a decrease in the normal amount of potassium in the serum and may occur as the result of either renal or extrarenal losses. As previously noted, the concentration of potassium is related to the intracellular fluid in the same manner that sodium is related to the extracellular fluid. It is the most abundant electrolyte within the cells, and its concentration there is thirty times greater than its extracellular concentration. Unfortunately it is difficult to measure the amount of potassium within the cells. It is possible, however, to measure the amount of potassium that exists in the serum, and in the clinical situation the serum determination is accepted as a close reflection of the cellular potassium value.

Potassium exists normally in the serum within a very narrow range, 3.8 to 5.0 mEq per liter (or 5.5 mEq per liter according to some laboratory standards). Small deviations in either direction can lead to serious consequences for the person.

Nursing Assessment

Population at risk DISEASE STATES

primary or secondary aldosteronism and **Cushing's syndrome** produce excessive amounts of adrenal steroids and directly stimulate the sodium-cation exchange mechanism in the kidney, resulting in urinary potassium loss.

renal diseases such as renal tubular acidosis and Fanconi's syndrome increase urinary potassium loss, although it is not known whether this is due to defective reabsorption or accelerated excretion.

congestive heart failure increases aldosterone levels and the kidney excretes potassium in its effort to conserve sodium.

SITUATIONAL OR THERAPEUTIC FACTORS

therapeutic diuretic agents such as the mercurials, thiazides, furosemide (Lasix), and ethacrynic acid (Edecrin) increase the exchange of sodium for potassium in the distal tubules with a resulting loss of potassium. Carbonic anhydrase inhibitors such as acetazolamide (Diamox) impair sodium-hydrogen exchange and favor the exchange of sodium for potassium in the kidney tubule.

adrenal steroid therapy initiates the process described in primary or secondary aldosteronism.

drainage or suction of gastric contents removes large quantities of potassium that exist normally in the gastric secretions.

GENERALIZED SYMPTOMS

prolonged vomiting leads to loss of the gastric juices, which usually contain a concentration of potassium somewhat greater than that of plasma.

diarrhea fluid contains large amounts of potassium.

Subjective and objective data The effects of hypokalemia are primarily those related to a decrease in the potassium ion and a resulting loss of its normal functions, the most predominant of which is neuromuscular excitation. In addition, hypokalemia is rarely seen without a concomitant state of alkalosis. If the plasma concentration of potassium is low, the kidneys will excrete hydrogen ions instead of potassium in order to fulfill their electrochemical needs. Conversely, if alkalosis is already present the kidneys will endeavor to conserve hydrogen and will excrete potassium.

musculoskeletal system. Decreased reflexes, muscle irritability, weakness, and speech changes may indicate partial muscle paralysis. Abdominal distention, flatulence, vomiting, and paralytic ileus are evidence of diminished smooth muscle strength. **Paralysis** of the respiratory muscles beginning with the diaphragm and progressing to the intercostal and accessory muscles occurs only in profound potassium depletion but may lead to death. Muscle pains and tenderness may also be present.

cardiovascular system. Rapid, weak, irregular pulse; decreased blood pressure; postural hypotension; and cardiac arrythmias may occur in severe hypokalemia.

central nervous system. Lethargy, apathy, drowsiness, confusion, and irritability.

urinary system. Nocturia, polyuria, and polydipsia due to the inability of the kidneys to concentrate urine.

Nursing Diagnosis

The physician usually identifies and labels this clinical condition; the nursing diagnosis will add pertinent information. Some possible examples might be

Hypokalemia related to congestive heart failure.
Hypokalemia related to prolonged vomiting.
Hypokalemia related to renal tubular acidosis.

Or, alternatively,

Polydipsia related to hypokalemia.

Abdominal distention related to hypokalemia.
Postural hypotension related to hypokalemia.

Nursing Plan

The objectives of the nursing plan would be to prevent potassium deficit in patients known to be at risk, promote therapy directed toward reversal of hypokalemic state, and prevent secondary disabilities due to therapy or as a consequence of the pathologic condition.

Nursing Intervention

Closely observe for early signs of potassium deficit The most specific sign of hypokalemia is a serum potassium level below 3.8 mEq per liter. Muscle weakness and fatigue are the first signs usually noted by the patient. The physician must be notified of these changes.

Closely observe for signs of metabolic alkalosis The presence of alkalosis may signal the probability of hypokalemia or, conversely, the presence of hypokalemia may indicate the approach of metabolic alkalosis. Nausea, vomiting, and diarrhea followed by mental confusion and irritability are symptomatic of metabolic alkalosis. The physician should be notified of these signs.

Maintain accurate records of intake and output

Monitor pulse and electrocardiogram Cardiac arrhythmias may occur in a patient who is receiving digitalis and diuretics and who develops hypokalemia. Severe cardiac changes are usually seen only in advanced states of hypokalemia, but they are serious complications.

Administer potassium replacement If the patient is alert, potassium may be replaced orally either by means of diet or medicines. Foods that are rich sources of potassium are bananas, orange juice, meat, coffee, tea, cola beverages, whole grains, and leafy vegetables. Pharmacologically, potassium may be given either orally or intravenously. The patient should drink a full glass of water with the oral preparations, since potassium is highly irritating to the gastric mucosa. Small bowel lesions may occur and are evidenced by abdominal pain, distention, and gastrointestinal bleeding. When given intravenously, potassium must be diluted; the more usual concentration is 30 to 40 mEq per liter of fluid.

The nurse should be aware of the appropriate concentration of potassium required and the flow rate for infusion of the fluids as determined by the needs of the individual patient. Adequate renal function must be established before potassium is administered, since potassium is primarily eliminated by the kidneys. In severe deficiencies of potassium, higher concentrations of potassium may be necessary. Continuous monitoring of the ECG is then essential, to detect the onset of arrhythmias that could lead to ventricular fibrillation (see Chap. 4). Because potassium may be given too rapidly, increasing serum levels to the point of hyperkalemia, the nurse must carefully monitor the administration and observe for signs of hyperkalemia. In addition, the patient may experience a burning sensation at the site of administration. This burning sensation indicates that the concentration is too great for the patient's tolerance and the flow rate should be slowed. Prevention of infiltration of potassium solution is essential, since infiltration into subcutaneous tissues is very painful.

Nursing Evaluation

On assessment it may be found that the patient is having large losses of fluids from diarrhea. He is a potential candidate for hypokalemia, and one of the nursing objectives would be prevention of this complication. Nursing intervention would include replacement of potassium loss with dietary sources. The outcome criterion would be: Ingests a daily diet containing at least 4 gm of potassium. Analysis of the patient's dietary intake would provide evidence of whether this level was being attained.

HYPERKALEMIA

Hyperkalemia, an excess of potassium in the serum, does not usually arise because of a gross absolute excess of potassium in the body but rather because of maldistribution of potassium between the cells and extracellular fluid. Conditions that cause a shift of potassium from the cells to the extracellular fluid, such as acidosis, anoxia, and increased cellular catabolism, give rise to this maldistribution. In addition, although there may not be an increase in whole body potassium, factors that diminish potassium output lead to hyperkalemia.

Nursing Assessment

Population at risk DISEASE STATES

acute renal failure in which there is no effective means of excreting potassium.

Addison's disease and **adrenal insufficiency** wherein aldosterone is not present to facilitate potassium excretion.

hemorrhagic shock in which potassium is released from damaged cells and the drop in circulating blood volume leads to renal shutdown and a loss of the major excretory pathway of potassium.

myocardial infarction and massive crushing injuries in which damaged cells release their potassium into the plasma. In myocardial infarction, the conduction system of the heart muscle is jeopardized by these excessive cations.

SITUATIONAL OR THERAPEUTIC FACTORS

excessively rapid infusions of intravenous potassium.

spironolactone (Aldactone), a diuretic that is an aldosterone antagonist and leads to inhibition of sodium-potassium exchange in the renal tubule, may be administered in excess of therapeutic doses.

Subjective and objective data Hyperkalemia is seen as either a cause of acidosis or the result.

cardiovascular system. Cardiac arrythmias progressing to ventricular fibrillation or standstill may occur due to the stimulatory effect of potassium on the electrical impulse that propagates the heartbeat. This feature is the most important effect of hyperkalemia.

neuromuscular system. Ascending muscular weakness may occur, leading to flaccid paralysis, with very high serum potassium levels.

gastrointestinal system. Nausea and diarrhea as a result of the body's efforts to eliminate surplus potassium.

Nursing Diagnosis

Examples of possible nursing diagnoses might be

Hyperkalemia related to acute renal failure.

Hyperkalemia related to too rapid intravenous administration of potassium.

Or, alternatively,

Diarrhea related to hyperkalemia.
Cardiac arrythmias related to hyperkalemia.

Nursing Plan

The objectives of the nursing plan would be to support the medical treatment directed toward reduction of high serum potassium levels, and to prevent the occurrence of hyperkalemia in the population at risk and the disabilities that may arise as a secondary consequence of the pathologic condition.

Nursing Intervention

Limit oral intake of potassium and protein Provide the patient with a diet low in potassium and high in carbohydrates. Foods that meet this criteria are potatoes, white rice, tapioca, hard candy balls, and such vegetables as carrots, asparagus, onions, and corn. The high carbohydrate intake allows the body to utilize these carbohydrates for energy, thus preventing the catabolism of tissue protein, which would lead to the release of cellular potassium into the extracellular fluid.

Promote excretion of excess potassium from the body The most common cause of potassium excess is the inability of the body to excrete potassium in the urine. Measures that encourage urinary output—adequate fluid intake, privacy during voiding, and prompt assistance to the bathroom when needed—may help increase output. In patients who experience renal shutdown, however, only peritoneal dialysis or hemodialysis will effectively remove excess potassium.

Therapeutic administration of a "cation exchange resin" such as Kayexalate may be effective in lowering the serum potassium by its action in the gastrointestinal tract. Kayexalate, which is nonabsorbable, exchanges its sodium ions for potassium ions as it travels through the intestine and is finally excreted in the feces. A significant decrease in potassium concentration can be accomplished by this route within 24 hours. This medication may be administered either orally or by enema. If the patient is in renal shutdown, the amount of fluid given with Kayexalate must be measured closely.

Closely observe patients at risk for early signs of hyperkalemia The earliest symptoms may be fairly nonspecific. The electrocardiogram will show definite and specific changes that are diagnostic of hyperkalemia. Some patients may complain of paresthesias.

Limit potassium intake in population at risk for hyperkalemia Patients who are anuric or oliguric should not receive potassium in any form, either dietary or pharmacological.

Assist the patient when he is ambulatory and protect him from injuring himself when alone

Nursing Evaluation

The assessment data may reveal that the patient is experiencing renal shutdown. This patient is at high risk for hyperkalemia, and one of the nursing objectives should be designed to prevent it from occurring. A low potassium diet would be an appropriate nursing intervention to meet this objective. The logical outcome criterion would be: Restrict dietary potassium. Evaluation of the patient's daily diet would indicate the success or failure of this intervention.

HYPOCALCEMIA

A decrease in the serum level of calcium below 4.5 mEq per liter is identified as **hypocalcemia.** The calcium deficit may be due to several different conditions. Excessive diarrhea leads to large losses of calcium from the gastrointestinal tract before it can be absorbed. Vitamin D is necessary for the normal metabolism of calcium, and deficiencies of this substance result in inadequate absorption of calcium. Pancreatic insufficiency and acute pancreatitis both affect normal metabolism of calcium. During pregnancy and lactation, calcium requirements are increased and may not be met by dietary intake. Following a thyroidectomy, when the parathyroid glands, which are responsible for maintaining normal serum calcium levels, may have been removed, a calcium deficit will likely occur. The administration of citrated blood in large amounts or at a rapid rate leads to hypocalcemia because the citrate binds the calcium, rendering it inactive.

A deficit in serum calcium increases the excitability of nerve and muscle cell membranes and causes the contraction of the heart muscle to be weak. **Tetany** is the most characteristic sign of hypocalcemia and is the name given to a complex of signs and symptoms representing neuromuscular irritability. The patient may have any or most of the following symptoms: carpopedal spasms, which are called a positive Trousseau's sign, are determined by inflating a blood pressure cuff on the arm for 1 to 5 minutes and observing for involuntary "hand folding in"; a positive Chvostek's sign, which is elicited by tapping the facial nerve just below the temple and observing for a momentary twitching of the face; paresthesias of the hands; changes in mood; spasms of the bronchial muscles that resemble an asthma attack; and, in advanced stages, convulsions. It must be noted that these convulsions are often misdiagnosed as epilepsy.

The treatment for hypocalcemia will depend on whether the condition is a mild one or whether tetany is present. In mild situations, calcium lactate or gluconate can be given orally, and a high calcium diet encouraged. Vitamin D may also be administered to increase the absorption of calcium. When tetany is present, more immediate treatment is indicated, and a solution of 10% calcium gluconate is given intravenously.

The nursing care for a patient with hypocalcemia is primarily related to the neuromuscular irritability. Prevention of deformities or injuries due to the muscle spasms, observation for signs of tetany, and provision of a quiet, nonstimulating environment are indicated. If digitalis is part of the patient's total treatment regimen, the patient is particularly observed for signs of decreased cardiac contraction. The action of digitalis is enhanced by calcium, and in digitalized patients who receive calcium, digitalis intoxication may occur.

HYPERCALCEMIA

The concentration of calcium in the extracellular fluid is normally maintained within very narrow limits, at or near 5 mEq per liter. An elevation of serum calcium above the norm to a level of 5.8 mEq per liter is considered to be hypercalcemia. Calcium levels may become elevated as the result of bone diseases, malignant bone tumors, immobilization, or tumors of the parathyroid gland.

The major cause of hypercalcemia is overactivity of the parathyroid glands, hyperparathyroidism, usually caused by tumors that secrete excessive amounts of parathyroid hormone. This hormone's normal feedback relationship with calcium keeps the serum level constant. Its usual actions are to move calcium from bone into the extracellular fluid, from the lower gastrointestinal tract across the intestinal walls into the blood, and from the kidney tubules into the extracellular fluid. It is obvious that an excess supply of this hormone produces excess serum calcium. In addition, when calcium is being reabsorbed from the kidney, phosphorus excretion is increased with a resulting low serum phosphate concentration. Immobilization, malignant bone tumors, and bone diseases all cause the movement of calcium from bone tissue into the extracellular fluid.

Excessive levels of serum calcium depress neuromuscular excitability, resulting in hypotonicity of muscles, lethargy, and mental confusion; psychosis and coma may be seen in severe states. The resorption of calcium from bones causes bone pain and can lead to pathologic fractures. Large amounts of calcium are present in the parenchyma of the kidneys and may lead to the formation of kidney stones with corresponding infection and flank pain. The hypotonicity of the smooth muscles of the gastrointestinal tract gives rise to constipation.

The most significant treatment of hypercalcemia is to correct the underlying cause. Until that is accomplished, however, measures that increase urinary excretion of calcium, such as administration of isotonic saline and sodium sulfate, may reduce the serum calcium level. Steroid therapy usefully inhibits absorption of calcium.

Again, nursing intervention is directed toward the neuromuscular problems. Safety of the patient because of his weakness and, possibly, altered level of consciousness is paramount. Pain intervention, both psychological and physical, is indicated in bone or flank pain. Mobility is encouraged as much as possible to prevent further loss of calcium from the bones. Fluid intake is promoted to compensate for increased urinary excretion due to medications and to dilute urinary calcium. It is a common practice to strain all urinary output in order to detect the passage of stones.

HYPOMAGNESEMIA

Hypomagnesemia is seen when the serum level of magnesium falls below 1 mEq per liter. Several different clinical situations can lead to this deficit. The normal diet provides more than adequate magnesium, and the body is very efficient in conserving this mineral if the dietary intake is low. However, in severe protein malnutrition, starvation, or prolonged intravenous therapy without magnesium supplement, magnesium deficiency develops. In small bowel disorders or increased intake of calcium, the normal intestinal absorption of magnesium is decreased. Nasogastric suction and severe diarrhea both lead to large losses of magnesium with the gastrointestinal fluid. Excessive loss of magnesium via the urine may occur with the use of mercurial thiazide diuretics and ammonium chloride in diabetic acidosis and in hyperthyroidism. Hypomagnesium may be seen in chronic alcoholism as a result of inadequate dietary intake and increased urinary excretion. A magnesium deificiency is seen in patients with hypoparathyroidism, who have a decrease in parathyroid hormone. As with calcium, parathyroid hormone also increases magnesium absorption from the intestine.

Most authorities agree that it is difficult to identify specific symptoms of magnesium deficiency. Symptoms that seem related to it are increased neuromuscular irritability similar to that seen in hypocalcemia, muscle weakness, gross tremors, personality changes—especially irritability and aggressiveness, and convulsive seizures in severe states. Tachycardia and a tendency toward hypotension are cardiovascular expressions of hypomagnesium. In malabsorption syndromes, such as sprue and enteritis, the malabsorption is intensified by a decreased serum magnesium level.

When magnesium deficiency is associated with convulsions, intravenous administration of either magnesium chloride or magnesium sulfate is the indicated treatment.

Less severe states may be treated with intramuscular injections of magnesium sulfate. Oral magnesium, as magnesium hydroxide, may be given prophylactically in patients known to be at risk.

HYPERMAGNESEMIA

An excess of serum magnesium above 3 to 5 mEq per liter is called hypermagnesemia. It usually occurs in patients who have renal insufficiency or untreated diabetic acidosis and are unable to excrete the excess magnesium normally ingested in the diet. It may also occur with the excess administration of magnesium containing salts or antacid mixtures. Hypermagnesemia is also associated with hyperparathyroidism due to the increased absorption effect that parathyroid hormone exerts on magnesium levels.

The symptoms exhibited by the patient are due to the blocking of neuromuscular transmissions by excessive amounts of magnesium ions. The clinical evidence of increased serum magnesium occurs on a continuum of increasing toxicity, beginning with hypotension at a serum level of 3 mEq per liter and ending with cardiac arrest at 12 to 15 mEq per liter. The progression of illness between these two extremes is frequently the following: again, hypotension sometimes accompanied by a feeling of warmth; nausea and vomiting; drowsiness; decreased deep tendon reflexes; weakness; depressed respirations; coma; and finally, cardiac arrest.

The treatment is primarily directed toward the underlying cause. With renal insufficiency, hemodialysis is frequently used. In hypermagnesemia, parenteral administration of calcium gluconate may be used to increase calcium absorption in preference to magnesium absorption.

EDEMA

Edema is the presence of excess interstitial fluid in the tissues. Normally, fluids and proteins that leak from the arteriole ends of the capillaries and do not diffuse back into the venules are removed from the tissue spaces by the lymphatic system. This route is the only way in which proteins can return to the circulation; they are too large to pass through the venule capillary membranes. So long as this normal mechanism is functioning, edema will not occur. There are, however, four primary alterations in the normal capillary–interstitial fluid mechanism that enable fluid to collect in the tissue spaces: increased capillary pressure, decreased plasma proteins, lymphatic obstruction, and increased capillary permeability.

When there is an **increase in capillary pressure,** fluid is rapidly pushed through the capillary membrane and into the tissue spaces. Pressure may be increased by venous obstruction such as venous clots, or cardiac failure; arteriolar dilatation as a local allergic reaction such as with insect bites; and increased extracellular volume due to kidney retention of fluid. A **decrease in plasma proteins** results in a decrease in the colloid osmotic pressure of plasma and a loss of fluid from the capillaries into the tissues. The plasma proteins may be decreased due to a loss of albumin in burns, decreased albumin formation in liver disease, loss of protein in the urine in nephrosis, or to inadequate dietary intake of protein.

Any **obstruction** to the lymphatic drainage allows fluid and proteins to collect in the tissue spaces to such a degree that the pressure rises to a high level. Tumors that occlude the lymphatics, injuries, and surgical removal of lymph channels as in a patient who has had a radical mastectomy are all possible causes of obstruction.

If the endothelium of the capillaries is destroyed, the walls become highly permeable and protein loss can occur into the interstitial spaces. Such destruction may be seen in severe burns and allergic reactions. In disease states related to retention of sodium, as in congestive heart failure, the presence of excess sodium in the extracellular fluid increases the pressure of the tissue spaces and causes retention of fluid. A common description of this phenomenon is "salt holds water." **Pulmonary edema,** which is one of the most serious types of fluid retention in the tissue spaces, results from the increased capillary pressure. It may result from generalized, increased pressure most commonly associated with left heart failure, or from capillary injury associated with primary lung diseases.

Edema is sometimes described clinically as

"pitting" and is roughly evaluated on a four-point scale. Pitting edema means that, if you press your finger over an edematous area, a small pit will remain when you remove your finger (see color insert Figure 3 on page 1078A). A one plus (1+) pitting edema indicates that edema is barely detectable, a four plus (4+) means excessive fluid accumulation. If the edema becomes so excessive that there is no space for the fluid to be displaced to, the tissues will become rock-like and pitting will not be possible.

Alterations in Hydrogen Ion Concentration

Four major imbalances occur relative to hydrogen ion concentration and are a direct expression of a decrease in the body's ability to regulate acids and bases. **Respiratory acidosis** and **alkalosis** primarily involve alterations in carbon dioxide, and **metabolic acidosis** and **alkalosis** primarily involve alterations in bicarbonate.

RESPIRATORY ACIDOSIS

When the production of carbon dioxide in the body tissues exceeds the rate of its removal by the lungs, the partial pressure of carbon dioxide in the blood rises and the person is said to have respiratory acidosis. This state is also called hypercapnia and may occur either as an acute or chronic condition.

In terms of hydrogen ion concentration the excess carbon dioxide combines with water to form carbonic acid, which decreases the ratio of bicarbonate to carbonic acid and results in a fall in the pH of the serum. The body compensates for this increase in acidity in several ways. The first response is to chemically buffer the carbonic acid with hemoglobin, resulting in the formation of bicarbonate ions and deoxygenated hemoglobin and culminating in a decrease in carbonic acid. The kidneys react by increasing the secretion and excretion of hydrogen ions and by retaining bicarbonate and sodium. In addition, the kidneys excrete ammonium and chloride ions. The acidosis also causes a shift of electrolytes across the cell membranes. Hydrogen and sodium ions move into the cells and potassium ions move out of the cells with a resulting rise in serum potassium hyperkalemia. The net effect of these mechanisms is a rise in the pH toward normal. In acute conditions the compensation may be total and the patient will regain a normal state of hydrogen ion concentration. In chronic conditions even though carbon dioxide secretion may be equal to carbon dioxide production, the patient's body has adapted to a higher than normal level of carbon dioxide in the blood. Table 2-6 is a graphic description of the events of respiratory acidosis in the body.

Table 2-6
Diagrammatic representation of respiratory acidosis in the body

Development of respiratory acidosis	Response of body	Result in body
↑ Serum P_{CO_2} ↓ $CO_2 + H_2O \rightarrow H_2CO_3$ ↓ ↓ $\frac{HCO_3^-}{H_2CO_3}$ = ↓ pH	*Chemical regulation* $H_2CO_3 + Hb \rightarrow HCO_3^- + H^+$ Hb *Kidney regulation* ↑ Secretion H^+ ↑ Retention HCO_3^- ↑ Retention Na^+ ↑ Secretion NH_4^+ ↑ Secretion Cl^- *Cellular action* Extracellular Intracellular H^+ ⟶ NA^+ ⟶ ⟵ K^+	$\left. \begin{array}{l} ↑ HCO_3^- \\ ↓ H_2CO_3 \end{array} \right\} = ↑ \frac{HCO_3^-}{H_2CO_3}$ pH normal

↑ indicates that this substance is increased, ↓ that the substance is decreased.

Nursing Assessment

Population at risk for acute respiratory acidosis DISEASE ENTITIES

acute pulmonary lesions that interfere with normal ventilatory function and cause pulmonary edema; pulmonary infections such as pneumonia; bronchial obstructions such as asthma; atelectasis; and either traumatic or surgical open chest wounds.

central nervous system lesions interfere with the respiratory center in the medulla.

metabolic alkalosis limits carbon dioxide excretion as a compensatory mechanism.

SITUATIONAL OR THERAPEUTIC FACTORS

Following **surgical anesthesia** in which respiratory ventilation has been decreased.

drugs such as sedatives, morphine, and alcohol depress respirations centrally.

mechanical asphyxia inhibits adequate oxygen–carbon dioxide exchange.

GENERALIZED SYMPTOMS Paralysis of respiratory muscles as a complication of nervous system diseases such as poliomyelitis and myasthenia gravis or the electrolyte imbalance, extreme hypokalemia.

Subjective and objective data There may not be very specific signs of acute respiratory acidosis. The following signs have been observed in some instances:

respiratory system. Decreased rate and depth of respirations.

cardiovascular system. Ventricular fibrillation as the result of hyperkalemia.

hematologic system. pH at the lower level of normal; may reach 7 in a few minutes; Pco_2 is above the upper limit of normal; CO_2 content* rises to upper limit of normal; CO_2 capacity† remains normal; serum sodium may rise slightly; serum potassium may be elevated.

Population at risk for chronic respiratory acidosis Persons with chronic emphysema, asthma, and bronchiectasis are likely to develop chronic respiratory acidosis. Hypoventilation in the obese is another factor increasing susceptibility.

Subjective and objective data Chronic respiratory acidosis is always complicated by a usually severe underlying disease. The following subjective and objective data may be observed:

respiratory system. Chronic, productive cough; cyanosis; typical emphysematous breathing pattern; may develop acute respiratory acidosis with pulmonary infection.

GENERALIZED SYMPTOMS Weakness; dull headache.

central nervous system. Stupor or coma may develop with severe acidosis.

cardiovascular system. Cardiac arrythmias may occur.

CO_2 narcosis. A serious complication that may arise in patients with chronic respiratory acidosis is carbon dioxide narcosis, which may be either acute or chronic. Patients who have chronic carbon dioxide narcosis have adapted to higher than normal levels of carbon dioxide over a long enough period of time so that their respiratory center is no longer sensitive to it. Hypoxia, as recognized by the aortic and carotid chemoreceptors, has become the respiratory stimulus. If these persons are given high concentrations of oxygen, their respiratory stimulus is removed, ventilation fails, and carbon dioxide increases.

Acidosis becomes increasingly severe until coma and death occur. Early signs of carbon dioxide narcosis may be psychological disturbances and neurologic problems such as muscle twitching and tremors of the face or limbs. Slight respiratory depression or even apnea may appear.

Nursing Diagnosis

The nursing diagnosis can be stated in either of the two previously described ways, such as

---

*CO_2 content: a measurement of the concentration in millimoles per liter of total carbon dioxide in solution, bicarbonate (HCO_3^-) plus carbonic acid (H_2CO_3). The normal value is 24 to 30 mEq per liter.

†CO_2 capacity or "combining power": the bicarbonate content of blood or plasma saturated with 5.5% carbon dioxide at 25°C (77°F).

These values are useful in determining the chemical disturbances of hydrogen ion concentration. In conjunction with the pH, they can explain the relative concentrations of carbonic acid and bicarbonate in the body. The following equation demonstrates that any two of these values will permit derivation of the third:

$$pH = \frac{CO_2 \text{ capacity} = HCO_3}{CO_2 \text{ content} - CO_2 \text{ capacity} = H_2CO_3}$$

Acute respiratory acidosis related to pulmonary edema.
Chronic respiratory acidosis related to emphysema.

Or, alternatively,

Decreased respiratory rate related to acute respiratory acidosis.
Cyanosis related to chronic respiratory acidosis.

Nursing Plan

Specific objectives that may apply to most patients experiencing respiratory acidosis include

Facilitate normal breathing process or maximum ventilatory function.
Prevent dysfunctions that may arise as complications of the illness or of the therapy.
Maintain safety of the patient's person.
Promote patient's self-care activities.

Nursing Intervention

Encourage the patient to turn, cough, and breathe deeply at frequent intervals This intervention is used not only with patients who have respiratory acidosis but also with patients who are at risk for the illness because of a decreased ability to carry out the normal oxygen–carbon dioxide exchange process. The patient is taught the most productive way to cough and deep breathe, and he may be able to schedule these exercises for himself.

Facilitate removal of pulmonary secretions Excess secretions limit the ventilatory function of the lungs and may be removed by mechanical aspiration or, if the patient is capable, he can be taught to carry out postural drainage. Clapping and manual vibration of the chest may be used to loosen secretions prior to postural drainage or suction (Chap. 3). An adequate fluid intake is necessary to keep secretions as liquid as possible, and if not contraindicated, fluid intake is encouraged.

Administer mechanical ventilatory aids An intermittent positive-pressure breathing machine (IPPB), which increases lung expansion, may be used to improve ventilation. A tracheostomy may be performed to reduce the dead air space, facilitate the removal of secretions, or to accommodate the attachment of a mechanical respirator. Meticulous care must be used in caring for the tracheostomy to prevent introducing infections into the tracheobronchial tree.

Administer oxygen Oxygen may be given at a very low rate by nasal cannula or mask. It should be used cautiously; overadministration of oxygen can lead to carbon dioxide narcosis in patients with chronic respiratory acidosis. Specific care must be given to the patient's nose and mouth when he is receiving oxygen, because of its drying effect on the mucous membranes.

Support medical regimen The goal of medical therapy is reversal of the cause of the carbon dioxide retention. Antibiotics are usually administered in infectious diseases. Bronchodilators such as isoproterenol (Isuprel) and bronchial detergents such as tyloxapol (Alevaire) may be used in chronic conditions.

Monitor closely for changes in respirations and level of consciousness Any progression of symptoms, such as shallow respirations or drowsiness progressing to stupor, signals a severe acidotic state and the physician is notified immediately.

Nursing Evaluation

The nursing interventions for respiratory acidosis are all interdependent relative to outcomes. Together, they may or may not accomplish reversal of the patient's acidotic state. It is especially essential therefore to establish outcome criteria that will identify the most effective interventions. During assessment, for example, it may have been noted that the patient had excessive bronchial secretions and one of the interventions established was that of teaching the patient to carry out productive postural drainage four times per day. The outcome criterion for this intervention could be: Three days after admission the patient carries out postural drainage four times per day without assistance and produces at least 10 ml of sputum each time. If this finding is true, this intervention is effective. However, the patient may still have an excess of secretions. In such a case the other interventions aimed at decreasing secretions should be evaluated for their success, or the outcome criterion of 10 ml of sputum may be evaluated as being too low.

RESPIRATORY ALKALOSIS

Respiratory alkalosis is the least common type of hydrogen ion disturbance. It occurs when carbon dioxide is excreted from the lungs so rapidly that normal levels are depleted. As a result the bicarbonate value of the body predominates. This lowered partial pressure of carbon dioxide is also referred to as hypocapnia.

Nursing Assessment
Population at risk Respiratory alkalosis results from hyperventilation: rapid, shallow respirations that do not permit complete ventilation. It is observable in several conditions. The following situations can give rise to hyperventilation and thus respiratory alkalosis:

hypoxia as a result of congestive heart failure, pulmonary atelectasis, and failure to adapt to high altitudes.
psychogenic disturbances such as fear and anxiety.
hypermetabolic states such as fever and delirium tremens.
central nervous system lesions that disturb the respiratory center.
mechanical, assisted respiration.
bacteremia.
exercise. Persons who are not trained to breathe properly when exercising (usually people who exercise infrequently) may attempt to meet their energy requirements by increasing the rate of their respirations.
compensatory mechanisms in respiratory acidosis.

Subjective and objective data
respiratory system. Patients who have developed hypocapnia are able to maintain the reduced partial pressure of carbon dioxide with very little respiratory effort. In other words, hyperpnea may not be obvious. Other patients in an acute phase will exhibit rapid, shallow respirations.
central nervous system. Numbness of extremities and circumoral area; altered consciousness; carpopedal spasms; lightheadedness and tremulousness.
hematologic system. pH is increased, Pco_2 is decreased, HCO_3^- is decreased, and chloride is elevated.

Nursing Diagnosis
Respiratory alkalosis related to salicylate poisoning.
Respiratory alkalosis related to fever.
Respiratory alkalosis related to anxiety.

Or, alternatively,

Altered level of consciousness related to respiratory alkalosis.
Carpopedal spasms related to respiratory alkalosis.

Nursing Plan
Facilitate awareness in patient of cause if the alkalosis is self-limiting.
Support medical intervention.
Promote reversal or control of underlying disease.

Nursing Intervention
Teach patient to recognize situations that precipitate hyperventilation and to consciously breathe deeply when these situations arise. Teach the patient more appropriate breathing patterns (Chap. 3).

Nursing Evaluation
If the patient is able to control his tendency to hyperventilate via measures taught by the nurse, the intervention can be considered effective.

METABOLIC ACIDOSIS

Metabolic acidosis results from an excess of inorganic or organic acids other than carbon dioxide that are not adequately excreted by the kidneys, or by a loss of excess base from the body. The resulting decreased pH stimulates the respiratory center to increase the ventilatory function in order to rid the body of excessive acid. The kidneys then compensate as they did in respiratory acidosis; they increase the secretion and excretion of hydrogen ions, excrete ammonium ions, retain bicarbonate and sodium ions, and excrete chloride. The respiratory response to a fall in pH occurs within a matter of minutes; however, the renal response may take from several hours to a day or more.

Nursing Assessment

Population at risk Persons who experience an **increase in absolute amounts of acid in the blood.** Catabolism of proteins and nucleic acids produces amino acids, and phosphoric, sulfuric, and uric acids. Lactic, pyruvic, and succinic acids are produced by carbohydrate metabolism, and ketones and fatty acids are produced by hydrolysis and oxidation of fats.

diabetic ketacidosis due to incompletely oxidized fat.
starvation with increased catabolism of body protein and fat.
lactic acidosis in which lactic acid, the end product of glucose metabolism, accumulates due to the hypoxic state.

Patients who either ingest **excessive amounts of acids** or receive them therapeutically. Ingestion of salicylates, methyl alcohol, paraldehyde, and ethylene glycol may result in excess acids in the breakdown of these substances.

overadministration of ammonium chloride to patients with congestive heart failure; the ammonium converts to ammonia and releases hydrogen.
carbonic anhydrase inhibitors that prevent formation of carbonic acid in the kidney tubules cause large losses of sodium bicarbonate.

Patients who **cannot excrete normal amounts of acid.** Retention of the normally produced acids of metabolism by patients who have renal tubular disease or chronic pyelonephritis.
Persons who lose large amounts of base via increased intestinal secretions in severe diarrhea, small bowel fistulas, or severe biliary fistulas.

Subjective and objective data The clinical observations of metabolic acidosis are rather variable and are related to the underlying cause. A mild metabolic acidosis may be asymptomatic. The following symptoms may occur:

general systemic involvement. Weakness, lethargy, dull headache.
respiratory system. Very deep respirations with obvious air hunger known as Kussmaul breathing; respiratory rate is usually increased but may be slow. The increased depth of respirations is more significant than the increased rate.
cardiovascular system. Vasodilatation with a flushed face; bounding pulse with a large pulse pressure.
central nervous system. Muscle twitching, convulsions or drowsiness, stupor, coma.
gastrointestinal system. Nausea, vomiting, and abdominal pain due to gastric dilatation.
hematologic system. Before renal compensatory mechanisms develop: pH is low, Pa_{CO_2} is normal, CO_2 capacity and content are low, and serum bicarbonate level is low. After renal and pulmonary compensatory mechanisms: pH is still low though slightly higher than in uncompensated state, Pa_{CO_2} is low, CO_2 content rises, bicarbonate serum level is low, and the serum potassium is elevated.
urine. pH is very acid (4.6 to 6.2) and the ammonia content is high.

Nursing Diagnosis
Possible nursing diagnoses might be

Metabolic acidosis related to starvation.
Metabolic acidosis related to diabetes.

Or, alternatively,

Kussmaul breathing related to metabolic acidosis.
Weakness related to metabolic acidosis.

Nursing Plan
Objectives in caring for the patient with metabolic acidosis could be to promote the measures that correct the underlying cause of the metabolic acidosis, restore fluids and electrolytes lost due to the pathologic state, and maintain the safety of the patient.

Nursing Intervention

Support the medical therapy The physician directs his efforts toward treating the underlying cause of the metabolic acidosis. As noted, these causes are many and their treatment can be quite diverse. If the illness is due to overadministration of acids, it is a simple matter to discontinue them. If the acidosis results from uncontrolled diabetes, insulin, sodium chloride, potassium, and water are administered. When the patient is acidotic due to large intestinal losses of fluids and electrolytes, replacement of these constituents is the indicated therapy. Metabolic acidosis in patients with renal tubular disease is treated by restoring the bicarbonate that the kidney tubular epithelium is unable to reabsorb from the glomerular filtrate. In some instances of kidney failure, dialysis is used to rid the body of its accumulation of acid wastes.

Nursing interventions will also differ based on the underlying cause of the acidosis. The following measures, however, are indicated in almost all cases of metabolic acidosis.

Measure and record all intake and output If the patient is vomiting, his acidosis may rapidly become complicated by dehydration. Intravenous fluid replacement is based on fluid losses, and an accurate record is maintained. For a detailed description of this intervention, see under Dehydration on page 168.

Administer intravenous fluids and electrolytes as prescribed If the patient is unable to tolerate oral fluids, intravenous solutions composed of the necessary electrolytes will be prescribed by the physician. Emergency treatment of metabolic acidosis is sometimes accomplished by the intravenous administration of sodium bicarbonate. Sodium lactate may also be used to increase the amount of base ions in the body.

Provide measures to prevent the patient from falling or from injuring himself Assistance when mobile, siderails on the bed, and supporting straps when sitting in a chair all provide security for the patient who is weak or who may have a lowered level of consciousness. Equipment that may be dangerous to the patient should not remain on his bed or within his reach.

Carry out qualitative urine measurements frequently A determination of the specific gravity, pH, and glucose content of the urine should be made approximately every hour to provide an accurate picture of the body's response to therapy.

Nursing Evaluation

Evaluation of the nursing care given to a patient with metabolic acidosis proceeds on the same principles described in previous nursing evaluation sections. An example of the evaluation process might be: On assessment it may have been found that the pH of the patient's urine was 4.6, very acidotic. The objective toward correction of this deficit could be stated as: Restore fluids and electrolytes lost due to pathologic condition. *One of the nursing interventions directed toward this objective is*: Administer intravenous fluids and electrolytes as prescribed. Assuming the prescription is appropriate, the criterion to evaluate this intervention could be: pH of urine is 6.5 two days after therapy is started. The data obtained from the nursing intervention reflect qualitative urine measurements and can be used to evaluate whether the nursing intervention accomplished the objective of the nursing plan. This example also illustrates the interdependency that exists between nursing and medicine. In this instance both disciplines have the same goal, but they seek to attain it in a different way, and each discipline must rely on the other for the complete success of their interventions. Proper administration of fluids will not reverse the patient's acidotic state if the prescribed fluids are inappropriate; nor will the appropriate fluids be effective if they are not correctly administered.

METABOLIC ALKALOSIS

An excess accumulation of bicarbonate ions or loss of hydrogen ions from the body results in **metabolic alkalosis.** The pH of the plasma rises above the normal limit of 7.45 and the bicarbonate–carbonic acid ratio rises (see page 161). The partial pressure of carbon dioxide may be normal or slightly elevated as the result of hypoventilation, which is an attempt on the part of the body to minimize the high level of plasma bicarbonate. It is necessary to distinguish between primary metabolic alkalosis and renal compensation for respiratory acidosis, which presents nearly the same blood chemistry picture. In addition to the patient's history, the partial pressure of carbon dioxide gives the best information; a Pa_{CO_2} higher than 60 mm Hg almost always indicates primary respiratory disease.

Nursing Assessment

Population at risk SYMPTOMATIC OR THERAPEUTIC FACTORS
- **vomiting or gastric suction** leads to large losses of hydrogen ions normally contained in the gastrointestinal fluid and a concomitant increase in bicarbonate ion. Chloride ions are lost by this route, and chloride depletion affects the ability of the kidneys to reabsorb potassium ions and bicarbonate appropriately; potassium is excreted and bicarbonate is retained.
- **diarrhea** with loss of chloride in the intestinal fluid and the renal effects described above.
- **excess administration of alkali** such as sodium bicarbonate or calcium carbonate increases the amount of base in the body if the kidneys are unable to excrete these substances due to the rapidity of their administration or to renal disease.
- **diuretic therapy,** which results in the excretion of sodium, chloride, potassium, hydrogen ions, and water, leads to a volume reduction and a concentration of extracellular bicarbonate.

DISEASE ENTITIES The Cushing syndrome, ACTH-secreting tumors, and primary hyperaldosteronism result in an excess of mineralocorticoid and can lead to metabolic alkalosis and potassium depletion. The excess mineralocorticoid affects the kidney resorption of potassium and bicarbonate.

Subjective and objective data The symptoms and signs of metabolic alkalosis are closely related to the underlying cause of the alkalosis and are difficult to identify. The following symptoms and signs may be present:

gastrointestinal system. Anorexia, nausea, vomiting, or diarrhea.
central nervous system. Confusion, mental unreliability sometimes described as "difficult," convulsions, and coma. Symptoms of calcium imbalance such as muscle twitching and tetany may be present.
cardiovascular system. Sinus tachycardia.
hematologic system. The pH is high, the Pa_{CO_2} is normal or slightly elevated, the CO_2 capacity is high, and chloride and potassium serum levels are decreased.

Nursing Diagnosis
Possible nursing diagnoses might be

Metabolic alkalosis related to vomiting.
Metabolic alkalosis related to diuretic therapy.

Or, alternatively,

Confusion related to metabolic alkalosis.
Muscle twitching related to metabolic alkalosis.

Nursing Plan
The objectives of the nursing plan could be to promote measures toward removing the underlying cause of the alkalosis and provide for the safety of the patient.

Nursing Intervention

Maintain accurate intake and output records
Closely observe for signs of hypokalemia Muscle weakness and hypotension may be early symptoms of a low serum potassium level.

Prevent patient from falling or from injuring himself

Support the medical regimen If chloride deficiency is the cause of the alkalosis, chloride will be given as sodium chloride or potassium chloride. Potassium depletion is almost always present and is treated with potassium chloride. Ammonium chloride or hydrochloric acid may be given to increase the amount of hydrogen ions in the body. If excessive use of alkali agents is the cause, their use must be discontinued.

Nursing Evaluation
Criteria should be established for each nursing intervention designed for the patient. Previous evaluation sections in this chapter

have explored specific criteria and the process of evaluation. Many of the same criteria could be used for the patient with metabolic alkalosis; selection is based on the individual patient's needs.

Consideration of the patient's total status is important in caring for persons with fluid and electrolyte imbalances. Although the previous discussion of specific classifications of imbalance imply that a patient may experience a singular imbalance, in reality, the seriously ill patient has multiple imbalances. A singular, or pure, imbalance of a single electrolyte rarely occurs. An important concept as the basis of nursing care is that fluid and electrolyte balance is dynamic. Therefore correction of imbalances must be maintained continuously until the patient's condition has stabilized enough so that his normal regulatory mechanisms are functioning sufficiently well to carry on the continuous regulatory processes through the buffer systems and the respiratory and kidney functions.

External regulation of fluid and electrolyte balances must always be continuously monitored by evaluating the patient's signs and symptoms in conjunction with laboratory values for serum electrolytes, osmolality, and urine tests. The internal milieu of the patient's fluid and electrolyte status is estimated on the basis of these data. Overcorrection of deficits quickly leads to excesses, so that balance is difficult to achieve in persons whose conditions are unstable. For example, a patient who is in metabolic acidosis on a given day may later require treatment for metabolic alkalosis. In every event, the underlying cause of the fluid and electrolyte imbalance must be diagnosed and treated if return to normal regulatory function is to be achieved. The success of the treatment will also depend upon the accurate observations and interventions of the nurse.

TOTAL PARENTERAL NUTRITION

An essential component of nursing care is provision of fluids, electrolytes, and nutrients. For patients who are unable to ingest these substances orally or to absorb sufficient amounts through oral administration, alternative means for their provision is necessary. Intravenous therapy is one alternative for providing fluids and electrolytes; however, traditional intravenous "feedings" have been composed of dextrose, vitamins, and minerals prepared as an isotonic solution. This solution is still useful in many instances of short-term management, or as a supplement to oral ingestion, but it is not adequate for long-term nutritional replacement. For example, one bottle of 1,000 ml of 5% dextrose in distilled water yields only 200 calories (5% = 50 grams of dextrose × 4 calories per gram of carbohydrates). Administering 3,000 ml of such an isotonic solution over a 24-hour period would provide an adequate fluid intake but only 600 calories and no protein. People differ in their caloric requirements relative to their degree of activity or to unusual metabolic demands. Adult energy requirements increase to as much as 2500 to 3000 calories per day for postoperative conditions or even 10,000 calories per day in the severely burned patient.

It is not possible to provide adequate calories intravenously via isotonic solutions, because an excessive volume of fluid would be required; nor is it possible to provide adequate calories via hypertonic solutions for administration in a peripheral vein. Hypertonic solutions would cause severe pain, irritation, and phlebitis of peripheral veins. Protein cannot be administered by the usual methods because it renders a solution hypertonic also, and when given in peripheral veins it may lead to emboli.

Therefore in current practice **total parenteral nutrition (TPN)** is the choice for long-term fluid and electrolyte management and provision for adequate nutrients. This method of nutritional therapy has come to be known by a variety of names, such as parenteral alimentation, intravenous hyperalimentation, central venous alimentation, and total parenteral nutrition. The term total parenteral nutrition is the most accurate description of the method and intent of the therapy and is generally accepted as the most appropriate term.

Total parenteral nutrition overcomes the qualitative inadequacies of traditional intravenous feeding by using solutions of approximately 20% dextrose, 5% protein (protein hydrolysates or synthetic amino acids), and 5% mineral and vitamins. It overcomes the problem of delivery of hypertonic solutions by means of a catheter introduced into the superior vena cava via either the right or the left subclavian vein. Insertion into the large central vein provides adequate blood volume to rapidly dilute the hypertonic solution.

Candidates for TPN fall into three broad categories: (1) patients whose gastrointestinal tracts cannot adequately absorb nutrients, as in the following disease states: malabsorption syndrome, gastrointestinal obstruction, paralytic ileus, bowel resection, bowel fistulas, and ulcerative colitis; (2) patients who are physically or emotionally unable to take in food. Examples of the former are patients with neurosurgical problems or those who are comatose; the latter are patients with anorexia nervosa; and (3) patients with excessive nutritional needs that cannot be met under usual methods, including patients with burns, multiple fractures, carcinoma being treated with radiation or chemotherapy, and severe infections.

Prior to the initiation of TPN the patient's weight, baseline electrolytes, blood glucose, and blood chemistry levels are established. The appropriate solutions are then prescribed according to the needs of the individual patient. In most hospitals the solutions are prepared under laminar-flow filtered air hoods, using strict aseptic technique, to prevent contamination.

The patient is advised in detail about the purpose of the therapy and what is expected of him during the treatment regimen. His understanding of the therapy is essential in obtaining his cooperation, which is vital to the success of this form of prolonged therapy.

Procedure for Insertion of Subclavian Line

The patient is lying supine with his head down in a 15° Trendelenburg position to facilitate maximum dilatation of the subclavian vein. The skin is prepared by first shaving the entire area of the neck and the upper thorax. Acetone is then used to defat the skin prior to a sterile scrub of the area, generally with iodine solutions. A local anesthetic is usually used at the injection site. The right subclavian vein is preferred in order to avoid damaging the thoracic duct, which enters the left subclavian vein. The patient is asked to turn his head to the opposite side for better access to the vein. After the needle has been inserted and while the physician removes the syringe and threads the catheter through the needle, the patient is directed to perform a Valsalva maneuver to prevent the introduction of air during the threading procedure. After the needle is withdrawn, the catheter is attached to standard intravenous tubing (and a Millipore filter in most protocols) and isotonic solutions are administered through the catheter. The catheter is sutured to the skin, and the hypertonic solutions are initiated only after correct placement of the catheter tip has been confirmed by x-ray. Antibiotic ointment is applied to the insertion site and is followed by a sterile, occlusive dressing. Strict aseptic technique is maintained in the follow-up care of the solutions as they are being administered, as well as of the dressing site and the equipment being used. Procedures vary in different hospitals regarding recommendations for redressing the insertion site and changing the tubings utilized in the administration. When TPN therapy is used extensively, some settings utilize TPN teams that are specifically responsible for dressing changes, addition of solutions, and care of the tubing. The nurse caring for the patient must take particular care that the dressing remains secure and that there is no tension on the tubing, which might accidentally pull the catheter out of place.

Nursing Plan

The objectives for the nursing care of the patient receiving TPN are those of preparing the patient mentally and physically to receive total parenteral nutrition, maintaining the sterility of the insertion site, the catheter, and the fluid administration equipment, maintaining a constant and proper infusion rate of the solution, and preventing physical and psychological disabilities that might arise from the therapy.

Nursing Intervention

Explain to patient the need for TPN and the catheter insertion procedure The physician may describe the TPN therapy to the patient, but it is necessary for the nurse to also discuss it with him. This discussion provides the patient with an opportunity to bring up any questions or fears he may have. The nurse should stress the advantages of this therapy as nutritional replacement and that the patient can still move and turn in bed, and even ambulate, if his condition permits.

The exact procedure that will be followed for the catheter insertion is demonstrated to the patient with the actual equipment. Knowing beforehand what to expect will help allay his or her anxiety and contribute to cooperativeness. The patient is instructed in precautions to use to prevent loosening or contamination of the dressings, and to keep the dressing dry.

Care for the dressing   Sterile technique is used when redressing the catheter insertion site and changing the intravenous tubing. Previously, dressings were changed every 24 hours; however, it has been found that this care can be given at less frequent intervals (every 2 days) and still maintain the sterility of the insertion site. The tubing change should be accomplished as quickly as possible with the patient lying flat in bed in order to avoid the possibility of an air embolus. Because of the high protein and glucose content of the solutions, they are excellent culture media for bacteria and fungi and extreme care must be used to prevent septicemia resulting from contamination. When the dressing is changed, the skin should be examined for any broken areas, edema, or localized reactions, and any leakage of fluid at the insertion site. Cleansing of the skin around the catheter is essential, and the application of an antibiotic ointment at the site is indicated.

Administer parenteral fluids   The solution must be infused at a continuous and regular rate. This rate is determined by the physician and is based on normal daily water requirements and carbohydrate utilization in the body. If hypertonic dextrose is infused too rapidly, the renal threshold for glucose will be exceeded and it will be excreted. Excretion of glucose is accompanied by osmotic diuresis, with the result that the patient becomes dehydrated. Conversely the islet cells of the pancreas respond to the continuous input of carbohydrates by increasing insulin production; if the hypertonic solution is suddenly slowed or stopped, insulin rebound may occur with the result of a secondary hypoglycemia. The flow rate is monitored every ½ to 1 hour. If the volume of fluid being infused is irregular, the infusion rate is not increased or decreased more than 10 percent per hour to compensate.

The catheter used for TPN is not used for intermittent intravenous medications because of the danger of contamination and potential incompatibilities. Another intravenous site is used for these medications or for the administration of blood transfusions.

Monitor progress of therapy   Fractional urine determinations are carried out every 4 to 6 hours in order to assess how adequately the patient is metabolizing glucose. Glycosuria is managed with prescribed doses of insulin, and in some situations it requires adjustment in the solution prescription.

An accurate record of the patient's intake and output is maintained. Some patients will be able to ingest food and fluids by mouth, and not only the volume but the caloric value of these nutrients is measured and recorded.

The physician will order studies of serum electrolytes and nitrogen balance in order to determine the adequacy of the fluid administration in meeting the patient's biochemical needs.

The patient is weighed daily for evaluation of the nutritional adequacy of the therapy. Patients on TPN should experience a steady weight gain. To assure accuracy, the weighing is done at the same time each day on the same scale and with the patient wearing the same clothes.

Provide emotional support   Total parenteral nutrition has been administered to some individuals for as long as 4 years; however, 6 to 8 weeks is more usual. It is a long time to be "connected to a bottle." The patient should be encouraged to involve himself in as much activity as possible and carry out as much self-care as he is physically capable of doing. An understanding of the stresses of long-term therapy helps the nurse facilitate the patient's own efforts at coping.

Monitor for untoward reactions   Several untoward reactions can occur with the administration of TPN. The nurse will often be the first person to observe these reactions, and should notify the physician immediately if they occur and should intervene in the indicated manner.

Monitor for signs of hyperglycemia, which leads to hypertonic dehydration due to too rapid infusion of fluid   The early subjective signs are nausea, headache, increased lassitude, and, objectively, glycosuria. If not properly reversed, the hyperosmolar state will lead to mental confusion, convulsions, coma, and death. The daily fluid balance, rate of infusion, fractional urine determinations, and blood sugar and electrolyte levels all provide information indicating whether signs of dehydration exist. These signs can be reversed by decreasing the rate of infusion of the hypertonic solution or by the administration of extra "free" water, 5% dextrose in distilled water and specific amounts of insulin. Rapid administration can also lead to fluid overload with distended veins in the neck, arms, and hands and respiratory difficulties.

Monitor for fever Fever is symptomatic of several different problems: an allergic reaction to the nutrients; infection of the catheter or insertion site; contaminated intravenous fluids or tubing; or possibly the patient's underlying disease process. If the cause of the fever is not known, the nutrient solution and administration tubing are changed. In the face of persistent fever, the subclavian catheter is removed and a new one inserted. The tip of the catheter, on removal, is cultured for bacteria or fungi.

Observe for infiltration of nutrient solution Infiltration of nutrient solution into the tissue around the insertion site is due to a misplaced, broken, or defective catheter. The patient may complain of pain in the shoulder or arm on the side of the catheter insertion and edema is present at the insertion site, and possibly in the neck and face. The infusion rate should be slowed and the physician notified to reinsert the catheter.

Although TPN has proved to be effective, and in many cases a life-saving procedure, there are potential dangers involved in its use. Understanding the basic purpose of the therapy and the individual patient's specific problems and needs will assist the nurse in making sound judgments in the supervision and management of TPN therapy. Meticulous, conscientious nursing care of the patient on TPN is essential to the success of the therapeutic regimen.

References

1. Cannon, W. B. *The Wisdom of The Body.* New York: Norton, 1963.
2. Gebbie, K. M., and Lavin, M. A. Classification of Nursing Diagnosis. St. Louis: Mosby, 1975.
3. Helson, H. *Adaptation Level Theory.* New York: Harper & Row, 1964.
4. Mundinger, M. O., and Jauron, G. D. Developing a nursing diagnosis. *Nurs. Outlook* 23:94, 1975.
5. National Research Council. Food and Nutrition Board. *Recommended Dietary Allowances* (8th ed.). Washington D.C.: National Academy of Sciences, 1974.
6. Singer, S. J., and Nicolson, G. L. The fluid mosaic model of the structure of cell membranes. *Science* 175:720, 1972.

Bibliography

Beeson, P., and McDermott, W. (eds.). *Textbook of Medicine* (14th ed.) Philadelphia: Saunders, 1975.

Burke, S. R. *The Composition and Function of Body Fluids.* St. Louis: Mosby, 1972.

Black, D. A. K. *Essentials of Fluid Balance* (4th ed.). Philadelphia: Davis, 1967.

Carozza, V. Ketoacidotic crisis; mechanism and management. *Nursing '73* 3:13, 1973.

Cowan, G., and Scheetz, W. L. (eds.). *Intravenous Hyperalimentation.* Philadelphia: Lea & Febiger, 1972.

Dudrick, S., and Nallinger, J. A. *Intravenous Hyperalimentation.* North Chicago: Abbott Laboratories, 1969.

Ganong, W. F. *Review of Medical Physiology.* Los Altos, Calif.: Lange, 1969.

Goldberger, E. *A Primer of Water, Electrolyte and Acid-Base Syndrome* (4th ed.). Philadelphia: Lea & Febiger, 1970.

Grant, J. A. Patient care in parenteral hyperalimentation. *Nurs. Clin. North Am.* 8:165, 1973.

Guyton, A. C. *Textbook of Medical Physiology* (4th ed.). Philadelphia: Saunders, 1971.

Hardaway, R. M. *Clinical Management of Shock.* Springfield, Ill.: Thomas, 1968.

Heath, J. K. A conceptual basis for assessing body water status. *Nurs. Clin. North Am.* 6:189, 1971.

Lee, C. A., Stroot, V., and Schaper, C. A. Extracellular volume imbalance. *Am. J. Nurs.* 74:888, 1974.

Masoro, E., and Siegel, P. *Acid-Base Regulation: Its Physiology and Pathophysiology.* Philadelphia: Saunders, 1971.

Maxwell, M. H., and Kleeman, C. R. (eds.). *Clinical Disorders of Fluid and Electrolyte Metabolism.* New York: McGraw-Hill, 1972.

Metheny, N. M., and Snively, W. D. *Nurses' Handbook of Fluid Balance* (2nd ed.). Philadelphia: Lippincott, 1974.

Parsa, M., Thornton, B. H., and Ferrer, J. M. Central venous alimentation, *Am. J. Nurs.* 72:2042, 1972.

Pollock, J. H. *A Survey of Surgical Shock.* Springfield, Ill.: Thomas, 1966.

Reed, G. M. Confused about potassium? Here's a clear, concise guide. *Nursing 74* 4:20, 1974.

Rooth, G. *Introduction to Acid-Base and Electrolyte Balance*. New York: Barnes & Noble, 1968.

Shoemaker, W. C., and Walker, W. F. *Fluid-Electrolyte Therapy in Acute Illness*. Chicago: Year Book, 1970.

Singer, S. J., and Nicolson, G. L. The fluid mosaic model of the structure of cell membranes. *Science* 175:720, 1972.

Stroot, V. R., Lee, C. A., and Schaper, A. C. *Fluids and Electrolytes: A Practical Approach*. Philadelphia: Davis, 1974.

Thal, A. P., Brown, E. B., Hermreck, A. S., and Bell, H. H. *Shock: A Physiological Basis for Treatment*. Chicago: Year Book, 1971.

Tilkian, S. M., and Conover, M. H. *Clinical Implications of Laboratory Tests*. St. Louis: Mosby, 1975.

Travenol Laboratories, Inc. *The Fundamentals of Body Water and Electrolytes*. Morton Grove, Ill.: Travenol, 1971.

Vander, A. J. *Renal Physiology*. New York: McGraw-Hill, 1975.

White, P. L., and Nagy, M. E. (eds.). *Total Parenteral Nutrition*. Acton, Mass.: Publishing Sciences Group, 1972.

Williams, S. R. *Nutrition and Diet Therapy*. St. Louis: Mosby, 1969.

Williams, R. H. (ed.). *Textbook of Endocrinology* (5th ed.). Philadelphia: Saunders, 1974.

Yura, H., and Walsh, M. *The Nursing Process* (2nd ed.). New York: Appleton-Century-Crofts, 1973.

part II   Clinical Nursing Care

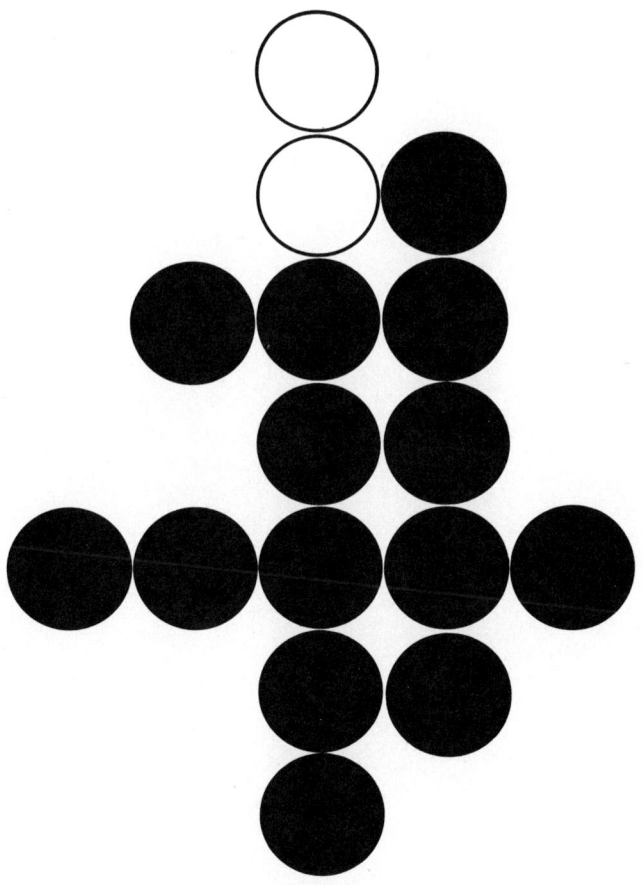

chapter 3
Patients with Respiratory System Dysfunction

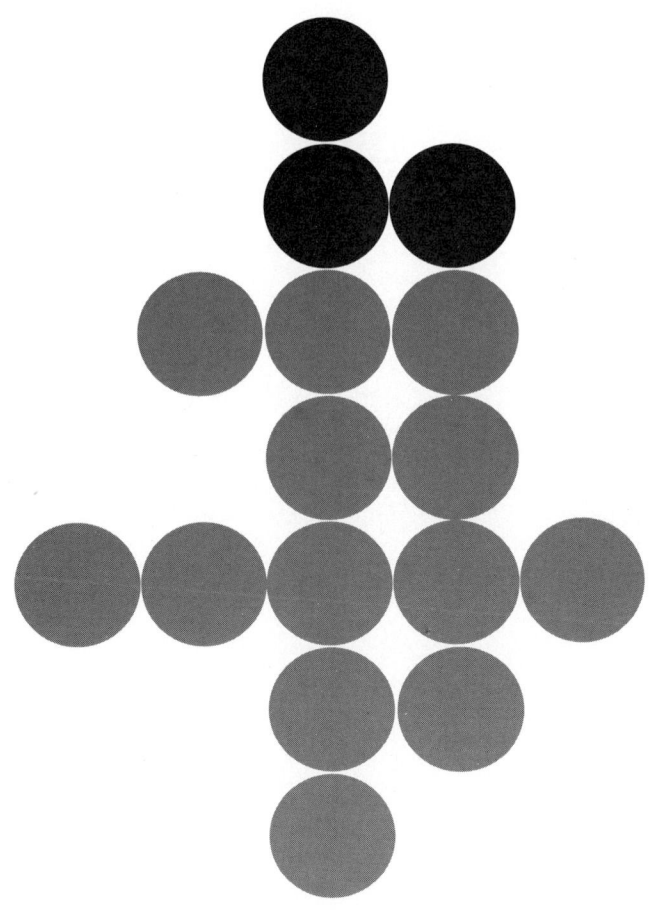

This chapter is concerned with nursing care of patients with dysfunction of the respiratory system. The respiratory system is one of the major body systems that are essential to life. Generally, one is unaware of the functions of this system; they occur easily and naturally without conscious effort in a well-integrated, healthy body. When respiratory functions are either temporarily or permanently impaired, however, as by a cold or chronic bronchitis, one can become acutely aware of the processes involved in respiration and the consequences of ineffective respiratory system functions.

Functions of the Respiratory System

VENTILATION AND PERFUSION

The primary function of the respiratory system is that of providing body cells with oxygen. The body can be thought of as a thermodynamic machine that requires energy for work. Most of this energy is produced by oxidation. All the cells in the body are dependent on oxygen; without sufficient oxygen, the body must restrict its work to the limits imposed by the reduced oxygen supply. If there is not enough oxygen available to the cells to supply the amounts needed for minimal work, the body dies.

In addition to supplying body cells with oxygen, the respiratory system functions to remove the waste products of oxidation, principally carbon dioxide. It is important that sufficient carbon dioxide be removed from the body to maintain the acid-base balance. Retention of carbon dioxide results in acidosis, whereas excessive loss of carbon dioxide results in alkalosis. An appropriate acid-base balance is essential in maintaining an optimal environment for cellular metabolism.

The two functions of the respiratory system, **ventilation** and **perfusion,** have special implications for nursing care. Because oxygen is essential to the body's biochemical processes for the production, storage, and release of energy to support life, the respiratory system functions influence all the major body systems; and because these energy-related functions depend on correct pH of the body's internal environment, ventilation and perfusion of oxygen and carbon dioxide are reciprocal processes influenced by other major body system functions, particularly the nervous, cardiovascular, endocrine, and urinary systems. Many reciprocal mechanisms take place automatically among the major body systems as the body adapts to internal and external changes. Dysfunction of the respiratory system will affect the other body systems, just as dysfunction of any other system affects the respiratory system.

In order to understand these processes better, the nurse must know how ventilation and perfusion take place. **Ventilation** is the passage of gases to and from the lungs; **perfusion** is the passage of gases between the circulatory system and the lungs. The respiratory zone in the lungs is comprised of secondary lobules, also called the acinus. This zone contains about three million alveoli, which line alveolar ducts. During inspiration, the ducts increase in size; during expiration, they decrease in size. The alveoli within the ducts appear as bubbles with thin walls about one micron thick. It is across these alveolar membranes that the transfer of oxygen and carbon dioxide to and from the pulmonary capillaries takes place.

Maintenance of the elasticity of the lung is essential for adequate ventilation and perfusion. Changes in pressure during inspiration and expiration cause movement of air into and out of the lung. The elastic recoil of the alveoli allows the lungs to passively become smaller after being distended during inspiration so that expiration may occur. During inspiration the pressure of air inspired must be greater than airway resistance and the elastic forces that cause collapse of the lung. **Compliance** of the lung defines the change in the volume of air per unit of pressure change in the lung. Compliance is increased when elasticity is decreased. Important in providing for the elasticity of the alveolar walls and in preventing their collapse is the secretion of surfactant, a phospholipid secreted by the alveolar membranes that stabilizes these thin membranes. Surfactant molecules spread apart on inspiration in conjunction with the expansion of the alveoli to raise the surface tension. On expiration, surfactant molecules become concentrated, lowering the surface tension to prevent collapse of the alveolar membranes [9, 11].

Function of the Alveoli

The total area available for gas exchange, which varies among different people, is about 50 to 100 square meters, and the capacity of the alveoli is about 3,000 ml [13]. Gases within the alveoli are constantly in motion so that the maximum amount of alveolar gas comes into contact with the membrane to allow diffusion to take place. In a healthy person the lung has considerable reserve capacity for ventilation and perfusion to meet the increased demands for oxygen during periods such as exercise or increased metabolism. Each alveolus makes up a very small part of this total space, being about 0.3 mm in diameter [17]. The alveoli change size and move in response to the changing pressures. If the pressure outside the alveoli is great enough to overcome the intra-alveolar pressure, atelectasis occurs; the alveoli collapse and cannot be ventilated. This situation is a possible postoperative complication and may also occur in certain types of lung dysfunction.

The alveolar membranes separate the alveoli from the pulmonary capillaries; perfusion of gases takes place through the thin alveolar membranes. The amount of oxygen and carbon dioxide exchanged depends on several factors: the differences between the partial pressures of oxygen and carbon dioxide in the arterial blood and within the alveoli; the total surface area over which diffusion takes place; the rate at which the blood flows through the capillaries; the volume of circulating blood; the hemoglobin content and the number of erythrocytes; and the thickness of the alveolar membranes. Any decrease in the total surface area available, increase in the rate of blood flow, or increase in the thickness of the alveolar membranes can decrease perfusion. Similarly, any change in the normal partial pressures of oxygen and carbon dioxide in either the intra-alveolar space or the blood, as well as a decrease in the number of erythrocytes or hemoglobin levels, will affect the rate of diffusion.

Hemoglobin is the major transporter of oxygen in the blood. When hemoglobin levels are decreased, the amount of oxygen that can be carried also decreases. Iron deficiency anemia is an example of a dysfunction in which the oxygen-carrying capability of the blood is low.

The exchange of oxygen normally differs in various parts of the lung. Ventilation is greater at the apex than in the base of the lung. Blood flow also varies in different parts of the lung, being less at the apex and greatest near the base of the lung, the flow rate being dependent on the pressure gradient between the pulmonary artery and the left atrium. Gas exchange depends on both ventilation and perfusion and the most ideal match of ventilation and perfusion occurs lower in the lung. Knowledge of ventilation-perfusion ratios is therefore important in determining therapy for patients with respiratory dysfunction. The ventilation-perfusion ratio is written as V_A/Q. Factors influencing the V_A/Q ratio are explained in the following discussion.

Dead Space

Air enters the alveoli through the airways, comprised of the main stem bronchus, bronchi, and bronchioles, which together make up the **anatomical dead space.** The capacity of the dead space is about 150 ml [17] and varies depending on the size of the person and his body position. A rule of thumb is that the amount of dead space in milliliters is equal to the person's weight in pounds. **Dead space** is the term used to describe the space containing air that is not involved in perfusion. Another way to refer to dead space is by the term **physiological dead space.** This term is the functional description of all the air in the lung that is not involved in perfusion [12]. Physiological dead space is important clinically because in disease states such as emphysema the physiological dead space increases as ventilation and perfusion are impaired; that is, larger amounts of air in the lungs cannot be perfused and the dead space increases. It is very difficult to measure actual physiological dead space, particularly when some lung tissue is destroyed, because the air that is not involved in perfusion is mixed with the air being exchanged. Normally, ventilation of the alveoli is greater when there are increased volumes of inspired air. In diseases such as emphysema, however, the volume of air is greater, but the overall ventilation and perfusion are impaired.

Pulmonary Circulation

Blood is brought to the pulmonary capillaries through the pulmonary circulation from the right side of the heart. The lungs are perfused with almost all the total cardiac output. Two percent of the cardiac output [9] is shunted from the right to the left side of the heart and does not go through the pulmonary vessels [17]. This process is termed **anatomical shunt.**

Pulmonary arterial pressure, in contrast with systemic arterial pressure, is very low and is maintained at a level just high enough to provide for the perfusion of the entire lung. Arteries and veins in the lung have thin membranes and expand along with the alveolar membranes. Any factor that causes smooth muscle contraction can increase the pulmonary vascular resistance by decreasing the caliber of the extra-alveolar vessels. Any vasoconstrictor, such as norepinephrine, histamine, or serotonin, may cause constriction. Conversely, methoxyphenamine (Orthoxine) and isoproterenol (Isuprel) relax smooth muscle. The result is that these substances have the effect of expanding the caliber of the vessels.

In disease states the pulmonary capillary blood volume can be reduced by any factor that decreases the ability of the right ventricle to deliver blood to the lungs. When there is resistance to blood flow in the pulmonary capillaries, the right ventricle compensates by increasing the pressure of blood flow to the lungs. If this increasing pressure continues for a long enough time and the work of the right side of the heart is sufficiently and consistently increased, right heart hypertrophy may result. This condition is called cor pulmonale. Impaired cardiac function, which reduces the heart's ability to maintain pulmonary pressure, can also impair diffusion. The effect of reduced rates of pulmonary capillary blood flow is increased diffusion in normal states because the time the blood is in contact with the alveolar membrane is longer. The pulmonary blood flow increases in response to the body's need for increased oxygen, as in exercise. The increase in flow rate actually reduces the time the blood cells are in contact with the alveolar walls. However, there is sufficient diffusion reserve in the normal lung to maintain adequate perfusion even with the more rapid blood flow. When ventilation is compromised as a result of lung dysfunction, this reserve may be minimal or nonexistent, so that a person with lung dysfunction may become dyspneic with moderate or mild exertion or even at rest.

Partial Pressure of Oxygen and Carbon Dioxide
During inspiration the volume of the thorax increases through contraction of the diaphragm and elevation of the ribs by the external intercostal muscles. Air enters the expanded thorax and flows downward into the lung and to the terminal bronchioles. Normally the **partial pressure of oxygen** in inspired air is decreased to 90 to 100 mm Hg by the time it reaches the respiratory zone. The **partial pressure of carbon dioxide** in the respiratory zone is normally 40 mm Hg [12]. New ambient air is supplied with each inspiration, but the perfused gases are continually mixing within the alveoli, which are not fully emptied of air on expiration. The partial pressure of oxygen delivered to the pulmonary circulation from the right heart can be varied, depending on the oxygen needs of the body. In a similar fashion, the carbon dioxide levels may also differ, depending on the metabolic processes going on within the cells. Blood returned through the pulmonary artery to the lungs for diffusion normally has an oxygen partial pressure of 40 mm Hg; the partial pressure of carbon dioxide is normally 46 mm Hg. Arterial blood leaving the pulmonary capillary bed for delivery to the left heart has a normal oxygen partial pressure of 90 to 95 mm Hg and a carbon dioxide partial pressure of 40 mm Hg. The purpose of diffusion is the replacement of oxygen and the elimination of carbon dioxide in the blood returning to the lungs from the systemic circulation (Figure 3-1).

The partial pressure of oxygen in ambient air at sea level is approximately 150 mm Hg and is affected by altitude and humidity (it is lower in high altitudes and in wet air). Alveolar hypoxia can be caused by insufficient partial pressure of oxygen in ambient air as well as by changes within the lungs. The partial pressure of oxygen in the alveoli can be affected by any factor that obstructs air flow to the alveoli, preventing delivery of a fresh supply of oxygen. Impaired ventilation can be caused by an obstruction to airflow or by any factor that renders the alveoli less able to take in the inspired air or to remove the air during expiration. The formation of fibrous tissue in the alveolar membranes decreases the elasticity of the membranes and impairs ventilation, just as the secretion or collection of exudate, secretions, or edema fluid prevents the entry of air so that ventilation is impaired.

The amount of oxygen that can be diffused from the alveoli to the capillaries is affected by the partial pressure difference between the two. When the difference in partial pressure is greater, oxygen diffuses more rapidly; when the difference is smaller, oxygen diffuses more slowly. Disease states that impair ventilation of some, but not all, the al-

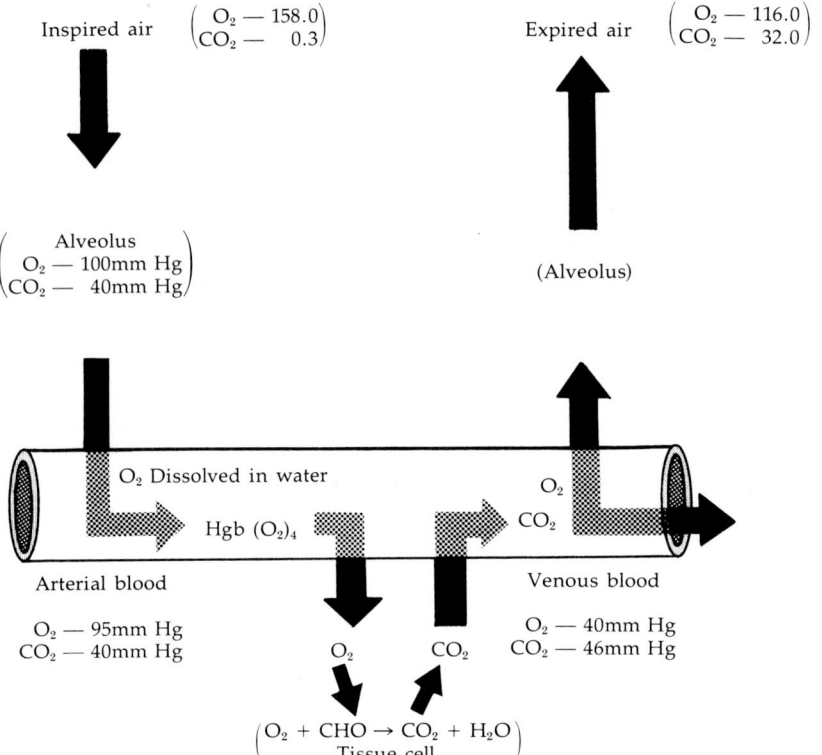

Figure 3-1
Gas exchange during respiration with average normal tensions in inspired air, arterial blood, venous blood, and expired air at sea level. (Adapted from E. Selkurt, *Basic Physiology for the Health Sciences*. Boston: Little, Brown and Company, 1975.)

veoli cause uneven distribution of air in the alveoli throughout the lung. Some alveoli may be well ventilated; others may be ventilated insufficiently or not at all.

Uneven Distribution of Oxygen
Uneven distribution of oxygen contributes to lower blood tensions because of the nature of the **oxygen dissociation curve.** This curve indicates the amount of oxygen that can be taken up by hemoglobin to form oxyhemoglobin. **Oxygen capacity** is the maximum amount of oxygen that is combined with hemoglobin [17]. The oxygen content in arterial blood, as well as the amount of hemoglobin present, determines the oxygen saturation level. (If there is a low oxygen content but hemoglobin levels are normal, the oxygen saturation will be lower. In the same manner, if the oxygen content is adequate but the hemoglobin levels are low, the oxygen saturation of blood will also be lower.) The oxygen saturation may vary from well to poorly ventilated alveoli; however, once the perfusion has taken place, these differences are equalized as blood with high levels of oxygen saturation mixes with blood with lower saturation levels from the impaired areas. This effects a decrease in the total saturation level of oxygen. Shunting of blood from poorly perfused areas in the pulmonary capillaries has the same effect.

Obstruction of ventilation as well as poor perfusion may also cause decreased oxygen saturation. When there is ineffective ventilation of certain alveoli, the oxygen tensions in these alveoli are reduced, followed by contraction of the smooth muscle in the arterioles to force the blood flow to the more effectively ventilated areas of the lung. As long as the poorly ventilated areas are not extensive, oxygen saturation in arterial blood can be maintained. In general there is a tendency for poorly ventilated areas to have decreased perfusion of blood and, similarly, poorly perfused areas tend to have a lower ventilation of air as the body attempts to conserve the energy used in ventilation and perfusion. Vasoconstriction can also occur in the total pulmonary vascular bed when the blood pH is lowered as a result of impaired ventilation. When this occurs, the pulmonary arterial pressure increases, requiring the right heart to work harder in order to deliver more blood to the lungs for oxygenation.

Fluid collection within the alveoli may be relieved via compensatory mechanisms. Fluid in the alveoli prevents the entry of oxygen and therefore must be removed if ventilation is to be improved or if perfusion is to be more effective. The fluid may be removed through two mechanisms. First, the perivascular space has a lower pressure than the alveoli so that the fluid drains into the perivascular spaces through action similar to that of a sump pump; second, the fluid may drain into the lymph system. When these mechanisms are not adequate, therapy is initiated to reduce the accumulation of fluid. If the impairment is caused by edema, measures are taken to reduce the edema. If the fluid accumulation has resulted from an infectious or inflammatory process, therapy is given to expel the secretions.

Carbon Dioxide and Oxygen Diffusion

Carbon dioxide diffuses more readily than oxygen because it is about twenty times more soluble than oxygen. The partial pressure of carbon dioxide in the capillaries (Pa_{CO_2}) is about 46 mm Hg in normal persons, and that in the alveoli is about 40 mm Hg. Even when oxygen diffusion is slow, carbon dioxide diffusion can be maintained at normal levels. The greater linearity of the carbon dioxide dissociation curve allows equalization of pressures, because the exchange of carbon dioxide can occur with a smaller difference between the capillaries and the alveoli.

Transport of Oxygen and Carbon Dioxide

A number of processes occur after oxygen is diffused in the blood. Some oxygen is dissolved in plasma. Most of the oxygen combines rapidly with hemoglobin to form oxyhemoglobin. The amount of oxygen attached to hemoglobin (oxygen saturation) cannot exceed 100 percent. The saturation level in arterial blood is normally about 97.5 percent with a normal pH and temperature; in venous blood it is normally about 75 percent. The normal hemoglobin level in the blood is approximately 16 gm per 100 ml for males and 14 gm per 100 ml for females [17]. The ability of hemoglobin to combine with oxygen is an important factor in oxygen transport, as is the volume of circulating blood. When the hemoglobin is reduced and contains little oxygen, it becomes purple. This low oxygen saturation of hemoglobin results in a dusky, bluish skin color called cyanosis, which is associated with hypoxia of tissues. Significant reduction in the volume of circulating blood can also result in hypoxia, as is seen in hypovolemic shock. Cyanosis is a late-occurring sign and is apparent when the superficial capillaries have at least 5 gm of reduced hemoglobin per 100 ml of blood. Its detection is dependent on the observer's perception of color, the light source, thickness and pigmentation of the patient's skin, and the status of the capillary bed.

Carbon dioxide is carried in the blood in several ways: it can be dissolved as bicarbonate, bound to procarbamino compounds, dissolved in plasma, or combined with hemoglobin. The Henderson-Hasselbalch equation is commonly used to interpret the ratio of carbon dioxide dissolved in bicarbonate to that in carbonic acid in relation to the pH, in order to determine the acid-base balance. Several mechanisms are involved in the formation of bicarbonate and in the release of H^+ ions from carbonic acid. One of these is the presence of the enzyme carbonic anhydrase in the erythrocytes, which increases the formation of carbonic acid. The carbonic acid readily dissociates into hydrogen and bicarbonate. The normal ratio of bicarbonate to carbonic acid is 20:1.

Oxygen-Hemoglobin Dissociation Curve

The Haldane effect is another mechanism in which hemoglobin releases oxygen in response to cellular need and takes up carbon dioxide from the cell in relation to the oxygen saturation levels. The oxygen-hemoglobin dissociation curve shifts to either the right or the left according to cellular needs. For example, when the pH is low and there is increased Pa_{CO_2}, the curve shifts to the right to release oxygen into tissue capillaries. Increased temperature also causes increased release of oxygen. The curve shifts to the left

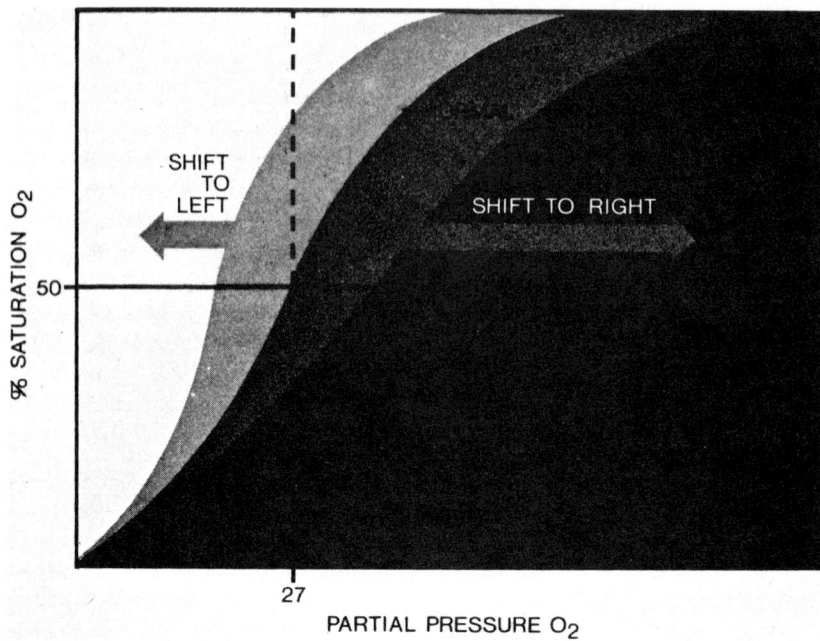

Figure 3-2
Hemoglobin affinity for oxygen. Increased oxygen affinity (shift to the left) means there will be a higher oxygen content at any given Po_2. Decreased oxygen affinity (shift to the right) means there will be a lower oxygen content at any given Po_2. (From B. A. Shapiro, R. A. Harrison, and C. A. Trout, *Clinical Application of Respiratory Care*. Copyright © 1975 by Year Book Medical Publishers, Inc., Chicago. Reproduced by permission.)

when the pH increases, when the Pa_{CO_2} levels are low, or when the temperature is low. A decrease in hydrogen ions causes oxygen to remain in combination with hemoglobin while an increase has the effect of releasing oxygen and taking up carbon dioxide [12, 17] (Fig. 3-2). A small amount of carbon dioxide combines with the blood proteins, particularly globin of hemoglobin, which can readily bind carbon dioxide when arterial oxygen (Pa_{O_2}) levels decrease. The carbon dioxide is then bound to the procarbamino compounds.

Oxygen binding is also influenced by the concentration of 2,3-diphosphoglycerate, a constituent of erythrocytes, which decreases the affinity and therefore the binding power of hemoglobin for oxygen [11]. 2,3-DPG concentrations increase in hypoxia, causing the O_2 dissociation curve to shift to the right [17].

The hydrogen concentration is measured as the blood pH and normally ranges from 7.35 to 7.45 (sometimes expressed as 7.4 ± 0.05). The pH is a negative log of the hydrogen ion, so an increase in hydrogen ions decreases the pH while a decrease in hydrogen ions increases the pH. There are a number of buffer systems in the body that function to maintain the pH within normal ranges for maximum body function. The hemoglobin buffer has just been described; other buffers have been discussed in Chapter 2.

HYPERVENTILATION AND HYPOVENTILATION

One of the important compensatory measures related to the lung's function in maintaining acid-base balance is hyperventilation.

Hyperventilation occurs in response to increased levels of Pa_{CO_2}. The chemoreceptors in the spinal fluid respond to increased levels of carbon dioxide to stimulate hyperventilation. The stimulus to hyperventilate is probably a result of the release of hydrogen ions, which decrease the pH of the cerebrospinal fluid. This decreased pH triggers the stimulus for ventilation so that the person breathes more rapidly and deeply in order to excrete the excess carbon dioxide. As the Pa_{CO_2} levels decrease, bicarbonate is excreted by the kidneys so that the levels of arterial pH return to normal. This process may take several days. People who are born in high altitudes tend to be less responsive to this compensatory mechanism and do not develop it even after moving to lower altitudes. On the other hand, people who live at sea level have this sensitivity and maintain it throughout their lifetimes. It is thought that this sensitivity is an early adaptive process occurring in children and that once formed, it does not change.

Although normally a compensatory mechanism, hyperventilation can be an abnormal state brought about by a feeling of nervousness that compels a person to breathe more rapidly and deeply because he feels that his lungs are not filling adequately. The onset may begin suddenly, at rest or during an emotional stress. Care includes use of a paper bag for rebreathing, exercises to regain normal respiration rate and depth and, in some cases, giving of tranquilizers.

As a normal compensatory mechanism, hyperventilation can be stimulated by hypoventilation, a decrease in the frequency and depth of respiration. This is particularly evident when lung dysfunction causes ventilation-perfusion inequality, thereby reducing the saturation of oxygen in arterial blood. This reduction causes respiratory acidosis in which the Pa_{CO_2} is increased above 40 mm Hg. In respiratory acidosis the ratio of HCO_3^- to Pco_2 is reduced; the result is a decreased pH or increase in hydrogen ion, or acidosis. The kidney responds by conserving HCO_3^- and excreting the excess hydrogen ions. For this reason, a base excess occurs in compensated respiratory acidosis.

Hyperventilation can also result in respiratory alkalosis. In this state there is a decreased Pa_{CO_2} because the increased rate of respiration serves to eliminate the carbon dioxide. There is then an increase in the HCO_3^- to Pco_2 ratio and the pH is elevated; the kidney responds by increasing the excretion of bicarbonate. In compensated respiratory alkalosis, there is a base deficit.

Among the causes of hypoventilation is depression of the respiratory center by narcotics, barbiturates, anesthesia, or impaired function of the respiratory center of the medulla. Obstruction to ventilation in the lung airway and traumatic injury or debilitating diseases that interfere with movement of the chest wall also cause hypoventilation. Hypoventilation causes hypoxemia (decreased oxygen saturation in arterial blood). The administration of oxygen is indicated in severe hypoxemia, whereas hypercapnia is treated directly by improving ventilation, perhaps by the use of a mechanical ventilator. If hypoxemia continues untreated, the resulting severe hypoxia may inhibit oxygen-dependent metabolism; the cells then resort to anaerobic metabolism with formation of lactic acid.

It is important that the nurse learn to interpret the meaning of the levels of Pa_{O_2}, Pa_{CO_2}, and the pH so that therapy and nursing care can be given precisely in relation to maintaining the narrow balances of oxygen, carbon dioxide levels, and pH. These values guide the use of oxygen therapy, mechanical ventilation, and medications and indicate the progress of the patient who is in respiratory insufficiency. In a healthy person, the mechanisms of respiratory control are seemingly automatic; when a patient is in respiratory insufficiency, however, the nurse must recognize how a given therapy will affect the respiratory function as a whole.

CONTROL OF RESPIRATION

The control of respiration is complex, involving a number of different response systems; their integration is not fully understood. It is believed that there is a relationship among all the neurons in the body that influence respiration. Both emotional and chemical stimuli affect the rhythm, rate, and depth of respirations, as does the mechanical movement of the chest wall. Strong emotions such as fear, anxiety, excitement, or anticipation stimulate respirations. The centers for voluntary control of inspiration and expiration are located in the cerebral cortex. Emotions that stimulate the cerebral cortex are thought also to stimulate the respiratory centers located there. Pain also stimulates respiration through reflex activity and perhaps through emotional stimulation as well. The spontaneous pattern of respirations can be altered through conscious effort to either increase or decrease respiratory rate.

Oxygen and carbon dioxide tensions in the

blood and the pH all affect the sensory neurons that automatically control respiration through chemical means. The sensory neurons are located in centers in the pons and medulla and in the chest wall, aorta, and carotids. In the pons, the apneustic and pneumotaxic centers respond to carbon dioxide levels. The cells of the pneumotaxic center inhibit inspiration while those of the apneustic center prolong and deepen inspirations. The medulla contains both inspiratory and expiratory centers, which can affect and be affected by the centers in the pons. The Pa_{CO_2} level is a very important stimulus to the medullary centers. Chemoreceptors in the medulla respond to changes in the pH of the cerebrospinal fluid (CSF); as the pH decreases (becomes more acid) respirations increase. Carbon dioxide readily diffuses into the CSF, causing liberation of H^+ ions.

The medulla receives impulses from the peripheral receptors (aortic bodies) through the vagus nerve and from the carotid bodies through the glossopharyngeal nerve. There are two types of receptors in the aortic and carotid bodies: the baroreceptors, which send inhibitory impulses, and the chemoreceptors, which send excitatory impulses. Peripheral chemoreceptor cells in the carotid bodies increase both the frequency and depth of respirations in hypoxic states when the oxygen tension is low; those in the aorta also increase the frequency of respirations. In the carotid bodies, increased levels of Pa_{CO_2}, decreased levels of Pa_{O_2}, and increased hydrogen ions increase the afferent impulses for stimulating ventilation. Decreased Pa_{O_2} levels stimulate ventilation when the body becomes sensitized to consistently increased levels of Pa_{CO_2}, as in chronic hypercapnia. When CO_2 retention is chronic, the medulla becomes refractory to the CO_2 stimulus. Although hypoxemia initially depresses respiration, an effect of prolonged hypoxemia is the development of cerebral acidosis, which eventually stimulates respiration. It is important to remember this when a patient with chronic hypoxemia is treated with oxygen therapy; giving increased oxygen will interfere with the stimulation of respiration that is triggered by low oxygen levels. The respiratory centers cannot immediately adapt to such changes by setting up new stimulation mechanisms; the result is further depression of respiration, which may cause death if the patient is in severe respiratory insufficiency.

A number of reflexes throughout the body can affect the rate of respiration, including reflexes in the joints and periarticular surfaces that stimulate respiration during muscular exercise. More important are the inflation and stretch reflexes from the chest wall, called the Hering-Breuer reflexes, which interact with the central nervous system (CNS) control of respiration. These inflation and stretch reflexes can control the frequency of respiration when CNS control is impaired, but usually they are integrated with the CNS control. Generally inflation of the lungs inhibits inspiration and collapse of the lungs stimulates respiration. The vagus nerve exerts an inhibitory effect on the Hering-Breuer reflex. In addition, the vagus nerve activates important protective reflexes from the trachea and the bronchi, such as vasoconstriction of the bronchi and production of cough when irritating substances are inhaled, so that airway resistance is increased.

Spindle cells in the diaphragm and the intercostal muscles are sensitive to the elongation of the muscles so that when muscle contraction is unopposed there is little increase in tension. The alpha motor neurons are excited when there is resistance to muscle contraction through such factors as airway resistance; as tension in the spindle cells increases, the muscles contract further. The gamma motor neurons stabilize ventilation when there is a reduction in the compliance of the lung, and it is thought that these neurons are responsible for the feeling of breathlessness known as dyspnea.

A number of reflexes throughout the body affect ventilation. A decreased blood pressure (as in hemorrhage) can stimulate reflex hyperventilation through stimulation of the carotid and aortic sinuses. Changes in temperature also affect respiration; hypothermia depresses the respiratory centers and decreases oxygen consumption. Ventilation is decreased in relation to temperature decreases and to the decreased work of metabolism. The opposite effect occurs with hyperthermia. Although the mechanisms by which ventilation is affected by temperature changes or by changes in blood pressure or in reflexes from joints during exercise are not understood, it is thought that the primary control is determined by the level of hydrogen ions present in the blood; therefore the acid-base balance is significant in the control of respiration.

The mechanisms that increase or decrease ventilation are normally dependent on effectively functioning lung tissue and on the integrity of the chest wall. When a decreased level of oxygen tension in the blood results from disease processes that alter lung tissue or the chest wall, the neuronal control of respiration cannot improve lung ventilation beyond the altered lung tissue's capacity to respond. The compensatory mechanisms for maintaining acid-base balance can be effective for some time after hypoxemia has been established, but even these mechanisms are ineffective if other components of the system are impaired.

Hypoxemia **Hypoxemia** refers to a low arterial oxygen tension; **hypoxia** refers to the inadequate oxygen tensions in the tissues [12]. As stated previously, any factor that decreases the diffusion of gases through the alveolar membrane will decrease the oxygen tension or partial pressure of oxygen. Increased levels of Pa_{CO_2} (hypercapnia or carbon dioxide retention) inevitably occur in hypoxemia as a result of hypoventilation. In long-standing hypoxia, administration of oxygen may increase the Pa_{O_2}, but it may also increase the carbon dioxide tension in the arterial blood. This is related to the dependency of the respiratory drive on the carotid and aortic chemoreceptor stimulation from the low Pa_{O_2}. Carbon dioxide narcosis then complicates the progress of patients with respiratory insufficiency.

Carbon dioxide narcosis The signs and symptoms of carbon dioxide narcosis range from headache and drowsiness to deep coma and increased intracranial pressure. Inability to concentrate, asterixis (flapping tremor), and vascular collapse causing flushed skin with sweating and tachycardia are predominant. Patients with carbon dioxide narcosis cannot tolerate the depression of respiration that occurs when oxygen is given in quantities high enough to diminish the mechanism of hypoxemia as the stimulus to respiration. The goal of therapy is then to give low concentrations of oxygen that are sufficient to increase the oxygen available to the tissues while also supporting the respiratory stimulus so that carbon dioxide can be expired.

The Work of Breathing
Many lung diseases affect the work of breathing and therefore increase the body's consumption of oxygen. The work of breathing is related to the amount of pressure required to overcome the elastic recoil of the lungs and the resistance to airflow in the airway so that air can be inspired and expired. Lung diseases that diminish that elastic recoil and cause obstruction of the airway therefore require additional work. Diseases that obstruct airflow reduce the vital capacity of the lungs, as do those diseases that restrict movement of the chest, inhibiting expansion.

Compliance Any factor that changes the compliance of the lung (the volume change per unit of pressure) increases the work of breathing. Extra work is required to move air out of the lungs when compliance is increased, with the result that the normally passive expiration becomes active. In this situation, the patient has frequent shallow breaths and increased physiological dead space. Decreased lung compliance as seen in atelectasis also increases the work of breathing. In this instance the hyperventilation occurs in response to hypoxemia.

Metabolic rate Some diseases affect the lung indirectly through their effects in increasing the metabolic rate or by causing changes in metabolism resulting in acid-base imbalances. In these diseases, the healthy lung can compensate for the changes to maintain adequate oxygenation of tissues and acid-base balance. If there is lung dysfunction present along with any of these other diseases, the patient's status may be seriously compromised. In any event, it is important to discover and treat the underlying cause of the dysfunction as early as possible.

Systemic diseases A number of diseases impair lung function through their effect on lung tissues or respiratory control mechanisms. Examples are the collagen diseases, associated with changes in connective tissue in various body locations, including in the lung, and neurologic and orthopedic dysfunction involving either the central nervous system (consequently affecting the respiratory centers) or the mechanical function of the lung (by decreasing muscle or nerve activity or impairing bone structure). In some instances the secondary lung dysfunction may be the cause of death.

The respiratory system, then, can be influenced by other body systems as well as exerting an influence on all body tissues. The provision of oxygen to the body cells and the maintenance of the body's acid-base balance are necessary functions for supporting life. When these energy-related functions cannot effectively meet the body's requirements for any reason, the patient is either in acid-base imbalance or respiratory insufficiency or both. These situations must be corrected by ascertaining the basic cause of the dysfunction and providing adequate treatment and nursing care. Careful assessment of the patient's status is necessary to obtain a data base for treatment and nursing care, and the care must be given precisely so that the patient's body reserves can be supported as much as possible while the cause of the dysfunction is being eliminated or allayed.

Assessment of the Patient's Condition

HISTORY

Because the causes of lung dysfunction are varied and because many environmental factors influence its occurrence, an important initial part of the nurse's assessment is that of obtaining a history from the patient. The history must be detailed enough to give the nurse important clues about what types of problems the patient perceives as well as the types of respiratory dysfunction that might be present in relation to risk factors.

Among the points to be covered in the initial assessment interview or history are the patient's work patterns, place of employment, and significant exposure to pollutants in either his home or work environment. The nurse should obtain a careful description of signs and symptoms of respiratory impairment (if present), including the time of onset, progression, and the relation of the occurrence of signs and symptoms to activity of various forms. These factors are significant in determining the degree of probable compensation in respiratory function that may have taken place since the onset of the disease or impairment. Methods the patient uses for intervention are also important in this description. Other pertinent points in the patient's history include the occurrence of infectious or inflammatory diseases, other diseases such as frequent colds, sinus problems, pneumonia, or tuberculosis, and any previous surgery, particularly involving the respiratory system.

As described in Chapter 1, the history or assessment interview should include a general overview of the patient's life status and life-style, in addition to a description of his previous medical history and perceptions of his present problems.

ASSESSMENT TECHNIQUES

Nursing care for patients with respiratory system dysfunction is challenging because the respiratory system influences the quality of functioning of the entire body. All the nurse's assessment skills are used when caring for these patients. Observation, measurement, examination, interpretation of laboratory and lung function tests and of x-rays, and careful documentation of the patient's progress throughout the duration of his illness are required. In the following pages, assessment techniques are described in detail along with the pertinent physiology. By understanding the relation of the assessment factors to physiology, the nurse can better interpret the importance of the assessment for both diagnosis and nursing care. Certain diseases are mentioned when appropriate with specific assessment techniques; these diseases are explained in more detail in later sections of this chapter, and reference can again be made to the assessment techniques as each disease is studied.

To a limited extent the effectiveness of respiratory system functions can be observed without special equipment or testing. It is possible, for example, to detect skin color, movement of the chest on inspiration and expiration, and the ease or difficulty the patient may be experiencing in breathing. The rate of respirations can be calculated. Observation of finger clubbing is also significant. Finger clubbing, usually representative of arteriovenous shunting, can be a diagnostic sign of respiratory disease; it is caused by formation of new bone along the finger phalanges. Finger clubbing is associated with pulmonary and suppurative lesions. In many cases it has been found that the primary source of the infectious process causing these lesions is an infection in the teeth or gums or a lung abscess.

Some aspects of the respiratory system function cannot be observed; they are felt only by the person with impaired respiratory function. Dyspnea is an example of a symptom that is experienced as a sensation of tightness in the chest or of smothering, which is not always obvious to an observer. Pain is another symptom a patient may experience but is not always detected by an observer. Skillful interviewing is necessary to obtain a history of the patient's perception of these symptoms, including their occurrence and duration and the conditions that cause them.

Certain other aspects of respiratory function can be assessed only by laboratory tests, chemical analysis, x-rays, and other special examination techniques such as bronchoscopy. The level of oxygen in arterial blood can be precisely determined only from a carefully handled blood specimen. The exact pathologic tissue changes that take place in certain areas of the lung can be seen with a bronchoscope within the limitations of visibility; they may be estimated from chest x-rays in certain diseases. Fractional concentrations of gases, oxygen, and carbon dioxide can be measured for inspired and expired air.

The respiratory system utilizes mechanical, chemical, and physical processes for the inspiration of ambient air, gas exchange in the alveoli, and the expiration of gas containing waste products. The processes through which the lungs are ventilated are primarily mechanical and physical in nature. Mechanical processes are those that change the size of the thorax, thereby producing changes within the lungs for inspiration and expiration of air. The physical properties of gases, such as the pressure gradients, the size of the lumen of the airway, the temperature of gases, and the volume and moisture content of gases, are also important determinations of lung ventilation.

EXAMINATION OF THE CHEST

Observation of Chest Movement

Changes in the size of the lungs result from the active contraction of the external intercostal muscles (elevating the ribs) and of the diaphragm (causing it to flatten); these actions expand the thorax, increasing thoracic volume, and stabilizing the chest. Passive relaxation of the intercostal muscles and diaphragm reduces the size of the thoracic volume. The volume of the right lung with its three lobes is greater than the volume of the left lung, which has two lobes. The elasticity of the lung tissue and the surface tension of the fluid lining the alveoli allow for distention and relaxation of lung tissue as the volume of the thorax increases and decreases.

During heavy exercise, the accessory muscles of respiration are normally used. The scalene muscle elevates the first and second ribs for inspiration, the sternomastoid muscles elevate the sternum for inspiration, and the pectoralis major muscle lifts the ribs and the sternum to expand the thorax in inhalation. Use of the accessory muscles at rest or during only moderate exercise indicates that there is increased work for breathing and gives the nurse a clue to the presence of respiratory dysfunction.

As mentioned previously, expiration is normally a passive process in which the intrapulmonic pressure increases, causing air to flow outward, and the thorax decreases in size. The abdominal muscles are under stress when expiration must be forced. As the nurse observes respiration, it is important to look either for retraction of the intercostal spaces or for bulging. Obstruction of the airways causes retraction on inspiration, while bulging is often seen in the presence of pleural effusion or in emphysema. The symmetry of the chest should also be noted; asymmetry of the chest wall may result from musculoskeletal dysfunction or from cardiac disease and certain types of respiratory dysfunction. The slope of the ribs should be noted. Normally the ribs are curved, but in chronic obstructive diseases such as emphysema they may be fixed in a more rigid, linear position.

Movement of the chest should be observed in relation to the rate and rhythm of respirations (16 to 20 respirations per minute is the normal adult rate) and the ratio of respirations to the pulse (the normal ratio is 1 : 4). The chest normally moves synchronously, and a healthy person may be able to expand his chest as much as four inches when voluntarily taking a deep breath. The ratio of inspiration to expiration should be fairly equal. Prolonged expiration is an indication that obstructive lung disease is present. In restrictive pulmonary disease, the inspirations are shallow and more frequent than normal. Short, panting breaths on inspiration may be an indication of hypoxia.

In addition to observing chest movement, the nurse can also examine the chest through inspection, palpation, percussion, and auscultation. When examining the chest, it is important to establish landmarks. Some of the commonly used landmarks are shown in Figure 3-3.

Inspection and Palpation

Inspection and palpation of the chest are carried out for a closer examination of the presence of any areas of tenderness or masses that can be observed or felt. A light pressure is used in palpation. Usually the examiner establishes a sequence beginning at one point and carefully examines the anterior, lateral, and posterior aspects of the chest bilaterally. The skin should be observed for lesions. The patient is asked to remain in a sitting position during this part of the examination; this position allows for observation of symmetry on both sides of the chest.

Percussion

Percussion of the chest involves listening to the sounds produced by gently striking the chest wall. Two methods may be used for percussion. In the first, the examiner strikes the body surface with the tips of the fingers, to percuss the chest wall directly. The second method involves placing the index or middle finger of one hand on the chest wall and striking the stationary finger with the middle finger of the other hand, close to the tip of the examining finger. The stationary finger is called the pleximeter and the striking finger is called the plexor.

Five types of sounds are usually described: flat, dull, tympanic, resonant, and hyperresonant. A **flat** sound is heard when a solid area is percussed; it implies the presence of pleural effusion or mass. **Dull** sounds are heard when there is air or fluid in the lung. The **tympanic** sound is usually musical with a long duration and is heard when air is present; tympany is normally heard only in the areas above the stomach and bowel and below the left hemidiaphragm. **Resonant** sounds are normal and are usually of long duration. **Hyperresonant** sounds occur when there is free air in the thoracic cavity.

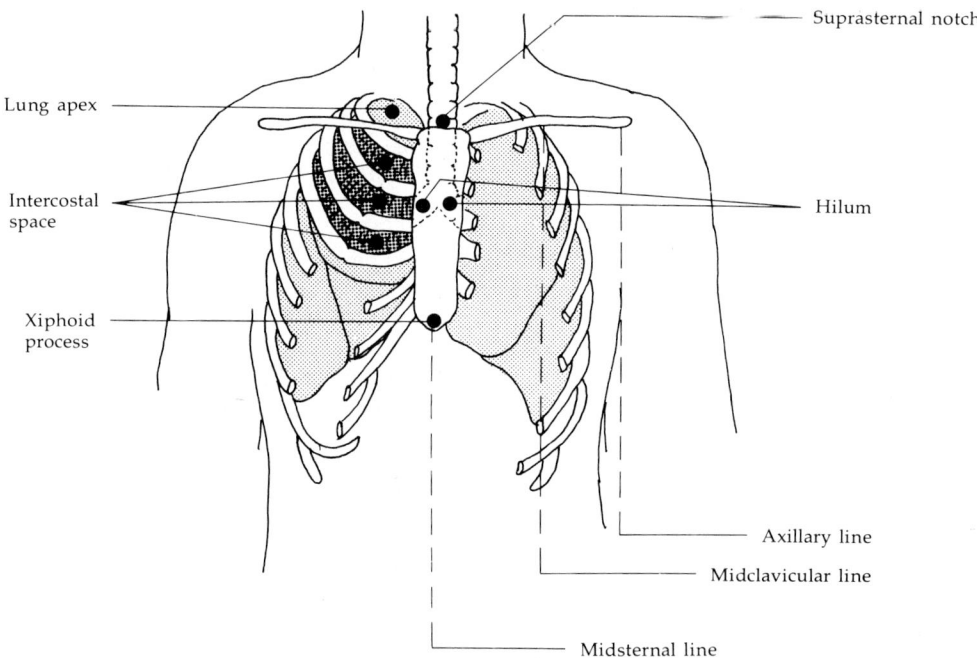

Figure 3-3
Structural landmarks for examination of the chest.

The quality of percussed sounds is described in relation to their intensity, pitch, and duration. The **intensity** is related to the loudness or amplitude and the **pitch** to the number of vibrations per second; the **duration** is the length of time the sound is heard. The excursion of the diaphragm can be percussed by first asking the patient to hold his breath following forced inspiration and then tapping downward to determine where the resonant sounds end at the margin of the diaphragm. This procedure is repeated following a forced expiration. As with palpation and inspection, percussion should be conducted in a sequential fashion so that changes in any portion of the thoracic cavity can be noted (Fig. 3-4).

Auscultation

Auscultation with a stethoscope is another important part of the chest examination. Breath sounds have characteristic changes that are related to certain disease processes. The patient is asked to take deep breaths through his mouth while the examiner listens and compares the sounds from one side of the chest to another. **Vesicular** breath sounds are normally heard over most of the lungs because of the air in the alveoli; they are soft and of low pitch, heard best on inspiration since they are almost inaudible on expiration. **Bronchovesicular** breath sounds are heard over the area of the trachea and bronchi and in the posterior right upper chest over the right main stem bronchus. They are heard better when the patient is thin and when the trachea and bronchi are close to the surface. These sounds are louder and higher pitched than vesicular sounds. When bronchovesicular breath sounds are heard in other parts of the chest, they indicate consolidation of the lungs.

Tubular (also called bronchial) breath sounds are heard when there is obstruction of flow to the alveoli so that the air remains in the larger airways. These sounds are high pitched with a hollow quality and may be accompanied by a whistling sound. **Cavernous** sounds are lower in pitch with a deep, hollow quality and indicate an abnormal cav-

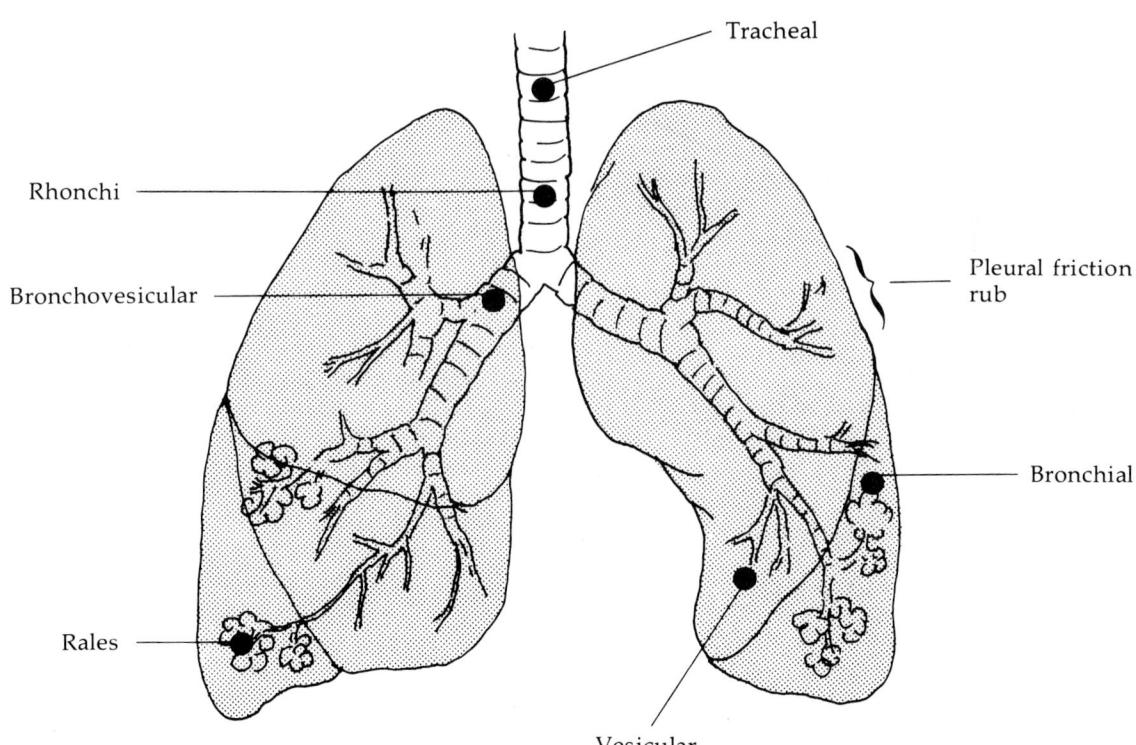

Figure 3-4
Breath sounds heard on auscultation.

ity or pneumothorax space. **Decreased** or **absent** breath sounds are indicative of a local obstruction to the passage of air in the alveoli.

Voice sounds can be heard by placing the stethoscope on the chest wall as the patient speaks. Normally voice sounds are not clearly heard through the stethoscope. The sound intensity of the voice decreases in the presence of fluid and increases over consolidated areas.

Adventitious sounds are rales, wheezes and rhonchi, and pleural friction rub that are superimposed on the breath sounds. They are considered abnormal sounds. **Rales** are described as fine, medium, or coarse. Fine rales are sometimes called crepitation and arise from the alveoli. Medium rales are heard over the bronchioles and have a rattling sound at midinspiration. Coarse, loud, clicking rales are heard over the bronchi and at the beginning of inspiration. Rales are produced when air flows through fluid in the alveoli and are heard best on inspiration. If rales are heard the patient is asked to cough, and the nurse checks to determine if the cough has cleared the rales.

Rhonchi and **wheezes** (mild rhonchi) are continuous musical sounds that can be heard on both inspiration and expiration. They differ in that rales tend to be constant and reproducible while rhonchi tend to vary with position changes, coughing, or drainage of respiratory passages. Rhonchi are formed when air passes through an obstruction in the bronchus or bronchioles. The obstruction can be caused by secretions, bronchospasms, or edema, all of which narrow the lumen of the bronchus and bronchioles. Rhonchi can be described as sibilant (high-pitched) sounds, which are generally heard over the bronchial branches, or sonorous (low-pitched) sounds heard over the trachea.

A **pleural friction rub** can be heard if the visceral or parietal pleura is inflamed. The sound is one of abrasive surfaces rubbing together; it occurs when there is an insufficient film of moisture between the pleurae. A pericardial friction rub has a similar sound and can be heard when the patient holds his breath.

The nurse can also make a rough determination of the presence of an airway obstruction by placing the stethoscope on the scapular region and asking the patient to breathe in and out. Normally the sound of expiratory breathing stops in three seconds. If it is prolonged, the nurse can assume that the patient might have an airway obstruction, and lung function tests should be obtained. During this part of the examination, the nurse also observes the excursion of the chest wall and notes any abnormalities or lack of symmetry.

Certain sounds can be heard without the aid of a stethoscope; these include wheezing and stridor. **Wheezing** is heard in patients who have an airway obstruction as the air passes through the narrowed lumen of the airway. This sound is frequently heard in either bronchitis or asthma and is related to the presence of secretions or bronchospasm. **Stridor** is actually a high-pitched wheeze produced in the trachea or larynx on inspiration when there is an obstruction.

SIGNIFICANT SIGNS AND SYMPTOMS

Pain

Another essential part of the nurse's examination is that of noting the presence of pain, cough, or sputum. Pleuritic, intercostal, and generalized thoracic pain are different types of chest pain that may occur as a result of respiratory dysfunction. **Pleuritic pain** is a catching, transient pain, produced when the thorax is moved. It is usually unilateral and is accentuated when the patient breathes deeply. There is often tenderness in the area of the pleuritic pain and the pain may be described as a stitch or catch in the side.

Intercostal pain is produced when coughing or straining causes compression of the intercostal nerves. It may be caused by herpes zoster or by fibrositis of the intercostal muscles. **Generalized thoracic pain** may be caused by cardiac disease, an aortic aneurysm, or a hiatus hernia. It is sometimes difficult to differentiate the exact cause, since the pain of each is similar. The pain of a hiatus hernia is most often a deep, aching pain. Sometimes the pain may be caused by costal chondritis, an inflammatory condition that causes pain similar to the typical cardiac pain; the difference is that costal chondritis causes a pain that tends to be localized in the area of the second and third intercostal spaces.

Cough

The presence or absence of cough is also diagnostic in the nurse's assessment of respiratory dysfunction. Cough can be described in different ways: chronic, paroxysmal, dry, or productive. A **chronic** cough is one that is experienced consistently in relation to irritation of the airway. Cigarette smoking is the most common cause of chronic cough; inhalation of polluted air, chronic upper respiratory infections, and sinus infections and allergies can also produce a chronic cough. A **paroxysmal** cough is one that occurs acutely and is difficult to stop. This type of cough is commonly observed in patients with asthma or chronic bronchitis and is often accompanied by wheezing respirations. A cough can be **dry,** without the production of sputum, or it can be **productive,** with expectoration of varying amounts of sputum. Since a cough is a normal protective mechanism for removing secretions from the airway, it is important to ascertain how much and what type of sputum the patient expectorates in relation to the cough.

Sputum

Sputum is a product composed primarily of mucus, which dilutes irritants that have come into contact with the mucosa of the air passages. The irritants are diluted by the mucus and can then be more easily expectorated. Therefore, sputum is actually excess mucus that forms in the presence of an infection or with irritation of the mucosa of the airways.

The nurse should, in addition to noting the effectiveness of coughing for removal of sputum, note the consistency, amount, and color of sputum expectorated with the cough. Because of the contact the nurse has with hospitalized patients, notations of sputum can be precise in terms of changes in cough patterns and sputum expectoration at different times of the day or night, and in terms of the relation of the occurrence of cough to events such as exercise or other stresses. Changes in the character and consistency of sputum should also be noted. When the nurse sees a patient periodically for short contacts, as in weekly clinic or home visits, notation of changes in cough and sputum production from visit to visit is important in assessing the patient's response to treatment or to other life factors.

Sputum is a product of many different disease processes; its character may vary with different types of pathology. Generally, it is described as mucoid, purulent, mucopurulent, rusty, black, or blood tinged. **Mucoid** sputum is clear and white, while **purulent** sputum may be yellow or greenish because of the presence of mucus and pus. **Mucopurulent** merely means that there is more mucus than pus in the sputum. **Rusty** sputum derives its color from exudate containing blood from capillary destruction. **Blood-tinged** mucus may occur in certain diseases such as bronchiectasis, tuberculosis, and pulmonary infarction or with carcinoma, all of which are discussed in detail in subsequent sections of this chapter. The presence of blood in mucus always indicates a disease process that should be further investigated by a physician without delay. In bronchiectasis, blood-tinged mucus may not be significant, particularly if it occurs infrequently. However, the blood in mucus may be the presenting sign of either tuberculosis or carcinoma. The term **hemoptysis** refers to the expectoration of blood, which may be mixed with mucus or may appear as gross blood and may arise from the nasopharynx or esophagus or from the airways of the lungs (it is important to discover the source in order to determine the meaning of the hemoptysis).

Sputum may also be examined for the presence of tumor cells or organisms that cause infection. Exfoliative cytology is used in the study of sputum when neoplasms of the lung are suspected. If an infectious process is present or suspected, sputum culture and sensitivity studies are done to determine the causative organism and the corresponding antibiotic(s) to which the organism is susceptible. Serum complement fixation tests may be done in order to determine the presence of viruses in sputum.

DIAGNOSTIC TESTING

Skin Tests

Skin tests may be performed to determine the presence of antibodies for some lung diseases; they are often done in association with sputum tests. Specific antigens are injected for tuberculosis, histoplasmosis, and several other organisms such as fungus. Disorders caused by these antigens are discussed in greater detail later in this chapter.

Special Diagnostic Tests

Examination of the respiratory system is supported by a number of additional diagnostic tests, including x-rays, fluoroscopy, tomography, pulmonary radiophotoscanning, pulmonary angiography, bronchoscopy, mediastinoscopy, and biopsy (which may be done in conjunction with bronchoscopy or mediastinoscopy). The nurse should understand how these tests are performed so that the patient can be prepared through teaching. Knowing what is expected is a significant factor in allaying anxiety, particularly in the patient with respiratory dysfunction, who does not have reserve energy because of oxygen deficit. In addition, the nurse should provide supportive care during and after the examination as well as observe for complications afterward.

Chest x-rays are commonly done on a routine basis for screening purposes. The chest x-ray shows the size of the lungs, heart, and diaphragm and the structure of the rib cage. Abnormalities such as masses, nodules, cysts, and areas of cavitation, filtration, or consolidation are seen on a chest x-ray. If an abnormality is suspected, additional and more specific diagnostic tests such as skin testing or sputum examination are performed; the x-ray serves as a guide to the type of additional testing indicated. Comparison of previous and current x-rays is useful in determining whether any changes have occurred and gives clues to the development of pathology. Most frequently a posteroanterior view is taken. Lateral or oblique views may be taken from either the right or left side.

Many times a screening x-ray is taken with a small x-ray machine. If pathologic changes are suspected via this smaller x-ray, a larger plate is taken with more sensitive radiographic equipment. Patients who are asked to have a repeat x-ray may be very fearful, thinking that their initial x-ray has revealed serious disease. It is important for the nurse to know that the smaller x-rays often have shadows that make reading it difficult; the larger x-ray will not be obscured by these smaller shadows and often turns out to be normal. However, there is always a possibility that the larger x-ray will reveal an abnormality, so it is important that the patient have the repeat x-ray without delay. The nurse can facilitate matters by making a definite appointment for the follow-up x-ray.

Fluoroscopy allows for multiple views of the lungs and can be used to diagnose the location of a tumor or lesion more precisely than with x-rays. Chest movements, including expansion and contraction of the lungs and the diaphragm, can be observed.

Tomography, or planigraphy, is a sequential filming of the lungs in planes at different depths. It is used diagnostically to examine lesions, hilar adenopathy, and the structures of the trachea and bronchi more closely.

Pulmonary **radiophotoscanning,** or lung scan, provides an image of the lungs from which data on ventilation and blood flow can be obtained. It is performed by injecting a radiosensitive substance. This test is useful for diagnosing embolisms and detecting decrease of or interference with blood flow, as well as for locating areas with decreased blood flow such as nonvascular masses.

Pulmonary **angiography** is a diagnostic test utilizing the injection of radiopaque materials into the veins; it provides for visualization of the systemic veins and pulmonary artery and is done primarily for the purpose of detecting emboli. Congenital or acquired lesions of the pulmonary artery can also be detected with pulmonary angiography.

Bronchoscopy utilizes a bronchoscope with a lighted mirror lens to observe the walls of the trachea, the main stem bronchus, and the major subdivisions of the bronchial tubes. Lesions such as carcinoma or benign lesions can be diagnosed by bronchoscopy. Either a rigid or a flexible fiberoptic bronchoscope may be used. The fiberoptic bronchoscope has fiberoptic bundles to transmit light and a lens connected to an external eyepiece which in turn can be connected to photographic equipment. The flexible fiberoptic bronchoscope is much smaller than the rigid bronchoscope and allows for increased visualization of the airways deeper in the lung. It can be inserted through the mouth or nose; however, when the patient's condition is such that complications are expected, the flexible fiberoptic bronchoscope can be inserted through an endotracheal tube. These methods provide for better control of the patient's airway if respiratory distress develops during the examination. Secretions can be removed more easily, and if hemorrhage occurs during the procedure, therapy can be instituted quickly. Insertion of the endotracheal tube or the rigid bronchoscope generally requires specific preparation of the patient with premedication and local anesthesia. In some instances general anesthesia is used according to the patient's condition and the physician's preference.

Both the rigid and flexible bronchoscopes can be used to obtain a biopsy, a bronchial brushing, or a bronchial washing. Biopsy forceps can be inserted through the bronchoscope and passed to the visualized area of the lung from which the biopsy is taken. In bronchial brushing, a small disposable brush is used to brush the areas of suspected abnormal cell growth to obtain cells for histologic examination. Some of the brushes have a small shield that prevents the cells from being dislodged as the brush is removed.

Bronchial washing is a technique in which saline irrigations followed by aspiration through the bronchoscope are used to collect specimens for histologic examination. Bacterial studies can also be done on the specimen. The advantage in collecting specimens by this method is that contamination by particles from the trachea, larynx, pharynx, or mouth is prevented because the specimen comes directly from the bronchus.

The patient who is scheduled for bronchoscopy should know what to expect during and after the examination. The nurse must explain the procedure to the patient and must make certain that he or she has signed a permission form prior to the examination. Bronchoscopy performed with a rigid scope is usually performed in an operating room or a special examining room containing equipment that might be needed if the patient develops respiratory distress. The patient is usually positioned on his back with his head hyperextended. Either general anesthesia or a local anesthetic is used; a sedative is given prior to the examination in either case. The smaller, more flexible fiberscope is sometimes used in examining rooms or in the patient's hospital room. Sedatives are often given prior to the examination, and the patient's position may vary from sitting to reclining, depending on the preference of the examiner. Some patients cannot tolerate the procedure without premedication.

Prior to bronchoscopy, the nurse discontinues postural drainage and medications that may affect the vessels or musculature of the air passages. It is important that the physician view the area without interference in order to make as correct a diagnosis as possible. Exact procedures for preexamination measures vary with the patient's condition, the physician's preference, and institutional policy, but generally food is restricted prior to the examination. If a general anesthetic is used, the patient is prepared as for surgery. The usual postoperative care, including recovery room measures, is followed after the examination, with particular attention to vital signs and respiratory status. The person cannot be given food or fluids until the gag reflex returns.

Depending on the patient's condition, the symptoms of existing respiratory disease may be aggravated by the procedure. Dyspnea and wheezing may be stimulated by the emotional stress of the examination or by irritation of lung tissue. Hemoptysis may occur because of irritation to fragile tissue or from obtaining a specimen. Bleeding is a serious complication that may occur during or after the examination. It is important that the nurse be prepared in the event of an emergency. The patient with compromised respiratory function may need specialized postbronchoscopy care in relation to his degree of respiratory insufficiency, as well as specialized care when he is in transit to and from the examining room.

A bronchogram is the insertion of radiopaque material into the tracheobronchial tree during bronchoscopy. The linings of the airway are coated with radiopaque material so that they can be seen on x-ray. This procedure is used to diagnose bronchiectasis or to ascertain the presence of airway obstruction from other causes, such as distortion or malformation of the airways.

Mediastinoscopy is a diagnostic test in which a mediastinoscope is inserted through an incision made between the laryngeal prominence and the sternum. The anterior and lateral sides of the external trachea are palpated prior to insertion of the scope. This procedure requires either general or local anesthesia. Mediastinoscopy allows for visualization and biopsy of lymph nodes, including the inferior tracheobronchial, the superior tracheobronchial, and the paratracheal nodes. Electrocoagulation is used to control bleeding.

Mediastinoscopy is primarily used to detect metastasis of carcinoma of the lung or related structures to the lymph nodes. Its value is in determining the most appropriate method of treatment. For example, if metastasis has not occurred, surgical intervention may be selected as the method of treatment, whereas palliative treatment might be selected if metastasis has occurred. Detection of sarcoidosis and tuberculosis can also be accomplished with mediastinoscopy in situations requiring differential diagnosis.

Complications of mediastinoscopy include bleeding, vocal cord paralysis, and pneumothorax. Cardiac dysfunction, including arrhythmias, or even myocardial infarction may occur. For this reason, the procedure is done in an operating room equipped for dealing with a cardiac emergency. Fortunately these complications do not occur frequently. All the usual treatment and nursing care measures for preoperative and postoperative care are required for the patient undergoing mediastinoscopy, with particular attention being given to monitoring for potential complications.

Biopsy of lung tissue and of surrounding tissues is important in the diagnosis of certain conditions. A scalene node biopsy can be taken from the paratracheal lymph nodes; the scalene fat pad is used as the site for this type of biopsy. A small incision is made in the anterior neck, the sternocleidomastoid muscle is divided, and the nodes near the fat pad are examined. The right lung and the lower left lung drain into the scalene lymph nodes. Although the scalene node biopsy does not give as extensive diagnostic information as mediastinoscopy provides, some physicians prefer the scalene node biopsy because there is less danger of spreading tumor cells than with mediastinoscopy and complications occur less frequently.

Biopsy of lung tissue can be obtained by using a cutting needle, an aspiration needle, or a trephine. Biopsy of the lung is contraindicated in patients with advanced lung disease, hypoxia, cardiac disease, or pulmonary hypertension. The cutting and aspiration needles are used with a local anesthetic, usually while the patient is undergoing fluoroscopy so that the needle can be placed in the desired position. The **aspiration needle** punctures the lung and allows for syringe aspiration of a small tissue sample; a larger core of tissue can be obtained by using a **cutting needle.** As with any biopsy obtained by cutting, bleeding may occur. When the biopsy is obtained from the lung through the pleura, there is a possibility of pneumothorax, particularly in restrictive lung disease. The **trephine biopsy** is obtained by making a small incision through the tissues, including the muscles overlying the area from which the biopsy is to be obtained. The trephine is attached to a drill, which powers the placement of the trephine into the lung tissue. A syringe containing physiologic saline solution is used to aspirate the specimen.

Lung tissue can also be obtained through **transthoracic lung biopsy,** a closed procedure, or through thoracotomy, an open surgical procedure. Bleeding and pneumothorax are complications, but they occur less frequently than with needle or trephine biopsy. Thoracotomy requires anesthesia, so the patient must be able to tolerate anesthesia. The advantage of a thoracotomy is that it enables the surgeon to visualize the lung tissue.

Because complications may occur, a biopsy is not performed unless it is required for differential diagnosis or for determining appropriate treatment. The term **biopsy** may be closely associated in the patient's mind with the term **cancer,** so the nurse must carefully explain the procedures and explore the patient's feelings and fears both before and after the biopsy.

Thoracentesis is the aspiration of fluid or air from the pleural cavity for diagnosis and treatment. A thoracentesis needle is inserted after the skin has been cleaned with an antiseptic and a local anesthetic has been administered. The amount of fluid removed is measured and examined in culture sensitivity tests and cytologic studies. During the procedure the patient is maintained in a comfortable sitting position, with arms and feet supported. Following the aspiration a pressure dressing or an adhesive strip is applied to the needle site. The patient must then rest on his unaffected side for at least 1 hour and is observed for faintness, tightness of the chest, cough, tachycardia, and expectoration of blood-tinged mucus.

Lung Function Tests

The effectiveness of the respiratory system may also be measured by lung function tests of the mechanical and physical aspects of ventilation for gas exchange. Although there is great variation among individuals, approximately 500 cc of air normally enters the lungs with each inspired breath; this is the **tidal volume** (TV). **Vital capacity** (VC) is the maximum amount of air a person can expel in a forced expiration following maximal inspiration. The amount of air remaining in the lungs at the end of a maximal expiration is the **residual volume** (RV). The two together, VC and RV, equal the total lung capacity.

The amount of air entering the lung (TV) can be increased in accordance with the **inspiratory reserve volume** (IRV). Similarly, the amount of air that can be expelled in a forced expiration is the **expiratory reserve volume** (ERV). These reserves enable a person to increase both the rate and depth of respirations to meet the body's requirements for increased oxygen during exercise, stress, or increased metabolism.

A person's ability to breathe effectively can be determined by a spirometer, which measures the volume of gas. A forced expiratory spirogram measures forced vital capacity, which is the maximum volume of gas the person has for adapting to increased requirements for oxygen when stress is placed on the respiratory system.

Maximum voluntary ventilation (MVV) is calculated by having the patient breathe as deeply and rapidly as he can for a period of 15 seconds. The **expiratory flow rate** (EFR) can be measured either as the **maximum midexpiratory flow rate** (MMEFR) or the **peak expiratory flow rate** (PEFR). Both are useful in estimating airway resistance. The first is measured at the midpoint of expiration; the second measures flow during the first 10 msec of a forced expiration. Normally the PEFR value is about 600 liters per minute for young men and 450 liters per minute in young women. The values fall with age or with respiratory dysfunction.

Forced expiratory volume (FEV) is the amount of air expired in measured seconds following a forced inspiration. A subscript is used to indicate the amount of time represented by each reading. For example, FEV_1 indicates the forced expiratory volume expired in one second; FEV_2 indicates the forced expiratory volume expired in two seconds, and so on. When lung dysfunction is present, both the VC and the FEV are decreased. The percentage of the VC that is expired within a second is significant. Patients with obstructive lung disease have prolonged expirations; the percentage of VC they expire in FEV_1 is significantly decreased. Patients with restrictive lung disease cannot expand their chest walls but usually do not have an airway obstruction. They have a decreased VC, but they can expire a greater percentage of the total VC in FEV_1 than those with obstructive disease.

The FEV is easily measured and is sometimes used as a screening procedure to evaluate lung function. It can also be used as a diagnostic test to determine the amount and type of impairment that exists. Another use of the FEV is to evaluate the effectiveness of therapy. For example, the FEV can be measured prior to administration of bronchodilators. Following therapy, usually after about a week, the FEV is repeated and the results are compared with the first test. If the FEV has increased, the therapy can be considered effective, giving evidence that the obstruction was reversible.

Forced expiratory time (FET) can be determined by having the patient first inspire as deeply as possible, followed by a forced expiration. Normally a forced expiration can be completed in six seconds; if the expiration time is prolonged, an obstruction of the airways is suspected.

Lung volume can be measured by diluting the inspired air, with the patient breathing either helium or nitrogen (the latter is used in the nitrogen washout test). The expired air is then analyzed at given time periods to determine the amount of helium or nitrogen that is expired until the values return to those of normal ambient air. The total lung capacity, functional residual capacity, and residual volume can be measured in the test; the values of all three are increased in diseases such as emphysema and bronchitis, which are associated with hyperinflation of the lungs. The ratio of the residual volume to the total lung capacity indicates the effectiveness of expiration. Restrictive lung diseases that diminish chest wall expansion decrease these values. The effectiveness of ventilation can be demonstrated by the amount of time it takes to completely "wash out" the helium or nitrogen.

Air normally flows through the airways with some turbulence. In obstructive lung disease the turbulence increases because the airways are narrowed, causing the velocity of the air to increase and the pressure to decrease. In diseases in which expiration is prolonged because of the increasing resistance to airflow, the pressure of air in the bronchioles weakens them and they tend to collapse before the alveoli can be emptied, a mechanism thought to be important in maintaining the volume of air in smaller airways in gravity-dependent lung areas. Gradually the resting levels of residual air increase so that there is an increasing functional residual capacity and residual volume. **Closing volume** is the amount of air trapped in alveoli during expiration. People with ventilatory failure are thought to have closing volumes greater than the functional reserve capacity.

Airways resistance is higher during expiration than during inspiration and greater when the lung volume is small. The resistance normally increases when irritants are inhaled or during forced expiration, as well as with obstruction of the airways caused by pathologic processes.

Pulmonary function studies are usually conducted in hospitals or clinics. It is important that the nurse recognize that changes in the values of lung function tests over a period of time are more significant for diagnosis or evaluation of progress than are specific values at any given time, because of the normal variations in lung capacities among individuals. The nurse should be able to interpret the results of the tests to the patient in terms of implications for self-care and treatment procedures.

All the assessment techniques just described are basic to planning and implementing nursing care of patients with respiratory dysfunction. Many common features in the nursing care of such patients are equally applicable to many different disease processes; these common nursing care measures are described in the following pages.

Nursing Care in Respiratory Dysfunction

The primary objective of nursing care for patients with respiratory system dysfunction is to provide the maximum amount of oxygen needed to meet the body's requirements for energy within the patient's capabilities for ventilation and perfusion. The ability of a person to function depends on sufficient oxygen to provide energy for his activities. The base level of respiratory functioning is the level that sustains the life of the cells; inadequate oxygen can be life threatening if the basic metabolic needs for oxygen cannot be met. Beyond this base level, oxygen is necessary to accomplish physical work. The amount of physical work a person can accomplish also depends on the amount of oxygen available to meet the body's metabolic requirements for energy production. People with severe oxygen deficits may be able to live only at rest or with minimal activity; the degree of limitation is directly related to the amount of oxygen available and the adequacy of the body's compensatory mechanisms for making the best use of the energy available. Nursing care plans are based on the patient's specific needs in relation to his capabilities and limitations and should be realistic and practical for the patient involved. The type of disease process is also significant in determining nursing care measures that will be effective in treating the basic cause of the dysfunction.

CLASSIFICATION OF LUNG DYSFUNCTION

Respiratory diseases may be generally viewed either as obstructing airflow or as restricting the mobility of the chest wall or the elasticity of the lungs. Some diseases, for example, pneumonia, both restrict mechanical breathing and obstruct airflow. The two broad classifications of respiratory dysfunction, then, are acute or chronic obstructive lung disease and restrictive lung disease. **Obstructive** lung diseases include those that partially or completely occlude the airways. Foreign bodies, increased secretions, and narrowing of the lumen of the airways all interfere with airflow. Bronchospasm, emphysema, and asthma are examples of three major lung diseases that obstruct airflow and are often chronic, leading to cardiopulmonary dysfunction in the later phases. **Restrictive** lung diseases limit the elasticity of lung tissue. Fibrosis resulting from hypersensitivity reactions or infections decreases the elasticity of lung tissue, restricting expansion. Nervous diseases may restrict respiration by impairing the nervous stimulation and inhibition of the chest wall. Diseases that impair the ability of muscles to move the chest wall for respirations can also restrict lung function.

Ventilation and perfusion abnormalities constitute the major source of symptoms in both obstructive and restrictive lung diseases. In obstructive diseases the **total lung** capacity (TLC) is increased but the FEV$_1$ is decreased. Restrictive diseases cause decreased TLC, decreased VC, and decreased inspiratory capacity with subsequent alveolar hypoventilation. These differences imply different treatment modalities and nursing care.

NURSING CARE IN CHRONIC OBSTRUCTIVE LUNG DYSFUNCTION

Chronic airway obstruction is a major cause of disability and death. The severity of the acute or chronic obstruction is directly related to the effectiveness of alveolar ventilation and perfusion at the level of alveolar gas exchange; this is the point at which oxygen is delivered to the blood for transportation to the body cells. The nurse should recognize that the patient with obstructive lung disease experiences an increased work load in breathing (see color insert Figure 12 on page 1078C). Usually expiration is prolonged and the patient has exertional dyspnea as a result of the uneven distribution of ventilation and perfusion. In caring for these patients, the nurse is concerned with their accommodating to the loss of alveolar structure and support. Anything that narrows the airways such as inflammatory reactions, hypertrophy of mucous glands, or accumulation of secretions will cause further impairment of ventilation. Avoidance of these processes or minimizing their effects is an important aspect of care.

Helping the Patient to Stop Smoking

The nurse should teach the patient to avoid anything that irritates the airways. Cigarette smoke is one of the primary irritants that increase the production of mucus; thus smoking is contraindicated for any person with impaired lung function. While it is imperative that the patient with respiratory insufficiency (as well as all others) stop smoking, nursing care must be based on an understanding of the patient's feelings and attitudes about himself. Of prime concern is the importance of smoking as a coping mechanism. Smoking is a habit, and withdrawal from smoking, while causing few side effects, is similar to withdrawal from opium. The nature and extent of the dependency on nicotine are important factors in helping the person recognize what is involved in stopping the habit of smoking. In order to break the habit, the person should be helped to understand why the habit is important to him; he can then determine whether the benefits of the habit outweigh the consequences of that habit. Knowing that continued smoking will reduce one's mobility is sometimes sufficient impetus to discontinue smoking. Recognizing that the consequences of smoking will hinder or impede other values and goals, particularly one's self-concept and health status, is helpful in intellectualizing the need to discontinue smoking. Techniques such as behavior modification employ the concept that if a person has positive reinforcement in breaking a habit or making a change, he will be more likely to accomplish the change. For this reason, people who are close to the person who wants to stop smoking can be of great assistance in providing positive reinforcement.

It is easier to intellectualize about stopping smoking than to actually accomplish it, particularly if the person is a long-term smoker. Even though one knows what the consequences of continued smoking will be, it is easy to rationalize and say, "That happens to other people, not to me." Nurses who care for patients who need to stop smoking should recognize that the patient must first make a commitment to stop smoking and second must be given the positive support necessary to reinforce the resolve to break the habit. It is helpful if other family members or associates do not smoke in the patient's presence. Joining a group such as an "I Want to Quit" group is one way to reinforce the resolve to stop smoking; however, many people begin smoking again after the group meetings have been completed either because of the wave of desire to smoke that is a recognized aspect of dependency or because of the fact that the reinforcement to stop is not available. Thus the patient must make a commitment to stop smoking and then develop the self-determination to carry out that resolve.

Emphasis is placed on prevention of smoking through campaigns to reach children and young adults who have not yet begun the habit. If one does not start smoking in the first place, there is no need to stop. The American Lung Association, the American Heart Association, and the American Cancer Society have teaching aids and materials that can be used in community programs explaining the hazards of smoking for the purpose of preventing people from beginning the habit of smoking. Nurses can and should become actively involved in these community programs.

The incidence of chronic lung disease may decrease significantly if people who are susceptible to lung dysfunction do not smoke. However, the nurse should recognize that even though a person does not smoke, he may acquire lung dysfunction. A number of other factors including environmental pollution, industrial pollution, individual susceptibility, and general state of health are also important factors in the incidence of lung disease. Unfortunately, there is no assurance that one will not have lung diseases even if he follows positive health practices. It is perhaps this knowledge that keeps people who smoke from actually accepting the fact that smoking is potentially harmful to them.

Instructing the Patient in Bronchial Hygiene
When nurses teach patients with chronic lung dysfunction how to care for themselves, attention should be given to avoiding infections. When a patient has compromised lung function, an infection can cause further dysfunction. Infection causes increased secretions, and the increased viscosity of secretions creates great resistance to ciliary action so that the expectoration of mucus is slowed. Infections also lead to further damage of lung tissue through fibrosis. Fibrosis can result from intra-alveolar exudate or interstitial exudate. The end result of fibrosis is that the involved lung tissue is less elastic and lung expansion is consequently restricted, which effects a decreased lung compliance. Generally the fibrosis is not evenly distributed throughout the lung, so there is unequal ventilation and perfusion in the alveoli.

Methods for increasing the effectiveness of respirations for patients with chronic lung disease include liquefying and removing secretions and improving control of respirations through a bronchial hygiene program. Bronchial hygiene involves a routine for the use of bronchodilators, moisture, and postural drainage. The routine may be implemented by the nurse or taught by the nurse so that the patient learns to conduct his own bronchial hygiene program.

Use of the nebulizer Nebulizers are used to pump bronchodilator medications deep into the airways. The medications used with a nebulizer include isoproterenol (Isuprel) and racemic epinephrine (Vaponefrin). These medications reduce the edema of the mucosa and dilate the airways; in addition, they improve ciliary motion and promote clearance of mucus from the airways. The aerosol bronchodilators are usually diluted, the dosage depending on the amount required by the patient. Usually one part aerosol and two parts water are used. Among the many nebulizers available are hand bulb devices and powered positive-pressure devices. Both operate by compressing air, which forces the medication against a jet that separates the particles. The particles of medication must be small enough to reach deeply into the airways, since smaller particles are carried further. Aerosols provide these finer particles that penetrate deeply into the airways.

The nurse must teach the patient how to use the nebulizer for maximum effectiveness. The patient first exhales and then, using the nebulizer, breathes in slowly. The aim is to achieve the best distribution of the aerosol possible, and inhaling slowly provides for the best contact of the aerosol with the deep airways. The nebulizer should be held in position at, not in, the mouth. The effort of pumping a hand bulb nebulizer sometimes causes a tendency to grasp the end of the nebulizer with the teeth for stability. It is necessary to instruct the patient to place the nebulizer so that air can enter the mouth around the tip of the nebulizer. This inspired air can help distribute the aerosol medication within the airways. Once the inspiration is completed, the patient should pause momentarily before expiring the air. A slow, controlled expiration through pursed lips also helps to maintain maximum distribution of the aerosol.

If the patient has difficulty managing a hand bulb nebulizer because of either muscle weakness or inability to coordinate the nebulizer action with inspiration, a pump nebulizer can be used. When the patient cannot breathe deeply enough for the nebulized aerosol to be effective, positive-pressure devices are used. These are available in both hand driven or pump driven models. Positive-pressure devices increase the flow of air so that distribution of the aerosol is greater. Another type of nebulizer is a small metered dose device, which is handy to use.

This device is simply a container of medication that is attached to a mouthpiece for directing the spray into the mouth. These devices do not have the ability to split the particles into very small sizes and therefore are not as effective for bronchodilation of the smaller airways.

Humidification The patient is taught to humidify the airways following nebulization. Humidification can be accomplished by many different means. A facial sauna is a good way of supplying heated air to the airways. The warm air carries more moisture than cold air and is therefore more effective if the patient can tolerate the heat (heat causes bronchospasm in some patients). Other devices for humidification may be as simple as a singing teapot or a small room humidifier, or they may be more complicated and expensive. Some patients find cold steam more beneficial than warm steam. The water is necessary to make secretions less viscous, since water both wets and thins the secretions, promoting their removal. As mentioned previously, continuous attention to adequate fluid intake is important and also contributes to the effectiveness of bronchial hygiene. (It should be noted that fluid intake should be carefully monitored in patients who also have cardiac disease.)

Postural drainage Having completed nebulization and humidification, the patient is instructed to use postural drainage to promote removal of the now thinned secretions via the use of gravity to drain secretions toward the main stem bronchus and to the trachea; from that point they can be removed by coughing. The patient's ability to tolerate postural drainage depends on his condition. Debilitated patients may not be able to use this method for draining secretions because they are unable to assume the positions comfortably.

The anatomy of the lung is such that different postures or positions are necessary to drain different parts of the lung. The most affected areas of the lung should be drained first. The lower lobes and posterior basal segments are best drained when the patient bends at the waist and places his head at a level below his waist. This position can be maintained by placing pillows on a bed in such a way that the patient can lie prone on the pillows, bending the hips and placing the head and legs below the level of the hips. The lateral segment of the left lower lobe is drained by having the patient remain in this position but with his left side turned upward. The lingula (which is the lower part of the upper lobe of the left lung) and the right middle lobe can be drained by having the patient change position so that the right side is upward. The anterior basal segments of both lower lobes are best drained when the patient lies supine with the head lower than the feet (Fig. 3-5).

The upper lobes can be drained with the head elevated; the anterior apical segments are drained when the patient leans backward and the posterior apical segments when he leans forward. The posterior segment can also be drained by having the patient lie in a side position with the head elevated. The right and left anterior segments of the upper lobe are drained by having the patient lie flat with the knees elevated. The apical segments of the lower lobes can be drained by having the patient lie prone on the bed with pillows placed under the head, abdomen, and feet.

Positions for postural drainage vary according to the site of the patient's lung pathology; the nurse should advise him which position is most conducive to drainage for his particular condition. The patient is advised to select a place for postural drainage that is convenient and that lends itself to the varying positions he must assume. He should be advised not to use the floor or any place that might be dusty, since the dust and dirt could easily be inspired into the lungs. Usually a bed or a heavy piece of furniture best supports the correct drainage positions with the aid of properly placed pillows. The frequency and duration of postural drainage depend on its effectiveness.

Postural drainage, in addition to being used in home care, can be used for different reasons with hospitalized patients. It is beneficial in any disease associated with increased lung secretion, such as pneumonia, cystic fibrosis, or a lung abscess, and for patients who are unable to cough adequately following surgery. Postural drainage is used to remove secretions that have the potential for infection if retained. Preoperative and postoperative care may include postural drainage to remove secretions; the patient who experiences post-

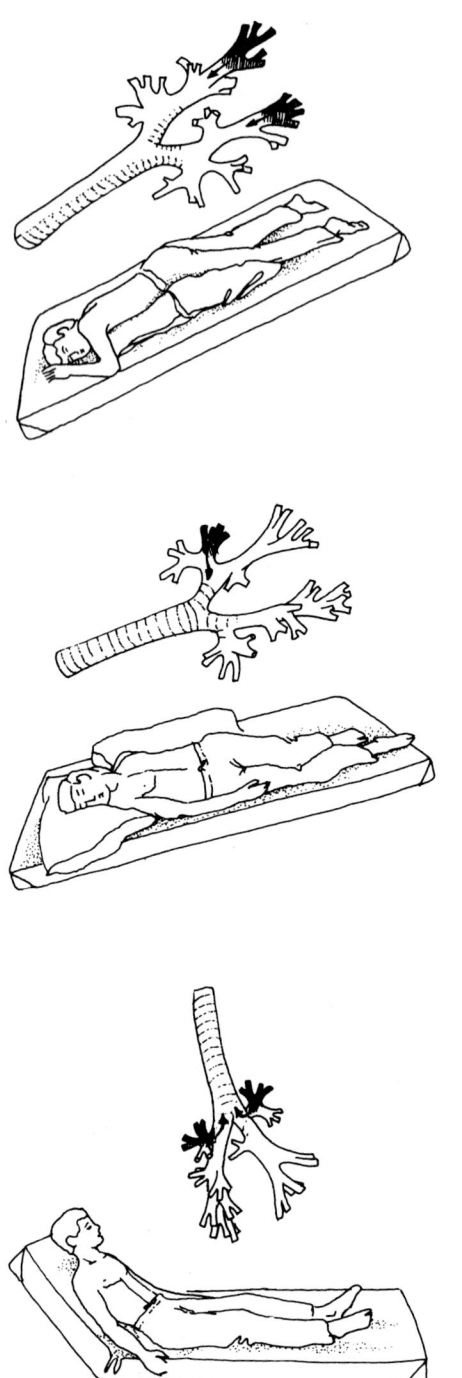

Figure 3-5
Common postural drainage positions. (From B. A. Shapiro, R. A. Harrison, and C. A. Trout, *Clinical Application of Respiratory Care*. Copyright © 1975 by Year Book Medical Publishers, Inc., Chicago. Reproduced by permission.)

operative pain may not cough sufficiently to remove the mucus. Patients who are treated with mechanical ventilation may also have postural drainage to remove secretions, thereby improving ventilation and making the mechanical ventilation more effective. There are limitations in the type of postural drainage that can be accomplished with mechanical ventilation, however, because the pressure-cycled respirators are far less effective when the patient's head is placed below his hips (because the abdominal contents exert pressure, thereby increasing pulmonary resistance). If postural drainage is necessary, mechanical ventilation can be interrupted or temporarily supplied by manual means, as with an Ambu bag.

Patients with neurologic dysfunction, including quadriplegics and paraplegics, also benefit from postural drainage, as do comatose patients. The frequent position changes required for the care of these patients help mobilize secretions and improve circulation to dependent body parts. Infection or increased secretions from any cause will require careful postural drainage associated with the total bronchial hygiene program.

Percussion Often postural drainage is carried out in association with percussion. In the hospital setting this is often performed by the respiratory–physical therapist. The purpose of percussion is to loosen secretions by applying pressure alternating with relaxation to the chest wall, which has the effect of changing pressures in the lung and facilitating the removal of mucus and secretions. A "cupped-hands" position for percussion creates an air cushion so that striking the chest wall is not painful. It is important that percussion be performed with care in order not to damage the skin, soft tissues, or underlying structures; there should be a layer of material, such as pajamas or a gown, between the patient's bare skin and the therapist's cupped hands. Percussion is performed using mild pressure while rhythmically striking the chest wall over the area of consolidation. The cupped hands remain stable as they are moved through alternate flexion and extension of the wrist. The duration of the procedure is usually 1 minute but not longer than 1½ minutes. The cupped hands exert a pressure known as clapping, which changes the air pressure

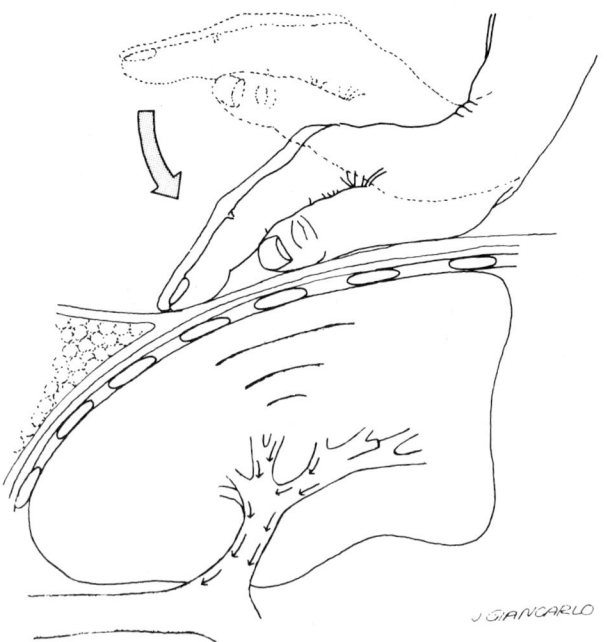

Figure 3-6
Principle of therapeutic chest percussion. The cupped hands create air vibrations that transmit to lung tissue. (From B. A. Shapiro, R. A. Harrison, and C. A. Trout, *Clinical Application of Respiratory Care.* Copyright © 1975 by Year Book Medical Publishers, Inc., Chicago. Reproduced by permission.)

within the airways so that mucus plugs can be dislodged. If effective air is allowed to pass distal to the mucus plugs, it promotes movement of the plugs to the trachea (Fig. 3-6).

The advantage in using percussion with postural drainage is that more mucus can be moved in a shorter amount of time. Not every patient responds favorably to percussion; however, this technique is not effective in obese patients and should not be used for those who have pneumothorax, fractured ribs, debilitating diseases with calcium-phosphorus imbalances, or chest pain. Patients with chronic lung disease sometimes cannot tolerate percussion because it may cause bronchospasm.

Vibration Vibration is a technique in which the flats of the hands are placed on the chest wall over the area that has been percussed. The hands are then vibrated as pressure is applied toward the direction of rib movement while the patient is exhaling. The action is similar to shaking and clapping a catsup bottle. The vibration is usually done for only three or four expirations and may be used in instances when the patient cannot tolerate percussion.

Another technique that can be used to mobilize mucus is teaching the patient to use the accessory muscles of respiration. This can be done by having the patient sit in a straight chair with a pillow in his lap and lean slightly forward, which facilitates the use of the accessory muscles. The person bends forward as he expires air from his lungs, then sits up as he inspires. Repeating this several times loosens secretions. The person is then asked to take a deep breath and to cough gently to expectorate secretions.

Coughing Coughing follows postural drainage. The patient should be taught to cough effectively by having him first take a deep breath with his mouth closed. The cough should be controlled and should begin with expiration, since the cough reflex is greatest during the expiration of air. It is important to prevent harsh, barking coughs or explosive coughs; instead the patient should be taught to use the force of expiration by placing his tongue forward in his mouth and coughing gently for maximum benefit of the cough with the least irritation to the airway. The patient should have the feeling of "rolling the cough out."

A cough is normally a protective response to irritation of the airways. The reflex is triggered by sensations arising in the afferent fibers of the pharyngeal branches of the glossopharyngeal nerve and the sensory endings of the vagus nerve in the larynx, trachea, and bronchi. These impulses are transmitted to the medulla, where the cough center is located, and from there to the muscles of the chest and larynx. The cough begins with inspiration; the glottis then closes and the cough results on expiration. Although the inspiration preceeding a cough can be controlled, the expiration is much more difficult to control. An explosive cough represents a contraction of the expiratory muscles with air under high pressure being exhaled. Control of cough, then, must begin with control of the inspiration. Coughing correctly is important for the patient who has increased secretions, and he must learn and pratice the mechanism of coughing productively. The aim is to remove secretions and to eliminate the need for explosive reflex coughing as much as possible.

For patients with chest pain, abdominal pain following surgery, or dysfunction of the muscles, assistance in coughing can be provided. This assistance is given in the form of supporting the chest wall with the palms of the hands so that the patient can exert his energies in coughing. The hands should be placed with mild pressure to provide a slight compression at the peak of inspiration, and the pressure should be maintained during expiration.

Effectiveness of bronchial hygiene program
In summary, the bronchial hygiene program advised for patients with chronic lung disease includes the use of nebulizers, humidification, postural drainage, and coughing to remove secretions. This is usually done at least twice daily. Each patient has to determine his own routine so that the pattern of bronchial hygiene becomes as natural as brushing teeth or tying shoes. The actual amount of time spent on bronchial hygiene varies from one person to another, but it usually does not take more than 20 to 30 minutes each time. It is important that the patient keep the program in perspective. A positive program of bronchial hygiene does not cure; more correctly it improves ventilation and helps prevent infection resulting from retained secretions. Generally the patient who follows the routine notices the improved ventilation and appreciates the positive effects achieved. Increased duration or frequency of the bronchial hygiene program does not necessarily promote better ventilation. Bronchial hygiene is effective only in that it facilitates maximum use of the lung function remaining; it cannot change a disease that is irreversible.

Breathing exercises are another form of treatment that improves remaining function but does not change irreversible lung dysfunction. These exercises are particularly useful for the person who notices dyspnea on exertion. In many people with lung dysfunction, periods of dyspnea cause anxiety; this is a normal response since it is frightening not to be able to breathe. By teaching the patient to know and anticipate his response, the nurse can then show him how to avoid anxiety by concentrating on prelearned techniques to improve breathing. The patient can sometimes reduce the severity of the dyspneic periods through these techniques [3]. This kind of teaching applies to the care of asthmatic patients and those who have emphysema or bronchitis in which periods of bronchospasm occur and in whom desensitization to dyspnea is important.

Care of the Patient with Bronchospasm
A bronchospasm is essentially a prolonged contraction of the smooth muscle of the bronchus. It often occurs in response to an inflammatory reaction, to irritation by noxious fumes or irritants such as pollutants, or to hypersensitivity reactions. It can occur at any point in the airways. The result of bronchospasm is narrowing of the airways. The causes may be edema of the mucosa, increased and immobile secretions, and impaired cough mechanisms, all of which result in increasing the resistance to airflow. A sign of narrowing is the characteristic wheezing sound that can be heard as the air passes through the narrowed airways. The nurse should recall that muscle tone in the airways is maintained by a balance between the parasympathetic and sympathetic nervous systems. When spasm occurs, the normally smooth bronchial walls

become ridged and develop folds of mucosa that retain secretions. The nurse should explain this mechanism to the affected patient; if he is able to anticipate the effects of bronchospasm and to recognize early symptoms he may then be able to act to reduce some of the effects.

The nurse will be called upon to offer support and counseling to the patient who experiences bronchospasm. An important aspect of this counseling is teaching the patient to recognize that emotions affect respirations. When one becomes upset, the consequences can often be seen in increased dyspnea, perhaps resulting from bronchospasm and cough. There are several techniques that can be used in this instance, the goal being to decrease the work of breathing while increasing its effectiveness, not only during or after bronchospasm but for the dyspneic patient in general.

Techniques of Breathing

Usually the dyspneic patient feels most comfortable in a sitting position, using a chair that supports his body in good alignment. A relaxed position is more conducive to controlling breathing, since tenseness further increases muscular work and contributes to anxiety. The spine should be straight and the feet should be firmly placed on the floor to stabilize the body.

In addition to assuming a comfortable and supportive position, the patient may also develop skill in the technique of abdominal-diaphragmatic breathing, which is most helpful in attaining effective respirations. The patient must expend effort to learn the control necessary to master this technique; it is difficult because one must learn to overcome the normal compensatory tendency to breathe in short, rapid, gasping breaths. When one is dyspneic, the short breaths are usually shallow and do not provide enough air for adequate ventilation because the dead space ventilation is actually increased. When the breathing is controlled, more air can be delivered to the alveoli, thereby reducing the dyspnea.

Normally, breathing is a rhythmic pattern of inspiration and expiration. The patient who is aware of his breathing may need to consciously coordinate it. The technique of a full inspiration followed by a slow expiration provides for more forceful flow and minimizes collapse of the small airways. Another benefit of this technique is that it decreases the work of breathing, thus reducing the need for oxygen. Exhalation can be further controlled by teaching the patient to contract his abdominal muscles while exhaling.

The specific technique used depends on the patient's response to cues that make him more comfortable. The nurse can help the patient find the most comfortable technique through observation and experimentation. If the patient sits in a stable, upright chair, with a pillow in his lap, he can comfortably lean forward. The relaxation of abdominal muscles afforded by this position is augmented by keeping the shoulders down, the arms in a side position, and the knees bent. This posture minimizes upper chest elevation in the inspiratory phase, and as previously described, abdominal-diaphragmatic breathing can be taught in this position (Fig. 3-7). To

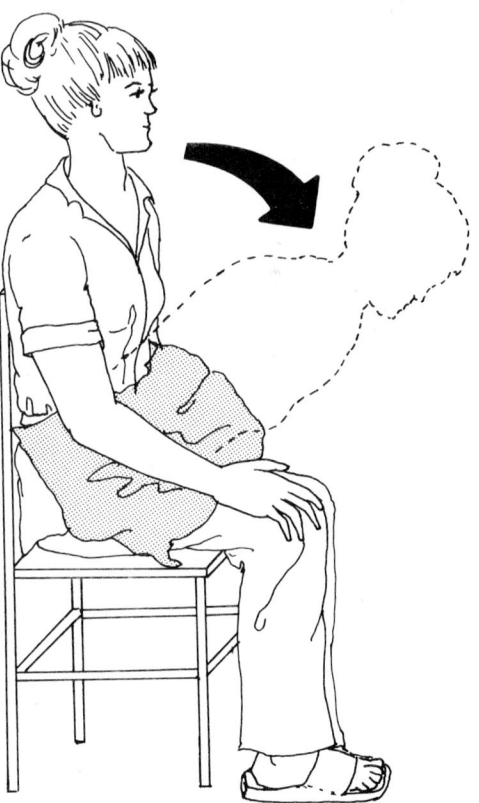

Figure 3-7
Position for relaxation of abdominal muscles and for teaching abdominal diaphragmatic breathing.

teach this exercise, the nurse places one hand on the epigastric area to supply mild pressure during inspiration. As the patient gets the feel of breathing with the abdominal muscles, he can place his own hand in position to feel the movement of air along with the downward movement of the diaphragm during inspiration.

Pursing of the lips is another method the nurse can teach to help the patient control a prolonged expiration by increasing the resistance to airflow. At the end of the expiration, the patient can consciously tighten his abdominal muscles, thus helping to force as much air as possible from his lungs to achieve maximum expiration.

Once the patient has learned to coordinate breathing, he or she can better control periods of dyspnea. When the patient consistently has exertional dyspnea, it is necessary that the nurse teach the patient to coordinate breathing with the performance of any activity. To do this, the nurse must make the patient aware that it is natural to tense up when doing anything that requires concentration, and this tendency must be overcome. People often do not realize that they become tense when performing routine activities such as cooking, cleaning, shaving, or walking; therefore, coordination of breathing with the activity must be based on an awareness of the tensing of muscles that normally accompanies these activities. The patient must learn to relax and breathe slowly with full inspirations and prolonged expirations while also moving to perform the activity. For some, this is similar to learning to juggle several items, but with practice and support from the nurse, movements can be learned so that they are coordinated with the breathing pattern. This coordination enables patients with chronic lung disease to be more mobile than they could otherwise be. Gorman [5] suggests that it may be possible for man to ". . . redirect an illness-producing pattern to a health-maintaining one." This has particularly pertinent application to the patient with respiratory dysfunction who must consciously synchronize all activity with breathing for maximal energy use. It should be recognized, however, that this synchronization can only be accomplished within the limits of the patient's oxygen supply.

Exercise Stress Tests

The ability to exercise is a major concern of people who become breathless on exertion. In the early stages of repiratory dysfunction, the patient may notice an inability to perform active sports; as the disease progresses, the breathlessness increases so that it is present during performance of normal daily activities or even at rest. There is great variability among individuals in the amount of exercise that can be tolerated in relation to the degree of tissue hypoxia. The degree of hypoxia is not necessarily an indication of the amount of exercise a person can tolerate because some people have a greater capacity for exercise than others.

The patient can test his own tolerance by measuring the amount of exercise he can perform. This can be used as an indication of progress and may be as simple as measuring the distance he or she can walk without becoming "breathless" from one time to another. More precise tests can be done, however, to test the tolerance of a given patient for exercise. These tests are **exercise stress tests** and may be accomplished in different ways; one method involves the use of a stationary bicycle equipped with a meter to measure distance and resistance. Exercise stress tests are useful to the nurse not only in counseling the patient about adjusting daily living activities to the limits of his or her dysfunction, but also for measuring the improvement of function resulting from therapy, such as the bronchial hygiene program.

Sputum Examination

Another measure of progress is the examination of sputum, which serves many purposes. As previously mentioned, sputum can be examined during an initial diagnosis for culture and sensitivity and for cytology studies to determine the presence of an infecting organism or of abnormal cells. For the patient with chronic lung disease, careful examination of sputum can provide clues to his status. The color, amount, and consistency of sputum are included in the observation. Changes in color are significant in determining the presence of infection. For example, if the sputum becomes yellowish, the patient may suspect that he has an infection; sputum that becomes increasingly clear following an infection indicates resolution of the infection. The amount of sputum produced increases during periods of bronchospasm, irritation, and inflammation, or in response to hypersensitivity reactions or emotional stimulation. The consistency of the sputum is a guide to the effectiveness of bronchial hygiene, to the state of hydration, and to the presence of secondary disease processes. Sputum becomes more viscous when the patient is dehydrated or when an infection is present.

In many cases the patient can use observation of the color, amount, and consistency of sputum as a guide to treating himself. Most patients with chronic lung disease learn to adjust their treatment to their needs at any given time. The patient is often given a supply of antibiotics by his physician, which he takes either routinely (one week per month) or if he feels an infectious process is pending, as determined by yellowish sputum. When sputum is more viscous, the patient knows he must increase his oral fluid intake and provide more humidity in his inspired air. Increased sputum production may indicate that the patient should pay more attention to the bronchial hygiene program. When the sputum increases in amount, the patient can evaluate what factors precipitated this event and can learn to some extent to control the factors that lead to bronchospasm or irritation. Knowing the reasons for the symptoms he or she experiences can help the patient in managing the dysfunction on a day-to-day basis. It is important, however, that the patient have regular, periodic medical checkups to determine his status and progress; these ensure that the patient is not undertreating or overtreating himself and that if changes do occur, treatment can be initiated to minimize their ill effects if possible.

Another reason for routine checkups is that most patients with chronic diseases require continuing support from other people. Knowing that there is someone who is willing to listen and answer questions is important to the patient with a chronic illness. Being examined periodically is sometimes a positive motivating factor for the patient to be careful about treatment and bronchial hygiene. Most people want to have "positive" results when they are examined for any reason; this is also true of patients with chronic diseases who are actively involved in their own treatment regimen. They often need to have their ability to manage the therapeutic plan evaluated by the physician or nurse practitioner, and they benefit from the sense of independence this self-management gives them.

Medication

A number of drugs are used in the treatment of chronic lung disease. The actions of these drugs should be understood by both the nurse and the patient to ensure their appropriate use. Bronchodilators are given to prevent bronchospasm and to dilate the bronchi. One of the factors that contribute to contraction of the bronchi is parasympathetic stimulation of the vagus nerve; this causes the release of acetylcholine at the myoneural junction which in turn causes the contraction of the smooth muscle of the bronchi. The effect of acetylcholine is counteracted by ephedrine. Atropine also blocks or hinders the reaction of acetylcholine at the myoneural junction. Other factors producing bronchospasm are the antigen-antibody response and the release of histamine.

Bronchodilation can be achieved by use of adrenergic and theophylline groups of medications, which may be given singly or in combination. Best results are often achieved by giving a combination of the adrenergic and theophylline drugs. Adrenergic drugs that act on the bronchial smooth muscle beta receptors causing relaxation are most useful and are available in oral, sublingual, aerosol, or injectable forms. Side effects of adrenergic drugs are associated with disturbances of cardiac rhythm and rate or central nervous system stimulation symptoms of nervousness, excitability, and insomnia. Dizziness, lightheadedness, nausea, and vomiting may occur with their use. Theophylline drugs tend to act directly on bronchial muscle to relax spasms. They also increase cardiac output, increase coronary blood flow, and cause a mild diuretic action. The side effects of theophyllines include gastrointestinal irritation and central nervous system stimulation. Barbiturates or sedatives are given to counteract the central nervous stimulation symptoms.

Epinephrine hydrochloride is the most frequently used of the adrenergic drugs and is most often given for anaphylactic reactions. In addition to relaxing smooth muscle of the bronchi, the adrenergic drugs also decrease production of mucus through alpha receptor stimulation and for this reason are often prescribed in bronchitis. Adrenergic drugs are contraindicated in people with arrhythmias. Tachycardia, increased blood pressure, and dryness of the mouth are common side effects. Rebound bronchospasm may occur after the effect of the drug disappears. With repeated use, the bronchial muscle becomes refractory to the drugs.

Other adrenergic drugs include ephedrine and isoproterenol. Ephedrine is used in aerosol inhalations for its bronchodilation effect. It may also be given at bedtime to prevent nocturnal wheezing. Pseudoephedrine hydrochloride (Sudafed) is similar to ephedrine in action. Isoproterenol (Isuprel) is a beta-adrenergic stimulator that results in relaxation of smooth muscles of the blood vessels in the gastrointestinal tract and increases the force and rate of the heart. Through its action on the blood vessels, it relieves vasoconstriction in the bronchial tubes. Isuprel may cause palpitation, tachycardia, or arrhythmias.

Aminophylline is one of the more frequently used bronchodilators in the theophylline group. It is believed that the therapeutic effect of the theophyllines results from bronchial relaxation and from increased cardiac output so that both ventilation and perfusion improve with their use. The response to their use is individual. The most apparent side effect is a result of dilatation of the cutaneous vessels, which causes flushing and hypotension. When drugs are given via the intravenous route, as in acute asthma attacks, they may decrease blood flow to the brain, resulting in headache, dizziness, nausea, vomiting, or toxicity. Intravenous administration of aminophylline must be monitored carefully and the medication must be administered slowly to prevent hypotension. The theophyllines may also cause palpitations because they affect cardiac muscle. When taken orally, they may cause gastric distress which can be alleviated by taking them either with or immediately after meals. Some people require antacids to counteract this side effect. Aminophylline can also be given rectally in retention enemas or in suppositories.

Mixtures of theophylline drugs or their derivatives with sedatives to counteract central nervous stimulation and, sometimes, an expectorant as well, are given. Examples are Amesec, which contains aminophylline, ephedrine hydrochloride, and amobarbital; and Marax, containing theophylline, ephedrine sulfate, and hydroxyzine hydrochloride.

Aerosol drugs are used to relieve bronchospasms whenever needed as well as during nebulizer treatments as part of a regular bronchial hygiene program. These are sympathomimetic drugs and it is important that the person using them knows that they should not be used too frequently. The sympathetic nervous system alpha receptors primarily found on arteriolar vascular smooth muscle cause constriction of the muscle when stimulated. These drugs must be used discriminately to prevent hypertension, which can result from continued and frequent use. Sympathomimetic drugs are also associated with the incidence of thyroid disease and diabetes when used indiscriminately. It is also important that the patient know that they may cause side effects if the dosage is too great. These side effects include tachycardia and palpitations and may be followed by a feeling of nervousness and dizziness. When these side effects occur, the dosage is usually decreased and the person is cautioned to decrease the frequency of their use.

Racemic epinephrine (Vaponefrin) is a commonly used aerosol. Other agents used with nebulizers are those that liquefy mucus. These agents act on the bronchial mucosa to decrease mucus production. Acetylcysteine (Mucomyst) acts to liquefy mucus and is often given with racemic epinephrine. It is effective only when given in sufficient volume with adequate nebulization. Side effects of acetylcysteine include nausea and increased coughing. Iodines (sodium or potassium iodide) are also commonly used to liquefy sputum [7]. They may be taken orally or used in aerosols. The iodines are thought to act by imitating the gastric mucosa so that there is reflex stimulation of secretion in the airways. The iodine drugs are given in diluted form. Side effects include gastric irritation and, in some cases, skin eruptions or anaphylactic reactions. A more serious effect is the development of iodism, which occurs with long-term use of iodine and causes inflammation of the lining of the tissues of the respiratory tract.

Expectorants are used to thin the secretions of the respiratory tract. It is very important that the patient be well hydrated because expectorants depend on adequate hydration for their effectiveness. Expectorants act by increasing ciliary activity to remove secretions from the airway. In this action they augment the normal response of the cilia in cleaning the airways by removing mucus and entrapped particles.

Cough suppressants are also given to patients with paroxysmal coughing spells, such as those who have chronic bronchitis. They are given only when indicated for relieving the fatigue and increased metabolic work of ineffective coughing. Excessive coughing also tends to irritate and dry the mucous membranes. When deciding whether or not to use cough suppressants, one must take into account the need for cough as a protective mechanism and the other forms of therapy employed to reduce and remove secretions. It is necessary that the cough be supported and not suppressed when coughing is the major source of removing secretions, since retained secretions can lead to infection or can further impair lung ventilation by blocking the passage of air in the alveoli. The major classifications of suppressants are narcotics and antihistamines; other suppressants provide for local anesthesia of the mucous membranes. Narcotics act on the medullary cough control center to suppress the cough reflex, while antihistamine suppressants act locally. Local anesthetic agents inhibit the vagus nerve endings and also the medullary control sites to suppress the cough reflex. The cough suppressants may cause generalized symptoms. The narcotics and antihistamines may cause drowsiness and promote sleep. Nausea is a common side effect of all the cough suppressants.

Often antibiotics are given prophylactically in chronic lung disease. Tetracycline is most frequently given for this purpose. Generally the patient is given a supply of antibiotics to be taken when he notices signs of an impending infection. Sometimes antibiotics are given prophylactically during high infection risk periods such as during the winter and when exposure to crowds or to infected persons cannot be avoided. Careful use of antibiotics is necessary to reduce development of resistance. Changing the antibiotic periodically helps reduce the possibility of developing resistance if they are taken over a long period of time. A usual course is antibiotics one week per month.

NURSING CARE IN RESTRICTIVE LUNG DYSFUNCTION

The care of patients with restrictive lung diseases differs from that required by those with obstructive lung dysfunction. The restrictive lung dysfunction results from a decreased ability to expand the lung because of neurologic or neuromuscular abnormalities or because of decreased elasticity of lung tissue. In neuromuscular dysfunction, the chest and lung structure may be normal, but the chest wall cannot be mechanically moved to promote respirations; this results in decreased pulmonary compliance. The compliance is also decreased when lung tissue becomes stiff as a result of pathologic change. When pulmonary compliance is decreased, there is a concomitant increase in the work of breathing to overcome the loss of elasticity. The patient with restrictive lung dysfunction typically has a pattern of shallow breathing and tachypnea. The volume of air inspired is decreased as a result of the mechanical defect, and there is usually no obstruction to the airflow on expiration as occurs in obstructive lung diseases. Therefore alveolar ventilation is normal, even though the total lung volume is decreased.

Restrictive lung diseases do cause decreased alveolar ventilation when the vital capacity is reduced sufficiently to cause alveolar hypoventilation (as measured in decreased Pa_{O_2} and increased Pa_{CO_2}). In this situation, hyperventilation compensates for the decreased lung compliance, which in turn causes excessive excretion of carbon dioxide so that the initial hypercapnia is reduced. The kidneys respond to increased carbon dioxide levels by retaining HCO_3^-, and since the excessive carbon dioxide is blown off more quickly than the kidneys can eliminate the excess base, a state of respiratory alkalosis develops and is associated with increased kidney excretion of chloride.

Initially, the respiratory center compensates for increased carbon dioxide tensions with hyperventilation. In chronic hypercapnia, however, the respiratory center does not respond to this increased tension, and hypoxia then becomes the stimulus for respiration. The neurologic signs of alveolar hypoventilation may include increased cerebrospinal fluid pressure and papilledema. A later sign is Cheyne-Stokes respirations, which are periodic respirations in which the patient hyperventilates for about 20 seconds and then is apneic for about 20 seconds. The cycles of periodic breathing are fairly regular and result from respiratory center depression in situations in which the blood flow to the center, such as in hypoxemia, is impaired. Cheyne-Stokes respirations are seen in many different types of disease processes with vasoconstriction of the brain vasculature, or vasodiuresis, such as diabetic ketoacidosis, uremic failure, and congestive heart failure.

Care for patients with restrictive lung diseases is based on treating the cause of the restriction to improve ventilation. If normal lung tissue has been replaced by fibrous tissue, lessening normal elasticity, or if the amount of lung tissue has been decreased because of a surgical procedure such as a pneumonectomy, the lung function is irreversibly restricted. Both of these situations result in decreased lung volume, and care focuses on making the best use of the remaining function. When the cause of the restriction is a reversible disease process such as pneumonia or pulmonary edema, care focuses on reducing the consolidation of lung spaces by removing excess secretions, controlling the excess fluid production, and attempting to resolve or halt the progress of the disease. When the restriction results from pleural effusion or pneumothorax, as found in certain disease processes such as cancer or severe infections or in the event of crushing injuries or other types of trauma to the chest, care focuses on improving function through the insertion of chest tubes to remove excess drainage and facilitate reexpansion of the lung as much as possible.

Patients with Reduced Lung Volume

A number of disease processes cause infringement on lung expansion, thereby restricting the volume; these include abdominal distention, ascites, pain, and edema associated with abdominal surgery and obesity. In these situations the pressure of the abdominal contents on the diaphragm prevents normal movement. The patient's respiratory status is improved when the underlying disease process is resolved. The **pickwickian syndrome** is experienced by patients who are severely obese and have congestive heart failure; these patients develop respiratory distress marked by hypoventilation with subsequent hypoxemia. The compensatory mechanism of increasing pulmonary artery pressure to improve perfusion leads to right heart hypertrophy, resulting in cor pulmonale. Obesity tends to cause respiratory distress when the weight gain takes place in a short amount of time. People who gain weight over an extended period of time usually have less respiratory distress because they have a longer period in which to adapt to the increased metabolic demands and pressure changes.

Neuromuscular dysfunction causes hypoventilation because of either impaired nervous stimulation and inhibition or impaired muscular activity. When the brain stem is involved in the disease process, respiratory dysfunction occurs in association with disturbances in swallowing and coughing, and there is a disturbance in the reflex control of breathing in the respiratory center. However, the patient often retains control of voluntary breathing. Another source of respiratory dysfunction may be disease affecting the respiratory center in the medulla, which results in hypoventilation. The patient may be able to compensate by voluntary hyperventilation. The respiratory center can also be depressed by narcotics and barbiturates. Anesthesia has the effect of depressing respirations so that hypoventilation occurs. In these situations there is no obstruction to airflow, and alveolar ventilation may be adequate unless additional stress is placed on the respiratory functions (for example, an infection may limit ventilation enough to cause respiratory insufficiency).

Diseases in which there is impaired skeletal muscle function (e.g., muscular dystrophy) also impair the mechanical function of the chest wall so that there is a reduction in vital capacity. In this situation, lung function is not impaired but the ability to change intrathoracic pressure is affected and volumes of air cannot be exchanged effectively. Paresis of the respiratory muscles may occur in many diseases that involve the nervous control of respiration. Myasthenia gravis is an example of a disease that can be complicated by respiratory insufficiency.

Care of patients with reduced lung volume includes a prophylactic program of routine bronchial hygiene and early treatment of infections; it is even better to avoid the occurrence of infection altogether if at all possible. When respiratory insufficiency develops, controlled oxygen flow, based on blood gas analysis, may be given to relieve hypoxemia.

Adult Respiratory Distress Syndrome
The adult respiratory distress syndrome (ARDS) results from a number of different conditions, including hemorrhagic shock in which fluids, blood, and electrolytes have been replaced in excessive amounts, narcotic overdose, pulmonary fat embolism, neurologic trauma, severe pneumonia, and oxygen toxicity. The syndrome is characterized by dyspnea and tachypnea and an increase in the mechanical work of breathing. Lung compliance is decreased, and the lungs are said to be stiff. **Shock lung** and **stiff lung** are two names that are used interchangeably with ARDS. ARDS leads to a decrease in arterial oxygen saturation, which occurs as a result of shunting in the pulmonary capillary bed [6].

ARDS is thought to be caused by damage to the pulmonary capillary membrane, resulting in edema and hemorrhage, as well as by microatelectasis due to decreased surfactant in the alveoli. Once the alveoli close, they remain closed so that oxygen therapy to maintain arterial oxygen tension and the maintenance of ventilation are priorities, even during diagnosis and treatment of the initial cause of the ARDS.

Continuous positive airway pressure (CPAP) system is used to improve oxygen transport and thereby increase oxygen tension. With CPAP, the patient inspires oxygen at a fixed positive pressure of 10 cm H_2O to produce a high end-expiratory pressure [6] to obtain increased functional residual capacity. Perfusion improves because more alveoli remain open, and as a result, Pa_{O_2} tensions increase. Corticosteroids are also given; their effect is probably to stabilize lysosomes, which prevents the added destruction of capillary membranes. Other treatment measures for ARDS are specific to the underlying cause (e.g., shock, excess fluid, septicemia).

The positive end-expiratory pressure (PEEP) technique is also used in some cases. This technique provides a constant positive pressure of 5 to 15 cm H_2O in the expiratory cycle and requires a ventilator. It achieves the same results as CPAP, which does not require a ventilator. It is important to observe the patient for signs and symptoms of tension pneumothorax when using the PEEP technique because of the constant use of high pressure [10]. When the increased airway pressures are conveyed to the intrathoracic space, cardiac functions may be compromised. The use of PEEP is contraindicated in hypovolemic shock until the shock state is corrected because the high pressure may affect the vascular system and interfere with venous return. The inspired gas tension ($F_{I_{O_2}}$) as compared to the arterial tension indicates the effectiveness of perfusion with PEEP.

Narcotic overdose One cause of respiratory distress syndrome that is acute but reversible is overdose of narcotics. This occurrence is increasing in frequency and may be terminal if treatment cannot be instituted soon enough. Narcotic overdose can result from intravenous, subcutaneous, or oral drugs that cause analgesia and produce sleep. Heroin is the most frequent cause of overdose, but morphine, barbiturates, and methadone are also commonly found in cases of overdose.

The classic symptoms of drug overdose are miosis (pinpoint pupils), stupor or coma, and depression of respirations. Since the patient is often in a coma when brought to the emergency room, the nurse or physician may have to search for the signs of drug usage, including the equipment for administration of drugs in the patient's belongings or track marks on the patient's arms, between the toes, or on the heels from repeated intravenous injection of a drug. Often the overdose may be a result of taking more than one kind of drug through different routes, or of mixing drugs with alcohol ingestion. The use of one or more drugs with alcohol can potentiate the overdose and prolong the recovery period.

Initial treatment in drug overdose includes the administration of oxygen (usually 100% concentration), insertion of an artificial airway, and tracheal suctioning to remove secretions or to prevent aspiration. Many physicians prefer to use an Ambu bag rather than intubation initially. Arterial blood gases are drawn and blood samples are obtained for the determination of barbiturate, alcohol, aspirin, or glutethimide levels and glucose levels. Hypoglycemia may be present in heroin overdose, particularly if the patient is addicted, because a prior state of malnutrition may exist since heroin addicts tend to have no hunger or desire for food. Obtaining glucose levels also helps in the differential diagnosis of diabetic coma. Both a narcotic antagonist (naloxone hydrochloride) and glucose (50 ml of 50% glucose) are given intravenously. Blood pressure and pulse should be checked, and if hypotension is present, volume expanders are given. Central venous pressure is used to monitor fluid therapy. If the cause of the coma is drug overdose, administration of naloxone generally elicits a response. (Naloxone is used because it does not cause respiratory depression as do other narcotic antagonists.) The patient becomes more alert and oriented if the naloxone is effective. If the patient is addicted to drugs, the naloxone may cause symptoms of withdrawal, including dilated pupils, nausea and vomiting, and chills. When these symptoms are noted, the patient should be given follow-up care for the treatment of addiction.

The complications of narcotic overdose include aspiration pneumonia and pulmonary edema. Aspiration pneumonia often results if attempts have been made to revive the patient with beverages such as water or milk. Pulmonary edema may result if hypoxia has been acute. Treatment for pulmonary edema, confirmed by chest x-ray, includes the administration of oxygen with ventilation, guided by blood gas levels. Initially the patient with drug overdose has a combined respiratory acidosis and metabolic alkalosis (or metabolic acidosis if the Pa_{O_2} is low enough) with an elevated Pa_{CO_2} and a low Pa_{O_2} and pH. After administration of oxygen, the Pa_{CO_2} and the pH return to normal. If either aspiration pneumonia or pulmonary edema is present the pH and Pa_{O_2} levels will continue to be low following treatment. Other symptoms of pulmonary edema include lethargy, tachypnea, abnormal breath sounds, and cyanosis.

Acute Respiratory Failure

Acute respiratory failure is characterized by a Pa_{O_2} of less than 50 mm Hg. Often there is a corresponding hypercapnia associated with the hypoxemia. The patient in respiratory failure may or may not have an increased carbon dioxide retention. A level of Pa_{CO_2} of more than 50 mm Hg is **acute ventilatory failure** [16]. Initially in the acute situation, emphasis is placed on increasing the levels of oxygen in arterial blood, which is accomplished by oxygen therapy. The importance of controlling oxygen therapy cannot be overemphasized. A result of giving oxygen in high concentrations to achieve high oxygen tension over a period of time is progressive pulmonary tissue damage causing stiffness of lung tissue. In patients with hypercapnia the administration of high concentrations of oxygen may cause further retention of carbon dioxide and lead to carbon dioxide narcosis. Patients with chronic lung disease may be dependent on the respiratory stimulation of hypoxemia; giving high concentrations of oxygen can eliminate this stimulus to respiration so that the oxygen only serves to depress respirations further. Hypoxemia always coexists with acute ventilatory failure.

Respiratory acidosis occurs when hypercapnia exists. The normal body compensation is retention of bicarbonate by the kidneys with excretion of H^+ ions; this process of renal compensation extends over a period of days to weeks. Levels of hypercapnia as high as 60 to 65 mm Hg of Pa_{CO_2} can be compensated for by the kidneys. The arterial pH drops when the Pa_{CO_2} levels exceed 65 mm Hg. A normal pH with elevated Pa_{CO_2} levels is indicative of chronic respiratory acidosis. In this condition the patient has adapted to the high levels of arterial carbon dioxide, and signs of neural involvement are usually not present; in acute respiratory acidosis, however, increased arterial carbon dioxide levels quickly cause neurologic signs.

Treatment for respiratory failure differs if there is chronic or acute hypercapnia, or if there is hypoxemia without hypercapnia. If the patient is in acidosis, care involves measures to decrease the amount of carbon dioxide produced through metabolic activity. Bed rest is important to achieve reduction in metabolic activity. Another important goal of therapy is to increase carbon dioxide excretion by the lungs, which is accomplished by reducing or relieving the factors that have precipitated the respiratory insufficiency and subsequent failure. Removal of secretions, reduction of the work of breathing, and treatment of infections are measures that reduce or relieve respiratory insufficiency and are also important in resolving respiratory failure.

The patient with acute respiratory failure has symptoms directly related to the effects of the failure and the underlying disease processes, which often makes immediate diagnosis difficult. For example, when respiratory failure is associated with trauma, the patient may be in shock and may have cranial damage or any number of other problems. The signs and symptoms specifically related to respiratory failure include tachycardia, restlessness, and confusion. Diaphoresis and headache may be present. Although the patient may initially be hypertensive as a result of compensatory responses, he becomes hypotensive, and respirations are depressed. Cyanosis is usually a later symptom. Chest expansion may be reduced. Neurologic signs of severe respiratory failure include asterixis (the flapping tremor associated with carbon dioxide narcosis) and unconsciousness.

Differentiation between respiratory insufficiency and respiratory failure is made by arterial blood gas studies and determination of the pH. In respiratory insufficiency the Pa_{O_2} levels may be as low as 60 mm Hg at sea level. At this point the chemoreceptors in the carotid and aortic bodies are stimulated and ventilation is increased. Hyperventilation is then a compensatory mechanism, which has the effect of increasing the inspired oxygen so that alveolar hyperventilation results. In this situation carbon dioxide is excreted more rapidly, and respiratory alkalosis develops. In addition to hyperventilation, the hypoxemia causes an increased heart rate through action on the chemoreceptors that stimulate the vasomotor centers. A compensatory mechanism that aids the perfusion of lung tissue in the presence of unequal ventilation and perfusion is the constriction of alveolar capillaries in the hypoventilated alveolar spaces, which conserves blood flow for the hyperventilated alveolar spaces; this explains why tachycardia occurs early in respiratory insufficiency and continues in respiratory failure. If the myocardium can respond to the increased load, this compensatory mechanism is temporarily adequate. If respiratory insufficiency is allowed to progress, however, the result is increasing fatigue, which is related both to the increased myocardial load causing hypertension and to the increased work of breathing. Normally the work of breathing uses only about 2 percent of the metabolic oxygen consumption; with increased work of breathing the percentage of the total metabolic consumption of oxygen to accomplish the work of breathing may account for as much as 40 percent of the total. When hypoxia continues, the oxygenation of body cells is impaired. The brain, which uses about 20 percent of the total oxygen supply, responds to hypoxia. Restlessness, irritability, and the inability to make decisions are early signs of hypoxemia in which cerebral circulation provides inadequate oxygen. Later there may be confusion and impaired motor function. Eventually, if the Pa_{O_2} is reduced below 30 mm Hg, coma ensues along with lactic acidosis, a condition discussed more fully in Chapter 16.

In view of these changes, treatment is based first on increasing the supply of oxygen to the body cells. Generally, moderate concentrations of oxygen (sometimes as high as 32%) are given. The oxygen reduces the hypoxemia and decreases both the myocardial work load and the work of breathing. Oxygen is given in conjunction with bed rest, which is important to reduce the metabolic requirement for oxygen consumption as much as possible so that the pattern of breathing can be restored to normal and the compensatory mechanisms can be effective until oxygen tensions are increased.

Causes of Respiratory Failure

The factors that have contributed to respiratory failure must be identified and treated as well. In pneumonia, for example, elevated temperature increases the metabolic work load, increasing oxygen requirements. The secretions associated with pneumonia can obstruct ventilation, and the cellular changes in the alveoli restrict alveolar movement and diffusion of gases across the alveolar membranes so that both restrictive and obstructive elements of dysfunction are involved in creating the hypoxemia. Resolution of the disease process, with reduction of fever and removal of secretions during the resolution, is an important adjunct to improving ventilation and perfusion throughout the lung.

Pulmonary edema or postoperative atelectasis may result in right-to-left shunting, which is caused by inadequate ventilation and perfusion in some alveoli so that poorly perfused blood mixes with the adequately perfused blood in the arterial system. The end result is a lower oxygen tension which, if severe enough, leads to hypoxemia.

General determination of a patient's ability to compensate in hypoxic states includes assessment of health status prior to the development of respiratory insufficiency or failure and the patient's age. These factors are related to the perfusion of oxygen. Oxygen tension in arterial circulation decreases with age, being approximately 95 mm Hg up to age 30 and decreasing to about 80 mm Hg by age 60 [9]; thereafter the oxygen tensions are reduced by 1 mm Hg per year because of aging. Therefore the compensatory mechanisms for hypoxia are less effective with increasing age, and respiratory failure may result more quickly.

Two other factors important in the perfusion of oxygen are the hemoglobin level and the hemoglobin dissociation curve. Hemoglobin is the principal carrier of oxygen. The oxyhemoglobin is then related to the total amount of hemoglobin available to transport the oxygen. In hypoxic states, the nature of the oxyhemoglobin dissociation curve is important. The curve shifts to the right in response to hypoxia, decreasing the amount of oxygen bound to hemoglobin so that increasing levels of oxygen can be released to the body capillaries. This mechanism is dependent on erythrocyte levels of 2,3-diphosphoglycerate; in hypoxia and alkalosis (high pH) the level is increased and in acidosis (low pH) it is decreased.

Another factor related to the patient's physical state is the adequacy of the cardiovascular system. Delivery of oxygen to the cells depends on an adequately functioning cardiac pump and adequate peripheral circulation. Factors that impair the function of the pump, such as cardiac disease, or that impair peripheral circulation must be assessed to determine the effects of hypoxia on the tissues. If the patient has an infection with increased temperature, the metabolic work load is increased, which also presents difficulties in reinstating adequate oxygenation.

Oxygen Therapy

Treatment for respiratory failure focuses on providing oxygen and humidification. The methods used for administering oxygen include nasal cannulas, catheters, closed masks, face tents, and hoods. These methods are classified as either high flow systems, which are closed systems that limit the patient's gas for breathing to that delivered from the oxygen administration device, or low flow systems, in which the patient breathes oxygen concentrations in addition to room air. The Venturi mask, which covers both the mouth and the nose, is an example of a high flow system that can be set to provide either high or low concentrations of oxygen in percentages at a determined F_{IO_2}; these masks are available for administering 24, 28, 35, or 40% oxygen [10]. Both the temperature and humidity of the gas can be controlled with a Venturi mask. Positive pressure devices may be used when it is desirable to force air into the lungs, as in restrictive diseases such as pneumonia. Generally, it is difficult to manage the air mix with positive pressure devices, and it is important to measure blood gas levels periodically to ensure that the oxygen concentration is not too high or too low.

Nasal cannulas and catheters Nasal cannulas and nasal catheters are examples of low flow systems. In these systems, the anatomic reservoir (nose, nasopharynx, and oropharynx) is filled with oxygen in the required concentration. This gas is mixed with the flow of inspired room air, providing the total concentration of oxygen that the patient receives. These systems do not provide a specific concentration of oxygen, such as a closed system can deliver, and the concentration of oxygen the patient receives can only be estimated.

A nasal cannula or catheter gives an approximate F_{IO_2} of 44 percent at a rate of 6 liters, while a mask gives an F_{IO_2} of approximately 50 percent at the same flow rate. When a reservoir bag is used with the oxygen delivery system, an F_{IO_2} of 60 percent can be achieved with a flow rate of 6 liters [12]. The reservoir bag consists of a mask with the bag attached. These devices vary according to the manufacturer, and the nurse should know that the size of the oxygen reservoir provided by the bag determines the percentage of oxygen that can be given. When a mask is used over the nose and mouth, it is necessary to have a flow rate of at least 5 liters so that the expired air will be flushed from the system; otherwise the patient will be rebreathing the expired air.

The nurse should be aware that tidal volume directly affects the F_{IO_2} received with a nasal cannula or catheter. When the tidal volume decreases, the F_{IO_2} increases. Therefore, when a patient takes short or shallow breaths when receiving oxygen via nasal catheter, the F_{IO_2} being delivered is increased. This means that at a given flow rate of oxygen, the patient is receiving a higher concentration of oxygen when his tidal volume is smaller than he would receive if his tidal volume were greater.

It is also important for the nurse to ascertain whether the patient's nares are patent when inserting a nasal catheter or prongs, since air will not flow through obstructed nares. Correct technique should be used when inserting the catheter. Insertion of the catheter is easier if it is first moistened in a water-soluble lubricant. The distance from the top of the nose to the ear lobe is measured to determine how far the catheter should be inserted. Placement should be checked, using a flashlight as a light source to make certain that the tip of the catheter is just above the uvula. After insertion, the catheter is taped to the side of the face in a comfortable position, so that the catheter does not tug or pull at the nares. Nasal cannulas are more comfortable and are sometimes selected in preference to catheters because it is easier for the patient to eat and talk with a nasal cannula. The nasal catheter, when used, should be removed and reinserted in the opposite nostril every 6 to 8 hours.

Nursing care of patients receiving oxygen therapy in any form requires attention to the feelings they may have in regard to the interference with communication and eating, since they must adjust to the continual presence of catheters and cannulas or masks. Nursing care must be supportive, and the nurse must provide for alternate modes of communication (particularly when masks are used) to promote the understanding and trust important to the patient's sense of security. The nurse should also be aware that patients who are hypoxemic or who have hypoxia often fight the oxygen therapy. The ability to breathe in cooperation with the oxygen therapy improves as the patient's condition improves.

Monitoring blood gas levels Blood gas levels are an important guide to oxygen therapy. The collection of arterial blood samples involves the use of a heparinized solution, which is first drawn into a syringe to fill the needle before the blood sample is drawn. The sample is then placed in ice. Glass syringes are used to prevent the diffusion of gases that occurs with plastic syringes. The site of injection should be covered with pressure for 5 minutes after the sample is drawn. When it is necessary to measure a patient's blood gases repeatedly as a guide to oxygen therapy, an arterial line may be inserted to eliminate the need for repeated needle injections.

When oxygen therapy is required, it is desirable to maintain Pa_{O_2} levels of at least 70 mm Hg and Pa_{CO_2} levels at normal values of 40 mm Hg or less, according to the patient's normal levels. Having the patient breathe 40 to 50% oxygen for 20 or 30 minutes will differentiate between hypoxemia caused by a diffusion block and that caused by shunting. High concentrations of oxygen will increase Pa_{O_2} tensions if a diffusion block is present but will not improve Pa_{O_2} tensions in the presence of a right-to-left shunt.

Concentrations of oxygen Oxygen concentrations appropriate to the care of specific patients are determined by the cause of respiratory failure. Oxygen in low concentrations (F_{IO_2} below 35 percent) is indicated when the hypoxemia is a result of chronic lung disease. Moderate concentrations (F_{IO_2} of 35 to 60 percent) are given when there is acute respiratory dysfunction, such as in pneumonia. High concentrations of oxygen (F_{IO_2} of 60 to 100 percent) are administered with controlled flow devices, such as a ventilator that supplies oxygen in a closed system; these high concentrations are given for short duration when the patient is in acute reversible respiratory failure [12]. Carbon monoxide poisoning and apnea are examples of reversible conditions requiring high concentrations of oxygen for short periods.

The nurse must observe the patient carefully to ascertain the effectiveness of oxygen therapy. In any case, high oxygen concentrations are not given for extended periods (more than 24 hours) because they may cause oxygen toxicity. Among the observations related to hypoxemia are tachycardia, dyspnea, metabolic acidosis, and arrhythmias, and determination of the presence of pulmonary hypertension. The inspired oxygen concentrations are measured by an oxygen analyzer to determine the effectiveness of the equipment being used. The nurse must make careful and periodic checks of the equipment to ensure that the closed system required when giving high oxygen concentrations is maintained.

An increase in the Pa_{CO_2} and a concomitant fall in the pH are significant, because these values may indicate ventilatory failure.

Humidification Oxygen is a dry gas and must be moisturized to prevent dehydration of the mucosa of the airways. The humidification of oxygen can be provided by vapor or particulate water or by the addition of aerosolized water. The relative humidity should be maintained at 60 to 65 percent of body temperature when oxygen therapy is given. When a nasal cannula is used to administer oxygen, humidification is provided by a water nebulizer. The use of heated sterile distilled water (127°F; 53°C) is considered more beneficial in providing moisture. Increasing the temperature increases the amount of water vapor in the air; the temperature decreases in transit so that by the time the oxygen reaches the patient's airways, the air temperature is similar to the body temperature.

Aerosol delivers minute liquid particles to the mucosa of the airways. Ultrasonic nebulization is most effective because the particles are smaller. The amount of fluid used every 24 hours should be carefully recorded and evaluated by the nurse since the amount of water being delivered, if in excess, may cause congestion in the lungs. Aerosol is helpful in diluting secretions so that they can be more easily removed. In addition, it helps maintain normal ciliary activity, which is also important for removing secretions. Usually a mixture of one-half distilled water and one-half saline solution is used because distilled water alone tends to irritate the respiratory mucosa. It is important to check the nebulizer for both condensation of water and formation of crusts. All tubing, catheters, or cannulas, and the water should be changed completely at least once every 24 hours. Because heated water is a good medium for bacterial growth, careful cleaning of nebulizers is important. Equipment must be cleaned routinely between use for the patient and should always be thoroughly cleaned between patients. Disposable humidifiers and nebulizers are valuable in preventing nosocomial infections.

Intermittent positive pressure breathing Intermittent positive pressure breathing (IPPB) may be used for patients with hypercapnia, atelectasis, and lung infections, as well as in generalized postoperative care. It is usually prescribed for a given period, such as 15 minutes, three times per day. IPPB is frequently used in the administration of bronchodilator drugs for patients with chronic lung disease. IPPB uses pressure greater than atmospheric pressure during inspiration so that air is forced deep into the air passages. It is important that the patient learn to breathe with the machine, taking slow, controlled inspiratory breaths to overcome the natural tendency to hyperventilate with IPPB. Expiration is controlled by the patient. When IPPB is used in conjunction with oxygen therapy, it is necessary to continue the oxygen flow by using a blender device so that the desired oxygen tension is maintained.

Importance of flow rate and concentration It is most beneficial to administer oxygen continuously, since experimentation has shown that intermittent oxygen therapy may be more harmful to the patient. Giving high levels of oxygen concentration for a period of time and then discontinuing the oxygen causes the patient's Pa_{O_2} to decrease further than before the administration of oxygen because of the slope of the oxygen dissociation curve. It is best to give the appropriate concentration consistently to maintain the desired level of oxygen. Patients with chronic lung disease who depend on hypoxia for the stimulation of respiration respond best to a flow rate of 0.5 to 4 liters of oxygen; at this flow rate they usually do not develop hypercapnia. Rates higher than 4 liters cause respiratory depression with retention of carbon dioxide and can lead to carbon dioxide narcosis.

A basic concept of oxygen therapy is that the patient must be given only sufficient oxygen to maintain tissue perfusion. During oxygen therapy the percentage of oxygen administered is based on this level. Lower flow rates are given initially; blood gas analysis demonstrates the effectiveness of the low flow rate, and adjustments are made by increasing the flow rates if the Pa_{O_2} continues to be low. In ventilatory insufficiency the Pa_{CO_2} is used to determine the effectiveness of therapy. Normal levels of 40 to 46 mm Hg are desirable, although some authorities prefer arterial tensions of 50 to 60 mm Hg in patients habituated to increased levels [10]. Evidence of the effectiveness of oxygen therapy is measured by the reduction of tachycardia, arrhythmias, dyspnea, and cyanosis and through blood gas analysis.

Oxygen toxicity can cause inactivation of pulmonary surfactant, increasing the possibility of atelectasis or pulmonary edema or both and creating the potential for further decrease in the diffusion rate of gas in alveolar circulation. The nurse should recognize the signs and symptoms of oxygen toxicity, which include nausea, vomiting, malaise, and discomfort in the substernal area. Later symptoms are the same as or similar to those previously described for respiratory insufficiency. Pulmonary congestion and loss of elastic recoil of the lungs may result in permanent damage to the lung tissue.

Shapiro [12] states that a concentration of 50 to 60% oxygen seems to be the threshold below which there is little evidence of oxygen toxicity. A healthy person can tolerate 100% oxygen at one atmosphere of pressure for 24 hours. However, there is always a risk of oxygen toxicity, and the threshold at which it occurs varies among patients. It seems that the rate of onset of the oxygen toxicity disease process is proportional both to the tension of oxygen and to the duration of the exposure [12].

The use of cannulation (intubation or tracheostomy) or mechanically assisted ventilation when hypoxia exists without carbon dioxide retention is controversial. These methods are used when the Pa_{O_2} levels are not maintained with oxygen therapy or when carbon dioxide retention results. Fatigue, which is caused by the inability to reduce the metabolic consumption of oxygen or is related to cardiac dysfunction, indicates the need to use assisted ventilation to prevent the patient from further fatigue and deterioration.

Mechanically assisted ventilation During emergency care, ventilation is assisted with an Ambu bag or similar device. The Ambu bag provides a higher concentration of oxygen than other types of hand-operated assisting devices. Mechanically assisted ventilation is necessary if the patient is apneic, if he or she has hypercapnia or a pH of less than 7.25 or both, when a neuromuscular disease or trauma precludes adequate mechanical functions of the respiratory system, and in the presence of atelectasis. There are many different types of ventilators and devices that can be used in conjunction with the ventilator. Essentially, all ventilators deliver air under pressure into the lungs. Their functioning depends on establishing a closed system from the ventilator to the lungs so that the pressure is not lost in transit; this is accomplished by inserting an endotracheal tube or by attaching the ventilator to a tracheostomy tube. The latter method is used when assisted ventilation is anticipated for more than five days. Intubation allows for better removal of secretions.

The different types of ventilators include time-cycled, pressure-cycled, pressure-limited, volume-cycled, and volume-limited ventilators. The time-cycled ventilators usually deliver a fixed inspiratory-to-expiratory ratio with constant volume ventilation; these ventilators frequently have PEEP devices. Pressure-cycled ventilators usually do not provide for a constant tidal volume because the volume varies according to the airways resistance. Volume-cycled ventilators generally deliver a constant tidal volume and can be cycled by the patient's respiratory rate.

Pressure-limited ventilators have air mix devices that can be used to dilute 100% oxygen. Inspiratory pressure is directly related to the percentage of oxygen inspired; as the flow rate is decreased, the oxygen tension increases. Nebulizer lines decrease oxygen tension. Volume-limited ventilators allow for more precise determination of oxygen, because the percentage of oxygen is directly related to the oxygen flow rate.

Mechanical ventilators may be used with or without oxygen. Without oxygen, the ventilators deliver room air. The concentration of oxygen may be increased over that of room air either by adding oxygen or by using a ventilator powered by an oxygen source. Air mix devices provide for mixed concentrations of oxygen with room air. There are also devices that can be used with ventilators to monitor the tidal volume and rate and to estimate the minute volume; they have an alarm system in the event apnea occurs. An important adjunct to mechanical ventilation is humidification; many ventilators have a humidifying system or provide for the attachment of humidification devices. Modern ventilators have a "sighing" mechanism that allows for periodic deep breaths to inflate the lungs, which is necessary to prevent atelectasis. If the ventilator does not provide for periodic deep breathing, this may be accomplished by using a self-inflating bag such as the Ambu bag. Hourly sighing using this method is desirable to aerate the alveoli and to activate surfactant.

Nursing care for patients with mechanically assisted ventilation includes maintaining an open airway, monitoring blood gases, providing for comfort, and adjusting the ventilators as necessary. Managing the care of patients on ventilators is a nursing practice specialty. In general, the nurse must be careful to suction the airways periodically or as necessary to keep them clear and to turn the patients frequently to provide for drainage of lung segments. When the patient has copious amounts of mucus, therapeutic bronchoscopy may be necessary. The nurse's observations are important in determining changes that may necessitate bronchoscopy. In addition, precise attention to routine changes of tubing, hoses, and masks (a source of gram-negative bacteria causing nosocomial infections), is a vital aspect of care [12].

The nurse should also make periodic notation of the placement of the endotracheal tube if one is used. It is important to know that the cuff may obstruct the airway. The cuff is inflated with low pressure so that there is minimal leakage of air around the cuff. Ongoing measurements of arterial blood gases and pH determine the ventilator adjustments. Usually ventilators are set for the desired tidal volume (approximately 10 ml per kilogram and a respiratory rate of 12 to 14 per minute), and the tidal volume is determined by the desired alveolar ventilation. The duration of inspirations should not exceed that of expirations, and the degree of humidification and the inspired oxygen concentration should be measured periodically.

Initially the patient may be hyperventilated (unless chronic lung disease is present) to increase the Pa_{O_2} and decrease the Pa_{CO_2}; thereafter the tidal volume is adjusted to maintain the Pa_{CO_2} at 35 to 46 mm Hg and the Pa_{O_2} at 70 to 100 mm Hg. In hypercapnia it is very important to lower the Pa_{CO_2} gradually to prevent the occurrence of rebound metabolic alkalosis. A general rule is to lower the Pa_{CO_2} 5 to 10 mm per hour until the Pa_{CO_2} is about 50 mm Hg and the pH is about 7.50. The ratio of Pa_{CO_2} to pH is important since rapid reduction of Pa_{CO_2} levels may rapidly increase the pH.

In addition to measuring the blood gases, the nurse should also observe the patient for changes in pulse rate, blood pressure, comfort, and patterns of breathing. It is not unusual for the patient to fight the respirator; this may occur when the rate of the ventilator is different from the patient's rate, as in tachypnea. Skillful regulation of the ventilator rate can minimize this discomfort. The ventilator rate can initially be set at a more rapid pace and then decreased as the patient's ventilation improves. It may be necessary to give the patient a sedative, but this should be carefully considered because sedatives depress respiration. Curare drugs are often used. The patient often fights the respirator when he is underventilated, or when he feels pain or is anxious. The nurse must learn to assess the patient's needs and provide the required support. Increasing ventilation may be essential, along with dealing directly with the patient's fears and anxieties about his dysfunction, care and treatment, and his future.

When the patient demonstrates improved

ventilation he may be weaned from the ventilator. Weaning may begin by changing from controlled to assisted ventilation and then from assisted ventilation to oxygen administration until the patient can breathe comfortably in room air. Different methods are used to determine the patient's readiness for weaning. In some hospitals a respirometer reading of the forced vital capacity (FVC) is made; if the FVC has increased to 1 liter, the patient is considered ready for weaning. Another measure is that of determining the spontaneous minute volume. Following a long period of mechanically assisted ventilation, the patient may have become dependent on the ventilator and sometimes loses diaphragmatic coordination. The nurse must provide psychological support for the patient who is being weaned so that the effects of losing the ventilator's security can be minimized. If this support is not adequate, the patient's emotional response to being weaned may augment his respiratory insufficiency and can be a factor in prolonging hospitalization. Intermittent mandatory ventilation and intermittent demand ventilation are newly developing techniques directed toward allowing the patient to gradually resume the work of breathing.

Results of oxygen therapy The outcome of oxygen therapy depends on whether the therapy was initiated early enough to prevent tissue damage related to lack of oxygen, and whether the patient's condition is reversible. If the initial cause of the oxygen insufficiency is reversible, the patient may recover following acute failure and may be able to conduct normal daily activities; this is typical of the patient who was in good health prior to failure and who has a disease process such as pneumonia that can be resolved. For patients with chronic lung disease or irreversible lung dysfunction, oxygen therapy may be continued indefinitely. This is accomplished by the use of portable oxygen equipment that the patient can take with him wherever he goes. Such a person is dependent on oxygen for activity but has increased freedom of movement; without oxygen, he might have to remain in bed or have very limited activity such as sitting up in a chair since none of the body's compensatory mechanisms, such as polycythemia, can increase oxygen supplies sufficiently to support mobility. With oxygen therapy the work load of breathing is reduced and the person is able to be more active with less respiratory insufficiency.

Polycythemia, even though it is a compensatory mechanism to improve cellular oxygenation, can also influence increased hypoxia. The increased red cell volume that occurs with polycythemia increases the viscosity of the blood, thereby increasing the incidence of hypertension and right heart failure.

Hypoxemia

Hypoxemia associated with hypercapnia in respiratory failure has implications for nursing care. If the patient is seen initially in the emergency room with respiratory distress, the cardiovascular complications may be diagnosed and treated first. Respiratory failure involving both hypoxemia and hypercapnia may cause cardiomegaly, arrhythmias, pulmonary edema, and hypertension (in some patients, hypotension rather than hypertension results). In long-standing respiratory insufficiency there is concomitant enlargement of the right heart. The patient may have peripheral edema. It is important to ascertain the kinds of symptoms the patient has experienced; questioning the patient or his family about the presence of paroxysmal nocturnal dyspnea will help differentiate between respiratory failure and cardiac failure. Paroxysmal nocturnal dyspnea is a symptom of right heart failure and is usually not a previous symptom if the patient has developed acute respiratory failure from primary pulmonary pathology. Hepatomegaly, which is a symptom of congestive heart failure, can also occur when the Pa_{O_2} is below 80 or 85 mm Hg. This is related to the development of pulmonary hypertension from hypoxemia; the right ventricle must work harder in the presence of pulmonary hypertension that is complicated by respiratory acidosis.

Cardiac arrhythmias can also result from hypoxemia, when the myocardium has insufficient oxygen. Production of adenosine triphosphate is decreased and muscle contraction is consequently impaired. Another factor that contributes to the development of cardiac arrhythmias is the acid-base imbalance that occurs with respiratory failure. Sinus tachycardia often results from impaired membrane potential from changes in the pH; other arrhythmias may also occur. It has been noted that beta-adrenergic stimulating drugs used with nebulizers can be absorbed through the mucous membranes, causing sinus tachycardia and ventricular ectopic heartbeats. The procedure of rinsing the mouth following inhalation of nebulized aerosol reduces the occurrence of arrhythmias.

Establishing an Airway in Respiratory Failure

Overdose of narcotics or heroin may result in pulmonary edema, causing acute respiratory failure. Whatever the cause, respiratory failure is an emergency. Initial treatment consists in establishing an airway by the use of an airway tube or an endotracheal tube. Airway tubes may be inserted through either the nose or the mouth and extend to the pharynx; they allow for suctioning or for mouth-to-mouth resuscitation. Endotracheal tubes may also be inserted through the mouth or the nose and are required for patients who are in a coma or who may require mechanically assisted ventilation. The presence of a gag reflex is determined prior to the selection of an appropriate tube. Either nasopharyngeal or oropharyngeal airway tubes may be used if the gag reflex is adequate. Endotracheal intubation is used if the gag reflex is diminished or absent, and if the patient has copious secretions.

It is imperative to remove secretions from the airway prior to inserting either an airway tube or an endotracheal tube; this may be accomplished with oropharyngeal or nasopharyngeal suctioning. If this is not successful, IPPB may be used. Bronchoscopy is required to remove secretions if the IPPB is not effective; when bronchoscopy is not successful, a tracheostomy is performed. Airway tubes or endotracheal tubes are used for short-term intervention of 48 to 72 hours; complications such as laryngeal trauma with edema may occur if the tubes are left in place for longer than 72 hours. A tracheostomy requires a surgical procedure and is performed when long-term intervention is anticipated. Both endotracheal and tracheostomy tubes can be used with or without mechanically assisted ventilation. Both are supplied with or without cuffs to prevent aspiration and air leaks around the tube in the event mechanically assisted ventilation is used. Generally oropharyngeal approaches are easier and allow for insertion of tubes with larger diameters while nasopharyngeal approaches are better tolerated. Both interfere with coughing because the vocal cords cannot close normally as the tube is inserted between the cords. Mouth care is important with both types of tubes and it is necessary to change the site of taping of the tubes to prevent tissue irritation.

Endotracheal intubation Prior to insertion of an endotracheal tube the patient's dentures or bridges are removed. The insertion is facilitated by local anesthesia. A laryngoscope blade is used as a guide to insert the tube between the vocal cords into the larynx and then into the trachea. The endotracheal tube is inserted far enough so that the cuff can be inflated in the trachea. After the cuff is inflated, the tube is marked at the point of insertion and the tubes are taped to the cheek to prevent pulling. It is important that the lumen of the endotracheal tube be large enough to maintain the pressure gradients between the alveoli and the air passage and that the cuff be inflated sufficiently to prevent air leaks but not so much as to cause injury to the mucous membranes of the trachea. The patency of the tube is checked by feeling for the exhalation of air and by spirometric studies.

Complications of endotracheal intubation are prevented by careful attention to routine care. The placement of the tube should be noted, since the tube can be displaced and travel to one of the major bronchi, often the right stem bronchus. The tube can also erode the carina. Notation of the mark at the point of insertion at the nose or mouth is used to monitor this displacement of the tube. Breath sounds in both lungs should be checked. Attention to suctioning is essential to avoid plugging, which can cause obstruction of the airway. Other complications are related to overinflation of the cuff. The mucosa in the area of the overinflated cuff can be damaged, causing bleeding or erosion of tissue. Later complications may include either fistulas that form at the site or stenosis of the trachea in the area of injury (Fig. 3-8).

The effectiveness of intubation is measured crudely by feeling the air pressure at the end of the tubing. Precise measurement of the tidal volume is accomplished by using a spirometer. A vital capacity of about 10 ml per kilogram of body weight is necessary to provide for adequate gas exchange. Blood gases give the most definitive measurement of the effectiveness of ventilation and perfusion. The nurse should also note subtle changes in the patient's skin tone or color; these changes are not precise measurements, however, because cyanosis occurs when hypoxemia is well established, and a patient's skin color may appear different in different light.

Tracheostomy As previously mentioned, a tracheostomy is performed when intubation is necessary for more than 3 to 5 days because of continued respiratory failure or paralysis of the trachea. It is sometimes difficult to determine whether a tracheostomy should be performed, but many authorities believe that if there is a question, it is better to perform the tracheostomy. The tracheostomy provides for more controlled ventilation and oxygen therapy and for suctioning when long-term care is needed to prevent respiratory fatigue. However, tracheostomy increases the patient's susceptibility to pulmonary infection. The procedure is best performed as a planned surgical procedure in which adequate attention is given to technique and to postoperative care to prevent complications. Generally, a tracheostomy should not be done on an emergency basis; the procedure that is performed to provide an airway in an emergency is a **cricothyreotomy.** In this procedure a small transverse incision (2 to 2.5 cm) is made through the cricothyroid membrane between the thyroid cartilage and the cricoid cartilage. A cricothyreotomy can be performed easily and provides for a temporary airway until a standard tracheostomy can be done.

The incision for a tracheostomy is usually placed at the second cartilaginous ring below the cricoid cartilage. At this point the trachea is close to the skin surface and there are fewer blood vessels. Correct placement is important to avoid the isthmus of the thyroid. Complications of tracheostomy are bleeding, infection, and tracheal stenosis. The bleeding may occur immediately or several days following surgery. Infection may result from failure to use sterile technique when giving tracheostomy care or from inadequate cleaning of tubes and hoses and ventilator or oxygen equipment. Organisms from the equipment or from the site of the tracheal incision can

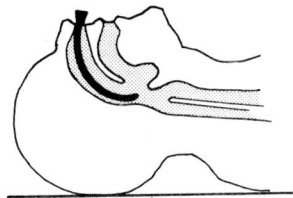
Nasopharyngeal airway

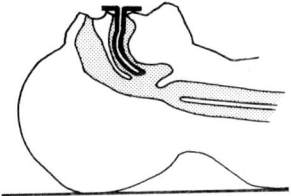
Oropharyngeal airway

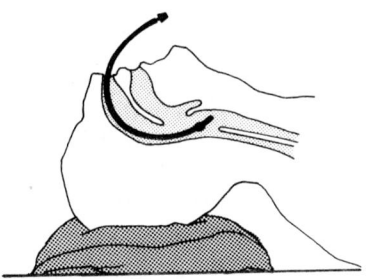
Nasotracheal intubation

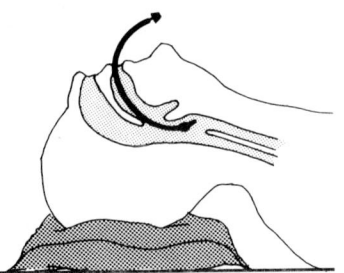
Orotracheal intubation

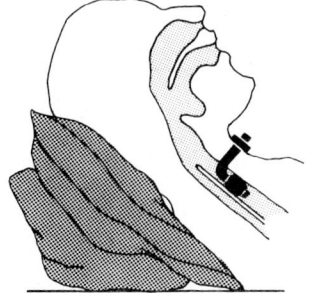
Tracheostomy tube

Figure 3-8
Comparison of devices used to establish an airway.

cause pulmonary infection. Another complication is tracheal stenosis, which follows injury to the tracheal mucosa resulting from performing the tracheostomy, the pressure of endotracheal or tracheal tubes, or forced suctioning.

An important result of a tracheostomy is that it precludes talking; the patient can form words but cannot produce sound. The tracheostomy opening must be covered if the person is to speak. The nurse must be sensitive to the patient's expressions and, if the patient is well enough, should provide paper or a slate so that he can write short messages.

Most hospitals have a specific protocol for tracheostomy care; it incorporates the principles of sterile technique along with the use of careful suctioning to prevent infection and injury to the tracheal mucosa. Suctioning should be done only when necessary, whereas tracheostomy care should be done on a routine basis, at least once every 8 hours. Sterile equipment and sterile technique should be used for both tracheostomy care and suctioning. It is essential that the nurse's hands be washed prior to giving tracheostomy care, and sterile gloves must be worn during the procedure [2, 12].

CARE OF EQUIPMENT Tracheostomy tubes may have either single or double cannulas. A double cannula tracheostomy tube consists of an inner and outer cannula. The outer cannula stays in place while the inner cannula can be removed for cleaning. Single cannulas made of plastic conform more to the shape of the trachea; however, tracheostomy tubes with an inner cannula are easier to clean. Plastic tracheostomy tubes cause less damage to the tracheal stoma and to the mucosa at the site of the cannula tip; this damage generally occurs as the tracheostomy tube is moved about while in place [7].

Tracheostomy care includes cleaning the skin immediately around the tracheostomy incision, using hydrogen peroxide and sterile water, with careful attention to sterile technique. The dressing around the tracheostomy tube is changed and an antibiotic ointment is applied around the incision. Cotton or fluff dressings are never used because particles can be inhaled. It is important to secure the tracheostomy tube with twill tape, which is attached to the tube and fastened around the patient's neck and which prevents accidental removal of the tube when the patient moves or coughs.

If a double cannula tracheostomy tube is used, the inner cannula is removed using aseptic technique and is cleaned with hydrogen peroxide and sterile water; sterile adapters are used to remove dried crusts that may have accumulated around the sides of the tube. If the patient is also receiving oxygen or is on a ventilator, these treatments are continued through the outer cannula, which remains in place while the inner cannula is removed for cleaning. Secretions are sometimes cultured weekly to monitor the presence of infection. This procedure varies among institutions, however, and sometimes cultures are done only when an infection is suspected.

The nurse should maintain suction catheters so that they remain free of bacterial contaminants, which is best accomplished by using a new sterile catheter for each suctioning. If catheters cannot be discarded following each suctioning procedure, the suction catheter should be disinfected so that it is ready for the next use. Disinfection between procedures may be accomplished by flushing the catheter either with a 1% solution of acetic acid or with 70 to 90% alcohol (ethyl or isopropyl). The catheter is then rinsed with freshly poured sterile water using a sterile container and finally wrapped in a sterile towel. The solution used for rinsing and the sterile containers should be changed completely every 8 hours. Another effective procedure consists in using hydrogen peroxide to soak the catheter, followed by rinsing with 70% ethyl or isopropyl alcohol and then rinsing the catheter with sterile water and wrapping it in a sterile towel [2]. In addition to taking care of the catheters, the nurse should completely change the suction bottles every 12 hours, replacing them with new sterile bottles and sterile water [2].

TECHNIQUES OF SUCTIONING Suctioning the tracheostomy tube should be done carefully, using sterile technique. The suction catheter is moistened prior to insertion, using sterile water. Sterile soft catheters, usually made of clear materials, are used and inserted without suction into the tracheostomy opening. The negative pressure of suction is applied only when the catheter is inserted and ready for withdrawal and should be used minimally. Some catheters have a thumb vent that can be used for controlling the suction with the thumb. Placing the thumb over the vent starts the suction, and by only partially occluding the vent opening with the thumb, one can reduce the negative pressure of the suction. If the catheter does not have a vent, a Y tube may be inserted in the tubing. Both intermittent suctioning and rotation of the catheter as it is removed also reduce the negative pressure effect (Fig. 3-9). Presuctioning and postsuctioning ventilation with a sigh volume at 100% oxygen is important in reducing the effects of the obstruction to the passage of gases in the airway before, during, and after suctioning. Ventilation given in between insertion of the suctioning catheter also prevents hypoxemia [1]. The lungs should be auscultated both before and after suctioning to determine the effectiveness of suctioning.

The catheter should be long enough to extend to the main stem bronchus, and attempts are also made to reach both the right and left stems. A curved catheter is used in some cases to facilitate suctioning of the right and left stem bronchus. This catheter is often less pliable, however, and may injure the mucosa; for this reason it is not used frequently. The catheter should not be larger than one-half the diameter of the tracheostomy tube. Suctioning is thought by some authorities to cause bronchospasm, and the use of negative pressure for suctioning can affect the intrapulmonary pressure; for this reason, the diameter of the tube is important. A No. 14 or 16 French catheter is frequently used. It is very important that the nurse observe the patient's tolerance of the suctioning procedure. Cardiac arrhythmias may be triggered by suctioning, so the vital signs should be monitored.

Determining when suctioning is necessary is important in view of the potential complications. A study conducted by Amborn [1] shows that the most effective and sensitive indicator of the presence of tracheobronchial secretions is an increased or decreased systolic and diastolic blood pressure. In this study, increases of more than 5 mm Hg were significant. Other indications of the presence of tracheobronchial secretions, according to the study, include increases in temperature, pulse, respiration, tidal volume, and coarse and prolonged expiratory breath sounds. The total number of signs present at any one time seems to be an indicator of the amount of

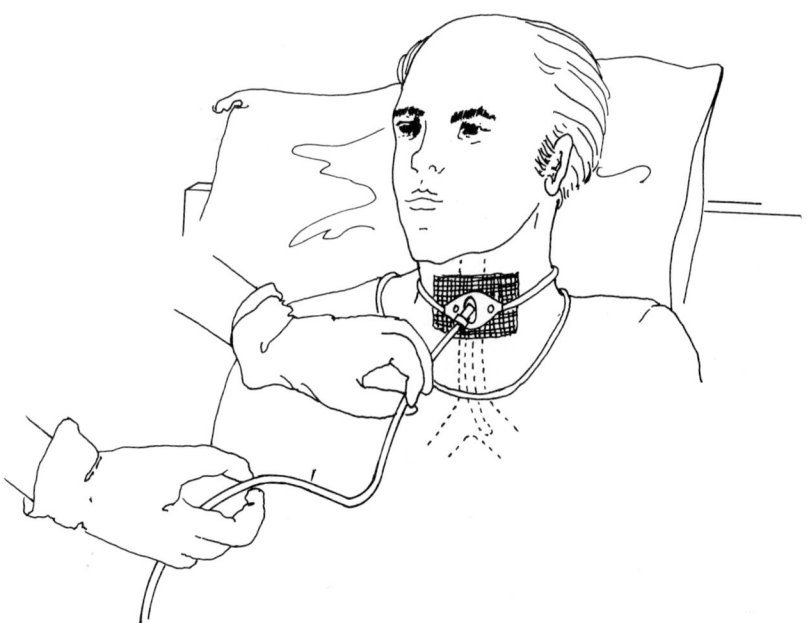

Figure 3-9
Tracheostomy suctioning. The nurse controls negative pressure with the thumb on the air vent. Sterile gloves are worn when suctioning with a tracheostomy tube. Note twill tape attached to the tube and tied securely around the patient's neck.

secretions present. The nurse must learn to detect the signs and symptoms of the presence of tracheobronchial secretions in order to determine when suctioning is necessary and when it is not necessary. As previously mentioned, unnecessary suctioning should be avoided.

A controversial issue in the care of patients with tracheostomy tubes is deflation of the cuff. Although procedures vary in different hospitals, the nurse should understand that the cuffs of certain types of tracheostomy tubes may cause airway obstruction by herniating over the end of the tube. If this occurs, the cuff should be deflated.

When it is accepted procedure to periodically deflate the cuff, it is usually done for 5 minutes or less every 1 to 2 hours to relieve the pressure on the tracheal mucosa and to allow for suctioning of secretions that may have pooled around the cuff. Some authorities, however, believe that periodic deflation of the cuff does not provide for improved circulation to the mucosa and that the interference with closed system ventilation caused by cuff deflation can cause instability in cardiopulmonary function [12]. If used, this procedure is usually also followed for the cuffs of endotracheal tubes. It is very important to reinflate the cuff correctly so that the tube is secure but does not press against the trachea. Some authorities believe that a tiny air leak is desirable to prevent pressure and subsequent injury to the mucosa. A minimal occluding volume is preferably used to create an airtight seal without occluding the mucosa. Postural drainage and pharyngeal suctioning prevent pooling of secretions at the cuff site. The nurse should be aware that the placement of the tracheostomy tube (or endotracheal tube) and the inflation of the cuff at the initial insertion must be checked carefully to maintain the closed system. As the patient's lung function changes, the inflation of the cuff may have to be adjusted to accommodate to the need for either more or less inflation to provide for a minimal occluding volume. The area around the cuff should always be suctioned if the cuff inflation is changed for any reason.

It is important that the nurse develop skill in suctioning. It has been shown that having the patient tilt his head to one side or the other does not facilitate suctioning of the right or left stem bronchus. Instead, the person suctioning must develop a feel for insertion of the suctioning catheter so that it is placed as deeply as possible and is guided to the right or left bronchus with gentle movement that does not traumatize the mucosa. Once the catheter has been inserted as far as it will go, it is withdrawn slightly to make certain that the suction tip is not against the wall of the airway. Suction is then applied as the catheter is withdrawn with a rotating movement; this clears the airway from the point of deepest insertion upward. The suctioning should be limited to periods of 10 or 15 seconds. As previously mentioned, ventilation is given between insertions of the catheter. The catheter is also cleaned before each insertion by placing its tip in sterile water, which allows the maximum negative pressure to draw the water through the catheter.

Prolonged suctioning can cause hypoxia, so care should be taken to perform the procedure as quickly and effectively as possible. If secretions are viscous, it may be necessary to insert 3 to 5 ml of normal saline into the tracheostomy tube immediately prior to suctioning to help liquefy secretions and facilitate the removal of any crusts or mucous plugs that may form. It is very important that adequate humidification be provided so that the secretions do not become viscous and difficult to remove. Water and salt depletion may also cause increasing viscosity of secretions.

When the patient has copious secretions, nasotracheal suctioning is performed. If the patient is conscious and able, he should rinse his mouth and throat prior to suctioning of the nasopharynx. If he is not able to do this for himself, the nurse should carry out meticulous oral hygiene. In every instance, the patient is encouraged to remove as much of the secretions as possible by effective coughing and blowing of the nose. The comatose patient cannot employ these normal protective mechanisms and therefore requires suctioning and positioning for removal of secretions.

When suctioning is necessary, the catheter is inserted during the inspiratory phase. Suction is applied after the catheter has been inserted as far as it will pass without force, and after the catheter has been withdrawn slightly. A rotating movement is used along with intermittent application of suction as the catheter is withdrawn. If the patient is receiving oxygen by nasal catheter or cannula, it may be necessary to increase the flow rate while suctioning. Humidification is also important for keeping the mucosa of the upper air passages moisturized, lessening the possibility of injuring the delicate mucosa during suctioning.

REMOVAL OF THE TRACHEOSTOMY TUBE Tracheostomy tubes interfere with the cough and gag reflexes as well as with the swallowing reflex; these must be checked carefully when the tubes are removed since aspiration may occur if the reflexes are impaired. (Most hospitals have a specific protocol for decannulation, which takes these problems of decreased reflexes into account.)

After a tracheostomy tube has been in place for 48 hours, a tract forms, which facilitates replacing the tube. A stoma also forms at the incision site as epithelial cells form. If the tracheostomy tube remains in place for a long period of time, surgical repair of the incision site may be required for closure. However, if the tracheostomy tube is in place for a shorter amount of time, the stoma closure heals without intervention. Tracheostomy tubes are removed as soon as possible because their presence in the trachea causes thinning of the tracheal mucosa around the tube. After the tracheostomy tube has been removed, sterile dressings are placed over the incision; they must be changed periodically to prevent the accumulation of secretions and to promote healing.

Patients often have to be weaned from the tracheostomy tube. When the tube is removed, dead space increases and there is an increase in breathing volume. The tidal volume–dead space ratio may increase if the patient cannot adjust to the increased breathing volume required. This factor and the depressed cough, gag, and swallowing reflexes make it necessary that the patient be prepared adequately for tube removal. The nurse should follow the decannulation procedure used in the institution or prescribed by the physician, with careful attention to monitoring for possible signs and symptoms of the complications of tube removal.

To determine whether the patient can tolerate removal of the tracheostomy tube by breathing without assisted ventilation, the nurse can use various devices to temporarily close the tube. The devices are usually referred to as "corks" and are placed carefully to occlude the tube opening in such a way that the patient is breathing without the aid of the tube. If the patient cannot tolerate removal of the tube, it can easily be "uncorked." Another method used is replacement of the tube with one that is fenestrated, that is, one that has an opening cut into the outer cannula so that the patient can "breathe around the tube." This type of tube allows the patient to talk and provides a means for evaluating his ability to breathe without the aid of the tube [12].

Indications for removal of the tracheostomy tube include the ability to cough effectively and to remove secretions, the ability to swallow, and the ability to maintain a sufficient vital capacity without the assistance of mechanical intervention. If the tracheostomy stoma must remain intact so that the tube can be replaced quickly if necessary, a tracheal "button" may be inserted. If a button is used, the nurse should maintain the cleanliness of the surrounding skin and should make certain that the button aperture is carefully corked. Following removal of the tracheostomy tube, the nurse should be watchful for indications of any of the complications associated with the inability of the patient to maintain adequate ventilation.

Complications of Treatment

Infection Infection can be a complication of any of the techniques used to maintain an open airway, to provide oxygen, or to assist ventilation. Very careful technique and attention to hand washing prior to giving care as well as the use of sterile equipment are essential elements of care. Antibiotics are usually given prophylactically to prevent infection. Care of ventilator devices, including changing tubes and cleaning nebulizer bottles or other humidification devices, is also essential. Nebulizers with reservoirs are a source of bacterial contamination, so the reservoirs should be changed or disinfected daily. Nebulizer bottles are completely emptied before refilling, and any fluid remaining after 24 hours is discarded (this is often the function of inhalation therapists but may be done by nurses in some institutions).

Aspiration Another complication that may occur in respiratory failure is aspiration, which is a particular problem in acute respiratory failure resulting from trauma, the aftereffects of anesthesia, or drug overdose. Any person who is ill has the potential for developing gastrointestinal symptoms, including nausea and vomiting; the effects of hypoxemia or hypoxia and subsequent acid-base imbalances may precipitate gastrointestinal symptoms as well. Careful positioning of the patient's head to the side after insertion of an airway and careful suctioning can help prevent aspiration. A nasogastric tube is inserted to decompress the stomach and to prevent aspiration pneumonia. It is imperative that the patient in respiratory failure have constant attention to prevent aspiration leading to pneumonia.

Acid-base imbalance The acid-base imbalances that occur with respiratory failure vary considerably from one person to another. The patient's status depends on his prefailure condition, the cause of his illness, the therapy he has received, and his response to the therapy. The patient may have chronic or compensatory imbalances along with acute imbalances of either respiratory or metabolic origin. The type of acid-base imbalance directly related to respiratory failure also differs for those with chronic lung disease and those with acute respiratory failure with no prior lung dysfunction. The acid-base imbalances in respiratory failure may cause significant complications that can compromise the patient's life.

In ventilatory failure, hypercapnia is increased as the work of breathing is increased. Both infection and the patient's anxiety may also contribute to hypercapnia. Intubation or tracheostomy may increase the anatomical dead space because of the length of the tubes attached to oxygen or to ventilators. It is important for the nurse to recognize that the increase in anatomical dead space caused by the tubes increases the total physiological dead space. In ventilatory failure the physiological dead space is also increased.

When the Pa_{CO_2} rises, the pH initially decreases. The hemoglobin buffer first functions to bind the carbon dioxide, forming H_2CO_2. Acidemia results, with shifts of chloride, sodium, and potassium. As the Pa_{CO_2} continues to rise, the kidneys compensate by retaining bicarbonate. Rapid removal of carbon dioxide through mechanical ventilation may cause rebound alkalosis because the kidneys cannot excrete the bicarbonate as rapidly as the carbon dioxide has been excreted; in this case the pH rises. If the patient is also receiving diuretics or corticosteroids, the potassium balance is further affected. Both types of drugs cause potassium loss and increase the renal excretion of potassium. Although the serum potassium may be near normal, the intracellular potassium may be depleted, and with increased renal excretion of potassium and replacement of cellular K^+ the patient develops hypokalemia. Chlorides may also be excreted so that replacement of chlorides, potassium, and fluids is necessary. Alkalosis can be severe enough to cause shock or neurologic symptoms or both.

Metabolic acidosis may result from hypoxia because anaerobic metabolism must provide the energy requirements in the absence of sufficient oxygen. Lactic acid is the major product of anaerobic metabolism, which depletes the buffers.

General Patient Care

Nutrition The nurse should carefully monitor the patient's state of nutrition. During respiratory failure, the intake of nutrients is severely hindered. It is important that the patient be encouraged to eat according to his tolerance as soon as possible. The diet selected should be suitable to the patient's physical and energy limitations and appropriate in nutrients. A high-carbohydrate, high-protein diet is given to provide for energy and tissue synthesis. Ingestion of carbohydrates is important because the body's stores of carbohydrates are quickly depleted. Fats and proteins are utilized when insufficient carbohydrates are provided, which further depletes the body's reserves. If the patient is unable to eat because he is comatose or because of his respiratory difficulty, total parenteral nutrition (TPN) may be started; this provides for infusion of carbohydrates and proteins so that tissue synthesis can be maintained. It is important that the patient receiving TPN be monitored carefully. A more detailed discussion of TPN can be found in Chapter 2.

Rest and exercise Rest and exercise are important aspects of nursing care for the patient with respiratory failure. While the patient is in severe failure, passive exercises should be done routinely by either the nurse or the physical therapist. It is necessary to provide passive exercise to maintain circulation and function of the joints. As soon as the patient's condition permits, ambulation and active exercise should be started, with gradual increases in the duration and amount of exercise. Both oxygen and ventilator equipment can be adapted to the patient's ambulation, with portable equipment being used if necessary.

The provision of rest is very difficult for the patient with respiratory insufficiency or failure because of the need for continuous monitoring and hourly routine care measures. Metabolic activity decreases during sleep, and periods of sleep are necessary for the patient's emotional and mental functioning. Lack of sleep may contribute to the patient's anxiety and inability to cope with the implications of his physical status. For the patient with respiratory dysfunction, providing for sleep and rest periods is even more difficult because sedation is contraindicated since it depresses the respiratory drive. Narcotics and barbiturates depress respirations and must be given with extreme caution.

Emotional support of the patient The nurse's challenge is to manage the patient's care so that he is as physically and emotionally comfortable as possible. Efficient management of care to allow for periods of uninterrupted rest between periods of care activities is essential. Every contact with the patient should incorporate emotional support to promote a feeling of being cared for and of security. The nurse must be aware that the patient is experiencing disruption not only of his normal routines but also of his ability to sustain life independently. Loss of independence may be crucial for the patient, and he may exhibit this stress in his behavior.

The nurse should recognize that the symptoms of respiratory failure, including those related to hypoxia and hypercapnia and those related to acid-base imbalances, are different in each patient. The nurse can expect the patient to experience mental confusion, restlessness, and even combativeness. Because the patient is experiencing symptoms from many different causes, it is important to observe his responses carefully in order to interpret their meaning. Reversal of hypoxemia and hypercapnia improve the patient's ability to think and to communicate. With experience, the nurse learns to differentiate among nuances of the patient's behavior and to respond to changes by validating them with blood gas analysis and by providing the appropriate intervention. The intervention may be suctioning, adjusting oxygen flow rates and concentration, adjusting the ventilator, providing for ingestion of nutrients and fluids, or dealing with the patient's fears and anxieties about himself and his care.

Communication with the patient The nurse who cares for patients with respiratory dysfunction, particularly respiratory failure, must recognize that the exertion of communicating increases the work of breathing. It is important that the nurse establish a sense of trust and understanding as early as possible to minimize the patient's frustration in being unable to communicate his needs or feelings. Obtaining information about the patient that will be helpful in anticipating his needs and in responding to him as an individual is an important aspect of nursing care; this information can be provided by the family or by others who are close to the patient or who have known him previously. Reading nursing care notes from previous hospital admissions or contacting community health workers who may know the patient can be helpful in learning about his response patterns and needs.

Initially the patient may be too sick to respond. Gradually as his condition improves he may become intimidated by all the equipment: the machines, the tubes, the intravenous lines, and the monitors. As he becomes accustomed to this equipment and learns its purpose the patient may develop a feeling of dependency on the equipment that is sustaining his life.

The patient with a tracheostomy has a particular problem in communicating because he cannot produce vocal sounds, since the opening of the trachea prevents the airflow through the vocal cords that is necessary for producing sound. Endotracheal tubes separate the vocal cords so the patient cannot talk. It is therefore important that the nurse communicate with the person effectively, developing a pattern of signs and signals that can be mutually understood. Some patients adjust to this type of communication better than others. The nurse must initiate the communication and must deal actively with the issues of care and the implications of the patient's illness without waiting for him to become increasingly anxious and frustrated because of his worries. The nurse should always attempt to communicate with the patient even when he is nonresponsive, since a patient can often hear and understand what is being said even though his ability to participate or respond to the communication is negligible.

As the patient's condition improves and he is able to tolerate increasing exercise and independence, the nurse should involve him to a greater extent in care decisions. Preparation for weaning the patient from the equipment begins as soon as he is able to respond to his own needs for independence. The nurse gives positive reinforcement to the patient's ability to resume independence at every opportunity: during positioning and during routine care such as in ambulation and eating. The most difficult problem the nurse must deal with in giving this positive reinforcement is that of uncertainty about the patient's progress and about the long-term effects of his illness. The nurse cannot give the patient false hopes or inaccurate information about his future; at the same time, the nurse cannot be so noncommittal about the future that the patient is increasingly aware of his precarious state.

Active involvement of the patient in his care implies that he or she can follow his or her own progress and knows the significance of the changes that occur. For example, having intravenous feeding discontinued and eating more normal meals is an indication of "getting better" that the patient can evaluate for himself. The changing dials on ventilators and oxygen equipment are observed by the patient, but he depends on the attitudes and expressions of those caring for him to interpret their significance.

If the patient is mentally alert, he tends to either subconsciously or consciously evaluate what is happening to determine the meaning of events in terms of his own status. The nurse must respond directly to the patient's need for information. False assurances should not be given; an honest appraisal of events tends to be more helpful to the patient than not knowing at all what is happening to him. At the same time, the nurse must provide information and evaluation of the patient's progress in such a way that he does not lose hope if there is a regression or delay in recovery.

Surgical Nursing Care in Respiratory Disease

Surgical intervention as a mode of treatment for respiratory diseases has specific implications for nursing care. The types of surgical procedures that may be performed include a wedge resection, a segmental resection, a lobectomy, and a pneumonectomy. The anatomy of the lung lends itself to these specific procedures. Each lung can be divided into lobes and segments; a wedge is a portion of a segment and is removed when the disease is localized. **Segmental resection** refers to the removal of one segment, a **lobectomy** is removal of one lobe, and **pneumonectomy** refers to removal of an entire lung. In addition to these procedures chest surgery may also be performed for repair of any of the lung structures, including the bronchus, the trachea or the mediastinal structures, and the pleura. When an opening is made in the chest wall, the procedure is termed a **thoracotomy. Thoracoplasty** is a permanent collapse of a portion of or an entire lung; it is performed by removing ribs and dividing muscles, so that postoperatively the patient needs physical therapy to overcome posture changes and to prevent contractures. Diaphragmatic breathing is taught to improve respiratory mechanical function following surgery.

Surgery may be performed in an emergency situation, as when trauma to the structures within the chest requires immediate repair, or it may be performed on an elective basis for removal of lesions, treatment of carcinoma, or repair of the pleura. Precise determination of lung function is always done prior to chest surgery performed on an elective basis; if there is insufficient function to sustain life following surgery, the procedure is contraindicated. Lung function studies are necessary to determine the exact amount of function the patient has. Generally it is necessary that the patient have at least 75 percent of the normal lung function in order to provide for the body's oxygen requirements. Because of the variability of each person's normal lung function, precise determination of the percentage of remaining function is difficult. It is very important to measure changes in lung function over a period of time to determine a base line for any one individual, since the same results may indicate respiratory insufficiency in one person and yet be normal for another.

Lung function studies are an important index of the patient's ability to tolerate surgery; other important considerations are the patient's physical health status, prior disease states, and the cause of his lung dysfunction.

When the surgery is elective, the patient must make the decision as to whether or not he wants to have the operation. It is necessary to know why the operation is being considered, what the possible consequences are of either having or not having the operation, and what the long-term effects of the operation may be for the patient. Because of the patient's involvement in making the decision about having the operation, the nurse must be aware of his perceptions and interpretation of the operative procedure. Knowing that the patient's decision should be based on thoughtful decision-making, awareness of the patient's emotional reaction to making such an important decision, and knowing that the patient's family may also be involved in the decision-making process are all important factors when the nurse plans preoperative teaching and care.

PREOPERATIVE CARE

Both preoperative and postoperative care are essential. Many of the complications that can occur in the postoperative phase can be prevented or minimized if the patient has a good understanding of how he is expected to feel and what he is expected to do to maintain his ventilatory function after surgery. In addition it is essential that the nurse ascertain exactly what the patient knows about the surgical procedure he is about to undergo. Many patients are concerned about their ability to breathe postoperatively, particularly if lung tissue will be removed. Sometimes they may think that it is safer to live with known pathology than to go through an operation and its unknown sequelae. The nurse should explore these thoughts with the patient and should clarify the expected effects of the operation for improved respiratory status or the reasons why the operation is advised. Preoperative lung function tests can also be used to help the patient understand that his lung function has been found to be adequate and that he will be able to adapt to the reduced lung tissue postoperatively.

The nurse should work closely with the patient preoperatively to prepare him for his postoperative condition and care; this involves informing him about the type of incision that will be made, teaching him to cough and do deep breathing effectively, preparing him for the presence of chest tubes, and informing him of the need for exercise that will be anticipated. The patient who is prepared for his postoperative care is more likely to continue to be an active participant in that care. He should be aware of the effects of anesthesia, the need for active removal of secretions through chest physiotherapy and through his own coughing and deep breathing, and the ways that he can expect to cope with postoperative pain. The teaching sessions should be carefully conducted so that the patient will be able to remember what to do during the postoperative period as well as to ensure that he has every opportunity to deal with his fears and misgivings.

Teaching the patient to cough and take deep breaths is an important aspect of preoperative care. Proper coughing to make the most efficient use of the body's normal protective response for removal of secretions is essential in maintaining a clear airway postoperatively and preventing atelectasis. Taking deep breaths is important in reducing the dead space that is present following surgery and immobilization. When the patient is able to practice these techniques prior to surgery, he is better able to carry them out even though he is experiencing the aftereffects of anesthesia and postoperative pain.

POSTOPERATIVE CARE

The patient must have a vital capacity of about 15 ml per kilogram of body weight to be able to breathe deeply enough to generate an effective cough. If the patient cannot effectively clear the airways with coughing and deep breathing, suctioning with catheter aspiration may be necessary. Some authorities prescribe IPPB for postoperative secretion removal while others feel that its value is questionable. IPPB is contraindicated with certain types of pathology and following certain types of surgery when pneumothorax is a probable complication.

Immediately after surgery it is important to maintain an open airway and to reestablish the negative pressure in the intrapleural space. Measuring the rate, depth, and pattern of respirations as well as the blood gases and pH is important to monitor the patient's lung function following surgery. Bradypnea may result from depression of the respiratory center by narcotics or anesthesia, and tachypnea may result from hypoventilation. Following anesthesia there may be increased viscosity of secretions, making them difficult to remove. Maintenance of hydration and provision for humidification, coughing, deep breathing, and suctioning when necessary are all important aspects of postoperative care. The patient who has undergone chest surgery is particularly prone to the development of atelectasis, which may lead to postoperative pneumonia. Pulmonary edema may result either from trauma to the lung tissue during surgery or from hypoxia following surgery. These complications can often be prevented by expert nursing care. If the patient develops respiratory failure following surgery, he will require longer term intensive care with oxygen and ventilator therapy.

Following surgery the patient is usually placed in Fowler's position, and his position is subsequently changed every hour to facilitate full expansion of the lungs. When a pneumonectomy has been performed it is necessary to position the patient in such a way as to drain the bronchial stump on the operative side as well as draining the unaffected lung. Following a lobectomy it is important to provide for maximum ventilation of the affected side. After a lobectomy the affected side is better ventilated when the patient is positioned on the unaffected side. The person should be supported while turning to minimize the incision pain and to promote a sense of security, which facilitates movement. The presence of chest tubes sometimes makes turning awkward for the patient unless the nurse is able to manage them deftly. (The care of chest tubes is discussed more fully on page 249.)

Thoracotomy

Recovery following a thoracotomy is usually rapid unless the patient develops complications. Ambulation is begun on the day of operation and increased gradually thereafter. The patient usually resumes oral intake of food by the second postoperative day and increases his diet to normal in a short time. Early ambulation and independence in performing personal hygiene tasks such as combing hair, brushing teeth, and assisting with one's bath contribute to the early resumption of normal activities; these tasks are also important in providing exercise for the shoulder and arm on the affected side. This exercise is very important following a thoracotomy to avoid stiffness of the shoulder joint (Fig. 3-10).

Certain patients—those with chronic lung disease, those who are obese or elderly, and those who have underlying cardiovascular disease—may be expected to have a slower recovery from chest surgery. Special attention to turning, coughing, and deep breathing and to providing additional support for ambulation and daily care measures according to the patient's capabilities is very important in the prevention of postoperative complications. Patients in this group have more frequent postoperative complications of respiratory insufficiency following surgery and should be monitored very carefully for any signs or symptoms of respiratory distress. Early intervention is imperative to prevent tissue hypoxia in all the major body systems, since the central nervous system effects of hypoxia may be irreversible.

Pneumonectomy

In a pneumonectomy, the space occupied by the lung is emptied. A major complication that may follow this procedure is mediastinal shift. The great vessels, the lymphatic vessels, the trachea and bronchus, and the esophagus, thymus, and heart may all be compromised if a mediastinal shift occurs. Symptoms of mediastinal shift include abrupt onset of dyspnea, tachypnea, restlessness, and anxiety. The pulse is irregular, and cardiac failure may result with pulmonary edema. Normally the space occupied by the lung fills with serosanguineous pleural fluid so that the pressures on each side of the chest are equalized, preventing shift of the mediastinal structures. Infrequently a chest tube may be inserted following pneumonectomy so that intrathoracic pressure readings can be obtained and to provide for the insertion of air if required to equalize pressures.

Excessive air in the mediastinum may also cause symptoms. The occurrence of a paradoxical pulse is an indication that venous

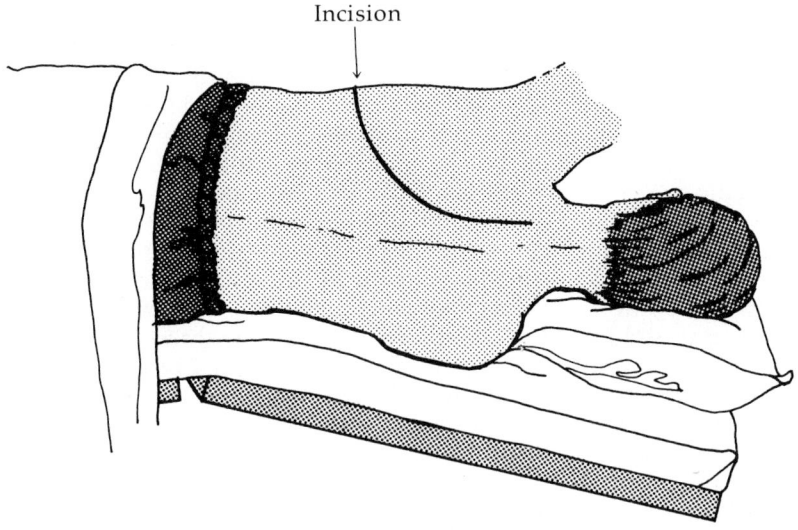

Figure 3-10
Site of thoracotomy incision indicates the need for exercise of the shoulder and arm on the affected side following surgery.

return to the heart is hindered because of the increased pressure of air around the heart. The paradoxical pulse is characterized by a change in the pulse on inspiration with weakening of the pulse and changes in systolic blood pressure.

Other Postoperative Complications
Another complication following chest surgery is **hemorrhage,** which is noted by an increased pulse and decreased blood pressure. The symptoms of hemorrhagic shock must be treated immediately. Often the patient is given an emergency blood transfusion and is taken to surgery for repair of the site of hemorrhage.

Pulmonary edema may develop following surgery because of trauma or hypoxia of the lung tissue or as a result of excessive fluid replacement. In severe cases, the patient will have rales and frothy, pink-tinged sputum. Pulmonary edema may precipitate right heart failure. Central venous pressure measurements should be monitored following surgery if pulmonary edema is an expected complication. An increase in central venous pressure is an indication that the right heart is not functioning adequately.

Cardiac tamponade may also be a complication of chest surgery if there is drainage of either fluid or blood into the pericardial sac. This accumulation places pressure on the vena cava and the atria so that myocardial failure can result from decreased venous return and subsequent decreased cardiac output. The central venous pressure should be monitored to detect early changes in venous return. Treatment involves removal of the fluid by needle aspiration. The electrocardiogram is also monitored.

Chest Drainage
Because the negative intrapleural pressure is disrupted during a thoracotomy, normal negative pressures must be reestablished following surgery. This is done through closed chest drainage. Any thoracic surgery in which the pleura is incised allows air to enter the pleural space. Normally the pressure in the intrapleural space is subatmospheric; this negative pressure is essential for lung expansion. Following the surgical procedure, a chest tube is inserted in the intrapleural space to provide for removal of air and secretions until the normal negative pressure is attained. Generally a single tube is used to remove air and provide for minimal drainage. When there is considerable drainage, two chest tubes are placed. The tube for air removal is placed in the upper lung spaces while that used to drain accumulated secretions is

placed in the lower lung spaces according to the patient's pathology (Fig. 3-11).

In order to reestablish negative intrapleural pressure, the chest tubes must be attached to a closed drainage system, which is usually referred to as water seal drainage. The water seal system may be a single bottle that provides for drainage by gravity or a two- or three-bottle system that provides for suction. In the one-bottle system, a glass tube is placed below the level of the water in the bottle to establish a water seal, and a second short tube serves as an air vent. The amount of intrapleural air that can be removed is determined by the depth at which the tube is placed under the water. The pressure of the water in the tube equalizes the pressure in the intrapleural space. The tube must be placed far enough into the water to prevent loss of the water seal by evaporation of water in the bottle. The water in the glass tube fluctuates with inspiration and expiration, rising on inspiration and falling on expiration. The water level is marked by a tape or other means so that the amount of drainage can be measured.

In a two-bottle system, the first bottle is the same as that in a one-bottle system except that the short glass tube that serves as the air vent in the one-bottle system is attached to a short tube in the second bottle. Altogether there are three outlets in the second bottle of the two-bottle system: the first is the short tube attached to the first bottle, and the second is a long glass tube that is open to atmospheric air at the top and that is submerged below the water level. The distance at which this tube is placed under water controls the amount of pressure exerted on the intrapleural space; the pressures equalize, with that of the water in the water seal tube being the same as that of the intrapleural space. The third tube in the two-bottle system is attached to suction.

The three-bottle system is the same as the two-bottle system except that there is an additional bottle between the chest tube and the water seal bottle; this third bottle collects drainage. Air is removed through a short tube attached to the water seal bottle, which is the second bottle in a three-bottle system.

The Pleur-evac is a commercially prepared disposable suction system that allows for removal of air and drainage from the pleural cavity; it is essentially the same as a three-bottle seal system that is attached to suction. It consists of a water seal chamber, a suction control chamber, and a collection chamber, all of which are neatly arranged in a single unit. As with the bottle system, the pressure is

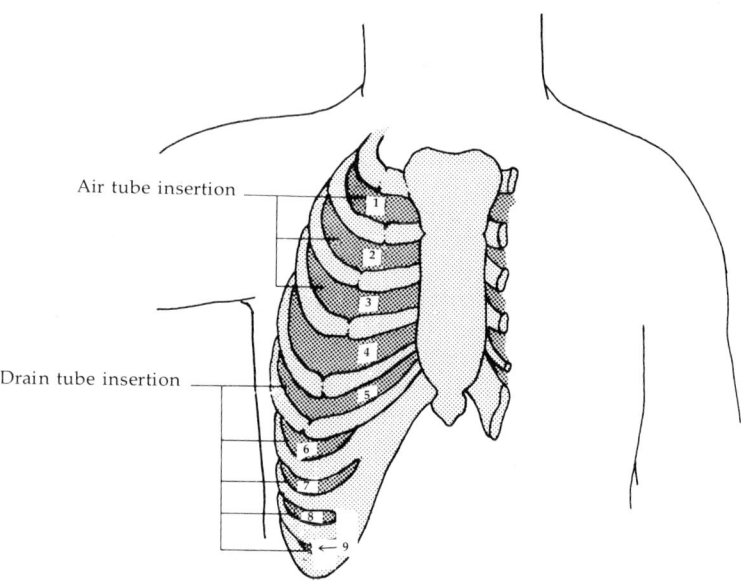

Figure 3-11
The precise placement of chest tubes depends on the patient's pathology.

established by the water level. The Pleur-evac provides for measurement of air pressure and the amount of air removed. It also has a float valve that preserves the water seal and that closes off the negative pressure if the intrapleural pressure is decreased more than 30 cm H_2O than the suction. The collection chamber of the Pleur-evac is calibrated so that drainage can be easily measured. It is also possible to remove drainage specimens for laboratory investigation without interfering with the suction (Fig. 3-12).

It is important that the chest tubes attached to the water seal drainage system be long enough to allow for movement of the patient but not so long as to interfere with effective drainage. Because exercise, turning, coughing, and deep breathing are so important for the patient, the chest tubes should be arranged to provide maximum comfort and motion without disrupting the patency of the tubes. The nurse should observe the rise and fall of water in the water seal bottle and should monitor the tubes at the site of attachment. Kinking of the tubes should be avoided and can be prevented by attaching the tubes to the bed linens so that the flow of air and drainage is not hindered by loops. Enough slack should be left so the patient can move freely without loosening the tube connections. For safety, the connections are taped securely. When the bottle system is used, the bottles should be attached to a holder or taped to the floor to prevent accidental jarring or upsetting of the bottles.

An indication that the negative intrapleural pressure has been reestablished is the cessation of fluctuations in the water seal tube. In

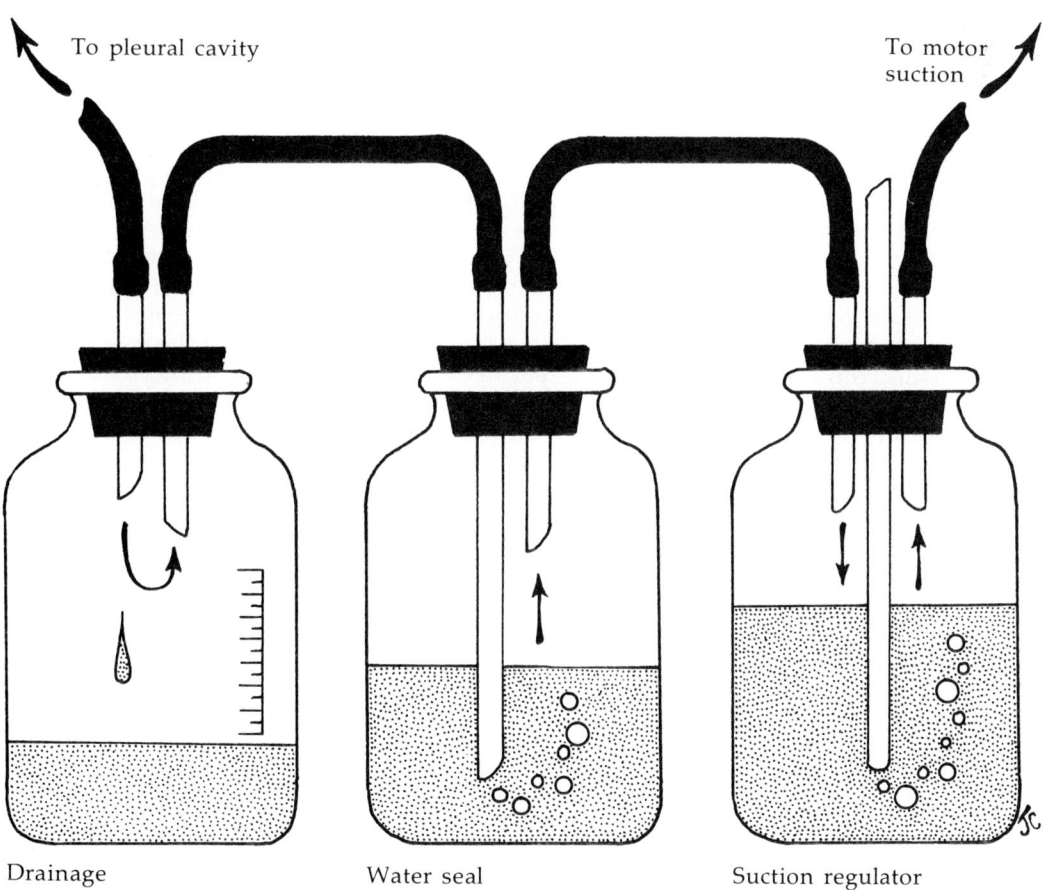

Figure 3-12
Water seal drainage system.

some cases an x-ray is taken to determine the degree of lung reexpansion prior to removing the chest tubes. Removal of the tubes is done quickly and is not painful. The opening is immediately covered with a sterile Vaseline dressing to close the incision site and to prevent air from entering the chest wall. If there is drainage on the dressing, it is reinforced and not changed for two or three days to prevent breaking the seal; after two or three days the site of insertion will have healed sufficiently to allow for dressing changes.

In current practice chest tubes are not clamped for any reason, since clamping may cause a tension pneumothorax which results when air enters the pleural space during inspiration and cannot escape during expiration. During the surgical procedure both the visceral and parietal pleurae may have been disrupted. Air entering the lungs enters the pleural space on inspiration, and the closed chest drainage system provides for removal of this excess air on expiration. However, if the route of escape via the chest tubes is closed, the pressure in the pleural space and the intrathoracic space increases, which may be sufficient to displace the structures of the mediastinum. The negative intrathoracic pressure is essential for the changes in intrapulmonary pressures, that is, expansion of the chest wall to increase the intrathoracic volume with concomitant decrease in pressure. When the intrathoracic space is in communication with atmospheric air, there are no pressure changes and the lung bellows cannot function. The lung responds to this increased pressure by recoiling because of its elastic recoil properties, and the air fills the space that the lung would normally occupy. The resulting tension pneumothorax may be mild or severe, depending on the amount of pressure. In pneumothorax, the unaffected lung is also subject to the pressure and may be unable to expand sufficiently for ventilation. If the pressure is sufficient, the mediastinal structures may be abruptly displaced so that both respiratory and cardiac function are severely impaired.

Controversy also exists about the milking of chest tubes. This has been done to maintain the patency of the chest tubes by facilitating removal of the fibrin and clots that may accumulate along the walls of the tube. When a chest tube is milked or stripped, the tube is compressed firmly near the chest wall while the tube distal to the site of compression is milked with a sliding, downward motion. Occluding the tube is considered by some authorities to be unsafe. Just as clamping prevents removal of excess air, occluding the tube for stripping prevents suction or gravity drainage from the intrapleural space and disrupts the pressure. The application of suction for more rapid removal of air and drainage may make milking chest tubes unnecessary. The patient's mobility is also important for facilitating drainage and for keeping the secretions and drainage mobile.

In summary, surgery can be performed for many different types of respiratory dysfunction. The outcomes of the surgery are, of course, dependent on the reasons for which the surgery was performed. However, the nurse has an essential role in the entire surgical experience, and the quality of nursing care is instrumental in the patient's recovery from the surgery.

Care of Patients with Specific Respiratory Diseases

In this section specific respiratory diseases are discussed in relation to pathologic processes. Nursing care measures previously described are referred to but not repeated because each patient's care will differ according to his unique response to the dysfunction and in relation to the presence or absence of other pathology, particularly cardiovascular dysfunction. The effects of any disease process cannot be predicted because of the many factors that influence the course of a disease, including genetic inheritance, personality characteristics, and coping mechanisms.

Obstructive lung diseases are a significant cause of death and disability. Some obstructive lung diseases may be either acute or chronic (e.g., asthma and bronchitis), others are chronic (e.g., emphysema). It should be noted that the term **chronic obstructive pulmonary disease** (COPD) refers to several different diseases—emphysema, bronchitis, and asthma—which may be complicated by either right or left heart failure. These three diseases are discussed separately in the following section. COPD consists of chronic inflammation of the bronchial passages with airway obstruction and stressed bronchial walls, impairment in the ability to clear the lungs of secretions, and collapse of the small air passages on forced expiration. Physiologically, the volume of the total lung capacity is increased, but forced expiratory flow volumes are decreased with airflow resistance on forced expiration.

EMPHYSEMA

Emphysema is an irreversible condition that represents a person's adaptive response to a number of different pathology-producing factors. The term **emphysema** may be defined differently by different authorities; some refer to emphysema as a specific disease that may be either primary or secondary, while others consider it to be a syndrome. There is some question as to whether or not a person can develop acute emphysema without having previously experienced lung dysfunction. Many authorities believe that emphysema is always preceded by episodes of lung disease or long-term exposure to pollutants. They feel that episodes of primary emphysema are actually acute events in a person who has had changes in lung function that were undetected until the acute illness made the person seek medical care, usually because of shortness of breath.

Emphysema is frequently described according to the anatomic changes in the lung parenchyma in which the elastic structure around the alveoli dissolves, with the result that the lungs become stiff and compliance decreases. It has been observed that many people who have emphysema also have chronic bronchitis. Both conditions are progressive and chronic, and diagnosis of a primary disease is not always possible in the person who seeks treatment only after lung dysfunction has beome moderate or severe. The person with asthma or chronic pneumoconiosis also has a high incidence of emphysema. Since not every person with these diseases develops emphysema, one can speculate that there must be some other reason why emphysema occurs. Again, in advanced disease, it may be difficult to determine the primary cause of the lung dysfunction. In light of this, it seems most appropriate to refer to emphysema as a syndrome that occurs as a result of a combination of factors, including progressive obstructive lung disease, in the presence of other predisposing factors such as age, cold and damp climates, weather or temperature changes, barometric pressure changes, exposure to air pollutants, and emotional stress. Not just one but a combination of these factors is generally present in the development of emphysema.

The common factor among the chronic progressive changes in lung function resulting from chronic bronchitis, asthma, or some of the diseases classified as pneumoconiosis is the obstruction of ventilation. The term **chronic obstructive lung disease** describes the physiologic changes that occur as the obstruction increases and is therefore a functional definition of the disease process. Treatment and nursing care for patients with impaired ventilation from any cause is similar because of this common functional disorder.

The cause of emphysema is unknown. It can occur in any age group and in both sexes. Men over the age of 50 have the highest incidence of emphysema. Cigarette smoking, a self-imposed form of pollution, is considered a significant factor in the development of emphysema. Any infectious process that leaves a residual of fibrotic tissue, thereby reducing the elastic recoil of the lung, chronic irritation that causes increased mucus production and hyperplasia of tissues, and hypersensitivity reactions to inhaled dusts and other foreign bodies all result in lung tissue changes that predispose to emphysema. A deficiency of alpha$_1$-antitrypsin may also be a genetic factor related to the incidence of emphysema, which usually occurs during the third or fourth decade.

Traditionally, emphysema has been described as enlargement of any part of the acinus with destruction of tissue and loss of elastic recoil. More recently it has been shown that the larger bronchial passages may be affected as well. In emphysema, the lungs are overinflated with air that the person cannot expel, even with forced expiration. The overinflated alveoli may then lose their structure as the alveolar walls coalesce. When this occurs, the pulmonary capillaries may be torn or fibrosed so that perfusion is impaired.

Classifications of Emphysema

Three major anatomic classifications commonly used to describe emphysema are centrilobular, panlobular, and focal. A person may have one type of emphysema exclusively, or he may have a combination with one type predominating. People who have had bronchial disease over a long period of time generally have more diffuse emphysema, which is difficult to classify.

Centrilobular emphysema refers to destruction and dilatation of specific bronchioles located in the secondary lobules of the lung. There is a corresponding dilatation of the alveoli supplied by the affected bronchioles. This type of emphysema is localized, and there may be unaffected units of lung tissue surrounding the affected areas.

Panlobular emphysema describes a process of destruction and dilatation of the bronchioles and alveoli within a lobule in which the entire acinus is involved. **Destructive emphysema** is another term used to describe the progressive destruction of the bronchioles and alveoli in aging people. In destructive emphysema, the alveolar walls become thin and atrophied from continued distention so that eventually there are large spaces with no structure. Emphysematous blebs and bullae are formed as the lung tissue is destroyed. Blebs are small areas of destruction, while bullae appear as cystic areas ranging in size from 1 cm in diameter to very large areas. Destructive emphysema is sometimes termed **paraseptal emphysema.**

Focal emphysema is the destruction of lung tissue around a focal point of residual dust that has caused the development of fibrosis of lung tissue. **Pneumoconiosis** is the term for diseases associated with the inhalation of toxic dusts. Coal workers' pneumoconiosis causes dilatation emphysema in the terminal bronchioles. Inhaled dusts are carried into the lung passages to the point where the velocity of air flow decreases; they then settle out in the regions where the velocity of flow falls the most rapidly in the terminal bronchioles. It is possible for people to have focal emphysema with no pulmonary dysfunction.

Emphysema may also be classified as overdistention emphysema and panacinar dilatation emphysema. The first type, **overdistention emphysema,** is considered a compensatory process in which lung tissue responds to a need created by a foreign body or tumor. The presence of either causes partial obstruction because air is trapped during expiration as the narrowed bronchus becomes more completely obstructed. This condition is not truly emphysema unless destruction of lung tissue with permanent dilatation occurs. **Panacinar dilatation emphysema** is also a compensatory type of emphysema that follows surgical removal of lung tissue or shrinking of lung tissue for any reason. In this type of emphysema, lung tissue expands to fill the empty space. Again, this condition is not correctly called emphysema unless destruction has occurred.

Yet another term, **aging emphysema,** is used to describe alterations in pulmonary function resulting from loss of elasticity in lung tissue. This loss of elasticity leads to dilatation of the alveoli so that there is hyperinflation of the lung as well as airway obstruction. A certain amount of alteration in lung tissue with concomitant dysfunction is an expected part of the aging process, and almost every person has some irregular emphysema with aging. The appearance of the lungs on x-ray films shows that the lungs become smaller with old age, whereas the lungs of people with emphysema who are in their middle years tend to be large and overinflated.

Some authorities also refer to **senile emphysema,** in which the change in cartilage tissue of the spine causes kyphosis of the thoracic segments of the spinal column. The ribs then rotate and the anterior chest is pushed forward, forming a barrel shape. Emphysema has traditionally been associated with a typical "barrel chest." However, not every person with a barrel chest has emphysema, and not every person with emphysema has a barrel-shaped chest.

Familial emphysema is a disease in which there is an alpha$_1$-antitrypsin deficiency, genetically transmitted. It is not fully understood, but it is thought that the lack of the alpha$_1$-antitrypsin, an enzyme inhibitor, may predispose a person to changes in lung tissue.

Progression of Emphysema

The onset of emphysema may be so gradual that the person who is experiencing the symptoms is not aware of the disease or of the progressive changes that have occurred over a long period of time. Initially, the person becomes aware of his breathing. An increased amount of work is required for breathing because of the increased airway resistance and loss of elasticity of lung tissue, so that expiration must be forced. During inspiration there is normally an increase in the intrathoracic pressure, which causes compression of the airway. The pressure within the alveoli and the intrathoracic pressure are greater than the pressure in the bronchioles. In emphysema, the bronchioles lose some of their supporting structures as the parenchyma is destroyed and the elastic recoil of the lungs is diminished. Pressure within the bronchioles is reduced and they tend to close more easily than is normal. The increased airway resistance and the pressure change between the alveoli and the mouth both augment the pressure drop, so that the pressure in the bronchi is further decreased and airflow is hindered. The loss of elasticity increases lung compliance, which causes a concomitant decrease in the air pressure because lung volume is expanded. For the person with emphysema, the overall effect is felt as a need to work harder to expel air. This initiates a cycle in which the more the person pushes with his chest wall, the greater is the intraalveolar pressure and the greater the turbulence of airflow, which increases the resistance. Consequently, as the syndrome becomes progressively more severe, the person is increasingly conscious of the work of breathing, and he works harder to accomplish less effective ventilation and perfusion. The ventilation-perfusion ratio changes because the decreased alveolar area causes physiologic shunting.

In emphysema, the areas of obstruction occur unevenly throughout the lung in the majority of cases. This means that some alveoli have more air than they can use while others have insufficient air and are underventilated. Some of the alveoli may be totally collapsed, and if there is fibrosis of the alveoli there may be perfusion without ventilation. When the alveolar capillary bed is damaged, there may be ventilation without perfusion. Uneven distribution of air causes a drop in the saturation of arterial oxygen. In the alveoli that are well ventilated, the P_{O_2} is normal (90 mm Hg) at sea level; those that are not well ventilated have lower levels of P_{O_2}, and those with destroyed capillary beds may be ventilated but cannot perfuse oxygen from the lung to the arterial system. This inequality of oxygen saturation reduces the arterial P_{O_2} and increases the arterial P_{CO_2}. The efficiently functioning alveoli cannot compensate for those not functioning because they have reached their saturation point for oxygen perfusion.

The pathologic process gradually extends. For a time, the Pa_{CO_2} can be maintained at normal levels even though the oxygen saturation is decreased. Any measures that decrease ventilation, such as increased exertion, infections, or bronchospasm (which may be related to exposure to irritants or emotional stress or both), will increase carbon dioxide retention. Likewise any measures that improve ventilation will increase the carbon dioxide elimination. For this reason, the blood gases and pH will differ depending on what is happening to the person with emphysema. The nurse should know that oxygen saturation is initially decreased but that carbon dioxide excretion may be adequate until the obstruction to ventilation becomes more severe. The reason for this is that the P_{CO_2} dissociation curve is linear rather than flat as is the oxygen dissociation curve; thus the carbon dioxide levels do not increase as rapidly as the oxygen levels decrease. However, as ventilation becomes so impaired that carbon dioxide cannot be effectively eliminated, the carbon dioxide levels will increase. When the Pa_{CO_2} levels are high enough for sufficient time to decrease the pH, the person develops respiratory acidosis. Hyperventilation triggered by increased arterial P_{CO_2} then provides for increased expiration of carbon dioxide. If alveolar ventilation improves, the carbon dioxide will return to normal. This compensatory mechanism may be needed only during periods of increased exertion in mild or moderate emphysema. The obstruction to ventilation is somewhat reversible at this point because rest or medication may significantly improve ventilation and the ability to eliminate carbon dioxide. As the emphysema progresses, however, hyperventilation occurs more consistently. It is important to note that with hyperventilation the ratios of oxygen to carbon dioxide return to normal, but the oxygen saturation continues to be lower than normal. When acute hyperventilation occurs as a result of exertional demands for more oxygen, the pH is high but returns to normal after adequate therapy, which causes the P_{CO_2} levels to decrease.

Hyperventilation may not appreciably increase P_{O_2} levels because only the poorly ventilated areas benefit from increased oxygen uptake; those that are functioning adequately cannot take up additional oxygen because their saturation levels have already been reached. The benefit of hyperventilation as a compensatory mechanism is primarily excretion of the excess arterial carbon dioxide, which is important in maintaining acid-base balance. The fact that the person's oxygen saturation is less than normal is significant. The relation of breathlessness to the Pa_{O_2} level varies, since some individuals can tolerate levels as low as 50 mm Hg and have no dyspnea while others may be markedly dyspneic with the same low level. The reason for this variation in the adaptive process is not understood, but it is influenced by both tissue oxygen needs and erythrocyte production.

When the lungs are overinflated, with uneven ventilation and impaired perfusion, the dead space increases. In emphysema, the total dead space may be as much as 50 percent of the volume of inspired air because of the inefficient ventilation. As the dead space increases in relation to the increasing impairment of ventilation, more carbon dioxide is retained in the body, which causes an increase in H^+ ion concentration of the blood. After a point, hyperventilation can no longer provide for compensation. When the ratio of bicarbonate to carbonic acid falls, decreasing the pH, hydrogen ions are released. These H^+ ions stimulate the chemoreceptors, the most important ones being located on the ventral surfaces of the medulla near the point of exit for the ninth and tenth cranial nerves. The central chemoreceptors are in the cerebrospinal fluid. Carbon dioxide readily diffuses to the cerebrospinal fluid and causes the liberation of H^+ ions. The resulting change in the pH of the cerebrospinal fluid causes hyperventilation, reducing P_{CO_2} levels and consequently reducing further H^+ ion stimulation. After a period of prolonged P_{CO_2} retention or hypercapnia, however, the pH of the cerebrospinal fluid is not altered by the increased P_{CO_2} levels. For some reason, the pH of the cerebrospinal fluid is no longer sensitive to H^+ ion stimulation and is maintained at a normal level despite the high carbon dioxide levels. It is not fully understood why cerebrospinal fluid chemoreceptors become sensitized to high carbon dioxide levels and establish new norms or higher tolerance to increased levels. However, the result is that a person with long-standing hypercapnia may have an increased Pa_{CO_2} with a normal pH. When this occurs, renal compensation provides for excretion of excessive H^+ ions and for conservation of base. As the increased level of arterial carbon dioxide no longer stimulates hyperventilation, the low arterial oxygen level then becomes the major stimulus to ventilation. Generally this happens when the carbon dioxide level is increased to 60 to 70 mm Hg. Low oxygen levels stimulate ventilation through the effect on the aortic and carotid chemoreceptors. Giving oxygen to relieve hypoxia can interfere with this stimulation of ventilation, which is not dependent on decreased P_{O_2} levels in arterial blood. Since removal of this stimulation may further decrease ventilation, oxygen must be administered in low concentrations to patients with severe chronic emphysema.

Symptoms of Advanced Emphysema

During the later stages of emphysema, so much carbon dioxide can be retained that the increased Pa_{CO_2} is no longer a stimulus to respiration. The increased levels of carbon dioxide may then have an anesthetic effect (carbon dioxide narcosis). Neurologic symptoms associated with late emphysema include occipital headache, a decreased ability to concentrate, and drowsiness. The hands are warm, the pulse may be bounding, and the Pa_{CO_2} is greater than 75 mm Hg. Asterixis (the flapping tremor), confusion, and coma are later signs.

In addition to renal compensation, hypoxemia is somewhat compensated for by increased erythropoiesis, with the result that the patient with chronic emphysema may develop secondary polycythemia. Prolonged hypoxemia or hypoxia creates a state in which the impaired ventilation and perfusion of oxygen causes right-sided cardiac hypertrophy with myocardial anoxia and increased pulmonary vascular resistance; the distended neck veins and peripheral edema that can be noted in patients with advanced emphysema are indicative of this process. This condition, known as **cor pulmonale,** may often be the cause of death.

Patient Assessment

The signs and symptoms of emphysema, then, may vary depending on the severity of the ventilation impairment and the individual response to the disease. Assessment of the severity of the emphysema involves obtaining a history of the symptoms, level of exercise, work history, and environment, as well as observing present status, obtaining blood gas and pH levels, and measuring ventilation capacities. Diffusion studies and x-ray examinations are diagnostic in the very late stages. The patient with emphysema usually has a history of frequent respiratory infections and chronic bronchitis; during periods of infection he may have a temperature and will have an increased production of purulent sputum. These respiratory infections interfere with ventilation so that the person can tolerate less exercise than usual. Because exercise normally increases oxygen requirements and consequently ventilation requirements, the person with emphysema will have exaggerated needs for increased ventilation during exercise and will therefore note increased breathlessness on exertion. In emphysema, the oxygen uptake cannot be increased in relation to the demands for increased oxygen necessitated by exercise. Pulmonary blood flow decreases, and the pulmonary capillaries may collapse. Exercise stress tests can be performed to determine the person's level of tolerance, which implies the adequacy of alveolar ventilation.

Breathlessness commonly increases during winter when the relative indoor humidity decreases, causing drying of the air passages. The occurrence of infection is also greater in the winter. Both the increased secretions and bronchospasm that are related to infections contribute to dyspnea, which is also greater during the winter than during the summer. The ventilation impairment may be somewhat reversible if the ventilation improves when infections subside or as other factors such as cold air are eliminated. However, as the obstruction of ventilation increases and becomes more irreversible, the person will notice that the dyspnea on exertion is increased and is more consistent throughout the entire year. When this feeling of breathlessness becomes persistent, the person usually has visible signs and symptoms of emphysema.

Usually emphysema follows a course of progressive worsening so that the person is continually adjusting to impaired ventilation; it may become his normal pattern to experience breathlessness. The person generally seeks medical care when he develops pneumonia or bronchitis that impairs his already decreased ventilation enough so that he is very uncomfortable or very dyspneic. When the pneumonia or bronchitis is never really "cured" following therapy, a diagnosis of emphysema may then be made. Often the person cannot recall previous episodes of respiratory disease or discomfort; such people often relate that they have attributed the breathlessness to increasing age and excessive smoking, together with smoker's cough, inconsistent exercise, and weight gain. (Many people with emphysema experience weight gain in the early stages.) In this way, the syndrome of emphysema seems to creep up on them, and they suddenly realize that their health may be seriously impaired.

The person may worry about his cardiac function, thinking that the breathlessness indicates cardiac disease. Questioning the person about his most comfortable sleeping position helps to differentiate between the breathlessness caused by cardiac dysfunction and that caused by emphysema. Persons with cardiac disease have a greater total vital capacity in the sitting or standing position and are more comfortable sleeping with the head of the bed elevated; those with emphysema are more comfortable sleeping in a flat position since their total vital capacity is greater in the supine position.

In other instances, emphysema is first noticed following a respiratory problem associated with another disease. Surgery with intubation or the administration of morphine or atropine may precipitate the emphysema in these people.

Two medical problems associated with emphysema—the development of inguinal hernias and the occurrence of peptic ulcers—are significant in detecting emphysema. The first is related to increased pressure and strain because of the frequent hacking cough of emphysema; the second is not fully understood. About 20 percent of people with emphysema have ulcers, most commonly duodenal ulcers. Among the factors thought to contribute to ulcer formation are cigarette smoking, prolonged hypoxia, and the emotional factors that are related to the occurrence of both emphysema and ulcers.

Assessment of the patient with emphysema is facilitated by looking for certain common signs. If the patient is a heavy smoker (40 pack-years) his fingers may have the yellowish brown stains of tobacco. Clubbing of the fingers may also be noted. The neck veins will generally distend on expiration, and the eyes tend to be prominent. There is also a characteristic sinking of the tissues around the neck and supraclavicular spaces. The chest is usually fixed in a position of hyperinflation because of enlarged chest volume resulting from air trapping and the decreased movement of the chest during respiration. If the emphysema is moderately severe or severe, the patient may be thin or even emaciated in appearance, will have a loss of vigor and energy, and may be suffering from protein starvation.

During the early stages of emphysema, the blood gases may be normal. As the syndrome progresses, the Pa_{O_2} first decreases, the Pa_{CO_2} rises, and the Pa_{O_2} then continues to decrease. As the body compensates for the respiratory acidosis first by hyperventilation and later through renal mechanisms, the pH becomes stabilized and the oxygen saturation is progressively lower. Both cardiac and respiratory energy are wasted in emphysema. There is increased dead space in the lung, with air entering but not undergoing gas exchange, so that ventilation is ineffective for the amount of work that must be done to accomplish ventilation. The work of ventilation increases the need for oxygen. Similarly, the cardiac work is partially ineffective because the lung tissues may not be adequately perfused in some areas of obstruction. There is an increase in pulmonary artery pressure with increased resistance to blood flow from the heart to the lungs; this may result in congestive failure. The person breathes deeper and harder with little return for his effort. Consequently he is tired, and his blood gases reflect the inefficiency of perfusion and ventilation as they become progressively more inadequate.

One of the mechanisms involved in the increased work of breathing is the use of the accessory muscles of respiration because of the necessity of forcing air from the lungs. The large sternocleidomastoid muscles are enlarged and active, and the scalene and pectoral muscles are also used. The trachea can be observed to move downward on inspiration. In addition, the abdominal muscles may be used to assist respiration, although they may be lax in emphysema. Other changes include the outward flaring motion of the lower rib margins and widening of the subcostal angle. Some people will also have dorsal kyphosis from the strain of the work of breathing.

Normally, the chest moves rhythmically in segments from bottom to top during inspiration. The person with emphysema tends to have singular chest movements because the accessory respiratory muscles are activated. Rather than moving in segmental rhythm, the chest moves in one piece with little upward movement of the flattened diaphragm. Both the diaphragm and the liver are low. Expiration is prolonged, and the typical "blowing" or "pursing" motion of the lips can be observed as the person exerts an effort to expel air. The term "pink puffer" is commonly used to refer to the person with emphysema because of the blowing on expiration. The pink puffer usually has no cyanosis because compensatory mechanisms have provided for adequate oxygenation of the tissues. The person with emphysema is seemingly very conscious of the need to work for ventilation. Wheezing may be noticed if there is irritation or narrowing of the bronchi, and the person may have a hacking cough that interferes with the rhythm of breathing and increases the work. The person is hungry for air and inspirations tend to be short and rapid.

Because of lung changes, the chest sounds will be different from normal. Breath and heart sounds may be absent, distant, or dull. Wheezing on expiration can be heard if the person has either bronchospasm or excessive secretion, while inspirational rales may be heard occasionally at the base of the lung. Breath sounds may be bronchovesicular.

Diagnostic Tests

In the early stages of emphysema, x-ray studies are generally insignificant. As the syndrome progresses, the x-ray will confirm the visible signs. For example, the size of the thoracic cage will be increased and the dorsal kyphosis will show, as will the flattened, low diaphragm. The heart is often elongated and narrow on x-ray. The ribs will be separated with wider than normal intercostal spaces and the rib cage will appear to be box-shaped rather than curved as normally. There may be blebs and bullae in the lung apexes and bases, and the bronchioles may be dilated. Fluoroscopy may reveal both the decreased movements of the diaphragm and air trapping in the alveoli.

Ventilation capacity is evaluated through lung function tests to determine both the diagnosis and the severity of emphysema.

The forced expiratory volume (FEV) is decreased in emphysema, and the expirations are prolonged. The test of FEV is repeated after a week's treatment with bronchodilator medication. The FEV increases after treatment in both bronchitis and asthma but remains decreased if the patient has emphysema.

Another indication of emphysema is a decrease in the maximal voluntary ventilation; the lungs remain inflated so that the volume of residual air increases. A nitrogen washout test reveals prolonged times for the washout in patients with emphysema. The time is often increased as much as twice the normal time.

Treatment

Because the ventilation impairment in emphysema becomes increasingly irreversible as the syndrome progresses, treatment is aimed at preventing further impairment of function and maintaining current function. This is accomplished by maximizing the patient's ventilation as much as possible and helping him adjust his life pattern to the diminished ventilation-perfusion capacity. Maximizing ventilation is provided for through medications such as bronchodilators and by keeping the secretions thin with adequate hydration and humidity. The patient should learn to recognize what brings about bronchospasms so that he can learn either to avoid them or to treat them. An important aspect of maintaining maximum ventilation and preventing further impairment of function is avoiding infection as much as possible. Bronchitis and pneumonia as well as complications such as atelectasis and bronchospasm significantly diminish ventilation.

Depending on the severity of emphysema, intermittent positive pressure breathing (IPPB) may be required during episodes of infection or exertion that place a strain on the impaired ventilation. IPPB provides for more effective ventilation and for drainage of secretions. Another positive result of IPPB treatments is an increase in alveolar ventilation and, therefore, increased carbon dioxide elimination. Bronchodilator drugs can be given with the IPPB treatments to distribute the drug more effectively throughout the lungs. IPPB treatments may be needed more regularly as the disease progresses; however, their use is controversial since some authorities believe that the patient should learn to use his own resources rather than depending on IPPB.

It is essential that the patient avoid pollutants in the air he breathes as much as possible. Of primary concern in this regard is smoking. The high level of pollution achieved by smoking contributes to irritation of lung tissues and an increase in symptoms and further impairs ventilation in patients with emphysema. However, it may be extremely difficult for the patient to stop smoking, particularly after years of habitual smoking. An important aspect of nursing care is counseling the patient about smoking and helping him find ways to stop. The nurse should recognize that smoking for some people is a habit or an addiction that is important in their coping mechanisms, and they cannot stop without adjusting to a new coping pattern to replace the smoking. The person with emphysema already has a number of restrictions in his daily life: He usually has a decreased ability to tolerate exercise; he must reduce his weight or avoid weight gain; and he may be faced with having to find a less physically taxing means of making his living. In the face of all these restrictions, stopping smoking may seem impossible. There are a number of clinics for people who wish to stop smoking and, depending on the individual, personal counseling may also be necessary. There are many ways to approach the problem of stopping smoking with the patient who has emphysema; however, it should be done with recognition of the reason the person smokes in the first place and with appreciation for the fact that a lecture or even detailed examples of the poor effects of smoking may serve only to make the patient more anxious about his condition.

The patient with emphysema can be taught to become more aware of his breathing by the use of spirometric evaluation to help the patient find more effective ways to expire air in order to maximize expiration, since he can measure the effectiveness of his own breathing. Breathing exercises can be taught to help the patient learn to use manual compression of the subcostal area in conjunction with slow and relaxed breathing to reduce the dead space. Some people breathe more easily when their torsos are bent forward. It is important for the nurse to know that the breathing exercises will not improve the patient's condition by decreasing the lung pathology; all that can be accomplished with more effective and efficient breathing is improvement of ventilation.

Eating patterns are another area of concern for the patient with emphysema. Breathing is more effective if a person is of normal weight or underweight, since excess weight can interfere with movement of the diaphragm and also increases the oxygen requirements. Another aspect of diet is the patient's tolerance of eating. Those with moderate or severe emphysema may not be able to tolerate eating large meals, and they must learn to eat small, nutritious meals more frequently to decrease the oxygen consumption needs related to metabolism at any one time as well as the oxygen need related to the physical activity of eating.

The patient with emphysema may have to make great changes in his daily life. In addition, he may need to support his family, and loss of work can be a serious emotional trauma not only for the patient but also for the entire family.

Because the demands on any person change almost daily, the patient with emphysema must learn how to use medications, particularly bronchodilators, when needed. Either oral or aerosol medications can be used. Their effects and side effects should be understood so that the patient will know when to use them, how much to use, and how to recognize when they are not effective so that he can seek medical attention. In addition to medication, it is important that the patient understand the need for adequate humidity in his environment as well as the need for an adequate fluid intake. The patient with emphysema is often dehydrated and needs an adequate oral intake of fluids. He usually has copious secretions with a hacking cough and expectoration of sputum, but may produce no sputum. The ambient humidity should be maintained at a level that keeps the secretions thin and less viscous. Adequate hydration is also essential.

It may be necessary for the patient to have a supply of antibiotics that he can use if he feels he is getting a cold or other type of respiratory infection. As previously mentioned, many patients learn to use antibiotics prophylactically so that they can avoid bouts of infection; this usage should be monitored by the physician. While important in preventing infection, the prophylactic antibiotic may not be the drug of choice if an infection does occur. Therefore, when an infection occurs, the patient should have the sputum examined by culture and sensitivity tests and receive appropriate antibiotic therapy for that particular infection.

When the patient has episodes of severe hypoxia, he will probably require hospitalization. At this time he may be in respiratory acidosis, and if his condition is severe enough, he may also be in cardiac failure. Therefore, careful evaluation of the patient's status is imperative to guide nursing care. All the measures required for less severely disabled patients are carried out during hospitalization, including the use of bronchodilators, removal of secretions, adequate hydration and humidity, and a bronchial hygiene program for improvement of ventilation. These measures are often carried out with the assistance of machines for suctioning in conjunction with a tracheostomy, if necessary, to ensure more efficient delivery of medications such as bronchodilators and provision for oxygen through mechanically assisted ventilation. Important values in evaluating the patient's status are the arterial blood gases, concise partial pressures of oxygen and carbon dioxide, and the pH; these values are a guide both to the severity of hypoxemia and respiratory acidosis and to the effectiveness of the therapy. It is important for the nurse to remember that the patient with severe emphysema may not tolerate high concentrations of oxygen if his stimulus to respiration is a low Pa_{O_2}. Oxygen therapy must therefore be carefully monitored and the concentration of oxygen should be low to prevent interference with this mechanism. Low controlled oxygen flow is used.

If the hospitalized patient also has right-sided cardiac involvement, the cardiac condition must be treated. If digitalis is used the nurse should observe for signs of digitalis toxicity, since the patient with emphysema is very sensitive to this condition. Diuretics, which are commonly used in many instances of cardiac failure, may be contraindicated in the patient with emphysema because he may be in respiratory acidosis and may have low levels of serum potassium and chloride. If the respiratory acidosis is successfully treated by improving ventilation, the patient may begin to develop metabolic alkalosis, requiring replacement of electrolytes. Aspects of treatment for fluid and electrolyte balance dysfunction are discussed in Chapter 2.

Corticosteroids are sometimes used to relieve severe bronchospasm in patients who do not respond well to treatment. They are usually prescribed for a minimal amount of time, and the nurse should carefully observe the dosages that are prescribed to provide for increments and decrements in dosage and to watch for any indications of complications. Steroid therapy may mask infection and may not be desirable for use in those who have infectious processes. If the steroids will preserve life, however, they are usually used. The patient with emphysema is particularly susceptible to the complications of steroid therapy, since he may have a peptic ulcer or edema.

Because one of the compensatory mechanisms in decreased ventilation is increased erythropoiesis, the patient with severe emphysema often develops polycythemia. This is treated by reducing the blood volume through phlebotomy to diminish the work of the heart. The nursing care for patients with polycythemia is discussed further in Chapter 5.

Another complication of emphysema can be rupture of the pleural blebs or bullae that appear as cystic spaces in the lungs. When rupture occurs, pneumothorax results and the patient is in severe respiratory distress. Treatment and care for patients with pneumothorax are discussed later in this chapter.

The prognosis for patients with emphysema is variable. Some people have the syndrome for years and seem to adapt to the activity restrictions and special care measures imposed by the dysfunction. In some people the syndrome does not become severe, while others experience a steady, progressively increasing severity in which the symptoms become more difficult to manage and medical intervention is required with increasing frequency. The terminal events can be varied; for some patients it is pneumothorax caused by rupture of blebs or bullae. Cor pulmonale, characterized by right heart failure, is the most frequent cause of death. A number of patients die from causes other than the emphysema.

The nurse will find great differences among patients with emphysema in terms of the symptoms evidenced and the adaptations they are able to make. One is often amazed to see a patient with emphysema whose blood gases show very low oxygen saturation but whose physical appearance is that of a relatively healthy person. Others with similar or even higher levels of oxygen saturation can appear extremely debilitated and dyspneic. The nurse will also find great variations in the ability of patients to adjust to the treatment and preventive regimens. Some patients learn to carry portable oxygen for use when exercise requisites require supplementary oxygen, so they will not be restricted as much; others prefer to remain quietly in a secure environment and do not choose to use portable oxygen to increase the scope of their activities.

Because of all these variations, it is necessary that patient care be determined by a sound data base of blood gas levels and pulmonary function tests. It would be harmful to encourage a seemingly well-adjusted, non-dyspneic person to increase his exercise levels if his Pa_{O_2} is low. Likewise, it would be inappropriate to encourage a dyspneic person to rest if he is able to tolerate exercise, which he needs, and if his arterial oxygen level is adequate. In practical terms, people usually adapt to the emphysema in the best way possible for them according to the resources they have available. The nurse must deal with the patient's total response to the emphysema in teaching, counseling, and guiding him to maintain the maximum amount of ventilation possible. It is necessary for the nurse to remember that any changes in the patient's behavior must come from his own commitment to change.

CHRONIC BRONCHITIS

Chronic bronchitis, another obstructive pulmonary disease, may be called an environmental disease in that its incidence is related to pollution, cold and damp air, and industrial dusts. Environmental pollution has been recognized as a factor in both the occurrence of primary respiratory disease and the aggravation of symptoms in patients with known respiratory dysfunction. Continued exposure to polluted air and cigarette smoke brings about further changes in lung function as the protective mechanisms are placed under constant stress.

The lung surface area ranges from 50 to 100

square meters. This entire surface is exposed to environmental air inhaled through the airway passages, so it is inevitable that some undesirable particles will reach the bronchus. There are goblet cells and mucous glands in the bronchial walls that secrete mucus. Millions of cilia function as the transport system for this mucus as they move rhythmically to push mucus with trapped inhaled particles out of the bronchi and up to the trachea and epiglottis. When the cilia are exposed to inhaled toxins, cold and damp air over long periods, or large amounts of undesirable inhaled particles, their work is hindered. Although the exact cause of bronchitis is unknown, the major physiologic event is overproduction of mucus in the bronchi. Excessive mucus production requires increasing numbers of goblet cells, which replace cilia-producing cells. Both the decreased number of cilia and the viscous mucus contribute to inefficient clearing of undesirable particles from the bronchi; this in turn creates a situation in which the bronchi are susceptible to infection.

Bronchitis is a progressive situation, as continued overproduction of mucus is further accelerated by the infectious process. The glands in the bronchi eventually become enlarged and the bronchial ducts are distended with mucus until the finer air passages are also involved. Resultant enlargement of the bronchial muscles and plugs of mucus cause obstruction of air passages. Bronchopneumonia may develop in the alveoli served by the involved terminal bronchioles. Fibrosis of tissues occurs during the healing process, leaving the bronchioles dilated or perhaps destroyed. The peripheral airways then become increasingly involved in the development of chronic bronchitis so that there is extensive airway obstruction. Airway resistance in chronic bronchitis, then, is related to several factors: the enlarging of the bronchial mucous glands, the presence of mucus, the destruction or narrowing of the peripheral airway passages from fibrosis or inflammation, and hypertrophy of the bronchial muscles in those patients with asthmatic bronchitis. Air may be trapped in the finer air passages, causing their dilation so that the lungs are overinflated.

As with emphysema, there is uneven distribution of ventilation, and perfusion is not efficient in the damaged portions of the lung. Cyanosis from inadequately perfused arterial blood indicates the severity of chronic bronchitis. Unlike patients with emphysema, who are usually able to compensate for the ventilation deficit, those with chronic bronchitis tend to have constriction of the pulmonary arterioles, which leads to inadequate ventilation and ineffective perfusion. The term "blue bloater" is derived from the symptoms of cyanosis and edema that ensue when cardiac involvement becomes marked; the cardiac muscle hypertrophies from hypoxia as pulmonary artery pressure increases to compensate for the pulmonary arteriole constriction. The severity of damage to lung tissue in chronic bronchitis is related to the degree of hypoxia that is present.

Progression of Signs and Symptoms

Usually the person with chronic bronchitis first experiences the symptoms of an early morning cough that he relates to smoking too much. As the bronchitis progresses he also notices coughing late at night and eventually may be awakened during the night by a coughing spell. The cough is usually accompanied by mucus, which initially is thick, white, and ropy. When periods of infection begin to occur with increasing frequency, the mucus may change in color to yellowish or greenish and become purulent. In regions where smoke pollution is great, the mucus may be black or grayish, becoming purulent during infections. The mucus may be streaked with blood in some instances. The amount of mucus varies among different people.

The characteristic pattern of the development of chronic bronchitis involves more persistent infections that last for longer periods of time. The American Thoracic Society defines bronchitis as a syndrome of persistent cough and sputum production that occurs during at least 3 out of 24 consecutive months. Wheezing may be noticed during severe infections in people who also have asthmatic tendencies; this wheezing may gradually become a persistent symptom. The person with bronchitis also experiences breathlessness, which increases in severity and duration over a period of time. Bronchospasms may also occur, particularly during times of infection. The episodes of infection, wheezing, dyspnea, and bronchospasms may occur with greater frequency during cold weather, finally becoming the person's "normal" or usual pattern all year as the disease worsens. Along with these symptoms, the person becomes progressively more inactive. He is able to maintain sufficient ventilation and perfusion to accommodate his normal activities at first, but as the disease progresses and infections are more difficult to overcome, he must adjust to decreased activity. Often the person with chronic bronchitis becomes discouraged about his loss of physical energy and may also suffer economic distress from loss of work.

Chronic bronchitis becomes debilitating when the person cannot perform his daily routine of activities. In this instance loss of work or inability to function effectively may cause true emotional depression, which may be further accentuated if oxygen perfusion is so inadequate that the person also has decreased mental alertness.

Patient Assessment

Assessment of the patient with chronic bronchitis includes a history of the frequency of infection, wheezing, breathlessness, and cough. Musical wheezes can be heard on auscultation. The patient's description of the pattern of mucus production and its color are significant in determining his status. Laboratory studies of the sputum during periods of infection identify the causative organism. X-ray studies generally do not show pathologic changes but do demonstrate the changes in the diaphragm and rib cage. As with emphysema, the lungs become hyperinflated as their elasticity is decreased. The diaphragm is low and flat and the chest movement is diminished. Some patients with chronic bronchitis have long, narrow chests while others have chest forms similar to those of patients with emphysema. Bronchography reveals narrowed bronchi with fewer branches than normal. The Reid index measures mucous gland enlargement in relation to the thickness of the bronchial wall; chronic bronchitis is associated with the gradual enlargement of mucous glands.

The patient with chronic bronchitis usually reports that the symptoms are more predominant in cold weather. He usually does not tolerate changes in humidity and barometric pressure very well and notices increasing symptoms when exposed to dusts or polluted air. Talking for extended periods of time and increased alcohol intake also increase the symptoms in most patients with chronic bronchitis. As the bronchitis becomes more severe, the cough becomes more persistent and is associated with varying amounts of mucus production. The patient may have chronic sinusitis with a postnasal drip, to which he attributes the bouts of coughing that awaken him from his sleep. The cough is often paroxysmal and productive. The nurse should teach the patient to avoid the factors that produce symptoms.

Bronchitis is considered reversible when the airway obstruction is caused by overproduction of mucus. When the bronchi become narrowed as a result of the mucus production and fibrosis following inflammation, the disease is usually irreversible. In some patients, the bronchitis extends to the bronchioles and destructive emphysema results, with air trapping distal to the affected bronchioles. The time period for the destructive process varies considerably among different patients. Those with advanced chronic bronchitis begin to lose weight and experience the symptoms of hypoxia and hypercapnia as the disease becomes severe.

Respiratory failure in patients with severe chronic bronchitis may be precipitated by any factor that further impairs the compromised ventilation and perfusion. Frequent causes of death are infection, taking barbiturates or narcotics, anesthesia, or cardiac failure, because the patient cannot tolerate any stress that increases the work of the already impaired lung function. Nursing care depends on the patient's needs and may include any combination of the measures previously described for obstructive pulmonary dysfunction.

ASTHMA (REVERSIBLE AIRWAYS DISEASE)

Asthma is an obstructive pulmonary disease that typifies the complex interrelationships between a person's physiologic processes and his environment. Persons with asthma have attacks of breathlessness that are paroxysmal in nature. The breathlessness is caused by obstruction of the bronchioles because of bronchospasm, edema of the mucous membrane, and production of mucus. Although the differences are not precise, asthma can be referred to as **extrinsic** or **allergic** and **intrinsic** or **idiopathic**.

Causative Factors

Allergic asthma attacks are precipitated by environmental stimuli. Allergens (which are usually proteins) in the environment that stimulate the attacks include such items as house dust, food particles, mites that feed on skin scales in bed linens, mattresses, and pillows, and food allergies. Among the foods known to precipitate asthmatic attacks in some people are wheat, milk, chocolate, nuts, and shellfish; other substances include synthetic drugs, such as aspirin, horse serum, and certain antibiotics. Irritating fumes from gasoline, kerosene, paint, glue, or mothballs may also trigger the allergic response. The allergic response is most commonly caused by pollens, mold spores, dander, lint, feather dust, powder, and inhalants such as aerosol sprays and insecticides. The response may occur at the time of contact or may be delayed, occurring some time after the contact with the allergen. Asthmatic patients frequently have a history of hypersensitivity to allergens, as evidenced by dermatitis, hay fever, rhinitis, hives, or migraines. There is often a family history of hypersensitivity to allergens, which supports the theory that there is genetic predisposition to allergy. Therefore, when the nurse obtains a patient history, questions about allergic responses in family members are significant.

The asthma attack is actually a local anaphylactic reaction. It is believed that asthmatic patients have increased bronchial muscle tone all the time, and when the allergen stimulates the hypersensitive bronchial muscle, it shortens and narrows in contraction. Because the bronchi are normally shortened and narrowed during expiration, this further reduction in the size of the bronchi causes increased airway resistance, obstructing the flow of air. This inflammatory response includes both edema and increased production of mucus, which further decrease the amount of space available for airflow.

The reason for the susceptibility of certain people to allergens is not known. The local anaphylactic reaction is primarily due to IgE antibodies, which cause the release of mediators including histamine and slow-reacting substance A (SRS-A). These mediators stimulate the contraction of the smooth muscle of the bronchi, the mucosal edema, and the increased mucus production. The inhaled antigens combine with specific IgE antibodies and the effector cell membranes release the mediators in this process. Allergic asthmatic attacks are sometimes accompanied by skin reactions, usually wheals and erythema.

Asthmatic patients with idiopathic asthma may have an attack without exposure to a specific stimulus such as an allergen. Factors that seem to precipitate such attacks are increased exercise, fatigue, changes in the temperature and humidity, exposure to environmental pollutants, cigarette smoke, cold air, industrial smog, and fog. Psychosocial stressors, such as worry, stress, anxiety, and emotional upsets, are often related to asthmatic attacks. However, it is probably true that no single factor but rather a combination of stressors is causative. Asthma may be precipated by infections because of the inflammatory process and bronchospasms; bacterial or viral debris can also function as antigens. The direct relationship between asthma attacks and the infection has been demonstrated even though the role of bacteria in causing the attacks is not understood. The nature of the hypersensitivity response is related to the asthmatic's total resistance and in part to the intensity of the irritant and the duration of exposure as well as to the combination of stressors.

Many studies have been conducted to identify the personality characteristics common to asthmatic patients; they often show that dependent, sensitive people with low self-concepts tend to have asthma. These traits are not peculiar to asthmatics, however, as many people with similar traits do not have asthma. It is interesting to speculate about the relationships between artistic creativity and sensitivities and the development of asthma. At any rate, the emotional factors that may precipitate asthma attacks may or may not be significant as a primary cause.

Identification of the precipitating factors of attacks and the coping patterns of the asthmatic patient are important in nursing care. If the asthmatic can isolate the stresses that tend to precipitate attacks, he can be helped to learn how to avoid the stresses at any given time; thus self-knowledge is an essential prerequisite of learning to cope more effectively.

Counseling can be a valuable adjunct to therapy for the asthmatic patient in helping him to explore his own action-reaction patterns.

Asthma Attacks

Asthma usually begins in childhood and decreases with maturity. However, a person may experience his first asthma attack after the age of 40. An asthma attack is usually very distressing for both the person and his family. Breathlessness gives rise to anxiety, and the attack itself may stimulate anxiety because the asthmatic must "get through" the attack. It is frustrating to watch a person with an asthma attack and not be able to help him immediately; by the same token, it is difficult to relax and let the attack take its course if one is the person who is breathless.

An asthma attack usually begins suddenly with breathlessness. The attack may occur at varying lengths of time following the exposure to an allergen. In some cases the attacks begin with mild wheezing, becoming more severe in an hour or two. The characteristic wheezing expiration occurs as the person makes an effort to force air from the lungs through narrowed bronchi. Although the obstruction to ventilation may be predominantly expiratory, in severe attacks it can also involve inspiratory obstruction to ventilation. The lungs become hyperinflated because of either air trapping or the increased residual volume and forced residual capacity. Wheezing can be heard throughout the chest, as can high-pitched rhonchi that disappear after the attack has ceased. Inspiration is more difficult because of the work required to inhale air into distended lungs with greater elastic tension.

Blood gases can be particularly affected in attacks of long duration. If ventilation and perfusion are ineffective there is first a decrease in arterial Po_2, and if the attack lasts long enough there will be a decrease in oxygen saturation because of the uneven distribution of ventilation and perfusion that occurs when some of the bronchioles become plugged with mucus. In mild or moderate attacks the arterial Pco_2 will be either normal or decreased. In severe attacks of long duration there may be carbon dioxide retention.

The person experiencing an attack of asthma is restless. He or she has to concentrate on the work of breathing and struggles to find a position that facilitates breathing. He or she may sit up or stand, or lean on an object for support, but no position gives comfort. The position may have to be changed frequently in efforts to alleviate the feeling of suffocation. Because of the necessity to force expiration, the chest accommodates by assuming a hyperinflated position similar to that seen in emphysematous patients. The accessory muscles of respiration are activated, and in moderate or severe attacks the neck veins are distended on expiration. Following the attack breathing becomes more normal and the chest resumes normal mechanical function. As the attack begins to subside there may be expectoration of mucus; the person is compelled to cough and gradually expectorates thick mucus. When this occurs he actually feels that his airway is clearing and the attack is diminishing. Following an asthma attack the person is fatigued and requires rest because of the extra work that has been required to oxygenate his tissues. He is also dehydrated to some extent because of the water lost through hyperventilation and to a lesser degree through excessive perspiration. Since the accessory muscles for breathing have been strained during the attack, the person may have muscle soreness for a day or two.

Status Asthmaticus

Asthma attacks lasting more than 24 hours are called **status asthmaticus** and must be treated as medical emergencies. The person with this condition has severe respiratory difficulty. He is not only uncomfortable but is also extremely fatigued from the effort of breathing under duress for a length of time and may actually die from exhaustion during the attack if medical intervention is not successful. The continued attack is emotionally wearing as well, and the person may become very frustrated and anxious when his breathlessness does not subside. As the attack continues for a period of time, the person may lose control of the conscious effort to relax and can only work to breathe. Ventilation and perfusion are more severely impaired as the attack continues, resulting in decreased oxygen tensions and retention of carbon dioxide, and then symptoms of hypoxia, cyanosis, hypotension, and tachycardia. Venous blood return to the heart is interfered with because of the increased intrathoracic pressure. Considerable fluid can be lost with hyperventilation so that symptoms of dehydration may ensue. Eventually some degree of hypovolemia and heart failure may occur. Heart failure is a major concern in monitoring patients during an acute attack of status asthmaticus.

Treatment and Nursing Care

Treatment for asthma attacks is determined by the severity of the attack and its duration. If the attack is mild the patient may not receive any specific treatment other than oral bronchodilator medication, ingest fluids if possible, and wait for the attack to subside. With slightly more serious attacks prompt treatment is desired. Inhalers or nebulizers may provide quick relief so that the attack subsides within about an hour. If the nebulizer is ineffective, epinephrine is given subcutaneously. Expectorants such as SSKI (saturated solution of potassium iodide) may be given. Aminophylline may be given intramuscularly or intravenously along with the epinephrine or if epinephrine is ineffective. If the patient continues to be breathless and wheeze with this treatment, as in status asthmaticus, corticosteroids are given. Since corticosteroids take from 6 to 12 hours to be effective, they are generally used only when the other medications have not relieved the symptoms of the attack. It is important that the nurse recognize and carefully evaluate the symptoms of drug ineffectiveness. Bronchodilators should not be continued if the asthma attack does not respond to the usual dose. Aminophylline can be toxic when given in excess. Attention should be given to the observation of pulse and blood pressure since the catecholamine bronchodilators can cause arrhythmias, adding further stress to the asthmatic patient's dwindling energy reserve.

The patient with status asthmaticus may require oxygen to assist him in the work of breathing. The route of administration should be selected to provide controlled oxygen in a manner that does not increase the patient's anxiety. Masks tend to make a breathless patient feel further suffocation. Adequate humidity is very important because the patient is dehydrated from hyperventilation. If oxygen is being given and the patient continues to show signs of inadequate perfusion, endotracheal intubation may be performed; this allows for suctioning of mucus and for assisted respiration until the corticosteroids can take effect. The use of IPPB is controversial in asthma attacks; some authorities believe it is helpful, whereas others believe that IPPB is contraindicated because mechanical ventilation may be required if the patient tends toward respiratory failure.

Assessment of the patient's condition during status asthmaticus involves continuous monitoring. The arterial Po_2, Pco_2, and pH should be measured every 4 hours to evaluate the ventilation-perfusion ratio. The early signs of heart failure, described in Chapter 4, should be watched for. Tachycardia is a danger signal that alerts the nurse to impending cardiac involvement. If hypoxia and hypercapnia are present, the asthmatic patient may show signs of confusion. He will probably already demonstrate fatigue from the effort of breathing and will have little vigor for activities and yet may be extremely restless. Tranquilizers may be given during the attack; antihistamines, sedatives, narcotics, and depressant drugs should not be given even though one might be tempted to use them to help the asthmatic rest.

Ingestion of food and fluids may be impossible for the patient, even with assistance. Nausea and vomiting may occur during the attack. This presents a challenging nursing care situation not only in terms of facilitating breathing while the patient vomits and is given hygienic care, but also in terms of maintaining adequate nutrition for the fatigued patient. Fluids are provided through intravenous infusion; the type of fluid used is determined by the pH. If the patient is in metabolic acidosis, sodium bicarbonate may be given with the intravenous fluid. An asthma attack may be fatal if the patient goes into respiratory failure; thus the nurse should watch for signs of increasing fatigue, gradual loss of consciousness, diminishing breath sounds, wheezing, increased carbon dioxide retention and decreased oxygen perfusion, increased sternal retraction, and diminishing movement of the chest wall. Mechanical ventilation is then necessary.

Once the attack has finally subsided the patient will require rest and further observation to determine the effects of the strain he has undergone. If the patient had some respiratory and cardiac dysfunction prior to the attack, the fatiguing work required by the attack and the perfusion imbalances may have effects lasting for several days. The effects of asthma on lung tissue may be reversible if the attacks are mild and subside completely, or the effects may be progressively more serious through changes that occur following each attack and subsequent bout of infection. Among the progressive changes is the response of the bronchial walls, which may have increased numbers of goblet cells, hypersecretion of mucus, and areas of destroyed bronchial epithelium. The bronchi and bronchioles may be plugged with desquamated cells and mucus, and the bronchial walls tend to be thick from hyperplasia resulting from muscle contraction. The alveoli are enlarged and distended from overinflation, which causes their walls to be thin.

Assessment of the patient's status depends primarily on the history of the timing, frequency, and duration of the acute asthma attacks. There are no significant x-ray findings, and laboratory studies may be negative. Eosinophils may be found in the sputum of asthmatic patients, and specific organisms may be found in the event of an infection. Skin testing to determine the asthmatic's hypersensitivity to given antigens is frequently done to enable the asthmatic to know what substances should be avoided. The trial and error method for determining sensitivities may be used instead of skin tests by some patients; in this method the asthmatic keeps a record of his experiences and relates specific events or exposures to his periods of attack. These factors are then considered to be the ones that precipitate the attacks.

Teaching the Patient to Adapt
On the basis of information provided by the skin tests or through the trial and error method, the asthmatic patient may act to become desensitized to allergens or change his habits or environment. For example, patients with allergies to animal dander should not have pets, particularly household ones, and those who are allergic to certain foods can eliminate them from their diets. The patient must learn to read labels on packaged foods. Changes in life patterns may mean moving to a drier climate, if this is possible, or moving from a highly polluted area to one with less pollution. If moving is impractical the patient may be advised to purchase air filtering systems or air conditioners for his home, although this may be expensive and perhaps out of range for some persons. Changing one's daily habits may mean establishing meticulous care in cleaning one's home and adjusting to new products in order to eliminate aerosol sprays and many of the convenience products used for household cleaning and for cosmetic purposes. All of these changes are geared to avoid the allergens that may precipitate asthmatic attacks.

Depending on the adjustment or adaptation required, the asthmatic patient may require assistance in learning to change. Food allergens are particularly difficult to avoid, as one tends to want the things he cannot have. Essentially the asthmatic must deal with giving up something he wants. When one makes changes in daily habits or life patterns because of a disease process, he may strongly react to the disability that such restriction or change implies. Accepting one's own condition is a primary focal point for patients who must make these adaptations, and nursing care must deal with this issue directly.

For asthmatic patients who are hypersensitive to a number of different substances, it is important for the nurse to remember that there are countless difficulties involved in a person's avoidance of allergens. Teaching must be practical and reflect the person's condition and state in life. It is not sufficient to tell the asthmatic to avoid household dusts; while a person might be able to control dust in his own home he would be very restricted in his activities if he avoided household dusts in the homes of his friends. It is not always possible to screen the places one visits to ensure that no allergens will be encountered. Likewise, it is difficult to avoid environmental air pollutants and pollens if one wishes to go outdoors. Therefore, teaching must be kept in the realm of reality for the asthmatic, since meticulous avoidance of all allergens could create a sense of psychological deprivation.

Certain aspects of daily life are not too difficult for the asthmatic patient to control. He can replace all feather and kapok pillows with foam rubber ones; he can ensure that his house is dusted daily with a wet cloth and that the floors are damp mopped or vacuumed daily; and all unnecessary furniture and dust-catching items such as heavy drapes can be eliminated from his house, as can aerosol sprays, paint, and other substances that are a source of allergens. To some extent, the patient can avoid changes in temperature and exposure to damp, cold air. He can arrange his periods of exercise and rest to avoid overexertion, and he can avoid ingestion of foods that precipitate asthma attacks. However, there are some aspects of life that the asthmatic cannot avoid. For this reason, one of the important aspects of therapy is teaching the patient to cope with the hypersensitivity. Since drugs are useful in controlling asthma attacks, the patient can be taught to use bronchodilator drugs appropriately. If the attacks are frequent, he can take bronchodilators on a prophylactic basis; this is advisable when the ventilation obstruction is consistent. Cromolyn sodium (Intal or Aarane), a prophylactic bronchospasmolytic agent, is currently being used for patients with allergic asthma. The drug is thought to act by stabilizing the cellular membranes of the mast cells. The patient should be taught the side effects of drugs and must also know how drugs interact so that he does not inadvertently develop tachycardia and perhaps arrhythmias from using both bronchodilators and nebulizers in multiple doses.

Recognition of one's own symptoms and early treatment when the patient feels an attack "coming on" are critical in avoiding severe attacks. In addition, the asthmatic patient should be aware that he must seek medical attention when the usual treatments are not effective. Sometimes the severity of the asthma attack can be lessened by early treatment, since the patient then does not have to undergo the exhausting breathing work, dehydration, and perfusion alterations that can accompany severe attacks.

Some authorities advocate desensitization for specific allergens, although the value of this is not clear since desensitization is not always effective for the total number of allergens that a given person might be sensitive to. Desensitization seems to be most beneficial for those with pollen, household dust, or fungus hypersensitivities and less useful with many of the other allergens. The asthmatic patient may choose to have the desensitization even though its value has not been proved because some patients do benefit. Possibly the fact that the patient is taking positive action to treat or prevent the disease is of great psychological benefit and results in the reduction of the frequency of allergic reactions.

Other aspects of long-term care for the asthmatic patient are similar to those for patients with other types of respiratory dysfunction. Hydration should be emphasized, with as much as 3,000 ml of fluid ingested daily to prevent dehydration. (The hydration level is determined relative to cardiac status. Patients who have had long-standing asthma with resultant congestive heart failure may not be able to tolerate this much fluid.) One extremely important aspect of care is avoidance of infections, since the incidence of infection may precipitate an asthmatic attack and may further damage vulnerable lung tissue.

BRONCHIECTASIS

Bronchiectasis is a disease resulting from congenital or acquired anatomic variations that make one susceptible to respiratory dysfunction. In bronchiectasis, the bronchi become dilated following inflammation and subsequent ulceration. There are several therories about the etiology of bronchiectasis; one theory is that a congenital weakness in the bronchi makes the person vulnerable to the dilatation that usually follows an infection. Another theory is that bronchiectasis follows an obstruction with consequent infection that damages the bronchial wall. The obstruction can be caused by anything that occludes the air passages distal to the eventual dilatation, including mucus plugs, foreign objects such as peanuts that are inhaled, pus produced in an infectious process, gastric juice aspiration that causes inflammation and edema, or the presence of a tumor. However, the incidence of bronchiectasis has decreased with the increased use of antibiotics to treat infections.

There is a relationship between bronchiectasis and sinusitis. Kartagener's syndrome is a disease in which this relationship is evidenced; in this syndrome there may be a congenital absence of the frontal sinuses or variation in sinus formation. The syndrome generally begins in childhood with repeated sinus infections. The infectious materials from the sinuses are aspirated, infecting the bronchi (most often those located in the dependent positions in the lung). In children, the bronchi are softer and smaller and are more easily plugged by mucus. Whether or not there is a preexisting susceptibility to the destruction of tissue has yet to be proved.

The occurrence of bronchiectasis can often be traced to childhood respiratory infections, particularly pneumonia or bacterial infections. Measles and pertussis may be complicated by an aftermath of bronchiectasis. Tuberculosis may also predispose to bronchiectasis when the tubercular lesions destroy normal bronchial tissue with formation of scars. In general, middle or lower lobe infections of the lung more frequently predispose to bronchiectasis because infectious materials do not drain as well from the middle and lower lobes as they do from the upper lobes.

When an obstruction forms in the bronchi, the portion of the lung served by the plugged bronchi collapses and negative pressure distends the bronchi above the obstructed area. If the distention can be relieved early enough, the bronchi return to normal. However, if the distention lasts long enough to destroy the elasticity of the bronchial walls, the bronchi remain distended and thereafter are increasingly susceptible to infection. The mucosa of the bronchial walls is replaced with scar tissue, and the loss of elasticity interferes with the normal bronchial clearing mechanisms.

Diagnosis

Characteristic changes of the bronchial wall in bronchiectasis include the formation of sacs containing mucus and pus. The sacs are found in the form of rounded or elongated pockets, and these dilated areas can be seen on a bronchogram when they are outlined with a radiopaque substance. The bronchogram is the diagnostic tool used to confirm the diagnosis of bronchiectasis. The mucus- and pus-filled sacs are often referred to as cystic, saccular, fusiform, or cylindrical, depending on the shape and placement on the dilated bronchi. The peripheral bronchi are most often affected.

Other factors significant in the diagnosis are a cough and expectoration of sputum. Usually the patient with bronchiectasis has had a persistent cough since childhood. Depending on the extent of the involved areas and the amount of infection, the patient may have sputum production varying from copious to minimal. The sputum is composed of mucus, desquamated mucosa, and granular products of the inflammation and necrosis that occur. The patient may have an infrequent acute inflammation or may develop chronic inflammation with more or less constant production of mucus and debris, causing an acute flare-up and infection as a result of their accumulation in the lung. The sputum production usually increases in times of infection, although expectoration of sputum may be consistent throughout the year. Lesions in the upper lobes are usually associated with less sputum because of their better drainage. Patients with upper lobe lesions and little sputum expectoration are said to have "dry" bronchiectasis.

Assessment of bronchiectasis is facilitated by the patient's description of coughing patterns and sputum expectoration. The sputum has the characteristic purulent quality associated with infections. Expectoration is increased when the patient changes positions, particularly when lying down or arising, because of the change in position of the affected bronchi in relation to the large bronchus and trachea, which promotes drainage from the involved areas of the lung. Because the capillaries are sometimes dilated from increased blood flow to the inflamed areas, the sputum may contain blood streaks or larger amounts of gross blood. This hemoptysis is frequent in bronchiectasis and often frightens the patient, since it implies a very serious lung infection.

In addition to the typical sputum and cough, the patient with bronchiectasis has the generalized symptoms of an infection. Anorexia, weight loss, low grade fever, increased susceptibility to stress, and anemia are commonly found generalized symptoms. Night sweats are not uncommon, so tuberculosis is often suspected. Since bronchiectasis is a chronic infectious disease these symptoms may vary in severity according to the patient's current physical status. Patients with bronchiectasis tend to have increasing numbers of infections during the winter months as well as a propensity for developing pneumonia. Some patients have mild cases with few symptoms while others have more severe discomfort and more frequent periods of infection.

Chest sounds vary in bronchiectasis. It is common to hear both rhonchi and rales even after the patient has coughed effectively. There may be localized crepitations in affected areas, and breath sounds may be diminished. In other instances the chest is clear.

Another important sign in diagnosing bronchiectasis is the clubbing of the fingers and toes associated with cyanosis. Cyanosis and orthopnea are observed in more advanced chronic cases.

Treatment and Nursing Care

Treatment for bronchiectasis is both symptomatic and curative. The symptomatic measures include provision for bronchial drainage through the use of expectorants and postural drainage; the latter should be done with knowledge of the infected area so that the positions for postural drainage provide for the most efficient clearing of mucus and pus. When infections occur, sputum is cultured and antibiotics are given to treat the specific organisms found. The more commonly found organisms include staphylococci, pneumococci, and species of *Escherichia* and *Hemophilus*. Care is taken to avoid repeated infections when possible. Precise oral hygiene and treatment of sinus infections are important for the patient with bronchiectasis.

If the bronchiectasis is localized, surgery can be performed to remove the involved bronchi. The procedure used is determined by the amount of lung tissue involved. Many authorities prefer surgical treatment because the bronchiectasis is progressive in its development, spreading to involve areas of lung tissue surrounding the initially damaged bronchi. Another indication for surgical intervention is that of repeated bouts of hemoptysis.

The overall goal of nursing care is to assist the patient in minimizing the extent of the bronchiectasis if medical therapy is employed. For patients with mild cases, this care and attention to positive health practices may be sufficient to alleviate further symptoms. If the patient has a more severe case of bronchiectasis, the signs of increasing respiratory dysfunction should be anticipated, including symptoms of either restrictive or obstructive respiratory disease with concomitant changes in ventilation and perfusion. Because of extensive tissue necrosis in bronchiectasis there may be anomalies of the pulmonary and alveolar capillaries, inducing pulmonary hypertension. This pulmonary hypertension interferes with adequate ventilation and perfusion, and cardiac involvement usually ensues and may even be the cause of death. Complications of bronchiectasis include increased bouts of pneumonia and the development of lung abscesses.

The nurse should encourage the patient with bronchiectasis to follow through with routine physical examinations and to contact the physician when infections occur. People often tend to adjust to the symptoms of a chronic disease and come to expect that they will not feel well on many days; the symptoms may increase in severity so gradually that the person is sometimes not aware that he needs medical attention. Teaching the patient to recognize changes and to be aware of their gradual occurrence so that early treatment can be initiated is a nursing function. The presence of blood in the sputum often motivates the patient to seek medical attention; however, this in itself may not be an indication of a serious change. A severe infection could compromise ventilation and perfusion most acutely and is therefore a very serious event in the patient with bronchiectasis.

RESPIRATORY TRACT INFECTIONS

Respiratory tract infections may cause dysfunction that is a combination of restrictive and obstructive mechanisms. These infections represent the relation between the quality of a person's immunologic defense mechanisms and his ability to protect himself from potential disease-producing agents within the environment. The range of infections experienced may vary from acute to chronic, mild to severe, and localized to generalized. Respiratory tract infections are usually caused by airborne microorganisms that are present in ambient air to a greater or lesser degree all the time.

Why some people are susceptible to respiratory tract infections while others can sustain long contacts with infected persons without having an infection is not fully understood. Observations have been made about the incidence of infections, however, so that some generalizations can be made about them. Overcrowding or grouping of large numbers of people in one place is considered a factor in the increased incidence of respiratory infections. Classrooms, offices where many people work in one room, meetings, and other types of large gatherings increase the possibility of the transmission of microorganisms from person to person. Poor ventilation and inefficient cleaning of rooms, as well as inadequate washing of clothes and linens such as napkins, are other contributing factors.

A person's suceptibility to respiratory tract infections may vary at different times in his life. Fatigue, depression, periods of anxiety, changes in one's environment (including weather and temperature changes), and emotional and physical stress are all important determinants of a person's ability to resist infections. Increasing evidence is being found that certain individuals may have impaired immunologic responses, making them particularly susceptible to repeated infections. As more is discovered, it is hoped that the impairment or dysfunction, if it does exist, will provide the basis for therapy to augment the individual's immunologic response and thereby reduce the incidence of infections. Certain disease states also make one susceptible to infections, which can be secondary to almost any other disease process that places a strain on the body's resources to cope with infection.

Another important consideration in the incidence of respiratory tract infections is that of the strength or nature of the microorganism. A number of microorganisms are known to be highly virulent and therefore have a high rate of associated infections or cause more serious disease, or both. Some viruses and bacteria are elusive, changing strains frequently and thus making prevention of infection through vaccines or controlled or natural stimulation of antibody production difficult. A person may develop antibodies for one strain of a virus, only to have another illness caused by a new strain for which he has no antibodies. The influenza virus is an example of a rapidly changing, elusive microorganism.

Certain microorganisms have been identified and specific preventive vaccines have been devised to limit their infection rates in the population. Measles is an example of a viral infection that can be prevented through use of a vaccine. On the other hand, as many as 50 percent of microorganisms or causes of respiratory tract infections are unknown. Another group of microorganisms is known, but there is no definitive treatment for attenuating the life of the microorganism. Yet another group, particularly bacteria, can be identified and their sensitivity to antibiotic therapy can be determined, allowing for definitive treatment.

To some extent, the microorganisms that infect the respiratory tract can be discussed as a group of infecting agents that, although different in and of themselves, cause similar symptoms. Both a common cold and a sore throat are frequently self-diagnosed because the symptoms are generally known. However, this cold or sore throat may have been caused by any one of the known microorganisms or by an unidentified organism, irritant, or disease-producing agent, which complicates definitive treatment. Of necessity the focus of therapy is on the symptoms in order to relieve the patient of the ill effects of the disease process. Of great concern is whether or not minor or mild infections should be treated. In many instances the symptoms eventually disappear spontaneously. Repeated infections, however, may lead to tissue damage or destruction that can eventually alter respiratory function. When such conditions become chronic, the altered function could become irreversible. This destructive process could often be prevented if mild illnesses were treated effectively in the early stages. Some seemingly "normal" and expected mild infections can later be recognized as the cause of a more serious chronic or acute disease that follows the mild infection. The relationship of group A β-hemolytic infections, causing sore throats and the potential for subsequent glomerulonephritis, demonstrates this phenomenon.

There is a natural tendency to treat minor illness with patent medications available in many variety, drug, and grocery stores. There are many reasons for this. Many people do not want to bother their doctors, who are very busy, for minor problems. The patent medications are considered to be less expensive than a visit to the doctor and are often effective in alleviating or diminishing the uncomfortable symptoms. People expect that they will normally have at least one cold or bout of influenza, particularly during the cold winter months, if they live in a geographic area with a variable climate. It is generally accepted that these minor illnesses wear themselves out, and consequently many individuals will let them "run their course" because no specific treatment is known anyway. Some people feel that a visit to the doctor gives them no additional information or assistance and they already know the common remedy; this may be true in uncomplicated, mild infections.

The nurse is often asked to give advice and counsel, officially or unofficially, regarding minor or even major illnesses. A critical requirement in this role is that the nurse should make an assessment before giving information or advice. For example, someone may ask the nurse what to do about a cough. The appropriateness of the nurse's response depends on knowing if the cough is persistent, productive, or related to any other dysfunction, or if it is associated with a mild cold in a person who has one cold every other year and who has no other evidence of disease. Screening one's responses through the assessment is imperative. The nurse should be aware that a number of people treat themselves according to the advice they receive from their friends in the "health professions" as well as by reading the labels on patent medications in an effort to match the cure with their particular symptoms. It is very important that the nurse refer the person to a qualified nurse practitioner or physician for diagnosis and treatment if any serious illness is suspected.

Patent medications are often similar to medications one obtains through prescriptions in that they contain some of the same ingredients in varying amounts. Many patent medications do not contain sufficient pharmacologic ingredients to be therapeutic. Their use becomes inappropriate when a person takes them indiscriminately or becomes dependent on them for relief of symptoms, thereby delaying medical attention for serious preventable dysfunction in the early stages. Indiscriminate use of medications without symptoms may also be harmful and should be discouraged.

Respiratory tract infections may be localized or they may be extensive, involving the entire respiratory tract. They are often named anatomically according to the area of the respiratory tract involved; for example, rhinitis, laryngitis, tracheitis, bronchitis, and pneumonia are the names of localized infections. The term **nasopharyngolaryngotracheobronchial pneumonia** refers to a condition in which the entire respiratory tract is involved. While the infectious process most often begins in the upper respiratory tract and spreads downward, it may begin with a lung infection and can be carried upward to the trachea and the rest of the upper respiratory tract.

The Common Cold

The common cold is so called because of its frequency among populations and its association with changes in weather toward colder climates. **Coryza** is another name for the common cold. It is known that there are approximately eighty to one hundred different viruses that can cause the common cold. Because there is little cross-reacting immunity for these viruses, it is impossible to develop an immunity for the common cold. Typical symptoms are a runny nose, congestion of the nasal passages with sneezing, and perhaps a sore throat. The person may have a slightly elevated temperature or none at all.

Colds with a known causative microorganism are most often due to rhinoviruses in the fall and winter months and to coronaviruses in the spring. There are about one hundred different antigenic types of rhinoviruses. Treatment is symptomatic, including rest, increased fluid intake, aspirin or decongestants as required, and adequate nutrition. Antibiotics may speed up the resolution of the cold, but their use may lead to complications by masking the primary or a secondary problem.

Pharyngitis and Tonsillitis

Acute pharyngitis and tonsillitis have similar symptoms: The person with these conditions experiences a sore throat and either an inflamed, edematous pharynx that may have yellowish patches, or inflamed tonsils that appear reddened and swollen. Discomfort when swallowing is bothersome, as is the dry, scratchy feeling of the sore throat. The person may have an increased temperature, often low grade, and the cervical lymph nodes are generally tender and sore and may be enlarged in varying degrees. There may be exudate as a result of the inflammatory process, and the person usually experiences hoarseness.

Laboratory examination of the white cell count shows leukocytosis. A throat culture is done to isolate the invading organism and to determine its sensitivity to antibiotics, which are then the definitive treatment. A follow-up culture is done about two weeks after the initial culture to ensure that the microorganism has been attenuated and that it is not merely masked by the antibiotic therapy. A number of microorganisms can cause pharyngitis or tonsillitis. Group A β-hemolytic *Streptococcus* is probably one of the most important because it can lead to complications of renal or cardiac disease, particularly in children. Either rhinitis or laryngitis or both may occur simultaneously with pharyngitis or tonsillitis.

Streptococcal infections may be caused by many different strains of *Streptococcus,* each of which seems to produce different diseases. The streptococcal organisms are classified according to their colonization and their patterns of hemolysis. Group A β-hemolytic *Streptococcus,* as previously mentioned, is particularly important in respiratory tract infections. This organism may normally reside in the upper respiratory passages of certain people without causing symptoms of disease; these people are known to be carriers who spread the organism to other people who may be vulnerable to bacterial invasion. The average incubation period is three to five days.

Perhaps the most frequently occurring upper respiratory tract infection caused by *Streptococcus* is streptococcal pharyngitis, commonly known as "strep" sore throat. In this condition, the person suddenly develops a sore throat associated with headache, chills, malaise, and sometimes severe dysphagia and a high temperature. The pharynx appears glistening and reddened with a grayish white exudate. A culture should be done prior to giving any antibiotics, since the streptococcal organism is known to be resistant to tetracycline. β-hemolytic *Streptococcus* may be followed by rheumatic fever in children as well as by glomerulonephritis; it is therefore imperative that careful diagnosis and appropriate drug therapy with antibiotics be carried out for the duration of the prescription.

An important aspect of nursing care is to make certain that the patient follows through with having a repeat throat culture after resolution of the pharyngitis. If the drug therapy has not been adequate either in amount or in duration, the patient may feel better but may still have the potential for developing another more serious disease.

Acute lymphonodular pharyngitis is thought to be caused by coxsackievirus A-10. This disease is characterized by nodular lesions that are raised, white or yellow, and surrounded by erythema. The symptoms are the same as those of pharyngitis from other causes: sore throat, hoarseness, and dysphagia.

Diphtheria

Diphtheria is an example of an infectious disease with a known causative organism, *Corynebacterium diphtheriae,* for which there is a commercially available preventive toxoid. This disease is characterized by the formation of a pseudomembrane covering the posterior pharynx; the membrane is formed of fibrinous exudate resulting from the toxins produced by the organism. The membrane can extend to the trachea, larynx, and bronchi in severe cases, causing obstruction of the airway that must be relieved by tracheostomy. As the membrane first forms, it appears white and then gradually becomes gray and finally black.

In addition to the formation of the membrane, there may be paralysis of the palatal and pharyngeal muscles, further compromising the ability to swallow and the passage of air. A significant number of people with diphtheria caused by *C. diphtheriae* also develop myocarditis resulting from the toxins of the organism. Since the ill effects of *C. diphtheriae* are caused by the toxins, the exudate is cultured as early as possible so that antitoxin can be given. The antitoxin is most effective if initiated prior to the proliferation of the toxin so that the ill effects can be reduced. The antitoxin for *C. diphtheriae* is a horse serum; because many people are sensitive to horse serum, a skin test is given before administration of the antitoxin to determine sensitivity.

In the early stages of diphtheria, a priority is obtaining a culture. When the patient has respiratory stress, maintaining an adequate airway and observing for symptoms of myocarditis are important priorities; it is hoped that the causative organism can be identified before the patient becomes this severely ill. When myocarditis occurs, it is treated by bed rest, and antibiotic therapy may be effective. Neural symptoms can also develop in severe cases of diphtheria. Maintaining fluid and electrolyte balance and adequate nutrition presents a major challenge for the nursing care of severely ill patients with diphtheria. As with any disease, an important nursing measure is prevention of the disease through proper immunization.

Influenza

Influenza, commonly referred to as "flu," can be caused by a number of different viruses, which have an incubation period of approximately 48 hours. The influenza virus type A is capable of mutation and thus has the ability to vary its composition. Influenza is anticipated as much as possible by tracing the progress of the disease throughout the world and by observing the development of new strains. Each year vaccines are prepared for the strain expected, and the people most susceptible to the development of serious viral infections are given priority in receiving the vaccines. This group includes children, elderly and debilitated people, pregnant women, people with chronic respiratory disease, those receiving immunosuppressive and cytotoxic drugs, those receiving radiation treatments, and those with chronic systemic diseases, heart disease, or renal disease. In some health agencies, all personnel are encouraged to obtain the vaccine.

Although the effectiveness of the vaccines and therefore their value are controversial, it should be noted that a given vaccine immunizes a person only against the specific strains of viruses for which it is prepared; it does not provide immunity to all viruses. To expect that one is immune to all viruses after receiving the vaccine is a misconception that leads to loss of faith in the positive value of vaccines if one develops a viral infection after taking the trouble to receive the vaccine for the current year. The influenza vaccine is actually effective in about 50 to 70 percent of those receiving it. Some people develop the symptoms of influenza when they take the vaccine, and others may develop allergic symptoms from the vaccine. The vaccine must be given in appropriate dosages, in order to be adequate for immunization; in addition it should be administered via the appropriate route. The timing of vaccine administration is also important: It should be given early in the fall, well before the epidemic period for the virus begins. Much experimentation is underway to develop more effective vaccines. It is desirable to develop a vaccine that will provide for long-lasting systemic immunity for the strains people are most likely to be subjected to, and one that can be prepared early enough each year to be useful for prevention.

Viral infections produce symptoms similar to those of the common cold: general malaise and headache. The person with a virus may have a low-grade temperature, chills, muscle soreness, and cough. Treatment is symptomatic, and if possible the causative organism is isolated.

It is interesting to note that although viruses are responsible for illnesses resulting in significant loss of productivity among people of all age groups, are known to occur in epidemic proportions, and are also communicable, they are not reportable communicable diseases. The virus is most potent in the nasal passages and has a relatively short lifetime. It does remain viable long enough to be infectious following coughing, sneezing, or blowing one's nose so that another person in close contact may be exposed. Therefore, care should be taken either to isolate the infected person or to minimize his contacts during the first 24 hours of an infection or during the time when the virus is most potent. Thereafter, the person should take care not to spread the virus. Good personal hygiene and careful handling of contaminated articles, such as handkerchiefs, are essential.

Pneumonia
Viral pneumonia Viral pneumonia is associated with generalized symptoms. The involved portions of the respiratory tract are inflamed and edematous and there is usually production of exudate, which is the basis for the feeling of congestion in the early stages as well as the productive cough in the later stages. Headache may be severe, with retro-orbital pain and conjunctival congestion. Some people experience photophobia. Flushed skin, chilliness alternating with extreme warmth, varying degrees of diaphoresis, and muscle soreness are also characteristic symptoms. The person may have a harsh, paroxysmal cough on activity or movement and may be breathless. If the pneumonia is extensive, cyanosis may be apparent. The pneumonia may also be associated with symptoms of gastrointestinal disturbance including vomiting, diarrhea, and anorexia.

Viral pneumonia usually progresses in stages. In the initial stage of infection, auscultation reveals dull breath sounds and rales in the involved lung areas with no localization of congestion. The person feels as if he has a common cold, which, however, begins to increase in intensity of symptoms. In the next stage, a paroxysmal cough that is most often nonproductive results in headache and muscle soreness from the strain of the coughing. These bouts of coughing may be so severe that the person becomes breathless, has tachycardia, and even appears cyanotic.

The pneumonia may be resolved in a week

or ten days or may advance in severity. If it advances and consolidates in the lung, shadows of the consolidated areas will appear, contrasting with the previously normal x-ray of the chest found in the early stages. Repeated x-rays may demonstrate movement of the shadowed areas from one part of the lung to another; these areas appear as veils or lacy shadows on the x-ray. In other instances, the consolidation may be stabilized and localized in a portion or an entire lobe of the lung. Symptoms increase in severity according to the amount of lung tissue involved. Emphysematous areas may be observed in some patients with viral pneumonia, depending on localization of the infection and the subsequent degree of airway resistance. Atelectasis is also noted in some patients.

If possible, the virus is identified through viral studies, which take a long time to complete. Not every health care facility is equipped to perform viral studies, making it necessary to transport specimens to a designated laboratory. Public Health laboratories provide this service as well as some large medical centers. The Public Health Service provides a kit for proper transportation of specimens. The specimen, whether sputum, nasopharyngeal washings using Ringer's solution, or a throat culture, is frozen to preserve the virus. If the laboratory is available within a health facility, the specimens are quickly taken there so that testing can be initiated without delay. Blood serum samples may also be used for viral studies; it is necessary to obtain two samples, the first during the acute stage of the infection and the second two to three weeks following the first, when the patient is in the convalescent stage. If there is a fourfold rise in the antibody titer between the acute and convalescent serum samples, it is assumed that a virus is present. More specific tests such as virus neutralization, complement fixation, or hemagglutinin-inhibition tests require one week to ten days for completion. These tests are performed using specimens obtained during the early stages when the infection is most virulent. A given patient may be found to have more than one virus. One purpose of the viral study is to ascertain that the disease has in fact been caused by a virus; this is important because other diseases such as cancer of the lung and tuberculosis have symptoms similar to viral pneumonia, and their diagnosis is delayed when the assumed viral pneumonia is resolved. If viral studies are not done and the patient develops a second case of viral pneumonia, the presence of other pathology is almost a certainty. Viral pneumonia is also known to be part of the disease condition for certain communicable diseases, including measles, variola, and varicella as well as infectious mononucleosis.

The treatment for viral infections and viral pneumonia remains symptomatic. Resolution of the viral pneumonia is generally marked by a productive cough with expectoration of sputum, a gradual decrease in symptoms with improved appetite, and increased energy levels. Antibiotics to shorten the period of illness and to prevent secondary infection have proved effective. Because of the stress of the illness, the body's physical energy reserves are depleted; rest is continued until a feeling of well-being is sufficiently restored for the patient to conduct his daily tasks without fatigue. Gradual return to normal activities is often recommended according to the patient's tolerance. A secondary bacterial infection may occur following a viral infection.

Pneumonia caused by other microorganisms Pneumonia can be classified according to the anatomic location of the disease or according to the causative organism (it may be caused by microorganisms other than viruses). Anatomic classifications include bronchopneumonia and lobar, segmental, and lobular pneumonia; pneumonias classified according to the causative organisms include Friedländer's pneumonia (caused by *Klebsiella pneumoniae*), streptococcal pneumonia, staphylococcal pneumonia, and tuberculosis pneumonia, as well as atypical pneumonia and viral pneumonia.

People are particularly susceptible to developing pneumonia either when they are exposed to events that place stress on the mucous membranes of the respiratory system or when they are debilitated for other reasons. Factors that interfere with the normal protective mechanisms of the respiratory system, such as exposure to pollution, cold and dampness, or previous infection, may predispose a person to pneumonia. The capacity of the cilia to clear the airways of the trapped microorganisms that are always present in the airways is an important protective mechanism. Production of excessive mucus can protect the bacteria from phagocytosis while also providing a medium for bacterial growth. The presence of edema or of a foreign object in the bronchi or bronchioles can also predispose a person to pneumonia. Aspiration of infected exudate from upper respiratory tract infections introduces bacteria into the lungs, which may cause pneumonia. Debilitating diseases and taking immunosuppressive drugs or corticosteroids tend to lower a person's resistance to pneumonia.

The anatomic location of the pneumonia is often related to the virulence of the organism, with those of lower virulence being associated with localized infection and those of higher virulence infecting extensive areas of the lung. Lobar pneumonia is the most serious because it involves extensive amounts of lung tissue, and it is usually caused by more virulent organisms. In contrast, segmental pneumonia is associated with a virus of lower virulence and therefore has more localized and less severe symptoms. Resolution of segmental penumonia is usually slower but more complete than that of lobar pneumonia, with less possibility of prolonged complications. Bronchopneumonia is caused by microorganisms of even lower virulence, with the infection located in the smaller bronchioles. Bacterial pneumonia is suspected when polymorphonuclear leukocytes are found in the sputum. Although the initial infection is less severe in bronchopneumonia, the lesions can cause serious lung impairment because of airway obstruction similar to that in acute bronchitis. The bronchioles tend to become obstructed with exudate, causing collapse of the lung areas they serve. Sputum is usually purulent and may be difficult to raise. Breath sounds are those of air passing through fluid with crepitations at the base of the lungs. The inflammatory toxins ulcerate the mucosa of the bronchioles so that fibrosis occurs in the healing process; emphysema may then develop because the bronchioles, when fibrosed, lose their capacity for elastic recoil. Pleurisy may occur with either lobar or lobular pneumonia.

Progression of pneumonia The progress of the inflammatory process and its resolution vary according to the virulence of the organism and the patient's capacity to withstand the infection. Except for segmental pneumonia, just described, and viral pneumonia, which causes congestion of the entire respiratory mucosa, pneumonia is essentially a restrictive lung disease. The inflammatory response occurs primarily in the alveoli and may be either intra-alveolar or interstitial; in the former, the microorganisms damage the epithelial cells, and in the latter they damage the connective tissue. Actually both types of inflammation may occur simultaneously, and it is difficult to differentiate between the two because their appearance on x-ray does not differ.

Changes in the alveoli with either intra-alveolar or interstitial pneumonia are somewhat similar. When microorganisms infiltrate the alveolar epithelial cells and damage them, macrophages gather. In the healing process, fibrinous exudate is produced, which is incorporated into the alveolar membrane. In milder pneumonias, the inflammatory process may be limited to the intra-alveolar space, and the fibrinous exudate may be completely resolved so that the alveoli can return to normal. When microorganisms invade the connective tissue of the alveoli, they cause interstitial damage that initiates the formation of edema and eventually leads to deposits of fibrinous tissue in the interstitial membrane. **Lymphedema** occurs when a large amount of fibrinous exudate is present, indicating that the lymph flow cannot carry away all of the exudate from the site of infection. As with intra-alveolar damage, the permanent lung tissue damage results from incorporation of nonresolved fibrinous exudate into the interstitial tissue of the alveolar membrane, loss of elasticity of the alveoli, and narrowing of the associated small bronchioles. The long-term effects of this damage can include bronchiolectasis, metaplasia of the alveoli cells, anastomosis of bronchopulmonary arteries of the capillary bed, or honeycombing of lung tissue in which fibrous tissue replaces the normal alveolar walls.

Certain typical characteristics differentiate lobar pneumonia from other pneumonias. **Lobar pneumonia** begins with the production of exudate and dilatation of the capillaries. The serous exudate is a product of the increased permeability of the dilated capillaries, which release fibrinogen, plasma proteins, and erythrocytes. The production of serous fluid not only interferes with leukocytes and diapedesis but also can spread. The second stage, referred to as the red hepatization, is a continuation of the inflammatory process in which the alveoli are filled with fibrin and degenerated red cells. The third stage, gray hepatization, follows with the digestion of the exudate by enzymes from the phagocytosed organisms and the clearing of infectious debris by coughing and expectoration. Finally, phagocytosis of the microorganisms is completed, capillary dilatation disappears, and the debris of the inflammatory process is cleared through both lymph flow and expectoration. If the infection is resolved successfully through the inflammatory process, the alveoli resume their normal color and consistency.

Signs and symptoms The signs and symptoms of lobar pneumonia include those of an inflammatory process. The patient may appear flushed and usually has chills, a high temperature, and malaise. Leukocytosis with polymorphonuclear leukocytes is diagnostic for bacterial pneumonia. Mononuclear lymphocytes, plasma cells, and macrophages are usually found with viral pneumonia. The inflammatory process in the lung produces specific symptoms of cough, breathlessness and pain, pallor, and perhaps cyanosis. The patient often experiences a sharp pain that is accentuated on exertion and when coughing. Pleurisy with a pleural friction rub is observed in about half of the patients with pneumonia. The expression of surprise noted when the patient experiences a sudden catching pain as he takes a deep breath is indicative of pleurisy. When this occurs, the nurse either helps the person splint his chest in the affected area, or if he is well enough, teaches him how to support his side to minimize discomfort when coughing or moving about.

Because of the congestion, breath sounds may be dull or absent in the affected area, and breathing is generally rapid and shallow. At first the patient's cough is dry and painful; then as the stages of the inflammatory process ensue, the patient begins to expectorate a typical rusty-colored sputum during the phase of red hepatization. This sputum is viscous and difficult to expectorate. Coughing continues to be painful. The chest is found to have dull sounds when the affected area is percussed, and vocal fremitus is exaggerated in the pleural areas. If the inflammatory processes follow a normal course, there is crepitation that increases with the resolution. The chest x-ray will usually show a hazy film over the lungs. Shadows may be uniform or patchy, and the areas of consolidation may appear as areas of increased density.

As stated earlier, pneumonia may be caused by a number of common causative microorganisms, each of which has certain characteristics. Viral pneumonia is usually milder than bacterial pneumonia, and the sputum is usually nonpurulent. Friedländer's pneumonia occurs most frequently in adult males from 40 to 60 years of age who are alcoholics, because of the increased probability of aspiration secondary to vomiting. Symptoms are chills and thick, jelly-like, brick-red sputum, anorexia, nausea, vomiting, and delirium. In streptococcal pneumonia, the sputum is thin, mucopurulent, and may be blood streaked; this type of pneumonia is frequently complicated by empyema. Staphylococcal pneumonia occurs mostly in children. The sputum is thick, purulent, and yellow, and the pneumonia may be complicated by the formation of cysts and abscesses. Tuberculosis pneumonia occurs in young adults and is associated with weight loss, night sweats, chills, and irregular fever. The onset is usually more gradual than with other pneumonias.

Pulmonary function changes The pulmonary function changes associated with pneumonia are primarily a decreased vital capacity and hypoventilation. Tachypnea is a predominant symptom and is a response to the lowered Pa_{O_2}. The low Pa_{O_2} in pneumonia is most always associated with a lowered Pa_{CO_2}. An x-ray does not demonstrate whether the alveolar changes are specifically intra-alveolar or interstital or both, but an air bronchogram will reveal the changes most specifically.

Dysfunction caused by the varying types of pneumonia may be different according to the anatomic region. Lobar pneumonia in the initial stages causes hypoventilation, which results in ventilation-perfusion imbalances and decreased levels of oxygen blood saturation. The high temperature displaces the oxygen dissociation curve with shifts to the right, further reducing the arterial saturation of oxygen. Depending on the amount of lung involved, the ventilation reserve may be either increased or decreased. If the unaffected areas of the lung have the capacity to increase ventilation in response to the hypoxia or if the pulmonary stretch receptors are stimulated, the Pa_{CO_2} is usually decreased.

Blood gas changes in bronchopneumonia also depend on the extent of the interference with ventilation. This condition is frequently associated with preexisting bronchitis and the ventilation may be already impaired; in this instance the Pa_{O_2} will be decreased and the Pa_{CO_2} will be increased. It is important that the nurse remember that bronchopneumonia is an obstructive lung disease, which means that oxygen should be given with care and no narcotics should be given. Aspirin taken in the initial stages masks the increase in temperature and may delay accurate diagnosis. Sedatives should be given with extreme care. Oxygen might interfere seriously with the patient's compensated breathing stimulus of hypoxia, while narcotics and sedatives further depress ventilation.

Nursing care It is important that the nurse provide for maximum rest for the patient to promote resolution of the inflammatory process and facilitate healing. Exercise should not be increased until the patient's temperature has remained normal for 2 or 3 days. After that time, exercise may be increased according to patient tolerance. Specific medical therapy must be relevant to the causative organism to be effective. Antibiotics are given according to the culture and sensitivity results, usually for a period of 2 weeks. An important aspect of nursing care is monitoring the patient's response to antibiotic therapy. Usually the response is visible in the first 24 hours; delayed response may indicate that the microorganism is resistant to the antibiotic being taken or that there is more than one microorganism present. In this instance the response may be one of increasing severity of symptoms. It sometimes happens that the sputum culture has been contaminated by the upper respiratory tract microorganisms; therefore the correct collection of sputum specimens as described earlier is essential to the accuracy of the culture and sensitivity. It is also important to observe for signs of patient reaction to the antibiotics. Following resolution of the infection, breathing exercises are taught to facilitate the patient's return to normal respiratory function.

In addition to the comfort measures required by any person who is ill, the patient with pneumonia may require oxygen. In this event, care should be taken in its administration. The nurse should be familiar with the patient's medical history and should know if any previous lung disease exists that might affect the appropriateness of oxygen therapy.

Pneumonia may lead to complications, including abscess formation and empyema (particularly in bacterial infections) as well as associated pathology in other systems. Certain microorganisms have an affinity for the valves of the heart, kidneys, brain, and joints; dysfunction in any of these areas can be a complication of lobar pneumonia.

Other types of pneumonia Other types of pneumonia include chemical, radiation, and hypostatic pneumonia. Chemical pneumonia is caused by the inhalation of irritants such as ammonia, nitrous fumes, and certain insecticides containing phosphorus or chlorine. Radiation pneumonia results from changes in the tissues that lie in the path of radiation for lung diseases or mediastinal tumors, or even for the treatment of breast cancer. Hypostatic pneumonia occurs when immobility prevents the normal clearing of the lungs.

Chemical pneumonia is usually caused by inhalation of gases that are toxic to lung tissue. If the gases are readily soluble in water they can be absorbed; those that are not as soluble cause changes in tissue. The upper respiratory system provides a great deal of protection for the lower respiratory tract. When a person is exposed to irritating inhalants the first response is a conjunctival, nasal, and pharyngeal reaction. The response to the inhalation of ammonia illustrates this; the fumes first cause the eyes to water and a tightened feeling in the throat. This response gives the person time either to go away from the irritant or to remove it from his environment. Irritating gases with a high degree of solubility in water can generally be absorbed in the oropharynx, the trachea, and the larynx. Laryngospasm and bronchospasm may result, which decrease airflow resistance for a short period of time. The less soluble gases often reach the alveoli, where the local response is edema. The serous fluid of edema is conducive to bacterial growth so that pneumonia ensues.

Lipoid pneumonia results from the inhalation of oils. The oils also stimulate a reaction in the alveoli. The alveoli fill with macrophages, which in turn fill with fat droplets, polymorphonuclear leukocytes, and lymphocytes. The alveolar walls may be irreversibly damaged by fibrinous tissue formation. An important application of this information in nursing care is that the use of oils should be avoided for lubricating Levin tubes or nasal oxygen catheters prior to their insertion, since these oils could easily be aspirated.

Aspiration pneumonia is associated with the inhalation of foreign bodies, fluids, or other substances not normally inhaled. Gastric juice is probably one of the most common substances aspirated by seriously ill people; because of its high acidity, gastric juice causes consolidation in the lung followed by necrosis of tissue. Aspiration of any foreign body can cause the same result. When aspiration occurs, immediate measures should be taken to remove the foreign substance from the lung—by postural drainage if no other method is available, or preferably by suction aspiration if the person can be quickly taken to a health care facility. Steroids may be given to reduce inflammation.

The changes in lung tissue resulting from **irradiation** are those of edema followed by hyperplasia of alveolar membranes, with the incorporation of fibrinous materials in the regeneration process.

Hypostatic pneumonia can be a complication of any debilitating disease that restricts mobility. In this condition, secretions are retained, especially in the dependent areas of the lung. Bacteria grow readily in the stagnant secretions, and the infection that results can seriously compromise ventilation and perfusion. Hypostatic pneumonia is often seen as segmental pneumonia in the most dependent lung areas. When a patient is confined to bed, the dependent areas are the lateral segment of the middle lobe, the apical segment of the lower lobe, and the axillary portions of the anterior and posterior segments. Hypostatic pneumonia is best prevented by good nursing care, which includes frequent position changes to facilitate drainage of dependent lung areas, coughing and deep breathing to stimulate clearing of secretions, and careful monitoring of the patient's ventilation status and respiratory hygiene as well as watching for the signs and symptoms of an infection.

Atypical pneumonia usually occurs in young adults and middle-aged people and is known to have an epidemic occurrence. *Mycoplasma pneumoniae* is the causative organism, which is larger than a virus but smaller than bacteria. This disease is associated with elevated titers of cold hemagglutinins. Typical symptoms include mucoid sputum and a variable fever with no chills. The onset is usually gradual.

Summary Pneumonia has been described according to its anatomic locations and its causative agents. Because there are so many different types of pneumonia, and because pneumonia in different anatomic locations causes varying signs and symptoms, the nurse should understand the implications of these differences. Both the nursing care and the patient's prognosis are determined to a large extent by the specific treatment for each type of pneumonia.

INFECTIOUS MONONUCLEOSIS

Infectious mononucleosis, commonly known as "mono," while not specifically classified as a respiratory system disease, often presents with the symptoms of a respiratory tract infection and makes a differential diagnosis necessary. Symptoms are extremely variable among individuals, and the severity of the disease ranges from very mild to serious with complications.

Initially the person with mononucleosis notices a sore throat that usually is followed by a headache, generalized malaise, and increased temperature in a few days. Pain or soreness in the back of the neck and enlargement of lymph nodes and spleen are common physical signs, as well as orbital edema. The person's throat is sore, and an exudate of grayish or greenish color is common. On observation, the tonsils may appear inflamed with whitish or yellowish patches, and a petechial type rash is often seen on the soft palate. Both the palate and uvula may appear shiny red in color.

A number of laboratory tests are used in differential diagnosis when infectious mononucleosis is suspected. The presence of mononuclear cells comprising more than 10 percent of the peripheral white cell count is indicative of mononucleosis. A heterophil antibody test is positive in about 20 percent of cases. The mononucleosis spot test uses the index of heterophil antibodies to screen the presence or absence of the disease. The serum bilirubin may be elevated, whether or not jaundice is evident. Nursing care and treatment of infectious mononucleosis is discussed in Chapter 5.

TUBERCULOSIS*

The causative organism of tuberculosis, the tubercle bacillus, was discovered in 1882. After years of experimentation and remarkably accurate clinical observation, the first major advance in the control of tuberculosis occurred in the 1950s with the use of isoniazid. The closest today's generation could come to realizing the effects of this once consuming communicable disease would be to come upon the "TB isolation huts" deep within Mammoth Cave or to visit the Trudeau Sanatorium in the Adirondack Mountains of New York State. The fear and death produced by the disease once called "galloping consumption" or known in ancient times as "captain of the men of death" have been replaced with an almost indifferent acceptance of the disease or an ignorance of the importance of today's known methods of prevention and treatment. It must be stated clearly that tuberculosis can be arrested only by chemotherapy; the disease will run its fulminating course to certain death if left untreated. Today the incidence of tuberculosis is rapidly becoming accepted, and rightly so, as just another part of a person's medical history. However, health workers must continue to stress that everyone should have certain essential information and act to ensure continued resistance to the tuberculosis infection.

Causative Factors

Tuberculosis is an infectious disease caused by *Mycobacterium tuberculosis* that predominantly involves the lungs (it may occur in other parts of the body). There are other mycobacteria (e.g., *M. kansasii, M. intracellularis* [Battey bacillus], *M. fortuitum*) that can produce similar pulmonary disease in man; these diseases, while not communicable, as is tuberculosis, require treatment.

The ability of a person to control tuberculosis once the invasion has occurred is not completely understood. It is known that resistance is lowered in those with conditions that interfere with internal nutrition; some obvious examples are alcoholism, uncontrolled diabetes mellitus, gastrectomy, and poverty with resultant poor nutrition. Resistance is also lowered in persons with diseases associated with immunosuppression, such as Hodgkin's disease and leukemia, and in patients being treated with corticosteroid and immunosuppressive drugs. Patients with silicosis tend to also develop tuberculosis, but other lung diseases do not seem to promote tuberculosis. Resistance to infection and to tuberculosis may be lowered during the first two years of life, during puberty and adolescence, in the postpartum period, following some infections and vaccinations, and during prolonged stress. The placenta serves as an effective barrier to the tubercle bacilli.

When tuberculosis is diagnosed, it is essential that the patient be given a regimen of chemotherapy adequate for treatment of his specific case, and the chemotherapy regimen must be completed as prescribed without interruption. It is also necessary that control of the tuberculosis be documented by both microscopic examination and x-ray examination.

Rate of Occurrence

In 1974, 30,122 new cases of tuberculosis were reported (a decline of 2.8 percent from 1973). The death rate figures for tuberculosis in 1974 show that 3,770 people died from the disease, which is a rate of 1.8 percent per 100,000 population [15]. This statistic refers to the primary cause of death as listed on the death certificate. Reactivated cases tend to occur in older people, the median age being 54 as compared to 49 for new cases. Most reactivated cases are pulmonary. In 1973, 93 percent of reactivations were pulmonary infections of tuberculosis compared to 87 percent for all new cases. In 1973, tuberculosis registers also showed that 86 percent of active cases were not hospitalized in tuberculosis hospitals; this demonstrates the current trend of closing specialized tuberculosis hospitals and treating patients with tuberculosis on an outpatient basis after short stays in general hospitals [13, 15].

These statistics are very generalized, and it must be kept in mind that statistics are only as accurate as the reporting system that supplies the data. The statistics do however provide a basis for prevention programs. Also, any health care person responsible for developing

*By Mary Marrs.

preventive programs must study the information available in the area in which the programs will be located. For example, the overall picture shows a decline in tuberculosis activity in the United States. However, the decline in the incidence of tuberculosis is not evident in all areas of the United States. In some areas there is actually an increase in the incidence of new cases. In order to establish preventive programs, the nurse must gather all the available data about the disease process, its mode of transmission, its rate of occurrence in the community, and the population groups most affected before beginning a program.

Action of the Tubercle Bacillus
The tubercle bacillus is a microscopic aerobe which is incapable of multiplication except under laboratory conditions. It is acid-fast and reproduces slowly in 18 to 24 hours. It may remain dormant in human tissue for long periods of time. Tubercle bacilli are transmitted through the air by droplet nuclei and are inhaled; both inhalation of these bacillus-laden droplet nuclei and their implantation on lung tissue are necessary for the transmission to be complete. The moisture portion of the large droplets evaporates, leaving droplet nuclei that are 1 to 5 microns in size. The droplet nuclei are expelled into the air through coughing, sneezing, singing, laughing, or talking by people with active disease. Infection occurs when droplet nuclei are inhaled by susceptible hosts. Usually, the host has been in close daily contact with a person with untreated or inadequately treated active tuberculosis; close contacts may be household members, friends, or working acquaintances.

The tubercle bacilli are implanted in a peripheral alveolus of the lung. The reticuloendothelial and lymphatic systems are involved, just as with any other infection. If the person has normal resistance, the bacilli are either killed within phagocytes or walled in by other cells to form tubercles. This process usually causes no apparent illness or symptoms. Occasionally, a person with altered immunologic responses is not able to resist the invasion, and the disease process then continues. Within 3 to 10 weeks, the tuberculin reaction develops in the cells and persists as long as any living bacilli are present; from this point, the tuberculin test will usually produce a positive reaction. An x-ray may show enlarged hilar nodes at the onset of the infection. Primary infection is usually followed by a latent phase that lasts through most of the person's life.

Pulmonary tuberculosis usually arises in the right apex of the lung. However, tubercles sometimes break down in the center, allowing bacilli to pour out into the bronchial tree and leaving a cavity. A breakthrough into a vein may then occur, allowing the infection to spread through the blood stream, lymph system or bronchi, which may result in miliary tuberculosis.

The tuberculous lesion may heal by absorption of the inflammation (resolution) or by scar formation (fibrosis), or a granuloma may result. Tuberculous lesions may become reactivated during the individuals' lifetime. However, the tubercles may not be able to contain the bacilli, which may escape and go through the same process again, starting daughter cells. The center of the tubercle has no blood vessels, so sometimes lack of blood and violent reaction to the concentrated tuberculin proteins cause death of the defensive cells as well. Necrosis and caseation in the center of the tubercles eventually leave a cavity from which tubercle bacilli may be released from the body. Healing of cavities usually requires chemotherapy to help the breathing lung calcify the area by lime deposits or to close the area by fibrosis. Cavities more than 4 cm in diameter almost certainly require chemotherapy to heal.

A few people have unusual resistance and healing may take place without chemotherapy, although massive scarring results and the lung area is greatly decreased. These people probably share their tubercle bacilli with many other people before significant healing is accomplished.

Control of Disease Transmission

The person with a newly developed tuberculosis infection usually has no symptoms. In the later stages fatigue, weight loss, anorexia, a productive cough, blood-streaked sputum, and a general feeling of malaise may develop. Because there are often no symptoms in the early phases of the tuberculosis infection, it is possible for the affected person to spread the disease without being aware of having done so. Therefore, close contacts of the affected person may have been exposed prior to his diagnosis and treatment. Hospitalization is not required for diagnosis and treatment.

A new system of classification of tuberculosis has been developed and accepted by the Conference of the State and Territorial Epidemiologists, effective January 1, 1975 [4]. All American states and territories will use the new classifications, which take into account the advances of chemotherapy in treating the disease. This classification system relates tuberculosis transmission to appropriate treatment, facilitates documentation of each patient's medical history for record keeping, and improves communication concerning the disease among health personnel and agencies. The classifications apply to both children and adults. In this classification **O** is no exposure and a negative skin test, **I** is exposure and a negative skin test, **II** is tuberculosis infection with a positive skin test and no symptoms, **III** is tuberculosis infection with active evidence of disease. Subclassifications of II and III indicate the patient's status in tuberculin tests, in x-rays, and during chemotherapy.

Every case of tuberculosis must be reported (by law) to the local health department and to the State Board of Health according to the local reporting requirements. The community health nurse and the nurses employed in hospitals pursue the following information to translate the classifications into meaningful data for patient follow-up.

The **tuberculin test** is used to determine the presence of an infection. It must be remembered that the body requires 3 to 10 weeks after infection occurs to develop the allergic reaction to tuberculin used in the test (delayed sensitivity reaction). Therefore the timing of testing should take into account the possibility of recent infection in persons who have been in contact with a newly diagnosed tuberculosis patient. The skin test is repeated in 90 days following the initial test, when initial test results are negative, to give the body time to develop the allergic reaction to the tuberculin.

The **Mantoux test** is the skin test of choice. Guidelines for its administration are available from Tuberculosis Control sections of State Boards of Health and should be kept current and followed precisely. Mantoux tests should be performed only by qualified persons, who know how to correctly administer and evaluate the results. Record keeping of results is essential for assessing new infection or reinfection in any one person, and to determine the status of the population as a whole.

Currently 5 TU (tuberculin units) of PPD (purified protein derivative of tuberculin) is given intracutaneously. The test is read in 48 to 72 hours; the reaction is recorded in millimeters. **Positive** reactions are those 10 mm or more of induration; **doubtful** is 5 to 9 mm, and **negative** is 0 to 4 mm. Persons with a reaction of 10 mm or more of induration should have a chest x-ray. Those with doubtful reactions should be retested unless they have had known contact with persons with active tuberculosis. It should be noted that false positives may result; the larger the reaction, the more likely there is a tuberculous infection. Less strong reactions may be indicative of cross reactions (see color insert Figure 1 on page 1078A).

People with radiographic evidence of disease compatible with tuberculosis should have sputum tests performed both to confirm the diagnosis and to determine the therapy. Acid-fast bacilli can be seen on a smear; a positive smear establishes the possibility of tuberculosis but is never conclusive. Cultures are necessary to establish positive identification of the tubercle bacilli, and sensitivity tests are done concurrently with cultures to determine which drugs will be effective in controlling the growth of the bacilli. It is essential that the drugs prescribed be appropriate according to the sensitivity studies. The concentration of the organisms in the sputum culture indicates how infectious the patient is and the extent of the follow-up of contacts required. After the patient is placed on chemotherapy, culture and sensitivity tests are repeated to determine the patient's response to treatment and whether the prescribed therapy is controlling the organism.

Chemoprophylaxis prevents the development of overt clinical disease in the infected individual. People with active tuberculosis include those not on chemotherapy as well as those who have insufficient medication either because they have not taken the drugs over the specified length of time or because they are resistant to the drugs. Four to 6 weeks is the minimum time for attenuation of the tubercle bacillus. Depending on the virulence of the organism and the patient's response to chemotherapy, the patient with tuberculosis may no longer be actively infective as early as 2 to 3 days after chemotherapy is initiated. With patients who have cavitation or moderately advanced disease, a longer time is required for chemotherapy to be effective, sometimes up to 3 months.

Preventive therapy includes the use of drugs. Isoniazid (INH), the drug of choice, is given in a dosage of 300 mg per day for adults and 10 mg per kilogram of body weight per day for children. Administration for 12 months will usually prevent development of active disease. INH diminishes the bacterial population in the tuberculous process that may not even be visible on x-ray. It also prevents infection from occurring in exposed persons, thus the term **chemoprophylaxis**. Although not effective 100 percent of the time, INH has about an 85 percent success rate and causes few side effects when given in the normal therapeutic dose. Prophylactic administration of INH, in order of groups important in prophylaxis, is used in (1) closely associated contacts of patients with active tuberculosis, (2) people who have recently converted from a negative to a positive tuberculin test or who have had an increase of 6 mm or more in a positive reaction, (3) tuberculin positive reactors with pulmonary lesions of unknown etiology compatible with tuberculosis and not sufficiently stable to be classified as inactive disease, (4) persons with inactive tuberculosis or residual fibrotic pulmonary disease presumed to have been tuberculous in origin, and (5) persons with a positive tuberculin reaction who have medical conditions such as leukemia or lymphoma or who are receiving immunosuppressive drugs.

A number of drugs are used in the treatment of active tuberculosis. They are divided into two groups, primary and secondary. **Primary drugs** are used in initial treatment of tuberculosis and are always given in combination so that resistant strains of bacilli have less chance of developing; they include Isoniazid (INH), streptomycin, para-aminosalicylic acid (PAS), ethambutol, and rifampin.

INH is the most effective drug available today with the least side effects. It is also the least expensive. One severe side effect is peripheral neuritis, which is controlled by the use of pyridoxine. Mild side effects include dryness of the mouth, constipation, visual disturbances, and headache. Orthostatic hypotension and mild anemia may occur. More severe side effects include peripheral neuritis and convulsive seizures. People with epilepsy should not be given INH. There are reports of drug-associated hepatitis occurring in 10 out of 1,000 patients. Hepatitis is more prevalent in persons over 35 years of age and has not been noted to develop in children. The effects disappear when the drug is discontinued or decreased in dosage. A history should be obtained prior to prescribing INH. If the patient has had hepatitis or any liver disease, INH is contraindicated. The risk of developing active tuberculosis with inadequate chemotherapy is 1 in 75. It is necessary to weigh the risk of developing tuberculosis against the threat of hepatitis. Monthly follow-up visits are recommended to determine the presence of symptoms consistent with those of liver damage, peripheral neuritis or other toxic effects. Any person who has fatigue, weakness, paresthesia of the hands and feet, nausea and vomiting, dark urine, icterus, rash, or an elevated temperature should be suspected of having hepatitis and should be treated.

Streptomycin is given intramuscularly for a short time until the desired effect is obtained; it is usually given with two other drugs which are continued. The side effects involve the eighth cranial nerve and the kidneys. Vertigo and renal toxicity are usually the first signs; these problems diminish when the drug is discontinued. Para-aminosalicylic acid is the least well tolerated of the primary drugs and its use is now being replaced with ethambutol.

Ethambutol is often used in conjunction with INH. The major side effect is reduced visual acuity. An eye examination should be done prior to giving the drug and then monthly thereafter. The first sign of side effects is usually decreased ability to perceive green color with either eye.

Rifampin is a new drug in the treatment of tuberculosis. Good results have been obtained with its use; it is expensive and should always be used in conjunction with another drug. It has the advantage of being useful in persons with renal failure. Rifampin is also a good agent for use in retreatment if persons cannot tolerate other primary drugs or are unresponsive to them.

Secondary drugs are used when people fail to respond to primary drugs. They are more toxic, have more side effects, and are less effective than the primary drugs. The secondary drugs are ethionamide, pyrazinamide, cycloserine, kanamycin, and viomycin. The drug regimen is usually continued for 2 years, depending on the extent of the disease and on the patient's response to therapy. Effectiveness of drug treatment is determined by how rapidly the sputum cultures become negative.

Patient Care

In addition to chemotherapy, the hospitalized patient also requires instruction for the proper handling of sputum. Other isolation measures are not indicated; it is not necessary for either the patient or the nurse to wear masks if sputum and coughing are handled correctly. (This is also true if the patient is being treated on an outpatient basis.) However, if the patient is unwilling or unable to cooperate in isolating the organisms through correct disposal of sputum, gowning and masking of personnel may be necessary. The infected patient should be in a well-ventilated room that does not have recirculation of air, to prevent air contamination.

The major hazard from tuberculosis actually occurs when patients are not initially suspected of having tuberculosis and the disease is diagnosed later. However, the nurse who teaches all patients to handle sputum and disposable tissues properly is practicing good preventive nursing and should feel more secure when these procedures are always carried out as a matter of course. When a patient who has been hospitalized for some time is diagnosed as having tuberculosis, all personnel who may have become infected must be identified. The success of this procedure and of subsequent management is facilitated by an active tuberculosis surveillance program. Those persons with negative reactions to tuberculosis skin tests are evaluated, and therapy is initiated for those who have become infected. Hospital personnel are usually tested immediately, unless they already have a positive reaction as determined on preemployment or subsequent testing, and again 10 weeks after exposure.

The nurse should be aware not only of the methods used for diagnosis and treatment but also of those used to protect others from infection by the tubercle bacillus. As previously mentioned, the tubercle bacillus is transmitted by airborne contamination from infected persons who have not begun chemotherapy. The tubercle bacilli that appear on fomites such as linen, furniture, books, and floors do not constitute a significant infection hazard, so these objects do not require special handling. The reason for this is that the tubercle bacilli are nonmotile organisms that are readily killed by heat, drying, sunshine, or ultraviolet light. Hand washing is an efficient method of removing those organisms that are picked up from fomites or by direct contact with infected sputum.

The primary method for preventing secretions from becoming airborne and contaminating the environment is teaching the patient how to isolate the organism. He should be taught specifically how to cover his nose and mouth with disposable tissues when coughing, raising sputum, sneezing, or laughing (Fig. 3-13). All contaminated tissues should be placed into bags for subsequent

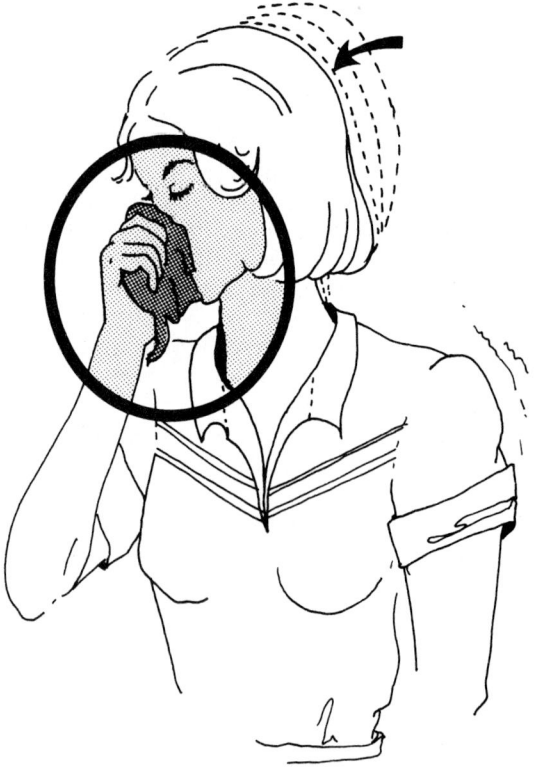

Figure 3-13
The patient should cover his nose and mouth with disposable tissues when coughing or sneezing.

burning. (Some hospitals have special containers and flush the contents into the sewage system.)

The initiation of appropriate chemotherapy, as previously described, readily eliminates the tubercle bacilli from the sputum and also reduces both the cough and the amount of sputum expectorated. This usually occurs within several days to two weeks in most patients, unless they prove to be drug resistant.

Follow-up Care
Once chemotherapy has been started, the infected patient may be discharged from the hospital. In fact, many patients with tuberculosis who are diagnosed in a physician's office or in an outpatient clinic are not hospitalized at all. The emphasis in nursing care following discharge focuses on ensuring that the patient continues to take the prescribed medications on an outpatient basis. The personnel in the local health department or in the visiting nurse association are often responsible for follow-up and have the responsibility of encouraging and supporting the patient who is taking the medication. Some patients do discontinue the drugs because they experience side effects.

Follow-up care also involves classifying tuberculosis patients as potential transmitters, probable nontransmitters, and nontransmitters. Potential transmitters have a positive smears with numerous acid-fast bacilli and require a culture to confirm the diagnosis. Included in the classification of potential transmitters are patients who have just begun chemotherapy and patients who are not responsive to chemotherapy because of drug resistance. Probable nontransmitters are those who have begun chemotherapy. The patient becomes a nontransmitter when he has had three consecutive negative smears, is on continued chemotherapy, and has no symptoms. The nurse should be aware of the importance of continuing chemotherapy when patients taking the chemotherapeutic drugs are admitted to the hospital for other reasons.

One of the most important reasons for treatment failures and continued development of new active cases of tuberculosis is lack of adequate patient education and follow-up to assure continuance of drug therapy to completion. The most important role of any nurse who deals with a patient in the initial stages of tuberculosis is that of helping him understand the nature and extent of his illness, that the illness is chronic and that medication will be required for approximately 2 years. The patient should be frequently reminded of the importance of taking his medication regularly and that failure to do so can only result in deterioration of the healing process and the possibility of the development of resistant organisms that are very difficult to treat. The patient is monitored monthly, if possible, for side effects; if any are noted, immediate referral is made to the physician. The patient should be supported in maintaining health and in pursuing his treatment regimen to completion. His tuberculosis then ceases to be a matter of public health concern and becomes a part of the patient's medical record. The major benefit is to the patient himself, who is then able to lead an active and productive life without the threat of tuberculosis, which can be a very debilitating disease. The event of tuberculosis should be recorded on the patient's medical record so that when other illnesses or respiratory problems occur, the possible implications of reactivated tuberculosis will be considered.

SARCOIDOSIS

Sarcoidosis is an example of a hypersensitivity that is often closely associated with tuberculosis when it affects the lungs. It is an environmental disease found in temperate climates; little is known about its cause. **Sarcoidosis** is a granulomatous reaction, associated with type IV hypersensitivity reactions, and can involve any organ of the body, although thoracic sarcoidosis is the most common form. Persons with active sarcoidosis may have increased IgG antibodies.

Sarcoidosis most frequently affects women between the ages of 30 and 40. Initially there may be no symptoms, and a routine chest x-ray may show changes in the lungs typical of sarcoidosis before the person actually experiences symptoms. In some persons the onset is acute. Sarcoidosis usually runs a course in which the acute phase lasts for 1 or 2 years and then resolves completely. If the disease does not resolve after 2 years, the condition is called chronic sarcoidosis. This condition is serious in that chronic sarcoidosis results in fibrosis of tissues with subsequent impairment of the organ involved. In thoracic sarcoidosis, fibrosis of lung tissue is followed by impairment of function, which eventually causes right heart failure.

The Nickerson-Kveim test is specific for sarcoidosis in the acute stage but is most often negative in the chronic phase. Intradermal injection of 0.1 to 0.2 ml of human sarcoid tissue suspended in saline results in the development of a purplish-red nodule at the site of injection if the test is positive. The nodule does not appear until 2 to 3 weeks following the intradermal injection. After the nodule appears, another 2 or 3 weeks is allowed to elapse and the site is then biopsied. Sarcoid granuloma found on histologic examination confirms a positive reading of the Nickerson-Kveim test. Because the results cannot be determined for several weeks, the tuberculin test is often given as an interim measure to rule out tuberculosis. If the response to tuberculin is negative or mild, it is assumed that the disease is not tuberculosis but sarcoidosis.

Changes in x-rays may be characteristic of sarcoidosis or may resemble the changes that are observed in either pneumonia or tuberculosis. The changes characteristic of sarcoidosis include hilar lymph node enlargement or linear infiltrated areas that extend from the hilum. Many persons have no symptoms at first; others have polyarthralgia of the joints, with the knees, ankles, and wrist and elbow joints being most frequently affected. Patients with thoracic sarcoidosis often have dermatologic evidence of the disease as well. Transient maculopapular skin eruptions as well as skin plaques, keloids, and chilblain can occur. The lesions are not painful, but they may be distressing to the patient because of the change they bring about in physical appearance. The lesions may resolve or may fill in with granulomatous tissue in the chronic stages. Chronic bone cysts are also associated with the lung lesions and are suspected if the patient has subcutaneous swelling of the fingers and toes.

A patient with sarcoidosis may have symptoms related to only one body organ or may have multiple symptom involvement. Eye lesions are particularly serious, since blindness can result. Typical eye lesions are uveitis, which develops with sudden pain and misty vision, conjunctivitis, and retinal lesions. The lacrimal glands may be enlarged as well. The disease can affect the salivary glands and the parotoid glands (swollen parotid glands may resemble mumps), and facial palsy can result from this form of sarcoidosis. Bone destruction may occur, with the cortical and medullary bones most commonly affected. There is associated swelling of the hands and feet, most often affecting the phalanges. Nasal granulomas may be associated with laryngeal plaques, the cervical nodes may be enlarged, and the nervous system may be affected as evidenced by peripheral neuropathy, encephalitis, or transverse myelitis. Space-occupying brain lesions may develop. The list of organs that can be involved continues with the spleen, which may be enlarged, and the kidneys, which may be affected either directly by formation of granulomatous tissue or indirectly by the deposition of calcium in and around the renal tubules. There may be an increased sensitivity to vitamin D, which causes increased absorption of calcium from the gastrointestinal tract so that hypercalcemia and hypercalciuria result. This condition may be transient or it may so severely damage the kidney that renal failure results. Cardiovascular function can be compromised by pulmonary fibrosis, which leads to pulmonary heart disease with arrhythmias, heart failure, and death. Finally, the endocrine system is involved, primarily in the posterior pituitary, and there may be diabetes insipidus.

Diagnosis of sarcoidosis is easier if the symptoms are obvious. However, if the diagnosis is obscure, a biopsy of the involved organ can be performed to identify the presence of granulomatous tissue. Treatment depends on the site of the disease and focuses on maintaining the function of the organ involved. Sarcoidosis often resolves itself with no treatment. If the condition tends to become chronic, corticosteroids are given for a period of 3 to 6 months. Some authorities prefer to treat sarcoidosis aggressively in the acute phase because the effects of the chronic disease are serious impairment of organ function; they feel that therapy should be instituted to prevent changes such as blindness, renal failure, and cardiovascular disease. Remissions in the chronic disease have been noted in the later months of pregnancy, but the symptoms return following delivery.

There is no specific nursing care for the

patient with sarcoidosis. These patients, however, require careful and attentive care when a body organ or system is impaired by the disease. The patient requires careful monitoring over the long run to determine the involvement of other organs. In general, the nurse's contacts with the patient during follow-up care focus on giving supportive care and honest reassurance.

FUNGUS INFECTIONS

Fungus infections of the lung may also cause lung dysfunction. A number of fungi can cause lung infections resembling tuberculosis in manifestation of symptoms. The most common route of entry is inhalation of dusts containing the fungi. Histoplasmosis, aspergillosis, coccidioidomycosis, blastomycosis, cryptococcosis, nocardiosis, and mucormycosis are among the fungus infections that can occur as primary infections of the lung. Usually the infections occur in people who are susceptible because of debilitating diseases. Long-term treatment with corticosteroids or immunosuppressive drugs and the presence of systemic diseases, diabetes mellitus, or uremia make people more susceptible to the occurrence of fungus infections. Unlike tuberculosis, fungal infections are not communicable but are contracted by exposure to infected objects in the environment.

Histoplasmosis

Histoplasmosis is caused by *Histoplasma capsulatum,* which is a fungus associated with birds and found in soil. The growth of the fungus follows different patterns; it is mild in some people and spreads through the reticuloendothelial system in others, causing enlargement of the spleen and lymph nodes. Pulmonary changes resemble those caused by tuberculosis, and the signs and symptoms of the disease are also similar to those seen in tuberculosis. Skin tests are available for histoplasmosis, and complement fixation tests are positive in those who are infected.

Aspergillosis

Aspergillosis is diagnosed by sputum culture. This fungus infection is associated with pigeons and occurs most commonly in debilitated people who have other diseases. Pulmonary changes include the formation of an aspergilloma, which appears as a tumor on x-ray. These lesions may spread to other major organs.

Coccidioidomycosis

Coccidioidomycosis (valley fever) is caused by *Coccidiodes immitis* and is found in desert areas. It causes pulmonary changes, with a sequence of inflammation followed by the development of granulomas. The disease may be self-limiting or may cause long-term chronic pulmonary dysfunction because of necrosis of lung tissue followed by fibrosis. In advanced disease, spread of the fungus through the circulatory system may cause involvement of other body organs and tissues; the disease may then be fatal.

Blastomycosis

Blastomycosis, which is caused by *Blastomyces dermatitidis,* causes a pulmonary disease similar to tuberculosis or pneumonia. This disease may be mild or fulminating, involving other organs, particularly the skin. Multiple pustules form and eventually ulcerate with formation of abscesses.

Cryptococcosis

Cryptococcosis, caused by *Cryptococcus neoformans,* is associated with birds and pets and has the ability to spread throughout the body before the signs and symptoms of an inflammation are evident. Often a diagnosis of meningitis is made because the central nervous system may be the first system in which symptoms are demonstrated. The disease may occur insidiously or may follow a more acute form. Positive cultures of sputum or spinal fluid confirm the diagnosis.

Nocardiosis and Mucormycosis

Nocardiosis and mucormycosis occur infrequently. If the primary infection occurs as a pulmonary infection, it may spread to other organs, particularly the nervous system.

Treatment

For all of these fungus infections, treatment usually consists of giving amphotericin B. Because fungus infections are tenacious, treatment must be continued for a period of months to ensure that the fungus has been attenuated. During the initial acute phase the drug may be given intravenously, and the dosage is often given in increments until a maximum desired dosage has been reached.

Amphotericin B can be toxic, causing side effects of nausea, vomiting, thrombophlebitis, or electrolyte imbalance. Other treatment modalities are specific to the manifestations of the disease, which vary greatly. The central nervous system is frequently affected in fungus infections that are either fulminating from the outset or that have not been diagnosed and treated and eventually invade other organs or body tissues. The person's immune response is probably one of the most important factors not only in the occurrence of the fungus infection but also in response to treatment.

PNEUMOCONIOSIS

The term **pneumoconiosis** refers to diseases that result from the inhalation of dusts. This type of lung disease is associated with environmental hazards present in certain types of employment; people who work in mines, foundries, agriculture, and certain types of industry have considerable continuous contact with dusts. Among the diseases classified as pneumoconiosis are silicosis, asbestosis, berylliosis, siderosis, byssinosis, bagassosis, and coal miner's pneumoconiosis. Pneumoconiosis, which may also be referred to as hypersensitivity pneumonitis, causes signs and symptoms of both restrictive and obstructive lung dysfunction.

Standards for the protection of employees exposed to occupational dusts are determined by the United States National Institute of Occupational Safety and Health and the Occupational Safety Division in the Department of Labor. People working in coal mining, copper mining, the mining of any ore embedded in quartz, glass and pottery works, sand blasting, polishing with silicone, and certain types of agriculture involving exposure to vegetable dusts are included in these standards. Both government agencies conduct studies to determine levels of safety and to make recommendations for positive health practices. A number of workers who experience lung dysfunction as result of employment also apply for disability insurance benefits; for this reason insurance companies are also very interested in establishing standards on which to base payments. Spirometry is used to assist in determining the amount of lung damage, which directly influences Social Security disability payments.

The Disease Process

The normal respiratory tract has protective mechanisms for the removal of inhaled dusts. Much filtration occurs in the nose. The production of mucus and ciliary action in the large air passages remove most of the larger particles of dust that get beyond the nares. Dusts that reach the alveoli are engulfed by macrophages and are then transported to the bronchi to be expelled as sputum. When large amounts of dust are present, the excess is removed by the lymphatic system. Dust particles less than 1 micron in size can be inhaled into the lung periphery; those from 1 to 7 microns can reach the bronchi; and those of larger size rarely pass into the lung beyond the upper respiratory tract.

Some of the dusts are highly fibrogenic and in the long run cause lung dysfunction through the development of fibrous tissue that replaces normal lung tissue. This destruction of normal tissue usually impairs ventilation, often in an unequal manner. If the periphery of the lung is involved, perfusion is also impaired; thus the symptoms associated with pneumoconiosis may be varied, including those of both obstructive and restrictive lung disease. In the situations where there is more dust inhaled into the lung periphery than can be accommodated by the macrophages, there is liberation of toxins from the nonviable macrophages. It is believed that these toxins lead to fibrosis. In other instances, as with silica, the particles of dust work their way into the alveolar interstitium and cause fibrosis.

Other dusts cause disease through the formation of granulomas in the lung; these granulomas may eventually coalesce to form areas of nonfunctioning lung tissue or to obstruct ventilation. Dusts such as hay, silage, and other vegetable dusts are thought to cause a hypersensitivity reaction and in many instances may be the source of fungi that infect the lung.

The inhalation of any foreign body, whatever the size, stimulates a response of increased mucus production in the bronchi. Irritation of lung tissues by dusts over a long period of time constantly increases mucus production; this mucus creates a culture medium that supports bacterial life, making the person susceptible to infections. As a result, people who are continually exposed to dusts often develop chronic bronchitis.

Role of the Industrial Nurse
The amount of lung dysfunction experienced by persons in continuous contact with dusts is determined first by the individual's susceptibility. Susceptibility cannot always be measured in advance unless the person has previous episodes of infection with residual lung dysfunction from the scarring of fibrosis. People who plan to work in industries or jobs that will expose them to large amounts of inhaled dusts should have lung function tests prior to employment to determine the presence of any dysfunction that would make them particularly susceptible to disease. These preemployment physical examinations are often conducted by health service personnel employed by the industry. The occupational health nurse has an important role in employment physicals and is often the person who establishes a system of routines to ensure that the necessary examinations are completed before employment is begun as well as making certain that there is a plan for follow-up. Another important role of the nurse in industry is monitoring the health standards within a place of employment. Teaching the employees about the necessary health protection practices, such as the use of masks or hoods to filter air and reduce the level of inhaled dusts, is another function of the occupational health nurse. The purpose of these practices may seem obscure to the employees, especially when they are stated as rules without an explanation of their protective purposes.

Several important components of follow-up are part of the occupational health nurse's role. Once a person begins employment, the nurse must conduct a continuous assessment of the effectiveness of the safety rules and the extent to which the rules are being followed and reinforced, which often means frequent meetings with supervisors and those responsible for management practices within the industry. Periodic follow-up examinations of the employee comprise another component of the nurse's role. If the periodic follow-up is conducted on a regular basis, any changes in the employee's lung function can be detected so that treatment measures or prevention can be initiated early. Concise records are important to detect the occurrence of frequent respiratory infections, however minor; these infections are significant and can be used to alert the health team to the lung damage that a given employee may be experiencing. Records are also important sources of data in broad-scale studies of the incidence of diseases.

Observation for symptoms is another area of the nurse's responsibility. Cough, sputum production, breathlessness, decreased exercise tolerance, and demonstration of lowered diffusion capacities within the lung as found in lung function tests during the physical examination are important. Increased areas of density in the lung will be seen on x-ray films if sufficient dust has collected. These changes are progressive and occur over a period of time, so comparison of x-rays from one examination to another is important. The nurse should know that the changes in x-rays are not directly related to the amount of lung dysfunction the person may have. Some people with x-ray changes have few symptoms, and in pneumoconiosis the symptoms often occur after changes on the x-ray are observed.

Types of Pneumoconiosis
A number of different types of dusts can induce respiratory dysfunction. Important factors to consider are the levels of dusts in the air, the size of the particles of dust, the duration of the exposure a person has to the dusts, and the person's susceptibility to lung damage caused by the dusts. Everyone is exposed to some dusts in the environment, but it is the continuous occupational exposure to high levels of dusts that is of concern in the development of the diseases known as pneumoconiosis. When there is visible evidence of the accumulation of dusts as patches of density on x-ray films without evidence of symptoms, a person is said to have **benign pneumoconiosis.**

Silicosis Silicosis is one of the most commonly occurring diseases in this group. The threshold of silica dust that is considered safe is 5 million particles per cubic foot; this is the standard that must be maintained for the protection of employees. Many cleaning agents contain silica, as well as abrasives and the sand that is used to make ceramics and pottery. Silica is a natural deposit in the earth and is found extensively in mining for almost any kind of ore.

Although most silica is removed through the protective mechanisms of the lungs, the silica that is embedded in lung tissue is not soluble by phagocytosis. The fine particles can work their way into the interstitial tissue of the lung, where they can be embedded, causing fibrosis in the form of grayish nodules. This fibrosis causes changes in lung function by exerting pressure on the bronchioles and increasing airway resistance, thus interfering with alveolar work so that either ventilation or perfusion or both can be impaired in later stages. Either ventilation or perfusion seems to occur in greater degree than the other in people with silicosis, with emphysema occurring as secondary to the silicosis in many cases.

Eggshell nodes are a characteristic finding on the chest x-rays of people with silicosis. The small nodules gradually grow, eventually coalescing to form larger eggshell nodes. These nodes tend to "draw up" the lung tissue toward the hilus, leaving damaged alveolar tissue in the lung periphery. The resulting lesion resembles that found in tuberculosis, and in fact there is a direct relationship between silicosis and the occurrence of tuberculosis in advanced silicosis. This condition is termed **silicotuberculosis.** People who are diagnosed as having silicosis are also given diagnostic workups for tuberculosis.

The symptoms of silicosis are progressive, beginning with a cough that is usually nonproductive at first and then produces increasing amounts of purulent sputum that collect during sleep, causing severe coughing bouts. Breathlessness on exertion gradually becomes more severe. The person begins to have frequent bouts of bronchitis and may have hemoptysis during the periods of infection or in bouts of paroxysmal coughing. Rales, wheezing, and rhonchi can be heard. Eventually there are changes in the lung tissue that lead to emphysema. As the disease progresses, heart failure resulting from ventilation and perfusion abnormalities occurs.

There is no specific treatment for silicosis. The patient must avoid further exposure to the continuous inhalation of dusts with high levels of silica. Drugs effective in treating tuberculosis are given in the event that silicotuberculosis occurs. Otherwise, the treatment is the same as for any obstructive or restrictive respiratory disease. The patient is often given isoniazid.

Siderosis Siderosis is caused by the inhalation of ferric oxide and resembles mild silicosis in its symptomatology. It is found in workers who handle hematite, welders, silver polishers, and those who work in iron foundries. Usually the upper half of the lung is affected.

Asbestosis Asbestosis is another commonly occurring disease that is found in people working in industries in which asbestos is used extensively. These industries manufacture products such as fabrics, fireproof shingles, floor tile, wallboard, and many other products containing asbestos. Rather than appearing as particles of fairly even size, asbestos appears as filaments or fibers, which vary considerably in size. These fibers find their way into the lung (usually the lower lobes) and are distributed unevenly. Asbestos bodies, which are fibers coated with protein, can be expectorated and located in sputum. Those that remain in the lung seem to undergo a chemical change, gradually losing their internal asbestos core and becoming a granule of iron oxide. The asbestos bodies are located within the bronchi and alveoli and accumulate proteins, gradually extending to include the alveolar membranes and forming fibrous tissue. There may be formation of adhesions between the lung and pleura as well as formation of calcified plaques. Cysts and honeycomb formations replace the normal alveoli. There is also formation of plaques in the pericardium in some people.

Cough and sputum production are typical early symptoms of asbestosis. There may be crackling rales in the base of the lungs. Certain types of asbestos fibers are capable of absorbing hydrocarbons, so there is a high incidence of carcinoma in patients with asbestosis. Treatment is symptomatic, and cortisone drugs are often effective. Weakness, weight loss, and finger clubbing are seen in this disease since there is interference with the ventilation and perfusion capabilities of the lung. Each patient tends to develop the symptoms of chronic lung disease in a different way. Bronchiectasis, chronic bronchitis, tuberculosis, pleural effusion, and especially bronchogenic carcinoma are all possible complications of asbestosis. There is no determined pattern relating the length of exposure to the occurrences of these complications. People may develop the lung dysfunction even though they do not work in the asbestos industry; for example, washing clothes containing asbestos dust or living near an asbestos factory can be sufficient contact for sensitive people to develop the disease. On the other hand, some people with long exposures to asbestos over a period of years do not develop any significant disease.

Berylliosis Berylliosis is actually a systemic disease that begins with the inhalation of beryllium dusts. It is one of the pneumoconiosis diseases that develops as a result of toxic hypersensitivities. Formation of granulomas, which may be found in the skin, liver, spleen, and lymph glands as well as lung, is typical of the disease. The first indication of the disease is often bronchopneumonia with a paroxysmal cough; some authorities believe that this is the acute stage of the disease, which is either resolved or which can become chronic, causing restrictive lung disease. The patient develops progressively and increasingly severe breathlessness, and x-ray changes show hilar adenopathy. The cough is typically nonproductive. Beryllium can be found in both lung tissue biopsy and in the urine. The patient may have skin lesions caused by a local reaction to beryllium. Treatment is symptomatic, with cortisone being the most useful drug. The prognosis is variable; early treatment will minimize the long-term effects of further fibrosis of lung tissue.

Coal miner's pneumoconiosis Coal miner's pneumoconiosis occurs primarily in anthracite coal mines where workers are exposed to coal dust, which also contains silica. Coal dust is carbonaceous material which, when inhaled, fills the interstitium and lymphatic vessels in a diffuse manner. Usually the upper two-thirds of the lung is involved, and a focal emphysema resulting from the collection of dust forms mainly in the bronchioles. The collection of coal dust forms into nodules, the nodules coalesce as the inhaled particles increase, and eventually there is a progressive massive fibrosis. The lesions may create cavitation similar to that found in tuberculosis. The patient has a productive cough with expectoration of black sputum, and there may be hemoptysis. The patient often experiences chest pain, which may be caused by intercostal myalgia or pleurisy. Sputum is frequently cultured for the tubercule bacillus since the incidence of tuberculosis in coal miner's pneumoconiosis is high.

The symptoms vary with the stage of disease and are progressive. If the patient is a heavy smoker, chronic bronchitis may be the first evidence of the disease. Later there is an increased ratio of the residual volume to the total lung capacity, and the disease progresses as an obstructive lung disease. As with the other diseases in this category, there is no specific treatment; the patient gradually requires an increasing amount of medical intervention as the lung dysfunction progresses. X-rays reveal collections of dust. Large collections of coal dust are known as anthracomas.

Byssinosis Byssinosis is a disease that occurs in people who work with cotton, hemp, and flax. It creates a hypersensitivity reaction to the inhaled dusts that sometimes appears years after the continuous exposure. The symptoms may be similar to those of bronchial asthma. Some authorities believe that byssinosis is caused by some factor in the cotton dust that results in bronchoconstriction. The symptoms of chest tightness and wheezing are more predominant on the first day of the working week and often diminish on successive days, occurring again after the worker's days off. Other manifestations of byssinosis are increased airway resistance, decreased ventilation, and unequal distribution of gas perfusion. Chronic bronchitis occurs frequently and seems to be the major problem of the disease.

Farmers' lung **Farmers' lung** is a term that applies to many of the vegetable dust inhalation diseases. The hypersensitivity reaction occurs in the alveoli, which are infiltrated with the inhaled dusts; this initiates an inflammatory response. The alveolar interstitial tissues are filled with polymorphonuclear leukocytes, lymphocytes, and plasma cells that have extravasated from the capillaries. Most often the symptoms occur 5 to 6 hours after exposure, with cough, chills, fever, malaise, wheezing, and breathlessness. Gradually the person may become anorexic and may also begin to lose weight. In some people the symptoms do not occur as abruptly but rather develop insidiously over a long period, often years. In this case the delay between exposure and the evidence of symptoms often obscures the diagnosis because the person may not remember having been exposed to the dusts. Eventually decreased ventilation and perfusion and decreased lung compliance occur; the symptoms are then treated according to the regimen for any restrictive lung disease. A precipitin test may reveal the specific antigen.

In some instances farmers' lung refers to the disease caused by exposure to the dusts from hay or silage or to vegetable dusts. Actinomyces is usually considered the most important of the microorganisms that cause the disease. The spores are inhaled into the lungs, and the ensuing reaction may be one of inflammation that abates or may progress to fibrosis, causing chronic lung disease with changes in lung compliance and ventilation-perfusion ratios. Treatment is specific to the type of lung disease the person develops: emphysema, chronic bronchitis, or asthma. Honeycombing in the lung is common, with its typical multiple cysts that can be found on x-ray.

Treatment of farmers' lung is symptomatic; cortisone is useful in treating the symptoms. People who work in areas where they will be exposed to vegetable dusts should wear masks. If they are particularly susceptible, they should be advised to avoid contact with the dusts.

There are many other diseases that cause hypersensitivity pneumonitis, and as new antigens are identified the list becomes longer. For example, contaminated air conditioners have been found to have organisms that cause a hypersensitivity reaction similar to that of farmers' lung. Most of the antigens causing this hypersensitivity reaction are found in molds.

LUNG ABSCESS

A lung abscess can be a complication of infectious processes. It can occur in association with infections of the lung such as pneumonia or tuberculosis, in conditions in which the blood supply to an area of the lung is markedly decreased, causing necrosis of tissue, such as in tumor growth, or in response to the inhalation of a foreign body or pus from upper respiratory tract infections. The abscess formation in the lung is no different from that found in other parts of the body. In the lung, the abscess appears as a cavitated lesion.

A number of different pyogenic organisms can cause lung abscesses. The source of the organism is most commonly an infection in the upper respiratory tract from infected teeth, pyorrhea, or sinusitis. The organisms gain entry to the lung when the normal defense mechanisms of the respiratory tract are impaired. Factors such as alcoholic intoxication, anesthesia, or toxins that depress the action of the cilia and the smooth muscle of the airway predispose to abscess formation. An abscess may also form following aspiration of foreign bodies or substances, including food particles, objects such as pins placed in the mouth that are inadvertently inhaled, or debris from dental or oral surgery. Inhaled objects generally follow the path of least resistance, so they enter the right main bronchus and then the right lung, often lodging in the upper lobes. Abscesses occurring with other lung infections are generally caused by stagnant secretions that harbor infections; this occurs in diseases such as pneumonia or tuberculosis. Another source of abscess formation in the lung is septic emboli, which travel to the lung from the lower extremities or pelvis.

The symptoms of lung abscess are similar to those of pneumonia, with chills, fever, malaise, and perhaps cyanosis and dyspnea. The pain may be a deep, dull ache or it may be the typical pleuritic pain, depending on the location of the abscess. The cough is dry at first and then becomes productive, with expectoration of foul-smelling, purulent, and sometimes blood-stained sputum. Leukocytosis, organisms in the sputum culture, and visualization of the cavity on x-ray are significant findings for the diagnosis of lung abscess. Chest sounds are dull over the abscessed area, and there may be crepitations or pleural friction rub if fluid has collected.

Causative organisms can be any of those commonly found in the nose, mouth, or throat, including streptococci, staphylococci, pneumococci, or even *Proteus*. Therapy for lung abscess includes prescription of the appropriate antibiotic, which the patient must take in adequate amounts for a long enough time to attenuate the microorganism. Rest and antibiotic therapy are usually effective in resolution of the abscess, which heals by marginal fibrosis and scar formation. However, if resolution does not occur as expected and symptoms persist for more than a week or so, bronchoscopy may be necessary. The bronchoscopy is performed both to confirm the diagnosis of abscess and as therapy to drain the abscess mechanically. Other methods used to facilitate drainage of the abscess include postural drainage and percussion. If the abscess still does not respond to these measures to facilitate drainage, surgical removal may be required.

If untreated, abscesses may become chronic. The patient with a chronic lung abscess usually has fever, persistent cough, expectoration of purulent sputum, and hemoptysis. If the abscess ruptures, pleuritic pain and dyspnea usually increase. Complications of ruptured abscess may be either empyema or pneumothorax (these conditions are discussed later in this chapter). Finger clubbing, which is associated with suppurative infections, may occur in patients with chronic abscesses within three weeks. The presence of finger clubbing, then, is a clue to the possibility of a lung abscess; it may indicate that an abscess has been established in the lung or that an abscess is becoming chronic rather than being resolved. Untreated lung abscesses can eventually spread to the pleura, causing empyema. From the pleura the abscess can spread to the brain, resulting in meningitis or a cerebral abscess.

PULMONARY THROMBOEMBOLISM AND INFARCTION

Pulmonary thromboembolism and infarction often occur as complications of other diseases that influence the blood vessels either directly or indirectly. Pulmonary thromboembolism is often the result of thrombus formation, most frequently in the lower extremities. The triad of causative factors consists of injury or pathologic changes of the blood vessel wall, changes in the coagulation properties of the blood, and stasis of blood. These factors, particularly stasis, are pertinent to the nursing care of all patients, and many nursing functions are directly related to their prevention. Thrombus formation should be prevented if at all possible; if one does form, nursing care should focus on resolution of the thrombus so that it disintegrates and is not carried through the systemic circulation.

Thrombus Formation

Thrombi are carried to the pulmonary vessels, where they tend to lodge because of the small diameter of those vessels. Small thrombi often occur in multiples. If they do not interfere with perfusion of the lung, they cause few if any immediate symptoms. Sometimes a small thrombus lodges in a vessel and causes transient symptoms of pain and perhaps dyspnea, which disappear as collateral circulation takes over to perfuse the lung tissue involved. When multiple thrombi of small size lodge in numerous vessels in the pulmonary bed, they cause narrowing of the lumens of the vessels. The multiple thrombi may be recurrent, so the overall result is gradual decrease in pulmonary blood flow. Pulmonary hypertension then develops as a compensatory measure to increase the blood supply to the lung. As the hypertension develops the patient will have dyspnea on exertion, syncope, and angina pain. Eventually the emboli narrow the vessel lumen because of local stasis of blood; the narrowing extends proximally to block the larger pulmonary arteries so that ultimately pulmonary infarction can result.

Larger thrombi can lodge in larger vessels, completely obliterating the lumen so that blood perfusion in the area of lung served by the affected vessels ceases. The resulting hypoxemia causes severe pain, generally resulting from myocardial ischemia and dyspnea. Embolus in a moderate size vessel is the most frequent cause of infarction. Perfusion of an area of the lung is impaired in accordance with the decreased blood supply, and the lung responds by constricting the alveoli in the affected area to conserve ventilation for the better perfused lung areas. In approximately 2 to 3 hours following infarction of a pulmonary vessel with subsequent impairment of blood flow, the alveoli in the affected area collapse; this is thought to result from the decreased production of surfactant that occurs when the blood supply to the alveoli is insufficient. Without surfactant, the alveolar surface tension cannot be maintained, and atelectasis then results as the alveoli collapse.

Pulmonary Infarction

Nursing care for patients with pulmonary infarction involves measures to facilitate resolution of the embolus and prevention of the complications of infarction, as well as prevention of additional thrombus formation. It should be noted that lung tissue is not infarcted by emboli unless the collateral circulation is not sufficient to supply the perfusion requirements of the lung. The bronchial arteries and the pulmonary arteries adjacent to the affected vessel supply this collateral circulation. If infarction does occur because of insufficient collateral circulation, the area of the lung involved undergoes progressive changes. Infarction of the lung usually occurs at the lung periphery since the distal vessels in the lower lobes are most often affected. Following infarction there is engorgement of the pulmonary capillary bed, which can be extensive because of the elasticity of the lung tissue and the distensibility of the capillary bed. The overdistended capillaries may rupture so that hemorrhage occurs along with necrosis of tissue. Granulation tissue gradually absorbs the infarct, and a fibrinous scar remains. Because the infarcted areas are usually located in the lung periphery, there is often pleural involvement, which may lead to pleurisy with pleural effusion and subsequent formation of adhesions. Bacteria may enter the infarcted area either from the systemic circulation or from inhalation via the bronchi so that the area of infarct may become infected, particularly during the necrotic stage. Lung abscess formation may occur in the area of the infarction.

Pulmonary infarction may occur in women who are taking oral contraceptives. Its incidence is sometimes preceded by an unexplained elevated temperature following childbirth or abdominal surgery, particularly gynecologic surgery. Symptoms of pulmonary infarction include leukocytosis with a low grade temperature, tenderness of the chest wall, and pleuritic pain with dyspnea. The diaphragm is often elevated, and a pleural friction rub may be heard. Hemoptysis occurs in about half of the cases, and the patient may be cyanotic if there is cardiac impairment. An x-ray of the infarcted area shows pleural effusion and opacity. The x-ray changes in infarction may be difficult to differentiate from lung changes observed in pneumonia, postoperative atelectasis, or carcinoma.

When infarction occurs following multiple recurrent thrombi, the patient will have developed pulmonary hypertension prior to the incidence of the infarct. In this case, the symptoms of infarct will also include weakness, syncope, angina pain, and dyspnea on exertion. The blood pressure is usually normal, and it is often difficult to determine if the patient has pneumonia or an infarct; for this reason, therapy usually involves treatment for both. Antibiotics are given for the pneumonia and anticoagulant therapy is instituted to treat the infarct. These patients may be severely ill and may be in respiratory acidosis because of hypoxemia. In this event oxygen in high concentrations is given at high flow rates to relieve the hypoxemia. Bed rest is continued for at least 10 days or perhaps longer if the patient's condition does not improve rapidly.

If the thrombus is large enough to occlude either one or both branches of the major pulmonary artery, the blood supply to the entire lung is severely decreased. Adequate lung perfusion can be maintained if as much as 50 percent of the pulmonary artery capacity is preserved. A massive pulmonary embolism causing cessation of blood flow results in sudden death. When the embolism reduces the blood flow below the limits necessary for sufficient perfusion, the patient may survive the massive pulmonary embolism but will require emergency care to prevent serious hypoxemia and extension of the embolus. Immediate care is the same as that for a patient with a myocardial infarction. The electrocardiographic changes often indicate right heart strain.

Treatment for Pulmonary Embolism

A massive pulmonary embolism is often difficult to differentiate from a myocardial infarction, and the diagnosis is often dependent on lung scans or pulmonary angiography. The lung scan gives information about the perfusion of the lung and may be used either for initial diagnosis or for determination of prognosis and treatment. Pulmonary angiography, described on page 212, is the most specific diagnostic test and gives information about the size of the obstruction. Injection of the contrast medium into the pulmonary artery or through the right heart gives the best results for diagnosis of the presence of a pulmonary embolism. Angiography is considered essential prior to surgical removal of the embolus if this method of treatment is being contemplated.

Surgical intervention for removal of the embolus is generally performed if the situation is life threatening and if the patient can tolerate the surgical procedure. An emergency pulmonary embolectomy is done with the cardiac bypass procedure. The value of surgical intervention is sometimes questionable or controversial, since many patients who develop a massive pulmonary embolus already have compromised systemic circulation because of vascular pathology; their prognosis is not as favorable as that for patients who have a pulmonary embolus following an acute event such as surgery and who have no underlying disease process. Some authorities prefer to use thrombolytic agents to dissolve the embolus. Streptokinase and urokinase are frequently used for the enzymatic dissolution of emboli in this method of treatment.

Nursing care in the initial phases of the illness is primarily concerned with relieving hypoxemia and concomitant pain. Oxygen therapy is essential in relieving hypoxemia. Aminophylline is given intravenously to decrease the bronchoconstriction that occurs in response to the decreased perfusion. Morphine is often given to relieve the severe pain. If pleuritic pain resulting from an infarcted lung periphery is not relieved by narcotics, an intercostal block may be performed. Administration of heparin is begun with an initial dose followed by a measurement of the clotting time or partial thromboplastin time. Different schedules of dosages and times for heparinization can be used, but it is important that the anticoagulant therapy be continued long enough to prevent possible recurrence of thrombus formation and in adequate doses to promote embolus dissolution and maximum circulation in the compromised lung areas. The heparin should be given either intravenously or subcutaneously. If given subcutaneously, the injection should be in the abdomen rather than in the buttocks to minimize the possibility of bleeding and subsequent formation of a hematoma. Care of the patient with a myocardial infarction and further discussion of anticoagulant therapy can be found in Chapter 4.

Nursing Care for Patients with Thrombosis

In addition to thrombi that travel to the lung from the systemic circulation, thrombosis of the pulmonary vessel can occur. This is largely the result of atheroma and consequent hypertension and occurs most frequently in the right pulmonary artery, although it may occur in the left artery or bilaterally. Atheroma causes a decrease in pulmonary artery flow, which eventually decreases blood flow in the pulmonary vein so that thrombi form. Certain diseases such as carcinoma, tuberculosis, and especially polycythemia vera may lead to the formation of pulmonary venous thrombosis.

Many nursing care measures are extremely important in preventing thrombosis at any location in the body. Prevention of blood stasis is essential, and the nurse should recognize the potential for thrombus formation. In addition to people with chronic respiratory insufficiency, certain people can be placed in a high-risk group for developing thrombosis, including the elderly, the obese, the debilitated, people with decreased mobility, and those with cardiac dysfunction. Thrombosis is also a complication of surgery and of childbirth. Early ambulation following the surgery or childbirth helps prevent stasis of blood. Venous drainage should be promoted as much as possible. Other nursing measures include monitoring fluid and electrolyte balance and providing for ease in defecation. Dehydration and hyponatremia may result in concentration of the blood and therefore may contribute to the formation of thrombosis. Although defecation is not directly related to thrombosis formation, it is important that measures be taken to prevent straining during bowel movements for people in the high-risk group. Straining during bowel movements places stress on venous circulation and can be prevented by giving stool softeners or a diet that provides for softer stools, and by adequate fluid intake. Both adequate hydration and ease in defecation may be difficult to achieve for people with respiratory insufficiency.

Every nurse should check for Homan's sign automatically when giving patient care. Localized warmth, tenderness in the calf, dilatation of a superficial vein, and edema are all significant signs. Intravenous injections should never be given in the saphenous veins unless it is absolutely necessary in a severely traumatized patient, such as one who has burns and both respiratory and circulatory insufficiency. Care should be taken when medications are administered through the intravenous push route, since many medications are particularly irritating to the blood vessels.

DYSFUNCTION AFFECTING THE PLEURA

Normally the smooth movement of the lungs is facilitated by a thin layer of lubricating fluid between the visceral and parietal pleura; this thin fluid is maintained by both capillary filtration and lymph drainage. The visceral pleura covers the lungs and adheres tightly to the lung surfaces. The parietal pleura covers all aspects of the chest wall that encase the lungs; it is a continuous thin sheet of connective tissue well supplied with lymphatic vessels, blood vessels, and nerve fibers. Anatomically the parietal pleura may be divided into the costal pleura, lining the ribs; the cervical pleura, covering the area over the apex of the lung; the diaphragmatic pleura, covering the diaphragm; and the mediastinal pleura. The parietal and visceral pleura are continuous at the hilus of the lungs. The pressure between the parietal and visceral pleura is negative, being -2 to -4 cm H_2O at the end of expiration and -4 to -8 cm H_2O at the end of inspiration. This negative pressure in the pleural space is essential to prevent collapse of the lung.

A number of different types of dysfunction can cause impairment of the pleural movement. These can be categorized broadly into any factors that change the balance and amount of pleural fluid, infection, trauma, and congenital malformations. Because the pleural cavities are separated during embryonic life, defects that occur in embryonic development may cause the pleura to be weakened or improperly formed. Affected persons are therefore susceptible to formation of fissures and are less able to resist stress to pleural walls.

Pleurisy

Pleurisy is an acute inflammation of the pleura or lining of the lungs. It may be caused by a virus or by bacteria and is often associated with pneumonia and tuberculosis. Although the visceral pleura is not sensitive to pain, the parietal pleura is highly sensitive. Pleural pain in the costal and cervical areas is directly referred to the chest wall and causes tenderness to touch in the affected areas. The typical pleuritic pain is described as a stabbing or acute pain felt on movement of the chest wall. Taking deep breaths, coughing, or any exertion that strains the muscles of the chest wall accentuates the pain, and the affected person has a tendency to restrict his movements to avoid pain. When the pleurisy is located in the diaphragmatic area, the pain is referred to the shoulder through the phrenic nerve from the anterior area and to the abdomen through the spinal nerve segments from the posterior area.

If there is a decrease in the amount of parietal fluid, **dry pleurisy** may result. It is sometimes referred to as **fibrinous pleurisy** and is associated with pulmonary diseases and trauma. A pleural friction rub can be heard on auscultation, and the patient experiences pleuritic pain. Patients with pleurisy associated with pneumonia have short respirations and seem to grunt when breathing. Treatment for dry pleurisy consists of applying local heat and providing support for the chest wall. Strapping the chest wall usually provides support and minimizes the pain experienced when the patient coughs, bends, or stretches. It is often difficult for the patient to find a comfortable position. The nurse should encourage the patient to experiment in order to find the most satisfactory position; usually lying on the affected side provides support and stabilizes the pleura somewhat. Pleurisy may resolve with the disease process that caused it in the first place, or it may continue, particularly if pleural adhesions have formed.

Pleural Effusion

Wet pleurisy or **pleural effusion** is a condition in which there is accumulation of fluid in the pleural space. The effusion is either transudate or exudate. Transudates are associated with excess pleural fluid resulting from other conditions such as congestive heart failure, the nephrotic syndrome, or malnutrition. The fluid is clear or faintly yellow and watery, with less than 3 gm per 100 ml of protein. The pleurisy is usually bilateral when caused by transudation of fluid. In comparison, exudates are darker yellow or even amber in color and clot when standing. Because the exudates are formed primarily from bacterial growth that causes infection and inflammation, the protein count is high—more than 3 gm per 100 ml. Pleurisy with exudate is more often localized on one side.

Pleural effusion may be generalized, with fluid accumulating freely in the pleural space, or it may be located in association with a fissure. Pulmonary infarction, pneumonia, and metastatic tumors are often associated with pleural effusion and fissure formation. If a fissure is present, the effusion may not be detectable on x-ray, although it may be seen more easily from a decubitus position on x-ray, which better demonstrates the fluid level. The localized accumulation of fluid predisposes to empyema, which is purulent pleural effusion caused by pyogenic organisms. Empyema is prevented by aspirating the excess fluid and by antibiotic therapy.

As little as 100 to 300 ml of excess pleural fluid can be seen on x-ray, but the clinical symptoms of pleurisy usually do not occur until the excess reaches 500 ml of fluid. When sufficient amounts of fluid have accumulated to cause pathology, the patient is said to have **hydrothorax.** Different terms are used to describe hydrothorax depending on the cause of the excessive fluid. **Hemothorax** indicates the presence of blood and **chylothorax** indicates the presence of chyle, which is a product of digestion transported via the lymphatic vessels to the thoracic lymph duct. Chylothorax is most often associated with trauma that causes injury to the thoracic duct at the point where it passes through the posterior mediastinum. Chyle has a typical milky appearance, a high protein content, and a fat content of 1 to 4 gm per 100 ml.

Pleural effusion with transudate is most often secondary to a number of conditions; carcinoma of the lung is perhaps the most common. In this case, the transudate is usually clear, yellow, or blood stained, and cancer cells can frequently be found on cytologic examination. Effusion is also common in association with other types of tumors located in the breast, stomach, pancreas, and uterus. Meigs' syndrome is pleural effusion that disappears after removal of an ovarian tumor, a relationship that is not understood. The occurrence of pleural effusion in association with tumors often indicates that metastasis has occurred.

Immunologic disorders affecting connective tissue are also associated with pleural effusion. Some of the more commonly occurring relationships are pleural effusion with rheumatic fever, rheumatoid arthritis, and lupus erythematosus. In rheumatic fever the effusion may be transient, and the parietal fluid contains polymorphonuclear leukocytes and leukocytes. In rheumatoid arthritis, pleural effusion results in a pale or dark yellow fluid that may appear grayish, and empyema is a frequent complication. Pleural effusion is thought to be related to taking corticosteroids, which suppress the body's immune response, as well as to the rheumatoid arthritic nodule development and the general debilitation of patients with rheumatoid arthritis. Lupus erythematosus, polyarteritis nodosa, systemic sclerosis, and dermatomyositis may all be associated with pleural effusion.

Another cause of pleural effusion can be the spread of an inflammatory process extending from a perforated peptic ulcer or following intra-abdominal surgery, particularly appendectomies or cholecystectomies. Usually when the infection in the primary site (the appendix, stomach, or gall bladder) is controlled, bacteria do not reach the pleura, and the inflammatory process is resolved as the patient's condition improves.

Primary pleural effusion occurs very infrequently. Mesothelioma, a condition in which pleural effusion occurs with asbestos inhalation pneumoconiosis, is one of the few types of primary pleural effusion. This condition is described as malignant pleural effusion, since it recurs.

The signs and symptoms of pleural effusion vary with the site and the degree of infection or inflammation. The patient's typical tendency to protect the affected side by restricting movement and pleuritic pain is a consistent symptom. On auscultation breath sounds are found to be either dim or absent, and fremitus or vocal resonance increases. Bronchial breathing can be heard in some instances. X-ray examination is helpful in making the diagnosis, with the affected areas appearing dense and opaque. Pleurisy may be difficult to diagnose through x-ray, however, since it may appear as a mass which is thought to be a tumor. The areas of pleurisy may alter in size, shape, and placement in the lung in repeated x-ray examinations. The patient is usually fatigued and may have diaphoresis and weight loss.

Diagnosis of the cause of pleural effusion is facilitated by examining pleural fluid obtained through a pleural tap. Aspiration can be both therapeutic, in draining the fluid, and diagnostic, in examining the fluid. Generally, blood in the fluid indicates malignant disease; however, it is important for the nurse to recognize that blood seen initially may be from a vessel that has been punctured in performing the tap, whereas blood appearing consistently in the fluid is indicative of hemothorax. Pleural fluid is examined in the laboratory for red blood cells, white blood cells, and differential blood cell count, hematocrit, protein, glucose, and amylase and lactic dehydrogenase concentrations and is cultured for microorganisms. Pleural exudate may be differentiated from transudate by comparing the ratio of serum protein to pleural fluid protein, and comparing the serum lactic dehydrogenase concentration to the pleural lactic dehydrogenase. Higher than normal ratios indicate exudate as does a high level of lactic dehydrogenase in pleural fluid.

Nursing Care for Pleurisy

Treatment and nursing care follow some consistent patterns that are the same for all types of pleurisy, including giving antibiotic therapy if microorganisms are found on culture of the pleuritic fluid, giving analgesics to relieve the pain and chest discomfort, and primarily managing the disease that has caused the pleurisy. When pleurisy occurs following pneumonia, the treatment is resolution of the pneumonia; the same is true of the other conditions causing pleurisy. Patients with systemic or immunologic diseases who have poor prognosis have many other problems in addition to the pleurisy. These patients present challenging needs to the nurse in terms of both general comfort and support and relief of symptoms.

An important part of the nurse's role is monitoring the patient's prognosis in relation to the pleurisy, which includes precise observation of the amount and color of sputum, the type and frequency of cough, and the type and degree of pain the patient experiences. Gradual reduction in cough, sputum production, and pain indicates resolution of the pleurisy. The nurse should watch for the signs and symptoms of infection, since in pleurisy resulting from inflammation there is always the potential for developing an infection. Fever is present in pleural effusion caused by infection. It is important to take the patient's temperature carefully, especially if therapy for his total condition includes taking corticosteroids. These drugs may mask the patient's symptoms, making detection of the progress of pleurisy resolution difficult. The patient may have a low grade temperature even if the symptoms seem to be diminishing.

Comfort measures include the application of heat to localized areas of tenderness and splinting the chest, which provides some measure of comfort by minimizing the amount of pain the patient experiences on exertion. Splinting should be secure enough to stabilize the chest wall without restricting respiration. In many cases the patient is already taking short breaths; he should be encouraged to breathe as deeply and slowly as he can with comfort. Giving analgesics can assist in making the patient comfortable enough to breathe effectively, but the nurse should carefully assess the patient's total condition when deciding when to administer analgesics. Certain obstructive lung diseases associated with pleurisy are most difficult to manage because pain medication may further depress respiration. The overall goal is to make the patient as comfortable as possible to facilitate effective respiration without further impinging on his ability to breathe effectively.

EMPYEMA

Empyema can complicate many different types of lung infections and may be a complication of pleural effusion. It is most common following infection of the lung, as previously described, and may occur when there is a cyst in the pleural space. Empyema may be a complication of thoracic surgery or of a subphrenic abscess following abdominal surgery. Rupture of the esophagus as occurs in cirrhosis can result in empyema, as can systemic pyemia or septicemia.

The symptoms of empyema are similar to those of pleural effusion: fever, pleuritic pain, and leukocytosis. The patient may also experience weight loss. When the empyema is not controlled, it can become chronic; the patient then experiences a persistent cough with purulent sputum. Pain and discomfort in breathing are consistent. Finger clubbing is a sign that the infectious process may be chronic, and secondary amyloidosis occurs in long-term chronic empyema.

Treatment for empyema involves aspiration of the pus, with injection of an antibiotic following aspiration. Antibiotics may also be taken orally. When there is a large amount of pus, water seal drainage may be used for continuous aspiration. If the pus is very thick and does not drain easily, surgical removal of the pus may be required. However, patients with severe empyema usually have other disease conditions as well and may not be able to withstand the stress of a surgical procedure. A rib resection might be performed in these cases, and antibiotic therapy is continued for several weeks in an attempt to control the empyema. When empyema is associated with tuberculosis, it is important that the patient maintain antibiotic therapy for at least 18 months.

Nursing care for the hospitalized patient with empyema is similar to that for pleurisy. A major goal is making the patient comfortable while monitoring his progress through temperature changes, determination of the amount of chest pain or discomfort and description of the site of the pain, and examination of the color and consistency of expectorated sputum. Coughing patterns and tolerance of chest movement are significant factors in the patient's response to therapy. Analgesics should be given to relieve pain and discomfort; however, this may be complicated if the patient has obstructive lung disease, in which case pain medications should be given with care to prevent further depression of respiration.

SPONTANEOUS PNEUMOTHORAX

Spontaneous pneumothorax usually occurs in healthy adults, most often in slender young men, during a period of exertion or following unusual stress. The pneumothorax is caused by disruption in the integrity of the pleura, which allows air from the lung to enter the pleural spaces. The disruption is thought to be rupture of a bleb (or small air cells) in the lung that has formed either during embryonic growth or as a result of an infectious or inflammatory process. Spontaneous pneumothorax often follows an infection such as pneumonia or sarcoidosis.

The immediate symptom of spontaneous pneumothorax is usually acute chest pain, localized to one side of the chest; however, pneumothorax may occur without any pain or discomfort in some people. The person who experiences this sudden, sharp pain is apprehensive and may be dyspneic from the emotional stress as well as from the impairment of respiration caused by the pneumothorax. The extent of impairment is related to the degree of collapse of the lung following the reduction of negative pressure in the pleural space and to the amount of pulmonary reserve the person has. Both the presence of fluid in the pleural space and the presence of pleural adhesions increase the symptoms.

Assessment of the degree of pneumothorax involves observation of chest movements and a chest x-ray. The chest x-ray is used to determine the presence as well as the extent of the pneumothorax. The person who has a pneumothorax usually compensates by breathing more deeply and more frequently so that the excursion of the chest is decreased on the affected side. Patients with chronic lung disease are unable to tolerate spontaneous pneumothorax as well as can healthy people, and pneumothorax in these patients may constitute an emergency situation and require critical care for respiratory insufficiency.

Treatment of pneumothorax is aspiration of the air from the pleural space, usually by inserting a chest catheter attached to a closed drainage system, which allows the lung to expand gradually as the negative intrapleural pressure is reestablished. Insertion of the catheter usually relieves the shortness of breath and cyanosis because it improves the ability to breathe deeply.

Spontaneous pneumothorax has a tendency to recur in about half of the cases. If a patient has repeated incidences of spontaneous pneumothorax, a thoracotomy may be performed. This procedure is most often performed to resect blebs or to accomplish abrasion of the pleura so that the visceral and parietal pleura adhere to one another.

THORACIC TRAUMA

Thoracic trauma may occur in many different ways. Automobile accidents, falls, impact with moving objects, gunshot wounds, and stabbings are among the most common incidents in which people sustain thoracic trauma. Generally trauma to the chest results in three types of dysfunction: airway obstruction, ventilation and perfusion abnormalities, and impaired mechanical function. The extent of trauma cannot always be determined immediately following injury; for this reason all people who have sustained thoracic trauma should have a thorough physical examination. Thoracic trauma is very often associated with multiple injuries. The patient's ability to survive the trauma depends on his physical condition prior to the injury, the type and extent of injury sustained, and the adequacy of care received immediately following the traumatic incident. In any emergency situation evaluation of the circulatory status and stopping blood loss are the prime concerns, along with ascertaining the adequacy of the patient's airway. Obstruction of the airway should be dealt with temporarily at the scene of the trauma. Assuring sufficient airway is of import until more sophisticated care can be given.

Airway obstruction is dealt with by a qualified health professional (physician, nurse, or paramedic) who either removes the cause of the obstruction or performs an emergency cricotracheotomy. The airway may be obstructed by blood clots from upper respiratory tract injury, secretions from the GI tract, compression of the airway, or by the tongue if the patient is comatose. If no suction is available, inhaled foreign objects or debris must be removed manually. If this is not possible, an emergency tracheostomy should be performed, using any sharp object available. The object must bypass the obstruction in order to allow air to enter the lungs.

Impairment of the mechanical functions of the chest wall should also be evaluated and dealt with immediately. One of the more commonly found mechanical injuries is fractured ribs, which can cause changes in the thoracic pressure or can contribute to piercing wounds. Any piercing wound destroys the integrity of the pleura, the degree of severity being related to the size of the wound. If a piercing wound is present, the lung or a major vessel may also be pierced or punctured. Measures should be taken to stabilize the chest wall to prevent further trauma until the patient can be given more adequate treatment for the fractured ribs. Usually fractures can be felt or seen in the uneven movement of the chest wall that results when a rib is broken in several places or when several ribs are fractured. The patient with severe rib fractures usually has severe pain, and ventilation is decreased both because of the pain, which limits respiration, and because of the loss of the chest wall integrity. In the case of a piercing injury, it is important to stop loss of air from the lungs. Plugging the site of the wound and applying mild pressure provides significant prevention of air exchange between the intrathoracic space and the atmosphere until further treatment can be given.

Ventilation-perfusion abnormalities may not be immediately apparent at the time of the injury and may require further examination with evaluation of blood gases and pH. Bruising, contusion, hemorrhage of the lungs, and the ineffective respiration resulting from mechanical injuries all cause ventilation-perfusion abnormalities, which may not result in blood gas changes for as long as 12 hours after the injury. When the lung is contused, edema forms in the alveolar walls and fluid moves into the intra-alveolar spaces. In compression injuries there is often interstitial hemorrhage as well. The total collection of fluid in the lungs is similar to that seen in pulmonary edema or in pneumonia.

Since congested alveoli cannot be ventilated, physiologic shunting is common in chest injuries. Shunting occurs when areas of lung tissue are perfused but not ventilated; this has the effect of limiting gas diffusion, with oxygen diffusion being affected most seriously. Carbon dioxide diffuses at a rate 20 times greater than does oxygen, so carbon dioxide diffusion continues when oxygen diffusion is limited. Mixture of the poorly ventilated blood with that from more adequately ventilated lung areas decreases the oxygen saturation of the arterial blood, with resulting hypoxia to the tissues. The response of lung tissue to hypoxia is vasoconstriction of the pulmonary capillary bed, which in turn further impairs perfusion. If the patient has had normal lung function prior to the injury, the lungs compensate through hypertension resulting from the vasoconstriction and through increased frequency of respirations; this results in increased cardiac output and tachycardia. Patients who have compromised lung function from chronic lung disease such as emphysema or bronchitis or compromised vascular capabilities from heart disease may not be able to compensate for the hypoxia. These patients may have severe respiratory insufficiency as a result of the added stress of the injury.

Hypovolemic shock can complicate the lung's ability to compensate for the injury since it has the effect of further reducing perfusion of the lung and contributes to hypoxia. If there is no great blood loss or other major injury, the respiratory hypotension may be sufficient to perpetuate systemic hypotension because of pulmonary vasocontriction. Changes in blood gases may not be evident until respirations are no longer effective in eliminating carbon dioxide; the amount of time this takes depends on the patient's respiratory reserve and its adequacy in accommodating to the body's oxygen needs. The increased work of breathing needed to overcome the dysfunction of the mechanical injury and the alveolar congestion contribute to the total amount of stress that is placed on the respiratory system. When hypoxemia and hypercapnia result, intervention through mechanical ventilation is necessary. It is important that the impending respiratory failure be anticipated and that measures be taken before carbon dioxide retention ensues.

Types of Injuries

Specific injuries that may be sustained include fracture of ribs consisting of a simple, single fracture of one rib or multiple fractures of one or more ribs. The stability of the chest wall is greatly compromised if there are multiple fractures, and this type of event is usually associated with severe contusion of the lungs as seen in crushing injuries. Tension pneumothorax, flail chest, rupture of the major organs or vessels in the mediastinum, and contusion of the lung are other specific injuries.

Fracture of the ribs A simple, single fracture can cause sharp pain, which is similar to pleuritic pain in that it is aggravated by movement or deep breathing. A chest x-ray often confirms the diagnosis of fractured rib and also reveals the presence of pneumothorax. The chest x-ray should be taken with the patient in the upright position to obtain the best view of the chest and to ensure visualization of any other injuries such as damage to the spinal canal or rupture of the diaphragm. Uncomplicated fractures are allowed to heal spontaneously. The patient is given analgesics for pain. Some authorities prefer to strap the rib with tape to stabilize it during the healing process, while others feel that this method of treatment is contraindicated. Strapping the rib may limit chest movement and impair respiration. Patients with emphysema or chronic lung disease of any kind may not be able to tolerate the pain of a fractured rib, and a simple, single rib fracture may cause respiratory insufficiency in such patients.

Tension pneumothorax Tension pneumothorax occurs with a puncture wound of the pleura that can be made by any sharp object, including a fragment of a fractured rib, a knife, or sharp debris. It can also be caused by puncture of the bronchi. If small enough, the opening allows air to enter the pleural space during inspiration when intrathoracic pressure is decreased, on expiration as the intrathoracic pressure is increased, the pleura closes the opening so that air does not escape. The lung eventually collapses as air pressures gradually equalize. As the lung collapses, the heart and trachea are pushed away from the site of the puncture wound and shift to the opposite side (Fig. 3-14). The opposite lung is not able to expand further because of loss of negative pressure in the pleural space and the increase in intrathoracic pressure. Treatment includes aspiration of air from the pleural space.

Pain is treated with analgesics. In mild cases aspiration may be sufficient to restore the intrathoracic pressure. Insertion of a chest catheter with continuous drainage of air and fluid, using a closed drainage system, is required when there is continuous production of fluid and when pressures are more nearly equal. The catheter is usually inserted between the ribs below the clavicle or behind the anterior axillary fold.

In more severe cases of tension pneumothorax, larger puncture wounds into the pleural space allow free exchange of air so that the intrathoracic pressure very quickly equalizes with the atmospheric pressure. Air moves in and out of the opening instead of through the trachea, causing severe respiratory distress. The patient cannot breathe because the essential pressure differences among the intrathoracic space, the pleural space, and the atmosphere have been altered. The mediastinum is pushed back and forth with respiration, and this causes a decrease in cardiac output.

Emergency care requires immediate closure of the opening by plugging it with an airtight dressing using the cleanest cloth

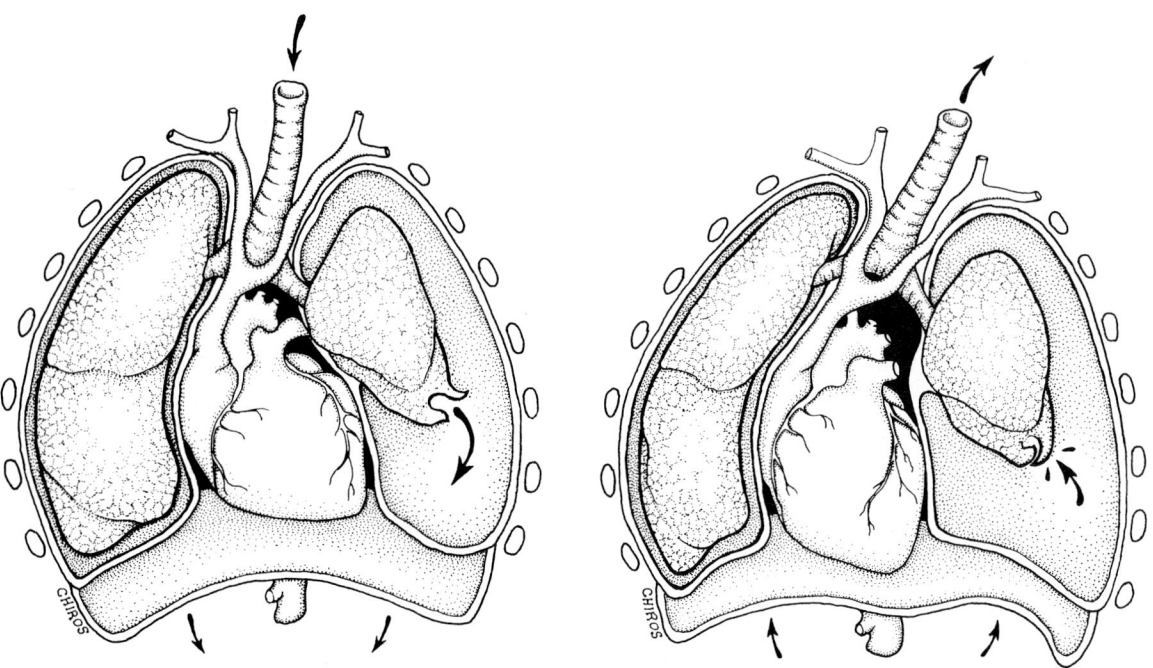

Figure 3-14
In tension pneumothorax the intrapleural pressure has increased because there is free passage of air during inspiration but minimal or no return of air during expiration resulting in mediastinal shift, decreased cardiac output, chest pain, dyspnea, cyanosis, and shock.

available; sterile dressings can be used if available. Light pressure should be placed over the wound. Insertion of a chest catheter attached to a closed drainage system for decompression is done as soon as possible. The wound is then sealed around the catheter to prevent further loss of air. The injury must be surgically repaired if there is tearing of the tissue or if the wound is too large to seal around the chest catheter. Repair requires a thoracotomy, which in itself can be life threatening if the patient's status is critical because of other injuries.

Flail chest Flail chest refers to paradoxical movement of the chest wall resulting from multiple rib fractures. It often results from the action of floating segments of ribs that have been fractured in two or more places; the floating ribs move inward during inspiration and outward with expiration. The patient with a flail chest has marked overbreathing, and asymmetry can be observed. Flail chest is frequently complicated by contusion of the lung and by pneumothorax, especially if a crushing injury has been sustained. Respirations are ineffective because the chest wall stability is decreased and the patient cannot cough effectively. Increased secretions and fatigue result, and the patient may be dyspneic or cyanotic. Emergency treatment involves compression of the fracture, which can be done by placing sandbags or some other similar object over the area until the patient receives further treatment. Many different forms of treatment are used for flail chest. If the fractures are extensive, surgical repair for stabilization is done. Other methods involve compression or application of external traction to stabilize the chest wall. External traction is difficult to apply and usually restricts the patient's movement considerably; for this reason some authorities prefer treatment by other methods.

When flail chest results from deceleration injuries (sometimes referred to as impact injuries) there may be compression without fractured ribs. These patients have congestion of the lungs because of increased fluid in the alveolar spaces. With this type of injury complications may not appear during the immediate posttrauma period but may appear months or years later. Complications include the development of aneurysms of the large blood vessels and formation of cysts of the lung. Periodic follow-up x-rays should be scheduled to check for the presence of these complications.

Positive pressure breathing helps to maintain lung function in the event of flail chest and prevents hypoxia. Endotrachial intubation or a tracheostomy may be performed; these techniques provide for more precise control of respiration and facilitate suctioning of the upper air passages. The use of a ventilator with positive end-expiratory pressure (2 to 5 cm H_2O) for a prescribed period is advocated by some authorities.

It is important that treatment be started as early as possible to prevent changes in the lung that result from compression. These changes include increased lung congestion, atelectasis, and pulmonary hemorrhage, all of which are difficult to reverse once they have been established. Generally treatment instituted within the first 24 hours posttrauma will prevent the occurrence of these conditions.

Nursing care for patients with flail chest is very important and includes continuous monitoring of the mechanical ventilation and maintaining clear airway passages through removal of secretions. Prophylactic antibiotics are given because of the potential for infection that exists with any loss of tissue integrity. Both pneumonitis and tension pneumothorax may occur to complicate the patient's progress. The tension pneumothorax can develop as the lungs expand. If there are rib fragments, the expanding lung rubs against the fragments, and the pleura can be damaged as a result. If there has been an open wound that is partially healed, a small amount of pressure can reopen the wound. A chest catheter should be available for emergency treatment if tension pneumothorax occurs.

Other injuries caused by thoracic trauma
Trauma to the chest wall may also cause injury to the structures within the mediastinum, to the trachea or bronchi, or to the sternum. Injury to the sternum generally requires no emergency treatment, and care usually includes the use of analgesics to relieve pain. Injury to the heart can be in the form of contusion causing myocardial injury, arrhythmias, and heart failure. There may be hemorrhage into the pericardial sac, or the patient may develop aneurysms long after the injury. Monitoring the electrocardiogram and central venous pressure is important to discover mediastinal injuries in the patient with multiple injuries. The presence of heart failure complicates treatment for the other injuries the patient may have sustained.

Deceleration injuries may cause trauma to the trachea or to the bronchi. These injuries may be severe and life threatening, or they may not be diagnosed until much later when the patient develops an infection. If the trachea is involved, a tracheostomy is usually performed to prevent the leakage of air into the mediastinal space. Air in the mediastinal space is called **mediastinal emphysema** (or subcutaneous emphysema), and this condition can impair ventilation of the lungs. Bronchial injury may vary from complete severance of the bronchi to a small hole. When the bronchus has been severed, surgical repair is necessary. Tension pneumothorax occurs with this type of injury and may necessitate the insertion of a chest catheter into the intrathoracic space. The surgical repair can be either a direct anastomosis or bronchoplasty.

If the bronchus is ruptured, the dysfunction may not be observed during the posttrauma period. Healing usually takes place spontaneously, but the remaining scar tissue can constrict the bronchus, making the patient susceptible to infection. Collection of mucus in the narrowed area of constriction causes coughing. Pneumonia or pneumonitis may occur later as the constricted area impedes the airflow and decreases the resistance of the distal lung area to infection. A completely obstructed bronchus as a result of healing causes atelectasis. If the lung area involved is small this may be asymptomatic; however, if the area of the lung served by the obstructed bronchus is great or if the patient already has compromised lung function, there may be more severe respiratory distress.

Injury to the diaphragm In certain types of trauma the diaphragm may be ruptured. If this occurs the abdominal fluids may contaminate the intrathoracic space, so there is always the potential of developing an infection such as abscess, pleural effusion, or empyema. Other injuries to the diaphragm are associated with trauma to the abdominal contents or the intrathoracic contents. These injuries are often caused by penetrating objects that cause ripping of tissue that must be surgically repaired. If they are puncture type injuries, hemothorax may result, requiring the insertion of a chest catheter. An important therapeutic measure is immediate removal of blood or secretions from the chest cavity since these contribute to the incidence of infection if allowed to remain. Usually puncture wounds of the lung seal off spontaneously with expansion of the lung. However, if bleeding continues after the chest catheter is inserted, it may be necessary to perform an exploratory thoracotomy to discover the source of the blood. In this case an important nursing function is monitoring the drainage from the chest catheter as well as the patient's total condition.

Summary

Even though the lungs may not themselves be injured, they can be affected by injuries in other body systems. It is thought that metabolic alterations following injury may be responsible for the respiratory insufficiency that follows massive injuries. It has been found that many patients actually die from pulmonary edema, embolus, pleural effusion, or pneumonia even when the lungs are not involved in the injury. The reasons for this are not understood.

Trauma to the chest, then, requires immediate evaluation of the extent of the injuries and immediate care to minimize their effects until further treatment can be given to the injured person. Trauma can be very mild or very serious, ranging from a simple, single fractured rib to multiple body injuries, and its effects on a person depend to a large extent on his state of health at the time of the injury. Respiratory system functions must be maintained to support life and are therefore a priority along with the maintenance of adequate circulation in the emergency situation. Nursing care related to thoracic injuries is the same as for any patient with respiratory insufficiency. It should be remembered that even though the injury may seem mild on initial examination, the person may have sustained an injury that can have consequences either within hours or years later. For example, ventilation-perfusion abnormalities do not occur until 12 hours or so after the injury; aneurysm formation may occur years later.

NEAR-DROWNING ACCIDENTS

Near-drowning accidents are respiratory emergencies. The water inhaled may be either hypertonic or hypotonic; sea water is hypertonic while fresh water is usually hypotonic. In hypertonic drowning, salt water in the lungs causes water to move from the circulation into the pulmonary alveoli with resultant hemoconcentration and hypovolemia. In hypotonic drowning, water is absorbed rapidly from the lungs into the blood stream. Hypervolemia and hemolysis then follow, resulting in myocardial failure. Finally hyperkalemia and dilution of electrolytes occur, with ventricular fibrillation as a consequence.

Resuscitation of people who have nearly drowned should begin at the scene of the accident to prevent hypoxia. Pulmonary edema, infections, and fluid and electrolyte imbalances are treated in accordance with the signs and symptoms. Patients are observed for 48 hours following the accident.

CARCINOMA OF THE LUNG

The majority of lung carcinomas originate in the bronchi. Although there is some controversy as to the cause of lung carcinoma, its incidence has been directly related to cigarette smoking. A number of studies have been conducted that demonstrate that people who smoke two or more packs of cigarettes a day have the highest incidence of death from carcinoma of the lung. Environmental polutants have also been linked to the incidence of lung cancer, but asbestos fibers seem to be the only industrial pollutant with a direct relationship to the development of carcinoma.

It is believed that the inhaled carcinogens become lodged in the mucus of the bronchi, predominantly at the bronchial bifurcations, where the flow of mucus is the slowest. The carcinogens stimulate metaplasia in these sites with eventual growth of carcinoma. Other areas of the lung previously scarred as a result of infection, bronchiectasis, or hypersensitivity reactions may be the site of carcinoma. For this reason it is assumed that people who have had previous lung disease and who smoke cigarettes are more susceptible to the development of carcinoma than those who do not smoke. Cancer of the lung causes more deaths among men than other sites of cancer and has a very high mortality rate. The incidence of lung cancer in women is increasing. The greater percentage of women who smoke are now approaching their fifth or sixth decade, and it is thought that this is the major cause of the increase. This statistic gives further credibility to the direct relationship between cigarette smoking and cancer.

Types of Cells

The types of cells identified in carcinoma of the lung include squamous or epidermoid, undifferentiated, adenocarcinoma, alveolar or bronchiolar, and bronchial adenoma cells. The symptoms caused by each of these cell types differ somewhat in terms of the point of origin for each type. The different types of cells also have different growth rates and different patterns of metastasis.

Epidermoid or squamous cell carcinoma Epidermoid or squamous cell carcinoma occurs the most frequently, making up about one-half of all cases of lung cancer. This type of cancer originates in the large bronchi and is the type most directly related to cigarette smoking. Metastasis occurs early, with the cells spreading through the lymphatic system and the systemic arterial circulation. Because of the point of origin, symptoms are related to obstruction of the bronchus. These symptoms include wheezing, if the bronchus is partially obstructed, and frequent infections. Often the carcinoma is discovered when a patient is being treated for pneumonia. The infections occur distal to the tumor because of the partial obstruction, which does not allow complete drainage of the area the lung serves. The symptoms of the infection, usually cough, pleurisy, and elevated temperature, may bring the affected person to medical attention, and the carcinoma is then often found on a diagnostic x-ray. Completely obstructed bronchi lead to atelectasis with subsequent loss of ventilation capability. When atelectasis occurs there is often a mediastinal shift toward the involved areas, which can be seen on x-ray.

Undifferentiated cell carcinoma Undifferentiated cell carcinoma includes different cell types: small round cells, large cells, and oat cells. The point of origin is similar to that for epidermoid cell types. Oat cells often have a point of origin between the periphery of the lung and the hilus. The undifferentiated cell types spread early via the lymphatic vessels and invade the pulmonary veins so that metastasis occurs through the arterial system. Some authorities believe that the oat cell is not one of the undifferentiated cell types, but a separate type. The oat cell is named for its form, which is similar to oat grains, and is highly metastatic. It is anaplastic, as are the small round cell and large cell.

The symptoms associated with the undifferentiated cell types include inflammation and ulceration of the bronchial wall. The inflammatory response is the same as that occurring in other forms of lung irritation. The ulcerations have a tendency to hemorrhage. Patients with undifferentiated cell type carcinoma have an unproductive cough. Their x-rays may be normal or in some cases may show bronchial obstruction. Diagnosis often depends on bronchoscopic examination and histologic examination of the cells.

Alveolar or bronchial cell tumors Alveolar or bronchiolar cell tumors originate in the epithelium of the bronchioles. The tumors tend to follow alveolar lines and frequently originate in lung scars. There may be many small tumors that grow slowly, consolidating large areas of the lung; the consolidation can be seen on x-ray and resembles pneumonia. The alveolar or bronchiolar cell types secrete large amounts of mucin. Metastasis occurs through the bloodstream and lymphatic system, most frequently to the opposite lung.

Adenocarcinoma Adenocarcinomas are the cell types that occur most frequently in women. They tend to originate in the periphery of the lungs, in both bronchial glands and epithelium. Tumors caused by adenocarcinoma are often asymptomatic. The lesions, sometimes called coin lesions, are small and appear on x-ray as localized lesions not unlike tuberculosis. A tuberculin skin test is often negative. The adenocarcinoma tends to invade the pulmonary veins and is associated with Pancoast's syndrome. In this syndrome, the tumor cells invade the bronchial plexus, causing pain and muscle wasting of the hand. The appearance of this phenomenon is sometimes the first indication that a patient may have carcinoma of the lung.

Bronchial adenoma has its origin in the mucus cells in either the bronchus or trachea. Bronchial adenomas are not always malignant but have the potential for becoming so. There are two main types, cylindroma and carcinoid. The cylindromas are similar to the adenoid cystic cancer that originates in the salivary gland and tend to invade locally; they metastasize through the lymph nodes and the bloodstream. Carcinoid tumors resemble those in the gastrointestinal tract and originate in the bronchial mucus membrane cells.

Mesenchymal tumors In addition to the bronchial and mucous gland tumors, there are also several different types of mesenchymal tumors, including fibrosarcomas and lymphomas. Fibrosarcomas arise in the connective and fibrous tissue of the lung. Lymphomas may occur singly in the lung or they may occur in combination with lymphomas elsewhere in the body, in lymphosarcoma. Lymphoma cells tend to originate in the peripheral portion of the lung and spread through the lymph nodes by direct extension.

Silent tumors Lung cancer has also been associated with cancers that are "silent" elsewhere in the body. The usual sites for growth of silent tumors are the kidney, the colon, the stomach, and the pancreas. Sometimes the finding of a lung tumor on a routine x-ray alerts the physician to the possibility of a silent tumor elsewhere.

Diagnosis of Carcinoma

Diagnosis of carcinoma of the lung is complicated by the fact that the early symptoms are similar to those caused by many respiratory infections. The tumor growth can actually predispose a person to infections because of obstruction of the airway or impairment of ventilation. Lung abscesses frequently occur in lung cancer and are most prevalent when tissue necrosis is present. Usually the person first notices a persistent cough but may fail to recognize its significance as a symptom of cancer. It is natural to attribute a chronic cough to cigarette smoking or a transient cold or to disregard it.

The tumor is often found on a routine chest x-ray. Many tumors can be seen on regular posteroanterior and lateral views. The mediastinum may be shifted, and consolidation can be heard on auscultation. If it is not evident that the patient has a tumor on the basis of these findings, more extensive examinations are performed. Bronchoscopy is one of the most important diagnostic tests used to differentiate carcinoma from other lung diseases. It is possible to obtain a biopsy of the tumor cell for cytologic examination through bronchial washings. Bronchoscopy is most useful in diagnosing epidermoid and undifferentiated cell carcinoma because these cells originate in the bronchus. Sputum examination is another important diagnostic tool. However, sputum examinations do not always reveal the cancer cells on cytologic examination even in the presence of a tumor; therefore a negative cytology does not exclude the diagnosis of cancer. Another diagnostic method is obtaining a biopsy. There is controversy as to the best method of obtaining a biopsy, with some authorities preferring mediastinoscopy and others the scalene node biopsy. Usually a lymph node biopsy is done if the cervical lymph nodes are enlarged.

Signs and Symptoms of Carcinoma

A number of different phenomena occur in association with carcinoma of the lung. One of these is vascular proliferation of the bone, which is usually observed in the terminal phalanges with ballottement of the nail base. Ballottement refers to the convex, raised nail bed that occurs with reddened skin at the tips of the fingers. Another associated set of symptoms includes periarticular edema and swelling of the hand, ankle, and knee joints. There may also be periosteal proliferation of the long bones. Resection of the lung tumor provides relief of these symptoms. The associated lung lesions are generally small and do not cause symptoms in the lung.

Oat cell types produce a substance like adrenocorticotropic hormone, which may be overtly demonstrated in the symptoms of Cushing's syndrome; one of the major symptoms of this syndrome is mental confusion. Squamous cell types may produce parathyroid hormone; in squamous cell types the mental changes are prominent and there is a rapid onset of symptoms, the calcium levels are extremely high, and if untreated the patient develops nephrocalcinosis, which can result in renal failure. The musculoskeletal and nervous system can also be involved.

Pancoast's syndrome may expand to include the superior cervical ganglion. It is then known as Horner's syndrome and can extend further to invade the ribs, causing pain in the arm, hand, fingers, and shoulder as well as the scapular region and jaw. The pain typically becomes more severe at night. In some cases degeneration of the brain is associated with lung tumors; it is thought that the tumor cells produce antigens, which then stimulate the formation of antibodies that cause a response in the brain. In addition to the brain, there may be involvement of the posterior and lateral columns of the spinal cord nonmetastatic carcinoma of the lung also associated with the myasthenia syndrome, gynecomastia, peripheral neuritis, and dermatomyositis. It is obvious that one should always consider the diagnosis of carcinoma when caring for patients who have a variety of symptoms that occur suddenly without any previous disorder.

The fact that lung tumors cause changes in respiratory function is helpful in achieving early diagnosis if people who notice changes do seek treatment. The cure rate of tumors diagnosed early before metastasis has occurred is very good. If the tumor is localized it can be removed. However, if there is lymph node involvement the possibility for complete cure decreases. In advanced tumors, the only plausible treatment is palliation.

Treatment and Nursing Care

There are three major forms of treatment for carcinoma of the lung: surgery, irradiation, and chemotherapy. Surgery involves removal of the tumor and all of its extensions; essentially this means that all traces of the tumor cells are removed if possible. This can be accomplished with a pneumonectomy, a lobectomy, or a segmental resection. A pneumonectomy is usually performed for lesions that originate in the stem bronchus or in the lobar branches of the bronchi. **Pneumonectomy** means removal of a complete lung, which is done by amputating the bronchus as close to the trachea as possible and closing the end of the bronchus so that a stump is formed. A radical pneumonectomy includes removal of all the lymph nodes that drain the lung with the lymphatic vessels and fatty tissue. A **lobectomy** is removal of one lobe of the lung and is the procedure preferred for peripheral carcinoma that is localized in a lobe. A portion of surrounding tissue can also be resected if the tumor has extended. The lymphatic vessels are removed in the hilus of the lung adjacent to the lobe that is removed. A **segmental resection** is removal of one segment of the lung and is performed when the lesion is small and well contained within a segment of the lung. Surgical treatment for bronchial adenoma is local excision if the tumor has not invaded the bronchial cell wall. Resection with anastomosis or bronchoplasty is performed if the tumor has invaded the cell wall.

Nursing care following resection of lung tissue is discussed on page 246 of this chapter. Essentially the most important aspect of postoperative care is maintaining an adequate airway. Patients who are about to undergo chest surgery are taught to turn, cough, and do deep breathing. Prior to chest surgery, lung function studies are performed with thoroughness to determine the patient's ability to ventilate adequately after the surgery. However, the particular nature of chest surgery places a stress on the respiratory system even if it has been deemed adequate through pulmonary function tests. First, the patient has had an operation, which may traumatize the airway; second, the anesthesia may depress respiration; and finally, surgery may have caused some residual edema or hemorrhage in the lungs that would decrease ventilation.

Mechanical ventilation may be required to maintain adequate oxygenation during the postoperative period, and a tracheostomy may be needed if the patient develops respiratory insufficiency. In addition, the patient who has undergone a lobectomy or segmental resection will return from surgery with a closed drainage system for removal of air and secretions from the operative site. The patient who has had a pneumonectomy usually does not have a chest tube since the entire lung has been removed.

Just as important as maintaining the airway is providing emotional support for the patient who is having chest surgery for carcinoma of the lung. The fact that carcinoma of the lung is associated with a high mortality rate is well advertised in the media with antismoking campaigns, and usually the patient is well aware that his condition is serious and his chances for recovery are variable. At times when the tumor is diagnosed early and resection seems complete, the patient may have to be convinced that his prognosis is statistically very good. The psychological trauma of knowing that one has cancer may contribute to the stress of surgery and can alter the patient's response to anesthesia as well as to postoperative care. The nurse should be aware of this and should help the patient deal with his feelings; family members should also be included in this process. There can be considerable guilt felt by family members when a person has carcinoma of the lung. In some cases it is difficult for the family members not to experience feelings related to prophesy fulfillment because they have conducted anti-smoking campaigns in their own homes with little success. In addition to these feelings there is often concern about how a person can live effectively with less than the normal amount of lung tissue. Fortunately a number of prominent people have had resection of lung carcinoma and are still very active; these people can be cited as models of success. An even better model is a person who is known to the family and who is willing to discuss his adjustment to the loss of a lung.

It is important that the patient who has undergone a lung resection for carcinoma have routine follow-ups with chest x-rays and sputum examinations. These examinations are usually every three months at first, and then after the first year the sputum examination is alternated with the chest x-ray so that there is consistent monitoring of the patient's progress. Some authorities prescribe radiation therapy before and after surgery; however, there is limited evidence that the prognosis improves as a result of radiation therapy, and its benefits are controversial.

For patients who have metastases to the lymph nodes, choice of the method of treatment is often a difficult decision. Some physicians allow the patient to make the choice if the situation is borderline. However, if the patient has compromised lung function, cardiovascular disease, and metastases to the lymph nodes, his prognosis is poor and surgery is often contraindicated. Radiation therapy and chemotherapy are the treatments of choice for these patients.

Carcinoma of the lung metastasizes most frequently to the adrenal glands; there can also be distal metastases to the central nervous system and the bones, joints, liver, and pleura. Cure is not possible if metastases have occurred. Another ominous sign is invasion of the pleura. This is usually demonstrated by the presence of hemothorax, which may result from multiple tumors in the pleura. Diagnosis can be made by a needle biopsy of the pleura and by cytology examination of the pleural fluid. When paralysis of the recurrent laryngeal nerve or the phrenic nerve occurs, the prognosis is usually poor, as it is if Horner's syndrome is present.

Complete lung function studies are often the data base used to determine if a patient can withstand surgery. If the values of these studies indicate that the patient does not have at least 50 percent of the normal lung function remaining, surgery is contraindicated. If a pneumonectomy is to be performed, it is generally expected that a patient should have at least 75 percent of normal lung function. In addition to the lung function studies, ventilation is evaluated through the blood gas levels. It is important that the patient's cardiovascular status also be carefully evaluated because dysfunction of this system is another contraindication for surgery.

Radiation therapy is preferred by some authorities in providing palliative treatment. If there is a great deal of pleural effusion, chemotherapy may be used. Nitrogen mustard is one of the more effective chemotherapeutic agents for treating lung cancer; many of the other chemotherapeutic agents are not effective in lung tumors. Radiation therapy is usually successful in diminishing or relieving the major symptoms of cough and pain experienced by patients with advanced carcinoma of the lung. Cobalt therapy is often given. Although the procedure differs with the physician and the patient's tolerance, the irradation treatments are generally given in two separate time periods at least 2 or 3 weeks apart. Each time period may vary in number of days, but the maximum dose given usually does not exceed 5,500 to 6,000 rads. Radiation pneumonitis may result following the therapy. The reaction is characterized by two phases, the first occurring within the first 5 months and the second as long as 2 to 8 years after the therapy. A dry, hacking cough that lasts a few weeks is the prominent symptom in the early reaction. The chest x-ray will show pneumonitis, and the illness subsides after a week or so. The later reaction is associated with dyspnea and cough and is thought to be caused by hyalinization of pulmonary tissue with fibrosis and formation of chest deformities. Cor pulmonale resulting from vascular obstruction is frequently the cause of death.

The patient with incurable cancer has very special needs. His ability to cope with death and the relationships he has with supportive family members are very important at this time. The nurse can do much not only to facilitate the patient's physical comfort within the limits of his condition but also to work with the patient and his family to explore and evaluate their resources for ongoing support. Despite foreknowledge and preparation, death is always a crisis.

References

1. Amborn, S. A. Clinical signs associated with the amount of tracheobronchial secretions. *Nurs. Res.* 25:121, 1976.
2. American Lung Association. *Introduction to Lung Diseases*, 5th ed. New York: 1973.
3. American Lung Association. *Diagnostic Standards and Classification of Tuberculosis and Other Mycobacterial Diseases*. New York: 1974.
4. American Lung Association. *The Tuberculin Skin Test*. New York: 1974.
5. Center for Disease Control, Bacterial Disease Division, Bureau of Epidemiology. *The Control of Pulmonary Infections Associated with Tracheostomy*. Atlanta: 1975.
6. Christman, M. Dyspnea. *Am. J. Nurs.* 74:643, 1974.
7. Gorman, M. L. Conscious repatterning of human behavior. *Am. J. Nurs.* 75:1752, 1975.
8. Gracey, D. R. Adult respiratory disease syndrome. *Heart Lung* 4:280, 1975.
9. Greenbaum, D. M. Decannulation of the tracheostomized patient. *Heart Lung* 5:119, 1976.
10. Mountcastle, V. B. (ed.). *Medical Physiology*, 13th ed. St. Louis: Mosby, 1974.
11. Petty, T. L. *Intensive and Rehabilitative Respiratory Care*. Philadelphia: Lea & Febiger, 1974.
12. Selkurt, E. *Basic Physiology for the Health Sciences*. Boston: Little, Brown, 1975.
13. Shapiro, B. A., Harrison, R. A., and Trout, C. A. *Clinical Application of Respiratory Care*. Chicago: Year Book, 1976.
14. U.S. Department of Health, Education and Welfare, Public Health Service. *Tuberculosis Programs*. 1973.
15. U.S. Department of Health, Education and Welfare, Public Health Service. *1974 Tuberculosis Statistics: States and Cities*.
16. Wade, J. F. *Respiratory Nursing Care*. St. Louis: Mosby, 1973.
17. West, J. B. *Respiratory Physiology: The Essentials*. Baltimore: Williams & Wilkins, 1974.

Bibliography

Adler, R. H. Guide to diagnosis and treatment of pneumothorax. *Hosp. Med.* 12:69, 1976.

Alexander, M. M., and Brown, M.S. Physical examination: Chest and lungs. *Nursing 75* 5:44, 1975.

Balsley, M., Brink, M. D., and Speckman, E. F. Nutrition in disease and stress. *Nurs. Dig.* 3:27, 1975.

Behnke, H. D. (ed.). *Guidelines for Comprehensive Nursing Care in Cancer Patients With Lung Cancer*. New York: Springer, 1973.

Bennett, R. M. Drowning and near drowning: Etiology and pathophysiology. *Am. J. Nurs.* 76:919, 1976.

Bergesen, B., and Goth, A. *Pharmacology in Nursing*, 12th ed. St. Louis: Mosby, 1973.

Blancher, G. C. Caring for the patient with advanced emphysema. *R.N.* 37:41, 1974.

Blanco, G. Spontaneous Pneumothorax. *Hosp. Med.* 11:40, 1975.

Bone, R. C. Compliance and dynamic characteristics curves in acute respiratory failure. *Crit. Care Med.* 4:173, 1976.

Brach, B. B., Yin, F., Timms, B., Moser, K., et al. Reduced inspiratory effort during intermittent mandatory ventilation with PEEP. *Crit. Care Med.* 4:142, 1976.

Buckingham, W. B., Sparberg, M., and Brandfonbrener, M. *A Primer of Clinical Diagnosis*. New York: Harper & Row, 1971.

Burrows, B., Knudson, R. J., and Kettel, L. J. *Respiratory Insufficiency*. Chicago: Year Book, 1975.

Busey, J. F. Modern concepts in the diagnosis and management of the pulmonary mycoses. *Clin. Notes Respir. Dis.* 14:4, 1976.

Bushnell, S. S. *Respiratory Intensive Care Nursing*. Boston: Little, Brown, 1973.

Center for Disease Control, Bacterial Disease Division, Bureau of Epidemiology. *Recommendations for the Care of Tracheostomy*. Atlanta, 1973.

Chetty, K. G., and Davidson, P. T. A guide to management of hemothorax. *Hosp. Med.* 11:25, 1975.

Clarke, E. B., and Niggeman, E. R. Near-drowning. *Heart Lung* 4:946, 1975.

Comer, P. B. Airway maintenance in patients with long-term endotracheal intubation. *Crit. Care Med.* 4:211, 1976.

Crelin, E. S. In R. K. Shapter (ed.), Development of the lower respiratory system. *Clin. Symp.* 27:4, 1975.

Egan, D. F. *Fundamentals of Respiratory Therapy* (2nd ed.). St. Louis: Mosby, 1973.

Evans, A. S. Diagnosis and prevention of common respiratory infections. *Hosp. Med.* 10:31, 1974.

Fink, J. N. Hypersensitivity pneumonitis due to organic dusts. *Clin. Notes Respir. Dis.* 13:1, 1974.

Fosburg, R. G. Help your patients become nonsmokers. *Clin. Notes Respir. Dis.* 14:30, 1975.

Goldstein, D. H., and Benoit, J. N. Occupational safety and health. *Am. J. Nurs.* 75:1759, 1975.

Kudla, M. S. The care of the patient with respiratory insufficiency. *Nurs. Clin. North Am.* 8:183, 1971.

Lagerson, J., and Ayres, S. M. Chronic airway obstruction: Essentials of care. *Hosp. Med.* 9:38, 1973.

Le Bow, M. D. *Behavior Modification: A Significant Method in Nursing Practice*. Englewood Cliffs, N.J.: Prentice-Hall, 1973.

Mackel, D. C. Sterilization and decontamination of inhalation therapy equipment. Presented at meeting of the American Society for Microbiology, Minneapolis, 1971.

Mostow, S. R. Diagnosis and treatment of bacterial pneumonia. *Hosp. Med.* 11:36, 1975.

Oakes, A., and Murrow, H. Understanding blood gases. *Nursing 73* 3:14, 1973.

O'Dell, A. J. Emergency care in establishing an effective airway. *Nurs. Clin. North Am.* 8:413, 1973.

Passmore, R., and Robson, J. S. (eds.). *A Companion to Medical Studies*, vol. 3, part 1. London: Blackwell, 1974.

Petty, T. L. Complications occurring during mechanical ventilation. *Heart Lung* 5:112, 1976.

Petty, T., and Nett, L. *For Those Who Live and Breathe* (2nd ed.). Springfield, Ill.: Thomas, 1975.

Piehl, M. A., and Brown, R. S. Use of extreme position changes in acute respiratory failure. *Crit. Care Med.* 4:13, 1976.

Riker Laboratories. *Living with Asthma, Chronic Bronchitis and Emphysema*. Northridge, Cal.: 1971.

Sabiston, D. C. *Davis–Christopher Textbook of Surgery* (10th ed.). Philadelphia: Saunders, 1972.

Shontz, F. C. *Psychological Aspects of Physical Illness and Disability*. New York: Macmillan, 1975.

Sodeman, W. A., and Sodeman, W. A., Jr. *Pathologic Physiology: Mechanisms of Disease*, 5th ed. Philadelphia: Saunders, 1974.

Soloway, H. B. Adult respiratory distress syndrome. *Hosp. Med.* 11:76, 1975.

Stephens, G., and Parsons, M. C. A delicate balance: Managing chronic airway obstruction in a neurosurgical patient. *Am. J. Nurs.* 75:1492, 1975.

Taylor, C. M. Pneumococcal pneumonia: Your patient's second threat? *Nursing 76* 6:30, 1976.

Tinker, S. J. Understanding chest x-rays. *Am. J. Nurs.* 76:54, 1976.

Traver, G. In E. Beland, and J. Y. Passos (eds.), *Clinical Nursing* (2nd ed.). New York: Macmillan, 1975. Chapter 10.

Traver, G. A. Living with chronic respiratory disease. *Am. J. Nurs.* 75:1777, 1975.

Traver, G. A., ed. Symposium on care in respiratory disease. *Nurs. Clin. North Am.* 9:97, 1974.

U.S. Department of Health, Education and Welfare, Public Health Service. *Suggested Tuberculosis Nurse Functions in a Nurse Directed Clinic*. 1974.

U.S. Department of Health, Education and Welfare, Public Health Service. *1974 Tuberculosis Statistics: States and Cities*.

Wilson, R. F., and Sibbald, W. J. Acute respiratory failure. *Crit. Care Med.* 4:79, 1976.

Wyper, M. A. Pulmonary embolism: Fighting the silent killer. *Nursing 75* 5:30, 1975.

chapter 4
Patients with Cardiovascular System Dysfunction

Eileen Mulqueeny

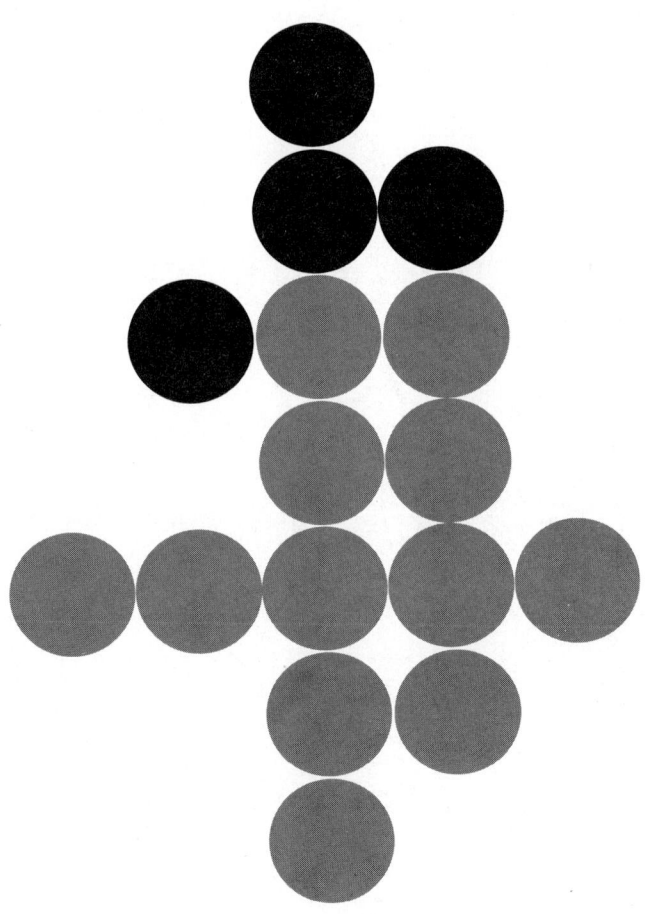

The purpose of this chapter is to review aspects of the basic anatomy, physiology, and functions of the cardiovascular system; to describe the assessments needed for a thorough evaluation of a patient's cardiovascular status; and to apply this information to nursing practice. Nursing practice should focus on measures to promote, maintain, and restore the cardiovascular function of each patient to the highest homeostatic level possible.

Anatomy and Physiology

The cardiovascular system transports and distributes life-supporting nutrients in the blood to the body tissues and removes unneeded substances. It is also important in body temperature regulation, humoral communication, and the adaptations necessary to supply body cells with nutrients and oxygen in various physiologic states. The **cardiovascular system** consists of the heart and its peripheral vascular system (with its principal functional unit, the capillaries; Fig. 4-1).

The heart is referred to as a pump and consists of four chambers that function in a cycle of diastole and systole. The **right atrium** (chamber) and the **right ventricle** propel blood through the pulmonary system for the exchange of oxygen and carbon dioxide; the **left atrium** and the **left ventricle** direct blood to all the other tissues of the body. The right atrium is a small, thin-walled, low-pressure compartment, and during **diastole** (the resting, or noncontracting, state) the right atrium serves as a reservoir for the deoxygenated venous blood returned to the heart. During **systole** (contraction of the atria) the stored blood is propelled through the tricuspid valves to the right ventricle. The atrial reservoir is responsible for approximately 25 percent of ventricular filling, while approximately 75 percent of the blood flows directly into the ventricles even before the atria contract. When the atria do not function effectively, ventricular filling and cardiac output are reduced and the heart becomes a less efficient pump.

After right ventricular systole, blood flows through semilunar valves into the pulmonary arteries and arterioles, and it eventually reaches the capillary beds of the lungs. The capillaries surround the alveoli of the lung and provide for the exchange of oxygen and carbon dioxide. The blood then returns to the heart through the pulmonary veins to the left atrium. The left atrium also serves as a reservoir and contributes to left ventricular filling. During left atrial systole, blood flows through the mitral valve into the left ventricle, which is the strongest and most important compartment of the heart. Circulation then continues through the semilunar valves into the aorta and subsequently throughout the peripheral vessels. Pressure changes within the chambers of the heart are synchronized with the opening and closing of the heart valves to assure propulsion of the blood. The atrioventricular (AV) valves (the mitral valve, with two cusps, and the tricuspid valves, with three cusps) prevent the backflow of blood from the ventricles to the atria during systole, and the semilunar valves (aortic and pulmonary valves) prevent backflow from the aorta and pulmonary arteries into the ventricles during diastole.

The heart receives its blood supply from the right and left coronary arteries, which arise from the aorta, just beyond the aortic semilunar valve. Perfusion of the coronary arteries occurs predominantly during diastole of the left ventricle, since blood flow through the myocardium is obstructed during ventricular systole. The left coronary artery divides into the anterior descending artery, which in most patients supplies the anterior part of the left ventricle and portions of the right ventricle, and the circumflex artery, which supplies the lateral, lower posterior walls of the left ventricle and the left atrium. The remaining portions of the myocardium are supplied by the right coronary artery and its branches. Blood is returned from the myocardium, via the coronary sinus, to the right atrium.

Although the **cardiac cycle** (systole and diastole) results in the intermittent cardiac output of approximately 5 liters of blood per minute, blood flow to the peripheral circulation is continuous. The distention of the aorta and its branches during systole and the elastic recoils of the large arteries during diastole propel the blood from the elastic structure of the aorta to the more muscular arteries and to the predominantly muscular arterioles.

The **peripheral vascular system** includes all of the circulatory system except the heart. This system can be divided into five main subsystems which are (1) the aorta and the large arteries, which form a **distributing system;** (2) the arterioles, or the resistance vessels, which **regulate arterial pressure;** (3) the **microcirculation** (capillaries and venules), through which passage of metabolites to and

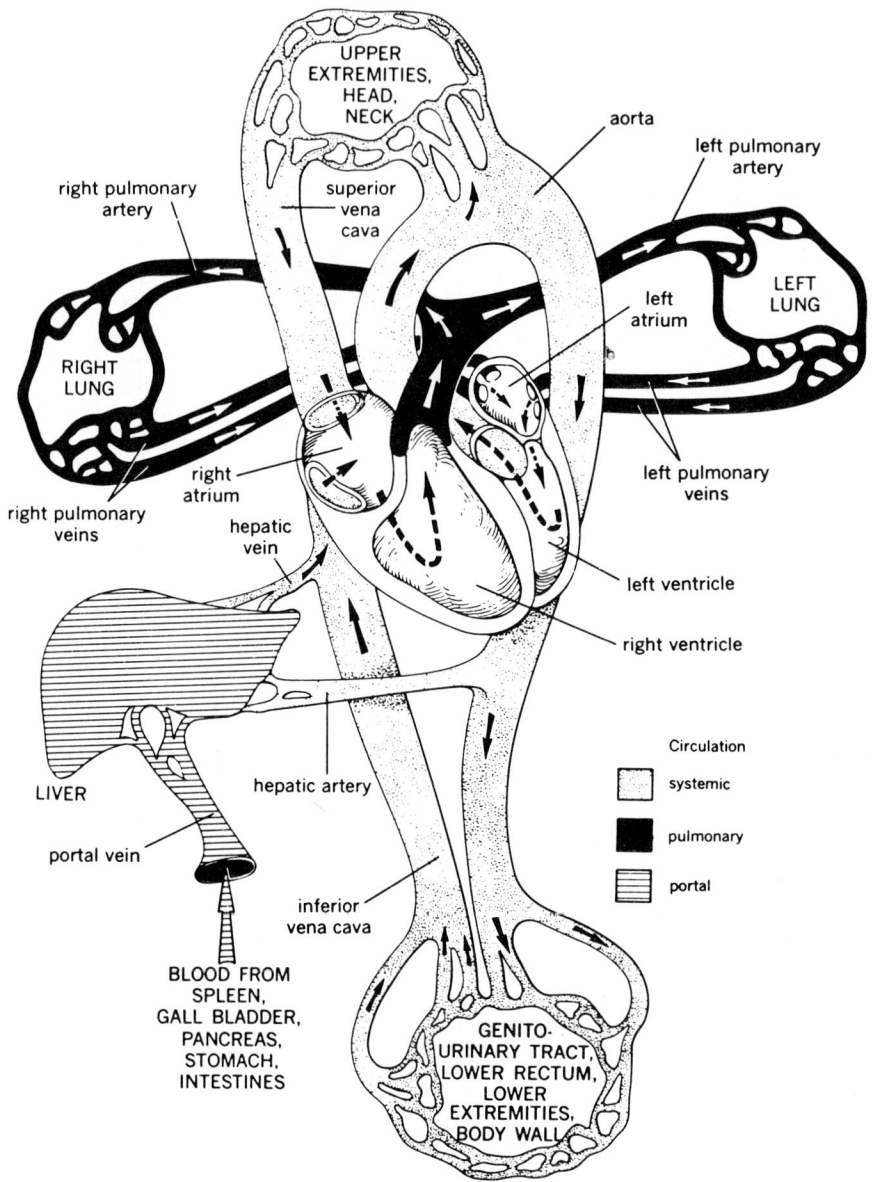

Figure 4-1
The systemic, pulmonary, and portal circulation of the circulatory system. (From W. Beck, *Human Design: Molecular, Cellular, and Systematic Physiology*. New York: Harcourt Brace Jovanovich, 1971. Reproduced by permission.)

from tissue takes place; (4) a **collecting system of veins** that carries blood toward the heart; and (5) the **lymphatic system.**

The ability of the heart to maintain a functional state, allowing the continuous and effectual movement of blood, is dependent on a number of factors that affect the entire cardiovascular system.

THE HEART

The heart has three layers: (1) the pericardium, (2) the myocardium, and (3) the endocardium. The **pericardium** is the fibroserous sac that encloses the heart. The inner, serous portion of the pericardium consists of two layers (visceral and parietal), which en-

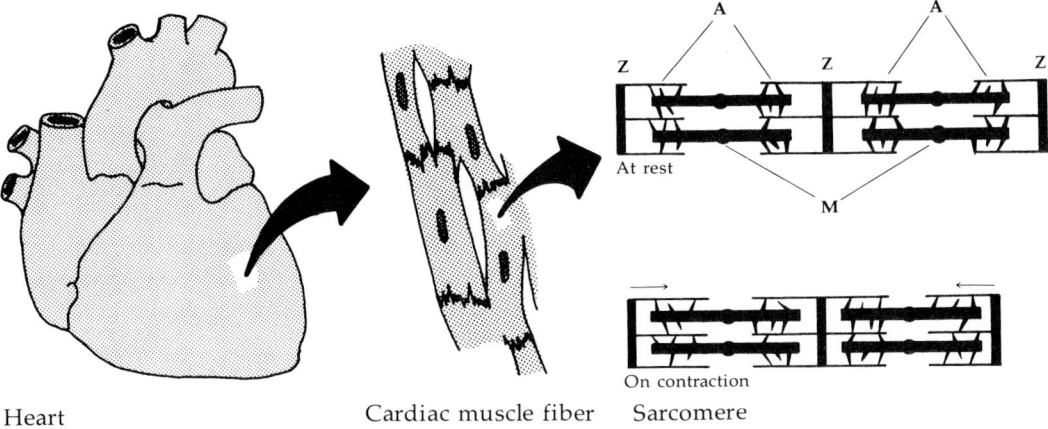

Figure 4-2
The sarcomere is the basic contractile unit of the muscle fiber in the heart. It is composed of Z bands (Z), which are attached to thin filaments of actin (A). Myosin (M) lies loosely among the actin fibers while at rest. On contraction, the actin slides over the myosin which, in turn, shortens the muscle fiber.

close a potential space, the pericardial cavity. The **myocardium** is the muscular layer of the heart, and the **endocardium** is the smooth endothelial lining of the heart chambers and the covering of the valves. The endocardium is continuous with the lining of the blood vessels entering and leaving the heart.

The cardiac muscle itself, although similar in many ways to skeletal muscle, has many unique properties. The basic unit of the myocardium is the muscle fiber, which consists of the basic contracting unit, the sarcomere. These sarcomeres can be identified by means of an electron microscope. As illustrated in Figure 4-2, the sarcomere is composed of filaments of actin and spiny myosin situated longitudinally and adjacent to each other. Actin is attached to Z bands while myosin, by its spines, is attached to the actin at various points along its length. The actin and myosin are movable over each other and their lengths are shortened through the movement of actin filaments toward the myosin. The greater the overlap of actin on the myosin, the shorter the muscle fibers become. When all the muscle fibers of a given heart chamber shorten at the same time, the chamber becomes smaller, forcing blood out into the passageway of least resistance. The valvular system of the heart prevents the backflow of blood into the preceding chamber, thus allowing the blood to continue on its designated pathway.

The stimulus for the actin to move over the myosin results from the electrical activation transmitted to the muscle cell. At this time, sodium enters the cell while potassium leaves the cell and calcium is released into the sarcoplasm, the fluid filling the cardiac cell. It is theorized that the calcium, by combining with the enzyme adenosine triphosphatase (ATPase), helps in the formation of electrochemical bonds between the spines of the myosin and the actin filaments. These filaments of actin move progressively inward as successive bonds are formed and broken. It is at this phase that systole will occur, if all the sarcomeres shorten at the same time. Once shortening has occurred, the calcium is actively pumped away from the sarcomere. Without available calcium to form bonds, actin slides back, resulting in a lengthening of the sarcomere with a lesser degree of overlap. Diastole results as blood flows into the chamber.

Knowledge of the mechanisms of contraction and lengthening of muscle fibers, and specifically of the sarcomeres, facilitates the understanding of abnormal functioning of the heart in cardiovascular disease. It is clear that the proper exchange of electrolytes is essential for maintaining the ability of the heart muscle to function. When dysfunction exists, the ability of the myocardium to pump effectively is compromised and cardiac output is jeopardized.

Cardiac output can be calculated by multiplying the stroke volume (the amount of blood ejected with each ventricular contraction) times the heart rate. Cardiac output therefore reflects the amount of blood pumped by the left ventricle per minute. The normal cardiac output is 5,000 ml of blood per minute but may vary from 3,000 ml per minute at rest to 25,000 ml per minute in a well-trained athlete during strenuous activity.

The ability of cardiac tissue to adjust cardiac output in accordance with the needs of the body tissues is dependent on three major cardiac properties: (1) the ability to change the heart rate, (2) the Frank-Starling principle, or the length-tension relationship, and (3) the variable contractility of the heart, or the force-velocity relationship. These three properties will now be discussed separately.

The Heart Rate

The normal range of heart rate is 60 to 100 beats per minute. The ability of the heart to vary its rate in accordance with the needs of the body tissues is a vitally important mechanism and is influenced by many factors. When there is an increased need for oxygen and the elimination of carbon dioxide (during exercise or when there is fever), a compensatory increase in heart rate results. **Bradycardia** is a heart rate slower than 60, and **tachycardia** is any rate above 100 beats per minute.

The heart can control its own rate and can also be influenced by external stimuli. The heart's ability to change its rate is a function of the cardiac cell's ability to respond to stimuli. The electrophysiologic characteristics of the heart are indeed unique. To understand this uniqueness, it is important to look at the electrical potentials of the cells of the heart in comparison to the cells of other organs in the body.

All cells have a variety of transmembrane differences, or differences between intracellular and extracellular compartments, that help to create a resting electrical potential. A **resting potential** is created by differences in concentration of substances or by electrical changes between two physical areas. For example, a dam in a river creates an enormous difference between two levels of water, resulting in a resting potential. When this potential is transformed into usable energy, entire communities are supplied with electricity.

The cell membrane can be compared to the dam because it, too, helps to maintain different levels of substances. As explained in Chapter 2, the cell membrane is responsible for the active transport of sodium ions to the extracellular compartment while actively keeping potassium in the intracellular compartment. It also helps to create the electronegativity of the intracellular compartments.

The electronegativity of a cell can be measured in the laboratory and recorded at rest, during excitation, and during recovery through the insertion of a microelectrode into the cell. Figure 4-3 illustrates the resting and action potential recordings of a living cardiac cell. The **action potential** can be defined as the change of potential that occurs when the cell is depolarized. When any living cell is at rest, the interior electrical charge of the cell is approximately -90 mv in comparison to the cell's exterior electrical charge. This phase is labeled phase 4. When stimulated initially, sodium (a cation) rushes into the cell, causing the interior to become electropositive, and an action potential begins. This activity is commonly described as **depolarization** and is labeled phase 0 of the action potential. Phase 1 is a brief, rapid (and often absent) change of potential toward **repolarization**. Repolariza-

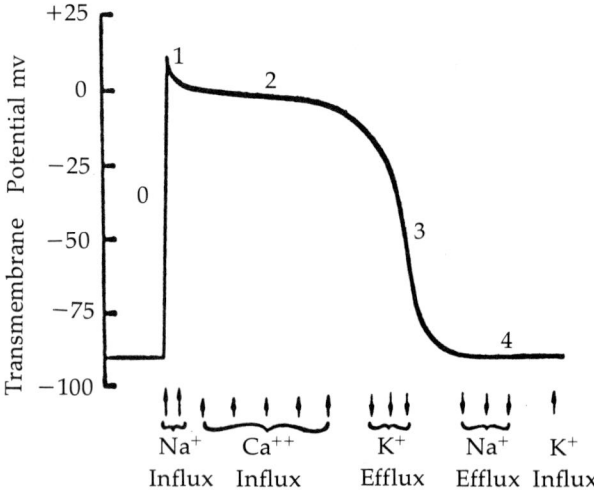

Figure 4-3
The resting and action potential recordings of a living cardiac cell. [From J. W. Hurst, *The Heart* (3rd ed.). Copyright © 1974 by McGraw-Hill Book Company. Used with permission.]

tion then slows into the **plateauing period,** or phase 2. **Active repolarization,** or phase 3, begins as the cell membrane again actively ejects sodium and retains potassium as it returns to the **resting phase,** 4.

Through observation of the action potential recording (Fig. 4-3) it can be seen that the electronegative differences in phase 4 create a potential that allows the cell to respond to a stimulus. Once this transcellular difference is eliminated after depolarization, the cell can no longer respond to a stimulus, regardless of the strength of the stimulus, because there is no significant difference between the two compartments. During phases 0, 1, 2, and the beginning of phase 3, the cell is said to be in an absolute refractory period and cannot respond to a stimulus. As the cell becomes more electronegative in phase 3, it enters a relative refractory period and a stronger-than-threshold stimulus is capable of exciting the cell and sending it into another action potential. As the cell approaches phase 4, a supernormal or vulnerable period develops in which a lower-than-threshold force can stimulate the cell. It has been discovered that a single strong stimulus at this time often elicits a high-frequency train of repetitive contractions or even fibrillation, which is an uncoordinated ineffectual contraction. Various types of fibrillation will be discussed later in this chapter.

The **noncardiac cell** is dependent on an outside stimulus, such as from the nervous system, hormonal substances, heat, cold, or pressure changes of a threshold strength, in order for it to depolarize. Therefore the phase 4 resting state is flat until stimulation occurs. When the potentials of **cardiac cells** are recorded, phase 4 appears to have a gradual incline, becoming less electronegative until it initiates its own action potential, referred to as **automaticity** and evident in cardiac cells only. Sodium is gradually leaked into the cell until the cell membrane no longer can maintain its function and rapid depolarization occurs.

The **conductive system** (Fig. 4-4) has precise and exact pathways composed of automatic cells. The usual initiating pacemaker of the heart, the sinoatrial (SA) node, is located in the upper left section of the right atrium, near the opening of the superior vena cava. Nervous tissue pathways are distributed throughout the atria and come together at the atrioventricular junction (AV node). Electrical conduction is delayed as it moves through the AV node (to allow for atrial emptying before ventricular contraction). At the bundle of His, conduction speeds up and is directed into the right bundle branch (RBB) and the left bundle branch (LBB). The bundle branch system then subdivides into smaller terminal divisions called **Purkinje fibers,** which directly excite the myocardial contractile fibers of the ventricles.

The electrocardiogram (ECG) is a vector (line) recording of the electrical potentials generated by the cardiac cells. Electrodes placed on the skin detect and record the size of the electrical current moving toward or away from the positive electrode. If electrical activity moves toward the positive skin electrode, the vector (ECG tracing) moves upward from the isoelectric baseline. If electrical current moves away from this electrode the vector deflects downward. The size of the vector (or ECG wave) is dependent on the magnitude of the electrical current and on the size of the particular muscle involved, due, for example, to the small size of the atria in comparison to the ventricles, the magnitude of the atrial electrical current is smaller and results in a small ECG wave. The P wave of the ECG represents the total depolarization of the atria (Fig. 4-4).

After the P wave is recorded the ECG vector returns to the baseline; it shows no electrical activity for a period of approximately 0.10 second, accounting for the time it takes for the depolarization wave to travel at a slower rate through the AV node and through the bundle system until it reaches the ventricular cells. The QRS wave of the ECG represents ventricular repolarization. Since the anatomic size of the ventricle is greater than that of the atrium, the size of this wave is larger. The majority of conduction pathways are directed downward and toward the left (toward the positive electrode) so that the QRS wave is primarily deflected upward, except for a small Q and S wave. The T wave of the ECG represents ventricular repolarization and is deflected upward since repolarization follows in the same direction as depolarization (as shown in Fig. 4-4). Additional information on the diagnostic value and interpretation of the ECG is given in a subsequent section in this chapter.

Almost all cardiac cells have automaticity,

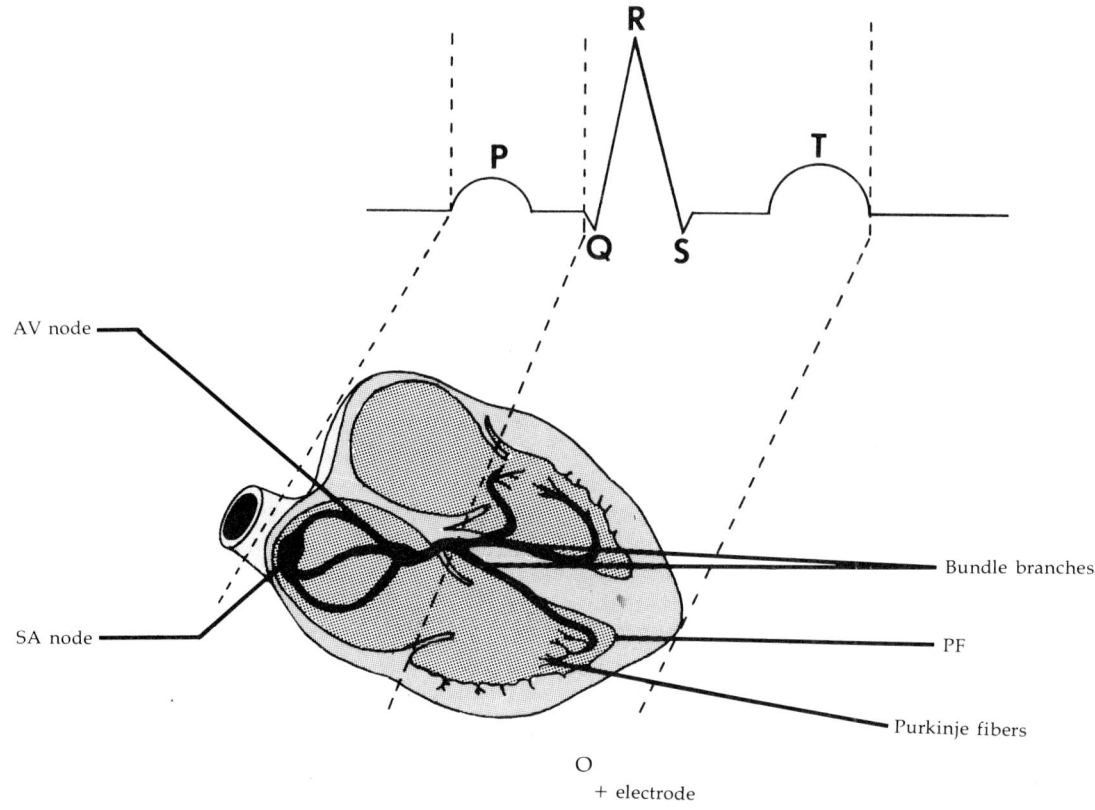

Figure 4-4
The cardiac conduction system in relation to the electrocardiogram. Note that the positive electrode for this tracing is placed at the lower left of the heart, resulting in an upward deflection of the P, R, and T waves.

but the automaticity rates vary with the anatomic location of the cardiac cells. The action potential recording of the SA nodal cells demonstrates a short, rapidly rising phase 4. The atrial cells have a slower automaticity than the SA cells but faster automaticity than the cells in the AV junctional area. The automaticity rate continues to decrease in the Purkinje cells and the ventricular cells.

The automatic cell that depolarizes first stimulates all adjacent cells, and the wave of depolarization continues until all responsive cells are stimulated. Normally the SA node, which has the most rapid automaticity rate (approximately 60 to 100 cycles per minute), is the pacemaker of the heart. If the automaticity rate of the SA cells is decreased for any reason, the automatic cell with the next fastest automaticity rate takes over as the pacemaker. Occasional beats originating elsewhere in the atria are common and may be a normal occurrence. The AV nodal rhythm produces a rate of 40 to 60 cycles per minute. Ventricular cells have a very low automaticity rate (about 30 to 40 cycles per minute) and therefore are not usually effective as a pacemaker to support normal daily activities.

The heart rate is dependent on the sinus automaticity rate, but is also affected by external influences. The autonomic nervous system, external physical stimulants (such as trauma), fluid and electrolyte changes, oxygen deficiencies, and circulation abnormalities also directly affect automaticity. A variety of drugs including antiarrhythmic agents are used specifically for the purpose of changing the sinus rate.

The autonomic nervous system originates in the central nervous system. It is composed of two branches: the sympathetic nervous system (SNS) (the fight, flight, or fright branch), which results in generalized body excitation and increased heart rate; and the parasympathetic nervous system (PSNS), which is the recuperative division resulting in a generalized slowing of body systems, including a decreased heart rate.

The structures of the SNS and the PSNS are similar. The major distinction between the two branches is the type of neurotransmitter at the myoneural junction. At this junction the SNS is activated by norepinephrine, a catecholamine, whereas the PSNS is dependent on acetylcholine to transmit electrical impulses across its synapses.

Another important part of these systems is the receptor sites on the target muscles themselves. The PSNS has one identified type of receptor site. The SNS has three major types of receptor sites: the alpha, beta I, and beta II. The heart has only beta I receptor sites while alpha and beta II receptor sites are scattered throughout the body. It is apparent that any stimulus affecting the autonomic nervous system will affect the cardiovascular system. Various drugs are used to influence the autonomic nervous system by either enhancing or inhibiting the neurotransmitters or the various receptor sites. Examples of these drugs include atropine sulfate, which is a PSNS vagal blocker resulting in a more active SNS effect on the body, and propranolol (Inderal), which blocks the beta receptor sites and thus causes a strong PSNS response. Reference will be made to other drugs throughout this chapter.

Table 4-1 illustrates the cardiac effects of stimulation of the PSNS and the SNS. An **inotropic effect** influences the strength of myocardial contraction. A **chronotropic effect** influences the heart rate, while the **dromotropic effect** influences the electrical excitability or conductivity of the nerve fibers. Anything that enhances the SNS, either by blocking the PSNS or by directly stimulating the SNS, will result in increased cardiac strength, increased heart rate, and increased nerve conductivity, possibly causing arrhythmias. Atropine sulfate blocks the PSNS and thus is often given to treat bradyarrhythmia. Isoproterenol (Isuprel) is a beta receptor stimulator. Since there are beta receptor sites throughout the heart, the entire myocardium has a positive SNS effect when stimulated by isoproterenol.

In addition to specific drugs, psychological entities such as anxiety and fear cause an SNS effect. Pain and an increased metabolic rate resulting from fever, infection, hyperthyroidism, respiratory distress, various fluid and electrolyte disturbances, exercise, and other, not all unpleasant, stimuli can increase the heart rate. Thus heart rate can be controlled initially by the intrinsic automaticity rate of the cardiac cells, especially of the SA node. The autonomic nervous system has a direct effect on the heart, and in response to bodily stresses or demands can cause either an increase or a decrease in heart rate.

An important hemodynamic effect resulting from heart rate is the degree of perfusion available to the coronary arteries. The right and left coronary arteries are the first branches of the aorta. Although the coronary arteries perfuse continually, the most effective perfusion occurs during diastole. During systole, blood is forced through the aorta so quickly and forcefully that only minimal blood is routed into the coronary arteries. During diastole the pressure and the flow rate are decreased and the greatest coronary perfusion takes place.

Tachycardia results in increased cardiac output to the body tissues. Over a long period of time, even if the tachycardia is functional, it can lead to myocardial ischemia due to the shortened periods of diastole. These shortened periods cause a decrease in coronary perfusion when the heart is doing more work and requires an increased blood supply. Decreased perfusion is an especially detrimental factor in a patient with previous cardiac ischemia, injury, or infarction.

The Frank-Starling Principle

Cardiac output is dependent not only on the heart rate but also on the force of muscle contraction. A basic principle that describes a major effect on contraction strength is the Frank-Starling law, the length-tension relationship. This law states that the force of contraction of the ventricles during systole is a function of the total blood volume within the

Table 4-1
Cardiac effects of autonomic nervous system stimulation

	SNS stimulation	PSNS stimulation
Ionotropic effect	+	−
Chronotropic effect	+	−
Dromotropic effect	+	−

+ = positive effect; − = negative effect.

ventricles at the end of diastole (also known as the preload, or the force applied prior to onset of the contraction). Thus the longer the length to which the muscle (or more specifically the sarcomeres) is stretched, up to a limit, the stronger will be the following contraction. When the amount of blood in the ventricles at the end of diastole becomes greater than normal, the following contraction will at times be noticeably stronger, and may be described as **palpitations.** When ventricular filling is incomplete and heart muscle is minimally stretched, the next beat will be weak or thready and at times not even palpable at the radial artery. Any condition that causes hypovolemia, such as shock, dehydration, burns, diarrhea, vomiting, and excessive use of diuretics, or other causes of dehydration will thus affect ventricular filling and cardiac output. Long-term overstretching of the sarcomeres can also eventually affect the integrity of the contractile muscle and result in progressive heart failure. Stretching, especially in arterial tissue, can initiate cardiac arrhythmias.

The Force-Velocity Relationship

Laboratory experiments initially demonstrated that a change in the contractile state is related to a qualitative change in the force generated by the muscle sites themselves regardless of muscle length. As described in the Frank-Starling law, increased preload or muscle strength increases the force of the contraction, but the velocity or speed of the contraction is not necessarily changed. The **force-velocity relationship** refers to the phenomenon in cardiac muscle that the heavier the pressure load, the more slowly the muscle contracts or shortens. Therefore, increased physical tension on the cardiac muscle can slow the speed of muscle contraction. When norepinephrine is applied to the cardiac muscle, the muscle-shortening velocity is increased, greatly enhancing the contractility state, which increases the cardiac output. This sequence of events is the inotropic effect.

Other positive inotropic drugs that favorably affect the force-velocity relationship include other catecholamines such as epinephrine (Adrenalin), isoproterenol (Isuprel), and dopamine; digitalis; calcium; and thyroid hormone. Drugs having a negative inotropic effect include barbiturates, alcohol, quinidine, propranolol (Inderal), procainamide (Pronestyl), and possibly lidocaine to a small degree. Hypoxia and myocardial injury also have a negative inotropic effect.

THE PERIPHERAL VASCULAR SYSTEM

When combining basic knowledge concerning the anatomy of the heart, the determinants of heart rate, and the contraction force and velocity, it becomes apparent that there are many physiologic controls in each of these factors. These physiologic controls can be affected by pathologic conditions and they can be manipulated by drugs and other interventions. These manipulations or interventions should not be made unless the effect on the peripheral vascular system is taken into consideration.

The cardiovascular system is a closed system whose efficiency is dependent on the pressure, total surface area, and circulation velocity of all of its divisions. The highest pressure can be recorded in the left ventricle, and this pressure only gradually diminishes until circulation reaches the arterioles and capillaries. The aorta and large arteries have the highest vascular pressure and velocity and they have the lowest surface area. The aorta and large arteries are composed of three layers: (1) the intima, a smooth endothelial lining; (2) the media, a muscular layer; and (3) the adventitia, the outer covering. The middle layer, composed of smooth muscle and elastic fibers, enables these vessels to be extensible and elastic. These two properties allow the vessels to withstand the high pressure of the blood flow sent with each heartbeat and also enable them to serve as a reservoir.

The arterioles, due to their increased muscular layers, are capable of quick and continuous constriction or dilatation resulting in a continuous flow through the microcirculation (the capillaries). When tissues require less blood, the vasoconstrictor nerves become activated and arterial vasoconstriction occurs, shunting (or diverting) the circulation to areas of greater need. Conversely, when tissues require more blood flow, vasodilatation occurs through the control of the vasodilator nerves. Since arterioles are normally in a state of partial contraction, the vasoconstrictor nerves act continuously, contributing to the maintenance of blood pressure by providing an optimum peripheral resistance. Hormonal regulation and local tissue response also contribute to the triggering of vasoconstriction or dilatation. Arterial blood pressure is dependent not only on the degree of peripheral resistance, but also on cardiac output and the elasticity of the arteries. More specific information about blood pressure is given later in this chapter.

When blood leaves the arterioles and passes into the capillaries, flow is regulated by arteriolar pressure, viscosity of the blood, and precapillary sphincter control. The precapillary sphincter (a smooth muscle fiber encircling the capillary) controls the blood entering the capillaries or diverts blood through the thoroughfare channels to the venules.

The filtration of blood from the capillaries to the surrounding tissue results from differences between capillary pressure and tissue pressure. Osmotic or colloidal pressure created by the nondiffusible protein in the blood creates a counterforce, which opposes the hydrostatic pressure of the circulating blood. As blood enters the capillaries the hydrostatic pressure is approximately 30 mm Hg but the opposing osmotic pressure is 25 mm Hg, resulting in an outflow force of 5 mm Hg into the tissues. Tissue hydrostatic pressure is 10 mm Hg and osmotic pressure is 15 mm Hg, resulting in a 5 mm Hg force to pull in capillary fluid, resulting in a 10 mm Hg pressure flow into the tissues [1, 2]. Hydrostatic pressure diminishes at the venule end of the capillary whereas the osmotic pressure remains the same. These pressure differences favor inward filtration from the tissues, accounting for uptake of tissue waste products.

Although large molecules such as protein can filter into the tissues to a certain degree, there must be a system to deliver the tissue proteins and other macromolecules back into the circulation; inward filtration pressure is not capable of this transfer. The lymphatic system carries out this function and transports tissue protein, iron, lipoproteins, and antibodies. Like the venous system, the lymphatic system has valves and depends on the muscular pumping action for movement of lymph against gravity.

The peripheral lymphatics join with larger lymphatics and filter lymph through regional lymph nodes before passing it into the circulation. Lymph is emptied into the blood mainly where the thoracic duct opens into the venous system, near the left subclavian-jugular junction. Lymph is also emptied into the blood in other regions of the venous system.

The venous system collects the deoxygenated circulating blood with tissue waste products from the microcirculation. Veins are relatively thin walled and have a progressively lower pressure as they approach the right atrium. Valves in the larger veins prevent even a temporary backflow of blood toward the capillary circulation. Backflow could result in a resistance to capillary outflow, causing tissue edema. Valves are particularly numerous in the lower extremities, where blood flows against gravity. Adequate valvular functioning as well as compression of the veins during skeletal muscle contraction provides for return of the blood to the right atrium.

Resistance to blood flow is negligible in the larger veins, but there is greater resistance through the postcapillary venules. Venous constriction can elevate capillary pressure by increasing outward filtration into the tissues while venous dilatation, accompanied by precapillary constriction, can increase reabsorption from the tissues.

Assessment of the Cardiovascular System

The assessment of the cardiovascular system requires a thorough history, physical examination, and analysis of pertinent diagnostic data. The physical assessment should include inspection, palpation, auscultation, and also percussion when indicated. An initial accurate assessment is essential both in planning care and in providing a baseline for evaluating the progress of the patient. The nurse must communicate assessment data accurately to all members of the patient's health team to assure continuity of care.

THE HISTORY

It should be remembered that in spite of the increased sophistication and number of diagnostic tools being developed, the patient's history is still the single most important tool in the assessment of cardiovascular disease. How the information is obtained will vary according to the nurse's individual style and the tools used for data collection (handwritten or computerized forms) in a given care setting. The information should be communicated in written form so that others who are caring for the patient need not repeat the same questions.

During the history-taking procedure, the nurse should be cognizant that many patients with cardiovascular problems are in an older age group and require sufficient time to think about questions before answering. The nurse also should be aware of the presence of anxiety or discomfort and should adapt the history procedure accordingly.

The initial cardiac screening history should record the known cardiac condition as described in the patient's own terms. Listening to the patient describe his condition may give clues to the patient's level of understanding of his condition as well as information about previous cardiac problems. It should be recognized that the patient with cardiovascular disease may be hypoxic.

The presence of anorexia, fatigue, dizziness, and fainting spells should be determined also. An evaluation of the patient's intellectual functioning can be made while the patient proceeds with his history. The patient's behavior and his attention span are noted; cerebral hypoxia, for example, may be reflected in lethargy, mental confusion, and apathy. Anxiety may also interfere with concentration, so a thorough assessment should be made before assumptions about the presence of hypoxia are made. If the presence of a heart condition has been established, the patient should provide information about the medications he is receiving. Again, the way he describes this information will give clues to his level of understanding of his medications and to his ability to manage the regimen. Medications being taken for noncardiac conditions also should be listed. The female patient with a potential cardiac problem, for example, should be asked about the use of oral contraceptives (oral contraceptives are associated with thromboembolic phenomena and hypertension). A history of cardiac problems in other members of the family (parents and siblings) also should be explored.

If the patient has experienced chest pain, he should describe the pain in terms of location, radiation, type and intensity, precipitating factors, and measures taken for relief of pain. Abdominal pain should be investigated in relation to location, duration, and food intake. (On occasion, epigastric distress has been erroneously attributed to indigestion when anginal pain was actually the cause).

The nurse should determine whether the patient is aware of any palpitations. Although palpitations are painless, they may be a troublesome source of concern for the patient who is anxious about any potential cardiac problem. The relation of palpitations to the excessive use of tobacco, coffee, or stimulating drugs should be determined. Some patients suffer from "cardiac neurosis," which is an overwhelming fear of heart disease even in the absence of any ECG abnormality. The patient's perceptions of his symptoms and his emotional state during the history-taking procedure should be noted.

Besides observing the patient's rate and depth of respiration, the nurse should ask the patient if he has experienced any shortness of breath or dyspnea, either related to exercise or occurring at rest. If the patient acknowledges the presence of dyspnea, the nurse should inquire about the number of pillows used for sleeping, when the dyspnea tends to occur, and how the dyspnea is relieved. The presence of cough or excessive sputum (as well as characteristics of the sputum) should be noted.

In addition to these observations and questions, the nurse should note the patient's posture and his breathing to detect any signs of anxiety, discomfort, or difficulty in breathing.

The patient should be asked about the incidence of **edema** (swelling), in addition to later being examined for the presence of swelling. The nurse should ask the patient specifically about the occurrence of any swelling in his ankles or feet, especially after standing for any period of time. The presence of swelling in relation to the menstrual cycle is a normal finding in the female patient.

The presence of other circulatory symptoms should be ascertained by asking the patient about exercise tolerance, the presence of varicosities, cold extremities, numbness, or pain in the legs after walking.

Information on the patient's normal weight (and comparison to current weight); social habits regarding smoking, tobacco, alcohol, or drug use; dietary patterns; and exercise patterns (as well as type of occupation) should be obtained. This information is important as a baseline for planning a teaching program for the patient if cardiovascular disease is confirmed.

If the patient has a history of cardiovascular disease, it is important to obtain the chief complaint in his own words, as well as a chronologic history of the symptoms of cardiovascular disease. Medical treatment sought, as well as response to treatment, should be briefly described. Precipitating events and other significant data should be included in this chronicle, which should end with the description of the patient's current illness.

CARDIAC ASSESSMENT

Inspection

An evaluation of the general appearance of the patient can provide a wealth of information concerning the cardiovascular system. The nurse should consider the following points during the general inspection of the patient. Is the patient comfortable or is he experiencing pain, dyspnea, or any other sign of inadequate cardiac output? Is there any evidence of edema; clubbing of the fingers; cyanosis of mucous membranes, nail beds, hands, feet, tip of the nose, ear lobes, or lips? Observation of poor tolerance to exercise may also give clues to a cardiovascular problem.

The general appearance of the patient is noted by observing the skin color and evaluating it for the presence of pallor, flushing, cyanosis, petechiae, or jaundice. Evaluation of pallor or cyanosis in dark-skinned patients may be difficult. Inspection of the mucous membranes of the mouth, under the tongue, the lobes of the ear, and the fingernail beds may be necessary to accurately detect the presence of cyanosis. The nurse should note also the temperature of the skin, observing for coolness and clamminess, which reflect either poor circulation or the effects of anxiety.

The neck veins should be examined closely for engorgement of the external jugular veins. Engorgement of neck veins while the patient is raised in a 45° position is an important sign of congestive heart failure. The extremities should be examined for any sign of inadequate circulation or ulcerations.

These same questions and observations should also be used by the nurse in the daily assessment of the cardiac patient. After accurate baseline data are obtained, the patient can be evaluated for changes that reflect either an increase in symptoms with diminished cardiac function and poor response to therapy or a decrease in symptoms that reflects a positive response to therapy.

The quality, rate, and rhythm of the pulse are determined and the blood pressure is taken with the patient in the sitting and, if feasible, the standing position. Assessment of the pulse should include apical auscultation and radial artery palpation. The quality of the peripheral pulses (femoral, popliteal, and dorsalis pedis) also should be determined. The pulse may be described as strong, full, bounding, weak and thready, absent, or not palpable.

Some of the abnormal types of rhythm that may be noted by apical and radial pulse assessment include the paradoxical pulse (also called pulsus paradoxicus) and bigeminal rhythm. The **paradoxical pulse** is characterized by a rebound of the pulse during expiration resulting in a pulse that is weaker during inspiration. **Bigeminal rhythm** is described as a coupling rhythm that reflects a normal beat quickly followed by a premature ventricular contraction.

The presence of a pulse deficit may be determined by comparing the apical rate and the radial rate. The apical rate is more rapid than the radial rate, and the pulse deficit is recorded as the difference between the two. A pulse deficit is detected when bigeminal rhythm occurs, as well as when atrial fibrillation is present. In atrial fibrillation, inadequate ventricular filling causes an absence of some radial beats and may also result in pulsus alternans, a variation in the force of ventricular systole. The pulse in pulsus alternans alternates between weak and strong beats.

Auscultation

If one follows a regular routine, listens to one thing at a time, and knows what to listen to, auscultation of the cardiovascular system can elicit valuable information about each event in the cardiac cycle. A stethoscope with a bell and diaphragm is necessary to appreciate the variety of sounds of the system. The bell detects low-pitched sounds while high-pitched sounds are heard best with the diaphragm.

The stethoscope is used to detect abnormalities of heart sounds and lung sounds, and vascular abnormalities such as bruits. An explanation of the purpose of auscultation and what is involved is warranted because one cannot assume that all patients understand or have had experience with this procedure. The explanation often relieves anxiety and promotes relaxation during the examination.

Although it is customary to describe heart sounds as "lub-dub," one must become accustomed to listening to a vast variety of heart sounds in order to analyze and recognize their character, quality, and pitch. A great deal of time and experience are required to achieve skill in accurate auscultation. (Students and beginning practitioners should not be misled to think that auscultation techniques can be readily learned in a simulated laboratory setting with minimal practice sessions.) It is also important to stress the value of a quiet environment before beginning auscultation. Heart sounds normally heard in auscultation and the more frequent abnormalities will be discussed. Although specific pathologic conditions are alluded to, they will be defined and discussed in subsequent sections of this chapter.

The first heart sound (S_1), heard best at the apex, results from the closure of the mitral and tricuspid valves as well as tensing of the myocardium and AV valve-supporting structures, and changes in blood velocity. It lasts about 0.8 second and is relatively low pitched. It may have two recognizable component sounds if there is asynchronous closure of the two valves, which is termed **splitting**. S_1 splitting usually has no clinical significance. Accentuation of S_1 is pathological and may be indicative of mitral stenosis, while dulling can be related to myocardial infarction or myocarditis.

The second heart sound (S_2) is due to the closure of the semilunar valves of the pulmonary arteries and the aorta. At the base of the heart (the aortic or pulmonic area) S_2 is usually louder than S_1. Physiologic splitting of S_2 into the louder aortic component and the softer pulmonic component can usually be accomplished during prolonged inspiration by causing a delay in pulmonary valve closure. Splitting may be abnormal when it is fixed or has a paradoxical pattern.

The term **paradoxical split** refers to splitting during expiration and is associated with any condition that delays left ventricular emptying, such as left ventricular hypertrophy, hypertensive heart disease, and left bundle branch block. These conditions will be described in more detail in subsequent sections of this chapter.

S_3 (ventricular gallop), an early diastolic extra sound, occurs during rapid ventricular filling and is often heard in mitral regurgitation, constrictive pericarditis, and ventricular failure. It is generally thought that the S_3 sound is caused by blood entering the left ventricle when it is already stretched and under tension. It is therefore associated with congestive heart failure. When the S_3 sound is heard, the examiner should always follow cardiac auscultation with chest auscultation for the detection of rales. (**Rales** are abnormal breath sounds produced when air flows through fluid.) Often difficult to detect due to its low pitch, the S_3 sound is best heard with light application of the bell of the stethoscope, while the patient lies in the left ducubitus position (lying on the left side).

S_4 (atrial gallop), a presystolic extra sound, is caused by vigorous atrial contraction in patients with any condition causing decreased left ventricular compliance, such as left ventricular hypertrophy or myocardial ischemia. It is a dull, low-pitched sound, increasing with inspiration and best heard with the bell over the apex with the patient rolled onto his left side.

Murmurs are subdued, continuing sounds resulting from abnormal turbulence of blood flow due to three major factors: (1) discrepancies between strength of the flow and the cross-section size of the passageway; (2) reversal of blood flow; or (3) abnormalities of intravascular structure (e.g., atherosclerotic plaques). Murmurs are described in terms of timing (diastolic or systolic), location, quality (blowing, rough, musical, rumbling, coarse), intensity, pitch, location, radiation (transmission), and change with position.

The intensity of a murmur may be graded as follows:

Grade 1	Very faint
Grade 2	Quiet but easily heard
Grade 3	Moderately loud; no thrill
Grade 4	Loud; thrill may be detected
Grade 5	Very loud; thrill present, heard with stethoscope partially off chest
Grade 6	Heard with stethoscope off chest

To auscultate the heart thoroughly, a systematic pattern of assessment is followed. Initially the heart rate and rhythm are determined. The examiner determines the sequence of any rhythm irregularities as well as whether the irregularity is related to respiratory movements. Then the examiner listens in the aortic area and pulmonic area (the base), Erb's point (the third left interspace close to the sternum), the tricuspid area, and the mitral area (the apex). Figure 4-5 identifies the reference points for localizing heart sounds. In each area it is essential to systematically listen to the first heart sound for intensity and splitting; then the second heart sound for similar characteristics. Finally, the examiner listens for extra heart sounds in systole and in diastole, noting timing, intensity, and pitch. Auscultation for systolic, then diastolic, murmurs follows.

The examiner also listens for friction rubs over the precordium that are synchronous with diastole and systole. These rubs may be described as soft and scratchy, loud and leathery, or low and grating sounds. Friction rubs are associated with pericarditis.

Readers are advised to utilize other resources, including audiotapes, for additional specific information about abnormal heart sounds and their significance.

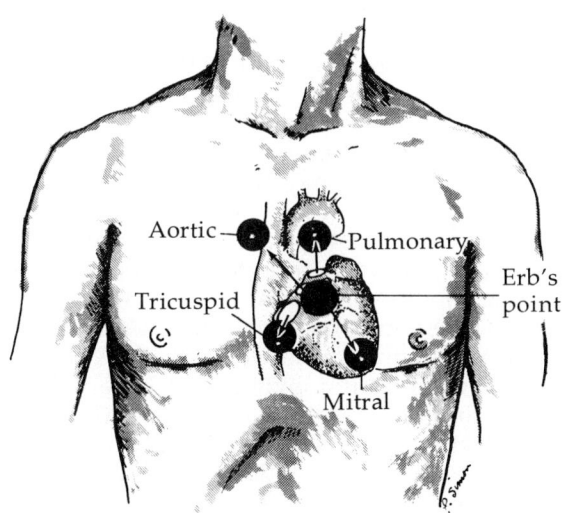

Figure 4-5
Reference points for localizing heard sounds. Diagram demonstrates actual valve locations and the points to which their sounds are usually referred. [Adapted from R. D. Judge and G. D. Zuidema (eds.), *Methods of Clinical Examination: A Physiologic Approach* (3rd ed.). Boston: Little, Brown and Company, 1974. Reproduced by permission.]

Palpation
The heart is palpable at the point of maximum impulse at the apex or mitral area. If this point is rotated laterally, hypertrophy of the heart is suspected. Intense palpitation, often of enough force to lift the hand off the chest, is also indicative of hypertension.

Percussion is seldom used in cardiac assessment. The technique, however, may be used to determine the size of the heart by comparing the dull sound obtained over the heart to the higher-pitched sounds heard in lung percussion. Normally the heart size is determined by locating the apex, as noted previously, by chest x-ray, and ECG tracing.

Diagnostic Tests
There are a variety of tests used in evaluating the status of cardiac function. Some tests are noninvasive, others require blood analysis, and still others require complicated invasive surgical techniques. Selection of specific tests depends on the presenting signs and symptoms.

Erythrocyte count and hemoglobin concentration These tests are done to evaluate the oxygen-carrying capacity of the blood. Severe anemia, for example, can result in dyspnea, especially on exertion. The hematocrit and hemoglobin values along with the electrolyte values are necessary in the interpretation of fluid and electrolyte status. (Normal red blood cell counts are 4.8 to 5.4 million per cubic millimeter for men and 4.5 to 5 million for women. The normal hemoglobin is between 14 and 18 gm per 100 ml of blood for men and between 12 and 16 gm per 100 ml for women.)

Leukocyte count The leukocyte count will indicate whether an inflammatory process is present. After a myocardial infarction, for example, there may be a rise in the leukocyte count in response to the inflammatory process. Leukocytosis also occurs in rheumatic fever and bacterial endocarditis. (The white blood count normally ranges from 5,000 to 10,000 per cubic millimeter.)

Electrolyte levels Routine electrolyte levels (along with the hematocrit) are necessary to determine the fluid and electrolyte status of the patient. With cellular injury, potassium (K^+) is released into the serum, causing an initial elevation of K^+, which is eventually excreted by the kidneys. Decreased levels of intracellular K^+ occur after myocardial infarction, often requiring supplements of the electrolyte to prevent hypokalemia and associated arrhythmias. This is especially important if the patient is receiving digitalis, since low K^+ levels precipitate digitalis toxicity, resulting in serious cardiac arrythmias. The effects of hypokalemia and hyperkalemia on muscles are discussed more fully in Chapter 2. Sodium retention is associated with congestive heart failure resulting in elevated serum levels of sodium. Sodium chloride levels or potassium levels or both may be dangerously decreased in persons who have been receiving excessive dosages of diuretics and restricted sodium diets for treatment of edema and congestive heart failure.

Erythrocyte sedimentation rate A sedimentation rate is done to determine the rate at which erythrocytes settle in a column of blood. An increased rate is associated with an inflammatory process such as rheumatic fever, or with postmyocardial infarction, as well as many other non-cardiac conditions.

Serum lipids and plasma lipoprotein patterns A total blood cholesterol (one of the components of the lipoprotein molecule) of more than 250 mg per 100 ml suggests the presence of atherosclerosis. Phospholipids and triglycerides are also lipid fractions that are evaluated. Lipoprotein patterns are determined to classify types of hyperlipoproteinemia. The significance of these tests and the dietary control methods used to correct different types of hyperlipoproteinemia are discussed in a subsequent section on coronary artery disease and atherosclerosis.

Enzyme studies A sample of venous blood is drawn to determine the serum levels of three major enzymes when cardiac damage is suspected. These enzymes, which are present in large amounts in cardiac cells, are (1) lactic dehydrogenase (LDH), which catalyzes the conversion of lactic acid to pyruvic acid; (2) serum glutamic oxaloacetic transaminase (SGOT), which is important in carbohydrate and protein metabolism because of its catalytic action in the synthesis of oxaloacetic acid; and (3) creatinine phosphokinase (CPK), which acts as a catalyst in providing energy for cardiac contraction. A fourth enzyme, serum alpha hydroxybutyrate dehydrogenase (HBD), is also evaluated in some institutional protocols. (Several laboratory methods are available with widely varied values for specific enzymes. It is important for the nurse to be knowledgeable of the values used in the specific institutional setting.)

These enzymes are released into the blood when there is cellular damage. After a myocardial infarction for example, serum levels of these enzymes are commonly elevated. Interpretation of these enzyme levels should be made cautiously since these enzymes are also located in other tissues of the body (skeletal muscle, brain, liver, skin, kidney, and red blood cells). The CPK level is considered a more specific indication of myocardial damage than are the LDH and SGOT levels, because it is found only in cardiac muscle, skeletal muscle, and brain tissue [3]. However, the CPK level may increase after frequent intramuscular injections and thus cause false results; therefore the use of intramuscular injections is avoided during this diagnostic period, if possible.

Electrophoresis has made possible the identification of five different components (isoenzymes) of lactic dehydrogenase. Various tissues have different compositions of these isoenzymes, so that specific isoenzyme levels and ratios are even more significant than total LDH levels. For example, the isomer LDH_5 is the major component of cardiac muscle; elevation of LDH_5 is therefore highly suggestive of cardiac damage and is considered a very significant diagnostic tool in myocardial infarction [3]. Isoenzymes of the CPK enzyme may also be measured.

Elevation of each enzyme occurs at a different time after injury, and repeated enzyme tests are necessary to determine patterns of changes. Other coexisting conditions that could cause enzyme elevations should be recognized. In myocardial damage, the CPK and SGOT are the first enzymes to become elevated and fall rapidly to normal within 2 to 7 days, whereas the LDH may take several days before an elevation is detected and may not return to normal for several weeks. Figure 4-6 illustrates a characteristic pattern of the rise and fall of enzyme levels after myocardial infarction.

Blood urea nitrogen A decreased blood supply to the kidneys related to inadequate cardiac function may result in elevations of blood urea nitrogen.

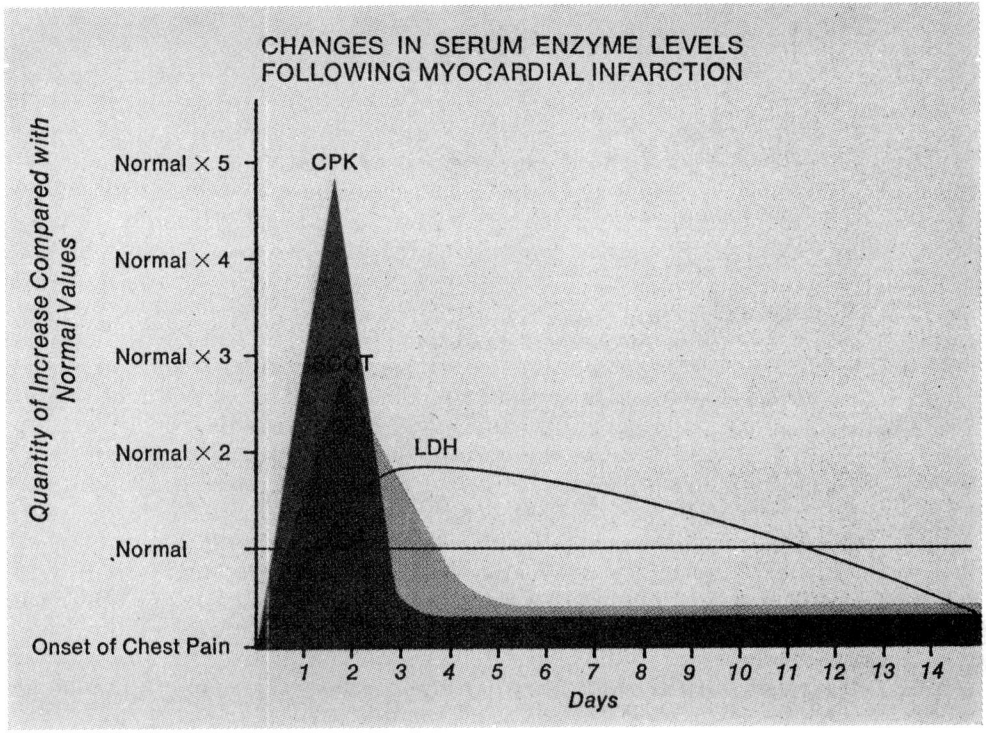

Figure 4-6
Characteristic pattern of serum enzyme levels after myocardial infarction. (Copyright © February 1973, The American Journal of Nursing Company. Reprinted from the *American Journal of Nursing* 73(2): 277, 1973, with permission.)

Blood glucose There is a higher incidence of coronary heart disease with diabetes and elevated blood glucose levels than with normal glucose levels. Often, glucose metabolic disorders are found when the patient is undergoing diagnosis for suspected cardiac disease.

Prothrombin time and clotting time When cardiovascular disorders are diagnosed, anticoagulant therapy may become necessary in thrombotic or embolic complications. Individual baseline data for normal clotting mechanisms are necessary. Patients admitted with a definitive cardiovascular diagnosis may already be on anticoagulants.

Blood culture A blood culture to detect the presence of bacteria in circulating blood is indicated when bacterial endocarditis is suspected.

Antistreptolysin O titer This test measures the presence and amount of antibodies against the streptococcal enzyme, streptolysin O, which destroys erythrocytes. It is done to determine whether a patient with possible rheumatic heart disease has had a recent infection.

Arterial blood gases Arterial blood is drawn to analyze oxygen, carbon dioxide, and pH levels. This is especially important when pulmonary edema, decreased cardiac output, or shock is a complication of the underlying cardiac disease. The significance of arterial blood gases is discussed in Chapter 3.

Urinalysis In addition to analysis of blood, urinalysis is indicated when cardiac disease is suspected. Abnormal amounts of albumin in the urine, for example, may be present in congestive heart failure.

Chest x-ray A **standard posteroranterior (PA) chest x-ray** and a lateral film are routinely done on patients suspected of having cardiac disease. Such films demonstrate the size of the heart, and examination of the lung fields gives valuable information about the status of the vascular bed. Cardiac views via fluoroscope are obtained when cardiac abnormality is suspected. In some settings, cardiac fluoroscopy is ordered routinely prior to cardiac catheterizations.

Noninvasive diagnostic procedures Noninvasive diagnostic procedures in cardiac assessment include the ECG, vectorcardiography, echocardiography, phonocardiography, ballistocardiography, and exercise testing.

The ECG is an essential tool in the evaluation of cardiac status. It can give information about arrhythmias and cardiac tissue ischemia, injury, and infarction. Drugs such as digitalis and quinidine influence interpretation. A requisition for an ECG should always include information about any drugs affecting cardiac rhythm that the patient is receiving. The ECG does not give hemodynamic information related to cardiac output.

The ECG is a comparatively simple device that requires the placement of electrodes on the body to pick up electrical current through the heart. The ECG transforms the electrical events of the cardiac cycle into visible form on a printout or on an oscilloscope. Voltage variations are caused by depolarization and repolarization of individual muscle cells. It is used so frequently in medicine that nurses and other personnel tend to assume that all people are familiar with the ECG and they tend to forget to prepare the patient. Although the ECG does not cause discomfort, some patients, having the test for the first time, are extremely fearful of electrical shock or of pain during the procedure.

As explained previously, the normal electrical flow moves downward toward the left. If electrodes are placed on various locations of the body, a recording can be made to detect disturbances of the normal conduction from the heart to that point. The electrodes placed on the limbs and chest create a specific plane and are described as "leads." A standard ECG is a 12-lead recording. This standard recording provides a comprehensive view of the electrical activity of the heart, as each lead allows the heart to be viewed from a different direction. The leads are of three types: bipolar limb leads, unipolar limb leads, and chest, or V, leads. The three bipolar limb leads (leads I, II, and III) record the electrical potential on an imaginary axis between two points on the frontal plane of the body. This axis of the bipolar limb leads forms a triangle with its tip at the lower part of the body and its center at the heart.

Nine body sites (plus a tenth site, the right leg, which is used for grounding purposes only) are used in the standard 12-lead recording. These sites include the right arm, the left arm, the left leg, and six different sites on the chest and are paired in 12 different ways. A switching network in the ECG machine is used rather than shifting lead wires and electrodes to record each successive lead. Lead I is conventionally recorded from the right arm to the left arm, with the left arm electrode being called positive. Lead II records from the right arm and the left leg, with the left leg electrode being positive. In monitoring patients in intensive care, a variety of lead placements are used, but the most common are leads II and MCL1 (a modified V1 lead or modified chest lead). However, lead placements will vary, depending on the specific determination of the physician or the protocol of the given unit. The reader is referred to the bibliography for more information about the details of ECG tracings.

The ECG can also detect disturbances in rate and rhythm. The normal ECG (Fig. 4-7) shows a series of P, Q, R, S, and T complexes, each regularly spaced from the other, indicating that the ECG tracing is a normal sinus rhythm (originating at the SA node). Irregular rhythms occur mainly from a disturbance in the SA node, a heart block with irregular conduction and competitive pacemakers, especially premature beats from any source. Ectopic beats are those caused by a pacemaker other than the SA node. The common arrhythmias are discussed later in this chapter.

To supplement the information obtained from the ECG, the **vectorcardiogram** has proved useful in the diagnosis of electrophysiologic abnormalities. The procedure is similar to that of a conventional ECG and takes approximately 15 minutes to complete. Six electrodes are used, and a simultaneous recording of the three standard limb leads is taken. The vectorcardiogram is a spatial recording of the electromotive field forces generated during cardiac activity. A graphic plot of the pathway of instantaneous vectors is made, using one cardiac cycle. The graphic plot utilizes a loop concept to visualize cardiac conduction. Three planes (frontal, sagittal, and horizontal) are used to create a three-dimensional picture of the conduction

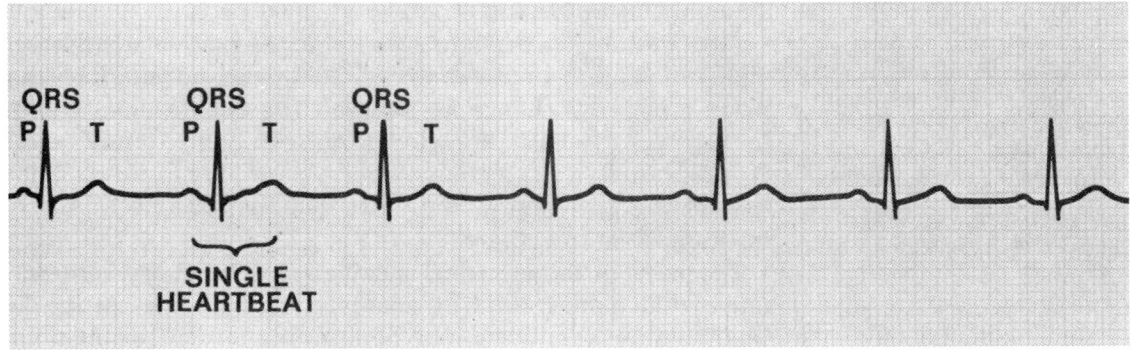

Figure 4-7
A tracing of a normal electrocardiogram. (From "How to read an ECG: Basic interpretations for nurses and other health workers." Reprinted from *RN* January 1973, p. 35, with permission.)

of the heart. Distorted loops with irregular shapes and abnormal sizes indicate pathologic changes. The vectorcardiogram allows a more detailed look at the QRS component, but it does not permit an appreciation of the time factor since it is a tracing of one cycle. The vectorcardiogram, therefore, cannot be used to determine cardiac rhythm.

Echocardiography is a recording of sound waves that reflect from interfaces between the heart wall and surrounding tissue or cardiac valves and blood. A transducer is placed against the patient's chest, through which pulsing, high-frequency sound waves are discharged as they are reflected off target cardiac structures. Movements and dimensions of structures such as valve leaflets and the chamber walls are reflected via the returning echo in terms of time and intensity on an oscilloscope or permanently on Polaroid pictures or stripchart recordings. Polaroid photography to record results and studies of correlation of graphs with hemodynamic data have enabled detection of latent or unsuspected cardiac dysfunction and evaluation of therapy. Echocardiography can be used to assess myocardial contractility, to calculate ventricular volumes, and to detect mitral or aortic stenosis and insufficiency. The patient, prior to the examination, should be advised that, although the test may take 30 to 60 minutes and may be tedious, it is a painless procedure.

Phonocardiography is the recording of audible vibrations from the heart and great vessels, allowing study of heart sounds in relation to murmurs, and is useful for documentation of physical findings. It can be considered an extension of cardiac auscultation. The phonocardiogram provides a permanent graphic record of the occurrence, timing, and duration of the sounds in the cardiac cycle. It cannot be considered a substitute for cardiac auscultation because the technique cannot assess subtle changes in the character, frequency, and quality of the heart sounds. However, the phonocardiogram is capable of recording low-frequency sounds (typical of murmurs and other significant sounds) that may not be audible via the stethoscope. It is useful in giving definitive information about the cardiac cycle and it is especially important when sounds on auscultation may be interpreted differently by different examiners.

The phonocardiogram requires no special preparation other than orienting the patient to the procedure and the purpose of the test. While the patient lies in a supine position, a transducer and microphone are applied to the apical region to obtain an apical impulse tracing that is recorded via a galvanometer. The transducer is then moved to the tricuspid, pulmonic, and aortic areas of the heart.

The **ballistocardiogram** is a graphic recording of the mechanical activity of the left ventricle. It reflects the recoil of the body following the ejection of blood into the aorta and provides information on the strength and coordination of the cardiac contraction.

Exercise testing is a valuable screening and evaluation tool. Exercise results in increased myocardial demands for oxygen. This fact is the basis for the screening and diagnostic procedure known as the stress test, exercise electrocardiography, or the treadmill test. Exercise testing evaluates physical performance capacity under a controlled setting via ECG monitoring *during* exercise. It is used to detect ECG abnormalities associated with myocardial ischemia. Studies have shown that exercise testing can reveal up to a 12 percent incidence of previously unrecognized coronary artery disease.

A motor-driven treadmill and an ergometer are methods used for exercise testing. In the treadmill test the speed and inclination are increased at regular intervals to produce a graded work load within predetermined protocols. The test is discontinued if any serious ECG changes, shortness of breath, or claudication occurs. In most settings, a consent form is required prior to the exercise testing procedure because risks are involved.

This type of graded exercise testing has generally replaced the Master's two-step test. The latter test consisted of taking a preselected number of trips up and down 9-inch steps within a prescribed time period, followed by an ECG reading to detect depression of the ST segment of the cycle, a sign of myocardial ischemia. The Master's test is not considered as accurate as the graded-exercise testing.

Arterial Blood Pressure Measurement

Blood pressure (B.P.) may be defined as the pressure exerted on the walls of the blood vessels. At any point in the vascular system, the blood pressure is dependent on ventricular contractility, cardiac output, elasticity of the arteries, and the peripheral resistance.

Blood pressure measurement at the brachial artery is the most frequent type of B.P. assessment that is done. It can be determined indirectly by auscultation via a stethoscope and a sphygmomanometer (of either the aneroid or mercury type). In critically ill patients, the arterial pressure may be measured directly with an intra-arterial catheter connected to an external manometer.

The procedure for taking a B.P. reading is one of the earliest procedures learned by nursing students. Many factors, however, affect the B.P. assessment, and certain precautions to assure accuracy warrant repeating. In addition, many lay persons are being taught to take their own pressures. The techniques used by the nursing staff should be explicit and accurate to serve as proper demonstrations.

A cuff of the proper size for the patient should be used. The inflatable bag within the cuff should be about 20 percent wider than the diameter of the extremity on which the B.P. is to be taken, and it should be long enough to encircle the limb. Wider cuffs should be used on persons with obese arms or if B.P.s are to be taken on the lower extremity. Using cuffs that are too narrow may result in false high readings. If the cuff is too large, false low readings may result [4]. The B.P. is usually taken in the arm unless arm injuries or other conditions mandate the need for lower-extremity readings.

The patient should be comfortable and in a stable position for at least 5 minutes prior to taking the B.P. The brachial artery should be approximately at heart level when it is used for B.P. assessment. The palpation technique is generally recommended as an initial step in order to avoid being misled by auscultatory gaps and to prevent excessive inflation of the B.P. cuff during auscultation. In the palpating technique, the cuff is inflated only until a palpable pulse at the brachial artery disappears. During auscultation the stethescope should be placed firmly, without excessive pressure, over the brachial artery. The cuff should be inflated only 20 to 30 mm Hg above the palpated systolic pressure. The cuff should be released slowly at a rate of approximately 2 to 3 mm Hg at a time to assure detection of changes. The eye of the observer should be at the level of the meniscus when a mercury sphygmomanometer is used. The level at which the first sounds (Korotkoff sounds) are heard is recorded as the systolic pressure (the pressure produced by ventricular systole). The diastolic pressure is usually considered the level at which the sounds become suddenly muffled. There has been controversy about the use of the muffling sound or the disappearance of sound as indications of the diastolic pressure. The latest American Heart Association recommendation for screening is to use the last sound heard as the diastolic reading. Some cardiologists advise that the level of the muffled sound should be recorded as the diastolic pressure. The nurse should record the diastolic pressure according to the policy of the institution in which he or she practices, in order to assure consistency. Some authorities advise the recording of all three sounds (the first sound, muffled sound, and disappearance of sound) to assure accuracy and consistency in interpretation

[4]. If the Korotkoff sounds are too feeble and difficult to hear, elevation of the arm before inflation, and inflation of the cuff during elevation, may reduce venous pressure. This technique may make the sounds louder, after the arm is returned to the horizontal position.

On initial assessment of a patient, the B.P. should be taken in both arms. A difference of from 5 to 10 mm Hg in pressures between the two arms is a usual finding. Comparisons between pressures in upper and lower extremities should demonstrate a significantly higher systolic pressure in the lower extremity. It is an important diagnostic sign (e.g., as found in coarctation of the aorta) to find lower systolic pressures in the legs. When assessment of the leg pressures is indicated, a wide cuff is applied to the lower third of the thigh. The popliteal artery is used for auscultation, preferably with the patient lying in a prone position.

The actual reading obtained via the auscultatory method can be affected by a great many factors (particularly by the technique used and variance in the hearing acuity of the person taking the B.P). In certain situations, therefore, as when a patient is receiving vasopressor drugs and accurate assessment of the B.P. is essential to safe therapy, a more objective means of assessment is required. Critically ill patients, such as the patient in shock with weak and thready pulses that produce poor Korotkoff sounds, also require an alternative means for blood pressure assessment.

The intra-arterial technique of B.P. measurement provides an accurate, objective, and continuous recording of arterial pressure and is therefore used in the care and monitoring of the seriously ill patient. A catheter is placed in an artery (usually the radial or brachial) and is connected to a transducer, which converts the pressure into an electrical signal that can be viewed on an oscilloscope. A fluid source for flushing the catheter is another essential component of the system. Special care must be taken to assure that the equipment is functioning appropriately. The transducer, for example, must be balanced to assure accurate readings. The puncture site must be observed for bleeding and for potential thrombosis of the artery. Monitoring of the pulses of the involved extremity is imperative. Intra-arterial readings are found to be higher than those obtained by the auscultatory method for patients in shock, with arteriolar vasoconstriction or vasodilatation, or in persons with peripheral artery obstruction.

Venous Pressure Measurements

Venous pressure assessment measures the amount of pressure exerted against the venous walls. Central venous pressure (CVP) reflects the competence of the right heart and is used primarily as a means for early recognition of congestive heart failure and shock.

Venous pressure may be measured by examination of the neck or cervical veins, by examination of the veins on the dorsum of the hand for assessment of filling and distention, by means of a manometer connected to a needle inserted directly into a vein for a single reading, or by a CVP technique for continuous monitoring.

Observation of the jugular veins provides a method for estimating CVP. The patient is positioned with his or her head slightly elevated on a pillow (usually about 30°) and should be relaxed and comfortable, with no constricting clothing about the neck. Tangential (oblique) lighting is used to examine both sides of the neck. The external jugular vein on each side is identified, and the pulsations of the internal jugular vein are then determined. Areas for location of the internal jugular vein pulsations are the suprasternal notch, between the attachments of the sternomastoid on the sternum and clavicle, or just posterior to the sternomastoid. The distance between the highest point at which pulsations of the internal jugular vein can be seen and the sternal angle is measured in centimeters. This distance is recorded, noting the position of the patient at the time of examination. Venous pressure greater than 3 cm above the sternal angle is considered abnormal and may be indicative of congestive heart failure, constrictive pericarditis, or superior vena cava obstruction [4].

A gross assessment of increased venous pressure can be made by noting that the neck veins remain distended when the head of the patient is elevated at 45°. It is also possible to make a rough estimate of the venous pressure by examining the veins of the dorsum of the hand. When the hand is elevated above the level of the heart, the venous pressure is reduced and the veins on the dorsum of the hand collapse. If the venous pressure is elevated, the veins remain distended for a prolonged period, even when the hand is raised.

Checking for a hepatojugular reflux may also be done to assess jugular venous pressure. Firm and sustained pressure of the examiner's hand over the patient's right upper quadrant for 30 to 60 seconds will cause a rise in the jugular venous pressure. A rise over 1 cm is considered abnormal [4].

A single measurement of venous pressure may be taken by inserting a needle into a vein and connecting it to a manometer via a syringe of normal saline and a three-way stopcock. The pressure is recorded when the level of fluid stabilizes.

More commonly, a catheter is inserted through the subclavian vein or other vein (such as the basilar, brachial, or cephalic) and threaded into the superior or inferior vena cava or right atrium. It is connected to a manometer and three-way stopcock and an intravenous infusion and the CVP is monitored at hourly (or more frequent) intervals. Normally, the CVP range is from 5 to 11 cm of water [10].

An original reference point for measuring the CVP should be established. It is generally advised to have the patient lying flat so that the zero mark on the manometer scale is level with the right atrium (the midaxillary line) (Fig. 4-8). Occasionally, the patient's condition may require that the head of the bed be elevated continuously. The measurement technique may be adjusted to this requirement, but the reference point and position for measurement should be clearly indicated so that all succeeding measurements are taken in the same manner.

The patient should be instructed not to hold his breath, cough, or strain during the reading. This precaution is necessary because voluntary muscle movement influences the reading, and increased intrathoracic pressure during these actions can give a false high reading. Mechanical respirators also must be discontinued while these measurements are being made, if not contraindicated.

Venous pressure in excess of normal may indicate cardiac insufficiency or an excess of intravascular volume associated with intra-

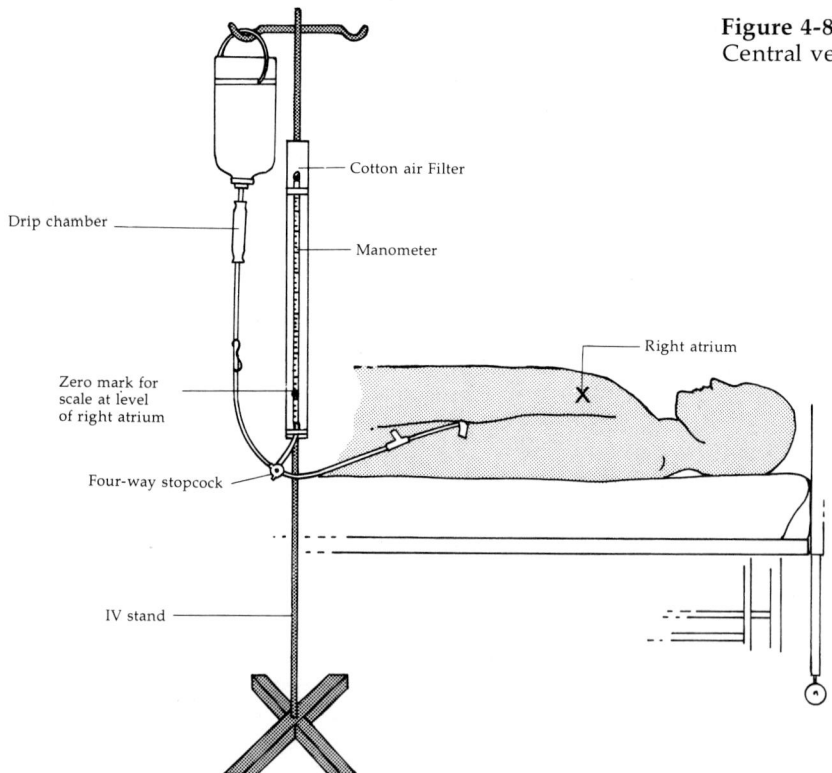

Figure 4-8
Central venous pressure monitoring.

venous fluid administration. A venous pressure below the normal range reflects hypovolemia and shock.

The patient who is to have a CVP catheter inserted must be carefully instructed both as to its purpose and the technique. After a surgical cleaning to prepare the site and the instillation of a local anesthetic, a needle (through which the catheter is threaded) is inserted into the selected vein. The patient should be in a supine position with the head lowered when either the jugular or subclavian veins are used for entry. The Trendelenburg position promotes distention of the vein, which facilitates insertion. The patient is asked to perform the Valsalva maneuver (to expire against a closed glottis) during insertion of the catheter, to prevent air emoblism. The catheter is then connected to an intravenous fluid administration set with a three-way stopcock and a manometer vertically attached to an intravenous pole. A chest x-ray may be taken with a portable unit to verify the position of the catheter in the vena cava. To obtain a CVP reading, the stopcock is turned to allow the fluid to flow up the manometer, and the reading is taken when the fluid remains at a relatively stationary level. Following the recording, the stopcock is readjusted to allow the intravenous solution to flow into the patient.

Attention to asepsis is essential in the care of the injection site. Antibiotic ointment usually is applied over the site and the site is covered securely with a gauze dressing. Dressing care is given the wound site on a regular basis (daily or every third day, depending on institutional protocol). Care must be taken to prevent traction on the catheter. The intravenous tubing is changed at least daily as a further preventive measure against infections. Infection of the wound site can lead to septicemia or bacterial endocarditis.

The CVP reading does not reflect left-sided pressure, except indirectly. A special balloon-tipped catheter (Swan-Ganz) can be inserted in the right heart (via an antecubital vein) and floated into the pulmonary artery to obtain pulmonary artery pressure and the wedge pressure of the pulmonary capillaries. The pulmonary wedge pressure reflects the left heart pressure. Once the catheter tip is in the pulmonary artery, the balloon is inflated and the wedge pressure is recorded. The catheter is advanced so that the tip is wedged in a branch of the pulmonary artery. The patient is connected to an ECG monitor prior to catheter insertion because of the potential complication of cardiac arrhythmia during insertion and manipulation of the catheter.

The catheter is attached to an intravenous fluid and manometer setup similar to the equipment used for a CVP line. The pulmonary artery pressure may also be measured by a transducer–oscilloscope method that permits continuous visualization of the pressure. With the latter method, heparinized saline is used periodically as a flushing mechanism to maintain the patency of the line.

The potential dangers associated with measurement of the pulmonary artery pressure are those related to the measurement of central venous pressure such as microemboli and air emboli, as well as infections at the insertion site. In addition, air emboli may occur if the balloon should rupture during inflation. The balloon is therefore not inflated with more than a standard amount (0.8 ml) of air after checking for any residual air, and it must be deflated immediately after the pressure reading is taken. Prolonged inflation of the balloon may cause ischemic damage to the lung. The deflated catheter is left in place for subsequent measurements.

Cardiac Catheterization

Cardiac catheterization is done to obtain multiple pressure measurements in the four chambers of the heart, to obtain samples of blood from the various chambers for analysis of oxygen content, and to inject contrast material for selective angiocardiography to determine the presence and location of obstructive vascular lesions (e.g., coronary artery disease). In the last procedure, usually an organic iodine medium such as diatrizoate sodium (Hypaque) or diatrizoate methylglucamine (Cardiografin) is used. Cardiac catheterization is usually done prior to open heart surgery and is used postoperatively to evaluate the effects of the surgical procedure.

The procedure is carried out in a cardiac catheterization laboratory and generally requires 1 to 3 hours. The patient is forewarned of the unique setting with its complicated equipment (x-ray table, fluoroscope, monitors, and resuscitation equipment). Baseline values for the patient's vital signs are obtained. A history of any allergies should be noted and a skin test with an iodine-containing solution is often done to detect potential reactions to the contrast medium. A consent form for the procedure, signed by the patient after he is advised of potential risks, is required.

The patient is told that a catheter will be inserted into a vessel and that a contrast dye will be instilled and that a hot flushed feeling is experienced as the dye is injected. The patient's cooperation is required during this rather tedious examination, especially because he will have to lie still on an x-ray table for a prolonged period. The patient is strapped to the table for security during the changes in position required during the examination and is advised that a nose clip will be applied at certain times in order to obtain accurate oxygen consumption measurements.

Food and fluids (except for medications) are usually withheld from 6 to 8 hours prior to the test, to prevent vomiting and possible aspiration and to provide a basal metabolic rate during the procedure. General anesthesia is not required for the examination, although a sedative or a narcotic is usually given. Atropine or phenergan or both and sometimes an antibiotic may be prescribed prior to the procedure. The patient should urinate prior to being transported to the cardiac laboratory.

The patient is awake and conscious during the entire procedure and thus requires emotional support and frequent explanations as the examination progresses. Too often personnel in the cardiac laboratory become so involved in the technical aspects of the procedure that minimal time is provided for comforting and talking with the patient.

The site of entry of the catheter (via a cutdown or a percutaneous method) depends on whether right-heart or left-heart catheterization is to be done, on the area to be studied, and on the preference of the cardiologist. A surgical scrubbing and shaving of the site is done prior to anesthetizing the site of the incision or puncture.

Right-heart catheterization utilizes a venous approach, usually via the brachial vein or the femoral vein. The catheter is then advanced through the vena cava to the right atrium and into the right ventricle from where it can be manipulated into the pulmonary artery. Left-heart catheterization can be achieved by either a venous or an arterial approach. In the venous approach (transseptal), the femoral vein is used for entry. The catheter is advanced via the inferior vena cava to the right atrium and through the interatrial septum to the left atrium and the left ventricle. The arterial approach for left-heart catheterization utilizes the femoral or brachial artery for entry of the catheter, which is advanced to the aorta and the left ventricle in a retrograde manner.

In selected cases, cardiac catheterization is accomplished by entry directly into the left atrium via bronchoscopy or by needle puncture at the apex of the heart directly through the chest wall.

Cine coronary arteriography (or selective coronary arteriography) enables visualization of coronary arteries and collateral circulation. The technique will delineate the severity and distribution of occlusive lesions of the coronary arteries, the status of collateral circulation, and the condition of the myocardium. There may be poor contractility, fibrosis, or aneurysm formation in the myocardium. A catheter is passed through either the brachial (Sones technique) or the femoral artery and the catheter tip is introduced into one coronary artery and then the other while pressures are continuously recorded. Multiple injections of contrast media are given and, with the use of the tilt table, the patient's position is changed from left to right anterior oblique while a variety of spot films and high-speed motion pictures are taken of each coronary artery as it is perfused.

Complications are associated with the different approaches to contrast visualization of the heart. The nurse must know the exact procedure that is to be done, the method and site of entry, and the route of the catheterization. Observations during and after the procedure are concerned with the potential complications. These complications include the following: bleeding due to trauma at the site of entry or related to anticoagulants generally used during the procedure; thrombophlebitis or arterial occlusion due to mechanical trauma; arrhythmias due to manipulation of the catheter within the heart chambers; cardiac perforation; myocardial infarction; embolic phenomena resulting in stroke or pulmonary embolism; and allergic reactions due to hypersensitivity to the dye.

Postcatheterization, the nurse must caution the patient to lie quietly in a supine position and to avoid any activity that would cause stress or strain on the puncture site. The affected extremity should be in an extended position to avoid any increase in pressure. The length of time for bed rest and limited activity will depend on which approach was used (a longer period of bed rest is required when the lower extremity site is used), the physician's preferences, and the individual's reaction to the procedure. Usually the bed rest restriction applies for 3 to 6 hours; the patient usually is fatigued after the procedure and prefers temporary bed rest.

The pressure dressing over the puncture site is checked for bleeding or any evidence of hematoma formation. Firm pressure over the entry site is used if any bleeding occurs. In some institutions sand bags are used for additional pressure. Vital signs are taken regularly to determine any cardiac arrhythmias, impending shock, or respiratory distress. Apical pulses are taken for a full minute to detect arrhythmias accurately. Continuous cardiac monitoring may be indicated, although it is not routinely used. Chest pain should be reported immediately to the cardiologist. Symptoms of extreme pain at the injection site or in the extremity and complaints of palpitations or unusual sensations are also reported. The pulses distal to the injection site are palpated at regular intervals to assure that arterial flow is not obstructed by thrombosis or emboli. The color and temperature of the extremity are checked frequently; severe pain or impairment of motion or sensations of tingling or numbness in the extremity are reported to the cardiologist.

After cardiac catheterization the patient is usually anxious and concerned about the results of the examination and requires appropriate explanations of the cardiologist's findings and emotional support and information about the implications of the findings. Confirmation of the need for open heart surgery is usually extremely anxiety provoking. On the other hand, the patient may be equally anxious if the cardiac catheterization results demonstrate that open heart surgery is not feasible and that his prognosis is grave. Appropriate counseling and psychological comfort measures are imperative in both cases.

Epidemiology and Prevention of Cardiovascular Disease

Cardiovascular disease afflicts over 28 million Americans in a variety of ways. One of every six adults has hypertension while 4 million have coronary artery disease. The average healthy adult male has about one chance in five of having a heart attack before age 60 to 65. Rheumatic heart disease and stroke each affect more than 1.7 million persons. Fifty-three percent of all recorded deaths are caused by cardiovascular disease. One-fourth of those who die are under 65 years of age.

In spite of the evolution of sophisticated diagnostic techniques and advances in medical and surgical treatment of cardiovascular disease, the morbidity and mortality rates have not changed significantly, especially in coronary artery disease. Certainly deaths during the first three days after a myocardial infarction have been decreased, but more than one-half of the victims of a heart attack die before they reach the hospital. One out of every five victims who die suddenly never had obvious early symptoms of heart disease. Numerous studies have shown that cardiovascular problems begin to develop, asymptomatically, at a very young age. By the time symptoms appear, destructive processes in the cardiovascular system have already taken their toll.

It should seem obvious that all health personnel must be involved in the prevention of cardiovascular disease in order to combat this threat to the health of the population.

The nurse has many opportunities to assist in the prevention of cardiovascular disease, in addition to providing direct care to hospitalized cardiac patients. The nurse has a significant role in case-finding (whether in the hospital, home, clinic, school, or in industry) and should take advantage of opportunities to teach about promoting cardiac health to persons who are without clinical symptoms. These opportunities to intervene with appropriate teaching may arise, for example, when the nurse observes families or young adults with eating habits that include excessive consumption of fats and cholesterol. Other opportunities arise when educating young mothers about the importance of the rubella vaccine in preventing the incidence of maternal rubella and its consequences of congenital heart defects. The use of LSD and other drugs is discouraged in order to prevent birth defects. The hazards of smoking are reinforced for long-term smokers, as well as adolescents who may wish to start the habit.

The school nurse has a significant role in the prevention of rheumatic heart disease by detecting children with pharyngitis and referring them for adequate medical therapy. The use of throat cultures for the detection of streptococcal infection should be enforced. The school nurse also is responsible for educating children, parents, and teachers about adequate surveillance and prophylactic medications to prevent recurrence of streptococcal infections. The nurse also can participate in B.P. screening programs and other programs sponsored by the American Heart Association in conjunction with community health agencies. All nurses should be resource persons about the risk factors for coronary heart disease and for information about factors that place excessive burdens on the heart.

Long-term studies of the risk factors in cardiovascular disease have resulted in the identification of people who are likely to develop cardiovascular disease. The Framingham study, a longitudinal study conducted over a period of 20 years, has resulted in the identification of hypertension, hypercholesterolemia, and smoking as the major risk factors in the incidence of cardiovascular disease. In addition, other risk factors have been identified: obesity, sedentary living, psychological tensions, a positive family history of premature atherosclerotic disease, hyperglycemia, and a habitual diet high in saturated fat, cholesterol, and calories. It is clear that the more risk factors a person has, the greater his or her risk for cardiovascular disease. It is also clear that these factors should guide the nurse in educating the public about the prevention of cardiovascular disease. The particular significance of hypertension and hypercholesterolemia requires more detailed discussion as follows.

Disorders of the Cardiovascular System

HYPERTENSION

During the past decade, hypertension has become recognized as a major health hazard in the United States that warrants the name "silent killer." Hypertension is usually an insidious condition with no specific perceptible symptoms in the early stages. Yet it is the most prevalent cause of cerebrovascular accidents and congestive heart failure and is also frequently complicated by coronary artery disease and renal failure.

It is estimated that 23 million people (approximately 1 of every 7 persons) in the United States suffer from hypertension. The nonwhite population is more frequently affected by hypertension [5].

The normal blood pressure ranges from 115 to 120 systolic and 75 to 80 mm Hg diastolic. The normal pulse pressure, which is the difference between the systolic and diastolic levels, is approximately 40 mm Hg. The World Health Organization has classified pressures of 140/90 mm Hg or less as normal and 160/90 or more as hypertensive. About 85 percent of the cases of hypertension are not associated with a specific or known cause. These people who have hypertension with no identifiable cause are categorized as having essential hypertension. The remaining 15 percent have hypertension secondary to other diseases such as renal vascular occlusion, pheochromocytoma, coarctation of the aorta, polycystic renal disease, glomerulonephritis, pyelonephritis, and eclampsia.

Prior to a discussion of the current approach to therapy and control of hypertension, it is important to review the basic concepts related to blood pressure and the factors that cause it to become elevated.

The pressure in the arteries is the result of the pumping action of the left ventricle of the heart. Maximal arterial pressure occurs during left ventricular contraction (systolic pressure). The arterial pressure falls during the resting stage of the cardiac cycle (diastolic pressure). The circulatory factors that influence arterial pressure are cardiac output, peripheral resistance, blood volume, viscosity of the blood, and elasticity of the arteries. Patients with hypertension have an increase in peripheral resistance because the arterioles (the terminal branches of the arterial system) are constricted. In addition, blood pressure rises if cardiac output, or total blood flow, increases and the peripheral resistance does not fall. This relationship of pressure, flow, and resistance is based on a fundamental principle of hydraulics: the flow through a tube is proportional to the pressure inside the tube and inversely proportional to the resistance in the tube [6]. Persistent elevation of the blood pressure causes increased cardiac effort, which results in hypertrophy of the cardiac muscle. According to the Frank-Starling law (discussed earlier in this chapter), the more the muscle is stretched in diastole (due to the preload or the volume of blood filling the ventricles during diastole), the greater it will contract in systole. However, increased pressure in the arteries increasingly impedes the ejection of blood by the heart (known as increase of the afterload) and may surpass the ability of the heart to stretch and contract adequately [6]. This limitation leads to the development of congestive heart failure. Sustained hypertension places the elastic tissue of the aorta under prolonged and abnormal stretching and leads to rupture of the fibers. The upper aorta loses its distensibility as fibrous collagen tissue replaces the elastic tissue. These changes result in elevated systolic pressure.

As noted previously, peripheral resistance is affected by constriction of the arterioles. Smooth muscle layers of the arterioles are supplied with sympathetic nerves that cause constriction upon being stimulated. Constriction of the arterioles is also affected by oxygen concentration, metabolic products, hormones, and drugs. These factors all are considered in the management of the patient with hypertension [6].

In current practice, there is much emphasis on screening programs to detect persons with asymptomatic stages of hypertension. The impetus for this approach has stemmed from studies showing that early treatment of hypertension is helpful in preventing complications such as cerebrovascular accidents. The diagnosis of hypertension, however, is not made on the basis of a single elevated B.P. reading. Persons with diastolic pressures that average 100 mm Hg on three or more office or clinic visits are considered candidates for treatment. Examination of the eyes with an ophthalmoscope should be included as part of the diagnostic procedure. Thickening of arteriolar walls, small retinal hemorrhages, soft exudates, and papilledema may be detected. Earlier signs of vascular changes include increased arteriolar tortuosity, increased light reflex, and narrowing and irregularity of the arteries.

The Veterans Administration study, reported in 1967, cited the beneficial effects of antihypertensive drugs on reducing morbidity in patients with moderately severe hypertension. This study involved patients with initial diastolic B.P.s of 115 to 129 mm Hg [7]. Subsequently, an extension of this study had an even greater impact on the current approach to treatment of patients with mild hypertension. A controlled trial of drug therapy was initiated to determine the effect on morbidity and mortality in persons with mild or moderate hypertension, designated as those with diastolic pressures averaging 90 to 114 mm Hg. The study showed that drug therapy decreased the estimated risk of morbidity over a 5-year period from 55 to 18 percent and confirmed that adequate B.P. control could improve health and prolong life. Treatment proved to be most effective in preventing congestive heart failure and stroke, but less effective in preventing complications of coronary artery disease [8].

Treatment for hypertension actually includes the control of many aspects of life in addition to the use of drug therapy. Basic to the long-term management of hypertension is the understanding and cooperation of the individual patient. The patient will more willingly accept responsibility to participate in management of the condition if he or she understands the disease, its cause, treatment, and prognosis. Acceptance may be difficult, however, particularly if the patient is asymptomatic at the time of diagnosis.

Much attention has been given to the role of counseling in working with patients with hypertension for the promotion of compliance with the prescribed regimen. The major goal of compliance is to have the patient accept a lifelong illness requiring medication and control. Having accepted this basic concept, the patient is usually more willing to comply with the regimen if it is perceived to be beneficial. It is helpful to include a member of the family or some other significant person in planning for long-term management so that support and encouragement for compliance to the therapeutic regimen is reinforced.

The nurse must ascertain what the patient perceives as possible, according to the demands of his or her daily life. The nurse and the patient together can explore ways that the patient can effectively and realistically incorporate care practices into the daily schedule. Depending on the necessary limitations indicated by the severity of the condition, the treatment regimen should enable the patient to retain as normal a life style as is possible. This approach will encourage cooperation with long-term management.

Although it is sometimes difficult for the

patient to identify with complications of the disease, especially when he is feeling fairly well, the dangers of prolonged and uncontrolled hypertension should be emphasized. The patient should be aware of the danger of irreversible damage to blood vessels, especially in the eyes, heart, kidney, and brain, if hypertension is not adequately controlled.

Weight reduction with a low caloric diet is indicated if the patient is overweight, in order to decrease the workload on the heart. A sodium-restricted diet is usually prescribed to assist in decreasing plasma volume, and thus to assist in decreasing the blood pressure. Adequate rest is important, and avoidance of emotional stresses is essential. Adherence to regular medical checkups is vital to the management of hypertension. Another aspect of both prevention and treatment is to avoid stimulants such as coffee, tobacco, and stimulating drugs. The patient should be given an opportunity to ask questions about all aspects of his or her condition and treatment. Supportive attitudes in the health personnel who educate the patient about the implications of hypertension are important in long-term management.

Patients are often taught to take their own B.P. readings. This is a common trend, as professionals recognize that the person who is more actively involved in his therapeutic program is more likely to follow prescribed regimens. The patient who monitors his B.P. is able to identify factors that affect his B.P. and to avoid those that cause elevations. The patient is also better able to observe the positive effects of proper diet, appropriate activities, and medications. The patient is usually instructed to take his B.P. in the morning before rising, at noon, and in the evening. Some patients, however, may become preoccupied with observing their B.P. and may become anxious about even normal variations. The use of self-measurement of the B.P. is indicated for persons who will be able to manage the responsibility without experiencing undue anxiety or stress. Some people reject taking their own B.P. for a variety of reasons. For example, patients may refuse to take their B.P. because they view it as a responsibility of the health professionals and may perceive their assumption of the function as an abdication of the doctor's or nurse's responsibility. Others welcome the opportunity to learn to control the disease. The advantage of having fewer doctor visits may be viewed as an important economic factor. However, the patient should understand the importance of regular follow-up visits with the physician even if they are monitoring their own B.P.

Teaching is vital in the care of patients with hypertension. A major component of the educational program is the orientation to medications, their purpose, anticipated therapeutic effects, and side effects. This is important in gaining the patient's cooperation to follow the prescribed regimen. There is a high rate of noncompliance (e.g., altering the prescribed medication regimen) with hypertensive drug therapy programs. Noncompliance is probably related primarily to the patient's asymptomatic or only mildly symptomatic status at the time of diagnosis and occasional troublesome or severe side effects of the medications. The nurse should regularly evaluate the patient's compliance and provide opportunities for discussion of his feelings and attitudes toward the regimen. Another reason for noncompliance in long-term medication regimens is the economic factor related to the expense of the required medications. Economic problems may require referral to agencies that can provide financial assistance.

When drug therapy is utilized, combinations of two or three different drugs are generally prescribed to obtain optimal effects while at the same time minimizing the side effects of individual drugs. The nurse must understand drug interactions and factors that potentiate drug interactions, such as foods and alcohol. Certain foods have been implicated in causing blood pressure elevation and should be avoided by patients with hypertension, in order to avoid competing with drug therapy. These foods include pickled herring, chocolate, chicken liver, licorice, canned figs, yeast products, beer, wine, and strong or aged cheese.

Cold and cough medications such as nasal decongestants that are sold over the counter generally have vasoconstrictive actions that also tend to increase the B.P. Patients should be warned against their use without proper medical direction, particularly when they are taking antihypertensive drugs. Oral contraceptives also have been implicated in the development of elevated B.P.s; alternatives to oral contraceptives may be necessary for the person receiving antihypertensive medications.

Most of the antihypertensive drugs cause side effects of drowsiness, light-headedness, lethargy, and orthostatic (postural) hypotension. The latter condition is characterized by a drop of at least 20 mm Hg in both the systolic and diastolic B.P.s upon assumption of an upright position. This drop in pressure decreases venous return, peripheral resistance, and cardiac output. The patient may be dizzy and faint. Patients should be advised that these symptoms are usually temporary and can be controlled by adjustment of dosages. These effects, however, have implications for the patient's safety, and precautions should be emphasized. The nurse should monitor the patient's B.P. in both the supine and standing positions and should substantiate that the patient understands the importance of moving slowly when changing positions in order to avoid sudden changes in blood pressure. Another aspect of safety is the potential danger in driving a car or participating in other activities in which drowsiness or lethargy may affect the safety of the patient or other persons. Discussion should include the warning that alcohol, barbiturates, and narcotics also potentiate orthostatic hypotension and other untoward effects and therefore should be avoided. Impotence is another possible side effect of some of the drugs, and the patient, regardless of age, should be prepared for this potential problem.

The major drugs used in the treatment of hypertension are (1) diuretics, (2) agents, such as methyldopa, that block the synthesis of norepinephrine, (3) agents, such as reserpine and guanethidine, that displace norepinephrine at the adrenergic endings, and (4) ganglionic-blocking agents such as pentolinium and mecamylamine [9]. When hypertension is associated with high plasma renin levels it is treated with renin-suppressing agents such as methyldopa (Aldomet) and reserpine (Serpasil). Patients with hypertension may be admitted to the hospital or clinic for other conditions, so that all nurses should be aware of the actions of these drugs and the precautions or contraindications related to their administration.

Thiazides are often utilized for initial therapy. These diuretics appear to alter the sodium-potassium ratio and decrease the responsiveness of arteriolar smooth muscle to catecholamines [9]. The effect is then to decrease peripheral resistance. Hydrochlorothiazide (Hydrodiuril) is usually started at a dose of 25 mg twice daily and maintained with total doses of 25 to 100 mg daily. The diuretic action of these drugs causes polyuria, dry mouth, and thirst, and may cause symptoms related to electrolyte (particularly potassium loss) and fluid disturbances such as weakness, lethargy, drowsiness, muscular fatigue, and gastrointestinal disturbances. Laboratory baseline data are obtained and evaluated during therapy to prevent the development of hypokalemia, hyponatremia, hyperglycemia, and hyperuricemia. Usually dietary sources of potassium such as orange juice or bananas, potassium supplements, or potassium-sparing diuretics such as spironolactone (Aldactone) are prescribed when thiazides are used. Persons with known sensitivity to sulfonamide-derived drugs are not candidates for thiazide therapy. Thiazides are also contraindicated in patients with impaired kidney function. Other diuretics such as furosemide (Lasix) and ethacrynic acid (Edecrin) may be used in lieu of the thiazide diuretics. The latter drugs, although potent and rapid-acting, do not reduce peripheral resistance as the thiazides do.

Reserpine, a *Rauwolfia* compound, actually acts at several levels of the nervous system including the limbic center of the brain and the vasomotor centers. Reserpine primarily seems to deplete norepinephrine from the adrenergic neuronal stores. The drug is usually started at doses of 0.25 to 0.50 mg daily and 0.1 to 0.25 mg daily is used for maintenance. The drug is seldom used alone, but is combined with other drugs, particularly the thiazide diuretics. Because the drug may cause mental depression, the patient is advised of the potential for decreased libido, dizziness, and mood changes. The drug is contraindicated in patients with a history of mental depression or with active peptic ulcer or ulcerative colitis. Weight gain, nasal stuffiness, peptic ulceration, postural hypotension, drowsiness, sedation, and constipation are all potential side effects of reserpine.

Hydralazine (Apresoline) primarily acts directly on the arterioles, causing a decrease in peripheral vascular resistance. It is usually started at doses of 10 to 12.5 mg two times daily and slowly increased to a total of 100 to

200 mg daily. The lowest effective dose is used for maintenance. It must always be administered along with a diuretic medication. Although the drug is usually well tolerated in small doses, headache, palpitation, flushing, and dyspnea may occur. Symptoms of angina may also be aggravated. The drug is therefore contraindicated in coronary artery disease, mitral valve disease, and hypersensitivity states. Long-term use of hydralazine may produce a lupus-erythematosus-like syndrome.

Methyldopa (Aldomet), which blocks the synthesis of norepinephrine, is usually started at a dose of 250 mg twice daily and is maintained at 750 mg to 2 gm daily. The patient should be warned of potential postural hypotension, sleepiness, bradycardia, and nasal stuffiness. The drug has caused hemolytic anemia and jaundice and therefore is contraindicated in the presence of hepatic disease. It is also contraindicated in pregnancy.

Spironolactone (Aldactone) blocks the action of the sodium-retaining effects of aldosterone on the renal tubules, thus causing sodium excretion but retention of potassium. The usual maintenance dose is 25 mg two times daily. Hyperkalemia and other electrolyte imbalances, such as hyponatremia, and an elevated blood urea nitrogen are potential complications. Monitoring of serum electrolytes at regular intervals is indicated. Patients should be warned that drowsiness, lethargy, headache, and diarrhea and other gastrointestinal symptoms may occur. The drug is best tolerated after meals. Urticaria, mental confusion, ataxia, and gynecomastia are other side effects that have been associated with the drug. The drug is contraindicated in patients with impaired renal function. Triamterene (Dyrenium) is another potassium-sparing diuretic with similar side effects (except for gynecomastia) and similar contraindications.

Guanethidine (Ismelin) is thought to displace norepinephrine at the adrenergic nerve endings. It does not cross the blood-brain barrier, so that mental depression is not associated with its use. The drug is administered initially at 10 mg daily, with gradual increases to a total of 25 to 50 mg daily as maintenance doses. Guanethidine is a potent drug and is used in moderate and severe hypertension. Venous pooling, decreased cardiac output, and decreased pulse rates are hemodynamic effects of the drug, resulting in postural hypotension. The patient should be cautioned, therefore, to change positions slowly, particularly when getting out of bed. Monitoring of the blood pressure in the supine and standing position is necessary. Support stockings may be indicated. The patient should avoid standing for long periods and should be particularly cautious of postural hypotensive effects when using alcohol, when exercising, or during hot weather. Sexual dysfunctions such as loss of the ability to ejaculate are associated with the use of guanethidine, as are dyspnea, fatigue, diarrhea, nausea, nocturia, and occasional urinary incontinence. The drug should not be used with tricyclic antidepressants and is contraindicated in pheochromocytoma.

The adrenergic blocking agents include pentrolinium (Ansolysen), and mecamylamine (Inversine). These drugs tend to be used for severe hypertension or in patients who are nonresponsive to other drugs. These drugs cause both sympathetic and parasympathetic blocking, which may precipitate varying side effects, including orthostatic (postural) hypotension, rapid hypotension, impotence, urinary retention, intestinal paralysis, constipation, and loss of visual accommodation.

Pargyline hydrochloride (Eutonyl) is a monoamine oxidase inhibitor that is sometimes used in treating hypertension. The action of this drug is not known, and its use is limited to persons who do not respond to other regimens.

Propranolol (Inderal), a beta adrenergic blocker, has recently been shown to be effective in some cases of hypertension associated with high plasma renin levels. Its exact role in treating hypertension has not been established and, at this writing, it has not received FDA approval for this use.

Other drugs that are utilized in short-term management are diazoxide, parenteral reserpine, trimethaphan camsylate (Arfonad), and sodium nitroprusside (Nipride). Diazoxide (Hyperstat IV) is given intravenously as a rapidly acting antihypertensive agent in the treatment of hypertensive crises. (Oral hypertensive agents are instituted as soon as the hypertensive state is controlled.) The rapid action of diazoxide requires close monitoring of the patient's B.P. at frequent intervals to prevent hypotensive reactions. The site of the injection also should be monitored closely, because extravascular injection causes inflammation and pain due to the alkalinity of the solution. Trimethaphan camsylate also requires close monitoring of the B.P. and observation for other potential problems associated with ganglionic-blocking agents. Parenteral (intramuscular) reserpine (Serpasil) may cause significant postural hypotension. Its effect begins within 1 to 3 hours after administration.

The reader is referred to pharmacology textbooks for more detailed information on antihypertensive drug therapy.

Sympathectomy may be attempted when the B.P. cannot be decreased effectively by drug therapy or when the patient is unwilling to follow a medical regimen. Currently, this surgical procedure is utilized less frequently, but it may be indicated when severe kidney involvement exists or cerebral dysfunction occurs. The procedure consists in resection of the tenth thoracic ganglion on through the first or second lumbar ganglion. Benefits from the surgery have varied widely, and it is difficult to predict the results. The purpose of the surgery is to block stimuli from the sympathetic nerve fibers to the blood vessels. Sympathectomy may cause the untoward effects of postural hypotension, neuritis, loss of perspiration in the areas innervated by the severed sympathetic fibers, and loss of ejaculation in male patients. As indicated previously, the wide range of medications currently available has reduced the number of sympathectomy surgeries being done.

Postoperative management of the patient who has had a sympathectomy includes supervision to prevent problems associated with orthostatic hypotension. Abrupt changes of position from supine to standing should be avoided by the patient. Elastic stockings are worn to decrease pooling of the blood in the lower extremities during sitting. Ambulation is initiated slowly and carefully. The patient may have difficulty adjusting to the excessive perspiration from areas of the body that were not surgically denervated by the sympathectomy. Extra coverings may be necessary to prevent undue loss of body heat or fluids.

The clinical course of hypertension may be described as benign or malignant, depending on the rate of progression of the condition. **Benign hypertension** implies a gradual onset and a prolonged course with no obvious effects of the mildly elevated B.P. The term is somewhat misleading, however, and is being used less frequently. The current emphasis on treating asymptomatic hypertension appears to make "benign" an inappropriate term in hypertension. The terms mild, moderate, or severe hypertension are more commonly used.

Malignant hypertension is an accelerated severe form of hypertension, characterized by acute vascular changes. Acute fibrinoid and necrotizing vascular changes are the major features of the condition, which can be fatal unless treatment is initiated promptly and effectively. Papilledema is an important diagnostic finding; retinopathy with hemorrhages and exudates is also present. Diastolic pressure generally exceeds 120 mm Hg and rapidly progressive renal insufficiency, resulting from fibrinoid necrosis of the renal arterioles, is usually present. The patient with malignant hypertension usually develops the condition as a complication of preexisting essential hypertension. Renin levels are generally elevated. (The significance of renin is discussed in Chapters 2 and 8.) Usually the patient's complaints are headache, dizziness, weight loss, and visual impairment. Renal involvement is demonstrated by the presence of proteinuria, microscopic hematuria, and elevated blood urea nitrogen levels.

Immediate hospitalization and prompt parenteral therapy with potent antihypertensive drugs are indicated to rapidly reduce the B.P. for the patient with malignant hypertension. The use of these drugs, which include parenteral reserpine, diazoxide, ganglionic-blocking agents, hydralazine, and guanethidine, requires close monitoring of vital signs during administration. Sodium nitroprusside (Nipride) is an antihypertensive agent used intravenously for rapid reduction of B.P. in patients with hypertensive crisis. It must always be diluted and given as an intravenous infusion. It has a short effect, causing peripheral vasodilatation by a direct action on the blood vessels. Vasopressor drugs should be available in case of excessive hypotensive reactions.

Untreated malignant hypertension may result in hypertensive encephalopathy, which causes neurologic changes such as changes in personality, severe headache, lethargy, convulsions, coma, and death. The changes are associated with cerebral edema and vascular insufficiency caused by marked cerebral vasoconstriction in response to high arterial pressure.

Secondary Hypertension

As mentioned previously, hypertension may be secondary to other diseases, such as coarctation of the aorta, pheochromocytoma, aldosteronism, and renal vascular disease. (Renal disease is the most common cause of secondary hypertension.) Hypertension is often relieved when the primary cause is treated. If hypertension is caused by coarctation of the aorta or pheochromocytoma, for example, surgical intervention may be curative. Renal artery stenosis may be treated by either bypass grafts or nephrectomy as another example of secondary hypertension that is potentially curable. If the primary disease is chronic, prolonged secondary hypertension may become irreversible because of adaptive vascular changes. In these chronic states, treatment is similar to that used in the treatment of primary hypertension (essential hypertension).

Except for coarctation of the aorta, the various types of secondary hypertension are discussed elsewhere. (The role of renin in the incidence of hypertension, for example, is discussed in Chapters 2 and 8.)

Young adults with long-standing mild hypertension should be evaluated for the presence of coarctation of the aorta, which is a stricture or narrowing of the aorta. Femoral pulses should be palpated; if they are not full and bounding, the B.P. should be taken in both the upper and lower extremities. Stricture of a segment of the aorta results in diminished pressure beyond the narrowed segment. Thus the presence of coarctation of the aorta is suspected when reduced B.P.s in the legs are detected. In addition, the patient's back should be inspected for pulsating intercostal arteries. A chest x-ray should be examined for the presence of notching of the ribs, which is characteristic of coarctation of the aorta. Surgical intervention involves the removal of the malformed segment of the aorta with direct anastamosis or replacement of long segments with a synthetic arterial graft.

When secondary hypertension is suspected, an extensive diagnostic work-up is required, which can be discouraging, fatiguing, and anxiety provoking. The patient requires thorough explanations of the various tests and their purpose. The diagnostic work-up may be a source of concern in relation to the expense involved; financial concerns should be referred to appropriate personnel for assistance.

In assisting with the diagnostic work-up, the nurse must be knowledgeable about the purpose of biochemical analysis of urine specimens for catecholamines; the importance of obtaining accurate and total volumes of urine during specific time intervals; and the purpose of each test used in the diagnosis of the specific primary disease. These tests, as well as the significance of plasma renin tests, are discussed in Chapter 8.

ATHEROSCLEROSIS

In this discussion, **arteriosclerosis** is used as a general term to include a variety of entities that cause "hardening" of the arteries. Typically, arteriosclerosis refers to conditions that lead to decreased blood supply to body tissues. The term generally refers to thickening of the muscular coats of the arteries that results from aging and hypertension. **Atherosclerosis** is the most common type of arteriosclerosis and is characterized by a sequence of changes in the intimal layer of the arteries, chiefly affecting the aorta and the coronary, cerebral, and lower-extremity arteries. The changes in the intima result from initial fibrous proliferation and consequent thickening of the intima of the affected vessel; fragmentation of the internal elastic membrane; accumulation of lipids in the form of plaques; and increased deposits of cholesterol crystals, debris, and calcifications known as atheromas [10]. As the atheroma continues to grow, it may occlude the vessel entirely or it may rupture and incite the formation of a thrombus at the site.

Atherosclerosis is more common in males than in females, but the rate in women rises after the menopause, so that both sexes are fairly evenly affected in the older age group. Coronary atherosclerosis and its complications are considered to be directly responsible for more than 50 percent of all deaths due to cardiovascular disease. Prevention of atherosclerosis is therefore an essential part of any approach to the prevention of the overall problem of cardiovascular disease.

Atherosclerosis is a disease process that

appears to be related to many factors in addition to elevated blood lipids. Therefore, efforts to prevent atherosclerosis must be concerned also with the other risk factors, such as control of hypertension, appropriate exercise, weight reduction for obesity, elimination of smoking, and the avoidance of stress. An example of the relationship of one of these factors and the development of heart disease was brought out in the Framingham study, which showed a high correlation between cigarette smoking and death from coronary artery disease. Cigarette smoking affects the cardiovascular system by functional changes produced through stimulation of the sympathetic system by nicotine and by hypoxemia resulting from changes in pulmonary function. It has been found that men smoking more than one pack of cigarettes per day have twice the risk of developing a myocardial infarction and more than three times the risk of sudden death. Another example of a risk factor is that of limited physical activity. Although physical activity has not been proved to decrease the development of atherosclerosis, it has been demonstrated to enhance collateral circulation.

HYPERLIPOPROTEINEMIA

Although the exact cause of atherosclerosis has not been identified, there is sufficient evidence to implicate a disorder of lipid metabolism in the onset of the pathological process. Cholesterol, in particular, has been implicated, because high contents of cholesterol are found within atherosclerotic lesions and elevated levels of serum cholesterol are found in populations with a high incidence of atherosclerosis and coronary artery disease. People with other metabolic diseases such as hypothyroidism and diabetes also have a high incidence of atherosclerosis. In addition, atherosclerosis has been produced experimentally in animals fed high cholesterol diets. However, cholesterol does not exist in the serum in free form, but rather in combination with other lipids and protein molecules, and current therapies therefore have been concerned with hyperlipoproteinemia (an excess of lipoproteins in the blood) rather than hypercholesterol levels alone. Hyperlipoproteinemia is a more inclusive term and is generally accepted as the appropriate approach in the study of atherosclerosis.

Cholesterol, phospholipids, and triglycerides are the major lipid fractions of the blood. These lipids are actually components of complex lipoprotein molecules; various combinations of protein and lipids form different types of lipoproteins. (Lipids are insoluble in water and therefore cannot be transported in plasma unless they are bound to protein in the form of water-soluble lipoprotein molecules.) Each of the major lipid fractions will be discussed separately.

The liver is the major site of **cholesterol biosynthesis;** the intestinal tract (particularly the small intestine) is also a site of cholesterol production. Most of the cholesterol in serum is in the form of cholesterol esters, rather than free cholesterol. Enzymes (cholesterol esterases) change the cholesterol esters from ingested cholesterol-containing foods to free cholesterol. A considerable portion is converted to steroid hormones by the adrenal glands and the gonads. The usual rate of synthesis of cholesterol is between 1,000 and 1,500 mg per day. Cholesterol is primarily excreted by secretion into the bile duct, with about 90 percent as bile acids and about 10 percent as sterol. **Phospholipids,** which compose more than 50 percent of the lipids, are produced primarily in the liver, although most cells synthesize this particular lipid. There are many phospholipids, but the majority in plasma are phosphatidylcholine (lecithin). Phospholipids have a role in blood coagulation, cell permeability, and fat absorption and are an important component of the neural myelin sheets. **Triglycerides** are esters of glycerol with three molecules of fatty acids. They are a source of energy and are stored in adipose tissue. Free fatty acids are released from these fat deposits and are oxidized as required by energy needs of the body. In addition, the liver may synthesize triglycerides from nonlipid precursors such as glucose. Nonesterified fatty acids may also be transported to the liver and re-esterified into triglycerides. Thus, high carbohydrate diets may provoke an increase in the biosynthesis of fatty acids by the liver and increase the triglyceride levels. Sugar, for example, has been found to elevate triglyceride levels and is described as lipogenic.

Blood samples may be analyzed to determine the individual patient's lipoprotein pattern. Electrophoresis techniques have also facilitated the classification of primary hyper-

Table 4-2
Characteristics of types of hyperlipoproteinemia and recommended therapies

Type	Plasma appearance	Cholesterol	Triglycerides	Recommended therapy
I Rare Appears to be genetically based—absence of lipoprotein lipase.	Cream layer over clear plasma	Normal or elevated	Grossly elevated (over 5,000 mg/100 ml in some cases)	Low fat diet Antilipemic drugs *not* effective in this type Alcohol restricted
II Common type—genetically and exogenously induced. Familial and nonfamilial types. Associated with nodular xanthomas.	Usually clear; may be slightly turbid	Elevated	Normal or slightly elevated	Cholesterol restricted to less than 300 mg daily Decrease of saturated fats; increase in polyunsaturated fats Drug therapy for familial type
III Less common than II and IV	Usually turbid	Elevated	Elevated	Low cholesterol. CHO and fats controlled Drug therapy used
IV Common type—endogenously and exogenously induced. Xanthomas may be present.	Usually turbid with no cream layer	Normal or elevated	Elevated	Emphasis on weight reduction Restriction of CHO and alcohol (possibly cholesterol) Drug therapy may be used
V Uncommon	Creamy top layer over turbid plasma	Elevated	Elevated	Caloric restriction Restrict fat and CHO Alcohol restricted

Modified from D. S. Fredrickson et al. *The Dietary Management of Hyperlipoproteinemia. A Handbook for Physicians.* Washington, D.C.: DHEW, USPHS, 1970.

lipidemia, which is not obviously caused by another known disease, such as obstructive liver disease, hypothyroidism, insulin-dependent diabetes, or the nephrotic syndrome. Table 4-2 describes the generally accepted classification of hyperlipoproteinemia, including some of the pertinent characteristics and some of the prescribed therapies for the individual types. Specific treatment depends on the type, but the first step is always dietary management; in fact, weight reduction alone will lower glyceride levels in most types of hyperlipidemia.

A dietary history taken by the nurse may give valuable information about tendencies to develop hyperlipidemia. If the dietary history reveals unusually high intake of calories, saturated fats, and dietary cholesterol, nutritional counseling is indicated. Any prescription for dietary management, however, must consider the individual's life style and must be planned with the individual patient to assure compliance.

Diets rich in cholesterol and saturated fats may elevate serum cholesterol levels. It has been recommended that dietary cholesterol be reduced to less than 300 mg per day and that caloric intake be adjusted to achieve and maintain optimal weight [11]. It has also been shown that mono-unsaturated fats have almost a neutral effect whereas polyunsaturated fats tend to lower the cholesterol levels in some patients. The degree of saturation reflects the consistency of the fat; for example, highly saturated fats such as hydrogenated vegetable oils are solids. These have relatively high melting points in contrast to unsaturated fats, which usually are liquids. Thus, foods may be classified according to their fat content.

Foods containing saturated fats include beef, lamb, pork, veal, whole milk, hydrogenated shortenings, cream, margarine, butter, ice cream, and chocolate. Intake of these foods is avoided, or at least restricted in amounts.

Foods containing mono-unsaturated fats include chicken, duck, turkey, almonds, pecans, olive oil, and peanut oil.

Foods containing polyunsaturated fats include fish, corn oil, sunflower oil, soybean oil, safflower oil, herring oil, and walnuts.

When dietary management is not adequate to control lipid levels, drug therapy may be indicated. Although the long-term effect of drug-induced lowering of lipid levels on morbidity due to atherosclerosis has not been clearly established, antilipidemic drugs are being used as adjuncts to diet therapy in all types of hyperlipoproteinemia except type I. Clofibrate (Atromid-S), 500 mg four times daily, is prescribed most often. The action of clofibrate is thought to be primarily that of inhibiting the hepatic release of lipoproteins and of inhibiting cholesterol biosynthesis. The drug frequently causes nausea and may be associated with vomiting, diarrhea, dyspepsia, and abdominal distress. When the patient is receiving coumarin anticoagulants, the anticoagulant dose is lowered, since clofibrate increases the action of coumarin. The drug is contraindicated in the presence or history of jaundice or hepatic disease; serum transaminase levels and other liver function tests may become abnormal. Serum lipid levels and liver function are monitored during the use of this drug. Clofibrate has also been associated with a variety of malabsorption phenomena, including malabsorption of vitamin B_{12}, iron, and electrolytes.

Niacin (nicotinic acid), which is actually a vitamin, has been shown to lower blood cholesterol and triglyceride levels. Studies suggest that niacin reduces the rate of synthesis of beta lipoprotein. Side effects of the drug are intense flushing, headache, and pruritus. Jaundice and abnormal liver function tests have occurred with the use of the drug; it is therefore contraindicated in the presence of liver disease.

Other antilipemic agents include sitosterols suspension (Cytellin), which inhibits cholesterol absorption; cholestyramine resin (Cuemid, Questran), which decreases bile absorption (and may decrease absorption of fat-soluble vitamins); and dextrothyroxine (Choloxin), estrogens, and heparin-sodium, which lower blood lipid levels.

As mentioned previously, many factors are involved in the development and the consequences of atherosclerosis, namely, cardiac and vascular diseases. Atherosclerosis, for example, impedes blood flow to the heart and results in angina pectoris and myocardial infarction.

ANGINA PECTORIS

Angina pectoris describes the chest pain associated with transient myocardial ischemia (diminished supply of blood to the heart muscle). Angina refers to the nature of the pain and pectoris to the pectoralis muscles, the general location of the pain. Angina is characterized by the sudden occurrence of substernal pain that is provoked by exertion, emotional crises, or ingestion of large meals. The pain is described as a pressure or heaviness, constriction, tightness, or squeezing sensation over the sternum. It may radiate to the precordium, the arms (particularly the left shoulder and down the inner side of the arm), the neck, the jaw, or teeth. The pain usually lasts 3 to 5 minutes and is relieved by rest and administration of nitroglycerine.

Angina pectoris commonly results when the coronary arteries are partially occluded by atherosclerosis and degenerative arteriosclerotic changes. Blood flow may be sufficient during rest, but it may be inadequate to meet the increased demands for cardiac output during exercise, emotional states, or eating. Aortic valve disease and anemia may also be predisposing factors in angina pectoris. Hyperthyroidism may cause angina pectoris by placing additional demands on the heart due to increased metabolic needs.

The exact cause of the pain has not been established. It is thought that inadequate oxygen results in anaerobic metabolism and the pain reflects the response of myocardial neural receptors to the irritation of acidic end products of the anaerobic metabolism. It is important to differentiate ischemic cardiac pain from that associated with esophagitis or musculoskeletal pain, such as intercostal neuritis or myositis. Pain associated with gallbladder disease has also been mistaken for angina pectoris. The history of the onset of angina in relation to increased activity and its relief with rest and nitroglycerine are the most important aspects of the diagnosis.

The therapeutic regimen for the person with angina pectoris is focused on averting anginal attacks and progression of the atherosclerotic process. Without preventive measures, the likelihood of a myocardial infarction occurring within five years (after onset of angina) is increased. Treatment is focused on educating the patient (in words appropriate to his level of understanding) about the myocardial blood flow in terms of supply and demand. Emphasis is placed on avoiding the factors that precipitate attacks of angina. Control of anxiety, anger, tension, and excitement should be emphasized. The patient is encouraged to engage in moderate exercise, such as regular walking, until increased levels of tolerance are attained to permit more activity. He or she is also taught the importance of avoiding hurried and rushed activity, and is advised to undertake work more slowly. Short rest periods after meals are generally helpful. Patients with angina are advised to avoid sudden exposure to cold and to limit activity in the cold. Breathing cold air, for example, may produce generalized reflex vasoconstriction, putting an additional work load on the heart and precipitating an attack of angina. In addition, since people tend to breathe through the mouth in the cold air, the air-warming effect of nasal breathing is therefore lost.

The use of nitroglycerine and other medications that result in coronary vasodilatation requires thorough understanding of their purpose, limits, and appropriate dosages. Nitroglycerine may be prescribed in dosages from 0.3 to 0.6 mg. The tablet is taken sublingually and should be completely dissolved. Within 1 to 2 minutes, it produces dilatation of the coronary blood vessels. If there is no relief, the dosage is repeated. Generally, if the pain is not relieved after resting and taking a nitroglycerine tablet every 5 minutes for three doses, medical assistance should be obtained. Patients need to be assured that there is no danger of addiction with the use of repeated administration of nitroglycerine; this is a frequently expressed concern.

The patient should always carry the nitroglycerine tablets for immediate use when indicated. Tablets lose their potency after 6 months, so their dates of effectiveness should be monitored. Deterioration of the drug should be suspected when a previously effective dose suddenly becomes less effective or when a tingling sensation under the tongue is no longer detected on taking the drug. (Nitroglycerine tablets are inactivated by heat, light, and moisture.) The patient should be advised about potential side effects of nitroglycerine, which are headache, hypotension, dizziness, and flushing. Nitroglycerine may be used prophylactically as well as at the onset of an acute attack. For example, the drug may be taken prior to exercise, participating in sexual intercourse, or engaging in an emotionally stressful situation.

Amyl nitrite, in the form of pearls or ampuls that are crushed or broken into a handkerchief and then inhaled, may be prescribed in lieu of the tablets. (However the ampuls are more difficult to handle than are the tablets.) The usual dosage of 0.3 mg results in a rapid action but of shorter duration than that of nitroglycerine tablets. Repeated dosages may cause syncope.

Long-acting nitrite preparations may also be used to maintain coronary artery vasodilatation. The more common preparations include pentaerythritol tetranitrate (PETN; Peritrate), trolnitrate phosphate (Metamine), erythrityl tetranitrate (Cardilate), and isosorbide dinitrate (Isordil). The last two drugs may be administered sublingually for an acute attack of angina as well as orally for their long-acting action. The use of the long-acting nitrates has been controversial. Tolerance appears to develop readily, and the actual effectiveness of the drugs in managing the anginal syndrome has been difficult to evaluate. Isordil, however, appears to be effective for 3-hour intervals. Nitroglycerin ointment, 2%, for cutaneous absorption also has proved effective in combatting angina. It can be reapplied every 6 hours.

Propranolol hydrochloride (Inderal), a beta-adrenergic blocking agent, is being utilized in selected patients with moderate to severe angina who have not responded to conventional methods of treatment. Abrupt withdrawal of the drug is to be avoided because it may exacerbate the angina. The drug, by decreasing sympathetic stimulation of the heart, apparently decreases myocardial oxygen demand and thus increases exercise tolerance. Inderal is contraindicated in people who have congestive heart failure, bradyarrhythmias, asthma, or other chronic pulmonary diseases.

Sedatives and tranquilizers often help to lessen the frequency and severity of anginal attacks. Small amounts of whiskey or brandy also may be prescribed to promote vascular dilatation and general relaxation.

The patient's ability to control the events that precipitate attacks of angina is probably the major factor in the successful management of angina. Increased tolerance developed through therapeutic cardiac rehabilitation programs has also helped in the management of angina by the increased development of collateral circulation. The use of coronary bypass surgery as a mode of therapy to control angina pectoris is discussed in another section of this chapter.

Patients with angina may be admitted to the hospital or clinic for conditions other than their cardiac problems. Nurses should utilize these opportunities to assess the patient's knowledge about the proper use of nitroglycerine and about methods to prevent attacks of angina, and to reinforce this information as indicated. All nurses should be aware of the significance of angina and the symptoms and changes that distinguish angina pectoris from an actual myocardial infarction.

MYOCARDIAL INFARCTION

In myocardial infarction (MI) morphologic damage results from complete occlusion of a coronary artery or its branches. The occlusion deprives the myocardium of its normal blood and oxygen supply, resulting in an area of necrosis termed **infarction.** The character, location, and even the severity of the pain associated with myocardial infarction may be identical to that experienced by the patient with angina pectoris. The major difference in the character of the pain in MI is that it is not necessarily brought on by exertion nor is it relieved by nitroglycerine or rest.

Chest pain is the major symptom associated with MI. It is usually described as a steady and constrictive substernal pain that may or may not radiate to various parts of the body, such as the jaw, neck, and upper extremities (especially the inner left arm). Although unusual physical activity (shoveling snow, for example) has been implicated in precipitating acute myocardial infarction (AMI), the majority of episodes do not occur during unusual physical activity. In contrast to angina pectoris, the onset of chest pain in MI may occur during rest or sleep. It is thought that the pain is due to the accumulation of metabolites resulting from diminished oxygen in the heart muscle. Apprehension and restlessness are usually present to a marked degree as the sensation of impending death is experienced by the patient. There is usually profuse diaphoresis; the skin is moist and clammy and the patient is very pale. Vital signs demonstrate hypotension, with initial rapid and thready pulse rates, which may change to bradycardia at a later stage. Rapid and shallow respirations or dyspnea may be observed. Fainting and weakness also may be present. Rapid onset of shock with tachycardia and peripheral vasoconstriction and lowered blood pressure may occur. Nausea and vomiting may occur in some patients, as a result of vagal reflexes initiated by the infarction. In some patients, rapid onset of pulmonary edema and congestive heart failure may be the predominant symptoms.

In contrast to the above acute symptoms, some patients suffer myocardial damage without showing such vivid symptoms, because a highly developed collateral circulation has compensated for the occluded vessel. In fact, myocardial damage may be detected later on a routine examination without any history of acute episodes of chest pain (these are termed "silent coronaries"). MI has also been first detected during autopsies of patients who did not have frank coronary artery obstruction. In these cases, a state of shock with decreased blood supply to the heart muscle may have caused the infarction.

Over 90 percent of the patients with MI demonstrate atherosclerotic changes in the coronary arteries. The onset of MI may occur as part of a well-established anginal pattern, demonstrated by an increase in frequency and severity of the pain. Other times, the MI may occur in the apparently healthy person who develops chest pain and dies suddenly. Prognosis after an MI depends on the amount of functional collateral circulation that is able to compensate for the occluded artery, as well as on the site, extent, and severity of the atherosclerotic process itself and of the infarction. The major areas of the heart that are sites of MIs are the anterior wall, the inferior wall diaphragm, and the lateral and posterior walls; the most serious site and that involving the highest mortality rate is the anterior wall infarct. Transmural infarction involves the entire width of the myocardial wall.

MI is the leading cause of death in the United States, and thus the threat of sudden death is a very real one. The threat of death is greatest during the first 24 to 48 hours, so that constant surveillance of the patient is particularly imperative during this period. Therefore, patients with symptoms characteristic of MI are usually admitted to the CCU. Even if a CCU is not available, the approach to nursing care and treatment of a patient with an acute myocardial infarction is the same. Nursing measures center on reducing the workload of the heart by decreasing the demands on the heart, relieving the acute pain associated with the condition, and observing the patient closely for complications.

Since 1962, CCUs have been developed in the majority of hospitals. The original purpose of the units was to provide appropriate resuscitation correctly and rapidly for patients susceptible to cardiac arrest. The purpose of the units, however, has changed to that of close monitoring of the patient to prevent the onset of fatal arrhythmias.

The CCU provides an environment for close monitoring of critically ill patients (or those who are potentially acutely ill) through the use of specialized equipment and a specially trained staff of sufficient numbers to provide constant surveillance. Essential equipment within the CCU includes cardiac monitoring systems (with an automatic alarm system with individualized preset parameters), defibrillators, resuscitative equipment, appropriate medications, and equipment to facilitate nursing care. Most monitors have the capacity for memory tape loops that play back the ECG tracing that preceded the alarm situation.

The primary personnel in the CCU are the nurses who utilize various resources in continuous observation of the patients within the unit; extensive electronic equipment is no substitute for a nurse. Pinneo [12] cautions that these monitors and electronic equipment "serve as tools that extend human observations of the heart's activation" and that "the nurse utilizes the unique combination of clinical assessment and cardiac monitoring," and emphasizes that by deliberately and systematically seeking clinical signs and symptoms of cardiac problems through direct observations, the nurse correlates the findings with those of the cardiac monitor [13]. The nurse's presence is probably the most important resource for providing a sense of security and comfort to the patient and his family, who are often overwhelmed by the equipment and the implications of the condition. The atmosphere of the CCU is often intense in light of the critical nature of the patient's condition; the need for warmth and understanding combined with simple and pertinent explanations of the environment cannot be overestimated.

Proper orientation to the purpose of the monitoring equipment as a means of assuring constant surveillance will generally reassure the patient. The patient should, however, be warned that the alarm system may go off if electrodes become detached from the skin or if there is excessive interference and activity; otherwise the patient may become frightened rather than reassured when the nurse quickly comes to check on him when the alarm is activated.

The complex array of electrical equipment within the CCU places another responsibility on the nurse, that of providing an environment free of electrical hazards. The nurse should be conscientious about checking that all the staff are well oriented to using only properly wired and grounded equipment. Extension cords are prohibited; only three-pronged plugs (that fit securely into the outlets) are utilized. Any person who has even a slight electrical shock when handling any equipment should realize the importance of discontinuing use of that equipment. This precaution also applies when tingling sensations are felt on touching electrical equipment, since the tingling indicates a problem of leakage of current. The CCU should be free of unnecessary electrical equipment such as electric shavers. Nursing personnel should be cognizant that the potential for electroshock hazards increases if there is simultaneous use of intracardiac catheters (pacemaker catheters) and ECG monitoring.

It is well known that a great number of deaths from MI occur even before admission to the hospital. About 40 percent of the cases of AMI occur within one hour of the onset of symptoms. Mobile CCUs, which are designed to rapidly deliver intensive care to the patient in the home or at the location where the attack took place, are being used to combat this aspect of the problem. The mobile units are furnished with the usual CCU equipment and a trained staff and are able to provide emergency treatment prior to transport to the hospital under a constant monitoring system. In addition, emergency rooms and admission procedures of hospitals have been modified to allow direct admission to the CCU or to provide intensive care in specially equipped emergency rooms.

After initial emergency or symptomatic treatment is provided, diagnostic measures are initiated to either confirm or rule out the presence of a myocardial infarction.

Diagnosis of Acute Myocardial Infarction

The diagnosis of acute myocardial infarction (AMI) is made on the basis of the presence of chest pain as well as ECG changes and laboratory findings.

ECG changes usually appear within 24 hours after onset of symptoms but may be delayed as long as 5 to 6 days [10]. A recent MI is characterized by ST elevation and T wave inversion. An enlarged Q wave indicates an old infarction. ST elevation reflects the formation of an ischemic area of the myocardium. The inversion of the T wave generally reflects the development of inflammation. The changes in the Q waves indicate necrosis formation. Observation of these changes requires serial ECGs to detect evolution of the change in the myocardium. The ECG is of significant value in determining prognosis when it is considered with the patient's clinical status.

Laboratory findings supporting the diagnosis of AMI are leukocytosis (usually with an onset on the second day and disappearing within a week as the inflammatory reaction subsides) and an elevated sedimentation rate that reflects the inflammatory process. The release of important enzymes from the injured muscle results in elevations of the serum levels of these enzymes. The rate of the serum enzyme elevations is probably more meaningful than the absolute level of the enzymes, indicating the necessity for serial determinations of enzyme levels. The degree of the rise in enzyme activity is directly related to the extent of the infarction. (Refer to Figure 4-6 to review the significance of the serum enzymes and the typical enzyme pattern associated with MI.) The SGOT level generally rises within 6 to 12 hours and reaches a peak in 24 to 48 hours. It may reach as high as 300 units in severe cases of MI, but is normal within 2 to 4 days in uncomplicated cases or within 7 days after severe infarction. (These estimates demonstrate the importance of an evaluation of the SGOT level shortly after the acute attack.) The LDH usually rises during the second to the fourth day and decreases to normal levels by the eighth to the fourteenth day. The CPK rises within 3 to 6 hours with a maximum peak usually within 12 to 24 hours. Its decreasing pattern follows that of the SGOT pattern. These enzyme levels are important not only in the diagnosis of AMI, but also in the management of the patient as he progresses through the stages of recovery. (For example, if the enzyme levels again rise after activity is increased, the change may reflect myocardial ischemia related to inability of the heart to tolerate the increased demands on the heart and activity may again be restricted).

Tissue changes in the myocardium result in a zone of tissue necrosis, which is the actual infarcted area and is surrounded by an area of inflammation and an outside area of ischemia. During the first 12 hours after the onset of the symptoms, the cardiac tissue actually appears grossly normal, but the necrotic area begins to be defined within 2 to 4 days and by the fourth to the tenth day is distinctive. By the tenth day, granulation tissue begins to form and fibrous tissue begins to replace the necrotic tissue. The formation of scar tissue continues for 6 to 8 weeks.

Nursing Care

The patient with an MI requires constant observation whether he or she is in the CCU setting or in a general unit. Significant changes in the B.P. or pulse, or the onset of dyspnea or any other type of respiratory distress, are reported immediately. An intravenous infusion is usually started on admission, to provide a vehicle for emergency medications that may be needed and as a means of supplying fluids in case of nausea and vomiting or shock. Heparin is usually initiated intravenously on an intermittent schedule. Anticoagulant therapy with heparin requires observation for bleeding (usually in body excretions, such as urine and stools), and evaluation of coagulation laboratory data prior to administration of subsequent doses.

The relief of pain should have a high priority in the nursing care activities. Usually meperidine (Demerol) or morphine sulfate is given to relieve pain, thereby decreasing apprehension, stress, and the work of the heart. To be most effective, narcotics are administered judiciously, without compromising the respiratory status of the patient, and prior to the onset of extreme pain. Vital signs are checked before and after the narcotic is administered.

The nurse's calm and competent manner is extremely important in relieving anxiety. Simple but pertinent explanations should be given to the patient about the monitoring equipment, the routine of the unit, and about notifying the nurse of any distress or needs. The family also should be oriented to the patient's status and the planned therapy.

Restlessness is evaluated as to whether it is caused by pain or by cerebral hypoxia. Regardless of cause, restlessness should be avoided because it only increases the metabolic demands on the heart. The administration of oxygen to increase oxygen arterial tension may also help to relieve the pain and thereby have a beneficial psychological effect on the patient. If oxygen is not being administered (some authorities do not routinely prescribe oxygen therapy), the nurse should observe for signs of hypoxemia that would indicate its need. Oxygen is administered if restlessness, dyspnea, or cyanosis occurs, or if the patient has a low Po_2 level according to arterial blood gases. If oxygen is being given, arterial blood gas levels are the most precise indicators of the effectiveness of the oxygen therapy. Regulation of oxygen flow is guided by the changes in arterial blood gas levels.

Sedatives, hypnotics, or tranquilizers (sometimes in combination) are often administered to control some of the cardiovascular responses to the stresses imposed by the MI and by the atmosphere of the CCU itself. These drugs must be used judiciously since they may mask symptoms or changes in the patient's mental status that are an important indication of low cardiac output or adverse reactions to other drugs being administered. Drugs should not be considered a substitute for dealing with the patient's anxiety and fears.

Other medications in AMI will vary according to the severity of the cardiac status and the ensuing complications. Antiarrhythmic drugs (particularly lidocaine by intravenous infusion or bolus injections) may be administered; nitroglycerine may be at the patient's bedside for use if symptoms of angina develop (if the MI is a mild one and narcotics are not needed); diuretic therapy may be initiated, particularly in the presence of impending heart failure. Although not used routinely, digitalis may be indicated in AMI if supraventricular tachycardias or congestive heart failure occurs. The use of digitalis is generally contraindicated because of the increased risk of producing arrhythmias and the possible increased metabolic needs brought about by the effects of the drug.

Electrolyte balance is monitored carefully, particularly when diuretics are utilized. Potassium replacement is indicated for the potassium loss caused by cellular destruction. In some settings, a polarizing treatment is utilized, consisting in a continuous intravenous infusion of dextrose in water, potassium, and insulin. The name **polarizing therapy** derives from its purpose to treat the MI at a cellular level by restoring polarization in the ischemic cells by forcing potassium (with the aid of insulin and glucose) into the cells. This is a controversial therapy, although its proponents claim it can rectify biochemical and electrical abnormalities at the cardiac cellular level and make the cell less likely to act as a focus of arrhythmia [14].

Depending on the patient's circulatory status and whether nausea and vomiting are present, oral intake may be restricted. The diet is generally that which is tolerated by the patient, either liquid or soft. Sodium restriction may be prescribed, cholesterol is usually restricted, and sometimes both measures are required. In vulnerable patients iced drinks can cause cardiac arrhythmias [15]. However, a recent study challenges the practice of restriction of ice water [16]. Hot drinks and stimulants, like coffee, are also usually restricted.

The patient is placed on complete bed rest for approximately 2 to 5 days to decrease the metabolic demands for oxygen and thus to decrease the work of the heart. Complete bed rest, which implies the need for assistance in feeding, hygienic care (including shaving), and position changes, may be necessary, depending on the patient's status and tolerance. In some instances, hygienic care may be contraindicated in order to conserve the patient's energy. The restriction of complete bed rest with total assistance may be so intolerable to some patients that the anxiety caused by the restrictions may be viewed as more dangerous for the patient's welfare than the activity itself. The major intervention in obtaining the patient's compliance with restrictions is to achieve an effective interpersonal relationship with the patient, developed on trust and effective communication about the significance and importance of rest for the healing of the damaged heart. It is helpful to have the patient participate in decisions about how to conserve energy; for example, if one activity may be allowed, the patient may be more cooperative if he is able to select which activity it will be.

It has been found that strictly enforced bed rest is more taxing to the patient with an MI than a sitting position in a comfortable chair. In addition, prolonged bed rest exposes the patient to the hazards of immobility, particularly respiratory and vascular complications. Nursing measures to prevent the complications associated with immobility are described in Chapter 10. The armchair treatment permits the patient to be out of bed even on the second day postinfarction, depending on the patient's physiologic status. The patient is assisted to the chair at the bedside, or in some cases is lifted onto the chair. A bedside commode is generally utilized in preference to the bedpan. Stool softeners are often needed, since inactivity contributes to constipation, which may precipitate straining during defecation and result in excessive workload on the heart. The early use of the bedside commode and the armchair treatment should not, however, be construed to mean that the patient can readily begin ambulation.

The patient is taught to avoid using the Valsalva maneuver during movements in bed. The Valsalva maneuver refers to the action of holding the breath and keeping the chest fixed while straining. The action pushes air against the closed glottis, raising the intrathoracic pressure and interfering with venous return to the heart. In addition, when air is exhaled, the increased intrathoracic pressure falls, resulting in a sudden increase in venous return to the heart. The maneuver frequently occurs when the patient is in bed as when moving or pulling himself up in bed, getting on and off the bedpan, or straining during defecation. The dangers of the Valsalva maneuver require the nurse to teach the patient about the action and how to prevent it. He should be taught to breathe through his mouth when moving in bed and when doing any of the other activities that precipitate a Valsalva maneuver.

If the patient remains in a chair for long periods of time, the nurse should ensure that there is no pressure on the popliteal arteries. The legs should be elevated at intervals during prolonged sitting in order to prevent venous stasis. Increases in activities are allowed as vital signs stabilize, diagnostic evaluative data show no progression in damage, and as the patient's tolerance for activity increases. To detect the patient's tolerance, vital signs are observed before, during, and after the activity. Excessive changes in the vital signs as well as the incidence of pain or elevations in the enzyme studies all imply that activity is excessive or that myocardial damage has increased. These changes also indicate the need for strict enforcement of bed rest.

The psychological state of a patient with AMI is one of anxiety and fear related to the sensation of impending death during the attack of acute pain. Usually during the early period of hospitalization, the patient is concerned primarily with survival and obtaining relief from the pain. But soon, concerns about helplessness, dependency, inactivity, and possible incapacity come to the forefront. These concerns are devastating ones for any patient. To help cope with these fears and the insult to the body image, the patient frequently manifests denial of the cardiac disease. Refusal to adhere to restrictions is the most obvious sign of a denial mechanism. In some situations the masculinity of a male patient is so threatened that the patient expresses his anxiety in overt sexual overtones to the female nurses. It is the responsibility of the nurse to recognize the patient's psychological response to the crisis and respond to it in a therapeutic manner. The patient must be made aware that denial, anger, and periods of depression are common and normal reactions to a heart attack and that the nurse will be available to talk about the feelings and to help find more therapeutic means of coping with these feelings. In the case of the male patient who is showing aggressive sexual behavior, the nurse should consider such behavior as a sign of anxiety and fears related to sexual inadequacy or impotence resulting from the heart condition, as well as anxiety about potential changes in his image as the breadwinner and strong figure in the family. Rather than becoming flustered or embarrassed and withdrawing from the patient or becoming punitive, the nurse should attempt to determine the patient's understanding of his restrictions related to sexual activity after the heart attack. Depending on the patient's cardiac status and extent of myocardial damage, a return to prior sexual activity is generally permitted on an average of 8 to 10 weeks after the infarction. Suggestions for less strenuous techniques for intercourse and avoidance of intercourse when fatigued or after a heavy meal are important. Prophylactic use of nitroglycerine prior to intercourse may be helpful. If angina or other cardiac symptoms occur during intercourse, it may be necessary to modify techniques to avoid excitement and exertion. In some cases, abstinence may be necessary. Posthospitalization conferences with the physician and the patient, spouse, or both are indicated to determine the appropriate degree of sexual activity if sexual problems continue, or if the patient or spouse is still uncomfortable or anxious about the sexual activity.

In some patients, withdrawal is the mechanism that is used to cope with the stress of having an AMI. Fear of the implications of the illness may be manifested by the patient's reluctance to participate in any activity even when it is safe or therapeutic. The nurse's approach to most patients (depending on their general cardiac status) is based on the knowledge that the majority (50 to 80 percent) of patients who have had an AMI return to work and to their preinfarction level of physical activity. Reinforcing the patient's feelings of competence and importance is extremely important to his well-being. Sufficient time should be provided for the patient to express his fears prior to initiating a plan for increased activity.

Ambulation and activities can be increased as the patient progresses satisfactorily. If there are no complications, the patient is often transferred from the CCU in 3 to 5 days. In many hospitals, the patient is transferred to an intermediate care unit that utilizes telemetry monitoring. This portable monitoring system involves the transmission of ECG tracings to a monitor via electrodes attached to a patient through a battery-operated transmitter (no electric wire connects the patient to a monitor). This method allows continuous cardiac monitoring as the patient ambulates and increases activities. Several varieties of telemetry systems are available. They are being continually improved to overcome the disadvantages (increased frequency of false alarms and more signal interference with telemetry than with conventional hardware equipment) of this method. These disadvantages are being counteracted by improved antenna systems and the use of different radio frequencies to lessen interference. Electrode products are also being prepared with improved adhesives and conducting gels to withstand the increased activity of the patient. Electrodes are changed at least every other day (some factory-prepared gel pads need to be changed only every 5 days) to allow for cleaning and inspecting the skin in order to reduce the incidence of skin irritation. Anxiety often occurs when monitoring equipment is discontinued. Patients feel more secure during continuous monitoring and they fear that important signs will be missed. The patient may be extremely anxious when he is transferred from the intensive care setting of the CCU and may question whether he will continue to receive proper care. Emotional support and reassurance are imperative. Recurrence of chest pain, dyspnea, fatigue, or cardiac arrhythmias are assessed carefully and appropriate interventions are initiated. A significant number of deaths still occur after transfer from the CCU, and proper monitoring of the patient's vital signs and tolerance of activity is still necessary.

Patient teaching must continue for both the patient and his family about the significance of the heart attack, the coronary risk factors, physical activity and evaluation of the patient's tolerance for activity, the prescribed diet, and medications. The patient and his family should clearly understand the significance of angina; the use of nitroglycerine; when to notify the doctor; have a thorough understanding of the names, purposes, dosages, proper administration, and possible untoward effects of all the medications he will be receiving after discharge from the hospital; and be aware of the signs and symptoms that require medical assistance. The patient should weigh himself daily and should contact his doctor if rapid weight gains occur (more than 2 pounds in 24 hours or 4 pounds in a week). The observance of scheduled rest periods, the avoidance of fatigue, and the importance of regular medical checkups and adherence to the medical regimen cannot be overemphasized.

The nurse must help the patient and his family accept a realistic appraisal of his limitations. Modifications in life style, depending on the patient's cardiac status, may be required. In some situations, early retirement may be necessary; in others, a change of occupation. Most patients are able to return to their prior employment, although in some cases it is on a part-time basis. All patients should avoid heavy lifting after an MI and driving is restricted for about 6 weeks postdischarge.

The goal in long-term care is to restore the patient to an appropriate level of activity and to prevent recurrence of MI. Coronary clubs are being formed as a resource for patients and their families to cope with the stresses of having an MI. The local chapters of the American Heart Association are resources for pertinent written materials that are helpful in learning more about cardiac disease. The local heart association may also be a resource for information about vocational counseling. A public health nurse referral can be arranged to help the patient and his family in the transition from hospital to home care.

Active rehabilitation programs are being initiated to restore and improve cardiovascular function. These programs emphasize the prevention of recurrence of MI and the promotion of a high level of physical fitness. Preexercise testing and evaluation of the patient's cardiac status are carried out prior to prescribing an individualized activity program.

Currently, a nationwide survey is being conducted by the National Heart and Lung Institute, National Institutes of Health, to determine whether aspirin, which has an effect on blood clotting by altering platelet function, will decrease the risk of recurrent heart attacks in patients who have had a previous heart attack. The study is known as the Aspirin Myocardial Infarction Study (AMIS).

Complications of AMI

As stated previously, one of the goals of nursing care in AMI is to protect the patient from the complications associated with the condition. The complications to which the patient is particularly susceptible in this period include arrhythmias, shock, congestive heart failure, ventricular rupture, ventricular aneurysm, and thromboembolic phenomena.

One of the most frequent complications associated with MI, as previously cited, is the onset of arrhythmias such as AV block (the blocking of conduction through the AV node) and the potentially lethal ventricular arrhythmias. Some of the factors that precipitate the onset of arrhythmias are related to pain, anxiety, hypoxia, acidosis, hypokalemia, congestive heart failure, and activities that increase the workload of the heart. These precipitating factors, therefore, require nursing interventions that provide adequate control of pain, relief of anxiety by the use of appropriate sedatives or tranquilizers and psychological comfort measures, adequate oxygen administration, accurate intake and output records as a basis for fluid and electrolyte replacement, and the prevention of additional burdens on the heart, including the avoidance of straining during stool elimination and the avoidance of the Valsalva maneuver. Specific types of arrhythmias and indicated interventions, as well as the specifics in interpreting ECG tracings for monitoring cardiac function, are discussed later in this chapter, as are congestive heart failure and cardiogenic shock.

The patient with an extensive MI is particularly susceptible to ventricular rupture during the first or second week after the attack. Scar formation is initiated by the second week, so that rupture rarely occurs after that time. Ventricular rupture is most often associated with hypertension or with the inability to rest adequately. Excessive straining or excessive activity, especially before fibrosis begins, may lead to ventricular rupture, which is an immediately fatal complication. The intraventricular septum may also rupture if this is the site of infarction; however, it is a potentially repairable lesion, if recognized early.

When MI involves the papillary muscle, rupture of the muscle may result. This complication, although rare, may occur in the first week after the MI occurs. It is detectable by the presence of an apical systolic murmur associated with mitral valve incompetence.

Transmural infarction (involving the entire ventricular wall) is frequently complicated by the formation of ventricular aneurysm (dilatation). In addition to compromising the ventricular contraction and effectiveness, the aneurysm is a potential site for rupture.

Thromboembolic complications arise from mural thrombi or from circulatory stasis associated with the therapeutic regimen of obligatory bed rest. The use of an anticoagulant, usually initiated with heparin and later substituted by oral coumarin drugs, is the usual prophylactic measure utilized to combat this complication. (The management of patients receiving anticoagulants is discussed in relation to the use of anticoagulants in thromboembolic phenomena in peripheral vascular conditions later in this chapter and in Chapter 5.) In addition, cerebral emboli may result from MI and should be suspected when changes in sensorium occur without an evident decrease in blood volume or cardiac output. Pulmonary embolism usually associated with pelvic or leg thrombosis formation or with right-heart thrombosis is another type of complication following MI. This complication also warrants the use of prophylactic anticoagulant therapy in the early stages of MI. Controversy continues as to the value of long-term anticoagulant therapy after MI.

Pericarditis (inflammation of the pericardium) is evidenced by pericardial pain or a friction rub. The condition appears most frequently on the second or third day after the onset of symptoms of MI. Recurrent and continuing chest pain associated with pericarditis may be suggestive of recurrent ischemia and may be a source of concern for the patient who fears another attack. The patient should be advised that this is a fairly common finding after MI, but that the condition is a transient one and lasts a maximum of several days. The pain associated with the pericardial friction rub is aggravated with deep inspiration or by lying in a supine position. Although usually self-limiting in these situations, pericarditis may require treatment with antibiotics and pericardiocentesis.

Late complications of MI are those of postmyocardial infarction syndrome and the shoulder-hand syndrome. Postmyocardial infarction syndrome (also known as Dressler's syndrome) generally occurs 10 days to 3 months after the acute infarction. The condition is generally considered to be an autoimmune process. Fever, chest pain, and a pericardial friction rub are the presenting symptoms. The chest pain, which is usually pleuritic in nature (varying in intensity with changes in position or with deep breathing), can frighten the patient and initiate fears of a new infarction. The condition is usually benign and generally disappears spontaneously within 1 or 2 weeks. It is treated symptomatically and bed rest is usually required. On occasion, serious arrhythmias and cardiac tamponade may occur.

An unusual complication of MI is the shoulder-hand syndrome, which is characterized by the onset of pain and swelling in the shoulder or hand or both about one week to several months after infarction. Movement or palpation of the shoulder and hand may be quite painful. The skin of the involved area may even become atrophic. Although it is usually a benign condition that is treated symptomatically, it may on occasion result in muscular atrophy. The major complication associated with myocardial infarction is that of disturbances in cardiac rhythm, which will now be discussed.

ARRHYTHMIAS

Normally, the rate and rhythm of the cardiac contractions originate from impulses generated in the SA node. Efficient cardiac function, which responds appropriately to physiologic demands of the body, is dependent upon the orderly spread of the impulse through the heart. Cardiac arrhythmias (or dysrhythmias) are disorders of the rate or rhythm or both that may jeopardize cardiac function. The severity of resultant circulatory alterations depends on the type of arrhythmia, the underlying cause, the associated disease of the heart, the duration and frequency of the arrhythmia, the psychological reaction of the patient, and the availability of appropriate intervention.

Arrhythmias may affect both normal and diseased hearts. Exercise, infections, drugs, emotional states, and stimulants such as coffee and cigarette smoking, for example, may cause arrhythmias in normal hearts as well as in diseased hearts. Arrhythmias may also be associated with disturbances of other organ systems such as sympathetic and vagal stimulation due to central nervous system disease, pulmonary disease, endocrine disease, anemia, and renal disorders. Some arrhythmias that occur fairly frequently will be discussed in this section. Sinus and atrial arrhythmias will be discussed first, followed by arrhythmias of the AV node (including treatment by cardiac pacing) and ventricular arrhythmias.

The diagnosis of an arrhythmia is confirmed with an ECG, but is suspected when pulse changes are detected on palpation of the radial pulse or during auscultation of the apical pulse. Palpitations, dizziness, angina, faintness, edema, shortness of breath, dyspnea, and other signs of congestive heart failure also may indicate the presence of an arrhythmia. Patients who are susceptible to arrhythmias (such as the patient with a recent MI) and those with potentially dangerous cardiac alterations, as well as those already demonstrating arrhythmias, are generally placed on continuous cardiac monitoring for varying prolonged periods.

Before a discussion of individual types of arrhythmias, it is important to review some of the components of an ECG tracing and the characteristics of normal sinus rhythm. The reader is referred to Figures 4-4 and 4-7 for information on the normal conduction of the heart and its relation to the normal ECG. ECG paper is marked so that voltage in millivolts is measured vertically and time in seconds is measured horizontally. The fine lines on the ECG graph are 1 mm apart both horizontally and vertically, and the heavier lines are spaced at 5-mm intervals both horizontally and vertically (Fig. 4-9). The speed of the paper through the machine is 25 mm per second, so that each fine line represents 0.04 second and each heavy vertical line represents 0.20 second. The standard setting is usually such that 1 cm (two large boxes) is equal to 1 mv. The diagram in Figure 4-9 is a normal ECG cycle and indicates the normal duration of the various component waves and complexes. When evaluating a particular tracing, the nurse should determine whether artifacts that might cause misinterpretation of the ECG are present. Artifacts result from alternating-current interference (reflected by regular deflections at 60 cycles per second), from muscle tremor (reflected by irregular jerks on the tracing), and a wandering baseline on the tracing. Artifacts may be mistaken for arrhythmias (even ventricular fibrillation) by the inexperienced evaluator. Examination of the patient and reevaluation of the ECG tracing will assist the nurse in validating the presence of artifacts; for example, an alert patient with palpable pulse is obviously not in ventricular fibrillation.

The heart rate is determined by identifying the P waves and counting the number of small squares between two P waves. If the rhythm is regular, 1,500 (1,500 small squares equals 60

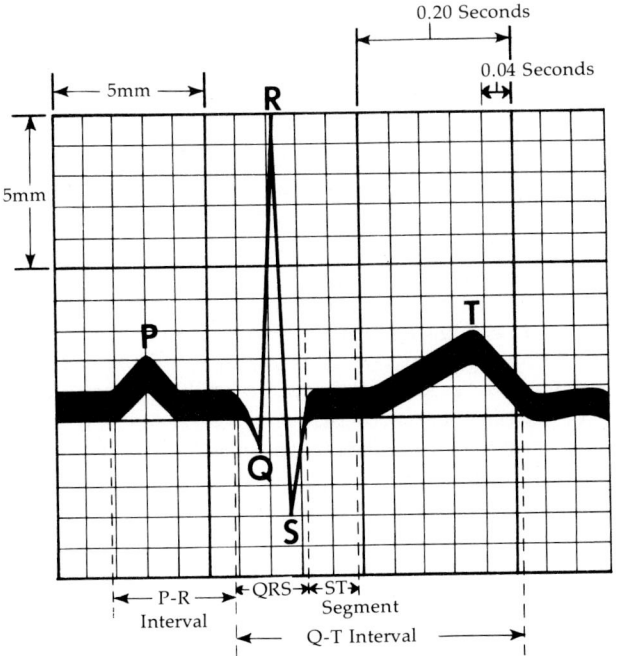

Figure 4-9
Typical lead II tracing. Normal ranges of intervals as well as segments and waveforms are identified.

seconds) is divided by the number of 0.04-second squares between two P waves to determine the atrial rate. Ventricular rate may be determined in several ways. If the rhythm is regular, 1,500 is divided by the number of 0.04-second squares between two QRS complexes (that is, between the R waves). Another method is to divide the number 300 (300 of the 0.20-second squares in 60 seconds) by the number of 0.20-second squares between two QRS complexes. If the rhythm is irregular, the number of cycles in 6 seconds (15 cm) is counted and multiplied by 10 to determine the ventricular rate. If the rhythm is regular, the distance between the R waves is identical. Measuring the distance between R waves with calipers is done to confirm this. (If calipers are not available, a paper and pencil method may be used; that is, the space between two P waves is marked on a paper which is then used to check the space between other sets of P waves.) The same techniques are used for measuring the regularity of ventricular rhythm.

A narrow QRS segment implies supraventricular origin; a broad, widened QRS complex implies ventricular origin or supraventricular origin with abnormal ventricular conduction. In most leads, the positive deflection in a QRS complex is an R wave and is preceded by a negative deflection, which is the Q wave, and followed by an S wave, which is also a negative deflection. The QRS complex is examined for symmetry in configuration and the presence of any premature QRS complexes, which are broad and different in configuration.

Atrial complexes are examined for abnormal configurations, rhythms, or rates. The examiner should also note whether every P wave is followed by a QRS complex. The PR interval is measured; normally it is 0.16 to 0.20 second (from the onset of the P wave to the beginning of the QRS complex). The QRS complex is usually 0.08 second and the ST segment is usually 0.12 second. Normally the ST segment of the cycle is neither elevated nor depressed. ST segment displacement, however, is diagnostic in MI. A small wave may follow a T wave, which is ordinarily the last large deflection in the cycle. This small wave is identified as a U wave, which may or may not be related to heart disease. U waves are especially prominent in the ECGs of patients with hypokalemia. From these examinations and measurements, and with practice in a simulated and actual setting, the nurse should be able to describe the ECG pattern, determine whether arrhythmia is present, and ascertain whether it is supraventricular or ventricular in origin or a conduction defect.

Sinus Arrhythmias

Arrhythmias are classified according to their location and their mechanism. When a normal P wave is followed by a normal QRS (and a normal PR interval), it can be assumed that the SA node is the pacemaker and the rhythm is described as normal sinus rhythm. The SA node is sensitive to sympathetic nervous stimuli, which increase the heart rate, and to parasympathetic stimuli, which slow the rate. These changes may occur during emotional states, blood chemistry changes, or as the effect of drugs, heart disease, and changes in metabolic rates. Thus arrhythmias originating in the sinus node have normal ECG patterns, but vary in their rates such as in sinus tachycardia (above 100 per minute) and sinus bradycardia (below 60 per minute). Deep breathing and respiratory cycles may also result in sinus arrhythmias. Although sinus arrhythmias are usually not of major significance and sinus tachycardia may in fact be a compensatory mechanism, prolonged sinus tachycardia may cause a strain on the myocardium and result in ineffective contractions. Sinus bradycardia, which in vulnerable persons may lead to a severe decrease in cardiac output resulting in congestive heart failure and insufficient cerebral blood flow, may be a normal occurrence in athletes or manual laborers who maintain adequate cardiac output with a slowed rate. It may also be the result of digitalis toxicity, hyperkalemia, or vasovagal attacks associated with gagging, forceful vomiting, and trauma to the eye. Treatment requires correction of the underlying cause. Atropine is indicated to counteract vagal stimulation; isoproterenol (Isuprel) is given to increase the heart rate; electrolyte imbalances are corrected; digitalis is discontinued; and cardiac pacing may be indicated in some cases.

Sick sinus syndrome is a term that describes a variety of arrhythmias and symptoms associated with malfunctioning of the SA node. The symptoms are caused by decreased cardiac output. Circulatory changes, congestive heart failure, and arteriosclerotic heart disease, as well as a variety of other conditions, are precipitating factors of the syndrome.

When the SA node is suppressed or is impaired or when a normal impulse is blocked through failure of conduction, ectopic foci outside the normal sinus node pacemaker (the atria, AV junctional tissue, or ventricle) are able to initiate impulses. The term **escape beats** describes the ectopic rhythm that develops as a result. The term **supraventricular arrhythmia** refers to an arrhythmia that originates in the SA node, atria, or AV junction.

Sinus arrest occurs when another pacemaker does not escape and take over immediately when the sinus node fails. One or more entire cycles may be missed. The seriousness of this arrhythmia is determined by the duration of the resulting pause and by the ability of an escape pacemaker to temporarily assume heart control. If no other pacemaker takes over, ventricular standstill and unexpected death result. In other situations, sinus arrest is so short that no symptoms result or, in some instances, syncope and dizziness may result when asystole is prolonged.

Sinus arrest is usually the result of ischemic necrosis of the SA node, increased vagal tone, or the effects of myocardial depressant drugs or electrolyte disturbances such as hyperkalemia. Temporary transvenous cardiac pacing is the preferred treatment, especially in patients who are on myocardial depressant drugs. Persistent sinus arrest obviously requires cardiopulmonary resuscitation techniques.

Atrial Arrhythmias

Any abnormal pacemaker will change the direction of the current and the shape of the wave on the ECG. Impulses that originate within the atrial walls are characterized by an abnormally shaped P wave (either inverted, diphasic, or notched). The QRS complex, however, continues to be initiated in a normal manner.

Extrasystoles are **premature atrial contractions.** An irritable focus in the atrium initiates this impulse and stimulates ventricular contraction before the next normal impulse is due. Generally a compensatory pause in the rhythm occurs until the next normal SA impulse arrives, because the ventricles have to recover from the contraction associated with the abnormal atrial impulse. **Paroxysmal atrial tachycardia** occurs when an irritable focus in the atrial wall beats at a rapid but regular rate of 150 to 250 per minute. A rapid onset and short duration are characteristic of this arrhythmia. It is commonly seen in young adults with normal hearts, but may be a sign of cardiac irritability that may proceed to persistent atrial tachycardia and seriously jeopardize a vulnerable heart. Treatment is by vagal stimulation via carotid massage, the Valsalva maneuver, or by stimulating the gag reflex with a tongue depressor. Digitalis may be utilized; propranolol (Inderal) and metaraminol (Aramine) have been used in other protocols. When antiarrhythmic drugs are contraindicated, direct-current synchronized electrical shock (cardioversion) may be used.

The **Wolff-Parkinson-White syndrome** (also referred to as "accelerated conduction syndrome" or the W-P-W syndrome) is characterized by sudden attacks of supraventricular arrhythmias, particularly atrial tachycardia. It is a preexcitation syndrome in which the SA node impulse bypasses the normal conduction pathway, resulting in early ventricular activation. Although it is often found in normal hearts, frequent episodes of the syndrome may cause myocardial weakness. Various antiarrhythmic drugs are used to treat this syndrome.

Atrial flutter is characterized by an atrial rate of about 250 to 350. The rate may be so rapid that the AV node is able to transmit only some of the impulses, resulting in a slower ventricular rate (a 2:1 or 3:1 or 4:1 ratio, or block). The ventricular rate may be a normal rate as a result. The P waves on the ECG tracing are uniform in configuration but have a sawtooth appearance (Fig. 4-10). Digitalis has been the classic treatment of atrial flutter, but cardioversion may be utilized as a

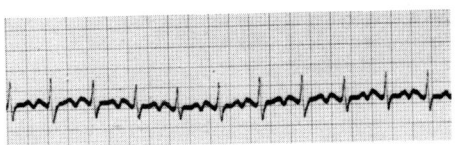

Figure 4-10
Electrocardiogram depicting atrial flutter. (From G. H. Whipple et al., *Acute Coronary Care*. Boston: Little, Brown and Company, 1972. Reproduced by permission.)

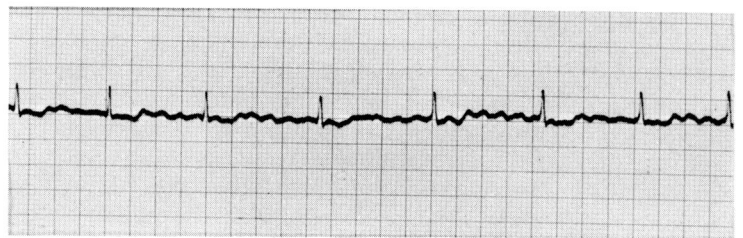

Figure 4-11
Electrocardiogram depicting atrial fibrillation. (From G. H. Whipple et al., *Acute Coronary Care*. Boston: Little, Brown and Company, 1972. Reproduced by permission.)

more rapid technique for terminating the arrhythmia.

In **atrial fibrillation** the irritable focus is so rapid that the atrial rate may be over 400. In contrast to premature atrial contractions and paroxysmal atrial tachycardia, the impulses in atrial fibrillation come from different foci and cause irregular contractions and P waves that are different in configuration. Effective atrial contraction is thus replaced by fibrillatory waves, sometimes designated as *f* waves (Fig. 4–11). Not all of these P waves are transmitted through the AV node, so that the ventricular rate is irregular, although normal in configuration. The condition is usually found in older patients with arteriosclerotic heart disease, which has caused scarring of the atrium. Atrial fibrillation generally causes a pulse deficit, which can be determined by comparing the apical and radial pulses. The rate and volume of the ventricular contraction are such that the apical rate is higher than the radial rate (that is, all contractions do not result in a palpable radial pulse).

If the atrial fibrillation is not caused by excessive digitalis, which occasionally is the precipitating factor, the drug is usually indicated. Digitalis is given to increase the refractory period of the AV node, thus reducing the number of impulses that reach the ventricles. Quinidine and procainamide have also been used to combat atrial fibrillation. Atrial fibrillation may result in cardiac enlargement and failure, embolic phenomena, and susceptibility to sudden death. Therefore, if atrial fibrillation is a life-threatening situation, cardioversion is indicated. If the patient has been receiving digitalis, cardioversion may result in lethal arrhythmias. Generally, digitalis is discontinued for several days prior to attempting elective cardioversion.

The cardioversion procedure usually includes the administration of diazepam (Valium) 10 mg intravenously unless it is contraindicated by the urgency of the clinical situation. Monitoring electrodes are applied if they are not already in place. Two large electrodes are applied with electrode jelly to the chest. One electrode is usually applied to the apex and the other to the right side of the upper sternum (anterior approach). An anteroposterior approach utilizes one electrode under the left lower scapula and a second electrode over the left midprecordium. Cardioversion for treating atrial fibrillation usually is started with 50 to 100 joules (wattseconds). The cardioverter is synchronized so that the shock is not applied during the vulnerable period of the T wave. No one should touch the patient or the bed during the cardioversion procedure in order to avoid receiving a shock. The nurse should provide emotional support for the patient as well as observe vital signs and be prepared for emergency treatment of complications.

In some protocols, anticoagulants are initiated prior to anticipated conversion of atrial fibrillation (either by drugs or electrocardioversion). There is a risk of embolization when cardiac contractions become coordinated and strengthened, because uncoordinated contractions typical of atrial fibrillation interfere with forward propulsion of the blood and thus predispose to thrombus formation. It should be noted that there is a risk of embolism from the atrial fibrillation itself due to increased turbulence in the atria.

Atrioventricular Node Arrhythmias
The atrioventricular (AV) node may take over as pacemaker of the heart, causing distinct characteristics of the so-called nodal rhythm.

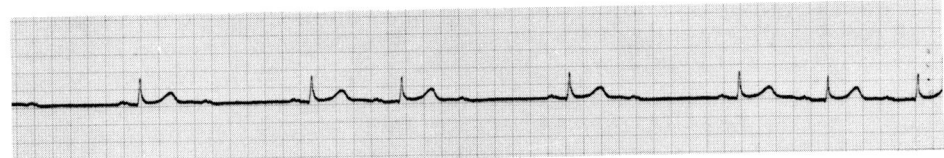

Figure 4-12
Electrocardiogram depicting second-degree heart block (Wenckebach). (From G. H. Whipple et al., *Acute Coronary Care*. Boston: Little, Brown and Company, 1972. Reproduced by permission.)

Nodal stimulation alters the spread of the impulse through the atrium, usually causing an inversion of a P wave or causing it to be nondetectable within the QRS complex that rapidly follows nodal stimulation. The PR interval also is usually less than 0.12 second. Premature nodal contractions and nodal tachycardia also may occur. Nodal tachycardia is managed according to protocols used for atrial tachycardia. AV block involves an impairment in the conduction of electrical impulses between the atrium and ventricle. The condition, which may be either a partial or complete heart block, is most commonly caused by arteriosclerosis and MI. The degree of impairment of AV conduction is described as first-, second-, or third-degree AV block.

First-degree AV block is characterized by an increased length of the PR interval on the ECG. The P wave, however, is normal and is consistently transmitted through the ventricles. The PR interval exceeds 0.20 second, the upper limit of the normal range. The condition is associated with damage of tissue around the AV node such as in coronary artery disease or rheumatic fever, but may also result from the effects of digitalis or quinidine. It may be the precursor to a more serious heart block.

Second-degree heart block is characterized by impulses being blocked at varying intervals, as conduction is slowed and the PR interval becomes more prolonged. There are two types of second-degree block, classified by their pattern of blockage of atrial impulses. Type I is called Mobitz I, or the Wenckebach phenomenon, and type II is called Mobitz II. **Mobitz I** is characterized by progressive prolongation of the PR interval until a point at which a P wave is not conducted through the AV node (Fig. 4-12). The QRS complex is normal, however, and not broadened. **Mobitz II** is considered more ominous than type I because it often progresses abruptly to third-degree block. Mobitz II is characterized by a fixed PR interval, which may or may not be within normal time limits, but which blocks every second, third, or fourth impulse from the atria.

In **third-degree block,** also known as complete heart block, atrial electrical current is not transmitted to the ventricles. The automatic cells of the ventricle must take over, usually at a very slow rate of 30 to 40 beats per minute. The atrium continues to depolarize, so P waves appear on the ECG tracing, but they have no consistent relation to the QRS complexes (Fig. 4-13). In addition, the QRS complexes are often grossly abnormal as in premature ventricular contractions. Third-degree heart block is associated with rheumatic fever, fibrosis (resulting from MI), digitalis toxicity, and congenital anomalies.

The seriousness of heart blocks increases as

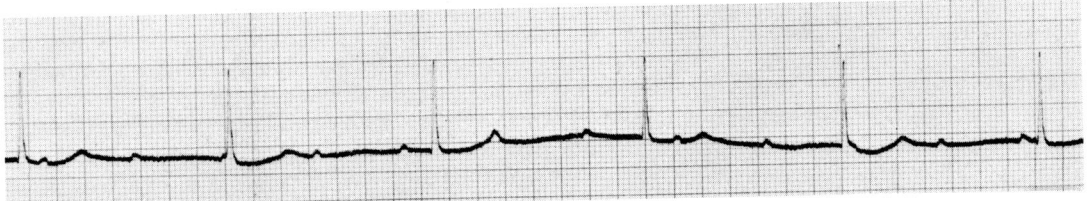

Figure 4-13
Electrocardiogram depicting third-degree (complete) heart block. (From G. H. Whipple et al., *Acute Coronary Care*. Boston: Little, Brown and Company, 1972. Reproduced by permission.)

the cardiac rate decreases. Serious bradycardias below 50 beats per minute cannot support normal daily activities and cardiac ischemia can result. A slowed heart may cause a deficient cerebral flow resulting in the **Stokes-Adams syndrome.** This syndrome is characterized by transient syncope, dizziness, and convulsions; cardiac arrest or shock may result. Stokes-Adams syndrome may occur with ventricular asystole when AV conduction ceases and before an idioventricular focus begins to assume the pacing of the heart. An idioventricular focus may also stop forming impulses in an established complete heart block, resulting in ventricular asystole and loss of consciousness. Patients who have suffered from an episode of Stokes-Adams syndrome are candidates for cardiac pacing. In the interval until pacing becomes initiated, isoproterenol (Isuprel) usually is indicated, to stimulate the heart action. The patient should be assisted to conserve energy and reduce the demands on his heart. The vital signs are monitored and the patient is observed for effects of reduced cardiac output, such as disorientation, syncope, oliguria, dyspnea, or angina. Attention to safety measures is essential.

First-degree block usually is not treated, but the patient is observed to detect advancement to more serious blocks. If the condition is caused by digitalis effects, a change in dosage or withdrawal of the drug is indicated. Second-degree block often responds to atropine or to isoproterenol, the latter being diluted and administered by slow intravenous infusion. Some cardiologists insert a pacemaker when second-degree block occurs, to facilitate rapid initiation of the pacemaker if and when the pulse rate falls to dangerously low rates.

As mentioned previously, complete heart block may be treated with isoproterenol, but its effectiveness cannot be relied upon for long periods of time. A temporary or permanent pacemaker is indicated.

Bundle-Branch Block

When the specialized conducting tissue of the Purkinje fibers is impaired, the impulse must instead travel through the ventricular muscle itself. In contrast to atrial tachycardias, which do not distort the QRS complexes, bundle-branch blocks (BBBs) result in some widening of the QRS. Compared to a normal QRS width (usually 0.10 second), complete BBB causes a QRS width of 0.12 second or more. BBB may be in either or both subdivisions of the left bundle branch or in the right bundle branch. In general, LBBB is considered more serious than RBBB, because the latter is usually associated with left ventricular disease. BBB may also be the result of digitalis toxicity [17].

Because cardiac pacing is most frequently used to treat heart block, this aspect of therapy will be discussed prior to a discussion of ventricular arrythmias.

CARDIAC PACING

Pacemakers are used in the control of intermittent or complete heart block, particularly in the Stokes-Adams syndrome, for control of arrhythmia associated with MI, following open heart surgery, and also in an attempt to suppress tachyarrhythmias.

Artificial cardiac pacemakers are available for temporary and permanent pacing. The artificial pacemaker is an electronic device that initiates electrical stimuli to the heart for control of heart rate. Temporary pacing utilizes internally fixed electrodes but the generating power source (the battery packet) remains outside the body, either strapped to the patient's waistline or attached to the arm with a compressive bandage. In permanent pacemakers the electrodes are either myocardial electrodes directly implanted in the ventricle (during thoracotomy) or catheter electrodes. A transistorized power source is implanted subcutaneously either in the right or left axilla–subclavicular space or subcutaneously in the upper abdomen (Fig. 4-14).

The most frequent method for inserting either a temporary or a permanent pacemaker is the transvenous route for endocardial pacing. This method involves the insertion of an electrode catheter either percutaneously or by cutdown through a vein leading to the vena cava (either the antebrachial, jugular, femoral, or subclavian vein) into the atrium and down into the ventricle. An attempt is made to stabilize the catheter in the trabecula of the heart. The catheter may be the "semifloating" type or the less flexible and heavier standard type [14]. It is usually inserted under fluoroscopy, but may be inserted under electrographic control.

There are other less frequently used approaches to inserting either temporary or

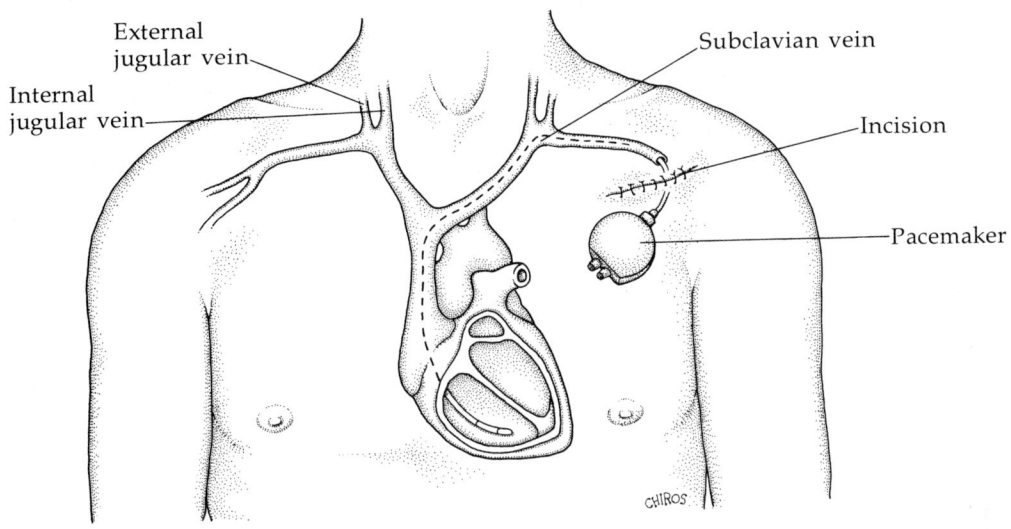

Figure 4-14
A permanent pacemaker; note site of insertion and location of power source.

permanent pacemakers. A permanent pacemaker may be inserted in a transthoracic approach via thoracotomy, under general anesthesia. It may be done, for example, if dislodgement has occurred several times when the transvenous approach has been used. The electrodes are sutured into the myocardium at the left ventricle. Such a procedure makes the patient vulnerable to all the complications associated with chest surgery and anesthesia.

During cardiac surgery, temporary epicardial pacing may be facilitated by suturing three very thin wires in place (one in the atrial epicardium, one in the ventricular epicardium, and one as a subcutaneous lead) and bringing them out through the chest wall. The external wires are usually enclosed in a gauze dressing. Care should be taken that no tension is applied on these wires in order to avert displacement. If pacing becomes necessary, the wires can be attached to a pulse generator. The wires are usually pulled out through the skin several days postoperatively when the patient's condition has stabilized.

Other emergency approaches for pacing are the transthoracic and external types, which are rarely used in current practice. In the emergency transthoracic approach, a thin wire electrode is inserted directly into the myocardium through a needle in the chest wall. This blind approach, however, may cause arterial trauma and pericardial tamponade and is therefore used infrequently. External emergency pacing involves the use of electrodes and electrical current applied directly to the skin to deliver impulses through the chest wall. Local pain and skin burns may result because large amounts of current are required to penetrate the chest wall.

Cardiac pacemakers are of three types according to the rate of pacing activity: (1) fixed rate, (2) synchronous, and (3) demand. A **fixed-rate** type functions with the generation of impulses at a predetermined rate (about 60 to 70 beats per minute). The fixed-rate type is of limited value because there is no way to alter the rate if physiologic demands warrant an increase. The fixed-rate type may also compete with the intrinsic rhythm of the heart. It may be used, however, in complete heart block when competition is less likely to occur.

A **synchronous pacemaker** utilizes a sensing device in the atrium that triggers impulses to the ventricles after a predetermined interval. An atrial synchronous pacemaker provides the most normal heart activity of the three types. Its disadvantage, however, is that any atrial arrhythmia or atrial disease that might develop will interfere with its function.

A **demand pacemaker** is the most common

type used currently. It triggers a ventricular impulse only when the patient's own heart rate falls below preset limits (usually below 60 to 70 beats per minute). If ventricular standstill occurs, the demand pacemaker will discharge at a fixed rate. This type is particularly useful for patients with intermittent heart block or bradycardia. It has the advantage of not competing with the intrinsic rhythm.

A **temporary pacemaker** is generally placed during an emergency or semiemergency type of situation. Temporary pacing may be done for hours, days, or weeks, depending on the needs of the individual patient. It often is continued until a permanent pacemaker can be installed. Temporary pacing allows an opportunity to determine the patient's response and the optimum pacing rate. Temporary pacemakers may also be inserted prophylactically and activated only when needed. They are powered by external generators that vary in sensitivity controls and sensing mechanisms. (The nurse is advised to read the literature provided with the individual pacemaker regarding its specific functioning and maintenance.)

Problems associated with temporary pacemakers are related to the necessary continued immobilization of the extremity involved with the insertion site and pulse generator. If an antecubital vein is used, the arm should be extended and secured on an arm board to prevent any tension on the electrode or generator. Finger exercises and some range-of-motion exercises of the shoulder are indicated to prevent venous stasis, but they should be done cautiously. Other problems are related to the potential for infection at the site of insertion. There is also a potential for electrical hazards because of the exposed external wires, which can come in contact with improperly grounded equipment, oil, or water. Electric shavers or other unnecessary electrical items are therefore contraindicated [18]. Only three-pronged, properly grounded equipment should be used in the vicinity of a patient with a temporary pacemaker.

The placement of a permanent pacemaker is generally a scheduled procedure that allows time for thorough preparation of the patient. The patient and his family are oriented to the purpose of the pacemaker, how it works, the anticipated results, and the procedure itself. The physiologic reasons requiring the pacemaker and its anticipated benefits are explained in terms of the patient's own symptoms and at the level of his understanding. The opportunity to hold and see a pacemaker model is usually helpful in understanding how it functions and the need for replacement of its power source. One of the most frequently asked questions by patients anticipating a permanent pacemaker is related to the length of battery viability. Batteries usually last from 18 to 20 months. Patients are advised that batteries can be replaced readily in a minor surgical procedure under local anesthesia. Researchers are attempting to develop batteries that will be more reliable and will last a decade or longer; pacemakers powered by a small capsule of plutonium 238 have recently been developed.

When a pacemaker is inserted, the nursing care plan or record should indicate the date of insertion, the type of pacemaker, and the rate for which it has been set. Usually a note is also added stating the amount of current being administered (milliamperes; mA).

Nursing care of the patient immediately following a pacemaker insertion centers on measures to prevent displacement of the catheter, preventing arrhythmias, initiation and maintenance of the pacemaker, providing an electrically safe environment, prevention of infection, and orientation and preparation for management of the pacemaker by the patient and his family.

Arm activity on the side of the pacemaker insertion is limited postoperatively. Coughing and vomiting should be prevented to avoid any sudden jerking of the body that might dislodge the catheter electrode. The patient is generally restricted temporarily to a supine position with the bed elevated to a maximum 30° angle. Deep breathing, leg exercises (unless femoral insertion has been done), and use of elastic stockings will help prevent pulmonary and vascular complications. In addition, turning to the side is generally restricted for a period of 1 to 3 days (depending on institutional protocols) to allow fibrosis to form around the pacemaker. In some protocols, the patient is less restricted and may turn on the left side. The nurse must observe for signs of displacement of the pacemaker electrode. These signs include hiccoughs (which may indicate perforation of the ventricle), an ECG tracing demonstrating that the pacing stimulus does not cause ventricular contraction, or disconnection of the electrode wire from an external pulse generator. Cardiac tamponade may occur as the result of perforation of the ventricle by the catheter.

The patient who has had catheter manipulation of the heart is vulnerable to cardiac irritability and arrhythmias. Continuous monitoring is indicated after pacemaker insertion. The nurse should observe for a pacemaker artifact (noted as a spike) before the QRS complex on the ECG when a demand pacemaker has been inserted. In such a case, the artifact will occur only when the patient's heart is not beating within the predetermined rate. If the patient's pulse is below the preset rate and no spike is observed, the demand pacemaker is obviously not functioning and the rate and amplitude of the pacemaker may need adjusting. In the temporary pacemaker, adjustments are made on the dial of the generator. In the permanent pacemaker, adjustments are made by the physician using a magnetic switch, an electrical induction control, or a screw needle inserted through the skin [19].

Observation for bleeding, discoloration, pain, and hematoma at the insertion site is necessary. Wound care involves cleaning the insertion site with an antiseptic and applying an antibiotic ointment and a sterile dressing once the original pressure dressing is removed. Wound care varies according to institutional protocols from twice daily to daily or every other day schedules.

The patient with a permanent pacemaker and his family need a teaching program to assure proper management of the pacemaker. Some type of identification (such as a Medic-Alert bracelet) should be worn at all times with information about the pacemaker (date of insertion, type, and preset rate).

The patient should avoid causing pressure or strain over the insertion area of the pacemaker. Arm activity (excessive stretching or lifting) on the side of insertion is restricted. For example, hanging clothes on a clothesline is contraindicated. Clothing should fit loosely around the area of the implant. Both male and female patients may be concerned about ways to disguise the protrusion on the chest that is evident from the implanted pulse generator.

Household electrical appliances, except microwave ovens, will not interfere with a pacemaker. Caution is taken, however, to avoid close contact with running lawnmowers and boat or automobile engines. Persons with pacemakers should advise dentists and hospital personnel that they have a pacemaker. They also need to show medical proof of the presence of a pacemaker when passing through airport monitoring devices. No danger is associated with bathing or showering because the system is completely enclosed in the body, but caution is required around electrocautery, diathermy, and other large electrical equipment.

Following pacemaker insertion, activities are resumed gradually and often exceed the level of tolerance prior to pacemaker insertion. The patient and a member of his family are taught to take the patient's radial pulse for a full minute at least once daily. Return demonstrations are essential to assure the nurse that the procedure has been learned appropriately and that the patient is able to recognize irregularities in rhythm. The patient should know how to detect pacemaker failure; he should notify his physician immediately if signs of failure occur. These signs include (1) a significant change in the pulse rate—a decrease of 5 or more beats—for a demand pacemaker and either a decrease or increase of 5 or more beats for a fixed-rate pacemaker; and (2) a return of symptoms such as dizziness, faintness, edema, shortness of breath, and palpitations.

The patient requiring a pacemaker is usually an older person. He will need sufficient time to ask questions and to discuss his fears about the pacemaker and his cardiac problem. Sufficient time for practicing pulse-taking should be allowed. Often a public health nurse can help the patient and his family in the adjustment to the pacemaker after discharge from the hospital. The family (or a friend or neighbor) also should be taught how to monitor the pulse and observe for significant signs of battery failure. However, overconcern with the pacemaker may cause as many problems as denial or inadequate concern, and appropriate guidance and counseling are necessary.

Battery replacement is likely to be needed about 18 to 24 months after insertion. The procedure is done under local anesthesia and

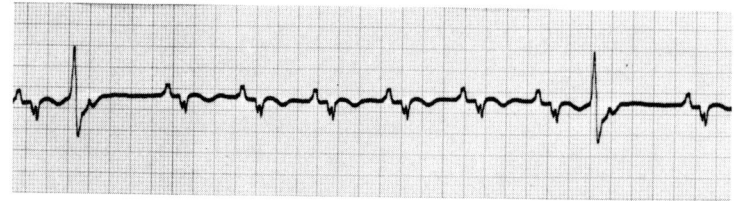

Figure 4-15
Electrocardiogram depicting premature ventricular contraction. (From G. H. Whipple et al., *Acute Coronary Care*. Boston: Little, Brown and Company, 1972. Reproduced by permission.)

involves reopening of the incision to remove the old power source and replacement with a new power source. The same electrode, however, is utilized. Usually the patient is discharged from the hospital the next day.

The patient requires periodic medical follow-up care, including ECGs at regular intervals and chest x-rays to monitor the function and integrity of the pacemaker.

Ventricular Arrhythmias

Ectopic foci in the ventricle cause ventricular arrhythmias that result in distorted and prolonged QRS complexes.

Premature ventricular contractions (PVCs or VPCs), also known as ventricular extrasystoles, occur when an ectopic ventricular focus stimulates a premature contraction of the ventricles, followed usually by a compensatory pause in the cycle until the next normal beat arrives (Fig. 4-15). A PVC is not preceded by a P wave, since the beat does not originate in the sinus node. In addition to a broadened and distorted shape, the voltage (height) of the QRS complex is greater than normal.

Premature ventricular contractions may occur in normal persons secondary to cigarette smoking, drinking excess coffee, and alcohol. The sensations may be described as palpitations. In patients with MI or chest pain, PVCs indicate potential ventricular tachycardia and fibrillation. PVCs are considered particularly dangerous and require aggressive treatment when they occur more frequently than 6 per minute, in groups of 2, 3, or more, when they land close to the vulnerable period of the preceding T wave, or when they have multiple shapes, indicating more than one irritable ventricular focus. In these situations, lidocaine, usually 50 to 100 mg, is given as a bolus injection, or it may be incorporated into an intravenous solution to provide 1 to 4 mg per minute. If sinus bradycardia is present, however, the PVCs may actually be a compensatory mechanism and lidocaine may be contraindicated. In this situation, atropine may be given in lieu of the lidocaine, which would depress myocardial excitability and cause further slowing of the cardiac rate. Procainamide HCl (Pronestyl) and quinidine, as well as propranolol (Inderal), are other drugs used to control PVCs.

Ventricular tachycardia is characterized by a sudden onset of rapidly recurring extrasystoles with widened and bizarre configurations, at a rate of 150 to 250, and with no normal beats in between (Fig. 4-16). This is a dangerous arrhythmia that must be corrected immediately to prevent decreased cardiac output and ventricular fibrillation. Lidocaine 75 to 100 mg as a slowly administered intravenous bolus is given and repeated

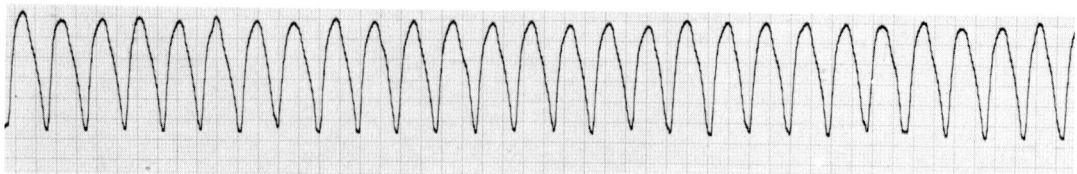

Figure 4-16
Electrocardiogram depicting ventricular tachycardia. (From G. H. Whipple et al., *Acute Coronary Care*. Boston: Little, Brown and Company, 1972. Reproduced by permission.)

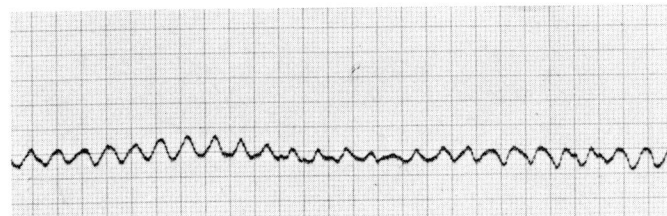

Figure 4-17
Electrocardiogram depicting ventricular fibrillation. (From G. H. Whipple et al., *Acute Coronary Care*. Boston: Little, Brown and Company, 1972. Reproduced by permission.)

in 2 to 3 minutes, followed by a continuous infusion (usually 5% dextrose in water) that delivers 1 to 4 mg per minute. Caution is required in avoiding circulatory overload if the patient is susceptible to congestive heart failure. Procainamide or quinidine may also be used as antiarrhythmic therapy in ventricular tachycardia.

Cardioversion, beginning with 100 to 200 joules, is initiated if lidocaine therapy is ineffective or if the patient's clinical condition deteriorates. The electrical impulse is synchronized with the QRS complex so that ventricular fibrillation is not induced by a stimulus during the vulnerable phase of the cardiac cycle (the upstroke of the T wave). A sedative or light anesthetic usually is given to minimize the discomfort of the patient.

Ventricular fibrillation causes a bizarre pattern of electrical activity that is erratic and uncoordinated (Fig. 4-17). It may be a sequel to ventricular tachycardia or it may occur spontaneously. Complete disorganization of the heartbeat results in the absence of any effective cardiac contraction and, functionally, ventricular fibrillation is equivalent to cardiac standstill or asystole. Without immediate treatment, ventricular fibrillation produces cardiac arrest and death. In ventricular fibrillation, there is no palpable or audible pulse or B.P. Within 4 minutes, cardiopulmonary resuscitation must be initiated. If the arrhythmia occurs in a hospital where defibrillation equipment is available, external defibrillation is indicated immediately (Fig. 4-18). Direct-current countershock (electrical discharge to the patient's chest wall) is used to cause simultaneous depolarization of the heart muscle and to halt ectopic impulse formation; as a result, all the myocardial fibers are brought into the same refractory period [14]. The normal pacemaker then becomes able to resume its usual sequence of excitation. In adults, a defibrillation charge of 400 joules, or less if the patient is on digitalis, is utilized. Electrode paste is applied to two paddle electrodes, which are firmly placed on the chest, one to the right of the upper sternum in the second interspace and the other just below the left nipple at the apex. No one should touch the patient or the bed during the defibrillation in order to prevent receiving the shock also. The paddles are removed immediately after the shock is administered, but defibrillation is repeated until organized cardiac excitation occurs. Intracardiac injections of epinephrine or intravenous injections of lidocaine or procainamide may be used to facilitate electrical conversion. (The use of intracardiac injections is controversial due to the hazard of causing cardiac trauma.)

When a defibrillator is not immediately available, the nurse should first pound on the chest once and then initiate resuscitation by external cardiac massage and mouth-to-mouth breathing to maintain effective circulation and ventilation. Acidosis is inevitable and requires correction with administration of sodium bicarbonate.

Nursing care of the patient with an arrhythmia requires a thorough knowledge of the drugs commonly administered to reverse arrhythmias, as well as of the other measures utilized, such as cardioversion and defibrillation. The names of the more common drugs used to reverse arrhythmias are given in Table 4-3. Digitalis is not included in this list, although it is often used in supraventricular arrhythmias such as atrial fibrillation. It is, however, often the cause of other arrhythmias. The specific drug(s) selected will depend on the type of arrhythmia, the clinical status of the patient, the underlying cause, the types of drugs the patient is already using, and the anticipated electrocardiographic and

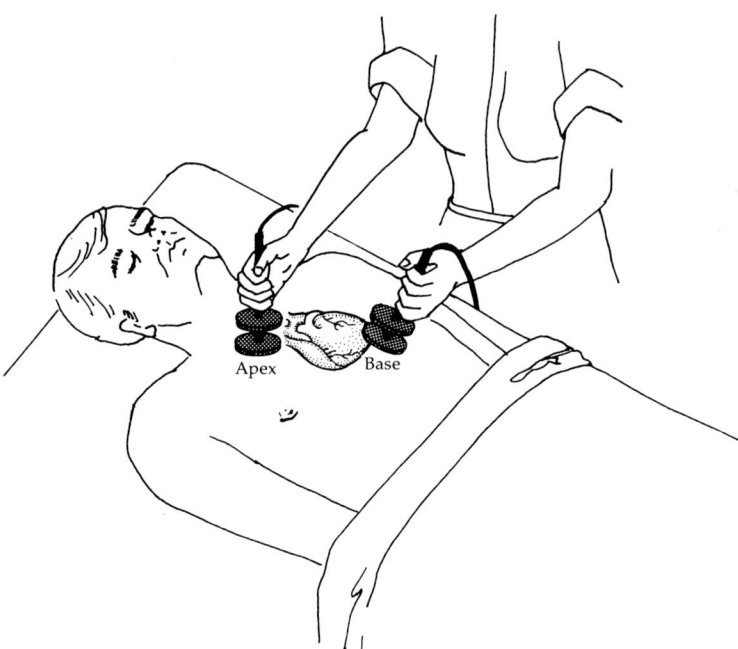

Figure 4-18
The use of the defibrillator in ventricular fibrillation. One electrode paddle is applied to the apex of the heart and the other at the base. The physician or nurse must not touch the bed or the patient when the electric current is applied.

Table 4-3
Drugs commonly used in the care of patients with arrhythmias

Drug	Action and indications	Dosage and route of administration	Side effects and contraindications
Quinidine	Depresses myocardial contractility; decreases myocardial excitability; prolongs refractory period and PR interval	Oral: 200–400 mg/3–4 hr, but not exceeding 2.4 gm/24 hr	Nausea; anorexia; vomiting; diarrhea Hypersensitivity reactions: rash; fever Hypotension (due to impairing myocardial contractility)
	Useful for supraventricular arrhythmias and premature ventricular contractions; ventricular tachycardia	May be given as IV bolus of 100–200 mg (rarely) Continuous infusion not advised IM: 400 mg	CNS symptoms: headache, tinnitus, diplopia, delirium Cardiac arrhythmias Thrombocytopenia Contraindicated in heart block, rheumatic fever, subacute bacterial endocarditis
Procainamide HCl (Pronestyl)	Similar action to quinidine, but does not depress AV conduction in usual doses	Oral: 250–500 mg/4–6 hr IM: 0.5–1 gm/6 hr	Same as quinidine May cause lupus erythematosus-like syndrome in long-term administration
	Useful for both atrial and ventricular tachycardia and premature ventricular contractions Useful for digitalis-induced arrhythmias	IV: 0.2–1 gm—very slowly. (To be used only in emergencies, very cautiously, due to danger of hypotension.)	Severe hypotension with parenteral use Excreted primarily by kidney; caution required in patients with renal insufficiency

Table 4-3 (Continued)

Drug	Action and indications	Dosage and route of administration	Side effects and contraindications
Lidocaine (Xylocaine)	Rapid-acting anesthetic agent; useful for decreasing ventricular excitability, conduction	IV bolus: 50–100 mg. May be repeated after 5 min (no more than 200–300 mg/1 hr)	CNS changes: blurred vision; irritability; somnolence; coma; convulsions. Fewer adverse circulatory effects than quinidine or Pronestyl
		Continuous infusion: 1–4 mg/min. Diluted in minimum of 250-ml solutions; 1,000-ml preferred	Contraindicated in heart block (may abolish idioventricular rhythm); hypersensitivity; severe hepatic dysfunction. (Drug is metabolized in liver.)
Propranolol HCl (Inderal)	Beta-adrenergic blocking agent; decreases heart rate; decreases ventricular irritability	Oral: 10–30 mg tid or qid	May result in sinus bradycardia and bronchospasm
	Used for digitalis-induced arrhythmias and atrial tachycardia	IV: 0.5–1 mg; may be repeated in 5 min	Contraindicated in heart block, bronchial asthma, cardiogenic shock, or heart failure. May cause nausea, vomiting, diarrhea
Phenytoin sodium (Dilantin)	Suppresses myocardial irritability; useful in digitalis-induced arrhythmias	Oral: 100–300 mg 3 times daily	Hypersensitivity reactions. Nystagmus, ataxia, slurred speech; nausea; vomiting
		IV bolus: 100 mg/5 min to 1 mg total	Contraindicated in hepatic disease (drug metabolized in liver)
Atropine	Counteracts excessive vagal nerve stimulation	IM or IV: 0.5–1.0 mg	Dry mouth; blurred vision (from dilated pupils); urine retention
		Subcutaneous: 0.6–0.8 mg	Contraindicated in glaucoma
Isoproterenol (Isuprel)	Increases cardiac output; increases heart rate; increases stroke volume and coronary blood flow	IV by infusion only; must be diluted: usually 1 or 2 mg in 500 ml D5W. (Speed of IV adjusted as heart rate and B.P. change.)	Tachycardia; palpitations; weakness; sweating; nausea; angina; headache
	Used in Stokes–Adams syndrome; sinus bradycardia; sinus arrest; heart block		Caution is necessary when used in patients with glaucoma
	A synthetic sympathomimetic amine structurally related to epinephrine	Oral: sublingual dose of 10–15 mg 3 times daily	Contraindications: tachycardia due to digitalis toxicity
Epinephrine (Adrenalin)	Cardiac stimulant; used in asystole and cardiac arrest.	Intravenous: 1–2 ml of 1:1,000 solution	May produce ventricular tachycardia, fibrillation
	Metabolic acidosis must be corrected before drug can be effective	Also given directly into cardiac muscle	May cause striking increase in B.P.

Bretylium tosylate is another antiarrhythmic drug being used experimentally. It has not been approved by the Food and Drug Administration. It appears to have an inotropic effect without myocardial suppression. *Digitalis glycosides* are not listed here, although they are utilized for certain supraventricular arrhythmias such as atrial fibrillation. However, digitalis also causes arrhythmias. Information on digitalis is found on page 379. *Potassium* can be considered an antiarrhythmic drug also. Information on potassium is found in Chapter 2.

hemodynamic effects of the drug. Drug therapy is not effective unless acid-base balance, fluid and electrolyte balance, and adequate oxygenation are achieved.

Effective intervention for patients with arrhythmias requires understanding and attention to other psychological and physiologic factors. The presence of an arrhythmia may be a critical and life-threatening situation. As mentioned previously, anxiety, fear, pain, and depression may produce or aggravate arrhythmias. The patient should be given clear explanations and emotional support to withstand the stress. Providing for safety measures, psychological and physiologic comfort, adequate rest, and conservation of energy are essential in the total care of the patient.

Ventricular Asystole

Ventricular standstill or asystole occurs when there is an absence of electrical activity from any pacemaker site. Death results unless cardiac automaticity is reestablished spontaneously within 2 to 4 minutes, unless cardiopulmonary resuscitation is initiated, or a pacemaker is inserted. **Cardiac arrest** (another term for cardiac standstill or asystole) means that the patient's heartbeat, circulation of blood, and respirations have suddenly and unexpectedly ceased. This problem may be the result of many causes, including but not limited to AMI, anoxia due to airway obstruction, anesthesia depression, hypotension; electrical shock, anaphylactic reactions, sensitivity to insect bites, digitalis and other drug sensitivities or toxicities, and carbon monoxide poisoning.

The absence of femoral and carotid pulses and the absence of heart sounds and respiration confirm the diagnosis of cardiac arrest. Other signs of cardiac arrest are dilatation of the pupils, abrupt and complete unconsciousness, and apnea or gasping respirations.

CARDIOPULMONARY RESUSCITATION

The purpose of cardiopulmonary resuscitation (CPR) is to restore and maintain oxygenation by artificial ventilation and to restore circulation by external cardiac massage. This emergency procedure is indicated in persons who have become victims of cardiac arrest. CPR, however, is not indicated in patients in the last stage of an incurable illness or in persons whose heartbeat and respirations have ceased functioning for over 4 to 6 minutes. Irreversible central nervous system damage will have occurred after 6 minutes without adequate circulation.

Cardiac arrest may occur anywhere—in the home, street, general hospital ward, or in a CCU or ICU unit of a hospital. Both professional and trained lay persons are capable of performing emergency CPR measures until appropriate medical assistance is available for definitive therapy. Familiarity with CPR techniques is the responsibility of every professional medical person, as well as of auxiliary staff. Usually CPR teams are appointed at institutions, but all nurses should maintain their skills in CPR by regular practice sessions and supervised demonstrations.

When a witnessed arrest occurs, the nurse should immediately strike one sharp blow with the fist to the midsternum. Although this technique is considered controversial by some, these blows have been effective in some instances in terminating transient ventricular tachycardia or in restarting cardiac action in the case of temporary asystole. If the arrest has occurred in a hospital setting, help is summoned according to the system established in the particular setting; if outside a hospital, assistance is summoned as available and appropriate to the situation. The resuscitator often must initiate CPR as a single rescuer until assistance arrives.

As Figure 4-19 indicates, the first step in CPR is the clearing of the airway, followed by rapid inflation of the lungs prior to initiation of external cardiac massage and definitive therapy. In clearing the airway, the head is hyperextended and the jaw is pulled forward to lift the tongue off the back wall of the pharynx. In some cases, this single act may terminate the cardiac arrest by opening the airway and permitting spontaneous respiration. If there is any obvious foreign material (including dentures) in the mouth or throat, it should be removed immediately.

If the victim still does not breathe spontaneously, the lungs are inflated by 4 rapid mouth-to-mouth ventilations, which should

Figure 4-19
Cardiopulmonary resuscitation. (Copyright © 1973 by American Heart Association. Reproduced by permission.)

CARDIOPULMONARY RESUSCITATION IN BASIC LIFE SUPPORT

Place Victim Flat On His Back On A Hard Surface

IF UNCONSCIOUS, OPEN AIRWAY

LIFT UP NECK
PUSH FOREHEAD BACK
CLEAR OUT MOUTH IF NECESSARY
OBSERVE FOR BREATHING

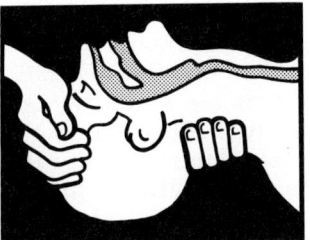

IF NOT BREATHING, BEGIN ARTIFICIAL BREATHING

4 QUICK FULL BREATHS

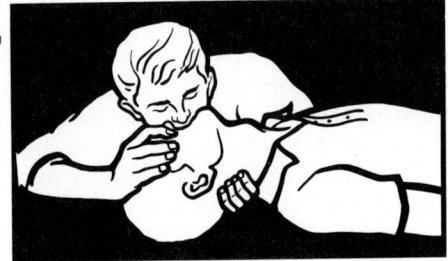

CHECK CAROTID PULSE

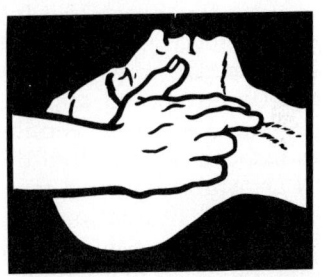

IF PULSE ABSENT, BEGIN ARTIFICIAL CIRCULATION

DEPRESS STERNUM 1½" TO 2"

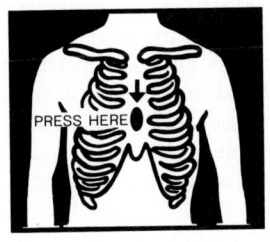

ONE RESCUER
15 compressions
rate 80 per min.
2 quick breaths

TWO RESCUERS
5 compressions
rate 60 per min.
1 breath

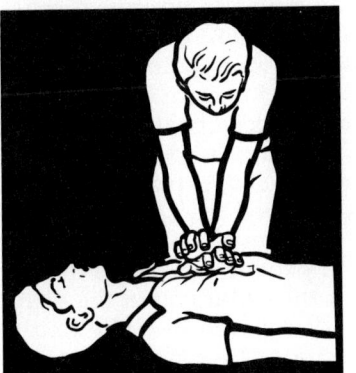

CONTINUE UNINTERRUPTED UNTIL ADVANCED LIFE SUPPORT IS AVAILABLE

American Heart Association

cause the chest to rise. If the chest still does not rise, it is necessary to open the mouth and to check again for airway obstruction. It is possible that the airway has not been cleared deeply enough. It may be necessary to roll the victim on his side toward the resuscitator and give 2 to 3 sharp blows to the back to release any mechanical obstruction. To promote effective mouth-to-mouth resuscitation, the resuscitator opens his mouth widely, takes a deep breath, and then makes a tight seal with his mouth around the patient's mouth, blowing the air into the patient's mouth. Removing his mouth, the resuscitator allows the patient to exhale passively. During mouth-to-mouth resuscitation, the patient's nose is pinched together to create a complete seal. When it is impossible to open the patient's mouth, mouth-to-nose ventilation may be used. After 4 successful ventilations (confirmed by rising of the chest), the resuscitator palpates the carotid artery to determine the presence of cardiac activity. If the carotid pulse is absent, cardiac massage is instituted at a rate of 60 to 80 compressions per minute. (The rate depends on the number of resuscitators present.) If alone, the resuscitator should compress the heart 15 times, alternating with 2 successful ventilations. If two resuscitators are present, one ventilation should be interposed after every fifth chest compression. Artificial ventilation (via mouth-to-mouth or nose-to-mouth) is continued until an Ambu bag and mask can be substituted or until intubation can be performed or until spontaneous respiration results. It should be noted that laryngectomized persons must be given mouth-to-stoma resuscitation. This procedure is discussed more fully in Chapter 13.

External massage is initiated with the patient on a solid surface (for example, on the floor or on a special board for resuscitation or even by placing a food tray between the thorax and the bed) to facilitate each compression forcing the blood from the heart to the arteries. The resuscitator stands facing the side of the patient and places the heel of one hand over the lower half of the sternum. The other hand is placed over the first hand and the resuscitator then exerts pressure almost vertically downward so that the pressure is adequate to depress the sternum (of an adult) about 1½ to 2 inches. This can be accomplished only if the resuscitator is positioned high enough over the patient so that his arms are kept straight during compression. Sequential compression should be regular, smooth, and uninterrupted, and compression and relaxation should be of equal duration to allow cardiac filling to maintain blood flow. Compression must not be interrupted for more than 5 seconds.

Care is taken during the procedure that injury to the patient does not occur as the result of the technique. The fingers of the hand must not touch the patient's rib cage, and the area of the xiphoid process of the sternum must not be compressed. The former situation may result in fractured ribs and the latter may result in a fractured sternum or laceration of the liver. Gastric dilatation may occur as the result of exhaled air ventilation, especially when excessive pressures are used for inflation or when the airway is not clear. Excessive gastric dilatation may cause regurgitation and aspiration and may also initiate vagal reflexes. Gastric dilatation also interferes with pulmonary ventilation by pressing on the diaphragm. Another rescuer, therefore, should place one hand with moderate pressure over the patient's epigastrium (between the umbilicus and rib cage) during CPR.

Periodic palpation of the carotid or femoral pulse is carried out to determine the effectiveness of the external cardiac compression or to check for the return of a spontaneous and effective heartbeat. The pupils will constrict (a major sign of adequate cerebral oxygenation), the color will improve, and spontaneous gasping respirations will start when the resuscitation is successful. Ineffective resuscitation is characterized by the absence of pulsations, persistence of dilated pupils, and continuous coma. Resuscitation may be ineffective if the technique is done incorrectly, if chronic lung disease interferes with adequate oxygenation, or if aspiration of vomitus occurs. Open cardiac compression may be necessary when cardiac arrest is associated with penetrating chest wounds, a crushed chest, or tension pneumothorax.

Cardiac arrest results in metabolic acidosis, and acidotic hearts are resistant to resuscitation and to vasopressor agents used in definitive therapy. Therefore, definitive therapy requires continued ECG monitoring of the patient to evaluate resuscitative efforts and the effects of drug therapy, laboratory analysis of arterial blood gases, and determination of pH levels. Sodium bicarbonate (1 mEq per kilogram) is given intravenously at 5 to 10 minute intervals. Other drugs utilized during CPR are those that increase perfusion pressure and stimulate myocardial contraction. Epinephrine (1 : 1,000) 0.5 ml diluted to 10 ml is administered intravenously or by an intracardiac route. Calcium chloride or calcium gluconate (2.5 ml of a 10% solution) is given intravenously to increase the force of cardiac contraction. Dopamine (Intropin) may be used for its vasopressor effect. Although it stimulates the heart by a beta-adrenergic action and constricts resistance vessels by acting on alpha receptors, it has a direct vasodilating action on the renal and splanchnic vascular bed [20]. Metaraminol bitartrate (Aramine, 200 mg in 500 mg of 5% dextrose in water) or levarterenol citartrate (Levophed, 4 ml of a 0.2% solution in 500 to 1,000 ml of 5% dextrose in water) is started to maintain systolic blood pressure above 80 mm Hg. Isoproterenol (1 to 3 mg in 250 to 500 ml of 5% dextrose in water) for continuous infusion may be used to increase myocardial irritability and contractility. If ventricular fibrillation is the cause of cardiac arrest, lidocaine 50 to 150 mg may be administered.

Unconsciousness, absence of spontaneous respirations, and fixed, dilated pupils for 15 to 30 minutes indicate that cerebral death has occurred and that further resuscitative efforts are usually futile. Nonetheless, successful resuscitation has been possible even after 2 hours of effective external cardiac massage and artificial ventilation.

Patients who have been successfully resuscitated are usually transferred to the CCU for several days for continuous cardiac monitoring and close observation. Vital signs are monitored closely; elevated temperatures, for example, may indicate cerebral damage and cerebral edema. Oxygen is administered and blood gas and pH levels are analyzed regularly. The patient is observed for postresuscitation convulsions, which may occur as the result of cerebral edema or acidosis. Amobarbital sodium or phenytoin sodium (Dilantin), or both, are used to control convulsions. A retention catheter is generally inserted to monitor urine output after resuscitation and determine the adequacy of renal circulation and function in case decreased tissue perfusion has resulted in renal damage. Treatment is centered on correcting the underlying cause of cardiac arrest; the length of hospitalization will depend primarily on the success in treating the underlying cause as well as on any untoward effects of the arrest itself.

During the postarrest phase of care and the remainder of the hospitalization, the nurse should observe the patient for both psychological and physiologic effects of the cardiac arrest and resuscitation. Nurses and physicians should provide opportunities for the patient to discuss his feelings about the experience and its implications. These measures are important also for patients who have observed the cardiac arrest. Providing for these discussions is a preventive measure against the onset of long-standing emotional problems related to cardiac arrest, as substantiated in a study by Druss and Kornfeld [21]. Their study demonstrated that the unique experience of "having been dead" caused patients to utilize various defense mechanisms, particularly denial and isolation, to protect themselves from the overwhelming anxiety associated with the implications of a cardiac arrest. Although denial is often necessary during the crisis period, the potential for long-term maladjustment must be recognized. Druss and Kornfeld also emphasize the importance of telling patients that their bodies were alive during the time their hearts had stopped, rather than saying that they had been dead and brought back to life.

Patients who have been resuscitated often require particular support during the transfer from CCU to the general unit. The fear of recurrence of the arrest may create such anxiety that the patient is fearful of being left alone and of increasing his activities. The danger that the patient will become a cardiac invalid is real unless appropriate emotional support and counseling are provided. The families of these patients also require guidance and counseling about realistic limitations on the patient's activities and realistic appraisals concerning the potential for recurrence of the cardiac arrest. These measures are necessary to assure a successful posthospitalization adjustment.

Disorders of Specific Cardiac Structures

Lesions of the specific structures of the heart, the myocardium, the pericardium, the endocardium, and the heart valves, may result from various factors. Only one structure may be affected, or, in some cases, all structures undergo pathophysiologic changes (e.g., pancarditis refers to a general inflammatory state of the entire heart). The factors affecting cardiac structures include infections (of viral or bacterial origin), toxins, tumors, trauma, and changes associated with various systemic diseases such as systemic lupus erythematosus.

Rheumatic fever, bacterial endocarditis, syphilis, and pericarditis are the diseases most commonly resulting in destruction of cardiac tissue. Of these, rheumatic fever is the most frequently occurring disease in persons under 45 years of age. The exact cause of rheumatic fever is not known, but it almost always is a sequel to an upper respiratory infection by the beta-hemolytic group A streptococcus. The disease primarily affects children between the ages of 5 and 15, but may also occur in susceptible individuals of any age group. A major impetus to the prevention of rheumatic fever is the early detection of a positive throat culture for the presence of the streptococcal organism and prompt treatment with penicillin or erythromycin, bed rest, and the use of salicylates (and sometimes steroids) to suppress rheumatic activity. Rheumatic fever is considered a hypersensitivity collagen disease and is characterized by fever, tachycardia, migratory polyarthritis, carditis, chorea (convulsive disorder with involuntary and irregular jerking movements), and subcutaneous nodules on the extensor surfaces of certain joints. Erythema marginatum is often present; this is the recurrent and transient pink rash often associated with the disease. Aschoff bodies, which are microscopic focal lesions consisting of fragments of muscle fibers and strands of collagen and fibrinoid material, are also found on the myocardium. The presence of rheumatic fever is confirmed by an elevated sedimentation rate, an elevated antistreptolysin titer, and an abnormal C-reactive protein test.

Cardiac involvement resulting from rheumatic fever is evidenced by tachycardia and the onset of murmurs associated with endocardial and valvular inflammation. Symptoms of congestive heart failure and arrhythmias may occur, depending on the site, number, and severity of valvular defects present. The most common site of valvular involvement with rheumatic fever is the mitral valve, followed by the aortic, tricuspid, and pulmonary valves. Inflammatory effects result in edema and inflammation of the connective tissue, the appearance of Aschoff bodies, and healing with scar tissue. Healing of the vegetations on the involved valves leads to mechanical deformity that results in hemodynamic disturbances. The scar formation results in thickening around the edges of the cusps of the valve(s) leading to fusion of the cusps and stenosis of the valve. Mitral stenosis is the classic lesion in rheumatic fever. Restriction of valvular motion reduces the effectiveness of the orifice and impedes the blood flow through it. The cusps may also be shrunken and deformed by the scarring process resulting from inflammation, so that there is an inadequate closure of the cusps. This defect, which leads to backflow or regurgitation of blood, is known as valvular insufficiency. The valvular defect may be one of either stenosis or insufficiency and often consists of both. Symptoms associated with valvular disease may be so mild that the lesion is not detected until a distinct heart murmur is noted in a physical examination. The symptoms, however, may be extremely debilitating immediately and necessitate restricted activity for a prolonged period until surgical repair is possible. (If severe myocarditis results in myocardial deficiency, surgical repair of the valve defects may not be possible.)

Symptoms will vary, depending on which valves are affected and on the type of defect. Mitral stenosis, for example, causes an increase in left atrial pressure and a decrease in cardiac output. Increased pulmonary pressure leads to failure of the right ventricle. Atrial fibrillation is often associated with mitral stenosis also. The murmur associated with mitral stenosis is of a late diastolic type with a rumbling quality.

Mitral insufficiency causes compensatory cardiac activity resulting in left ventricular enlargement and cardiac insufficiency. Aortic stenosis results in decreased cardiac output and left ventricular enlargement and is often associated with dyspnea on exertion. It is characterized by a very loud, harsh systolic murmur. Aortic insufficiency is associated with a higher-pitched diastolic murmur and may be undetected for many years; the onset of symptoms may occur suddenly with rapid development of congestive heart failure.

Surgical repair of the valvular lesions is indicated when symptoms interfere with functional ability. However, the elective repair may be indicated earlier in order to prevent other complications that result from valvular disease. In addition to congestive heart failure and arrhythmias, neurologic defects may occur if emboli break off the scarred valves and travel to cerebral arteries. Patients with rheumatic valvular disease are susceptible to the onset of subacute bacterial endocarditis, which tends to occur on previously damaged valves. Prevention is important for the patient who has suffered rheumatic heart disease. Parenteral long-term prophylactic therapy of using penicillin or sulfa is indicated to prevent recurrence of active carditis and bacterial endocarditis.

Surgical repair of valvular lesions depends on whether the lesion is singular or multiple. Mitral commissurotomy (a valvotomy technique to rupture the fused commissures of the mitral valve under closed heart surgery) may be indicated in selected cases. Open heart surgery may be indicated to replace the mitral valve with a prosthetic valve. Other valvular lesions are corrected by valvular replacement also, either by the ball-valve prosthesis or by homografts. The Starr-Edwards valve is designed so that the ball moves to the apex of the cage of the valve during forward flow of the blood, uncovering the valve orifice. When forward flow ceases, the ball recedes to the rim of the orifice to prevent backflow. More recent modifications of the basic Starr-Edwards design (a metal type originally) have lightweight disks or lens-shaped elements. In addition, leaflet valves made of soft, rubbery Silastic molded over a thin layer of polypropylene mesh have also been developed. The long-term durability and value of the synthetic valves (as well as heterografts currently being used in some settings) have not been determined. It is felt that the tendency to form blood clots is minimal or absent with the synthetic or grafted valve replacements. Thus long-term anticoagulant therapy is not required, as is the case for persons with the conventional types of valvular replacements. Care of the patient who requires open heart surgery is discussed on page 385.

Although valvular lesions have been discussed in relation to rheumatic heart disease, the reader is reminded that these lesions may also occur as the result of congenital heart defects, syphilitic infections, and trauma. Aortic stenosis may also be associated with arteriosclerosis.

BACTERIAL ENDOCARDITIS

Bacterial endocarditis is a bacterial infection of the valves and endocardium leading to deformities of the valve leaflets. Acute bacterial endocarditis most often follows an infection of staphylococcal, pneumococcal, streptococcal, or gonococcal origin elsewhere in the body. An increasing number of cases of acute bacterial endocarditis are found in addicts who use drugs intravenously. It may also result from infections associated with intravenous lines, especially CVP monitoring. The aortic valve is most often affected, and cardiac failure may occur suddenly in this potentially fatal condition. Postoperative patients may develop acute endocarditis due to exposure to virulent resistant organisms, lowered resistance, and inappropriate use of antibiotics. Acute endocarditis is suspected when cardiac dysfunction occurs with a high fever and chilling after an episode of an acute infection.

Subacute bacterial endocarditis is usually caused by *Streptococcus viridans* and tends to involve valves that are already defective from congenital disease or previous infection such as rheumatic fever. Symptoms are similar to the acute form (which is why some authorities do not differentiate between the two types), but symptoms are not as acute. They may be intermittent and mild and generally include fever, chills, diaphoresis, anorexia, and weight loss. (The fever may be a fulminating one in acute bacterial endocarditis.)

The diagnosis is confirmed by blood cultures that verify the presence of bacteremia. Sensitivity studies are done to determine the appropriate antibiotic therapy. Most often, the antibiotic used is penicillin administered by intermittent or continuous intravenous infusion. Long-term therapy is required and dosages must be sufficiently adequate to maintain high serum levels of the antibiotic. Therapy is evaluated by frequent blood cultures. Hospitalization is prolonged, at least for 4 weeks. The prolonged hospitalization and intravenous therapy can be extremely discouraging for the patient. The nurse is challenged to provide psychological support and appropriate diversional activities for the patient on prolonged bed rest. Attention to details of asepsis and the prevention of phlebitis are imperative to prevent complications from the therapy itself.

Complications of bacterial endocarditis include drug sensitivity and recurrent or persistent fever related to inadequate drug therapy. Fragments of the vegetations may break off and act as an embolus. The patient is observed closely for any signs of the onset of emboli (e.g., pain, and signs of malfunction of the specific organ), which may occur in an extremity, cerebral vessels, the kidney, or the spleen. Congestive heart failure or renal involvement also may result from the disease; surgical repair of the affected valves may be necessary.

PERICARDITIS

Pericarditis is an inflammation of the pericardium and may be either acute or chronic. It may be of infectious origin (bacterial, viral, fungal, or parasitic) or it may be associated with collagen vascular diseases (rheumatic fever, systemic lupus erythematosus) or with AMI, chest trauma, and metastatic tumors.

Symptoms associated with acute pericarditis are precordial and substernal pain, fever, chills, anorexia, and malaise. Dyspnea may also be present. Often the patient describes the pain as a very sharp one that "takes his breath away." The pain is accentuated on deep breathing or when the trunk is rotated. Patients with acute pericarditis tend to assume a sitting position, leaning forward to relieve the pain. This position alleviates the pain somewhat because the heart recedes from the anterior chest wall in this position. Pericardial pain is typically made worse when the patient lies down. Occasionally the pain may simulate anginal pain and may be difficult to differentiate from that of AMI. More often, however, the pain is diversified in its location and its referral to other areas.

A major finding is that of a pericardial friction rub detected on auscultation. The rub, however, tends to disappear as fluid accumulates in the pericardial sac. Pericardiocentesis, the aspiration of fluid from the pericardial sac, may occasionally be performed to determine whether the fluid is purulent. The procedure is also done as a therapeutic measure to remove excess fluid. Normally the pericardial sac holds approximately 50 ml of fluid. In pericarditis with effusion, the fluid may accumulate to such amounts that cardiac tamponade may occur.

Cardiac tamponade is the restriction of normal heart action due to compression of the heart by blood, effusion, or a foreign body in the pericardial sac. Cardiac filling is restricted and contraction is impaired, leading to a decreased cardiac output. Symptoms of cardiac tamponade are increased venous pressure, decreased arterial pressure, dyspnea, and cardiac arrhythmias. A diagnostic finding is the presence of a paradoxical pulse, characterized by a decreased amplitude during inspiration and a stronger pulse on expiration. In many settings, the nurse is expected to assess for a paradoxical pulse in patients suspected of impending tamponade. This assessment is done by pumping the B.P. cuff to 10 points above the patient's systolic pressure. The top level of the paradoxical pulse is that which occurs during the first couple of beats, as they vary with respiration. The point at which the pressure no longer varies is the lower level of the paradox. The paradoxical pulse is recorded as the difference between the two; a paradoxical pulse over 10 cm is considered abnormal.

To prevent cardiac tamponade, pericardiocentesis may be indicated. The procedure is performed under a local anesthetic after the patient is premedicated with a sedative or narcotic. Atropine is also given to prevent a vasovagal reaction during the procedure. The patient is connected to an ECG monitor and emergency equipment should be available. The patient is positioned in a sitting position (with the head of the bed elevated about 60°) to help the heart recede from the anterior chest wall. The apex is the site for the puncture with a needle that is connected to the precordial lead of the ECG. If the needle tip contacts the myocardium, an elevation of the ST segment of the ECG is observed and the needle is withdrawn a few millimeters. Electrocardiographic monitoring has reduced the incidence of complications associated with pericardiocentesis; these complications are vasovagal reaction (in which profound bradycardia or even asystole may accompany puncture of the pericardium) and laceration of the myocardium. Removal of the fluid (less than 500 ml is removed at any one time) should decrease venous pressure and provide relief from some of the symptoms; the underlying disease that initiated the pericarditis must be treated also. In addition to appropriate antibiotic therapy, corticosteroids may be given to combat the inflammatory process.

Chronic pericarditis, a chronic inflammatory condition, is characterized by formation of thick fibrous tissue that compresses the heart and compromises ventricular filling. Cardiac failure eventually results. The disease is often associated with tuberculosis. Medical treatment is focused on relieving symptoms of congestive heart failure with digitalis, diuretic therapy, and low sodium diet. **Pericardectomy,** which is the surgical removal of the constricting pericardium, may be indicated in the majority of patients with constrictive pericarditis.

MYOCARDITIS

Myocarditis is an inflammatory process in the myocardium and is usually associated with a bacterial, viral, or syphilitic infection, as well as those of fungal or parasitic origin. The most common cuase is rheumatic fever. Symptoms vary, depending on the type of infection, the extent of the myocardial damage, and the presence of other pathologic processes. On occasion, myocarditis may be so mild that the diagnosis is made on ECG tracings, in the absence of symptoms. It is more often diagnosed, however, in the presence of ventricular enlargement and sudden heart failure. Fever and tachycardia are present and cardiac murmurs, as well as a gallop rhythm (a tripling of the heart sounds), are often detected.

Bed rest is absolutely essential as the onset of stress or overexertion may result in sudden death. Appropriate antibiotics are given. Digitalis is administered in the management of the patient with myocarditis. Convalescence is prolonged and the prognosis is guarded.

CARDIOMYOPATHY

Cardiomyopathy is a form of myocardial disease that is caused by a variety of factors. The specific etiology is unknown but is thought to be related to viral infections, injury from toxic effects of alcohol, and malnutrition. **Primary cardiomyopathy** refers to conditions in which the heart alone is involved. **Secondary cardiomyopathy** refers to involvement of the heart as a manifestation of a systemic disease process, usually of a metabolic nature. These systemic diseases include, for example, both hypothyroidism and hyperthyroidism and beriberi (malnutrition due to thiamine deficiency). Myocardial contractility is reduced in these diseases and symptoms of congestive heart disease become evident. Alcohol is recognized as having negative inotropic effects and is contraindicated in patients with cardiomyopathy. In addition to congestive heart failure, arrhythmias are frequently present as a complication of the disease. Bed rest and supportive therapy similar to that for the patient with congestive heart disease are the usual therapeutic regimen.

CARDIAC TUMORS

Primary tumors of the heart are extremely rare. The most common cardiac tumor is **myxoma,** which is a soft mass of connective tissue covered by thrombus formation and often attached to the endocardium by a pedicle. It is most often found in the left atrium. The disease is suspected when an apparently healthy individual develops dyspnea, pulmonary edema, and congestive heart failure. Symptoms depend on the location, size, and consistency of the tumor; in some cases, the tumor obstructs venous blood return into the atrium and may interfere with valvular function. Surgical removal is usually possible and results in relief of the cardiac symptoms.

CONGESTIVE HEART FAILURE

Congestive heart failure (CHF) is a state of diminished cardiac function resulting in circulatory congestion and failure of the heart to pump sufficient blood to meet the metabolic needs of the body. The term **pump failure** is used to reflect both congestive heart failure and cardiogenic shock. This discussion, however, will be concerned with CHF; cardiogenic shock is discussed in a subsequent section.

CHF may be present as an acute condition or as a progressive and chronic condition. Therefore the nurse may work with CHF patients in an acute setting of a hospital or in a clinic, or in the home situation. The symptoms may be similar in both the acute and chronic stages, but will differ primarily in the degree of severity and in the presence of complications.

Virtually all cardiac diseases can lead to CHF; therefore, prevention of CHF is important in the care of patients with all types of cardiac disease. CHF may result when the workload required exceeds the capability of the pump; when the heart's ability to pump effectively decreases; or when blood flow through the heart is impeded and compensating mechanisms for cardiac function fail. Conditions that may result in CHF include AMI, an infectious process such as bacterial endocarditis or myocarditis, congenital and acquired valvular and septal defects, arrhythmias, hypertensive cardiovascular disease, and cardiomyopathy. In all these conditions, CHF is a consequence of excessive stress on an impaired heart. As explained previously, cardiac output is dependent on the strength of contraction as well as on the heart rate. Whatever the cause in CHF, the heart can no longer pump effectively. Signs and symptoms of CHF are related to the inability of the heart to pump blood to tissues throughout the body. Compensatory mechanisms within the heart to augment the cardiac output are tachycardia, hypertrophy, and dilatation of the myocardium. Eventually these compensatory mechanisms are no longer effective. Excessive dilatation overstretches the muscle fibers and compromises contractility and stroke volume. Hypertrophy increases the need for oxygen while coronary blood supply is limited. (The reader will recall that the coronary arteries are perfused during diastole of the cardiac cycle. Thus, tachycardia interferes with perfusion of the coronary vessels.)

CHF may be described as either right- or left-sided failure, depending on which clinical problems predominate initially, although symptoms of both right- and left-sided failure may occur simultaneously. If the left side of the heart is unable to adequately pump the blood in its chambers, the blood is backed up in the pulmonary circulatory system. For example, left-sided failure is the type most likely to occur after MI. Signs and symptoms of left-sided heart failure reflect the increased congestion and pressure within the pulmonary system and the symptoms associated with decreased blood supply to the body tissues and organs. These symptoms of left-sided failure include dyspnea on exertion, orthopnea, paroxysmal nocturnal dyspnea, coughing, pulmonary rales, fatigue, mental confusion, decreased urinary output, and decreased tolerance to exercise. **Orthopnea** is the inability to lie in a supine position without becoming short of breath due to the shift of blood to the heart from the veins in the lower part of the body. **Paroxysmal nocturnal dyspnea** is the sudden onset of dyspnea that awakens the patient and requires him or her to sit up or stand in order to breathe more easily and to become comfortable. This symptom results from a shift of fluid from the base to the top of the lungs when the person is in a horizontal position. The shift of fluid from the extravascular to the vascular space also results in an increased venous return and an increased plasma volume that exceeds the cardiac workload capabilities and leads to pulmonary congestion.

Right-sided failure is manifested by dependent edema, coolness of the extremities, ascites, hepatomegaly, aching abdominal pain, neck vein engorgement, and increased venous pressure. **Anasarca** is the term used to describe the accumulation of excessive amounts of fluid in all body tissues. These symptoms of edema are attributable to the pooling of blood in the venous system throughout the body and the extravasation of fluid into the interstitial spaces. Normally the colloidal osmotic pressure exceeds the hydrostatic pressure of the blood and interstitial fluid moves into the capillaries. With increased venous pressure due to the pooling within the venous system, the hydrostatic pressure of the blood exceeds blood protein osmotic pressure and does not permit movement of interstitial fluid into the capillaries. Thus, in CHF, reduced renal blood flow interferes with renal function and the resultant retention of sodium and water contributes to edema formation. An increased secretion of aldosterone also promotes reabsorption of sodium in the kidneys.

Right-sided failure most often follows left-sided heart failure since the right side must pump against the increased resistance in the pulmonary system that results from left-sided heart failure. Right-sided failure may result from obstructive pulmonary disease; emphysema, asthma, and chronic bronchitis resist blood flow through the lungs, causing the right heart to beat more forcefully. Right-sided heart failure that results secondarily to lung disease is **cor pulmonale.**

In addition to the presence of the signs and symptoms listed, heart failure is suspected when an enlarged heart is visualized on chest x-rays or when ECG changes indicate left ventricular hypertrophy. Arterial blood gas analysis demonstrates decreased oxygen tension and increased levels of carbon dioxide. Electrolyte levels demonstrate increased sodium retention and other electrolyte imbalances. The blood urea nitrogen level is usually elevated, and the urinalysis usually shows albuminuria. The CVP is elevated.

The treatment and nursing care of the patient with CHF is basically focused on restoring balance in the demand for blood and the supply of the blood to the tissues. This effort necessitates measures to increase cardiac output by improving the pumping action of the heart to reduce the body's need for oxygen and thus reduce the cardiac workload, and to decrease sodium and fluid retention. The use of digitalis is aimed at improving cardiac output by improving the pumping action of the heart. When the pumping action is improved, circulation to the kidney is improved also; this assists in increased urine output and a secondary diuretic action. In addition, the circulating blood volume and the edema formation in the tissues are reduced via medications to promote diuresis and the restriction of sodium in the diet and, in some cases, the restriction of fluid intake.

Providing physical and psychological rest is the major means for decreasing the demands on the heart. Increased metabolic activity increases the need for oxygen; therefore, activity is restricted in CHF. In addition, depending on the pulmonary status, oxygen may be administered to combat the hypoxia associated with decreased oxygenation. Oxygen is given cautiously if the patient has chronic hypoxia with increased CO_2 tensions due to chronic lung disease. As explained in Chapter 3, giving oxygen may interfere with the stimulus for ventilation. A low calorie diet may be indicated to initiate weight reduction if obesity is a contributing factor to the increased cardiac workload. Severe edema, however, may mask malnutrition, so the nurse must make an accurate assessment of the patient's nutritional status. Nursing measures are planned to conserve the patient's energy. In severe CHF, the mechanical work of breathing may be so difficult that energy resources for the activities of eating and elimination may be extremely limited. Providing for frequent rest periods is a major aspect of the plan of care.

Any activity by the patient that increases exertion or straining, such as pulling himself up in bed, reaching for articles, or straining during defecation, is contraindicated. The nurse should plan to position the patient at regular intervals, anticipate his needs, and provide essential items within easy reach. The administration of a stool softener is important in reducing the problem of constipation and straining. Permitting the use of the bedside commode rather than the bedpan also facilitates defecation and reduces strain during the activity. Patients in severe CHF are extremely uncomfortable until therapeutic measures effect improvement in their condition. These patients are extremely restless and the nurse often finds it difficult or impossible to relieve their discomfort. Position changes may provide some comfort. The patient with CHF is often more comfortable sitting in a chair with his legs elevated rather than lying in bed. The sitting position permits maximum lung expansion because there is less pressure from the abdominal organs. The patient should not misunderstand the purpose of the chair privileges, however. Some patients assume that sitting in the chair means that ambulation can also be increased. Patients should either be lifted into the chair or be moved with minimal activity to the chair in order to prevent excessive burden on the heart by increased metabolic activity.

The nurse, through constant reassurance and control of the patient's environment, can help to insure optimum rest. Many patients will have problems adjusting to the dependent role required in the treatment of CHF. Anxiety can be controlled by tending to the patient's smallest needs so that he or she does not need to ask for assistance frequently. These patients require time for perceptive listening and discussions with the nurse to better understand the need for rest and the consequences of excessive strain on the heart. Although rest is important and pain and discomfort should be relieved, the nurse should be cognizant that hepatic congestion associated with CHF may limit the efficiency of the detoxifying functions of the liver. Caution in the administration of barbiturates or sedatives is necessary and effects of drugs should be evaluated carefully.

Prolonged immobility requires nursing measures to prevent the occurrence of decubitus ulcers. The patient with tissue edema is particularly vulnerable to trauma and pressure with resultant necrosis due to the poorly nourished tissue. Alternating-pressure mattresses, frequent massage, frequent assessment of skin condition, and assisted position changes should be instituted early.

Although the prevention of fluid congestion within the pulmonary system is desirable to prevent the onset of pulmonary edema, this should not be at the expense of causing increased venous congestion in the peripheral circulation. Active exercises (or at least passive exercises) should be accomplished regularly and elastic stockings may be indicated to prevent the formation of thrombi in the peripheral system.

As mentioned previously, the use of digitalis constitutes a major aspect in the treatment of CHF. Digitalis has a direct inotropic effect on the heart, increasing the force of myocardial contraction. This effect results in increased cardiac output and increased blood flow to the body tissues. In addition, digitalis prolongs the refractory period and thereby reduces the frequency of transmission of impulses from the atria to the ventricles. Thus the heart rate is reduced. This effect is especially important in the presence of tachycardia and atrial fibrillation. However, digitalis may also result in AV dissociation and sinus bradycardia. There is often a narrow margin between the therapeutic and toxic doses of digitalis preparations, due to variations of absorption and excretion and the effect of dosages in different persons. These facts place more responsibility on the nurse for accurate observations and assessment of the patient and his response to digitalis therapy.

Digitalization is the term used to describe the administration of the amount of digitalis required to produce the blood level necessary to achieve an optimal cardiac effect in a given patient. The rate of digitalization may vary from rapid digitalization (by repeated dosages every 4 to 6 hours until an optimum effect is reached, usually within 12 hours) to gradual digitalization over several days. Once the appropriate blood level and optimal effect are achieved, a maintenance dose is prescribed. Rapid digitalization may be required with the use of intravenous administration of the drug, when symptoms of congestive heart failure are severe. The need for accurate observation of the effects of the drug is increased during rapid digitalization. Potassium levels must be maintained well into the normal limits. The danger of digitalis toxicity is increased in the presence of hypokalemia. Recognition of digitalis toxicity is imperative to prevent the onset of dangerous arrhythmias such as premature ventricular contractions or bradycardia. Potassium replacement is particularly significant if diuretic therapy results in potassium depletion. Phenytoin sodium (Dilantin) may be given to treat digitalis-induced arrhythmias or lidocaine and other antiarrhythmic drugs may also be used. The latter drugs, however, are contraindicated if bradycardia exists with AV dissociation. Digitalis toxicity may also be monitored by analysis of blood samples for digitalis levels. (Digoxin levels below 2.0 mg per milliliter and digitoxin levels below 2.0 mg per milliliter are generally considered safe levels in most persons.) The drug is generally withdrawn, or at least decreased in dosage, when signs of toxicity are present.

Other signs of digitalis toxicity are nausea, vomiting, diarrhea, anorexia, blurred vision, visual color disturbances, headache, lethargy, restlessness, and other central nervous system symptoms. Close monitoring is essential to detect these signs before severe symptoms develop. The nurse should assess the patient for the presence of these symptoms prior to administering the medication. The apical pulse should be taken to detect a pulse rate that is excessively slow (below 60) or any significant rise in the pulse rate. (Other arrhythmias may result due to increased latent automaticity.) Any sudden change in cardiac rhythm should be reported to the physician. One of the most distinctive arrhythmias associated with digitalis toxicity is the bigeminal pulse, which may be detected by radial artery palpation as well as by apical auscultation. Bigeminy is characterized by "coupling" of the cardiac contractions.

The patient who is being maintained on digitalis is taught to monitor his pulse and is advised when to notify his physician regarding pulse changes as well as when to withhold the medication. He is also advised of signs of impending heart failure that require medical evaluation. Table 4-4 lists the various digitalis glycosides and their usual dosages and routes of administration. Except for intravenous administration of digitalis glycosides, these drugs are rarely used parenterally due to their local irritating effects and the uncertainty of

Table 4-4
Digitalis glycosides

Glycoside	Usual digitalizing dose	Usual maintenance dose
Ouabain	0.4 mg in 100 cc D5W given over 10–20 min (0.4–0.8 mg total)	—
Deslanoside (Cedilanid-D)	0.4–0.8 mg IV initially, followed by 0.2 mg; 1.2–2.0 mg in some protocols	—
Digoxin (Lanoxin)	IV: 0.5–1.0 mg initially, followed by 0.25 mg in 2–4 hr Oral: total digitalizing dose of 2–3 mg (in divided dosages)	0.25–0.5 mg orally or intramuscularly daily
Digitoxin	Total average digitalizing dose is 1.2–1.5 mg (in divided dosages) Oral administration only; 2- to 4-hr action	0.1–0.2 mg daily
Digitalis Leaf (Foxglove)	Digitalization dosage 1.0–2.0 gm (in divided dosages) Not available in parenteral form	0.15 gm average maintenance dose

absorption. The two preparations most commonly utilized are digitoxin and digoxin. The latter preparation is most often used when rapid digitalization is indicated due to its rapid excretion, which facilitates easier adjustment of dosage. The nurse must be extremely cautious in administering the digitalis glycosides; the names of the different preparations are similar but the dosages vary widely.

Diuretic therapy is indicated in CHF to decrease the fluid accumulation in the body. Diuretics that primarily decrease tubular reabsorption of sodium may be selected from a variety of drugs available. (Table 4-5 lists common drugs utilized for diuretic therapy.) Rapid-acting diuretics such as furosemide (Lasix) and ethacrynic acid (Edecrin) are initially given intravenously, but oral administration is utilized in long-term management. Rapid diuresis may be desirable but may also result in complications by causing depletion of electrolytes, particularly potassium. (Symptoms of hypokalemia are discussed in Chapter 2.) Serious arrhythmias (especially if the patient is being digitalized) associated with electrolyte depletion may result. The patient who is receiving drugs for rapid diuresis should be closely monitored for effects of the drug therapy. Serum electrolyte levels should be used also to guide the diuresis regimen. Daily weights (using the same scale at the same time each day) and accurate intake and output records are essential for proper evaluation of the patient's response to diuretic therapy. The patient should be forewarned to expect both an increase in volume of urine and increased frequency of urination.

The patient with CHF is frequently anorexic and therefore is likely to tolerate smaller, frequent meals rather than three large meals. (Oxygen needs are increased during digestion of a large meal.) The diet should be low in sodium and generally low in calories. Gas-forming foods should be eliminated to prevent abdominal distention, which causes pressure on the diaphragm and decreased lung capacity.

The amount of sodium restriction prescribed will depend on the severity of the heart failure and the response to diuretic therapy. The diet prescribed should specify the precise amount of sodium to be permitted. In contrast to the usual sodium intake (more than 3 gm daily), the diet may be restricted to only 200 to 600 mg if warranted by the clinical state of the patient. The most common source of sodium in the diet is table salt; omitting the use of salt added to the food is the initial means of restricting sodium intake. Foods that are high in sodium and that should be omitted or restricted (depending on the type of diet prescribed) include smoked meats, fish, frozen and canned foods (due to the sodium used in the preservative), milk, beer, soft drinks, potato chips, olives, pickles, salad dressings, breads, and crackers. In addition, the patient is advised about the sodium content of other less common sources such as certain medica-

Table 4-5
Drugs used in diuretic therapy

Drug	Usual dose	Precautions and side effects
Rapid-Acting		
Furosemide (Lasix)	IV bolus: 40–80 mg IM: 20–40 mg Oral: 40 mg once or twice daily	K^+ depletion; alkalosis; circulatory collapse in excessive diuresis
Ethacrynic acid (Edecrin)	IV bolus: 50 mg (or 0.5 mg/kg weight) Oral: 50–100 mg twice daily	Electrolyte depletion: K^+, Na^+, and Cl^-. GI symptoms: nausea and diarrhea; agranulocytosis
Thiazides		
Chlorothiazide (Diuril)	Oral: 250–1000 mg once or twice daily	K^+ depletion may occur (also Na^+ and Cl^-). Controlled with dietary or K^+ supplements or both
Hydrochlorothiazide (Hydrodiuril)	50–100 mg once or twice daily	Hyperuricemia in some patients
Chlorthalidone (Hygroton)	Oral: 50–100 mg daily or every other day	Nausea and vomiting
(also Esidrex, Naturetin are other forms)	Oral	Insulin antagonistic
Potassium-Sparing		
Spironolactone (Aldactone)	Oral: 25 mg 4 times daily	Aldosterone antagonistic. K^+ supplement or K^+-rich diet contraindicated. Danger of hyperkalemia. Often used with other diuretics
Triamterene (Dyrenium)	Oral: 100 mg daily or twice daily	Tends to conserve K^+. Potential danger of hyperkalemia. Often used in combination with other diuretics. May cause nausea; vomiting
Organic Mercurials		
Meralluride sodium (Mercuhydrin) Mercaptomerin sodium (Thiomerin)	IM: 1–2 ml	Used less frequently due to other drugs available; may cause hypochloremia and alkalosis
Carbonic Anhydrase Inhibitors		
Acetazolamide (Diamox)	Oral: 250 mg daily	May cause paresthesia; acidosis in long-term therapy

tions (e.g., sodium salicylates, laxatives, sedatives, and alkalizing drugs), baking powder, and baking soda.

The purpose and principles of sodium restriction are explained to the patient and guidance in selecting appropriate foods is initiated as soon as the patient is able to understand and tolerate such discussions. Anxiety, decreased oxygenation, and a decreased attention span associated with CHF may interfere with learning if detailed instructions are given too soon in the acute phase.

The nurse can reinforce knowledge of the sodium content in certain foods while assisting the patient in eating. Patients should have the opportunity to discuss the planning of diets and selection of low sodium foods. Lists of high sodium foods to avoid are provided the patient, as well as lists of foods that are permitted on the diet. Low sodium diets can be made more palatable by adding salt substitutes such as Diasol, Cosalt, and Neocurtasal, if they are not contraindicated by the patient's condition. Excess use of potassium salt substitutes, for example, should be avoided in the presence of renal dysfunction. The patient will also benefit from suggestions on ways to season foods to make them more palatable without the use of salt. (These suggestions might include the use of lemon and lime juice, bay leaves, paprika, mushrooms, and wine.)

Low sodium diets in combination with diuretic therapy may, on occasion, result in sodium excretion beyond therapeutic levels. Manifestations of weakness, nausea, vomiting, and lethargy warrant evaluation of the sodium content in the blood to determine the presence of a sodium deficit. An increase of sodium in the diet or drug adjustment may be necessary.

Fluids also may be restricted depending on the status of the individual patient and his response to sodium restriction and diuretic therapy. Fluids may be limited to a total of 1,500 ml daily. The patient is more likely to cooperate if allowed to schedule fluid intake as well as the amounts and types of fluid to be taken.

Due to the decrease in fluid intake and the diuresis, thirst is a frequent complaint of the patient and needs frequent attention. Mouth wash and the use of glycerine swabs may help to alleviate thirst for short periods of time. The nurse must understand the patient's extreme physical and psychological discomfort and the anxiety that fluid restriction and resultant thirst may initiate. Frequent mouth care and prompt provision of allotted fluid can keep the anxiety at a minimum.

Although the medical treatment of CHF may be highly effective, particularly if the underlying disease can be controlled, many patients continue to have chronic heart failure with varying degrees of limitation. The American Heart Association previously classified the degrees of cardiac disease on the basis of functional and therapeutic classifications, but this classification is no longer recommended. The new classification, Cardiac Status and Prognosis, which was developed by the New York Heart Association [3a], replaces the Functional and Therapeutic Classification, which utilized only symptoms as a basis for determining appropriate physical activity. Because patients may be asymptomatic even in the presence of anatomic or physiologic abnormalities, the new classification reflects assessment based on etiologic, anatomic, and physiologic aspects.

Cardiac Status	Prognosis
1. Uncompromised	1. Good
2. Slightly compromised	2. Good with therapy
3. Moderately compromised	3. Fair with therapy
4. Severely compromised	4. Guarded despite therapy

Thus the plan for rehabilitation and prescribed activity of the patient with cardiac disease should be individualized, based on various sources of data on the patient's physiologic and psychological status. The aim of the care of the cardiac patient is to enable him to live as useful and as satisfactory a life as possible within the resultant physiologic limits. In some instances, the nurse may have the goal of encouraging rather than restricting activity. Some patients may become incapacitated, not by their decreased cardiac function, but by their fear of another episode of CHF. Appropriate guidance and counseling are required to assist the patient in combating this fear in a more realistic manner.

Heart failure may become **refractory,** a term used to describe a state of the disease that does not respond to therapy. Fluid restriction to less than 1,000 ml per day or even 500 ml per day may be necessary in patients with CHF who do not respond to dietary sodium restriction and diuretics. When a patient with CHF does not respond to the usual treatment of bed rest, diet, drugs, and other measures, a thorough review of the patient is indicated to determine whether other conditions, such as hyperthyroidism or severe anemia, may be interfering with the effectiveness of therapy (that is, increasing the metabolic demands of the tissues).

In addition to the treatment measures already described, paracentesis and thoracentesis may be required. Paracentesis (the removal of fluid from the peritoneal cavity) is indicated when severe ascites compromises the respiratory function by compressing the diaphragm and restricting lung expansion. Thoracentesis (removal of fluid from the pleural cavity) is often required when fluid accumulation within the pleural cavity compromises respiratory function.

The nurse is responsible for providing effective nursing measures to enhance the therapeutic regimen and should evaluate carefully the effects of these measures and of the specific medical therapy. The patient is observed for symptoms of deterioration and complications. These complications are primarily the onset of acute pulmonary edema and cardiogenic shock, which will now be discussed.

PULMONARY EDEMA

Sudden failure of the left ventricle or abrupt increases in the cardiac load beyond the capacity of the left ventricle may lead to acute pulmonary edema. The condition results from extreme left ventricular failure. It is a medical emergency that requires prompt treatment to prevent a fatal outcome.

Pooling of the blood with increased pressure in the left ventricle results in increased pressure in the pulmonary veins and capillaries, leading to transudation of fluid into the alveoli. Symptoms associated with the condition are therefore related to decreased oxygenation of the blood and fluid accumulation in the alveoli. Symptoms are vivid and devastating in this life-threatening situation. The patient is dyspneic, cyanotic, panting, and coughing. Gurgling respirations are audible and the patient expectorates a pinkish or bloody frothy sputum. The patient is always apprehensive, agitated, and restless as he gasps for air. The patient is profusely diaphoretic and tachycardia is present.

Prompt medical and nursing intervention is essential. The primary goal of all treatment is to decrease the blood flow to the heart and thereby decrease the workload of the heart. An upright position is most comfortable; the patient may even wish to sit in a chair. Morphine sulfate 10 to 15 mg is given to relieve anxiety, relieve the forceful respirations, dilate the peripheral veins, and thus decrease the intrathoracic pressure. The nurse must reassure and calm the patient to prevent any increase in dyspnea and hypoxia. Humidified oxygen under pressure is instituted to prevent further transudation of serum from the pulmonary capillaries by exerting pressure on the pulmonary epithelium during expiration. If the patient is conscious and cooperative, positive-pressure oxygen via a snug face mask may be adequate. Otherwise intubation with a volume-cycled respirator may be necessary to increase intra-alveolar oxygenation (ventilation) and arterial oxygen tension (perfusion).

If the patient has not been previously digitalized, rapid digitalization is often indicated. A rapid-acting diuretic such as furosemide (Lasix) or ethacrynic acid (Edecrin) is administered intravenously to decrease the intravascular fluid volume and the workload on the heart. Aminophylline (usually 500 mg intravenously) may be administered for its bronchodilating action, but must be used with caution. It has caused ventricular arrhythmias and toxicity. The drug is given slowly by intravenous injection in order to prevent circulatory collapse; it may be given rectally.

The prompt use of diuretics may control the condition so that symptoms are relieved. In some situations, rotating tourniquets, or less often phlebotomy, may be necessary. In phlebotomy, approximately 500 ml of blood is removed via venipuncture to decrease intravascular fluid volume. In order to decrease venous return to the heart, rotating tourniquets may be utilized to temporarily store a volume of blood in the extremities. Tourniquets are systematically rotated on the extremities, at 15-minute intervals, so that three of the four extremities are compressed at any one time, but no single extremity is compressed continuously for more than 45 minutes. (The procedure may be modified in the elderly patient by rotating the tourniquets at 5-minute rather than 15-minute intervals.) Sphygmomanometer cuffs may be utilized to compress the extremities. Equipment (such as the Danzer apparatus) is available to inflate and deflate B.P. cuffs automatically. Whatever system for compression is used, the nurse must ensure that arterial pulses are not obliterated by the pressure. The patient should be draped so that the extremities are exposed to facilitate assessment of peripheral circulation and the transfer of the tourniquets. If compression is not monitored appropriately and if the rotation system is not clearly understood and followed exactly, there is danger of phlebothrombosis or fatal pulmonary embolism. The time of rotations, the pattern to follow, and the clinical response to the technique are recorded. An illustration of the procedure is found in Figure 4-20.

The use of rotating tourniquets may increase the patient's anxiety. A careful, calm explanation is necessary. Vital signs are monitored closely. There is a danger of hypotension developing in some patients when this procedure is utilized. When the procedure is to be discontinued, only one tourniquet at a time is removed according to the time-interval schedule. If all tourniquets are removed at the same time, the sudden increase in circulatory blood volume creates a circulatory overload and original symptoms recur.

In addition to monitoring vital signs, the nurse carefully observes intake and output. Rapid-acting diuretics may cause sudden re-

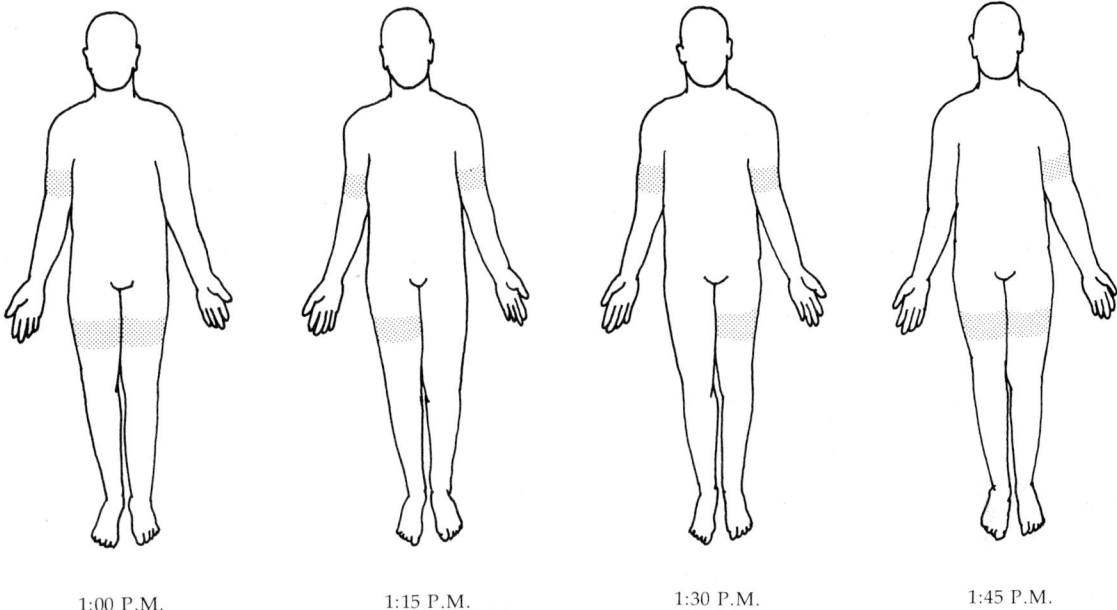

1:00 P.M.   1:15 P.M.   1:30 P.M.   1:45 P.M.

Figure 4-20
Pattern and timing for rotating tourniquets. When discontinuing the treatment, the nurse should remove only one tourniquet at a time according to the schedule being followed.

duction in plasma volume that may result in hypotension, oliguria, and other fluid and electrolyte imbalances. Once the crisis state is controlled, the nurse's role centers on measures to assist stabilization of cardiac function and to decrease demands on the heart. Bed rest is necessary and sedation is indicated to promote adequate rest. The patient needs assurance that the crisis is controlled and needs to understand how to prevent recurrence. Patients with potential pulmonary involvement from cardiac failure should be observed for early signs of impending pulmonary edema. These signs include diffuse bilateral crepitant rales, cardiac arrhythmias, increasing orthopnea, tachycardia, distended jugular veins, and tachypnea. The primary treatment of pulmonary edema should be the prevention of its onset.

CARDIOGENIC SHOCK

About 10 to 20 percent of patients with AMI develop cardiogenic shock as a result of pump failure. Symptoms associated with this critical state are related to decreased cardiac output and decreased tissue perfusion, as well as to initial compensatory sympathetic mechanisms. These common symptoms are decreased B.P. (systolic B.P. below 80 mm Hg or a drop of more than 30 mm Hg systolic pressure from the patient's "normal" B.P.) and symptoms of cerebral hypoxia such as restlessness and confusion progressing to apathy, lethargy, and eventually coma. Generalized vasoconstriction results in cool, clammy skin and ashen color. Tachycardia is present and oliguria results from decreased renal flow.

The onset of cardiogenic shock in the presence of AMI is an ominous sign. It may reflect extensive myocardial damage that prevents effective pumping action or it may reflect the metabolic disturbances (related to myocardial ischemia) that inhibit effective pumping action. Because the heart is no longer able to pump an adequate supply of blood, blood is backed up into the lungs where oxygen–carbon dioxide exchange is thus inhibited. There is also a backing-up into the vascular system and body tissues. The normal pressure systems initially attempt to adapt to this stress through various mechanisms. Vasoconstriction occurs, increasing peripheral resistance in order to increase the arterial pressure but also causing the already-failing heart to work harder. The baroreceptors in the heart and aorta and carotid arteries trigger the release of aldosterone from the adrenal glands. Aldosterone causes the kidneys to retain sodium and water. In addition, when low B.P. threatens kidney perfusion, renin is secreted by the kidneys. The renin angiotensin system also stimulates the adrenal cortex to secrete aldosterone, which may initially increase circulating blood volume. The B.P. increases and eventually, due to the inadequate pumping of the heart, fluid volume is backed up into the tissues and edema results. The liver also suffers because the fluid congestion interferes with important metabolic functions. Aldosterone is destroyed in the healthy liver, but this process is inhibited when the liver is affected by fluid congestion and inadequate circulation. Thus, aldosterone continues to influence decreased urinary output. In addition, urine output is decreased due to the low cardiac output and the diminished B.P. Coronary artery perfusion is also diminished by low cardiac output. In an effort to preserve cellular function, the body's defense mechanisms maintain perfusion of vital organs at the expense of peripheral tissues, causing anaerobic metabolism. Anaerobic metabolism results in accumulation of lactic acid, resulting in acidosis. Compensatory mechanisms of hyperventilation in this state are inadequate, and acidosis results in cellular death and arrhythmias.

The basic therapeutic plan for treating patients in cardiogenic shock must be aimed at supporting the systemic circulation by improving the cardiac action and thereby improving tissue perfusion. The pathologic events contributing to myocardial damage and failure must be interrupted.

Absolute bed rest and conservation of energy are imperative. Oxygen is administered to increase arterial oxygen tension. Continuous monitoring is essential to evaluate accurately the patient's status and the effects of treatment. Intra-arterial B.P. monitoring is particularly important when vasopressor drugs are used because this method is more accurate than the auscultatory method. A retention catheter is inserted for monitoring hourly urine output.

Drug therapy varies according to various protocols. Digitalis or isoproterenol (Isuprel) may be given for its inotropic effect. However, myocardial irritability with potential for dangerous arrythmias exists with the use of these drugs, particularly in the presence of extensive myocardial damage, so that their use may be controversial. Controversy also exists regarding the use of vasopressor drugs, which increase vasoconstriction in order to increase arterial B.P. Levarterenol (Levophed) or metaraminol (Aramine) may be prescribed, but require continuous monitoring to avoid prolonged vasoconstriction and to avoid rapid acceleration of B.P. beyond therapeutic levels. (For example, excessive elevations in B.P. increase the workload of the heart.) In addition, tissue necrosis and damage may result if intravenous solutions with Levophed are allowed to infiltrate into the tissue. Currently, in many settings dopamine, another catecholamine, is preferred as an agent to increase cardiac output because it is less likely to restrict renal blood flow.

In other protocols, vasodilating drugs, such as phenoxybenzamine (Dibenzyline) and nitroprusside, are used in cardiogenic shock. (It is thought these drugs also decrease the afterload.) The basis of this approach is that excessive vasoconstriction and subsequent ischemia of the tissues results in release of toxins that aggravate the status of shock. This approach, therefore, utilizes adequate fluid volume replacement with the vasodilating drugs. Observations for hypotension and arrhythmias are essential when these drugs are utilized.

The pancreatic hormone, glucagon, has been used experimentally to increase myocardial contractility in the treatment of cardiogenic shock. It appears to increase myocardial contractility without sacrificing systemic vascular perfusion and without inciting arrhythmias.

Appropriate volume expansion is a crucial aspect in the treatment of the patient in shock. Use of laboratory data such as the hematocrit, hemoglobin, blood volume, arterial blood gases, blood pH level, and serum electrolytes is essential for determining proper fluid and electrolyte replacement and acid-base balance. Hypertonic solutions, such as low-molecular-weight dextran, may be utilized as volume expanders. CVP readings, pulmonary artery pressures, and observation for signs of pulmonary edema should be closely monitored during fluid challenge procedures. Auscultation for rales and abnormal lung sounds and interpretation of hemodynamic data contribute to accurate evaluation of the effects of this mode of therapy. (The reader is referred to Chapter 16 for additional information regarding the significance of volume expansion and other methods used in the treatment of shock.)

Counterpulsation techniques, which decrease the workload of the left ventricle and thus decrease oxygen requirements while increasing diastolic perfusion, have proved to be helpful in the treatment of cardiogenic shock. The intra-aortic balloon-pumping technique uses a ballooned tube that is threaded into the femoral artery and positioned in the thoracic aorta. The balloon is synchronized to inflate at the onset of diastole and to deflate during systole, thus facilitating ejection of blood from the left ventricle. Thus the balloon (which is inflated with helium) provides an extra pulse after each heartbeat and increases systemic blood flow. An external pump machine, which synchronizes the inflation and deflation, requires proper maintenance to assure adequate functioning of the system. Would care is required for the large femoral incision used for insertion, and monitoring of circulation in the extremity distal to the femoral incision is essential.

In severe cardiogenic shock, emergency infarctectomy may be attempted to resect large infarcted areas that interfere with adequate cardiac-pumping action. Ventricular septal defects resulting from MI may also be repaired in this manner.

In spite of the increased knowledge concerning the causes and consequences of cardiogenic shock, about 85 percent of the patients with this condition die. The mortality rate has not changed in the past decade despite different treatment modalities. When the patient does recover from cardiogenic shock, a long hospitalization ensues. Management is similar to that for the patient with CHF (long-term digitalis and diuretic therapy, low sodium diet, and restricted activity).

Cardiac Surgery

Surgical intervention is another mode of therapy for certain types of cardiac disease. Among the conditions that are treated surgically are congenital heart defects, such as tetralogy of Fallot, transposition of the great vessels, pulmonary stenosis, patent ductus arteriosus, and atrial and ventricular septal defects. All these conditions are usually corrected during infancy or early childhood. Certain congenital defects, however, such as atrial septal defects, may not present symptoms until adolescence or adulthood, when surgery becomes necessary. (The reader is referred to a pediatric nursing textbook for review of surgical procedures for correction of congenital defects.)

Valvular defects, either congenital or acquired, are generally corrected surgically by valvular repair or valvular replacement. Prosthetic valves may be of the metal ball-in-cage type or a homograft or heterograft. **Homograft** is a graft of tissue from another person, while **heterograft** is a graft of tissue from an animal. Currently the rings of the older prosthetic valve models are being combined with porcine (pig) heterograft valves. Recent problems with infections and delayed rejections of these heterografts may result in restricted use, however. Valve replacement requires the technique of cardiopulmonary bypass (which will be discussed shortly) in contrast to the technique of mitral commissurotomy, which can be done by means of a conventional thoracotomy. Mitral commissurotomy involves palpation and valvulotomy using an indirect, finger-probing method to release the stenotic valve cusps.

One of the most recent developments in cardiac surgery is that of myocardial revascularization procedures for the treatment of coronary artery disease. Several different approaches have been used. Endarterectomy, which involves incising an obstructed vessel and removing the atherosclerotic plaques or thrombosis or both, has proved to have a high mortality rate and is being used less frequently. Reconstruction procedures utilizing patch grafts and pericardial tissue also have proved of limited value. Single or double mammary artery implantation procedures may also be accomplished for myocardial revascularization by implanting the mammary artery into the wall of the left ventricle. The artery is inserted directly into a small tunnel created surgically in the myocardium. Mammary implantations are done rarely as a singular approach. They are more often done in combination with more current revascularization procedures, when indicated. The most commonly used revascularization procedures are those of interposed vein grafts or bypass procedures, which provide instant revascularization.

A segment of an autogenous saphenous vein is resected and interposed for an excised obstructed segment of a coronary artery. In a saphenous vein bypass graft, the segment of the saphenous vein is reversed on one end and is anastomosed to the ascending aorta, and the other end is attached to the affected coronary artery beyond the site of the obstruction (Fig. 4-21). (The segment is reversed to prevent the valves in the vein segment from impeding blood flow through the artery.)

Revascularization procedures may also be performed in combination with repair of functional defects such as in the excision of a ventricular aneurysm. This defect is the result of extensive transmural infarction and consists of a flaccid, noncontractile sac. Ventricular aneurysms hamper the effectiveness of the cardiac pump and serve as a reservoir for blood clots, sediments, and infection.

Prior to cardiac surgery, a thorough history, physical examination, and various diagnostic procedures including cardiac catheterization and blood coagulation profiles are essential. In the case of myocardial revascularization procedures, coronary cinearteriography is necessary to demonstrate obstructions of the coronary arteries and to determine the extent of the atherosclerotic process within the entire myocardial circulatory system. In addition to coronary cinearteriography, ventricular angiography also is done to determine the functional ability of the left ventricle. Surgery is indicated when the atherosclerotic process is confined to segments that are relatively short and are accessible surgically. The best candidate for myocardial revascularization is the patient with an undamaged or salvageable myocardium, but with blockage of one, two, or more coronary vessels. Patients with generalized fibrosis and diffuse scar tissue are not candidates for the surgery.

There continues to be controversy as to the value of myocardial revascularization. Many studies have shown that although a high percentage of patients benefit from the surgery and are relieved from anginal

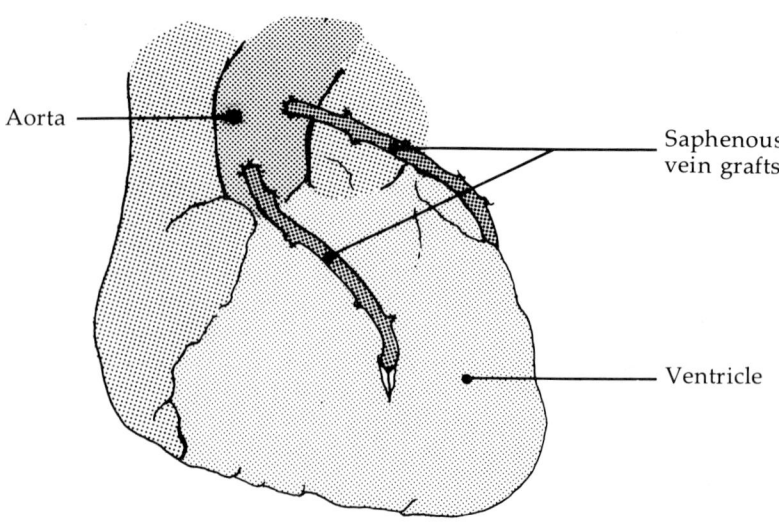

Figure 4-21
Myocardial revascularization procedure utilizing the saphenous vein bypass graft.

pain postoperatively, a high number of patients have no significant relief of symptoms (angina) and some even become worse and die within a year or two after surgery. The National Heart and Lung Institute of the National Institutes of Health has recently initiated a long-term study to determine the effectiveness of the surgical technique in significantly lengthening the life of patients with coronary artery disease.

Techniques of cardiac surgery are evolving as technology expands and provides improved heart-lung machines, physiologic monitoring, mechanical heart valves, and improved surgical and anesthetic techniques. In the broadest sense there are two possible approaches to cardiac surgery: (1) closed heart surgery, via a conventional thoracotomy (which is described in Chapter 3 in relation to chest surgery); and (2) open heart surgery, which utilizes extracorporeal circulation (ECC). The latter approach, which allows for direct visualization of the heart during the surgical procedure, was initiated in 1953. Previously, hypothermia was utilized for cardiac surgery, but has been replaced almost entirely by cardiopulmonary bypass techniques. However, some surgeons continue to use hypothermia in combination with ECC. Among the disadvantages of hypothermia is that its use is restricted to short-duration surgery (that is, when used as a single technique) and also is thought to contribute to complications such as ventricular fibrillation, cardiac arrest, and cardiac failure.

CARDIOPULMONARY BYPASS

Extracorporeal circulation, also known as cardiopulmonary bypass, is maintained by the heart-lung machine. The technique permits the diversion of venous blood out of the body through the heart-lung machine for oxygenation prior to being pumped back into the patient. The technique bypasses the heart and lungs, permitting prolonged intracardiac surgery under direct vision.

All heart-lung machines include three basic parts, although there are various types available (Fig. 4-22). The three essential components are the oxygenator, the arterial pump, and the arterial filter. The oxygenator may be a membrane, stainless steel screen, disk, or bubble type. All of these provide for oxygenation and removal of carbon dioxide by direct contact of a film of venous blood with a ventilating gas (oxygen or an oxygen and carbon dioxide mixture). An arterial pump maintains the flow of oxygenated blood returned to the patient. The flow rate produced by the pump is determined by the rate that is necessary to provide for the patient's normal resting cardiac output. The arterial filter is used to remove air emboli, fat emboli, tiny clots, or any particulate matter that may have been introduced into the arterial line during the oxygenation process.

To prevent clotting of the blood as it contacts the cannulas, oxygenator, and tubing, the patient is given an anticoagulant (heparin) prior to use of the bypass. Heparin is also added to the fluid used to fill the extracorporeal system. Currently, a technique known as hemodilution is used to "prime" (fill the machine with appropriate fluid) the bypass machines. Varying proportions of electrolyte solution, Ringer's lactate, albumin, or low-molecular-weight dextran are used to dilute whole blood. In addition, osmotic diuretics such as mannitol (Osmitrol) may be added to the fluid to increase kidney perfusion.

Venous cannulas are usually placed into the superior and inferior vena cava and the total venous return from the body is drained by gravity into a reservoir, prior to being passed into the oxygenator. The blood is passed into the heat exchanger, which can be regulated to cool, warm, or maintain the blood at normal body temperature. Oxygenated blood of the desired temperature then is passed via a roller pump through a filter and bubble trap. The blood enters the arterial circuit through an arterial cannula placed in the femoral artery (or in the ascending aorta in some situations), from where it perfuses the patient's body.

After the surgical procedure on the heart is completed, the heart begins to take over the circulation as the rate of blood flow from the heart-lung machine is gradually decreased. After the heart-lung machine lines are all clamped and the cannulas are removed, protamine sulfate is administered to neutralize the anticoagulation effects of heparin.

Problems associated with extracorporeal circulation include postoperative bleeding and hemorrhage (due to destruction of coagulation factors by the heart-lung machine or by incomplete neutralization of heparin) and

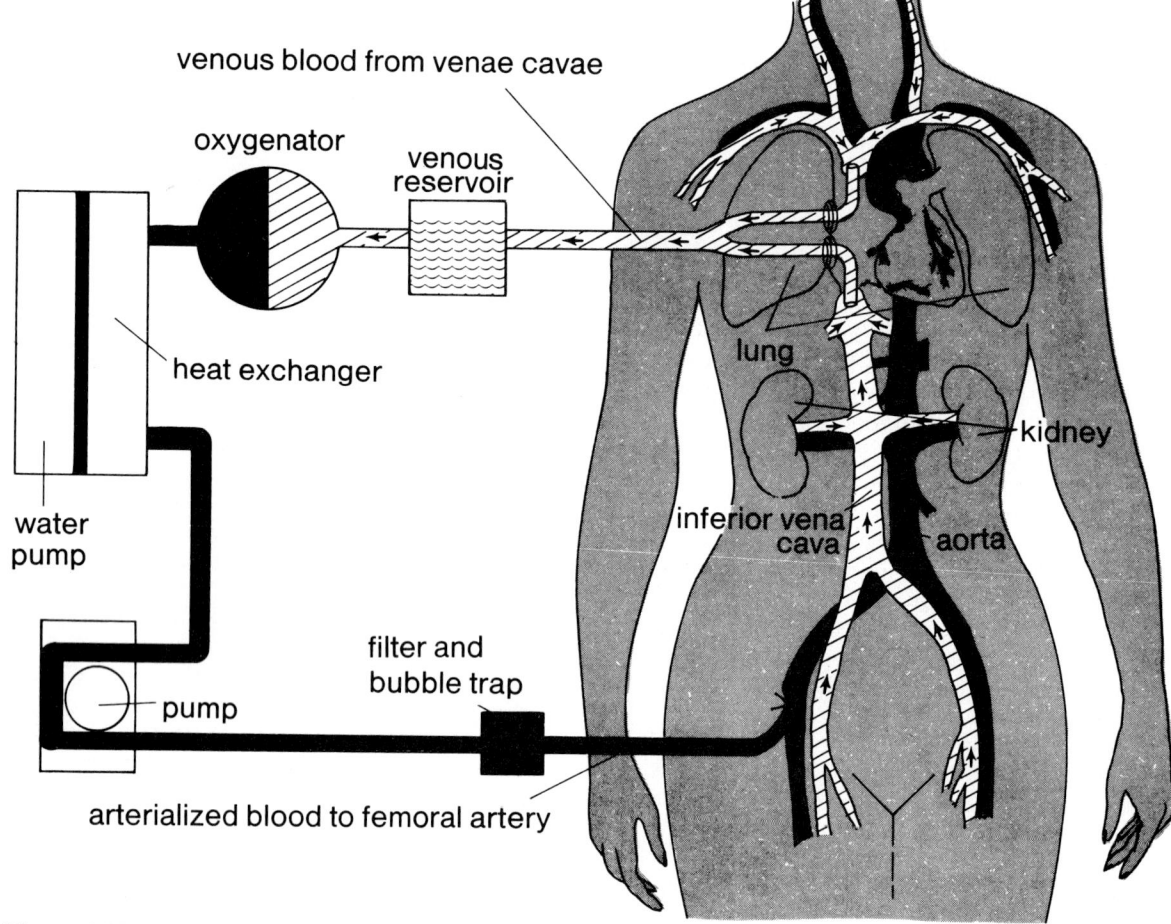

Figure 4-22
Cardiopulmonary bypass technique. (From *American Journal of Nursing* 74:861, 1974. Reproduced with permission.)

hemolysis of the red blood cells. The latter condition results from the trauma of the machine on the blood cells or from reactions with the donated blood used for priming. Hemolysis may be excessive and beyond the capacity of the liver and the kidneys to metabolize and excrete the free hemoglobin. Intratubular obstruction may occur leading to acute tubular necrosis and renal failure. Prolonged and inadequate perfusion may result in tissue anoxia and metabolic acidosis leading to the "low cardiac output" syndrome (decreased cardiac output with deficient tissue perfusion). This shock-like state is treated with the administration of sodium bicarbonate or tromethamine (THAM) and electrolyte replacement to correct the acidosis, the administration of inotropic drugs to improve cardiac function, and oxygen therapy. Pulmonary complications are fairly common because the lungs are not continuously ventilated during cardiopulmonary bypass, and the system therefore predisposes the patient to the development of atelectasis and pneumonitis. Onset of fever frequently occurs following use of ECC. Postoperative nursing measures must be concerned with the improvement of respiratory functioning. The importance of the respirator, endotracheal intubation, adequate suctioning, and deep breathing and coughing cannot be overemphasized. The heart-lung machine has also been implicated in the occurrence of emboli to the brain resulting in cerebral edema, hypoxia, and brain damage. The relation of cardiopulmonary bypass to the incidence of postcardiotomy psychoses is discussed in another section of this chapter. The body's reaction to the trauma of the surgery may be mild fever during the first few postoperative days without a significant rise in the leukocyte count or without signs of infection.

Preoperative Care
Whatever the reason for cardiac surgery and whatever the approach utilized, the need to prepare the patient and family for the life-threatening procedure is imperative. Optimal physical and psychological stability is the underlying goal of the preoperative period. The nurse should be aware that the patient and family have already undergone an anxiety-provoking experience during the diagnostic workup and previous episodes of cardiac pain.

The initial step involves an explanation to the patient about the pathologic condition present, the planned surgery, and the benefits anticipated. The risks in the procedure as well as in the cardiopulmonary bypass must be reviewed with the patient to ensure an informed consent for the surgical procedure. With revascularization surgery, the patient must understand that the operation can relieve the current symptoms but that the basic mechanism causing atherosclerosis is not altered by the surgery [22]. Most cardiac surgeons prefer to utilize precise diagrams for teaching their patients exactly how the operation will be accomplished.

Patients are usually admitted to the hospital at least 3 days prior to the operation to complete preoperative diagnostic measures and to obtain other baseline data. An electrocardiogram and extensive laboratory work are done to determine baseline data and to detect other conditions that might interfere with a satisfactory response to the surgery and anesthesia. Preoperative coagulation profiles, for example, are essential when a bypass procedure is expected. The patient continues on his prescribed diet (low calorie, or low cholesterol). If the patient is a smoker, he is usually required to discontinue smoking because the effects of nicotine may cause spasms of the coronary arteries. In revascularization surgery, surgeons may be unwilling to operate unless the patient has agreed to stop smoking.

Any infectious process in the body, including active dental infections, is a contraindication for cardiac surgery. Weight reduction is accomplished before surgery is scheduled, and pulmonary function is improved with therapeutic measures for patients with respiratory dysfunction.

Anxiety stimulates the release of catecholamines and causes arterial spasms and increased sympathetic action. Preoperative anxiety has also been implicated in the development of postoperative delirium. A major emphasis, therefore, during the preoperative period, is on decreasing anxiety and assisting the patient to cope with the stress of open heart surgery. The family is also included in the preoperative preparations as much as possible, as they may be a resource for emotional support to the patient. Family members can be a resource only if they are aware of the expected preparations, results, and purposes of all steps in the preoperative period. In addition, the anxiety of the family, if not dealt with, can be conveyed to the patient.

Medications may be initiated preoperatively and prescriptions should be followed explicitly to assure that cardiac function is optimal for surgery. In some protocols patients may be digitalized prior to the cardiac surgery; in others, digitalis preparations may be discontinued preoperatively. Patients may be started on prophylactic antibiotic therapy; sedatives or tranquilizers may also be administered. A patient's behavior and comments should be observed closely during this preoperative period.

It has been found that patients manifesting considerable anxiety or depression have a lesser chance of surviving surgery and a greater morbidity after surgery than other patients. Kimball [23] stresses the importance of finding objective ways, other than interviewing, for evaluating preoperative anxiety, depression, and poor coping responses and evaluating the need for limited psychotherapeutic intervention for patients identified as poor psychological risks for surgery.

When possible, several teaching sessions should be conducted with both the patient and his family. In some institutions, group classes for cardiac surgery patients may be held; patients who have recently experienced cardiac surgery may be included in the classes. These former patients are useful in reinforcing the importance of cooperating in the postoperative care. Regardless of the method used for teaching the patient and the family, a record that preoperative teaching has been carried out must be documented. A check list of essential content must be provided for each patient, to assure that important aspects are not omitted. The patient's acceptance and understanding of the information must be evaluated to determine the need for reinforcement of specific items.

The patient is also instructed by physical therapists and inhalation therapists, and by the nursing staff, in the proper techniques for deep breathing and coughing. This instruction should also include orientation to the use of the intermittent positive-pressure machine (as well as practice sessions) to assure its proper use postoperatively. The patient should be advised that an endotracheal tube will be in place postoperatively and that it will be connected to a respirator for proper ventilation. He should be warned that he will not be able to speak, eat, or drink until the endotracheal tube is removed, usually within 24 to 48 hours. Other ways of communicating are established during this preoperative period.

Dial soap or pHisoHex showers are prescribed often twice daily for several days preoperatively. Daily weight and data on vital sign recordings are obtained for baseline information for postoperative evaluation. In addition to the respiratory assistance devices, the patient is advised about the various usual types of equipment that will be used postoperatively. Equipment that should be discussed includes the nasogastric tube, Foley catheter, chest drainage tubes, and intravenous and arterial lines for monitoring and administering medications and fluid therapy. The patient is also advised that his heart rate will be continuously monitored and that he will therefore be wearing electrodes on his chest. If the patient is not familiar with the monitoring procedure, he is shown the electrodes preoperatively. The patient is advised that frequent blood analysis (for arterial gases and other laboratory data) will be drawn. If not forewarned, the patient may fear that complications have occurred when blood specimens are drawn frequently.

A visit to the ICU will prepare the patient for what to expect postoperatively. He is advised that staffing is planned to provide a one-to-one, or similar, ratio. On occasion, some patients may prefer not to see the unit. The visit to the ICU may increase their anxiety, so the visit is made when patients can meet some of the ICU staff as well as have an opportunity to discuss their feelings and concerns after seeing the unit. The patient is warned about the types of sounds normally heard in the ICU so that he will realize that these are usual and anticipated. For example, the typical swooshing sound of the respirator can be very disturbing. Ample time for answering questions of both the patient and family should be provided.

Postoperative Care

To provide for appropriate postoperative care, the nurse must understand the preoperative condition of the patient, the purpose of the surgery, the type of surgical procedure, the implications of the surgery and the cardiopulmonary bypass, and potential complications [22].

Postoperatively, there are many areas of concern when assisting the patient to optimal recovery. Adequate cardiac output is achieved by maintenance of adequate blood volume, and prevention of cardiac failure or arrhythmias by accurate and continuous monitoring. Hemodynamic monitoring utilizing CVP measurements and pulmonary wedge and intra-arterial pressure has facilitated early detection of pump failure. Arterial blood gas levels, hematocrit, hemoglobin, and blood volume analysis are obtained at regular intervals. The pulse, temperature, respirations, skin color, and urinary output are consistently monitored to detect complications. Drainage from chest tubes is observed for excessive blood loss. The chest tubes usually are retained for 24 to 48 hours and their patency is carefully maintained. The reader is referred to Chapter 3 for more detailed information on the care of patients with chest tubes.

If cardiac output begins to diminish and inotropic therapy is indicated, catecholamines such as norepinephrine (Levophed), isoproterenol (Isuprel), epinephrine (Adrenalin), and dopamine (Intropin) are used in conjunction with digitalis, diuretics, and antiarrhythmic drugs. Dopamine is increasingly being used because it is less likely to constrict renal arteries, which is a distinct advantage over other inotropic drugs.

Arrhythmias are treated according to their type and cause. Lidocaine is usually the drug of choice in controlling ventricular arrhythmias. Digitalis, propranolol, and quinidine are other drugs used for tachyarrhythmias. Direct-current countershock is indicated for tachyarrhythmias that are nonresponsive to drug therapy.

Fluid and electrolyte imbalance is a common cause of arrhythmias. Accurate intake and output records are essential, and serum levels of major electrolytes must be routinely monitored. Due to the cellular destruction and loss of potassium during surgery, its replacement is crucial, especially if the patient is receiving digitalis. Low potassium levels are a common cause of digitalis toxicity. If urine output diminishes, however, potassium dosages must be modified, since the kidneys are responsible for excreting up to 80 percent of circulating potassium. Renal function is monitored via hourly urine outputs. Daily weights are usually taken to detect sodium and fluid retention, as well as to evaluate nutritional intake.

The patient with open heart surgery may have considerable pain. Judicious use of analgesics must be practiced in order to make the patient comfortable enough to cooperate in the coughing and deep-breathing exercises without jeopardizing respiratory function by excessive depression of the respiratory center. Pain is assessed carefully, distinguishing incisional pain from angina pain that might indicate an impending MI.

Circulatory status is evaluated by also assessing the quality of peripheral pulses (the femoral, posterior tibial, and dorsalis pedis) and of the radial pulse, in order to detect thrombi or emboli. Neurologic status is monitored to detect cerebral ischemia or damage.

As discussed previously, patients who have had cardiopulmonary bypass are vulnerable to pneumonia, atelectasis, and pneumonitis in relation to limited lung ventilation during the surgical procedure. Endotracheal intubation and the volume respirator are utilized only until the patient is able to resume his own respiratory control and his blood gas levels indicate adequate ventilation. The nurse must be persistent in encouraging coughing and deep breathing and in encouraging turning and active range-of-motion exercises in order to prevent pulmonary and vascular complications. Evaluation of the effectiveness of coughing techniques is done by chest auscultation. Splinting the chest incision is important to prevent incisional pain and to facilitate coughing. Patients tend to immobilize the left arm and shoulder, so gentle passive movements gradually increasing to active exercise are encouraged.

Postoperative complications include those already discussed as related to cardiopulmonary bypass or those occurring after any type of surgery or anesthesia. In addition, cardiac tamponade is a potential complication. Blood clots may accumulate within the pericardial sac, restricting cardiac function and resulting in hypotension and shock. Cardiac tamponade should be suspected in the presence of a fluctuating pulse pressure (e.g., when the systolic B.P. drops more than 10 mm Hg during inspiration). Treatment consists in the insertion of a drainage tube into the pericardial cavity via pericardiocentesis.

The psychological status of the patient and the family is an important aspect in total assessment of the cardiac surgery patient. The fear of dying along with unrelieved postoperative pain and discomforts, as well as the deprivation of sleep during the initial critical phases, often leads to depression or to periods of delirium or "cardiac psychosis." It has been shown that the highest incidence of postoperative delirium occurs in cardiotomy patients. Postoperative psychological reactions are usually demonstrated initially by restlessness, apprehension, and confusion that lead to impairment of orientation, memory, judgment, sensory discrimination, and intellectual functioning. Disorientation, visual and auditory sensory disturbances, delusions, and paranoid behavior also have been observed. Symptoms tend to develop after an initial lucid period and progress to delirium by the second or third postoperative day.

A specific cause of postoperative reactions has not been determined; it is likely that multiple factors contribute to the reactions. Preoperative anxiety, sensory overload, sleep deprivation, hypoxia, electrolyte disturbances, effects of prolonged use of cardiopulmonary bypass, anesthesia, drugs, and unfamiliarity with either monotonous or ambiguous stimuli have all been identified as predisposing factors [25–27]. Various studies done on cardiotomy patients have cited implications for nursing care of the patient in combating physiologic and psychological stresses during the preoperative and postoperative periods.

Budd and Brown [25] found that a specific reorientation procedure for orienting the patient to time, place, person, and physical status was helpful in significantly lowering the incidence of delirium and complications, and reducing the length of hospitalization. Teaching systemic relaxation techniques has also proved to be helpful in decreasing the number of untoward postoperative reactions.

Ellis studied postcardiotomy patients in relation to the development of intermittent stimulus experiences for which there are no apparent stimuli within the environment. She found that significant numbers of patients associated these experiences with pain that was not adequately controlled. Her study reinforced the importance of skillful management of postoperative pain, the recognition of discharge from the hospital as a time of anxiety, the management of sleep, the importance of allowing patients to express their fears of falling asleep, the importance of reality-orienting devices, and the vital measure of providing adequate communication about any of the patient's unusual sensory experiences [26].

Woods also studied sleep patterns of patients who had open heart surgery to determine whether sleep deprivation actually occurs. She found that none of the subjects studied obtained more than four sleep cycles per postoperative night. Direct and indirect monitoring as well as measures to promote respiration were the most frequent causes of potential interruptions. Her study verified the importance of planning for incorporating sleeping needs into nursing care plans. Her study also cites the need for a more active role of the nurse in controlling environmental stimuli [27]. Nurses have a vital role in improving preoperative and postoperative care of cardiotomy patients by assisting them to better cope with the stresses associated with the surgery.

As the patient's vital signs and cardiac status stabilize, progressive ambulation and activity are planned, depending on the individual's tolerance and on the type of surgical procedure performed. For example, the patient who has undergone surgical repair of coarctation of the aorta or multiple valve replacement will progress more slowly than the patient with myocardial revascularization. Careful observation of vital signs and the patient's response to activity is essential. Any shortness of breath, chest pain, or edema is reported, and activity is restricted until the patient is evaluated by the surgeon. Often cardiotomy patients are ambulated the first postoperative day and walking is encouraged; one week postoperatively, patients may already be walking up and down 10 stairs, depending on the status of the patient and the type of operation. If tolerance is achieved the patient, soon after discharge, takes 15- to 20-minute walks daily and increases these either in length or briskness. Patients are cautioned about walking in cold weather, however, for reasons given on page 346. It should be emphasized that activity schedules and planning are individualized and no set pattern can be determined without consideration of the individual's needs, tolerance, and concerns. Although ambulation is encouraged, the patient should not assume that his progress is such that other types of activity are readily assumed. Heavy lifting is not permitted; cardiac surgery requires a sternal incision which requires adequate healing. Lifting also encourages the patient to use the Valsalva maneuver (holding the breath and straining) while lifting, which is contraindicated for the cardiac patient. The Valsalva maneuver causes a rise in B.P. and an increase in intrathoracic pressure.

In addition to all these precautions and aspects for teaching, the patient requires instruction in diet and medication management. The diet may be one restricting salt, cholesterol, or calories, or another special diet. The patient who has been placed on anticoagulants requires specific instruction regarding safety aspects in the utilization of the medication. The patient who has had a prosthetic valve replacement is likely to be maintained on long-term anticoagulant therapy because of tendencies for blood to clot from contact with the metal prosthesis. These patients are also susceptible to prosthetic valve endocarditis. Other types of invasive procedures may lead to this complication, so that prophylactic antibiotics are usually indicated for dental procedures, cardiac catheterizations, and biopsies.

Depending on the type of surgery and the recovery rate of the individual patient, discharge from the hospital may be within 10 to 14 days. This period allows for adequate preparation for discharge, assuming that attention to discharge planning is a nursing priority early in the postoperative period.

Gradual increase in activity continues during the home recovery phase; assuming no complications, 8 to 10 weeks is the normal length of time for recovery, and return to work is generally possible after 8 weeks postoperatively. Emphasis continues on maintenance of normal weight, avoidance of activities and habits considered risk factors, and moderation in activity. Successful cardiac surgery generally results in increased capacity for activity and a renewed spirit if secondary gains from cardiac disease are not essential to the psychological makeup of the patient. Patients are often anxious about the long-term results of the surgery, even though the immediate results are favorable. They often fear initiation of each progressive step in convalescence because of the perceived possibility of sudden death. Participating in the care and management of patients during and after cardiac surgery is therefore a challenging and satisfying experience for the nurse.

HEART TRANSPLANTATION

The first human heart transplantation was done in 1967; the procedure continues to be a controversial one in the management of cardiac disease. Although the procedure is not an established mode of therapy and the number of long-term survivals has been minimal, the surgical procedure has raised the potential for modern cardiac surgery. Even with the increased number of risks involved with the surgery, persons with deteriorating advanced heart disease are willing to withstand the procedure in order to survive a few years longer. (The procedure has also been significant in requiring a redefinition of death; formerly death was defined as the absence of the heartbeat and respirations, with clinical death defined as the cessation of these functions.)

Problems associated with human heart transplantation have been related primarily to immunologic rejection by the recipient. Histocompatibility with the donor heart is determined by leukocyte typing as well as by customary typing and cross-matching both the recipient and the potential donor. When surgery is anticipated, immunosuppressive drugs such as azathioprine (Imuran), corticosteroids, and antilymphocytic globulin are initiated. Postoperatively the patient is placed in reverse isolation for protection from infections. Postoperative management is similar to that for any patient having open heart surgery, with the added component of reverse isolation technique and observations and monitoring for symptoms of infectious processes or donor rejection. Early signs of a rejection crisis include temperature elevation, a narrow pulse pressure, tachycardia, signs of congestive heart failure, and often symptoms similar to postoperative depression, including malaise alternated by restlessness.

Other problems associated with heart transplantation are related to the advanced age of most of the patients with terminal heart disease, the presence of secondary complications in other vital organs such as the kidneys, and the lack of suitable artificial circulatory support devices such as an adequate artificial mechanical heart. The intra-aortic balloon pump has been used to assist circulation during and after cardiac surgery. Some ventricular assisting devices such as air-driven diaphragm pump systems for temporary pumping assistance are currently being used experimentally in some heart centers. The lack of alternative approaches to external energy sources to power artificial hearts is a major limiting factor. Research on methods of implantable power sources such as high capacity, long-life batteries and miniature nuclear power is currently under way. The satisfactory development of materials that do not damage red blood cells or promote clotting and which are compatible with body tissue is necessary to construct adequate artificial hearts. Continued research in these areas and in improving surgical techniques may result in more effective transplant surgery or artificial mechanical heart replacement.

The Peripheral Vascular System

The **peripheral circulation,** which is generally defined as the circulation other than that in the ventricular and atrial chambers of the heart, includes the arteries, veins, capillaries, and their subdivisions to the other organs of the body. This discussion is limited to diseases that occur in the aorta and its branches, and in the arterial, venous, and lymphatic circulation in the periphery, that is, in the extremities. (Extracranial vascular disorders associated with neurologic problems are discussed in Chapter 11. The pulmonary circulation is discussed in Chapter 3, and the portal circulation is discussed in Chapter 7.)

The role of the cardiovascular system is to maintain homeostasis at the cellular level. Physiologically the total network of the cardiovascular system must be evaluated because the system functions interdependently with the rest of the body. The reader will recall that inadequate perfusion of the heart results in cardiac dysfunction and damage; in a similar way, tissues of the extremities are damaged when blood flow to the peripheral vessels is disturbed in peripheral vascular disease.

An earlier section of this chapter described the anatomy and physiology of the peripheral vascular system and stated that the contractile properties of the arteries are under the influence of several stimuli, including local metabolic products, neural factors, and the concentration of catecholamines. The sympathetic nervous system richly supplies the arteries and causes vasoconstriction when stimulated. Epinephrine, specifically, constricts superficial blood vessels, but dilates cerebral, cardiac, and muscular vessels. Norepinephrine, which affects all blood vessels, particularly affects peripheral vessels. Other substances contained in the systemic circulation also act on blood vessels. These substances include the following: histamine, which is a potent vasodilator of small blood vessels; bradykinin, a potent vasodilator of cutaneous vessels; acetylcholine, a transient vasodilator; serotonin, a strong dilator of cutaneous arterioles; and the antidiuretic hormone (ADH) which can increase B.P. by causing constriction of arterioles. Angiotensin is also related to arterial constriction.

Another factor that affects the diameters of vessels is temperature change; heat dilates arteries and cold constricts arterial segments. Injury to an artery also causes vasoconstriction as a compensatory mechanism to combat hemorrhage.

ASSESSMENT OF THE PERIPHERAL VASCULAR SYSTEM

The history of a patient with peripheral vascular disease will vary according to the cause and the site of involvement. It is important, however, to determine the patient's knowledge of any previous injury to the extremities, the presence of hypertension, or any other major disease (such as diabetes mellitus) and any history of thrombophlebitis or varicose veins.

The patient is asked to describe any pain that occurs in the extremities and the factors that precipitate or relieve the pain (e.g., rest, elevation of the legs). When the patient describes the presence of pain, it should be determined whether the pain is aggravated by cold weather, or exercise, or if it occurs even during rest. If walking results in pain, the patient is asked how far or how long he or she can walk before pain develops. The patient is also asked (in addition to the examiner's subsequent physical examination) about the nature (incidence, duration, contributing factors, and the length of time the symptom has been noted) of color or temperature changes in the extremities and about the presence of any sensory changes, such as numbness or tingling. Any episodes of leg swelling, leg ulcers, or problems in the healing of sores on the legs or feet are also determined.

The physical examination includes inspection, palpation, and auscultation, as well as specific diagnostic tests as indicated by the patient's presenting symptoms. The patient is observed for the presence of any gross abnormalities as he walks and carries out activities. The extremities are examined for coldness, numbness, pallor, loss of hair, and trophic changes in the skin that demonstrate a decrease in blood flow and cellular nutrition. Atrophy of muscles and varicosities are also noted. In chronic obstructive vascular disease, decreased hair growth and thickened nail beds are frequently evident. In prolonged venous insufficiency, a brown discoloration of the skin around the ankles is frequently observed.

Inspection is done after specific exercise and postural changes are accomplished. Determination of retarded arterial filling is made by raising an extremity for a period of time and then lowering it. This determination can also be accomplished by physically obliterating circulation temporarily, releasing the obliteration, and then observing the return of arterial flow to determine obstruction in the flow. If arterial circulation is markedly impaired, the return of color may require 45 seconds or longer. When ischemia is severe, dependent extremities may develop a cyanotic redness, which is termed **rubor.** Capillary filling defects are tested simply by applying a small amount of pressure on the tip of the patient's toenail to produce blanching. Slow return of color upon releasing the pressure indicates diminished circulation.

Palpation is an important procedure in evaluating the vascular system. The skin is felt for temperature abnormalities and for the quality and extent of edema. Palpating for the presence and quality of major peripheral pulses, and comparing the pulses bilaterally, are essential procedures. The major pulses that are evaluated are the radial, brachial, carotid, popliteal, femoral, and dorsalis pedis, before and after exercise (Fig. 4-23). The pulses may be recorded as bounding, full, strong, weak, or absent.

Pain response to palpation is also evaluated. The presence of tenderness when the gastrocnemius muscle is compressed anteriorly against the tibia but not when the muscle is pulled away from the tibia is significant when deep vein thrombosis is suspected. A positive Homans' sign is also a significant finding. This sign is the occurrence of calf pain on sharp dorsiflexion of the foot. The extremities are also checked for symmetry. Unilateral swelling may be determined by comparing the circumference measurements of the extremities at the thigh and calf. This technique can be used by the nurse in subsequent assessment of progress and changes in the extremity after therapy has been initiated.

Skillful abdominal palpation may detect the presence of an abdominal aneurysm. Mesenteric arterial insufficiency may be suspected when abdominal pain is severe, especially after meals.

Auscultation is used to determine the B.P. in both the upper and lower extremities. The stethoscope is also used to detect the presence of bruits, which are vascular murmurs, or extracardiac blowing sounds, that are often detected at the sites of narrowed vessels.

Diagnostic tests to evaluate the peripheral vascular system include oscillometry, skin temperature studies, angiography, the Trendelenburg test, and in some cases a lumbar sympathetic block.

Oscillometry provides a record of arterial pulsations in an extremity to determine the extent of arterial occlusions. A pneumatic cuff, wrapped around an extremity, is inflated and pressure readings are taken; an oscillometric index is determined. Readings are taken at various levels of the extremity.

Skin temperature studies may be accomplished in a variety of ways to compare limb response to temperature changes. One leg is immersed in warm water and the temperature

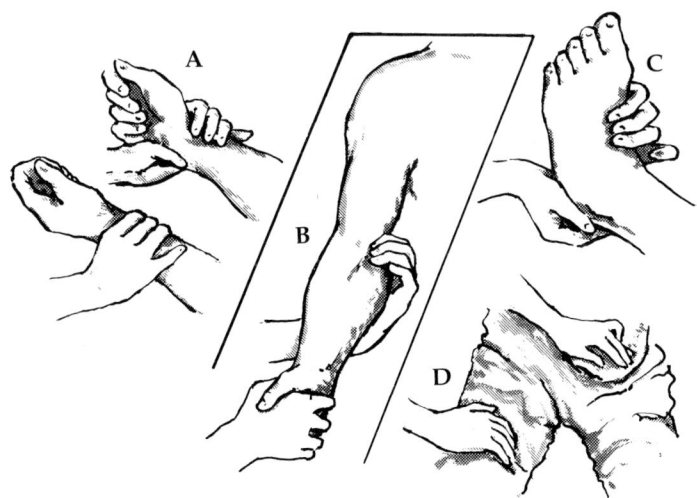

Figure 4-23
Palpating the arterial pulses of the extremities. **A.** Radial pulse. **B.** Brachial pulse. **C.** Dorsalis pedis pulse. **D.** Femoral pulse. [From R. D. Judge and G. D. Zuidema, *Methods of Clinical Examination: A Physiologic Approach* (3rd ed.). Boston: Little, Brown and Company, 1974. Reproduced by permission.]

of the other leg is noted. Normally the skin temperature of the opposite leg should rise within 30 minutes. Placing a heating pad on the abdomen to determine bilateral temperature responses in the legs is also done. The reliability of temperature studies is questionable, however, because the patient's emotions may influence vasomotor tone.

Angiography is an x-ray visualization (utilizing contrast media) of specific vessels to determine the location and extent of vascular occlusion and narrowing.

The **Trendelenburg test** is a procedure to determine the competence of the valves and venous filling in relation to body position and constriction.

A **lumbar sympathetic block** involves the injection of a local anesthetic (procaine) to block the sympathetic ganglion fibers that control the affected leg. Vasodilatation should occur since the controls of vasoconstriction are eliminated. The test is often done to determine whether sympathectomy might benefit the patient with impaired circulation to an extremity.

MEDICAL AND NURSING CARE

Peripheral vascular conditions are generally chronic conditions with frequent recurrences. The conditions, which occur most often in the elderly, are generally painful and the treatment is complicated by slow healing. Patients with peripheral vascular disease are often discouraged because of prolonged hospitalization and chronic disability. In addition, economic problems related to long-term medical care and hospitalization often contribute to chronic discouragement and depression. The nurse should take these aspects into consideration when working with the patient who has peripheral vascular disease.

General principles in the care of patients with peripheral vascular disease are, for the most part, similar, whether the primary problem is in the arteries, veins, or the lymphatic system. Positioning of the extremity is based primarily on determination of whether increased arterial flow is desirable or whether increased venous return is most important. This determination is based on the presence of either arterial or venous insufficiency. In the patient with arterial disease, for example, it is especially important to increase blood flow by utilizing the dependent position more extensively, and in patients with venous deficiency the elevation of the extremity is more likely to be required. However, the nurse should remember that, except in those cases where no movement, or minimal movement, is desirable (such as gangrene, cellulitis, ulceration, or in early stages of deep thrombosis), varying the position of the extremity is indicated.

For arterial insufficiency in the lower extremities, the Buerger-Allen exercises may be prescribed. These exercises improve blood flow by utilizing gravity to alternately fill and empty arteries. The exercises, which are repeated about five times, are usually done three times daily. The technique is illustrated in Figure 4-24. (A special board or a chair may be used if an electrically operated bed is not available.)

A passive approach to the use of postural exercises for emptying and filling the blood vessels requires the use of an oscillating bed. A rocking motion is produced by a motor that is set to tilt the bed longitudinally at a rate determined by the patient's need and tolerance. In some cases, the oscillating bed is used day and night; in other cases it is used only at intervals.

Vasodilatation is encouraged in most conditions, except when increased metabolic demands may be contraindicated. Vasodilatation is accelerated by drug therapy and moist heat, and surgical sympathectomy in selected cases. Warmth is most appropriately provided by control of the environmental temperature and the use of adequate clothing to prevent chilling. Direct heat to the extremities is contraindicated unless specifically prescribed by the physician. Because decreased sensory perception related to neurologic involvement is frequently associated with peripheral vascular disease, the possibility of burns and thermal damage to an extremity is a potential hazard. Cigarette smoking should be discontinued by patients with peripheral vascular disease; the nicotine in cigarettes contributes to vasoconstriction of vessels. For the same reason, avoidance of emotional stress and chilling is necessary.

Vascular obstruction is prevented by educating the patient about factors that constrict vascular flow, such as obesity, standing for prolonged periods, wearing of constrictive garments, and crossing the legs at the knee. Prevention of venous stasis is also important in preventing venous thrombosis and potential embolic phenomena. The use of compression supports (elastic stockings, elastic bandages, support hose) may be indicated for some patients to prevent venous stasis. Directions for applying the different varieties of support devices should be followed specifically; the proper size and the prevention of wrinkles are essential factors in their use. Vascular obstruction is also combated by the use of anticoagulant therapy, which will be discussed later in this chapter.

The relief of pain is an important aspect of care. Increasing the blood flow to the part is generally more effective in relieving pain than is the use of analgesics. Narcotics are contraindicated in chronic peripheral vascular disease because of the danger of addiction.

A major aspect of care involves education of the patient concerning the prevention of tissue damage and infection. Proper foot care and measures to prevent trauma are given later in this chapter with the discussion of chronic arterial deficiency. The principles in the protection of the extremity are applicable to all types of vascular disease.

ANTICOAGULANT THERAPY

Anticoagulant therapy is used extensively in the presence (or potential development) of thromboembolic phenomena to prevent thrombosis formation by decreasing the level of blood coagulability. A **thrombus** is an abnormal clot that forms in a blood vessel and partially or completely occludes the vessel. An **embolus** is a clot (or fragment of a clot, or a fat, gas, or air embolus) that breaks from its attachment and travels to another part of the body. When it reaches a narrow point in the circulatory system it then obstructs the vessel. The formation of thromboembolic phenomena is promoted by three processes: (1) endothelial surface damage of the vessel, such as in arteriosclerosis, infection, and trauma; (2) a decreased rate of blood flow, such as occurs in venous stasis; and (3) an increase in blood coagulability. The two major types of anticoagulant drugs are heparin and the coumarin derivatives such as warfarin so-

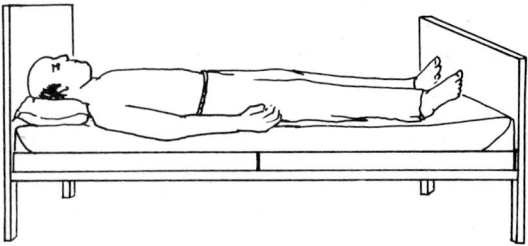
To start: Patient lies flat on his back.

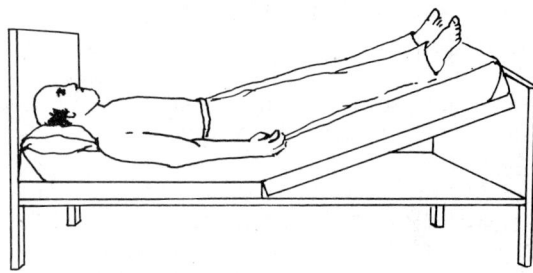
Position 1: Patient elevates and rests his legs for about 2 minutes, or until his legs become pale.

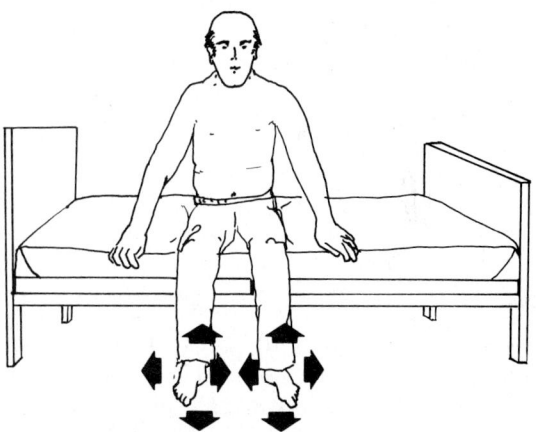
Position 2: Patient lowers his legs, sits up, and dangles them for about 3 minutes or until his legs become pink. While dangling, he moves his feet through six positions: toes down, up, in, out, spread, and return to neutral. He then repeats these positions. The feet should become entirely pink.

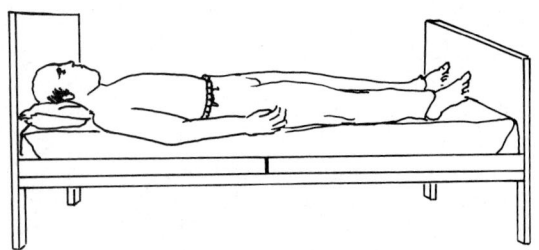
Position 3: Patient returns to flat starting position for about 5 minutes and then repeats the exercise.

Figure 4-24
Positions indicated for use of the Buerger-Allen exercises in the treatment of arterial insufficiency.

dium (Coumadin). Heparin is used when rapid effects are desirable and warfarin is generally used in long-term management.

It is generally felt that heparin prevents the activation of thrombin and inhibits thromboplastin formation. (It is important to clarify that heparin does not dissolve the fibrin of formed clots.) It also prevents platelet agglutination.

Heparin must be given parenterally because it is not absorbed from the gastrointestinal tract. Heparin is generally administered intravenously by continuous infusion or by intermittent administration every 4 to 6 hours through a **heparin lock** (a scalp vein needle with a special rubber plug to facilitate repeated injections). Less often heparin is administered subcutaneously. When it is administered subcutaneously, precautions are necessary to avert the formation of hematomas. Usually the lower abdominal fat pads are the preferred sites. (It is advantageous to make a chart of the patient's abdomen to record the sites where injections are given so that the sites of previous injections will not be repeatedly used. Repeated injections in the same site predispose to hematoma formation.) A very sharp and short needle (5/8 inch long) is used for the subcutaneous injection which is given at a 90° angle. The puncture site is *not* massaged after withdrawal of the needle. The area approximately 5 cm or 2 inches around the umbilicus is avoided as a site for injections.

Usual intravenous doses of heparin are 5,000 to 10,000 units every 4 (or sometimes every 6) hours. Continuous infusions are usually prescribed at 10,000 to 20,000 units in 1,000 ml of fluid. Subcutaneous heparin is usually prescribed at 10,000 to 20,000 units every 8 hours or 14,000 to 20,000 units every 12 hours.

To evaluate the effect of heparin, the patient's blood is tested for the clotting time before therapy is started and at regular intervals (according to institutional protocol as well as the status of the patient) during heparin therapy. Usually the Lee-White coagulation method is used, but the activated partial thromboplastin time is preferred by some authorities. The clotting time is ordinarily maintained at 2 to 2½ times the normal time (which in the Lee-White method is 5 to 10 minutes).

In spontaneous bleeding, or a prolonged clotting time, heparin is neutralized by protamine sulfate, which is administered at a dosage determined by the amount of heparin that was given in the preceding dose. Hypersensitivity reactions have occurred with heparin administration; mild fever, urticaria, rhinitis, and a burning sensation in the feet are noted.

The action of the coumarin drugs is to interfere with the action of vitamin K, which is necessary for the synthesis of clotting factors II (prothrombin), VII, IX, and X. The major coumarin drugs include warfarin sodium, bishydroxycoumarin (Dicumarol), acenocoumarol (Sintrom), and phenprocoumon (Liquamar). Another type of anticoagulant that is used less often is phenindione (Hedulin), which is a derivative of indanedione.

Warfarin sodium (Coumadin) is available for parenteral (IM or IV) injection, but is mainly given orally. Coumadin is probably the most commonly used of the coumarin drugs. It may be started at the same time heparin is initiated. Coumadin has a slower onset of action (3 to 6 days); the overlapping of the drugs may facilitate a smooth transition when heparin is discontinued (usually in 3 to 7 days). The prothrombin time is used to measure the effectiveness of Coumadin therapy, and is usually maintained at 1½ to 2½ times (18 to 30 seconds) the normal activity time (which is usually 11 to 13 seconds in most controls).

If the prothrombin time is prolonged excessively or if spontaneous bleeding occurs, vitamin K (e.g., Synkayvite or AquaMephyton) is administered. A refractory period usually follows for about a week after the vitamin K is given.

When patients are on anticoagulants, large painful hematomas may form at intramuscular injection sites. For this reason, intramuscular injections are contraindicated during anticoagulant therapy. Other signs of bleeding complications include nasal or mucous membrane bleeding, hemoptysis, hematuria, increased menstrual bleeding, joint pain, abdominal or flank pain, purpura, ecchymosis, and black tarry stools.

The action of anticoagulant drugs, particularly the coumarin derivatives, may be influenced by the simultaneous administration of certain other drugs. Drugs that potentiate the effect of anticoagulant drugs include indomethacin (Indocin), salicylates, phenytoin sodium (Dilantin), chloral hydrate, phenylbutazone (Butazolidin), and clofibrate (Atromid S). Antibiotics, quinidine, and adrenocorticosteroids also prolong the anticoagulant effect. Drugs that inhibit the anticoagulant effect include oral contraceptives, barbiturates, furosemide (Lasix), and glutethimide (Doriden). Diabetic patients may require changes in insulin or tolbutamide therapy when receiving anticoagulants; warfarin may potentiate the action of tolbutamide, and heparin may potentiate the action of insulin.

Patients on long-term anticoagulant therapy must understand the purpose of the therapy, the exact dosage and schedule, the signs of bleeding complications, and the need for regular monitoring. Patients must understand the importance of informing other physicians and their dentist that they are receiving anticoagulants. These drugs potentiate or antagonize the effects of many other drugs.

AORTIC AND ARTERIAL DISEASES

The aorta, the major artery of the body, is composed predominantly of elastic tissue in its upper portion in order to withstand the increased pressure during cardiac systole. Distensibility is diminished, however, during aging and especially in the presence of atherosclerosis and hypertension.

The aorta consists of three sections: (1) the ascending aorta, which has two branches, the right and left coronary arteries; (2) the arch of the aorta, with its branches, the brachiocephalic, common carotid, and subclavian arteries; and (3) the descending aorta. The upper extremity receives its blood supply via the subclavian artery, the axillary artery, and then the brachial artery, which branches into the radial and ulnar artery. As the descending aorta descends through the aortic opening in the diaphragm, it becomes the abdominal aorta and later divides into the right and left common ileac arteries. The major branches of the abdominal aorta are the celiac, superior mesenteric, renal, and inferior mesenteric arteries. This review of the aortic structure is important, to emphasize the importance of diseases of the aorta, which jeopardize the systemic circulation.

Aortitis is inflammation of the aorta; it particularly involves the arch of the aorta. The major causes are arteriosclerosis and syphilis. The condition may lead to aortic insufficiency and aortic aneurysm. Syphilis is suspected as the cause when aortitis occurs before the age of 50; the arteriosclerotic type more often occurs after 60. Penicillin is the agent used to treat syphilitic aortitis. Surgical treatment may be necessary when aortic insufficiency or aortic aneurysm results. Although chest pain may be present in some patients, occasionally the condition is diagnosed by the incidental finding of dilatation and calcification of the ascending aorta.

Problems with the aorta and large arteries usually are manifested by **aneurysm,** which is a localized abnormal dilatation of the vascular wall, and **obstruction,** which is usually associated with atherosclerosis. The aneurysm may occur at different levels of the aorta and its branches, most often in the ascending portion and then the arch of the aorta.

There is a higher incidence of aneurysm among older men than women, and the mortality rate is high if surgical correction is not performed. The major cause of death is spontaneous rupture of the aneurysm. Aneurysms, which may be singular or multiple, occur in several forms: saccular, fusiform, and dissecting. A **saccular aneurysm** is characterized by an outpouching from one side of an artery, caused by localized stretching of the medial layer. A **fusiform aneurysm** is one in which the entire segment of the artery is distended, with tapering at both ends. A **dissecting aneurysm** is one in which the blood is forced between the layers of the arterial wall; it generally originates with a tear in the intima.

Arteriosclerosis is the major cause of aneurysm formation. Other causes include syphilis, infections within and around the vessel, and trauma. Congenital defects, such as cystic medial necrosis, also may predispose to structural changes that cause aneurysms.

Symptoms, when present, result from compression or erosion of the surrounding structures by the aneurysm. These symptoms vary according to the location and size of the lesion. For example, pain may result from pressure on the spine, intercostal nerves, or various organs. Cough and dyspnea may occur due to tracheobronchial compression. Hoarseness may result from pressure of an aneurysm on the recurrent laryngeal nerve, or dysphagia may result from esophageal compression. Often the aneurysm may be asymptomatic and may be detected as a thoracic mass on x-ray. In some cases, a large aneurysm may be palpable as a localized bulge or mass.

Diagnosis is made by a thorough history and physical examination, roentgenography to detect the location of masses, and fluoroscopy to determine pulsations of the lesions. Aortography is helpful in outlining the aorta, especially to differentiate a pulsating aortic aneurysm from a mediastinal tumor. Abdominal aneurysms, when symptomatic, are often associated with persistent or intermittent pain in the middle or lower part of the abdomen that is often referred to the back. A pulsating mass may be evident and a bruit may be audible over the site. Although some aneurysms are asymptomatic and may not be discovered except incidentally during exploratory laparotomy for other conditions, other aneurysms may rupture suddenly and cause immediate death.

Symptoms of dissecting aneurysms often simulate coronary occlusion, due to the presence of severe and persistent chest pain. It is often described as a "tearing" pain and may be referred to the back. The dissection usually originates in the ascending aorta and may involve a small segment of the vessel, or it may extend into the ileac artery. The condition is associated with severe hypertension, as well as with cystic medial necrosis and coarctation of the aorta. Prompt reduction of the B.P. and the use of myocardial depressants such as propranolol are indicated before surgical therapy. Surgical intervention is indicated to prevent further dissection, prevent external rupture, and to correct associated aortic valve damage (usually by aortic valve replacement).

Elective repair of aneurysms is the usual approach to treatment, because of the ever-present threat of rupture. Most aneurysms require removal of the involved segment of the aorta and replacement with a nonporous, synthetic Dacron or Teflon graft (Fig. 4-25). When aneurysms are small and saccular, they may sometimes be closed by simple suturing. When the aneurysm is of the dissecting type, repair of the intimal layer of artery is necessary and the false lumen of the artery also must be corrected. Cardiopulmonary bypass is utilized in surgical treatment of lesions of the ascending aorta. Nursing care is similar to that with open heart surgery. Such patients are susceptible to vascular and other postoperative complications as well as to those related to the cardiopulmonary bypass procedure.

Postoperatively, routine postoperative assessment and nursing care measures are carried out. In addition, attention is given to the circulatory status, particularly distal to the graft site. Evaluation of the presence and quality of the peripheral pulses (femoral, popliteal, and dorsalis pedis pulse) and assessment of the temperature of the extremities are absolutely essential. Monitoring of renal function, with accurate measurement of intake and output, is vital to determine that no renal complications have resulted from the cross-clamping of the aorta required during the surgical procedure. The patient who has had repair of an aneurysm is also susceptible to hemorrhage and peripheral arterial occlusion due to emboli formation. These same observations and complications should also be nursing concerns when renal artery, subclavian artery, or popliteal artery aneurysms are involved or when there is trauma or penetrating injury to the abdominal aorta.

The patient has an impaired vascular system and lives with the potential for development of other aneurysms. The patient requires continued follow-up care and management of dietary and activity restrictions.

CHRONIC ARTERIAL INSUFFICIENCY

As mentioned previously, atherosclerosis and arteriosclerosis are systemic pathological processes of the arterial vessels. Associated changes result in lesions that cause narrowing of the arterial lumen and reduce the blood flow through the vessel, thus promoting stasis and stimulating thrombus formation. Gradual occlusion, however, may allow for development of collateral circulation so that distal tissues may still obtain some blood supply.

Chronic arterial insufficiency of the peripheral vessels occurs more commonly in the lower extremities than in the upper, and men are more often affected than women. The condition is characterized by pallor and coldness of the extremity, intermittent claudication, and pain, even at rest in later stages. **Intermittent claudication** refers to the sensation of pain, fatigue, or cramping in a lower

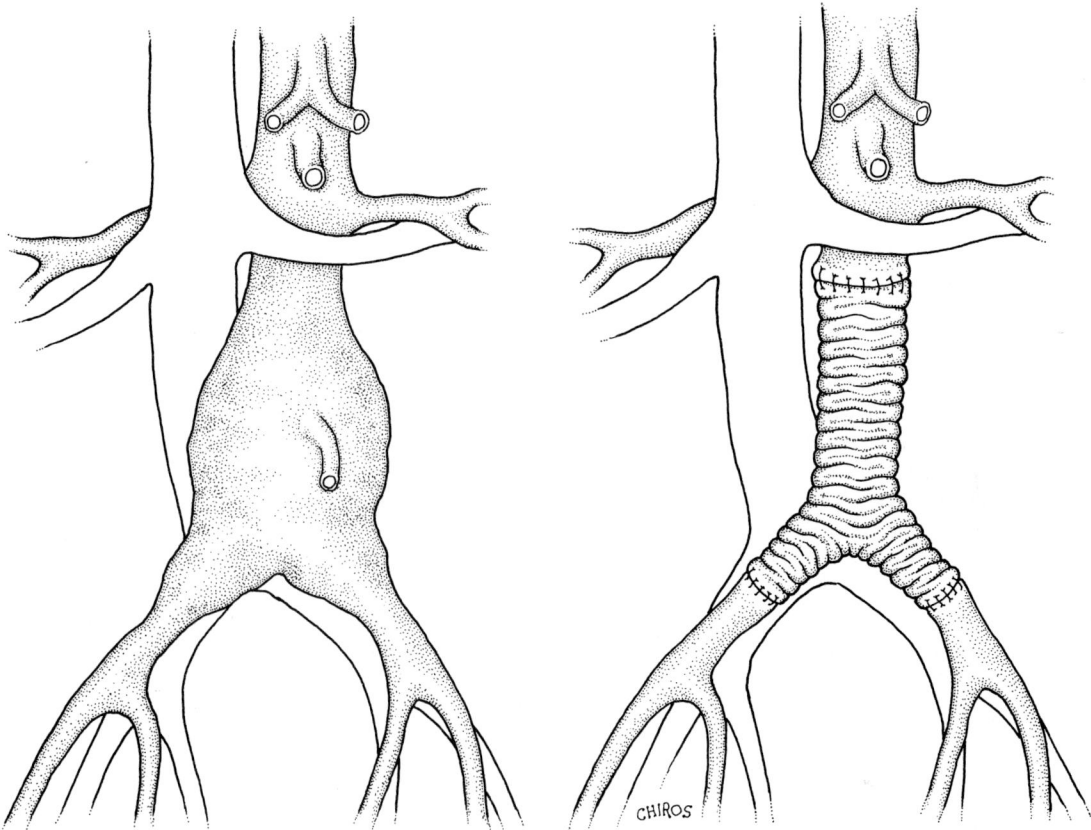

Figure 4-25
Graft replacement for an aneurysm of the abdominal aorta.

extremity (particularly the calf muscles) that occurs on walking, but is relieved with rest. Decrease in the size of the extremity and tingling and numbness of the toes are other symptoms. Alterations in the extremity that reflect inadequate blood supply and consequent inadequate nutrition are thickened and opaque nails, shiny and atrophic skin, and decreased hair growth. Ulcers of the legs, toes, and feet are often present. Auscultation over the main arteries may reveal a bruit over involved arteries. Probably the most important sign is the absence or diminishing of a normally palpable pulse, such as the posterior tibial, dorsalis pedis, popliteal, or femoral pulse. Chronic arterial insufficiency may be unilateral or bilateral, so that comparison of the pulses in the two extremities is important. The toes are often very tender to touch; the nurse therefore should take care in handling the extremity during assessment or treatment. Raising and then lowering the involved extremity will result in delayed filling, as detected by delay in the return of normal color. The patient also complains of being cold most of the time. The inadequate circulation to the extremities is compromised in a cold environment. Therefore, these patients tend to overdress for the weather.

Chronic arterial insufficiency can result in further complications and deterioration unless the nurse initiates specific measures. Nursing measures should focus on the prevention of further progress of the condition, on prevention of infections, ulcerations, or cracking of the skin, and on increasing the blood supply to the extremity while also reducing or limiting the demands of the tissues within an appropriate balance of exercise and rest. In addition, the extremity is protected from trauma. Not only do these measures require scrupulous attention while the patient is hospitalized, but a thorough program of education to assist the patient in coping with the long-term management of this chronic condition is required.

Because nicotine is a potent vasoconstrictor and causes vasospasms, smoking is contraindicated. Generally dietary restriction of total fat intake is prescribed and weight reduction diets are also recommended when indicated. Meticulous cleanliness is emphasized in order to prevent infections. The patient is advised to wash his feet daily with soap and warm water and is also advised of the danger of burns when hot water is used and the problems of constriction caused by cold water. Instructions are given on drying the feet thoroughly, but not roughly, creaming the feet with lanolin, keeping the toenails trimmed straight across, and seeking the assistance of a podiatrist for appropriate foot care. The feet are to be examined regularly for blisters, ingrown toenails, or any type of infection or skin breakdown.

In order to prevent trauma to the extremity, the patient should not go barefoot, should wear properly fitted shoes and clean socks, and should avoid wearing constricting garments that would jeopardize arterial blood flow. Women are warned about the dangers of wearing tight girdles, garters, or constricting hosiery. The dangers of local heat (hot water bottles, heating pads) cannot be overemphasized. Prolonged sitting or standing or sitting with the legs over each over further retard arterial and venous circulation.

Walking is encouraged as an exercise to stimulate the development of collateral circulation, but exercise should not exceed the patient's tolerance nor be excessive. Increased metabolic demands only aggravate arterial insufficiency. Adequate rest is therefore emphasized.

Vasodilating drugs may also be prescribed to increase blood flow in arterial insufficiency. Although their value is questionable and their use controversial, they are often utilized. Their limitations are related to their lack of specificity and postural hypotension may occur with their use. Other adverse effects associated with vasodilating drugs are palpitations, headache, vertigo, nausea, and other gastrointestinal symptoms. Patients should not expect improvement as a result of the use of the drugs, but rather should understand that the drugs are prescribed to prevent or minimize complications associated with arterial insufficiency. Some of these vasodilator drugs include phenoxybenzamine (Dibenzyline), isoxsuprine (Vasodilan), nylidrin (Arlidin), niacin (nicotinic acid), and tolazine hydrochloride (Priscoline). The use of vasodilators is felt by some authorities to be limited to relieving vasospasms and therefore more appropriate for Raynaud's disease than for chronic arterial insufficiency.

Surgical intervention is not generally indicated for chronic arterial insufficiency unless intermittent claudication becomes incapacitating or unless localized areas of diseased arteries are identified. Lumbar sympathectomy may be done to relieve pain of intermittent claudication, although the results are unpredictable. **Endarterectomy,** or bypass grafts, may be done in select situations. Endarterectomy involves the removal of arterial obstructions localized in short segments of an artery. Constriction of small vessels tends to occur at the suture line so that patch grafts are often used. Autogenous grafts (usually from the saphenous vein) may also be used.

ACUTE ARTERIAL OCCLUSION

Acute arterial occlusion most often originates from a thrombus in the chambers of the heart, associated with atrial fibrillation, MI, or aneurysm, as well as rheumatic heart disease after mitral commissurotomy. The underlying cause of the embolus must also be treated. Arterial occlusions may also result from thrombosis or injury.

Symptoms are the result of severe ischemia and include acute pain in the extremity with loss of both sensory and motor function of the part. Pallor and coldness are evident and the patient complains of numbness in the extremity distal to the obstruction. Cyanosis and mottling become rapidly evident. Arterial pulses are absent below the level of occlusion, but the pulse is often strong above the occlusion. Ischemia is particularly severe in acute arterial occlusion because of the lack of development of collateral circulation. The emboli are most often located at bifurcation points of the aorta, ileac, femoral, or popliteal arteries.

Treatment involves the use of anticoagulants (heparin) to prevent the expansion of the embolus or the formation of a distal embolus. Embolectomy is indicated to prevent further deterioration of circulation and the potential loss of the extremity or even death in complicated cases. Femoral embolectomy may be done under local anesthesia, which lessens the risk to a patient who already may have a complicating cardiac problem. When the occlusion is extensive, however, a bypass or prosthetic graft may be necessary, which requires more prolonged surgery and anesthesia. Fibrinolytic agents are being used experimentally as a means to remove occluding lesions; however, their use remains controversial.

When irreversible gangrene ensues, amputation is required (see color insert Figure 6 on page 1078B). Signs of irreversible gangrene are necrosis of the skin and of the digits. A cold, blanched extremity without capillary filling tends to indicate impending loss of the limb. Nursing care of the patient requiring an amputation is detailed in Chapter 10.

Postoperatively the nurse is concerned with those observations and nursing care measures previously mentioned with surgical repair of the aortic aneurysms. Observation of the wound for bleeding (especially when heparin has been used) and observation of the circulatory status distal to the level of the incised vessel are absolutely essential. Associated cardiovascular disease requires close monitoring of cardiac and circulatory status. Extremity movement is encouraged to prevent stasis of the extremity. When vascular grafts have been used across areas of flexion, such as the groin and knee, precautions are taken to prevent flexion of the site for about 2 weeks postoperatively.

Embolism to the visceral arteries, particularly mesenteric emboli and potential infarction, requires early abdominal exploration in order to avoid bowel necrosis. Without surgery, mesenteric embolism is a fatal condition. Surgical postoperative care requires attention to the circulatory status, as previously described, and to potential complications related to gastrointestinal function.

THROMBOANGITIS OBLITERANS

Thromboangitis obliterans, also known as Buerger's disease, is a chronic occlusive disease of unknown etiology. It is characterized by inflammation in the arteries with thickening of vascular walls leading to occlusive thrombosis, usually of the lower extremities. Venous or arterial thrombosis or both are often present and ulcers are frequently evident. When the upper extremity is involved, digital pain with numbness and fatigue are characteristic symptoms. Without medical attention and patient compliance in several restrictions, gangrene is the eventual outcome.

The condition occurs primarily in young males between the ages of 20 and 45 and the patients are almost always heavy smokers. Treatment requires abstinence from smoking.

Pain is the predominant symptom. Intermittent claudication is commonly found in the arch of the foot and the calf of the leg. The extremity is usually very tender and painful to touch. Coldness and sensitivity to cold are common symptoms. The peripheral pulses (popliteal, dorsalis pedis, and posterior tibial) are impaired or absent. Edema and thrombophlebitis are often associated with the condition.

As mentioned previously, treatment requires complete abstinence from smoking. If this is not accomplished, prognosis is poor, with eventual development of gangrene requiring amputation.

Avoiding mechanical, chemical, or thermal trauma to ischemic areas is absolutely essential. Treatment is also centered on preventing disease progression by promoting vasodilatation, relieving pain, and treating associated ulcers and gangrene. Exercise regimens, following the Buerger exercise regimen, are also prescribed.

RAYNAUD'S DISEASE

Raynaud's disease is characterized by episodes of excessive vasoconstriction and digital ischemia, which may involve all extremities but predominantly the hands. The condition occurs most often in females between the ages of 20 and 40. The episodes are precipitated by exposure to cold or by emotional stress. Raynaud's disease is distinguished from Raynaud's phenomenon, which is a symptom not only of Raynaud's disease but of other conditions such as neurologic lesions, certain occlusive diseases, lupus erythematosus, and polyarteritis.

The diagnosis of Raynaud's disease often

rests on the long history of sensitivity to the cold. The symptoms are variable. Intermittent changes in the fingers or toes cause a blanched and white appearance with numbness, changing to cyanosis as the capillaries become dilated because of the increased metabolites. When circulation is reestablished after the vasospasm, a period of hyperemia occurs with evident rubor followed by return of normal color in the digits.

Treatment requires the avoidance of exposure to cold and the elimination of smoking. If the condition is severe, the patient is advised to move to a warm climate. Vasodilators may be indicated. Avoidance of stress is a major factor in the control of the condition; emotional support and reassurance are imperative for these persons. Cooperation in therapy is required to prevent potential thrombosis and gangrene related to arterial wall changes from frequent vasospasms.

Variations of Raynaud's syndrome include acrocyanosis and livedo reticularis. **Acrocyanosis** is characterized by a persistent cyanosis of the hands and feet, even present to some degree in a normal environment; the condition occurs most often in young women. Except for concern with the cosmetic appearance of the hands, the patient does not usually suffer any other serious consequences. No underlying organic disorder is usually found; the patient requires reassurance of the generally benign nature of the syndrome.

Livedo reticularis is an angiospastic disorder that also occurs predominantly in young women. The condition is characterized by mottled skin, particularly in the lower legs. Cessation of smoking is advisable, but generally no other measures are needed.

THORACIC OUTLET SYNDROME

The syndromes of the thoracic outlet and cervicoaxillary canal (cervical rib, scalenus anticus syndrome) are treatable problems, usually occurring in women in the fourth and fifth decades. Scalenus anticus syndrome causes symptoms related to vascular and neurologic changes due to the compression of the subclavian artery, its sympathetic nerve supply, or the nerve trunks of the brachial plexus by a cervical rib or the scalene anticus muscle. Symptoms of Raynaud's phenomenon may be present and a bruit may be heard over the subclavian artery. Pain is generally located in the shoulder but may radiate down the inner surface of the arm, simulating angina pectoris. Forceful downward pressure on the shoulders or abduction and rotation of the shoulders may obliterate or diminish the quality of the radial pulse; these techniques may be used to diagnose the condition. Heavy lifting or activities requiring that the arms be held above the head should be avoided. Surgical intervention may be necessary to remove the cervical rib or to transect the scalene muscle.

ARTERIOVENOUS FISTULAS

Arteriovenous fistulas result in direct communication between arteries and veins. They may be singular or multiple and are most often the result of congenital anomalies or trauma. Traumatic fistulas most commonly result from stab or bullet wounds, especially in the axillary or inguinal region. An iatrogenic fistula may occur as an injury during surgery for an intervertebral disk repair. The aorta, inferior vena cava, or iliac vessels may be injured. An iatrogenic fistula may be purposefully constructed to provide easy access for repeated hemodialysis.

Symptoms and signs of arteriovenous fistulas depend on their location and size. Large fistulas may result in heart failure. Pulsating veins, rapid development of varicose veins, continuous murmur over the vessel, and edema formation after a local injury or surgery are significant symptoms. Patients with a single acquired or congenital fistula generally have a good prognosis if arterial and venous continuity can be restored by surgical repair (arterial and venous grafts). Reconstructive and multiple surgeries may be necessary to correct multiple fistulas. Diffuse involvement prohibits surgical repair, and symptomatic treatment may be the only recourse. Amputation may be necessary for large inoperable fistulas that result in vascular complications or deformity.

VENOUS DISORDERS

The function of the venous system is that of returning blood from the capillaries to the heart. Within the venous system, blood must flow against gravity and is therefore dependent upon the competence of valves located within the veins and the pumping action of the muscles surrounding the veins, as well as the B.P. gradients within the cardiovascular system. The valves, most commonly found in the lower extremities, facilitate the flow of blood against gravity. The valves, when open, permit flow in one direction and close to prevent the backward flow of blood as surrounding muscles relax. The contracting muscles provide for partial or complete emptying of both the deep and superficial leg veins. Flow of blood to the heart is also facilitated by the change in pressure gradient between the thoracic and abdominal cavities during inspiration. The negative intrathoracic pressure and the descent of the contracting diaphragm displace the abdominal organs and compress the veins in the abdominal and thoracic cavities. Thus blood flow into the thoracic cavity is increased.

It should be clear, therefore, why standing or constriction on the lower extremities impedes the return of venous blood flow and results in an increase in venous pressure and subsequently an increase in hydrostatic pressure of the capillaries. Edema formation occurs when fluid is not readily reabsorbed from the tissues as the venous pressure rises and blood accumulates in the dependent veins. When the veins are overstretched by excessive venous pressure for a prolonged period (as in obesity, pregnancy, or an occupation that requires standing for long periods), the veins distend and prevent the valve leaflets from closing tightly. Thus venous insufficiency is promoted by the incompetence of the valves.

Chronic edema of the subcutaneous tissue predisposes the patient to inflammation, fibrosis, and atrophy, due to inadequate diffusion of nutrients from the capillaries to the cells of the skin. These factors promote stasis dermatitis and cellulitis and eventually ulcerations.

Chronic venous insufficiency leads to distinct changes in the skin of the extremity. Initially the edema is soft and can be compressed, but later it becomes firm and disappears less rapidly, if at all, with elevation of the extremity. This type of firm edema gives a sensation of a "wooden feeling" and is described as brawny induration. The skin is often darkly pigmented, dry and scaling, especially around the ankles, the most common site of venous ulcer formation (see color insert Figure 7 on page 1078B). The patient with chronic venous disease presents with symptoms of aching, particularly experienced at the end of the day after periods of relative inactivity such as sitting or standing.

Treatment and nursing measures in chronic venous insufficiency require techniques to counteract gravity pressure, prevention of leg ulcers by meticulous skin care and prevention of trauma. Counseling and emotional support help the patient cope with discouragement brought on by the nature of the chronic condition.

VARICOSE VEINS

Varicose veins are abnormally elongated, dilated, and tortuous superficial veins of the lower extremities (the saphenous veins). The varicosities, which are a common disorder, result from dilatation of the veins and valve incompetence, as previously described. Congenital weakness of the veins, pregnancy, obesity, and prolonged standing are causes of varicose veins. They may also be associated with thrombophlebitis of the deep veins, arteriovenous fistulas, or pressure from a tumor pressing on the inferior vena cava or the femoral veins.

The condition may cause minimal discomfort and only slight edema, although the tortuous veins may be quite evident. Usually, symptoms of aching, muscle cramps, and muscle fatigue are described. The symptoms are generally relieved by elevation of the leg, which increases the return flow of blood to the heart. The condition may be bilateral or unilateral. Valvular incompetence of both the superficial and deep veins is evaluated by means of the Trendelenburg test, by observing venous pressure changes during walking, and by phlebography (roentgenography of the veins after injection of a contrast medium). Increased venous pressures, as evidenced by distended veins, generally decrease markedly during walking as muscular contraction increases the flow of blood in the deep veins and facilitates increased blood flow from the superficial to the deep veins. A gradual return of venous pressure to normal levels should occur as exercise is discontinued. The extremities of patients with varicose veins do not have as marked a decrease in venous pressure on walking and the superficial veins fill rapidly (due to incompetent valves) when exercise ceases.

The competence of the valves can be evaluated by the Trendelenburg test. The patient lies down and elevates the involved leg about 70° to allow the veins to empty. A tourniquet is applied on the upper thigh, but only to constrict the superficial veins and not the deep veins. The patient is then asked to stand, the tourniquet is taken off, and the filling of the superficial veins is observed. Rapid distention of the varicose veins implies valvular incompetence as the veins fill from above. In addition, venography or, specifically, phlebography is done to visualize both normal and abnormal veins and valves by injection of radiopaque contrast material into the deep and the superficial veins.

The patient with varicose veins must be instructed in measures to prevent venous stasis. Sitting or standing for prolonged periods, crossing the legs at the knees for prolonged periods, and sitting in chairs that cause excessive popliteal pressure are avoided. Wearing of tight girdles or garters is discouraged. Weight reduction diets are prescribed when appropriate. Frequent elevation of the legs is encouraged and, in some situations, elevation of the legs at night while sleeping is prescribed. The use of elastic stockings may be prescribed to help prevent deep calf thrombosis by compressing the superficial veins and forcing blood into the deep veins, thus increasing circulation and lessening the likelihood of clot formation in the larger veins and subsequent formation of an embolism. Elastic stockings such as the Jobst antiembolism stocking claim to provide smoothly tapering gradient pressure. The proper use of these elastic stockings must be ensured. They should be of the proper size, and measured according to the directions of the specific manufacturer. They should be washed properly and should not be hung up for drying because they will be stretched out of shape. Elastic stockings should be removed regularly to provide for adequate inspection of the underlying skin. They should be applied prior to standing up in order to prevent stagnation of blood in the lower extremities; if the patient has been standing, he should sit in a chair for 15 minutes with his legs elevated before applying the elastic stockings. The stockings should be wrinkle-free when used, in order to prevent any strictured areas, particularly at the knee when full-leg stockings are utilized. There is some controversy over the use of elastic stockings; when improperly used, they can actually stimulate the conditions that should be prevented (constricting forces on the veins of the extremity).

Surgical treatment of varicose veins may be done, as long as the deep veins are patent (as demonstrated by modifications of the Trendelenburg test). The patient should not feel that the surgery will cure the problem. Varicosities may recur. Vein ligation involves the ligating of the saphenous vein at the saphenofemoral junction and stripping the saphenous vein system from that point to the ankle. The stripping is done using a vein stripper inserted from the ankle superiorly to the groin. Alternate incisions may also be required along the pathway of the saphenous vein to remove varicosities of the smaller branches of the veins. Remaining dilated veins may be sclerosed by injecting 5% sodium morrhuate or 1 to 3% sodium tetradecyl sulfate (Sotradecol) into the vein. These substances produce a localized phlebitis and thrombosis of the veins.

Postoperatively the legs are wrapped in pressure bandages or elastic stockings and are elevated while the patient lies in bed. The nurse must emphasize the importance of (as well as supervise) walking for at least 5 minutes at regular intervals (often scheduled hourly) and lying in the bed with the legs elevated. The patient should not sit or stand in one position. When up, he should be walking. The circulation of the extremity is observed for any constriction, which is evidenced by swelling, pain, or coldness of the distal extremity. The dressings are examined for signs of bleeding. Gradual increase of activity is encouraged. Measures previously described to prevent increases in venous pressure must continually be followed.

VENOUS ULCERS

Most ulcers formed on a lower extremity are the result of varicose veins or postphlebitic syndrome. They may also be associated with burns, neurogenic disorders, diabetes, and arterial disease. They are particularly common in the elderly patient. Associated vascular disease, which accounts for the occurrence of the ulcer, also contributes to poor healing and chronicity of venous ulcers.

Treatment includes bed rest with elevation of the affected extremity. Various cleaning agents may be utilized (such as hydrogen peroxide, saline, soap and water). Gentleness should be emphasized in cleaning the ulcer. Cultures and sensitivity tests are indicated when the wound is infected; appropriate systemic or local antibiotics or both are prescribed. Continuous, warm and moist compresses of normal saline or boric acid may be prescribed to stimulate granulation and relieve discomfort. Debridement and the application of enzymatic ointments may also be prescribed. (More information on the management of superficial ulcers is found in Chapter 14.) Dry dressings covered by sponge rubber and held in place with elastic bandages may also be the type of management utilized. When the ulcer is free of infection and necrotic tissue, the foot and leg may be enclosed in a "boot" made of Unna's paste. This paste, composed of gelatin, zinc oxide, and glycerin, is applied to the leg and then covered with an elastic bandage. A commercially prepared gauze bandage impregnated with these substances (such as Gelocast or Dome-Paste) is available. The Unna boot protects the ulcer and provides even pressure to the veins. The paste dries quickly (within ½ hour), and the patient should be observed for any sign of circulatory impairment. Usually the "boot" is not applied until after about 2 days of bed rest to reduce any edema in the extremity. The boot is changed in about 4 days to check the underlying ulcer and the condition of the skin; it may be reapplied and then changed every week or every 2 weeks depending on the status of the patient.

If the ulcer does not heal with conservative treatment, excision of the ulcer with skin grafting may be necessary. Regardless of the approach used, the patient must be encouraged to practice meticulous skin care and to adhere to the measures that prevent venous stasis in order to prevent recurrence of venous ulcers.

THROMBOPHLEBITIS

Phlebitis is an inflammation of the wall of a vein; it is associated with injury, prolonged pressure on the vein, infection, or mechanical or chemical irritation (such as from intravenous medications or fluids). When the endothelial lining is damaged, a **thrombus** may develop at the site of inflammation leading to thrombophlebitis.

Thrombophlebitis is characterized by three cardinal symptoms: (1) increased local temperature, (2) edema of the calf muscle, and (3) tenderness along the vein. In addition, the Homans sign may be present. **Homans' sign** is the presence of pain in the calf upon dorsiflexion of the foot. Additional signs associated with thrombophlebitis are restlessness, fever, and tachycardia. Thrombophlebitis is also often associated with varicose veins and often related to hypercoagulability of the blood or slowing of the blood flow, such as occurs in immobilization. Thrombophlebitis has been found frequently in women who have been taking oral contraceptives.

The threat of embolization of the thrombus to the pulmonary artery is a constant danger in thrombophlebitis and requires preventive measures and adequate treatment of the thrombophlebitis. Absolute bed rest is required for several days in order to foster adherence of the thrombus firmly to the vascular wall. (This may vary from strict bed rest for 7 days to bed rest with bathroom privileges according to varying protocols.) Any massaging or rubbing of the calf is contraindicated and the patient must be advised of this precaution. Often the patient may wish to rub the leg in order to relieve the pain. The patient should be advised of the danger of fragmenting the clot and causing embolus formation. Elevation of the affected leg will promote venous return and avert stasis. Elevation also relieves edema and pain. Some physicians recommend the use of elastic stockings for additional support of superficial veins, particularly when ambulation is started. Currently there is controversy over the use of elastic stockings and over elevation of the extremity (some physicians feel that elevation may precipitate release of the embolus). Anticoagulation therapy is initiated to prevent extension of the thrombus by reducing platelet adhesiveness and inhibiting thromboplastin formation. Heparin is usually administered initially and then oral anticoagulants are started. Moist warm compresses to the extremity may also be ordered. The purpose of moist warm compresses is to decrease edema and discomfort by dilating the blood vessels and improving circulation; heat also relieves accompanying muscle spasm. The compresses are removed regularly to examine the underlying skin, and care is taken to prevent burns or injury from the treatment. The nurse should remember that cold compresses will combat the intended effect, so that the compresses must be changed regularly or provision must be made for maintaining the temperature of the compresses.

Surgical measures may be necessary if anticoagulant therapy is not effective and there is a threat of pulmonary embolism, and also when extreme thrombosis threatens gangrene. Thrombi, for example, may be removed from major veins such as the subclavian, femoral, or iliac veins. Plication of the inferior vena cava may be indicated to partially impede blood flow, thus allowing normal flow but trapping emboli from traveling to the pulmonary system. Either the iliac vein or the vena cava itself may be plicated, although generally the vena cava is the preferred site. The procedure involves the partial suturing of the vena cava or insertion of a special grid-like clip or umbrella-like prosthesis into the lumen of the vena cava. Another approach is to suture a special filter in the vessel, allowing blood to flow through, but emboli to be retained. The major complication with this surgery is that new thrombi form at the surgical site.

Phlebothrombosis is distinguished from thrombophlebitis in that clot formation is not associated initially with an inflammatory process. Phlebothrombosis is often described as a "silent" thrombus because signs of its presence may not be evident until pulmonary embolism suddenly occurs. Stasis of venous circulation of the deep veins related to prolonged bed rest, and inactivity is the most important precipitating factor. Actually, both phlebothrombosis and thrombophlebitis of the deep veins are often clinically similar. More importantly, they are both treated aggressively to prevent the onset of pulmonary embolism. In addition, phlebothrombosis and thrombophlebitis are both prevented by providing for some activity when a patient is immobilized. Postoperative exercises and early ambulation are the major factors in the prevention of these vascular problems, which often occur in relation to surgery.

PULMONARY EMBOLISM

Pulmonary embolism is the most serious complication of peripheral venous thrombosis. Signs and symptoms are often vague when emboli are small enough to reach the periphery of the lung; the symptoms may be dramatic and life-threatening when larger emboli occlude pulmonary arterial branches. Pain in the midchest and radiating to the back may simulate an MI. Tachycardia, cyanosis, dyspnea, and rapidly developing hypotension may lead to death in a few minutes or several hours, despite supportive therapy.

Anticoagulant therapy with IV heparin is started immediately, after oxygen, intravenous lines, and life-saving measures are initiated. The patient is obviously frightened and apprehensive during the crisis and requires psychological support through verbal assurances and a calm atmosphere.

When smaller arteries are occluded by the pulmonary embolus, symptoms of fever, cough, hemoptysis, a pleural friction rub, and pleuritic pain may occur. A lung scan is helpful in confirming the diagnosis. A chest x-ray often is nondiagnostic, initially. Bed rest and supportive measures, as well as the use of anticoagulants, are indicated for all types of pulmonary embolism.

LYMPHATIC DISORDERS

The **lymphatic system** is a network of vessels that drain the intracellular fluid from the interstitial spaces back into the circulation. Lymph nodes located along the course of the lymphatic vessels filter the lymph before it is returned to the bloodstream.

Lymphatic disorders are generally either inflammatory or obstructive. Inflammatory lymphangitis (acute inflammation of the lymphatic channels) may be caused by puncture wounds of the skin or spread of infection from a focus of infection in an extremity. Symptoms include chills, fever, local swelling, and enlarged and tender regional lymph nodes. The infecting organism is usually the β-hemolytic streptococci. Penicillin is usually given to resolve the infectious process. This infectious process may be recurrent in persons susceptible to streptococcal infections of the skin and the symptoms often mimic those of thrombophlebitis.

Acute cervical adenitis is an acute infection of the lymphatic glands of the neck, usually secondary to an infection of the mouth, pharynx, or scalp (particularly pediculosis). Swelling usually occurs on one side of the neck; the area is markedly tender. Treatment includes the use of appropriate antibiotics, determined by culture and sensitivity analysis of the original source of the infectious process. This condition, although more commonly found in children, is also found in adults.

Lymphedema

Lymphedema is the result of an obstruction to the lymph flow in an extremity. Stasis of the tissue fluid results in persistent edema. It may be a primary disorder affecting younger females, in which case it is often unilateral. The development of edema is usually gradual over a period of months or years. Elastic bandages or elastic stockings are prescribed. Bed rest with elevation of the involved extremity is indicated. The use of diuretics may be indicated also. When both the skin and the subcutaneous tissues are involved, the extremity becomes enlarged and often grotesque. The name associated with primary lymphedema, elephantiasis, is derived from the fact that the subcutaneous changes resemble pigskin or the hide of an elephant. In addition to the unsightly appearance, which often leads to psychological distress, ulcers and dermatitis further complicate the condition. Surgical treatment of massive lymphedema involves removal of the epithelium without removing any lymphatic tissue in the skin. After the fat (thickened fibrosed subcutaneous tissue), excess skin, fascia, and the lymph are excised, the same epithelium is sutured back directly on the muscle without any underlying layer of the removed tissues. This type of surgery is performed in several stages over a period of several months. Successful surgery of this type eventually returns the extremity to normal size and normal function. Postoperative care involves protective measures to promote adherence of the grafts, prevent excessive strain or movement in the extremity, and minimize trauma. Also, encouragement and emotional support are essential to promote psychological comfort during the long and tedious therapy.

References

1. Beck, W. S. *Human Design: Molecular, Cellular, and Systematic Physiology.* New York: Harcourt Brace Jovanovich, 1971. Pp. 283-327.
2. Guyton, A. C. *Textbook of Medical Physiology* (4th ed.). Philadelphia: Saunders, 1971.
3. Smith, A. M., Thierer, J., and Huang, S. Serum enzymes in myocardial infarction. *Am. J. Nurs.* 73:277, 1973.
3a. Criteria Committee of the New York Heart Association. *Nomenclature and Criteria for Diagnosis of Diseases of the Heart and Great Vessels* (7th ed.). Boston: Little, Brown, 1973.
4. Bates, B. *A Guide to Physical Examination.* Philadelphia: Lippincott, 1974.
5. Cooper, T. The national hypertension program. *J. Am. Pharm. Assoc.* 513:135, 1973.
6. Freis, E. D. *Introduction to the Nature and Management of Hypertension.* Bowie, Md.: Robert J. Brady Co., 1974.
7. U.S. Veterans Administration Cooperative Study Group on Anti-Hypertensive Agents. Effects of treatment on morbidity in hypertension. Results in patients with diastolic blood pressures averaging 115 through 129 mm Hg. *J.A.M.A.* 202:1029, 1967.
8. U.S. Veterans Administration Cooperative Study Group on Anti-Hypertensive Agents. Effects of treatment on morbidity in hypertension. II. Results in patients with diastolic blood pressure averaging 90 through 114 mm Hg. *J.A.M.A.* 213:1143, 1970.
9. Hartshorn, E. Factors to Consider in the Drug Therapy of Hypertension. In *Pharmacy Horizons, The Role of the Pharmacist in the Overall Management of the Hypertensive Patient.* Summit, N.J.: Ciba Corp., 1972.
10. Whipple, G. H., Peterson, M. A., Haines, V. A., Learner, E., and McKinnon, E. L. *Acute Coronary Care.* Boston: Little, Brown, 1972.
11. McIntyre, H. M., and Mason, D. T. The prevention of heart disease: A greater challenge. *Cardio-Vasc. Nurs.* 7:77, 1971.
12. Pinneo R. Concepts in cardiac nursing. *Nurs. Clin. North Am.* 7:411, 1972.
13. Pinneo, R. Cardiac monitoring. *Nurs. Clin. North Am.* 7:457, 1972.
14. Meltzer, L. E., and Dunning, A. J. *Textbook of Coronary Care.* Philadelphia: Charles Press, 1972.
15. Pratte, A. L., Padilla, G. V., and Baker, V. Alterations in cardiac activity from ingestion of ice water. *Commun. Nurs. Res.* 6:148, 1974.
16. Houser, D. Ice water for MI patients? Why not? *Am. J. Nurs.* 76: 432, 1976.
17. Winsor T. *The Electrocardiogram in Myocardial Infarction.* Clinical Symposia Reprint. Summit, N.J.: Ciba Corp., 1968.
18. Cortes, T. S. Pacemakers today. *Nursing 74* 4:22, 1974.
19. Belling, D. I. Nursing care of patients with mechanical cardiac pacemakers. *Nurs. Clin. North Am.* 7:509, 1972.
20. AMA Department of Drugs. *AMA Drug Evaluations* (2nd ed.). Acton, Mass.: Publishing Sciences Group, 1973.
21. Druss, R. G., and Kornfeld, D. S. The survivors of cardiac arrest. *J.A.M.A.* 201:75, 1967.

22. Brogan, M. R. Nursing care of the patient experiencing cardiac surgery for coronary artery disease. *Nurs. Clin. North Am.* 7:517, 1972.
23. Kimball, C. P. Psychological responses to open heart surgery. *Am. J. Psychol.* 126:348, 1969.
24. Long, M. L., Scheuhling, M. A., and Christian, J. L. Cardiopulmonary bypass. *Am. J. Nurs.* 74:860, 1974.
25. Budd, S., and Brown, W. Effect of a reorientation technique on postcardiotomy delirium. *Nurs. Res.* 23:341, 1974.
26. Ellis, R. Unusual sensory and thought disturbances after cardiac surgery. *Am. J. Nurs.* 72:2021, 1972.
27. Woods, N. F. Patterns of sleep in post cardiotomy patients. *Nurs. Res.* 24:347, 1972.

Bibliography

Aagaard, G. N. Treatment of hypertension. *Am. J. Nurs.* 73:620, 1973.

Abdellah, F. G. The physician-nurse team approach to coronary care. *Nurs. Clin. North Am.* 7:423, 1972.

Aiken, L. H., and Henrichs, T. F. Systematic relaxation as a nursing intervention technique with open heart surgery patients. *Nurs. Res.* 20:212, 1971.

Baden, C. A. Teaching the coronary patient and his family. *Nurs. Clin. North Am.* 7:563, 1972.

Bergan, J. J., and Yao, J. S. T. Modern management of abdominal aortic aneurysm. *Surg. Clin. North Am.* 54:175, 1974.

Berman, L. B., and Vertes, V. *The Pathophysiology of Renin.* Clinical Symposia Reprint. Summit, N.J.: Ciba Corp., 1973.

Berne, R. M., and Levy, M. N. *Cardiovascular Physiology* (2nd ed.). St. Louis: Mosby, 1973.

Bortz, W. M. The pathogenesis of hypercholesterolemia. *Ann. Intern. Med.* 80:738, 1974.

Boyd, J. M. L. Understanding and treating cardiogenic shock. *RN* 38:53, 1975.

Boylk, N. What heart patients want to know—and what to tell them. *Nursing 72* 2:38, 1972.

Brener, E. R. Surgery for coronary artery disease. *Am. J. Nurs.* 72:469, 1972.

Castaneda, A. R. *Surgical Treatment of Cardiac Valvular Disease.* Clinical Symposia Reprint. Summit, N.J.: Ciba Corp., 1969.

Chucker, F., Fowler, R. C., and Hurley, C. W. Raynaud's disorders revisited. *Am. Fam. Physician* 10:70, 1974.

Clark, N. F. Pump failure. *Nurs. Clin. North Am.* 7:529, 1972.

Cobey, J. E., and Cobey, J. H. Chronic leg ulcers. *Am. J. Nurs.* 74:258, 1974.

Cogen, R. Cardiac catheterization: Preparing the adult. *Am. J. Nurs.* 73:77, 1973.

Col, J., and Weinberg, S. Factors affecting prognosis in acute myocardial infarction. *Heart Lung* 1:74, 1972.

Cole, J. S., and McIntosh, H. D. Electroshock hazards in the coronary care unit. *Heart Lung* 1:481, 1972.

DeVillier, B. Preoperative teaching of the cardiovascular patient. *Heart Lung* 2:522, 1973.

Dorr, K. S. The intra-aortic balloon pump. *Am. J. Nurs.* 75:52, 1975.

Drake, J. J. Locating the external reference point for central venous pressure determination. *Nurs. Res.* 23:475, 1974.

Duncan, J., et al. A program for the teaching of cardiovascular patients. *Heart Lung* 2:508, 1973.

Effler, D. B. *The Surgical Treatment of Myocardial Ischemia.* Clinical Symposia Reprint. Summit, N.J.: Ciba Corp., 1969.

Effler, D. B., and Sheldon, W. C. Revascularizing the myocardium: The saphenous vein bypass. *Hosp. Pract.* 8:65, 1971.

Engleman, K. Diagnosis and management of pheochromocytoma. *Hosp. Med.* 6:112, 1970.

Exercise Testing and Training of Apparently Healthy Individuals: A Handbook for Physicians. New York: American Heart Association, 1972.

Finnerty, F. Aggressive drug therapy in accelerated hypertension. *Am. J. Nurs.* 74:2176, 1974.

Forrester, J. S., and Swan, H. J. C. Direct Assessment of Cardiac Function in Acute Myocardial Infarction. In Meltzer, L. E., and Dunning, A. J. (eds.), *Textbook of Coronary Care.* Philadelphia: Charles Press, 1972.

Foster, S. Pump failure. *Am. J. Nurs.* 74:1830, 1974.

Foster, S., and Andeoli, K. Behavior following acute M.I. *Am. J. Nurs.* 70:2344, 1970.

Fredrickson, D. S., et al. *Dietary Management of Hyperlipoproteinemia. A Handbook for Physicians.* Bethesda, Md.: National Heart and Lung Institute, NIH, 1970.

Friedman, B. Cardiac surgery: Skilled nursing during the critical postoperative period. *Nursing 74* 4:37, 1974.

Germain, C. P., and Minogue, W. F. Precoronary care: Nursing considerations. *Cardio-Vasc. Nurs.* 8:11, 1972.

Griffith, G. C. Sexuality and the cardiac patient. *Heart Lung* 2:70, 1973.

Harken, D. E. Postoperative care following heart-valve surgery. *Heart Lung* 3:893, 1974.

Heart Facts 1975. New York: American Heart Association, 1974.

Holling, H. E. *Peripheral Vascular Diseases.* Philadelphia: Lippincott, 1972.

Hurst, J. W. *The Heart* (3rd ed.). New York: McGraw-Hill, 1974.

Hypertension: Office Evaluation. New York: American Heart Association, 1972.

Introduction to Arrhythmia Recognition. San Francisco: California Heart Association, 1968.

Jackson, B. S. Chronic peripheral arterial disease. *Am. J. Nurs.* 72:928, 1972.

Judge, R. D., and Zuidema, G. D. (eds.). *Methods of Clinical Examination: A Physiological Approach* (3rd ed.). Boston: Little, Brown, 1974.

Kampmeier, R. H., and Blake T. M. *Physical Examination in Health and Disease.* Philadelphia: Davis, 1970. Pp. 301-360.

Kannel, W. B., and Dawber, T. R. Contributors to coronary risk implications for prevention and public health: The Framingham Study. *Heart Lung* 1:797, 1972.

Kones, R. F., and Benninger, G. W. Digitalis therapy after acute M.I. *Heart Lung* 4:99, 1975.

Koprowicz, D. G. Drug interactions with coumarin derivatives. *Am. J. Nurs.* 73:1042, 1973.

Krupp, M. A., and Chatton, M. J. *Current Medical Diagnosis and Treatment.* Los Altos, Calif.: Lange, 1974. Pp. 151-169.

Lamberton, M. M. Cardiac catheterization: Anticipatory nursing care. *Am. J. Nurs.* 71:1718, 1971.

Leonard, J. J. *Examination of the Heart. Part IV: Auscultation.* New York: American Heart Association, 1967.

Lindeman, C. Influencing recovery through preoperative teaching. *Heart Lung* 2:515, 1973.

Logue, B., and Dorney, E. Answers to questions on acute pulmonary edema. *Hosp. Med.* 6:20, 1970.

Marchiodo, K. CVP: The whys and hows of central venous pressure monitoring. *Nursing 74* 4:21, 1974.

Mayer, G., and Kaelin, P. Arrhythmias and cardiac output. *Am. J. Nurs.* 72:1597, 1972.

Moyer, J. H., and Millis, L. C. Vasopressor agents in shock. *Am. J. Nurs.* 75:620, 1975.

Muller, O. F., and Schelbert, H. Management of acute emergencies associated with myocardial infarction. *Hosp. Med.* 8:88, 1972.

Nielsen, M. A. Intra-arterial monitoring of blood pressure. *Am. J. Nurs.* 74:48, 1974.

Norris, R. M. Prognosis in myocardial infarction. *Heart Lung* 4:75, 1975.

Oliver, M. F. The metabolic response to a heart attack. *Heart Lung* 4:57, 1975.

Palmer, E. M., and Griffith, E. W. Effect of activity during bedmaking on heart rate and blood pressure. *Nurs. Res.* 20:17, 1971.

Pitorak, E., et al. *Nurse's Guide to Cardiac Surgery and Nursing Care.* New York: McGraw-Hill, 1969.

Powell, A. H., and Winslow, E. H. The cardiac clinical nurse specialist: Teaching ideas that work. *Nurs. Clin. North Am.* 8:723, 1973.

Pranulis, M. F. Loss: A factor affecting the welfare of the coronary patient. *Nurs. Clin. North Am.* 7:445, 1972.

Pribble, A. H., and Tyler, M. L. Emergency, part I: On the spot cardiopulmonary resuscitation. *Nursing 75* 5:45, 1975.

Rhoads, J. E., et al. *Surgery, Principles and Practice.* Philadelphia: Lippincott, 1970.

Robinson, A. M. The R. N.'s goal: Under 90 mm Hg diastolic. *RN* 37:43, 1974.

Roberts, S. L. Skin assessment for color and temperature. *Am. J. Nurs.* 75:611, 1975.

Rombelt, D. Physical signs in acute myocardial infarction. *Heart Lung* 2:74, 1973.

Rose, M. A. Home care after peripheral vascular surgery. *Am. J. Nurs.* 74:260, 1974.

Rushmer, R. F. *Cardiovascular Dynamics* (3rd ed.). Philadelphia: Saunders, 1970.

Sana, J. M., and Judge, R. D. *Physical Appraisal Methods in Clinical Practice.* Boston: Little, Brown, 1975.

Schmitt, Y., Hood, W. B., Jr., and Lown, B. Armchair treatment in the coronary care unit: Effect on blood pressure and pulse. *Nurs. Res.* 18:114, 1969.

Sczekalla, R. M. Stress reaction of CCU patients to resuscitation procedures on other patients. *Nurs. Res.* 22:65, 1973.

Shapiro, R. M. Anticoagulant therapy. *Am. J. Nurs.* 74:439, 1974.

Sovie, M. D., and Fruehan, C. T. Protecting the patient from electrical hazards. *Nurs. Clin. North Am.* 7:469, 1972.

Spence, M. E., and Lemberg, L. Modalities of pacing. *Heart Lung* 3:820, 1974.

Spence, M. E., and Lemberg, L. Cardiac pacemakers: Complications of pacing. *Heart Lung* 4:286, 1975.

Strandness, D. E. Evaluation of the patient for vascular surgery. *Surg. Clin. North Am.* 54:13, 1974.

Stude, C. Cardiogenic shock. *Am. J. Nurs.* 74:1636, 1974.

Tharp, G. D. Shock: The overall mechanisms. *Am. J. Nurs.* 74:2208, 1974.

Tyzenhouse, P. Myocardial infarction: Its effects on the family. *Am. J. Nurs.* 73:1012, 1973.

Undue apprehension in heart patients. *Nursing 72* 2:35, 1972.

Ungvarski, P. J., Argondizzo, N. T., and Boos, P. K. CPR: Current practice reversed. *Am. J. Nurs.* 75:236, 1975.

Viewpoints: What do you tell post coronary patients regarding sex activity? *Med. Asp. Human Sex.* 2:22, 1968.

Walker, B. B. The postsurgery heart patient: Amount of uninterrupted time for sleep and rest during the first, second, and third postoperative days in a teaching hospital. *Nurs. Res.* 2:164, 1972.

Warner, H. F., et al. Heart muscle: Clinical applications of basic physiology. *Heart Lung* 1:494, 1972.

Walton, C. A. A Review of Physiological and Pharmacological Principles Fundamental to Rational Antihypertensive Therapy. In *Pharmacy Horizons, The Role of the Pharmacist in the Overall Management of the Hypertensive Patient.* Summit, N.J.: Ciba Corp., 1972.

Wenger, N. K., and Mount, F. An educational algorithm for myocardial infarction. *Cardio-Vasc. Nurs.* 10:11, 1974.

Wiley, L. (ed.). The threat of thrombophlebitis: Nursing grand rounds. *Nursing 73* 3:40, 1973.

Wiley, L. Staying ahead of shock. *Nursing 74* 4:19, 1974.

Wilkins, R. W., Hollander, W., and Chobanian, A. V. *Evaluation of Hypertensive Patients.* Clinical Symposia Reprint. Summit, N.J.: Ciba Corp., 1972.

Winsor, T. Bedside diagnosis of coronary heart disease. *Hosp. Med.* 6:63, 1970.

Winslow, E. H. Digitalis. *Am. J. Nurs.* 74:1062, 1974.

Winslow, E. H., and Mareno, L. B. Temporary cardiac pacemakers. *Am. J. Nurs.* 75:586, 1975.

Wise, D. J. Crisis intervention before cardiac surgery. *Am. J. Nurs.* 75:1316, 1975.

Wooley, A. S. Excellence in nursing in the coronary care unit. *Heart Lung* 1:785, 1972.

chapter 5
Patients with Hematopoietic and Lymphatic System Dysfunction

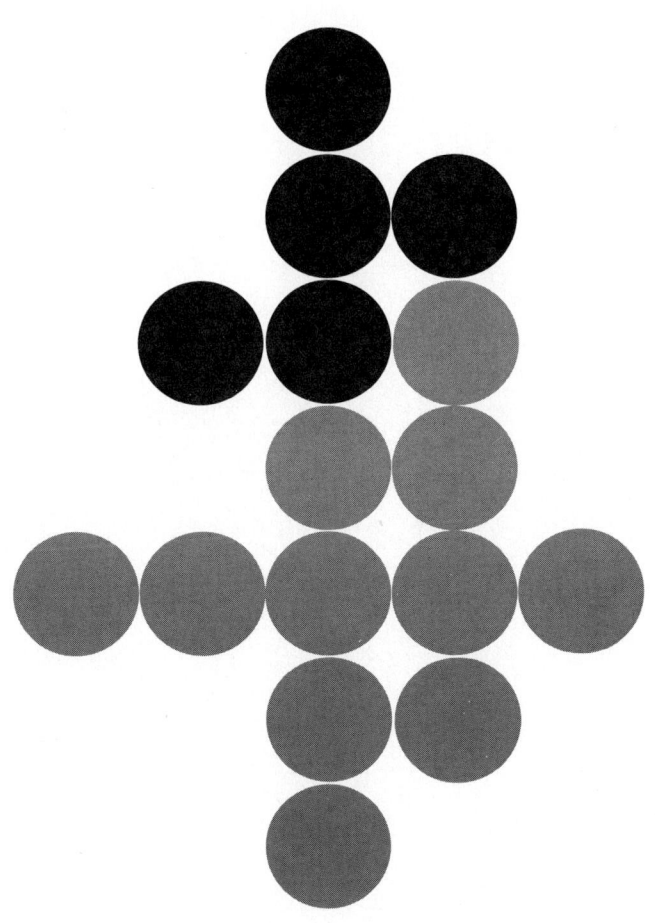

The hematopoietic and lymphatic systems are responsible for the formation of the cellular elements of the blood. Some of these elements, the **erythrocytes** (red blood cells), the **granulocytes** (granular leukocytes), and the **megakaryocytes** (precursors of thrombocytes, or platelets), are formed in the bone marrow. In the adult, the bone marrow is concentrated in the sternum, iliac crest, vertebral bodies, ribs, base of skull, and pelvic girdle, and in the proximal epiphyses of the long bones [25]. The **lymphocytes** are formed in the lymphoid tissue, which is found primarily in the lymph nodes, but also in the spleen, liver, thymus gland, and submucosa of the gastrointestinal tracts [15].

Composition and Function of Blood

The cellular elements include the erythrocytes, the leukocytes (including granulocytes, lymphocytes, and monocytes), and the thrombocytes. These elements make up approximately 45 percent of the blood and are suspended in the straw-colored fluid, **plasma,** which constitutes the remaining 55 percent. The average volume of blood in the adult is 5 to 6 liters.

Blood has a major role in **homeostasis**—that of assisting in the maintenance of a relatively constant environment for optimal cellular activity. Blood carries out its homeostatic functions by transporting oxygen from the lungs to the tissue cells. It also transports nutrients and electrolytes absorbed from the gastrointestinal tract to various body tissues and distributes hormones and enzymes that regulate body activities. Blood transports waste products like carbon dioxide, urea, uric acid, and excess body water to the organs of excretion; the kidneys, skin, and lungs. The blood also transfers heat from the site of production to the body surface, from which it can be eliminated.

Blood functions in body defenses in both the inflammatory and immune responses. Blood, which normally has a slightly alkaline reaction with a pH of 7.35 to 7.40, assists in providing chemical buffers of acids and bases, and it transports acid and base substances to the organs of excretion.

The constituents of plasma are 90 percent water and a variety of solutes. In addition to various nutrients, gases, electrolytes, and cell products, the plasma contains blood proteins, anticoagulants, clotting factors, and antibodies.

Four types of plasma proteins—serum albumin, serum globulin, fibrinogen, and prothrombin—are the major components of the plasma solutes. The plasma proteins have a large molecular structure and therefore do not readily diffuse through the capillary membranes. The normal concentration of plasma proteins is approximately 6 to 8 gm per 100 ml and accounts for the colloidal osmotic pressure of the plasma. This pressure prevents plasma fluid from leaking out of the capillaries into the interstitial spaces. Edema results when there is an abnormal decrease in the plasma proteins, particularly the albumin.

Serum albumin, fibrinogen, and prothrombin are formed by the liver from amino acids of ingested foods. They may also be synthesized from tissue protein in protein starvation. Fibrinogen and prothrombin are essential for blood coagulation; fibrinogen also has a role in tissue repair at sites of inflammation or injury.

Serum globulin is produced by the liver and reticuloendothelial cells. The three fractions of serum globulin include the alpha and beta globulins, which are synthesized in the liver, and the gamma globulin fraction, which is synthesized in the reticuloendothelial cells. These factors contain antibodies against microbes and their toxins, thereby providing the body with mechanisms of immunity.

Erythrocytes (Red Blood Cells)

The blood normally contains approximately 4.5 to 5.0 million erythrocytes per cubic millimeter in women and 4.8 to 5.4 million in men. The normal erythrocyte is an elastic, biconcave disk, a shape that provides the maximum surface for diffusion. The integrity of the cell membrane of the normal erythrocyte adapts to circulatory stresses and permits a normal life span of 120 days.

Table 5-1 indicates the stages of development of the erythrocyte. Normal erythrocytic and hemoglobin development is dependent on adequate amounts of protein, vitamin B_{12} (cyanocobalamin), folic acid, iron, pyridoxine, copper, and cobalt. Various pathologic states or deficiencies may interfere with normal erythrocytic development, resulting in varied sizes, shapes, and hemoglobin content. **Poikilocytosis** is defined as an abnormality in the shape of cells. **Anisocytosis** refers to cells of unequal size.

Vitamin B_{12} is one of the elements that are essential for normal erythrocyte formation and maturation. It is absorbed only in the

Table 5-1
Stages of erythrocyte development

Stages	Characteristics
Hemocytoblast	A primitive cell that is large, undifferentiated, and nucleated
Basophil erythroblast	A cell with a slightly clumped, nuclear chromatin and basophilic cytoplasm; it has no hemoglobin
Polychromatophil erythroblast	A cell having increased chromatin clumping and the earliest appearance of pink cytoplasmic hemoglobin
Normoblast	The nucleus becomes fragmented and disintegrates; hemoglobin content in cytoplasm increases
Reticulocyte	A non-nucleated cell with increased amounts of hemoglobin; grossly indistinguishable from erythrocyte; on staining, shows granules or diffuse network of fibrils
Erythrocyte	Mature red blood cell; nucleus remnants have disappeared; consists mainly of hemoglobin and a supporting framework

presence of the intrinsic factor that is secreted by the gastric mucosa. Minimum daily requirements for vitamin B_{12} have been reported as from 0.6 to 1.2 mg daily, with a range to approximately 2.8 mg. The National Academy of Sciences–National Research Council, in 1974, revised its recommendations to a daily intake of 3 mg to allow for individual variances [11]. Animal foods such as liver, kidney, lean meat, milk, eggs, and cheese are rich sources of vitamin B_{12}. It is important to remember that an adequate intake of these foods will not promote erythrocyte production unless the intrinsic factor is present. Deficiencies of vitamin B_{12} inhibit the rate of erythrocyte production and also result in the formation of larger than normal cells, called megaloblasts. These cells are oval-shaped, rather than biconcave, and they have a weakened membrane. Both of these characteristics of megaloblasts result in shortened life spans of the cells.

Folic acid (pteroylglutamic acid) is also concerned with the maturation of erythrocytes. The richest sources of folic acid are fresh, green vegetables, liver, and kidney. The 1974 recommendations of the National Research Council for folic acid were set at 400 μg daily with increases to 800 μg daily in pregnancy and 500 μg in lactation [11]. It is believed that both folic acid and vitamin B_{12} act as coenzymes at different stages in the synthesis of nucleic acids. Folic acid and vitamin B_{12} are both required for formation of deoxyribonucleic acid (DNA), and vitamin B_{12} is required for the production of ribonucleic acid (RNA). Maintenance of the integrity of the central nervous system requires RNA rather than DNA [16]. This fact is the probable explanation for the presence of neurologic symptoms associated with B_{12} deficiency.

A daily adult dietary intake of 10 mg of iron for men and 18 mg for women during the childbearing years is the recommended allowance of the 1974 revisions of the National Research Council [11]. This intake should provide for absorption of the 1 to 3 mg needed to maintain normal hemoglobin levels. Iron is absorbed slowly from the small intestine, in the ferrous form, the result of the action of the acid medium of the stomach on the ferric form that is usually ingested. When iron is absorbed from the small intestine, it combines with a beta globulin to form the compound transferrin for transportation in the blood plasma. Excess iron in the blood is deposited in all cells of the body, especially in the liver, where it combines with the protein apoferritin to form ferritin. When iron deficiency occurs, iron can readily be released from ferritin and is carried throughout the body in the form of transferrin, to be used where it is needed [15].

About two-thirds of the iron in the entire body is located within the hemoglobin of the blood. **Hemoglobin,** the major constituent of the erythrocyte, is the vehicle by which oxygen is carried to the cells. The normal concentration of hemoglobin is approximately 12 to 16 gm per 100 ml of blood for women and 14 to 18 gm per 100 ml for men. Hemoglobin is composed of the protein globin and an iron-containing pigment called heme, which is formed by the union of iron and the pigment porphyrin. The pigment content gives the red color to the blood. Oxygen combines loosely with hemoglobin to form oxyhemoglobin, so that it can be freed readily from the erythrocyte and diffused into the plasma. Adequate transportation of oxygen therefore is dependent upon a sufficient amount of hemoglobin within an adequate number of erythrocytes. Several forms of hemoglobin have been found in the blood, but only type A in adults and type F in the fetus are considered normal. Hemoglobins S and C, for example, are abnormal forms. (Hemoglobins S and C are associated with sickle cell disease, which is discussed on page 438.

Under normal conditions, the rate of production and maturation of the erythrocytes matches the rate of erythrocytic destruction. The physiologic stimulus for **erythropoiesis** (the production of erythrocytes) is a reduction in the oxygen tension of arterial blood. For example, erythropoiesis is increased at high altitudes where oxygen concentration in the atmosphere is low, and during extensive exercise. Renal hypoxia stimulates the kidneys to release renal erythropoietic factor (REF) into the plasma; this factor reacts with a plasma globulin produced by the liver to form erythropoietin, which stimulates an increase in erythrocyte production in the bone marrow [23]. Erythropoietin production is increased by androgenic hormones. The higher production of androgens in the male may account for the higher red blood cell count of men as compared to women [34]. Although most of the aged erythrocytes are destroyed by the reticuloendothelial tissues of the spleen, some are destroyed by phagocytes from the liver; this process is known as **phagocytosis**. When erythrocytes are destroyed, hemoglobin is broken down and free iron is liberated and transported to the bone marrow for formation of more hemoglobin or it is stored in the ferritin pool of the liver. Porphyrin molecules are converted to bilirubin and are excreted in the bile through the liver into the feces [16]. (The functions of bile and bilirubin are discussed in Chapter 7.)

Leukocytes (White Blood Cells)

Leukocytes normally number from 5,000 to 10,000 per cubic millimeter of blood and are divided into the major groups on the basis of their characteristic cytoplasm, being granular or nongranular. **Granulocytes** are formed in the bone marrow and are of three mature types—neutrophils, eosinophils, and basophils. Lymphocytes and monocytes have the **agranular** type of cytoplasm. Most authorities agree that both lymphocytes and monocytes are formed in the lymphoid tissues. Table 5-2 indicates the stages of development in **leukopoiesis** (the production of leukocytes).

Leukocytosis indicates an increase above the normal leukocyte count and **leukopenia** indicates a decrease below normal. A differential white blood cell count determines the percentage of the various types of leukocytes and indicates the specific cells involved in leukocytosis. The normal percentages of the leukocytes are: neutrophils, 60 to 70 percent; eosinophils, 0 to 5 percent; basophils, 0 to 3 percent; lymphocytes, 30 to 40 percent; and monocytes, 0 to 5 percent [13]. These percentages may vary slightly in different laboratory methods. Leukocytes have an important function in defending the body against infections and the products of degenerated tissue. Leukocytes are mobile and perform these functions by the processes of phagocytosis, diapedesis, and chemotaxis.

Phagocytosis, which involves the engulfing and digesting of foreign particles (including bacteria and products of tissue breakdown),

Table 5-2
Stages of leukocyte development

Granulocytes			Agranulocytes	
Myeloblast → Megakaryocyte*			Stem cells	
↓ ↗			↙ ↘	
Promyelocyte			Lymphoblast	Monoblast
↓			↓	↓
Myelocyte			Prolymphocyte	Promonoblast
↙ ↘			↓	↓
Neutrophil	Eosinophil →	Basophil	Lymphocyte	Monocyte

*Platelets are derived from this leukocyte (megakaryocyte).

is the principal function of the neutrophils. Neutrophils are therefore increased in acute infections and in severe tissue damage. The function of the neutrophils is facilitated by the ameboid movement of these cells. **Chemotaxis** occurs when tissue is injured. Chemotaxic substances (such as bacterial or cellular products) are released from the tissues with the highest concentration at the site of damage. These substances attract neutrophils to the areas of injury. **Diapedesis** is the passage of leukocytes through capillary membranes into the tissues.

Monocytes initially move slowly through the tissues, but change into the large phagocytic cells called **macrophages.** Macrophages are more powerful than neutrophils because they can engulf larger particles. After initial stages of inflammation, an acid environment develops at the site of injury; macrophages thrive in an acid environment, in contrast to neutrophils, which cannot live in an acidic environment. Monocytes are therefore more important for resisting long-term, chronic infections while neutrophils are most important in resisting acute infections [15].

Eosinophils are increased in allergic reactions, apparently to detoxify the foreign proteins entering the body. Eosinophilia also occurs in the presence of parasitic infections. The precise function of the basophils is not known, since they exhibit mild ameboid motion, minimal phagocytic activity, and minimal chemotaxis. It has been postulated that basophils may have a role in preventing intravascular blood coagulation by releasing small quantities of heparin [15]. The function of the lymphocytes primarily is to wall off chronic infections and to produce antibodies. As mentioned previously in the discussion of immunity, there are two major types of lymphocytes: T lymphocytes, derived from the thymus gland, and B lymphocytes, derived from the bone marrow (refer to Chapter 1 for information on immunity and the role of the lymphocytes).

Plasma cells are responsible for almost all antibody formation. Before exposure to an antigen, the plasma cells are in a dormant state and are known as **plasmablasts.** Upon entry of a foreign antigen into the lymphoid tissue these plasmablasts divide rapidly, becoming mature plasma cells. During this process, maturing plasma cells rapidly produce antibodies specific against the foreign antigen.

Thrombocytes (Platelets)

The platelets, which are the smallest of the formed elements of the blood, are produced in the bone marrow by the fragmentation of the giant cell megakarocytes. The average number of platelets is 150,000 to 300,000 per cubic millimeter of blood [15]. Platelets adhere to foreign substances; they also adhere to the vessel wall when it is injured. In this way, platelets promote coagulation at the site of injury and help prevent hemorrhage. Hemostatic mechanisms and their relation to coagulation and hemorrhagic disorders will be discussed in more detail later in this chapter. It is important, however, to remember that certain bone marrow diseases affect erythrocyte and leukocyte production and also affect the platelet levels, resulting in bleeding problems.

Assessment of the Patient

Assessment of the hematopoietic and lymphoid systems of the patient requires a thorough history and physical examination. Important physical signs associated with hematologic disorders may be caused directly by changes in the lymph nodes, spleen, or liver. Other indirect signs include those involving the skin and mucous membranes. No organ, however, is immune to the effects of the various blood dyscrasias.

Clinical assessment of the patient's nutritional status is essential in evaluating the status of the hematopoietic system. Because normal erythrocyte development is dependent upon adequate intake of certain essential nutrients, the patient's dietary habits must be determined. A question worded, "Do you eat a normal diet?" is inappropriate in this situation; what is "normal" for a given individual may not be a nutritious diet, although it is viewed as normal by the person. A better approach is to ask the person to describe his meals on a typical day. Ingestion of fad diets or omissions of vital nutrients may then be detected more readily. Alcohol ingestion should also be determined; malnutrition is often associated with chronic alcoholism. People who live alone, who are elderly, or who live in poverty are most vulnerable to nutritional deficiencies resulting in anemia. Previous surgery should be investigated, because subtotal or total gastrectomy, or resection of segments of the small intestine, may result in malabsorption and deficiency states.

The skin is examined carefully, because many blood disorders are manifested by cutaneous changes. Pallor and skin coldness may be present. A good light source must be utilized to determine pallor. Pallor may be a normal characteristic in fair-skinned persons, and may be difficult to assess in dark-skinned persons. Pallor of certain parts of the body, such as the nailbeds, conjunctiva, mucous membrane of the mouth, and lips, is a better indicator of anemia than skin pallor.

The nails are also examined to determine normal contour. The nail base normally is firm to touch and the nails have a convex curve. Koilonychia, a concave or spoon-shaped curve of the nails, is the most advanced type of nail abnormality. It is a very rare sign, but may be associated with severe iron deficiency anemia and severe malnutrition. Mild nail changes in anemia may be observed as thin, brittle, longitudinal ridges, and nails that lack any luster.

The skin should be examined for the presence of purpuric lesions, either petechiae or ecchymoses. **Petechiae** are small, superficial, cutaneous or mucosal hemorrhages that are less than 5 mm in size. **Ecchymoses** are larger than 5 mm and are purplish in color with irregular borders [21]. The location, distribution, and size of these lesions should be noted. Epistaxis, bleeding of the gums, and frank hemorrhages are very significant signs in assessing the status of the hematopoietic system, because they may indicate dysfunction of hemostatic mechanisms.

Rapid hemolysis associated with certain blood dyscrasias may be demonstrated by the presence of jaundice. (Jaundice is discussed in detail in Chapter 7.) With excessive erythrocytic production (polycythemia vera), the superficial veins and venules may be dilated; the face and neck may typically present rubor. Cyanosis may also be present as a result of excessive concentration of reduced hemoglobin in the blood.

Dermatitis may be associated with certain blood disorders. Pruritus is often associated with jaundice in patients with hemolytic disorders. Pruritus may be so intense that the skin actually has excoriated areas from excessive scratching.

The mouth and mucous membrane are examined for the presence of glossitis (inflammation of the tongue) and stomatitis (inflammation of the mucosa of the mouth). These are common characteristics of the deficiency anemias. The tongue may be pale and smooth when atrophy of the glossal papillae occurs, as in pernicious anemia. Bleeding of the gums may be noted. Ulcerations of the gums, mouth, and pharynx may be present in leukemia, as well as in other conditions of agranulocytosis.

Localized bone tenderness is evaluated, particularly in the sternum, since this symptom is frequently associated with blood disorders. During the physical examination particular attention is given to the status of the lymph nodes, spleen, and liver, which are often enlarged in certain blood dyscrasias. Ocular examination with the ophthalmoscope is also indicated, since changes in the fundus are often associated with blood disorders. These changes may include retinal edema, hemorrhages, exudates, and dilatation of the veins [21].

Lymph nodes are normally flat, bean-shaped, and generally not palpable. They are examined by simple inspection and palpation. Asymmetry should be noted. Light palpation with slow and gentle movements, using the middle and index fingers to oscillate up and down, back and forth, in a rotary motion, is the proper technique. When the deep cervical nodes are palpated, however, the thumb and fingers must be hooked around the sternocleidomastoid muscle. Both sides of the neck may be palpated simultaneously to compare corresponding nodes [20] (Fig. 5-1).

Characteristics of the nodes that should be evaluated are the following: size and shape (diameter in centimeters or descriptive terms as almond-sized, size of split-pea); tenderness; degree of fixation (movable, matted, fixed); and texture (hard, soft, firm). When enlarged or tender nodes are detected, the region and structures drained by the node(s) must be carefully examined. Lymph node enlargement may be an indication of localized infection in the region drained, an infectious process elsewhere in the body, a neoplastic disease, or a systemic disease [20].

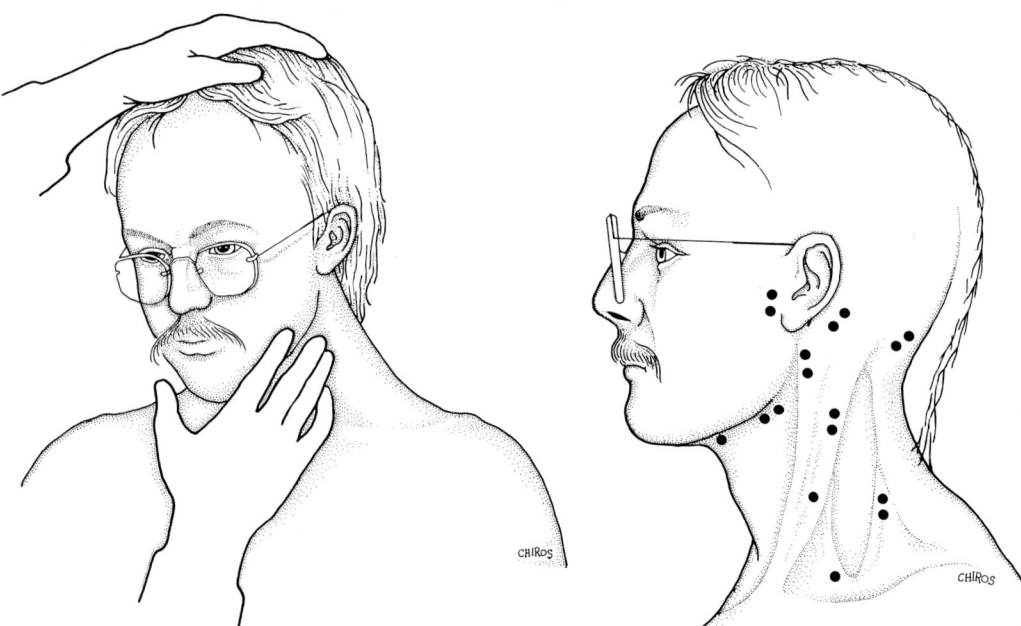

Figure 5-1
Palpation of the cervical lymph nodes.

Figure 5-2
Location of lymph nodes in the head and neck.

The ten groups of nodes to be examined in the head and neck region include the following: preauricular nodes; posterior auricular nodes; occipital nodes; tonsillar nodes; submaxillary nodes; submental nodes; superficial cervical nodes; posterior cervical chain of nodes; deep cervical chain of nodes; and supraclavicular nodes [4, 20]. Figure 5-2 indicates the location of these nodes.

When the axillary nodes are being examined, the patient should be sitting or in a supine position. The examiner reaches as high as possible into the apex of the axilla and then moves down, using the fingertips to exert gentle pressure against the thorax. This is repeated several times to check the lateral posterior group of nodes, the central group, and the pectoral group. The axillary nodes include five or six small groups lying at the lateral edge of each pectoralis major muscle in the armpit.

The epitrochlear nodes are located on the medial aspect of the arm just above the elbow, and drain the hand and arm. It is important that the arm be relaxed during examination of the epitrochlear nodes. The examiner uses one hand to support the patient's arm at the wrist while examining the epitrochlear nodes.

The inguinal nodes lie along the inguinal ligament and the saphenous vein. These nodes and the femoral nodes are palpated by the fingertips in the groin area, moving the fingertips from side to side with firm pressure, moving downward toward the thigh to check if femoral nodes are palpable. Inguinal lymph nodes are commonly palpable without having clinical significance. Femoral lymph node enlargement, however, is more significant. Figure 5-3 illustrates the location of lymph nodes throughout the lymphatic system.

Since the spleen and liver are examined as part of the abdominal examination, the technique for examining these organs is described in Chapter 7.

HEMATOLOGIC MEASUREMENTS

Observations made during the physical examination and the history-taking may lead the examiner to suspect the presence of some type of blood dyscrasia. Laboratory analysis follows to confirm the suspicion. Several blood tests are done routinely and have particular significance in the diagnosis of hematologic diseases. The general blood tests that are frequently used to distinguish blood

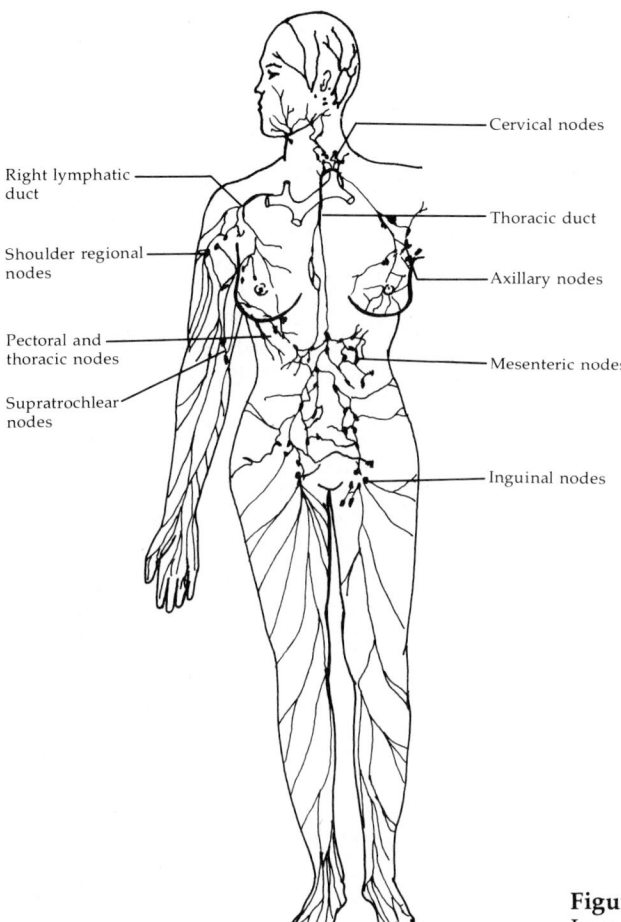

Figure 5-3
Location of lymph nodes in the lymphatic system.

dyscrasias will be discussed. Specific tests related to certain disorders will be discussed with the specific disease entity.

The **erythrocyte count,** or red blood cell (RBC) count, measures the concentration of erythrocytes per cubic millimeter of blood. The body maintains a fairly constant number of erythrocytes; a decreased number occurs as one form of anemia.

The **hemoglobin concentration** measures the hemoglobin content of the erythrocytes. The hemoglobin pigment gives blood its red color. Hemoglobin determinations are used in diagnosing the different types of anemia.

The hematocrit demonstrates the relation of formed elements to plasma and is used to determine the volume of erythrocytes. A sample of whole blood is centrifuged until the erythrocytes separate from the plasma. Normal values range from 45 to 50 volumes per 100 ml of blood for men and from 40 to 45 volumes per 100 ml for women. The hematocrit is elevated in dehydration and polycythemia, and is decreased in anemia.

The **corpuscular indices** include the mean corpuscular volume (MCV), the mean corpuscular hemoglobin (MCH), and the mean corpuscular hemoglobin concentration (MCHC). These classic tests aid in determining the type of anemia present, and they are based on the patient's predetermined RBC, hemoglobin, and hematocrit levels.

MCV is computed to determine the volume of the average erythrocyte in cubic microns. This figure is obtained by multiplying the hematocrit by 10 and dividing this number by the total number of erythrocytes. MCV designates the cells as normocytic, microcytic, or macrocytic. This analysis, plus MCHC, is used to determine normochromic or hypochromic erythrocytes. The normal size of the erythrocyte is 82 to 92 cubic microns.

MCH measures the average amount of hemoglobin per erythrocyte. The normal is 29 to 32 micromicrograms. In megaloblastic anemia, MCH is elevated to about 50 μg. It can be diminished to about 15 μg in microcytic hypochromic anemia.

MCHC is used to determine the average number of grams of hemoglobin in 100 ml of packed cells. The normal value is 30 to 38 gm per 100 ml of **packed red cells.** The value is more commonly expressed as a percentage, reflecting the ratio of hemoglobin concentration to the volume in which it is contained (30 to 38 percent). In megalocytic anemia, it may be normal or diminished. In microcytic hypochromic anemia, it is decreased to as low as 22 percent.

The **reticulocyte count** measures the percentage of circulating erythrocytes that are reticulocytes. The count reflects the activity and rapidity of erythrocyte formation and the ability of the bone marrow to respond to a decrease in the number of mature circulating erythrocytes. It is an important test to determine whether the anemia results from underproduction, excessive destruction, or from loss of erythrocytes. The normal value is 25,000 to 75,000 reticulocytes per cubic millimeter of blood. Reticulocyte counts are usually reported as a percentage of the total erythrocyte count, with normal values being 0.5 to 1.5 percent of the total erythrocytes. If reticulocytes are persistently elevated but without an associated rise in hematocrit, the anemia is probably a result of excessive destruction or excessive loss of erythrocytes requiring an abnormal increased activity.

Erythrocyte fragility may be evaluated by observing the reaction and hemolysis of erythrocytes in a series of graded hypotonic sodium chloride solutions. Physiologic saline solution is a 0.9% solution of sodium chloride and water and has the same osmotic pressure as blood serum (isotonic). Some normal cells begin to hemolyze in a solution of below 0.5% (0.44 to 0.42%) saline and almost all are hemolyzed in 0.34% saline solution [13]. Certain hemolytic anemias (e.g., spherocytosis) are characterized by increased erythrocyte fragility.

The **Coombs** tests are agglutination procedures done on a suspension of the patient's erythrocytes. A direct Coombs test is done to determine the presence of antibodies (agglutinins) that adhere to the erythrocytes. The direct test is significant in identifying types of hemolytic anemias and is also used to detect possible development of erythroblastosis fetalis. An indirect method is done on serum to test for the presence of antibodies to the erythrocyte antigens.

Bilirubin, the product of hemoglobin catabolism, undergoes conjugation in the liver. Serum bilirubin levels are used to evaluate hemolytic anemias and liver function. **Direct bilirubin** refers to that which is conjugated with glucuronide and is soluble in water; **indirect bilirubin** refers to that which is not conjugated (free) and is not soluble in water.

Urobilinogen is a compound produced in the intestinal tract by the bacterial breakdown of bilirubin excreted in bile. Only approximately 1 percent of the total urobilinogen excreted is eliminated by the kidneys in the urine. The other 99 percent is normally excreted in the feces. Urinary urobilinogen is increased, however, in hemolytic anemia because of excessive destruction of erythrocytes and breakdown of hemoglobin. Urine specimens may be either 24-hour collections or a 2-hour afternoon collection. This procedure requires that the patient empty his bladder just prior to the initiation of the test; this urine is discarded. It has been found that the peak of urinary excretion of urobilinogen occurs between the midafternoon and early evening. The volume of the specimen is critical in determining accurate results; the entire urine specimen collected during the specified time should be sent for examination.

Fecal urobilinogen is normally 50 to 300 mg in 24 hours. The amount of urobilinogen excreted in the feces is increased in excessive erythrocyte destruction.

Erythrocyte life span can be determined by tagging the erythrocytes with radioactive chromium (^{51}Cr) and determining their life span [13]. The life span is shortened in hemolytic anemia.

The leukocyte count is normally 5,000 to 10,000 per cubic millimeter. A differential leukocyte count is done to determine the percentages of the various types of leukocytes that comprise the total leukocyte concentration.

The blood platelet count is normally 150,000 to 300,000 per cubic millimeter of blood. The platelet count and coagulation tests are done frequently in diagnosing blood dyscrasias. The most common coagulation tests include the bleeding time, prothrombin time, and the coagulation, or clotting, time. The significance of these tests is discussed later in this chapter in the section on disorders of hemostasis.

Bone marrow aspiration and **biopsy** are valuable diagnostic tools for the study of bone marrow function. Aspiration is indicated when peripheral blood abnormalities require further investigation. Examination of films of the specimen permit evaluation of the number of cells, their various developmental and maturational phases, and their size, shape, and cellular characteristics. (Films, rather than smears, are generally used because films provide a more uniform distribution of cells across the slide.)

Aspiration procedures can be done readily on an outpatient basis or at the bedside of a hospitalized patient. A signed permit for the procedure is usually required. Preparation of the patient regarding the procedure and its purpose is essential in order to allay apprehension and also to gain his cooperation in lying still during the procedure. The patient is likely to be fearful of having the needle inserted into his sternum or iliac crest, and should be warned that he may experience pain at the time the specimen is being aspirated; otherwise, the procedure should not cause pain.

Either the sternum (between the second and third ribs) or, preferably, the iliac crest is used as the site of the puncture. There is a danger of injury to the underlying structures in the mediastinum in sternal puncture if penetration is too deep. The site is shaved and cleaned with an antiseptic. After anesthetizing the puncture site, the physician inserts a short, thick needle into the marrow. The stylet from the needle is removed and 1 to 2 ml of marrow is removed by means of a syringe. (Some authorities remove only 0.2 to 0.3 ml marrow in iliac crest aspiration.) The specimen is placed immediately in a jar containing a preservative such as sodium oxalate. A small dressing or Band-Aid is placed on the site. The patient may complain of slight soreness at the puncture site for several days; this is normal. The patient, particularly if thrombocytopenic, is instructed not to remove or wet the dressing for 24 hours.

Transfusion Therapy

Whole blood and its components are used widely in the treatment of diseases of the hematopoietic and lymphoid systems. It is advantageous therefore to discuss transfusion therapy as a basic treatment measure, prior to the discussion of the specific disease entities.

Transfusion is the introduction of whole blood or any of its components directly into the circulation to correct deficiencies of blood volume or deficiencies of specific components. Before blood can be given to a recipient, compatibility of the blood with that of the donor must be established. Incompatibility results in hemolytic transfusion reactions. The universally accepted ABO classification system is used to determine blood types and is based on the presence of specific antigens, called agglutinogens, in the erythrocytes and the presence or absence of antibodies (called agglutinins) in the plasma. The individual's blood is typed A, B, AB, or O, depending on the presence or absence of the agglutinogens, A and B. This typing is established by adding specially prepared sera which contain either anti-A or anti-B agglutinins to any given sample of blood. Clumping of the erythrocytes when anti-A serum is added to the blood sample indicates that the blood is type A. Type B blood is that which results in clumping of the erythrocytes on addition of anti-B serum. If clumping of the erythrocytes occurs with the addition of both anti-A and anti-B serum, the presence of both A and B agglutinogens is indicated and the blood is classified as type AB. If a person has A or B or both A and B agglutinogens, his plasma will not contain antibodies that will agglutinate his own erythrocytes. When the addition of either anti-A or anti-B serum causes no agglutination of the erythrocytes, the blood is labeled as type O. Type O reflects an absence of both A and B agglutinogens in the erythrocytes; however, the plasma contains both anti-A and anti-B agglutinins.

These factors are the basis for determining the appropriate type of blood to be used for transfusion. If no other compatibilities are present, persons with type O blood can donate their blood to recipients in all four blood groups because their erythrocytes do not contain either A or B agglutinogens. (For this reason, persons with type O blood have been called universal donors; however, this term is no longer appropriate as more antigens are being identified.) Persons with type O blood, however, cannot receive any other type of blood except type O; their serum contains both anti-A and anti-B antibodies, which will agglutinate erythrocytes in A, B, and AB blood.

If no other compatibilities are present, persons with AB type blood can receive blood from donors in all four blood groups because their plasma contains no anti-A or anti-B antibodies. (For this reason, persons with AB type blood have been called universal recipients.) About 60 additional commonly occurring antigens besides the A and B agglutinogens have been identified on erythrocyte membranes, and other agglutinins in the plasma have also been identified. For this reason the terms *universal donor* and *universal recipient* are no longer appropriate. The blood groups and their constituent agglutinogens and agglutinins are summarized in Table 5-3.

In addition to the ABO classification, blood is tested for the presence or absence of the Rh factor in the erythrocytes. There are at least eight different types of Rh agglutinins. In contrast to the ABO system, in which agglutinins responsible for causing transfusion reactions occur spontaneously, the Rh system requires prior exposure to some antigen in the system before enough agglutinins are developed to cause significant transfusion reactions. This same principle explains why erythroblastosis fetalis (a blood dyscrasia of the newborn resulting from incompatibility between the infant's blood and the mother's blood) is not likely to occur in the first pregnancy of an Rh-negative mother who delivers a fetus which inherits Rh-positive blood from an Rh-positive father. The hemolytic condition is likely to occur in succeeding pregnancies, after the mother has developed antibodies to the Rh agglutinins.

The Rh blood groups are determined by a series of three closely linked genes, C, D, and E, of which the D factor is the most important clinically. It is the presence or absence of the D antigen (also expressed as Rh_o type blood) that determines whether the person's blood is Rh-positive or Rh-negative. The determination of Rh type is done by testing with anti-Rh_o (D) typing serum. Approximately 85 percent of the white population and 99 percent of the nonwhite population are Rh-positive.

After the blood is typed, blood from the potential recipient is crossmatched with the blood from the potential donor. Serum from the recipient's blood and the donor's erythrocytes are mixed together and incubated to rule out any agglutination process. This procedure is called a **major crossmatch,** in contrast to the **minor crossmatch,** which is an optional step in the crossmatching process [29]. The latter procedure consists in crossmatching the cells of the recipient with the serum of the donor. If no agglutination occurs, the donor's blood and the recipient's blood are considered compatible and safe for transfusion.

Before blood is even accepted for donation, there are several precautions and procedures that are necessary to promote the safety and protection of both the recipient and the donor. The American Association of Blood Banks lists the minimum requirements to detect prospective donors with disease of the heart, kidneys, lungs, liver, or other organs, as well as those with a history of cancer, infectious disease, abnormal bleeding tendencies, or allergies that would exclude them from donating blood. The interval between donations of a full unit of blood is at least 8 weeks. These points are covered in a short history form. In addition, the temperature, pulse, respirations, and blood pressure and a hemoglobin (or hematocrit) are taken to detect any abnormalities. Blood specimens from the donated blood are tested for syphilis and for hepatitis antigen (HB_sAg), and blood is rejected unless these tests are nonreactive.

Once the blood is received on the unit, the nurse is responsible for its administration and proper handling. The expiration date on the blood label should be checked first. Blood collected in acid citrate dextrose (ACD) or citrate phosphate dextrose (CPD) anticoagulant solution has a 21-day expiration period [29]. The patient's name, room, hospital number, the container number, the patient's blood group and Rh status, and the donor's blood group and Rh status should be checked. (Many institutions have policies requiring

Table 5-3
The blood groups and major agglutinogens and agglutinins

Blood Groups	Agglutinogens	Agglutinins
O	—	Anti-A and anti-B
A	A	Anti-B
B	B	Anti-A
AB	A and B	—

that this check be done by two registered nurses prior to administration.) If any discrepancy is found, the blood is not given.

Specific identification of the patient should be confirmed. At the bedside the patient, the patient's identification bracelet, and hospitalization number should again be verified with the identification information on the blood label. Vital signs are taken to establish baseline data prior to beginning the blood transfusion so that changes can be accurately evaluated during and after the transfusion.

An infusion of physiologic saline is started with a large-gauge needle (usually an 18-gauge, but a 15-gauge needle may be used in some cases) to allow infusion of the viscous blood. Only isotonic saline solution is used in starting a blood transfusion or to flush the tubing on completion of the transfusion. Solutions such as 5% dextrose in water contain no electrolytes and can cause hemolysis of erythrocytes when mixed with the blood. Therefore, other solutions are not to be used to start blood transfusions. After entrance into the vein has been confirmed, the blood unit is then added to the infusion set. Blood must be administered via an infusion set that contains a filter within its drip chamber. The filter is capable of retaining precipitates and coagula potentially harmful to the recipient [29]. Blood is not routinely warmed before its administration except to remove it from the refrigerator for several minutes prior to administration. In rapid or massive transfusions, exchange transfusions, or for patients with potent cold agglutinins, however, warming of the blood is indicated; it is done by means of a warming device during passage of blood through the infusion set. The American Association of Blood Banks recommends that "no medication shall be added to the blood prior to, or during, a transfusion" [29].

BLOOD TRANSFUSION REACTIONS

After the blood has been started, the nurse remains with the patient while the first 50 ml of blood is transfused because hemolytic reactions occur even after only a small amount of the blood has been transfused. Vital signs are taken periodically during the transfusion, so that changes can be evaluated. The major symptoms associated with hemolytic reactions are headache, back pain, fever, dyspnea, chills, cyanosis, decreased blood pressure, and an overwhelming feeling of apprehension. Oliguria and jaundice are later signs. If a hemolytic reaction occurs the nurse should immediately discontinue the blood, change the IV tubing, and allow the saline to flow. It is important to maintain the patency of the intravenous infusion to provide a means for administering additional fluids and drugs as ordered by the physician. Both the physician and the laboratory are notified immediately when hemolytic reactions occur. The blood container, remaining blood, and tubing are returned to the laboratory for analysis and another type and crossmatch verification. Vital signs are taken every 15 minutes to observe for impending hypotension and shock. Intake and output are recorded to observe for oliguria or anuria, which may result from hemoglobin precipitation in kidney tubules and subsequent renal failure. Oxygen and epinephrine are often necessary if hypotension or shock occurs; sedation to counteract restlessness and apprehension is often indicated, but is administered judiciously in light of other symptoms. Mannitol (an osmotic diuretic) may be ordered to counteract oliguria. Other vasopressor drugs may be indicated if severe shock develops. The onset of hemolytic reactions is an emergency situation and requires prompt action on the part of the nurse; however, the nurse should remember that the patient is very anxious and apprehensive as these critical changes occur, and should provide calm explanations and psychological support.

As the antibodies in the recipient's plasma react with antigens carried in the donor's erythrocytes, resulting in agglutination, the clumped cells block the patient's capillaries and interfere with blood flow and oxygen to the vital organs. Macrophages devour the agglutinated cells after a few hours; the resulting hemolysis releases free hemoglobin into the plasma and the urine. The free hemoglobin may plug the renal tubules, disrupting nephron function and causing renal failure. Some patients die from renal failure and shock after hemolytic transfusion reactions. Patients may recover if the plugs in the renal tubules are disintegrated. It is necessary to send urine specimens to the laboratory for examination of hemoglobin content. Serum bilirubin determination should also be done within 5 to 7 hours after the transfusion reaction [29]. Treatment is centered upon preventing renal damage caused by hemoglobin precipitation in the kidney tubules. Diuresis is promoted by the use of intravenous fluids, diuretics, and methods to alkalinize body fluids, because alkaline tubular fluid dissolves hemoglobin more readily than acid tubular fluid [16].

Circulatory overload with development of pulmonary edema may develop during blood transfusion therapy. Elderly or debilitated patients or those with cardiac problems are vulnerable to such complications if fluid is infused too rapidly or in too great a quantity. Severely anemic patients are highly susceptible to cardiac failure from circulatory overload, because their weakened hearts may not be able to cope with the additional volume. Signs of circulatory overload are cough, dyspnea, edema, tachycardia, and hemoptysis. The transfusion is stopped and the physician is notified. At times, a digitalis preparation is indicated; phlebotomy to remove excess fluid from the general circulation may be necessary. Rotating tourniquets may also be utilized. (The use of rotating techniques is described in Chapter 4.) Circulatory overload can be prevented by cautious administration of transfusions to vulnerable patients and by a slowed rate versus a rapid transfusion. Packed cells (which provide the cellular elements with minimal plasma) rather than whole blood are therefore indicated for patients susceptible to circulatory overload.

Bacterial transfusion reactions may occur from the administration of contaminated blood. Signs of this reaction include fever, chills, lumbar pain, headache, malaise, flushed skin, and diarrhea. Although this complication is rare as a result of modern aseptic blood-banking techniques, the nurse should observe for the signs and discontinue the blood if they occur. Although the skin is typically flushed in patients experiencing bacterial transfusion reactions, vital signs are observed for impending shock. The remaining blood and the container are sent to the laboratory for culture and sensitivity tests. As in hemolytic reactions, it is important to maintain fluid administration, diuresis, and intake and output records. Antibiotics, in high dosages, are utilized, and corticosteroids are often indicated for their anti-inflammatory action. Temperature changes are observed; cooling measures such as alcohol sponges and cooling blankets are indicated for the control of elevated temperatures.

Allergic reactions result from the presence of proteins in the donor plasma to which the recipient is allergic or from the presence of breakdown products in old, deteriorating donor blood [16]. In some cases the reaction may be related to drugs or foods the donor has ingested and to which the recipient is allergic. The allergic reactions cause chills, urticaria, vertigo, mild edema, and headache, but they may also cause severe dyspnea, bronchial wheezing, bronchospasm, and shock. Antihistamines and antipyretics are given to the patient with a mild allergic reaction. Bronchodilators, vasopressors, corticosteroids, and oxygen therapy, as well as other respiratory support therapy, are indicated in severe allergic reactions. If the reaction is mild, the transfusion rate may simply be slowed while other interventions are carried out. If the reaction is severe, the blood is discontinued and other intravenous fluids are used to maintain the infusion site.

Other complications that can occur with transfusion therapy include air embolism, hyperkalemia, hypocalcemia, hypothermia, and infectious disease transmission. **Air embolism** is rare, but it can occur, particularly when blood is being transfused under pressure. When air embolism is suspected, the patient is positioned on his left side in a slight Trendelenburg position to divert air from the pulmonary system. (It is felt that this position allows the air to rise into the right atrium and away from the pulmonary artery.)

When banked blood is stored until nearly the end of its expiration period, there is danger of causing **potassium intoxication** because the erythrocyte breakdown in the stored blood increases the level of potassium in the blood. This complication is most likely to occur in patients made vulnerable by existing cardiac or renal disease. The nurse should consider these factors in determining whether the blood is safe to administer when it is nearing the expiration period and the patient to receive the blood is a person susceptible to potassium intoxication.

When large quantities of ACD blood are used for multiple transfusions over a short period of time, the sodium citrate anticoagulant in ACD blood binds with the calcium ions and removes them from the circulation. This condition is sometimes described as **citrate intoxication.** Prophylactic treatment usually consists in the intravenous administration of calcium gluconate or other calcium salts.

Hypothermia may occur when cold blood, particularly in large amounts, is administered. Blood should be about room temperature when it is administered. Usually, removing the blood from the refrigerator for several minutes prior to its administration will be sufficient to prevent discomfort or dangerous reactions. Blood can be warmed in specific situations, as previously described.

Although potential donors are carefully screened before donating blood, delayed complications of transfusion therapy may include transmission of hepatitis, malaria, and syphilis. Although the transmission of malaria and syphilis rarely occurs, the incidence of post-transfusion hepatitis continues to be a problem. The frequency and severity of post-transfusion hepatitis can be reduced by routine testing of all donor blood for hepatitis B antigen. The incidence of hepatitis appears to increase when donors are paid for their blood because paid donors are less likely to be in good health, when they participate in blood programs only for the money.

Whole-blood usage has been limited to situations of acute hemorrhage (a decrease in volume as well as erythrocytes). Shortages of whole blood and the fact that whole-blood transfusions are contraindicated in situations in which increased fluid volume is a potential hazard are two reasons for limiting usage of whole blood. It is estimated that at least 80 percent of all transfusions currently given as whole blood could in fact be given in the form of packed red cells [14]. The specific component required by the individual patient should be determined and then administered in lieu of whole-blood transfusions. For example, elderly patients with anemia have a normal or increased total blood volume and are susceptible to fluid overload if whole-blood transfusions are given. Such patients are more appropriately given packed red blood cells.

BLOOD COMPONENT THERAPY

Packed red blood cells are erythrocytes that have been separated from citrated whole blood that has been cross-matched with the recipient's blood group and Rh type. Five types of packed cell preparations are in current use; these include sedimented cells, centrifuged cells, washed cells, frozen red cells, and thawed resuspended cells. Sedimented cells contain all the cellular elements of blood. Most of the fluid element is withdrawn, but the antigenic potential of leukocytes, platelets, and plasma proteins remains. These cells must be used within 24 hours after donation. Centrifuged cells reduce the amount of fluid in the cells and permit longer storage; if a closed method of separation has been used, these cells can be stored for up to 21 days. Centrifuged cells contain less antigenic material than the sedimented cells [30].

Antigenic material is removed more completely in the preparation of washed cells. These are prepared by centrifugation with removal of plasma and the buffy coat. **Buffy coat** is a term used to describe the white layer that settles between the erythrocytes and the plasma after a blood specimen has been centrifuged. The white layer is basically the leukocyte layer. The erythrocytes are suspended and washed three times in sterile saline. Frozen erythrocytes have the advantage of being viable for many years, and they are essentially leukocyte-free. All plasma can be removed in this preparation so that there is a significant reduction in the incidence of hepatitis. The freezing method allows for storage of rare blood and also facilitates the use of autologous transfusions (the removal and storage of blood or blood components from a donor for subsequent reinfusion). Thawed resuspended cells provide the safest preparation, since they contain the least amount of antigenic material [30].

Plasmapheresis is the withdrawal of blood to obtain plasma or platelet products (plateletpheresis) with subsequent reinfusion of the erythrocytes and/or platelet-poor plasma [29]. Plateletpheresis or plasmapheresis is a tedious procedure and an uncomfortable one for the donor. A large 14-gauge needle is necessary, making the initial injection a painful one. The donor must be ABO-compatible with the recipient because of the potential erythrocyte contamination of the leukocyte collection. HL-A (human leukocyte antigen) typing is done to determine histocompatibility. Large volumes of platelets from a single HL-A-compatible donor can be collected by means of continuous-flow centrifugation (such as the IBM cell separator). This procedure can be done so that there are no side effects for the donor, although boredom, stiffness of the arm, and the prolonged immobilization for approximately 4 hours can be very disturbing to the donor. Platelet transfusions are done for the control or prevention of bleeding in patients with aplastic anemia, leukemia, and other malignant conditions treated with intensive chemotherapy or radiotherapy [14].

Leukapheresis and the use of leukocyte transfusions are still considered primarily experimental [14]. Various instruments have been developed to facilitate the collection of large numbers of leukocytes from single donors for transfusion to patients with severe bone marrow depression, as an adjunct to treatment of life-threatening infections. Continuous-flow separation techniques via filtration leukapheresis are used to concentrate granulocytes selectively from whole blood as it is propelled through the system [14]. Histocompatibility testing in the HL-A system is done in selecting donor-recipient pairs for leukocyte transfusions, as is done in platelet collection.

Plasma components are preparations of plasma that can be separated from whole blood. These components include albumin, fibrinogen, gamma globulin, and the antihemophilia factor. Human plasma is used to increase plasma volume in patients suffering from hypovolemia, such as in shock, burns, and in initial hemorrhage while typing and crossmatching are being done for whole blood replacement. When replacement of blood-clotting factors or proteins is required, the plasma can be further separated to provide concentrates of these substances.

Single-donor fresh-frozen plasma is prepared within 4 hours of collection and is frozen within 6 hours to ensure retention of factors V and VII, which are lost during storage. The danger of frequent hepatitis transmission has resulted in recommendations that the use of pooled plasma be discouraged.

Cryoprecipitated antihemophilic factor is the cold, insoluble fraction of plasma protein obtained by centrifugation when frozen fresh plasma is thawed. The cryoprecipitated fraction contains about 56 percent of the original factor VIII globulin, along with trace amounts of all plasma constituents. It is used in the treatment of classic hemophilia and von Willebrand's disease, which are discussed later in this chapter.

Human fibrinogen is a sterile, freeze-dried fraction of normal human plasma, which in solution has the property of being converted into insoluble fibrin when thrombin is added [30]. It has a 5-year expiration date, even though it contains no preservative.

Normal human serum albumin is a sterile preparation of serum albumin that is obtained by fractionation of whole blood. It is readily stored in its concentrated form and is quite stable. It is used primarily in renal or liver disease to reduce edema by increasing the serum protein levels in hypoproteinemia.

Immune serum globulin (gamma globulin) is a sterile solution for intramuscular administration of globulins containing the antibodies normally present in adult human blood. Serum globulin may be used as a prophylactic immunizing agent against measles and hepatitis. It is also used for preventing recurrent infections in acquired or congenital deficiency of gamma globulin.

Disorders of the Erythrocytes

Disorders of the hematopoietic and lymphatic systems include a wide variety of diseases that primarily affect the erythrocytes, the leukocytes, and the hemostatic mechanisms. Disorders of the erythrocytes will be discussed first.

The physiologic basis of the diseases underlying the erythrocytic disorders are related either to a deficiency of normal circulating erythrocytes or to an increased number above normal of circulating erythrocytes.

ANEMIA

The most prevalent condition resulting from disorders of the hematopoietic system is anemia. **Anemia** indicates a reduction below normal levels of hemoglobin concentration or of erythrocytes, or both, resulting in decreased oxygen-carrying capacity of the blood. Anemia is considered a symptom of an underlying disease process and is caused either by decreased production of normal erythrocytes or by increased losses or abnormal destruction of erythrocytes.

Hypoxia of body tissues and cellular dysfunction result from an inadequate supply of oxygen carried by the blood. The classic symptoms of anemia, regardless of the underlying cause, therefore, are related to tissue hypoxia. The severity of the symptoms depends on the rapidity of development of anemia, the degree of anemia, the effectiveness of adaptive mechanisms of the patient, and the status of the circulatory system. Weakness and fatigue are common symptoms related to the oxygen deprivation of the muscle cells. Persons with anemia often describe an increased need for sleep and rest. Persons with moderate anemia often describe symptoms of unexplained lethargy and loss of productivity. Dyspnea on exertion related to inadequate oxygen during activity may also be a presenting symptom. Tachycardia and tachypnea are compensatory mechanisms for decreased levels of oxygen being transported to the cells. In severe anemia, congestive heart failure may result from increased demands on the heart to transport more oxygen to the tissues.

Central nervous system symptoms include dizziness, light-headedness, irritability, and depression. Often normal thought processes are also affected, with slowing and dullness in responses being notable. Pallor, which formerly was considered a reliable sign of the state of anemia, may be minimal or profound. The extent of pallor, however, is affected by other factors, such as the normal skin pigmentation of the individual. Pallor of the mucous membranes in the oral cavity or the conjunctiva of the eyes is a more reliable criterion of anemia. The person with anemia tends continually to feel cold. A warm environment must therefore be provided. Feeling cold is related to the decreased metabolism, which is the body's effort to conserve the limited oxygen available. Other symptoms, such as neurologic changes or jaundice, are associated with specific types of anemia and are discussed later in this chapter.

The classic symptoms associated with anemia have general implications for nursing care, regardless of the cause of the anemia. These care aspects relate to alleviating the cause of the anemia, alleviating the symptoms, and preventing complications. Careful observation of the patient's tolerance for activity and his energy level is essential to determine the individual's needs for adequate rest. In mild anemia, patients usually are ambulatory; patients with severe anemia, however, require hospitalization with complete bed rest. Nursing care is planned to conserve the energy of the patient and to provide for the safety of the patient, who is typically quite weak.

Dietary instruction is indicated, particularly when anemia relates to dietary deficiencies. Emphasis is placed on including the essential nutrients—protein, iron, and vitamins—that support the production of erythrocytes. Because inadequately oxygenated tissues are more susceptible to invasion by microorganisms, the patient with anemia must be protected from infection. Therefore, patients with anemia should not be in rooms with patients with infectious diseases. Ambulatory patients should be instructed to avoid exposure to sources of infection. Patients with aplastic anemia, associated with leukopenia, cannot withstand even usual or normal exposure to microorganisms; they often require protection by means of reverse isolation. A "life island" or laminar-flow room is used in some settings. (This therapy was described on page 128.)

Anemia is associated with poor wound-healing, so that protection from injury must be included in nursing care measures. Anemia associated with thrombocytopenia requires protection from any source of trauma that might incite bleeding. The severely anemic patient requires complete bed rest and is likely to develop decubitus ulcers unless preventive measures are initiated.

Inadequate cerebral oxygenation may result in dizziness leading to falls and injury, particularly when the person moves too quickly, changes positions too rapidly, or is already handicapped with cerebral arteriosclerosis. Patients with anemia may have associated neurologic disturbances that limit sensory perception. Such persons must be taught to avoid the use of hot water bottles or heating pads as external sources of heat, but should apply additional clothing or covers instead. The danger of burns from externally applied heat is a real threat for such persons.

In aplastic anemia associated with leukopenia, necrotic lesions develop in the mouth and pharynx due to increased susceptibility to infections. These lesions may also occur in persons with anemias associated with nutritional deficiencies. The gums tend to bleed either spontaneously or with slight trauma. Therefore, there is difficulty in keeping the mouth clean and in providing adequate intake. Careful and frequent (after every meal and at the hour of sleep) mouth care with diluted mouthwashes and the use of soft toothbrushes (or cotton swabs or Toothettes) are indicated for oral hygiene to avoid mechanical or chemical trauma to the oral lesions. These persons are particularly sensitive to either hot or cold foods, as well as spicy foods. A bland diet, with an increase in liquid protein supplements, is more palatable to them.

With any type of blood dyscrasia, including anemia, frequent venipunctures are required to determine the diagnosis as well as to evaluate the effectiveness of therapy. This requirement contributes to physical discomfort and psychological stress. The frequent venipunctures may become the focus of the patient's feelings of frustration or irritability. The patient may become annoyed, angry, and discouraged with repeated venipunctures. Emotional support and understanding must be extended to the patient as he expresses his anger about frequent blood tests, or when, on occasion, he may refuse to permit further venipunctures. Physical discomfort can be limited by preventing excessive puncturing through careful scheduling of blood examinations.

Major aspects of the care of the patient with chronic anemia are the teaching and supportive measures required to assist the patient to understand the necessity for continued treatment. The patient is more likely then to cooperate in long-term management of his or her condition.

Anemias may be classified morphologically, by etiology, or on a pathophysiologic basis. **Normocytic, normochromic anemia** indicates erythrocytes that are normal in size and content of hemoglobin; however, there is a reduction in the number of erythrocytes and therefore a reduced hemoglobin and hematocrit. Sudden blood loss with hemorrhage is an example of normocytic, normochromic anemia.

Microcytic, hypochromic anemia is characterized by a reduction in the size of the erythrocytes and in the quantity of hemoglobin in the cells. Iron deficiency anemia is the most common cause of this type of anemia.

Macrocytic, normochromic anemia indicates abnormally large erythrocytes which, because of the size, may contain increased concentrations of hemoglobin. Formerly these cells were described as hyperchromic, due to their appearance on a stained blood film. This term, however, is incorrect, because the increased hemoglobin concentration is proportional to the increased size of the cells. There is a reduction in the total erythrocyte count, however, as well as a reduced total hemoglobin concentration. Therefore normochromic is a more accurate term. Vitamin B_{12} deficiency, as present in pernicious anemia or malabsorption syndromes, and folic acid deficiency, result in macrocytic anemia. Anemias related to these deficiencies may also be classified as **megaloblastic,** referring to the abnormally developed precursors that may be present in the patient's bone marrow.

In the following discussion, the various types of anemia will be discussed separately according to the basic etiologic classifications. Table 5-4 lists the types of anemia.

Iron Deficiency Anemia

Iron deficiency anemia is the most prevalent type of anemia. It results from inadequate iron intake, defective iron absorption, increased iron requirements, or improper utilization. Some groups of persons—for example, those in underdeveloped countries with extremely poor nutrition—are particularly vulnerable to this type of anemia. Even in the developed countries, poverty and the increased use of fad diets may contribute to the lack of adequate iron intake. Pregnant women, who must furnish iron to the fetus, and infants whose only nutrient is milk which is deficient in iron are vulnerable to iron deficiencies. Women of childbearing age may develop iron deficiencies as a result of chronic blood loss in the menstrual flow. The average monthly loss is about 30 ml, but some women with excessive menstrual flow may lose between 60 and 100 ml. Iron deficiency anemia in men or postmenopausal women may reflect the presence of some condition causing chronic blood loss. This disorder is often of gastrointestinal tract origin, as in hemorrhoids, peptic ulcers, ulcerative colitis or cancer. Gastrointestinal x-rays or sigmoidoscopy or both are indicated in in these situations to determine the underlying cause.

Table 5-4
Etiologic classification of types of anemia

I. Anemias resulting from decreased erythropoiesis
   A. Deficiency anemias (deficiency of factors essential to normal production)
      1. Iron deficiency anemia
      2. Vitamin B_{12} deficiency
      3. Folic acid deficiency
   B. Aplastic anemia (resulting from depressed bone marrow activity)
II. Anemias resulting from excessive rate of hemolysis (hemolytic anemias)
   A. Intracorpuscular defects (inherent defects of the erythrocytes)
      1. Inherited defects
         a. Hereditary spherocytosis
         b. Hemoglobinopathy
            (1) Sickle cell anemia
            (2) Thalassemia
         c. Glucose 6-phosphate dehydrogenase (G-6-PD) deficiency
      2. Acquired defects
         a. Paroxysmal nocturnal hemoglobinuria (PNH)
   B. Extracorpuscular factors (erythrocytes damaged by external factors)
      1. Infections
      2. Industrial toxins
      3. Immune bodies
         a. Erythroblastosis fetalis
         b. Idiopathic autoimmune hemolytic anemia
         c. Drug reactions
III. Anemia resulting from excessive blood loss

When chronic blood loss is suspected, the nurse should ascertain whether the patient has had tarry stools or has passed bright red blood from the rectum, and should also determine the frequency of these events. The presence of blood cannot always be observed. Therefore, stool examinations via the guaiac method are indicated to determine the presence of occult blood. Because a patient's bleeding may not be continuous, and because a patient may lose more than 300 ml per day without making the stool overtly black, daily examinations of at least three stool collections are required [12]. These collections are generally initiated after a regimen of a meat-free diet for 3 days and restriction of iron medication and salicylate drugs.

When chronic blood loss is suspected, the nurse also questions the patient about medications he or she is taking. Bleeding, for example, may be related to aspirin intake or to certain antirheumatic drugs such as indomethacin (Indocin) and phenylbutazone (Butazolidin).

As discussed previously, a daily intake of 10 mg of iron in men and 18 mg in women will provide an adequate iron absorption of approximately 1 to 3 mg. Approximately 1 mg of iron is lost daily, mostly in desquamated epithelium and in secretions from the gastrointestinal tract and skin [8]. The major sources of iron are liver, lean meats, egg yolk, whole wheat bread, dried fruits, and certain vegetables, such as spinach. The body may be able to compensate for chronic losses by increasing the absorption of iron or limiting the excretion of iron. In severe states of iron deficiency anemia, however, iron supplements are necessary to restore iron balance.

In the presence of adequate dietary intake, iron deficiency anemia may reflect inadequate absorption. The most frequent causes of inadequate absorption are chronic diarrhea, malabsorption syndromes such as celiac disease, tropical and nontropical sprue, and total or subtotal gastrectomy. The latter conditions cause a decrease in both the assimilation and absorption of iron.

The diagnosis of iron deficiency anemia is confirmed by the identification of microcytic and hypochromic erythrocytes, a decreased hemoglobin concentration, and a reduction in all three of the erythrocyte indices (MCV, MCH, and MCHC). The MCV may be as low as 50 cubic microns and is often between 50 and 80 cubic microns. The reduction of the MCH to below 27 μg is an excellent index of the degree of iron deficiency. The MCHC usually is below 30 percent in this type of anemia. The diagnosis is further substantiated by a reduced serum iron level (below 30 μg per 100 ml), an elevated iron-binding capacity, and a very low percentage of saturation. Depletion of iron stores normally present in bone marrow is reflected by the absence of hemosiderin in bone marrow aspirations. Severe iron deficiency may result in hemolytic disease, since hypochromic cells are abnormally brittle and fragment easily [8].

Patients with iron deficiency anemia may be asymptomatic or may demonstrate classic symptoms of anemia in severe degrees. Cheilosis (cracking of the skin at the corners of the lips) is often observed; dysphagia is often present, as are glossitis and atrophy of the papillae of the tongue. Tongue changes, however, are not specific for iron deficiency anemia; they are also associated with vitamin B_{12} and folic acid deficiencies.

Some patients with iron deficiency may develop the syndrome known as **pica,** which is an abnormal craving for and ingestion of such nonfoods as starch and sand [8]. Clay-eating, for example, is a common symptom in women and children in deprived areas of the world. This abnormal craving disappears within several days after iron replacement has been initiated.

The treatment of iron deficiency consists in determining the cause and restoring the body's iron content to normal. The patient is usually started on oral iron preparations, which are the safest, cheapest, and most readily accepted type of preparation. Ferrous iron is better absorbed than ferric iron; ferrous sulfate, 300 mg three times per day is frequently ordered. Children usually receive liquid ferrous sulfate preparations in dosages determined by body weight. Persons taking liquid iron are advised to take the medication through a glass tube or straw to avoid injury or staining of the teeth. The patient should be forewarned that black stools will develop as a side effect of iron administration.

Iron is best absorbed on an empty stomach when the absorption surface is likely to be in an acid state, which supports iron absorption [31]; however, it may cause epigastric distress with abdominal cramps, nausea, diarrhea, and constipation. It may then be necessary to administer the iron with food to reduce side effects until tolerance has become adequate to administer iron between meals. Alternative preparations may be attempted to determine whether the patient is able to tolerate other preparations better. Iron absorption is aided by vitamin C; therefore, ascorbic acid can be combined with the iron preparation or it can be given in the form of orange juice with the medication.

When iron is not tolerated by mouth, when the patient is unreliable in taking the medication, or when there is a need for more rapid repletion of iron, parenteral iron administration may be necessary. The major parenteral preparations include iron dextran (Imferon) for intramuscular and intravenous use, and iron sorbitex (Jectofer) for intramuscular use only. When either of these is administered intramuscularly, special precautions are necessary to prevent tissue discoloration or damage and pain. The Z track technique is used to minimize staining of the tissues from the iron medication. In this technique, the skin is pulled to one side as the needle is injected deep into the muscle of the upper outer quadrant of the buttocks. (Iron should not be administered into other muscles.) Figure 5-4 illustrates the Z track technique. Other measures to decrease the likelihood of staining the tissues include the use of one needle for the withdrawal of the medication from the vial and another needle for the actual injection. To clear the needle of any iron that might leak out during withdrawal of the needle, 0.5 ml of air is drawn into the syringe and is injected after the medication is given.

Anaphylactic reactions, evidenced by hypotension, headache, urticaria, and shock, have been reported during administration of iron. These have occurred particularly with intravenous injections. The nurse should therefore always aspirate the needle prior to injection of the medication. Patients with histories of allergies may possibly not be candidates for parenteral iron therapy; allergies should be verified when obtaining the patient's history.

After iron therapy has been started, the reticulocyte count, serum iron levels, and hemoglobin are monitored within several days. The reticulocyte count rises generally within 3 days and will continue to rise for 8 to 10 days. The hemoglobin levels rise more slowly. Although iron therapy typically results in a favorable response within several days, patients require iron therapy for 3 to 6 months or longer to replenish iron stores, even after the hemoglobin levels return to normal. Patients must be encouraged to

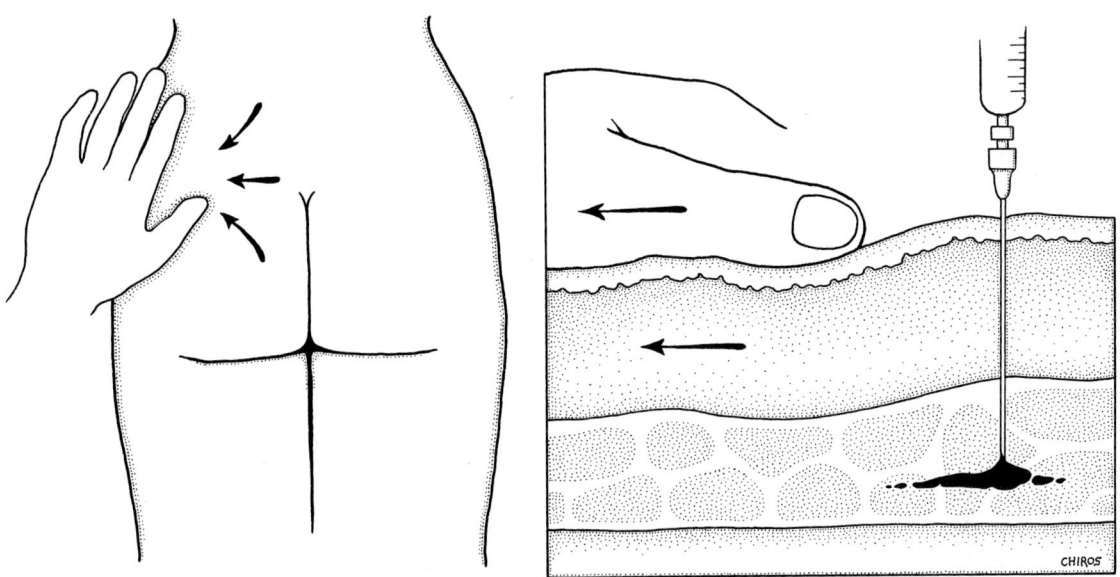

Figure 5-4
The Z track technique used for the intramuscular administration of iron.

cooperate in this long-term therapy and must understand the chronic nature of their illness as well as the ways to prevent recurrence of the deficiency. People often think of iron as being a harmless drug and may be careless in handling or storing it. Toxicity can occur with excessive dosages of iron; this is especially true if children accidentally mistake iron for candy and ingest excessive amounts. The dangers of toxicity must be emphasized. The signs and symptoms of iron toxicity include gastrointestinal distress and tissue destruction.

If iron therapy does not result in any improvement, the physician must evaluate the patient for another cause of the iron deficiency; however, it must first be established that the patient has been reliable about taking the medication before a decision is made that the treatment was ineffective.

Vitamin B_{12} Deficiencies

Pernicious anemia is the most common result of vitamin B_{12} deficiency. This type of chronic, progressive, macrocytic anemia is caused by failure to absorb vitamin B_{12} (cyanocobalamin) from the intestinal tract because of the absence of the intrinsic factor. The **intrinsic factor,** a mucoprotein normally produced in the gastric secretions, combines with B_{12} that has been ingested in the diet to make it more soluble for absorption in the small intestine. The absence of intrinsic factor is associated with atrophy of the gastric mucosa. Persons who have had a total gastrectomy and have lost the source of the intrinsic factor will eventually develop pernicious anemia unless replacement therapy is given.

Vitamin B_{12} deficiency may also occur with malabsorption diseases, such as sprue, which affects the small intestine and particularly the ileum, where vitamin B_{12} is normally absorbed. Competition for available vitamin B_{12} may occur with bacterial or parasitic infections (such as fish tapeworm) in the gastrointestinal tract; these infections deplete the amounts of stored B_{12}. In this situation, vitamin B_{12} deficiencies will not be corrected until the underlying infection or parasitic infestation has been treated.

Iatrogenic malabsorption syndromes may result from surgical resections of the small intestine as associated with the treatment of ulcerative colitis or Crohn's disease, or with jejunal bypass surgery for obesity. Vitamin B_{12} deficiency is rarely caused by dietary deficiency alone, because only small amounts of animal protein are necessary to provide the required amounts of B_{12} [25]. Plant foods, however, are poor sources of the vitamin, and deficiency may occur when persons follow a strict vegetarian diet.

Vitamin B_{12} deficiency affects the maturation of the erythrocytes. Diagnosis is confirmed by a reduced erythrocyte count and a peripheral blood smear that demonstrates megaloblastic maturation. Confirmation of the megaloblastic, macrocytic type of anemia is established by an increased MCV above 94 microns (because of abnormally large erythrocytes), an increased MCH above 30 μg (because of abnormally large volumes of hemoglobin), and a normal MCHC (because the erythrocytes are oversized). A bone marrow aspiration demonstrates hyperplasia.

Upper gastrointestinal tract x-rays may demonstrate gastric atrophy. Gastric analysis will usually show a persistent hypochlorhydria or achlorhydria even after injection of histamine, which should normally cause an increase in gastric secretions. Absence of hydrochloric acid may be an indication of either pernicious anemia or cancer of the stomach; gastroscopy with biopsy may be indicated to differentiate the two conditions.

A Schilling test may be ordered to determine whether the vitamin B_{12} deficiency is a result of the absence of the intrinsic factor or is caused by some other malabsorption problem. The Schilling test requires a 12-hour fast before initiation. Vitamin B_{12} is tagged with radioactive cobalt and is given orally to the patient. A 24-hour urine collection is then started. Two hours later (or longer in some institutions), an intramuscular dose of nonradioactive B_{12} is given. If the intrinsic factor is present, oral B_{12} is absorbed, and large amounts of the radioactive dose are eliminated into the urine. In the absence of the intrinsic factor, little oral B_{12} is absorbed and nonradioactive B_{12} is utilized so that the urine contains minimal radioactive B_{12}. Pernicious anemia is confirmed by repeating the test and utilizing a dose of intrinsic factor preparation as well as the radioactive B_{12}. (Intrinsic factor preparations are commercially available concentrates of hog stomach or normal human gastric juices [22].) After receiving the intrinsic factor, the patient with pernicious anemia excretes normal amounts of radioactive B_{12} in the urine. The test is long and tedious, and the lengthy fasting period may be annoying to the patient. The test must be fully explained to the patient to gain his cooperation. The need for an accurate collection of all the urine voided in the 24-hour collection period cannot be overemphasized. The accuracy of the test results upon measurement of radioactive B_{12} in the entire 24-hour specimen.

As established earlier in this chapter, vitamin B_{12} is required for the production of RNA, which is required for maintenance of central nervous system integrity. Therefore, in addition to varying degrees of the classic symptoms of anemia (fatigue, weakness, and pallor), the patient with pernicious anemia will demonstrate symptoms of neurologic disturbances. These disturbances may vary from numbness and tingling of the extremities, described as "pins and needles" sensations, to symptoms of spinal cord degeneration, such as paresthesia and gait disturbances. Patients may describe problems in holding small objects in their fingers and problems related to a loss of finer movements.

Personality changes and behavior problems will often be present, not only related to decreased cerebral oxygenation, but also associated with the neurologic changes. On occasion, neurologic changes may precede other symptoms, so that delays in diagnosis may occur; sometimes these changes have resulted in diagnosis of a psychiatric nature before the organic cause is detected.

A symptom commonly associated with pernicious anemia is **glossitis,** characterized by a beefy red tongue, which has a glazed appearance. It is associated with complaints of a "sore tongue." Tongue changes, such as a smooth tongue, are related to atrophic glossitis with loss of the filiform papillae. Consequently, anorexia is a usual symptom that requires careful planning of meals and snacks to entice the patient to eat. A distinctive lemon-yellow hue to the skin may be associated with pernicious anemia and is related to the increased hemolysis of the abnormally large cells that are characteristic of the disease.

Pernicious anemia primarily affects middle-aged or elderly persons. It is felt that pernicious anemia may represent an autoimmune defect related to the production of chronic inflammation and gastric atrophy associated with the condition [25]. There appears to be a genetic predisposition to the disease in persons of northern European descent (fair-skinned, blue-eyed persons, often Scandinavians) [17]. Some authorities disagree with this claim of racial predisposition, however, since the disease has been reported in all racial and ethnic groups [9].

Nursing care of the patient with pernicious anemia involves consideration of the general aspects of care of anemic patients as previously described. In addition, constant vigilance is required to provide for safety and to prevent trauma or injury, for these persons are vulnerable to such problems because of the associated neurologic changes. Pressure or trauma to the lower extremities, particularly, should be avoided because of circulatory changes effecting impaired sensation. For some patients, even the pressure of a heavy blanket will not be tolerated, so that a bed cradle over the legs may be necessary. These patients complain of being cold; a warm, well-ventilated room is essential. The use of external heating pads should be avoided. Sensory deficits in these persons increase susceptibility to burns and further nerve damage. Ataxia may be present; ambulation requires supervision in order to prevent accidents.

The patient may show signs of behavioral changes and decreased tolerance to noise and activity. Expressions of irritability, annoyance, and impatience may alienate them from their families and from the nursing staff. The nurse should understand the pathology of the patient's condition and demonstrate patience and acceptance of such behavior. Provision of a quiet, nonstimulating environment will contribute to the patient's rest and psychologic comfort.

Parenteral administration of vitamin B_{12} is essential to treat the anemia as well as to control the associated neurologic changes. Initially 100 μg of vitamin B_{12} is given intramuscularly three times a week for 2 weeks, then two times a week for 2 weeks, and followed by monthly injections. Parenteral administration of vitamin B_{12} on a monthly schedule is required for the rest of the patient's life. Generally, there is a fairly rapid, favorable response in pernicious anemia. Hematologic symptoms improve, the appetite increases, and tongue soreness rapidly disappears. Neurologic improvement is less predictable. Abnormal behavioral changes and confusion disappear readily, but spinal cord and peripheral nerve involvement may improve only slightly or may remain static. During the first 48 hours after vitamin B_{12} therapy has been initiated, a temporary lowered serum potassium level tends to occur [28]. Patients, particularly those with associated cardiovascular disease, should be observed for any adverse changes possibly related to hypokalemia.

Folic acid, if administered in pernicious anemia as a single treatment, may correct the hematologic abnormalities, but will have no effect on the neurologic changes. Some authorities claim that folic acid may actually aggravate the neurologic symptoms; they feel that folic acid is contraindicated in pernicious anemia [24]. Some physicians, however, prescribe small doses of folic acid, along with parenteral B_{12}.

There is no way in which the atrophied stomach cells can recover the ability to secrete the intrinsic factor. Therefore, replacement therapy is required for the rest of the individual's life. Parenteral administration is necessary because oral vitamin B_{12} cannot be absorbed in the absence of the intrinsic factor. This prolonged therapy will be difficult to accept, especially by persons who dislike injections of any type. Elderly persons may be forgetful and unreliable in obtaining the monthly injections, or they may have difficulty obtaining transportation to a clinic or physician's office on a monthly basis. Teaching someone in the home to give the injection or referring the patient to a public health agency may be more appropriate.

The control of the disease is dependent on the understanding and cooperation of the patient in the continued management. The patient must accept this fact and realize that if he omits the injections, the classic symptoms of anemia will recur and the neurologic symptoms may become irreversible. Untreated pernicious anemia will terminate in death.

Folic Acid Deficiency

Another fairly common form of anemia is **folic acid deficiency,** which is also associated with a macrocytic megaloblastic anemia. Folic acid is necessary for the maturation of erythrocytes because it promotes the formation of nucleotides required for DNA synthesis [16]. This condition is most often caused by intake of a diet that is deficient in such foods as green vegetables, whole grains, citrus fruits, and liver. The condition is commonly found in alcoholics because of associated poor nutritional intake. In addition, high levels of alcohol in the blood may interfere with erythropoiesis by directly suppressing the bone marrow response to folic acid [17]. Folic acid deficiency is also found in women during late pregnancy, as fetal requirements for folic acid increase, and in persons with malabsorption syndromes.

Folic acid deficiency is also associated with certain drugs, some of which are used as chemotherapeutic agents in the treatment of cancer. These drugs include methotrexate, a major drug in cancer chemotherapy utilized for its action as a folic acid antagonist, purine analogues such as 6-mercaptopurine, and pyrimidine analogues such as 5-fluorouracil. Phenytoin sodium (Dilantin) and some oral contraceptives have also been implicated in folic acid deficiency.

The cause of megaloblastic anemia (confirmed by peripheral smear and bone marrow aspirations) must be differentiated between folic acid deficiency and vitamin B_{12} deficiency. Folic acid deficiency, in contrast to vitamin B_{12} deficiency, is not associated with neurologic manifestations, nor is it associated with hypochlorhydria. The best way to confirm a folic acid deficiency is by serum assay. Normal folate is 5 to 22 mg per milliliter and the normal serum level of vitamin B_{12} is 300 to 400 μg per milliliter [12].

Oral folic acid up to doses of 1 mg daily is prescribed. This regimen is continued indefinitely if the patient is malnourished or is a known alcoholic. If the folic acid deficiency is related to pregnancy, usually therapy is continued for only 6 months. Vitamin C can be prescribed along with the folic acid, because ascorbic acid supports the activity of folic acid in erythropoiesis.

Aplastic Anemia

Aplastic anemia indicates a deficiency of circulating erythrocytes resulting from insufficient bone marrow activity. Other terms used to describe this condition, or phases of the disease, include **hypoplastic anemia,** or **primary refractory anemia.**

Aplastic anemia rarely occurs alone; when it does, it generally is a congenital absence of erythrocyte precursors and is called **congenital pure red cell aplastic anemia** [12]. Usually **agranulocytosis** (a reduction in granulocytes) and **thrombocytopenia** (a reduction in platelets) are also present. Because the bone marrow is responsible for production of granulocytes and platelets, as well as erythrocytes, all three types of cells are affected in bone marrow disease. **Pancytopenia** is the term used to describe depression of all three cellular elements.

Aplastic anemia may be caused by the toxic action of certain drugs, industrial chemicals, excess exposure to radiation (x-rays, radium, radioactive isotopes), or space-occupying lesions that destroy bone marrow tissue. Leukemia and metastatic carcinoma can cause such lesions. Chromosomal defects and thymomas (tumors of the thymus gland) have also been implicated. Hypoplastic anemia may be associated with chronic infection, such as miliary tuberculosis, and with uremia. Milder forms of marrow suppression, probably based on erythropoietin deficiencies, are related to endocrine diseases such as hypothyroidism and hypopituitarism. The cause of aplastic anemia is often difficult to determine and is classified as idiopathic in about 50 percent of the cases. Drugs appear to be the most common offending agent. Drugs that are capable of suppressing bone marrow function include, but are not limited to, the following: chloramphenicol (Chloromycetin, the most common offender); sulfonamides; quinacrine (Atabrine); phenylbutazone (Butazolidin); the anticonvulsants, phenytoin sodium (Dilantin) and mephenytoin (Mesantoin); and gold salts. In rare cases, streptomycin and meprobamate (Equanil, Miltown) have been implicated. These drugs cause bone marrow deficiencies only in certain persons, apparently when there is an idiosyncratic reaction to the drug. There also appears to be a genetic predisposition to aplastic anemia [28].

Alkylating drugs and antimetabolites used in cancer chemotherapy consistently cause bone marrow depression by the very nature of their therapeutic action. These drugs are toxic to cells that reproduce rapidly, which, unfortunately, also includes the normal blood cells.

Benzene is an organic solvent that is frequently implicated in aplastic anemia. Carbon tetrachloride, aniline dyes, and DDT, as well as other insecticides, are causative agents also. Glue-sniffing, because of the presence of toluene, has been associated with the condition [28].

Diagnosis of aplastic anemia is made primarily on the basis of bone marrow aspiration and biopsy. Cellularity may vary from complete aplasia, with only lymphocytes present, to hypoplasia, with hypocellular activity. Normocytic anemia is usually below 1 million per cubic millimeter, and the reticulocyte count is also decreased. Granulocytopenia is confirmed by a leukocyte count often less than 2,000 per cubic millimeter. The platelet count may be less than 30,000 per cubic millimeter.

The onset of aplastic anemia may be insidious or rapid. The symptoms of anemia are present in a severe degree with increased fatigue, lethargy, and dyspnea. The onset may be of an explosive nature with a fulminating bacterial infection resulting from granulocytopenia. Cutaneous bleeding and bleeding of the mucous membranes are the result of the decreased platelet levels.

The first step in treatment is to evaluate the patient's history and environment for all possible causes and to withdraw the apparent offending drug or agent. It may be difficult to determine the specific cause because of the large number of drugs, assorted sprays, and chemicals currently in use.

Treatment modalities include the use of androgens and corticosteroids, splenectomy, or transfusion therapy. In mild forms, androgens or anabolic steroids may be beneficial in increasing bone marrow function by stimulating production of erythropoietin. Corticosteroids and splenectomy are used particularly in severe thrombocytopenia; these procedures appear to potentiate the effectiveness of platelet transfusion. Antibiotic therapy is indicated when infection occurs from granulocytopenia. Transfusion therapy of platelets, packed red cells and leukocytes is used for supportive therapy. Early bone marrow transplantation has been increasingly utilized.

The patient with pancytopenia is critically ill. In addition to suffering from severe hypoxia, the patient is susceptible to infections and to bleeding tendencies. Nursing care measures are related to conservation of the patient's energy, protection from infection by reverse isolation methods, and protection from trauma that might incite bleeding. Close observation for increased hypoxia, impending infection, or hemorrhage is absolutely essential. Periodic, thorough assessment of the patient is necessary to detect impending complications in their early stages.

The severity of the disease process, as well as the necessary isolation required as a protective measure, is a source of increased anxiety for patients and their families. The nurse is challenged to provide adequate psychological support as well as to provide physical comfort measures.

The course of the disease is precarious. Mortality is high in pancytopenia, particularly in the older age group and in those with profound leukopenia and thrombocytopenia. Half of the deaths occur within the first 2 years from hemorrhage or infection [28]. Partial or complete spontaneous remissions may occur. Prognosis is good if a specific causative agent can be determined and if the withdrawal of the agent is made before aplasia has progressed very far. The patient is warned to avoid further contact with the agent because reexposure may be fatal.

The incidence of aplastic anemia can be reduced by preventive measures to reduce the unnecessary exposure to drugs and chemicals. Public education regarding the dangers of certain chemicals, pesticides, insecticides, and nonprescription drugs is imperative. When a patient is receiving a drug that is likely to cause aplastic anemia, laboratory evaluation of effects on the bone marrow function must be made regularly, comparing baseline data obtained prior to initiation of the drug. Patients should be advised of signs and symptoms (lethargy, frequent infections, fever, and bleeding tendencies) that indicate bone marrow depression, because early detection is essential. When drugs implicated in aplastic anemia are being administered, nurses have a responsibility to contact the physician if prolonged medication therapy is no longer indicated by the patient's condition.

Hemolytic Anemias

Normally, the production of erythrocytes by the bone marrow balances the destruction of erythrocytes. As described previously, most of the aged erythrocytes (approximately 120 days old) are destroyed by phagocytosis by the reticuloendothelial tissues, particularly the spleen. On breakdown of the erythrocytes, hemoglobin is broken down, but some components, like the iron molecules from the heme portion, are conserved for reuse by the bone marrow. Remnants of heme are converted into bilirubin, which is normally excreted by the liver.

The rate of hemolysis is increased and the life span of the erythrocytes is shortened in all the types of hemolytic anemias. Hemolysis increases as fragility or permeability of the erythrocyte membrane increases. Associated anemia occurs when the bone marrow is no longer able to compensate for the increased destruction. The liver may not be able to excrete the increased bilirubin that results from excessive erythrocyte destruction. Consequently, bilirubin becomes elevated in the plasma and jaundice develops. Jaundice may be barely perceptible or it may be profound. Hemolysis may develop slowly or rapidly.

Examination of the bone marrow of persons suspected of having hemolytic anemia usually shows hyperplasia with an increase in the proportion of erythrocyte precursors. Persistent reticulocytosis without a rise in the hematocrit level indicates anemia is from either hemorrhage or hemolysis [12]. Indirect bilirubin levels are usually elevated, but the elevation does not necessarily reflect the intensity of the hemolytic process. The status of the liver and its ability to handle the excess bilirubin are factors, as is the amount of hemoglobin being released. The direct Coombs test can be done to detect the presence of antibodies on the erythrocyte surface to determine antiglobulin reactions. The direct Coombs test, however, is not specific for hemolytic anemias. Other laboratory findings that support the diagnosis of hemolytic anemia are increased fecal and urinary urobilinogen and hemoglobinemia.

Hemolytic anemia may result from inherent defects of the erythrocytes (intracorpuscular defects) or from the influence of external factors that damage or destroy the erythrocyte membrane (extracorpuscular defects). Intracorpuscular defects, which are generally congenital defects, include hereditary spherocytosis, the hemoglobinopathies (sickle cell anemia and thalassemia), and enzyme defects, such as glucose 6-phosphate dehydrogenase (G-6-PD) deficiencies. Paroxysmal nocturnal hemoglobinuria is an example of an acquired intracorpuscular defect. Extracorpuscular abnormalities that result in hemolysis include infections, toxins, transfusion reactions, and hypersplenic states. Mechanical hemolysis may be associated with prosthetic heart valves; immune hemolysis may be associated with certain autoimmune diseases, or may be drug-induced.

Hemolytic anemias are often characterized by splenomegaly, as well as hepatomegaly in some situations. Splenectomy is indicated, particularly in hereditary spherocytosis, but it may also be done in treating other types of hemolytic anemias. Therapy for patients with hemolytic anemia is directed toward the underlying disease. When there is no solution to the underlying problem, supportive therapy is the only recourse. Careful administration of blood transfusions is often indicated. Associated jaundice may cause pruritus, a source of great discomfort in these patients. Avoiding use of soap and applying calamine lotion to the skin may provide relief.

Hereditary Spherocytosis

Hereditary spherocytosis is a disorder of abnormal hemolysis that is transmitted as an autosomal dominant trait [9]. The disease primarily affects whites of northern European ancestry, but may affect all races. The trait is present at birth, but the disorder usually does not become clinically evident until adulthood.

Although the exact pathogenesis is not known, it is thought that excessive accumulation of sodium in the erythrocytes results in dilatation and eventual rupture of the cells. This increased osmotic fragility causes an abnormal spherical shape of the erythrocytes, in contrast to the normal biconcave shape. In addition, the spleen appears to have an overactive role in direct destruction of the cells or making them susceptible to destruction [25]. An enlarged spleen is very characteristic of the condition, and splenectomy may give permanent improvement.

The severity of the disorder varies. It may be asymptomatic in persons with slight or moderate spherocytosis. Acute crises may occur and may be fatal. The more usual form is a chronic course with mild subicterus and anemia [9]. These persons may develop gallstones as a consequence of the bilirubinemia associated with the disorder.

Sickle Cell Disease

Sickle cell disease is a term used to identify hereditary disorders with clinical and hematologic characteristics related to the presence of abnormal hemoglobin (hemoglobin S) in the erythrocytes. These conditions include homozygous sickle cell anemia, sickle cell–hemoglobin C disease, and sickle cell thalassemia. The latter two are modifications of sickle cell disease, with simultaneous presence of other abnormal hemoglobins. Sickle cell trait is not included within this classification, because it is felt by many authorities that it is technically not a disease. This is because persons who have the sickle cell trait have normal hemoglobin and hematocrit levels, and predominantly normal hemoglobin (hemoglobin A). Consequently, they are usually asymptomatic, unless oxygen tension falls below physiologic levels.

A mutant gene is considered responsible for the synthesis of hemoglobin that is different from normal hemoglobin. In sickle cell anemia, hemoglobin S differs from hemoglobin A in the substitution of one amino acid, valine, for another, glutamic acid, in the beta polypeptide chain. When there is a decrease in oxygen supply, hemoglobin S will not readily dissolve in fluids; long, pointed, rigid, and crystal-like structures form within the cell. It is this process that causes the normally biconcave disks to develop the abnormal crescent shape for which the disease is named.

The abnormal cell is more fragile than the normal cell, so that its life span is shortened to from 26 to 35 days, in contrast to the normal 120 days. The production of new blood cells to replace the sickled cells that are rapidly destroyed may not keep pace with the destruction, resulting in the state of anemia. Mechanical stagnation of the blood in the capillaries tends to occur, contributing to thrombotic formation and vascular occlusion. Extreme pain and swelling, therefore, result from the decreased oxygenation of surrounding tissues and organs. These events lead to the development of sickle cell crisis.

The disease is found predominantly in the black population; however, it has been found among whites, particularly those from the Mediterranean countries. The diagnosis is made on finding sickle cells on peripheral blood smears. Sickle cell slide preparations, sickle-turbidity tube test (Sickledex), and hemoglobin electrophoresis are the other diagnostic examinations utilized. The diagnosis is generally made during the preschool period, although improved screening methods have facilitated earlier diagnosis. Signs observed in infants and children are swelling of the hands and feet, abdominal distention, pallor, jaundice, irritability, and fever. The symptoms may simulate rheumatic fever or appendicitis, so that diagnostic errors may be made unless the examiner is alerted for sickle cell disease. Hepatomegaly, splenomegaly, and cardiac enlargement may also be discovered along with the presenting sign of lowered hemoglobin, generally under 9 gm per cubic milliliter. Hypoxic tissue damage of the spleen, resulting from splenic erythrostasis, causes fibrosis and shrinkage of the spleen, a process that is termed **autosplenectomy.** It is seen in adults with longstanding disease.

There is no known cure for sickle cell anemia. Treatment is supportive and symptomatic; patients and parents are taught preventive measures to avoid situations that predispose to crisis states. In addition to lowered oxygen tension, other events promoting the sickling process include elevated temperatures, lowered pH levels, and increased osmolarity. The potential hazards of riding in unpressurized airplanes and going to high altitudes of lowered oxygen concentration are emphasized. Drugs that cause vasoconstriction, such as some classic cold remedies (for example, ephedrine and other decongestants) should be avoided. Also, special precautions should be taken to avoid infections. Chronic hemolysis may cause a relative deficiency of folate; supplementary folic acid may be necessary. With proper management, life expectancy has been prolonged. Nurses will often see adolescents or young adults in the hospital or clinic situation who have sickle cell anemia but who are being treated for other conditions. The nurse must be aware of special precautions in the care of these persons. For example, when patients with sickle cell anemia are admitted for surgical procedures, the use of medications such as barbiturates may depress the respirations and lead to hypoxia; anesthesia increases the patient's susceptibility to crisis states. Monitoring of blood gases is therefore indicated to prevent respiratory problems, including acidosis. Tachycardia and restlessness are classic signs of hypoxia, while cyanosis may not occur in the patient with sickling until late stages of hypoxia.

Nursing measures should focus on prevention of situations that can cause intravascular sickling. Maintenance of adequate oral intake or the intravenous administration of fluids is essential. Monitoring of vital signs for indications of hypovolemia and hypotension is necessary before initiating treatment. Shock may occur too rapidly in these patients to enable them to be treated successfully. Many persons with sickle cell anemia have cardiomegaly. Although fluid administration is important to combat sickling, fluid overload and pulmonary edema must be prevented. Provision for adequate rest and activities within the tolerance of the individual patient is an essential component of nursing care. These same measures apply when the patient is admitted in a state of sickle cell crisis. In addition, the judicious management of the associated severe pain is essential. Analgesics are necessary, and often narcotics are prescribed. The effect of these drugs on the respiratory status must be carefully evaluated. In patients with pneumonia or pulmonary emboli, exchange transfusions may be required to prevent exacerbation of the sickling process [28]. Generally, therapy of the crisis states has been unsatisfactory and not definitive. Currently, urea and potassium cyanate are being studied as potential agents for combating the sickling process [18, 28].

Because treatment of the crisis states is still unsatisfactory there is greater responsibility for the medical and nursing staffs to identify persons with the disease and to avoid placing them in situations that predispose to crises. Many hospitals now perform routine sickling tests for blacks prior to surgery as a method of preventing complications from general anesthesia. Regardless of the presenting diagnosis, the nurse should be aware of the incidence of the disease. The adult with sickle cell anemia, for example, may complain of aching bones and swollen joints; these may be associated with arthritis, but may also be symptoms of sickle cell disease. Body contour may suggest to the careful examiner the presence of the disease, for adults with sickle cell anemia typically have thin, short trunks and long extremities; kyphosis of the upper back and lordosis of the lower back; a tower-shaped skull; and increased anteroposterior diameters of the chest [10]. Persons who have sickle cell anemia should wear a Medic-Alert identification tag in case of emergency.

The nurse may become involved in counseling prospective parents who either have the trait (that is, they are heterozygous for the gene for sickling) or have sickle cell disease (the homozygous state). Couples should be advised of the risks involved, so that they can make informed decisions about having children. They should be informed of the meaning of the trait versus the presence of the disease and should also realize that sickle cell anemia can incapacitate a person and shorten his life and may be fatal during a medical crisis. Many people have been given much misinformation, which creates unwarranted anxiety. Often persons with the trait have felt that they are unable to have children or that their trait carries a severe personal health hazard.

The following information is used to provide appropriate teaching regarding the transmission of the disease. Two persons with sickle cell anemia may have difficulty producing a child; if they do have children, all will have sickle cell anemia. If one parent has sickle cell anemia and the other parent has normal blood, all the children will have the trait, but none will have sickle cell anemia. If one parent has sickle cell anemia and the other parent has the trait, all the children will have either sickle cell anemia or the trait. If one parent has the sickle cell trait and the other parent has normal blood, the children may have either normal blood or the sickle cell trait, but none will have sickle cell anemia. If both parents have the trait, the child may have normal hemoglobin, the trait, or sickle cell anemia. This usually means that the child has one in four chances of being normal; one chance in four of having sickle cell anemia; and two in four chances of being a carrier.

Sickle cell mass screening programs have been developed in increasing numbers in recent years. The usual mass screening test used for the detection of sickle cell hemoglobin is the sickle-turbidity tube test. This test involves pricking the finger and mixing the blood with Sickledex solution in a test tube. The specimen is observed for cloudiness after 5 minutes. The Sickledex solution becomes turbid in the presence of hemoglobin S, but will remain clear when mixed with normal hemoglobin. The test, however, does not differentiate between sickle cell disease or sickle cell trait, and further follow-up is required.

In order to be successful in disseminating accurate information about the disease and its genetic transmission, screening programs for sickle cell anemia should be integrated into an ongoing health-care and proper counseling setting. (In May 1972 Congress passed the National Sickle Cell Anemia Control Act to provide programs for information, educating, screening, counseling, and treatment.) Vocational guidance should also be available for persons with sickle cell anemia. Information on the management of sickle cell anemia is available from the National Association for Sickle Cell Anemia. Various chapters of the organization are being initiated throughout the country.

Thalassemia

Thalassemia is a type of anemia characterized by an inherited defect in the rate of synthesis of the globin chains (either alpha or beta) in hemoglobin. The name is derived from the Greek *thalassa,* which means sea, because originally the disease was most commonly found in persons from the Mediterranean area. The disease is also found, however, in persons from central Africa, southern Asia, and in American blacks. β-**thalassemia** is much more common than α-**thalassemia.** The disease occurs in two forms, major and minor. β-thalassemia occurs in a homozygous form, known as thalassemia major and also known as Cooley's anemia.

Thalassemia major is characterized by severe microcytic hypochromic anemia, reduced MCV and reduced MCHC. There is marked splenomegaly, marked hepatomegaly, and jaundice. The blood picture is characterized by many stippled target cells (abnormally thin and fragile cells), as well as polychromatic and nucleated erythrocytes [8]. The disorder usually causes abnormal mental and physical development; afflicted children rarely reach adulthood. Treatment is usually supportive, although splenectomy may be done in some cases.

Thalassemia minor is the heterozygous and benign form of the disease. Persons with thalassemia minor are usually asymptomatic; however, mild microcytic and hypochromic anemia may be discovered on a routine blood examination. These persons have a normal life expectancy.

Glucose 6-Phosphate Dehydrogenase Deficiency

Enzyme deficiencies within the erythrocyte cause various types of hemolytic anemia. The most common deficiency is that of **glucose 6-phosphate dehydrogenase** (G-6-PD), an enzyme that has a role in glucose metabolism. This disorder is a sex-linked defect that is primarily found in the black population as well as in persons from the Mediterranean countries.

The disorder is usually asymptomatic until the person is exposed to certain oxidant drugs and foods. These substances include, but are not limited to, drugs such as quinine, aspirin, phenacetin, chloramphenicol, probenecid, sulfonamides, and the thiazide diuretics, and certain foods, particularly fava beans (a broad bean common in Europe). One of the most serious forms of G-6-PD deficiency hemolysis occurs with exposure to fava beans and is termed **favism** [9]. When erythrocytes are exposed to oxidative drugs and foods, increased glucose metabolism is required. A deficiency in G-6-PD prohibits adequate glucose metabolism in these instances and hemolysis occurs. Infections can also cause hemolysis in G-6-PD deficiency. The condition is usually self-limiting, because hemolysis only affects the older erythrocytes, and bone marrow usually replaces the hemolyzed cells fairly readily. Blood transfusions may be required in severe hemolytic episodes. Persons known to be G-6-PD-deficient should avoid substances that are likely to precipitate hemolytic episodes; they should also be protected against serious infections.

Acquired Intracorpuscular Defects

Paroxysmal nocturnal hemoglobinuria (PNH) is an acquired intrinsic abnormality of the erythrocyte (of idiopathic origin) characterized by chronic hemolytic anemia, repetitive nocturnal intravascular hemolysis with morning hemoglobinuria, and a tendency to thrombotic complications [17]. Associated anemia is normocytic and normochromic, but may be hypochromic if sufficient hemoglobin has been lost in the urine to deplete iron stores. In addition to the usual symptoms associated with hemolytic anemia (chronic fatigue, jaundice, splenomegaly), the patient will report the passage of dark urine upon awakening in the morning, a result of the acute hemolytic episodes during sleep.

Patients with PNH may have a relatively benign type or they may have a type that is severely incapacitating. The course of the disease is rather unpredictable and the prognosis is guarded. Treatment is supportive and requires transfusions of erythrocytes during hemolytic states. Transfusions must be given very cautiously, however, because of the danger of further stimulating the hemolytic process. Androgens may be administered to promote erythropoiesis. The major cause of death in patients with PNH is thrombosis; attempts to prevent thrombosis with anticoagulants or infusion of dextran have not been successful.

Other types of paroxysmal hemoglobinuria are less common; they may be related to exposure to cold temperatures (paroxysmal cold hemoglobinuria) or extreme exertion.

Extracorpuscular Factors in Hemolytic Anemia

Infections, certain chemicals, drugs, and immune bodies are extracorpuscular factors that can cause hemolytic anemia. Treatment of hemolysis requires treatment of the underlying cause, as well as treatment to increase erythropoiesis.

Severe infections, such as those caused by the hemolytic streptococci, *Staphylococcus aureus*, and pneumococci, may result in increased hemolysis. Control of the infection is necessary for the control of the hemolysis, which is caused either by the microorganisms or by their toxins. **Malaria** is an infectious disease caused by a protozoan parasite, which is transmitted by the *Anopheles* mosquito. The protozoa are harbored in the human in the blood, where they cause rupturing of the erythrocytes and hemolytic anemia.

Industrial poisons such as benzene, trinitrotoluene (TNT), or aniline have been implicated in hemolytic anemias. Industrial workers may also develop hemolytic anemia from prolonged daily exposure to lead vapors. Lead poisoning (plumbism) also occurs in children who chew on furniture, toys, or wall-peelings covered with lead-base paint or in persons who ingest lead during attempts at suicide. Lead has an inhibiting effect on hemoglobin synthesis, which results in anemia. Erythrocytes become fragile and are readily destroyed as their cell membranes are damaged by lead salt coating. In addition to the hematopoietic effects, lead ingestion may cause neurologic degeneration and gastrointestinal damage.

Diagnosis of anemia caused by lead intoxication is confirmed by identification of lead in the urine, the presence of basophilic stippling, and the presence of the "lead line." This latter sign is the line of discoloration at the dental margins of the gingivae in the mouth. In children, there is increased x-ray density of epiphyseal ends of the bone, caused by deposits of lead. Removal of the lead from the body is hastened by the use of chelating agents such as British anti-Lewisite (BAL) and edetic acid (EDTA) [17]. Educating parents to the danger of their children nibbling on furniture and paint chips is extremely important. (Awareness of the hazards of lead has promoted the passage of protective laws. The Federal Hazardous Substances Act, administered by the Consumer Product Safety Commission, governs the standards on lead content in household paint and for spraying furniture, toys, etc.)

Immune Hemolysis

Erythroblastosis fetalis is the hemolysis of fetal erythrocytes. Fetal erythrocytes that carry a blood group antigen lacking in the mother may cross the placenta and enter the maternal circulation, causing an immune reaction. Antibodies produced by the mother then enter the fetal circulation; they attach to the antigenic site on the surface of the fetal erythrocytes and cause hemolysis [9]. Fetal hemolysis most often is caused by ABO incompatibility; hemolysis related to Rh incompatibility, though less common, is more severe.

Rh incompatibility is rare in a primiparous Rh-negative mother, unless previous sensitization by Rh-positive blood transfusions has occurred. The prognosis for the infant worsens, however, in succeeding pregnancies.

$Rh_o(D)$ immune globulin (RhoGAM) is used to prevent the formation of active antibodies in Rh-negative mothers after delivering an Rh-positive infant or abortion of an Rh-positive fetus. The medication, which is given intramuscularly, must be given within 72 hours after the delivery or abortion.

A Coombs titer is done in early pregnancy to determine whether the mother has been immunized. The test is repeated at later stages of the pregnancy to determine significant rises in the titer, indicating that the fetus is susceptible to hemolytic disease. Rising titers indicate the need for amniocentesis and spectrophotometric analysis of the amniotic fluid to predict the severity of fetal disease and to determine the appropriate intervention. Exchange transfusions are usually indicated.

Early recognition of the disease in the newborn is essential. The newborn may initially appear normal or slightly pale, but within 24 hours may develop jaundice. A severe form of congenital jaundice of the newborn, known as **fetal hydrops,** is associated with congestive heart failure and massive hepatosplenomegaly and hemorrhagic phenomena [9]. **Kernicterus** indicates the central nervous system damage that results from toxic accumulation of unconjugated bilirubin in the brain tissue.

Autoimmune hemolytic anemias result from the presence of an antibody that causes increased erythrocyte destruction. Most often the disorder is spontaneous with no known cause and is known as idiopathic autoimmune hemolytic anemia. It may occur secondary to other diseases, such as malignant lymphomas, ulcerative colitis, and lupus erythematosus. **Lupus erythematosus** is a systemic collagen disease that primarily involves the smaller blood vessels and connective tissue. The blood characteristically contains an abnormal globulin which increases susceptibility to breakdown of the erythrocytes, as well as of the leukocytes and platelets.

Ingestion of drugs such as methyldopa (Aldomet), penicillin, quinidine, and the sulfonamides can result in autoimmune hemolytic anemia. Hemolytic anemia secondary to ingestion of these drugs usually subsides after the drug has been discontinued. The hemolytic anemia will also subside after the primary disease has been controlled. Corticosteroid therapy may be beneficial in certain types of autoimmune hemolytic anemia; splenectomy may be indicated when steroids do not produce a remission.

Other conditions associated with increased hemolysis of erythrocytes include severe thermal injuries. Severely burned patients are predisposed to develop anemia. Mechanical hemolysis may occur associated with disease caused by faulty prosthetic heart valves or abnormal microvasculature. Toxins from snake and spider venoms may cause hemolytic anemia that is usually fatal. Persons exposed to insecticides, arsenic, and coal tar products have also developed hemolytic anemia.

All patients with hemolytic anemia, regardless of the cause, suffer from the classic symptoms of anemia. Hemolytic crises are associated with malaise, chilling, fever, backaches, and hemoglobinuria. The major complication in hemolytic crisis is acute renal failure.

Anemias Caused by Blood Loss

Excessive blood loss results in **normocytic** and **normochromic anemia.** The rate of bleeding, the site of the hemorrhage, and the volume of blood loss all influence the severity of the symptoms. For example, a gradual loss of a large amount of blood allows for some compensatory mechanisms to relieve the symptoms of anemia. The bone marrow becomes hyperactive as the body attempts to replace the lost erythrocytes. A rapid loss, however, can be a life-threatening situation because of the rapid decrease in blood volume. A blood loss of 20 percent or more of the total blood volume requires rapid replacement with whole blood.

Acute hemorrhage results in restlessness; thirst; hypotension; pallor; diaphoresis; a rapid, thready pulse; headache; dizziness; and disorientation. Emergency treatment requires controlling and stopping the hemorrhage, restoring the blood volume, and treating shock. When hemorrhage is uncontrolled, hypotension becomes more severe and shock develops. Death may result from irreversible shock.

After an acute hemorrhage, the severity of the anemia is not readily detectable by laboratory findings, since the total intravascular volume is reduced. Loss of plasma volume may cause a misleading elevation of the red blood cell count and hematocrit until a day or two after the hemorrhagic episode. Reticulocytosis is evident as the bone marrow attempts to replace the loss of erythrocytes. The plasma, when replaced, dilutes the blood and reduces the hematocrit. Blood restoration begins within 4 to 5 days and if there is no further bleeding, the erythrocyte count and hemoglobin return to normal within 4 to 6 weeks. When blood is lost (either in chronic or acute types), the body's store of iron is lost as well, since two-thirds of the body's iron is contained in the hemoglobin. Iron stores depleted during hemorrhage require replenishment with a diet high in protein, iron, and vitamins. Thus, iron supplements may be necessary to bring the hemoglobin concentration back to normal.

Polycythemia

Polycythemia is an excess of erythrocytes, which may be a response to a physiologic need, as in people who exercise excessively or who live at high altitudes with low oxygen pressure, or it may be secondary to pathologic conditions associated with tissue hypoxia, as in chronic lung disease.

When the rate of erythrocyte production becomes much greater than normal, even when there is no apparent physiologic need for the increased production, the condition is termed **polycythemia vera.** The condition is viewed as a neoplastic proliferation of erythroblastic tissues in the bone marrow; normal regulatory mechanisms are unable to control the production. The etiology is unknown. In many ways, polycythemia vera is similar to the leukocytic proliferation characterizing leukemia; it has often terminated in **myelogenous leukemia** [23].

The onset of polycythemia vera is usually insidious and is most frequent during the late middle years. The condition is characterized by an increased erythrocyte mass and an increased hemoglobin content. Erythrocyte counts may rise as high as 8 to 10 million per cubic millimeter. The increase in total blood volume and viscosity impedes the flow of blood throughout the circulatory system. Hypertension often results, and the increased load on the heart results in congestive heart failure. Hyperplasia of all the cellular elements is demonstrated by bone marrow biopsies. The increased platelets and erythrocytes augment viscosity and predispose to formation of venous and arterial thrombi. Intermittent claudication is a frequent finding; coronary thrombosis, cerebral vascular accidents, and gangrene are also associated with the disease.

Patients with polycythemia vera often have symptoms of headache, dizziness, pruritus, fatigue, dyspnea, and lowered heat tolerance. These patients are often recognized by their dusky complexion, and are often described as somewhat cyanotic.

Treatment is centered on decreasing the activity of the bone marrow and on reducing the volume and viscosity of the blood. Radioactive phosphorus may be utilized to depress the bone marrow. Irradiation of the long bones and certain chemotherapeutic drugs such as nitrogen mustard and cyclophosphamide (Cytoxan) can be used to inhibit erythrocyte production. (These drugs are discussed in Chapter 1.) Phlebotomy can be done periodically to reduce blood volume.

These patients are not usually hospitalized for the primary disease, unless complications develop. They are taught to prevent circulatory complications by exercising appropriately within their tolerance levels. Factors enhancing venous stasis are avoided. Glandular meats and foods high in iron are limited in the diet because of existing elevated hemoglobin concentrations. Signs and symptoms of potential complications are emphasized so that the patients will seek early treatment.

Disorders of the Leukocytes

The physiologic basis of the diseases underlying the leukocyte disorders is related to either a deficiency of the normal circulating leukocytes or above-normal levels of circulating leukocytes or their precursors. Disorders may also affect the quality of the leukocytes produced.

Leukopenia is a reduction in the number of leukocytes below the normal values of 5,000 per cubic millimeter. Usually there is a decreased production or excessive destruction of the neutrophil category of leukocytes. This condition is termed **agranulocytosis** or **neutropenia.**

Agranulocytosis is most often the result of toxic effects of certain drugs. The drugs most often implicated are gold salts, sulfonamides, aminopyrine (Pyradone), phenylbutazone, chlorpromazine (Thorazine), and the thiouracil preparations utilized in the treatment of thyroid conditions. The condition may also be associated with miliary tuberculosis, typhoid fever, malaria, uremia, and septicemia. Agranulocytosis is also associated with bone marrow depression that results from radiation and cancer chemotherapy. Benzene exposure also has resulted in agranulocytosis.

Because neutrophils have an important role in defending the body against infection, agranulocytosis always results in a lowered resistance to infection. Overwhelming infections make this condition a potentially fatal one.

Early invasion of the mucous membranes and skin by pathogenic organisms, with development of ulcerations on the mouth and pharynx, is a common initial sign. Lesions may also occur in the rectum and vagina. A sudden onset with chills, fever, and prostration characterizes the condition; respiratory infections are frequent complications.

Diagnosis is based on finding total leukocyte counts as low as 500 to 3,000 per cubic millimeter, with an extreme reduction in the polymorphonuclear cells. Bone marrow examination reveals an absence of polymorphonuclear leukocytes.

To prevent complications of agranulocytosis, the nurse should observe those patients on chemotherapy or other predisposing drugs for signs of infection (sore throat, sore mouth, or fever) and should check the blood count reports regularly for early leukopenia. Antibiotics are given after a blood sample for culture and sensitivity has been drawn. Causative agents of the agranulocytosis are discontinued, and corticosteroids are often indicated. Emergence of infection with resistant organisms frequently complicates the condition, making therapy difficult. Leukocyte transfusions have been used in short-term episodes of neutropenia. (Their use is controversial, however, and they are not readily available in most settings.)

The patient with leukopenia must be protected from further infection. Bed rest is essential. Frequent and thorough mouth care is instituted to prevent oral infections. A high-protein, high-vitamin, and high-caloric diet is indicated. Mouth lesions may be present and interfere with adequate food intake. Protein concentrates and liquids may be more readily taken in these situations.

The patient may be placed in reverse isolation in order to reduce his exposure to infectious organisms. A plastic isolater (life island) or laminar-flow room may be necessary in severe neutropenia (see Chap. 1). Usually, gastrointestinal "sterilization" using antibiotic therapy is also indicated, because many times the infectious process in these patients may be caused by an organism of the person's own normal body flora.

The mucous membranes of the gastrointestinal tract, which are constantly exposed to large numbers of bacteria, are susceptible to invasion by bacteria normally present in the body. Ulcers appear in the mouth and colon; special attention to these areas is therefore required. Mouth care must be meticulously done to remove necrotic exudate from the oral and pharyngeal mucosa by frequent and thorough irrigations with warm normal saline solution. Constipation should be avoided, since hard stools can damage the intestinal and rectal mucosa and cause infection. Stool softeners are usually indicated.

The patient is usually diaphoretic, requiring frequent linen changes, comforting sponge baths, and alcohol sponges to lower elevated temperatures.

Leukemia

Leukemia is a condition of neoplastic proliferation of either leukocyte cells or their precursors, impairing maturation and functional capability [24]. It is a disease of the bone marrow that is reflected by abnormal changes in the blood. Like malignant neoplasms, leukemic cells may occur in various stages of maturity from the most primitive to the almost normal state and may infiltrate other blood-forming organs as well as other vital organs.

Although the specific cause of leukemia is not known, ionizing radiation, viruses, and genetic mutations have all been implicated. The increased incidence of leukemia in radiologists and in survivors of atomic bombings has established its relation to ionizing radiation. Genetic factors have been implicated because of the increased incidence of leukemia in the identical twins of leukemic patients and in persons with Down's syndrome (mongolism) and other congenital conditions. Evidence such as the identification of virus-like particles in human leukemic cells has increasingly implicated the role of viruses in the etiology of leukemia. In addition, certain chemicals, chiefly benzene, and the drugs phenylbutazone and chloramphenicol have also been implicated in the development of leukemia. Certain hematopoietic disorders can terminate in leukemia. Although the cause of this development has not been established, iatrogenic causes have been implicated. For example, terminal leukemia may occur after radioactive phosphorus therapy has been administered in polycythemia vera and after prolonged administration of L-phenylalanine mustard in multiple myeloma.

Leukemia is classified as **acute** or **chronic** and is also categorized by the primary type of cell involved. The two major types of cellular categories are myelogenous and lymphocytic. **Myelogenous leukemia** (also known as granulocytic or myelocytic) is the overgrowth of leukocytes formed in the bone marrow and originating from the myeloblasts. Neutrophils are usually the particular cells involved, although in rare instances, the eosinophils and basophils may be involved [25]. **Lymphocytic leukemia** is the proliferation of leukocytes produced in lymphoid tissue. In most cases, the total leukocyte count is elevated; on occasion, however, the total count may be normal. **Subleukemic** is a term used to identify normal or decreased leukocyte counts with at least some of the circulating cells being abnormal. Diagnosis is confirmed by a bone marrow aspiration or a biopsy that demonstrates abnormal proliferation and abnormal cells. A differential count may identify a predominant type of leukocyte, but in some cases the values may be normal.

Clinical manifestations and the incidence vary according to the type of leukemia. Susceptibility to anemia, hemorrhage, and infection, however, is characteristic of all types of leukemia. Nursing-care measures are therefore oriented primarily to preventing complications related to these three aspects of the disease. These symptoms result from the displacement of bone marrow with reduction in the normal production of erythrocytes, platelets, and leukocytes. Not only does the disease process itself interfere with normal production of these elements, but chemotherapeutic agents also depress bone marrow activity and make the patient vulnerable to complications.

Table 1-5 in Chapter 1 lists the various agents (and their side effects) that are used in cancer chemotherapy. Of these drugs, prednisone, cyclophosphamide, nitrogen mustard, vincristine (Oncovin), L-asparaginase, cytarabine, methotrexate, 6-mercaptopurine, daunomycin, doxorubicin (Adriamycin), procarbazine hydrochloride (Matulane), and chlorambucil (Leukeran) are often used in the treatment of various types of leukemia. Complete remissions (the disappearance of all abnormal cell forms in the bone marrow and peripheral blood) and prolonged survival rates are being accomplished through the use of combinations of specific chemotherapeutic agents according to carefully planned protocols.

Examples of these drug combinations include VAMP, POMP, and COAP. The VAMP protocol utilizes vincristine, Amethopterin, 6-MP, and prednisone. The POMP protocol utilizes prednisone, Oncovin, methotrexate, and 6-MP. The protocol termed COAP includes Cytoxan, Oncovin, Ara-C, and prednisone. These drugs are given on a cyclic schedule, alternating the drugs according to the specified protocols. Management of leukemia also involves the use of supportive therapy to counteract hemorrhage and infection and blood component transfusions to replace deficiencies.

To achieve remissions, the dosages of the chemotherapeutic agents are given to levels of toxicity. The toxic effects cause much physical and psychological discomfort for the patient and the family. Nursing care of patients with leukemia, therefore, emphasizes measures to counteract the effects of drug toxicity and of the disease itself. This places a responsibility on the nurse to be knowledgeable about the anticipated therapeutic effect of the drugs as well as about their toxic effects. Nursing care is directed toward preventing complications related to the side effects of these drugs. For example, proper mouth care will be indicated because ulcerations tend to develop with the use of methotrexate and certain other agents. The use of frequent and gentle mouth care is also indicated because of associated bleeding tendencies that affect the gums. Anorexia, which is a symptom of the diease, is aggravated by chemotherapy and requires much ingenuity on the part of the nurse to devise ways to tempt the patient to eat. A high-caloric and high-vitamin diet is indicated to combat weight loss, weakness, and debilitation. Rapid destruction of normal protein tissues of the body by the leukemic cells, as well as the massive destruction of leukocytes during chemotherapy, results in elevated serum uric acid levels which may lead to obstructive nephropathy. In addition to the administration of allopurinol (Zyloprim) to combat this complication, good hydration and alkalinization of the urine are indicated.

One of the most distressing symptoms of toxicity caused by vincristine (or other agents) is alopecia. Even though patients are forewarned of this event, they become discouraged and anxious when alopecia occurs. Selection of attractive wigs and the assurance that the alopecia is a temporary effect of the drug therapy are measures to counteract this concern. The use of a rubber tourniquet applied to the scalp during and after vincristine administration for a period of 10 minutes has been reported as a measure to limit the extent of alopecia. (This is used to limit the distribution of the agent to the hair follicles.) With the use of vincristine, there are frequent occurrences of numbness and tingling in the fingertips, and loss of fine movements. Unless preventive measures are taken, vincristine may cause neuropathy resulting in foot drop.

The frequent administration of intravenous drugs causes sclerosed veins, which make intravenous administration increasingly difficult for the patient. Rectal temperature should be avoided in persons on methotrexate, which tends to cause rectal fissures that might be traumatized during insertion of the thermometer. There are many other symptoms for which the nurse should watch when patients are receiving chemotherapeutic drugs. As patients are being treated increasingly on outpatient regimens, the nurse has the added responsibility of teaching both patients and family about the specific toxic effects of each of the agents. On each visit to the treatment center, the patient should be examined for the presence of any infections, ulcerations, and hemorrhagic tendencies. Any lesion, no matter how small, should be noted and treated because it is a potential infection site for the susceptible leukemic patient.

The diagnosis of leukemia is a shocking one for a patient of any age and for the family. Treatment and management emphasize support of the patient and family in the emotional impact of the diagnosis and the prolonged, expensive, and intensive treatment regimens. The course of the illness, despite aggressive treatment, often is one of irregular periods of relapses and remissions, with an eventual fatal outcome. The major goal of medical and nursing therapy is related to providing as long and as normal a life as possible. For this reason, management of patients on an outpatient basis during most phases of the disease is generally preferred in lieu of frequent hospitalizations for treatment regimens. Teaching about the disease and the required treatment, particularly the specifics of chemotherapy, is an essential element of the nursing care of leukemic patients and requires a thorough understanding of the various types of leukemia and the specific therapy for each.

Acute leukemia includes those types in which the affected cells are predominantly immature (the blast forms of the respective type of cells) or poorly differentiated. When cells are so immature that classification is not possible, these cases are designated as **stem cell leukemia**. Acute leukemias include **acute lymphocytic leukemia** (ALL), which is predominantly a disease of childhood (peak ages from 3 to 4 years), and **acute myelogenous leukemia** (AML), which is seen in nearly equal frequency at all ages.

ALL is the most common type of malignant condition that occurs in children. Clinical symptoms are primarily malaise, fever, lymphadenopathy, and gingival, cutaneous, and nasal bleeding. Osseous and articular symptoms are more frequently found in ALL than in other forms of leukemia [19]. The presence of blast cells is almost always detectable in the blood of children with ALL, which is confirmed by the finding of bone marrow replaced by lymphoblasts. When the child is diagnosed as having ALL, induction therapy is started to achieve eradication of all leukemic blast cells, rendering the patient free of the disease (a state of remission). It is assumed that such induction will then allow regrowth of the normal hematopoietic cells that were suppressed by the leukemic activity.

Induction involves the use of combinations of the chemotherapeutic drugs mentioned previously. Combination therapy is preferred to using a single drug, in order to limit the toxicity of individual drugs as well as to assure destruction of cells sensitive to various agents. The difficulty in determining exactly when all the leukemic cells are destroyed contributes to the development of levels of toxicity that damage normal tissues. A "tolerable" level of toxicity is therefore often the criterion for limitation of the induction phase. The patient and family should be forewarned of the toxic effects that are likely to occur with the various drugs.

Once remission has been achieved, maintenance therapy is initiated, often with drugs different from those used in the induction phase. A considerable number of children with ALL develop meningeal infiltration, so that intrathecal administration of chemotherapeutic drugs is frequently indicated. (This procedure was described in Chapter 1.) Systemic administration of the drugs does not permit perfusion beyond the blood-brain barrier. It is felt that minute or occult foci of the disease are present even at the time of diagnosis, so that treatment of the meninges is necessary early in the course of therapy [5]. Chemical arachnoiditis may occur, and it results in severe headache, nausea and vomiting, and fever. In intrathecal administration, usually a volume of cerebrospinal fluid equal to the amount of drug to be administered is removed to reduce the incidence of chemical arachnoiditis.

Even during the periods of remission, the child is susceptible to infections. Constant vigilance is necessary to avoid the patient's exposure to infections. When infections are present, antibiotic therapy is initiated. Supportive therapy such as blood, platelet, and leukocyte transfusions may be indicated during various stages of the disease and therapeutic regimen. Bone marrow transplants may be done. Bone marrow transplantation is the intravenous administration of bone marrow which has been surgically removed via multiple aspirations of the iliac crest of a donor with proved histocompatibility. Immunization therapy with the BCG vaccine is also being studied.

With remission induction, most of these children will have about 3 years of near-normal health; however, even during the periods when the child is able to attend school and lead a fairly normal life, monthly examinations and close observation for recurrence of the disease are essential. Therefore, even during remission, there is an ever-present threat of recurrence, which is a burden for both the child and parents.

In AML, clinical symptoms are related to the effects of the reduction or absence of normal hematopoietic cells. This type of leukemia primarily affects young adults. Classic symptoms of anemia are present. The presence of thrombocytopenia is evidenced by petechiae, purpura, epistaxis, gingival bleeding, gastrointestinal bleeding, or urinary tract bleeding. The onset of symptoms may be very abrupt, but most patients have a prodromal period of 1 to 6 months [19]. Total leukocyte counts can be low, normal, or markedly elevated. Peripheral blood smears demonstrate the presence of increased percentages of myeloblasts. The presence of Auer rods, which are rod-like azure cytoplasmic inclusions, is helpful in differentiating AML from ALL [19]. Hyperuricemia is also a common finding in AML, as in ALL, because of the rapid turnover of nucleoprotein.

Intensive therapy is indicated to suppress leukemic proliferation to allow return of normal hematopoiesis. The resultant bone marrow depression during therapy, therefore, requires a protective environment (to limit exposure to infections) and the administration of appropriate transfusions. Often, protection against the patient's own flora is required; antibiotics such as neomycin are used for gastrointestinal sterilization. Chemotherapy utilizes protocols that include cytosine, arabinoside, mercaptopurine, thioguanine, and antibiotics such as daunomycin. Adjuvant drugs include methotrexate and cyclophosphamide. Death in AML is usually caused by overwhelming infections. Use of intensive therapy, however, has increased the median survival of 2 months to 13 months [19]. The survival rate in acute leukemia has also been lengthened by the use of platelet transfusions to counteract the bleeding episodes related to thrombocytopenia. To prevent autosensitization and refractoriness to platelet therapy, transfusions of platelets from HL-A matched donors are utilized. In some settings, frequent transfusions of platelets (2 to 3 times weekly) are given to maintain the level above 20,000 per cubic millimeter to prevent serious hemorrhage [1]. In other settings the platelet count is not used for determining the need for transfusions, but rather platelets are given according to clinical symptoms, because not all patients with low platelet counts bleed. In addition, fresh-frozen plasma transfusions are required by patients with liver involvement to provide clotting factors normally synthesized in the liver.

In **chronic myelogenous leukemia** (CML), the onset is usually insidious, with symptoms of malaise, fatigue, sweating, and heat intolerance. Abdominal discomfort is a frequent symptom and is generally related to splenomegaly, which is a frequent finding in CML. The disease is rarely encountered in persons under the age of 20. Leukocytosis can reach levels above 300,000; mature forms of the granulocytes are the predominant cells.

X-ray therapy, either with total irradiation or splenic irradiation, has been utilized. Radioactive phosphorus has also been utilized in CML. The use of busulfan (Myleran), an oral alkylating agent, is the current drug of choice in CML [19]. Busulfan can cause serious side effects of marrow aplasia, pulmonary fibrosis, and skin hyperpigmentation, however. It is generally felt that rapid, intensive treatment is rarely warranted, but new treatment modalities to determine the effects of early splenectomy and intensive treatment are being studied. Eventually, patients with CML have an alteration in the course of the disease, with increased anemia and thrombocytopenia and increased numbers of immature cells. These patients then respond poorly to busulfan and enter the terminal phase of the disease.

Chronic lymphocytic leukemia (CLL) generally has an insidious onset and often is diagnosed incidentally during routine laboratory examinations. It occurs most often in persons 50 to 70 years of age. Although many patients with CLL are asymptomatic at diagnosis, others present with classic signs of anemia, weight loss, abdominal discomfort with hepatomegaly and/or splenomegaly, and palpable lymph nodes. Lymphocytosis is present with counts above 10,000 per cubic millimeter and over 100,000 per cubic millimeter in 25 percent of the patients [19]. CLL is similar to lymphosarcoma, and errors in diagnosis have been made. Median survival is approximately 7 years after the diagnosis has been made. Drugs that are used in CLL include chlorambucil or cyclophosphamide as well as glucocorticoid steroids. Rubin and others, however, feel that premature exposure to cytotoxic agents and corticosteroids can aggravate and even induce complications by compounding the immunologic deficiencies [26]. Splenectomy may be indicated in certain cases. Leukapheresis is used in some settings; and extracorporeal irradiation and total body irradiation in CLL are also being studied. Lichtman states that "although lymphocytic accumulation can be controlled, death is often related to recurrent infections due in part to the acquired immune deficiencies that are not improved by therapy" [19].

Regardless of the type of leukemia, the patient is always fearful and anxious about the disease and the therapy, as well as the outcome. Schumann and Patterson [27] recommend an environment of hopefulness to help direct the patient's energy toward adapting to the situation. They also acknowledge that the redefining of hope is a continuous process that changes as the possibilities of recovery are reduced. This means that initially the person may hope for a cure, but if and when relapses occur, the person then hopes for another remission. When relapses occur with increased pain and discomfort, the person then redefines hope for periods of comfort and freedom from pain. The importance of listening to the patient as he works through this adaptive process cannot be overemphasized. The supportive role of the nurse during these periods is critical.

Hodgkin's Disease

Disorders affecting the lymphoreticular system include the malignant lymphomas and nonmalignant infectious mononucleosis. The malignant lymphomas are often classified under six categories: (1) lymphocytic, well-differentiated, also known as lymphosarcoma; (2) lymphocytic, poorly differentiated, also known as lymphosarcoma or lymphoblastic; (3) stem cell (including Burkitt's lymphoma), known as reticulum cell sarcoma; (4) histiocytic, also known as reticulum cell sarcoma; (5) mixed (histiolymphocytic); and (6) Hodgkin's [2]. Hodgkin's disease, which is the most common of the malignant lymphomas, will be discussed first. Hodgkin's disease has some unique clinical features, so that it is advantageous to discuss it separately.

Hodgkin's disease, one of the primary lymph node diseases, is characterized by enlarged lymph nodes. Occurring more often in men than in women, the disease is most often found in persons between the ages of 20 and 40. The fact that it primarily affects young adults is probably the reason the disease creates so much public interest.

The etiology of Hodgkin's disease is not definitely known, although viral, neoplastic, environmental, genetic, and immunologic causes have been implicated. A particular epidemiologic study received considerable publicity when it suggested an infectious etiology. This study was based on finding an increased incidence of Hodgkin's disease in certain groups with moderately close contact, but it has been considered nonconclusive [32].

The condition generally has an insidious onset, manifested by painless and progressive enlargement of lymph nodes and lymphoid tissue. The most common initial site is in the upper half of the body, particularly the cervical lymph nodes. The disease usually spreads in a contiguous manner, affecting the adjacent lymph node tissue. Although some patients present with generalized disease at diagnosis, involvement of retroperitoneal nodes, the liver, spleen, or the bone occurs later in the disease process in the majority of cases.

Fever, night sweats, weight loss, malaise, and pruritus are other symptoms that may be associated with the disease. Pruritus is an unexplained symptom. Generalized itching may be severe and only partially relieved by the use of antihistamine drugs. The pruritus usually disappears, however, when treatment is initiated. Another interesting symptom is the occurrence of nodal pain on ingestion of alcohol; the etiology of this relationship is not known either.

The disease may spread to other lymphoid tissues throughout the body, and other organs may be affected either by infiltration or by pressure from adjacent enlarged nodes. For example, dyspnea, cough, and dysphagia may occur when mediastinal lymphadenopathy is present. Ascites and edema of the lower extremities may occur with inferior vena cava obstruction related to intraabdominal lymph node enlargement.

The diagnosis is established by excision and biopsy of an enlarged lymph node with identification of the Reed-Sternberg cells, (large atypical cells with distinctive enlarged dark nuclei). (Although Reed-Sternberg cells are diagnostic, they are not always present.) The pathologic determination must be carefully done to differentiate the cells accurately from those of infectious mononucleosis, which causes similar histologic changes and symptoms. Phenytoin (Dilantin) therapy has also been known to cause similar histologic changes. Four histologic patterns are associated with the Reed-Sternberg findings in Hodgkin's disease and usually help clarify the diagnosis. (These patterns include lymphocyte predominance, mixed cellularity, lymphocyte depletion, and nodular sclerosis.)

Persons who have painless enlargement of lymph nodes as their only symptom are usually quite shocked when the diagnosis of Hodgkin's disease is made. The role of the nurse is to support the patient during this period, clarifying what the diagnosis means to the patient, and allowing the patient to express any fears he may have. Clear explanations of the intent of therapy and the anticipated effects must be made in order to gain the patient's understanding and cooperation. With more generalized symptoms, supportive therapy is necessary and the patient must be protected from becoming overly tired.

In 1971 the Ann Arbor Symposium on Staging in Hodgkin's disease recommended the following system of pathologic and clinical staging to facilitate universal communication, exchange information, appropriate therapy, and determination of the prognosis [6]. The system is currently used as the basis for describing the status of the disease. Clinical staging is based on information from the history, physical examination, laboratory tests, and x-rays. The pathologic staging is dependent upon surgical biopsy of the bone marrow, the spleen, liver, and additional lymph nodes obtained by abdominal staging laparotomy.

Stage I Involvement of a single lymph node region (I) or a single extralymphatic organ or site (I_E).

Stage II Involvement of two or more lymph node regions on the same side of the diaphragm (II) or localized involvement of extralymphatic organ or site and of one or more lymph node regions on the same side of the diaphragm (II_E).

Stage III Involvement of lymph node regions on both sides of the diaphragm (III) which may also be accompanied by localized involvement of extralymphatic organ or site (III_E) or by involvement of the spleen (III_S) or both (III_{SE}).

Stage IV Diffuse or disseminated involvement of one or more extralymphatic organs or tissues with or without associated lymph node enlargement. The involved extralymphatic site should be identified by symbols used for pathologic staging: H+ for liver, L+ for lung, M+ for marrow, P+ for pleural, O+ for osseous, and D+ for skin [6].

Each stage is divided into A and B categories: A for those without certain general symptoms and B for those with general symptoms of (1) unexplained weight loss of more than 10 percent of the body weight in the 6 months prior to admission; (2) unexplained fever with temperatures above 38° C (100°F); or (3) night sweats. The single symptom of pruritus no longer qualifies for B classification [6].

The most important step in the diagnostic and staging procedure is a thorough history and physical examination of the patient, noting all palpable lymph nodes and pertinent constitutional symptoms. A routine blood count, hemoglobin and hematocrit, leukocyte count, differential, and an erythrocyte sedimentation rate are indicated. The erythrocyte sedimentation rate has been found to be a reliable and inexpensive indicator supporting the presence of Hodgkin's disease. Most of the laboratory tests, however, are nonspecific. Liver function tests, including serum alkaline phosphatase levels, a blood urea nitrogen (BUN) level, and urinalysis are indicated to determine the extent of the disease and to help differentiate the diagnosis from other diseases. Liver, bone, and spleen scans are also often indicated.

Posteroanterior and lateral chest x-rays are indicated to evaluate the status of the mediastinal-hilar lymph nodes. Intravenous pyelograms are indicated to determine renal function and abnormalities related to adjunct lymph node disease. Bone marrow biopsy may be done routinely in some settings, or it may be done only on patients with very abnormal blood profiles or with extensive disease.

Lymphangiography and inferior venacavagram are procedures that are done to determine involvement of retroperitoneal lymph nodes, since these are not accessible for palpation. **Lymphangiography** involves the injection of a dye solution intradermally in the first interdigital space in each foot. When the lymphatic vessels can be visualized, a vessel in each foot is cannulated, and radiopaque contrast material is injected. Patients must be instructed to lie very still during the procedure so that the needles are not displaced. Films are taken of the abdomen and chest immediately and during the next 48 hours at intervals. The dye remains in the system for several months and is slowly eliminated through the kidneys. Patients should be forewarned that their urine will turn blue for several weeks after the test. Because there is a danger of embolization of the oily medium in this procedure, only a small volume is used.

Venacavagraphy is done about 24 to 48 hours after lymphangiography, when retroperitoneal lymph nodes are filled with the soluble oil from the previous test. This procedure makes it possible to visualize the right iliac vein, inferior vena cava, and the ureters. A radiopaque dye is injected into the right femoral vein, and posteroanterior and lateral films of the abdomen are taken immediately and at intervals over a period of 30 minutes.

The **staging laparotomy** is indicated for all stages except stage IV, when it can be diagnosed histologically without laparotomy. Although some authorities do not emphasize laparotomies as part of the staging process, others emphasize the necessity of laparotomy to determine the presence of unsuspected stage III or stage IV disease. These latter authorities, therefore, do routine laparotomy staging except where surgical risks contraindicate the use or if the findings would not change the course of treatment.

Diagnostic laparotomy has made possible the histopathologic verification of retroperitoneal Hodgkin's disease that is demonstrated radiographically. It is felt by some authorities that removal of the spleen at laparotomy is important to avoid unnecessary radiation to the lower left lung and portions of the left kidney, which might occur if the spleen were to be radiated later. It is also felt that splenectomy increases hematopoietic tolerance to radiotherapy and perhaps to chemotherapy. This is in contrast to other authorities who feel that a splenectomy is not always indicated because of the possibility of severe bacterial infections postsplenectomy.

Liver involvement is difficult to assess, even with the diagnostic laparotomy, and therefore it is felt that liver biopsies have been only somewhat helpful in evaluating Hodgkin's disease of the liver. There is a possibility however, that liver involvement can be predicted when the presence of splenic involvement is confirmed.

Biopsies of the liver and of various nodes that appear to be involved are taken during the laparotomy. Metal clips are customarily used to mark the sites of biopsy specimens and the apparent boundaries of the disease to enable x-ray evaluation of the treatment.

In the young female, ovarian transposition (ovariopexy) may be done during the exploratory laparotomy when follow-up radiation therapy of abdominal lymph nodes is deemed necessary. Ovariopexy is done to move the ovaries from the direct line of subsequent irradiation of the pelvic lymph nodes in the hope of minimizing radiation damage to the ovaries. There is a risk, however, of temporary or permanent sterility despite the preventive surgery or shielding of the gonads during therapy.

The young adult is frequently concerned about the effect of Hodgkin's disease on fertility and pregnancy. There is no known effect of the disease on these; however, treatment does affect fertility and pregnancy. Spontaneous abortion or delivery of stillborns is the usual reaction of persons undergoing therapy for Hodgkin's disease.

After staging has been determined, treatment and prognosis can be more specifically determined. Excellent prognosis is usually given to those with stage I or stage II disease. Although complete remission has been known for some persons with stage IV, the prognosis is generally less favorable.

It is widely believed that adequate radiotherapy delivered to all sites of the disease can cure most persons with Hodgkin's disease. Use of supervoltage radiation techniques is necessary, however, to provide effective therapy. Persons with stages IA, IB, IIA, IIB, and IIIA are usually treated with intent to cure.

For patients with Hodgkin's disease, there are generally two approaches to treatment with radiotherapy. Some authorities advise total lymphoid (including the spleen) radiation. This procedure implies radiation to all lymph-node-bearing areas from the mastoids to the femoral triangles, to make certain that both the obvious and occult nodal disease is destroyed for patients with stage I, II, or III disease. Other authorities, who feel that Hodgkin's disease usually is unifocal in origin and then spreads in an orderly manner to contiguous lymphatic sites, do not feel that total lymphatic irradiation is necessary. They believe in the use of the staging procedure to determine that the disease is still localized; then they use radiation to treat only the locally involved areas.

The treatment approach to stage IIIB is still controversial. Some authorities use intensive total nodal radiotherapy, whereas others substitute or add combination chemotherapy. Intensive radiotherapy, however, does not prove beneficial to patients with stage IV disease and in fact may hamper the individual's tolerance to necessary chemotherapy. This is why lymphangiography and the staging laparotomy are considered necessary to determine the presence of undetected stage III or IV disease. Treatment with a systemic combination chemotherapy such as the MOPP program is usually the choice for stage IV disease. The MOPP protocol uses Mustargen (nitrogen mustard), Oncovin (vincristine), procarbazine hydrochloride (Matulane), and prednisone administered on a set schedule and set cycles.

Although Hodgkin's disease has been thought of as a fatal disease, this grave picture has changed to a great degree within the last few years. With early diagnosis and appropriate and aggressive treatment, the majority of patients with localized disease can now be cured. It is important therefore for the nurse to understand the significance of staging, which determines the treatment as well as the prognosis for the given patient. A fatalistic attitude is inappropriate for the patient who has stage I or stage II disease and is seeking reassurance that the extensive therapy he is undergoing is the correct approach. The nurse can also be supportive during the period when the patient becomes reconciled to the need for a staging laparotomy, which may be difficult to understand.

Even with stages I and II of the disease, however, patients will be exposed to the effects of aggressive therapy measures that may cause side effects of nausea, vomiting, and fatigue as well as other personal discomfort and loss of free time. At this point, nurses must be very supportive and emphasize the potential for cure in these early stages. Too often nurses themselves have a fatalistic attitude about Hodgkin's disease, regardless of the stage, and they may reflect this attitude to the patient. An understanding of the implications of staging for a particular individual and a particular response to therapy are the important factors for each nurse to consider. Thus, all patients with Hodgkin's disease should not all be viewed in the same manner or with the same prognosis.

Therapy is often administered on an outpatient basis, so prolonged hospitalization is not necessary. Radiation therapy and chemotherapy cause symptoms that often make the patient feel that the treatment is worse than the disease. Measures must be instituted to limit the side effects of these drugs. For example, nausea and vomiting associated with nitrogen mustard therapy are controlled with antiemetics; alopecia associated with vincristine is anticipated and is temporarily handled with the use of wigs until treatment is discontinued and the alopecia ceases; antacid therapy may be indicated to control the gastric symptoms that may occur with the administration of prednisone.

Pneumocystis carinii pneumonia may occur in patients on long-term chemotherapy. The condition is a protozoal infection in severely immunosuppressed patients and is diagnosed by open lung biopsy. Nursing care is directed toward providing respiratory support for patients with this complication.

The patient with Hodgkin's disease who is on chemotherapy is susceptible to herpes zoster and other monilial infections. Examination of the mouth and skin is essential each time the nurse assesses the patient who is receiving chemotherapy.

The therapeutic phase of Hodgkin's disease can be traumatic and discouraging, but when it results in a cure or a remission, it is successful in terms of helping the patient to lead a normal life again. The patient with Hodgkin's disease requires medical follow-up, especially in the first years following the diagnosis and initial treatment. He or she will be advised to notify the physician of any signs of recurrence of clinical signs or symptoms. Consequently, even though he is in a stage of remission, the patient fears the recurrence of the disease. If and when a relapse occurs, the patient is extremely discouraged and fearful, knowing that his prognosis is poor, as the disease is obviously spreading. The need for emotional support from understanding nurses cannot be overemphasized during these periods.

Non-Hodgkin's Lymphomas

The non-Hodgkin's lymphomas represent a spectrum of lymphoproliferative disorders that range from well-differentiated lymphocytic to more malignant, poorly differentiated, and histiocytic varieties. Proliferation of primitive reticuloendothelial cells, histiocytes, and lymphocytes is characteristic of the involved lymph nodes. The well-differentiated lymphocytic type is usually seen in older patients. The undifferentiated features are characteristic of Burkitt's lymphoma, a type of lymphoma that occurs most frequently in children in certain low, humid parts of Africa. The Burkitt's tumor has been closely linked to a viral etiology; a herpes-like virus has been implicated.

Lymphosarcoma is a malignant tumor of lymphoid tissue, characterized by a proliferation of lymphocytes. Lymphosarcoma has often been used as a general term to include all non-Hodgkin's lymphoma. The term **lymphoma,** however, is more appropriate for general use. In contrast to Hodgkin's disease, lymphosarcoma has a peak incidence after the age of 50. It is similar to Hodgkin's disease in that males are affected more frequently.

The symptoms of the non-Hodgkin's lymphomas are similar to Hodgkin's disease. There is an earlier tendency for widespread disease in the former group, however. There is earlier involvement of oropharyngeal lymphoid tissue, the skin, the gastrointestinal tract, and the bone. Eventually, lymphomas invade the bone marrow; it is sometimes difficult to distinguish between lymphosarcoma and chronic lymphocytic leukemia because the disease processes closely resemble each other.

The diagnostic procedures are similar to those used in Hodgkin's disease. Evaluation of the disease requires obtaining a specific diagnosis by biopsy and establishing the anatomic extent of the disease. Localized disease is less common among these patients, so that laparotomy for diagnostic purposes is a less frequent procedure in cases of non-Hodgkin's lymphoma.

In the staging of lymphomas, the method is the same as that used for Hodgkin's disease. Patients with clinical stages I and II disease, however, more often have positive lymphangiograms. Dissemination of the disease is more often seen at diagnosis, and extension of the disease by widespread dissemination (rather than by contiguous lymph nodes) is more common in non-Hodgkin's lymphoma.

Radiotherapy is the treatment of choice in early stages. Combination chemotherapy utilizing cyclophosphamide, vincristine, and prednisone is currently the most effective treatment [3]. Total body irradiation may be effective in controlling stage IV disease if marrow invasion is the only extranodal site. Cyclophosphamide has proved to be an effective single agent in the treatment of Burkitt's tumor. Localized gastrointestinal involvement is treated by surgical excision.

The prognosis depends on the stage of the disease at the time of discovery and the type of treatment initiated. The course of the disease, unless cure has been attained in early localized disease, is generally one of remissions and exacerbations leading to a fatal outcome. The importance of early detection and treatment therefore cannot be overemphasized.

Infectious Mononucleosis

Infectious mononucleosis is a benign disease of probable viral etiology and linked to the Epstein-Barr virus (EBV) of the herpes group. It is primarily found in adolescents and young adults between the ages of 15 and 24. The disease is spread through close personal contact. Outbreaks of the disease are frequently reported on college campuses, and kissing has been implicated as a means of transmission of the disease. Presenting subjective signs include sore throat, headache, and malaise associated with fever ordinarily under 40° C (104° F) and lymphadenopathy. The lymphadenopathy is generally of a bilateral and nontender nature, affecting the cervical nodes primarily. Other physical signs include eyelid edema and palatal enanthema (round, sharply circumscribed red spots found on the roof of the mouth), pharyngitis, and tonsillar exudate. Varying degrees of splenomegaly and transient impairment of liver function also occur.

The diagnosis is based on the clinical, hematologic, and serologic findings. Hematologic signs include the presence of atypical lymphocytes and the presence of lymphocytosis usually peaking 12 to 18 days after onset. Histology may resemble lymphocytic leukemia and requires differentiation. In fact, there are similar clinical aspects of infectious mononucleosis and the lymphoproliferative disorders. The fear of a diagnosis of leukemia may be present in patients who have a prolonged course of the disease.

Serologic findings include a positive Paul-Bunnell heterophil agglutination test. Characteristic heterophil antibodies can almost always be demonstrated in the second and third weeks after onset of the illness. Heterophil antibodies in the serum are capable of agglutinating sheep erythrocytes. A heterophil titer of 1:56 or greater supports a diagnosis of infectious mononucleosis. A biologic false positive VDRL (Venereal Disease Research Laboratories) test for syphilis may also be present in infectious mononucleosis.

Treatment is symptomatic, with bed rest indicated until the temperature returns to normal. Throat gargles and the use of aspirin usually relieve the symptoms of sore throat. A high-caloric, high-protein, and high-vitamin diet is indicated, although anorexia may be present. The course of the disease is usually limited to 2 to 3 weeks, but convalescence varies and may require several months. Fatigue prevails for a period of time and necessitates gradual return to previous activities. Although conservative treatment is the routine, small doses of corticosteroids may be utilized when the course begins to worsen or if the natural course of the disease is prolonged or severe. The period of communicability lasts from some time prior to the onset of symptoms until fever and sore throat cease.

Complications of infectious mononucleosis are not common; however, hemolytic streptococcal pharyngitis may occur, and infiltration of the atypical mononuclear cells into various organs may result in hepatitis and neuropathies. Rarely, splenic rupture with hemorrhage results in death.

Multiple Myeloma

A neoplastic proliferation of plasma cells characterizes this primary malignant tumor of the bone marrow. It occurs most commonly in persons over 50 years of age and more often in men. Normal plasma cells produce the globulins associated with immune mechanisms of the body (antibody production), but myeloma produces an abnormal plasma protein that may be detected in the blood and in the urine. Back pain or chronic fatigue associated with normochromic, normocytic anemia may be the presenting symptom. Progressive development of bone pain is the usual pattern of the disease process. Metastasis may occur in extraosseous sites such as the spleen, liver, or lymph nodes.

The disease is diagnosed by detecting the Bence Jones protein in the urine. (The Bence Jones protein is a low molecular weight protein found in many patients with multiple myeloma.) X-rays reveal the sharply punched-out areas of bone destruction that result from the expanding mass of plasma cells in the underlying marrow. Osteolytic lesions are most often observed in the skull, spine, ribs, and pelvis and may be located in any part of the skeletal system. Bone scans using radioactive strontium are used to detect the disease even before bone erosions are detected by x-ray. Bone marrow biopsies demonstrate the presence of abnormal plasma cells.

With increased deposits of plasma cells in the bone marrow, pain becomes constant and agonizing, predominantly in the ribs, sternum, and skull. The inability to produce normal gamma globulins increases the susceptibility to bacterial infections; coagulation defects result in bleeding tendencies.

Renal insufficiency may result from the effects of the Bence Jones proteinuria, as well as of the associated pyelonephritis and hypercalcemia. Hypercalcemia results from excessive bone destruction with excretion of excessive amounts of calcium in the urine. Adequate hydration, diuretics, corticosteroids, and oral phosphates are measures used to counteract effects of hypercalcemia. Mobilization prevents further bone resorption, so maintaining mobility as long as is feasible is an important aspect of nursing care of these patients.

Treatment consists in radiation and chemotherapy to relieve local painful lesions. Chemotherapy generally includes the use of alkylating drugs alone or in combination with prednisone. L-phenylalanine mustard (melphalan, Alkeran) and cyclophosphamide, used in intermittent high-dose courses, are often used in the treatment of multiple myeloma. When these drugs are given, observation for bone marrow depression is an essential component of medical and nursing management. There have been reports of some patients with multiple myeloma who eventually developed acute granulocytic or lymphocytic leukemia as a result of an iatrogenic cause such as treatment with L-phenylalanine mustard.

The prognosis is poor. These patients are prone to infections, particularly pneumonia. Care in the late stages, when every movement becomes painful and difficult, is centered on keeping the patient as comfortable as possible. Analgesics are necessary for pain relief. Blood transfusions may be required. Extreme caution in preventing falls and possible fractures of affected bones is an important component of the nursing care. Pain and pathologic fractures can be caused by improper handling during transfers, but may occur in debilitated patients despite extreme care. The spinal cord may become compressed because of perforation of osseous tissue, leading to paralysis unless surgical decompression by laminectomy or irradiation is accomplished.

Other plasma cell dyscrasias include Waldenstrom's macroglobulinemia and amyloidosis. **Waldenstrom's macroglobulinemia** is a relatively rare disorder associated with uncontrolled proliferation of lymphocytoid cells. These cells are intermediate between lymphocytes and plasma cells. Other symptoms, the prognosis, and treatment are similar to that of multiple myeloma. Cardiovascular and neurologic symptoms are related to serum hyperviscosity.

Amyloidosis is a rare disorder characterized by accumulation of a protein-polysaccharide substance in nearly all tissues of the body. Bone marrow plasmacytosis is frequently found in these patients. Symptoms vary according to the organ most severely involved such as cardiomegaly and congestive heart failure with cardiovascular involvement and the nephrotic syndrome with renal involvement. Patients usually experience weakness, anorexia, and weight loss. Amyloidosis is usually associated with a chronic inflammatory disease or an overt platelet cell dyscrasia and is a progressive disease that usually terminates in death from cardiac or renal failure.

Disorders of the Spleen

The precise function of the spleen remains obscure. In embryonic life, the spleen participates in blood formation; in the adult, extramedullary hematopoiesis is an abnormal state that may be associated with bone marrow depression. The spleen's function in the destruction of aged erythrocytes has been described. Its function in producing lymphocytes, plasma cells, and antibodies is in conjunction with other tissues that have a similar function. The spleen is the primary source of antibody production in the infant and small child, however.

The normal spleen (150 gm) is not palpable and must be enlarged to about 500 gm before it can be felt under the left costal border. Diseases affecting the spleen generally cause some enlargement of varying degrees. The spleen is often enlarged in Hodgkin's disease, lymphoma, leukemia, metastatic neoplasms, portal hypertension, and in certain acute infections. Structural changes other than enlargement may occur including cystic development or atrophy of the spleen, as found in late stages of sickle cell anemia.

The spleen is not an essential organ since many or perhaps all its activities are carried out by other organs also. Splenectomy usually is followed by mild but persistent leukocytosis and thrombocytosis. Thrombocytosis may predispose the patient to thrombus formation postoperatively. To prevent thrombus complications, bed exercises, early ambulation, and adequate hydration are therefore particularly important after splenectomy. A frequent complication postsplenectomy is pneumonia and atelectasis, caused by the reduced expansion of the left lung and related to the close location of the spleen to the diaphragm. Therefore, deep breathing and turning are particularly important nursing measures in preventing respiratory complications after splenectomy. For children, it is felt by most hematologists and pediatricians that splenectomy should be deferred until after the age of 6 to 8 years, so that the child's immune status is not compromised. (Splenectomy may increase the frequency and seriousness of infectious diseases in children.) The value of splenectomy is determined carefully in individual cases in children under the ages of 6 to 8 years.

Rupture of the spleen, complicated by hemorrhage, usually resulting from traumatic accidents, is the most frequent indication for splenectomy. Splenectomy may also be indicated in hypersplenism, particularly to treat hereditary spherocytosis. Splenectomy is also beneficial in some cases of idiopathic uncontrolled acute hemorrhagic thrombocytopenic purpura. Splenectomy may be done during the staging laparotomies for Hodgkin's disease and lymphoma; it has been found that the tolerance to subsequent x-ray and chemotherapy is increased after splenectomy. Splenectomy is also done before renal transplantation, in order to reduce the likelihood of host rejection of the transplanted kidney.

Disorders of Hemostasis

Hemostasis is the process of preventing blood loss whenever a blood vessel is ruptured or severed. The hemostatic mechanisms include local vasoconstriction, formation of a platelet aggregate, formation of a clot, and eventual formation of scar tissue.

When a vessel is damaged, spasms of the smooth muscle of the vascular wall, sympathetic reflexes, and release of vasoconstrictor substances (such as serotonin) by the platelets stimulate vasoconstriction. This process reduces blood loss even before a clot can form at the site of injury.

As platelets come in contact with the damaged vascular wall, they adhere to the surface. This process of platelet adhesiveness is facilitated by the release of adenosine diphosphate (ADP) from the damaged cells. The platelet aggregate (a viscous plug) serves to prevent further bleeding. The formation of platelet aggregates results in a temporary hemostatic plug and accounts for the cessation of blood flow from a standard puncture (the bleeding time) within 6 minutes. Therefore, if platelets are decreased in number, or if they are defective, bleeding time will be prolonged [33].

The precise mechanism of blood clotting is still unknown. Although most authorities agreed that there are three essential steps to the clotting mechanism, there is much disagreement on the details of the mechanism.

First, **prothrombin activator** is formed when a vessel is ruptured. (This step is sometimes referred to as the stage of formation of a prothrombin-converting factor.) Second, the prothrombin activator serves as a catalyst in the conversion of prothrombin into thrombin. Third, the **thrombin** acts as an enzyme to convert fibrinogen into fibrin threads that entrap the erythrocytes and plasma to form the clot itself [16].

The classic theory for initiation of coagulation describes two means by which blood coagulation is initiated; the extrinsic system and the intrinsic system. Guyton describes the **extrinsic system** as that which is initiated by the damage of a vessel wall and surrounding tissue [16]. This system causes a tissue extract containing thromboplastin to be released into the tissue fluids, which mixes with blood and normally causes clotting in about 15 seconds. Thromboplastin contains several phospholipids, one of which is cephalin, an active promoter of clotting. Tissue thromboplastin then interacts with several different procoagulants (factors V and VII and calcium ions) in the plasma to form extrinsic prothrombin activator [15] (also known as extrinsic prothrombinase).

The **intrinsic system** for initiating blood coagulation when a vessel surface becomes roughened or if blood becomes traumatized is started by two procoagulation factors, XI and XII. These factors form a contact activation product when they come in contact with a roughened or wettable surface. The product then reacts with factors V, VIII, and IX, and calcium ions and platelet factor 3 to form an intrinsic prothrombin activator [16]. (This activator is called intrinsic prothrombinase by some authorities.)

Platelet factor 3, which is either secreted by plasma or released from platelets on their disintegration, is a major factor in this process. If there is an inadequate number of platelets in the blood, the intrinsic system for initiating blood coagulation is greatly inhibited.

Calcium ions, although not actively involved in these reactions, are necessary for both the intrinsic and extrinsic system. The role of calcium ions, which are almost always present in adequate amounts, is to serve as a cofactor to cause the reactions to take place.

The second phase in coagulation involves the conversion of prothrombin to thrombin, a protein enzyme with proteolytic capabilities. Prothrombin is a plasma protein produced by the liver and requires vitamin K for formation. Prothrombin levels are therefore reduced in vitamin K deficiency or in liver disease that prevents its synthesis.

The third stage involves the polymerization of fibrinogen molecules into fibrin threads. Thrombin acts on fibrinogen, a protein of high molecular weight, to form a molecule of activated fibrin, also known as fibrin monomer. Guyton states that "many fibrin monomer molecules polymerize rapidly into long fibrin-threads that form the reticulum of the clot" [16]. The stability of the clot is influenced by calcium and the protein-stabilizing factor by strengthening the bond between the fibrin monomer molecules. The clot comprises a meshwork of fibrin threads going in all directions and entrapping the blood cells, platelets, and plasma. The fibrin threads adhere to damaged surfaces of the blood vessels. The blood clot becomes adherent to any vascular opening and thus prevents blood loss.

After it has been formed, the blood clot quickly begins to contract, and within 30 to 60 minutes expresses most of its plasma. This process, which consolidates or tightens the clot, is **clot retraction.** The yellow-colored plasma released from the clot is **serum;** it no longer has fibrinogen, and most of the other clotting factors have also been removed. A large number of platelets are also necessary at this time for clot retraction to occur.

The process of fibrinolysis, the eventual lysis or dissolution of the fibrin clot, is facilitated by an inactive enzyme, plasminogen (profibrinolysin), which becomes active on its conversion to a proteolytic enzyme called plasmin (fibrinolysin).

Disorders of hemostasis include those that are a result of (1) vascular abnormalities, (2) defects in the clotting mechanism (resulting from absence of one or more of the essential clotting factors), and (3) excessive anticoagulants (such as iatrogenic hemorrhagic situations in the excess intake of anticoagulant drugs).

To obtain data related to a bleeding disorder, and to determine the cause, a thorough patient history is the most important initial step. The history often provides clues regarding the nature of the bleeding disorder, particularly in the family history, and in the identification of the age at which the bleeding disorder was first noted. A thorough discussion of the bleeding pattern and the predisposing factors is necessary. A thorough physical examination (with particular attention to petechiae or ecchymoses) is essential. This is followed by the most common tests of coagulation and hemostasis. These tests include the following: bleeding time, clotting time, prothrombin time, platelet count, capillary fragility, partial thromboplastin time, thrombin time, and clot retraction.

COMMON TESTS FOR HEMOSTASIS

The bleeding time is a gross evaluation of vascular integrity; it measures the time it takes to stop bleeding naturally. Using the ear lobe puncture technique, the normal range is 2 to 6 minutes.

The clotting time is a gross evaluation of the formation of intrinsic thromboplastin. This test measures the time it takes for a blood specimen in a chemically clean glass tube to clot [16]. The normal range is 10 to 20 minutes, but it will vary with the temperature of the reaction, the number of test tubes used, the diameter of the tubes, and the size of the needle used [17].

The prothrombin time is used to evaluate factors V, VII, and X and prothrombin. An exogenous source of thromboplastin is added to the test plasma, and calcium is introduced. The results are expressed in the number of seconds required for a clot to form; this is then converted to the percent of normal [17]. This will vary in different institutions according to the technique used. Generally, the normal prothrombin time is between 11 and 13 seconds.

The platelet count has been described earlier as being normally within a range of 150,000 to 300,000. The capillary fragility test is a relatively crude estimate of vascular integrity. A blood pressure cuff is placed around the upper arm and the cuff is then inflated midway between the systolic and diastolic pressures (not to exceed 100 mm Hg) and maintained for 5 minutes. Normally, no more than one petechia forms below the pressure cuff. The number and speed of the development of petechiae are noted. The test is discontinued if petechiae are being developed too rapidly [21].

The partial thromboplastin time evaluates the formation of intrinsic thromboplastin, and thus factors XII, XI, IX, and VII. The test measures the clotting time of citrated plasma after the addition of cephalin and calcium chloride [17]. Thrombin time is used to measure the concentration of fibrinogen by adding a solution of thrombin to plasma and recording the clotting time. A prolonged time indicates a low concentration of fibrinogen, the presence of an inhibitor, or a structurally abnormal fibrinogen molecule [21]. Clot retraction normally occurs in 30 to 60 minutes after a clot has formed at the bottom of a test tube. Clot retraction depends on the number and quality of the platelets.

VASCULAR DISORDERS

Vascular abnormalities include the following disorders: idiopathic simple purpura, allergic purpura, infections that cause an increase in capillary fragility, ascorbic acid deficiency, hereditary hemorrhagic telangiectasia, and senile purpura.

Idiopathic simple purpura is a fairly common and usually mild disorder characterized by the appearance of easy bruising and spontaneous ecchymoses.

Allergic purpura, also known as Schönlein-Henoch disease, is apparently a hypersensitivity reaction (with an accompanying vasculitis) to one of a large number of possible antigenic stimuli. Antibiotics, thiazide diuretics, and sedatives have been implicated, although in many cases the causative agent is not known. The characteristic clinical findings include a symmetrical petechial rash occurring in clusters. The limbs and trunk are more often involved in this type of purpura; often there are urticarial and erythematous components [17]. Treatment is primarily supportive; the possible causative agent is withdrawn.

Increased capillary fragility is often seen in certain infections, such as rheumatic fever, sepsis, and Rocky Mountain spotted fever. No specific treatment is required other than that for the underlying infection.

Vitamin C deficiency, known as scurvy, causes a loss of vascular integrity, manifested by a bleeding tendency in the mouth and in the skin. Spongy, bleeding gums are the hallmark of the disease [17].

Hereditary hemorrhagic telangiectasia is a rare bleeding disorder associated with dilated, thin-walled vessels that lack normal muscular tissue. Normal vasoconstriction does not occur in the affected vessels, and angiomas appear on the skin and mucous membrane surfaces. The management is local hemostasis, often difficult in some cases. Some patients may be profoundly anemic as a result of chronic recurrent blood loss, although other persons have very infrequent bleeding episodes.

Senile purpura is not of importance clinically, since there is no generalized hemorrhagic diathesis associated with the condition, and there is no predisposition to bleeding following surgical procedures. The condition may be the source of confusion in detecting other causes of abnormal bleeding, however. Usually there is recurrent intracutaneous bleeding on the dorsal surface of the hand and the extensor surfaces of the forearms. The hemorrhage often leaves a permanent mark of dark brown pigmentation.

COAGULATION DISORDERS

Coagulation disorders are the result of a deficiency of a plasma protein necessary for normal blood coagulation. The known factors necessary for the clotting mechanism are listed in Table 5-5. Only the more common factor deficiencies (hypoprothrombinemia, hemophilia, and von Willebrand's disease) and thrombocytopenia will be discussed.

Hypoprothrombinemia

Hypoprothrombinemia results from a deficient supply, an impaired absorption, or an impaired utilization of vitamin K, which is essential for the liver to produce prothrombin. Vitamin K, a fat-soluble vitamin, requires the presence of bile salts in the intestine for proper absorption. Obstruction of the flow of bile from the biliary tract into the intestine is thus a common cause of prothrombin deficiency. Intrinsic hepatic disease can interfere with the production of prothrombin. Ulcerative colitis, steatorrhea, malabsorption syndrome, and extensive intestinal resections are also associated with vitamin K deficiency. Sterilization of the bowel by oral administration of antibiotics may produce a vitamin K deficiency by interfering with the normal flora of the gastrointes-

Table 5-5
Blood-clotting factors

Factor	Synonym	Characteristics; Sources
I	Fibrinogen	Formed in the liver; converted into fibrin by thrombin; human fibrinogen available as a fraction for replacement therapy
II	Prothrombin	Vitamin K necessary for its synthesis in the liver; forms thrombin when acted upon by thromboplastin Vitamin K is indicated in depressed prothrombin activity
III	Thromboplastin	Converts prothrombin to thrombin
IV	Calcium	Serves as catalyst in conversion of prothrombin to thrombin (may be administered as calcium gluconate, e.g., when large amounts of stored blood are given and calcium may bind with the citrate in blood)
V	Labile factor	Accelerates conversion of prothrombin to thrombin Fresh whole blood, fresh citrated plasma, or fresh-frozen plasma is used in factor V deficiency
VI		Active form of factor V
VII	Stable factor (also proconvertin)	Produced in liver; vitamin K necessary for synthesis; accelerates conversion of prothrombin to thrombin; is replaced by use of banked blood, freeze-dried plasma, stored serum, or commercially available concentrates; also available in cryoprecipitate
VIII	Antihemophilic factor, AHF (antihemophilic factor globulin, AHG)	Necessary for formation of active platelet thromboplastin; available commercially as a concentrate; therapy may require combination approach: packed cells, factor VIII concentrate or packed cells plus cryoprecipitate; fresh-frozen plasma may be used if erythrocyte replacement is not needed
IX	Christmas factor (plasma thromboplastin component, PTC)	Requires vitamin K for synthesis in liver; is similar to factor VIII Available as concentrate; also replaced by fresh or fresh-frozen plasma, or cryoprecipitate
X	Stuart factor (Stuart-Prower factor)	Vitamin K is essential for synthesis in liver; promotes action of thromboplastin; available in concentrate form
XI	Plasma thromboplastin antecedent (PTA)	Promotes release of thromboplastin; deficiency is corrected with fresh or fresh-frozen plasma or cryoprecipitate
XII	Hageman factor	Physiologic function not known; factor deficiency corrected by use of citrated blood, normal plasma, and normal serum
XIII	Fibrin-stabilizing factor (FSF)	Maintains firm clot after it is formed; deficiency is associated with mild bleeding tendency; deficiency corrected with use of fresh-frozen plasma

tinal tract through which vitamin K may also be synthesized. Salicylates, propylthiouracil, and many other drugs have been implicated in inducing or intensifying hypoprothrombinemia states.

Overdosage of oral anticoagulants such as bishydroxycoumarin (Dicumarol) and warfarin sodium (Coumadin) may result in hypoprothrombinemia. These drugs act by interfering with the conversion of vitamin K to prothrombin within the liver cells.

The prudent nurse is aware of the conditions that predispose to bleeding tendencies related to hypoprothrombinemia and will be alert for the major symptoms. These symptoms include ecchymosis following minimal trauma; epistaxis; prolonged bleeding from a venipuncture; hematuria; gastrointestinal tract bleeding, noted as vomitus with blood or as tarry stools; and postoperative hemorrhage from an incision. The major laboratory finding is a prolonged prothrombin time. The nurse will thus take special precautions in administering parenteral medications to these susceptible persons and will protect the patient from situations that predispose the patient to trauma.

Synthetic preparations of vitamin K may be administered orally, but are usually given parenterally to patients with hypoprothrombinemia. Correction of the underlying cause is necessary for conditions in which the cause of diminished prothrombin is evident, as in patients with biliary tract obstruction. Blood transfusions to supply prothrombin are needed at times for patients with prothrombin deficiencies related to liver disease.

The Hemophilias
The hemophilias are a group of inherited coagulation disorders characterized by prolonged bleeding and related to the deficiency of one of the clotting factors necessary for hemostasis. Classic hemophilia, the most common type, is **hemophilia A** and is related to the deficiency of factor VIII, the antihemophilic factor (AHF). **Hemophilia B,** also known as Christmas disease, is transmitted as a sex-linked recessive trait, and is caused by a deficiency of factor IX. It is clinically indistinguishable from hemophilia A. **Hemophilia C,** which is caused by a deficiency of factor XI, differs from hemophilia A in that it is transmitted as a mendelian dominant trait in both the male and female.

Hemophilia A is an abnormality of coagulation which is transmitted by females as a sex-linked recessive mendelian trait contained in the X chromosome. If a male hemophiliac has children, none of his sons will have the disorder, but his daughters will carry the trait, although they do not manifest symptoms of the disease. If the carrier marries a nonhemophiliac, there is a 50 percent chance that her daughters will be carriers and there is a 50 percent chance that her sons will be hemophiliacs. Occasionally, some generations remain free from the disease, so that when the disease occurs, the family may not be aware of a particular ancestor from whom the disease was inherited.

Hemophilia is usually diagnosed at infancy, when prolonged bleeding occurs after circumcision, or during the crawling stages, when minor injuries cause bleeding. There is a wide range of severity in hemophilia. Bleeding may occur spontaneously or may result from trauma. Laboratory findings in hemophilia include a prolonged coagulation time, increased partial thromboplastin time, and decreased prothrombin consumption. The bleeding time is normal, since there is no platelet deficiency in this disorder. The prothrombin time is also characteristically normal. The primary arrest of bleeding thus may be normal, but hemostasis is defective because of the delayed evolution of thrombin.

Patients with hemophilia characteristically have delayed periods of bleeding after an injury or surgery. For example, dental extractions or tonsillectomies are precipitating events leading to bleeding episodes that may occur several hours later. Because inadequate fibrin is formed, a clot that normally begins with primary hemostasis is unstable in hemophilia and causes rebleeding later. Bleeding is demonstrated by hematomas and bleeding into the muscles and into the joints (hemarthrosis). The knees, ankles, elbows, and wrists are most often affected with acute pain, swelling, and limitation of movement. Severe incapacitation may occur with hemarthrosis.

Topical bleeding can usually be controlled temporarily by applying pressure to the injured site, packing the area with Gelfoam or fibrin foam, and applying topical hemostatic preparations such as thrombin. Cold compresses and Ace bandages may be used to limit the joint complications and deformities that otherwise may occur. To halt the bleeding episode permanently, the plasma clotting factors must be replaced. AHF must be administered by means of fresh plasma, fresh-frozen plasma, cryoprecipitate, and/or commercial concentrates. Fresh whole blood is generally not used unless the patient requires blood volume as well as the factors.

Until recently, the only treatment available to control bleeding episodes was whole-blood transfusions and fresh or fresh-frozen plasma, both of which are expensive and difficult to obtain in sufficient amounts. Another problem was the danger of hypervolemia, since excessive volumes of these products are required to provide adequate amounts of the deficient factor.

AHF levels may also be raised by the administration of commercial AHF concentrates such as cryoprecipitate, hemophil, and fibro-antihemophiliac globulin (AHG). The advantage of the AHF concentrates is that the small volume of the concentrates avoids the danger of hypervolemia. The concentrates are being used in the management of bleeding episodes as well as in prophylactic management of hemophilia. Some persons with hemophilia are being taught to administer infusions of the concentrates to themselves at home in order to facilitate rapid therapy in case of bleeding episodes. Early treatment not only reduces the trauma and limits development of hemarthroses and joint deformities, but also limits the need for frequent hospitalizations.

The major disadvantage of the AHF concentrates or plasma therapy for treatment of hemophilia is that the incidence of hepatitis is increased in hemophilic adults and adolescents who receive frequent transfusions. In addition, some hemophiliacs become sensitized to AHF and apparently develop autoimmune anticoagulants (anti-AHF factor); consequently, they are then unable to respond to transfusion therapy. Research is being done on these inhibitor factors, however; a product, Auto-9, is currently being used on an experimental basis to inhibit sensitization. Other problems related to this therapy are those of difficulty of intravenous administration and the expense of the substances.

In addition to deep hematomas and hemarthrosis, hemophiliacs can develop spontaneous hematuria, and life-threatening gastrointestinal, retroperitoneal, or intracranial hemorrhage. Pressure of a hematoma on a vital structure or excessive loss of blood can result in death if adequate intervention is not available. Persons with hemophilia should always carry or wear a Medic-Alert card or bracelet so that their condition is made known in emergency situations.

The person with hemophilia must completely understand his condition, his needs, and his limitations. Some hemophiliacs are overprotected and lead unproductive lives, fearing any type of activity. Others may be almost self-destructive in their unrealistic approach to life. The hemophiliac can lead a normal productive life if he realistically considers the physical limitations and engages only in appropriate activities. When hemophilic patients are admitted to the hospital or clinic for treatment of their major condition, or for some other medical or surgical problem, nurses should be aware of the special needs of these patients.

The nursing care plan is formulated so that measures are taken to help the patient avoid physical trauma. Intramuscular injections should be avoided, since they can result in severe muscular hemorrhages. Injections may be given intravenously or subcutaneously if proper compression is carried out after the injection. Nurses should be aware of common drugs that interfere with platelet function or prolong bleeding; these drugs are contraindicated in the patient with hemophilia. These drugs include, but are not limited to, aspirin, phenacetin, phenylbutazone, and indomethacin.

Nursing goals are oriented to protection of the hemophilic patient from trauma or injury, but this should not be done by instilling fear and anxiety. The usual pattern of independence and activities should not be altered, any more than necessary. Genetic counseling is important for families of hemophiliacs and may also be a part of the nursing care plan, if appropriate at the time.

Von Willebrand's Disease

Von Willebrand's disease, in contrast to classic hemophilia, is a bleeding disorder that is transmitted by an autosomal dominant trait. This condition involves not only a deficiency of the antihemophilic factor (as in classic hemophilia) but also a defective platelet adhesiveness. Therefore, in addition to an abnormal prolonged coagulation time, these patients will demonstrate prolonged bleeding times. Patients with von Willebrand's disease have symptoms associated with classic hemophilia, but in addition, they have symptoms of petechiae and ecchymoses related to the platelet dysfunction. The condition is characterized by bruising and a tendency to bleed from the mucous membranes.

The disease may present initially in adulthood as excessive bleeding during surgery or as a spontaneous gastrointestinal hemorrhage. Treatment consists in administration of the normal plasma fractions, as utilized in classic hemophilia, and in some rare cases, whole-blood transfusions. Platelet transfusions may also be necessary. Surgical intervention for the control of gastrointestinal hemorrhages is often necessary.

Thrombocytopenia

The term **thrombocytopenia** refers to a reduction in platelets caused by decreased marrow production, increased platelet utilization, or increased destruction. Signs of thrombocytopenia generally become apparent when the platelet count falls below 50,000 per cubic millimeter, and gross bleeding such as epistaxis and genitourinary and gastrointestinal hemorrhage occurs with greater frequency in patients with platelet counts of 20,000 per cubic milliliter or less [14]. Small punctate hemorrhages occur throughout the body tissues. The skin characteristically has many small, purplish blotches, from which the name thrombocytopenia purpura is derived [16].

Idiopathic thrombocytopenic purpura (ITP), also known as immune thrombocytopenic purpura, has been shown to be caused by a circulating humoral factor, which accelerates the destruction of platelets. Platelet survival in ITP may be 1 to 3 days or less, compared to the normal 8 to 10 days. The disease is found primarily in children in the acute form; the chronic form affects persons of all ages and is more common in females. Easy bruising, ecchymoses, prolonged bleeding after minor trauma, and bleeding from the nose, gastrointestinal tract, or bladder are common symptoms. Complications of ITP include cerebral hemorrhage; severe hemorrhages from the nose, gastrointestinal tract, and urinary system; and bleeding into the diaphragm, resulting in pulmonary complications.

Diagnosis is confirmed by the presence of a reduced platelet count, prolonged bleeding time, inefficient clot retraction, and increased capillary fragility. The coagulation time is normal. Steroid therapy is often utilized for the treatment of idiopathic thrombocytopenic purpura because glucocorticoids stimulate erythropoiesis and platelet production. Prednisone is the steroid most commonly used. Splenectomy is often indicated, and may result in complete and permanent remission. It is felt that the spleen probably contributes to the premature destruction of sensitized platelets. Spontaneous remissions occur in some instances without specific therapy. Immunosuppressive drugs have also been used.

Secondary thrombocytopenic purpura results from primary viral infections, bone marrow depression, the defibrination syndrome, lupus erythematosus, and infectious mononucleosis, as well as from hypersensitivity to certain drugs. Drugs that are commonly associated with thrombocytopenia include, but are not limited to, quinidine, quinine, sulfonamides, phenylbutazone (Butazolidin), and chlorothiazide derivatives.

Treatment in secondary thrombocytopenia requires the control of the primary cause and control of bleeding. Drugs that are potentially toxic are discontinued. If the primary cause is treated or eliminated, the platelet count begins to rise within a few days. Corticosteroid therapy may be utilized. Platelet transfusions are usually given when hemorrhage is severe, but platelet transfusions are a means of supportive therapy rather than a curative measure. Splenectomy is contraindicated in secondary thrombocytopenia.

EXCESSIVE ANTICOAGULANT THERAPY

Heparin, a sulfated mucopolysaccharide, is often used as an effective anticoagulant in the treatment of intravascular thrombosis. It inhibits thrombin as well as the early stages of coagulation. Coagulation tests are done at appropriate intervals to evaluate the therapy; excessive dosages can result in bleeding. Heparin is cleared rapidly from the blood so that rather frequent administration is required to promote an active therapeutic effect (every 4 to 6 hours intravenously). If major bleeding occurs, protamine sulfate, which is a heparin antagonist, is prescribed.

Oral anticoagulants such as bishydroxycoumarin (Dicumarol) and warfarin (Coumadin) may be prescribed as prophylactic or therapeutic measures to decrease the incidence of thrombi. Both of these drugs inhibit the production of prothrombin and in excess doses may lead to bleeding. The effects of these drugs are usually monitored by periodic prothrombin tests. Patients may not understand the dosages or the purpose of the drug and may take excessive doses. Patients may also take some other drug that potentiates the effect of the anticoagulant so that the prescribed dose results in bleeding tendencies. Some of the many drugs that increase the effect of coumarin are antibiotics, quinidine, quinine, propylthiouracil, tolbutamide (Orinase), salicylates, reserpine, phenylbutazone, and phenytoin (Dilantin). Patients should be oriented to these dangers and should be taught to avoid some of the common drugs that might affect the anticoagulant therapy. Rather than aspirin, for example, the patient should take acetaminophen (Tylenol) for headaches; this drug does not cause a prolonged bleeding time. The patient should be taught to observe for bleeding tendencies, such as bleeding gums, hemoptysis, tarry stools, hematuria, and ecchymoses. The importance of regular laboratory evaluation of the prothrombin time to determine the adequacy of the prescribed dosages of the anticoagulant cannot be overemphasized in the teaching of these patients. If and when bleeding does occur, alterations in dosage are necessary and vitamin K administration is indicated.

The patient who is receiving anticoagulant drugs for therapy must be aware that certain drugs may interact with the anticoagulants and decrease their effect. These drugs include (but are not limited to) barbiturates, chloral hydrate, oral contraceptives, thiazide and mercurial diuretics, antacids, and diazepam (Valium).

DISSEMINATED INTRAVASCULAR COAGULATION

Disseminated intravascular coagulation (DIC) is a condition characterized by diffuse intravascular fibrin deposits, principally in arterioles and capillaries, as a result of activation of the clotting mechanism. Occlusion with microinfarctions and tissue necrosis in various tissues and organs are associated with the process. Activation of the clotting mechanism causes a depletion of clotting factors and platelets, so that a bleeding diathesis also occurs. The onset is usually acute; the patient is critically ill.

It has been postulated that thromboplastin material enters the circulation causing intravascular consumption of clotting factors [17]. Other factors that have been implicated include endothelial damage to blood vessels, hypoxia, and blood stasis.

DIC, also known as consumption coagulopathy or defibrination syndrome, has been associated with surgical complications and obstetric complications such as sepsis (usually of gram-negative origin), abruptio placentae, amniotic fluid embolism, and intrauterine fetal death. It may occur secondary to liver disease, leukemia, disseminated cancer, septicemia, shock, anaphylactic reactions, hemolytic transfusion reactions, massive and rapid transfusions with banked blood, severe dehydration, and other conditions.

Diagnosis is confirmed by a decreased platelet count (thrombocytopenia), prolonged prothrombin time, usually a prolonged partial thromboplastin time, and decreased fibrinogen levels (12.5 percent compared to the normal 30 to 36 percent). An important sign is the presence of fibrin degradation products (split products) in the plasma of affected patients [17]. The degradation products result from the breakdown of fibrin. Spontaneous bleeding, signs of thrombocytopenia such as cutaneous petechiae, and pain related to bleeding into the joints are the predominant clinical symptoms. Hemorrhages also occur in internal organs, particularly the brain, kidney, lungs, pituitary gland, and the gastrointestinal mucosa. Dyspnea, cyanosis, oliguria, convulsions, coma, and shock are other symptoms related to the complications of DIC. It is often complicated by renal failure and damage to the heart, lungs, gastrointestinal tract, and the central nervous system.

The basis of treatment of DIC is related to treating the underlying disease, reversal of pathologic clotting, and control of bleeding and shock. Fresh-frozen plasma, fibrinogen, clotting factor concentrates, packed red cells and/or platelet transfusions are utilized in supportive therapy. Although it is still considered a controversial therapy by some authorities, heparin has frequently been used for the treatment of DIC. Heparin has antithrombic and antithromboplastic effects that can inhibit the activation and consumption of the clotting factors utilized in the coagulation process. Heparin also prevents further deposits of fibrin thrombi in the tissues. Heparin must be used cautiously, however, especially when platelet counts are very low or when patients have associated liver disease. Monitoring of coagulation tests and the partial thromboplastin time is essential to evaluate the effects of therapy. Sometimes DIC is diagnosed erroneously; if signs of increased bleeding occur after a dose of heparin, the nurse must contact the physician immediately. Protamine sulfate, an antidote for heparin, may be required. Epsilon aminocaproic acid (EACA) has been used to control DIC, also; its effect is the inhibition of fibrinolysis [7]. Its effect, however, has not always been beneficial, and it may be harmful in some types of DIC.

Nursing care of the patient with DIC involves close observation, appropriate interventions required in an acute and usually life-threatening situation, and emotional support and comfort measures. The excessive bleeding that occurs in DIC is an extremely frightening event that causes much anxiety for the patient and family. Relief of stress is an important component of nursing care of the patient with DIC, particularly since it is well known that stress plays a significant role in DIC, as it activates the fibrinolytic system. Protection of the patient from trauma is essential, because the patient with DIC bleeds easily when bruised or injured. Injections must be administered cautiously. Mouth care is given gently with a soft toothbrush and diluted mouthwashes. The patient is very weak and conservation of energy is imperative. An accurate record of intake and output is necessary to recognize impending acute renal failure. Relief of pain is managed with appropriate analgesics after careful evaluation of respiratory and cardiac status.

Prognosis is variable for patients with DIC. An increased awareness of the incidence of DIC in critically ill patients has resulted in earlier detection and intervention. Although DIC may be self-limiting, with complete recovery for some patients, uncontrolled hemorrhage and organ damage may result in death.

References

1. Al-Mondhiry, H. Disorders of hemostasis in acute leukemia, part II. *Clin. Bull.* 5:51, 1975.
2. Bakemeir, R. F. The Malignant Lymphomas. In Rubin, P. (ed.), *Clinical Oncology for Medical Students and Physicians. A Multidisciplinary Approach* (4th ed.). New York: American Cancer Society, 1974.
3. Baldy, C. M. The lymphomas: Concepts and current therapies. *Nurs. Clin. North Am.* 7:1763, 1972.
4. Bates, B. *A Guide to Physical Examination.* Philadelphia: Lippincott, 1974.
5. Berry, D. H. The child with acute leukemia. *Am. Fam. Physician* 10:128, 1974.
6. Carbone, P. P., Kaplan, H. S., Musshoff, K., Smithers, D. W., and Tubiana, M. Report of the committee on Hodgkin's disease staging classification. *Cancer Res.* 31:1860, 1971.
7. Colman, R. W., Robboy, S. J., and Minna, J. D. Disseminated intravascular coagulation (DIC): An approach. *Am. J. Med.* 52:679, 1972.
8. Crosby, W. H. (ed.). *Iron.* New York: Medcom, 1972.
9. Custer, R. P. *An Atlas of the Blood and Bone Marrow* (2nd ed.). Philadelphia: Saunders, 1974.
10. Doswell, W. M. Sickle cell disease. *Nursing '74* 4:18, 1974.
11. Food and Nutrition Board, National Academy of Sciences—National Research Council. *Recommended Daily Dietary Allowances* (rev. ed.), 1974. Washington, D.C.
12. Fowler, A. (ed.). Update: Diagnosing anemia; a three-step approach. *Patient Care* 8:70, 1974.
13. French, R. H. *Guide to Diagnostic Procedures* (4th ed.). New York: McGraw-Hill, 1975.
14. Graw, R. G., and Yankee, R. A. Principles of hematologic supportive care. *Med. Clin. North Am.* 57:441, 1973.
15. Guyton, A. *Function of the Human Body* (3rd ed.). Philadelphia: Saunders, 1969.
16. Guyton, A. *Textbook of Medical Physiology* (4th ed.). Philadelphia: Saunders, 1971.
17. Harvey, A. M., Johns, R. J., Owens, A. H., and Ross, R. S. *The Principles and Practice of Medicine* (18th ed.). New York: Appleton-Century-Crofts, 1972.
18. Jackson, D. E. Sickle cell disease: Meeting a need. *Nurs. Clin. North Am.* 7:727, 1972.
19. Lichtman, M. A., and Klemperer, M. R. The

Leukemias. In Rubin P. (ed.), *Clinical Oncology for Medical Students and Physicians: A Multidisciplinary Approach* (4th ed.). New York: American Cancer Society, 1974.
20. Mechner, F. Patient assessment: Examination of the head and neck; programmed instruction. *Am. J. Nurs.* 75:1, 1975.
21. Meyers, M. C. Hematopoietic System. In Judge, R. D., and Zuidema, G. D. (eds.), *Physical Diagnosis: A Physiologic Approach to the Clinical Examination* (2nd ed.). Boston: Little, Brown, 1968.
22. Passmore, R., and Robson, J. S. *A Companion to Medical Studies*, Vol. 3. London: Blackwell, 1974.
23. Peery, T. M., and Miller, F. N. *Pathology: A Dynamic Introduction to Medicine and Surgery* (2nd ed.). Boston: Little, Brown, 1971.
24. Reich, C. The cellular elements of blood. *Clin. Symp.* 14:79, 1962.
25. Robbins, S. L., and Angell, M. *Basic Pathology*. Philadelphia: Saunders, 1971.
26. Rubin, A. D., and Davis, S. The role of the lymphocyte in producing the clinical manifestations of chronic lymphocytic leukemia. *Med. Clin. North Am.* 57:463, 1973.
27. Schumann, D., and Patterson, P. The adult with acute leukemia. *Nurs. Clin. North Am.* 7:743, 1972.
28. Spivak, J. L., and Barnes, H. V. *Manual of Clinical Problems in Internal Medicine*. Boston: Little, Brown, 1974.
29. *Standards for Blood Banks and Transfusion Services* (7th ed.). Chicago: Am. Assoc. Blood Banks, 1974.
30. *The Use of Blood: A Practical Guide to the Clinical Applications of Blood and Blood Derivatives*. North Chicago: Abbott Laboratories, 1971.
31. Vaz, D. S. The common anemias: Nursing approaches. *Nurs. Clin. North Am.* 7:711, 1972.
32. Vianna, N. J., Greenwald, P., Brady, J., Polan, A. K., Dwork, A., Mauro, J., and Davies, J. N. P. Hodgkin's disease: Cases with features of a community outbreak. *Ann. Intern. Med.* 77:169, 1972.
33. Weiss, H. J. Bleeding disorders due to abnormal platelet function. *Med. Clin. North Am.* 75:517, 1973.
34. Wintrobe, M. M. *Clinical Hematology* (7th ed.). Philadelphia: Lea & Febiger, 1974.

Bibliography

Bitheel, T. C., and Wintrobe, M. M. The hemorrhage prone patient. *Hosp. Med.* 6:96, 1970.
Bolin, R. H., and Auld, M. E. Hodgkin's disease. *Am. J. Nurs.* 74:1982, 1974.
Davidson, I., and Henry, J. B. (eds.). *Todd-Sanford Clinical Diagnosis by Laboratory Methods* (15th ed.). Philadelphia: Saunders, 1974.
Desser, R. K., Moran, E. M., and Ultmann, J. E. Staging of Hodgkin's disease and lymphoma. *Med. Clin. North Am.* 57:479, 1973.
DeVita, V. T., Jr., and Carbone, P. P. Chemotherapeutic implications of staging in Hodgkin's disease. *Cancer Res.* 31:1838, 1971.
Eisenhauer, L. Drug-induced blood dyscrasias. *Nurs. Clin. North Am.* 7:799, 1972.
Kaplan, H. S. Formal discussion of paper by F. Teillet et al.: A reappraisal of clinical and biological signs in staging Hodgkin's disease. *Cancer Res.* 31:1730, 1971.
Keaveny, M. E., and Wiley, L. Hodgkin's disease, the curable cancer. I: Diagnosis and treatment. *Nursing 75* 5:49, 1975.
Laboratory assessment of nutritional status. *Am. J. Public Health* 6[Suppl.]:28, 1973.
Levin, W. C. (ed.). Symposium on Hodgkin's disease. *Arch. Intern. Med.* 131:331, 1973.
Mayer, G. G. Disseminated intravascular coagulation. *Am. J. Nurs.* 73:2067, 1973.
McCurdy, P. R. Sickle cell trait. *Am. Fam. Physician* 10:141, 1974.
McFarlane, J. M. The child with sickle cell anemia. *Nursing 75* 5:29, 1975.
Miale, J. B. *Laboratory Medicine: Hematology* (4th ed.). St. Louis: Mosby, 1972.
Patterson, P. C. Hemophilia: The new look. *Nurs. Clin. North Am.* 7:777, 1972.
Rogers, J. M. Hodgkin's disease: Hope is the key to nursing care: II. Nursing Needs. *Nursing 75* 5:55, 1975.
Schick, P. K. Hemophilia. *Med. Clin. North Am.* 57:1095, 1973.
Schumann, D., and Patterson, P. Multiple myeloma. *Am. J. Nurs.* 75:78, 1975.
Seedor, M. M. *The Physical Assessment: A Programmed Unit of Study for Nurses*. New York: Teachers College Press, 1974.
Selkurt, E. *Basic Physiology for the Health Sciences*. Boston: Little, Brown, 1975.
Sergis, E., and Hilgartner, M. W. Hemophilia. *Am. J. Nurs.* 72:2011, 1972.
Showfety, M. P. The ordeal of Hodgkin's disease. *Am. J. Nurs.* 74:1987, 1974.
Smith, L. G., and Louria, D. Infectious disease problems in various hematologic disorders. *Med. Clin. North Am.* 57:409, 1973.
Warren, B. Maintaining the hemophiliac at home and school. *Nursing 74* 4:73, 1974.
Widmann, F. K. *Goodale's Interpretation of Laboratory Tests* (7th ed.). Philadelphia: Davis, 1973.
Williams, S. *Nutrition and Diet Therapy* (2nd ed.). St. Louis: Mosby, 1973.
Williams, W. J. (ed.). *Hematology*. New York: McGraw-Hill, 1972.

chapter 6

Patients with Kidney and Urinary Tract Dysfunction

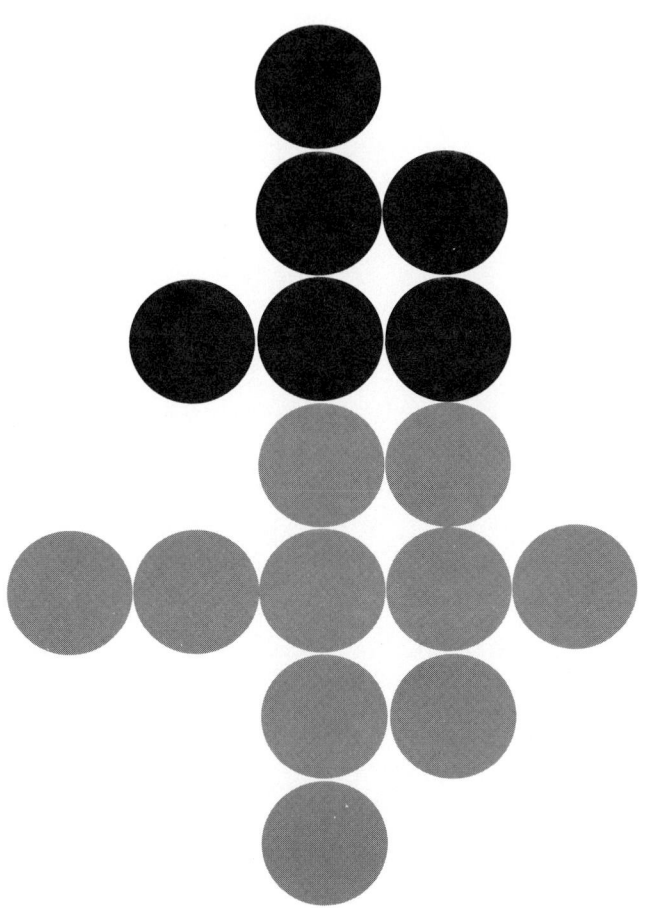

In this chapter, the urinary tract and kidney will be discussed in terms of dysfunction and related nursing care. The kidney and urinary tract can be compared to a filtration plant and a plumbing system that provide for "processing" a liquid and then for passage of that liquid from one place to another. Urine, the end product of renal function, is comprised of the water, electrolytes, metabolic waste products, and other substances that are not required by the body. Elimination of urine is provided for by the parts of the urinary system concerned with flow: renal calyces, ureters, the bladder, and the urethra.

Nursing care of patients with urinary system dysfunction must take into account the aspect of the urinary system people are most aware of—the act of voiding. Each person has a habitual pattern of voiding. Idiosyncrasies associated with this pattern may be of either physiologic or emotional origin. These idiosyncrasies are first learned and then evolve from the age of 3; at this age, the act of voiding can be voluntarily controlled. Physiologic voiding patterns are related to eating and fluid intake patterns, as well as to the special way a given person's urinary tract functions. Family attitudes and cultural mores influence a person's development of attitudes and concerns about voiding. The very act of voiding is generally a private function that a person learns to conduct in designated places. Voiding is also associated with feelings about modesty and, for many people, it has sexual overtones.

An awareness of each person's sensitivities about voiding is part of the nurse's role when caring for patients. How a person views elimination is particularly significant in the event of urinary system dysfunction; attitudes not only affect a person's readiness for learning how to manage dysfunction but also influences that person's participation in treatment and care. Some people are consciously aware of their own patterns of elimination and their feelings related to elimination, whereas others have never thought about either until a disturbance arises. Therefore the nurse may need to help the patient explore these areas in order to assist him in establishing habits that are conducive to attaining the most effective urinary system function possible.

Functions of the Urinary System

A brief review of normal urinary system function is helpful in understanding dysfunction.

Urine is produced by the kidney via a process termed **renal function.** Effective renal function depends on adequate blood flow through the renal artery. About 20 to 25 percent of the cardiac output flows through the kidney at a rate of up to 1,200 ml per minute in a normal young adult at rest [21]. The kidney has millions of nephron units, which function to retain or reabsorb substances required by the body and to eliminate those not required. The glomerulus of the nephron filters the blood, and the tubules reabsorb water and substances needed by the body. The excess water and the waste substances make up the urine that collects in the renal calyces, where the outflow of urine begins.

From the renal calyces, urine flows to the renal pelvis and into the ureters. Urine flow through the ureters is accomplished by the pressure of the urine volume and by peristalsis. The peristaltic action of the ureters helps prevent reflux or backward flow of urine toward the kidney. The ureters deliver urine to the bladder in spurts. **Micturition,** the emptying of the bladder, does not normally occur until a sufficient amount of urine is collected in the bladder.

Emptying of the bladder occurs as a result of both sympathetic and parasympathetic nerve influences, which provide for both voluntary and reflex control. The sympathetic nerve supply to the bladder wall (made up of the body, the neck, and the internal sphincter of the bladder) arises from the upper lumbar segments of the spinal cord and passes downward to the hypogastric nerves, made up of both preganglionic and postganglionic fibers. Sympathetic fibers inhibit micturition by causing contraction of the internal sphincter and relaxation of the bladder wall. The parasympathetic nerve fibers supplying the bladder arise from the second, third, and fourth sacral segments of the spinal cord and unite to form the pelvic nerves. Parasympathetic innervation causes contraction of the bladder, relaxation of the sphincter muscles, and reflex micturition.

When the bladder fills with urine up to the threshold point (usually 400 to 500 ml) the intravesical pressure abruptly increases and initiates the micturition reflex. Normally bladder distention beyond this point cannot be tolerated. Bladder volumes up to 700 ml can cause both pain and loss of control [16]. When the intravesical pressure is great enough to stimulate the micturition reflex, the detrusor muscle of the bladder contracts, the internal sphincter relaxes, and urine flows through the urethra. The external sphincter, controlled by the pudic (pudendal) nerve, then relaxes, and urine continues to flow outward through the urethra.

If the micturition theshold is reached and the person becomes aware of the need to void, but cannot appropriately void at that time, the cerebral cortex inhibits voiding by causing the detrusor muscle to relax and the external sphincter to remain closed. In this way, voiding can be voluntarily inhibited. Several factors assist inhibition, including contraction of the striated muscle of the urogenital diaphragm and the levator ani muscle surrounding the midurethra and the distal prostatic and membranous urethra in males. Both perineal and abdominal muscles are important in the inhibition of voiding.

In the event innervation to the bladder is interrupted, as occurs in spinal cord injury, the effects on the bladder will depend on the level of the cord injury. When the injury occurs above the level of the sacral cord, the reflex arc for micturition may still take place. (The reader is referred to Chapter 11 for a more detailed discussion of reflex arcs.) In this case, the bladder distends as urine volume increases until intravesical pressure thresholds are reached, causing the stretch receptors in the bladder wall to initiate impulses to the pelvic nerves and on to the spinal cord. The efferent portion of the reflex arc comes into play, causing a reflex contraction of the detrusor muscle and internal sphincter relaxation. In an **automatic bladder** (one in which the upper motor nerve supply is impaired) bladder capacity is usually much lower than normal, being only 150 to 200 ml as compared to variable normal capacities of 500 to 600 ml, because the bladder becomes hypertonic without inhibitory impulses from the upper motor neurons. An **autonomous bladder** results from lower motor neuron lesions affecting the second, third, or fourth sacral segments of the spinal cord. There is no inhibition of bladder function, bladder contractions are weak, and the bladder tends to contain large amounts of residual urine.

The amount of urine required to initiate micturition not only varies among individuals but also changes from one time to another in any one person. Individual bladder capacities are lessened by factors such as emotional stress [16] and cold temperatures. Nervous people tend to have smaller bladder capacities, as do those with impaired detrusor muscle function or impaired innervation. It is therefore necessary to ascertain a person's usual or normal patterns in order to evaluate the significance of measurements or changes in the volume of urine output.

Knowledge of bladder function is helpful in understanding the effects of parasympathetic depressants. Synthetic atropine-like drugs, belladonna alkaloids, including atropine and scopolamine, antihistamines, monoamine oxidase inhibitors (which are psychic energizers), meperidine hydrochloride, and morphine all exert an effect on bladder function. Patients who are taking any of these drugs should be informed that changes in normal voiding patterns are expected.

The urinary tract is like a continuous tube from the kidney to the bladder. The bladder is a reservoir that connects with another tube, the urethra. Urine flow flushes the tract of foreign bodies and microorganisms. Although the urethra does have some normal flora, the ureters and the bladder are considered sterile. This sterility is maintained because reflux (back flow) of urine from the bladder to the urethra is prevented. The flow of urine and concomitant pressure gradients associated with urine flow, as well as the external sphincter and the urogenital muscle, prevent reflux.

The effectiveness of the urinary system can be altered by (1) anomalies or acquired cellular changes in the kidneys, ureters, bladder, and urethra, (2) obstructions within the urinary tract such as foreign bodies, (3) externally applied pressure from surrounding organs that impinge on the kidney or the urinary tract, causing obstruction, (4) trauma causing disruption of the integrity of the kidney or the urinary tract, (5) drugs that impair urinary function by their effect on parasympathetic nerves, (6) damage or impairment to the nerves supplying the tract or to the muscles controlling micturition, and (7) infection. Whatever the cause, dysfunction is characterized by changes in urine secretion if the kidneys are affected, and impairment of urine flow if the urinary tract is affected. Retention of urine and concomitant infection are two complications of almost all disorders of the urinary tract that progress without treatment or that do not respond to treatment. Because the urinary system is anatomically continuous from the kidney to the urethra, any changes in the function of one portion of the urinary system will eventually affect the function of the entire system; thus untreated dysfunction in the ureters, bladder, or urethra will eventually affect the kidney. Impaired kidney function may result in changes in the character, consistency, or amount of urine.

Assessment of the Patient with Urinary System Dysfunction

Assessment of urinary system functions includes taking a history of the patient's signs and symptoms, in both current and past experiences, and performing a physical examination and diagnostic tests, including laboratory and x-ray examinations. The significance of diagnostic tests for diagnosis and treatment plans is explained later in this chapter at the point of application. In general, the diagnostic tests for urinary system function are extremely important because the system is not directly visible, and abnormalities cannot be felt easily on physical examination. Therefore the various measurements of function, and visualization through instrumentation and x-ray studies, become the major source of data used to confirm the presence of dysfunction. Assessment factors and specific tests are described in this section. The nurse should be familiar with these tests in order to prepare the patient correctly for the examinations as well as to advise him or her about what to expect.

In assessing urinary system function, the nurse should be aware of risk factors. Certain groups of people are subject to urinary system dysfunction. Women, particularly those who are sexually active or pregnant, and men over the age of 70 with prostatic hypertrophy, have a high incidence of infection. Young men or those who participate in contact sports tend to have a high frequency of trauma causing injury to the urinary system. People with congenital anomalies of the kidney or urinary tract are vulnerable to dysfunction, as are people with systemic diseases that impair renal function. People who are immobilized, such as those with debilitating neuromuscular diseases, are subject to both infection and formation of stones, usually referred to as calculi.

There are two major reasons why assessment of urinary tract function and dysfunction is difficult. First, the urinary tract is anatomically associated with the genital system and is closely aligned with the intestines in the pelvis. Many symptoms of urinary tract dysfunction may be ambiguous (e.g., nausea or abdominal pain) and are similar to symptoms caused by disturbances of any of the other organs in the pelvis. Second, the majority of symptoms presented in urinary system dysfunction, particularly those related to the urinary tract, are subjective and cannot be observed objectively. Therefore the patient's history and description of his symptoms are important assessment tools. Laboratory examination of the urine and visualization of the urinary system by x-ray and cystoscopy (bladder visualization) are the most definitive means of assessment.

TERMS USED IN URINARY SYSTEM ASSESSMENT

A number of terms are used to define urination for assessment purposes. These terms are used to ensure common understanding of the patient's symptoms. During the interview when the patient's history is taken, the nurse may need to explain what is meant by each term and ask the patient to describe his symptoms according to these terms to obtain more precise data. When the patient is able to describe clearly how he feels, the nurse can evaluate his statements and interpret them according to this terminology when writing the history and when recording nursing observations.

The terms commonly used are frequency, nocturia, polyuria, oliguria, anuria, urgency, dysuria, hesitancy, intermittency, dribbling, incontinence, and pain. **Frequency** refers to the number of times a person voids and is usually estimated over a 24-hour period. People normally void during the hours when they are awake. **Nocturia** is the need to void frequently during usual sleeping hours. The terms polyuria, oliguria, and anuria refer to the amount of urine voided. **Polyuria** is a larger than normal amount of urine and occurs in certain metabolic disorders such as diabetes, when renal function is impaired, or when a person drinks greater than normal quantities of fluid. **Oliguria** is a urine volume of 400 ml or less in a 24-hour period. **Anuria** refers to absence of urine output.

Urgency is the term used to define the feeling that all of a sudden one has to void and cannot wait. **Dysuria** is a more general term and means difficulty in urination; this condition includes discomfort and sometimes pain. **Hesitancy** describes the feeling that one has to void but cannot start the stream; there is a delay before urination actually occurs. **Intermittency** describes urination that occurs with interruptions in the stream. **Dribbling** is a condition in which small amounts of urine are eliminated in drops either continuously or at the end of the stream. **Incontinence** means the inability to inhibit micturition. **Pain**, sometimes included in the term dysuria, may be located either perineally or may occur along the line of the urinary tract (Fig. 6-1).

The nurse should ascertain the presence of pain and its location and should obtain a description of the type of pain. Renal pain is most frequently dull and aching or severe and acute, as in colic.

EXAMINATION OF URINE

Examination of the urine and laboratory urinalysis are important in assessment of urinary system dysfunction and of many other body disturbances, because they reflect the body's electrolyte and metabolic status in a general way. The constituents of the blood are "processed" through renal function for maintenance of acid-base balance and elimination of metabolic wastes. Table 6-1 gives the normal and abnormal values significant in urinary tract assessment.

The nurse should routinely observe the appearance of the urine when collecting urine samples for urinalysis or when emptying bed pans or urinals. It is also important for the nurse to ask the patient to describe the appearance of his urine when gathering data for the patient history. Normally urine is straw colored or clear yellow. The intensity of the yellow color is related to the concentration, the more concentrated urine being a deeper yellow. **Hematuria** (blood in the urine) is frequently present in urinary tract pathology involving obstruction or infection. When gross hematuria is present, the urine is red or brownish from the change of hemoglobin to hematin. Smaller amounts of blood in the urine give it a smoky appearance, while very small amounts can be seen only with a microscope. Hematuria may be present in the entire voided urine sample, or it may appear

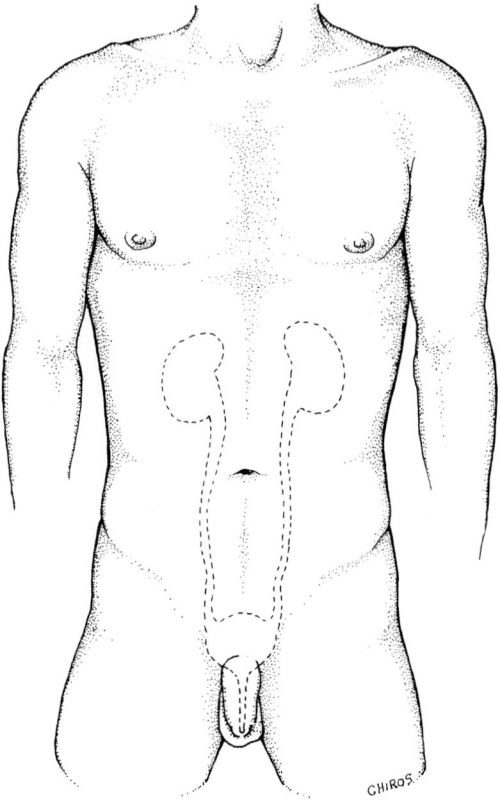

Figure 6-1
Location of pain felt along the urinary tract.

only at the start or completion of the urinary stream. If it appears only at the start, the patient may have a urethral lesion such as a urethral caruncle, which is a polypoid growth. Uniform hematuria in the entire specimen indicates pathology above the urethra. Hematuria appearing at the end of the urinary stream implies a problem in the bladder or urethra.

If **pyuria** (pus in the urine) is present, the urine will appear whitish or foamy; this type of urine sample may also have a foul odor. Contamination of the urinary tract from the genital system (due to the proximity of the urinary tract orifices to those of the genital system) is suspected in this instance. The presence of bacteria in the urine gives it a hazy or cloudy appearance. Ketone bodies in the urine have a peculiar fetid smell.

Simple urine tests can be conducted by patients in their homes, if necessary for monitoring the progression of a dysfunction or for evaluating the effectiveness of therapy.

Table 6-1
Normal urine values measured in urinalysis with interpretation of abnormal values

Urinalysis Measurement	Normal Values	Interpretation of Abnormal Values
Specific gravity	1.003–1.030	Decreased in inflammation; interference with concentration capabilities as in pyelonephritis. Increased in dehydration
Protein	Small amounts	Increased in severe infection and glomerular disease; increased in primary renal disease. Increase indicates need to investigate renal function
Leukocytes	Occasional (3–5)	Slightly increased in most renal diseases. Largely increased in tuberculosis of the kidney, glomerulonephritis, pyelonephritis, and inflammation of the urinary tract. Increases indicate need for culture
Erythrocytes	1–3	Increased in most renal disease and urinary tract diseases: infection, stones, and tumors
Casts		Increase in all casts indicates presence of renal disease
Hyaline	Occasional	Presence indicates inflammation and need to culture
Granular	Occasional	Presence indicates degenerated cells, as in glomerulonephritis
Epithelial	Few	Presence indicates contamination of specimen or cellular destruction as in tubular degeneration
Red blood cell casts	0	Present in glomeruli and lower urinary tract lesions
White blood cell casts	0	Present in pyogenic infection, usually involving the kidney
pH	4.5–8.0 Usually acid	Urine is acid in renal tubule acidosis, urinary tract infection, or tuberculosis of the kidney. Alkaline urine indicates urea metabolism, *Proteus* infection
Bacteria	Few	100,000 per ml of urine indicates infection
Glucose	0	Presence indicates renal glycosuria (may indicate diabetes)

Nursing care includes teaching patients to perform these tests correctly. The patient who must observe his urine in order to monitor important changes or to determine progress can purchase the materials for some of these tests, such as urine tests for glucose and those for urinary pH, at a drugstore. The patient who is monitoring his own urine output is usually asked to record his observations of the color, consistency, and volume of the urine. On the other hand, testing the urine for bacteria and for metabolic constitutents and cells requires sophisticated laboratory equipment. Even this equipment is useless, however, if the urine samples being tested are not collected correctly.

Urine samples must be as free of contamination from other sources as possible to be of value. A midstream urine collection is used by women to eliminate possible contamination from the genital area. This method involves cleaning the perineal area with soap and water or a mild antiseptic. One hand is used to spread the labia, and attention is given to thorough cleaning of the urinary meatus. The woman then voids, discarding the first portion of the stream and collecting the remainder in a sterile urine container. Males use a two- or three-specimen sequence to collect urine. Cleaning of the penis and particularly of the urinary meatus precedes urine collection. The first part of the urinary stream is collected in one container; usually 15 to 30 ml of urine is sufficient. The midstream is collected in the second container, and the remaining urine is placed in the third container. The three-specimen sample is preferred because males have a longer urethra than females, and prostatic secretions are mixed with urine. Therefore, the first specimen contains the urine from the urethra and prostatic secretions (Fig. 6-2), and the second, urine from the bladder. There is controversy about the source of urine in the third specimen. The second or midstream specimen is used for cultures. This three-specimen method of collection enables the examiner to compare specimens. Abnormal findings in all three containers imply bladder or kidney dysfunction; abnormal findings in only the first specimen imply urethritis or prostatic dysfunction.

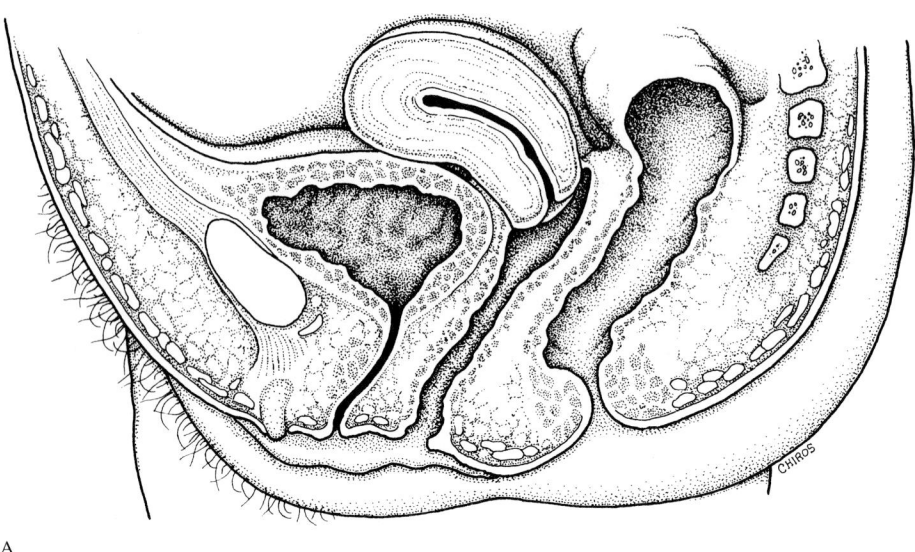

A

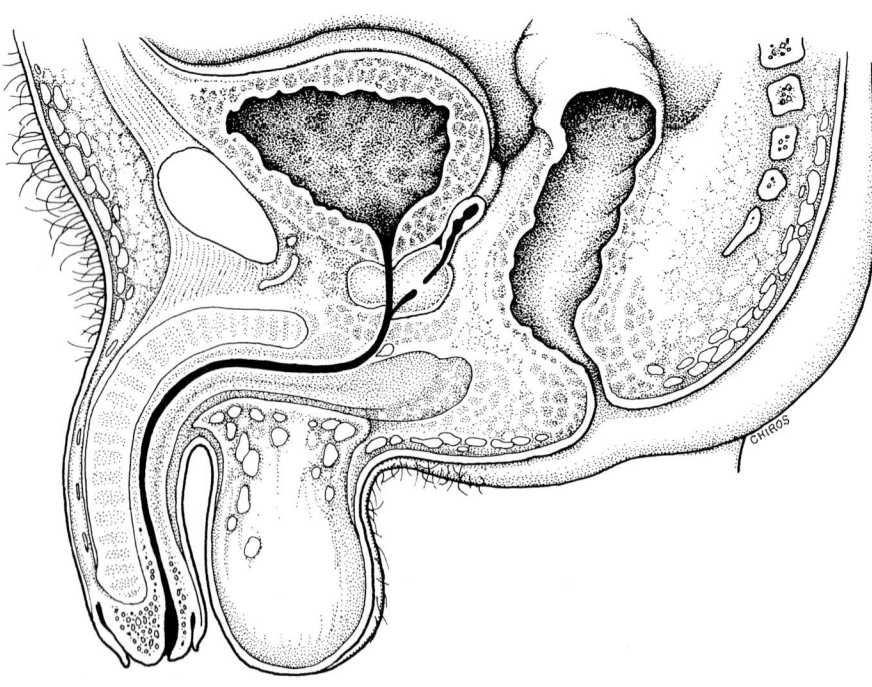

B

Figure 6-2
Comparison of male and female urethras and surrounding structures.

PHYSICAL EXAMINATION

Physical examination of the kidneys and urinary tract includes palpation and percussion to detect abnormalities. The kidneys are protected by the rib cage and the deep muscles of the back. Normally only the lower pole of the right kidney can be felt by deep palpation. The urinary tract cannot be palpated, with the exception of a distended urinary bladder, which can be determined by palpation or percussion. Tumor masses and engorgement of the kidney by hemorrhage can usually be felt.

The pole of the right kidney is palpated with the patient in the supine position. The examiner places his right hand between the rib cage and the iliac crest anteriorly and his left hand posteriorly just below the costal margin. The left hand is used to support the body from below and the right hand is used for deep palpation as the patient takes a deep breath. Because the left kidney is slightly higher than the right, it cannot be felt in ordinary circumstances. Sometimes the pole of the right kidney can be felt better if, as the patient takes a deep breath, the examiner places downward pressure on the palpating hand and upward pressure on the supporting hand. The patient is instructed to exhale and then hold his breath. When this is done the kidney pole may be felt as the examiner slowly releases pressure (Fig. 6-3).

Tenderness of the kidney is felt with the patient in a sitting position. The examiner's left hand is placed over the costovertebral angle and percussion is done with the fist [3]. The lightly striking motion of percussion by the right fist should result in a dull sound. Pain is an abnormal finding and usually implies infection.

A distended bladder may be felt in the suprapubic area, using the pads of the fingers for light palpation. The distended bladder feels soft and elastic. When the abdominal examination has been completed, the patient is asked to empty his bladder for subsequent examination because a distended bladder may be mistaken for a mass. Figure 6-4 indicates the area to be percussed to detect bladder distention. In addition to distention from normal urine collection, a bladder may be distended because of obstruction at the neck of the bladder, because of loss of tone of bladder musculature causing urine retention, or when there is prostatic hypertrophy or disease. Masses in the bladder can be felt as solid formations.

DIAGNOSTIC TESTS

Further examination (often termed a **urologic workup**) is performed for any patient who has symptoms of urinary system dysfunction. A urologic workup includes tests that visual-

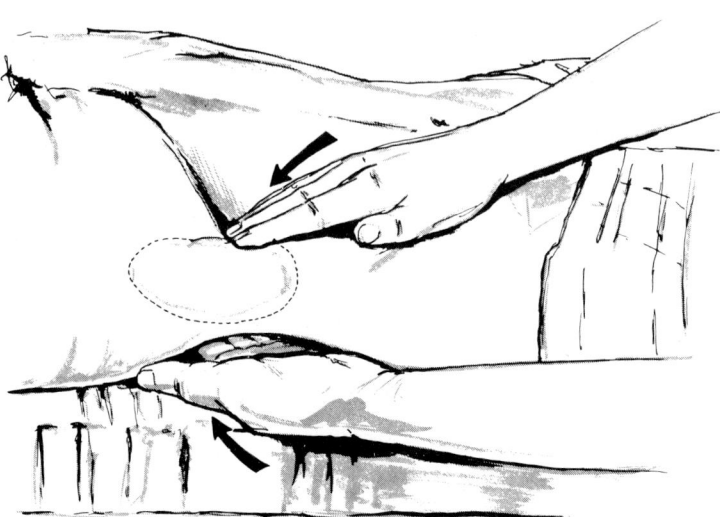

Figure 6-3
Palpation of the kidney. (From J. Sana and R. D. Judge, *Physical Appraisal Methods in Nursing Practice*. Boston: Little, Brown and Company, 1975. Reproduced by permission.)

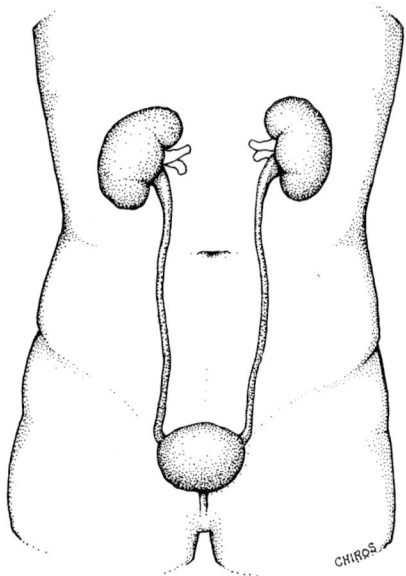

Figure 6-4
Area for palpation of the bladder.

ize the kidney and urinary tract and those that measure renal function. X-rays and cystoscopic examinations provide for visualization; urine and blood tests and concentration, dilution, and clearance tests are used to measure renal function.

The nurse often prepares the patient for examination, both giving him directions about preparation so that test results will be accurate and giving him information about what to expect. When possible these instructions are given to the patient in written form so he can refer to them when it is time to carry out the actual preparation.

Urine Tests

Explicit instructions are given for the collection of urine samples according to the requirements of the test the patient is to have. Urine tests are either qualitative or quantitative or both; this means that the collections must be controlled so that variables in time do not skew the test results. Qualitative tests are performed to measure the kidney's ability to filter or reabsorb certain substances. These substances may be endogenous or they may be given to the patient orally or intravenously. Creatinine is an example of an endogenous substance with a fairly consistent filtration rate; thus comparison of blood levels with the amount of creatinine excreted in the urine in a timed urine collection will demonstrate renal function.

Many urine collections require 24-hour urine specimens. It is imperative that the collection be precise. The first morning specimen is discarded and the remaining specimens are collected for a 24-hour period beginning at the time the first specimen was discarded. Inclusion of the first specimen will cause inaccurate test results since the specimen will then consist of urine collected in the bladder prior to the beginning of the 24-hour period. This should be carefully explained to the patient in order to gain his cooperation.

For tests of kidney function that depend on knowing the time required for the kidney to filter or reabsorb a certain substance, the timing for collection of specimens must also be precise. This is of particular importance when a blood sample is to be compared to a urine sample obtained at the same time. Clearly marking all specimens so that they will not be mixed up in transport to the laboratory is essential. The nurse must consider the time and effort the patient expends in collecting specimens and the laboratory costs in analyzing specimens and must obtain specimens correctly for accurate diagnosis.

Urine specimens should be sent to the laboratory promptly if they are single specimens. When 24-hour samples are collected, it is necessary to refrigerate those in which substances to be measured are degraded through standing or exposure to warmth. Degradation of these substances may lead to a prolonged hospitalization or an inaccurate diagnosis or both.

One of the major concerns of the nurse when a patient has a urologic workup is the patient's comfort. The preparation for many of the tests requires fasting, drinking large amounts of water or none at all, or physical discomfort from sitting or lying on uncomfortable examination tables for an extended period of time. The patient may not feel well in the first place, so these discomforts may further distress him. Attention should be given to the patient's comfort before, during, and following the tests. As soon as the tests are completed food, fluid, rest, or whatever relief the patient requires should be made available.

Catheters are sometimes inserted into the bladder to provide for continuous urine flow in the event of incontinence. They are not inserted unless absolutely necesssary, however, because their use is related to a high incidence of infection. If catheters are placed, care must be taken to keep all tubing patent and to place the collection bag below the level of the patient to facilitate drainage by gravity and to prevent reflux of urine from the collection bag to the bladder. The catheter should be secured by taping so that movement does not dislodge the catheter and the flow of urine is not interfered with by kinking of the catheter or drainage tubes.

Measurement of Intake and Output

A record of fluid intake and urine output over a period of time is an important diagnostic measure that can be used to monitor the patient's progress. Intake and output records are sometimes neglected, and in an effort to catch up, the nurse may estimate the calculations, which are therefore not accurate. Involving the patient whose fluid intake and output are being measured in the process of measurement is sometimes very helpful in maintaining the accuracy of the record. This is also a good technique to use when the patient is being taught to monitor his own output in order to estimate the success of forcing fluids. As described in Chapter 2, loss or retention of fluid is important in assessment of dysfunction.

One precise measure of fluid retention is body weight. When fluid is retained, the weight will be increased; when fluid is lost, the weight will decrease. Body weights are accurate if they are taken on the same scale at the same time each day while the patient has the same weight of clothes on. A commonly used measure of the weight of clothes is 5 pounds; however, this obviously varies considerably. A better method is to teach the patient to form a habit of weighing daily after his bath or shower and before dressing; the variable weight of clothing will then not be a factor.

Fluid loss includes both sensible and insensible fluid loss. Sensible fluid loss is that of urine excretion. Insensible fluid loss includes that lost in perspiration, vomitus, drainage, or routes other than urine. Insensible fluid loss through perspiration can only be estimated. Liquid emesis or drainage should be accurately measured. Solid particles of undigested food or other substances are generally measured along with the liquid component. The patient must be observed closely and often can be taught to observe his own sensible and insensible fluid loss. The patient who is forcing fluids must drink more than usual if he participates in an activity that causes excessive perspiration.

Yet another factor in fluid output measurement is loss of urine through incontinence or leakage around tubes. In situations requiring precise measurement of output, the bed linen is weighed and the weight of the wet linen compared to that of dry linen. One gram of fluid in the linen or dressing is equal to 1 milliliter for purposes of calculation.

When the patient has special needs related to urine incontinence, the nurse should make provisions for his care and comfort when he has diagnostic tests such as x-ray studies. The nurse's role in this regard is often facilitated by institutional policy and is frequently influenced by the physician's preferences in conducting test procedures. If the patient is incontinent, the nurse should be aware of his special needs. The nurse should understand that incontinence usually causes a feeling of helplessness and often embarrassment in the patient. In addition, incontinence can lead to skin irritation, so it is essential to keep the patient clean and dry. The methods used will depend on the reasons for the incontinence; it may be caused by the inability to inhibit micturition, or it may result from leakage around drainage tubes such as urinary bladder catheters or suprapubic tubes. Often bladder spasms are the cause of incontinence around suprapubic tubes.

X-ray Studies

X-ray studies include the KUB (kidneys, ureters, and bladder) study, tomography, intravenous pyelogram, and retrograde pyelogram. A **KUB** is a flat plate x-ray of the abdomen. The x-ray film outlines the kidneys, ureters, and bladder, demonstrating their size, shape, and position in relation to the structures in the pelvis and the lumbar spine. Radiopaque calculi, calcified areas of renal tissue, and soft tissue masses can be observed on a KUB.

Tomography is a body sectioning x-ray technique that is useful for diminishing the shadows of other organs on the x-ray. It is performed to determine kidney size and the presence of masses. (The normal kidney is about 12 cm in length.)

The **intravenous pyelogram (IVP)** utilizes an organic iodine such as Conray-400 or

Hypaque, which is excreted by glomerular filtration, as a contrast medium to visualize the size and shape of the renal calyces and pelvis. It is contraindicated if the patient is hypersensitive to iodine or has myeloma. In the latter, proteins can be precipitated in the collecting ducts of the kidney, which can result in renal failure. Iodine sensitivity skin tests are done prior to the use of iodine dyes. However, the nurse should be aware that negative skin tests do not always ensure that hypersensitivity reactions will not occur.

Preparation for an IVP consists in restricting fluids from at least midnight on so that the patient will be somewhat dehydrated; this restriction facilitates concentration of the contrast medium and results in better visualization. A laxative or enema is given the night before to remove flatus and fecal material from the bowel that might interfere with visualization. The test begins with intravenous injection of the contrast medium, followed by x-rays at intervals of 2, 5, 10, and 15 minutes. X-rays are taken for longer periods of time if there is a delay in concentration of the contrast medium. If effective renal function is questioned, a double dose of contrast medium is given to ensure concentration. If only faint shadows can be determined on x-ray it can be assumed that the medium has been poorly concentrated, and it may indicate an impairment in renal function. Sometimes the patient is so nervous about having the IVP that his degree of stress reaction causes diuresis. The IVP may then be repeated at a later time with normal results. A delay of the appearance of contrast medium on one side is indicative of renal artery disease. An IVP cannot effectively be used to visualize the urinary tract in uremic states and may in fact be contraindicated if there is kidney pathology.

A **timed sequence IVP** involves filming every 5 minutes following injection of the contrast medium. Normal kidneys concentrate the dye more quickly than diseased kidneys. **Retrograde pyelography** involves injection of contrast media into each kidney via a catheter inserted into the uretha for x-ray visualization of the renal pelvis calyces, the ureter, and bladder.

Renogram

A renogram or scan is a qualitative examination of the kidney's functional status. Radioactive substances selectively concentrated in the kidney, such as ^{131}I orthoiodohippurate (Hippuran) are given intravenously. After injection of the radioactive substance, the radiation emitted is recorded on a time curve. The resulting renogram gives information about the rate at which the substance is secreted into the proximal tubule fluid. This demonstrates renal blood flow to the kidney, the secretory capacity of the proximal tubular cells, and urinary output. Because the radioisotopes are readily circulated through functioning renal tissue, normal tissue will show up on the renogram. Cysts, calculi, and necrotic tumors with no blood supply cannot concentrate the isotope. The renogram can be used, to some extent, to differentiate between vascular and nonvascular lesions, as well as to define the size, shape, and position of masses. The nonvascular lesions are often called "cold spots" on the renogram.

Renal Angiogram

Angiography is performed to visualize the renal arteries. The patient must sign a consent form for this procedure. A renal angiogram can demonstrate stenosis, distortion of the vessels by either tumors or cysts, and opaque vascular tumors. A radiopaque medium is injected into the aorta above the renal arteries or directly into the renal artery through the femoral artery. X-rays are taken after injection. This is one of the most uncomfortable and hazardous tests for determining renal dysfunction. Care must be taken to observe the patient for allergic reactions, since anaphylactic shock could ensue from the radiopaque medium. There is also the possibility that the arterial system might be damaged during angiography, particularly if the patient has diseased kidneys. Following a renal angiogram the patient should remain in bed for 2 to 3 hours. Pulses in the lower extremities should be frequently checked to determine whether circulation has been impaired, and the patient should be carefully monitored for other signs of circulatory distress such as tachycardia and hypotension.

Cystoscopy

Cystoscopy is a procedure that uses instrumentation to examine the urinary tract. The patient is prepared as for surgery and must sign a consent form prior to cystoscopy.

It can be combined with x-ray studies to examine the urinary tract, the renal pelvis, and calyces. Cystoscopy is particularly valuable as a diagnostic tool when an IVP is contraindicated or is ineffective. As with the IVP, preparation for a cystoscopy includes giving enemas so that fecal material and flatus are removed. The patient is premedicated before cystoscopy and may have a general or local anesthetic. A general anesthetic is often given because it is important that the patient remain quiet during the examination, since jerking or moving about could result in damage to the urinary tract by the instruments. The patient is placed in the lithotomy position on a cystoscopy table with his feet in stirrups, and the cystoscope is inserted through the urethra to the bladder. The cystoscope is a hollow metal tube with both a light and a magnifying lens so that the internal bladder and urethra can be examined. The bladder capacity can be measured and the presence of diverticuli (sacs formed by herniation of the bladder wall) can be observed. Sterile water can be used to irrigate and distend the lower portion of the urinary tract, demonstrating obstructions or ureteral reflux. Ureteral catheters can also be inserted to remove urine directly from the kidneys or to insert a contrast medium for retrograde pyelography of the kidney calyces, pelvis, and ureters. This procedure is contraindicated if the patient has allergies or renal function pathology.

A cystoscopy becomes a therapeutic procedure when done to fulgurate bleeding areas, to excise diverticula or tumors with a resectoscope, or to remove stones. Antibiotics can be inserted directly into the kidney or bladder during cystoscopy. Catheters may be left in place for purposes of draining urine if there is an obstruction, or for flushing the urinary tract. The patient may have both a Foley and a ureteral catheter. A ureteral catheter can easily be recognized because it is a very small, fine catheter similar to a guitar string. The catheters are carefully secured to prevent pulling or tension so that they are not dislodged.

Following a cystoscopic examination, the patient may be very uncomfortable. Back pain and bladder spasms may be experienced following instrumentation. In addition the patient may have a feeling of fullness or burning in the bladder and the urine will probably be lightly pink tinged. He may have muscle soreness from the lithotomy position, which places pressure on the back. Care involves comfort measures and general postanesthetic care. Fluids should be forced following a cystoscopy. When catheters are left in place, the nurse should know where they are placed and their purpose in order to give appropriate care. The nurse should be aware that the kidney pelvis only holds 5 ml of fluid; damage can result to the tissues from irrigation with more than 5 ml, and the risk of infection is great. Therefore ureteral catheters should not be irrigated, because of their proximity to the kidney, whereas Foley catheters placed in the bladder may be irrigated. One problem encountered with a cystoscopic examination is that infection can be spread throughout the urinary tract by instrumentation. The nurse should be watchful for the symptoms of infection. Bleeding and perforation are two other complications requiring careful monitoring. Urine should be carefully checked periodically to ascertain changes in color. Hematuria and pain in the bladder area are significant symptoms that require immediate attention.

Renal Function Tests

A number of other forms of testing can be included in a urologic workup, including divided renal function tests, biopsy, and cystometry. Divided renal function tests are performed to measure glomerular filtration rates, renal blood flow, and sodium excretion. This procedure is done when stenosis of the renal artery is suspected. A catheter large enough to fill the entire lumen of the ureter is inserted to collect the urine from each kidney. The procedure may be dangerous if the patient has renal pathology.

Biopsy

Renal biopsy for histologic examination of tissue can be done via a skin puncture (percutaneous puncture) or an incision through the flank; the latter is generally safer because bleeding can be better controlled. The incision also allows for inspection of the kidneys, and a larger specimen can be obtained. When the skin puncture technique is used, an IVP is done prior to the biopsy to locate the kidneys and to set out guidelines for placing the needle by marking the skin. Because hemorrhage is a complication of biopsy, the patient's platelet count and bleeding and clotting times are obtained before the procedure. Patients with hypertension, disturbances in hemostatic mechanisms, and those with a single kidney should not have a biopsy. Other contraindications are the presence of tumors, hydronephrosis, and infection. Complications include the formation of arteriovenous fistulas, which generally heal spontaneously, and perinephric abscesses, which may form at the biopsy site. Follow-up care includes provision for rest and observation of the patient for indications of hemorrhage.

Cystometry

Cystometry is a procedure that is performed to measure bladder function. The bladder capacity, pressure, and sensation can be noted as well as the efficiency of micturition. This procedure is often used to measure bladder contractions in response to the pressure of urine when innervation to the bladder is impaired or when the detrusor muscle is damaged. A two-way urethral or suprapubic catheter is inserted, and water is placed into the bladder in measured amounts. The patient's first desire to void and his subsequent sensations of bladder fullness are noted in relation to the amount of water inserted. Accurate timekeeping is essential in making evaluations of bladder contractions in response to pressure.

Clearance, Concentration, and Dilution Tests

A number of additional diagnostic tests can be performed to measure renal function, including clearance, concentration, and dilution tests. Creatinine, urea, and inulin clearance tests are helpful in measuring glomerular filtration rates. The phenolsulfonphthalein (PSP) excretion test measures renal tubular excretion function. The PSP test is the easiest to perform and requires little time; the inulin clearance test is the most accurate and also the most complicated to perform. Creatinine and urea clearance tests are fairly accurate measures of glomerular filtration. These tests are explained in greater detail in the following paragraphs.

A blood urea nitrogen (BUN) test provides an approximate measure of renal function. The normal BUN level is 8 to 18 mg per deciliter [22]. It is not as accurate as blood creatinine levels because urea levels vary, the daily output being equal to the daily intake of dietary protein and protein catabolism. Creatinine production is more consistent.

Concentration and dilution tests measure the kidney's ability to concentrate urine when fluid intake is restricted and to dilute urine when intake is large. In the concentration test the patient prepares by ingesting a dry meal on the evening prior to the test and then taking no additional food or fluids until the test is completed. Fluid restriction is essential to the effectiveness of the test. On the morning of the test, urine samples are collected on consecutive hours, beginning with the time of the patient's first morning voiding. Accurate test results require that the time of voiding and the total amount of urine voided be recorded. The specific gravity of each sample should not be less than 1.024 if the kidneys are functioning normally. The dilution test is begun early in the morning. The patient voids and discards the first morning specimen and then drinks a liter of clear fluid such as water or diluted lemonade within a time span of 30 minutes. The urine samples are collected in hourly sequence. Again the time and amount of urine voided are both important. Normally the first specimen should have a specific gravity of 1.002, with the specific gravity increasing with each subsequent voiding.

Clearance tests, as previously mentioned, measure glomerular filtration rates and tubular excretion function. They are not accurate if the patient has residual urine that may have accumulated before the test was begun. Urea, creatinine, and inulin are used for clearance studies; they are all cleared by glomerular filtration and excreted by the tubules and can be measured in blood and urine. Urea, the end product of protein catabolism, is endogenous to the body. The urea levels vary as dietary protein is increased or decreased. Creatinine, which is also endogenous to the body, is produced primarily by musculoskeletal activity from creatine and phosphocreatine at consistent rates. Inulin, a polysaccharide, is exogenous to the body and must be given intravenously. Normal creatinine clearance is 115 ± 20 ml per minute; inulin clearance is normally 124 ± 25.8 ml per minute in men and 119 ± 12.8 ml per minute in women [22].

For urea clearance tests the patient usually has no breakfast and drinks at least 500 ml of water. The first voiding is discarded and a blood sample is taken. The time should then be noted. Exactly one hour later, the patient voids and another blood sample is taken. The serum and urine levels of urea are then used to calculate the amount of urea cleared by the kidneys in 1 hour.

Creatinine clearance tests are done over a defined time period, usually 24 hours. A blood sample is taken and a 24-hour urine specimen is collected. The blood sample may be taken at the beginning, middle, or end of the 24-hour period. In some protocols for this procedure the patient remains in bed during the test on the premise that the test results will be inaccurate if the patient is active, since muscular activity increases the production of endogenous creatinine.

The PSP test measures the function of renal tubules for excreting urine. The dye is given intravenously and is normally excreted rapidly by the tubules. A specified amount of water, usually 400 to 500 ml, is given and the patient then voids, discarding the urine. The dye is injected intravenously and urine specimens are then collected after 15 minutes, 30 minutes, 1 hour, and 2 hours. All urine from each voiding is saved. Timing is extremely important in determining test results; therefore, as with other tests, both the time of specimen collection and the amount of urine collected are significant. Normally 28 to 35 percent of the PSP is excreted during the 15 minute period following injection of the dye [22].

Pathology in the Urinary Tract and Kidney

All the assessment techniques just discussed are important in determining the presence or cause (or both) of pathology in the urinary tract and kidney. The different types of dysfunction are discussed more fully in the section that follows. This discussion is organized around the concept that almost all the causes of urinary tract dysfunction that interfere with the flow of urine do so because they obstruct the tract, either mechanically as with calculi, or because of inflammation, which narrows the tract. Other causes of obstruction include trauma or changes in the contour or structure of the tract from abnormal cell growth. Among the types of dysfunction included in this section are infection, urinary stone formation, and structural changes in the kidney, ureter, bladder, and urethra. The structural changes include those caused by changes in cell structure such as tumor growth, those caused by trauma, those that result from anomalies, and those related to either systemic or intrinsic renal disease.

Many types of urinary tract dysfunction are not noticed by the patient until the cumulative effects of the pathology result in infection or obstruction. In many cases the pathology is found on routine examination or when the patient receives treatment for another condition. As long as one kidney continues to function normally, the body's needs for elimination are met. This tends to hide asymptomatic conditions of dysfunction in the contralateral kidney. For this reason, irreversible kidney damage may have occurred before diagnosis is made. The end result of progressive urinary tract dysfunction is impairment of kidney function. As this progresses, the patient experiences renal failure. The kidneys gradually lose their ability to adapt to body needs for elimination of metabolic wastes. The retention of these wastes by the body requires that compensatory mechanisms come into play; when these are insufficient, the symptoms of renal failure ensue. Since chronic renal failure is life threatening, it is best to prevent its occurrence if at all possible. Knowledge about the possible causes of renal and urinary tract dysfunction makes the nurse alert to symptoms and signs of dysfunction that might otherwise go unnoticed.

INFECTIONS IN THE URINARY TRACT

There are many different causes of urinary tract pathology. Of all the different types that occur, infections are the most frequent. Infections may be iatrogenic or a result of any type of urinary tract dysfunction, or they may be independent of other pathology. Urinary tract infections are commonly encountered in all types of nursing practice since they can result from infectious processes that begin elsewhere in the body, or they may be a complication of systemic disease or immobility.

Infections that occur singly, without other diseases, are most commonly caused by entry of bacteria through the urinary meatus. Both the colon and perineum have similar flora, which can be a source of infection for the urinary tract. These microorganisms are primarily gram-negative [15]. Bacteria can enter through the urethra and can pass upward in the tract against the flow of urine. The infection is often preceded by some type of stress on the urethra, such as catheterization or other instrumentation that interferes with normal protective mechanisms. In women, intercourse, particularly initial experiences, makes the urethra prone to infection. The term "honeymoon cystitis" describes infection following initial intercourse. These initial infections may lead to recurrent infections, particularly during pregnancy (for example, acute pyelonephritis in the third trimester [13]). Other but less frequent sources of bacteria are the blood and lymph nodes. The capsular lymphatic vessels of the right kidney communicate with the right side of the colon so that bacteria can enter the kidney from the colon. Lymph flow from each kidney connects with the ureters, bladder, and external genitalia, allowing bacteria to spread along the urinary tract. Yet another source of bacteria is the left spermatic or ovarian vein, both of which drain in the left renal vein. The renal artery, which supplies the kidney with blood, can also be a source of bacterial invasion.

The patient's health status is a significant factor in the occurrence of urinary tract infections that accompany other diseases. Hypertension that is associated with renal disease as either a cause or a result, diabetes, collagen diseases, and kidney diseases all predispose to infection because of impairment of renal function. People with spinal cord injury or neurologic deficits such as myasthenia gravis and multiple sclerosis are subject to urinary tract infections because of the nervous and muscular impairment and the effects of immobility. Any condition that results in immobility predisposes a person to urinary tract infections.

Use of Catheters

Patients with debilitating diseases such as multiple sclerosis have associated urinary incontinence, particularly in the later stages of the disease, and require urinary drainage with a Foley or a coudé retention (indwelling) catheter (condoms may be used for males). Several factors must be considered by the nurse in caring for these patients. The patient should drink large quantities of water so that the urinary tract continues to be flushed from the inside out, so to speak. If the patient has a disease that alters mobility but does not preclude exercise, adequate oral intake of fluids is sufficient to flush the urinary tract. Indwelling catheters that are left in place for long periods of time may require irrigation if urinary sediments and mucus obstruct the catheter. Sterile technique must be observed when irrigating the catheter to minimize the possibility of introducing bacteria into the bladder. However, even with proper technique in irrigating the Foley catheter and with adequate fluid intake, the potential for urinary tract infection is high. For this reason, routine urine cultures should be done, sometimes as often as once a month for patients who are considered particularly prone to infection. Treatment is initiated if bacteriuria is present. If infections occur with frequency, prophylactic antibiotic therapy or urinary antiseptics are given for periods of 2 to 6 months, depending on the situation.

When a patient requires a retention catheter over a period of months or years, the frequency of changing the catheter depends on the patient's status and the function of the catheter. Care is always taken to ensure that sterile technique is observed when the catheter is inserted. Catheters that have been in place too long are difficult to remove from the bladder, since calcium deposits tend to form on the catheter so that it is covered with incrustations. In addition to holding the catheter in a fixed position in the bladder and urethra, calcium deposits can also lead to kidney stone formation. Male patients may develop urethritis if the catheter is left in place for long periods of time. The use of a retention catheter, particularly one that completely fills the urethra, impedes drainage of prostatic secretions so that they collect between the catheter and the lining of the urethra; these secretions augment the development of urethritis. This problem can be prevented by using a condom to provide for urine flow instead of a catheter. Care must be taken to fit the condom securely but not so tightly that circulation is impaired. The attachment of the drainage tube to the condom should be arranged so that there is at least 1 to 1½ inch of space between the distal end of the penis and the drainage tube. The condom is changed at least every 8 hours and the penis is carefully cleaned to prevent tissue irritation from accumulated secretions. Circulation and the integrity of the skin should be checked.

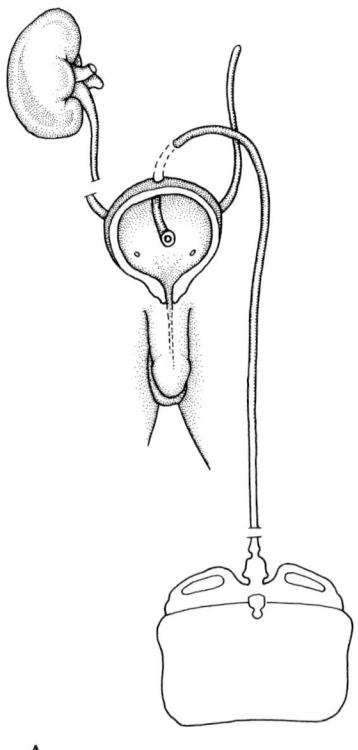

A

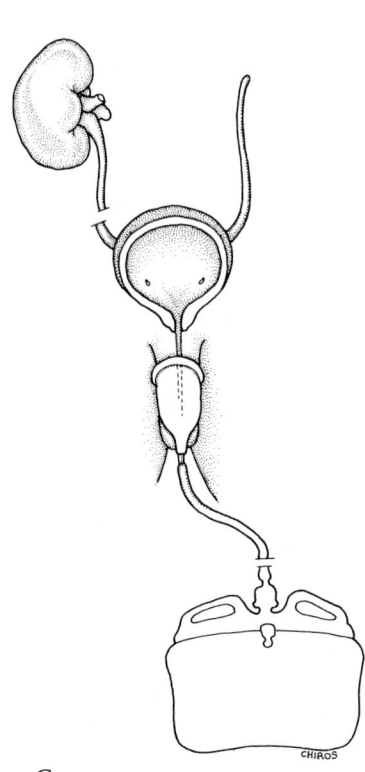

C

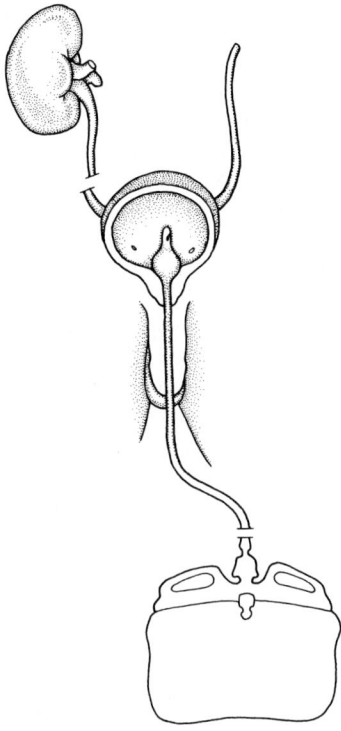

B

Figure 6-5
Three methods used to provide for urinary drainage: urethral catheter, condom, and suprapubic catheter. The drainage bag serves as a reservoir for urine.

Another method of providing for drainage from the urinary bladder is the insertion of a suprapubic tube. An opening is made in the bladder through the skin above the bladder and a tube is inserted to provide for drainage with less possibility of infection in males than with Foley catheter insertion. Sterile technique is followed when the suprapubic tube is irrigated. Drainage is generally better because the suprapubic tube has a larger lumen and there is less possibility of its becoming obstructed. Patients with a suprapubic tube should have a fluid intake of at least 3,000 ml per day to keep the urine dilute and to flush the urinary tract (Fig. 6-5).

Neurogenic Bladder

Bladder function is altered in many nervous system dysfunctions and in spinal cord trauma. **Neurogenic bladder** is the term used to describe loss of innervation of the bladder. When there is a lesion in the upper motor neurons, the bladder retains its reflex arc, and the detrusor muscle as well as the external sphincter may become spastic with the result that the muscles stretch and contract quickly and all of the urine may not be expelled (Fig. 6-6). Experimentation with implantation of electronic stimulators in the bladders of patients with upper motor neuron lesions is currently under way in some centers. Trauma or lesions of the lower motor neurons interrupt the reflex arc so that there is no way to provide for emptying the bladder. In this situation, the bladder expands and retains large amounts of urine in its flaccid state. Many nervous sytem diseases have localized effects that are not limited to either the upper or lower motor neurons, so there can be many variations of interruption in nervous innervation. For this reason, cystometric examinations are sometimes performed to ascertain the amount of control the patient has remaining. These data are then the basis for initiating a bladder training program that makes the best use of the patient's ability to control function.

A bladder training program makes use of the patient's remaining innervation, muscle activity, and bladder response to the pressure of urine. The training involves giving the patient a measured intake of 3,000 to 4,000 ml of fluid per day. A patient with upper motor neuron lesions can trigger the reflex arc by stroking sensitive zones. These zones are different for each person but usually are found on the inner thigh, the abdomen, or the genitalia. The triggering will activate the reflex arc and voiding can occur. The amount of residual urine is checked by catheter after the patient voids; if the residual amount is over 100 ml the catheter is replaced; if it is less than 100 ml, voiding is continued every 2 or 3 hours in a planned routine to "train the bladder."

If the patient has a lower motor neuron lesion, some form of assistance is required to substitute for the reflex arc. When the patient senses an urge to void, pressure is applied to the abdomen to contract the muscles. The Credé method is commonly used; this involves placing both hands at the level of the umbilicus and pressing downward toward the suprapubic area six or seven times in sequence. Then one hand is placed on top of the other just above the pubic arch, and firm pressure is applied to the bladder with an increase of pressure downward toward the perineal area as the bladder empties. This sequence is continued in a routine pattern to train the bladder.

Regaining control of bladder function is important to the patient's self-esteem and independence. Additional information about bladder training programs is found in Chapter 11. If feasible, the patient should be involved in monitoring his urinary tract function so that he becomes aware of the importance of adequate intake and output and actively participates in preventing urinary tract infection. Urine retention fosters the growth of bacteria with concomitant infections. Measures to prevent these infections include maintaining adequate fluid intake and output, taking acidifiers such as ascorbic acid to keep the urine acid, and using urinary antiseptics to minimize bacterial growth.

Reflux of Urine

A reflux of urine within the tract is another type of situation that has great potential for infection of the urinary tract. **Reflux** means backward flow; this generally occurs as a backward flow of urine from the bladder into the ureter and is known as vesicoureteral reflux. There may also be a flow of urine from the urethra to the bladder; in this instance, urine returns to the bladder, and the condition is called a urethrovesical reflux. The causes of reflux include congenital malformations in which the ureter or urethra is improperly attached to the bladder, changes in the cellular structure from disease so that the normal sphincter-like action does not occur, and changes that impair nervous or muscular function. A vesicoureteral reflux may occur as the urethra to the bladder; in this instance, a result of changes in the bladder that alter its size, shape, or capacity. Dilatation of the ureters or of the renal calyces may also contribute to loss of the control that prevents reflux. The backward flow of urine generally occurs when pressure in the bladder changes. Coughing or straining, as when having a

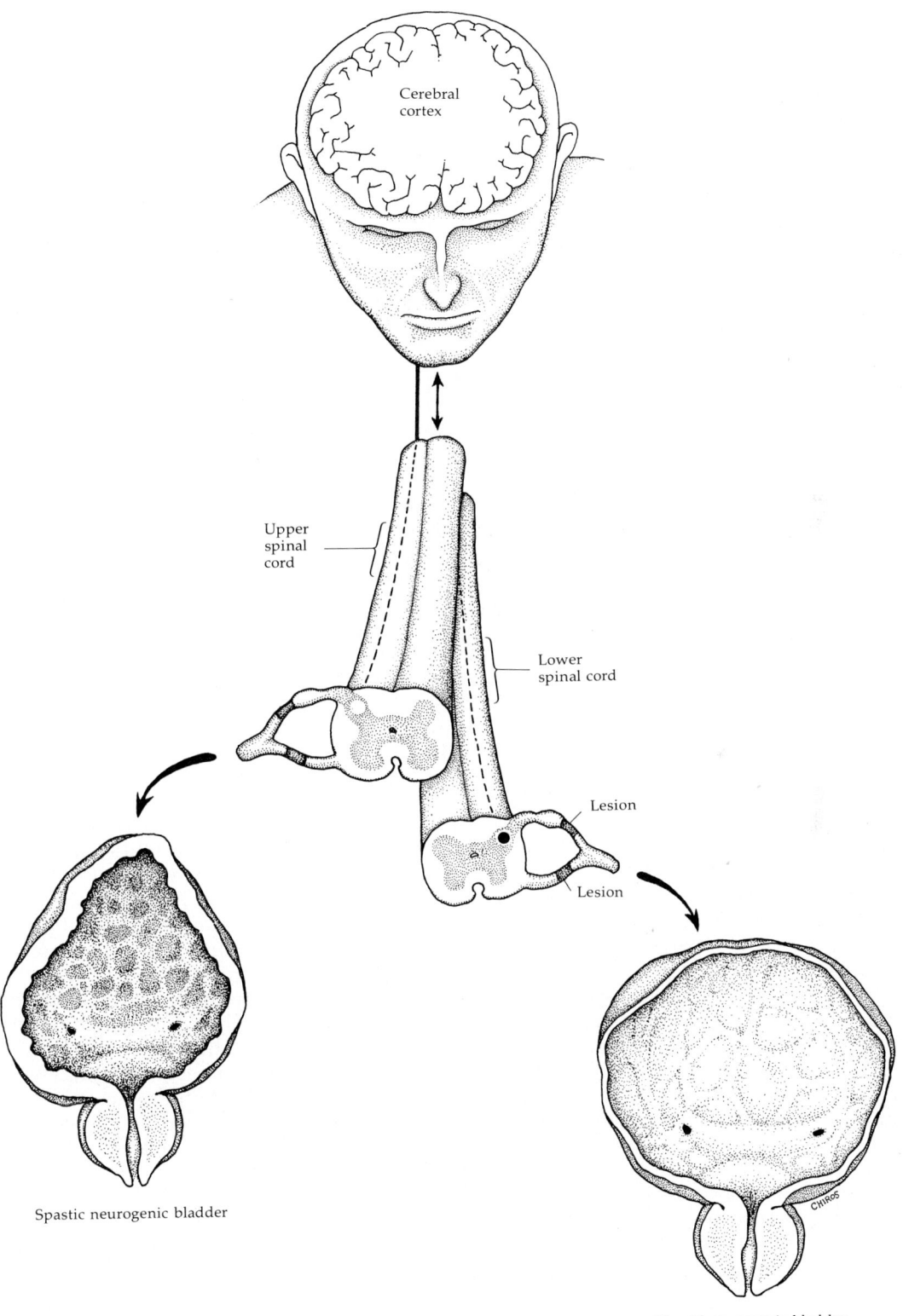

Figure 6-6
Comparison of site of lesion in upper and lower motor neuron bladders.

bowel movement or lifting heavy objects, exerts enough pressure to force the urine into the ureter or urethra. After the pressure in the bladder returns to normal, the urine flows back into the bladder; thus urine from the bladder has contaminated the ureters, or urine that has been in the urethra contaminates the bladder. In this way infection can spread through the tract.

Causative Organisms

Infections of the urinary tract are generally caused by gram-negative cocci. *Escherichia coli* is the most frequent causative organism; others are *Klebsiella, Enterobacteriaceae, Proteus,* and *Pseudomonas*. Enterococci, *Aerobacter, Staphylococcus,* and group B *Proteus* are usually the causative organisms when the abnormality is anatomic or a result of instrumentation. *Staphylococcus* infections are often related to focal infections in other parts of the body and may cause multiple abscesses or carbuncle formation within the urinary tract. Perinephric abscesses are frequently caused by staphylococci. *Proteus* can split urea, thereby liberating ammonia and resulting in alkalinization of urine, causing infections that are persistent and difficult to cure. Yeast infections occur in debilitated patients who have been treated with prophylactic doses of antibiotics so that the normal renal flora that would ordinarily prevent yeast growth is altered.

Certain factors either inhibit or increase the rate of bacterial growth. For example, bacteria grow more rapidly in concentrated urine than in dilute urine. Acid urine also inhibits growth; this is thought to be related to the diffusion of undissociated organic acids into bacterial cells, where a bacteriostatic action occurs. Optimal bacterial growth occurs with a pH of 6.0 to 7.0. Stagnant urine is an excellent medium for bacterial growth; for this reason urinary retention and infection are closely related.

Tuberculosis lesions may develop in the upper pole of the kidney when the tubercle bacillus spreads via the bloodstream. The tubercle bacillus can spread to the urinary tract, causing symptoms similar to those of other infections. In this case the urine will have an increased white blood count without bacteria.

Patient Assessment

Assessment of urinary tract infections is sometimes difficult because the symptoms are similar to those caused by other forms of dysfunction in the pelvic area. It is also difficult to ascertain the exact placement or extent of urinary tract infections because they can ascend to involve the entire tract. However, infections are often categorized according to the part of the tract that seems to be most involved; the terms used are **urethritis** (infection of the urethra), **cystitis** (infection of the bladder), **ureteritis** (infection of the ureters), and **pyelonephritis** (infection of the kidney pelvis). The majority of the symptoms are subjective, so a history and a confirming urinalysis or urine culture are the major assessment tools used in diagnosis.

The patient with a urinary tract infection is uncomfortable, the degree of discomfort often being a measure of the extent of the infection. Assessment of subjective symptoms is helpful in determining the site of the infection. For example, patients with urethritis will have dysuria, perhaps a urethral discharge, and burning on urination. Patients with cystitis may have all these symptoms together with a sense of urgency, frequency, nocturia, and pain. The pain is typically in the perineal and suprapubic areas and in the lower portion of the back. If the infection involves the ureters and the kidney pelvis, symptoms may also include pain in the flank, tenderness, and symptoms of systemic infection, including chills, fever, and malaise. Anorexia, nausea, and vomiting may also occur [15]. In pyelonephritis, the kidney pelvis is swollen and tense. The acute infection, which may be accompanied by tachycardia, requires attention to the patient's composite of symptoms, and the patient is often hospitalized. Pain is relieved with analgesics, fever is treated with antipyretics, and urine output is monitored. Measurements of all urine and body weights are important in monitoring output. In a few cases, bacteremic shock can be a complication of acute pyelonephritis.

It is possible, however, to have a urinary tract infection with either no symptoms or only minor discomfort. In some instances abnormal findings in a routine urinalysis are the first indication that an infection is present. Bacteriuria with a urine count of 100,000 bacteria per milliliter of urine is indicative of infection [13]. If an examination is done using spun urinary sediment, organisms of at least 30,000 colonies per milliliter are indicative of infection [15]; some authorities consider 10,000 colonies per milliliter significant of infection [13]. Urine culture and sensitivity tests identify the specific causative bacteria and the antibiotic that is most effective to treat that bacteria. Urine specimens for culture should be sent to the laboratory as soon as possible after they are obtained and should be refrigerated in the interim if there is a delay [15].

The presence of bacteria, protein, red blood cells, white blood cell casts, and pus in the urine indicates renal tubular infection.

Treatment

Treatment of urinary tract infections should begin as soon as the patient notices symptoms and must be carried out over a long enough period of time to ensure effectiveness. Nursing care includes management of the discomfort and teaching about medications and other measures that can be employed by the patient to prevent further infection. Because most patients with urinary tract infections care for themselves at home, the nurse's teaching role is vital.

The patient with a urinary tract infection should be well informed at the outset about the treatment procedures and about factors he can control to prevent reinfection or the recurrence of infection. Specific measures for relieving the discomfort of urinary tract infections include forcing fluids to flush the urinary tract, taking warm baths to relieve the pain, and taking analgesics if required for pain. Patients with systemic symptoms should rest in bed until the chills, fever, and general malaise disappear. Observation of progress toward recovery can be made by noting the frequency of voiding as well as discomfort related to voiding. Female patients with urethritis or cystitis should not use vaginal hygiene sprays and should abstain from intercourse until the symptoms subside.

Antibiotic therapy that is specific for the causative bacteria is started as soon as possible. The drugs most frequently used are streptomycin, kanamycin, neomycin, gentamicin, tetracycline, nitrofurantoin (Furadantin), methenamine mandelate (Mandelamine), ampicillin, and cycloserine (Seromycin). Urinary pH influences the effectiveness of all these antibiotics with the exception of ampicillin. The aminoglycoside antibiotics (given parenterally) including streptomycin, kanamycin, neomycin, and gentamicin are the most active in alkaline pH, whereas tetracycline, nitrofurantoin, and methenamine mandelate are more active in acid pH. In order to achieve the desired pH, ascorbic acid is given to acidify the urine or sodium bicarbonate to alkalize it. The cure rate is increased if the pH is appropriately monitored. In addition to the drugs just mentioned, nitrofurazone (Furacin) urethral suppositories are sometimes given along with a sulfonamide if the infection is localized in the urethra. Sulfonamides are often used for patients with initial urinary tract infections [13]. It is important that the patient have a high fluid intake when taking sulfonamides to reduce the deposition of sulfonamide crystals in the tubules.

There are variations in the routine used to give antibiotics for urinary tract infections, but usually the antibiotic is given for a period of 1 to 2 weeks. Seven days is the time span generally used for moderate infections. One week after the conclusion of the antibiotic therapy, the urine is recultured to evaluate the effects of treatment. If bacteria are still present, further antibiotic therapy is initiated. In acute infections, follow-up cultures are done at 3, 6, and 12 months following the infection [22].

The symptoms of urinary tract infections subside quickly once treatment is begun. There is a natural tendency for a patient to stop taking medication when he or she begins to feel well; however, a urinary tract infection can be evasive and very difficult to cure once started and unchecked. Even though the symptoms of an acute infection subside, the infection may be latent and can become chronic. If medication is discontinued before the infection has been cleared up, the infection has the potential for becoming chronic. Some infections, however, may disappear spontaneously. Chronicity usually develops over a period of time and is so gradual that the patient becomes accustomed to having occasional episodes of infection. Therefore very specific information should be given to the patient along with clear directions for follow-up cultures so that he or she continues taking medications and has follow-up cultures as prescribed.

Long-Term Consequences of Infection

The consequences of chronic urinary tract infections range from inconvenience and periodic discomfort over a long period of time to eventual serious disturbances in renal function. Chronic infection can cause cellular damage, resulting in the development of fibrous tissue; this may cause strictures in the urethra or the ureter or interstitial cystitis. Chronic pyelonephritis may lead to renal failure.

Interstitial cystitis is a condition most frequently found in older women. Localized patches of thickened plaques caused by chronic inflammation appear on the bladder wall; then ulceration and spread of the patches lead to fibrosis, which in turn causes contraction of the bladder tissue. The bladder capacity becomes smaller, affecting the flow of urine, and eventually renal insufficiency or hypertension may result. Chronic inflammation in the bladder is also the cause of two other conditions: cystitis cystica and malacoplakia. In the former, mucus forms in damaged deep tissues resulting eventually in the formation of cysts; in the latter condition, soft, yellowish, raised lesions are formed.

Chronic pyelonephritis causes progressive changes in the renal calyces and pelvis. The tissues of both become scarred, thickened, and fibrotic, and the entire kidney shrinks in size. In the late stages, the patient will have generalized symptoms of nausea, vomiting, muscle irritability, and gastrointestinal bleeding. These are the symptoms of chronic uremia; if the condition persists renal failure may develop, causing death. Patients with acute episodes of chronic pyelonephritis are often hospitalized and require exacting care in relation to the degree of infection and renal failure. In addition to comfort measures, specific treatment involves obtaining a culture from a ureteral urine sample obtained by cystoscopic examination. Antibiotic therapy given over a 6- to 8-month period is effective in reducing the frequency of acute attacks. Urinary antiseptics such as Mandelamine are also helpful. After the patient returns home, the nurse's role is one of supportive health teaching along with assistance to the patient in following the prophylactic measures that could prevent further attacks.

Because prostatic secretions seem to protect males from urinary tract infections, the occurrence of infections generally indicates the presence of an obstruction of the urinary tract, usually by an enlarged prostate. For this reason, a urologic workup and a rectal examination are performed after the initial infection has abated. The workup usually includes an intravenous pyelogram and perhaps a cystoscopic examination. A proctoscopic examination may be indicated to determine the presence of prostatic enlargement or of changes in the rectum and large intestine that may be impinging on the urinary tract, causing obstruction.

Urinary tract infections are expected in pregnant women, because the increasing size of the uterus can exert external pressure on the urinary tract so that infection results from obstruction. Another factor in the female's susceptibility to infection is the proximity of the urethra to the vagina and rectum. Sexually active women may have as many as three or four infections per year; more than this number generally indicates that there is some underlying pathology such as strictures or urinary stones. For this reason, a complete urologic and gynecologic workup is performed immediately after the second episode of infection has abated. The nurse should also be aware that urinary tract infections may be caused by systemic diseases. For example, an infection accompanied by vulvitis is an early indication of diabetes, especially when the urine contains albumin and glucose.

It is possible for a person to become reinfected with another organism or to have a recurrent infection caused by the same organism. Some people are particularly susceptible to urinary tract infections for unknown reasons; they must learn how to care for themselves in order to minimize the number of episodes. These infection-prone people may take a minimum dose of a prescribed antibiotic for a 3- or 4-month period (several different antibiotics may be given in sequence to prevent resistance to any one). The dosage is increased to therapeutic levels if the person begins to feel the onset of an active or acute infection. Another method of prevention includes the long-term use of a urinary antiseptic or medication to acidify the urine. Some women find that infections can be avoided by taking an antibacterial agent following intercourse. The prophylactic needs of patients with chronic infections and of debilitated or immobilized patients are met by taking routine urine cultures, sometimes as often as once a month, and by actively treating infections as they occur. Prophylactic antibiotic therapy may be used along with adequate fluid intake and attention to elimination to prevent retention of urine. The importance of maintaining adequate fluid intake cannot be overemphasized for anyone who is susceptible to a urinary tract infection. The nurse should remind the patient that fluid (urine) flushes the urinary tract and is thus an important mechanism in keeping the tract free from bacteria.

Infection in the pelvic organs can cause a perinephric abscess; this may also be caused by trauma during diagnostic procedures such as a renal biopsy. The symptoms of perinephric abscess arise from distortion of the renal collecting system and are therefore similar to those of pyelonephritis. Care generally includes rest and antibiotic therapy.

OBSTRUCTION OF THE URINARY TRACT

As with infection, obstruction of the urinary tract is a complication common to most of the pathologic conditions that impede the flow of urine. Urinary calculi can block the passage of urine. Tissue changes such as tumors, cysts, and strictures can change the size and shape of the ureters, the kidney pelvis and calyces, the bladder, or the urethra. Obstruction of urine flow can occur in any of these sites. External pressure caused by an abdominal mass or an enlarged prostate can impinge on the urinary tract, creating an obstruction. The effects of the obstruction depend on where it occurs in the tract, the degree to which it impedes the flow of urine, and the length of time it lasts. Initial effects of the obstruction are similar to those that occur when any tube conducting liquid is obstructed; when a liquid cannot flow freely through a tube, there is backup of the fluid. In the case of the urinary tract, urine collects above the obstruction and distends that area of the tract. Urine continues to be produced, and the pressure increases because of the increased volume. The muscles in the involved area exert increased pressure in an effort to overcome the obstruction. If the obstruction persists, the muscles will gradually hypertrophy, and the increased pressure of urine above the obstruction will cause tissue damage. As this damage progresses, normal tissue is replaced with fibrous tissue, impairing function even further. The urinary retention caused by an obstruction in the tract can lead to serious consequences, since any obstruction, if untreated, can lead to renal failure. The backup of urine eventually reaches the kidney, and the nearer the obstruction to the kidney, the greater is the seriousness of the effects.

An obstruction in the neck of the bladder or in the urethra first causes dilatation of the bladder. If long-standing, the dilatation leads to hypertrophy of the bladder wall, and diverticula may form in the weak areas of the bladder wall (a diverticulum is a small sac or pouch created by herniation of mucous membranes). Because of the obstruction, urine flow is impeded. The bladder responds by increasing the strength of contractions to push the urine through or around the obstruction. However, the bladder does not fully empty and some urine remains in the bladder. Eventually the muscle fibers of the bladder become overstretched, causing trabeculation (a basketwork-like appearance of the overlapping enlarged muscle fibers) so that the normal distensibility of the bladder is impaired.

When the obstruction is in the bladder, the symptoms are generally easier to assess than those in the upper urinary tract. There will be distention of the bladder, noted by dullness on percussion or by palpation, and the patient will experience hesitancy on urination despite a strong feeling that he needs to void. Urine may pass in an intermittent stream that is decreased in both size and force. If the obstruction is long-lasting, the dilatation will eventually extend to the renal pelvis and calyces, impairing renal function. The kidney changes can be reversed if the obstruction is eliminated. Renal blood flow can then increase to normal and the renal function improves.

When the obstruction occurs in the ureter, **hydroureter** or distention of the ureter above the obstruction results. When this distention progresses, **hydronephrosis** results. In this condition, the ureter, the renal pelvis, and calyces dilate and may in time merge into one another, losing their normal structure. The distended tissues that remain appear as a thin, atrophied capsule as the pressure or urinary retention gradually destroys the normal tissue. The kidney continues to produce urine even when hydronephrosis exists. Some urine retained above an obstruction can be reabsorbed at the pelvic-ureteral junction through the lymph nodes and veins and, if the pressure is great enough, through extravasation into kidney tissues. Reabsorption can prevent rupture up to a point. Only vascular endothelium and pelvic epithelium separate the blood and the urine at the pelvic-ureteral junction.

The symptoms of obstruction above the bladder can be minimal or severe. A "silent" hydronephrosis can exist without symptoms as long as the other kidney carries on normal renal function. A sudden obstruction causes colicky pain similar to that experienced in an "acute abdomen," while a gradually developing obstruction causes pain in the abdomen or loin. Drinking fluids aggravates this pain because of the increased dilatation above the obstructed areas. Presenting symptoms include infection or urinary stone formation related to the stagnation of urine blocked from flowing by the obstruction.

An acute obstruction in the kidney brings about an immediate increase in renal blood flow followed by a decrease. The decreased blood flow then results in anoxia and tissue destruction, with the renal tubules and glomeruli being damaged so that renal failure ensues. A complete obstruction of urine flow results in anuria.

Treatment of obstructions includes relieving symptoms and removing the cause of the obstruction. If the obstruction is at the level of the bladder, drainage of urine can be accomplished via a suprapubic cystostomy, which involves placing a catheter into an opening made in the bladder via the pubic area above the bladder. If the obstruction is higher, a nephrostomy or a ureterostomy may be performed by placing a catheter into the kidney or ureter respectively. These measures relieve the pressure and prevent further renal function disturbances while more definitive treatment is carried out. The final treatment depends on the underlying cause of the obstruction, which may include changes in structure because of tumors, the presence of stones, or congenital anomalies.

Tumors

Tumors are often the cause of urinary tract obstruction. Renal adenocarcinoma arises from mature renal tissue and is most common in adults, affecting males in the 50- to 70-year age group more than females. A renal tumor in immature renal tissue is called a nephroblastoma or Wilms' tumor [7]; the majority of these tumors occur in children under the age of 3. Renal adenocarcinoma includes all tumors arising from the renal epithelium. These are highly vascular tumors that metastasize through the bloodstream to the lung, bone, liver, and other organs. Renal tumors can be silent and are often diagnosed only when a chest x-ray shows scattered small tumor sites in the lungs. "Cotton ball" and "cannon ball" are terms used to refer to the tumors in the lungs that are associated with renal tumors. Transitional cell carcinomas arise from tissue in the renal pelvis and calyces. Often these tumors begin as transitional cell papillomas, which have a great tendency to become malignant. Approximately 95 percent of renal tumors are malignant [1].

In order to interpret pathology reports and to understand the patient's prognosis, the nurse should be familiar with the nomenclature used to describe tumors. Efforts are presently being made to standardize the classification of renal tumors, which are now evaluated in different ways. One method is to grade tumors from grades I to IV, with grade I being differentiated cell tumors and grade IV being undifferentiated cell tumors. Another classification is that of staging tumors anatomically; in this method **grade IA** tumors are intracapsular, **grade IB** tumors are intrarenal but extracapsular, **grade II** tumors are perinephric microscopic, **grade III** tumors are perinephric gross, and **grade IV** tumors include distant metastases. The patient's prognosis becomes increasingly grave in relation to the extent of the tumor. Yet another evaluation staging is the tumor, node, and metastasis (TNM) classification, which is based on radiography. **T** refers to the tumor itself, with **T0** indicating no primary tumor, **T1** indicating normal kidney size, **T2** indicating enlarged kidney without deformity or displacement, **T3** indicating enlarged kidney with either deformity or decreased mobility, and **T4** indicating enlarged kidney with no mobility. **N** refers to the lymph nodes: **N0** indicates no change in regional nodes and **N1** indicates changes in nodes. **M** refers to metastasis: **M0** means no metastasis and **M1** indicates that there is distant metastasis; **M1a** means single metastasis whereas **M1b** means multiple metastases.

When a tumor has extended to the renal veins, the prognosis is poor. A good prognostic factor is the degeneration and calcification of the tumor, which means that the tumor is localized. Renal carcinoma may regress spontaneously after removal of a primary tumor elsewhere in the body, or it can regress and then recur as long as 20 years after the primary tumor is removed. Because renal tumors can be silent for long periods of time, it is often difficult to ascertain where the primary tumor is—in the kidney or elsewhere in the body. Some renal tumors have rapid growth rates whereas others grow slowly.

The symptoms of renal tumors are first hematuria, then weakness, fatigue, malaise, anorexia, and weight loss, and finally flank pain. The patient may have fever, or anemia. All, some, or none of these symptoms may be present; if all are present, the tumor is usually advanced. Treatment for kidney tumors is surgical removal of the entire kidney and sometimes also the ureter and the cuff of the bladder in a procedure called nephroureterocystectomy. The adrenal gland, perirenal fat, and adjacent lymph nodes are removed in the radical surgical procedure. Renal tumors are resistant to irradiation.

Benign tumors of the kidney include hemangioma, leiomyoma, and lipoma, all of which originate in connective tissue. Again, hematuria is the most common symptom.

The bladder is the most frequent location of urinary tract tumors. Bladder tumors occur most frequently in males [19] and are usually malignant. It is sometimes difficult to differentiate between a bladder tumor and a prostatic tumor in males because the symptoms are almost identical. Initial symptoms are hematuria (the predominant symptom), enuresis, and dysuria. The three-phase urine specimen is a significant diagnostic test: if hematuria is present in all three phases, continuous bleeding is present. If hematuria is limited to the first phase, blood has collected in the bladder; if it is limited to the last phase, the bleeding is caused by contraction. The later symptoms are those of obstruction of the tract. Bladder tumors can be visualized by cystoscopy; some can be palpated rectally.

Bladder tumors can be benign or malignant and are generally transitional cell tumors. Benign papillomas in the bladder have a high incidence of recurring after removal and of becoming malignant. Sessile carcinomas and undifferentiated carcinomas are two other types of bladder tumors. The majority of bladder tumors are located in the trigone and obstruct the flow of urine leaving the bladder; the second most common site is the posterior wall of the bladder. The prognosis depends on the degree of infiltration of the tumor into the bladder wall. The incidence of bladder tumors seems to be greater in people exposed to certain chemicals such as betanaphthylamine from aniline dyes, in people exposed to rubber or pitch, and in people who smoke cigarettes.

Other Causes of Obstruction

Ureteral diverticula are another form of obstruction; they occur congenitally in females and usually result from injury in males. Diverticula cause dribbling of urine because they can fill during micturition and empty after voiding has been completed. They can become infected or contain stones. Treatment sometimes involves teaching the patient to empty the diverticula by pressure at the termination of voiding.

A growth that appears in the urethra of females is the urethral caruncle, which is usually a small swelling at the external meatus. These caruncles, which consist of vascular granulation tissue, appear red and are similar to polyps. Treatment usually involves excision.

A common cause of obstruction in males is hypertrophy of the prostate gland. This gland lies immediately beneath the bladder, and the urethra passes through it. An enlarged prostate gland (benign prostatic hypertrophy) can impair the action of the sphincter at the neck of the bladder, or it can impinge on the bladder externally. For this reason, the symptoms of bladder tumors and tumors of the prostate are similar. Both kinds of tumors can often be palpated in a rectal examination. Normal function of the prostate gland depends on androgens, particularly testosterone. These hormones cause a gradual enlargement of the prostate throughout life, and consequently men in the 70-year-old age group often have prostate enlargement great enough to impinge on the urinary tract. Carcinoma of the prostate is also a cause of urinary tract dysfunction. Early signs of prostatic hypertrophy include hesitancy and intermittency of urination. The man has difficulty beginning urination and feels the need to strain to urinate. The urinary stream may be narrow, and he may find that he has to get up from sleep several times to urinate. In addition to these symptoms, the man may experience pain in the kidney areas in the back as a result of the back pressure from the distended bladder. A prostatectomy is the desired treatment for benign prostatic enlargement. Hormonal therapy is usually employed to treat prostatic carcinoma because it often is too far advanced for surgical treatment by the time it is found. An indication of metastasis is an elevated serum acid phosphatase level or osteoblastic metastases or both. Prostatic carcinoma usually extends to invade the surrounding structure, including the neck of the bladder, the urethra, and the veins and lymphatic vessels in the area [18].

Treatment for Tumors

Surgery is the primary mode of treatment for tumors in the urinary system. Removal of tumors that invade the renal parenchyma or bladder tissue is desirable. There are several different approaches to selection of the type of surgery, depending on the individual patient. Radiation therapy is also used in treating bladder tumors in combination with surgical procedures. If the tumor is confined to the urethra, the amount of tissue surgically removed depends on the extent of invasion and the type of tumor. Squamous cell tumors that are localized are simply removed by a partial urethrectomy whereas adenocarcinoma requires more extensive surgery.

A nephrectomy is performed for renal tumors involving the nephrons. A ureterectomy is performed along with the nephrectomy for tumors involving the renal pelvis and calyces. These procedures are done only after the patient's total renal function has been thoroughly evaluated. If one kidney is functioning well and the other is diseased, the nephrectomy can be performed with no interference with renal function; the remaining functioning kidney will be able to carry the entire load of renal function for the body. In fact, when kidney disease has been progressive in the excised kidney, the contralateral kidney has probably already taken over the entire load for function. If, however, the extensive evaluation of the contralateral kidney's function reveals disease in this kidney as well, the decision about treatment becomes complicated. In situations in which function is borderline and there is a possibility of controlling tumor growth without excision, conservative measures are usually taken. When both kidneys are diseased and nonfunctioning, the patient's renal function must be provided for by dialysis. If the patient's health status permits it, renal transplant may be performed.

Nursing care with nephrectomy Preoperative care for patients undergoing a nephrectomy is similar to that required for any surgery, as described on page 82. The patient should be informed that the remaining kidney has an amazing capacity for adapting to the tasks of carrying out the body's total need for urine elimination. Careful monitoring of urine output postoperatively is important in ascertaining kidney function; an output of less than 30 ml per hour may indicate renal failure and is significant. Body weight is taken daily both preoperatively and postoperatively. Although it does not occur frequently, hemorrhage is another serious complication, and the patient is checked for signs of hemorrhage during the postoperative period. A decreased blood pressure, rapid and weak pulse, or the appearance of clotting or profuse drainage of blood at the incision site indicates hemorrhage.

Following nephrectomy it can be expected that the patient will have muscle soreness, since the surgical procedure generally requires the patient to lie on his side in a hyperextended position to provide maximum visibility of the kidney and its surrounding structures through a flank incision. If the operation involves extensive repair of the renal blood supply or includes radical excision of the kidney and surrounding structures, or if the patient has a respiratory or cardiac disturbance, a thoracoabdominal incision is made [4]. In this situation the patient will return from surgery with chest tubes and is observed for signs of respiratory distress. The possibility of pneumothorax or perforation of the pleura in this type of surgery is a concern postoperatively.

Care of the wound is an important nursing function following any type of surgery with skin incisions. Following renal surgery the wound must be observed. Depending on the procedure used, there may be drains in the wound. The nurse should monitor the amount and type of drainage and the wound should be kept dry through dressing changes as necessary.

In addition to monitoring the urinary output and watching for the signs and symptoms of hemorrhage and respiratory distress, the nurse should give the patient who has had a nephrectomy care similar to that required by any major surgery. Turning, coughing, and deep-breathing exercises and early ambulation are important to prevent postanesthetic complications. Because renal tumors occur most frequently in patients who are also susceptible to cardiac and respiratory diseases, and because the tumors are often located near the diaphragm, the patient's total condition must be considered in both preoperative and postoperative care.

Treatment of bladder tumors Bladder tumors can be excised during cystoscopy by fulguration or by excision with a resectoscope if they are localized and noninvasive. The size and shape of bladder tumors facilitate removal by these methods, since they often occur as either multiple fronds or as papillae on stalks that can be snipped off at the bladder wall. Bladder tumors have a high rate of recurrence so that excision may have to be repeated frequently. The patient is advised to have frequent follow-up examinations to monitor the recurrence. Benign tumors tend to become malignant, and bladder tumors "seed" readily so that implantation of tumor cells in the bladder wall may occur during surgery. If the bladder tumor has invaded the wall but has not extended to include the entire bladder, a segmental resection of the bladder may be performed; this procedure may require a ureteral reimplantation, depending on the location of the segments involved. Whenever possible, the function of the bladder as a storage area for urine is preserved.

Another procedure for removal of large bladder tumors is through a suprapubic incision. A patient who has undergone this procedure will have a Foley catheter in place postoperatively. To prevent pressure, this catheter in the bladder is not irrigated, although it sometimes becomes plugged. It is necessary to remove the plugs, which might obstruct urine flow to prevent retention of urine. Milking or squeezing the tubing may be sufficient to facilitate passage of the plug. If irrigation is necessary to maintain the patency of the catheter, only small amounts of normal saline solution are used, and care must be taken not to apply pressure when irrigating.

RADIATION THERAPY Radiation therapy for bladder tumors involves the destruction of tumor cells by contact with radium or isotopes or by supervoltage irradiation. The placement, size, and extent of tumor growth all determine the approach used. Internal radiation is prescribed for more localized tumors, whereas external radiation is generally used for tumors that have metastasized. Often external radiation is used for palliation rather than for cure. The number of treatments, the dosage, and the area radiated are determined by each patient's needs, which include the resistance of the tumor to irradiation. One complication of radiation therapy is radiation cystitis, which may later necessitate a cystectomy if the impairment is severe enough.

Internal radiation can be accomplished by placing radium in the bladder in proximity to the tumor. One method involves a suprapubic cystotomy; with this procedure, placement can be visualized to ensure that the radium is in best contact with the tumor. The radium is placed in the balloon of a Foley catheter, which remains in the bladder until the desired dose is achieved. The first application is usually followed by a second application of lesser dosage and shorter duration. Evaluation of the tumor by biopsy determines the duration of radiation required to destroy the tumor. Another method for internal radiation is implantation of radon seeds into the bladder wall. This method is used less frequently than formerly, having been replaced by the technique of inserting radium in the balloon of a Foley catheter. Another method for internal radiation involves instilling a solution of colloidal gold (^{198}Au) into the bladder and leaving it in place for 2 to 3 hours, depending on the desired dose. A Foley catheter is placed in the bladder so that the bladder neck is obstructed; this prevents drainage of the solution during treatment. Prior to instillation of the colloidal gold solution, the patient must abstain from fluids for at least 12 hours so that dilution of the gold solution by urine is minimized.

CHEMOTHERAPY There has been experimentation with chemotherapy to treat bladder tumors, involving the instillation of chemotherapeutic agents into the bladder. Instillations of thiotepa (an alkylating agent) have proved useful for some bladder papillomas, although the effectiveness of this procedure is variable. Generally chemotherapy is used following excision of tumors as a prophylactic measure.

SURGERY When tumors are advanced, having invaded the bladder wall and metastasized to surrounding tissues, a cystectomy may be performed. Depending on the extent of the tumor growth, a simple or a radical cystectomy may be performed. A simple cystectomy is removal of the bladder with a urinary diversion procedure. Many physicians believe that a radical cystectomy (removal of the lymph nodes and urethra as well as the prostate and seminal vesicles in males and the uterus, fallopian tubes, and ovaries in females) provides for the best cure. The urethra is the first site of recurrence of tumor growth following a simple cystectomy. Radiation therapy may be given either before or after the cystectomy, or both before and after, depending on the method of treatment the physician uses and on the patient's condition.

A cystectomy, particularly if it involves radical surgery, is a life-threatening procedure. The patient who is about to undergo this operation can be expected to be anxious. He or she will experience body image changes because of the need to divert urinary flow, and these changes may be difficult to accept. It is important that the nurse deal actively with the patient's emotions and feelings during preparation for surgery. The patient may realistically anticipate death as an outcome; although this is a possibility, care should be future oriented and the patient should be prepared during the preoperative period for the postoperative phase of treatment. Involving the patient in the preparation for surgery by explaining the importance of the preparatory measures and discussing these measures with the patient provides an opportunity for the patient to express anxieties and fears about the surgical procedure and the changes this procedure will bring about in his or her life.

URINARY DIVERSION PROCEDURES Different procedures can be used to divert the flow of urine when required for treatment of bladder cancer, invasive cancer of the cervix, radiation cystitis, or other nonmalignant pathology such as neurogenic bladder and congenital anomalies. Currently the most commonly used procedure is the **ileal conduit,** made from a section of the ileum. However, sigmoid colonic, or retroperitoneal jejunal conduits are other approaches. Nursing care in all these procedures is similar. Still another diversion procedure is ureterostomy.

In the ileal conduit procedure a 6- to 8-inch portion of the ileum is separated from the intestine (keeping the mesentery and nerve supply intact) and is used to form a conduit into which the ureters are implanted. The remaining small intestine is anastomosed to restore continuity of the bowel. The segment that forms the conduit is closed at the proximal end, the distal end of the conduit is brought to the skin, and a stoma is then fashioned to form an external opening for urinary flow. The conduit is constructed for urine flow and is not a reservoir for urine. Peristalsis of the segment of the ileum is directed to the skin to assist the flow of urine in that direction. A second procedure, **cutaneous ureterostomy,** involves direct implantation of the ureters into the skin, making either one or two small stomas on the skin with the terminal ends of the ureters. The ureters may be joined so that there is only one stoma, or each ureter may be brought to the skin separately, forming two stomas. A third procedure, **ureterosigmoidostomy,** involves implanting the ureters into the large bowel, which is left intact so that both urine and feces are eliminated rectally. A variation of this procedure is the formation of an isolated rectal pouch into which the ureters are implanted. Either a separate anal colostomy for urine elimination or a dry colostomy for fecal elimination (with urine elimination from the rectal pouch through the anus) may be part of the procedure.

In some instances when the tumor has metastasized and extensive removal of pelvic organs is required, a **wet colostomy** is performed; this involves implanting the ureters into the bowel and forming a stoma for elimination of both urine and feces (Fig. 6-7). A **vesicotomy** (cystostomy) provides for elimination of urine via a stoma fashioned from the bladder wall following suturing of the bladder wall to the abdominal wall. In **total pelvic exenteration** (Chap. 9), the patient may have two stomas—one for urinary diversion and the other for fecal diversion.

All procedures for urinary diversion are potentially dangerous because the normal protective mechanisms of the bladder and the urethra no longer exist. In these procedures the ureters are placed in nonsterile body parts, there are no pressure gradients as in the normal urinary tract, and urine flows in the direction of least pressure because reflux is not prevented. Therefore infection is a major concern, not only because of the possibility of reflux, but also because bacteria can travel from the skin or the bowel to the kidney. Each of the urinary diversion procedures has certain advantages and disadvantages for the patient, and each necessitates learning to perform what was previously a normal and automatic mode of elimination.

PREOPERATIVE PREPARATION Preparation for surgery with any of the diversion procedures involving the bowel requires the same kind of preoperative care necessary in any type of bowel surgery. This care includes antibiotics to reduce the bacteria in the bowel and cleaning the bowel of fecal material by taking cathartics and enemas. The patient reduces his food intake by ingesting a clear liquid diet during the 24 hours prior to surgery. The patient should actively participate in this bowel preparation if he is able, first by understanding the reasons for the preparatory measures, and then by participating in selection of appropriate foods for his diet and the scheduling of the cathartics and enemas in relation to his other activities and sleep habits.

An important aspect of preparation of the patient having an ileal conduit or a cutaneous ureterostomy is acquainting him or her with the appliances that will be used postoperatively for urine collection. The appliances may be applied preoperatively to orient the patient to their use if the patient is well enough to learn before the operation. Expectations for the postoperative period will be more realistic if the patient is oriented to appliances preoperatively. Preoperative selection of an appropriate stoma site is essential to ensure successful management postoperatively. Positive planning for the future may facilitate the patient's acceptance of the change in body image he or she is about to experience. The hope for life that the operation offers as well as the relief from pain or discomfort may serve as a motivating factor in the learning. Helping the patient become interested in the appliances to be used following the operation encourages more positive and future-oriented thoughts. If another patient is available who has already adapted to a urinary diversion procedure, an exchange of information and feelings about the operation and its effects between the patient who is using the appliances and the patient who expects to use them can be very supportive. Family members should also be included in this preoperative teaching so that they can learn to be supportive of the patient who is about to have the operation.

POSTOPERATIVE CARE Immediate postoperative care for patients who have had a urinary diversion procedure focuses on prevention of complications from the abdominal surgery and the maintenance of urine flow. Following surgery, it is imperative that the section of the bowel at the site of surgery be free from distention to promote healing of the suture line and to prevent pressure that could interfere with urine flow. The abdomen should be observed for any changes that might indicate inflammation. Paralytic ileus can occur as a result of manipulation of the bowel. There is a possibility of urine leakage at the suture lines, which allows urine to enter the peritoneal cavity; the resultant inflammation causes pain, fever, nausea, and vomiting. The patient's abdomen will be sensitive to touch postoperatively and will feel rigid. Peristalsis may return slowly following surgery, and a nasogastric tube is usually inserted to provide for decompression. Oral intake of fluids is restricted until peristalsis returns and the nasogastric tube can be removed. Complications following ileal conduit diversion proce-

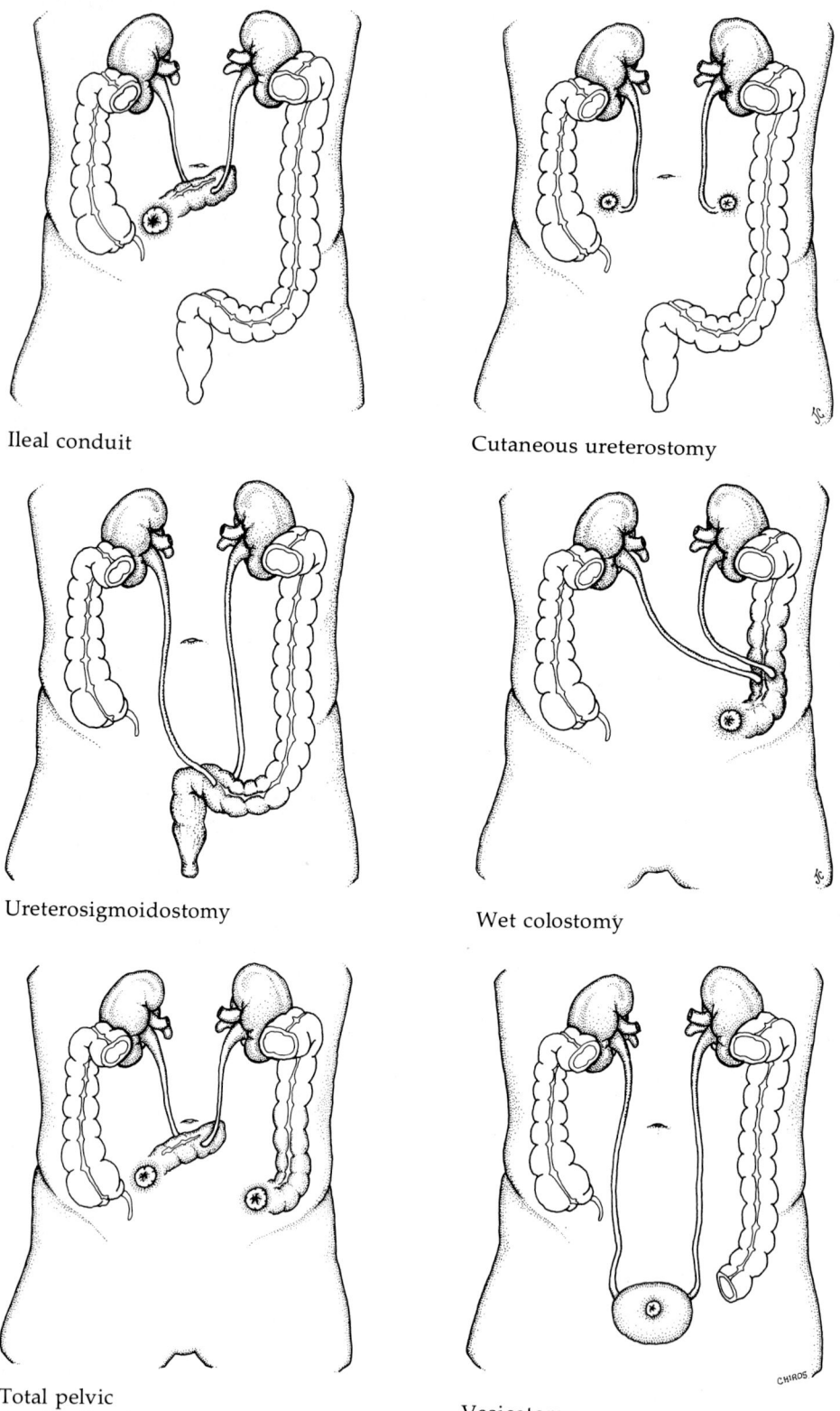

Figure 6-7
Surgical procedures used to accomplish urinary diversion. Note that the bladder is removed.

dures include small bowel obstructions secondary to intestinal adhesions, peristomal irritation, and infection of the remaining urinary tract from reflux of urine.

The patient who has had an ileal conduit will return from surgery with a catheter in place or with a temporary transparent appliance attached to the skin to collect urine. If the catheter is used, it is attached to a sterile gravity drainage system. The appliance is also attached to a drainage system to provide for the flow of urine, which will be continuous from the ileal conduit since the patient no longer has a bladder for storage of urine. Care must be taken to maintain the flow of urine by placing the drainage system correctly at a level below the patient and keeping it patent. The patient's position should facilitate drainage, and any pressure on the appliance or collection bag that might obstruct the flow of urine must be avoided. Reflux of urine to the kidney can cause damage because the kidney cannot tolerate pressure. Reflux is also a cause of infection.

An essential nursing function for these patients is that of monitoring fluid and electrolyte balance, particularly urinary output. In some hospitals, urinary output is measured hourly; an output smaller than 30 ml per hour indicates renal dysfunction. It is necessary to monitor renal function following the surgery to assess the status of the implanted ureters. Complications can include loosening of the ureters at the suture sites and kinking or twisting of the ureters, both of which must be corrected quickly. A baseline body weight is usually established prior to surgery, and the patient is weighed daily after surgery in similar circumstances to provide a measure of fluid elimination or retention. If a catheter is in place in the ileal conduit, sterile irrigation may be required to remove mucus. Only small amounts of normal saline solution are used for irrigation, with very gentle insertion of fluid to prevent the application of pressure to the surgical sites. The amount of fluid used to irrigate must be noted accurately so that the measurement of urinary output includes only the urine and not the irrigating solution.

The newly formed stoma of the ileal conduit becomes the focal point for the patient's perception of the surgery and for his attention in learning about self-care. Placement of the stoma is an important consideration prior to surgery. The patient's abdomen and its folds are inspected and a site is selected that will allow the patient maximum movement and will permit the best application of the drainage appliance. An appliance should be applied preoperatively to determine if changes of position will affect adherence of the appliance. The site may vary according to the contour of the abdomen. Folds and creases and any scars from previous operations are avoided because it is difficult to secure appliances to these sites. Care of the stoma postoperatively includes assessment of the status of the stoma and the surrounding skin. The condition of the stoma should be assessed regularly. Normally, the stoma should be smooth, cherry red, shiny, and moist. The presence of pallor, pedicles, lesions, or white encrustations indicate irritation from improper hygiene or from an improperly fitting appliance.

URINARY DRAINAGE APPLIANCES Because urine is irritating to the skin, the appliance used for urinary drainage must be selected to fit the patient's stoma since stomas can vary in size. An appliance that fits too tightly may cause formation of a fistula at the site of the stoma's attachment to the skin, whereas one that fits too loosely fosters unnecessary skin irritation. There are several different kinds of appliances: permanent (reusable) appliances, semidisposable appliances, and disposable, single-use appliances. Selection and fitting of a permanent appliance is delayed until the edema around the stoma has subsided following surgery. Various skin barriers, such as Colly-seels or Stomahesive, may be applied directly to the peristomal skin both to prevent irritation and to treat irritated skin areas. (Stoma care is discussed in Chapter 7.) When the appliance is changed, the peristomal skin should be examined carefully. Yeast infections may occur under the appliance; these are usually treated with application of nystatin (Mycostatin) powder.

The appliance used may be custom-made for the patient according to his individual specifications; however, the patient can usually obtain a suitable ready-made appliance. Permanent appliances have a faceplate, either firm or flexible, that is attached to the skin with cement or a double-faced adhesive. The collection pouch is attached to the faceplate. In order to ensure good contact between the plate and the skin, the skin must be completely dry. Since urine flow from the ileal conduit is continuous, a gauze sponge can be placed over the stoma or a tampon can be placed on the stoma to absorb urine while the appliance is being changed. A permanent appliance can be worn without changing for 3 to 7 days. If there is a leak between the faceplate and the skin, the appliance should be replaced to prevent unnecessary skin irritation. Each person develops his own habits, and the frequency of changing the appliance is related to his activity, the contour of his abdomen, and his rate of success in keeping the appliance in place. Because the person must provide for urine collection continuously and because the appliance needs to be properly cleaned and aired, it is recommended that two permanent appliances be purchased to enable the person to have one appliance ready for application while the other is washed, dried, and aired.

Semidisposable appliances are similar to the permanent ones in that they have a reusable faceplate or gasket; the difference is that they have disposable pouches attached to the faceplate. All appliances for urinary diversion have a spout for periodic emptying of urine. Disposable appliances are used only for single applications and are generally applied immediately after surgery since they provide for good visualization of the stoma. Some patients prefer this type rather than the permanent or semidisposable appliances and continue to use them after surgery.

Patients may have difficulty learning to change the appliance. It is helpful to teach the patient a systematic method of arranging supplies and preparing the appliance for application before removing the one he or she is wearing. Solvents can be used to dissolve the cement or adhesive so that the appliance can be removed easily. It is important that the patient learns not to pull the appliance from the skin, since this may cause irritation. Prior to placing the new appliance, the patient should clean the skin with soap and water, taking care to rinse well and dry thoroughly. Meticulous attention to the care of the skin around the stoma will minimize irritation. The patient will feel better about himself if the stoma and peristomal area heal well and remain in good condition. The patient tends to pattern his or her own care according to observations of the nurse's care procedures in the hospital. Therefore the care the patient is expected to learn should be carefully demonstrated by the nurse. As the patient learns to manage his or her own care the nurse should compliment the patient for preciseness in carrying out the details of the procedure.

LONG-TERM MANAGEMENT One problem that the patient may encounter is the formation of salts and crystals that settle out of the urine and collect on the stoma. These substances have an action similar to sandpaper and can cause bleeding of the stoma and irritation of the surrounding skin; they can also collect in the urine collection appliance. Diluted white vinegar is used to clean the stoma of crystals as well as to soak the appliance to dissolve the crystals. The patient should be advised to contact the physician in the event of sudden changes in the color of the stoma, abnormal cloudiness, or persistent foul odor of the urine or sudden changes in the quantity of urine output.

The patient's sleep patterns are important in determining management of the appliance during sleeping hours. It is recommended that the appliance be emptied every 2 to 3 hours. If the patient does not normally awaken periodically, the appliance can be connected to a urinary drainage system during sleep. The control valve that permits emptying of the appliance can be left open, and the spout is used to connect the appliance to the drainage system. The patient and family must be taught how to place the urinary drainage system to provide for drainage by gravity in order to maintain the patency of the system as well as how to disinfect it.

A well-planned teaching program is helpful for patients who are learning to care for their urinary drainage appliances. The patient who has had an ileal conduit should feel secure in his or her own ability for self care before going home. Teaching aids, written materials, and audiovisual materials can assist the patient in this learning process. Having the patient perform self care with gradual withdrawal of assistance and support by the nurse is a technique often used in preparing the patient for managing the techniques independently at home. Follow-up visits in the patient's home environment often facilitate the patient and family adjustment and prevent frustration by helping them solve problems that were not anticipated in the hospital.

Long-term care includes maintenance of

urine flow and prevention of complications. The urine is cultured periodically to make sure that the person does not have an infection. The culture specimen is obtained by aseptically inserting a French catheter no more than 2 inches into the stoma. Renal system function can be evaluated by x-ray since the contrast medium can be instilled through the stoma, using a loopography technique.

The person with an ileal conduit is very aware of the character of his or her urine. The urine will contain some mucus from the bowel, but other changes in the color or consistency of the urine are reported to the physician. The person should be informed that certain foods affect the odor of urine; for example, asparagus causes urine to have a pungent odor, and other foods such as beets can change the color of urine. Maintenance of an acid urine is helpful in preventing both odor and bacterial growth. This can be accomplished by taking acidifying medication or by drinking cranberry juice [45]. It is important that the person's fluid intake be at least 2,000 ml per day.

The person with an ileal conduit can lead a normal life and can accommodate his activities to the special requirements of the appliance. Clothing can be selected that will prevent pressure on the appliance and that will not interfere with the placement of the appliance on the abdomen. Some people recommend avoidance of contact sports in which there is a possibility of blows or trauma to the abdomen. Most people with an ileal conduit find their own level of activity, and some are very active in work and sports. The appliance can be removed for bathing or showering since the pressure of the continuous urine flow prevents fluid from entering the stoma.

The other type of urinary diversion procedure that requires wearing an appliance is **cutaneous ureterostomy.** There is a tendency for the ureters to close and for strictures to form with this type of surgery. Ureteral catheters will be in place postoperatively to support the ureters and to keep them open until healing occurs. If there are two stomas, there are two drainage systems for urine collection. Urine in each is measured carefully, and it should be noted with precise detail how much was emptied from each ureteral catheter. Each catheter and its respective drainage receptacle is labeled so that it is easier to keep them separate. Information about urine drainage is also recorded separately for the right and left ureter.

The stomas or stoma (if the ureters have been anastomosed before being brought to the skin) are smaller than the stoma of an ileal conduit because the lumen of the ureter is smaller than that of the ileum. Skin is sometimes used to form a larger stoma to facilitate application of the urine collection appliance; this procedure is also done because stomas made of the terminal ends of the ureters tend to slough. During the first week or so following surgery, the stoma must be kept moist with normal saline solution. This is usually discontinued when healing has progressed enough for the catheters to be removed. After the catheters are removed the patient begins to wear an appliance similar to those available for ileal conduits.

The patient who has had a ureterosigmoidostomy initially will have a catheter or a large rectal tube in place following surgery; this catheter or tube is attached to a drainage bag for collection of both urine and feces and prevents the accumulation of bowel contents that could distend the area of surgery and prolong or prevent healing of the suture lines. The catheter or tube may require irrigation to remove feces so that drainage is continuous. A small amount of fluid is used for irrigation. If the tube comes out, it should be gently reinserted no more than 4 inches to avoid damage to the rectum.

The measurement of output is essential in monitoring the effectiveness of the implantation. This is more difficult than with other methods of surgery because urine and feces will be mixed. For this reason, body weight is an important daily measurement. One long-term disadvantage of ureterosigmoidostomy is that hypochloremic acidosis may develop from reabsorption of urine by the bowel; this can be minimized if the bowel is emptied at 2- to 3-hour intervals. The patient can expect that the feces will always be soft, since dilution by urine occurs. It is usually necessary to insert a rectal tube into the rectum during sleep to provide for drainage unless the patient awakes periodically for elimination. The rectal tube will prevent distention. Perineal exercises are taught so that the patient develops more control of the anal sphincter, thereby better controlling elimination. These exercises consist merely of contracting and relaxing the muscles that control sphincter activity.

In addition to the development of hypochloremic acidosis, another common complication of ureterosigmoidostomy is infection. Because the ureters are implanted into the bowel, there is always the possibility of reflux of fecal material or bacteria normally present in the bowel to the kidney. Therefore, it is essential that these patients have a fluid intake of at least 2,500 and as much as 3,000 ml per day. An adequate fluid intake provides for flushing of the ureters and is extremely important in preventing infection and obstruction. If obstruction does occur, hydronephrosis readily develops because the urine backs up and fills the kidney calyces and pelvis.

FOLLOW-UP CARE Infection is always a serious potential hazard for patients who have had urinary diversion procedures. The possibility of infection is lower with the ileal conduit and greatest with the ureterosigmoidostomy. The signs of infection should be taught to the patient so that he can seek immediate therapy if they should occur. Fever, flank pain, and any of the generalized symptoms of infection are serious. One of the earliest indications of infection may be changes in the odor or color of the urine. Extremely cloudy or foul-smelling urine should be reported to the physician so that treatment can be obtained.

Throughout the entire period of preoperative and postoperative care the patient requires emotional support along with teaching to facilitate adaptation to the change in his method of elimination. Removal of the life-threatening tumor is the trade-off for adaptation to urinary diversion. The male patient may be impotent, depending on the extent of the surgery, and must deal with this change in his life as well. The female patient who has had a pelvic exenteration (as described in Chaps. 1 and 9) retains her vagina and thus can have normal sexual intercourse. In many instances, the attitude and support of the patient's spouse in coping with the changes in body image are the most important factors in his or her successful adaptation. Acceptance by others, particularly the people closest to the one having surgery, is therefore crucial, and the nurse's teaching plan should take this into account.

Follow-up examinations to determine the status of renal function are important for all patients who have had surgery for urinary diversion. Usually a plan for periodic x-ray examination, IVPs, cultures of urine, and testing for blood electrolytes is developed. The importance of this examination for early detection of any changes should be impressed on the patient so that he recognizes the need for the examination and follows through with appointments. If the urinary diversion is not functioning well, another operation for adaptation of the initial procedure or for performance of another procedure may be required. If urinary diversion has been performed as a palliative measure, the patient requires supportive care and treatment. In many instances, the patient must make the final decision about whether or not he wants further treatment. This is a difficult decision that requires honest and forthright support from the nurse.

Trauma to the Urinary Tract

Trauma to the urinary tract may also create obstruction to urine flow. The kidneys are protected by the rib cage and by the large back muscles. Trauma generally results from strong blows, falls (particularly on the abdomen or side), and splinters of bone from a broken pelvis. Any trauma followed by hematuria, oliguria, anuria, pain, a palpable mass, a fistula, or sepsis is considered an energency condition.

Among the types of trauma commonly occurring are contusion, laceration, and rupture. A bruised or contused kidney usually causes flank pain or aching. Bedrest and analgesics are used to treat this condition. Because of the possibility of internal hemorrhage or rupture the patient is kept in bed until all microscopic hematuria clears. A progressive drop in the hematocrit and an enlarging palpable kidney mass are indicative of hemorrhage. Penetrating injuries to the kidney may result in blood loss and extravasation of urine. Forceful blows may cause a whiplash to the kidney. Diseased kidneys are more prone to rupture than normal kidneys. Usually surgical intervention is delayed for 2 or 3 days and the progress of healing is observed. Bed rest may be sufficient treatment if the wound is small enough and can seal itself off. Drainage of fluid accumulation may be necessary and is accomplished by inserting a catheter in the area to be drained. The approach for insertion may be via the urinary tract or via a nephrostomy tube placed directly into the kidney. In severe trauma in which the kidney is damaged beyond repair, a nephrectomy is performed; this is done only after a careful urologic workup to observe the extent of the injury and the status of renal function.

Trauma establishes a potential for future kidney pathology. Follow-up urologic workups are conducted for several years after the trauma has occurred to monitor possible complications, which include cyst formation and calcification. Hypertension may also be a complication because of impaired renal function that affects the flow of blood. Ureteral injury is uncommon. However, if the ureters are severed, surgery is performed to reinstate continuity of the ureter. Several different procedures may be done to accomplish this.

The bladder is susceptible to trauma because of its position in the pelvis and because it is not as well protected as the kidneys. Perforation of the bladder may occur following a pelvic fracture, splinters of bone being the primary cause. This is always treated as a surgical emergency. The patient will experience severe abdominal pain, inability to void, muscular rigidity, tenderness, and perhaps shock. If urine from the bladder contaminates the bowel cavity, peritonitis can result.

Trauma resulting from infection can be another cause of obstruction; this usually involves the urethra and can involve the ureters. In the latter situation, strictures can be repaired surgically by removing the areas of fibrotic tissue resulting from damage to tissues by infection and restoring the continuity of the ureter. Strictures of the urethra are often treated by inserting sounds into the urethra. A **bougie** is the instrument used to measure the urethra; a **sound** is a small, metal, inflexible instrument that is made in different sizes so that the urethra can be increasingly dilated by passing the sounds. A **filiform** is a thin, threaded guide that is used to bypass very extensive strictures and to guide the larger, inflexible sound. The patient experiences slight discomfort after the passing of sounds, which is generally relieved by analgesics.

Urinary Calculi

A third type of pathology causing urinary tract obstruction is urinary calculi or stones. The formation of stones demonstrates the interdependency of dietary intake, metabolism, and urinary system function. Stones may appear singly or in multiples. They may be lodged at some point in the urinary tract and may never cause any symptoms if they do not impede urine flow; on the other hand, they may move within the tract and cause severe pain. Stones may be located in the kidneys, ureters, or bladder. A **staghorn stone** is so called because it fills the entire renal calyx and is shaped accordingly.

Symptoms and treatment The classic symptom of urinary calculi is renal colic, which occurs when stones are in the kidney or ureters and block the flow of urine. Colic pain has a sudden onset, usually beginning on one side and radiating downward to the testes in males and the labia in females. When the pain is severe the patient will be in extreme discomfort; he will be anxious and perspiring and may have nausea and vomiting. This pain can last for hours or days and subsides when the stone passes into the bladder. Colic pain may be intermittent, which usually means that the stone has moved, either before or after the attack of pain. It is thought that the ureter dilates above the site of the lodged stone, allowing passage of urine so that the pain abates. As the stone moves to a lower level it again causes obstruction, and the pain begins again as previously. The patient with ureteral or renal stones will generally have tenderness over the abdomen or along the line of the ureter.

The majority of small stones pass spontaneously. If this does not occur, removal of the stone is accomplished through cystoscopic examination and the use of catheters to remove the stone mechanically through manipulation. Large stones that can be moved into the bladder can be crushed and flushed out. If possible, the catheter is used to manipulate and guide the stone outward. If the stone cannot be removed in this manner, a ureterolithotomy is performed. Stones that are large enough to fill the kidney pelvis must be removed by pyelolithotomy. Those in the renal calyx are removed in a procedure called nephrolithotomy. A partial nephrectomy may be required if the stone is very large and if it has impinged on normal renal tissue. If kidney stones are bilateral and surgery is required, the less affected kidney is operated on first.

Patients with stones require special care related to their discomfort. Analgesics are given to relieve pain, and the degree of pain is noted. Changes in colic pain, tenderness, and the timing of intermittent pain including the duration are important observations. In addition, urine flow is monitored both for amount and for the presence of stones. All urine from patients who are suspected of having stones is strained by placing a strainer or a gauze square tightly over the urine measurement container. Small stones that are passed spontaneously in the urine can be recovered this way. Often the patient will pass gravel, which can mean that there are multiple stones, that a stone is breaking up, or that the stones are as small as gravel. Recovered stones are saved and sent to the laboratory for analysis.

Care required after a urologic workup is the same as for patients who have these tests at any time. Stone removal usually results in great relief for the patient. Convalescence is rapid because the inflammation caused by the stone subsides quickly. Following removal, the stones are analyzed and a long-term treatment plan is initiated according to the composition of the stones. The purpose of the long-term plan is to prevent recurrence of the stones, based on current theories of stone formation.

Causes of stone formation Much research has been done to determine why stones form. This question is still unanswered, although there are several theories about the causes and factors that predispose to stone formation. It has been found that systemic infections may influence stone formation, perhaps because of the fever. As previously mentioned, urinary tract infections may be associated with the incidence of stone formation. Stone formation may also be a family trait as in the case of cystinuria, which predisposes to cystine stone formation. Chronic diarrhea and certain medications such as acetazolamide (Diamox) and absorbable alkalis may influence the formation of urinary stones. Other factors that may predispose to stone formation include obstruction in the urinary tract, which causes stasis of urine; retention catheters, which have a precipitate of calcium salts on them when left in place for long periods of time; and changes in calcium metabolism associated with immobility. Males tend to form stones more frequently than do females.

Because of the composition of stones, there is also evidence that their formation may be related to dietary intake or to metabolism. In regard to this theory, it has been found that stones tend to form in people who live in areas where the water is hard (that is, where the water contains dissolved salts such as calcium and magnesium salts). Some authorities think that the use of biologic water conditioners to render water alkaline may influence susceptibility. People who live in areas where diets consist of high-carbohydrate, protein-poor foods tend to have a high incidence of stones. There is also a theory that a deficiency of vitamin A might be a causative factor. There is not enough conclusive evidence to establish modes of treatment through metabolic routes; therefore the emphasis of treatment is placed on relief of symptoms and analysis of recovered stones.

Types of stones The most commonly occurring type of stone is comprised of magnesium ammonium phosphate, calcium phosphate, and calcium carbonate. These stones are found in conditions in which there is hypercalciuria: namely, hyperparathyroidism, renal tubular acidosis, and bone tumors. Immobilization and steroid therapy also predispose to this type of stone formation. These are generally referred to as **phosphate stones.** Ammonium chloride is given to patients with this type of stones to acidify the urine. Surgery is not performed until the pain and inflammation have subsided.

Calcium oxalate stones form next in the order of frequency. These stones are thought to be formed because of an inborn error in metabolism. Oxalate excretion is increased because endogenous oxalate production is greater than normal. People with oxalate stones should avoid foods with high oxalate content, such as spinach and rhubarb.

Uric acid stones occur less frequently and are related to hyperuricemia. In some cases people who have these stones later develop gout, a condition in which purine metabolism is altered. Treatment for these stones usually involves elimination of foods such as sweetbreads, liver, caviar, and sardines from the diet. A low-purine diet may be prescribed for the treatment for gout.

Cystine stones occur when there is decreased urine excretion and high urine concentration of cystine. Excessive perspiration is thought to be a causative factor, since stone formation is related to dehydration. Treatment includes increasing fluid intake and giving medications to make the urine alkaline.

Preventive measures People who are prone to stone formation should drink large quantities of water to keep the urine diluted to flush the urinary tract and are advised to follow a low-calcium diet as a preventive measure. This can be done fairly easily; for example, if the person is a milk drinker, sufficient reduction of calcium can be accomplished by eliminating milk. The average adult's ingestion of calcium varies, with about one-half coming from milk. Calcium excretion is increased with immobility, so the low-calcium diet is particularly important for people who are immobilized.

Serum calcium, phosphorus, and uric acid levels are measured to determine the type of radiopaque stone. In addition, urinary calcium and uric acid tests are performed. The patient abstains from foods high in calcium for 2 days prior to and 2 days during the test. Urine is collected for two consecutive 24-hour periods following the 2-day abstention from calcium. If the amount of calcium ingested is less than 300 mg per day, the amount excreted in the urine should be less than 170 mg during a 24-hour period. An amount greater than 170 mg of calcium excreted is significant. It is important that the nurse remember that this is a qualitative test, so urine collection must be precise as to time if the test results are to be useful.

The urine is also tested to determine the presence of bacteria. Some bacteria, such as *Proteus* and some species of *Pseudomonas* [20], are capable of splitting urea and may cause "infection stones." A freshly voided specimen is collected for qualitative urine studies to determine the presence of uric acid and cystine. The pH of urine is also significant in both stone formation and in the treatment of stones. The patient can monitor his own urine pH at home with test tape to determine whether desired acidity or alkalinity is being maintained.

Anomalies of the Urinary Tract

Another cause of obstruction in the urinary tract is a congenital anomaly. There are many different types of anomalies, including the development of a supernumerary or double kidney with either complete duplication or a partial duplication of the urinary tract. A partial duplication generally includes just the kidney and the ureter. A **horseshoe kidney** is one in which both kidneys are connected by a band of tissue or a functioning isthmus of renal tissue. This type of anomaly causes the kidneys to be placed closer together and lower than normally placed kidneys. Another type of developmental or acquired kidney is called a **sponge kidney,** in which there is dilatation of the distal collecting tubules. These anomalies may be present without producing symptoms, if urine flow is effective. When urine flow is obstructed, symptoms of urinary retention and consequent infection result and are treated by surgical correction of the anomaly.

Other anomalies include an **ectopic kidney** with placement in either the pelvis or the thoracic region, and **ectopic ureters** and **bladders.** Among the anomalies that are found in the renal calyces and pelvis, obstruction of the ureteropelvic junction most commonly causes difficulty. In this condition urine cannot flow from the pelvis to the ureter. Sometimes this obstruction is caused by bands or strictures of the ureters, or it may result from a functional anomaly. Vascular anomalies may include malformation of renal vessels or a tendency to aneurysm formation; these conditions create serious problems when renal blood flow is impaired. Treatment involves surgical repair of the vessels.

Certain hereditary conditions predispose the kidneys to dysfunction. One of the most important of these conditions is **polycystic kidney disease.** Children with this disease have a poor prognosis. In the adult form the disease progresses very slowly, with hypertension developing over a period of time. The adult disease is autosomal dominant, whereas the disease is autosomal recessive when it occurs in children. Patients with polycystic disease are prone to infection. The polycystic kidney is removed if hemorrhage occurs; otherwise treatment is conservative.

Cysts may occur in any part of the kidney or urinary tract. They can cause no symptoms at all or they can be obstructive. **Ureterocele,** which is a cystic outpouching of the ureter, must be treated surgically.

The Kidney

Many references have been made in the preceding paragraphs to kidney failure. It must again be emphasized that kidney failure should be avoided if at all possible because effective kidney function is essential to life. The kidneys are amazing organs in that they can adapt to great variations in dietary intake, fluid intake, circulatory changes, and cellular needs. Blood that is transported to the kidney leaves with the appropriate constituents for the body's cellular needs and acid-base balance; the kidney takes care of eliminating substances and fluid that are not needed and that are harmful to the total body function.

STRUCTURE AND FUNCTION
OF THE KIDNEY

The **nephron** is the operational unit of the kidney. Each nephron begins with a **glomerulus** in its glomerular capsule, also called Bowman's capsule. This capsule narrows to form the **tubules,** which are divided into four segments: the proximal tubule, the loop of Henle, the distal tubule, and the collecting tubule. Each kidney has about one million nephron units, each one working independently of the others. The total ability of the kidney to accomplish its work is related to the number of nephron units that are functioning. In the event that some are damaged, the remaining functioning nephron units can increase their work load to compensate.

Blood is filtered by the glomeruli at an average rate of 120 ml per minute. The blood elements and large protein molecules are separated from the plasma that forms the filtrate. From Bowman's capsule, the filtrate passes into the tubule. The glomerular filtration rate depends on the number of effectively functioning nephrons and on the hydrostatic pressure in the glomeruli and in Bowman's capsule. As the plasma begins its route through the tubules, the reabsorption of sodium, potassium, chloride, glucose, creatinine, urea, phosphates, and bicarbonates, and water takes place. The mechanisms of reabsorption in relation to the body's fluid and electrolyte balance are described in Chapter 2. Reabsorption is a function of several factors: electrical potentials of electrolytes, concentration gradients, and active transport mechanisms. Water reabsorption is controlled by the concentration gradients. Reabsorption is facilitated by checks and balances throughout the tubules. The process of reabsorption is continuous throughout the four segments of the tubules until it is completed in the formation of urine.

A number of factors are important in understanding the effects of renal failure and the rationale for treatment and care of disturbances in the acid-base balance. Potassium and sodium reabsorption are dependent on the pH, with less potassium reabsorption occurring in alkalosis and more in acidosis. The renin-angiotensin system controls the exchange of potassium and sodium to a great extent. The enzyme renin is formed in the afferent arterioles of the glomeruli. The mechanisms of its release are not clearly understood but may be a response to decreased blood pressure or to low sodium concentrations in the distal tubule, which trigger sympathetic nerve stimulation for release. At any rate, renin converts angiotensinogen in the plasma to angiotensin I. Another enzyme converts angiotensin I to angiotensin II, which has vasoconstrictive powers and thus elevates the arterial blood pressure. Increased blood pressure stimulates the adrenal cortex to produce aldosterone. The aldosterone effects an increase in sodium reabsorption primarily along the distal and collecting tubules. Without aldosterone, potassium is reabsorbed and sodium and water are eliminated.

The antidiuretic hormone (ADH) from the posterior pituitary also functions to increase sodium reabsorption. This hormone accelerates water reabsorption by increasing the permeability of the distal tubule so that water is retained by the body. Stimulation of ADH secretion by the posterior lobe of the pituitary occurs when there are concentrated extracellular fluids with high osmolality. In the absence of ADH the tubules retain water and urine is more dilute. The relationship between ADH and aldosterone is such that large quantities of ADH increase the fluid volume of the plasma so that aldosterone is not secreted. When this occurs, sodium reabsorption along the tubules increases and potassium reabsorption decreases.

Two other factors are important in the regulation of acid-base balance: the secretion of hydrogen, which is very important in the kidney's participation in the maintenance of acid-base balance, and the secretion of ammonia. Hydrogen ion secretion is related to carbon dioxide levels in arterial blood and is accelerated when potassium levels are low. Hydrogen ion formation is basic to both ammonia secretion and reabsorption of bicarbonate (the hydrogen ions promote reabsorption of bicarbonate to maintain plasma concentrations). The enzyme carbonic anhydrase increases bicarbonate reabsorption, as does the arterial level of carbon dioxide. Reabsorption of bicarbonate is increased when arterial carbon dioxide levels are high. Hydrogen exchanges with sodium bicarbonate ($NaHCO_3$) to form carbonic acid (H_2CO_3) which can be further broken down into water and carbon dioxide. Phosphate buffers also provide for the exchange of hydrogen and sodium so that base can be reabsorbed.

An important buffer of hydrogen ions is ammonia. NH_3, a diffusible nitrogen, is formed in the renal cortex and is converted to NH_4, which is more stable and can be excreted. Glutamine in the plasma is the precursor of ammonia formation. Carbonic anhydrase is also important in the excretion of hydrogen and ammonia, both of which contribute to the acidity of urine. Ammonia is produced in greater amounts when there is a smaller supply of buffers.

RENAL FAILURE

With these facts about renal function in mind, the concept of renal failure assumes more meaning. The inability of the kidneys to carry out these processes will lead to alterations throughout the body, and symptoms will result. Renal failure means that both kidneys have lost their ability to adapt to the body's needs. The failure may occur progressively or it may be a sudden occurrence; the first condition is called chronic renal failure and the second is acute renal failure. An important step in the treatment of both chronic and acute renal failure is finding the cause.

Causative Factors

Chronic renal failure is the long-term result of urinary tract infections and obstructions that gradually involve increasing amounts of renal tissue in the destructive processes. In addition to the stresses of urinary tract dysfunction, the kidneys are also subjected to stresses from systemic diseases that affect renal function. Lupus erythematosus and diabetes are examples of systemic diseases that are associated with renal pathology; the former disease causes glomerular lesions whereas the latter affects the blood vessels by causing sclerosis. Generalized arteriosclerosis may also cause renal pathology, called nephrosclerosis. Yet another cause of renal failure is any disease that affects the kidneys directly; glomerulonephritis is the most frequently occurring disease in this category.

Some authorities classify renal failure according to prerenal, renal, and postrenal causes. **Prerenal** causes are the systemic diseases or changes that occur in the circulation before it reaches the kidneys. **Renal** causes are the primary renal diseases, and **postrenal** causes are those that involve urinary tract dysfunction.

Acute renal failure may also result from prerenal, renal, and postrenal causes [10]. Prerenal causes relate to the kidney's blood supply, blood volume, or electrolyte balance. Renal causes are any conditions that cause sudden alteration in the tubules so that the kidneys cannot function; examples are shock, trauma involving crushing injuries, acute glomerulonephritis, septicemia, blood transfusion reactions, surgery that temporarily interferes with blood supply, chemical toxins such as carbon tetrachloride and antifreeze, and drug overdose. Barbiturates in large doses, for example, cause depression of the medullary centers with subsequent depression of the respiratory center causing hypoxia and hypotension, and the cardiovascular effects on the kidney lead to oliguria. Postrenal causes include any factors that suddenly obstruct the flow of urine so that anuria results.

Symptoms of Renal Failure

The patient who is in renal failure, chronic or acute, usually feels sick and has a very limited capacity for daily activities. Perhaps the function of the kidneys is most understood and appreciated when lost. Because acute renal failure occurs suddenly, these patients will have fewer of the generalized body symptoms of kidney failure experienced by those with long-term chronic renal failure. However, patients with either acute or chronic renal failure experience similar symptoms of fluid and electrolyte imbalances.

Management of Acute Renal Failure

Acute renal failure follows a course of renal shutdown, called the oliguric phase, and a return to function, called the diuretic phase. Renal shutdown is first evidenced by increased blood serum levels of urea and then by changes in urine output. Oliguria, an output of 400 ml or less per day, and anuria, complete lack of urine output, are significant. For this reason urine output is an essential measurement for any patient following surgery, trauma, shock, or a transfusion reaction. Early detection allows for prompt treatment.

Acute renal failure is not fully understood; although it is known that renal changes involve the tubules. The terms used to refer to these changes are **tubular acidosis** or **tubular nephropathy**. **Tubulo-interstitial nephropathy** is the term preferred by some authorities [17]. Inadequate oxygenation of the kidneys is usually the common denominator of shock and trauma, but this in itself may not be the basic cause of tubular pathology. It is thought that there are toxins that cause tubular changes, but these have not been identified.

Nursing care for these patients is complex because they often have demanding care requirements for other conditions in addition to renal failure. For example, the patient who has been in an accident may have any number of other problems including fractures, contusions, and lacerations. If the patient has undergone an operation, he must receive appropriate care and must be monitored for wound healing and complications of the surgical procedure. The patient is usually placed in an intensive or special care unit and requires assistance for daily hygiene. Both physical comfort and emotional support are important so that the patient does not get lost in the maze of pacemakers, respirators, intravenous tubes, and perhaps traction.

Special concerns in caring for the patients with acute renal failure are related to fluid and electrolyte balances. Insensible and sensible fluid losses are carefully calculated so that the intake does not exceed the output. Metabolic water production (insensible fluid loss) amounts to about 300 ml of fluid per day. This amount plus the patient's total urine output should equal the total intake, which can be given orally, or if the patient cannot take oral fluids, via intravenous administration. Wound drainage, emesis, or gastric drainage must be calculated as insensible fluid loss. If no intervention such as dialysis is employed, it is extremely important that the fluid intake not exceed the total of sensible and insensible fluid loss. When the body cannot eliminate water, the excess intake is retained in the intracellular and extracellular spaces.

Analysis of the urine reveals some of the processes that are going on in the kidney. There is reduced urine flow, and the urine has a high specific gravity and contains red blood cells, casts, and protein. As oliguria continues, further changes include increasing acidosis and azotemia, which are measured in blood levels of the pH, urea, and creatinine. (**Azotemia** refers to the increased level of nitrogen products—urea, creatinine, and uric acid—in the blood; all of these are end products of protein metabolism that are normally eliminated from the body by kidney function.) Serum potassium levels rise in accordance with the acidosis so that cardiac function is affected. As the acidosis and azotemia progress, dialysis is performed, if possible, to limit the complications of altered fluid and electrolyte levels. This reduces the incidence of toxicity to the nervous system that is demonstrated in symptoms of coma and convulsions, as well as reducing the potential for death resulting from cardiac disturbances that are caused by increased serum potassium levels.

Another reason for the importance of dialysis is that wound healing is better if the effects of acidosis are minimized. Wound healing in states of renal failure is hindered because of the interference with protein metabolism. However, if dialysis is not available, precise and meticulous care in managing dietary or parenteral caloric intake (or both), fluid intake, and electrolyte balance is necessary if the patient is to survive acute renal failure. Cardiac monitoring is imperative in hyperkalemia since increased serum potassium causes irritability of cell membranes. Peaking of the T wave, disappearance of the P wave, and flattening of the QRS complex of the electrocardiogram signifies a serious degree of cardiac irritability. If hyperkalemia continues, the cardiac irritability may be sufficient to cause ventricular fibrillation.

When dialysis is not available for patients in acute renal failure, methods are employed to reduce the level of serum potassium. Sodium polystyrene sulfonate (Kayexalate), a resin, can be given orally or by retention enema. Sodium ions are exchanged with potassium ions in the intestine, with 1 gm of Kayexalate being able to remove 1 mEq of potassium. Oral administration of Kayexalate provides for more extensive contact of the resin with the gastrointestinal tract. If Kayexalate is given orally, sorbitol is often given to act as a cathartic because Kayexalate promotes constipation. When given by retention enema, Kayexalate is given after cleaning the bowel, and the patient is made comfortable so that he can retain the Kayexalate long enough to achieve the desired ion exchange.

The patient in renal failure, then, is in a state of metabolic acidosis in which there is an excess of acid and a deficiency of base. The body responds by using all the available buffers to diminish the acid levels. Bicarbonate and phosphate are the most significant of these buffers. In acute renal failure, the patient will require care related to physical comfort to minimize the effects of metabolic acidosis and to prevent acidosis as much as possible. The need for fluid intake and output monitoring with measured intake equal to output and insensible fluid loss has already been mentioned. In addition, care requires providing the patient with sufficient calories for cellular function without giving foods containing substances that the body does not need and that the kidneys cannot handle, such as protein, potassium, and salt. Dietary intake must also be considered in terms of the patient's ability to ingest foods and fluids. Depending on the total body disturbances the patient is experiencing, oral ingestion of foods may be impossible.

There are several methods of supplying calories during the oliguric phase. When the patient cannot tolerate oral fluids or foods, intravenous glucose may be given. Although the amount of glucose prescribed may vary with different treatment plans, about 100 to 150 gm of glucose is required to meet the body's daily requirements. One author [6] states that when eight essential amino acids, histidine, and vitamins were added to the glucose infusion, mortality was reduced. Commercial products have been prepared to provide calories in limited amounts of fluid for oral ingestion; examples are Controlyte* and Cal-Power†, which are protein-free, electrolyte-poor mixtures that contain carbohydrates to provide energy. Various homemade mixtures can be prepared as well. These usually contain glucose, water, and lemon juice to improve the taste. Specially bottled water is sometimes used to control the electrolytes, since water in different locations has different electrolyte values of sodium and potassium. If the patient can tolerate oral foods, hard candy or butter balls made of butter rolled in powdered sugar are given to increase the caloric intake. Potassium intake must also be controlled because in hyperkalemic states the presence of only a small amount of potassium can cause cardiac failure. As previously mentioned, potassium-binding substances are sometimes given to reduce the amount of potassium through its excretion from the gastrointestinal tract.

The oliguric phase of acute renal failure lasts for about 14 days. The procedure for calculating fluid intake according to output is continued at this point. As the nephron units begin functioning, the amount of protein ingested is generally increased according to the blood levels of urea. These levels remain high during the initial diuretic phase because high concentrations have built up in the body during the oliguric phase. As the kidneys begin to catch up with the backload, protein can be given. The amounts vary, but usually 20 gm of protein per day is the maximum amount allowed while the patient is in the diuretic phase. Diuresis is accomplished by loss of sodium and potassium in the urine. For this reason, blood levels of both sodium and potassium are monitored, and these electrolytes are given to restore normal levels.

The diuretic phase is one in which the patient's kidneys gradually resume normal function. The diet is returned to normal as the nephron units demonstrate increasing ability to maintain fluid and electrolyte balances and to eliminate metabolic wastes. It is estimated that about 50 percent of patients with acute renal failure recover completely. Those whose failure was caused by shock or injury usually recover, whereas those who have primary renal disease have a poorer prognosis and the dysfunction often becomes chronic. Continued treatment is then necessary in an effort to maintain as much renal function as possible.

Diseases Leading to Renal Failure

Glomerulonephritis Both glomerulonephritis and the nephrotic syndrome are examples of diseases that may lead to renal failure.

---

*Manufactured by the Doyle Pharmaceutical Co., Minneapolis, Minnesota.
†Manufactured by the General Mills Chemical Co., Minneapolis, Minnesota.

Glomerulonephritis is a disease that can be either acute or chronic; the term actually refers to a complex of diseases that cause pathology in the glomeruli. It can occur in different degrees, ranging from minimal lesions, which are the least serious, to lesions that involve the membranes and those that are proliferative and are therefore the most serious. The incidence of the disease is related to streptococcal infections anywhere in the body but primarily in the respiratory tract. Infection by group A β-hemolytic *Streptococcus*, strains 12, 4, 25, and 18, may be followed by acute glomerulonephritis, usually within 10 to 14 days after the respiratory infection. The symptoms result from the acute inflammatory response of the glomeruli, which is thought to be an antigen-antibody response. The patient will have edema, hypertension, and proteinuria. Hematuria is usually present.

Care for patients with acute glomerulonephritis includes bed rest together with monitoring of intake and output and of blood electrolytes. The edema, a function of salt and water retention, makes the patient uncomfortable. The patient also experiences malaise and anorexia, so attention must be given to helping him ingest sufficient carbohydrates to spare his protein stores. Initially small amounts of fruit juices are given and the diet is increased as the patient can tolerate more food. A high carbohydrate diet is then given, salt is restricted, and proteins are held to a maximum of 40 gm per day. The acute phase of the disease lasts for 2 to 3 weeks. Because of the edema and salt retention an important measure of fluid balance is daily weight, which is significant in determining fluid and salt intake. Another measurement that is important in planning the patient's diet is the blood urea level. Proteins are restricted until the kidneys can function. In some patients proteinuria continues for years, whereas in others function returns to normal. Diuretics and antihypertensives are sometimes prescribed to relieve both edema and hypertension. Acute glomerulonephritis has the potential for becoming chronic. In this case the disease may be latent for a period of time, reappearing months or years after the initial acute episode of glomerulonephritis.

Chronic glomerulonephritis is similar to the acute condition in that the symptoms are the same: hypertension, edema, and proteinuria. The glomeruli gradually become sclerosed and nonfunctioning, and the symptoms may occur in lesser or greater degrees as the disease progresses. In some situations chronic glomerulonephritis is discovered through the symptom of hypertension; in others, it is not found until the person demonstrates symptoms of the nephrotic syndrome. This syndrome is a complex set of metabolic changes that occur in relation to the proteinuria. The glomeruli are unable to retain the large protein molecules because of their increased permeability, with the result that large amounts of protein are lost in the urine and hypoalbuminemia occurs.

The nephrotic syndrome Another condition that may result in acute renal failure is the **nephrotic syndrome.** This condition, also known as nephrosis, is characterized by hypoalbuminemia and proteinuria with massive edema. As with renal failure, the mechanisms of the nephrotic syndrome are not well understood. There are theories that its occurrence is related to thyroid function. Fat metabolism is altered in the nephrotic syndrome, perhaps because albumin is important in the metabolic pathway of fats. If albumin is being lost in the urine in great quantities, the chain of metabolic reactions cannot proceed normally. There is a consequent increase in triglycerides; hyperlipemia and hypercholesterolemia occur; and there will be cholesterol esters and fat bodies in the urine.

As with glomerulonephritis, there is salt and water retention in the nephrotic syndrome. The reduced glomerular filtration rate leads to hypertension via the renin-angiotensin system, with angiotensin II causing vasoconstriction and therefore hypertension. Because the blood osmolality is decreased as proteins are eliminated in the urine, water and electrolytes pass into the interstitial tissue. The result is edema, decreased plasma volume, and subsequent decreased cardiac output; this in turn reduces the renal blood flow and stimulates aldosterone secretion. The patient can be given salt-poor albumin and diuretics that block aldosterone formation, such as furosemide (Lasix), ethacrynic acid (Edecrin), and the thiazides.

Patients with the nephrotic syndrome have a typical skin pallor that is accentuated by edema. The edema may be of varying degrees: if the degree is great, edema is generalized; when edema is of a lesser degree, it can be observed in the dependent areas of the body such as the ankles, feet, and the sacral area. White bands in the fingernails are another sign of the nephrotic syndrome. The patient has a general feeling of malaise, is tired, anorexic, and lethargic, and is often depressed with no interest in eating or activities. Nursing care includes improving the patient's outlook with comfort and dietary measures and closely monitoring the significant tests.

Because the kidneys are eliminating large amounts of protein, the diet should include high-protein foods. Salt is restricted because of the salt retention and edema formation. The usual diet varies, but it can contain about 100 gm of protein and is limited to 500 mg or less of sodium. Daily weights are important in monitoring fluid loss. Activity is restricted when edema is severe and is increased as edema is lessened.

Up to this point acute renal failure and the nephrotic syndrome have been discussed, and it was stated that many patients with acute renal failure will develop chronic renal failure. There is also a potential for renal failure in any pathology that affects the circulatory system because the kidney is a highly vascular organism. A condition called **nephrosclerosis** refers to fibrosis of the tubules following interference with blood flow to the kidney; this is a progressive condition which, like degenerative diseases, has no cure. Chronic renal failure also has no cure, but it can be managed in several different ways.

Management of Chronic Renal Failure

The first and most effective treatment for chronic renal failure is a renal transplant, which may be performed if the patient is otherwise healthy but has bilateral kidney disease. Another method of long-term treatment is routine hemocorporeal or peritoneal dialysis [9]. Dialysis provides for the functions of the normal kidney in a format that is very similar to the way the kidney operates. The third method of managing chronic renal failure is to restrict dietary intake of nutrients and fluids to levels that the kidneys are able to manage effectively. The dietary restriction does not cure the dysfunction but rather minimizes symptoms. As renal failure becomes more severe, the kidneys cannot handle even minimal dietary intake.

Chronic renal failure can be mild, moderate, or severe. The term **renal insufficiency** connotes moderate dysfunction and means that the kidneys are not able to maintain normal function, but they are able to manage a lighter load. However, even renal insufficiency is spoken of in terms of degrees. **Uremia** is a term that has been used for years to describe terminal renal failure; although it is less popular now than formerly, the term is still used.

Consider what your life would be like if you were faced with a choice of three options for its preservation. The first option, renal transplantation, offers great hope for recovery, but it also has inherent dangers. At best, deciding to have a renal transplant is deciding to take a risk. The risk is complex: Will you survive the surgery? Will the transplant "take?" Will the transplant last for only a short time, to be rejected later? How long will you have to wait for a kidney? The second option also offers great hope along with risks. Can you imagine yourself eating a restricted diet and watching your fluid intake for the remainder of your life? What will your weekly schedule be like if you must spend 5 to 10 hours three or four times a week constrained by a machine that is washing your blood? How do you think your family will respond to the constraints and restrictions of your life? However, the third option offers even less hope. Can you follow the very carefully controlled diet and fluid intake that you must have to feel better? How do you feel about the knowledge that you will gradually feel worse and worse and then eventually die? Do you imagine that all the researchers and experiments may come up with a magic cure before your symptoms are so serious?

These kinds of decisions are not easy to make, and yet this is exactly what the patient with chronic renal failure must do. The fact that there are these decisions to make, however, represents great advances in medical science. Prior to the 1960s there was only one option for the majority of these patients: to live with renal failure until death. As more is discovered about how the kidney functions and about factors related to kidney function, there may be even better options.

The nurse who works with patients who have chronic renal failure must deal with each patient's own motivation for selecting his or her options; this represents a complex relationship among the events of the patient's life, the nature of family and peer support, and primarily his or her own determination to select the option. The patient who selects dialysis or transplantation is essentially making a strong commitment to living. Even that strong commitment may waver, however, with the stresses of life, so the nurse must support the patient through the times of stress and provide for the most positive experiences possible in contacts with the patient and family.

Chronic renal failure formerly meant that a person would gradually withdraw from an active life as his energy diminished, and he would eventually become an invalid. Now the person with chronic renal failure can lead an active and longer life, pursuing the activities for an extended period of time. The patient's life has to be adapted to the need for dietary management and dialysis, but even these adaptations can be worked into a routine pattern of normalcy. This is accomplished best if the patient and family understand the dysfunction and the factors that make it either better or worse. The nurse has much teaching to do, initially in preparing the patient for self-care and then in helping him or her to adjust to changes resulting from the progressive renal failure. It is important that the nurse and other members of the health care team be realistic in dealing with the implications of dialysis with the patient and family. Dialysis is not a cure but a method for carrying on the kidney function, so the patient is dependent on it for life.

All the symptoms of chronic renal failure are the result of changes in fluid and electrolyte balance and in metabolism. Knowing why each symptom occurs will give the patient control in making adjustments to relieve the symptoms. Some symptoms do not change but must be accepted, whereas others can be managed. In addition to the dialysis and diet, the patient is increasingly subject to other stresses that he or she could normally cope with; one example is infection, which increases protein catabolism, a situation that the diseased kidney cannot manage. It is important for the patient to know the sources of problems so that they can be avoided.

Progression of the disease As chronic renal failure progresses there is retention of acid, and systemic acidosis ensues. In this state there is an excess of acid with the result that all of the available buffer systems are used. The major buffer system, that of bicarbonate (HCO_3^-), is inadequate to buffer the increased amount of acid. After the supply of bicarbonate buffers is exhausted, other intracellular and extracellular buffers that are not normally used are called into play; among these are bone salts (calcium and phosphorus) and the hemoglobin in red blood cells. Because bone salts are ionized and because phosphates are neither filtered effectively nor reabsorbed efficiently, the calcium-phosphorus equilibrium is disturbed. Some patients have particular problems in this regard if they develop hyperparathyroid-like states. A few patients also have dysfunction of vitamin D synthesis, which further complicates the picture. The use of hemoglobin as a buffer depresses the ability of the circulatory system to carry oxygen. The respiratory center also comes into play, responding to the decreased pH by causing hyperventilation to lower the partial pressure of carbon dioxide. In addition, there is an obligatory loss of sodium in the urine since the diseased kidney cannot reabsorb sodium effectively. In the later stages of renal failure there is hyperkalemia, which may be severe enough to cause cardiac arrhythmias. There is also an increased concentration of urea in the blood, because the urea load cannot be fully eliminated by the poorly functioning kidneys. Symptoms related to all of these changes are discussed in the following section.

Symptoms of chronic renal failure Patients with chronic renal failure have a characteristic skin color that can be described as dusky and yellowish, and their complexion appears pale. Both anemia and the accumulation of urochrome pigments give rise to this color, which changes only in degree, even with dialysis [17]. The patients are usually thin because of their restricted diet and because they are encouraged to maintain their weight as "dry" without excess fluid. Another symptom is generalized itching (pruritus), which is quite bothersome to the patient and is difficult to control even with moisturizing lotions. The patient is compelled to scratch, sometimes so much that the skin is excoriated and becomes subject to infection. Dialysis does relieve the pruritus. There is also a tendency to have ecchymoses and purpura. A symptom of the late stages is the formation of uremic frost on the skin, especially around the mouth; the body has such high concentrations of urea that it is excreted in the perspiration, where it then crystallizes and forms the frost.

Another set of symptoms involves the gastrointestinal tract. First, the patient may have stomatitis, which is caused by the action of the urea-splitting flora of the oral cavity on the increased urea. This also gives rise to a metallic taste in the patient's mouth, requiring meticulous oral hygiene to counteract it. Anorexia, nausea, and vomiting are commonly experienced early in renal failure; this contributes to an additional loss of sodium in a situation in which there is already an obligatory sodium loss. This loss further depletes the extracellular volume and can contribute to reduced renal blood flow because of the dehydration. Dysphagia is another symptom that bothers patients, making it difficult to eat, particularly if the patient does not feel hungry. The action of ammonia, formed when urea is metabolized by the intestinal tract, causes the formation of ulcers in the mucosa and submucosa of the gastrointestinal tract. Because there is a depression of platelet formation related to uremia, the ulcers may hemorrhage, causing melena.

Neurologic symptoms include a generalized feeling of lethargy. The patient feels progressively more tired and finds it difficult to concentrate. As uremia advances, the patient may become drowsy and then confused. Coma may occur in late stages. The reason for the neurologic symptoms is not known; it is thought that substances toxic to the central nervous system are no longer eliminated by the kidneys in uremic states. Various symptoms can be experienced in both sensory and motor functions. Initially burning sensations in the feet are experienced and may be followed by numbness, paresthesia, muscle cramps, and twitching. Another cause of muscle weakness is the high potassium level. Hyperkalemia increases the irritability of muscles; this is particularly significant because the increased irritability of the heart muscle may result in arrhythmias.

Another set of symptoms that can affect mobility results from changes in phosphorus and calcium levels. There is a great deal of variability in the symptoms of hyperphosphatemia and hypocalcemia among different patients. Some have no symptoms, whereas others have a generalized muscle irritability followed by tetany or convulsions if calcium levels are extremely low. In uremia the serum phosphorus increases because phosphate filtration is decreased in acidosis. Oral aluminum hydroxide gel antacids are given to decrease the intestinal absorption of phosphorus in an effort to restore the normal phosphorus-calcium balance by lowering serum phosphorus levels. This has questionable results, however, and these antacids tend to decrease the appetite of a patient who is usually already anorexic.

Some patients excrete large amounts of calcim in the feces, indicating that they have impaired ability to absorb calcium from the gastrointestinal tract. For some reason yet unknown, these patients are thought to have a failure of vitamin D activity, which is important for calcium metabolism. It is believed that the diseased kidney cannot convert vitamin D to its active form, and without vitamin D, ionized calcium cannot be absorbed from the gastrointestinal tract; hence calcium is eliminated in the feces. In this instance, high doses of vitamin D are given.

When serum calcium levels are low, a normal mechanism for restoring the phosphorus-calcium balance is the stimulation of parathyroid hormone secretion. Normally, the parathyroid hormone increases the tubular reabsorption of phosphorus in an attempt to reduce serum phosphorus levels. This does occur in renal failure to the extent allowed by the functional ability of the kidneys. However, renal function is insufficient to increase the reabsorption of phosphorus enough to lower serum levels, and the imbalance persists. The parathyroid hormone, in addition to its effect on the tubules, stimulates mobilization of calcium from bone. For this reason, bone demineralization may occur in patients who have renal failure, and they may have a tendency to fracture bones easily. Calcium and phosphorus in the bone are mobilized as one of the buffer mechanisms in the body's attempt to reduce acidosis. In some patients, the calcium and phosphorus may be equilibrated in the blood at high levels of concentration. When this situation occurs, the ionized calcium and phosphate are readily deposited, resulting in the formation of calcium phosphate deposits in soft tissues and in the bones.

Depletion of bicarbonate also occurs as the acidosis progresses, which stimulates the respiratory center to increase the respiratory rate. A deep, sighing form of breathing is therefore a symptom of renal insufficiency. In the very late stages of uremia, hyperventilation is so great that a typical form of breathing known as Kussmaul-Kien respiration occurs to compensate by ridding the body of carbon dioxide. It is not unusual for the patient to experience air hunger and a mild dyspnea; this is particularly noticeable when the patient is active. These respiratory symptoms are caused in part by the anemia that accompanies chronic renal failure. Belching and hiccups are also frequent and bothersome to the patient.

As anemia develops, the patient will experience cardiovascular symptoms including hypertension, which is a compensatory mechanism related to the decreased oxygen-carrying capacity of the blood in anemia. Retinopathy may occur in association with the hypertension. The kidney is thought to be one of the principal sites of formation of either erythropoietin or its precursor erythrogenin. Although the kidney's role in formation of either erythrogenin or erythropoietin is not known for certain, it is known that the formation of erythropoietin does not occur in renal failure. Blood transfusions are sometimes necessary. Care must be taken to use only washed donor cells; this is important particularly for those patients awaiting kidney transplants. Antigens should not be introduced into the body unnecessarily because the formation of antigen-antibody complexes may limit the patient's ability to receive a donor kidney. Anemia usually continues even if the patient is being dialyzed. Blood transfusions together with a combination of factors including hyperkalemia, fluid retention (which may lead to pulmonary edema), and hypertension may culminate in congestive heart failure. When treating congestive heart failure it is important to check the dosages of drugs that are normally excreted by the kidney (about one-half as much digoxin is required compared to usual dosages). Diuretics that depend on glomerular filtration for their action will not be effective.

All the symptoms just discussed appear in some degree as renal failure progresses and are present in the late stages when uremia occurs. Individual patients respond differently, but generally acidosis appears when the glomerular flow rate is 15 to 20 percent of normal. At this time the patient has early renal insufficiency, and a program of dietary management is instituted. The point at which dialysis is begun is usually determined by the patient's symptoms and evaluation of the degree of acidosis. The goal of nursing care is to help these patients become as independent as possible in managing their renal dysfunction.

Treatment Plans in Chronic Renal Failure
Patients with renal insufficiency must develop positive health habits, paying more attention to adequate rest and exercise than they might have done previously. They need to know how to avoid infections and must seek prompt treatment if an infection does occur in any part of the body. Because of renal failure, antibiotics normally excreted by the kidneys will be retained, so dosages are decreased considerably since blood levels of the antibiotics will remain high. The patients must also be aware of the effect of stress, the types of activities or life problems that are stressful to them and how to cope with the stressors. Those close to the patients—families and friends—must also make adjustments, and their support is important in helping patients adapt. All this must be accomplished in such a way that the patients have a positive self-image. They do not need to become fearful of things, places, or people; they do however need to learn how to protect themselves from those things that might have a negative effect on their condition.

There are many different approaches to treatment plans for patients with chronic renal failure, and each patient can adjust the given plan to his own life-style [2]. Whatever the approach, most plans provide for prevention of acidosis. Much is still not understood about the kidney and its functions. Many authorities believe that as renal function declines, toxins yet to be identified remain in the body; these toxins seem to be related to protein metabolism, which is affected by the kidney's inability to clear urea. Some believe that early intervention with dietary management may prevent or minimize the buildup of toxins, thereby enabling the kidney with impaired functional abilities to be more effective for a longer period of time.

Dietary management Normally the clearance of urea is directly related to protein intake. In chronic renal failure, the kidneys cannot handle elimination of a normal load of urea; they eliminate as much as they can, but much is still retained by the body. Urea excretion is a function of the glomerular flow rate, and urea is also reabsorbed according to the tubular flow rate, more being retained by the body when flow rates are low. When the blood urea nitrogen level is high, a proportional amount of urea is absorbed in the gastrointestinal tract where it is hydrolyzed by the urease-producing microorganisms and produces ammonia. This process is utilized in dietary management when ammonia is reused in the anabolism of proteins. Protein metabolism is then a significant factor in determining the type of diet that is most beneficial for patients with chronic renal failure.

It is necessary to give some protein to patients in chronic renal failure because in the absence of protein, tissue wasting occurs. On the other hand, too much protein increases the load for elimination of its metabolic end products. Protein intake, then, is one of the primary factors in dietary planning. Considerable attention has been given to protein metabolism in order to determine how much and what types of protein foods are most conducive to maintaining the body's nitrogen balance. Most plans in current practice make use of the Giordano-Giovannetti diet. This diet emphasizes that not only the quantity but also the quality of the dietary protein is important [5, 8].

The Giordano-Giovannetti diet is limited to the inclusion of only high-biologic proteins such as milk and eggs that contain the essential amino acids. All low-biologic proteins that contain nonessential amino acids are restricted or completely eliminated, depending on the patient's renal function. Adaptations can be made by substituting cereal products containing rice, which has little protein, for those containing wheat. Deglutenized wheat grains are used in making such items as low-protein breads, spaghetti, and cookies; these are available commercially and can be purchased in most health food or grocery stores. Other commonly used foods with low-biologic protein value are peas, beans, lentils, and corn. The amount of high-biologic protein allowed depends on the renal function as evaluated by the patient's symptoms. Several different guidelines are used; one reference cites the use of the creatinine clearance level as a guideline for determining the amount of protein allowed. Protein is replaced gram for gram of that lost in the urine, plus 50 gm if the creatinine clearance level is 20 to 30 ml per minute, 40 gm if it is 15 to 20 ml per minute, 30 gm if the creatinine clearance is 10 to 15 ml per minute, and 25 gm if it is 5 to 10 ml per minute [6]. It is important that the protein restriction be evaluated in terms of the patient's symptoms since not everyone has the same symptoms with the same levels of blood urea or creatinine clearance. As the patient's renal failure progresses, the amount of protein is decreased to as little as 20 gm per day. When the kidneys cannot handle even this reduced metabolic load, dialysis is required.

Another important factor in planning the diet for a patient in renal failure is the need to provide adequate calories to meet the body's energy needs. Carbohydrates and fats are generally given quite liberally, with at least 2500 or 3000 calories ingested daily. If sufficient calories are not ingested from carbohydrates and fats, glyconeogenesis occurs, thereby increasing the protein metabolic end products. Calories are frequently added by having the patient use foods such as jams, jellies, honey, and whipped cream liberally. A few calories can be taken in the form of alcoholic beverages such as whiskey, vodka, gin, or brandy.

As with acute renal failure, fluid balance is of prime importance for patients with chronic renal failure. The amount of fluids allowed in the diet is calculated the same way: The patient may have 300 to 500 ml to compensate for insensible fluid loss plus an amount equal to the fluid excreted in urine. The patient is encouraged to maintain a dry weight; fluids in excess of the amount that can be eliminated are retained in the body.

Other dietary restrictions are related to the degree of acidosis the patient has. Potassium is retained by the body in acidosis, so foods high in potassium should be restricted. Sodium intake is controlled at a level sufficient to replace the sodium loss without causing fluid retention. Table salt is almost always eliminated, and commercially prepared low-salt foods are used. Coffee, tea, nuts, dried fruit, fish, and certain fruits and vegetables have high potassium values. Boiling removes considerable potassium from vegetables such as potatoes, and canned fruits and vegetables have less potassium than fresh ones because of the processing.

Once the patient has begun dialysis, the diet can be more liberal. Again, there are no specific guidelines as to the amounts that should be given. Instead a number of factors should be considered, including the status of the patient's kidney function, the frequency and duration of dialysis, and the constituents of the dialysate. The diet should be planned with all these factors taken into account. Generally, the diet is less restrictive if the patient has more frequent dialysis. Some plans include a very controlled diet in conjunction with dialysis on the premise that the patient is not as likely to develop complications of the symptoms of uremia; the patient's prognosis is improved if these symptoms are not allowed to occur. Sometimes the protein intake is as low as 1 gm per kilogram of body weight, compared to the normal protein intake of 9 gm per kilogram. Fluid restriction is also maintained even if the patient has dialysis frequently. One of the measures of how well the patient has followed his diet is body weight; often he or she is expected to gain only one pound or less between dialysis treatments.

Dialysis The decision to begin dialysis as renal failure progresses is usually based on the patient's total status. Mental acuity is depressed in renal failure; the patient who begins to learn how to manage his or her disease early can therefore learn more effectively. Each patient is taught to manage renal failure according to individual requirements. If, for example, a patient is on the borderline between regulating his or her condition with diet or with dialysis, he or she might be dialyzed occasionally during periods either when the diet was not followed or when intervening factors such as infection or stress have altered the body's ability to cope. Other patients with no urine output or with very little urine output will need a routine plan for continued dialysis. Usually dialysis is accomplished in three sessions per week. The duration of the sessions varies from 4 to 12 hours; it depends on the patient's status and on the type of dialysis machine used.

EXTRACORPOREAL HEMODIALYSIS Extracorporeal hemodialysis stimulates kidney function by bringing the blood into contact with dialysate (blood and dialysate are separated by a porous cellulose membrane). The passage of metabolic wastes, electrolytes, and water (plus substances not yet identified as uremic toxins) into the dialysate is accomplished by concentration gradients and by the pressure of the blood flow. Substances that are in greater concentration in the blood pass to the dialysate and vice versa. The dialysate contains higher concentrations of sodium, calcium, magnesium, chloride acetate, glucose, and bicarbonate. Substances in high concentration in the blood are potassium, urea, creatinine, uric acid, phosphate, and water. Viruses and bacteria cannot pass through the membrane from the dialysate to the blood. **Membrane clearance** is the measure of waste products removed from the blood.

There are three types of dialyzers. The **flat-plate dialyzer** has a plate that channels blood in one direction and the dialysate in the opposite direction. The **coil dialyzer** channels blood through two cellophane tubes held in place between two layers of mesh while the dialysate circulates around the tubes. The **hollow-fiber dialyzer** has thousands of tiny tubes (capillaries) through which the blood flows while the dialysate flows on the outside. These machines must be primed with blood, saline, or colloid solution. In most dialyzers the flow rate of the blood and the dialysate can be controlled.

Patients are monitored carefully during dialysis; complications include loss of blood, hemorrhage from heparinization, either hypotension or hypertension, arrhythmias, and muscle cramps. Disequilibrium occurs when there is rapid removal of solutes from the blood so that the diluted water passing into the brain results in cerebral edema.

Dialysis tubing connects the patient's circulatory system to the dialysis machine. Blood from the artery is channeled into the machine and then returned to the vein. Repeated injections for this purpose would soon damage the patient's veins and arteries. One method used to overcome this problem is the use of an external cannula made of a material compatible with blood vessels to provide for a shunt so that there is access to both the artery and vein. The cannula can be placed in location on the arms or legs. The specific type of cannula used and its placement are determined according to the patient's vascular status, access, and activities. If the patient is right-handed, the shunt is usually placed on the right arm. One cannula lasts for four to nine months and usually has to be replaced because clotting occurs. These cannulas require care; clotting is minimized by careful cleaning of the cannula. There are two concerns when an external cannula is used. First, the patient may acquire an infection if the cannula is not cared for with strict aseptic technique, and this infection can lead to sepsis. Second, the circulatory system can be affected, either by clotting or by potential thrombosis. Hemorrhage may occur if the loop connecting the cannulas accidentally comes apart. If this occurs, emergency measures include the application of a blood pressure cuff inflated to systolic pressure above the shunt. Because the cannula can be so easily opened, the patient's emotional stability must be carefully evaluated since he or she could easily commit suicide by opening the cannulas. After the cannula has been inserted, the stitches remain in place for about a week. Bacitracin ointment or a similar antibiotic ointment is usually placed around the site of insertion. Ongoing cannula care includes cleaning with pHisoHex or another effective antiseptic. Crusts are removed carefully with cotton guard or application of a circular bandage such as Kling or an Ace bandage.

The other method used to attach dialysis tubing involves an arteriovenous fistula in which a vein is surgically anastomosed to an artery. The vein then becomes distended and the vessel wall thickens and can be palpated easily so that needles can be injected for dialysis hookup over a long period of time. When used, fistulas increase the blood supply to the limb. A bruit can be heard with a stethoscope over the fistula because of the increased blood supply. The extremity used should be carefully observed for any signs of inflammation or infection. (See Fig. 6-8.)

Because blood must be thinned and evenly

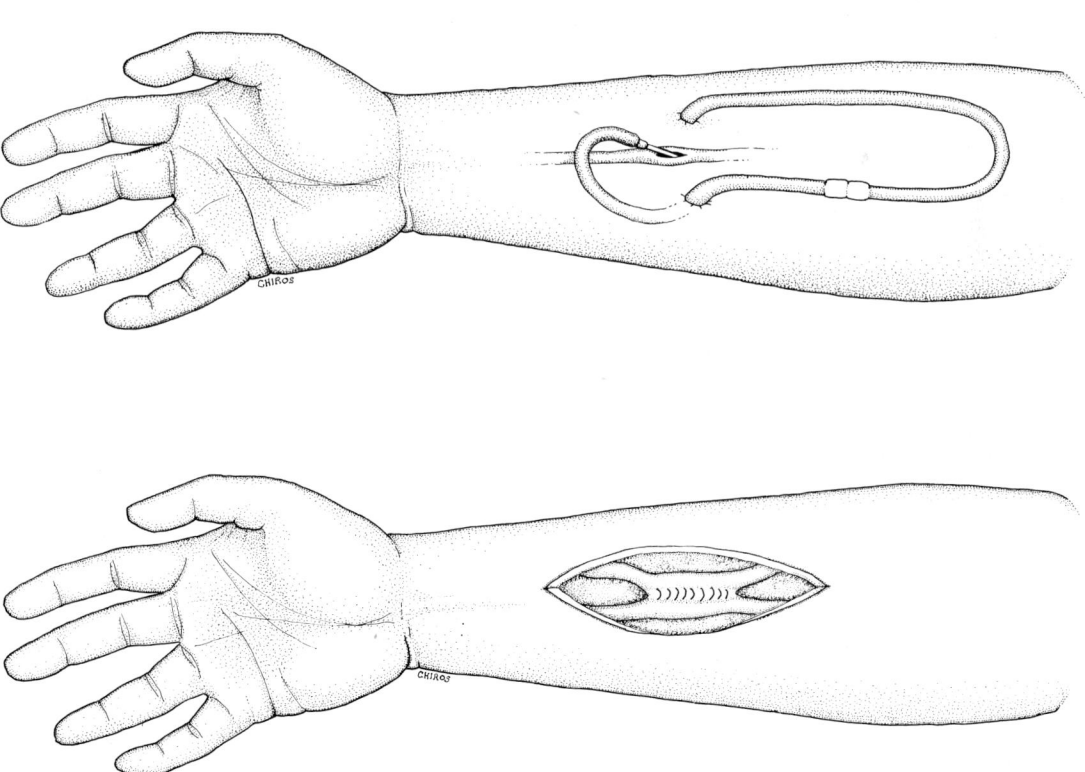

Figure 6-8
Arteriovenous shunt and arteriovenous fistula.

circulated in the dialyzer, it is necessary to use heparin. Either regional or systemic heparinization is used. With regional heparinization, heparin is added to the patient's blood at a point between the patient and the dialyzer; protamine is added after the blood leaves the dialyzer and before it is returned to the patient's veins. Systemic heparinization involves the administration of anticoagulants to the patient. The patient is monitored for bleeding and clotting times with both methods.

Patients with chronic renal failure have associated anemia and occasionally require blood transfusions. Repeated blood transfusions, together with the fact that the dialyzing machines must be primed with blood, make the patient susceptible to hepatitis. As the patient receives increasing numbers of transfusions over a period of time, there is also a possibility that blood cell antibodies will form, decreasing not only the compatible blood supply but also future donor kidneys.

Patients on dialysis are at risk for hypertension, stroke, and myocardial infarction and require treatment to control hypertension. Patients can conduct dialysis at home; teaching for home dialysis usually takes place in the dialysis center. The patient learns how to manage his own dialysis in a setting that simulates his home needs as much as possible. The nurse teaches him how to perform the dialysis, how to make routine checks of blood pressure and clotting time, and what to do to manage difficulties as they arise. The nurse also works with the patient's friends and family who will be helping him. Family members or friends begin to establish their roles in helping the patient. Gradually the nurse withdraws from active participation in the dialysis procedure as the patient becomes more capable. The length of the training programs varies according to the family's needs. It is generally felt that the home dialysis program is more convenient for the patient, and many think that those on home dialysis feel and look better than patients who have their dialysis at the hospital.

There are many different approaches to managing dialysis for the patient in renal failure. Home dialysis offers the patient the most options. Some physicians require strict adherence to diet and follow-up care between dialysis procedures, whereas others are more liberal in attitude and allow the patient some leeway in occasional splurging with restricted foods or liquid. Motivation to follow the plan of therapy closely is generally greater if the patient is aware of the body's responses to this splurging in terms of an increase in symptoms and the consequences of longer periods of time spent with the dialysis machine. Strict adherence to diet is often difficult, however, for the person who has trouble saying no to food and drink, particularly at social gatherings. Perhaps one of the most difficult aspects of care for the patient being dialyzed is that of helping him or her to accept and voluntarily follow the treatment regimen.

PERITONEAL DIALYSIS Peritoneal dialysis uses the same principles as hemodialysis. The patient's own peritoneum serves as the membrane (Fig. 6-9). Two to four liters of dialysate is infused into the peritoneal cavity through a catheter and remains there for a period of 15 to 30 minutes. Studies indicate that the maximum concentrated gradient occurs in the peritoneal cavity in the first 5 to 10 minutes, and equilibrium is reached in 15 to 30 minutes [21]. The dialysate is then removed and a fresh dialysate is infused. This can be accomplished with a machine that controls the timing of infusion and drainage, or by gravity flow. Either way, the process is continued sequentially to remove the desired waste products (usually in 24-hour cycles). The blood in closest contact with the peritoneum is that in the splanchnic vascular system, so the passage of substances to and from the blood takes place in this area. Urea is cleared most rapidly; then in order of clearance are potassium, phosphate, creatinine, and uric acid. Peritoneal dialysis requires a longer time than hemodialysis to achieve similar results, and it is difficult to control infection if the peritoneal dialysis is carried out over a period of months. Peritonitis may be a complication. The dialysate becomes cloudy on return if an infection is present [9]. Hemodialysis is more effective in purifying the blood because protein excretion cannot be as precisely controlled with peritoneal dialysis as it can with hemodialysis. Hypernatremia, hyperglycemia, or hyperosmolality may complicate peritoneal dialysis because fluid shifts from cells to blood change the concentration gradients of electrolytes.

Peritoneal dialysis is effective, however, for patients who are not admitted to a

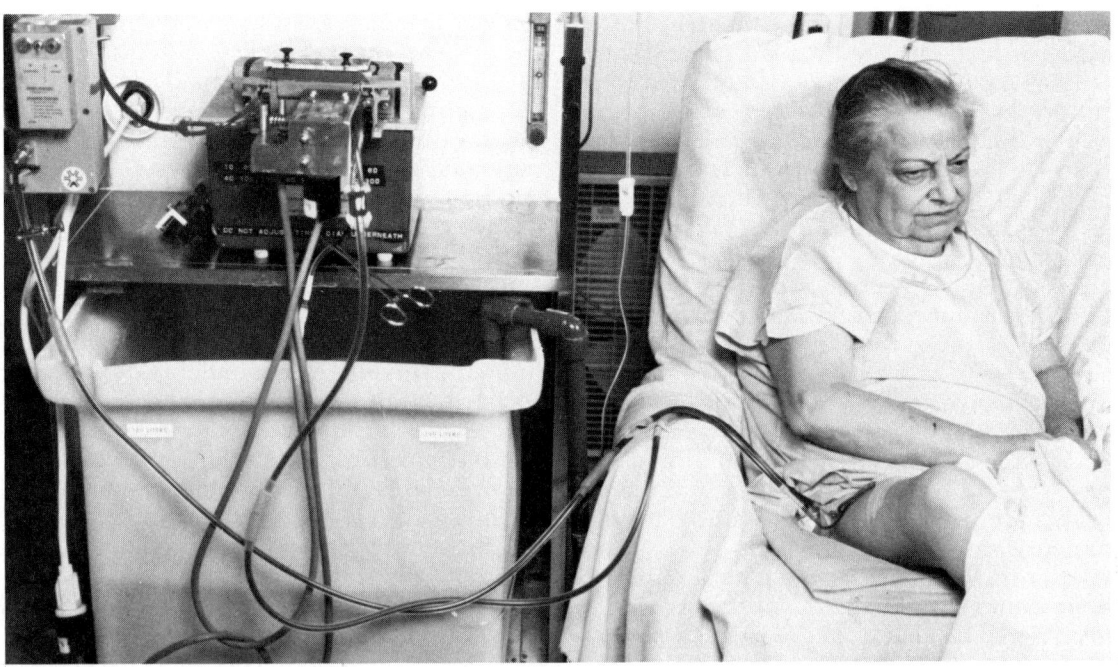

Figure 6-9
A patient receiving hemodialysis.

hemodialysis program or for those who cannot tolerate hemodialysis (this includes patients with cardiac or respiratory conditions whose adaptive resources to accommodate changes in blood volume or pressure are minimal). In observing the patient during peritoneal dialysis, the nurse must give attention to the symptoms of respiratory distress or to the occurrence of arrhythmias, particularly if there is respiratory or cardiac disease. This is essential because of the changing intra-abdominal pressure, which may exert increased pressure on the diaphragm. Vagal stimulation or excess K^+ loss can lead to arrhythmias. Perforation of the bowel may occur in patients who have adhesions. Signs of perforation are diarrhea following the instillation of dialysate or fecal return in the dialysate. In addition, comfort measures and monitoring the dialysis procedure are primary nursing concerns. Peritoneal dialysis is uncomfortable for the patient and takes a long time; therefore the patient tires easily, becomes restless, and requires a great deal of emotional support to tolerate the procedure.

USES OF DIALYSIS Dialysis, then, can be used for long-term care for patients with chronic renal failure, or it can be used as a temporary measure for treatment of acute renal failure. Toxins and the effects of drug overdose can be dialyzed out; for example, barbiturates, phenobarbital, and other drugs that are capable of being removed through a semipermeable membrane can be removed from the body via dialysis. Timing is important in dialyzing for removal of drugs and poisons since they can only be removed if they are still in the circulating blood. Dialysis is also used during the interim between bilateral nephrectomy and renal transplant. Patients awaiting transplant often have many anxieties that are never really resolved until the transplant is performed.

ROLE OF THE NURSE IN DIALYSIS Because there are so many different methods used in caring for patients requiring dialysis, there is no single approach to nursing care. The nurse must become familiarized with the method used in each dialysis center or hospital. It is very important that everyone involved in the care shares a common set of goals for the patient. This means that the patient receiving dialysis, the nurses, and all other personnel should know the rationale for the therapeutic plan and follow through with precision in their particular part of the plan. It is essential that whatever the plan, everyone involved support the same concepts and goals. The patient's diet, dialysis schedule, and medications all form a composite of activities, all of which are interdependent. When diet changes, the dialysis schedule may have to be altered accordingly.

Most dialysis centers require that nurses complete a training program before becoming actively involved in care. The nurse who decides to work with a dialysis program accepts the challenge of mastering the technical knowledge of the process as well as mastering and dealing with extremely complicated behaviors on the part of the family and the patient with renal failure. The nurse and the patient receiving dialysis form a very close relationship because of the long duration of their contacts in the treatment process. These behaviors emanate from the process of adaptation to dialysis, which is particularly difficult because of a combination of factors; among these are the problems of selecting candidates for dialysis, the expense associated with dialysis, the fact that dialysis may not prove to be effective for a particular patient, and the amorphous knowledge that the underlying issue that must be dealt with by the patient in renal failure is death.

Patients can receive assistance from the National Kidney Foundation, 11 East 27th Street, New York, New York 10016. At this writing, there are 57 regional or state affiliates of the Foundation. The Foundation has a program through which patients can buy drugs at 10 percent over cost and it provides free identification cards and many publications for patient and professional education. The National Association of Patients on Hemodialysis and Transplantation, Inc., 505 Northern Boulevard, Great Neck, New York 11021, publishes the *NAPHT News* and provides services such as giving patients information about where to obtain dialysis while traveling. Patients benefit from the support of these organizations as well as from contacts with other dialysis patients in their local areas. Patients must be motivated to participate in the dialysis program, and this motivation must be nurtured continually as renal failure is a chronic condition and the patient requires lifetime treatment.

For some patients, the financial aspects of dialysis present very grave problems. By having dialysis, the patient may be draining family finances that have been designated for other purposes and thus requiring sacrifices on the part of family members. If the patient's renal dysfunction has been associated with loss of work or the necessity to change the type of work, there may also be the added factor of reduced income for the family.

It is very discouraging for the patient who has made a commitment to long-term dialysis to find that he or she does not respond as hoped to the treatments. Some patients develop associated health problems such as cardiac problems, infections, or other dysfunction and have difficulty controlling the renal failure even when they follow the treatment regimen. The nurse shares this discouragement and must deal with feelings of guilt or sorrow experienced by the patient. Other patients find the long-term dialysis program and its associated regimen too taxing and decide that they no longer wish to continue. This also is difficult for the nurse who is working with the patient and family to accept. A feeling of failure on the part of the nurse is not uncommon, even if the nurse firmly believes in the right of the patient to choose his or her own fate.

The patient who continues with a long-term dialysis program will be expected to have crises. These may be of family origin, associated with the patient's increasingly weakened condition, or from other sources. Despite the fact that dialysis is maintaining the patient's life, the threat that complications might develop despite very meticulous care is ever present. This knowledge is a subtle form of stress. The nurse may be the recipient of the patient's feelings of anxiety, anger, hostility, or fear during the crisis periods. Because of the very close involvement between the family and the nurse, each is reacting to the crisis in an individual way. The nurse has to remain supportive of the patient and family. For this reason, staff members involved in the care of patients in renal failure often have weekly meetings ranging from planning sessions to group therapy sessions to provide support to the staff as each member experiences his or her own unique management problems. In some places these meetings are open to dialysis patients as well.

Kidney transplantation Kidney transplantation offers hope to many patients who have bilateral kidney disease and no renal function. Sources of kidneys to transplant are still scarce, and not every kidney that is available can be used in a patient who is awaiting transplantation. The most successful transplants are those done with a sibling or family member with the same blood type. By carefully matching the donor kidney with the recipient, kidneys from unrelated people and from cadavers are transplanted with fair success. In preparation for the transplant, the patient undergoes a bilateral nephrectomy so that he or she will be ready for the donor kidney whenever it becomes available. Since renal function is absent in these patients, dialysis is absolutely necessary until the transplantation can be accomplished. The major problem in transplantation is that of rejection. Prior to surgery the patient's immunologic responses are suppressed by the administration of azathioprine 24 hours before surgery is to take place. Steroid therapy is also used to suppress the immunologic response. (The mechanisms of the immune response are discussed in Chapter 1.) The rejection can occur soon after surgery, or it can be delayed for months or even years following transplantation.

Teaching is essential in the nursing care of patients who are dependent on dialysis. Jenrich [12] states that important variables in the types of problems patients have during dialysis include "diagnosis, stage of illness, age, emotional problems, and other medical problems." Wolf [24] studied perceived problems of patients awaiting kidney transplant who were being dialyzed in the interim. She found that they ranked as very important the problem of possible rejection and the medications required to decrease rejection. Of middle priority were factors such as postoperative diet, and of low priority were care needs in the operating room and intensive care unit.

Laatsch [14] studied time perception as a product of man's total interaction between internal cues and rhythms and the external environmental events in patients with chronic illnesses. She observed that people have an overwhelming need to be somewhat future oriented and hypothesized that hospitalized patients are in waiting situations. The waiting situations are defined in Laatsch's study as expectancy, waiting in uncertainty, and waiting for a dreaded outcome. She found that one way patients had of coping with waiting in uncertainty was definition of daily schedules to create structure in the "waiting in uncertainty" situations. This structuring allowed short-term goal attainment, even though the final outcome of the chronic illness remained uncertain.

Laatsch also noted that chronically ill patients became increasingly aware of internal cues, which provided a sense of certainty for them within the interval of uncertainty. Continual successful adaptation to these new cues by the patients required knowledge of treatment modalities; for example, one patient requiring periodic blood transfusions recognized the need for transfusion by the internal cue of ringing in the ears; this symptom was perceived as an internal cue signaling the need for a blood transfusion. Awareness of the cue, knowledge of the meaning of the internal cue, and information about the required care associated with the cue decreased the patient's anxiety and frustration during the period of uncertainty. Waiting in uncertainty then became more manageable for the patient, and less energy was expended in anxiety [14].

These studies, while dealing in a theoretical framework, imply that nurses must carefully assess the patient's feelings, attitudes, and important perceived symptoms as well as the visible signs of disease processes. These factors can be structured into a perceived reaction pattern in which the patient's care needs evolve. If the nurse can successfully deal with the foremost worries and concerns of the patient (which involve both present and future events), the nurse can use this information in planning ways to meet these priority needs. Nursing care managed in this way can both utilize and conserve the patient's energy for the care process as well as the cure process in a constructive manner. Enabling the patient to perform small tasks that are meaningful and that provide for a sense of accomplishment may be the crucial factor that determines whether a potentially chronic debilitating disease can be managed in accordance with a productive life. By the same token managing schedules for dialysis within the patient's daily or weekly schedule of events can facilitate maximum use of energy for activities meaningful to the patient. This seems to be vitally important for patients who are waiting in uncertainty.

References

1. Anderson, L., Dibble, M. V., Mitchell, H. S., and Rynbergen, H. J. *Nutrition in Nursing.* Philadelphia: Lippincott, 1972.
2. Anger, D., and Anger, D. W. Dialysis ambivalence: A matter of life and death. *Am. J. Nurs.* 76:276, 1976.
3. Bates, B. *A Guide to Physical Examination.* Philadelphia: Lippincott, 1972.
4. Bouchard, R., and Owens, N. *Nursing Care of the Cancer Patient* (2nd ed.). St. Louis: Mosby, 1972.
5. Burton, B. T. Current concepts of nutrition and diet in diseases of the kidney. *J. Am. Diet. Assoc.* 65:623, 1974.
6. Burton, B.T. Nutrition and diet in kidney disease. *J. Am. Diet. Assoc.* 65:627, 1974.
7. Camino, J. E. Diagnosis and management of urinary tract infections. *Hosp. Med.* 10:59, 1974.
8. Corea, A. Current trends in diet and drug therapy for the dialysis patient. *Nurs. Clin. North Am.* 10:469, 1975.
9. Freedman, P., and Smith, E. Acute renal failure. *Heart Lung* 4:873, 1975.
10. Glenn, J. F. *Urologic Surgery* (2nd ed.). New York: Harper & Row, 1975.
11. Hassett, M. Teaching hemodialysis to the family unit. *Nurs. Clin. North Am.* 7:2, 1972.
12. Jenrich, J. A. Some aspects of nursing care for patients on hemodialysis. *Heart Lung* 4:885, 1975.
13. Kunin, C. A. *Detection, Prevention and Management of Urinary Tract Infections.* Philadelphia: Lea & Febiger, 1974.
14. Laatsch, N. Time Perception in the Holistic Nursing Care of Individuals with a Nonlocalized Malignancy. M.A. Thesis, 1975.
15. Montague, D. K. Guide to the diagnosis of urinary tract infections. *Hosp. Med.* 11:6, 1975.
16. Mountcastle, V. *Medical Physiology* (13th ed.), Vol. 2. St. Louis: Mosby, 1974.
17. Netter, F. A. *The Ciba Collection of Medical Illustrations. Kidneys, Ureters and Urinary Bladder.* Summit, N.J.: Ciba Pharmaceutical Co., 1973.
18. O'Neill, M. (ed.). Symposium on care of the patient with renal disease. *Nurs. Clin. North Am.* 10:411, 1975.
19. Paulson, D. F. Carcinoma of the bladder and urethra. *Hosp. Med.* 11:11, 1975.
20. Roberts, J. A. A guide to the urologic examination. *Hosp. Med.* 12:6, 1976.
21. Selkurt, E. E. *Basic Physiology for the Health Sciences.* Boston: Little, Brown, 1975.
22. Tilkian, S. M., and Conover, M. H. *Clinical Implications of Laboratory Tests.* St. Louis: Mosby, 1975.
23. Watt, R. C. Urinary diversion. *Am. J. Nurs.* 74:1806, 1974.
24. Wolf, Z. What patients awaiting kidney transplant want to know. *Am. J. Nurs.* 76:92, 1976.

Bibliography

Bartecchi, C. E. When should peritoneal dialysis be considered in elderly patients? *Geriatrics* 30:12, 1975.

Beeson, P. B., and McDermott, W. *Cecil Loeb Textbook of Medicine* (13th ed.). Philadelphia: Saunders, 1971.

Berman, L. B., and Vertes, V. The pathophysiology of renin. *Clin. Symp.* 25:5, 1973.

Burke, E. *The Composition and Function of Body Fluids* (2nd ed.). St. Louis: Mosby, 1976.

Dossetor, J. B., and Gault, M. D. *Nephron Failure.* Springfield, Ill.: Thomas, 1974.

Dougherty, J. C. High protein diets and renal function. *J. Am. Diet. Assoc.* 63:392, 1973.

Favero, M. S., et al. Gram-negative water bacteria in hemodialysis systems. *Health Lab. Sci.* 12:321, 1975.

Fennell, S. E. Percutaneous renal biopsy. *Am. J. Nurs.* 75:8, 1975.

Goldberger, E. *A Primer of Water, Electrolyte and Acid-Base Balance* (5th ed.). Philadelphia: Lea & Febiger, 1975.

Hamilton, M. S., and Schlapper, N.B. Pelvic exenteration. *Am. J. Nurs.* 76:266, 1976.

Hepinstall, R. H. *Pathology of the Kidney.* Boston: Little, Brown, 1974.

Melber, S., Leonard, M., and Primack, W. Hemodialysis at camp. *Am. J. Nurs.* 76:938, 1976.

Murray, B., et al. The patient has an ileal conduit. *Am. J. Nurs.* 71:1560, 1971.

Nelson, W. E. *Textbook of Pediatrics* (9th ed.). Philadelphia: Saunders, 1969.

Paulson, D. F. Ureteral obstruction: Diagnosis and management. *Hosp. Med.* 11:85, 1975.

Pitts, R. F. *Physiology of the Kidney and Body Fluids* (3rd ed.). Chicago: Year Book, 1974.

Richard, C. Nursing implications in prevention of complications in renal dialysis. *Heart Lung* 4:890, 1975.

Romankiewicz, J. A. Factors influencing renal distribution of antibiotics a key to therapy of pyelonephritis. *Drug Intell. Clin. Pharm.* 8:9, 1974.

Rubin, P. *Cancer in the Urogenital Tract: Part I. Current Cancer Concepts: Multidisciplinary*

Views. New York: American Cancer Society, 1969. An AMA reprint.

Sabiston, D. C. *Davis-Christopher Textbook of Surgery* (10th ed.). Philadelphia: Saunders, 1972.

Santopietro, M.-C. S. Meeting the emotional needs of hemodialysis patients and their spouses. *Am. J. Nurs.* 75:629, 1975.

Schaffer, E. Do it yourself dialysis. *Can. Nurse.* 69:29, 1973.

Simon, N. M., Johnson, N. K., Lennor, R. G. Chronic renal failure. Part II. Treatment by dialysis and renal transplantation. *Cardiovasc. Nurs.* 12:11, 1976.

Smith, E. B., and Hill, P. Protein in diets of uremic patients. *J. Am. Diet. Assoc.*, 60:389, 1970.

Suke, W., and Eknoyan, G. *The Kidney in Systemic Disease.* New York: Wiley, 1976.

Taylor, G. H. *Fluid Therapy and Disorders of Electrolyte Balance* (2nd ed.). Edinburgh: Blackwell, 1970.

Zinner, S. H. Pyelonephritis: Guide to diagnosis. *Hosp. Med.* 12:54, 1976.

chapter 7
Patients with Gastrointestinal System Dysfunction

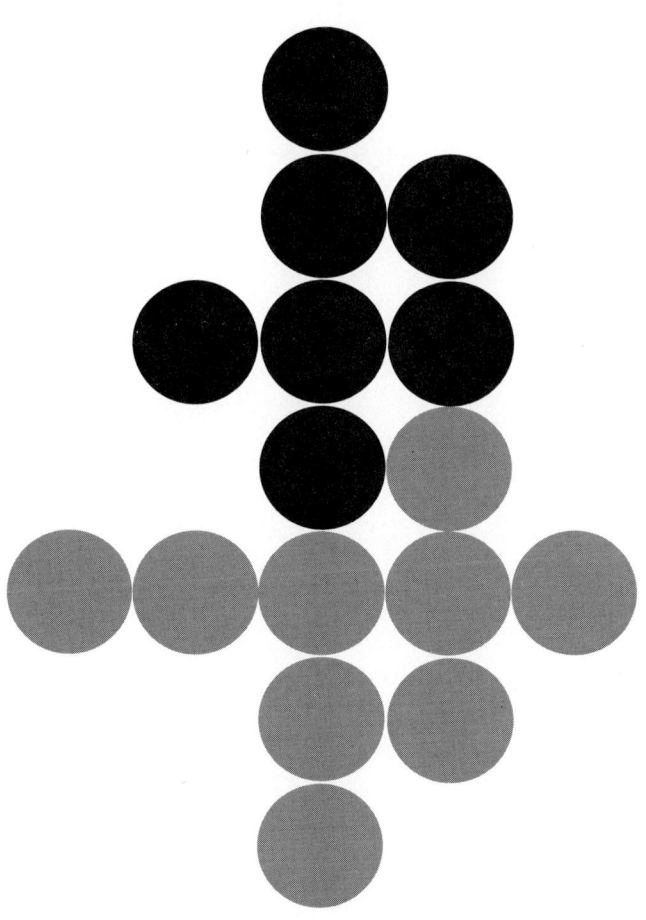

The primary function of the gastrointestinal system is to provide the body with fluids, nutrients, and electrolytes in a form that can be utilized at the cellular level. It must also dispose of the waste products that result from the digestive process. The gastrointestinal tract from the stomach to the anus is the site of major digestive, absorptive, and excretory activity, but the digestive system also includes the teeth, salivary glands, the esophagus, the gallbladder, the liver, and the pancreas. These accessory organs also have important functions in the proper ingestion, digestion, and absorption of nutrients.

The nurse must understand the location and function of the various parts of the gastrointestinal system in order to correctly assess and interpret the significance of signs and symptoms and to carry out therapeutic medical and nursing measures. Figure 7-1 shows the structural arrangement of the parts of the alimentary canal and accessory organs. The alimentary canal is a continuous tract of approximately 25 to 30 feet in length, through which food moves during the digestive process.

The adequate intake and alteration of nutrients so that they can be utilized by body cells are dependent on the integrity of the gastrointestinal tract, which provides for chemical changes of the digested food, the transportation of the food, and the absorption of the nutrients into the circulating blood. Saliva is produced by the secretions from three pairs of salivary glands (parotid glands, sublingual glands, and submaxillary glands) and the oral mucosa. Saliva keeps the mucous membranes moist and aids mastication and swallowing by moistening and lubricating food. Saliva also facilitates movement of the bolus of food through the pharynx and esophagus. Ducts of the three pairs of salivary glands open onto the surface of the mouth. The parotid glands, which lie in front of and below the ear, produce the digestive enzyme ptyalin. Ptyalin (salivary amylase) converts starch into maltose and dextrose.

The stomach is a reservoir for nutrients, where gastric juice is mixed with ingested food. Gastric juice is secreted in amounts of 1,500 to 2,500 ml daily. It contains mucus, hydrochloric acid, pepsin, rennin (in children), and inorganic salts. Hydrochloric acid and pepsin are the components in gastric juice that are potentially corrosive to the mucosa. Gastric juice is formed by secretions from three types of secretory cells: (1) the chief cells contain **zymogen granules**, which secrete and store pepsinogen, which is converted to active pepsin, an enzyme that hydrolyzes proteins; (2) the **parietal cells** secrete hydrochloric acid; and (3) the **mucous cells** produce mucus, which protects the gastric mucosa and serves as a lubricant. The hormone gastrin stimulates hydrochloric acid and pepsinogen secretion.

The small intestine, which is where the completion of digestion of foods and absorption takes place, is divided into three parts: (1) the **duodenum** receives the bile and pancreatic enzymes from the common bile duct and pancreatic ducts; (2) the **jejunum;** and (3) the **ileum.** The hormone enterogastrone is formed in the mucosa of the duodenum by the activation of fats or fatty acids and inhibits both gastric secretions and motility. (The enzymes entering the duodenum from the pancreas are discussed on page 608.)

The large intestine is divided into the **cecum, colon, rectum,** and **anal canal.** The colon is divided into the ascending, transverse, and descending colon; the latter is designated as the sigmoid colon as it curves through the pelvis. The appendix, which is a frequent site of inflammation and infection, is attached to the cecum. The mucosa of the large intestine secretes only mucus and no enzymes, since digestion is completed by this point. The function of the colon is to absorb only water and electrolytes, to some degree, and primarily to store and transport the feces for evacuation.

Several protective mechanisms serve to ensure the integrity and functioning of the gastrointestinal system. The digestive enzymes that chemically change the food, for example, do not normally attack the wall of the gastrointestinal tract. Cells in the gastrointestinal lining secrete mucus to lubricate and protect the lining of the wall and allow passage of the food. The tract has a high rate of cell regeneration since it has to withstand the mechanical contact and trauma of the passage of food. This high rate of regeneration, in addition to the absorption activity, requires a maximal blood supply and thus the tract has a rich vascular supply.

The mouth, tongue, and pharynx obtain their blood supply from the external carotid artery via the lingual and external maxillary arteries. The esophageal artery arises from the thoracic aorta. The stomach is supplied by many arteries; the left gastric artery is a branch of the celiac trunk, the right gastric

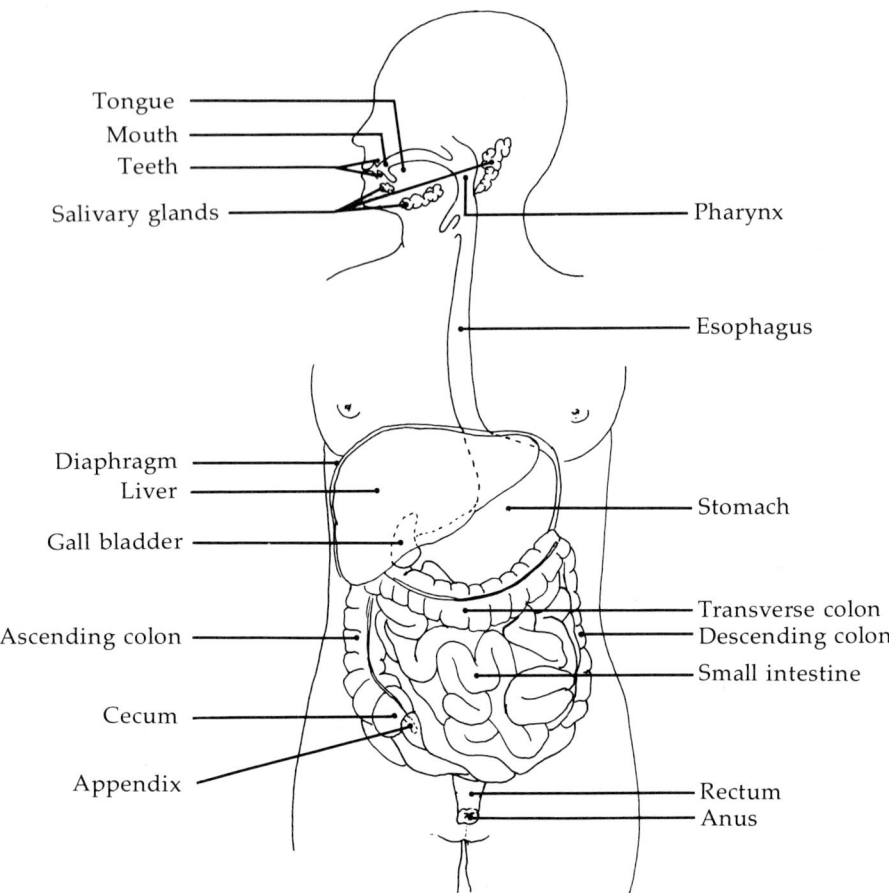

Figure 7-1
Structures of the alimentary system.

artery and the right gastroepiploic artery arise from the hepatic artery and the left gastroepiploic artery arises from the splenic artery. In addition, there are several small gastric arteries. The other parts of the gastrointestinal tract are supplied by the superior and inferior mesenteric arteries, which are direct branches from the abdominal aorta.

Blood that contains absorbed nutrients is carried from the gastrointestinal tract, particularly the small intestine, by the superior and inferior mesenteric veins into the portal vein, which carries the blood and nutrients to the liver for use in metabolism and other vital functions.

Along the gastrointestinal tract are muscular sphincters and valves at strategic points to provide for forward propulsion of the food bolus and feces at appropriately timed intervals. **Sphincters** are located at the opening of the esophagus into the stomach (cardiac sphincter) and the opening of the stomach into the small intestine (pyloric sphincter) as well as at the junction of the common bile duct and duodenum (sphincter of Oddi). The function of these sphincters is to control the one-way movement of substances in the alimentary canal. When functioning properly, they prevent reflux of contents. At the junction of the ileum and cecum, an ileocecal valve functions to pass contents from the ileum into the cecum. At the short terminal portion of the alimentary canal (the anal canal) the internal anal sphincter controls movement between the rectum and anus; the external anal sphincter promotes voluntary evacuation through the anus. The normally patent gastrointestinal tract has inherent motility, which provides for forward movement of food and for churning and mixing the food to allow maximal surface area contact for chemical reactions and absorption. The small intestine, as the site of most absorption activity, is the longest functional unit of the body. Duration of surface contact of the food with the gastrointestinal wall is important, because rapid movement interferes with adequate absorption while slowed movement results in increased absorption of fluids and problems with elimination.

The stomach and the intestines are protected by a serous membrane, the visceral peritoneum and the parietal peritoneum, which lines the walls of the abdominal cavity. These two layers of peritoneum enclose the potential space, the **peritoneal cavity.** A section of the peritoneum, the **great omentum,** is an apron-like structure that protects the intestines by walling off areas of infection or inflammation of the peritoneum (peritonitis). The **mesentery** is the portion of the peritoneum that supports the intestines and contains blood vessels, lymphatics, and nerves.

The gastrointestinal system, however, is not the sole system involved in digestion. Motility of the gastrointestinal tract and secretion of digestive enzymes and juices are governed by parasympathetic and sympathetic nerve fibers. The nervous system is also vital for the voluntary aspects of chewing and swallowing (via the cranial nerve fibers to the muscles of the mouth and the pharynx). Social and cultural attitudes toward food and excretory functions influence the integrative neural responses of the cerebrum for control of gastrointestinal function. The hypothalamus contains the centers of hunger, appetite, and satiety, and has a role in increasing the peristaltic activity of the intestinal tract. In addition to the nervous system, the endocrine system also has a vital role in activating different metabolic functions of the body, and the circulatory system delivers the nutrients to tissue cells and transports the waste products of metabolism.

Assessment of the Gastrointestinal System

A general survey of the patient gives clues to the status of the patient's nutritional state and the initial clinical assessment of the gastrointestinal system. The patient's posture and facial expression indicate relaxation, tenseness, or pain. The integrity of the skin, nails, and hair reflects the nutritional and hydration state and therefore the status of the gastrointestinal system. The amount of adipose tissue may reflect inadequate or excessive intake of food as well as the rate of metabolic activity.

HISTORY

The presenting symptoms as well as past illnesses or operations are included in the patient's history. The nurse should elicit information on dietary patterns, allergies, and social habits, which affect the gastrointestinal system. Information about medications being taken and known allergies is essential. The patient should be asked about the presence of major symptoms associated with gastrointestinal disorders such as dysphagia, pain, anorexia, melena, hematemesis, and changes in bowel habits. Pain is described in terms of onset, site, type, predisposing factors, and relation to eating.

When assessing symptoms and complaints, it is extremely important for the nurse to listen and observe closely as the patient describes them. The nurse needs to be careful in the use of terms, for some descriptive terms have different meanings for different individuals. For example, "diarrhea" may mean having two stools per day to one individual whose bowel pattern is usually one stool a day, whereas another person using the term may mean ten watery stools per day. In taking a history, the nurse needs to verify the meaning of terminology used by the patient and must also be specific in recording signs and symptoms. Accurate interpretation of progress notes and reports written by the physician also requires an appropriate understanding of some of the common terms used in evaluating the status of the gastrointestinal system. These symptoms are investigated in relation to their occurrence and to eating, elimination, position, and activity. Common terms used in describing gastrointestinal disturbance include the following:

achalasia Failure of a sphincter to relax.
anorexia Loss of appetite.
belching Expulsion of gas from stomach when the stomach is distended with excess food or gas.
borborygmi Waves of loud, gurgling, and tinkling sounds heard in hyperactive bowel activity.
cachexia Profound malnutrition and weight loss.

constipation Difficult evacuation of stool because of dry and firm consistency and relative to the individual. (The frequency or infrequency of evacuation is not the determining characteristic of constipation as is commonly thought.)

colic Acute, cramping abdominal pain.

dyspepsia Feeling of abdominal fullness, with nausea, belching, and heartburn sensation of "indigestion." It is characteristic of excessive acid in the stomach and is aggravated by spicy foods, excessive coffee, and cola drinks.

dysphagia Difficulty in swallowing. (The patient is usually able to cite the exact location of the difficulty.)

diarrhea Frequent passage of unformed stools with increased fluidity or volume. (The number of stools should be identified.)

eructation A normal phenomenon of raising gas, sometimes accompanied by gastric acid fluid. An important symptom if excessive or accompanied by discomfort.

flatulence Excessive accumulation of gas in the stomach or intestine.

flatus Passage of gas from the intestines.

guarding Voluntary or involuntary muscular rigidity or resistance in the abdominal musculature.

hematemesis Vomitus containing blood.

heartburn Burning sensation originating in the subxyphoid region, spreading upward into the chest.

hiccups Rhythmic contraction of the diaphragm, usually resulting from stomach disturbances due to excessive food. May indicate severe disease.

ileus Intestinal obstruction with dilatation of the bowel and obstipation; cause may be mechanical or neurogenic.

melena Black stool due to blood pigments; varies in color from deep maroon to tarry.

obstipation Persistent failure to pass any stool.

pyorrhea Pus formation of the dental periosteum resulting in necrosis of the alveoli and loosening of the teeth.

pyrosis Heartburn; a sensation of burning in the epigastrium and along the course of the esophagus.

vomiting Voluntary or involuntary excretion of stomach contents through the mouth. (Important signs to report include the frequency, time of occurrence, contributing factors, color, quantity, odor, and consistency.)

An adequate nutritional state is dependent on adequate and appropriate intake, digestion, and absorption. In almost all disease processes there is a threat to the ability to take in and utilize food. For the patient with disease of the digestive system, the inability to take nutrients may be the central problem.

Food habits are evaluated because they can give insight into potential nutritional problems during a disease state. Any recent change in dietary pattern and any food intolerances are recorded. Cultural and religious attitudes and beliefs frequently dictate food intake and should always be considered in the assessment phase of care as well as during the treatment phase. The vegetarian or the person who maintains a natural organic food diet may experience difficulties during hospitalization where so many additives and prepared foods are used.

The person who frequently ingests a low carbohydrate, unlimited protein diet in order to lose weight may develop nutritional imbalances and increased serum levels of uric acid. These effects are particularly dangerous in persons with potential, or existing, liver and kidney disease. The nurse frequently finds that the person on a self-prescribed low carbohydrate diet increases fat intake, resulting in increased cholesterol levels. Concern with weight control as determined during the nursing assessment requires a plan for health teaching in this area. A reduction of total calories while maintaining a well-balanced diet is emphasized. The importance of a slow, regular loss of weight as a means of avoiding potential health hazards from rapid weight loss is discussed with the patient.

Besides the initial interview to establish the food habits, allergies, likes, and dislikes, continual assessment of dietary habits is done by noting what foods the patient selects when hospital menus are provided. The nurse should be available at mealtimes to observe what the patient eats and to assist the patient if appropriate. This is an ideal time to evaluate nutritional habits and intake and the effect of diet instruction on the patient's nutritional habits. While the physician prescribes the diet and the nutritionist plans the diet, the nurse is responsible for ensuring that the patient ingests the food. It is the nurse's responsibility to note the patient's response to food and to be persistent in trying to find out what the patient will eat if there is inadequate intake. Feeding the patient may be necessary. The nurse should report to the physician when the intake is inadequate for the patient's needs. Alternative ways for providing nutrition should then be arranged.

Food intake can vary as widely as the emotional attitudes of patients can vary, as observed in states ranging from cachexia to obesity. The physiologic needs for nutrients can be insignificant to emotionally disturbed persons. The nurse must evaluate the adequacy of these patients' food intake and take measures to provide required nutrients to promote their well-being or recovery because these patients cannot be expected to take responsibility for their own nutrition.

Butterworth [4] recently published his criticism of hospitals and physicians regarding the neglect of nutritional health of hospitalized patients. He identified the failure to observe the patient's food intake as one of the undesirable practices affecting nutritional health. Citing malnutrition as a common accompaniment to the stress of illness among hospitalized patients, this author also listed the failure to record height and weight, the diffusion of responsibility for patient care, the prolonged use of glucose and saline as intravenous feedings, and failure to recognize increased nutritional needs due to injury or illness among the fourteen undesirable practices resulting in iatrogenic malnutrition. Such criticism only reinforces the potential dangers that result when nurses also neglect nutritional health evaluation.

PHYSICAL EXAMINATION

Physical examination of the gastrointestinal system includes assessment of the oral cavity, the abdomen, and the rectum. An initial step in efficient digestion is the proper mastication of food, which is dependent on healthy natural teeth or a functional dental prosthesis. Normally the crowns of the teeth have a white enamel surface and are regular in form. Discoloration is related to poor hygiene, surface stains as with heavy smokers, trauma, or disease. The healthy mouth has an absence of dental caries, or at least treatment of a minimal number of decayed teeth. To be functional, dentures must fit securely and should be worn regularly to prevent changes in facial contour. If dentures fit poorly, they may have to be realigned or the edges may have to be ground. When the condition of the mouth and teeth is assessed, the nurse may determine the patient's need for review of proper brushing technique, the importance of an adequate diet and fluid intake, and the need for regular dental examinations. All are important aspects of health teaching.

The gingivae are normally attached securely to the teeth, have a pale coral-pink color, a smooth glossy appearance, and show no evidence of bleeding or swelling. Reddening and swelling accompanied by bleeding may indicate inflammation. The gums in black persons may have bluish patches or may be normally bluish. Gingivae recessed to a low position on the tooth roots may indicate peridontal disease and pyorrhea.

The lips are examined for symmetry, color, activity in speech, facial expressions, and control of secretions. Normally lips are moist and pink. There should be no edema, drooling, numbness, ulceration, or hard firm lumps on the lips. During assessment, the nurse should remember that the lower lip is the most frequent site of lip cancer (see color insert Figure 9 on page 1078C).

During assessment of the oral cavity, the nurse is responsible for detection of oral cancer by noting any abnormality. The majority of oral cancers are squamous cell carcinomas that originate from the surface epithelium; they should be amenable to early recognition by inspection and palpation [15]. The nurse should also remember that susceptibility to oral cancer is increased when there is a history of heavy use of tobacco and alcohol. Any sore that has failed to heal, or any suspicious lesion, lump, or thickening should be reported. It is particularly important to observe for **leukoplakia** (whitish plaques in the oral cavity). These are premalignant lesions. Cytologic examination and biopsy are usually indicated for all suspicious lesions.

With the patient's mouth opened wide and the head tilted back, the hard and soft palates can be observed for lesions, swelling, irritated areas, malformations, and unilateral abnormalities. A tongue blade is used to depress the dorsum of the tongue, while the patient sounds the "ah" phonation, so that midline uvula elevation and coordinated pharynx constriction can be observed. Symmetry and muscle coordination of the tongue are assessed with the head erect while the patient protrudes the tongue to each side. (Lingual cancer is found most often on the lateral border in the middle third portion.) The mucosa of the tongue is examined for atrophy, hypertrophy, or elevated areas. Brown freckle-like pigmentation of the tongue borders is a normal phenomenon observed in blacks. There is some normal furring or coating of the tongue, but poor oral hygiene may be reflected in a heavily coated tongue. Normally, there is no unusual odor from the mouth. A plan for additional teaching of proper oral hygiene, including instruction in brushing the tongue as well as the teeth, is indicated when a heavily coated tongue is found on assessment.

The oral mucous membrane is normally pale, coral pink, moist, smooth, and shiny. It is free of bright red areas, pallor, cyanosis, ulceration, local deposits of brown pigment, or any bleeding. The oral mucosal surfaces should be moist, showing adequate salivary function. However, anxiety and tenseness can cause a dry mouth through stimulation of the autonomic nervous system.

Problems in swallowing, mastication, or appetite are asked about in order to substantiate other symptoms related to the gastrointestinal system. There should be no pain, crepitus, or restriction of mandibular movement when the patient is asked to make chewing movements. Movements of the mandible should be smooth and gliding in type. The parotid glands and cervical lymph nodes should be inspected and palpated.

Prior to examining the abdomen the patient is asked to empty the bladder, because a full bladder may be mistaken for an abdominal mass. The abdomen is examined with the patient in a recumbent position with knees slightly raised to relax the abdominal muscles. Using the umbilicus as a central point, the abdominal topography is identified as right and left upper quadrants and right and left lower quadrants (Fig. 7-2). The body build can modify the position of abdominal organs, but the topographic system allows for precise localizing of physical signs and symptoms. Another system divides the abdomen into nine sections, also illustrated in Figure 7-2. Most authorities advise a systematic examination in the order of inspection, auscultation, percussion, and light and deep palpation, although some practitioners suggest auscultation as the last step.

The contour of the abdomen may be flat (as in a person with good muscle tone), rounded (as in an individual with a lack of muscle tone or excessive fat), or scaphoid (as in a thin individual with a depressed center of the abdomen). The abdomen is carefully inspected for symmetry, skin integrity, color, texture,

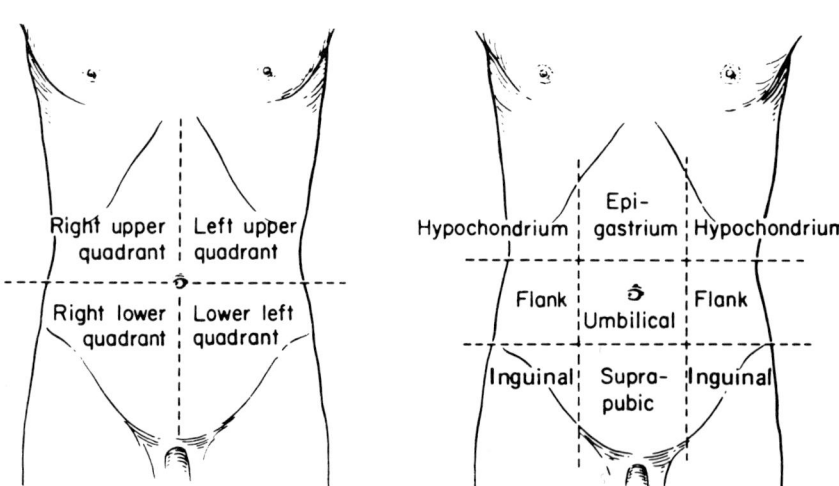

Figure 7-2
Topographic anatomy of the abdomen. (Reprinted by permission from J. M. Sana and R. D. Judge, *Physical Appraisal Methods in Nursing Practice*. Boston: Little, Brown and Company, 1975.)

abnormal markings, scars, visible peristalsis, localized swelling, distention, or masses. Protrusions of the abdomen should be described as general or localized, and they suggest ascites, organomegaly, or abdominal masses. When the patient is asked to cough or bear down, there should not be any bulging or pain in the abdomen.

Bowel sounds are caused by the peristaltic movement of air and fluid in the intestines. The presence and quality of the relatively high-pitched bowel sounds in the abdomen are determined by auscultation with a diaphragm type of stethoscope. Because the intestine is sensitive to touch, and palpation can alter the peristaltic sounds, auscultation is usually done prior to palpation. The intensity of the bowel sounds is determined and described as hypoactive or hyperactive. A gurgling and bubbling quality is normal with five or more sounds occurring per minute. The bowel sounds vary in intensity, frequency, and pitch in relation to the phase of digestion. For example, when the intestinal contents are passing in the area of the ileocecal valve 4 to 8 hours after the meal, sounds are more intense in the right lower quadrant. The examiner should therefore always question the patient regarding the time of the last meal.

When no peristaltic activity is heard, the examiner listens for 2 to 5 minutes in each of the other quadrants. It is easier to hear the bowel sounds in thin rather than in obese patients, so that the inexperienced examiner must be particularly careful in evaluating the absence of bowel sounds in the obese patient [3].

The absence of bowel sounds is an abnormal finding that occurs in peritonitis, ileus, and advanced obstruction. Waves of loud gurgling and tinkling sounds are also significant. Very active and loud peristaltic sounds are often heard in hypermotility conditions, including some functional disorders, as well as in areas proximal to an early obstruction.

Percussion involves the use of both hands to examine the abdomen to determine the sizes of solid viscera and the presence of gas, fluids, and masses. The fingers of one hand are partially flexed, serving as a hammer to tap the finger of the dependent hand, which is placed directly on the abdomen. Changes in sound are noted. The size of these organs can be determined by changes in percussion sounds. A dull, short, or high-pitched sound can be heard over the dense organs like the liver and the spleen. For example, the liver is normally percussed at about the fifth intercostal space for its upper boundary with a normal span of about 10 to 12 cm. The lower boundary is found at about 2 cm below the right costal margin. The spleen is percussed in the area of the tenth intercostal space [23]. A tympanic sound is low-pitched, of long duration, and is observed over a gas-filled organ.

Before the abdomen is palpated, the patient is asked to identify tender areas. These areas are avoided until the end of the examination to prevent stiffening of the abdomen during the entire examination. Light palpation is used to determine the general condition of the abdominal wall and to detect gross abnormalities, masses, areas of pain or tenderness, crepitus, and areas of reflex rigidity. The palmar surfaces of the fingers, which are extended and held together, are used with gentle pressure to just indent the skin (less than 1 cm). The quadrants are palpated systematically, exploring specific organs in each quadrant. The tone of the abdominal muscles is assessed as normal if the muscles are relaxed and the muscle tone is reduced. The palpation examination is considered normal if there are no areas of tenderness, no solid masses, no pain, no skin sensitivity, no edema, and no pathologic enlargement of organs. Both objective and subjective findings are reported. Having the patient take deep breaths through his mouth will help him relax during this stage. The examiner's hands should be warm to assure that there is no reflex tensing of the abdominal muscles, and a warm room will prevent involuntary muscle spasm that also can interfere with the examination.

Deep palpation, in contrast to light palpation, requires increased but steady pressure, pushing the organs toward the posterior abdominal wall to detect enlargement, abnormal masses, and swelling. As the patient breathes through his mouth, the depth of the probe of the fingers on the abdomen is increased with each successive expiration. In deep palpation, the small intestines are not palpable unless they are abnormally distended or enlarged. The bimanual technique, which is used particularly to detect an enlarged liver, gallbladder, or spleen, requires palpation with one hand and application of counterpressure with the other hand.

The liver is described in relation to firmness, smoothness or presence of nodules on its surface, and the regularity of its edge. The normal liver usually has sharply defined smooth edges. Although the gallbladder is generally not palpable, it may be felt as a small bulge under the edge of the liver. The spleen is not palpable normally, so it is considered enlarged if it is palpable in the bimanual technique. As the examination is carefully and slowly carried out, the patient's facial expressions are observed for winces and other signs of discomfort. Findings of the abdominal examination are recorded, indicating both normal and abnormal findings.

The rectal examination is also a part of the assessment of the gastrointestinal system. After inspection of the anal area for inflammation or excoriation, a digital examination is done with a well-lubricated glove. After inserting the index finger gently and slowly into the rectum, the examiner evaluates sphincter tone and palpates the anal wall for strictures, inflamed areas, or masses. The same technique is utilized to determine the presence of an impaction in a patient reporting obstipation on initial admission or during his or her hospital stay.

DIAGNOSTIC TESTS

The findings of the history and physical examination may indicate the need for additional examinations of the gastrointestinal system. The nurse should inform the patient about the purpose of the tests planned and what he or she is expected to do before and during the tests. A blood count is obtained to determine the presence of anemia related to bleeding in the gastrointestinal tract or to a suspected nutritional anemia.

Analysis of a stool specimen may be done for occult blood. Usually a series of three stool collections is required, after a period of 3 days on a meat-free diet. Iron and salicylates are not taken during this time. Stools may also be cultured for the presence of bacteria, ova, and parasites. Stool specimens must be fresh for these examinations.

Stool analysis can also be done to determine fecal weight, osmolality, and electrolytes. The stool examinations should be completed before barium x-ray studies are done since barium invalidates microscopical and chemical studies of the stool. The nurse should examine the stools of patients suspected of gastrointestinal disease and should describe the consistency, color, volume, odor, and the presence of blood, pus, or mucus.

A gastric analysis of the fasting contents of the stomach may be required. This analysis can be done indirectly (by a tubeless method) or directly by analysis of gastric contents obtained via a nasogastric tube. The tubeless gastric analysis (Diagnex Blue test) determines the presence or absence of free hydrochloric acid. After an 8- to 10-hour restriction of food and fluids, an initial urine specimen is obtained. The patient is then given a dose of caffeine or histamine as a gastric acid stimulant. One hour later, after emptying his bladder, the patient is given granules of Azure A in an exchange resin with water. One or two hours later a urine specimen is collected to determine the amount of dye absorbed and then excreted in the urine. The specimen will appear blue if hydrochloric acid is present in the stomach, since acid in the stomach displaces the dye from the exchange resin. Absence of hydrochloric acid can be an indication of pernicious anemia or cancer of the stomach.

In the second method, stomach secretions are aspirated via a nasogastric tube after 8 to 10 hours of fasting. The secretions are tested for acid content. No smoking is permitted prior to the test, and anticholinergic drugs are omitted for at least 12 hours. The amount of secretions obtained after the fasting period is also noted; an excessive amount of gastric secretions containing food ingested the previous night suggests a pyloric obstruction. Histamine or betazole hydrochloride (Histalog) may be given subcutaneously to stimulate gastric secretions. Histalog is preferred when there is a history of allergies. It is extremely important to forewarn the patient that he or she may feel flushed after the injection. The patient, however, is observed carefully at this time since an allergic reaction with potential shock is a danger with the administration of histamine preparations. The blood pressure and pulse are monitored for the onset of hypotension after histamine administration. Emergency equipment, including drugs such as epinephrine and diphenhydramine hydrochloride (Benadryl), should be available if needed. Gastric secretions are collected at specific intervals before and after the administration of the histamine and are carefully time labeled.

On some occasions a Hollander test may be utilized. Insulin is given as a stimulant for gastric secretion in this test. A Hollander test is sometimes used to evaluate the effectiveness of a vagotomy. Insulin, in causing a drop in the blood glucose, stimulates the vagus nerve, thereby increasing the gastric secretions. Glucose should be available in case hypoglycemia develops. A lavage done in conjunction with the gastric analysis can be used to obtain stomach washings for exfoliative cytology and Papanicolaou tests for cancer.

Roentgenographic examinations of the gastrointestinal tract, including a flat plate of the abdomen, may be indicated. Barium x-rays of the stomach are frequently necessary. A barium contrast medium, which is flavored to make it more palatable, is swallowed and fluoroscopic films are taken as the barium progresses to the stomach and duodenum. Six hours after the first films, more films are taken to determine the amount of barium remaining in the stomach, which should actually be empty by that time. The patency, caliber, and motility of the stomach are thus determined. Spasms, ulcerations, and anatomic abnormalities may be seen. Successful visualization of the stomach requires an empty stomach, so that the patient is given nothing by mouth for 6 to 8 hours prior to the x-ray. Because smoking can stimulate gastric motility, patients are discouraged from smoking the morning of the examination. The patient is forewarned that he or she will be placed in a variety of positions on the tilt table in the x-ray department to allow the barium to flow by gravity into the intestinal loops. This information will assist in decreasing the patient's anxiety and encouraging cooperation. Too often the nurse may forget that some patients may never have had a "GI series" and will not understand the procedure or the terminology. The nurse will need to adapt explanations in this situation as compared to an explanation given the patient who has had repeated x-ray examinations. After the x-rays, the patient is usually given a cathartic or a lubricant (mineral oil) daily for several days to help eliminate the barium remaining in the bowel, which might otherwise become impacted. A barium swallow may be done to visualize the duodenum, jejunum, and ileum.

If an ulcer, polyp, or any abnormality in the stomach is suspected, gastric endoscopy (gastroscopy) may be indicated. This procedure permits direct visualization of the stomach to observe for the presence of lesions. A biopsy of existing lesions can be taken during the endoscopic procedure. It is felt that the number of malignant ulcers that have been found via endoscopy warrants this procedure. Cooperation and tolerance are required of the patient who is to undergo gastroscopy. To pretend that a gastroscopy is not an uncomfortable procedure is to mislead the patient, and only increases his or her anxiety during the procedure. The gastroscopy procedure requires a permit to be signed by the patient. A realistic explanation of what the patient can expect and how he or she can help to facilitate the procedure is most desirable. Prior to gastroscopy the patient is restricted from food and fluids for 6 to 8 hours and is taken to the treatment room by cart (although the procedure can be done at the bedside). Dentures are removed. The patient is instructed to remain still during the passage of the gastroscope. Usually a narcotic or a sedative is administered. Diazepam (Valium) may be administered intravenously just prior to the insertion of the gastroscope. The posterior pharynx is sprayed with an anesthetic or an oral liquid preparation of ethyl aminobenzoate (Hurricaine) is gargled by the patient immediately before the tube is inserted to inactivate the gag reflex. The patient lies on his side, with the head supported and held perfectly still by the nurse to prevent sudden movement, which could cause perforation of the esophagus. Suctioning of oral secretions is necessary. The new fiberoptic gastroscopes are more easily handled and are more flexible, providing for easier insertion and examination. Attachments for photography can also be used with fiberoptic gastroscopes. Any lesion seen on gastroscopy is biopsied via open biopsy forceps or the brush technique; both methods can be utilized via channels of the gastroscope. Flexible fiberoptic instruments have increased the use of gastroscopy as a valuable diagnostic tool. Even if the x-ray series is normal, gastroscopy is indicated if the patient's symptoms persist because small lesions not seen on x-rays are frequently found on subsequent gastroscopy.

After the gastroscopy is completed, the patient cannot eat or drink until the gag reflex returns (usually 3 to 4 hours) in order to prevent aspiration into the lungs. The patient may be drowsy and fatigued from the medications and exhausted from the strain and discomfort of the procedure. The nurse should observe the patient for signs of perforation; these signs are pain and an elevated temperature. A sore throat may occur after this procedure and can be controlled with saline gargles, lozenges, and oral analgesic drugs.

A barium enema x-ray may be ordered when there are symptoms of abnormalities of the lower intestine. Adequate preparation of the bowel via cleaning enemas or cathartics or both is necessary in order to permit accurate visualization and interpretation of the x-ray. Barium enema x-rays are contraindicated when colonic perforation is suspected or when increased intra-abdominal pressure may be hazardous for the patient.

Proctoscopy involves direct examination of the anal canal, rectum, and sigmoid colon via a rigid instrument. The sigmoidoscope will reach only 25 cm and therefore limits the area that can be directly visualized. Nonetheless this examination is an important procedure for diagnosing cancer of the colon and the rectum, because about two thirds of the cancers found in the lower bowel occur within the reach of the sigmoidoscope. Proctoscopy is considered an important part of every annual physical examination in persons over the age of 40 as a means of detecting early malignant lesions in an asymptomatic stage. The examination is also indicated for anyone with symptoms of hemorrhoids, blood in the stool, unexplained anemia, or an unexplained change in bowel patterns.

Proctoscopy also requires adequate cleaning of the lower bowel by giving enemas until clear returns are obtained. (Usually no more than two enemas are given in order to prevent exhaustion of the patient.) The patient should also be advised that an awkward knee-chest position will be required during the procedure. This awkward position and the sensation of pressure from the instillation of air create considerable discomfort for most patients. Some physicians prefer doing the examination with the patient in a left lateral position.

A more recent adaptation of this procedure is colonoscopy, using a fiberoptic colonoscope. These flexible scopes can be inserted further into the rectum than can the sigmoidoscope, allowing visualization of the transverse colon, and often the ileocecal valve. Visualization of these areas makes possible direct examination and biopsy of lesions or polyps in the tract that are not reached by the sigmoidoscope. Lesions can be examined, photographed, biopsied, excised, and fulgurated all under direct vision. In the hands of an experienced gastroenterologist, the colonoscope has proved to be a valuable diagnostic tool. The procedure, however, is not considered part of a routine physical examination or a substitute for a barium enema. Bleeding, infection, and perforation are potential complications.

As with other examinations in which the colon is visualized, adequate preparation is essential; however, preparatory procedures vary in different institutions. Purgatives (castor oil) or enemas (or both) until clear returns are obtained are usually prescribed. Some physicians also require a clear liquid diet for 1 or 2 days before the examination. A thorough explanation is essential to prepare the patient and to obtain his or her cooperation during the procedure. The patient who has had previous experience with proctoscopy may require even more support. Recalling the discomfort of the rigid proctoscope, the patient may be reluctant to submit to an examination with a tube that goes farther into the colon. Being allowed to feel the flexible scope before colonoscopy may be reassuring to this patient. The procedure is usually done with the patient lying in a left lateral recumbent position with the knees flexed. Combinations of meperidine hydrochloride (Demerol), diazepam (Valium), and/or atropine sulfate may be given prior to the procedure, or Valium may be administered intravenously immediately before the colonoscope is inserted. Some physicians do not prescribe premedication, and their opinions vary as to whether the procedure should be performed using fluoroscopy, which provides visualization to guide insertion of the scope. It is important that the nurse remain with the patient and be available to provide emotional support during the procedure. When discomfort occurs, the nurse should advise the patient to take slow, deep breaths and relax the abdominal muscles. It is important to tell the patient that passing of flatus is expected and unavoidable. After the procedure, the patient is observed for pain, elevated temperature, or rectal discomfort, all of which may indicate perforation. Colonoscopy can be done on an outpatient basis, but hospitalization is required when a biopsy is needed so that the patient can be observed for signs and symptoms of bleeding and perforation.

An advantage of using the colonoscope is that many polyps may be biopsied or removed without resorting to general anesthesia and bowel surgery. If the lesion is benign, further surgery is not indicated. If the lesion is malignant and not completely removed by colonoscopy, bowel surgery is required.

Another serum examination that is increasingly being used in the diagnosis of gastrointestinal disease is the detection by radioimmunoassay of levels of the carcinogenic embryonic antigen. Serum levels have been found to be elevated in a significant number of patients with colonic cancer, especially with metastasis to the liver. Radioimmunoassay methods are also used to measure blood concentrations of the cancer-related protein, alpha fetoprotein. Other diagnostic tests will be discussed in subsequent sections of this chapter, when the indications for their use are discussed.

Disorders of the Gastrointestinal Tract

The integrity of the gastrointestinal tract and the nutritional health of a patient can be disturbed in the following ways: (1) inadequate intake, (2) excessive intake of nutrients, (3) loss of integrity of the lining, (4) interference with motility, (5) interference with patency, and (6) inability to absorb nutrients, all problems that can affect the digestive, absorptive, and eliminative functions of the gastrointestinal system, and consequently other systems and body functions. Causes of these changes include infections, neoplasms, trauma, inflammation, and congenital defects.

Examples of reasons for **inadequate intake** include anorexia, psychological aversion to food, and obstruction in the upper gastrointestinal tract.

The patient who is obese as a result of **excessive intake** may also have problems related to the functions of other body systems and is vulnerable to cardiovascular system complications. Although psychological aspects must be considered in controlling obesity, some attempts at controlling intake through surgically devised physiologic changes are now being attempted.

Peptic ulcer illustrates the type of problem that occurs with loss of the integrity of the lining of the gastrointestinal tract. Since the stomach is a highly vascular organ, ulceration may result in hemorrhage. Perforation of the gastrointestinal tract may also complicate ulcers. Perforation can occur at any level of the tract, and is always viewed as a surgical emergency. Many potentially pathogenic microorganisms are normally found in the gastrointestinal tract and are contained by the lining, which can withstand these organisms. If perforation occurs and the contents of the gastrointestinal tract, such as digestive materials or feces or both, are allowed to escape into the peritoneal cavity, the onset of infection is drastic. In the case of perforation of a gastric ulcer, the contents also contain chemical juices that may not ordinarily be destructive to the stomach lining, but that may be traumatic to the membrane of the peritoneal cavity and result in inflammation and destruction of the lining.

Interference with motility of the gastrointestinal tract can be illustrated by a neurogenic paralytic ileus or an esophageal hiatal hernia, when problems in motility increase heartburn and other symptoms. Hypermobility and hypomobility associated with functional disorders also illustrate interference with motility of the gastrointestinal tract.

Whether an obstruction occurs at the esophagus or at the intestinal level, the total function of the gastrointestinal system is altered when there is **interference with the patency** of the tract. An obstruction interferes with passage of food, fluids, and gas. The higher the level of the obstruction, the more likely the major problem will be that of vomiting, while with lower levels of obstruction the major problem will be obstipation. The patient with an obstruction in the esophagus and stomach will need surgical relief of the obstruction or adequate nutritional intake via alternative methods, or both. The patient with an obstruction in the colon or rectum will need surgical relief of the obstruction via a permanent or temporary artificial orifice for adequate elimination.

The small intestine, as previously stated, is the major site of absorption. When ulcerative colitis occurs, excessive diarrhea causes **inadequate absorption** of fluids and electrolytes. Fistulas, which are abnormal openings from an organ to the external body or to another body part, also result in loss of fluids and electrolytes and affect the individual's nutritional state. Some absorption of water takes place in the colon. When parts of the colon are removed, problems in absorption may result until adaptations of the body are completed. Problems in absorption also occur when the gallbladder is diseased and bile that is normally utilized in the absorption of fats is no longer readily available for this function.

When considering the nursing care of patients with disease states that affect the integrity of the gastrointestinal system, it is important for the nurse to remember that an intact tract is necessary for adequate digestion and absorption. Patients with diseases that result in the loss of secretions from various organs of the gastrointestinal tract are losing specific electrolytes as well as fluid. Gastrointestinal secretions vary in acidity and alkalinity, depending on their source, and loss of these secretions may result in acid-base imbalances. The particular type of imbalance that occurs depends on the pH of the secretions lost. A helpful guideline is that secretions from above the level of the pylorus of the stomach are generally acid in nature, whereas those from below the pylorus are generally alkaline in nature. Table 7-1 illustrates the various types of secretions, their normal volumes and pH. The nurse who appreciates the implications of loss of gastrointestinal secretions will be conscientious about the observation and recording of all secretions and drainage from the tract.

GASTROINTESTINAL INTUBATION

Patients with disorders of the gastrointestinal system as well as other diseases frequently require intubation of the gastrointestinal tract. Intubation of the stomach and small intestine may be necessary to decompress the tract by removing fluid and gas in **hypomobility** (such as postoperatively), to withdraw secretions from the stomach or intestine for diagnostic analysis, to administer feedings (gavage) or drugs, to wash the stomach of toxins or irritants, or to apply cold and pressure to the walls of the esophagus, stomach, or small intestine to control bleeding.

There are a variety of tubes available. Selection of the specific type is determined by the purpose of the intubation and by the individual physician's preference. The Levin tube, a rubber tube with a single lumen and several openings at the distal end, is used for gastric intubation and is introduced through the nostril. Variations of the Levin tube include plastic nasogastric tubes and the Salem sump tube, which is a double-lumen tube. The Salem sump has a primary lumen for drainage and a second lumen which is open to the air to prevent excessive negative pressure by allowing ambient air to enter the cavity continuously. The Ewald tube, which is a larger tube, is introduced through the mouth for withdrawal of gastric contents as well as for lavage. Withdrawal of contents is facilitated by manual pressure on the bulb portion of the tube.

Intestinal intubation requires a tube as long as 6 to 10 feet and one which usually has a modified distal end to permit easier passage. The Miller-Abbot tube, a double-lumen tube, has one lumen for fluid and gas aspiration and a second lumen with a rubber bag at the distal end. After the tube is passed into the stomach, the rubber bag is inflated with air or instilled with mercury. The balloon causes pressure which stimulates intestinal motility while the weight of the mercury assists the movement of the tube through the pylorus and along the intestine. The proximal ends must be identified clearly so that the inflated lumen is not inadvertently attached to the suction apparatus.

The Cantor tube, a single-lumen tube, also has a small rubber bag at its distal end. The bag is filled partially with 5 to 10 ml of mer-

Table 7-1
Approximate volume, pH, and electrolyte content of gastrointestinal secretions

Secretion	Volume per 24 hr (ml)	pH	NA$^+$	K$^+$	Cl$^-$	HCO$_3^-$
			(mEq per liter)			
Saliva	1,000–1,500	6.0–7.0	9–10	26	10	10–15
Gastric juice	1,500–2,500	1.0–3.5	60	9.2–10.0	84	0–14
Pancreatic juice	1,000–2,000	8.0–8.3	140–141.1	4.6–5	75–76.6	115–121
Bile	600–800	7.8	145–148.9	4.98–5.0	100–100.6	35–40
Small intestine	2,000–3,000	7.8–8.0	111.3–140	4.6–5	104.2	30–31

cury via a needle and syringe prior to insertion of the tube. The rubber seals itself over the puncture site, so that no mercury will escape from the bag. The Harris tube is a smaller tube but resembles the Cantor tube except that suction openings are at the end and sides, whereas the Cantor tube has openings on the side only, behind the rubber bag. The Blakemore-Sengstaken tube is a triple-lumen, double-balloon tube used for hemostatic effects. It is discussed later in this chapter.

Relaxation of the patient is extremely important to facilitate the passage of any of these tubes. A thorough explanation to the patient is thus essential. The nurse should check for any nasal obstruction or deformity before inserting the tube. A guide for determining the length of tube to be inserted for gastric intubation is to measure the distance from the ear lobe to the tip of the nostril and to the bottom of the xiphoid process. The tube, which is well-lubricated with water-soluble lubricant, is inserted through the nares (or mouth, as with the Ewald tube), while the patient's head is initially hyperextended. Then the patient sits erect with the head slightly flexed in a natural position to swallow the tube as it is gently pushed down to the stomach. Taking sips of water will facilitate swallowing the tube. The tube will curl in the pharynx or the patient will start gagging if the tube is pushed faster than the patient can swallow it. Aspiration of stomach contents verifies insertion into the stomach. If there is a question about the insertion, the free end of the tube can be placed under water. If air bubbles appear in the water or if coughing ensues, the tube is in the trachea and should be removed. Listening with a stethoscope over the epigastrium (for whooshing sounds) while 5 ml of air is rapidly instilled into the tube via a syringe also can verify that the tube is in the stomach. When the correct position is reached, the tube is taped to the face; pressure or tension on the nares is avoided.

During intestinal intubation (using Miller-Abbot or Cantor tube) the patient is placed in different positions after the tube reaches the stomach to facilitate the passage of the tube through the pylorus and duodenum. The directions provided with the tube should be followed precisely. Lying on the right side initially, for example, assists passage of the tube through the pylorus. Lying on the back and left side and ambulation, at specified times, also facilitates passage of the tube. The tube also passes by the motion of peristalsis and by gravity of the weighted bag filled with mercury or air. The tube is not taped to the patient's face, but rather hangs loosely from the nostril, until it reaches the desired level. It is advanced at specified intervals according to the physician's instructions, but it must not be advanced too quickly or it will curl and kink in the stomach. The tube has markings in centimeters so that its location can be determined, and location of the tube is also confirmed by x-ray or fluoroscopy.

When the patient is intubated, gentle suction is provided via a Wangensteen machine or through intermittent low-pressure suction, with the electric Gomco suction machine or similar apparatus. Patency of the tube must be assured to avoid accumulation of fluid and gas, which could result in pain, vomiting, or abdominal distention, and to avoid pressure and distention on a suture line postoperatively. Repositioning the patient also assists in facilitating drainage. Irrigation with specific amounts of normal saline (usually 30 ml) is necessary at intervals to release accumulations of thick secretions or clots. Irrigation is indicated when the gastric output is decreased and no drainage is observed through the nasogastric tube. In addition, the patient generally becomes uncomfortable and gags frequently. The color, characteristics, volume, and odor of the drainage should be recorded. Precise recording of intake and output, including those amounts utilized for irrigation, is necessary for determination of needed fluid and electrolytes. The nurse should remember that secretions from the stomach and the intestines vary in their electrolyte concentrations and pH and therefore should observe for signs of electrolyte imbalances (Chap. 2). Excessive loss of drainage fluid can also result in acid-base imbalances. Gastric suction results in loss of H^+ ions leading to alkalosis, whereas intestinal suction results in loss of HCO_3^- ions, leading to acidosis.

The nasogastric tube generally causes much irritation and discomfort. Restricted oral intake and mouth breathing contribute to mouth dryness that is not completely relieved even with frequent cleaning, gargles, and oral hygiene. Throat lozenges, ice chips, or hard candies may be permitted in some situations, but not during the 24- to 48-hour period following surgery. Lubrication of the lips and nostrils contributes to oral comfort.

Oral hygiene is required for patients with nasogastric tubes at least very 4 hours, and preferably every 2, to promote the patient's comfort and to prevent infections. Passos and Brand compared the effectiveness of three agents, hydrogen peroxide, milk of magnesia, and alkaline aromatic mouthwash, in similar circumstances for both the technique and frequency of oral hygiene. They found hydrogen peroxide to be the most effective agent [19]. **Parotitis,** which is an infection (usually staphylococcus) of the parotid gland, is a potential complication when oral hygiene is inadequate. Parotitis results in pain, swelling at the site of the gland, absence of salivation, fever, and purulent drainage from the duct of the gland. Adequate fluid intake and the frequency of oral hygiene is necessary to treat parotitis, and surgery is required for drainage of the gland if suppuration occurs. The importance of proper oral hygiene in all patients, but particularly in those with nasal intubation and restricted intake, cannot be overemphasized.

The nasogastric tube and suction are generally maintained until bowel sounds return or the passage of flatus indicates adequate gastrointestinal function. If discontinuation of suction is tolerated and after decompression is no longer necessary, the tube is removed. To remove the gastric tube the nurse clamps the tube and withdraws it gently and quickly while the patient holds his or her breath to avoid possible aspiration of fluid from the tube into the oropharynx. Intestinal tubes, however, are removed slowly, inches at a time, without any force. Air-filled balloons are deflated prior to removal of the tube. The mercury-filled bag is brought out through the mouth and the bag is cut off before the rest of the tube is removed through the nostril. If the tube has passed the ileocecal valve it is generally allowed to pass through the rectum. Thorough mouth cleaning is indicated following removal of the tube. The patient often complains of throat soreness from the tubes for several hours after removal.

Consideration of some of the more common medical and surgical disorders of the gastrointestinal tract will be discussed according to the six problem areas previously identified. It is recognized that most of the diseases cause more than one of these problems and that many diseases could be discussed in each of the six sections.

INADEQUATE INTAKE OF NUTRIENTS

The patient who has anorexia presents a genuine challenge to the nurse. The cause of the anorexia must be determined initially. On occasion, poor oral hygiene alone may be the primary cause of a lack of desire for food because of its effect on the taste of food. Anorexia may be a symptom of the patient's disease, reaction to various drug therapies (particularly in cancer chemotherapy), or emotional tension. Usually the patient with anorexia accepts several small feedings per day better than large feedings. Providing meals that include the patient's favorite foods may improve the desire for food. Drug therapy, including antiemetic and antinausea drugs may also be effective in controlling symptoms of anorexia and nausea.

Anorexia may be related to emotional upsets. An extreme form of anorexia related to emotional disturbances is **anorexia nervosa** which, on occasion, may have a fatal outcome. Usually the patient is a young woman or adolescent with an aversion to food, a loss of appetite, or an inability to eat adequate amounts. Although more prevalent in females, anorexia nervosa has also been described in young boys. Often there is a previous history of obesity with an abnormal preoccupation with eating. Ironically these patients claim that they are extremely hungry, although this serious disease of unknown cause results in malnutrition and debilitation.

The basic problem in anorexia nervosa often is viewed as the struggle for a sense of identity, security, and control over the body and life. The individual consistently denies being too thin and is extremely fearful of being overweight. Difficulty in swallowing, a dislike for certain foods, and guilt associated with eating are often additional presenting symptoms. Such persons have likely gone through extensive diagnostic tests and treatment where the initial goal is to interrupt the process of starvation, and they usually require psychotherapy in a pyschiatric setting to treat the basic underlying problem of insecurity and distorted body image. Operant conditioning has been utilized successfully as a therapeutic approach in some settings. Operant conditioning is predicated on the theory that abnormal eating is a specific learned behavior reinforced by the environment, and that eating behaviors can be controlled in individual and group situations. In these situations there is close observation and supervision of meal and snack times with immediate nasogastric tube feedings at times of inadequate eating, coordinated with psychotherapy and a program to develop social acceptance and self-esteem. Monitoring of the patient's weight changes is related to the increase or decrease of social privileges, and the patients often eventually respond to the treatment. The improvement in interpersonal relationships and basic security, as well as improved self-image, is reflected in these patients when they gain weight and begin to develop good, regular eating habits.

Anorexia may also be a symptom of organic disease. The patient with cancer of the esophagus or of the stomach, for example, may initially experience anorexia that progresses to dysphagia and finally to vomiting as the cancer obstructs the lumen of the esophagus or interferes with the digestive processes of the stomach.

Whatever the cause of the inadequate intake, provisions must be made for supplying essential nutrients. If the patient cannot ingest solids, blenderized foods may be tolerated. When blenderized foods are no longer tolerated, nasogastric feedings are given either by intermittent feedings via a syringe or a funnel attached to the tube or by a continuous drip method. (A Barron food pump with controllable motor speeds is another method of feeding patients liquefied foods in which the feeding is delivered via a nasogastric tube to the patient at a preset rate.) The feeding, which can be made of blenderized foods providing all essential nutrients, is kept in an insulated plastic container to prevent bacterial growth. The feeding rate can be regulated from 40 ml up to 200 ml per hour and can be adjusted for intermittent or continuous feedings.

Gavage feedings should not only meet the body's requirements for calories but should be balanced nutritionally. Either a well-balanced diet of selected ingredients may be blenderized or one of several different commercially prepared feedings can be given by gavage. Vivonex, for example, is an elemental standard food in a soluble powder form. The product comes in 80-gm packets and provides a balanced nutritional diet of 1800 calories. It comes in an unflavored form or in six palatable flavors. Vivonex high nitrogen preparation provides 3000 calories including vitamins and minerals in each 80-gm packet. Other commercially prepared feedings are Sustagen, Isocal, Precision LR, and Complement A8. The use of high protein concentrates for tube feedings can lead to the "tube feeding syndrome" characterized by dehydration, hypernatremia, and azotemia [9, 28]. Liquid prepared feedings should therefore be diluted according to the patient's fluid requirement and tolerance for volume in any given feeding. To prevent clogging of the tube and to maintain its patency, 50 to 100 ml of water is given after each feeding.

Tube feedings often cause changes in stool consistency and frequency (constipation or diarrhea) and also abdominal cramping, gastric dilatation, nausea, and vomiting. Although most authorities advise that tube feedings be given at room temperature in order to prevent diarrhea and other untoward effects, some investigators have demonstrated that the temperature of tube feedings is not a factor in the incidence of untoward effects associated with tube feedings [11, 26]. These studies indicate that warming of refrigerated tube feedings is probably an unnecessary procedure. Rapid and forced administration of feedings or intolerance to the lactose content of the feedings is more likely to cause these untoward effects [26–28].

Care of the patient who is being fed by nasogastric tube includes measurement of intake and output; daily weights; proper oral hygiene; observation for signs of diarrhea, constipation, or abdominal cramping; and prevention of aspiration pneumonia. Providing for the psychological comfort of the patient who is deprived of normal feeding patterns is extremely important. The nurse should make every effort to create a pleasant atmosphere and give the feeding slowly, by gravity. Feedings are generally better tolerated when the patient is in a normal sitting position. As soon as the patient is physically and psychologically able, he or she may be taught to administer his or her own feedings.

The intravenous administration of hypertonic solutions of glucose, nitrogen (amino acids and polypeptides), and other nutrients by means of total parenteral alimentation (hyperalimentation) is a method of maintaining a positive nitrogen balance for patients unable to ingest or digest sufficient nutrients. Total parenteral nutrition is discussed in detail on page 188.

EXCESSIVE INTAKE OF NUTRIENTS

In contrast to the patient with anorexia, the patient who is obese often has problems directly related to excessive eating. Considered by many authorities to often result from a neurotic attitude toward food related to a need to fill an emotional gap, or in some cases to prevent the development of relationships with others, obesity can also result from direct physiologic causes.

Obesity is a serious health problem because of its effect on the emotional integrity of the individual and its relation to the incidence of certain diseases such as diabetes and hypertension. Obesity also increases the risks in surgical procedures and is associated with increased mortality rates. Economic factors are also affected if working becomes difficult and clothing becomes more expensive. No single causal relationship has been identified with obesity, but genetic, metabolic, socioeconomic, cultural, and psychological factors have all been implicated.

Whether the cause is overeating due to excessive intake, to decreased caloric requirement by the body, or to disturbances in digestion, absorption, or utilization of foods, the treatment is to decrease food intake or to increase activity thereby increasing bodily requirements for nutrients. The treatment of obesity begins with a history and physical examination to determine endogenous causes of obesity. (Endogenous causes of obesity are discussed in Chapter 8.) Intake restriction and exercise programs are usually the basic elements of approved therapeutic programs to control obesity, and the benefits of group therapy in controlling obesity have been proved in the success of the various weight control clubs that have come into existence throughout the country. Psychotherapy may be indicated in some situations to assist the patient to handle underlying depression and hostility. Bariatric clinics are increasingly being developed to combat the problems of obesity. Drug therapy to decrease the appetite may also be utilized as an *adjunct* to intake restriction and exercise programs, although many physicians feel that drug therapy should not be part of the weight reduction regimen.

Medications to decrease the appetite include clortermine hydrochloride (Voranil), phenmetrazine hydrochloride (Preludin), diethylpropion hydrochloride (Tenuate), phendimetrazine (Plegine), fenfluramine (Pondimin), and mazindol (Sanorex). Sanorex, unlike most other anorexiants, does not contain the phenethylamine structure characteristic of amphetamine drugs, although it is similar in action to the amphetamines and can produce tolerance and psychological dependence. Dry mouth, tachycardia, constipation, nervousness, and insomnia are some of the potential adverse effects of the drug.

These drugs should be used only for short-term therapy, if at all, and only as an adjunct to caloric restriction. Long-term use is discouraged due to their tendency to produce tolerance and psychological dependence. The amphetamines are the prototype of drugs used to suppress appetite. All these drugs affect the central nervous and cardiovascular systems. Caution is necessary if the patient is also taking antihypertensive drugs. Safety precautions are necessary, because the drugs impair the ability to perform activities such as driving a car.

Fatness is considered socially unacceptable by many people who value appearance and is also detrimental to health. The difficulty encountered by people who have tried to lose weight and the positive social and physiologic value of weight loss have led to aggressive approaches to control the amounts of food ingested. Total fasting under medical and nursing supervision is being tried in various settings [25]. In total fasting, weight loss is rapid and reflects loss of salt and water in the first 48 to 72 hours of a fast. A decrease in plasma volume makes the person vulnerable to postural hypotension; safety precautions and careful observations are indicated. Vitamin depletion is possible during fasting so that thiamine in particular is administered to persons fasting more than a week. Total fasting results in elevation of serum fatty acids and urine acetone, both of which contribute to sensations of anorexia. Some investigators have reported fasting periods from 10 days up to 249 days without harmful effects and with a majority of successes [1, 25].

Increased numbers of obese persons, usually women, have submitted to surgical wiring of their jaws for several months until a satisfactory weight is attained. This method has been successful in some cases, and after treatment the patient's self-image has been enhanced to the point where interpersonal relationships have also been improved. Other patients, however, have immediately returned to previous eating habits after removal of the wires.

Jejunoileal bypass or intestinal shunt has been done in selected excessively obese persons who are not able to adhere to either prescribed dietary regimens or exercise programs. Though considered by some to be a radical and experimental surgical procedure, increasing numbers of excessively obese patients are undergoing this treatment. Selection of the patients is important, with consideration given to the absence of other diseases that would contribute to the obesity or would be contraindications to the surgery. Evaluation of the patient's endocrine, metabolic, and psychological status is essential. The patients are intellectually prepared by being informed of the risks and complications that may occur. Patients must understand the need for a prolonged recuperation and adjustment period. Thorough mechanical cleaning of the bowel and oral antibiotics are indicated. The surgery involves the bypass of all but 8 to 14 inches of the jejunum and 2 to 8 inches of the terminal ileum. The jejunum is divided 14 inches from the ligament of Treitz. The proximal jejunal end is anastomosed to the side of the terminal ileum 4 inches from the ileocecal junction while the distal end of the jejunum is closed and anchored to the transverse colon [5, 8, 13]. No part of the intestine is removed, so that if severe complications occur, the intestine can be reconnected. Postoperative pulmonary complications, wound infections, and incisional hernias are major problems. The jejunoileal bypass is done to limit the amount of small intestine that is exposed to digested food, thus limiting the amount absorbed by the body. The decreased absorption of fats and fluids in the small intestine, the rapid transit of food through the shortened small intestine, and the irritating presence of the gastric enzymes, which reach the large intestine quickly, result in an increase in the frequency and liquid consistency of stools. Monitoring of fluid and electrolyte status is of paramount importance. Eventually the frequency of the stools decreases and the consistency becomes more solid as the body makes its own adaptations; medications such as diphenoxylate with atropine, (Lomotil) and modification of dietary habits by limiting the amount of fat in the diet aid this process. A low fat diet is necessary to prevent the laxative effect and steatorrhea (fat in the feces) associated with decreased fat absorption. There is always a danger of fluid and electrolyte imbalance, and vitamin-B_{12} absorption may be particularly disturbed after this surgery, requiring replacement to prevent persistent anemia. Patients are instructed to eat foods high in potassium because of the decreased absorption of potassium associated with loss of absorptive tissue.

During the first year after surgery, patients usually lose 8 to 12 pounds per month, but then a plateau is reached within 2 years. The patient who has the surgery is exposed to many risks involved with abdominal and bowel surgery. In addition, impaired liver function and hepatomegaly have been associated with fatty accumulation of the liver after jejunal bypass surgery, evidently resulting from surgically induced protein malnutrition. Therefore, administration of amino acid supplements may be prescribed. Urinary calcium oxalate stone formation has also been reported. Regardless of these potential complications, however, increasing numbers of persons are consenting to this procedure as a treatment for excessive obesity.

LOSS OF INTEGRITY OF THE LINING OF THE GASTROINTESTINAL TRACT

The Oral Cavity and the Esophagus

The integrity of the lining of the oral cavity, esophagus, stomach, and intestines may be affected by various diseases. The integrity of the oral cavity may be disturbed by infections, ulcerations, or malignant lesions. Inflammatory lesions of the oral cavity include stomatitis, thrush, herpes simplex, and Vincent's angina. **Stomatitis** is an inflammation of the oral mucosa. It is caused by a variety of factors, including dental sepsis, dehydration, vitamin deficiency, blood dyscrasias, and toxic effects of chemotherapeutic drugs. Symptomatic treatment includes mild mouthwashes, vitamin therapy, analgesic lozenges to relieve discomfort, and a bland diet. (Stomatitis is discussed on page 127, under cancer chemotherapy.)

Thrush, a monilial infection (discussed in Chapter 14), is caused by the fungus *Candida albicans*. It occurs most often in debilitated adults, but may also follow the use of certain antibacterial drugs. Local application of gentian violet or an antifungal antibiotic solution such as nystatin (Mycostatin) is the usual therapy. In addition, the patient is encouraged to ingest a nutritious diet in order to improve his or her resistance to infection. **Herpes simplex,** the fever blister or cold sore found on the lips or on the skin around the lips, is caused by a dormant virus. The virus causes blister formation when the patient's physical state is weakened and resistance is lowered, as in fevers. The lesion appears as a small inflamed area, which then develops a vesicle and ruptures. There is no specific treatment. Ointments may be prescribed to prevent cracking and bleeding.

Vincent's angina (trench mouth) is an inflammation of the gums (gingivitis) that is followed by ulceration and necrosis. It is caused by fusiform bacilli and spirochetes. There is usually pain, associated with swollen gums that bleed easily, excessive salivary secretion, and offensive breath.

As indicated previously, the oral cavity is also a fairly frequent site of **malignant lesions;** they may occur on the tongue, the floor of the mouth, the buccal mucosa or tonsillar area, and the lips. Small superficial and localized lesions may be excised through the mouth. The surgical approach and the extent of the surgery is determined by the location and size of the lesion and its proximity to the mandible and the maxilla. Metastasis from oral cancer generally occurs in the jaw and cervical nodes.

Superficial lesions on the lateral border of the tongue may be treated by partial glossectomy and reconstruction. If the tumors are large or if metastasis has already occurred in the mandible and in the cervical nodes, intraoral excision, partial mandibulectomy, and radical neck dissection is accomplished. This procedure is the "Commando" operation. Depending on the residual defects of the oral cavity and on the facial structure, skin grafts and various prosthetic devices and implants are required.

The fear of disfigurement and potential swallowing difficulties and loss of speech because of vocal cord removal are significant problems with which the patient and family must cope in preparing for this type of surgery. Altered means of providing nutrition are required; tube feedings are temporarily necessary. Nursing care is focused on providing psychological comfort, respiratory support, adequate nutrition, fluid and electrolyte balance, meticulous suctioning to maintain a patent airway, and meticulous oral hygiene. Prevention of infection is of paramount importance. Because the patient is unable to communicate normally, alternate means, such as use of a Magic Slate, should be established prior to the surgery so that the patient can communicate postoperatively. Care of patients requiring laryngectomy is discussed in Chapter 13.

The **Mallory-Weiss syndrome** is characterized by mucosal lacerations and erosions of the gastroesophageal junction. Massive hematemesis is preceded by severe retching and vomiting from any cause. The syndrome usually occurs after ingestion of alcohol. Measures similar to those used in caring for patients with bleeding ulcers are used to control bleeding and prevent further irritation to eroded areas.

The Stomach and the Small Intestine

The lining of the stomach is protected by mechanisms that prevent the gastric juices from digesting the lining of the stomach itself, and irritation or injury of the tract from ingested substances. Mucus produced by glands in the mucous membrane lubricates the food to facilitate passage through the tract. The adequate blood flow and the rapid regeneration of gastrointestinal cells are two other mechanisms protecting the gastric lining. Nonetheless, pathologic states arise when the defense mechanisms are weakened, when the wall of the stomach is attacked by its own secretions, or when irritating substances or secretions or both are excessive and injurious to the lining.

Gastritis, an inflammatory or degenerative disorder of the stomach, usually involves only the mucosal layer of the stomach, but occasionally involves the entire thickness of the gastric wall. The condition may be local, diffuse, acute, or chronic in nature. Gastrointestinal or systemic infections, allergic reactions, food poisoning, or uremia may precipitate attacks of gastritis. While the direct cause may be obscure, ingestion of corrosive chemicals; chemical irritants such as salicylates, digitalis, and iodides; ingestion of alcohol; and staphylococcal toxins have been identified as irritants that injure the lining of the stomach. Symptoms generally include epigastric pain, bloating, belching, and nausea. Gastritis cannot be detected by x-rays, but is diagnosed during direct vision and biopsy with gastroscopy. Edema, hyperemia, and exudates are characteristic findings. Many authorities feel that chronic gastritis may be a precursor of cancer of the stomach. Although acute gastritis usually subsides within hours to days, some patients have severe vomiting and require bed rest and intravenous administration of fluids and electrolytes. In others with less severe gastritis, withholding food and administering sedatives may be the only treatment required. Gastritis may be diffuse, causing ulcerations and bleeding, and blood transfusions may be required to treat the hemorrhage.

Peptic ulcers involve the loss of tissue of the mucous, submucous, and muscular layers and occur in those sites. These areas are exposed to the acid-pepsin gastric juice. (Pepsin is the enzyme that splits and dissolves proteins.) Sites of the peptic ulcers include the lower portion of the esophagus, the stomach, the first portion of the duodenum, the duodenal bulb, and the jejunum. These sites are distinguished in the names given to the different types of peptic ulcers. Gastric ulcers, for example, are located most frequently on the lesser curvature near the pylorus, and may become malignant. The duodenal ulcer is located most commonly in the first 3 to 4 cm of the duodenal bulb. Jejunal ulcers, also called marginal ulcers, most often occur at the site of the surgical anastomosis after certain gastric surgical procedures. The name **peptic ulcer** is derived from the relation of the digestive action of hydrochloric acid and pepsin in the gastric juice. While excess acid in the stomach is frequently cited as the cause of ulcers, the defective protective and defensive mechanisms of the lining must not be negated as causative factors. Patients have developed ulcers, for example, in situations when there was not an excessive amount of acid in the gastric secretions. It is also well recognized that the administration of adrenal glucocorticoids may cause gastric ulcers, since the glucocorticoids reduce the resistance of the mucosa to the digestive action of the gastric juice. Esophageal ulcers, also, can result from a nonfunctioning cardiac sphincter that allows reflux of the gastric juices and acid chyme to the esophagus. The esophageal lining cannot withstand the action of the acid secretions and ulcers form.

The control of hydrochloric acid secretion is complex and not fully understood. It is theorized that this control occurs in three phases, the cephalic or neural phase, the gastric phase, and the intestinal phase. In each phase there are both inhibitory and stimulating factors resulting from synergistic neural and hormonal activity as well as from the gastric pH. Because therapeutic medical regimens and surgical therapy are directed at controlling specific phases of the hydrochloric acid secretion in treatment of peptic ulcers, these phases will be briefly described. The cephalic phase is initiated by the sight, smell, and taste of food and occurs even before food enters the stomach. Neural impulses arising in the cerebral cortex are transmitted to the stomach via the vagus nerves. Stimulation of the vagus nerves causes acetylcholine release, and acetylcholine mediates secretion of hydrochloric acid in relation to the gastric pH. Vagus nerve stimulation also causes release of the hormone gastrin from the endocrine cells in the mucosa of the antrum of the stomach. The hormone gastrin, in synergistic action with acetylcholine, also stimulates secretion of hydrochloric acid. The gastric phase of hydrochloric acid secretion continues as long as food remains in the stomach. An alkaline pH of the antral contents, mechanical distention of the antrum, and certain food substances such as caffeine, ethyl alcohol, and products of protein digestion stimulate the release of gastrin. The intestinal phase is regulated by neural and hormonal reflex mechanisms in the intestinal mucosa that act to inhibit or stimulate stomach secretion of gastric juices and motility.

While an imbalance between the protective mechanisms and the action of the gastric juices is generally identified as the major factor in the development of ulcers, there is no single basis for susceptibility in persons who develop ulcers. Specific factors that contribute to the incidence of peptic ulcers include hereditary factors, as demonstrated by the finding that persons with O-type blood tend to have duodenal ulcers more frequently than do other persons. Emotional factors and environmental factors that affect gastric secretion and motility as well as the blood supply to the gastric mucosa also play a part in ulcer development. Men are affected with duodenal ulcers more than women at a ratio of about 4:1. The stress factor is demonstrated by the development of ulcers after severe burns, or under other circumstances of acute stress, as well as in people who are anxious and tense. Drugs that have been identified as ulcerogenic include adrenal steroids, salicylates, phenylbutazone (Butazolidin), histamine, iron, antibiotics, reserpine, indomethacin (Indocin), and tolazoline (Priscoline). The increased numbers of patients with arthritis who developed ulcers was a factor in recognizing the ulcerogenic elements of aspirin and other salicylates. As mentioned previously, alcohol, also a direct irritant, and coffee cause increased secretion of hydrochloric acid. Smoking irritates the gastric mucosa.

The patient with peptic ulcer, which may occur in either the duodenum or stomach, has symptoms of pain caused by the action of the gastric juices on the exposed nerve endings of the inflamed or injured mucosa or alteration of motor activity or both. Therefore the pain is characteristic in its type and timing, location, and nature. The pain is usually described as gnawing, aching, burning, or dull, located in the epigastrium and possibly radiating around the costal border to the back. Pain is further distinguished in gastric ulcer by its location in the left epigastric area whereas that associated with duodenal ulcer is in the right epigastric area. Pain generally appears 1 to 2 hours after eating, when the stomach begins to empty, and it may disappear with ingestion of food or antacids. (Pepsinogen is not converted to active pepsin in a pH above 5.5.) In the case of duodenal ulcer, the pain may be delayed for 2 to 4 hours after eating. Pain may occur at night in both gastric and duodenal ulcers and is particularly characteristic of duodenal ulcer. Vomiting and hematemesis are complications of ulcers when obstruction occurs due to scarring or hemorrhage. Diagnosis is usually verified through x-rays, gastric analysis showing excess acid, and gastroscopy.

Nursing care of the patient with an ulcer includes the provision of mental and physical rest, emotional support, and relief of pain and discomfort to promote healing. (Neutralization and decrease of the digestive power of the gastric juices and diminishing of the motor and secretory activities of the stomach are also promoted through diet therapy and medications.) Helping the patient to adhere to the therapeutic program of relaxation, exercise and rest, diet therapy, and medications to prevent complications is a vital element of the medical and nursing care of a patient with ulcers.

Thorough explanation of the therapeutic program promotes the cooperation of the patient in following his or her therapeutic regimen and permits active participation. In a study done by Putt [21] on 36 male and female patients with known peptic ulcers, two experimental nursing approaches were compared with a control of routine hospital care. The two experimental approaches consisted of one with an emphasis on psychological and interpersonal nursing techniques and the second with emphasis on teaching and instruction. Interpretation of the data showed that instruction of the patient was more effective than psychological support, which in turn was more effective than routine nursing care in decreasing the discomfort after admission, in decreasing the length of hospitalization, and in altering the patient's perceptions of food, tension, and dependency as related to the illness. Though done on a relatively small population, this study supports the theory that the patient's knowledge about the condition and treatment enhances participation and cooperation in the therapeutic regimen.

Mental and physical rest may be achieved in part by removing the patient from the environment that is causing the stress. A vacation may be prescribed in some instances to isolate the patient from anxiety-producing events in a temporarily stressful home or work situation that may be resolved in the interval. When the ulcer patient is admitted to the hospital, nursing staff must realize that encouragement of an initial period of dependence is important in planning the care. Some authorities feel that a basic issue in the lives of patients with ulcers is an underlying dependency-independence conflict, which prevents acceptance of the dependent role even temporarily. This inability to allow others the responsibility for their care due to an unresolved dependency wish may be demonstrated in the patients' irritation and expression of hostility and helplessness when treatments are not given at the exact time prescribed. Impatience and irritation tend to alienate the patient from the staff and establish a cycle or pattern of inability to have the basic needs of security met. The nurse who recognizes these issues will make particular efforts to provide a nonthreatening environment by avoiding rush, confusion, and impatience on the part of the staff, and will promote an understanding and calm atmosphere for these patients. Avoiding punishment through alienation by staff is important when the patient actually vents his or her frustrations and worries. The nurse who recognizes that anxiety may play a major role in the development and antagonism of an ulcer will use thoughtful approaches in intervening in the patient's anxiety state. Helping the patient to recognize anxiety and to gain insight into the causes of the anxiety are initial steps in aiding the patient to cope with the actual or perceived threats. As soon as it is appropriate, the patient's participation in his or her own therapy is encouraged. When it is felt that the patient may need additional professional assistance, the nurse should confer with the physician regarding referral for psychotherapy, which is sometimes indicated for the ulcer patient.

In some cases continuous gastric suction and total food restriction are necessary. Other patients with acute symptoms of an ulcer may require a diet restricted to milk and cream administered hourly and alternated with an antacid to absorb the excess acid. The acid-combining power of food protein neutralizes the free acid secreted by the stomach and may be necessary around the clock. When hourly treatment around the clock is prescribed, the nurse will not be hesitant in awakening the patient, but will realize that the hourly administration of the antacid medications or milk is needed to prevent the occurrence of pain. In some instances a continual drip regimen of milk via a nasogastric tube is utilized to maintain continual contact with the stomach lining for constant neutralization of the acid.

Later, a bland diet that provides for protein and fat to neutralize the acidity and delay stomach emptying is usually prescribed. Some patients may begin their dietary regimen with a bland diet. Bland foods include cream soups, baked or steamed chicken, baked fish, soft cooked eggs, cottage or cream cheese, and stewed vegetables. Milk products, custard, ice cream, pudding, and gelatin are also allowed. Gastric contractility increases when the stomach is empty or is distended by a large volume of food; therefore small frequent feedings are indicated. The acid-buffering action of milk, cream, custard, and eggs makes them an important part of this diet. Milk and cream can be constipating and also may be contraindicated in patients with high cholesterol levels. Skim milk may be used for these persons. Since the initial small feedings of the initial bland or ulcer diets are low in vitamins and minerals, particularly thiamine, niacin, iron, and ascorbic acid, replacement of these may be needed during this time. There is a gradual progression to a nutritionally adequate diet, with observation for foods that tend to aggravate the symptoms and elimination of them from the diet. It is usually necessary to avoid chemical irritants like alcohol and caffeine (as contained in coffee, tea, and carbonated drinks), which stimulate the flow of gastric juices, as well as mechanical irritants that increase peristaltic action. The latter group includes coarse, fibrous foods such as raw vegetables, raw fruits, bran cereals, whole grain cereals, and fried foods. Thermally irritating and spicy foods are also avoided.

Medications to relieve pain and discomfort and to promote healing include antacids, anticholinergic drugs, and tranquilizers. The antacids are given to neutralize the acidity of the stomach and to protect the mucosa by their demulcent action. Anticholinergics may be given to suppress vagal action and decrease gastric motility and spasms, and to reduce the volume of gastric secretions. The use and effectiveness of anticholinergic drugs, however, is controversial. Ivey [14] considers the role of anticholinergics to be limited to use in persons with persistent pain or in those failing to show healing after several weeks. Particular attention is given to the manner of administering antacid medications and to their effects on intestinal motility. Aluminum and calcium antacids tend to be constipating whereas those with magnesium have a laxative effect. These medications are available in liquid or tablet form. Some of the antacid drugs in tablet form must be chewed completely to be effective. Proper instruction by the nurse about following the specific directions for particular antacids is indicated, for cases have been reported in which mechanical obstruction of the ileum has occurred from impacted antacid tablets that were obviously swallowed rather than chewed [20]. Instruction in the avoidance of excess use of soda bicarbonate is also particularly important. Alkalosis has resulted from excessive use of soda bicarbonate (Pepto-Bismol and Alka-Seltzer), which is readily absorbed in the system. Anticholinergic drugs are contraindicated in glaucoma, parotitis, urinary tract infections, or prostatic hypertrophy. These drugs cause dry mouth, dilated pupils, blurred vision, headache, tachycardia, and urine retention. Tranquilizing drugs are often used to promote relaxation and combat anxiety as an adjunct to therapy. The nurse should observe whether the patient is adhering to the regimen and whether the regimen is effective in promoting comfort and relieving pain.

Observation of the patient is necessary also to recognize early signs of complications of ulcers which may include hemorrhage, perforation, obstruction, and intractability (unrelieved pain and other symptoms). Testing stools for occult blood via the guaiac or Hematest methods and observing the color of stools facilitates early detection of bleeding. The patient may be admitted to the hospital in an acute, hemorrhagic state that rapidly progresses to a state of shock if untreated. Esophagoscopy or gastroscopy or both are often done to determine the site of bleeding, as is visceral arteriography. Either the patient may have neglected dietary and drug management for a known ulcer or some precipitating factor such as increased intake of alcohol or aspirin may have stimulated formation of the ulcer, resulting in the acute state. In some patients the acute hemorrhage may be the first sign of the presence of an ulcer. An acute ulcer or erosion of the lining of the tract due to acute stress may rapidly cause massive blood loss. Typically, a stress ulcer, for example, may occur a week after a major surgical procedure, intracranial injury, burns, or sepsis.

Excessive hematemesis may occur with a gastric ulcer; however, tarry stools (melena) will also occur when the bloody drainage is swallowed.

The nurse must monitor vital signs and hemoglobin, hematocrit, and blood volume levels in transfusion therapy, and must provide for maintenance of blood and fluid administration. Measuring and reporting of all bleeding via stool, emesis, or suction is absolutely essential. Enforcement of bed rest is necessary. This is usually not a problem, since the patient is generally too ill to attempt activity. Phenobarbital and other drugs to prevent restlessness are often indicated. Morphine may be given to relieve pain as well as to slow peristaltic activity. Vasopressin (Pitressin) may be administered via intra-arterial infusion for localized vasoconstriction. A nasogastric tube is inserted to remove acid secretions and to determine the amount of bleeding, and is usually maintained for 24 hours after bleeding stops. Iced saline is sometimes prescribed for hourly irrigations of the stomach via a large lumen oral tube or through the nasogastric tube.

Gastric freezing is one technique used to control bleeding. A modified nasogastric tube with a balloon at the end is introduced into the stomach. A mixture of alcohol and ice water is instilled into the balloon; the direct contact of the balloon to the gastric mucosa causes vasoconstriction and decreases bleeding and secretory responses. Gastric freezing may be used even in the absence of bleeding to relieve pain, promote achlorhydria, and promote ulcer-crater healing. Another approach is gastric lavage with ice water through the nasogastric tube. When blood transfusion, intravenous fluids, and total bed rest correct the immediate crisis or if bleeding is mild, the regimen of hourly milk and antacid administration may be prescribed. This conservative treatment may also be used until the patient can be better prepared for elective surgery. When massive bleeding cannot be controlled, emergency surgery is necessary. The bleeding vessels are ligated and usually a subtotal gastrectomy is done. Severe hematemesis of gastric ulcer must be differentiated from that caused by esophageal varices. However, symptoms of degenerative liver disease generally are evident when the esophageal varices bleed. The care of the patient with esophageal varices, though similar to the care of the patient with bleeding ulcers, is discussed on page 593.

Perforation of the ulcer is always considered a surgical emergency. The perforation is more likely to occur with a duodenal ulcer than with a gastric ulcer, since the intestinal wall is thinner. The classic symptoms include a sudden onset of agonizing epigastric pain, vomiting, epigastric tenderness, diminished or absent bowel sounds, apprehension, tachycardia, shallow respirations, and impending shock. As peritonitis develops, board-like rigidity, diffuse tenderness and distention of the abdomen occur. The patient is extremely uncomfortable and avoids position changes. Even jarring of the bed and body movement aggravate the pain.

A chest x-ray and an upright x-ray of the abdomen are taken to detect the presence of air below the diaphragm in the peritoneal cavity. Surgical intervention is necessary, with one of two approaches being utilized: a plication procedure or definitive surgery. **Plication** is simple closure of the perforation and aspiration of the gastric contents from the peritoneal cavity. An antibiotic solution may be instilled into the abdominal cavity via lavage, sump drainage is established, and Penrose drains are placed. Plication is indicated when generalized peritonitis or localized abscesses of the peritoneal cavity have already occurred prior to surgery and when the patient has serious associated disease, which increases the risk of extensive surgery in this emergency situation. Definitive surgery is postponed until the physical status permits.

If local and systemic conditions are favorable at the time of the emergency procedure, **definitive surgery** may be accomplished. This procedure may include vagotomy and antrectomy, or vagotomy and hemigastrectomy, depending on the extent of the disease process, and also includes closure of the perforation and aspiration of the gastric contents from the peritoneal cavity.

If the patient is critically ill or if the perforation occurred more than 24 hours prior to medical treatment, conservative treatment with nasogastric suction and supportive therapy and antibiotics may be the only intervention possible. Residual abscesses will require drainage at a later time.

Nursing care of the patient requiring surgery for perforation of an ulcer is similar to that required by other patients having major abdominal surgery. In addition, it is particularly important to detect early signs of peritonitis and abscess formation, which are demonstrated by increased pain, elevated temperature, tachycardia, and other signs of infection, as well as nausea, vomiting, abdominal distention, and muscular rigidity with rebound tenderness. Analgesics and antibiotics are utilized to control these symptoms. Daily girth measurement is helpful to monitor abdominal distention. The patient is usually maintained in a semi-Fowler's position to enhance maximal gravity drainage through the drains in the wound. This position also promotes better respiratory exchange. Observation of the drainage as to its consistency, odor, and amount is particularly important postoperatively.

Obstruction may occur when edema or scar tissue of a healed peptic ulcer partially occludes the pyloric sphincter and impedes food passage through it; vomiting is the prominent symptom. Surgical repair and revision of the pyloric sphincter in a procedure called pyloroplasty is indicated if antispasmodic drugs are not successful in improving the condition. In pyloroplasty, the pylorus is stretched or an incision is made into the sphincter muscle.

When ulcers are chronic and do not respond to medical treatment, they are classified as intractable. Surgical intervention may be indicated when intractability causes excess pain and interferes with maintaining comfort and employment. A long-standing ulcer may predispose to cancer, so that prophylactic elective surgery may be indicated.

The incidence of **cancer of the stomach** has been declining in the United States, but the reason for this decline is not defined. Some authorities feel that carcinoma does not develop in normal mucosa, but is often associated with chronic gastritis (atrophic gastritis) or chronic gastric ulcer. A high incidence of gastric cancer has been found in countries where high consumption of smoked food (particularly fish) is a cultural pattern. There is also an increased incidence among persons with a group A blood type.

Any region of the stomach may be involved, but the pylorus and the antrum are the most frequent sites. The cancer may cause ulcerating lesions or may infiltrate the mucosa of connective tissue, causing rigidity and affecting motility. Metastasis generally spreads by direct extension to the pancreas or invasion through the lymphatics, most frequently to the liver, but also to the peritoneum and cervical lymph nodes. The symptoms of carcinoma of the stomach vary according to the type and extent of involvement. If the lesion is an ulcerating one, for example, symptoms of occult bleeding with fatigue, weakness, and chronic anemia are usually present. Altered digestive activity in any middle-aged person should be investigated. Initial symptoms are usually insidious and often absent until the disease is far advanced. Nonresectable lesions are treated with chemotherapy, usually 5-fluorouracil. Cancer of the stomach is not radiosensitive within safe dosages.

X-rays with a barium swallow that show interference with peristaltic action necessitate further investigation with gastroscopy, biopsy, and cytologic examination. As discussed earlier, symptoms of carcinoma of the stomach may simulate those of gastric ulcer. A gastric analysis, however, will likely demonstrate low levels of hydrochloric acid in carcinoma as opposed to normal or elevated levels in gastric ulcer. Endoscopy is also performed to differentiate between benign and malignant ulcers.

In patients with severe, intractable ulcer pain who have not been candidates for surgery, irradiation of the body and fundus of the stomach has been done in conjunction with medical management to reduce gastric acidity. When repeated attacks occur, the Zollinger-Ellison syndrome should be suspected. In this condition, hypersecretion of acid gastric juice is due to excessive secretion of the hormone gastrin. A non-beta islet cell tumor of the pancreas stimulates the secretion of excess gastrin. The ulcer in this disease process is usually in an atypical location. Treatment of this syndrome requires surgical removal of the pancreatic tumor and resection of the ulcerated areas of the stomach. This treatment is discussed in more detail in the section on pancreatic diseases (page 613).

Several types of surgical procedures are utilized in the treatment of ulcers and their complications. These surgical techniques are also used in removing cancer of the stomach or duodenum. The surgical treatment, which is directed against gastric secretion of acid and pepsin, involves removal of the acid-forming cells (which are located in the distal two-thirds or three-fourths of the stomach), or removal of the acid-stimulating mechanism of the stomach by dividing the vagus nerve (vagotomy) or removing the antral portion of the stomach (antrectomy) or both vagotomy and antrectomy. The current emphasis in surgery is on reduction of the stimuli of acid secretion rather than on removal of the acid-secreting organ, although there is still considerable controversy over which approach is most effective. Vagotomy and hemigastrectomy are done to decrease both the nervous and hormonal activation of acid production [7]. Figure 7-3 illustrates some of these surgical procedures.

A subtotal gastrectomy may be indicated to remove the diseased portion of the stomach, usually the lower half or two-thirds of the stomach. In a gastroduodenostomy procedure, also known as Billroth I, the gastric remnant is attached to the duodenum.

Benign or malignant lesions in the stomach or duodenum may be surgically treated by a gastroenterostomy (Billroth II). The lower half or two-thirds of the stomach is resected and the duodenal stump is closed. The remaining segment of the stomach is anastamosed to a loop of the jejunum, thus bypassing the duodenum. Bile continues to flow from the duodenal stump into the jejunum.

Gastrojejunostomy (or gastroenterostomy) provides a permanent connection between the proximal jejunum and the anterior wall of the stomach without removing a segment of the tract. It is done usually to treat inoperable lesions of the pylorus, but can also be done to treat benign obstructions at the pylorus or to provide a larger opening for drainage when vagotomy is performed.

Pyloroplasty is a procedure to form a larger passage between the prepyloric region of the stomach and the duodenum as a treatment for pyloric obstruction or in gastric atony associated with vagotomy.

Vagotomy involves the segmental resection of the vagus nerve usually at 6 to 7 cm above the junction of the esophagus and the stomach to remove the main route of neural stimulation of gastric secretion. Vagotomy alters the motility of the stomach and intestine. It may result in decreased motility and de-

Figure 7-3
Types of gastric surgical procedures. A. Gastroduodenostomy (Billroth I). B. Gastrojejunostomy and vagotomy (Billroth II resection). C. Total gastrectomy.

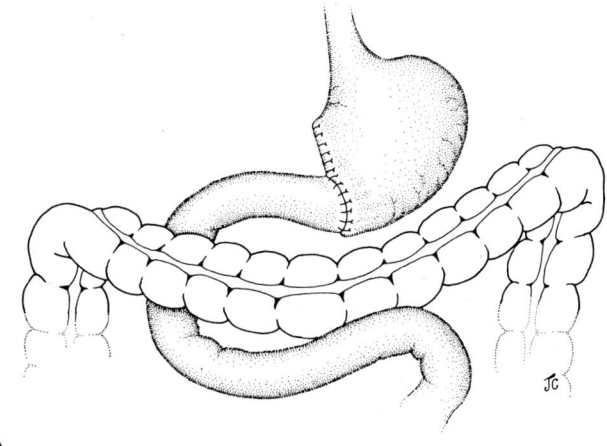

A

B

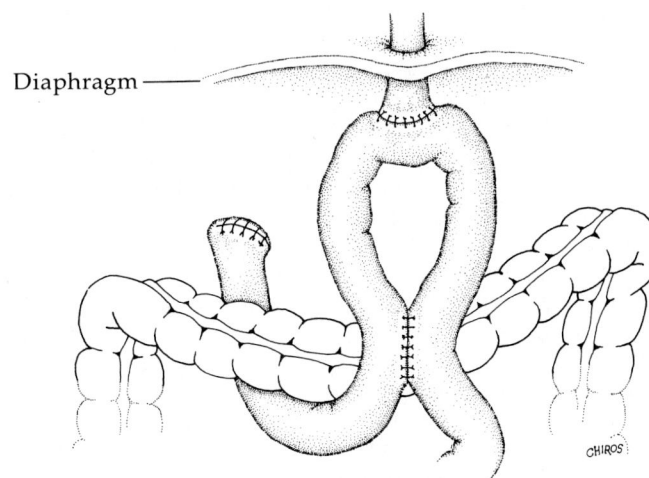

C

layed emptying of the stomach, causing sensations of fullness after meals with belching, abdominal distention, and intestinal flatus or diarrhea. Therefore vagotomy is usually done in conjunction with a corrective drainage procedure such as pyloroplasty to minimize gastric atony.

Selective vagotomy is a technique of selectively denervating the parietal cell mass (the corpus and fundus of the stomach) while preserving the innervation of the antrum. This technique is used to decrease the vagal influence on acid secretion without sacrificing normal gastric emptying function. Selective vagotomy thus may be done in some situations without a drainage procedure.

In **total gastrectomy** the entire stomach is removed and the jejunum is brought up and connected to the esophagus while the free end of the duodenum is closed. Postoperatively, weight loss and malnutrition often occur. Since there is a loss of the intrinsic factor (a substance essential for vitamin B_{12} absorption and normally secreted by the stomach), replacement therapy of vitamin B_{12} is necessary to prevent pernicious anemia. Hydrochloric acid is also often administered to aid digestion. Radical (total) gastrectomy is usually limited to cancerous lesions involving major portions of the stomach, while localized cancer may be treated by subtotal gastrectomy.

The patient who has had gastric surgery has a potential for developing any of the complications that can ensue after any type of surgical procedure. This patient is as vulnerable as or more vulnerable than others to cardiovascular complications, respiratory complications, and reactions to anesthesia. Because the site of the incision is in the upper part of the abdomen, the pain on coughing and deep breathing may be accentuated. The patient therefore may be more hesitant to deep breathe and cough and will tend to breathe shallowly to avoid pain. The nurse must pay particular attention to these aspects as well as those necessary to prevent thrombophlebitis, wound infection, dehiscence, and evisceration. (These complications are discussed on page 104.)

For several days postoperatively, the patient will receive nothing by mouth and will require a nasogastric tube connected to low intermittent suction. In some settings a gastrostomy is done in lieu of using a nasogastric tube, which causes much discomfort for most patients. The fluid restriction provides physiologic rest for the stomach by decreasing motor and secretory activity. The patency of the nasogastric tube must be maintained to ensure that the gastric stump is not distended with an accumulation of secretions, gases, or drainage, which could cause strain on the sutures and rupture of the gastric stump. Nasogastric suction also prevents distention due to edema or impaired peristalsis resulting from surgical trauma. The drainage from the stomach is expected to be bloody for approximately 12 hours; any fresh bloody drainage after that period should be considered unusual. Caution is taken to retain the patency of the tube, and irrigation of the nasogastric tube is often prescribed by the surgeon. To prevent pressure on the gastric suture line, the irrigating solution should be instilled with minimal pressure on the bulb of the Asepto syringe used for irrigation. Inability to recover irrigating fluid is reported. To keep instilling irrigating fluid without obtaining any returns causes distention of the already limited capacity of the stomach.

Oral hygiene and measures to combat the discomfort caused by the oral fluid restriction and mouth breathing caused by the use of the nasogastric tube are important elements in postoperative care. Frequent mouth washes and gargles, the application of soothing glycerine and lemon juice swabs to the lips, and brushing of the teeth or dentures can prevent further discomfort. Cetylpyridinium chloride (Cepacol) lozenges and ice chips are sometimes prescribed to provide sucking activities that prevent mouth dryness. The nurse should caution the patient to limit the amount of ice chips, since excessive amounts of water in the stomach from the melted ice chips will only be removed by the nasogastric tube, along with electrolytes, chiefly sodium and potassium, from the gastric contents. The withdrawal of electrolytes can lead to electrolyte imbalance. Precise measurement of nasogastric drainage and urine output is necessary for determining accurate prescription of intravenous fluid and electrolyte replacement. Fluid replacement, electrolyte status, and the hemoglobin and hematocrit reports must be carefully monitored postoperatively to detect complications.

Usually gastric motility is reestablished approximately 3 days postoperatively. When motility is verified by the passage of flatus per rectum, the return of bowel sounds, or the passage of stool, the nasogastric tube is removed. Usually the tolerance of the patient is first tested with the tube clamped for 4 hours; the gastric residue after this period is measured. If there is stasis of fluid with dilatation and excess gastric residue (more than 100 ml), an obstruction, edema, or spasm may be present and the nasogastric tube is not removed. Absorption of fluid and patency of the lumen at the operative site are assured when there is minimal gastric residue. If the clamping of the tube is tolerated without occurrence of pain, nausea, vomiting, or distention, and the gastric residue is minimal, the tube is removed.

The patient is started gradually on a progressive diet from clear liquid to full liquid to a bland diet of six small feedings. Initially, strained cooked cereal, custard, and cottage cheese are the foods usually served. The nurse observes and records the patient's tolerance of liquids and foods in monitoring intake.

Obstruction, paralytic ileus, and acute gastric dilatation are potential complications after gastric surgery. Obstruction may occur from inflammatory changes resulting from the trauma of the surgery. Paralytic ileus may occur when the motor activity of the intestinal tract does not return to normal due to surgical trauma or to leakage of gastric contents at the suture line. Paralytic ileus also may occur if hypokalemia is present. Distention of the abdomen is the initial symptom of paralytic ileus. Gastric dilatation results in a feeling of fullness, hiccoughs, retching, or vomiting. Providing for the maintenance of the patency of the nasogastric tube and gradual progression in the diet postoperatively will usually prevent gastric dilatation.

The **dumping syndrome,** a group of symptoms that may occur after a total or subtotal gastrectomy, is not clearly understood. The term dumping is used because the problem is believed to be due to the rapid emptying of gastric contents into the small intestine. The small intestine is then distended due to the sudden increase in intraluminal pressure. Symptoms of weakness, profuse perspiration, nausea, faintness, flushing, epigastric discomfort, vomiting, and palpitation occur usually within 15 minutes after eating (early dumping syndrome). Symptoms may be mild or so severe that the patient is forced to lie down.

Some authorities theorize that the symptoms are due to the considerable amount of extracellular fluid that enters the intestine to dilute the hypertonic fluid as large quantities of food enter the intestinal tract. The symptoms occur particularly after meals containing large amounts of sugars or carbohydrates. The subsequent lowering of the blood volume may result in shock-like symptoms.

Postgastrectomy hypoglycemic reactions may also occur. This hypoglycemic reaction results from rapid digestion and absorption of carbohydrates, which produce hyperglycemia, which in turn stimulates the secretion of insulin in excess of the quantity required, leading to hypoglycemic symptoms (late dumping syndrome). Eating frequent small meals rather than three large meals, taking rest periods after eating, drinking fluids between meals rather than with meals, and avoiding high carbohydrate foods are measures to prevent these symptoms, which usually disappear in time. When medical therapy is ineffective, surgical intervention may be necessary. An antiperistaltic segment may be interposed between the stomach and duodenum or the anastomatic opening from the stomach into the small intestine may be made smaller to control the gastric output.

Postoperative management for the patient with ulcers includes dietary instruction in types of foods to be eliminated and moderation or total avoidance of foods that aggravate symptoms. Identifying environmental and psychological stresses is important in devising plans to control or cope with these stresses. Although most patients recover from ulcer surgery without complications and without recurrence, one must recognize that recurrence is possible.

The Lining of the Large Intestine

Integrity of the lining can be lost in other parts of the gastrointestinal tract as well as in the gastric and duodenal areas. **Ulcerative colitis** is an inflammatory disease involving the mucosa of the colon and rectum and, in some cases, the terminal segment of the small bowel. The disease is most frequent in young adults and tends to occur slightly more often in females than in males and more often in the Jewish population than in the general population.

Several factors have been identified as contributing to the incidence of ulcerative colitis.

There is general agreement that emotional disturbances have a part in aggravating the physical symptoms of ulcerative colitis, but metabolic disturbances, infection, mucolytic enzymes, allergic hypersensitivities, collagen changes, and autoimmune processes have all been implicated. No definite cause has been isolated, but rather it is likely that the disease is the result of many factors.

Inflammation and ulcer formation of the mucosal, and sometimes the submucosal, layer occur. The mucosa initially is edematous with hyperemia and is friable. Diffuse involvement of both the colon and the rectum is common. Abscess and ulcer formation occur in severe cases of the disease. The mucosa may be completely stripped in some areas, with formation of mucopurulent exudate. These changes account for the classic symptoms of severe diarrhea with blood and mucus in the stools, accompanied by abdominal cramps (usually in the left lower quadrant), malaise, tenesmus, loss of appetite, and weight loss. In a severe attack of ulcerative colitis, the rectal discharge may be composed almost entirely of blood mixed with mucus and pus and no stool. The urge to defecate may come so suddenly that incontinence may result. Diagnosis is confirmed by proctoscopy and barium enema, both of which demonstrate distortion of the mucosa, filling defects, and loss of haustral markings in the colon. The patient with intractable ulcerative colitis or in an acute stage of the disease is hindered in all activities as the bloody and purulent diarrhea increases and the symptoms of pain, weakness, and subsequent discouragement become severe. The patient may become a chronic invalid, limiting social interactions and compromising family relationships.

The disease is usually characterized by phases of exacerbations and remissions. Control may be achieved through diet and medications, but surgery is necessary in life-threatening complications such as bleeding, unremitting anemia, excessive diarrhea, chronic malnutrition, fistula formation, and perforation. The latter condition is the cause of the majority of deaths associated with ulcerative colitis. Although the disease is usually insidious, it may be fulminating. The patient in an acute fulminating stage of disease presents with signs of hemorrhage, generalized sepsis and shock, and fluid and electrolyte imbalance due to loss of potassium and plasma proteins. Toxic megacolon (marked dilatation of the colon) may occur and cause marked abdominal distention, tenderness, and possibly perforation.

In progressive ulcerative colitis a variety of systemic disorders, such as arthritis, pyoderma gangrenosum, and hepatic disease, may accompany the disease. **Pyoderma gangrenosum** consists of cutaneous lesions that destroy all the layers of the skin; they are usually located on the extremities. Healing of the cutaneous lesions often reflects improvement in the colonic lesions.

Medical treatment depends on the type and severity of the disease. It consists in measures to correct nutritional deficiencies and fluid and electrolyte imbalance, to control diarrhea, and to prevent infection and control inflammation. Meeting the psychological needs of the patient is extremely important, as it is well recognized that emotional stress aggravates the disease process. A low fiber, high protein, and high carbohydrate diet is indicated; nutritional and vitamin supplements are often necessary.

Antidiarrhea agents, often combined with antibiotics, sedatives, tranquilizers, and corticosteroids, are used. Anticholinergic medications may be used to control colonic spasms.

Azulfidine, a brand of salicylazosulfapyridine, is often the drug of choice in ulcerative colitis. It is a combination of sulfonamide and salicylic acid and is given in doses of 2 to 6 gm orally per day. Unlike other sulfa drugs, it has a special affinity for connective tissue and is therefore useful for treating the marked changes that occur in the subepithelial connective tissue. The drug can cause side effects of headache, dizziness, and epigastric distress.

Corticosteroids may be administered orally, by enemas, by suppositories or by parenteral injection, for their anti-inflammatory effects. The nurse observes the patient for side effects that frequently occur with increased dosages and prolonged administration. Local administration of hydrocortisone or prednisolone suppositories or small retention enemas may be useful in localized disease. Medications such as diphenoxylate hydrochloride with atropine sulfate (Lomotil) are frequently used to help control intestinal motility. Recently, immunosuppressive drugs such as azathioprine (Imuran) have been used in treating ulcerative colitis.

Blood transfusions, intravenous fluids, and electrolytes are utilized in acute stages of the disease. Potassium depletion is common in excessive diarrhea, and magnesium deficiencies can also occur. Plasma or serum albumin transfusions may be necessary to replace protein loss.

Permanent **ileostomy** with total colectomy is the surgical procedure usually performed for the management of intractable ulcerative colitis. Previously, when an ileostomy was done, the colon was often left in the abdomen for potential reanastomosis. Statistics have shown that patients with long-term ulcerative colitis (more than 10 years) are more susceptible to malignancy of the colon. About 10 percent develop carcinoma. Therefore total colectomy including removal of the rectum currently is the more acceptable procedure. In this procedure, gastrointestinal elimination is provided for by creating an artificial orifice by bringing the ileum to the skin through the abdominal wall, creating a stoma. In some settings partial colectomy, sparing the rectum so that subsequent ileoproctostomy can be done, is the preferred surgical procedure.

Complications after ileostomy are those that can occur with any abdominal surgery. Drainage from the stoma must be accurately observed and measured in the early postoperative period to detect fluid and electrolyte complications. The patient not only will have to cope with the adjustment to the artificial orifice, but also will suffer the discomfort of an extensive perineal wound. In the patient with ulcerative colitis the inflammatory process of the disease tends to interfere with the healing of the perineal wound so that sometimes the healing process may take as long as 6 to 8 months. (Care of the perineal wound is discussed on page 576.)

Success of the surgery requires a functional stoma which can be readily cared for and which does not interfere with the patient's activities postoperatively. Therefore the stoma site should be selected preoperatively according to these functional requirements, and the site is marked for the surgeon. An inappropriate site might be selected while the patient is under anesthesia because the abdominal contours change as abdominal muscles are relaxed. There are several considerations important in selection of the stoma site. Ostomy appliances to be used by the patient postoperatively can be sampled preoperatively and the best site determined to avoid scars, bony prominences, the umbilicus, and skin folds. The stoma should be located on a flat abdominal surface, generally in the lower right quadrant. The site should have at least 2 inches (5 cm) of smooth skin around the stoma to facilitate good adherence of the appliance. Esthetic aspects are also taken into consideration; for example, if the patient anticipates being able to wear a bikini. Appliances can be sampled preoperatively and the site should also be evaluated as the patient sits, bends, and does other activities that might tax the appliance. An appliance may fit satisfactorily when the wearer is in a recumbent position but may cause excessive pressure or may be released easily on bending or sitting.

The ileostomy stoma is formed by incising the sheath of the rectus muscle, dilating the muscle fibers, and then pulling the ileum through the stoma to the skin. The mesentery of the ileum is sutured to the peritoneal wall to anchor it and to prevent prolapse or volvulus. The stoma is "matured" at surgery by everting the terminal ileum so that the serosal surfaces are opposed and the mucosa is exposed. The bowel ends are sutured to the skin, leaving a smooth, rounded, and everted ileum at the end of the ileostomy. The matured stoma heals readily with less likelihood of the occurrence of stenosis or stricture. The stoma should protrude about ¾ inch (2 cm); a flush stoma interferes with management of the ileostomy. Immediately postoperatively, the stoma has a velvety red appearance and is usually edematous; the edema usually subsides within 7 to 21 days, but may last 6 weeks postoperatively.

The ileostomy patient has almost continuous drainage once peristalsis is reestablished postoperatively. It is important that minimal peristomal skin be exposed to the drainage because it contains proteolytic enzymes. A leakproof transparent disposable appliance that is drainable is placed on the stoma in surgery or in the recovery room as an immediate measure to prevent skin excoriation and to provide for collection of drainage. The nurse should observe the color and size of the stoma and the amount and type of drainage. A healthy stoma is pink or reddish whereas a dark or somewhat bluish stoma reflects ischemia and can lead to necrosis of the stoma.

The ileostomy appliance must have an open end for emptying the drainage. Figure 7-4 illustrates how the appliance is rinsed to remove drainage. The bottom of the pouch is then folded over and closed with a clip or rubber band. Usually the pouch will have to be emptied four or five times per day. The entire appliance will have to be changed when it becomes loose. Reusable appliances are applied with cement or with double-faced adhesives, and there is a wide variety of opinion about the appropriate time intervals for changing the appliances. While some authorities advise changes every 24 hours, some ostomates retain appliances for 3 to 7 days or longer. Most authorities state that an appliance should adhere at least 48 hours without leakage and should be reapplied at least weekly so that the state of peristomal skin can be observed. The pattern for changing the appliance is best determined by the patient, assisted by the nurse and enterostomal therapist, after evaluation of adherence, skin care, and odor. Initially while adapting to the appliance the patient may feel relieved to have it hold for 24 hours without leakage. Reusable appliances are washed well with soap and water or a vinegar solution after use, and are air-dried thoroughly.

The specific type of appliance selected from the many varieties available should be suited to the individual patient and should be well-fitting and leakproof. Most patients' major concern is that the appliance be leakproof, odorproof, and concealable under clothing, as well as easy to handle. Disposable appliances may be used even after the early postoperative period, or the patient may prefer reusable (permanent) appliances because they may be more economical. The patient, the nurse, and the enterostomal therapist should consider all these factors in planning the long-term management of the ileostomy.

A reusable (permanent) appliance consists of a pouch for the collection of drainage and a face plate (mounting disk) that attaches to the peristomal skin. The reusable appliances may be of one piece or the face plate may be separate from the pouch. In this two-piece appliance, the face plate is attached to the skin and may be left in place for several days, while the pouch is removable and is changed as necessary. Generally, patients are discharged from the hospital with disposable appliances. If a reusable appliance is preferred, the appliance is usually ordered about 6 weeks after surgery when the stoma size has stabilized. A nurse or an enterostomal therapist should teach the patient how to use the reusable appliance correctly. In some institutions the reusable appliance is ordered while the patient is hospitalized and before the edema has completely subsided so that the patient may have assistance in learning to use the appliance under supervision. Another appliance, however, will be necessary within 6 weeks when the stoma is smaller, making the opening in the first appliance too large. This arrangement may create a financial problem for some patients.

Disks used for the face plates are made of a variety of materials, such as plastic, metal, and metal covered with rubber. These disks

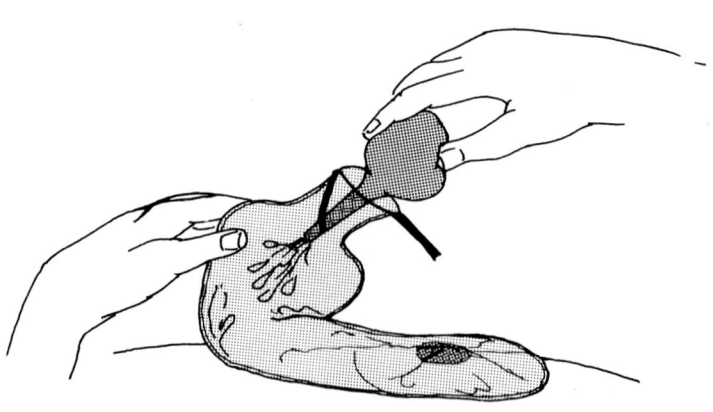

Figure 7-4
Rinsing the ileostomy appliance after emptying the drainage.

vary in weight, rate of deterioration, and odor resistance. A patient should always have two face plates and two appliances that can be alternated. As the stoma regresses in size after surgery, the face plate may become too large. To avoid having to buy a new appliance before the stoma has stabilized, a circular "closed-cell" foam pad may be inserted around the stoma to protect the exposed skin. The closed-cell foam does not shred or hold odors. Companies vary in policies regarding the reworking or modification of disks once they are purchased, but some companies custom-fit face plates when patients are having management difficulties.

Disks range in convexity to provide better fitting for varying types of abdominal contours. The adult with a firm, flat abdomen may be able to use a flat disk; a relatively slim adult will likely use an average disk. With a soft abdomen, however, a medium convexity is required. With a soft, deep, flabby abdomen, a deep convexity is necessary. The various types of convexity provide a means to cover a stoma that does not readily protrude and therefore could cause leakage problems. Too great a convexity can cause the face plate to pop off and result in leakage and skin problems. The particular face plate must be checked at regular intervals, particularly if the patient's weight increases or decreases, causing a change in the abdominal contour.

Some disks may adhere so snugly that no belt is needed to secure the appliance or the edges of the disk may be secured with adhesive. Other appliances come with belts or are attached to belts by patients who feel more secure with them. Several points should be stressed to persons who wear belts with their appliances. Belts should not be too tight, but should have a two-finger leeway to avoid skin ulcers from belt pressure. The nurse should observe for pressure lesions from a tight belt. The patient should purchase several elastic belts to permit daily changing, and a rubber belt should be used for water sports, since elastic belts lose elasticity in water.

A variety of substances are available to control odor. Table 7-2 lists the names of some of these substances and particular points re-

Table 7-2
Odor control methods for ostomy care

Agent	Administration	Uses
Oral Agents		
Bismuth subgallate (Devrom)	Taken orally as a chewable tablet (usually 5 grains tid or qid)	Useful for controlling fecal odors. Has constipating effect. (There have been reports of toxicity from the prolonged consumption of large amounts of bismuth salts of gallic acid.)
Bismuth subcarbonate	Taken orally. Usually 1 or 2 tablets (5 grains in each) after meals	Useful as a fecal deodorizer
Chlorophyll (Derifil)	Water-soluble chlorophyllin tablet; oral tablet, 100 mg	Adsorbs gas
Charcoal	Oral tablet	Adsorbs gas; leaves film or dark ring in toilet bowl
Cranberry juice	One glass several times daily	Prevents odor in urostomies; maintains urine acidity
External Agents	These are all placed in the appliance when emptied or changed. They should not be applied to the stoma.	
Banish	Liquid deodorant; 8 to 10 drops in appliance	Has no odor of own; no perfume added. Useful for all ostomies
Ostobon	Powder form; 2 puffs into pouch of appliance	Unscented; useful for fecal ostomies
Nilodor	1 gtt into pouch of appliance	Has distinct odor of its own; sometimes odor is offensive
Mouthwash	1 tablespoonful into pouch of appliance	Sometimes effective for fecal ostomies

Aspirin has sometimes been recommended for insertion into the appliance to neutralize odor. This use should be discouraged, because ulcerations of the stoma may be caused by contacts with the acidic solution.

garding usage. Dietary aspects are also important in controlling odor. Foods that are especially troublesome should be eliminated.

If leakage occurs frequently with the appliances, the appliance has probably not been put on correctly or is not suitable for the individual. Skin irritations develop when the disc is too large and the irritating discharge comes in contact with the skin. A face-plate opening should be only 1/16 to 1/8 inch (1.4 to 1.6 mm) wider than the stoma (Fig. 7-5). When the disk is too small, fistulas, bleeding, or mucosal swelling tends to occur.

The patient should avoid changing the appliance soon after eating because it will be difficult to keep the peristomal area free of drainage during the change. The ileostomy is more likely to be quiescent before meals or before retiring, or at least 2 to 4 hours after eating.

The fresh duplicate appliance should be readied before the used one is removed. Usually a solvent is used to remove the cement; double-faced adhesive is used to adhere the reusable appliance. The peristomal skin is patted, not rubbed, during removal of the appliance and during cleaning. Benzine (petroleum ether) is the common solvent and should not be confused with benzene, which is very irritating and toxic and which has been known to cause bone marrow depression. All solvents are flammable, and precautions are necessary in their use. To remove disposable appliances, only mild soap and water are necessary.

If cement is used for adhering the appliance to the skin, only thin coats are applied and sufficient drying time is allowed. Superfatted soaps and bath oils leave an oily residue on the skin that will hinder adherence; consequently, oily soaps are not used in cleaning peristomal skin. The peristomal area is cleaned with tissue or soft cloth.

When an appliance is being changed, a small piece of gauze (or small tampon) is placed on the stoma to absorb the effluent and prevent leakage while peristomal skin is being cleaned or while a skin barrier or cement is being applied. To reapply an appliance that is not translucent, a dissolvable guide strip should be used by the patient (or nurse) to center the appliance over the stoma. This paper will fall into the pouch and be dissolved or eliminated when the pouch is emptied (Fig. 7-6).

In place of cement, tincture of benzoin is preferred by some ostomates for peristomal skin appliance adherence. Skin Prep (an adhesive and protective preparation), karaya washers, or double-faced adhesives are applied for adherence or skin protection or both. Skin barriers are used to protect the peristomal skin from irritating drainage and to promote healing if lesions occur. The skin barriers also promote adherence of the appliance. Table 7-3 lists the most common barriers used in the care of stomas.

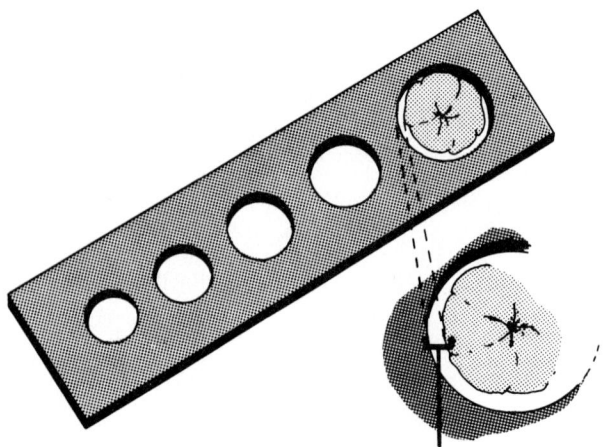

Area between stoma and measuring guide should be *no larger* than 1/8"

Figure 7-5
Measuring the stoma for application of an appliance.

and slowly instilling approximately 50 ml of normal saline via an Asepto syringe. The saline is instilled slowly and withdrawn, and instillation is repeated to break up the blockage if necessary.

In addition to food blockage, potential complications after an ileostomy include dysfunction of the ileostomy, fluid and electrolyte imbalance, prolapse of the stoma, adhesions, retraction, fistula formation, and hernia. **Ileostomy dysfunction** refers to altered sporadic functioning of the ostomy and is characterized by foul odor of the effluent and increased output of liquid effluent. It is usually caused by peristomal scarring and stenosis, which may require surgical intervention. Fluid and electrolyte imbalances occur quickly in the presence of vomiting or diarrhea or both, associated with a variety of gastrointestinal disturbances. The ileostomate readily loses sodium and water. Fluids with increased carbohydrate and electrolyte content, such as orange juice, tea, Gatorade, and bouillon are given when diets are not tolerated. If antidiarrheal agents are not effective, intravenous fluid and electrolyte administration is necessary.

Prolapse of the stoma generally results when the mesentery is not securely attached to the abdominal wall. Surgical repair is the treatment, but use of a prolapse guard or manual reduction may be a temporary solution. **Retraction** refers to a stoma that becomes flush with the skin. This retraction creates problems in the use of an appliance, and skin irritation occurs from leakage. The use of skin barriers and a convex face plate is a temporary measure until stoma revision can be performed. **Fistulas** may result from surgical damage to the ileum, mechanical trauma by an ill-fitting appliance, and recurrence of the disease. In addition to effluent leakage and skin excoriation, large amounts of fluids and electrolytes are lost through fistulas, requiring total parenteral nutrition to promote spontaneous healing or surgical intervention. **Hernias** at the stoma site most often occur in patients with weak abdominal muscles and inadequate healing. Surgical repair is indicated to prevent obstruction of the stoma and problems in appliance management. Appliances do not adhere well if there is a hernia at the stoma site, and problems with leakage and skin irritation frequently occur.

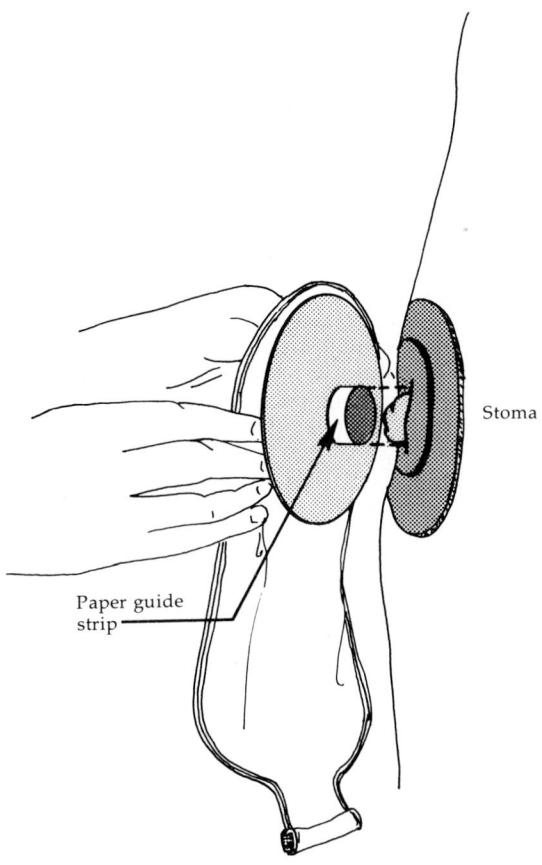

Figure 7-6
Placement of an ileostomy appliance using a paper guide strip. (Note skin barrier around the stoma.)

An ileostomy is not to be confused with a colostomy. The ileostomy drains continuously and initially drainage is liquid but later, as the body adapts to the loss of the colon and its water-absorbing activities, the ileum increases its absorption and the stools tend to become pasty in consistency. Drainage from a conventional ileostomy cannot be regulated as drainage from some colostomies can be. The only indication for irrigation of an ileostomy is when food blockage occurs, although food blockage occurs rarely. Usually fibrous foods like coconut, mushrooms, celery, nuts, seeds, or popcorn cause blockage. Irrigation (via gentle lavage) is done only after the cause of the obstruction is determined. For example, irrigation is contraindicated when obstruction results from volvulus or defects in stoma healing. Ileostomy lavage is performed by using a small French catheter

Table 7-3
Selected skin barriers for peristomal care

Agent	Uses, advantages, and techniques
Stomahesive (Squibb)	Useful on excoriated skin; will adhere to a weeping surface, but greasy substances will interfere with adhesion. Has effective skintight adhesion
	Fits under all types of face plates and appliances for long adherence. Useful for all types of ostomies and fistulas
	Dull side of wafer goes to skin (after removing parchment protective cover). Shiny side goes to appliance
	If karaya powder, Kenalog, or Mycostatin powder is used on irritated skin, it is helpful to spray Skin Prep (or other adhesive protective spray) before applying Stomahesive
Karaya	Prepared in powder, rings, washers, and paste forms. Washers fit snugly around the stoma helping to protect skin from irritation. Rings or washers can be adapted to the size of the stoma by molding and stretching to appropriate size. Rings or washers should be lightly moistened on the skin side before applying
	Karaya powder soothes peristomal skin; a protective base to which most appliances adhere if excess powder is brushed off. Should be sprinkled lightly. Useful for fecal ostomies
	Karaya washers tend to melt readily around urostomy stomas
	Few side effects in its natural form. May cause allergic reactions, depending on specific additive
	Causes burning sensation when first applied to skin
	Karaya wafers tend to retain their size and do not stretch as washers do. Allow 1/8 inch around stoma
	Karaya paste is useful to protect hard-to-seal skin areas; can be used to fill in scars, skin depression, or areas left exposed around irregularly shaped stomas. The paste should not be applied directly over open cuts or sores (contains isopropyl alcohol). It is applied by using a thin film on finger or tongue blade (allow few minutes for paste to dry before applying appliance)
Reliaseal (Davol)	Adhesive discs that adhere to dry or moistened skin. Useful for all types of stomas. Will not adhere to weeping surfaces
	To apply: adhere blue side to appliance, white side to skin; hold in place for 30 seconds after applying
Colly-seels (Mason Labs)	An amalgam with karaya gum as a base, but is not the same as a karaya seal. Useful for ileostomies and urostomies. The seel itself and the body heat seal the barrier to skin; does not have an adhesive. Should be used with belted appliance. Does not work over skin covered with powder, oils, ointments. Moisten smooth side of seal and position it around stoma after cutting hole to fit over stoma
	Functions even over irritated and partly denuded skin. Should be stored in dry, cool area
Skin Prep (United Surgical)	Sprayed on peristomal skin prior to applying appliance (cover stoma when spraying). Binds to skin and provides protective coating. Can be used over application of karaya powder and Amphojel in treating excoriated skin before applying appliance. Should be allowed to dry before applying skin barriers or appliances
Stoma Barrier Cream	Karaya gum and silicone. Applied around exposed skin at base of stoma
Skin Gel (Hollister)	A protective film. Spread very thinly. Should be completely dry before applying appliance. Useful to prevent irritation due to repeated use of adhesive appliances and tapes
Carbo zinc oxide (Osto Care)	A kneadable material that forms a protective stomal gasket to prevent peristomal irritation. Can be used to fill in scar areas and skin creases under appliance
Skin Care (Sween)	A white vanishing cream that can be used around stomal skin before attaching the appliance or face plate. Also useful for perianal care if irritated or frequent stools
Aluminum hydroxide (Amphojel)	Amphojel is applied in a thin coating after irritated skin is cleaned. Allow to dry until it becomes white and chalky. Sprinkle karaya powder over this film, but remove excess. Use adhesive spray before applying Stomahesive and appliance. (If tissue is weeping, more than one application of Amphojel is required before chalky consistency results.) Soothing to excoriated skin
Kenalog spray, powder	Prescription required. Useful for inflammatory skin irritations. May be used in combination with Mycostatin. Useful for controlling fungal infections
Mycostatin powder	Prescription required. Definitive treatment for monilial fungal infection under appliance
Tincture of benzoin	Applied to promote appliance adherence. Compound preparation is contraindicated; has irritating and toxic properties

Dietary management is essential and the patient should be given clear instructions so that he or she selects the appropriate foods. Postoperatively the diet should be well-balanced but foods are selected carefully to prevent blockage, watery or excessively heavy discharge, or excessive odor and gas. A low fiber diet is usually prescribed for 6 to 8 weeks, and additional foods are permitted according to the patient's tolerance. Low fiber diets limit fried foods, raw fruits, whole grain breads, nuts, condiments, milk, strong flavored cheese, and certain vegetables. Foods high in fibrous content (e.g., seeds and kernels) are avoided in order to prevent blockage. Some ostomates, however, are able to eat small quantities of these foods, taking care to chew them thoroughly, and thus retain them in their diet program. Green beans, broccoli, spinach, and highly spiced foods often cause diarrhea and may be restricted. Avoiding beans, carbonated drinks, onions, cabbage, garlic, asparagus, and certain cheeses may be necessary to control odor. Patients should be encouraged to experiment with foods gradually to determine which foods adversely affect them. Ileostomates should be instructed to ingest sufficient fluids and salt because both may be readily lost through the ileostomy, since the absorptive functions of the colon no longer are available. Patients should be instructed in the importance of notifying their physician in case of diarrhea or excessive ileostomy drainage and should be familarized with signs of electrolyte imbalance. Fluid and electrolyte imbalance can occur quickly in the ileostomate who no longer has a functioning colon.

An ileostomate is likely to be an adolescent or young adult, the ages most susceptible to ulcerative colitis. At a stage of development when intense peer dependency, conformity, and a struggle for self-identity are characteristic, the individual with an ileostomy has the additional burden of learning technical skills and adaptations in his or her life pattern and is likely to be distressed about his or her altered body image. Patience, understanding, and emotional support from significant persons in the family as well as from professional staff are of paramount importance as the individual experiences grief, depression, and loneliness in adjusting to the ileostomy.

The symptoms of ulcerative colitis may have interfered with a normal life pattern and although the ileostomy may have corrected the disease itself, the surgical procedure may emotionally handicap the patient if proper emotional support and teaching are not provided. The nurse can be a significant person to such patients by providing support, knowledge, and interest in assisting the ileostomate in rehabilitation. The operation is considered mutilating surgery by most patients, and sufficient time for verbal expression related to coping with adjustments to an altered body image is absolutely essential.

The major role of the nurse is to assist the patient in learning self-care and in adapting to the altered pattern of elimination. The patient's readiness for learning and the level and rate of instruction are major considerations. Besides dietary information, the patient is thoroughly prepared in stoma care, appliance changing, and how to handle the problems of diarrhea, skin excoriation, appliance leakage, odor, flatus, and food blockage. Information is also provided on how to obtain the appliances and other equipment from pharmacies or directly from the manufacturer. The patient is advised of any medications to continue or those to avoid, such as laxatives, and is cautioned to advise any physician or dentist who might prescribe medications that he or she has an ileostomy, since some medications may not be absorbed adequately. This problem is most likely to occur with enteric-coated tablets and time-released capsules. Diuretics can quickly cause fluid and electrolyte imbalance and must be used with caution.

The patient frequently has questions about clothing. If appliances are properly fitted, they are not detectable by others. Lightweight girdles and form-fitting elastic undershorts are useful in keeping the appliance in place and providing a smooth contour. If stoma sites are properly selected, women are able to wear bikinis and form-fitting slacks.

The patient is able to resume previous activities after ileostomy, and often increases his or her activities because of improved health. Contact sports may be contraindicated, although some ileostomates are known to participate in them without having complications.

Ileostomy groups have organized to provide mutual aid and information to facilitate physical, emotional, and social rehabilitation. Working with the medical and nursing professions to improve instruction on ileostomy care, the rehabilitated ostomates provide support and encouragement to new postoperative patients via a visiting program and ongoing activities. Addresses of local chapters of the United Ostomy Association can be obtained by writing the Association:

United Ostomy Association
1111 Wilshire Blvd.
Los Angeles, California 90017

One of the most frequent concerns of the ostomate is related to the effect of the surgery on sexuality. It is also one of the most neglected aspects of ostomy rehabilitation. Most ileostomies are performed in the adolescent or young adult age group; the nurse should be concerned with the special needs of this age group in aspects of sexuality. Appropriate counseling by the nurse and other professionals is indicated. Approximately 10 to 20 percent of male ileostomates suffer impairment of sexual function after removal of the rectum if the surgery has interfered with the nerve pathways controlling sexual functions of the male genitalia. In most cases the problems with sexual relationships are related to psychological rather than physiologic changes. The patient's attitude toward self, sex, and marriage before surgery is likely to be the most important factor affecting sexual relationships after an ileostomy. Sometimes the patient may perceive that the ostomy has resulted in poor sexual relationships when the problem of poor sexual experiences has actually been a long-standing one. There are several possible concerns regarding sexual relationships that should be explored with the patient. For example, in some instances, the mate may be concerned about hurting the stoma and may be hesitant in the sexual relationship because of concern for the ostomate, who may, in turn, interpret the hesitation as rejection. Some ostomates may be fearful that the appliance will dislodge during the sexual act, but this is not likely to occur if the appliance has been appropriately applied. Proper hygiene and an odor-free appliance promote acceptance of the stoma and the ostomate's sense of security. If desired by the ostomate, various garments are available to conceal or decorate the appliance. In some cases, the stoma actually may not cause difficulty. If the rectum has been removed, however, delayed healing of the perineal area may temporarily prohibit sexual activity. Successful sexual experiences result from cooperation and patience on the part of both the ostomate and the partner, and the nurse should include both in the teaching program [16].

The young female with an ileostomy may be concerned about the likelihood of pregnancy. An ileostomy itself is not a barrier to pregnancy, although most surgeons advise a delay of pregnancy for 1 to 2 years after an ileostomy is performed. The surgeon and an obstetrician should both be consulted during the pregnancy. A vaginal delivery is usual, though a cesarean section may be done in some situations. In the early stages, morning sickness with nausea and vomiting may precipitate electrolyte imbalance for the already vulnerable ostomate. As the pregnancy proceeds and the abdominal contours change, often causing stomal edema, appliances will need adjustments. Reusable appliances may temporarily have to be replaced by readily adjusted disposable bags, which are also lighter, when the pregnant woman has problems keeping the reusable appliance in place. A large fetus during the last trimester may interfere with the stoma and can cause prolapse of the stoma or obstruction due to kinking of the bowel.

An alternative procedure for control of ileostomy drainage is being utilized to avoid the necessity for a stoma that continually drains and requires a permanent appliance. The **continent ileostomy,** also known as Kock's continent ileostomy, utilizes a skin-level stoma but an internal reservoir is prepared from the distal ileum. The open end of the ileal pouch is brought between the rectus muscles to form a seal and then opens on the abdomen. A nipple valve is designed within the reservoir by intussusception of the distal ileum; this technique prevents leakage of gas or effluent. The internal pouch is emptied by means of a catheter inserted through the stoma to drain the contents. Postoperatively the initial capacity of the pouch is only 100 to 200 ml, but after 6 months, the internal pouch expands to hold as much as 500 ml of drainage. The pouch generally requires emptying two or three times a day, and catheter insertion must be done carefully to prevent perforation.

Some patients with conventional ileostomies have elected to convert to a continent ileostomy, even though the surgery is still considered experimental. Difficulties in the management of the continent ileostomy can occur; continence may not be achieved and an appliance may be required. Thick drainage may clog the catheter, and gentle lavage may be required. For persons who have achieved continence of both gas and effluent, the surgery has been exceptionally beneficial.

INTERFERENCE OF MOTILITY IN THE GASTROINTESTINAL TRACT

The normal motility of the gastrointestinal tract provides for peristaltic activity with forward propulsion of food and chyme through the upper tract, and forward movement of feces in the lower part of the tract. Extensive parasympathetic and sympathetic innervation supplies the entire muscular gastrointestinal tract. The vagus nerve carries the parasympathetic stimuli to the upper part of the tract, and the distal colon receives parasympathetic stimulation through the nervi erigentes (pelvic splanchnic nerves). Stimulation of the parasympathetic system nerves increases the activity of the intramural nerve plexus. Stimulation of the sympathetic nervous system inhibits activity in the tract, except at two points, the ileocecal sphincter and the internal anal sphincter.

Food is chewed in the mouth to form a bolus that is initially moved voluntarily into the pharynx and then is transported via the esophagus to the stomach in an involuntary phase of swallowing. Automatic control of swallowing arises in the medulla and lower portion of the pons. In addition to peristaltic movement controlled by vagal reflexes, gravitational pulling contributes to the passage of food through the esophagus when a person is in an upright position.

Food is mixed with gastric secretions in the stomach, forming the semifluid mixture called chyme. Emptying of the stomach is influenced by the fluidity of the chyme, the stimulation of the enterogastric reflex that inhibits gastric peristalsis when the small intestine contains excess chyme, and the stimulation of the inhibiting hormone enterogastrone in the presence of fatty acids in the chyme. In the small intestine, peristaltic movements propel the chyme toward the anus, and segmental contractions mix the chyme with intestinal and biliary secretions. Passage into the colon is controlled by reflexes from the cecum at the ileocecal valve. The first part of the colon has an absorption function, and the distal colon has a storage function, so that movements in the colon are normally sluggish. The stimulus for defecation arises from distention in the rectum, but there is voluntary control of the external sphincter until the person wishes to defecate.

Problems in motility can occur in any part of the tract, particularly at the sites of the sphincters. **Dysphagia** is the major symptom related to motility problems in the esophagus, which has the sole purpose of transporting food from the mouth to the stomach. There is a wide range of divergent causes of dysphagia, so that investigation is indicated not only of the structures directly involved with swallowing but also of systemic processes. Dysphagia may originate from emotional causes, as in globus hystericus, when the patient complains of a lump in the throat. Thorough investigation for physical causes of the symptom of dysphagia is necessary, however, since the same sensation can occur in patients with hypopharyngeal cancer. Mechanical obstruction due to intrinsic pathologic conditions such as inflammation, ulcers, or tumors (and neurologic conditions like myasthenia gravis) may cause dysphagia. The nurse who listens to the patient carefully will find that when mechanical obstruction is the cause he or she often can locate the exact site at which dysphagia occurs. When dysphagia is an intrinsic condition, the patient generally has difficulty in swallowing solids before difficulty in swallowing liquids occurs. Patients often take liquids in large quantities to help swallow the solids, which they describe as "needing to wash down the food." In dysphagia related to neuromuscular disease, the patient usually has less difficulty with solids than with liquids. The patient requires psychological support because of the fear of choking. The fear may cause avoidance of any attempts to eat.

Achalasia, also termed cardiospasm, is a generalized disorder of esophageal motility resulting in failure of the terminal esophagus and cardiac sphincter to relax at the gastroesophageal junction. The result is functional obstruction of the distal esophagus secondary to abnormal parasympathetic stimulation; regurgitation commonly occurs. Distention of the esophagus with sensations of retrosternal pressure is likely to occur. Esophagoscopy is indicated to rule out a malignancy at the site of the terminal esophagus, which may also cause similar symptoms. Treatment usually includes the use of pneumatic or rubber dilators to forcefully split the submucosal smooth muscle fibers in the contracted area. Esophagomyotomy may also be performed.

Vomiting is an example of reverse peristalsis with ejection of stomach contents through the mouth, which can be caused by a variety of reasons, ranging from emotional tension to pyloric stenosis. While the vomiting reflex is an essential protective mechanism by which the body attempts to eject harmful chemicals and drugs from the stomach before they are absorbed, the vomiting reflex can endanger life when excessive amounts of fluids are lost. Dehydration, exhaustion, and electrolyte imbalance can result. Supportive therapy by means of intravenous feedings and nursing comfort measures are necessary until the vomiting is controlled.

The vomiting center is located in the medulla oblongata. Sensory stimuli of the vomiting reflex may originate in receptor areas in almost any part of the digestive tract, other abdominal viscera, and the labyrinth of the ear (motion sickness). The chemoreceptor trigger zone located beneath the cortex also relays afferent impulses toward the vomiting center.

Antiemetic drugs to inhibit hyperactive vomiting reflex activity are administered to help control vomiting. These drugs make the chemoreceptor zone less sensitive to emetic stimuli or to nerve impulses from the motion receptors in the inner ear. The drugs may act locally or centrally. Phenothiazine and nonthiazine compounds are centrally acting antiemetics and are used more frequently than the locally acting agents such as topical mucosal anesthetics, antacids, and adsorbents. The more common central acting drugs include chlorpromazine (Thorazine), promethazine (Phenergan), trimethobenzamide (Tigan), prochlorperazine (Compazine), and dimenhydrinate (Dramamine). A more recent antiemetic drug, benzquinamide hydrochloride (Emete-con), has proved effective in the prevention and treatment of nausea and vomiting associated with surgery and anesthesia. Most of these drugs cause drowsiness as their major side effect.

Diagnostic measures related to evaluating the motility of the esophagus and the gastrointestinal tract include x-rays with single swallows of barium and observation of the swallowing mechanisms in different positions. These are used to detect both anatomic and motor abnormalities of the esophagus and the tract. A horizontal oblique position, for example, may be required to demonstrate hiatal hernia. A subjective test to determine acid reflux and esophagitis is the esophageal acid perfusion test, also known as the Bernstein test. After a 6- to 8-hour period of fasting and nonsmoking, a radiopaque nasogastric tube is inserted into the patient's stomach. The gastric contents are aspirated and the tube is withdrawn to the level near the junction of the upper and middle thirds of the esophagus as verified by fluoroscopy. The open end of the tube is then connected to test solutions located behind the patient so that he or she will not see when solutions are changed. (Otherwise the patient's reporting of different sensations may be influenced.) Initially, normal saline solution is administered by drip method and then a solution of hydrochloric acid is administered. The patient's descriptions of symptoms and their timing are recorded carefully. Extreme pain during the administration of the acid, which is run at specific rates for 5 minutes, warrants discontinuing the test. An antacid and water are given orally after the test. Relief of any symptoms and the timing of the relief are also recorded.

A motility test of the esophagus may be done to confirm the diagnosis of achalasia. After a 12-hour fast and a 12-hour abstinence from anticholinergic medication, narcotics, antacids, and smoking, thick barium is administered orally. The motility pattern of the esophagus is recorded by fluoroscopy. A prescribed dose of acetyl-β-methacholine chloride (Mecholyl) is administered and the motility is again recorded. Subjective responses of the patient to Mecholyl are also recorded to determine hypersensitivity of the esophagus to cholinergic stimulation. An exaggerated response to Mecholyl indicates that, at least in part, there is a loss of postganglionic neurons that normally innervate the smooth muscle of the esophagus. Normally the esophagus is so situated and constructed that it acts as a one-way channel to transport food. The cardiac sphincter resists reflux from the stomach at the cardiac orifice. Since the esophageal lining is not constructed to withstand frequent exposure to corrosive gastric juice, an effective gastroesophageal sphincter is essential. Constant irritation from the juice may lead to esophagitis, with constant heartburn. One of the most common causes of reflex esophagitis is a weakening of diaphragm muscles that normally retain the esophagus in its anatomic relation to the diaphragm and stomach. The esophageal hiatus, the opening in the diaphragm through which the esophagus passes, may widen and permit the abdominal esophagus and even the upper part of the stomach to prolapse through it into the thoracic cavity. This type of hiatus hernia is esophagogastric (diaphragmatic) hernia.

Hiatal hernia may be asymptomatic and is often incidentally diagnosed on x-ray. Symptoms are usually caused by the inappropriate motility and the regurgitation of acid gastric juices into the esophagus, resulting in heartburn, sensations of fullness, substernal discomfort, pain, dysphagia, and sensitivity to hot and cold foods. The symptoms often occur at night. Uncorrected esophagitis may eventually lead to fibrosis, resulting in esophageal stricture and interference with swallowing. Ulceration and hemorrhage may also occur from esophageal lesions.

The patient with hiatal hernia needs to take special precautions to reduce gastric regurgitation. Overeating tends to encourage regurgitation and pressure on the diaphragm. A bland diet of small frequent feedings is better tolerated. Belching, air swallowing, and a supine position after meals must be avoided. Bending over, heavy lifting, or wearing constricting garments increases intra-abdominal pressure. It is particularly important to stress to obese patients, who tend to wear tight girdles and undergarments, that these garments are not to be tight-fitting. Obese patients are also encouraged to reduce their weight. Sleeping with the head propped up or with the head of the bed elevated 6 inches rather than in a flat position will discourage regurgitation, which can also be prevented by eliminating bedtime snacks. Problems with gastric acidity and heartburn are usually treated with antacid medications. Anticholinergic drugs are contraindicated because they tend to delay gastric emptying and lower esophageal sphincter pressure. These effects aggravate symptoms.

If signs and symptoms continue despite conscientious medical regimens, or if complications occur, surgery to repair the hernia may be indicated. Surgical treatment may utilize one of two approaches to excise the sac, remove the hernia, and repair the site. The thoracic approach to repair the hernia is utilized if the hiatal hernia is the only lesion to be repaired, and if there is no cardiovascular disturbance present. The abdominal approach is utilized if there is a possibility of coexisting intra-abdominal disease that might also require surgical correction, or if cardiopulmonary disease is present. Postoperative care varies, depending on which approach is used. The prevention of respiratory complications by adequate deep breathing and coughing is a major focus of care in either approach. The high abdominal incision tends to cause the patient to take shallow breaths, so that he or she is as vulnerable to respiratory problems as when the thoracic approach is used. In the transthoracic approach the patient will have chest tubes requiring special nursing care measures. Nursing care related to thoracotomy is described on page 247.

Functional disorders of the gastrointestinal tract can occur in patients who have disorders such as duodenal ulcer, chronic ulcerative colitis, and cardiospasm, but functional disorders also can occur in the absence of any pathologic condition. Psychic influences are capable of altering intestinal functions, for example, by changes in secretion, vascularity, and tonicity. Functional disorders are often diagnosed in the presence of globus hystericus, functional vomiting, air-swallowing, constipation, and anorectal spasm. These symptoms may be indicative of pathologic states also, but in functional disorders there is generally a prolonged period of the symptoms without significant impairment of health. The symptoms are often related to an emotional or stressful event, or there is pain radiating to anatomically unrelated areas, which disappears at night. There may also be bizarre timing of the symptoms with no relation to causative factors, which rules out certain pathologic states. The patient with functional disturbances is likely to have vague symptoms such as nervousness, tension, headache, insomnia, palpitation, and other symptoms of emotional disorders. Even if there is no apparent physical basis for the symptoms, a thorough examination and diagnostic measures are indicated to rule out occult pathology. Functional symptoms, however, may be the only way some persons have for expressing a need for emotional and psychotherapeutic support.

Psychological, social, and somatic approaches are all used in the treatment of functional disorders. Dietary prescriptions and medications are also utilized. A diet adequate in proteins, calories, and vitamins is prescribed, with modification of the amount of roughage in the diet depending on the presence of diarrhea or constipation. Patients are encouraged to eat and drink slowly and moderately and to chew the food well. Excesses in hot or cold foods are avoided. Sedatives and tranquilizers are used to help the patient in coping with crises, and antispasmodic drugs are useful to control spasms of the tract. Management of underlying emotional problems may include psychotherapy when it is obvious that deep inner conflicts may be underlying the gastrointestinal problem.

Functional alterations of the digestive tract may result from hyperfunction or hypofunction. In **hyperfunction,** motor dysfunction occurs with hypertonicity, spasms at various points of the tract, hyperperistalsis and arrhythmia resulting in rapid gastric emptying and cardiospasm. Diarrhea, epigastric distress, pain, and dysphagia result. Gastric hypersecretion can occur with hyperacidity and regurgitation symptoms. At the level of the large intestine, hypersecretion of colonic mucus may cause excessive discharge of mucus as noted in neurogenic mucous colitis.

The **irritable bowel syndrome** (also called spastic colon) is a functional disorder that produces a group of symptoms including abdominal pain, flatulence, and constipation or diarrhea or both. Functional diarrhea is increased by stress; weight loss does not occur, however. The diagnosis is made by ruling out organic causes by various diagnostic tests. Although the syndrome does not involve structural changes, there is a potential for causing organic alterations. Symptoms of irritable colon are attributed to spastic and uncoordinated muscle contractions of the colon, usually related to emotional and dietary problems, such as ingestion of excessivly coarse or highly seasoned foods. Mild sedation and diphenoxylate hydrochloride (Lomotil) may be helpful. Diarrhea can also be caused by increased vagal stimulation with generalized hypermotility of the entire alimentary canal. The accelerated movement of contents through the intestine results in frequent or unformed stools.

Diarrhea may be associated with intrinsic disease such as infections, mechanical obstruction, obstructive neoplasms, ulcerative colitis, Crohn's disease, and malabsorption syndromes. The most common infectious agents associated with diarrhea are caused by salmonella, shigella, or staphylococcal organisms ingested with contaminated food or liquids. Lactase deficiency, food allergies, chemical irritants, antibiotics, and laxative abuse also cause diarrhea.

A long history of abdominal discomfort and recurrent attacks of diarrhea that are not relieved by diet or medication may indicate the presence of a carcinoid tumor. Hyperperistalsis is almost constantly present when this relatively rare tumor occurs. The tumor is usually located in the ileum, but may occur in other parts of the small bowel, colon, stomach, bronchus, or ovary [2]. It is usually a benign tumor, but some are malignant. Many carcinoid tumors secrete serotonin, which causes smooth muscle to contract and accounts for vasomotor disturbances, hyperperistalsis, and bronchoconstriction. Cutaneous flushing may occur several times a day, particularly in the face and neck. Treatment is generally medical with dietary and vitamin supplements; drugs to control serotonin synthesis are being investigated. Surgical excision of the tumor is rarely successful.

In observing the stools of patients with diarrhea, the nurse notes the color, odor, presence of foreign matter, consistency, frequency, and associated pain. When diarrhea continues, important nutrients, fluids, and electrolytes are lost, so that intervention is required to prevent dehydration by maintaining fluid and electrolyte balance. The cause of the diarrhea must be determined and corrected. Supportive therapy, including fluid and electrolyte replacement, antidiarrheal medications, and sedatives as well as rest and adequate nutrition are necessary. The diet prescribed eliminates iced fluids, carbonated drinks, whole milk, foods containing roughage, raw fruits, and highly seasoned foods. A bland diet, increased calories, and a high protein and high carbohydrate content are indicated. Drugs to decrease intestinal spasm and peristalsis are usually indicated; such drugs include camphorated tincture of opium (paregoric), diphenoxylate hydrochloride (Lomotil), and tincture of belladonna. Kaolin and pectin (Kaopectate), aluminum hydroxide gel (Amphojel), and bismuth subcarbonate may be used as adsorbents and to provide a protective mucosal coating. Antibiotics are indicated if diarrhea is of microbial origin.

Hypofunction may occur with muscle flaccidity and muscular relaxation so that esophageal stasis resulting in dysphagia, or gastric stasis resulting in anorexia, or epigastric fullness may occur. Functional achlorhydria may occur with gastric hyposecretion causing nausea and anorexia. In the colon, hypofunction is reflected by the onset of constipation.

Constipation is one of the most common problems in motility that the nurse encounters, whether practicing in the hospital, home situation, or clinic. **Constipation** is a term that is relative to the individual and must be clarified carefully by the nurse making the assessment. Some patients, for example, have a normal pattern of a bowel movement only two or three times a week without difficulty. Others state that they are constipated if they do not have a bowel movement every day. Prolonged retention of feces results in absorption of increased amounts of water, which accounts for the hard, dry consistency of the stools.

The hard fecal consistency causes difficulty and pain in passing the feces. Faulty elimination habits are generally considered one of the major causes of constipation. Occupational demands, carelessness, and neurotic delay in defecating may all hinder the response to the normal defecation reflex so that awareness of rectal fullness becomes dulled or disappears. A lack of adequate exercise and a sedentary occupation also are contributing factors. The loss of natural, normal bowel habits also occurs after chronic use of laxatives.

Lesions such as hemorrhoids and fissures make defecation painful and can also contribute to constipation. Medications such as narcotic analgesics, tranquilizers, anticholinergics, and bismuth compounds also are contributing factors. An atonic colon with weak musculature and inefficient peristalsis is a common cause of constipation in the aged or the chronically ill. When diets limited in bulk or fluid are ingested, peristaltic movement becomes sluggish because stimulation from normal distention is limited. Inadequate fluid intake also causes food residue to be hard, resulting in constipation.

Constipation can be controlled by appropriate intake of fibrous foods, to provide bulk in the large intestine and encourage evacuation. Raw fruits and vegetables, stewed prunes, dried fruits, and whole grain cereals are excellent sources of bulk. Regular exercise, adequate fluid intake, decreasing emotional tension, and the development of appropriate and regular schedules for defecation are important factors in preventing constipation.

When food and bowel hygiene are inadequate to establish defecation and proper bowel habits, laxative medications may be necessary. These drugs include several types of preparations such as stimulant cathartics, saline cathartics, lubricants and wetting agents, and bulk-forming laxatives. Stimulant cathartics increase motility by causing local irritation and include bisacodyl (Dulcolax), cascara and senna preparations, and castor oil. Castor oil is used primarily as a purgative and a bowel preparation for x-ray examinations and surgery. Saline cathartics, which cause contraction and movement by osmotic activity, include magnesium citrate, milk of magnesia, and sodium biphosphate with sodium phosphate (Phospho-Soda). Lubricating agents facilitate passage of the stool, and wetting agents soften the feces and lessen the strain of defecation. Mineral oil is a lubricant, and dioctyl calcium sulfosuccinate N.F. (Surfak) and dioctyl sodium sulfosuccinate (Colace) are commonly used wetting agents. Psyllium hydrophilic mucilloid (Metamucil) is a bulk-forming cathartic, which may also be classified as a stimulant cathartic.

The nurse should be familiar with the actions of these agents and should also discourage their long-term use by patients. The nurse must be responsible for noting when cathartics or purgatives are routinely used in x-ray preparations; these medications are contraindicated in the presence of intestinal obstruction.

Fecal impaction resulting from constipation usually has to be removed manually. Oil retention enemas are given to soften the stool. In elderly patients and those who are bedridden, observation of regularity of defecation as well as the size and consistency of feces is important to prevent fecal impaction. Stool softeners, increased fluid intake, dietary changes, and increased ambulation are indicated to promote intestinal function in these patients. Suppositories are an inefficient method of correcting fecal impaction.

Constipation in infants may be caused by **megacolon** or Hirschsprung's disease, the absence of parasympathetic nerve ganglia, particularly in the sigmoid colon, resulting in failure of peristalsis of the affected portion. Fecal content accumulates in the colon, adjacent to the affected portion, which is constricted and which does not participate in propulsion of the intestinal contents. Obstruction necessitates surgical resection of the aganglionic segments, usually in two stages. A temporary colostomy is the usual procedure prior to the subsequent resection and reanastomosis. Mild cases may be treated with enemas and laxatives, and surgery is postponed.

Peristalsis may be inhibited by **paralytic (adynamic) ileus,** the disturbed autonomic innervation of the intestine, resulting in neurogenic obstruction. Although the lumen of the bowel is patent, an obstruction occurs because the intestinal contents cannot be propelled forward. Distention of the inactive intestine on adjacent vessels may also result in impaired circulation to the tract. Impaired circulation may result from occlusion of the arterial blood supply to the bowel, which is normally supplied by the celiac and the superior and inferior mesenteric arteries. Any occlusion of the arterial blood supply will inhibit bowel function and result in gangrene of the bowel unless surgical intervention is accomplished. Acute mesenteric thrombosis is a surgical emergency. The ischemic tissue causes intense and diffuse abdominal pain and later fever, absence of bowel sounds, leukocytosis, and shock. A high mortality rate occurs unless surgery is done immediately to restore circulation. Necrotic segments of the bowel are resected and reconstruction of involved vessels is accomplished.

Partial occlusion due to atherosclerosis of the mesenteric arteries causes symptoms when the blood supply is increasingly interrupted and bowel function is decreased. The condition is often called abdominal angina. Pain after eating is the major symptom associated with the disease. Vascular or bypass grafts may be done to improve circulation to the affected portion of the bowel.

Paralytic ileus may develop in the presence of peritonitis, pancreatitis, severe toxemia, spinal cord lesions, or electrolyte imbalance (especially hypokalemia), or following administration of anticholinergic drugs or ganglionic-blocking agents. Extensive abdominal surgery with excessive trauma to the intestine may also be a contributing factor. The intestine and stomach become distended by gas and fluids, so that abdominal distention is the major significant finding in paralytic ileus. Absence of bowel sounds is further confirmation of the diagnosis; no peristalsis is seen, heard, or felt. Intestinal contents may be vomited or will be aspirated when a nasogastric tube is inserted. X-rays of the abdomen show air and fluid in distended loops of both the large and the small bowel. At first the distended bowel loops and the stretched abdominal wall cause pain, but the pain is steady in contrast to the sharp intermittent pain of mechanical obstruction.

Treatment consists in bed rest, intravenous fluid and electrolyte replacement, and the use of gastric intubation or intestinal intubation to aspirate secretions until the bowel begins to function. Physicians vary in their practice of pharmacologically stimulating the bowel by prescribing parasympathomimetic drugs. Prostigmine administered intramuscularly is recommended by some physicians while vasopressin (Pitressin) is recommended by others. Bethanechol chloride (Urecholine) may be prescribed in adynamic ileus when recent traumatic surgery is not the cause of the ileus and when the ileus is the result of a lack of acetylcholine. Urecholine, a potent cholinergic agent, is injected subcutaneously or given orally but cannot be given intravenously or intramuscularly. Many authorities recommend that no drug stimulation be utilized for paralytic ileus; they feel that if the primary disorder is reversible, paralytic ileus will be temporary and will generally be resolved through supportive therapy.

PROBLEMS OF ABSORPTION

The small intestine is the site of the major absorptive functions of the gastrointestinal tract and is affected in a variety of conditions that include organic causes and functional disorders.

Most absorption results from the churning action of the small intestine, which continually exposes the chyme to the mucosa, the circular folds of the mucosal surface which increase surface area; and the villi, which are small, thread-like mucosal projections from the intestinal wall. Each villus has a network of small capillaries and a central lymph channel through which nutrients are absorbed and carried into the systemic circulation. Absorption occurs by active transport and by diffusion. Adequate absorption depends on sufficient healthy tissue in the small intestine to allow sufficient surface contact and also depends on an appropriate length of time for surface contact. Therefore any loss of healthy tissue (such as occurs in ulcerative colitis, regional enteritis, ileostomy with the loss of some of the terminal ileum), inadequate preparation of the chyme in the absence of essential secretions and enzymes, or diarrhea when rapid movement through the small intestine prevents adequate absorption can lead to malabsorption.

As the chyme enters the small intestine, it is mixed and churned by sharp contractions of the circular muscle of the intestinal wall. Secretions from the liver, the pancreas, and the intestinal mucosa mix with the chyme to break it down into substances to complete the digestive processing so that nutrients can be absorbed into the blood. These secretions include bile (containing bile salts, cholesterol, and lecithin) secreted by the liver, which alkalinizes intestinal contents and emulsifies and absorbs fats. Pancreatic juices, containing bicarbonate and chloride, are rich in enzymes. The three major pancreatic enzymes are: **trypsin,** which breaks down proteins; **amylase,** which converts starch into sugar; and **lipase,** which splits fats into fatty acids and glycerol. Disease states of the liver, pancreas, and the biliary tract, therefore, interfere with the digestion and absorption of nutrients. Problems associated with disease of the biliary tract are discussed in a later section of this chapter (page 602).

Intestinal juice, secreted by the mucosa of the intestine, contains inorganic salts and mucin and some enzymes, mainly enterokinase and intestinal amylase. Enterokinase converts pancreatic trypsinogen to trypsin.

Absorption is the final step in obtaining sugars, fatty acids, amino acids, vitamins, minerals, and water and electrolytes to supply the body. Absorption of fluid and electrolytes occurs primarily in the small intestine, but some active absorption of sodium and water occurs in the proximal half of the colon. The fat-soluble vitamins A, D, E, and K are absorbed from the small intestine if bile salts are present. The water-soluble vitamins B complex (except for vitamin B_{12}, which depends on the intrinsic factor secreted by the stomach mucosa) and C generally are readily absorbed from the small intestine.

As described previously the small intestine, especially in the duodenum, can be the site of ulcer formation. When the small intestine is ulcerated and destroyed, absorption problems occur as the amount of healthy tissue is decreased. **Regional enteritis,** also known as Crohn's disease, transmural colitis, or granulomatous colitis, is a chronic disease of unknown origin. It results in inflammation, fibrosis, scarring, and ulceration of all layers (transmural) of the tract. Though it tends to involve primarily the terminal ileum, the disease process can affect any part of the bowel, including the colon. In some patients, the disease may involve the colon without any changes in the small intestine. It most often affects persons in the 15 to 30 age group. Absorption of toxins, and psychosomatic, autoimmune, and other factors have been implicated but not proved as causative factors.

As the name regional enteritis implies, only one segment of the bowel may be involved, or segments of healthy tissue may alternate with multiple segments of diseased tissue. Patients complain of intermittent attacks of cramping, pain in the mid or right abdominal area after eating, diarrhea ranging from three to ten stools per day, anorexia, fatigue, fever, and weight loss. Diarrhea rarely contains mucus, pus, or gross blood. Often, an initial observable lesion is a perianal fistula, often preceding other overt symptoms. There can be periods of exacerbations and remissions; symptoms vary depending on the location of the lesions in the tract. Malabsorption, however, is the major problem when the small bowel is involved. Megaloblastic anemia results from decreased absorption of vitamin B_{12}. Fluid and electrolyte disturbances with acid base imbalances can occur particularly with a depletion of sodium or potassium associated with diarrhea or with excessive small bowel drainage through fistulas that may be associated with the pathologic process. Diagnosis is confirmed by x-ray.

A nutritious low fiber diet, careful use of anticholinergic drugs and sedatives, and bed rest during exacerbations are symptomatic treatment measures. Sulfasalazine (Azulfidine), adrenocorticotropic hormone, and other corticosteroids are often used to control symptoms and prevent further pathologic changes. Complications of inflammation with fibrous scarring, obstruction, fistula formation in the small bowel, abscesses, or perforation are indications for surgical excision and anastomosis. Extensive colon involvement requires ileorectal anastomosis or ileostomy. Bypass procedures are sometimes done in colonic disease, followed by restorative surgery after healing of the bowel has taken place. Recurrence of Crohn's disease is frequent. Particular problems with inadequate vitamin B_{12} absorption result when the terminal ileum is resected; lifelong replacement of vitamin B_{12} is then necessary.

The **malabsorption syndrome** includes a group of disorders resulting in various forms of intestinal malabsorption of fats, proteins, carbohydrates, water, electrolytes, and fat-soluble vitamins. **Celiac disease,** also known as celiac sprue, occurs in juveniles or adults. It is considered a hereditary disorder with genetic transmission of a metabolic defect. The disease causes a characteristic lesion of the small intestine: flattened, distorted, or absent villi. Since the intestinal villus is the functional unit of the small bowel, there is a marked decrease in the absorptive function of the small intestine. Sensitivity to the ingestion of gluten (a fraction of wheat protein) is the basic malabsorption problem. Elimination of foods containing gluten, such as wheat, rye, barley, and oats, often improves the condition. Nursing care is supportive and centers on education of the patient regarding dietary restrictions and improved nutrition. The patient must be warned to avoid foods that may not obviously contain gluten, but contain additives that may include it, as in some brands of frozen foods, frankfurters, instant tea, coffee, gum, and candy. The patient should therefore learn to *check all food labels* carefully; commercially prepared gluten free foods are available. **Tropical sprue,** in contrast to celiac sprue, is of unknown etiology, though it is considered an infectious process and is related to nutritional deficiencies.

Symptoms of chronic malabsorption are anorexia, weight loss, weakness, diarrhea, muscle wasting, dehydration, and states of malnutrition. Variations in symptoms occur when different nutrients are particularly involved. Steatorrhea, the excessive loss of fat in the stool, affects the consistency of evacuation and is associated with a foul odor of the stool, which is bulky and pale. Impaired fat absorption also results in the loss of the fat-soluble vitamins A, D, E, and K. Vitamin K malabsorption can cause bleeding tendencies while muscle weakness and wasting are associated with vitamin E deficiencies. Hypocalcemia with neuromuscular symptoms of tetany occurs in vitamin D malabsorption and deficiency. Magnesium deficiencies and hypocalcemia may occur, since calcium and magnesium are primarily absorbed in the proximal section of the small bowel. Neuromuscular symptoms with neuritis and neuropathy, macrocytic anemia, glossitis, and stomatitis, are associated with vitamin B deficiencies.

The malabsorption of proteins can result in edema, hypotension, muscle wasting, and infections due to decreased levels of albumin, immunoglobulin, and gamma globulin (hypoproteinemia). Abdominal distention, acid, frothy stools, and excessive flatulence are present when there is an inability to digest carbohydrates. Inadequate digestion of carbohydrates promotes abnormal bacterial growth in the distal ileum and colon, resulting in infections.

Examination of the stool is indicated when malabsorption is suspected. A modified Schilling test to differentiate intestinal malabsorption of vitamin B_{12} from pernicious anemia is indicated. Xylose tolerance tests can demonstrate defects in intestinal malabsorption, since xylose is a substance that does not require digestion prior to absorption. Small bowel x-ray examinations and biopsy are also utilized for differentiating malabsorption problems. In small bowel biopsies, a weighted biopsy tube is inserted through the mouth to obtain specimens from the distal duodenum or proximal jejunum.

The **nursing care** of patients with malabsorption syndromes is centered on improvement of the nutritional state through the provision of an appropriate and nutritious diet, fluid and electrolyte management, and restriction of offending substances. Instruction in dietary management and explanations of replacement therapy must be thorough in order to obtain the patient's full cooperation in preventing continual problems. Therapy may include replacement of vitamins, minerals, human serum, albumin, or gamma globulin. The administration of some of these substances can be extremely painful when frequently administered parenterally, and the nurse is presented with the challenge of preventing discouragement and impatience with the therapy. Dietary changes, though necessitating the avoidance of either fats or carbohydrates, must still provide for adequate caloric intake, which presents a challenge to the nurse or the nutritionist who has to instruct the patient in dietary management.

Malabsorption problems also occur in **Peutz-Jeghers syndrome,** an inherited disease that results in multiple polyps of the small bowel primarily and in the colon. The gastrointestinal lesions are often found after other characteristic lesions, such as melanin spots of the mouth, lips, and fingers, are noted. (Increased pigment appears as round, oval, or irregular patches.) Bleeding, obstruction, and intussusception may occur as the result of these polyps. Surgical excision of the polyps is indicated. The surgical procedure decreases the length of the small intestine and thus can cause potential nutritional deficiencies unless nutritional intake is appropriate and sufficient. In contrast to other forms of polyposis, polyps in this disease rarely terminate in cancer. **Whipple's disease** is a disorder of the jejunum resulting in malabsorption. Progressive stages of the disease are dominated by effects of malabsorption. Intensive antibiotic therapy is used for this condition, which is bacterial in origin.

Other problems in malabsorption can occur in relation to other diseases, or in surgical procedures that affect absorption. For example, the patient with a recent ileostomy is particularly vulnerable to fluid and electrolyte imbalance, due to the resection of the proximal colon, where water and sodium are normally absorbed. Until the body adapts to the loss of this function, the patient is in danger of excess loss of water and sodium. **Fistulas,** abnormal tracts from one organ to another or to the external abdomen, may occur in the small intestine. Excessive drainage through the fistulas with loss of fluids, electrolytes, and nutrients may result in fluid and electrolyte imbalance and in malnutrition.

The nurse who is aware of the absorptive functions of various parts of the gastrointestinal tract will therefore be alert for potential problems that can also occur in patients with conditions not specifically identified as being malabsorptive. He or she will be observant in noting inadequate nutritional intake or excessive loss of nutrients, fluids, and electrolytes and will seek alternative methods of providing nutrition.

INTERFERENCE WITH PATENCY OF THE GASTROINTESTINAL TRACT

The patency of the gastrointestinal tract can be obstructed at any point in the tract. Adequate intake will be prevented by obstructive lesions of the mouth, esophagus, stomach, and small intestine. Elimination functions are prohibited by obstruction in the small and large intestines as well as the rectum and anus. Obstruction anywhere in the tract, however, eventually affects all parts of the digestive system.

Obstruction of any one of the three salivary glands may result from infection, neoplasms, or calculi. Inflammatory lesions may occlude the salivary ducts by swelling and edema, as well as by scar tissue. Swelling of the affected gland results when salivary stimulation increases, particularly during meals. Antibiotic therapy and dilation of the duct may be necessary.

The parotid gland is the most frequent site of salivary tumors, which are firm, fixed, and often involve the facial nerve. Surgical treatment of malignant tumors of the parotid glands may also require removal of the mandible and cervical lymph nodes if metastasis has occurred. The patient then has problems associated with disfigurement and fears associated with this surgery, as previously described for the Commando procedure (page 542). In addition, the proximity of the parotid gland to the facial nerve endangers facial nerve functioning after parotid surgery. Permanent facial paralysis may result, depending on the extent of the tumor and surgical damage to the nerve.

Cancer of the esophagus, which obstructs the lumen, results in dysphagia, anorexia, and eventually vomiting, weight loss, and dehydration due to inadequate intake. The vomitus typically consists of recently chewed particles. Pain, described as a "gnawing" retrosternal sensation, is a later symptom. Smoking and excessive ingestion of alcohol have been related to the development of cancer of the esophagus, which occurs predominantly in men over the age of 50. Verification of an obstructive tumor necessitates surgical resection with anastomosis, if possible. If the tumor is too extensive for resection, a gastrostomy is performed to bypass the obstruction and provide for nutritional intake. Intake and output recording, adequate nutritional intake via tube feedings, and oral hygiene are major aspects of care. Prognosis is poor due to early lymphatic spread; overt symptoms usually occur after the tumor has grown extensively. Cancer of the esophagus may erode into the trachea or bronchus and form a tracheoesophageal or bronchoesophageal fistula.

Obstruction of the esophagus can also result from the swallowing of caustic substances that cause inflammatory changes or ulcerations. Lye ingestion, for example, sometimes a method of attempt at suicide, causes severe ulcerations. Strictures result from scarring caused by the inflammatory process and may interfere with the patency of the tract by occluding the lumen.

Periodic dilations of the esophagus with bougie tubes may be attempted; if these dilations are unsuccessful in maintaining patency, surgical intervention is necessary.

When an extensive lesion of the esophagus is present, an anastomosis may not be possible after resection of the traumatized tissue. Additional tissue from another source is obtained. The colon, provided it is prepared as aseptically as possible, is often the source of needed tissue for transplantation to the esophagus. Prolonged restriction of oral intake is necessary to ensure healing for an intact anastomosis. A gastrostomy is initially done to provide adequate nutritional intake until resection and anastomosis are accomplished. If the lesion is nonresectable, a permanent gastrostomy is performed. In this situation a stomach flap may be formed around the gastrostomy tube to stabilize it.

The lumen of the esophagus may also be obstructed by an esophageal diverticulum, causing dysphagia and a sensation of a foreign body in the throat. Malnutrition and perforation of the diverticulum with contamination of the mediastinum are potential complications. A bland, nonirritating diet is indicated, or in some cases a gastrostomy, until surgical repair of the diverticulum is accomplished. In some patients, esophageal diverticuli are asymptomatic and nondetectable, only discovered during diagnostic testing for other conditions.

When cancerous lesions of the esophagus are extensive, fistulas may form a channel to the neck with problems of constant drainage. Fistulas in this location result in skin irritations from the secretions; protective skin barriers are indicated. When fistulas occur anywhere along the gastrointestinal tract, total parenteral nutrition is usually indicated to prevent malnutrition and electrolyte imbalance, and to promote healing by putting the tract at rest.

To remove strictures of the lower esophagus or tumors of the distal esophagus, a partial esophagectomy and intrathoracic esophagogastrostomy is done. The surgery requires a thoracotomy to resect the diseased esophagus and to anastomose the severed end of the esophagus to the stump of the remaining stomach after the cardia is resected.

Esophagomyotomy may be indicated to correct esophageal obstruction due to cardiospasm. In this procedure an incision is made through the muscular wall of the distal esophagus and proximal stomach to relieve the stricture. A similar technique, pyloromyotomy, is utilized when the pylorus is obstructed due to hypertrophied stenosis of the pyloric sphincter.

A malignant tumor may be the cause of an obstruction in the stomach. This condition has been discussed in the section on ulcers; surgical intervention is similar to that for ulcers. A gastrostomy or jejunostomy may be indicated when gastric lesions are nonresectable, in order to provide a means for long-term nutrition. A total gastrectomy is done to remove a malignant lesion of the stomach with metastases in the adjacent lymph nodes, and continuity of the tract is then established by anastomosis of the jejunum to the esophagus. Postoperative management requires diligent monitoring of fluid intake and output, maintenance of suction to prevent accumulation of fluid and drainage at the suture line, and gradual and careful adjustment of oral intake once intestinal function is restored. Replacement of vitamin B_{12} is necessary; hydrochloric acid may also be required, due to the absence of normal gastric juices.

Pyloric obstruction is yet another type of obstruction of the upper gastrointestinal tract. It may be caused by a congenital lesion requiring corrective surgery in the neonatal period, or it may be associated with scar tissue formation from healing of ulcerations in the adult patient. Pyloric obstruction is corrected by either pyloroplasty or by resection of the involved segment with anastomosis.

A variety of diseases can cause an obstruction in the small bowel and lower gastrointestinal tract. The obstruction may be a mechanical one that interferes with the normal flow of intestinal contents, or it may be a disturbance of the autonomic nervous system resulting in paralytic ileus, as described previously. Mechanical obstruction may be due to extrinsic causes such as adhesions or hernia, or to intrinsic causes such as neoplasms, hematomas, volvulus, intussusception, and strictures, as well as foreign bodies, fecal impaction, diverticulosis, and polyps. Rectal bleeding, changes in bowel patterns, and abdominal pain warrant investigation. In the absence of diarrhea, bright red blood that is not mixed with the fecal mass usually has originated from the anal area or from the colon distal to the splenic flexure. The blood is usually noted at the beginning of the stool, on the toilet tissue or in the toilet bowl. When no cause is found in the anus (e.g., hemorrhoids), the cause is usually a polyp or a malignant neoplasm in the rectum or sigmoid. Even in the presence of anal disease, a digital examination, x-rays, and sigmoidoscopy are indicated when rectal bleeding occurs to ensure that another lesion is not also present. Too often bright red blood from the rectum has been attributed to benign conditions such as hemorrhoids or fissures and patients have delayed seeking proper treatment only to discover that a malignancy was present and is now too advanced for curative treatment to be possible. In obstructive lesions, diarrhea may alternate with constipation. As the lumen of the bowel is decreased with enlargement of the tumor, liquid feces are moved past the site of obstruction and evacuated. Increased obstruction causes pain, obstipation, and eventually vomiting and weight loss.

When the obstruction occurs to a point that fluids and air collect proximal to the site, there is a temporary initial increase in peristaltic activity as the intestine attempts to force the material past the obstructed area. Depending on the level of obstruction, the intensity, persistence, and onset of vomiting vary. When the obstruction is mechanical, bowel sounds initially are typically active and high-pitched, usually come in rushes, and are accentuated during attacks of colic. This is in contrast to the absence of bowel sounds when the obstruction is due to paralytic ileus. When mechanical obstruction causes ischemia or peritonitis, however, bowel sounds diminish and disappear.

Within a few hours, increased peristalsis stops and the bowel becomes flaccid. Increased pressure within the bowel causes a decrease in absorption, so that fluid retention is increased. Intraluminal pressure rises, leading to the compression of the bowel wall and its capillaries; necrosis of the bowel wall results. If the obstruction occurs in the proximal small bowel, vomiting is likely to occur with severe loss of water and electrolytes and acid-base disturbances. Vomitus initially consists of gastric contents, then of bile and, finally, becomes feculent. Even if there is no vomiting but there is distention, fluid and electrolyte imbalance is a danger. Abdominal distention occurs early in lower bowel obstruction and results in diminished absorptive capacity. Fluids in the distended bowel are thus not available for use.

Symptoms that suggest an acute obstruction include acute abdominal pain, cramps, vomiting, and distention. The nurse should check for a history of gradually increasing constipation, sometimes alternating with diarrhea and a history of a hernia in the groin area, or of abdominal surgery (which might have caused adhesions), or of melena.

Abdominal tenderness is mild or moderate in early mechanical obstruction unless a strangulated hernia is the cause, a perforation with peritonitis has already occurred, or there is an infarction of the intestinal wall.

Laboratory examinations of blood counts for leukocytosis, serum electrolytes, hemoglobin and hematocrit values, and amylase levels are particularly essential for differential diagnosis. Immediate initiation of accurate intake and output measurements is necessary to determine appropriate fluid and electrolyte replacement.

Treatment requires intubation and fluid

and electrolyte replacement. Decompression of the gastrointestinal tract is necessary to eliminate some of the gas and fluid shadows that may prevent accurate subsequent x-rays. If the cause of the obstruction is not obvious and emergency surgery is not immediately indicated, x-rays are taken to determine the obstruction site by noting distribution of gas and fluid levels in the bowel, abdominal masses, and intraperitoneal gas. There is controversy about the use of a barium enema in suspected colon obstructions due to the danger of perforation, but the technique is used with suitable precautionary measures by some physicians.

In small bowel obstruction, gastric or intestinal intubation may relieve the symptoms caused by recurrent obstruction due to adhesions, so that surgery will not be necessary. When food is initiated after the intubation is discontinued, patients must be encouraged to eat slowly, take adequate fluids, and chew the food thoroughly to avoid recurrence of the symptoms.

Appropriate fluid and electrolyte replacement requires careful measurement of water and electrolyte loss through accurate intake and output records and monitoring of serum electrolyte levels. Table 7-1 indicates that with gastric suction an excessive loss of H^+ ions can lead to alkalosis and that with intestinal suction there is danger of acidosis due to loss of HCO_3^-. Antibiotic therapy is indicated when strangulation or perforation is suspected or in the presence of inflammatory processes associated with obstruction.

Emergency surgery is required for hernial strangulation or perforation, or when the undiagnosed obstruction does not improve with supportive therapy. Depending on the cause, the surgical procedure varies from a release of adhesions to a resection of diseased bowel or a preliminary colostomy in acute colonic obstruction.

Postoperatively, intubation is continued until bowel function returns and fluid and electrolyte imbalance is prevented by accurate monitoring and replacement. The patient is closely observed for abdominal distention and the prolonged absence of bowel sounds, since there is a tendency for paralytic ileus to develop after inflammatory processes or extensive surgery of the bowel.

The lumen of the gastrointestinal tract can also be altered by the presence of **polyps,** mucosal growths that protrude into the lumen of the colon and rectum. Polyps may occur singly or in multiple locations along the lower gastrointestinal tract. While many polyps are asymptomatic, some may cause rectal bleeding. There is controversy as to how aggressively polyps should be treated. However, polyps over 1 cm in size are generally resected because polyps of this size are more commonly malignant. Polyps are either sessile or pedunculated. **Sessile** polyps are flattened protrusions, whereas **pedunculated** polyps have a stalk and can be villous or adenomatous. **Villous** polyps generally have a soft velvety appearance and may be palpated on digital examination in some instances. Rhoads [21a] estimates that in villous adenoma, the incidence of carcinoma is 40 to 50 percent and it is therefore considered a premalignant lesion. Proctoscopic examinations, barium x-rays, and colonoscopy are helpful in detecting polyps. Polyps are biopsied and excised.

Patients with multiple polyps are more likely to develop cancer. **Familial multipolyposis,** for example, is a pathologic condition in which large numbers of adenomatous neoplasms arise from the epithelial mucosa of the colon. The condition is a hereditary disorder and produces cancer of the colon with predictable regularity, so that surgical resection and anastomosis or ileostomy are indicated in the early stages. Often the rectum can be retained and an ileorectal anastomosis may be possible.

Another disorder characterized by multipolyposis of the colon and rectum with potential for malignancy is **Gardner's syndrome,** a dominantly transmitted hereditary disease. Signs such as cutaneous cystic lesions, fibrous tissue tumors, osteomas, and dental anomalies are associated with the disease and are often the reason for seeking medical assistance. When these overt signs occur in any number or over a period of time, a sigmoidoscopy is indicated to detect the asymptomatic polyps. Surgical resection of the polyps is indicated because the malignancy potential is great. If the polyps are extensive, a total colectomy with ileostomy or a subtotal colectomy with an ileorectal anastomosis is performed. The **Peutz-Jeghers syndrome,** as previously discussed, is a hereditary disease that consists in polyps in the small intestine, particularly the jejunum, but occasionally in the stomach and large intestine. Melanin spots on the lips, fingers, and toes are characteristic cutaneous lesions associated with the condition, even before the polyps become symptomatic. Surgical treatment consists in resection of the involved segments of the bowel.

Adhesions, bands of fibrous scar tissue formed by peritoneal tissue after an inflammatory process or after surgical trauma, cause kinking and constriction of the intestine. Adhesions are the most common cause of obstruction of the small bowel in adults and are usually a result of previous operations. Surgical release of the adhesions or resection of diseased sections of the bowel are the types of intervention indicated.

Volvulus causes obstruction when the bowel becomes twisted upon itself and thus prevents normal forward movement of intestinal contents. Volvulus may occur in either the small or large intestine. **Intussusception** occurs mainly in infants and children. A segment of intestine is invaginated into a segment immediately below, causing compression and decreasing the blood supply of the attached mesentery. An **incarcerated hernia** with strangulation and interference with the blood supply is another cause of intestinal obstruction, necessitating emergency surgical intervention. Hernias and complications are discussed on page 580.

Patency of the gastrointestinal tract can be obstructed by **diverticulosis,** which may occur in the esophagus, but more commonly in the lower gastrointestinal tract. The outpouching of the intestinal wall is due to weakness of the muscular layers of the intestine and generally occurs in middle-aged or elderly persons. Diverticulosis may be asymptomatic until **diverticulitis** occurs. Diverticulitis can occur as the sacs fill with feces, causing obstruction and inflammation with danger of perforation. Symptoms include left lower quadrant pain, low back pain, changes in bowel habits, and blood in the stool. Surgery is often indicated before rupture occurs to prevent perforation and peritonitis. Perforations, fistulas, obstruction, and hemorrhage require surgical treatment. A temporary colostomy may be necessary to allow the distal inflammatory lesion to subside or to allow healing if a distal resection and anastomosis are accomplished. Medical management is primarily dietary, but there is controversy over the type of diet to be recommended. Some physicians feel it is necessary to use refined, low roughage foods to avoid irritation; others feel that a fibrous diet is indicated to avoid feces collecting in the pouches and causing inflammation.

When surgery requiring the bowel to be opened is anticipated, the patient requires particular preparation of the bowel to suppress microflora of the colon. A low fiber diet is prescribed for 2 or 3 days preoperatively to reduce the fecal contents. A liquid diet is usually ordered for the day before surgery and intravenous fluid therapy may be initiated at this time. Mechanical and chemical cleaning of the bowel are utilized to provide as clean and bacteria-free a bowel as possible. Purgatives and enemas are given at prescribed intervals until returns are clear. Antibiotics are administered orally or parenterally, or may be instilled per rectum or via a colostomy if it is present. Typically, surgical antibacterial preparation has included neomycin sulfate tablets at prescribed intervals for 1 to 2 days preoperatively or kanamycin sulfate and tetracycline or phthalylsulfathiazole (Sulfathalidine) for 2 or 3 days preoperatively. In some settings, neomycin and erythromycin base are given during the 24 hours prior to surgery to temporarily suppress anaerobic as well as aerobic organisms [17, 18]. (Anaerobic organisms are prevalent in the colon.)

Antibiotic administration and mechanical cleaning of the bowel affect the normal flow of the bowel and subsequently the absorption of certain fat-soluble vitamins. Parenteral vitamin K, for example, may be required due to interference with synthesis of the vitamin. The intensive procedures for bowel preparation may exhaust and dehydrate the patient, so that observations of fluid and electrolyte balance are essential.

Depending on the location and the type of pathologic condition found at surgery, several approaches may be utilized to control the disease process. If the pathology is localized, surgical resection with anastomosis is done. Postoperatively, healing of the anastomosis is assured by limiting bowel activity with fluid restriction and gastric or intestinal intubation.

The resection may be extensive, as in a right hemicolectomy and ileocolostomy. In this procedure the right half of the colon, including a portion of the transverse colon, ascending colon, and cecum and a segment of the terminal ileum and mesentery are resected. An anastomosis is then accomplished between the ileum and transverse colon. This procedure is usually done to remove a malignancy of the right colon or an extensive inflammatory lesion of the ileum, cecum, or ascending colon.

Cancer of the large bowel is generally classified by the Duke's system, according to the depth of anatomic involvement and the presence of nodal and distant metastases. Treatment of cancer of the colon is resection of the tumor and affected adjacent tissue and lymph nodes. If a resection and anastomosis cannot be performed, decompression of the colon, diversion of the fecal stream, and creation of an artificial anus are accomplished with a colostomy. There are several different types of colostomies, depending on the location and purpose, and whether the stoma is to be temporary or permanent (Fig. 7-7). Appliances used to collect fecal drainage vary according to the type of colostomy performed.

A **cecostomy** in the lower right abdomen is done when obstructing lesions of the right colon cannot be safely resected or bypassed. A rubber drainage tube is inserted in the stoma and is connected to either gravity or suction drainage, usually as a temporary diversionary procedure. If the drainage tube is not inserted, a drainable appliance is worn continually to collect drainage that is similar to that in ileostomy surgery.

An **ascending colostomy** is the least common type. It is usually temporary and is done in the presence of distal inflammatory or neoplastic disease. The stoma is located usually on the right lower quadrant of the abdomen and discharges liquid or unformed stool.

A **transverse colostomy,** of a double barrel or loop type, is usually done in acute obstruction to divert the fecal stream from a distal diseased segment that may be a potential or real perforation or from a distal surgical resection and anastomosis. A transverse loop colostomy can be carried out quickly and with minimal operative manipulation when the patient's condition warrants emergency decompression and diversion. A glass rod or plastic bridge is placed underneath the exteriorized intestine to immobilize and support the bowel and to prevent the bowel from returning to the peritoneal cavity. The glass rod is kept from slipping out by a short length of latex tubing connected to each end. The plastic bridge may or may not be sutured to the skin. Another means of supporting the bowel is the Cambridge loop colostomy, in which a subcutaneous rod segment is surgically secured [24]. The exteriorized bowel looks like one stoma, but when opened by cautery or scalpel there are actually two openings, a proximal loop and a distal loop. The bowel is usually opened by cautery 24 to 36 hours postoperatively and the glass rod (or other support) is usually maintained 5 to 8 days. The loop colostomy may be the first of either a two- or three-stage procedure to treat diverticulitis or cancer, the two most common obstructive diseases of the left colon. In the two-stage procedure, a subsequent distal resection and closure of the colostomy are accomplished in the second surgery. In the three-stage procedure, the distal resection is done in the second surgery and then closure of the colostomy is done after the anastomosis has healed.

A modification of a loop colostomy is the **Mikulicz procedure.** Although it currently is not used as often as in the past, it is still used by some surgeons in emergency situations. In this operation, a loop of bowel is delivered through the abdominal wound and a spur is formed after the bowel is resected. A crushing clamp is gradually applied to the spur several days later until the spur is broken down. Permanent closure and reestablished continuity are accomplished once the spur has been broken and the patient can tolerate the surgery.

A **double barrel colostomy** has two stomas, which may or may not be separated by skin; therefore no rod is required for this surgery. The proximal loop will discharge feces and the distal loop will discharge mucus. The diseased portion of the bowel is resected and the two ends are brought through the abdominal wall for a temporary diversion. The closure of the colostomy is usually accomplished within 6 months.

A **descending** or **sigmoid colostomy,** also called an end colostomy, is usually a permanent colostomy done when an abdominal perineal resection of the rectum is required. It is done to treat cancer of the sigmoid colon or rectum and in traumatic injury to the rectum or anal sphincter or in certain central nervous system diseases.

In **abdominal perineal resection,** the end of

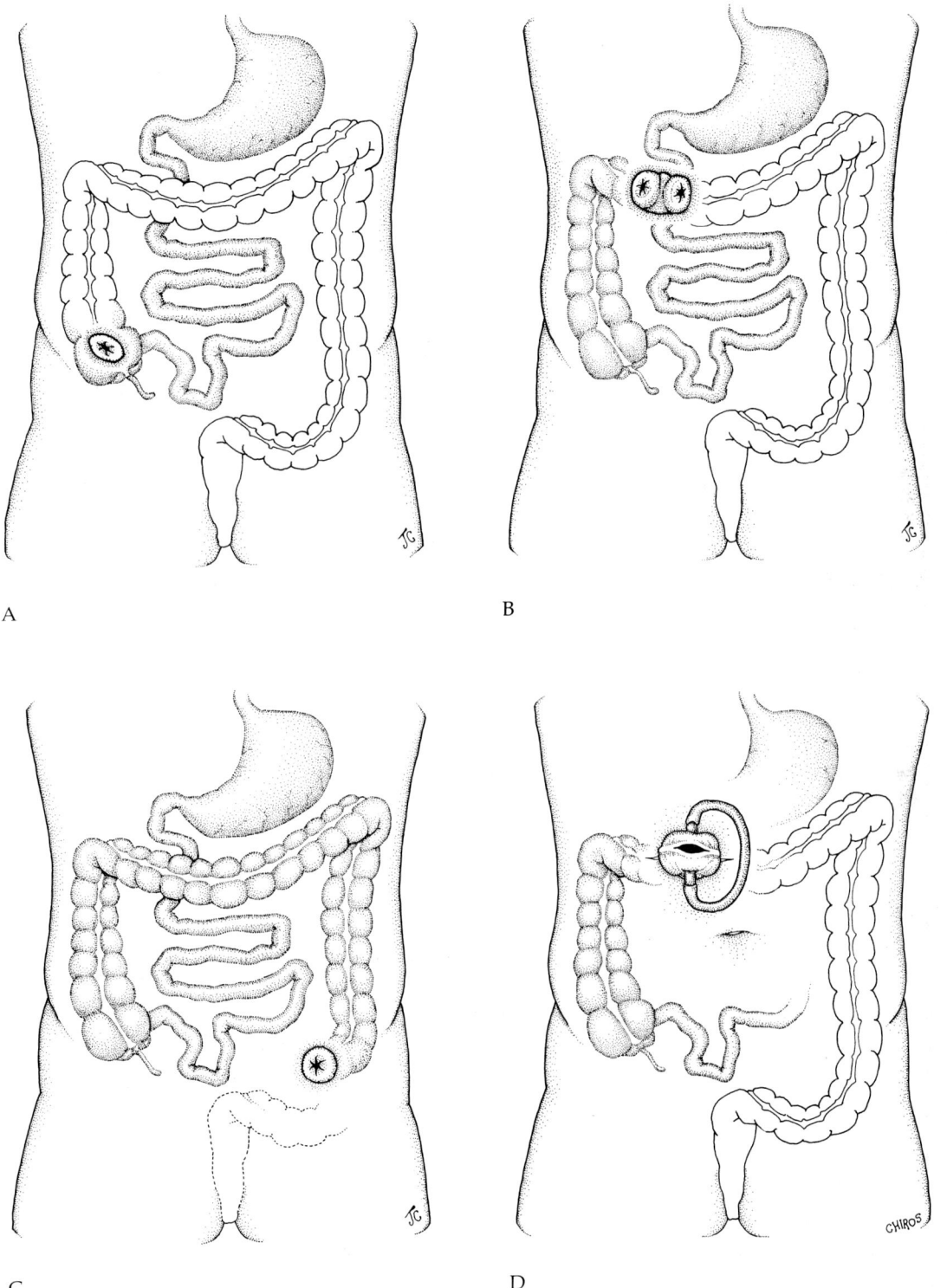

Figure 7-7
Types of colostomy procedures: ascending (A), double barrel (B), descending (C), and loop (D).

the remaining bowel is brought out as a stoma and the distal end is removed through the hollow of the sacrum with a wide resection of the perineum that is either closed primarily or is permitted to heal by secondary closure. Care of the perineal wound varies, depending on the type of closure performed.

The perineal wound, through which the anus, rectum, and lower colon are removed, creates a hollow space that eventually fills in with serum, plasma, and fibroblasts. The wound may be allowed to heal by either primary or secondary intention.

The perineal wound may be sutured at surgery and two catheters may be placed for subsequent irrigation with antibiotic solutions such as neomycin. The sump catheters are connected to low suction to remove serum and blood collecting in the pelvic space. Absorbent dressings are applied to the wound and changed when they become moist. Aseptic technique is essential to assure that clean wounds do not become contaminated. The wound is inspected regularly to determine type of drainage, erythema, or edema of the area, as well as to ensure that the catheters still are securely placed. The catheters are usually removed within 1 or 2 weeks postoperatively when drainage is minimal. In lieu of catheter drainage, penrose drains may be placed in the wound to promote drainage.

If the wound is left open to heal by secondary intention, a packing is placed at surgery. The packing may be removed within 48 hours, or small amounts may be removed daily. Hydrogen peroxide and normal saline solution (or antibiotic solutions) are used to irrigate the wound when the packing is removed; irrigations are continued several times daily.

The perineal wound requires meticulous care, and dressings should be changed often to prevent discomfort and odor. Positioning and movement may be difficult for the patient. Sitting on a soft foam pad and sitz baths several times daily are helpful to relieve discomfort.

Sitz baths are usually started about a week after surgery when packings, drains, and catheters have all been removed. The perineal wound may take several months to heal completely, especially if an inflammatory process has been the underlying disease process. Patients often complain of a sensation of wanting to evacuate their rectum. This distressing symptom results from packings, drainage, and the healing process itself.

If the perineal wound does not heal by either primary or secondary intention, skin grafts may be necessary.

If immediate decompression is necessary, colostomies may be opened at the end of surgery. In other situations the stoma may be opened a day or two after surgery to permit a more thorough seal of fibrin. The colostomy is opened with cautery or scalpel. Because there are no sensory nerve endings in the bowel tissue, bleeding points are easily ligated without pain. The opening of a colostomy is not painful, but it may be emotionally traumatic for the patient if drainage or flatus is suddenly expelled. The patient should be prepared for this potential event prior to the opening of the colostomy.

When the bowel has been opened surgically, postoperative care includes all the nursing measures required for abdominal surgery plus special nursing measures for the care of the colostomy and the perineal wound when the rectum is resected. The patient will usually have a nasogastric tube in place, and fluids and food will be restricted until bowel sounds are heard or until passage of flatus occurs, indicating that peristalsis has returned. Extensive abdominal surgery makes the patient vulnerable to hemorrhage, infection, and paralytic ileus, so that the nurse must be observant for initial signs of these complications. Urinary retention often occurs; an indwelling catheter is usually inserted for several days postoperatively. Some abdominal distention may be expected, but excessive and prolonged distention will cause pressure on the suture line. Prolonged distention may be the first sign of paralytic ileus. Nurses often insert rectal tubes in patients who have distention after abdominal surgery, but this practice should be avoided in patients who have had bowel surgery. If an anastomosis has been done in the lower bowel area, rectal tube insertion may traumatize the suture line. If rectal tube insertion is prescribed by the surgeon, the nurse should be aware of the location of the anastomosis and should take precautions by personally inserting the tube, rather than having ancillary personnel do it.

If a loop colostomy is performed, the stoma may be surrounded and covered with petroleum jelly- or neomycin-soaked gauze dressings. Some surgeons prefer immediate application of a disposable colostomy bag over the stoma. Using either technique, the nurse will need to prevent cross contamination of the separate abdominal incision by fecal drainage and will need to prevent skin irritation from the drainage. Even the large loop stoma with a glass rod or plastic bridge in place can be adapted for collection of drainage by the use of disposable bags with openings for the large stoma.

Disposable colostomy appliances are adhered to the skin or are attached to a belt. The appliances are clear and transparent so that the condition of the stoma and the drainage can be observed. Most of the appliances come in varying sizes and may be precut or nonperforated so that the size of the opening can be adjusted to the individual stoma. The appliances may be single use or drainable with an open end that is clamped between intervals of emptying.

Initially in the postoperative period, the drainage from any of the colostomies is likely to be more liquid, since dietary intake is limited. The patient will need a lot of support during this period, for the excessive liquid drainage can be distressing, especially if there is leakage from the dressing or from around the appliance. Prompt changing of the appliance and thorough cleaning of the peristomal skin are essential measures. When the patient begins to look at the stoma, he or she should be told that the stoma is the mucosal lining of the intestine and has the same type of tissue as that inside the mouth.

Adapting to a colostomy involves adjustment to the changed body image and to a different way of carrying out normal body function. Not only is the patient required to handle the stress of surgery and a diagnosis of cancer, but also the patient is faced with fears of fecal odor, soiling, flatus, and social isolation. Both the patient and nurse are members of a society that emphasizes cleanliness and codes of behavior related to body wastes. Each of them will have feelings about discussing changed body functions. Though the patient intellectually may acknowledge a colostomy as a therapeutic measure, he may find fecal incontinence a repulsive situation.

The adjustment to the changes in body function will be facilitated by the assistance of sensitive professional nurses who can be supportive during the grieving process associated with changes in body image. The sensitive nurse realizes that a radical change in elimination habits will be an emotionally disturbing event and that periods of discouragement, depression, and withdrawal can be anticipated.

An early assessment of the patient's perception of the surgery and the meaning it will have on his or her life is important for the nurse to accomplish. An assessment of the strengths and limitations of the patient and his or her family and their ability to cope with stressful situations is also important. The way the nurse approaches each patient in discussing the need for having a stoma for functions of elimination depends on the cause for the surgical procedure, the age and occupation of the patient, the personality of the patient, style of living, the kinds of experiences he or she has had, and the presence or absence of family support.

The patient brings to the situation the cumulative effects of his or her unique life experiences, so that his or her perception of the event rather than the realities of the event is most important. Some patients view the surgery as life-saving and readily adapt to the changes required. Other patients develop an extreme state of depression or dependency, especially when the colostomy begins to function. Still others refuse to look at the colostomy or to care for it or even to consent to the colostomy surgery. Early rapport and a therapeutic relationship with a nurse can help the patient cope with fears and feelings about having the colostomy. If the patient feels inadequate, the nurse should devise ways to make him or her feel adequate. The adjustment will also be facilitated by effective teaching in the postoperative management of a colostomy. Provisions for continuity of care after hospitalization are important because some patients are unable to master care of the colostomy before discharge.

Correct information as to what is expected of the patient postoperatively and the kinds of changes to expect in body functions is absolutely essential. Goals developed with the patient and family should be realistic ones, in light of information available concerning his or her individual situation. The nurse needs to be knowledgeable about the sites of the ostomies to properly teach the patient about realistic management. In teaching the patient how to manage the drainage, it is important to consider where the colostomy is and the type of drainage that will occur.

When the colostomy is in the ascending or in the transverse colon, it is misleading to discuss with the patient control of the drainage by irrigation. The drainage from the ascending colon is liquid, is likely to contain some proteolytic enzymes, and is more or less continuous and requires a drainable appliance to be worn continuously (similar to the appliance used for an ileostomy). The drainage from a transverse colostomy is semisolid and mushy and likely to be frequent so that a colostomy appliance is usually worn continuously. This appliance is preferably a drainable type, but if drainage is less frequent, an appliance with a closed-end pouch may be used. A patient with a transverse colostomy may, in some cases, be able to irrigate and have no drainage for varying periods of time. It may be a matter of convenience for some patients to avoid spillage temporarily for several hours and an irrigation might be then utilized. Nonetheless, it remains misleading to have the patient with a transverse colostomy think he or she will eventually control drainage by irrigation.

Since water absorption has been completed by the time the feces arrive at the sigmoid colon, the stool is formed; the drainage at this site can usually be regulated, depending on the individual patient's habits and preferences. There is controversy within the medical profession regarding irrigations (stimulation of the bowel to empty itself). Since a daily enema is not a normal occurrence for most persons, a daily irrigation of the colostomy is not considered a normal procedure by some authorities. While some persons prefer to eliminate daily irrigation in their colostomy management, other persons find it convenient and manageable. The patient's life style should be considered in the approach to colostomy management and the options for management should be discussed. Patients who had regular patterns of elimination preoperatively may be able to establish control of the colostomy simply by dietary management. However, the patient who had irregular and unpredictable elimination habits preoperatively is not likely to establish control of the colostomy even with irrigations. Patients who do not irrigate or who are not regulated by diet alone must wear a disposable appliance. It is helpful if the patient can decide on a schedule for doing the irrigation at home so that a similar schedule can be started at the hospital. If the home has only one bathroom for several members, the time of least demand for its use is selected. Colostomy irrigations are usually initiated about the sixth to the eighth postoperative day.

In irrigating the colostomy, the solution used is generally normal saline or water, but may vary as do solutions for rectal enemas. The temperature of the solution should be tepid or lukewarm; hot water may burn the mucosa and cold water causes spasms and cramping. The amount of solution for the average patient should not exceed 1,000 ml. The procedure is facilitated by the patient being in a normal upright position in the bathroom, but it can also be done in bed. (Initially the patient usually prefers to sit in a chair on a pillow facing the toilet, because of perineal discomfort, rather than sitting on the toilet.) The height of the irrigating container should be at a level with the bottom of the bag no higher than shoulder level when sitting or 1 to 1½ feet above the stoma of a bedridden patient. Various types of irrigating equipment are available; specific modifications and directions should be followed with each. If the nurse is doing the irrigation for the first time, the path of the bowel should be checked by inserting a lubricated gloved finger into the stoma. Most authorities no longer recommend routine dilation of the stoma, because it is felt that finger dilation of the stoma may cause mucosal tears. In addition, improved surgical techniques have decreased the number of constricting stomas and decreased the need for daily finger dilation. In some situations, however, dilation of the stoma may be prescribed.

To prevent trauma to the bowel, a well-lubricated soft latex catheter is used. The catheter should never be forced into the stoma because perforation could result from trauma. The catheter should be gently inserted only 2 to 4 inches (5 to 10 cm) into the stoma after air is expelled from the tubing. To prevent backflow of the solution, the irrigation is given slowly and the bag is lowered; if cramping occurs the flow of the solution is stopped temporarily. A cone-tipped tube has been developed to prevent backflow. It also requires lubrication before insertion and is inserted until it fits snugly in the stoma without pressure on the mucosa.

The usual length of time for evacuation to

take place is 25 to 45 minutes and all the solution usually returns within 15 minutes. Colostomy irrigation sleeves can be closed at the end, so that the patient can get up and move about while the solution and stool are returned into the collection appliance. When the returns are completed, either an adhesive-backed pouch or a simple gauze dressing is applied to the stoma. If no returns occur, a lubricated tube may be inserted 5 to 10 cm to siphon the drainage. The patient should also be checked for the presence of hard stool, which might be impeding the returns. Usually, patients use a schedule of daily or alternate days for irrigations. Some patients prefer to use another method of irrigation, the bulb-syringe technique, which utilizes smaller amounts of water instilled via a catheter attached to an Asepto syringe. This technique, however, requires manipulative skill in handling the bulb and filling it with water and may be difficult for the elderly patient to manage.

The person who is able to regulate the colostomy by diet and irrigation may only require a stoma shield as a cover between irrigations. Some patients prefer to wear an appliance between irrigations because they feel more secure if any spillage should occur.

Successful management of a colostomy by irrigation means that the individual's colon empties only in response to a stimulus of fluid. Some patients succeed at control by irrigating once every 24 hours, while others may have to irrigate only every 2 days.

When an irrigation of a transverse colostomy or double barrel colostomy is prescribed, as in a preoperative preparation, the purpose of the subsequent surgery must be understood before irrigations are instituted to clean the bowel. The surgeon may order irrigations of the proximal loop only, the distal loop only, or irrigations of both loops. The correct loop must be irrigated. If it is not clear which stoma is proximal and which is distal, this determination is best clarified by the surgeon. When the distal loop is irrigated, return of the fluid is expected from the rectum unless complete obstruction is present. The nurse should be cognizant of the pathology when irrigations are done, taking appropriate precautions. For example, excessive distention of the distal loop during a distal loop irrigation in the presence of diverticulosis could result in perforation.

The person with a recent colostomy when beginning to take food orally is often reluctant to eat because he or she hopes to limit the movements from the colostomy. This misconception and fear should be discussed thoroughly with the patient to clarify that eating regularly will facilitate more regular movements of more solid consistency. The patient should be weighed at regular intervals to determine that adequate food is being ingested.

After an initial diet of bland, low fiber foods for several weeks postoperatively, the diet becomes one generally similar to the preoperative diet. As the diet is gradually increased in variety, the individual patient can determine which foods cause constipation, gas accumulation, dyspepsia, or diarrhea. Moderation in the use of these foods or total avoidance of them may be indicated, depending on the individual's preferences. The patient with a colostomy should be encouraged to eat a normal, varied diet that includes fats, carbohydrates, and proteins, and one that promotes the proper consistency of the feces with the least amount of flatus. The patient with a colostomy no longer has sphincter control over the passage of flatus; it must be controlled by diet. Foods that caused the patient problems preoperatively may still produce the same effects, so that the patient is the best resource for planning dietary management. A low fiber diet can be taken in cases of diarrhea; increased ingestion of fluids, fruits, and vegetables will help counteract constipation. Eating balanced and regular meals in a leisurely manner, chewing food well, and avoiding the intake of cabbage, sauerkraut, corn, nuts, and carbonated beverages, or gum chewing will prevent flatulence. Onions, beans, cabbage, fish, asparagus, cheese, and eggs may cause odorous drainage.

Successful adaptation to a colostomy is achieved when the patient is free from odor, has an acceptable way of managing the elimination of the feces (either by irrigation or use of an appropriate appliance), has minimal problems with flatus expulsion, and feels comfortable and secure and begins to broaden his social interactions and activities. If problems with odor occur, various agents may be used (see Table 7-2), and if peristomal irritations occur, skin barriers are utilized to promote healing (see Table 7-3). The presence of a colostomy does not impede physical or social activities, unless the patient has failed to learn to manage the colostomy properly or is in poor physical health or if the patient has failed to adjust emotionally to the altered body image.

Resumption of previous patterns of sexual activity may not be entirely possible for all patients who have had an abdominoperineal resection. It is estimated that about 30 to 50 percent of male patients who require resection for cancer of the rectum are impotent after surgery. The duration of impotence varies; in some patients, impotence may be only a temporary problem. The meaning of impotence for the individual patient must be determined; appropriate referrals are made when necessary for counseling, if the nurse and doctor are unable to assist the patient in this adjustment. The female patient who has a colostomy also may be fearful of problems with her sexual relationship with her spouse. The spouses of patients with colostomies should be included in discussions on the effects of the surgery. (Refer to page 560 for discussion of ways for the ostomate to manage sexual intercourse.)

Patients react in individual ways to the need for a colostomy. Adaptation to an altered body image associated with alterations of excretory functions and loss of sphincter control is facilitated by proper teaching and supervision in learning to manage the colostomy. Adjustment is also facilitated by listening to the patient and supporting the patient in the grieving process associated with a change in body image.

OTHER DISORDERS OF THE
GASTROINTESTINAL TRACT

Other diseases and disorders of the alimentary canal, although not directly involved in digestive functions, can cause indirect interference and complications and thus affect the integrity and functioning of the gastrointestinal tract. These conditions—hernias, appendicitis, pilonidal cyst, and anorectal conditions—are discussed generally.

Hernia

A **hernia** is the abnormal protrusion of part of an organ through the structures that normally contain it. Although hernias may occur in various parts of the body they are most commonly found in the abdomen. An **abdominal hernia** occurs when the bowel, or any viscus, is displaced through a defect in the wall of the cavity, which forms a sac or peritoneal pouch. The defect may be congenital or acquired. Hernias may be inguinal, femoral, epigastric, umbilical, incisional, or diaphragmatic, depending on their location. Hernias may also be classified as reducible or irreducible. A **reducible hernia** is one in which the hernial contents can be replaced by manipulation into their normal position with the sac remaining in the abdominal wall. When the hernial contents cannot be replaced in their normal position, due either to adhesion formation or to a narrowing of the neck of the sac, the hernia is termed **irreducible,** or incarcerated. A diminished or absent blood supply to the hernial contents results in a **strangulated hernia.**

The most common type of hernia is the **inguinal hernia,** which may be unilateral or bilateral. Inguinal hernias can be direct or indirect. These terms refer to the relation of the hernia to the inguinal canal which is the passageway of the spermatic cord through the muscular structures in the groin area. The canal begins at the internal ring in the transverse muscle and ends in the external ring. A **direct hernia** is one that is due to the weakness of the fascial floor of the inguinal canal, but does not enter the canal through the internal ring. Rather it protrudes directly through the transverse fascia and comes out at the external ring. An **indirect inguinal hernia** is due to the weakness of the fascial margin of the internal ring and leaves the abdomen through the inguinal ring, passing through the inguinal canal and emerging at the external ring. The inguinal hernia is associated with sharp, steady pain in the groin which usually occurs when the person lifts heavy objects, coughs, or strains. The hernia is visualized as a small and slightly tender lump in the groin that usually disappears when the person returns to a supine position. Often a truss is used to contain the hernia, but surgical repair or herniorrhapy is the most appropriate treatment.

Femoral hernias occur in the abdominal wall where the femoral artery passes into the thigh and is observed as a swelling in the groin if a portion of bowel or omentum escapes through the femoral ring. There is a high incidence of incarceration and strangulation with femoral hernias.

The **umbilical hernia** is the result of an

abnormality of muscular structures about the cord and is thus fairly common in infants at birth. The hernia may disappear as growth of muscles and fascia correct the defect; a strip of adhesive tape may be used to keep the herniation in position. In some situations herniorrhaphy is necessary. Umbilical hernias in adults most often occur in women who have had several pregnancies or are obese. A congenital defect of the umbilicus is also a factor in the incidence of umbilical hernias.

An **incisional hernia** occurs at the site of a previous surgery. It is usually associated with infection, inadequate nutrition, extreme abdominal distention, or obesity. Surgical repair is indicated. If it is not possible to pull the layers of the abdominal wall together without creating tension, reconstructive methods are required. Prosthetics such as Teflon, marlex mesh, or tantalum mesh are utilized.

Herniorrhaphy (surgical repair of the hernia) is the dissection of the hernial sac and return of the contents to the abdominal cavity. Emergency surgical intervention is necessary for treating strangulated hernia resulting in intestinal obstruction if ischemia and necrosis of the bowel are to be prevented. Symptoms of strangulated hernia are colicky pain, nausea, vomiting, and obstipation. Postoperatively, the patient with an inguinal herniorrhaphy is generally allowed to ambulate as soon as he or she is recovered completely from the anesthesia. Herniorrhaphy may be done under local or spinal anesthesia or general anesthesia. Although early ambulation is encouraged, the nurse must prevent intraabdominal pressure, which could compromise the surgical repair. Respiratory infections are a contraindication to surgery, because coughing may cause undue strain on the suture line. Urinary retention is a fairly frequent complication postoperatively, especially in inguinal herniorrhaphy. Excessive distention of the bladder must be corrected promptly in order to prevent pressure on the surgical site. **Scrotal edema** may occur following inguinal herniorrhaphy. A scrotal support is often necessary to prevent tension on the spermatic cord and edema and swelling. The scrotum should be examined at regular intervals to detect any occurrence of swelling. Ice bags may be applied to the scrotum to relieve swelling and pain.

Hernial repair in the case of strangulation requires a bowel resection if gangrene of the bowel has occurred by the time surgery is initiated. An end-to-end anastomosis is accomplished after the involved segment is resected. These patients require a nasogastric tube and suction, fluid and food restriction, and fluid and electrolyte administration until bowel function returns postoperatively. (Care of the patient with bowel surgery was discussed on page 573.)

The patient who has had a herniorrhaphy must receive instructions about restrictions on strenuous activities, such as lifting heavy objects, and also should be advised of the importance of avoiding constipation and straining with defecation. Depending on the type of occupation, the patient may require an extended recuperation period prior to return to work. In some situations, an occupation that requires considerable lifting and straining is contraindicated for the patient with a herniorrhaphy due to the potential for recurrence. A change or modification in occupation is suggested by seeking machines or other people to perform the heavy lifting or by completely changing the nature of the person's work, if possible.

Appendicitis

Appendicitis is the acute inflammation of the appendix and is considered to start as an obstruction of the lumen of the appendix with a fecalith. Characteristically, the first symptom is epigastric discomfort, often mistaken for indigestion, but in some patients the pain originates as colicky pain in the periumbilical area. Within a few hours, pain shifts to the right lower quadrant. Frequently, McBurney's point becomes very tender on deep palpation; tenderness is an important finding. Anorexia, nausea, vomiting, fever, and leukocytosis are usually present. Surgery is indicated to prevent perforation and generalized peritonitis or periappendiceal abscess. Postoperative care involves early ambulation. Recovery is usually rapid unless the appendix becomes perforated.

Pilonidal Cyst

Pilonidal cyst is a lesion, often of congenital origin, that is located in the midline of the sacral region, overlying the junction of the sacrum and coccyx. The cyst rarely becomes symptomatic until the individual reaches adulthood, when infection generally causes severe pain and swelling in the area. The inflammatory process ranges from a mild, irritating, and draining sinus tract to an acute abscess. Treatment consists in drainage of the abscess during the acute phase; later, a total surgical excision is accomplished. The cyst is thought to result from an infolding of the skin in which hair continues to grow. Thus the cyst usually contains hair, and the sinus tracts must be completely excised in order to prevent recurrence. Usually excision and primary closure is attempted, but if the defect is too large for primary closure, the wound is left open to heal by granulation. Postoperatively a pressure dressing is in place. The patient may find it uncomfortable to lie on his back and is usually placed in a side-lying or prone position. Wound care is essential to prevent infection or trauma to the site.

Anorectal Conditions

The major function of the rectum is storage of the feces until defecation takes place. Pathologic conditions in the rectum are usually evidenced by difficulty in defecation with the occurrence of pain or bleeding or both. Itching of the perianal skin may occur due to irritation of the skin from organisms, mucous drainage, or fecal matter. Anorectal conditions include perirectal or ischiorectal abscess formation, anal fistula, rectal fissues, and hemorrhoids.

Perirectal abscess and **fistula formation** most often begin with an infection of the crypts, which are small recesses in the rectal mucosa. Pain and swelling in the area and leukocytosis are usually present. The only treatment is incision and drainage to provide adequate drainage of the abscess. Antibiotics may be indicated; a packing is usually necessary for the resultant wound.

An **anal fistula** is an abnormal opening or tract in the skin near the anus; it is usually associated with an infectious process. Surgery is indicated to cut the fistula open. A packing is inserted and the wound is allowed to heal from the bottom outward. A **rectal fissure** is a split in the skin lining the rectum and is usually associated with failure of the rectal muscles to relax. Acute local pain occurs on defecation and slight bleeding may also result. Dilation of the anal sphincter and excision of the fissure are indicated.

Hemorrhoids are varicose veins of the external or internal hemorrhoidal venous plexus. External hemorrhoids are found outside the external sphincter and can often be seen on examination of the anal area. Internal hemorrhoids are located above the internal sphincter. Hemorrhoids are associated with pain, itching, constipation, and bleeding with the stool. Symptoms increase in severity in constipation or diarrhea. Hemorrhoids may become thrombosed, resulting in severe rectal pain associated with a tender mass. Surgical removal of the clot is indicated. Chronic constipation, straining at defecation, pregnancy, sedentary occupations, and obesity are some of the predisposing factors. Increased hydrostatic pressure (portal hypertension) in the portal system also results in hemorrhoids.

Both internal and external hemorrhoids are common. Diagnosis is made by inspection, digital examination, proctoscopy, and barium enema. It is important to rule out the presence of carcinoma when bleeding is present. Too often it is assumed that rectal bleeding is caused by hemorrhoids when they are detected, and further investigation for other lesions is not continued.

Sitz baths, stool softeners, and dietary control to prevent constipation or diarrhea are the usual medical measures to treat hemorrhoids. Injections of sclerosing agents are used by some physicians; this technique causes shrinkage of the lesion. The usual treatment of hemorrhoids, when pain increases or when they become thrombosed, is hemorrhoidectomy. The procedure involves ligation and excision of the hemorrhoid(s) and leaves minimal scarring. The surgery does not interfere with the sphincter mechanism.

Postoperatively the patient's dressings are observed for bleeding; hemorrhage can occur. Although the surgery is considered minor the patient may have much discomfort and pain; relief of pain and comfort measures are necessary. Often the patient is unable to find a comfortable position. Either a prone position or a foam rubber pad to prevent pressure on the operative site is helpful. Once the wound packing is removed, usually the day after surgery, warm sitz baths are begun. In addition, witch hazel compresses or other astringents are applied to the wound to reduce swelling and promote healing.

Often, patients who have undergone hemorrhoidectomy have difficulty in voiding, and the nurse should observe for urine retention. Stool softeners are started in the early postoperative period. The patient should be prepared for a painful first bowel movement after surgery; bleeding may also occur. Analgesics may be necessary at this time.

When caring for the patient with anorectal conditions, the nurse should always be tactful and sensitive to the pain, discomfort, and embarrassment of the patient. Too often, anorectal conditions, and particularly hemorrhoids, are considered minor problems and inadequate attention is given to relieving the patient's discomfort. Consequently, patients may hesitate to ask for relief and also are embarrassed by examination of the surgical site. The nurse should instruct the patient in dietary management necessary to control constipation and prevent recurrence of hemorrhoids.

Disorders of the Liver, Biliary Tract, and Pancreas

The following discussion is concerned with the care of patients with disorders of the other organs involved in the functions of the gastrointestinal system. These organs include those of the biliary system (the gallbladder and the bile ducts), the liver, and the pancreas.

The **liver** is the largest organ in the body and is located predominantly in the upper right quadrant of the abdominal cavity, immediately below the diaphragm. Liver tissue is made up of its functional units, the lobules, which consist of rows of hepatic cells and blood vessels. At the center of each lobule is the central vein, which is a tributary of the hepatic vein. Blood enters the central vein from the sinusoids, which are small channels between the rows of cells to which blood is delivered from subdivisions of both the hepatic artery and portal vein. Thus the liver is a highly vascular organ, receiving its blood supply from two sources: the portal vein, which carries blood from the stomach, intestines, spleen, and pancreas and the hepatic artery, which delivers blood from the aorta. Blood leaves the liver via the hepatic vein, which joins the inferior vena cava.

Sinusoids are lined with two types of cells, endothelial cells and Kupffer cells. The Kupffer cells are reticuloendothelial cells capable of phagocytic activity on bacteria and other foreign matter in the blood and are involved in transforming the hemoglobin released by disintegrating erythrocytes into bile pigment. The parenchymal cells of the liver secrete bile into very small bile ducts, called canaliculi, which unite between the rows of liver cells, forming larger ducts similar in size to the blood capillaries. Larger ducts are formed between the lobules and eventually become the hepatic duct, which joins the bile duct from the gallbladder (the cystic duct) to form the common bile duct. The liver cells secrete 600 to 800 ml of bile daily. Bile is a yellowish-orange fluid that is strongly alkaline and is composed of 90 to 97% water. Bile pigments, bile salts, sodium, chloride, bicarbonate, calcium salts, cholesterol, fatty acids, mucin, conjugated bilirubin, lecithin, and traces of numerous other constituents are also present. The alkaline bile neutralizes gastric acid in the duodenum.

Bile pigments (bilirubin and biliverdin) result from the breakdown of erythrocytes. These pigments are affected by bacteria in the intestine and changed to urobilinogen (and then oxidized to urobilin), part of which is excreted in the feces and part of which is absorbed into the blood and carried to the liver. In the liver, urobilin is reconverted to bilirubin and secreted again in the bile. Urobilin excreted into the stool gives the color to the stool. Minute amounts are excreted in urine. The bilirubin secreted from the canaliculi is conjugated bilirubin. Indirect or unconjugated bilirubin, which is not water-soluble, is conjugated within the liver cells with glucuronic acid to form the water-soluble, direct or conjugated bilirubin.

Bile salts have an important function in digestion and absorption by emulsifying fats and assisting in the hydrolysis and absorption of fat. They also promote the absorption of the fat-soluble vitamins A, D, E, and K and activate intestinal and pancreatic enzymes.

Bile serves as an excretory vehicle for bilirubin and cholesterol as well as for sex, thyroid, and adrenal hormones, and also certain drugs (e.g., salicylates, phenol, and atropine), toxins, and excess minerals.

In addition to its secretory functions, the liver plays an important role in the metabolism of carbohydrates, proteins, and fats. The liver changes the simple sugars, or monosaccharides fructose and galactose, into glucose and converts glucose to glycogen for storage (glycogenesis). By the process of glycogenolysis, the liver converts glycogen into glucose and releases it into the blood when necessary to maintain adequate blood glucose concentration. Glycogen may also be synthesized from proteins or fats by the process of gluconeogenesis, and the liver also converts lactic acid to glycogen. Thus, maintenance of the normal blood glucose level is dependent on the liver's ability to store and release glucose as needed by the body.

The end products of protein digestion are primarily amino acids which, after absorption, pass into the liver via the portal vein. Amino acids are deaminized by the liver to produce ketoacids, and ammonia is released during deamination. Ammonia is converted into urea by the liver and is excreted in the urine. The liver also synthesizes plasma proteins such as prothrombin, factors V, VII, VIII, IX, and X, fibrinogen, albumin, and globulin. The role of the liver in the clotting mechanism of the blood and in the maintenance of serum osmotic pressure is an important one, as is its role in the metabolism of fatty acids. Most plasma phospholipids, cholesterol, and triglycerides (except those in the chylomicrons, the form entering the lymph) are synthesized in the liver. In addition to these metabolic and blood-related functions, the liver stores vitamins A, D, and B_{12} as well as iron in the form of ferritin, copper, cholesterol, and phospholipids.

The detoxifying functions of the liver render certain foreign and toxic substances more water-soluble so that they can be eliminated through the kidney. These substances include drugs such as barbiturates and nicotine, poisons, and heavy metals. Detoxifying functions are carried out by the processes of conjugation, oxidation, and hydrolysis.

IMPAIRED LIVER FUNCTION

Regardless of the cause of liver impairment, disorders in its physiologic functioning result in symptoms that are characteristic of liver disease and reflect problems of nutrition, metabolism, blood coagulation defects, inability to combat infection, and inability to detoxify harmful substances. It is important to remember that the liver has exceptional regenerative capacity, so that dysfunction of a marked degree reflects diffuse parenchymal damage. Diseases of the liver that are discussed include hepatitis, cirrhosis, and neoplastic disease. Because alcoholism is frequently associated with liver diseases it is also discussed generally in this chapter.

Symptoms common to hepatic disease include jaundice, bleeding tendencies, pain, gastrointestinal symptoms, ascites, generalized edema, portal hypertension, hepatomegaly, and skin changes. Because these symptoms are important in the nursing assessment of patients with liver disease, they are discussed prior to consideration of individual diseases.

Jaundice, also known as icterus, refers to the yellowish discoloration of the tissues, particularly in the sclerae, mucous membranes, and skin, that results from an excess of bilirubin in the blood. Jaundice is best detected in daylight, rather than in artificial light. Excess bilirubin may result from either intrahepatic or extrahepatic disease. Jaundice is classified as hepatocellular, obstructive (or posthepatic), or hemolytic, depending on the site and cause. Hemolytic jaundice may also be referred to as prehepatic jaundice. In this situation the liver may not be impaired but rather is unable to keep up with demands placed on it to remove bilirubin from the circulation due to excessive destruction of erythrocytes. (Hemolytic anemia is discussed on page 437.)

Hepatocellular or **hepatic jaundice** is caused by intrinsic liver disease which prevents the hepatic cells from conjugating, secreting, and excreting bilirubin. (It is important to remember, however, that jaundice is not always present in early stages of chronic liver disease, because regeneration of the hepatic cells may keep up with the damage as it occurs and bilirubin can be handled adequately.) **Obstructive** or **posthepatic jaundice** is caused by obstruction of the flow of bile in the extrahepatic ducts. It is most frequently associated with common bile duct obstruction by gallstones, but may also be caused by ductal strictures or neoplastic disease in adjacent structures, such as the pancreas.

In addition to the yellowish discoloration, the patient with jaundice often experiences pruritus, or itching of the skin, apparently due to the irritation of cutaneous sensory nerves by the bile salts. Urobilinogen content in the urine increases and causes dark urine. In severe hepatocellular jaundice, as well as in obstructive jaundice, the stools are pale gray due to the lack of urobilinogen.

Bleeding tendencies occur with liver disease as inadequate production of prothrombin and other coagulation factors interferes with the normal clotting process. Purpura, epistaxis, bleeding of the oral mucous membrane, and melena may all occur. **Pain** is often described in the presence of acute liver disease as a dull aching in the right upper quadrant or epigastric region. Pain is due to the stretching of the liver and its capsule. Palpation of the liver often demonstrates tenderness. Progressive liver disease results in **ascites**, which is an accumulation of fluid in the peritoneal cavity due to increased pressure within the portal vein. This increased pressure occurs as blood flow is obstructed by hepatic tissue damage and compression of the blood vessels.

Generalized edema may develop in patients who are unable to produce sufficient serum albumin to maintain the normal colloidal osmotic pressure of the blood. In addition, when the liver cannot inactivate the antidiuretic hormone and aldosterone, there is an increase in water and sodium reabsorption by the kidneys and further edema occurs.

Portal hypertension results in dilatation and varicosities of veins that drain into the portal vein. Gastric and esophageal varices are distended superficial veins and often rupture in the presence of portal hypertension. Esophageal and gastric hemorrhages result in extensive hematemesis or melena or both. The problem of portal hypertension and esophageal varices is discussed in greater detail in the subsequent section on liver cirrhosis (see page 593).

Hepatomegaly (enlarged liver) may be detected on physical examination and may indicate the presence of a variety of diseases, including cancer of the liver (either primary or metastatic), cirrhosis, hepatitis, and liver abscess. It is also frequently noted in patients with leukemia, lymphoma, or Hodgkin's disease. Hepatomegaly may also be associated with chronic congestive heart failure due to venous congestion within the liver; this type of hepatomegaly responds to digitalis, diuretics, and salt restriction. Hepatomegaly is often associated with splenomegaly due to the hyperplasia of the reticuloendothelial tissue as well as to venous congestion. (It is important to remember that severe hepatic necrosis results in atrophy of the organ.)

Liver disorders are usually associated with other generalized symptoms such as anorexia, vague digestive discomfort, weight loss, lethargy, and weakness. Muscle wasting is often present, as a result of impaired carbohydrate and protein metabolism. Various skin changes associated with certain types of liver disease are **palmar erythema,** characterized by mottled, red, and warm palms related to capillary dilatation and **spider angiomas** or nevi, superficial arterioles with radiating branches that are clearly visible on skin surfaces, particularly on the face, neck, arms, and chest. **Caput medusae** are varicosities in the abdominal wall near the umbilicus. In liver cirrhosis, a loss of axillary and pubic hair in both sexes and decreased facial hair in the male are frequent findings related to the effects on the sexual hormones resulting from liver dysfunction. Gynecomastia and testicular atrophy occur in males, due to elevated levels of estrogen.

Neurologic disturbances often occur in severe hepatic disease as a result of ammonia toxicity, because the liver is unable to convert ammonia to urea. Irritability, lethargy, apathy, memory defects, and disturbed behavior may all be demonstrated. Confusion and irritability may then lead to stupor and eventually coma. Asterixis reflects impaired central nervous system metabolism. Although asterixis, a tremor, is associated with other systemic diseases, it is termed "liver flap" because it is so frequently associated with liver disease. This flapping tremor is characterized by sudden flexion of the wrist, followed by extension of the wrist joint back to the original position. This tremor occurs when the patient extends the hand at the wrist, holding the fingers in a straight position.

Fetor hepaticus is an aromatic sweet-sour odor in the breath and urine, due to the presence of methyl mercaptan. It is apparently due to disorders of amino acid metabolism and abnormal intestinal bacterial action.

Diagnostic Tests of Liver Function

A variety of laboratory tests are used to evaluate the liver functions. Some of these tests are not specific to liver function but are helpful to confirm the presence of hepatic disease when combined with the patient's history, current symptoms, and test results.

The **serum bilirubin** (van den Bergh's) test is used to estimate the concentration of bilirubin in the blood and to determine whether the bilirubin is conjugated or unconjugated. As described previously, hepatic cells remove the pigment from the blood and convert the unconjugated bilirubin to bilirubin diglucuronide, a water-soluble compound, before excreting it into the bile. Unconjugated bilirubin (indirect) is normally approximately 0.7 mg per 100 ml, while conjugated (direct) bilirubin is normally less than 0.5 mg per 100 ml [46]. The total serum bilirubin is generally reported to be between 1.0 and 1.5 mg per 100 ml. Normal values differ among laboratories. Comparing direct (conjugated in the liver) and indirect (unconjugated) bilirubin levels is important to differentiate the etiology of jaundice and determine the site of pathology. For example, the direct bilirubin level is usually elevated in obstructive jaundice, whereas elevation of the indirect bilirubin reflects hepatocellular disease and the liver's inability to remove unconjugated bilirubin from the blood. The differentiation between direct (conjugated) and indirect (unconjugated) bilirubin is not always clear-cut in certain clinical situations. Jaundice is usually detectable, however, when the total bilirubin level is over 3 mg per 100 ml.

The **icterus index** indicates the degree of jaundice by comparison of the color of serum with a standardized color solution expressed in arbitrarily designated units and is a rough estimate of the concentration of bilirubin. Normal levels are 2 to 8 units [46]. The **cephalin-flocculation test** is also used to determine alterations in serum proteins; the test is normally negative or only 2 plus, but values are increased in liver disease. Thymol turbidity, the reaction of gamma globulin and lipids, may also be done to determine the degree of hepatic cell damage and gamma globulin concentration.

The liver is responsible for the production of serum albumin and minimal globulin (most of the latter is produced by the lymphoid tissues in the body). Plasma protein levels of albumin and globulin are measured and the albumin-globulin ratio (A/G ratio) is also determined. In liver disease, albumin production is decreased while the globulin is retained at usual levels, resulting in a reversal of normal ratios. Albumin levels are normally 3.6 to 5.5 gm while globulin levels are usually 1.5 to 3.0 gm per 100 ml. **Serum protein electrophoresis** is increasingly being used instead of A/G ratios for more accurate serum protein measurement because with electrophoresis, the globulins can be fractionated according to mobility, giving much more precise information than obtained with A/G ratios.

Serum alkaline phosphatase is normally excreted in the bile by the hepatic cells, but is elevated in liver disease or in obstruction in the bile ducts (as well as in other systemic diseases). Other enzymes that are elevated in the presence of liver disease are serum glutamic oxalacetic transaminase (SGOT), serum glutamic pyruvic transaminase (SGPT), and lactic dehydrogenase (LDH). Elevations of these enzymes, however, are also found in other systemic disorders.

When liver disease results in failure to produce prothrombin or vitamin K, a decrease in prothrombin levels in the blood occurs. Prolonged prothrombin times, over 11 to 12 seconds, may also result from vitamin K deficiency caused by the absence of bile salts, which are necessary for the absorption of fat-soluble vitamins in the small intestine. Thus, a prolonged prothrombin time reflects either hepatocellular or obstructive biliary tract disease.

Cholesterol levels are decreased in the presence of liver disease, but are elevated in obstructive biliary disease. Normal values vary but generally are within 160 to 330 mg per 100 ml in persons over 20 years of age [46].

Several of these tests (SGOT, LDH, alkaline phosphatase, bilirubin, cholesterol, total protein, and albumin) are included in the widely used screening test, the **sequential multiple analysis** (SMA), done on hospital admissions or in physical examinations. Blood ammonia levels are evaluated to detect impending hepatic coma and elevations associated with liver disease. Normal levels in whole blood are 75 to 200 μg per 100 ml. Blood levels vary with protein intake; fasting is required.

The **Bromsulphalein** (BSP) test consists in the injection of dye that is normally excreted by the liver cells in the bile. A dosage calculated by the individual's weight (5 mg per kilogram of body weight) is given intravenously in an arm vein. A venous blood specimen is collected from the opposite arm 45 minutes later. Normally only 5 percent or less of the dye remains in the blood within 45 to 60 minutes and reflects the liver's detoxification functioning ability.

The liver's ability to form hippuric acid by detoxifying benzoic acid and combining it with glycine is evaluated by the **hippuric acid test.** Sodium benzoate (usually in a dose of 6 gm) is dissolved in 250 ml of water and is given orally. Normally the hippuric acid is circulated in the blood and then eliminated in the urine. After the oral administration, urine is collected for 1 to 4 hours; normally 2.0 to 3.5 gm hippuric acid is excreted within 4 hours. A variation of this test is to administer the sodium benzoate (1.77 gm) intravenously, and to collect the urine for 1 hour after the injection. Normally, 0.7 gm hippuric acid appears in the urine within the hour after the intravenous injection [46].

Liver scans are usually accomplished with the use of rose bengal tagged with ^{131}I, which is administered intravenously and is followed by detection of the uptake of the radioactive isotope by the liver. This technique indicates areas of functioning and nonfunctioning liver tissue by the presence of "cold" or blank areas where the liver is nonfunctioning and unable to take up the isotope. Less often, radioactive gold or vitamin B_{12} tagged with radioactive cobalt is utilized. Because the liver scan is not associated with particular risks, other than reactions to the substances used, it is used often in suspected liver disease. As with other scanning techniques, a permit is usually required from the patient and the patient is given a thorough explanation of the procedure. It is important for the patient to lie still during the scanning technique; this factor should be emphasized in order to obtain cooperation.

Urine examinations for urobilinogen and bilirubin are often obtained to differentiate the type of pathologic condition in the presence of jaundice. For example, bilirubin is present in the urine in obstructive and hepatocellular jaundice, but not in hemolytic jaundice. In the presence of liver disease, urobilinogen is no longer adequately removed from the blood to be excreted in the bile, but is increasingly excreted in the urine. It is important to remember that bacterial action by the small intestine changes conjugated bilirubin to urobilinogen. Therefore in the presence of obstructive jaundice, when bile is not reaching the intestine, or when antibiotic administration has resulted in diminished bacterial content in the intestine, urinary urobilinogen may be decreased rather than increased. Normally, less than 4 mg of urobilinogen is excreted in the urine during 24 hours. Single specimens of urine for testing urobilinogen may also be collected. Urobilinogen is found in highest concentration in the afternoon and night. Voidings at specific times in the afternoon may be collected. Specimens should be protected from light, which destroys urobilinogen.

The **galactose tolerance test** may be done to evaluate the liver's ability to remove galactose from the blood and convert it to glycogen. This test requires an 8-hour fasting period, prior to the oral administration of 100 ml of a solution of 25% galactose. Blood samples are drawn in 1, 1½, and 2 hours after the solution is ingested to determine the presence of abnormal concentrations in the blood.

Liver biopsy is an important examination in diagnosing most hepatic disorders. A permit is usually required for this test; hemorrhage is a potential complication. A special liver biopsy needle is used to aspirate a specimen of liver tissue for subsequent microscopic examination. Because many patients have clotting defects, various tests of hemostasis are usually done prior to this test. The results of these tests, as well as baseline data on the patient's vital signs, should be ascertained prior to the procedure. It is important that the patient not move while the liver biopsy is being done and that he or she understands the importance of maintaining bed rest and a restricted position postexamination in order to prevent complications. Emotional support is of paramount importance because the thought of a liver biopsy and the potential for bleeding as well as the potential of a diagnosis of severe liver disease are anxiety-provoking.

The patient is positioned on his or her left side so that the right side is exposed. The site is aseptically prepared and infiltrated with a local anesthetic. The patient is asked to inhale and exhale deeply and then to hold his or her breath at the end of expiration in order to immobilize the chest wall and diaphragm until the needle is withdrawn. The physician then inserts the biopsy needle via the intercostal or transabdominal approach to penetrate the liver and aspirate a specimen. The needle is immediately withdrawn and pressure is applied to the site. The patient is then turned on the right side with a pillow placed under the costal margin to provide pressure to the site and is instructed to lie immobile in this position for 2 hours. Bed rest is usually maintained for 24 hours. Vital signs are measured every 10 to 15 minutes for 2 hours or until stabilized and then every 4 hours for 24 hours. Any signs of hepatic bleeding, as demonstrated by an increase in pulse rate or decrease in blood pressure, is reported immediately. The presence of pain, tenderness, and rigidity at the site may indicate bile peritonitis due to leakage of bile.

Laparoscopy (also called peritoneoscopy) is a fairly recent development in the diagnosis of liver disease. It permits selective biopsy and visualization of the liver without resorting to major surgery. However, an operative permit is required for this procedure. A small incision is made into the abdomen after infiltration with a local anesthetic, and a pneumoperitoneum is created. A fiberoptic laparoscope is inserted and the examination and biopsy are carried out by percutaneous techniques. Biopsy sites are cauterized. The dangers of the procedure are those of bleeding, air embolism, and perforation of the intestine. After the laparoscopy, the patient is usually allowed to be ambulatory within a few hours. If biopsies are done, the patient must remain in bed for approximately 24 hours as in conventional liver biopsy techniques.

Angiographic techniques may also be utilized for visualizing the vascular structure of the liver and the portal circulation. These techniques include the hepatic arteriogram and splenic portal venography. Both techniques require the use of a contrast medium; the danger of reactions to the dye must be anticipated. As in other angiographic techniques, a permit is required before the procedure can be done. The patient requires an explanation of the procedure and is warned of the warm sensation that occurs when the dye is injected into the artery.

Viral Hepatitis

Viral hepatitis is an inflammation of the liver that destroys the parenchymal cells and results in necrosis. Until regeneration of cells occurs, there is decreased ability of the liver to carry out its normal functions. Usually the patient recovers but has some residual liver damage. Although mortality from viral hepatitis is relatively low, fulminating types frequently are fatal. Regenerating cells may develop into nodules separated by bands of connective tissue and cause a type of cirrhosis known as postnecrotic cirrhosis.

Viral hepatitis occurs in two forms: hepatitis A (formerly called infectious or epidemic hepatitis) and hepatitis B (formerly called serum hepatitis). Recent information on the varied routes of transmission of both of these types has made the former classification of serum and infectious hepatitis no longer appropriate. Viral hepatitis is a reportable communicable disease. In 1975 approximately 55,000 cases were reported to the Center for Disease Control [33]. The incidence of hepatitis B appears to be increasing since 1966 when differentiation between hepatitis B and hepatitis A was first required.

The major differences between the two types of hepatitis appear to be primarily related to the incubation period, manner of onset, and the usual mode of transmission. The clinical picture in both types is generally similar and includes symptoms of anorexia, dyspepsia, nausea, and possibly vomiting, malaise, fever, hepatomegaly, abdominal tenderness, and jaundice. Dark urine and clay-colored stools are often reported by the patient.

The patient's history usually indicates contact with another person who has actually demonstrated jaundice or with others who are potential sources of hepatitis. Assessment of clinical symptoms and physical examination as well as abnormalities in liver function tests confirm the diagnosis. In type B hepatitis, the presence of hepatitis B surface antigen (HB_sAg) is usually detected on blood analysis; the antigen is absent in type A. The antigen appears even before jaundice becomes evident, and usually disappears within 2 months after the onset of illness. If the antigen is present after 3 months, the person is likely to be a chronic carrier [33]. This antigen was formerly identified as the hepatitis associated antigen (HAA) or Australian antigen but HB_sAg antigen is the currently accepted terminology. The antibody anti-HB_sAg (formerly anti-HAA) may also be detected. A core antigen known as HB_cAg may also be present.

Various liver function tests are important

not only in diagnosing the presence of hepatitis but also in evaluating the patient's progress. Particularly important are tests evaluating transaminase levels in the serum, alkaline phosphatase, serum bilirubin, and the prothrombin time, all of which are usually elevated. Other tests are the serum albumin, which is usually lowered, and ammonia levels, which are elevated in impending hepatic coma.

Hepatitis A is believed to be the cause of communitywide outbreaks of hepatitis. The causative agent, a filterable virus, is carried most often in the stools of infected individuals and is spread through contaminated food and water. Contaminated milk, various foods, shellfish, and polluted water have been implicated most often. Transmission occurs less often via inoculations and blood transfusions from infected persons and possibly via respiratory secretions. It is apparent that two different viruses are involved in the two types of hepatitis, because immunity to one of the types does not appear to provide immunity to the other. Recently scientists were able to visualize the causative virus in hepatitis A, using immune electronmicroscopy techniques.

The incubation period of hepatitis A is usually between 2 to 6 weeks, with an average of 4, and the onset is usually acute although the disease process is often mild. Mortality in this type of hepatitis is low. When people are known to have been in close and continuous contact with infected persons, prophylaxis with immune serum globulin (ISG) may be recommended. There is controversy over the value of prophylactic immunization; however, it does seem to lessen the severity of the disease even if it does not prevent its occurrence. Other characteristics of hepatitis A are its seasonal occurrence, predominantly in the autumn and winter.

Hepatitis B is characterized by a variable clinical picture and a mortality rate as high as 10 percent. The incubation period is 40 to 180 days, but commonly 60 to 90. There is no seasonal pattern and all ages are affected. Transmission is primarily via the parenteral route, and possibly via the feces, saliva, and various body secretions [45a]. The increased incidence of hepatitis B appears to be related to widespread drug use and the use of contaminated needles by groups of addicts. An increased incidence of hepatitis B occurs in renal dialysis and in cancer units in general hospitals, with hepatitis taking its toll on patients already weakened by disease. Hepatitis B also occurs often among hospital personnel, particularly those employed on dialysis units; the incidence appears to be related to puncture of the skin with needles or equipment contaminated by patients with clinical or subclinical hepatitis (or by introducing organisms into the mouth via inadequately washed hands contaminated with blood).

A high incidence of hepatitis is also reported in institutionalized patients with Down's syndrome. Ear piercing with inadequately sterilized instruments recently has been implicated [37]. Transmission of hepatitis B has also been reported in dental offices, where the disease has evidently been transmitted from small cuts or abrasions in the dentist's hands or from inadequately sterilized instruments [41]. Immune serum globulin administration is not generally considered useful in preventing or ameliorating effects of hepatitis B in persons who have come in contact with carriers or with the clinical disease [35].

Treatment and nursing care of patients with viral hepatitis is supportive and symptomatic. Currently, no specific chemotherapy, antiserum, or vaccine is available for either A or B viral hepatitis. Bed rest, or at least limited activity, is recommended until symptoms and signs of hepatic dysfunction have subsided. Monitoring of liver enzymes (alkaline phosphatase, SGOT, SGPT, and LDH), prothrombin, and bilirubin is done at least biweekly to evaluate the progress of the disease.

High carbohydrate diets to prevent glycogen depletion are indicated. Protein is necessary for nitrogen balance, but is usually not recommended over 20 gm daily due to the potential for hepatic coma. Patients often are unable to tolerate fatty foods. Anorexia is often present, and the nurse is challenged to encourage the patient to eat an adequate caloric intake. Antiemetics prior to meals may be necessary, and small frequent feedings rather than three large meals are usually better tolerated.

Fatigue is a lingering symptom; adequate rest periods and conservation of energy are encouraged. Mental depression is often present, especially if convalescence is prolonged; recovery from the disease may take as long as

4 months. The nurse must provide emotional support and diversionary activities as the patient is often discouraged with delayed progress and continued symptoms. The patient is often concerned about interruption of work or school. Economic and personal factors may be a source of constant worry and may interfere with needed rest. Although sedatives or tranquilizers may be indicated in some cases, barbiturates and tranquilizers such as chlorpromazine (Thorazine) and prochlorperazine (Compazine) are contraindicated, due to their known toxic effects on the liver. Many other drugs are also known to have hepatotoxic effects. Nurses caring for patients with hepatitis and other types of liver disease should develop the practice of checking drug information on all medications administered to these patients to determine their potential for hepatotoxicity. Ingestion of alcohol is also contraindicated.

Vitamin supplements, particularly vitamin K, may be necessary. Failure of vitamin K administration to correct prothrombin time abnormalities is a sign of severe hepatic injury and is considered a reliable index of potential hepatic coma [35a]. The nurse should take special precautions in avoiding trauma in patients with bleeding tendencies and prolonged prothrombin time levels. Patients should be observed for signs of bleeding through any orifice or of subcutaneous bleeding. Although controversial, steroids have been used in the treatment of viral hepatitis to hasten recovery and to relieve symptoms.

Pruritus can be an annoying symptom during the icteric stage of hepatitis. Calamine lotion applications and diluted soda bicarbonate soaks to the skin may be helpful. Soaps tend to aggravate itching. Antihistamines and diphenhydramine (Benadryl) may be prescribed. Cholestyramine (Questran) may also be prescribed. Questran binds bile acids in the intestine and prevents their reabsorption. Nausea and constipation are frequently associated with the drug. Questran comes in a dry powder form, which must be mixed with water or other fluids before ingestion. Since the drug may also bind other drugs, it should not be given at the same time with other medications. If pruritus is severe and scratching is persistent, the patient's nails should be cut short to prevent trauma to the skin.

Prevention of the spread of hepatitis is centered on preventing cross contamination and transmission of the causative organism. Control measures include the education of the patient, family, and personnel, about the disease and how it is transmitted.

Although a private room and separate toilet facilities are preferred for the patient with hepatitis, adults can be adequately isolated in multiple patient rooms if the patient and roommates are thoroughly instructed in good personal hygiene and meticulous hand-washing techniques. Gowns and gloves are usually worn by personnel when they are likely to come in contact with either blood or excreta of the patient with hepatitis. Respiratory precautions are indicated when caring for patients with viral hepatitis who have copious nasopharyngeal secretions or require frequent suctioning. Because the virus can be transmitted in the saliva, disposable dishes are preferred. If the patient is being cared for at home during the infectious period, a dishwasher will be adequate for cleaning dishes. Linens are changed as soon as they are soiled by either oral or fecal drainage and are placed in separate isolation bags. Patients should be taught how to use tissues properly for either coughing or spitting and how to properly discard them. The nurse should also instruct family members and friends who visit the patient about these measures and advise them to avoid kissing the patient because of the danger of transmission.

Disposable needles are used for any injections, and the nurse should take precautions to avoid accidental punctures. Needles are placed in puncture-resistant containers, and syringes into impervious bags for subsequent incineration or autoclaving prior to disposal [32].

It is important for obstetrical nurses to remember that both hepatitis A and B can be transmitted to the fetus through the placenta of an affected mother or one who is a carrier. In addition, transmission may occur during the delivery of the baby.

All these precautions are applicable to patients with either type of active hepatitis, since it has been proved that hepatitis B can also be transmitted by feces, urine, saliva, or semen as well as by parenteral inoculation. Feces from patients with hepatitis A are not usually infectious 2 to 3 weeks after onset of jaundice. Isolation precautions other than proper hand washing are usually not necessary after that time.

The incidence of transfusion-associated hepatitis B has been decreased by requiring the testing of every unit of blood for transfusions. Testing of all units of blood for the presence of HB_sAg antigen is one of the current requirements of the American Association of Blood Banks. Adequate surveillance of HB_sAg positive patients and staff personnel is necessary. A chronic carrier may not have overt evidence of hepatic disease. However, it is important to recognize that not all HB_sAg positive persons spread infection. Transmission of the disease is related to many factors including personal hygiene, aseptic technique, and the use of protective clothing.

Measures for control of hepatitis A are oriented to communitywide education regarding proper personal hygiene, public health monitoring of persons handling food, promotion of proper sanitation methods, and prevention of water pollution.

Although the majority of patients with viral hepatitis recover, some patients develop either persistent or chronic active hepatitis; a few develop fulminating hepatitis. **Chronic persistent hepatitis** varies in its pattern and severity. Some patients have prolonged jaundice, hepatomegaly, and elevated transaminase levels beyond 4 to 6 months. Liver biopsy is indicated and usually demonstrates inflammation limited to the portal tracts. Spontaneous recovery usually occurs eventually without specific treatment. **Chronic active hepatitis,** also known as chronic aggressive hepatitis, reflects necrosis, lymphatic infiltration, and fibrosis and may lead to cirrhosis. Liver biopsy shows a pattern of inflammation extending beyond the portal tracts with necrosis of surrounding hepatocytes [35a]. Corticosteroids have been useful in improving the prognosis in this type of hepatitis.

Fulminating viral hepatitis, also known as acute yellow atrophy, results in hepatic failure. It is an uncommon but very serious condition most frequently associated with hepatitis B rather than with hepatitis A. There is a high mortality rate in this disease, regardless of the mode of therapy used. Typically, hepatic failure occurs within 8 weeks of the onset of the illness; jaundice, hemorrhages (especially in the gastrointestinal tract), neurologic manifestations, and symptoms of renal failure become evident and the patient rapidly progresses into coma.

Treatment is generally supportive and symptomatic. Fluid and electrolyte replacement and nasogastric tube feedings are indicated to provide adequate caloric intake and to prevent fluid and electrolyte imbalance. Proteins are withheld as long as symptoms of encephalopathy are present. Purgatives, enemas, and neomycin therapy are utilized to decrease intestinal bacterial growth and thereby restrict formation of ammonia. Although use of steroids is controversial, many physicians prescribe intravenous hydrocortisone and later oral prednisone in fulminating hepatitis. Hyperimmune human gamma globulin has been prescribed in fulminating hepatitis, but recent studies have not substantiated its value in these situations [45].

When patients do not respond to conventional bowel sterilization and fluid and electrolyte replacement, exchange blood transfusions are indicated. The treatment is used to remove ammonia, bilirubin, and other toxic substances from the blood; fresh heparinized blood rather than citrated blood is used for this procedure. Plasmapheresis may also be used. In a few centers, extracorporeal liver perfusion (using pig livers) has also been utilized.

Nursing care is oriented to supportive nursing measures and protection of the patient who is in coma. These patients are highly susceptible to bacterial infections, especially in the urinary and respiratory tract. Position changes, adequate suctioning, prevention of decubitus formation, and meticulous oral hygiene as well as other important measures required for the unconscious patient are all necessary elements of nursing care. Even though these patients may have periods of agitation and extreme restlessness, sedation is avoided due to the liver's inability to detoxify these pharmacologic substances.

Toxic Hepatitis

Toxic hepatitis results in liver necrosis as a response to various toxic agents. These agents include halothane anesthesia, which has been found to cause a hypersensitivity reaction. Carbon tetrachloride is one of several industrial inhalants that have also been implicated in toxic hepatitis.

It is well recognized that alchohol is a hepatotoxic drug, although only 10 to 25 percent of chronic alcoholics develop cirrhosis. Alcoholic hepatitis develops in persons with a long history of heavy drinking. Alcohol is metabolized primarily in the liver, where it is converted to acetaldehyde and then acetate for oxidation to carbon dioxide and water in extrahepatic tissues. It has been shown that fat accumulation and ultrastructural changes occur with alcohol consumption. Genetic factors and other unknown factors appear to cause the liver to respond abnormally to alcohol and other agents.

A variety of drugs have proved to cause either a hepatic or cholestatic type of liver dysfunction. Erythromycin, chloramphenicol, sulfonamides, isoniazid (INH), and chlorpromazine (Thorazine) are only a few of the many drugs that have hepatotoxic effects. Although some patients develop only mild symptoms reflecting liver necrosis, others develop a fuminating form that can be fatal. Supportive and symptomatic treatment is the only approach currently available, in addition to elimination of the causative agent. Prevention of this disease process must be oriented to avoidance of drugs and agents known to be hepatotoxic to susceptible persons.

Liver Abscess

Liver abscess develops as a collection of leukocytes, liquefied liver cells, and bacteria usually resulting from abscess formation in other sites of the gastrointestinal tract, with transport of emboli via the portal circulation. High fever, chills, jaundice, painful hepatomegaly, and anemia are usually present. A toxic state may follow, and death results if adequate chemotherapy is not initiated. The type of chemotherapy is dependent on the causative organism. Surgical drainage of the abscess may also be indicated.

Liver Cirrhosis

The term **cirrhosis** refers to chronic degeneration of liver tissue with destruction of hepatic cells and formation of extensive dense fibrous scar tissue. Proliferation of fibrous tissue around the hepatic vessels causes compression of blood, lymph, and bile channels. These changes result in increased pressure in the portal circulation (portal hypertension), ascites, splenomegaly, hepatic encephalopathy, and jaundice. As fibrotic tissue forms, the liver becomes smaller and firmer. Its surface becomes rough as regenerated hepatic cells create small nodules on the liver.

Liver cirrhosis is most frequently associated with alcoholism, but also with malnutrition and protein deficiency, hepatitis, and other types of infectious processes, biliary duct disease, and chemical toxins. Cirrhosis due to nutritional deficiencies and alcoholism is referred to as **Laennec's cirrhosis** (portal or atrophic cirrhosis). Prolonged alcohol intake leads to fat accumulation in the liver and distortion of parenchymal cells, causing destructive alterations of the mitochondria and other ultrastructural changes [44]. Early fat accumulation is a reversible condition; if abstinence from alcohol and adequate protein intake is assured, accumulated fat is rapidly mobilized from the liver and further liver damage is prevented. Although the direct hepatotoxic effect of alcohol has been demonstrated, factors in the development of cirrhosis are still not clear. Many alcoholics do not develop cirrhosis whereas others develop cirrhosis even when maintaining an adequate and nutritious diet. Apparently genetic and hypersensitivity factors are also related to the onset of cirrhosis. Cirrhosis may also occur in the nonalcoholic after severe viral hepatitis, when there has been extensive necrosis and scarring. This type of cirrhosis is called **postnecrotic cirrhosis.**

Biliary cirrhosis is an uncommon type associated with cholestasis and obstruction to the flow of bile. It is usually associated with obstruction of the extrahepatic bile ducts by a stone or stricture. It is found primarily in middle-aged females with a history of gallstones and is associated with hypercholesterolemia. **Congestive cirrhosis** (cardiac cirrhosis) is associated with severe and prolonged hepatic congestion resulting from congestive heart failure, pericarditis, and rheumatic heart disease. Congestive cirrhosis improves if the underlying cause is corrected.

Regardless of the cause, an insidious onset of signs and symptoms of impaired liver function reflects the progression of cirrhotic changes over a period of years. Liver function tests demonstrate increasingly severe abnormalities. Commonly occurring symptoms include vague abdominal pain, nausea, vomiting, a palpable nodular liver, jaundice, splenomegaly, ascites, edema, hemorrhagic tendencies, palmar erythema, caput medusae, spider nevi, gynecomastia, and testicular atrophy. Symptoms will vary, depending on the severity of the disease.

Treatment and nursing care of the patient depend on the extent of liver damage. Care is supportive and symptomatic to promote liver cell regeneration and prevent complications. A diet high in calories, protein, and vitamins is indicated to improve nutrition; fluid and electrolyte replacement is usually necessary. Sodium is restricted if edema or ascites is present. Special skin care is necessary to prevent skin breakdown of edematous tissues. Daily weights, intake and output recording, and diuretic therapy are initiated. Total abstinence from alcohol is essential. Protein is eliminated from the diet in the presence of neurologic signs or elevated levels of serum ammonia. Prolonged prothrombin times require observation for bleeding and protection from trauma. Potentially toxic drugs such as barbiturates, opiates, and chlorpromazine are avoided because they require inactivation by the liver. The patient should be protected from sources of infection. Signs of impending coma, neurologic changes, and an increased tendency to bleed are reported promptly.

Limited ambulation and other activity are allowed in uncomplicated cirrhosis. Bed rest is required in advanced cirrhosis in order to reduce the metabolic demands on the liver and to conserve energy. Patients with advanced cirrhosis are easily fatigued and generally very weak. The success of the treatment and supportive therapy depends on the patient's adherence to the therapeutic regimen, including abstinence from alcohol. If the patient does not adhere to the regimen, or if hepatic damage is far advanced before treatment is initiated, many complications can occur.

Portal Hypertension

Portal hypertension is a major complication of cirrhosis of the liver. It results from any condition that impedes the flow of blood from the liver. Obstructions to blood flow may occur within the portal vein itself, sinusoidal or postsinusoidal channels, or the hepatic veins; the condition may also arise from obstruction of the inferior vena cava. Obstruction of the hepatic venous outflow due to thrombosis of the hepatic veins is referred to as the Budd-Chiari Syndrome. Obstruction within the hepatic vessels results from fibrosis, which compresses the sinusoids and hepatic vessels. Normally portal venous pressure is less than 20 cm of water, but is increased in varying degrees depending on the severity of obstruction to the flow.

Collateral circulatory channels develop to bypass the hepatic obstruction and to allow blood to empty into the systemic circulation. These channels usually occur at the cardia of the stomach, the esophagus, the periumbilical veins (resulting in caput medusae), and in the hemorrhoidal veins. These vessels become dilated, and since they are fragile, they are vulnerable to hemorrhage as pressure is increased.

Portal hypertension results in bleeding varices, ascites, congestive splenomegaly, and congestion in other organs of the gastrointestinal system. **Hepatorenal syndrome** refers to associated oliguria and azotemia.

Esophageal Varices

Esophageal varices result when normal channels for portal blood flow are compromised by liver disease and portal hypertension. They are frequently associated with liver cirrhosis, but also may result from thrombosis of the hepatic vein and veno-occlusive disease. The varices contain minimal elastic and supportive tissue and therefore readily become distended, fragile, and susceptible to rupture. Varices most frequently occur at the lower end of the esophagus, but may also occur in the upper esophagus and stomach.

Gastrointestinal bleeding from esophageal varices is usually distinguished from gastric ulcer bleeding by the absence of pain and epigastric tenderness. The presence of cirrhotic symptoms such as ascites, spider angiomas, and palmar erythema also supports the diagnosis of esophageal varices as the cause of bleeding. If the cause is not known, esophagoscopy may be indicated to determine the cause, unless the situation and the patient's condition do not permit delay of treatment for this procedure.

Variceal bleeding may be caused by increased abdominal venous pressure (associated with physical exertion), mechanical trauma (abrasions from swallowing poorly chewed food), coughing, nausea, and vomiting. Large amounts of blood are rapidly lost by hematemesis; a high mortality rate is associated with variceal hemorrhage. In addition to hemorrhage, anemia, and shock, bleeding varices further compromise hepatic blood flow and cause further hepatic necrosis. Blood from esophageal varices may reach the intestine and increased nitrogen absorption results, leading to hepatic coma.

Bleeding esophageal varices are a medical emergency requiring immediate intervention. Maintenance of a patent airway is a primary concern of the nurse caring for such a patient, as there is danger of aspiration during vomiting and accumulation of blood in the oropharynx. The most commonly used emergency measure for controlling massive hemorrhage from varices is esophageal tamponade with the Sengstaken-Blakemore tube. This tube has three lumens for (1) gastric aspiration, (2) inflation of esophageal balloon, and (3) inflation of gastric balloon. Each balloon is checked for leaks and patency prior to insertion. After insertion, each lumen is individually marked and identified to prevent accidental deflation or inflation of the wrong lumen. In some settings, a Linton tube, which has an integral lumen for aspiration, is preferred.

Prior to insertion of the tube, the patient is instructed in how to swallow the tube. The stomach is often lavaged through a Ewald tube first and then the lubricated Sengstaken-Blakemore tube is inserted via the nose into the stomach (Fig. 7-8). The gastric balloon is inflated with 200 ml of air after it is positioned at the gastroesophageal junction. Sometimes, ice water is instilled into the gastric balloon to further control bleeding. The esophageal balloon is inflated with air to a pressure of only 20 to 40 mm Hg. Pressure is usually maintained for 24 to 48 hours and then gradually decreased. Often the esophageal balloon is deflated within 24 hours, whereas the gastric balloon is deflated 24 hours later [6]. In some protocols even after deflation the tube is left in place for immediate reinflation if necessary. A primary responsibility of the nurse is to maintain the position of the tube and the prescribed pressure. The tube is carefully secured externally to prevent excessive traction or movement; one approach is by having the patient wear a rigid face mask or helmet, which is designed like a standard

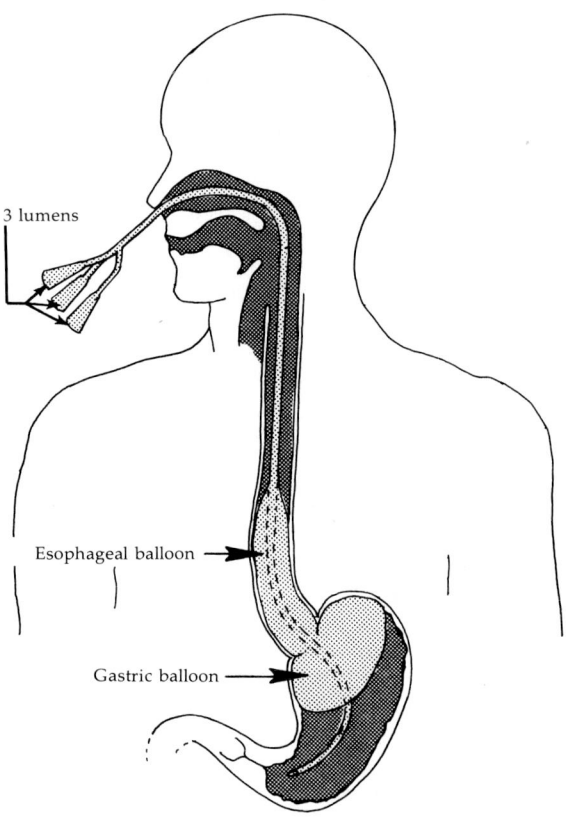

Figure 7-8
Placement of the Sengstaken-Blakemore tube.

football helmet and to which the tube is fixed [6].

Excessive and prolonged pressure causes great discomfort for the patient and may cause ulcerations of the esophagus and gastric mucosa. The manometers attached to the esophagogastric tube are checked frequently. There is danger of rupture of the balloon causing displacement and potential asphyxiation due to obstruction of the airway. If this complication occurs, both of the balloons are deflated by cutting the outside tubings and the entire tube is removed. Another Sengstaken-Blakemore tube is then inserted to prevent further variceal hemorrhage.

The third lumen of the tube facilitates aspiration of blood and gastric secretions. Accurate measurement and reporting of the amount and characteristics of the secretions are essential in determining blood loss. The inflated esophageal balloon prevents the swallowing of saliva, so the patient must be assisted in expectorating frequently. Frequent oral and pharyngeal suctioning is indicated if the patient is unable to expectorate the secretions. Often another small nasogastric tube is inserted in the opposite nostril to drain oral secretions that may collect just above the inflated esophageal balloon: this tube is connected to intermittent suction.

The nurse should place the patient in a semi-Fowler's position to promote ventilation and to combat gastric acid reflux. Frequent and thorough oropharyngeal suctioning to remove emesis and bronchial secretions is required to prevent airway obstruction. Vital signs are assessed frequently and accurate records of intake and output are maintained. Sedation is often necessary to counteract restlessness, but medications are used with caution because of the possibility of hepatic coma related to the diminished detoxifying ability of the liver. Oxygen therapy also may be indicated.

Breathing through the mouth and the accumulation of old blood cause oral discomfort and odor; frequent oral hygiene is necessary for the patient's comfort. Bed rest is maintained to prevent recurrence of bleeding and exhaustion. The patient requires assurance that his or her needs will be met. The critical and sudden onset of hemorrhage is a frightening experience, and the fear of choking and aspiration is ever present. The patient needs the psychological comfort and assurance of being observed closely. The patient is also observed for complications that may occur with the use of the Sengstaken-Blakemore tube. In addition to dislodgement and asphyxiation, aspiration pneumonia and esophageal perforation may occur.

Following insertion of the Sengstaken-Blakemore tube and control of esophageal bleeding, liver function assessment and fluid and electrolyte and blood replacement are continued. Vitamin K is usually administered to promote prothrombin synthesis. In addition the intestinal tract must be emptied of blood in order to prevent ammonia intoxication and hepatic coma; magnesium sulfate may be administered, and saline enemas are given as soon as the patient's condition permits. Intestinal antimicrobial agents such as neomycin are given to decrease intestinal bacterial action on the blood; they may be administered via the nasogastric tube while it is in place. But more commonly, these agents are initiated after the nasogastric tube is removed.

Vasopressin (Pitressin) may be prescribed to lower the portal venous pressure by promoting vasoconstriction of the splanchnic arterial system as an additional measure to control bleeding from esophageal varices. It may be administered via intravenous infusion or by selective angiography of the superior mesenteric artery. The nurse should observe the patient for abdominal discomfort, cramping, facial pallor, and involuntary bowel evacuation, which are anticipated effects of the drug.

If bleeding cannot be controlled by either of these two measures, emergency surgery may be indicated. Transesophageal ligation of varices has been used in some cases, but has not proved to be very effective. Emergency portocaval shunting may be required if bleeding cannot be controlled by other means. The weakened patient is, however, a poor surgical risk and emergency portocaval shunting carries a high incidence of mortality. The preferred method of treating esophageal varices is by preventive therapy and elective portocaval shunting after bleeding has been controlled and the patient's nutritional and physical status has improved. The surgical procedure is done to create systemic venous shunting and thus lower portal pressure. It is a complicated procedure and requires extensive preoperative and postoperative management to prevent hepatic failure and fluid and electrolyte imbalance.

Portasystemic Shunting Procedures

Several surgical approaches are utilized to divert blood from the portal system into the vena cava. Probably the most common is the **portacaval shunt,** in which an anastomosis is created between the portal vein and the inferior vena cava (Fig. 7-9). Portal decompression results in a decrease in portal pressure, an increase in hepatic arterial flow, and a reduction in the pressure within the collateral circulation channels. In this manner, recurrence of bleeding from esophageal varices is prevented. Another type of shunting procedure is the **splenorenal shunt,** in which splenectomy is accomplished and an anastomosis is created between the splenic vein

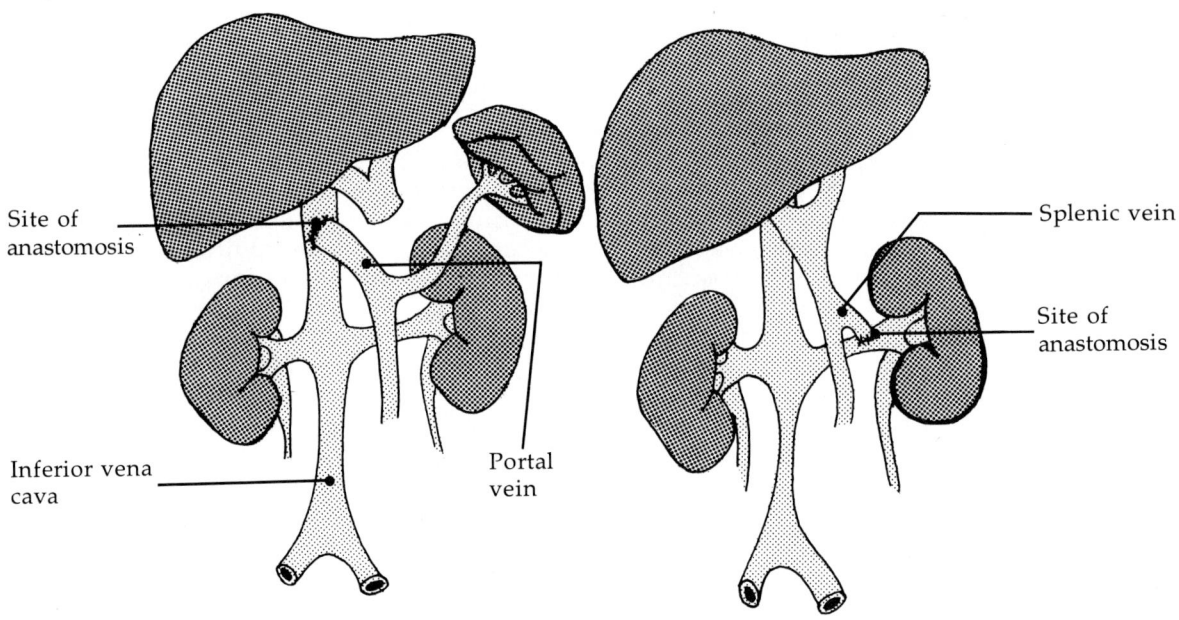

Figure 7-9
Portasystemic shunts.

and the left renal vein. Some surgeons prefer this latter approach because it is associated with a lower incidence of encephalopathy. Other variations are the portarenal shunt and the mesocaval shunt.

Careful nursing observation is important for detection of early signs of several complications that may occur postoperatively. Hemorrhage may occur due to leakage of the anastomosis or of other ligated vessels. Respiratory complications may occur due to the patient's reluctance to breathe deeply. Nursing care of these patients is similar to that described in Chapter 1 for patients having abdominal surgery. In addition, the nurse must be aware of the implications of the patient's impaired liver function and the potential for hepatic coma after shunting procedures. Hepatic encephalopathy is the most important complication of portasystemic shunt procedures. It is difficult to predict which patients are likely to develop the complication, so the nurse must observe the patient carefully for neurologic changes and increased lethargy typical of impending hepatic coma. Neomycin may be administered to prevent the onset of coma by decreasing the production of ammonia by the intestinal flora. The nurse should also observe the patient for the onset of jaundice, which indicates deterioration of hepatic function. Ascites may also appear postoperatively, but this is usually a temporary complication. Shunt thrombosis may occur, resulting in failure of the shunting procedure. Although shunting procedures reduce the incidence of recurrent variceal hemorrhages, they do not resolve the underlying liver disease nor prolong life expectancy, unless the patient strictly adheres to medical management and abstains from ingesting alcohol.

Ascites

Ascites is the abnormal accumulation of fluid in the peritoneal cavity (see color insert Figure 5 on page 1078B). It develops from transudation of fluid from the mesenteric veins and by lymphatic seepage from the liver. Transudation results from portal hypertension as well as from hypoproteinemia. Water and sodium retention also contribute to the condition. The latter phenomenon is related to the failure of the liver to inactivate the antidiuretic hormone and aldosterone.

The patient with ascites has marked abdominal distention and demonstrates symptoms of dehydration and fatigue. Dilated vessels are visible on the abdomen. Excessive distention causes respiratory disturbances, pain and discomfort, and compression of abdominal viscera. In these situations, the patient is most comfortable in a low or semi-Fowler's position, which tends to facilitate ventilation. The abdominal girth is measured daily to determine whether ascites is increasing in severity. To assure conformity in measurement, the abdomen can be marked to indicate the line of measurement. Daily weights are also taken to detect increased fluid retention.

The patient is usually placed on a low sodium diet as an initial means of controlling fluid accumulation. The nurse should teach the purpose of the diet and advise the patient of the types of foods to be eliminated. Lemon juice, vinegar, pepper, and parsley are substances that can be added to foods to make them more palatable in the absence of salt. The nurse should also be aware of medications or other sources of sodium that the patient might be receiving. Certain antacid medications, for example, contain sodium. Aluminum hydroxide gel (Amphojel) and other preparations with low sodium content are utilized.

Diuretic therapy may be instituted along with a low sodium diet in order to increase sodium and water excretion. However, serious side effects (such as precipitation of hepatic coma) due to electrolyte imbalances may occur in the patient with cirrhosis, and close observation of the patient is of paramount importance. Precise intake and output records, daily weights, and regular assessment of serum electrolyte levels are essential; potassium supplements may be necessary. The nurse should particularly watch for symptoms of hypokalemia and hyponatremia when a regimen of dietary sodium restriction and diuretic therapy is used.

When these measures fail to adequately control ascites and respiratory and abdominal distress increase, paracentesis may be required. This procedure is used as a last resort because of its many disadvantages. Each time fluid is removed in this manner, there is a loss of body proteins, sodium, and potassium via the ascitic fluid. Hypovolemia may also result from removal of large amounts of ascitic fluid, and paracentesis may predispose to the onset of hepatic coma, due to electrolyte losses and hypovolemia. If fluid is removed too rapidly, the decreased pressure may cause massive vasodilatation and shock. All these factors should be kept in mind as the nurse assists the physician in the procedure and cares for the patient during and after the procedure.

Prior to paracentesis the nurse should carefully explain the purpose and steps in the procedure and should obtain baseline data on vital signs. The patient is asked to void before the treatment is begun in order to prevent injury to the bladder with insertion of the trocar. The patient is then usually placed in a sitting position at the side of the bed with the feet supported on a stool and is draped to expose the abdomen. The puncture site is prepared with antiseptic solution and local anesthetic infiltration. A receptacle for receiving the ascitic fluid is made available. A small incision is made below the umbilicus, and a trocar with an obturator is inserted to penetrate the peritoneum. The obturator is then removed and a rubber tubing is attached for removal of the fluid by gravity flow. The fluid is removed slowly in order to prevent too rapid a decrease in abdominal pressure, which could result in circulatory and respiratory complications. The patient is observed closely during the procedure for symptoms of tachycardia, respiratory difficulty, and dizziness. When the procedure is completed the trocar is withdrawn and a dressing is applied to the puncture site. The amount of fluid removed is measured and the amount and characteristics of the fluid are recorded. Specimens of the fluid are sent to the laboratory for examination for protein, bacteria, electrolytes, and specific gravity.

The patient is kept on bed rest for several hours after the procedure and vital signs are monitored every 15 minutes for an hour and then at regular intervals for the next 24 hours. The patient is usually exhausted after the procedure and requires a quiet and restful environment. Usually the puncture site closes spontaneously, but in some instances leakage of ascitic fluid may continue.

Hepatic Coma

Important metabolic functions of the body are carried out in the liver, and hepatic failure affects almost every known synthesis and function. **Hepatic coma** is the state of severe liver disease in which the patient progresses from stupor to deep coma and usually death. The term **hepatic encephalopathy** is also used to describe cerebral dysfunction associated with liver disease. Cirrhosis of the liver is the most common cause of hepatic coma, but it may also occur as a complication of severe viral hepatitis, toxic hepatitis, biliary obstruction, or electrolyte imbalances, or after paracentesis or shunting procedures. The coma results from failure of the liver to detoxify harmful substances from the circulation. The major causative substances are ammonia, certain anesthetic agents, and drugs like morphine.

Normally the liver converts ammonia, one of the by-products of protein metabolism, to a less toxic form before it reaches the brain via the bloodstream. When the severely diseased liver is no longer able to carry out this function, ammonia entering the brain causes toxic effects on both glial and nerve cells. Coma may also be precipitated when certain events result in the formation of large amounts of ammonia in the bowel, such as excessive protein intake, massive bleeding into the gastrointestinal tract, and the ingestion of ammonium salts or diuretics.

The nurse should be alert for early symptoms of impending hepatic coma in susceptible patients and should report symptoms promptly so that appropriate treatment can be initiated. The nurse should become suspicious of impending hepatic coma even in the presence of minimal mental changes; these changes often progress to dulling of mental acuity, slurred speech, and altered behavioral patterns. Writing ability becomes impaired and can be used to assess neurologic changes. Muscular twitching and poor muscular coordination follow. Asterixis (liver flap) is a characteristic sign associated with impending hepatic coma. As the condition progresses, fetor hepaticus (a musty or sweetish odor) is detectable and the patient demonstrates confusion, restlessness, and irritability. It is at this point that sedation may erroneously be used, precipitating the onset of the coma.

Treatment in the early stages is focused on decreasing ammonia formation by reducing protein intake and inhibiting the bacterial action on protein substances in the bowel. (Ammonia is formed in the gastrointestinal tract by the action of bacteria on protein end products.) Fluid and electrolyte imbalances are corrected, with particular attention to glucose and potassium administration. Serum electrolyte levels are evaluated frequently. Administration of salt-poor albumin is often necessary as serum albumin levels decrease. Although exchange transfusions are used, they are less likely to be beneficial in advanced liver disease associated with hepatic coma. If oral intake is possible, concentrated fruit juices and other forms of simple carbohydrates are given. Colonic purges are instituted by ingestion of magnesium sulfate and by administering enemas; neomycin, kanamycin, or other bactericidal agents are administered to suppress bacterial action in the bowel. Oral purgatives and neomycin may be administered through a nasogastric tube, which is often placed when the patient develops hepatic coma. Lactulose, a nonabsorbable disaccharide, may also be prescribed. It reduces bacterial production of nitrogenous substances by acidifying the intestine and producing diarrhea [44].

The patient in hepatic coma requires intensive nursing care. Neurologic assessment is required at regular intervals and the nurse must provide for all supportive and protective functions required by an unconscious patient (see Chap. 11). The patient is aroused frequently to determine changes in the level of response as hepatic coma ensues. The patient is susceptible to skin breakdown due to inability to move as well as to edema, ascites, and jaundice. When coma is present more than 24 hours, the prognosis is poor and a fatal outcome is likely.

If the patient improves, fluid and electrolyte administration is continued, and dietary protein is slowly introduced but continually limited to 50 to 60 gm or less daily. Maintenance doses of neomycin are prescribed, and measures are taken to prevent constipation, by using stool softeners and appropriate dietary intake. Constipation may lead to increased bacterial action and ammonia formation. The patient is instructed about the importance of avoiding potassium depletion, and about the dangers of diuretics, sedatives, and opiates. Signs of impending hepatic coma are discussed, and in the event of these signs the patient and family are advised to promptly discontinue all protein intake and to seek medical assistance. Abstinence of alcohol, of course, is an essential component in any regimen of prevention of further hepatic damage. In selected patients, a colon-exclusion or colon-bypass procedure has been done to prevent recurrence of hepatic coma [31].

Hepatic Tumors
Although primary malignant tumors of the liver are rare, metastasis to the liver frequently occurs via the portal vein system, the

hepatic artery, and the lymphatics. Metastasis may also occur by direct extension from the ducts, gallbladder, stomach, and pancreas. Neoplasms may be of the parenchymal liver cells (hepatomas), of bile duct cells (cholangiomas), or both. Carcinoma and sarcoma may occur, although the former is more common. Metastases from primary hepatic tumors occur most commonly to the lung, but also to regional lymph nodes and the peritoneum. A fatal outcome within a year after onset of liver metastasis is the usual prognosis. A majority of patients with hepatic tumors have postnecrotic cirrhosis. Viral infections, hepatoxic agents (such as vinyl chloride), and nutritional factors are also considered predisposing factors.

Hepatoma is suspected in the presence of weight loss, extreme weakness, anemia, and hepatomegaly. Irregular surfaces and nodules of the liver may be detectable on palpation. Jaundice is present if biliary obstruction occurs; ascites results from portal obstruction as well as from neoplastic involvement of the peritoneal cavity. Abnormalities in the various liver function tests, as discussed earlier in this chapter, are usually present. Liver scanning, liver biopsy, and hepatic arteriography are valuable diagnostic procedures in detecting hepatic tumors. The last procedure is also helpful in defining the extent and location of the tumor and the vascular structure of the liver in preparation for surgical removal.

Hepatic lobectomy can be done when the hepatic tumor is localized or when metastasis is limited and the primary tumor can be completely excised. Total hepatic resection with liver transplantation can be done if a primary tumor is found in both the right and left lobes of the liver and other organs are not involved. (Hepatic resections and lobectomies are also done in liver trauma.) If the tumor is nonresectable, hepatic artery ligation with infusion of a chemotherapeutic agent is usually accomplished as a palliative measure. In this last approach, a catheter is left in place in the hepatic artery and is connected to an external pumping mechanism for subsequent instillation of a chemotherapeutic agent. Methotrexate and 5-fluorouracil are the agents commonly used.

Extensive and thorough preoperative preparation is essential. The patient needs much psychological support when considering the risks involved in this radical surgical procedure and also needs assistance in tolerating the extensive preparation required preoperatively. Extensive laboratory and roentgen studies are required. These tests must all be explained to the patient so that he or she will understand the techniques and the reasons they are necessary. The amount and type of information given depends on the desires, expectations and status of the individual patient.

Fluid and electrolyte and nutritional needs are identified and corrected. Mechanical and antibiotic preparation of the bowel is necessary to combat potential ammonia intoxication postoperatively. The patient is observed for bleeding tendencies associated with hepatic dysfunction. Measures to prevent trauma are instituted. The use of intramuscular injections should be minimized; adequate pressure must be applied to injection sites in order to prevent bleeding. Other aspects of preoperative preparation are those routinely accomplished and as described in Chapter 1.

Usually a thoracoabdominal approach is used for a right lobectomy whereas a large midline incision is usually made for a left lobectomy. A bilateral subcostal incision is used in some techniques. Adequate hemostasis is absolutely essential during the procedure; cold perfusion techniques and hypothermia are utilized. Hepatic resection has been done by the finger fracturing technique, which involves fixation of friable liver tissue with the fingers while isolating the vascular and ductal structures intrahepatically. A recently developed special hepatic clamp facilitates an almost bloodless field during the surgery. This clamp is used to crush the liver tissue and expose the vascular and ductal structures to direct vision [41]. Laser techniques have also been developed as another approach in managing hemostasis in hepatic surgery [34].

Hepatic surgery is radical surgery and requires intensive nursing care postoperatively. The patient is observed for complications related to increased hepatic dysfunction, hemorrhage, ammonia intoxication, and hepatic coma as well as to cardiopulmonary complications, infection, and bile peritonitis. The serum albumin level is markedly decreased for several days after extensive resection and requires daily replacement. Patency of the chest tubes connected to underwater seal drainage must be maintained. Patency of the nasogastric tube, and suctioning and the indwelling catheter must also be ensured. Coughing and deep breathing, position changes, and monitoring of vital signs, dressings, and essential equipment are all important aspects of nursing care. The patient needs much support to tolerate the discomfort, pain, and extensive equipment and monitoring associated with hepatic surgery. Depending on the status of hepatic function and vital signs, ambulation is increased gradually and postoperative care continues as for other major thoracic and abdominal surgery.

Liver transplantation is being done in several centers in the United States. Usually patients with primary brain tumors are preferred donors for liver transplants; discussion of this complicated procedure is beyond the scope of this book. In addition to intensive nursing care, as is required after any major thoracic or abdominal surgery, organ transplantation requires special preoperative and postoperative measures including protection of the patient from potential infections, complications related to immunosuppression therapy, and observations for rejection of the transplant.

Alcoholism

Because alcoholic intake is frequently associated with hepatic dysfunction and cirrhosis, it is necessary to discuss some general aspects of alcoholism. It is estimated that about 9 million persons in the United States are afflicted with alcoholism or problem drinking. Although alcoholism has frequently been considered a moral or criminal problem, it is increasingly being viewed as an illness and a complex medical, social, and environmental problem. A major impact for this change in attitude is the Comprehensive Alcohol Abuse and Alcoholism Prevention, Treatment, and Rehabilitation Act of 1970. This Act established the National Institute on Alcohol Abuse and Alcoholism within the National Institute of Mental Health and established a National Advisory Council on Alcohol Abuse and Alcoholism. It also required that comprehensive state health plans include services for the prevention and treatment of alcohol abuse and alcoholism and also prohibited discrimination by hospitals in regard to admitting alcoholics for treatment.

Alcohol abuse causes serious health problems. In addition to the nutritional deficiencies and hepatic effects already described, laryngitis, gastritis, chronic diarrhea, pancreatitis, neurologic disorders such as neuropathies, and cardiac disorders such as cardiomyopathy, are associated with chronic and excessive use of alcohol. The damaging effects of alcoholism on the alcoholic's psychological status as well as on that of the family cannot be overemphasized.

Sudden cessation of alcoholic intake for the habitual excessive drinker leads to withdrawal symptoms. Within 12 to 48 hours following abrupt cessation or lessened alcohol intake, anxiety and irritability and, eventually, delirium tremens occur. Medical intervention is essential to calm the patient and to specifically treat associated illnesses. **Delirium tremens** (DTs) is a serious and sometimes fatal condition characterized by confusion, trembling, fever, hallucinations, and sometimes convulsions. The use of tranquilizers, management of caloric and fluid and electrolyte balance, and supportive nursing care are important components of required intervention during the crisis period. The use of sedatives must be accomplished judiciously to avert complications related to the inability of the liver to detoxify these substances. Diazepam (Valium) and chlordiazepoxide hydrochloride (Librium) are the most frequently used sedatives for alcoholic withdrawal and in detoxification programs. Paraldehyde, once the standard drug for DTs, is still used in some settings. Phenytoin sodium (Dilantin) may also be used to prevent withdrawal seizures.

The nurse should convey a quiet, calm, and nonjudgmental attitude when working with a patient having withdrawal symptoms. A calm attitude is helpful in promoting a sense of security for the patient. During this time the nurse must observe the patient closely for increasing anxiety and agitation and other symptoms indicating the need for additional sedation. Safety must be provided because the patient is often confused and agitated and may become combative. Ataxia may interfere with the patient's ambulation and result in falls and injuries.

Alcoholic patients frequently have nutritional deficiencies requiring specific therapy and replacement. Protein supplements, electrolyte replacements including magnesium, and vitamin supplements (particularly thiamine) are essential. Adequate hydration and intake of carbohydrates are also important. The patient should be observed for hypoglycemia; orange juice, Gatorade, or other concentrated carbohydrates should be provided.

Withdrawal symptoms often occur unexpectedly in the hospital situation when the patient is being treated for other problems. Because the patient often denies he or she is an alcoholic, his or her pattern of drinking is not conveyed during history taking. The nurse must therefore learn to tactfully obtain information on alcoholic intake and must be alert to symptoms of alcoholism. Some of these symptoms include flushed face, trembling or sweaty hands, and signs such as palmar erythema and dilated peripheral blood vessels.

There are various approaches to treating the alcoholic person to correct his or her dependency on alcohol. The most successful incorporate a multidisciplinary approach with involvement of family members in the treatment program in order to elicit their support. Alcoholism is a family disease, and no member is immune to the deleterious effects of alcohol on family relationships.

Heavy drinking is viewed as a means by which an individual copes with severe underlying problems. Therapeutic programs are therefore most appropriately oriented to efforts in establishing other less destructive and more appropriate types of coping behavior. Special techniques sometimes used include the use of aversion therapy in which an emetic drug such as emetin hydrochloride or disulfiram (Antabuse) is used to establish aversion to the sight, smell, and taste of alcohol.

Long-term psychotherapy may be indicated. Support services are available from local Alcoholics Anonymous (AA) groups. These AA groups have proved to be effective resources for reinforcing the motivation of persons wanting to combat alcoholism. AA volunteers have assisted in helping alcoholics become sober in order to be able to use other services; the organization focuses on total abstinence as the basis of its program. A sponsor in the group provides support to the individual in avoiding temptation to indulge in alcohol. A strong group feeling is created with reward systems for avoiding alcohol. Some alcoholic persons require a completely structured environment, which is the basis for the development of various alcoholic rehabilitation centers.

Families should be advised of specific organizations such as Al-Anon, which provides support for family members, and Alateen, an organization oriented to assisting teenagers in a family with an alcoholic member. The nurse can be an important resource for providing encouragement and psychological support to both the alcoholic person and the family as well as being able to provide information on other resources.

Other Liver Disorders

Other less common forms of liver disease include those associated with disturbances in storage and deposits of substances in the liver. These include Wilson's disease, hemochromatosis, and amyloidosis.

Wilson's disease (hepatolenticular degeneration) is a familial disorder of copper storage. Copper, which is normally excreted in the bile, is retained in the liver, causing fibrosis. As necrosis occurs, copper is released into the serum and deposited in other tissues, particularly the kidneys and basal ganglia of the brain (lenticular). Copper deposits in the periphery of the cornea cause a classic sign known as Kaiser-Fleischer ring; a rusty brown ring visualized on the cornea. The wide variety of neurologic changes in Wilson's disease result in deformities, dysarthria, muscle wasting, and emotional disturbances. Early vague symptoms cause a delay in diagnosis, which is determined by measuring urine copper excretion and serum ceruloplasmin concentration. Specific treatment is the long-term administration of copper-chelating agents such as penicillamine.

Hemochromatosis is a rare disease of iron metabolism resulting in an accumulation of excess iron. It is associated with hepatic cirrhosis and pathologic changes in the pancreas, skin, and heart. Genetic and environmental factors such as prolonged administration of parenteral iron appear to predispose to increased iron absorption. Hemosiderosis is excessive deposits of iron on the liver due to prolonged use of parenteral iron.

Amyloidosis is the accumulation of amyloid in various body tissues including the liver, spleen, kidney, lung, and adrenal cortex. Amyloid is an almost insoluble glycoprotein. Amyloidosis is thought to be due to obscure metabolic disturbances. Although amyloidosis causes hepatomegaly, it may be of no consequence in some cases. On occasion, it is severe enough to cause jaundice and ascites. There is no specific treatment. Symptoms depend on the specific organ that is affected. When the heart is involved, death most often occurs from heart failure.

THE BILIARY TRACT

The biliary tract includes the hepatic duct, the cystic duct, the gallbladder, and the common bile duct. The **gallbladder,** a musculoelastic pouch with a capacity of 30 to 50 ml, is located on the undersurface of the liver. Its functions are to collect, concentrate, and store the bile that reaches it via the hepatic duct from the liver. Leading from the gallbladder is the cystic duct, which joins the hepatic duct to form the common bile duct. The latter duct joins the pancreatic duct at the ampulla of Vater, which opens into the duodenum. The sphincter of Oddi controls the opening at the ampulla of Vater and the flow of bile into the small intestine. The sphincter of Oddi is closed between meals, but opens during digestion as bile empties from both the gallbladder and the liver. Contraction of the gallbladder is stimulated by the release of the hormone **cholecystokinin,** which is secreted by the cells of the duodenal mucosa when food enters the duodenum. Other hormones that also stimulate bile flow are gastrin and glucagon.

The passage of bile into the duodenum is dependent on the tone of the sphincter of Oddi as well as on the regulation of pressure within the ductal system by the gallbladder. Contractions of the gallbladder and stimulation of the sphincter of Oddi are produced by epinephrine and cholinergic drugs such as neostigmine (Prostigmin). Morphine causes spasm of the sphincter and thus increases intraductal pressure. Anticholinergics such as atropine and propantheline bromide (Pro-Banthine) result in decreased tone of the gallbladder and decreased spasms of the sphincter of Oddi. In addition, psychic factors such as the sight, smell, or taste of food may stimulate the gallbladder. Decreased flow occurs with fear or excitement.

Assessment of the Patient

Nursing assessment of the patient is based on observing the patient for usual manifestations of disease of the extrahepatic biliary system. Signs and symptoms vary with the severity of the condition. Pain is a common symptom and is usually felt in the right upper quadrant or the epigastric region and is often referred to the subscapular region. The pain may be described as a persistent and dull ache or it may be severe and cramp-like. The latter type is termed **biliary colic.** The onset of pain in relation to food intake is usually characteristic of biliary tract disease. Digestive disturbances are associated with biliary tract disease and are demonstrated by the presence of anorexia, certain food intolerances (especially to fatty or fried foods), nausea, vomiting, eructation, flatulence, and distention; tenderness in the right side of the abdomen is often present. If the patient is not already jaundiced, the nurse should carefully examine the skin, sclera, and oral mucous membranes to determine the presence of impending jaundice and should note any complaints of pruritus. Obstruction of the biliary tract interrupts the flow of bile into the intestine and its reabsorption into the blood, resulting in obstructive jaundice. The color of the urine and the stool is noted, and the presence of steatorrhea is determined. Bile flow obstruction also results in disturbances in fat absorption, in the absence of bile salts in the small intestine. Fat-soluble vitamins, particularly vitamin K, are also ineffectively absorbed in the absence of bile. Vitamin K deficiencies result in reduced prothrombin levels and interfere with the normal clotting process. Thus the patient with obstructive jaundice frequently demonstrates bleeding tendencies. Fever and chills are frequently present when infection and inflammation occur within the gallbladder or bile ducts.

Diagnostic studies in suspected biliary tract disease are indicated to determine the patency of the tract and to determine the nature and degree of jaundice. Various roentgenographic techniques, as well as blood, urine, and stool examinations, are carried out.

Cholecystography is frequently indicated to detect gallbladder disorders. This x-ray procedure requires the administration of oral radiopaque dye (such as iopanoic acid tablets [Telepaque]) for visualization of the gallbladder. Since the gallbladder fills approximately 12 hours after the dye is ingested, the dye is given the evening before the examination. The tablets are taken at 5 minute intervals with minimal amounts of water; any emesis or problem in taking the tablets is reported to the physician. If the dye is not retained, the x-ray is cancelled. After a fat free diet given the evening before the x-ray, followed later by the oral dye administration, the patient is allowed nothing by mouth until the cholecystogram is completed in the morning. In addition, depending on institutional protocol, an enema or rectal suppository may be prescribed to facilitate visualization by adequate bowel preparation.

After the cholecystogram is completed, a fatty test meal may be given to stimulate the emptying of the gallbladder. This meal is followed by additional x-rays to check the patency of the ducts and gallbladder emptying. Other than this fatty test meal, when it is specifically ordered, no food or fluids are given the patient until the nurse has verified that the x-ray examination is completed.

In preparing the patient for this examination, the nurse should keep in mind that the iodine-based dye may cause reactions in susceptible persons. The history of the patient is checked for any indications of allergies, particularly to iodine. The physician and radiologist are notified if any problem is suspected. In addition, the nurse should keep in mind other tests that may be ordered for the patient and determine appropriate sequences for them. For example, the gallbladder x-rays should not be done until after tests involving measurement of iodine synthesis or metabolism such as thyroid function tests have been completed, if these have also been requested.

Cholecystography can demonstrate either a normally visualized gallbladder, a nonfilling of the gallbladder, obstruction of the bile ducts, or cholelithiasis. If the gallbladder cannot be visualized, the examination may be repeated to verify that inadequate preparation is not the reason for nonvisualization.

The gallbladder may also be visualized by means of intravenous injection of the radiopaque dye. This may be necessary if the patient cannot take the dye orally. In this case, the dye is injected intravenously about 10 minutes prior to the x-ray procedure.

Cholangiograms are used to visualize the biliary ductal system. The procedure is done by intravenous injection of the contrast medium with x-rays being taken as the liver excretes the dye through the bile ducts; excretion is usually completed within 4 hours. Preparation of the patient for intravenous cholangiography also requires fluid and food restriction to permit dye concentration. Cleansing enemas or laxatives are given the evening before the examination to empty the lower gastrointestinal tract. Cholangiography can also be accomplished during surgery and is usually indicated to detect residual filling defects or retained stones in the common or hepatic ducts during biliary tract surgery. The x-ray procedure may also be done postoperatively by injecting the dye through a T tube left in the common bile duct.

These two approaches to studying the gallbladder and biliary tracts are dependent on adequate functioning of the hepatic cells necessary to excrete the radiopaque dyes into the bile. Another technique, **percutaneous transhepatic cholangiography,** is effective regardless of the status of hepatic function, because the dye is injected directly into the biliary tract and permits visualization of the entire biliary system. The technique is also helpful in differentiating hepatocellular jaundice from extrahepatic jaundice and in locating biliary duct stones or neoplasms as well as for investigating gastrointestinal symptoms of patients who have had previous cholecystectomy.

Percutaneous transhepatic cholangiography requires a prior fasting period and usually sedation to prepare the patient. After local anesthesia and local disinfection, a spinal puncture type of needle is inserted into the liver below the right costal margin. The needle is withdrawn slowly until bile appears in the syringe; bile is withdrawn prior to injection of a radiopaque dye. Fluoroscopic examination is immediately done to determine filling of the biliary tract. After the x-ray films have been completed, care is taken to aspirate as much of the dye and bile as possible before removing the needle, in order to prevent leakage into the needle tract. The nurse should observe the patient closely for signs of bile leakage or hemorrhage from the puncture site. Vital signs are observed frequently for 24 hours. Pain, fever, chills, abdominal distention, bile leakage, or other signs of peritonitis are reported immediately. A variation of percutaneous transhepatic cholangiography is the transjugular approach for direct cholangiography [38a].

The patency of the bile ducts and pancreatic ducts may be determined by **duodenal intubation.** The presence of cancer of the pancreas or duodenum may be detected by this method. Specimens are obtained for microscopical examination including cytology. The color changes, volume, timing, and duration of bile flow are all noted during this procedure.

Endoscopic cholangiography is performed to determine possible biliary tract obstruction; flexible endoscopes make cannulation and contrast visualization of the biliary tract and pancreatic ducts possible. It is an extremely valuable technique in differentiating hepatocellular from extrahepatic jaundice, particularly when surgical exploration is anticipated. Accurate diagnosis is imperative, since surgery may be deleterious in a patient with hepatocellular disease. The procedure requires that the patient fast for at least 8 hours prior to the test. Sedation with diazepam (Valium) is often utilized. Atropine and dicyclomine hydrochloride (Bentyl) are usually used to obtain duodenal atony and relaxation of papillary smooth muscle. The fiberduodenoscope is introduced into the descending duodenum down to the ampulla of Vater, where a cannula can be directed into its orifice; a contrast medium is then injected retrograde into the biliary tract and the pancreatic ducts. The contrast medium commonly used is meglumine diatrizoate with sodium diatrizoate (Renografin-60) [42]. Radiographic study of the biliary tract is then accomplished.

Ultrasound, a noninvasive procedure, has also been performed for detecting abdominal masses and gallbladder dilatation, which may be the cause of biliary tract obstruction. **Echography,** which is reflected ultrasound imaging, is another approach to detecting biliary tract stones, because stones return fairly strong and readily detectable echoes [36].

Radioiodinated rose bengal has been used for scanning of the biliary tract. The substance is cleared from the blood by the hepatic parenchymal cells and is excreted normally through the biliary tract. Absence of intestinal radioactivity 90 minutes after injection suggests a biliary tract obstruction [36].

Tests for detection of levels of bilirubin in the serum have already been discussed. Elevation of conjugated bilirubin (direct bilirubin) levels supports a diagnosis of extrahepatic jaundice and biliary tract obstruction as the cause. Ordinarily bilirubin should not be present in the urine in significant amounts, but an increase occurs when direct bilirubin is elevated in the blood. Urine specimens for urine bilirubin evaluation must be collected in a dark bottle, since light causes bilirubin decomposition. It is also necessary to take the urine specimen directly to the laboratory rather than allowing it to stand, which also promotes decomposition.

Urine urobilinogen is normally excreted in only small amounts. As mentioned previously, urobilinogen is produced by the action of intestinal bacteria on bilirubin. Therefore an increased amount indicates the failure of the liver cells to reabsorb the urobilinogen as it is broken down in the intestine. Urine urobilinogen may be decreased if bowel sterilization or antibiotics are being given; it is important to note on the laboratory slip with the specimen that the patient is receiving antibiotics.

Stool specimens are examined for urobilinogen, which is normally present in the feces and is responsible for the color of the stools. Decreased amounts are reflected in clay-colored stools and are usually caused by biliary tract obstruction.

Disorders of the biliary tract include gallstone formation, inflammation, or neoplastic disease. The signs and symptoms associated with these diseases are related to interference with the normal flow of bile into the duodenum and vary according to the severity of the disease.

Cholelithiasis

Cholelithiasis is the term used to indicate stones in the gallbladder. It is one of the most common diseases of the gastrointestinal system. **Cholesterol,** which is a normal constituent of bile, is the major ingredient of most gallstones. Cholesterol is normally kept in solution by two other bile components, lecithin and bile acids. When cholesterol content increasingly exceeds that of lecithin and bile acids, **gallstones** are formed. Research continues on measures to increase the concentration of bile acids to make the cholesterol soluble and to dissolve gallstones. The most hopeful approach currently appears to be the use of chenodeoxycholic acid (chenic acid), which is a natural bile acid. The substance is administered orally to patients with gallstones and is under continued investigation. The patient receiving chenodeoxycholic acid should be observed for diarrhea, a side effect which is usually dose related. Potential serious side effects are hepatotoxicity and hyperlipidemia.

Gallstones vary in shape and size and may be single or multiple; they tend to occur more often in middle-aged females. In addition to changes in chemical composition of the bile, stagnation of the bile and infection, overeating, and other poor eating habits appear to be predisposing factors to gallstone formation. Cholelithiasis may not cause any symptoms (silent gallstones), but in other situations signs and symptoms range from mild digestive disturbances such as fullness, eructation, and dyspepsia following fat ingestion to more severe symptoms and signs such as severe pain, fever, jaundice, and bleeding. The pain is usually located in the right upper quadrant, often radiating to the back. The more severe symptoms and signs occur when the gallstone(s) cause(s) biliary tract obstruction in the common bile duct. Gallstones may be lodged in the cystic or common bile duct or be impacted in the ampulla of Vater, causing pancreatitis. Cholelithiasis may also cause acute or chronic inflammation of the gallbladder (cholecystitis) or stasis of bile within the liver (cholestasis) and lead to impaired hepatic function.

During an acute attack of biliary colic, bed rest is indicated. When nausea and vomiting are present, food and fluids are restricted and intravenous fluids are given. A nasogastric tube is placed and connected to intermittent suction. Antispasmodic drugs, such as atropine and propantheline bromide (Pro-Banthine), may be prescribed to relieve the painful reflex spasms that occur with stones within the ductal system. Analgesics are administered for the relief of pain. When the acute attack subsides and the nasogastric tube is removed, a liquid diet is initiated and gradually increased to a light, low fat diet. Adequate fluid intake is encouraged.

After the acute episode subsides, plans for surgical intervention may be indicated, because of the potential for acute cholecystitis or common bile duct obstruction. The surgical procedure is **cholecystectomy** (removal of the gallbladder) and exploration of the common bile duct for gallstones or strictures. Surgery may be indicated during the acute phase if obstruction of the common bile duct persists. Surgery of the biliary tract is discussed in a following section.

Cholecystitis

Inflammation of the gallbladder may be either acute or chronic. Acute upper abdominal pain, generalized signs of inflammation, and tenderness of the right upper quadrant of the abdomen are symptoms characteristic of **acute cholecystitis.** Fever, nausea, vomiting, and leukocytosis are usually present. Treatment includes bed rest, food and fluid restriction, intravenous fluid and electrolyte administration, analgesics, and antibiotic therapy. Ordinarily, surgery is postponed 6 to 8 weeks after an episode of acute cholecystitis to assure full recovery from inflammation. Evidence of deterioration such as increased pain, signs of worsening inflammation, mass enlargement, and involuntary rigidity in the right upper quadrant usually indicates the need for emergency surgery in order to prevent possible rupture of the gallbladder. If acute inflammation is far advanced, cholecystostomy with insertion of a drainage catheter that is retained as long as 6 weeks to 6 months is the preferred approach to relieve the intravisceral pressure. In these situations, cholecystectomy is difficult and dangerous.

Chronic cholecystitis is characterized by a long history of vague complaints related to digestive disturbances. Abdominal discomfort usually associated with ingestion of excess food and fats, flatulence, and dull aching pain are usual symptoms. The intensity and frequency of the symptoms tend to increase, as the chronic inflammation causes scarring and thickening of the gallbladder wall and eventually cholestasis. Cholecystectomy is the usual treatment in progressive chronic cholecystitis.

Cancer of the Gallbladder

Primary cancer of the gallbladder is a relatively rare occurrence and is found most often in females. It is usually asymptomatic in its early stages and may be found incidentally during surgery for cholelithiasis. Symptoms associated with cancer of the gallbladder are similar to those of chronic cholecystitis, gradually increasing in severity with persistent pain. Obstructive jaundice develops either from compression of the biliary ducts by the enlarging gallbladder or by direct extension of the malignant process.

The malignant process may spread to the common bile duct as well as to the lymph nodes and liver. In these situations a limited hepatic resection and regional lymphadenectomy as well as cholecystectomy may be accomplished if the cancer has extended to these sites. Other distant sites of metastases are the lung, peritoneum, and ovaries.

Bile Duct Disorders

Obstruction of the common bile duct may result from an obstructing gallstone that has traveled from the gallbladder (**choledocholithiasis**), from inflammation (**choledochitis** or **cholangitis**), or from a stricture of the duct formed by scar tissue from trauma or inflammation. As noted above, neoplastic disease may result in extension to the common bile duct or may cause obstruction of the duct by compression from the primary neoplasm. Obstructive jaundice follows, regardless of the cause of obstruction. Pruritus is often severe, requiring administration of cholestyramine (Questran) for control of itching.

Surgery of the common bile duct is usually accompanied by a cholecystectomy, because the gallbladder disease is often the original problem. Stones are removed from the common bile duct by choledochostomy. In this procedure an incision is made into the common bile duct and stones are removed. Operative cholangiogram and cholecystectomy are performed. A T tube is inserted at the site of entry into the duct for decompression to provide for biliary drainage while the tissues recover from the surgical trauma. The T tube provides a means for removing excess bile and prevents back flow and leakage. If the tube is not placed, edema may occur and obstruct the bile duct postoperatively. The stem portion of the T tube is brought out to the abdominal surface through a stab wound or incision and is attached to a drainage appliance for gravity drainage.

Surgery may also be accomplished to correct a stricture defect. If the stricture is minimal, a resection and end-to-end anastomosis may be accomplished over a T-tube splint. If the obstruction is neoplastic in nature, resection of the ductal tumor is accomplished and the remaining portion of the common bile duct is anastomosed to the duodenum (choledochoduodenostomy) or to the jejunum (choledochojejunostomy) to reestablish biliary flow into the intestinal tract. In cases of spasm or stricture at the sphincter of Oddi, drainage from the common bile duct and pancreatic duct may be improved by sphincterotomy.

Nursing Care in Biliary Tract Surgery

Preoperative preparation of the patient for biliary duct exploration includes care necessary for the preparation of any patient for abdominal surgery (discussed in Chapter 1). In addition, care includes measures related to disturbances resulting from obstructed biliary flow.

Pressure within the biliary system rises as the liver continues to secrete bile, in spite of obstruction to bile flow within the tract. The pressure stimulates the receptors in the wall of the biliary tract and causes severe pain. Therefore the patient who is scheduled for biliary tract surgery is often in considerable pain. This pain may hinder the patient's ability to learn preoperatively, so that the nurse must observe the patient closely to determine appropriate times for preoperative teaching.

Obstruction of bile flow promotes bleeding tendencies due to the vitamin K deficiency that results in the absence of bile salts within the intestine. The patient is observed closely for signs of bleeding, and prothrombin levels and blood clotting tests are monitored preoperatively. Vitamin K is usually administered preoperatively; blood transfusions are often indicated. Carbohydrates are given in large amounts either orally or intravenously in order to build up glycogen stores in the liver.

The patient should be prepared to expect various types of drainage apparatus postoperatively. Usually nasogastric suction is indicated. An explanation of the purpose of the T tube and important precautions related to maintaining its position and patency postoperatively must be given. The patient is taught to deep breathe and cough effectively, because patients having gallbladder and biliary tract surgery are prone to pulmonary complications.

Postoperatively the patient is placed in a low Fowler's position to facilitate lung expansion and to promote biliary drainage. Depending on the specific type of biliary tract surgery and the general status of the patient, ambulation is generally initiated early (the first postoperative day). Special attention is given to frequent coughing and deep breathing, because the patient tends to take shallow breaths to prevent pain and discomfort. Close observation for bleeding is necessary, particularly if the patient has low prothrombin levels.

The T tube and any other drainage apparatus must be checked regularly to observe the drainage as well as to determine patency of the tubes (Fig. 7-10). The T tube is secured to the dressing in a manner to prevent traction and dislodgement as well as to prevent kinking. The patient is reminded of the importance of not lying on the tube or accidentally pulling the tube. The drainage is observed frequently during the first 24 hours. The nurse should expect that a small amount of blood will be mixed with the bile during the first few hours, but persistent bleeding is reported to the surgeon. Assuming the T tube is kept patent, there is usually 300 to 500 ml of bile drainage in the first 24 hours, diminishing to 200 ml or less within 3 to 4 days. The character and volume of bile drainage is recorded precisely and included in the intake and output record. A cholangiogram is usually performed within 7 to 10 days postoperatively, and if no stones are identified, the tube is removed. In some cases the patient is discharged with the T tube in place and requires specific instruction in its management.

Prior to the removal of the T tube, a clamping schedule is usually initiated. The tube is usually clamped for 1 hour before and after meals to promote the flow of bile to the duodenum to aid digestion. The patient is observed closely for signs of discomfort, pain, and increased bile drainage around the tube, which indicate that the common bile duct is still not patent. The urine, stools, sclerae and skin, and mucous membrane of the mouth are checked for any indication of obstructive jaundice. Return of normal bile flow is indicated by a decrease in drainage from the T tube and a return of normal color in the stools.

Precautions are taken that dressings soiled

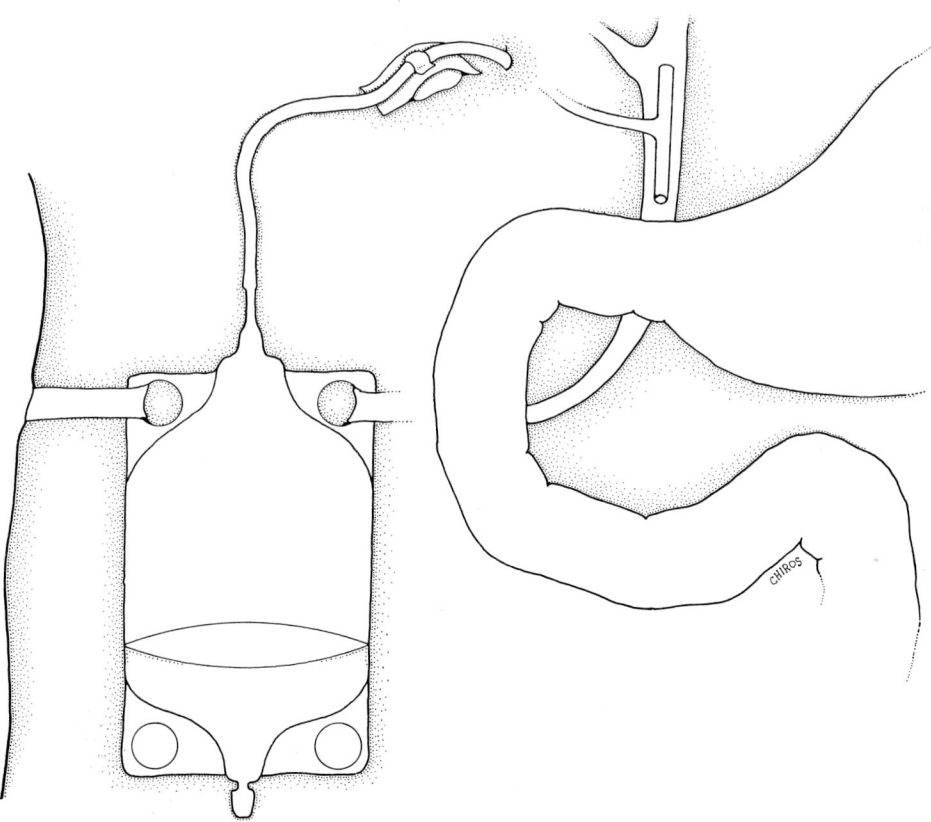

Figure 7-10
Use of the T tube in common bile duct explorations.

with bile are changed frequently to prevent excoriation of the skin. A skin barrier is utilized prior to application of new dressings. The patient is also observed for signs of peritonitis, which may result from bile leakage into the peritoneal cavity. Signs and symptoms of fever and abdominal pain, distention, and rigidity are reported promptly.

Immediately postoperatively, the patient is restricted from oral intake and a nasogastric tube is maintained for at least 24 hours. Oral fluids are then given, and increased to a soft diet if tolerated. The diet is high in protein and carbohydrates, but low in fat content. After cholecystectomy, some patients may tolerate a regular diet well. Other patients are encouraged to gradually increase the fat intake over a period of 4 to 6 months.

When the T tube cholangiogram is done and stones are found, cholic acid may be instilled via the tube to treat retained biliary stones [40]. In some cases another surgical procedure is necessary to remove the retained stones. In other situations, no treatment is given and stones may spontaneously pass into the duodenum. The patient is followed for potential recurrence of symptoms.

If prolonged T tube drainage is required or if bile drainage is excessive, bile may be returned to the patient by feeding it orally to the patient or by introducing the bile through a nasogastric tube. The bile is usually chilled and diluted with grape or apple juice for oral ingestion. Bile salts may be replaced by oral administration of florantyrone (Zanchol) or sodium dehydrocholate (Decholin Sodium), in order to facilitate fat absorption. Supplemental fat-soluble vitamins may also be given.

Another complication that may occur after biliary tract surgery is fistula formation along drain tracts. These fistulas usually result from bile leakage from the site of cystic duct ligation or from a defect in the common bile duct system. Infection control and maintenance of nutrition are of paramount importance. Prevention of skin irritation from bile drainage is an important component of nursing care. The use of skin barriers such as Stomahesive and application of disposable adhesive appliances facilitate skin protection as well as accurate observation and measurement of drainage. Sodium is lost with biliary drainage loss through fistulas. Accurate intake and output records are essential. Total parenteral nutrition may be necessary to maintain nutrition, to replace electrolytes, and to promote healing. Although the fistula may close spontaneously, surgery is often required.

Another complication that may occur after cholecystectomy is the **postcholecystectomy syndrome.** This syndrome occurs with the onset of preoperative complaints and symptoms. It is felt that errors in diagnosis before surgery may be a causative factor, in that the original cause of the symptoms may not have been gallbladder disease or that gallstones are still present in the remnant of the cystic duct or gallbladder or in the common bile duct. Intravenous cholangiography and consideration of other causative factors are indicated. Another operation may be necessary and may reveal an unsuspected common duct stone.

DISORDERS OF THE PANCREAS

The pancreas is an essential gland that has both endocrine and exocrine functions. It is located retroperitoneally, below and behind the stomach and liver, a factor that limits its accessibility to palpation during physical examination. Its endocrine function related to the production of insulin and glucagon by the islet cells is discussed in Chapter 8. The following discussion is concerned primarily with its exocrine function.

The pancreas is composed of acinar cells, which are arranged in groups known as acini. Minute ducts in the acini empty mainly into a larger duct, the pancreatic duct (duct of Wirsung) which joins the common bile duct at the ampulla of Vater to enter the duodenum. Acinar cells are responsible for producing an average of 1 to 2 liters of pancreatic juice each 24 hours [39]. The juice contains two components: the **aqueous juice,** which contains water and electrolytes but few enzymes, and a small amount of juice that contains essential **digestive enzymes.** The former juice is osmotically the same as plasma and contains a high bicarbonate content, to promote neutralization of the acid juices entering the small intestine from the stomach. The digestive enzymes secreted by the pancreas include the proteolytic enzymes that are activated by substances released by the intestinal mucosa on contact with chyme; trypsinogen is activated by the intestinal hormone enterokinase; chymotrypsinogen is converted to active chymotrypsin by trypsin;

procarboxypeptidase is converted to active carboxypeptidase by both trypsin and enterokinase. Other proteolytic enzymes include ribonuclease, deoxyribonuclease, cholesterol esterase, lecithinase, and elastase. The pancreatic enzyme amylase is secreted to hydrolyze starch and glycogen and most other carbohydrates into disaccharides. In the presence of bile salts and calcium, lipase hydrolyzes fats into glycerol and fatty acids. Although moderate amounts of pancreatic enzyme secretion are stimulated by parasympathetic impulses via the vagus nerve, two hormones, secretin and cholecystokinin-pancreozymin (CCK–PZ), which are released when chyme enters the small intestine, are responsible for the secretion of large amounts of pancreatic enzymes.

The pancreas is divided into three segments: the head, the body, and the tail. The head of the pancreas surrounds the common bile duct and is usually attached to the duodenum. The position of the head of the pancreas accounts for obstructive symptoms of the gastrointestinal tract that occur with certain pathologic states of this portion of the gland. The pancreas is a highly vascular organ, as circulation is important to both its endocrine and exocrine functions; it receives arterial blood via branches of the celiac, splenic, and superior mesenteric arteries. Disorders of the pancreas can affect exocrine or endocrine function or both, resulting in disturbances of digestion, nutrition, and carbohydrate metabolism. These disturbances result in symptoms that vary in severity, depending on the stage, type, and course of the pancreatic dysfunction. In assessing the patient with suspected or known pancreatic disease, the nurse should accurately describe the presence of pain, its cause, and its relation to meals. Often, pain is described as being relieved by a change in position. The presence of weight loss, weakness, anorexia, nausea and vomiting, food intolerance, and symptoms of malnutrition should all be noted during assessment and history taking. Information on discoloration of the urine, the color and characteristics of feces, and the presence of steatorrhea may be obtained from the patient as well as by direct examination of these excretions. A history of alcohol intake and drug ingestion should be investigated. Abdominal palpation is accomplished to detect abdominal distention, rigidity, and abdominal masses in the area of the pancreas. The sclera and mucous membranes of the mouth should be examined for jaundice, if jaundice is not readily detected on the skin. Jaundice is associated with disease of the head of the pancreas, which results in compression of the common bile duct. It is also important for the nurse to remember that endocrine dysfunction of the pancreas affects glucose metabolism; testing of a urine specimen may indicate the presence of glycosuria.

Pancreatic disorders may result in varied symptoms. Certain conditions have an insidious onset that complicates and delays diagnosis, while other pancreatic disorders produce severe and acute symptoms that are often life-threatening. It is estimated that 90 percent of the pancreas is destroyed before pancreatic insufficiency is produced. Reestablishment of functioning depends on arresting the disease process and preventing damage to the remaining viable tissue [39].

Diagnostic Tests

Various diagnostic tests help to evaluate pancreatic function. The endocrine function is evaluated by blood glucose determinations and by the glucose tolerance test, as discussed in Chapter 8.

Blood enzyme levels are determined to detect elevations of amylase and lipase levels. Normally, the **serum amylase** is 60 to 180 Somogyi units and **serum lipase** is 1.5 units; these levels are usually elevated in pancreatic duct obstruction and destruction of pancreatic cells. **Urinary amylase** excretion is normally 260 to 950 units in 24 hours. Analysis of 24-hour specimens can demonstrate increased excretion of amylase, a particularly important finding in the diagnosis of pancreatitis. **Calcium** levels in the blood are also affected in certain types of pancreatic disease, with a resultant decrease in the serum calcium level. **Alkaline phosphatase** levels may be increased when pancreatic tumors compress the common bile duct.

Stool examinations are indicated to determine the quantitative fat content. Specimens may be collected for 72 hours. Failure of the pancreatic lipase to reach the intestine results in excretion of undigested and unabsorbed fat (steatorrhea). Normally, less than 5 gm of fat is excreted in the feces during 24 hours.

A provocative **pancreozymin-secretin test** may be done to evaluate pancreatic exocrine function. After a fasting period of 8 to 12 hours, a duodenal tube is inserted to obtain baseline data on aspirated secretions. An intravenous dose of secretin, followed by an injection of pancreozymin, is given and then other aspirations of the duodenal secretions are obtained at timed intervals to determine the presence of pancreatic enzymes. The total volume is determined, as well as the concentrations of amylase and bicarbonate. Serum amylase values are also evaluated at regular intervals after stimulation with the hormones.

A **xylose tolerance test** may be done to distinguish pancreatic deficiency from intestinal malabsorption disease when steatorrhea is present. Normal results occur if the steatorrhea is due to pancreatic deficiency, because pancreatic secretions do not affect d-xylose absorption.

Roentgenographic examinations, such as barium x-rays of the stomach and duodenum, may give indirect information about the pancreas when they demonstrate compression of the duodenum or pyloric obstruction due to pancreatic disease. **Splenoportography,** which is the percutaneous injection of contrast medium into the splenic vein, may be used to detect tumors of the body and tail of the pancreas and sites of blockage in extrahepatic portal hypertension.

Pancreatic scans are also done when pancreatic disease is suspected. Usually an overnight fast and a fat-free breakfast are required pror to injection of the radioactive isotope. Selenium-tagged methionine (^{75}Se) is the radioactive substance most commonly used. Abnormalities of the pancreas are reflected by the failure to visualize the radioactive substance in the pancreas within 20 to 30 minutes after selenium-tagged methionine is administered. A lack of filling of all portions of the pancreas may also be demonstrated. This technique, while detecting abnormalities, does not define the etiology.

Selective **celiac arteriography** is used to demonstrate the pancreatic vasculature to detect abnormalities resulting from inflammation or tumor. In this test, epinephrine is often injected to contract normal arterioles, while tumor vessels remain dilated and readily visualized [22]. **Transhepatic cholangiography** is also used to demonstrate biliary obstruction due to cancer of the head of the pancreas. This procedure has been described in the discussion on biliary tract disease. Fiberoptic duodenoscopy techniques permit entrance into the duodenum and visualization of the ampulla of Vater and the pancreatic duct.

Pancreatitis

Pancreatitis is an inflammatory condition of the pancreas resulting from the escape of activated digestive enzymes into pancreatic tissue and autodigestion, particularly by proteolytic enzymes. Severe cases of pancreatitis are complicated by hemorrhage, necrosis, and abscess formation.

Acute pancreatitis may be mild or severe in onset, lasting for several days. The chronic form persists for years with recurrent acute episodes. Although the symptoms may be similar in the two types, they vary in degree of severity and there is concomitant variation in the treatment and prognosis. Other classifications of pancreatitis include interstitial and hemorrhagic pancreatitis. Chronic pancreatitis is also called relapsing pancreatitis. Some authorities distinguish between recurrent acute pancreatitis and chronic pancreatitis and indicate recurrent disease as being associated with gallstones. (Chronic pancreatitis is discussed in a later section.)

Acute pancreatitis is often associated with prolonged and heavy alcohol consumption, blockage of the ampulla of Vater by gallstones or spasm, and edema associated with inflammation of duodenum as well as with hyperlipemia. Pancreatitis is also associated with infections secondary to reflux ductal infections or from infections such as mumps, typhoid, and hepatitis. Nutritional deficiencies, prolonged use of certain drugs such as tetracyclines, chlorothiazides, and oral contraceptives, and surgical trauma to the pancreas have also been identified as causative factors.

Acute pancreatitis causes symptoms due to pancreatic edema. The most common symptom is the sudden onset of persistent epigastric pain, which may be dull, aching, or burning and pressing and severe enough to require frequent analgesics for relief. Pain is usually accompanied by nausea, vomiting, and low grade fever. The abdomen may be distended and tender, and a palpable mass may be present. Dehydration and shock may occur, and the patient may present in a life-threatening state. The patient may have a history of a recent onset of diabetes without a family history of the disorder, a history of increased or prolonged alcoholic intake, or the presence of gallstones. When assessing the pain, the nurse must ascertain the relation of pain to eating and position. Overindulgence of food may aggravate pain symptoms; restlessness and frequent changes of position may be noted as the patient tries to find a comfortable position.

The most important diagnostic tests in determining the presence of acute pancreatitis are those for estimating serum amylase and lipase levels and the urinary excretion of amylase. Serum amylase tests are done before any opiates are given to relieve pain, because these medications may increase the amylase levels. Serum amylase levels of 300 to 500 Somogyi (and often over 800) units suggest pancreatitis. These values rise within 2 to 6 hours after onset of symptoms but return to normal within 48 to 72 hours if no complications arise, even in the presence of continued clinical activity. Urine amylase levels rise later and tend to be elevated for a longer time than serum levels. Stool analysis may demonstrate excess fat excretion and excess nitrogen content. Metabolic disturbances result in mild hyperglycemia and glycosuria, hypocalcemia, and decreased sodium and potassium levels. Hypomagnesemia usually occurs to some degree in all patients with an alcoholic history.

Increased direct bilirubin is usually associated with biliary and hepatic involvement, and the prothrombin time may be prolonged due to decreased vitamin K synthesis and malabsorption of the fat-soluble vitamin. Cutaneous signs of acute pancreatitis may be present and include bluish discoloration of the flanks (Grey-Turner's sign) due to fat necrosis caused by pancreatic enzymes in the skin and discoloration of periumbilical area (Cullen's sign) [10].

The nurse should observe the patient for behavioral signs and changes in sensorium that may be related to alcohol withdrawal, as well as to sepsis or fluid and electrolyte imbalances.

The treatment of acute pancreatitis depends on the severity of the disease and on the underlying cause. Fluid and electrolyte replacement, albumin, and plasma expanders are necessary to correct hypovolemia, electrolyte imbalance, and shock. Vitamins, magnesium, electrolytes, and glucose are particularly indicated for the malnourished patient. Calcium gluconate is often administered to maintain calcium levels and prevent the onset of tetany. Hypocalcemia is thought to be due to removal of calcium from the serum and its being sequestered in areas of fat necrosis as insoluble calcium soap [12].

Other measures are directed at suppression of pancreatic juice secretion and the relief of pain. Continued secretion of pancreatic juices into the tissues increases tissue damage. Oral intake is restricted and nasogastric suction is instituted to minimize the acid content in the duodenum and to avoid stimulation of pancreatic secretion. (Food in the duodenum stimulates pancreozyme and pancreatic secretion.) Anticholinergic drugs are given to inhibit secretion and sphincter spasm; these drugs include propantheline bromide (Pro-Banthine) and atropine sulfate. Appropriate analgesics are given for relief of pain; meperidine hydrochloride (Demerol) is generally preferred to morphine sulfate, because the latter drug tends to cause spasms of the sphincter of Oddi.

Antibiotic therapy may be indicated and steroid therapy may be utilized to treat shock and to prevent further inflammation. In certain situations, surgery may be necessary to promote drainage of the pancreatic secretions and to provide decompression by cholecystostomy or choledochotomy. Because of its action on protein release from the cells and diminished acinar activity, 5-fluorouracil has recently been studied as an adjunct measure in the treatment of pancreatitis, but long-term evaluation is still forthcoming [38]. When nasogastric suction is discontinued, the patient is started on small feedings of high-protein, high-carbohydrate, and low-fat content. Large meals, which stimulate pancreatic secretion, are avoided. Antacids may be used to neutralize gastric secretions which stimulate pancreatic secretion.

Acute pancreatitis may be controlled and result in complete recovery, or the acute pancreatitis may become increasingly severe progressing to acute hemorrhagic pancreatitis. Fistula formation may occur when pancreatitis is the result of surgical injury to the pancreas. Pseudocyst formation, pancreatic abscess, or subphrenic abscess may also occur; the abscess may enlarge and perforate, causing peritonitis. Surgical drainage is required when abscess formation is detected. Pseudocyst formation is discussed in a subsequent section in this chapter.

Nursing care of the patient with acute pancreatitis requires careful observation for signs of complications, particularly those of hemorrhage, shock, and fluid and electrolyte imbalance. Accurate assessment and recording of vital signs and intake and output are essential. The nurse should observe for signs and symptoms of inadequate respiratory ventilation that may result from retroperitoneal edema and elevation of the diaphragm. The nurse should also observe for symptoms of tetany because of hypocalcemia and should examine hematocrit and electrolyte reports regularly to detect any changes.

In addition to observing for the presence and characteristics of pain and providing necessary analgesics, the nurse must also utilize measures to decrease the patient's anxiety. Both pain and anxiety tend to increase vagal stimulation and thus, pancreatic secretion. Bed rest is maintained to decrease metabolic activities, and fever is controlled. When administering anticholinergic drugs, the nurse should observe for side effects such as urine retention, dry mouth, and abdominal distention. Maintenance of nasogastric suction is essential, and the contents, volume, and characteristics are reported. Oral hygiene and care of the external nares are necessary measures to relieve discomfort of the nasogastric suction, fluid restriction, and the suppressed salivary secretion caused by anticholinergic drugs.

As acute pancreatitis begins to subside, prevention of other attacks is initiated by teaching the patient the importance of abstinence from alcohol as an essential requirement to prevent recurrence. Dietary instruction is necessary to explain the purpose of the low-fat, high-carbohydrate, and high-protein diet. Small, frequent feedings will be prescribed to limit pancreatic secretion. Coffee and other caffeine-containing drinks are restricted, as they stimulate pancreatic secretion. The patient is also advised of side effects that may occur with analgesic and anticholinergic therapy if these are continued.

Hemorrhagic Pancreatitis

Hemorrhagic pancreatitis is a more advanced stage of acute pancreatitis and may lead to hemorrhage with a fatal outcome due to extensive pancreatic destruction. Necrotic tissue extends to the vessels and causes blood to escape into the pancreas and retroperitoneal tissues. The patient with hemorrhagic pancreatitis is critically ill and has excruciating pain, often radiating to the back, and usually has abdominal rigidity. Nausea and vomiting, signs of paralytic ileus, and signs of shock are usually present.

Nursing care of these patients is similar to that described for the patient with acute pancreatitis. The nurse should be aware of the high mortality rate associated with this type of pancreatitis and should remember that patients who survive this phase will have chronic pancreatic insufficiency. The nurse should also observe for symptoms of impending fluid overload, which may occur in hemorrhagic pancreatitis as reabsorption of the fluids lost in the peritoneal and retroperitoneal spaces occurs.

Chronic Pancreatitis

Chronic pancreatitis results from recurrent attacks of acute inflammation that cause diffuse and progressive fibrotic changes and loss of functioning tissue. Diminished enzyme and insulin production results. Each attack causes increased damage and alteration in functions. Chronic pancreatitis is associated with a high risk of pancreatic carcinoma. Chronic pancreatitis may follow acute pancreatitis or may be the result of chronic fibrosis and atrophy due to gallbladder disease or to pancreatic and duodenal duct obstruction.

Chronic pancreatitis is characterized by metabolic disturbances due to pancreatic damage and results in diabetes, impaired digestion, azotorrhea (increased nitrogen in the stool), and steatorrhea (increased fat excretion in the stool, resulting in bulky, pale, and malodorous stools). Malnutrition and weight loss may be present. Often the patient is reluctant to eat because food intake provokes nausea, vomiting, and pain. Malnutrition is also frequently associated with alcoholism. Calcification of the pancreas and calcium stone formation may be detected on abdominal flatplate x-rays. Serum amylase and lipase levels may or may not be elevated, depending on the amount of remaining functioning tissue.

Treatment is similar to that of acute pancreatitis. Complete abstinence from alcohol and adherence to a low-fat, bland, high-protein diet are essential components of management. Anticholinergic drugs may be prescribed. Pancreatic extracts, such as pancreatin (Viokase) or pancrelipase (Cotazym), and insulin replacement are indicated in severe pancreatitis. Calcium supplements and bile salts may also be prescribed.

When a specific cause is identified in the etiology of chronic pancreatitis, surgical therapy according to the type of pathology may be indicated. Abscess formation is treated by incision and drainage. Pancreatolithotomy is accomplished when calculi are detected within the pancreatic duct. Cholecystectomy or choledochotomy is indicated in the presence of gallbladder disease when it is the causative factor. Sphincterotomy may be indicated to enlarge the pancreatic sphincter or the sphincter of Oddi or both if it is fibrotic and causing an obstruction. A Roux-en-Y type of pancreatojejunostomy is sometimes done to promote pancreatic drainage and relieve ductal obstructions. Surgical procedures to control pain include celiac ganglionectomy and splanchnic resection.

Pancreatic Cysts

Both true cysts and pseudocysts may occur in the pancreas. Pseudocysts are collections of fluid (pancreatic juice, blood, and debris) contained within a capsule formed by fibrous tissue of the pancreas. These cysts may be a complication of acute pancreatitis, or they may occur with chronic pancreatitis. They may also result from injury to the pancreas. Pseudocyst is suspected on finding persistent hyperamylasemia and an upper abdominal mass or ascites. At times the pseudocyst may increase in size and produce symptoms due to compression on adjacent structures or infection. The high protein content within the cyst draws fluid into it, which accounts for the increasing size. The cyst may decrease in size and clear up spontaneously in some cases. Usually, surgical drainage is accomplished either internally into the jejunum or externally through the skin surface. In the latter approach the nurse must take special precautions to protect the skin from excoriation by pancreatic enzymes. Skin barriers and collection into disposable adhesive pouches facilitate measurement of the drainage and also prevent skin trauma. Measurement of the drainage is important to monitor fluid and electrolyte losses, particularly of bicarbonate, sodium, calcium, and potassium in large amounts of pancreatic drainage. In some cases, suction is applied to a tube inserted in the cyst and continuous suction is maintained. It is important that the nurse maintain the patency of such tubes to assure adequate drainage. Cyst excision is usually curative in the case of pseudocyst formation, but removal of true cysts is often associated with fistula formation.

Tumors of the Pancreas

Although previously considered to be relatively rare, cancer of the pancreas appears to be increasing in incidence and is now the fourth leading cause of cancer death in men and the sixth cause for women. A major factor in this picture is that cancer of the pancreas is not readily diagnosed until far advanced. The tumors mainly occur after the age of 35, with a peak incidence about the age of 60.

The insidious onset of the disease with initial vague symptoms generally accounts for delays in diagnosis. These symptoms include anorexia, fatigue, weight loss, nausea, flatulence, and dull pain in the epigastrium or referred to the back. The back pain usually results from pressure on the nerve plexus around the celiac ganglia. The onset of diabetes and an abdominal mass or tenderness in the epigastric area as well as a palpable gallbladder in the jaundiced patient are significant findings. The head of the pancreas is the most common site for cancer of the pancreas and causes jaundice by compressing and obstructing the common bile duct. Biliary obstruction and gallbladder dilatation are subsequent complications.

Islet cell tumors may be either functioning or nonfunctioning tumors (insulin secreting or non-insulin secreting) and either benign or malignant. These tumors may occur in the head, body, or tail of the gland. Functioning islet cell tumors cause excessive insulin production with hypoglycemia and symptoms of fatigue, malaise, and untoward effects on the sensorium. Nonfunctioning tumors, termed the **Zollinger-Ellison tumor** or the ulcerogenic syndrome, cause excessive production of gastrin and result in fulminating peptic ulcer disease that is intractable to usual medical therapy. In the presence of this tumor, gastric analysis demonstrates an increased volume of gastric juice produced in overnight collections of gastric secretions.

Cystadenomas are rare tumors which are usually benign and are located in the body and tail of the pancreas. As mentioned previously, diagnosis of cancer of the pancreas is often delayed until the disease is far advanced. Metastasis generally occurs by direct invasion of the duodenum and by lymph node metastases to the liver and lungs. Metastatis to the pancreas occurs from cancer of the lung, stomach, duodenum, and common bile duct. Diagnosis at the early stages is being attempted by radioimmunoassay for circulating cancer embryonic antigen (CEA) and tumor associated antigen (TEA). Duodenal endoscopy is being utilized to obtain specimens for cytologic contents and to detect cancer of the ampulla of Vater. Other diagnostic tests are those used to determine the presence of pancreatic dysfunction and are not specific for diagnosing cancer of the pancreas.

Treatment of cancer of the pancreas is primarily surgical and has been associated with a high mortality rate. Cancer of the head of the pancreas is usually treated by pancreaticoduodenectomy, the Whipple procedure. This surgical approach consists in resection of the head of the pancreas, the duodenum, a portion of the jejunum, the lower portion of the stomach, the distal portion of the common bile duct, and a portion of the pancreatic duct. To reestablish the continuity of the gastrointestinal tract and the biliary and pancreatic systems, a gastrojejunostomy, choledochojejunostomy, and pancreatojejunostomy are accomplished. These procedures promote drainage of the alkaline bile and pancreatic juice into the jejunum to prevent jejunal ulcers forming from the acid gastric juice. The operation is a hazardous one with potential for hemorrhage at any of the sites of anastomosis.

The cancer often recurs, and the subtotal pancreatic resection often results in pancreatic fistulas postoperatively. Therefore, total pancreatectomy is being advocated by some authorities; others advocate regional pancreatectomy to control the highly malignant process. In the latter technique total resection of the pancreas plus a segment of the portal vein and regional lymphatics are accomplished.

Chemotherapy has generally been ineffective except for the use of streptozotocin for insulinomas. Combination therapy with 5-fluorouracil and BCNU (a nitrosurea) has also been proved effective in palliative approaches to pancreatic cancer [43]. Cancer of the pancreas with disseminated disease has also been treated with intensified radiation, using radon seeds combined with intraarterial infusions or systemic administration of floxuridine (FUDR).

In the presence of islet cell tumor and the ulcerogenic syndrome (the Zollinger-Ellison syndrome), removal of the pancreatic tumor is indicated. In addition, some authorities recommend total gastrectomy to remove the target organ of increased gastrin secretion and resection of as much of the tumor as is feasible. It is felt that parietal cell hyperplasia present in the ulcerogenic syndrome may continue to cause gastric hypersecretion even if the pancreatic tumor is removed [115], which in turn can cause formation of intractable ulcers. Gastrectomy is thought to reduce the incidence of metastasis.

Pancreatic surgery is radical surgery that requires critical care nursing. Fluid and electrolyte balance, prevention of hemorrhage and respiratory complications, and management of endocrine and exocrine functions of the pancreas are the major aspects of postoperative care. Maintaining the patency of gastrointestinal tubes is important to prevent distention and compression on the surgical site. Intake and output measurement and daily weights are important in assessing the patient's fluid and electrolyte and nutritional status. These patients are prone to develop pulmonary complications unless preventive measures are taken with particular attention to turning, coughing, and deep breathing. One of the most frequent and serious complications of pancreaticoduodenal surgery is pancreatic fistula formation due to breakdown of the pancreaticojejunostomy with associated erosion, hemorrhage, and infection [30]. The nurse must observe closely the vital signs and the drainage from the wound site in order to detect any complications in their early stages. Cutaneous pancreatic fistulas readily cause skin excoriation. The use of skin barriers and disposable postoperative collection pouches and appliances is indicated to prevent enzymatic contact with the skin and to facilitate accurate collection and measurement of pancreatic drainage.

The nutritional status of the patient requires close management. Exocrine function is controlled with the use of pancreatic extract (Pancreatin) or whole pancreatic preparation (Viokase) as well as by controlling intake of fats [30]. Depending on the amount of remaining pancreatic cells, it may be necessary to control endocrine function by insulin administration and dietary management.

The recently developed fiberoptic techniques for visualizing the pancreas as well as the various new approaches to pancreatic surgery and improved postoperative management are likely to contribute to changing the current poor prognostic picture of pancreatic disease.

References

GASTROINTESTINAL DISORDERS

1. Achord, J. L. Acute effects of fasting on gastrointestinal structure and function. *Med. Times* 95:441, 1967.
2. Armstrong, D., and Tedder, E. Care of patients with the carcinoid syndrome. *Nurs. Clin. North Am.* 4:171, 1969.
3. Bates, B. *A Guide to Physical Examination*. Philadelphia: Lippincott, 1974.
4. Butterworth, C. E. The skeleton in the hospital closet. *Nutr. Today* 9:4, 1974.
5. Craft, C. Body image and obesity. *Nurs. Clin. North Am.* 7:677, 1972.
6. Derezin, M. Laxatives and fecal modifiers. *Am. Fam. Physician* 10:126, 1974.
7. Dodsworth, J. M., and Fischer, J. E. Surgical therapy of chronic peptic ulcer. *Surg. Clin. North Am.* 54:529, 1974.
8. Fikei, E., and Cassella, R. Jejunoileal bypass for massive obesity. *Ann. Surg.* 79:460, 1974.
9. Gault, M. H. Hypernatremia, azotemia, and dehydration due to high protein tube feedings. *Ann. Int. Med.* 68:778, 1968.
10. Given, B. A., and Simmons, S. J. *Nursing Care of the Patient with Gastrointestinal Disease*. St. Louis: Mosby, 1975.
11. Hanson, R. L. A Study to Determine the Difference in Effects of Administering Cold and Warmed Tube Feedings. In M. Batey (ed.), *Communicating Nursing Research*, vol. 6, *Collaboration and Competition*. Boulder, Colo.: WICHE, 1973.
12. Harvey, A. M., Johns, R. J., Owens, A. H., and Ross, R. S. *The Principles and Practice of Medicine* (18th ed.). New York: Appleton-Century-Crofts, 1972.
13. Heydman, A. H. Intestinal bypass for obesity. *Am. J. Nurs.* 74:1102, 1974.
14. Ivey, K. J. Anticholinergics: Do they work in peptic ulcers? *Gastroenterology* 68:154, 1975.
15. Keough, G., and Niebel, H. Oral cancer detection—A nursing responsibility. *Am. J. Nurs.* 73:684, 1973.
16. Mooney, T. O., Cole, T. M., and Chilgren, R. A. *Sexual Options for Paraplegics and Quadriplegics*. Boston: Little, Brown, 1975.
17. Nichols, R. L., Broido, P., Condon, R. E., Gorbach, S. L., and Nyhus, L. M. Effect of preoperative neomycin-erythcomycin intestinal preparation on the incidence of infectious complications following colon surgery. *Ann. Surg.* 178:453, 1973.
18. Nichols, R. L., and Smith, J. W. Modern approach to the diagnosis of anaerobic surgical sepsis. *Surg. Clin. North Am.* 55:21, 1975.
19. Passos, J., and Brand, L. Effects of agents used for oral hygiene. *Nurs. Res.* 15:196, 1966.
20. Potyk, D. Intestinal obstruction from impacted antacid tablets. *N. Engl. J. Med.* 283:134, 1970.
21. Putt, A. M. One experiment in nursing adults with peptic ulcers. *Nurs. Res.* 19:484, 1970.
21a. Rhoads, J. E. The control of large bowel cancer. *Cancer* 36:2314, 1975.
22. Rubin, P. (ed.). *Clinical Oncology for Medical Students and Physicians* (4th ed.). New York: American Cancer Society, 1974.
23. Sana, J. M., and Judge, R. D. *Physical Appraisal Methods in Nursing Practice*. Boston: Little, Brown, 1975.
24. Schuler, J., and Aliapoulios, M. The Cambridge loop colostomy. *Surg. Gynecol. Obstet.* 137:281, 1973.
25. Stokes, S. A. Fasting for obesity. *Am. J. Nurs.* 69:796, 1969.
26. Walike, B., Padilla, G., Bergstrom, N., Hanson, R., Kubo, W., Grant, M., and Wong, H. L. Patient Problems Related to Tube Feeding. In *Communicating Nursing Research*, vol. 8, *Critical Issues in Access to Data*. Boulder, Colo.: WICHE, 1975.
27. Walike, B. C., and Walike, J. W. Lactose content of tube feeding diets as a cause of diarrhea. *Laryngoscope* 83:1109, 1973.
28. Walike, J. W. Tube feeding syndrome in head and neck surgery. *Arch. Otolaryngol.* 89:117, 1969.
29. Zollinger, R. M. Surgical management of the ulcerogenic syndrome. *Hosp. Pract.* 9:72, 1974.

LIVER, BILIARY TRACT, AND PANCREAS

30. Aston, S. J., and Longmire, W. Management of the pancreas after pancreaticoduodenectomy. *Ann. Surg.* 179:322, 1974.
31. Brown, H. Treatment of hepatic failure and coma. *J.A.M.A.* 201:137, 1967.

32. Center for Disease Control. *Isolation Techniques for Use in Hospitals* (2nd ed.). DHEW Publication No. (CDC 76-8314). Atlanta, 1975.
33. Center for Disease Control, Bacterial Disease Division, Bureau of Epidemiology. *Morbid. Mortal. Wkly Rep.* 25. Supplement: Perspectives on the control of viral hepatitis, type B. No. 17. May 7, 1976.
34. Fidler, J. P., et al. Laser surgery in exsanguinating liver injury. *Ann. Surg.* 183:74, 1975.
35. Garibaldi, R. A., and Panky, G. A. Who should receive gamma globulin? *Patient Care* 8:93, 1974.
35a. Gocke, D. J. Current status of viral hepatitis. *Hosp. Med.* 11:8, 1975.
36. Hawkins, I. F., et al. Radiologic approach to obstructive jaundice and pancreatic disease. *Med. Clin. North Am.* 59:121, 1975.
37. Johnson, C. J., et al. Ear piercing and hepatitis. *J.A.M.A.* 227:1165, 1974.
38. Johnson, R. M., et al. Treatment of acute pancreatitis: In search of a rationale. *Proc. Instit. Med. Chicago* 29:268, 1973.
38a. Kadell, B., and Weiner, M. Current status of the transjugular approach for direct cholangiography. *Surg. Clin. North Am.* 53:1019, 1973.
39. Klotz, A. Laboratory tests for pancreatic function. *Hosp. Med.* 3:42, 1967.
40. LaMont, J. T. Postoperative jaundice. *Surg. Clin. North Am.* 54:637, 1974.
41. Lin, T. A simplified technique for hepatic resection: The crush method. *Ann. Surg.* 180:285, 1974.
42. Loeb, P. M., et al. Endoscopic pancreatocholangiography in the diagnosis of biliary tract disease. *Surg. Clin. North Am.* 53:1007, 1973.
43. Lokich, J., et al. Chemotherapy in pancreatic carcinoma. *Ann. Surg.* 179:450, 1974.
44. Tumen, H. J. Alcoholic liver disease. *Hosp. Med.* 10:6, 1974.
45. Vittal, S., B. V. Fulminant viral hepatitis and hepatic failure. *Am. Fam. Phys.* 9(5):110, 1974.
45a. WHO Scientific Group. *Viral Hepatitis Report of a WHO Scientific Group.* WHO Technical Rep. Series No. 512. Geneva, 1973.
46. Widman, F. K. *Goodale's Clinical Interpretation of Laboratory Tests* (7th ed.). Philadelphia: Davis, 1973.

Bibliography

GENERAL AND GASTROINTESTINAL

A. H. Robins G. I. Series: *Physical Examination of the Abdomen.* Richmond: Robins, 1969.
AMA Department of Drugs. *AMA Drug Evaluations* (2nd ed.). Acton, Mass.: Publishing Sciences Group, 1973.
Anderson, B., et al. Topical ampicillin against wound infection after colorectal surgery. *Ann. Surg.* 176:129, 1972.
Anxiety, recognition and intervention, programmed instruction. *Am. J. Nurs.* 65:129, 1965.
Aquirre, A., et al. The role of surgery and hyperalimentation in therapy of gastrointestinal-cutaneous fistulas. *Ann. Surg.* 180:393, 1974.
Ballinger, W. F., Treybal, J. C., and Vose, A. B. *Alexander's Care of the Patient in Surgery.* St. Louis: Mosby, 1972.
Beahrs, O., et al. Ileostomy with ileal reservoir rather than ileostomy alone. *Ann. Surg.* 179:634, 1974.
Behnke, H. D. *Guidelines for Comprehensive Nursing Care in Cancer.* (Report of a Series of Continuing Education Seminars at Sloan-Kettering Cancer Center.) New York: Springer, 1973.
Behringer, G. E. Polypoid lesions of the colon—Which should be removed? *Surg. Clin. North Am.* 54:699, 1974.
Belinsky, I., et al. Colon fiberoscopy: Technique in colon examination. *Am. J. Nurs.* 73:306, 1973.
Braasch, J. W. The surgical treatment of obesity. *Surg. Clin. North Am.* 51:667, 1971.
Connors, M. Ostomy care: A personal approach. *Am. J. Nurs.* 74:1422, 1974.
Corman, M. L., et al. Cathartics. *Am. J. Nurs.* 75:273, 1975.
Cross, J. E., and Parsons, C. R. Nurse teaching and goal-directed nurse teaching to motivate change in food selection behavior of hospitalized patients. *Nurs. Res.* 20:454, 1971.
Curtis, C. Colonoscopy: The nurse's role. *Am. J. Nurs.* 75:430, 1975.
DeRisi, L. L. Starving in the midst of plenty—Adult celiac disease. *Am. J. Nurs.* 70:1048, 1970.
Donovan, C., and Lenneberg, E. S. *Guidelines for the Rehabilitation of Ostomy Patients.* Chicago: International Association for Enterostomal Therapy, 1975.
Dukes, C. E. *Cancer of the Rectum.* London: Livingstone, 1960.
Dyk, R. B., and Sutherland, A. M. Adaptation of the spouse and other family members to the colostomy patient. *Cancer* 9:123, 1956.
Escovitz, G., and Rubin, W. The malabsorption syndrome. *Med. Clin. North Am.* 57:907, 1973.
Ferguson, D. Intestinal obstruction and paralytic ileus. *Hosp. Med.* 9:8, 1973.
Fleshman, R. P. Eating rituals and realities. *Nurs. Clin. North Am.* 8:91, 1973.
Fry, W. A., and Daicoff, G. R. Principles in the selection of colostomy. *Hosp. Med.* 3:12, 1967.
Gallagher, A. Body image changes in the patient with a colostomy. *Nurs. Clin. North Am.* 7:669, 1972.

Gibbs, G. E., and White, M. Stomal care. *Am. J. Nurs.* 72:268, 1972.

Gutkowski, F. Ostomy procedure: Nursing care before and after. *Am. J. Nurs.* 72:62, 1972.

Guyton, A. C. *Textbook of Medical Physiology* (4th ed.). Philadelphia: Saunders, 1971.

Hallenbeck, G. A., and Gleysteen, J. Proximal gastric vagotomy without drainage. *Ann. Surg.* 179:608, 1974.

Hansky, J. Clinical aspects of gastrin physiology. *Med. Clin. North Am.* 58:1217, 1974.

Hilger, E. E. Developing nursing outcome criteria. *Nurs. Clin. North Am.* 9:323, 1974.

Hoerr, S. O., and Hertzer, N. R. Current concepts of diagnosis and management of cancer of the stomach. *Hosp. Med.* 8:58, 1972.

Jacoway, J. R., et al. Oral cancer. *Hosp. Med.* 8:69, 1972.

Jensen, V. Better techniques for bagging stomas. Part II: Colostomies. *Nursing 74* 4:30, 1974.

Jensen, V. Better techniques for bagging stomas. Part III: Ileostomies. *Nursing 74* 4:60, 1974.

Jordon, G. L., DeBakey, M. E., and Duncan, J. M. Surgical management of perforated peptic ulcer. *Ann Surg.* 180:628, 1974.

Judge, R., and Zuidema, G. *Physical Diagnosis: A Physiologic Approach to the Clinical Examination* (2nd ed.). Boston: Little, Brown, 1968.

Kaplan, B. J. Detection of early cancer of the anorectum and colon. *Hosp. Med.* 7:53, 1971.

Katz, J. Gastrointestinal hormones. *Med. Clin. North Am.* 57:93, 1973.

Keefer, C., and Wilkins, R. *Medicine: Essentials of Clinical Practice.* Boston: Little, Brown, 1970.

Kennedy, T. The vagus and the consequences of vagotomy. *Med. Clin. North Am.* 58:1231, 1974.

Kock, N. C., et al. The quality of life after proctocolectomy and ileostomy. *Dis. Colon Rectum* 17:287, 1974.

Krieger, H. Guides to electrolyte balance in the postoperative patient. *Hosp. Med.* 3:62, 1967.

Lenneberg, E. Role of the enterostomal therapist and stoma rehabilitation clinics. *Cancer* 28:226, 1971.

Letton, A. H., et al. Rehabilitation of the patient with a colostomy. *Cancer* 28:219, 1971.

Levine, S. M., and Rubin, W. Benign disorders of the esophagus: Presentation, diagnosis and treatment. *Med. Clin. North Am.* 57:907, 1973.

Matt, R., and Nundy, S. Rectal carcinoma, abdominoperineal and anterior resection. *Surg. Clin. North Am.* 54:741, 1974.

McGinty, C. P. Hiatal hernia. *Hosp. Med.* 7:133, 1971.

Metheny, N. M., and Snively, W. D., Jr. *Nurses' Handbook of Fluid Balance.* Philadelphia: Lippincott, 1974.

Musante, G. J. Obesity—A behavioral treatment program. *Am. Fam. Physician* 10:95, 1974.

Muto, T., Bussey, J. R., and Marson, B. C. The evolution of cancer of the colon and rectum. *Cancer* 36:2251, 1975.

Newton, M. E., Beal, M. E., and Strauss, A. L. Nutritional aspects of nursing care. *Nurs. Res.* 16:46, 1967.

Patient assessment: Examination of the abdomen, programmed instruction. *Am. J. Nurs.* 74:1679, 1974.

Peery, T. M., and Miller, F. N. *Pathology: A Dynamic Introduction to Medicine and Surgery.* Boston: Little, Brown, 1971.

Phillips, S. F. Diarrhea: Pathogenesis and diagnostic techniques. *Postgrad. Med.* 37:65, 1975.

Prudden, J. F. Psychological problems following ileostomy and colostomy. *Cancer.* 28:236, 1971.

Reitz, M., and Pope, W. Mouth care. *Am. J. Nurs.* 73:1728, 1973.

Rodman, M. J., and Smith, D. W. *Pharmacology and Drug Therapy in Nursing.* Philadelphia: Lippincott, 1968.

Rosillo, R. H., Welty, M. J., and Grahm, W. P. The patient with maxillo-facial cancer. II. Psychological aspects. *Nurs. Clin. North Am.* 8:153, 1973.

Rowbotham, J. L. Colostomy problems—Dietary and colostomy management. *Cancer* 28:222, 1971.

Schauder, M. R. Ostomy care: Cone irrigations. *Am. J. Nurs.* 74:1424, 1974.

Schmidt, M., and Duncan, B. Modifying eating behavior in anorexia nervosa. *Am. J. Nurs.* 74:1646, 1974.

Seedor, M. M. *The Physical Assessment: A Programmed Unit of Study for Nurses.* New York: Teacher's College Press, 1974.

Sheridan, J. L. Obstructions of the intestinal tract. *Nurs. Clin. North Am.* 10:147, 1975.

Sill, A. R. Bulb-syringe technique for colonic stoma irrigation. *Am. J. Nurs.* 70:536, 1970.

Smith, M. L. Parotidectomy. *Am. J. Nurs.* 76:422, 1976.

Southwick, H. Cancer of the tongue. *Surg. Clin. North Am.* 53:147, 1973.

Sparberg, M. *Ileostomy Care.* Springfield, Ill.: Thomas, 1971.

Spivak, J. L., and Barnes, H. V. *Manual of Clinical Problems in Internal Medicine.* Boston: Little, Brown, 1974.

Stemmar, E. A. et al. A physiological approach to the surgical treatment of the dumping syndrome. *J.A.M.A.* 199:159, 1967.

Swinton, N. W., and Samaan, S. T. Pilonidal sinus disease. *Hosp. Med.* 4:12, 1968.

Thorek, P. Acute obstruction of the colon. *Hosp. Med.* 3:53, 1967.

Trowbridge, J. E. Caring for patients with facial or intra-oral reconstruction. *Am. J. Nurs.* 73:1930, 1973.

Turnbull, R. B., Jr. Overviews of the problems following treatment of rectal cancer. *Cancer* 28:220, 1971.

Turnbull, R. B., Jr., and Weakley, F. L. *Atlas of Intestinal Stomas.* St. Louis: Mosby, 1967.

U.S. Department of Health, Education and Welfare. *Research Advances 1975*. Bethesda, Md.: DHEW (MH) no. 75–3, 1975.

Vukovich, V., and Frubb, R. *Care of the Ostomy Patient*. St. Louis: Mosby, 1973.

Walike, B. C. A Physiological and Behavioral Approach to Understanding the Mechanisms of Obesity and Anorexia. In M. Batey (ed.), *Communicating Nursing Research*, vol. 6, *Collaboration and Competition*. Boulder, Colo.: WICHE, 1973.

Walike, B. C., Jordon, H. A., and Stellar, E. Studies of eating behavior. *Nurs. Res.* 18:108, 1969.

Washington, J. A., Dearing, W., Judd, E. S., and Elveback, L. R. Effect of preoperative antibiotic regimen on development of infection after intestinal surgery. *Ann. Surg.* 180:567, 1974.

Watson, R. C. The whole body scan. Computed tomography (CT)—A major advance in the diagnosis of cancer. *Clin. Bull.* 6:47, 1976.

Welty, M. J., Grahm, W. P., and Rosillo, R. H. The patient with maxillofacial cancer. I. Surgical treatment and nursing care. *Nurs. Clin. North Am.* 8:137, 1973.

Weisburg, H. *Water, Electrolytes and Acid-Base Balance* (2nd ed.). Baltimore: Williams & Wilkins, 1962.

Wilkins, E. W., and Burke, J. F. Colon esophageal bypass. *Am. J. Surg.* 129:394, 1975.

Willacker, J. Bowel sounds. *Am. J. Nurs.* 73:2100, 1973.

Williams, S. R. *Nutrition and Diet Therapy* (2nd ed.). St. Louis: Mosby, 1973.

Winkelstein, C., and Lyons, A. S. Insight into the emotional aspects of ileostomies and colostomies. *Medical Insight Reprint*. New York: Insight Publishing, 1971.

Zakariai, Y. M., Quan, S. H. Q., and Hajdu, S. I. Carcinoid tumors of the gastrointestinal tract. *Cancer* 35:588, 1975.

LIVER, BILIARY TRACT, AND PANCREAS

Adson, M. A. Carcinoma of the gallbladder. *Surg. Clin. North Am.* 53:1203, 1973.

Ashkar, F. Clinical guide to pancreatic screening. *Hosp. Med.* 10:21, 1974.

Barone, R. M. Treatment of carcinoma of the pancreas with radon seed implantation and intra-arterial infusion of 5-FUDR. *Med. Clin. North Am.* 55:117, 1975.

Bauer, J. J., et al. The use of the Sengstaken-Blakemore tube for immediate control of esophogeal varices. *Ann. Surg.* 179:273, 1974.

Belinsky, I. Visualizing the pancreatic and biliary ducts. *Am. J. Nurs.* 76:936, 1976.

Berk, R. N. Radiology of the gallbladder and bile ducts. *Surg. Clin. North Am.* 53:973, 1973.

Center for Disease Control, Bacterial Disease Division, Bureau of Epidemiology. *Hepatitis Surveillance Report No. 37*. Atlanta, 1975.

Chey, W. Y., et al. Diagnosis of diseases of the pancreas and biliary tract. *J.A.M.A.* 198:167, 1966.

Criteria Committee National Council on Alcoholism. Criteria for the diagnosis of alcoholism. *Am. J. Psychiatry* 129:2, 1972.

Curtis, S. J. A guide to practical use of liver function tests. *Hosp. Med.* 10:51, 1974.

duPlessis, D. J., and Jersky, J. The management of acute cholecystitis. *Surg. Clin. North Am.* 53:1071, 1973.

U.S. Department of Health, Education and Welfare, National Institute on Alcohol Abuse and Alcoholism. *Facts About Alcohol and Alcoholism*. Rockville, Md., 1974.

Fortner, J. G. Recent advances in pancreatic cancer. *Surg. Clin. North Am.* 54:859, 1974.

Glenn, F. Retained calculi within the biliary ductal system. *Ann. Surg.* 179:528, 1974.

Goldsmith, H. S. Hepatic resection. *Surg. Clin. North Am.* 53:703, 1973.

Hayter, J. Impaired liver function and related nursing care. *Am. J. Nurs.* 68:2374, 1968.

Hofman, A., and Thistle, J. L. Chenodeoxycholic acid: The Mayo Clinic experience. *Hosp. Pract.* 9:41, 1974.

Howard, J. M. Problems associated with pancreatic surgery. *Hosp. Med.* 7:69, 1971.

Kaude, J. V., and Deland, F. Hepatomegaly. *Med. Clin. North Am.* 59:145, 1975.

Knoebel, L. K. The Gastrointestinal System. II. The Exocrine Pancreas, Biliary System and Small and Large Intestines. In E. Selkurt (ed.), *Basic Physiology for the Health Sciences*. Boston: Little, Brown, 1975.

Lahana, D., and Schoenfield, L. J. Progress in medical therapy of gallstones. *Surg. Clin. North Am.* 53:1053, 1973.

Leadbetter, A., et al. Carcinoma of the pancreas. *Am. J. Surg.* 129:356, 1975.

Leopold, G. R., and Sokoloff, J. Ultrasonic scanning in the diagnosis of biliary disease. *Surg. Clin. North Am.* 53:1043, 1973.

Levin, J. L., et al. Hepatitis B transmission by dentists. *J.A.M.A.* 228:1139, 1974.

Longmire, W. P., et al. Elective hepatic surgery. *Ann. Surg.* 179:712, 1974.

Midgley, J. W., and Osterhage, R. A. Effect of nursing instruction and length of hospitalization on postoperative complications in cholecystectomy patients. *Nurs. Res.* 22:69, 1973.

Mikkelsen, W. P. Portal hypertension. Part I. Clinical assessment. *Hosp. Med.* 9:56, 1973.

Mikkelsen, W. P. Portal hypertension. Part II. Management. *Hosp. Med.* 9:6, 1973.

Olsen, H. Pancreatitis: A prospective clinical evaluation of 100 cases and review of the literature. *Am. J. Dig. Dis.* 19:1077, 1974.

Overall, J. E., and Patrick, J. H. Unitary alcoholism and its personality correlation. *J. Abnorm. Psychol.* 79:303, 1972.

Peskin, G. W. The treatment of silent gallstones. *Surg. Clin. North Am.* 53:1063, 1973.

Peterson, H. (ed.). Round table—Alcoholism: No longer the impossible challenge. *Patient Care* 8:22, 1974.

Pfeffer, R. B. Acute hemorrhagic pancreatitis. *Hosp. Med.* 6:79, 1970.

Saypol, G. M. Post cholecystectomy syndrome. *Hosp. Med.* 6:91, 1970.

Scheig, R. Acute biliary disease. *Hosp. Med.* 6:52, 1970.

Schoenfield, L. J. Clinical aspects of the chenodeotycholic acid trial. *Hosp. Pract.* 9:53, 1974.

Simmons, S., and Given, B. Acute pancreatitis. *Am. J. Nurs.* 71:964, 1971.

Vennes, J. A., et al. Endoscopic cholangiography for biliary system diagnosis. *Ann. Int. Med.* 80:64, 1974.

Wareen, K., and Garabedian, M. Surgical management of chronic relapsing pancreatitis. *Hosp. Pract.* 9:72, 1974.

Warren, W. D., et al. The meso-splenal renal shunt procedures: A comprehensive approach to portasystemic decompression. *Ann. Surg.* 179:791, 1974.

Way, L. W. Retained common duct stones. *Surg. Clin. North Am.* 53:1139, 1973.

Webster, P. D., and Spainhour, J. B. Pathophysiology and management of acute pancreatitis. *Hosp. Pract.* 9:59, 1974.

Wheeler, H. O. Pathogenesis of gallstones. *Surg. Clin. North Am.* 53:963, 1973.

chapter 8

Patients with Selected Endocrine Disorders

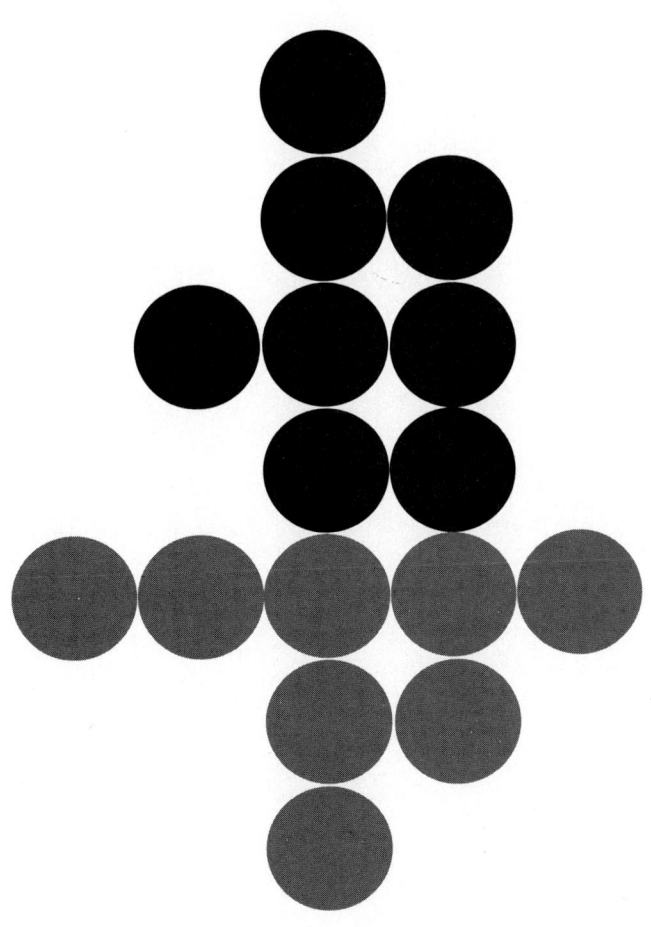

The endocrine system provides for both regulation and adaptation of body processes. Most endocrine dysfunction is not specifically physiologic or psychological. Instead, endocrine dysfunction demonstrates the relation between body and mind in total body functioning. Patients with endocrine dysfunction usually exhibit unique and individual signs and symptoms that cannot always be matched with an expected pattern for a certain type of dysfunction. Therefore, nursing care for these patients must include provisions for their unique and individual needs necessary for adaptation.

This chapter is concerned with the functions of the thyroid, pituitary, parathyroids, the adrenals, and the pancreas. The pineal and thymus glands are also discussed briefly. Hormonal control of reproductive function is discussed in Chapter 9. It should be mentioned that other body organs are thought to have endocrine function also. These include the lungs, which recently have been found to have endocrine functions in certain disease states. The intestinal mucosa has endocrine functions, as does the kidney in its ability to secrete erythropoietin, which is also considered an endocrine function.

For the most part, endocrine dysfunction is related to a failure or an inability to adapt. Nursing care and treatment are generally focused on helping the individual learn to control the effects of this failure or inability. Because this care requires that the nurse have a good understanding of the physiology of hormone secretion and activity in the body, this chapter includes considerable information about the mechanisms of hormonal activity in the body.

The action of hormones is biochemical in nature and therefore is dependent on an appropriate environment to be effective. There are three classes of hormones: polypeptides, steroids, and amines. Each class of hormone has certain requisites for activity, and different hormones have highly specific functions. It is fascinating to note that the hormones are capable of a great deal of adaptability within the confines of their specific functions and that the functions of different hormones are intertwined with the functions of not only other hormones, but also with those of many other chemical substances. The internal milieu of the cell and its various divisions are thus protected by having more than one means to accomplish some of the same activities.

The endocrine glands by definition are ductless glands that release their secretions (hormones) directly into the bloodstream (Fig. 8-1). These glands are highly vascularized, which is fitting, since the circulatory system provides the means of transport for hormones. Hormones are delivered to their target organs where they elicit specific responses. All hormones are subject to control by cells in their target organs. The receptor cells not only provide for receiving the hormone within the target organ, but protect the hormone's message substances from degradation long enough for the message to be acted on within the organ (Fig. 8-2). The concentrations of metabolites in the cells and stimuli from the nervous system may directly or indirectly influence a given cell's response to the message received, so that there is integration of function at a cellular level.

Regulation of hormones occurs via direct neural stimulation such as in the adrenal medulla and the posterior pituitary gland, by concentrations of metabolites as in the pancreas and parathyroid glands, and via feedback loops as in the anterior pituitary, the thyroid, the adrenals, and the gonads. Feedback loops may simply involve the endocrine gland and the target organ, or may include a group of interrelated endocrine glands. A hierarchy of function exists in some of these feedback loops in which the hypothalamus integrates body functions and neuroendocrine functions through secretion of releasing hormones. The hypothalamus both directly and indirectly influences hormone secretion in the anterior pituitary, the master gland. The anterior pituitary is called the master gland because it controls secretion of tropic hormones which in turn influence stimulation or inhibition of secretion of hormones in the gonads, the thyroid, and the adrenal glands. Tropic hormone secretion is influenced by concentrations of releasing factors and of hormones secreted by the specific endocrine glands. Most often this influence is accomplished through negative feedback loops in which decreases in hormonal levels stimulate secretion of releasing factors or of tropic hormones which in turn stimulate secretion of specific hormones. To some extent, hormone secretion is also controlled within the endocrine glands independently of the control of higher centers. Mechanisms for regulation of specific hormones are discussed in subsequent sections of this chapter.

Endocrine dysfunction may be caused by

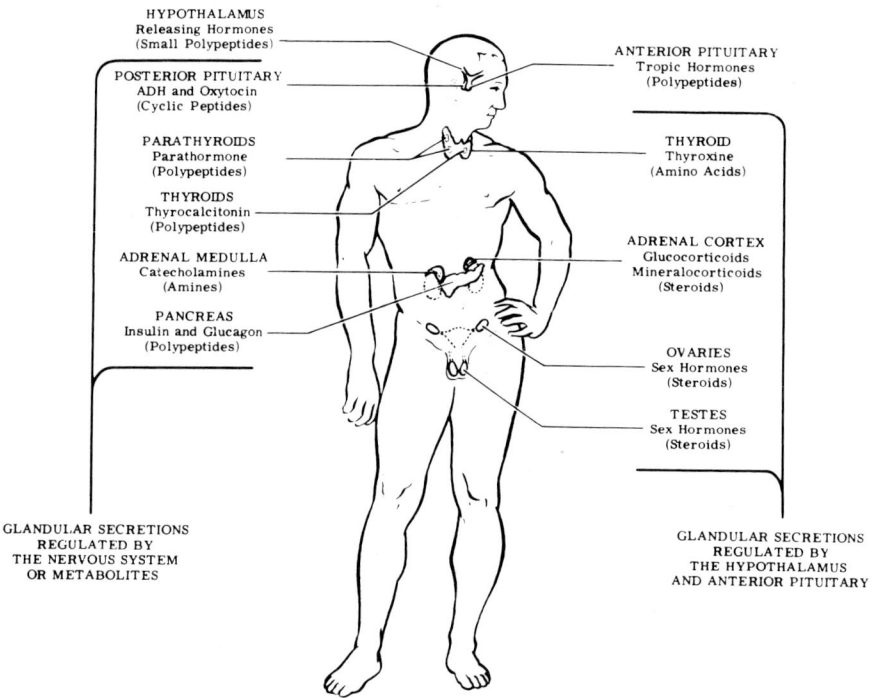

Figure 8-1
Relative location of the endocrine glands. (Adapted from E. Selkurt, *Basic Physiology for the Health Sciences*. Boston: Little, Brown and Company, 1975. Reproduced by permission.)

overproduction or underproduction or failure to secrete hormones. There is interdependency among hormone functions, so that dysfunction of one endocrine gland may cause reciprocal dysfunction in other endocrine glands. Some hormones are antagonistic to the action of other hormones whereas others support the action of still other hormones so that there are checks and balances in the regulatory processes. Treatment of dysfunction involves determining the nature of the imbalance and its cause, and then correcting the imbalance. It may be necessary to replace hormones not being produced by the body, or control may be achieved by regulating factors that influence the metabolic processes that affect hormone secretion. This regulation depends on knowledge of hormones, their activities in the body, their precursors, and substances that influence their action. The nurse must understand these processes in order to teach and counsel the patient receiving treatment for regulation of hormonal balance.

Hormones were first discovered in the 1800s and research for synthesis of hormones and causes of dysfunction of the endocrine system is ongoing. Since there is much theoretical information about how best to facilitate regulation of hormonal balance, the nurse will find that different physicians use different treatment plans with equal success. The nurse must understand the rationale of a given treatment plan for regulation of a patient's endocrine dysfunction to be able to effectively plan for nursing care. In many instances nursing care involves helping the patient learn to control factors that influence the metabolic processes that affect hormone secretion and activity. These factors often include diet, exercise, and medications and may also require changes in the patient's daily habits.

The Pituitary Gland

The pituitary gland can be considered as the "tower" at an airline terminal in its role of controlling and regulating the secretion of

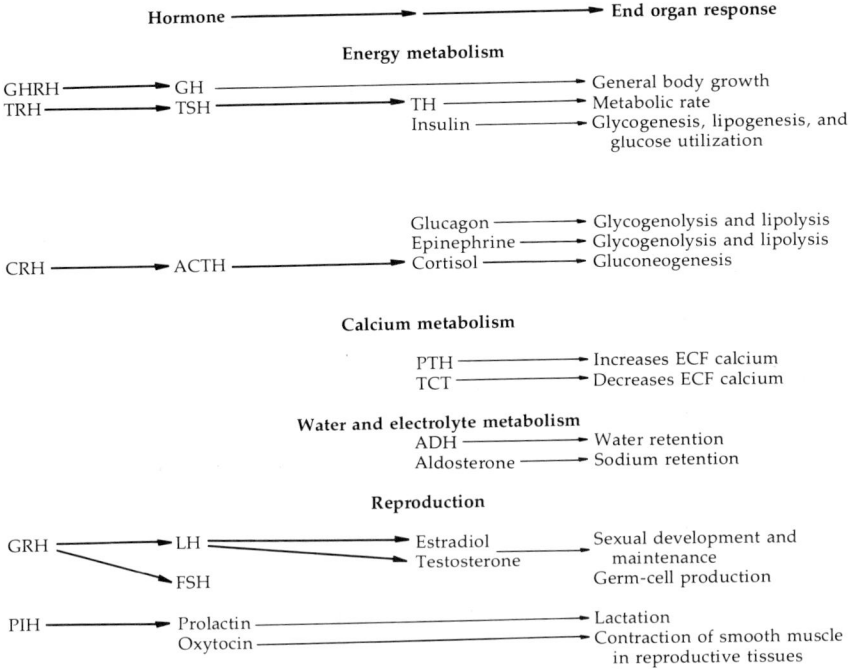

Figure 8-2
The hormones and the major end-organ responses. The hormones are divided into types depending on their end-organ effects. (Adapted from E. Selkurt, *Basic Physiology for the Health Sciences*. Boston: Little, Brown and Company, 1975. Reproduced by permission.)

body hormones. Neural transmissions from the hypothalamus are delivered to the pituitary gland in the form of releasing hormones or factors, which stimulate secretion of tropic hormones by the pituitary. Most of these tropic hormones in turn stimulate secretion of hormones in target structures—the thyroid, parathyroids, adrenals, pancreas, ovaries, and testes. Growth hormone and prolactin act directly on specified body tissues. The pituitary integrates information received through various types of feedback loops—open, closed, positive, and negative—from the target areas, the hypothalamus, and, in some instances, within the pituitary, either to secrete or inhibit the secretion of tropic hormones. In this way, conscious and subconscious input related to emotions and perceptions and body functions of physiologic origin are transmitted electrically through the nervous system and hypothalamus. From the hypothalamus, the electrical impulses are interpreted and converted to chemical transmitters or hormones, which are the communication medium of the endocrine system, and are conveyed by the circulating blood. At the level of the target structures, neural influences are primarily indirect, serving to increase blood flow in the structure specified for hormonal action such as the thyroid or adrenal.

The hypothalamus is bordered by the sulci of the temporal lobes on each side, by the optic chiasm anteriorly, and by the mamillary bodies posteriorly. The pituitary has two parts: the neurohypophysis and the adenohypophysis. The neurohypophysis is made up of three areas: the median eminence (located in the center of the base of the hypothalamus), the neural lobe, and the infundibulum (the funnel-shaped portion or stalk which connects the median eminence with the neural lobe). The adenohypophysis makes up 75 percent of the weight of the pituitary, and traditional classifications of its cell types are acidophils, basophils, and chromophobes. The pituitary is located in the sella turcica, a depression in the sphenoid bone. The diaphragma sellae separates the pituitary from overlying cranial structures.

The superior and inferior hypophyseal arteries, branches of the internal carotids, provide the blood supply to the pituitary. The posterior pituitary's blood supply from the inferior hypophyseal arteries is separate from that of the anterior pituitary. In the median eminence, the superior hypophyseal arteries divide into a system of capillary loops which communicate with the portal system of venules that pass through the infundibulum or stalk to the adenohypophysis. The inferior hypophyseal arteries also divide into capillaries at the lower part of the infundibulum, with shorter portal venules. The trabecular arteries also supply the adenohypophysis. The pituitary blood supply is considered crucial to integration of neuroendocrine function of the pituitary. Numerous nerve fibers are located in the median eminence. This rich nerve supply may be important in the transmission of central nervous system input to the pituitary, exercising control over the release of tropic hormones. TRH (thyrotropin-releasing hormone) was synthesized in 1970. Releasing and inhibiting factors have been isolated for MSH (melanin-stimulating hormone), GH (growth hormone), and CRF (corticotropin releasing hormone).

POSTERIOR PITUITARY DYSFUNCTION

The posterior pituitary is the storage area for two hormones secreted in the hypothalamus: vasopressin, commonly known as ADH, and oxytocin. After they are synthesized, these two hormones are bound to neurophysin, a protein, to be delivered to the posterior pituitary. Release of ADH and oxytocin is stimulated by nerve impulses along the neurohypophyseal tract from the hypothalamus to the pituitary. Calcium is important in release of the hormones from neurophysin. Experiments have shown that there are two forms of vasopressin: arginine and lysine. Arginine vasopressin is predominant in man.

ADH (vasopressin) is a potent antidiuretic hormone and is released from the pituitary to conserve body water when dehydration occurs. Osmoreceptors in the anterior portion of the hypothalamus are sensitive to the plasma osmolarity. ADH release is also stimulated by decreased blood volume. The mechanism for this response to ADH is not known; it is thought that the volume of blood in the thoracic vessels is important in this response. The mechanisms through which the hypothalamus responds to decreased osmotic pressure in the plasma and decreased blood volume are associated with the thirst response, which brings a person to conscious awareness of the need to drink fluids.

The action of ADH for conservation of water takes place in the kidney, in the distal tubule and in the collecting ducts. ADH increases permeability of the distal tubules and collecting ducts and, along with the osmotic gradient, is able to return water to the blood to expand blood volume and decrease blood osmolarity. ADH is inactivated in the liver and kidney and a small percentage is excreted in the active form.

When given in large amounts exogenously, vasopressin stimulates contraction of smooth muscle, causing an increased vascular resistance in both peripheral and visceral blood vessels. For this reason, it has a variety of therapeutic uses.

Diabetes insipidus results from insufficient ADH. This condition may be caused by trauma or destruction from neoplastic disease of the hypothalamus or the neurohypophyseal tracts. It may occur for a single short period following brain injuries in which the hypothalamus is injured. Secondary diabetes insipidus occurs from head injuries and from neoplasms most frequently. Primary or idiopathic diabetes insipidus occurs infrequently.

Idiopathic diabetes insipidus usually has an acute onset characterized by a sudden increase in urine volume (polyuria) and concomitant thirst (polydipsia). The thirst is an adaptive response to the increased loss of water. However, compulsive drinking of water can initiate polyuria that cannot be differentiated from that occurring in diabetes insipidus. Plasma osmolality usually is slightly higher than normal in diabetes insipidus and the glomerular filtration rate is normal or low.

The alert active person with diabetes insipidus is able to compensate effectively for the water loss of polyuria by drinking extremely large quantities of water. It is possible that the urinary output may be up to 10 liters within a 24-hour period. When diabetes insipidus occurs in an incapacitated or comatose person, it is necessary that urinary output be measured precisely and that fluid volume be restored. The nurse should carefully monitor fluid intake and output for critically ill patients at all times. This is particularly essential following brain injury, as diabetes insipidus may occur, usually within a 4-week period following the injury.

Diabetes insipidus is diagnosed by determining the cause of the polyuria. The causes may include excessive intake of water, insufficient ADH, or impaired renal function. Specific tests for diabetes insipidus include the water restriction test and challenge tests, which involve administering a substance to elicit secretion of ADH. These tests are performed differently in different places but the same general procedure is usually followed.

The water restriction test is conducted by withholding fluids for a 24-hour period. During this time, the urine from each voided specimen is measured and the osmolality is determined. Body weight is obtained at the beginning of the test and periodically during the test to ensure that no more than 3 to 5 percent of body weight is lost in fluid output. This is necessary to prevent sufficient decreases in blood volume to cause cardiovascular distress. Normally, urine flow is below 0.5 ml per minute and the concentration is 800 mOsm per kilogram. In diabetes insipidus urine volume is far greater and the concentration is less, usually below 200 mOsm per kilogram [10]. The specific gravity of the urine is often 1.001 to 1.007.

A challenge test to stimulate the secretion of ADH is that of giving nicotine acid tartrate intravenously. Urine volume decreases within about 3 hours following administration of nicotine if diabetes insipidus is present. Aqueous pitressin (an antidiuretic agent) may also be given intravenously or intramuscularly to determine ADH response. Fluids are restricted, and urine volumes and concentrations are measured for a 3-hour or otherwise specified period. Both polyuria and polydipsia decrease following administration of pitressin if diabetes insipidus is present.

Hypertonic solutions may be given intravenously to well-hydrated people to determine if ADH will be affected. Urine volume normally decreases with infusion of a hypertonic solution, but in diabetes insipidus the volume of urine continues to be great.

One of the greatest problems experienced by people with diabetes insipidus is the annoyance of having to urinate frequently. This has many implications, because it limits to some extent the freedom to go about unhampered (by having to find a bathroom) and it also interrupts sleep. The intense thirst is also distressing. Treatment includes use of pitressin inhaled through the nostrils or given intramuscularly. Vasopressin tannate in oil, made of posterior pituitary extracts, can be given in dosages of three to five units intramuscularly. The effects last from 36 to 72 hours. When this drug is used, the person is counseled not to give regular injections, but to wait until the symptoms of polyuria and polydipsia recur before taking another dose. This prevents retention of fluid. Lypressin (Diapid), a synthetic polypeptide, lysine-8-vasopressin, is available as a nasal spray. The effect is of shorter duration than that of vasopressin tannate in oil, lasting only from 3 to 8 hours, and it can be used singly or between injections.

Some persons develop allergies to the posterior pituitary preparation made from animal extracts and therefore find use of lypressin more satisfactory. It is suggested that, if the nasal spray requires more than two sprays, the medication should be used more frequently instead of giving a larger dose at one time. The nasal spray is not effective in those who have nasal congestion from any cause. It is also contraindicated in hypertension. The side effects of lypressin are fewer than those noted with use of vasopressin powder. The posterior pituitary powder is used as snuff, inhaled in dosages of 5 to 40 mg. People who have formerly used the powder need to be informed that the nasal spray lypressin should not be inhaled. It should be administered by holding the head in a normal upright position while the spray is placed in contact with the nasal mucosa.

Chlorothiazide sodium (Diuril) and chlorpropamide (Diabinese) has also been found useful in treating diabetes insipidus, although it might seem a contradiction that a diuretic reduces polyuria. It is thought that the action of inhibiting active transport of sodium in the distal tubules contributes to improved concentration of urine in diabetes insipidus.

Protein and salt are restricted. The purpose of these restrictions is to reduce the urine volume through decreasing the amount of solutes in the plasma.

Oxytocin, the second pituitary hormone stored in the posterior pituitary, is released independently of vasopressin. Oxytocin was the first hormone to be developed in a synthetic preparation. Du Vineaud and his associates discovered its structure in 1954 [10]. Oxytocin functions to contract uterine muscles and mediates the reflex mechanism of milk letdown or ejection in nursing mothers. There is no identified function of oxytocin in males.

Therapeutically, oxytocin has many applications. It is used to induce labor, to control postpartum hemorrhage, and to relieve the pain of breast engorgement. Very large doses are required to decrease peripheral vascular resistance. The effects of large doses include increased cardiac output from increased peripheral resistance, causing tachycardia and increased blood pressure.

ANTERIOR PITUITARY DYSFUNCTION

The anterior pituitary or adenohypophysis is the glandular portion of the pituitary and synthesizes a number of important hormones. These hormones are secreted by specialized cells, namely corticotropic, melanotropic, somatotropic, gonadotropic, lactotropic, and thyrotropic. The two major secretory cell types are the acidophils and the basophils. Chromophobe cells are nonsecretory. Because of this cell specialization, it is possible to have dysfunction of one type of cell with resultant hyposecretion. All the cells of the anterior pituitary can be involved in dysfunction; this condition is called panhypopituitarism.

The adenohypophysis is essential to life because it secretes the very important tropic hormones that influence body homeostasis. Endocrinology is a rapidly developing area in which new information is continually being brought forth by researchers. Although much is currently known about the mechanisms of biosynthesis of hormones, many questions remain to be answered. Of major interest is the integration of neural regulation and control with hormone synthesis and release through feedback systems. The tropic hormones synthesized by the anterior pituitary have specialized functions, either by acting directly on body tissues or by stimulating the biosynthesis of other hormones in target glands or organs. Neural input that influences release of adenohypophyseal hormones is delivered to the anterior pituitary through the hypothalamus. Plasma levels of hormones produced by the target glands and organs also influence the synthesis and release of adenohypophyseal hormones.

Somatotropin, or growth hormone (GH), is secreted by somatotropic cells that are located in the lateral aspects of the anterior pituitary. GH is essential to generalized growth from childhood to adulthood. It is thought that GH acts through mediation of somatomedin, but little is known about the source or specific activity of somatomedin. Among the activities of somatomedin are increased synthesis of DNA, of ribonucleic acids, and of collagen.

Growth hormone is thought to be necessary for repair of body tissues through its anabolic effects. It does not have a specific target organ, but acts directly on body tissues to achieve its effects. It is normally secreted most consistently during sleep. Its secretion is stimulated by decreased blood sugar levels, ingestion of proteins, exercise, and stress. It produces a positive nitrogen balance and fosters retention of sodium, chloride, potassium, magnesium, and phosphorus and promotes gastrointestinal absorption of calcium. Growth hormone is antagonistic to the activity of insulin, a function that protects the body from development of hypoglycemia.

Specific dysfunction from hypersecretion of GH is **gigantism** if the hypersecretion occurs prior to the closure of the epiphyses of the long bones. Hypersecretion of GH following epiphyseal closure results in acromegaly. Adenomas of the anterior pituitary are the major cause of hypersecretion of GH. Hyperplasia of the pituitary is another cause.

The onset of **acromegaly** is usually insidious, occurring most frequently in the age range of 30 to 60 years. The pattern of growth varies among individuals with acromegaly probably because of varying genetic factors and differences in the age of onset. Eventually, a plateau is reached. In children with hypersecretion of GH there is delayed epiphyseal closure and the growth period is extended. Gigantism is usually associated with hyposecretion of gonadotropic hormones, and giants are often sexually immature. Children with hypersecretion of GH may reach heights of 8 feet or more and tend to have short life spans, becoming debilitated early in life. They are subject to development of infections and, as adults, often have hyposecretion of growth hormone.

Acromegaly influences the soft tissues and

acral portions of the body (the extremities). Changes are evidenced by increased thickness of bones and increased mass of soft tissues. Facial features change progressively, and there is excessive growth of the skull bones. The entire face seems to become bigger and wider, with development of a lantern jaw, that is, growth of the mandible so that it protrudes. This is also called prognathism. If one extends the jaw so that the lower lip protrudes and the lower teeth reach beyond the upper teeth, one can somewhat experience the feeling of having a lantern jaw. The frontal and nasal bones and the frontal, mastoid, and ethmoid sinuses are enlarged. The teeth shift with the bony enlargement, so that spaces appear between them. The tongue is also enlarged.

The skin seems to stretch so that all the pores and markings of the skin become increasingly obvious, and the skin has a coarse appearance. Body hair increases in amount and also becomes coarse in texture. During the period of active growth, there is excessive sweating and the skin is oily, having an odor.

Changes in the joints include proliferation of the articular cartilage, causing increased spaces between joints. There are also changes in the articular plates, and arthritis may develop. In some persons with acromegaly, the arthritis is debilitating, whereas others have only mild symptoms. The hands thicken and a characteristic tufting of the distal phalangeal tips creates a spade-like appearance.

Most of the body organs are also enlarged, particularly the kidneys. As reabsorption of phosphorus is increased in acromegaly, hyperphosphatemia may occur. The heart is enlarged and cardiovascular symptoms may develop, including coronary arteriosclerosis, hypertension, and, eventually, congestive heart failure. Other body organs and glands, including the liver, spleen, pancreas, thyroid, and parathyroids, also enlarge. About 10 percent of the people with acromegaly have diabetes. The total amount of interstitial fluid increases because of the increase in the tissue mass.

Some people also develop symptoms of nerve compression, because the nerves are caught between enlarged bones and soft tissues. The carpal tunnel syndrome (pain, numbness, and tingling of the fingers caused by compression of the median nerve) is common, as are paresthesias and neuropathies.

The person with acromegaly may have all or a few of these changes. The enlargement of the sella turcica from hyperplasia of pituitary tissue or from growth of an adenoma may cause headache and impairment of vision to varying degrees.

Diagnosis of acromegaly comprises obtaining a history of the development of signs and symptoms and evaluating the level of growth hormone in blood plasma. Because the symptoms develop over a long period of time, the person with acromegaly often finds it difficult to relate the onset of symptoms to events with any degree of specificity. A comparison of pictures taken at various ages of the patient and talking with those who do not see him or her consistently to learn their perceptions of the changes in appearance are ways of determining the time span of the changes in growth of the acral portions of the body. As is true of anyone whose appearance changes, the nurse should recognize that people with acromegaly are often disturbed by their distorted or unpleasant body image.

Growth hormone levels from plasma are obtained in the fasting state and prior to activity, such as bathing or eating breakfast. Challenge tests using oral glucose, followed by drawing a blood sample 1½ hours after the ingestion of glucose, gives an indication of the activity of growth hormones. Normally, the level of growth hormone should decrease after the ingestion of glucose.

A number of people with acromegaly also have variations from normal levels of other adenopituitary hormones. Approximately 25 percent have hyperthyroidism with formation of goiter. Eventually, they become hypothyroid if suppression of pituitary tissue occurs. Prolactin levels are often high in persons with acromegaly. There is frequently a decrease in ACTH reserve, and many pituitary tumors are associated with decreased secretion of gonadotropin. As mentioned previously, giants may be sexually immature for this reason.

Treatment for acromegaly caused by pituitary tumors consists of a variety of options. These include surgical removal of the tumor, chemotherapy, or radiation.

Hyposecretion of growth hormone occurs as a single deficiency or in relation to hyposecretion of other anterior pituitary hormones. In children, hyposecretion results in **dwarfism.** Approximately one-third of all dwarfs have hyposecretion of GH as a single entity, while the remainder often have other hormone deficiencies as well. Growth deficiency may be noted in the first year of life or obvious symptoms may not occur until the ages of 1 to 3 years. In dwarfs, the rate of growth is slow, and adult dwarfs rarely achieve heights over 4 or 5 feet.

A very small percentage of dwarfs have an inherited recessive gene, which is specific to secretion of growth hormone. The involvement of somatotropin is postulated, as the concentrations of somatomedin are low in these people. These dwarfs grow into adulthood and, although their puberty is delayed, have normal sexual functions and the ability to procreate. The African pygmies have a polygenic inheritance defect which makes them resistant to both growth hormone and somatomedin. Their somatomedin concentrations are normal and they often have glucose intolerance. Approximately one-third of the dwarf population have tumors, either craniopharyngiomas or pituitary tumors. These dwarfs have diabetes insipidus and some have cleft palates. The deficiency of growth is often not noted until the child reaches toddlerhood, when skeletal growth becomes obviously slow in relation to normal growth patterns. Growth failure caused by isolated GH deficiency affects boys more frequently than girls. Indications of growth failure include prolonged immaturity of facial features and body size. The child-dwarf often has fat deposits over the iliac crests and abdomen, so that he appears pudgy. Fine wrinkles appear around the mouth and eyes and eruption of the secondary teeth is delayed. About 10 percent have hypoglycemia, while impaired glucose tolerance is common.

Diagnosis of the cause of dwarfism is often difficult, as many factors can lead to delayed growth. Among these are nutritional deficiencies, hypothyroidism in which bone maturation delay is predominant, and dysfunction of gonadal tissue, which is associated with a variety of anomalies as well as retardation of growth. Children who have severe chronic diseases or debilitating diseases, and who have received immunosuppressive therapy, may have delayed growth. Growth retardation is part of the malabsorption syndrome in children. When the retardation is related to nutritional deficiencies, ingestion of a proper diet causes the condition to reverse and the child then is capable of normal growth. Treatment of hypothyroidism also corrects the growth deficiencies, depending on the age of the child when treatment is initiated.

Buccal smears to detect genetic deficiencies, radioimmunoassay of GH levels, x-rays to detect pituitary or cranial tumors, and thyroid function studies are usually done in an extensive diagnostic plan to evaluate the cause of dwarfism. The plasma GH levels in children are normally low. Therefore provocative or challenge tests are done to determine the child's GH level. Administration of regular insulin in a dosage of 0.05 to 0.1 units per kilogram of body weight or arginine or L-dopa normally stimulates secretion and release of GH. When insulin is given, it is important to have glucose available to prevent severe hypoglycemic reactions. Arginine is usually not associated with side effects while L-dopa may cause nausea and postural hypotension. The latter is prevented by having the patient rest in a reclining position.

Treatment for children who have pituitary dysfunction consists in giving GH. Because no suitable synthetic GH has been developed and because GH from animals is not effective in humans, human GH must be used. The National Pituitary Agency, 210 W. Fayette St., Baltimore, Md., collects human cadaver pituitary glands so that GH can be made available to children with a firm diagnosis of pituitary dysfunction in preference to other uses, including research, or experimental treatment for other types of dysfunction. With treatment by human GH, the child has an initial rapid growth that may be as much as 6 inches. The rate of growth levels off after the initial spurt but is continuous according to normal growth patterns. In a few persons, there is a refractory response because of the high levels of antibodies they have for GH.

While hyposecretion or hypersecretion of GH occurs most frequently as a single entity, there can also be hypersecretion of other single hormones. **Forbes-Albright syndrome** describes hypersecretion of prolactin, which causes lactation at abnormal times, that is, at times other than during pregnancy or nursing. Usually there is associated amenorrhea. Nelson's syndrome describes a series of events that begin with an adrenalectomy as treatment for Cushing's syndrome. This results in the need for exogenous cortisol and often the corticotropin secretion increases because plasma cortisol levels are low. As a result, pituitary tumor growth occurs. It is not known if in persons who develop Nelson's syndrome pituitary tumors develop prior to adrenalectomy or if they occur after adrenalectomy. A predominant feature of Nelson's syndrome is pigmentation in concert with increased secretion of corticotropin because of the associated increased secretion of beta MSH.

Hypersecretion of gonadotropin is a rare occurrence and may be primary or secondary. The primary cause is associated with early development of the hypothalamus. Secondary hypersecretion most often results from cranial lesions that involve the hypothalamus. Precocious puberty results in children who then develop physically and sexually at an early age. The condition is benign and growth rates decline with age so that eventually the child reaches an adult height that is even slightly lower than normal. The child does have problems in that his level of physical maturation exceeds his emotional maturation. Adults tend to treat him as though he is older than he is because his physical appearance is that of an older child. The child also has problems with his peers because he is "older" in appearance. Hypersecretion of gonadotropin in adult women causes excessive menstruation.

Hypopituitarism may also involve one hormone or all the pituitary hormones. The latter is called **panhypopituitarism.** It is not known for certain but it is generally accepted that deficiency in a single pituitary hormone is probably caused by dysfunction in the hypothalamus.

Hyposecretion of a single hormone causes signs and symptoms related to the activity and function of the specific hormone involved. Hyposecretion of gonadotropin causes **amenorrhea** in women. The gonadotropin levels are decreased or absent in both plasma and urine. The gonadotropic cells include those for the follicle-stimulating hormone (FSH) and those for luteinizing hormone (LH) plus the chorionic gonadotropin hormone of the placenta (HCG). FSH activity causes stimulation of the development of the ovarian follicle in women, and formation and maturation of sperm in the seminiferous tubules in men. LH provides for luteinization of ovaries so that the mature graafian follicle ruptures. It is also known as interstitial-cell-stimulating-hormone (ICSH). In men, LH activity serves to promote the function of testicular Leydig cells, stimulating the synthesis and secretion of testosterone by the interstitial cells.

LH is easily measured by radioimmunoassay techniques, while FSH is not as easily measured because it interacts synergistically with LH. The levels vary with age and in cycles, increasing in puberty and after menopause in women. It is thought that LH also stimulates pituitary secretion of FSH. Stimulation of pituitary secretion is also influenced by plasma levels of estrogens and, to a lesser degree, of testosterone.

Corticotropin and melanotropin are secreted primarily in the anterior pituitary and probably, to some small degree, in the neurohypophysis. Corticotropin stimulates the secretion and release of adrenocortical hormones and prolongs the metabolic activity of cortisol. In addition, corticotropin affects metabolism through increasing the uptake of amino acids in muscle cells and lipolysis in fat cells, and it stimulates the beta cells of the pancreas to secrete insulin. Corticotropin functions in the pituitary to promote secretion of growth hormone.

The rate of secretion of corticotropin varies in a diurnal cycle with the highest levels occurring between 6 and 8 A.M. and the lowest levels between 6 and 11 P.M. in those who sleep at night. This diurnal cycle precedes the diurnal peaks and troughs of the cortisol secretion diurnal cycle. In stress, the levels may increase considerably. For example, the plasma concentration of ACTH may be less than 50 pg per milliliter and may increase to 600 pg per milliliter during stress.

Secretion of ACTH is controlled by the corticotropin-releasing hormone (CRF) in the hypothalamus and by the level of cortisol in plasma. Infections, pain, anxiety, and hypoglycemia all stimulate secretion of ACTH via the corticotropin-releasing hormone. The circadian rhythm also influences CRF release.

When hyposecretion of ACTH occurs as a single entity, the changes are similar to those of hyposecretion of cortisol, with weight loss, hypoglycemia, and generalized weakness.

These are discussed more fully in the later section on adrenal function.

MSH is similar to ACTH in its chemical composition, as the first thirteen amino acids of ACTH are also found in the sequence of alpha MSH. Beta MSH varies from alpha MSH and is the form stored in greatest quantity in the anterior pituitary. MSH is secreted in accord with cortisol levels and is active in promoting the synthesis of melanin.

Prolactin is secreted by the anterior pituitary by lactotropic cells. Increases in prolactin secretion are normal in pregnancy and during nursing. The action of prolactin is stimulation of mammary gland tissues for lactation. Adequate levels of estrogen and progestin are necessary to prepare the tissues for prolactin activity. The increased secretion of prolactin begins in the first trimester of pregnancy and continues to rise, increasing after the mother begins to nurse. The levels decrease only when nursing stops. The stimulus for prolactin secretion is derived from sensory receptors with specialized nerve endings in the nipple and areolae. When impulses from these receptors are transmitted to the hypothalamus, prolactin-releasing factors are secreted. There is no identified function of prolactin in males. Prolactin levels increase in stress, including such events as surgery and exercise. Increased prolactin levels cause intermittent lactation in the absence of pregnancy or nursing (Forbes-Albright syndrome). Decreased levels cause inability to nurse because the milk supply is not maintained.

Hyposecretion of thyrotropin may also occur as a single pituitary deficiency. The functions of thyrotropin are primarily those of stimulation of the secretion of thyroid hormone and of its release. As with other tropic hormones, regulation of the secretion of thyrotropin comprises both thyrotropin-releasing hormone from the hypothalamus and the levels of plasma thyroid hormones. Deficiency of TSH causes signs and symptoms of hypothyroidism.

Hyposecretion of pituitary hormones in **Sheehan's syndrome** results from hemorrhage and ischemic necrosis of the pituitary. This syndrome occurs in women who have hypertrophy of the pituitary gland during pregnancy. The stimulation of estrogens causes proliferation of the lactotropic cells. Postpartum hemorrhage, most commonly caused by coagulation abnormalities, then results in hemorrhage of the pituitary tissue. The amount of necrosis depends on the duration and on the extensiveness of the hemorrhage. Both the neurohypophysis and the adenohypophysis may be involved. The signs and symptoms usually become obvious when the mother cannot nurse her baby because of an inadequate milk supply. The affected mothers do not regain their strength and become apathetic and listless. Some of them may become too debilitated to be able to care for their babies or cope with ongoing responsibilities.

Hand-Schüller-Christian disease is caused by invasion of pituitary tissue with histiocytes full of cholesterol. Granuloma cells can also invade the pituitary as well as the thyroid and adrenal glands, causing dysfunction. Another cause of pituitary dysfunction can be hemochromatosis, in which sarcoidosis extends to the pituitary with formation of sarcoid granulomas.

Pituitary tumors include chromophobe adenomas, acidophilic adenomas, and basophilic adenomas. The highest frequency of chromophobe adenomas occurs in the age range of 30 to 50 years. Both men and women are affected. Chromophobe adenomas comprise about 85 percent of all pituitary tumors. Acidophilic adenomas occur in the same age range and in both sexes, as do chromophobe adenomas. Basophilic adenomas are the most infrequently occurring type and are thought to develop from the remnants of Rathke's pouch.

All these pathologic conditions occur as primary pituitary dysfunction and cause symptoms when significant amounts of tissue become nonfunctioning. Usually 75 percent of the gland must be destroyed before symptoms occur. The manifestations are those of hyposecretion of the cells involved. Gonadotropins are usually first involved and then somatotropins. Thyrotropin, corticotropin, and prolactin cell involvement follow in sequence.

Secondary pituitary dysfunction occurs from any disease process that involves the hypothalamus. These diseases may include infectious processes, trauma to the brain, congenital malformations or hydrocephalus, and autoimmune diseases. Meningiomas and chordomas often involve the sella turcica and cause enlargement of the pituitary, so that it breaks out of its borderlines on all sides (Chap. 11). Usually, this causes displacement of the optic nerves and loss of the visual fields in the superior temporal quadrant because of pressure on the medial segments of the nerves. As optic nerve damage progresses, the person has hemianopia and even later scotomas (areas of depressed vision in a visual field) with loss of vision in the nasal fields. Blindness may be the result of progressive damage. Intermittent headache, which can be very severe, is another common symptom.

The cranial nerves are not usually involved, with the exception of the third cranial nerve. If involved, damage to the third cranial nerve causes interference with the sense of smell. Symptoms related to hypothalamic involvement are dysfunction of the temperature-regulating mechanisms, sleep disturbances, and changes in appetite. Focal seizures may result from hypothalamic involvement. In addition to these signs and symptoms, there is always the possibility that blood vessels in the highly vascular site of the tumor may rupture. When blood vessels rupture, symptoms of headache, hypotension, hypothermia, and abrupt blindness may result. Sometimes, the tumor growth surrounds the normal pituitary tissue, encapsulating it. Hypopituitarism then occurs usually with hypogonadism becoming obvious first, and then hypothyroidism. ACTH reserves are decreased so that adrenal insufficiency results when the person is in stressful situations. If hypersecretion results, it usually involves somatotropin, prolactin, corticotropin, and melanotropin.

Treatment and Nursing Care of Pituitary Disorders

Pituitary tumors are treated by radiation, chemotherapy, use of isotopes, or surgery. Radiation is usually the treatment of choice if the tumor has not extended beyond the sella turcica. The dosage is evaluated to achieve decreased secretion of hormones without damaging pituitary tissue extensively if hypersecretion of growth hormone is the single dysfunction. Excessive radiation of the pituitary may cause long-term damage to the cranial nerves or to the hypothalamus. The format for radiation varies according to the equipment available. Generally, the radiation treatment, to be effective, is given in very small doses over a span of 1 to 2 years.

Surgical procedures include a craniotomy from the transfrontal approach, surgical resection from the sphenoid approach, and stereotaxic surgery. Each method has advantages and disadvantages.

A craniotomy may result in any number of complications. In people with acromegaly, bleeding may occur because of the excessive growth of frontal bones. The transfrontal approach is preferred if the tumor has extended upward, involving the optic chiasm. The sphenoid approach is often used for smaller tumors that are confined to the sella turcica. Microsurgery techniques have improved the procedure. The two major complications of this approach may be rhinorrhea and meningitis because of the interruption of cerebrospinal fluid flow during surgery. These complications can, however, be avoided, and since the tumor can be better visualized with microsurgery techniques, its resection can be accomplished with greater accuracy. Some prefer this method because the increased accuracy ensures that the pituitary tissue has been removed. Function continues when only a small portion of the tumor is left.

Cryohypophysectomy is the technique of inserting a probe through the transsphenoidal route. The probe is used to freeze the tumor, and its manipulation in the tumor tissue is monitored and guided by fluoroscopy to allow for the insertion of probes directly into the tumor so that the tissues can be destroyed, leaving the surrounding tissue intact. Freezing is accomplished by using liquid nitrogen. Heat from radioactive coils to destroy the tumor tissue can be used.

Postoperative nursing care should be based on the patient's dependence on hormone replacement to provide for hormones normally stimulated or secreted by the removed pituitary. Without this replacement, the person cannot live, because the pituitary is essential to life in that its hormones are essential to maintenance of body homeostasis. Therefore the immediate postoperative needs of a patient following hypophysectomy include nursing management of essential hormone replacement. Corticosteroids are critical to the patient's well-being. Adrenal insufficiency will ensue if cortisol levels are not maintained. In those with good kidney function, mineralocorticoids may not be required in either the immediate or long-term phases of care. The nurse must make certain that medications are given precisely in terms of both dosage and time.

Fluid and electrolyte balance must be monitored in the postoperative period. The person may have a transient requirement for ADH because of the incidence of diabetes insipidus. (Depending on the patient's response to surgery, ADH may be required in the long-term care. If the hypothalamus remains intact, the patient may not need exogenous medication.) During the first week postoperatively, the patient may have decreased osmolality of blood without hypovolemia, because of the action of vasopressin. If a cortisol insufficiency also is present, diuresis may be augmented. Fluid balance must be carefully maintained to prevent excessive intake of fluids, which can cause all the symptoms of water intoxication.

Because of these factors, careful nursing observation and monitoring of the patient's vital signs, fluid and electrolytes, and blood gases are essential to prevent complications in the postoperative care. Depending on the operative procedure used, care will vary. Further information about nursing care following surgical procedures involving the cranium is given in Chapter 11.

In both preoperative and postoperative care, the nurse teaches the patient the importance of hormone replacement. When the source of the tropic hormones is completely or severely limited, adrenal insufficiency, hypothyroidism, hypogonadism, and, in some instances, deficiency of ADH, all result. Following total hypophysectomy, the patient therefore requires replacement hormones. Since human pituitary hormones are not available in great supply and since no synthetic pituitary hormones have as yet been developed, there are two choices for replacement. The first is use of extracts from animal pituitary glands. The second is provision of exogenous hormones for cortisol, thyroid, androgens, and estrogens. Injections of pituitary hormones of animal extracts cause the development of antibodies in many people. Replacement of exogenous hormones of the specific adrenal, thyroid, and gonadal structures is usually the treatment of choice. The nurse should be aware that hormone replacement must be accompanied with development of routines and teaching for adjusting medication to cope with stressful events such as infection.

Cortisol preparations are supplied through many different brand names, all of which may be suitable for replacement. The dosage of cortisol required following hypophysectomy is usually less than is required in severe adrenal insufficiency of primary adrenal origin or following adrenalectomy. As with the event of adrenal insufficiency from primary causes, the person who has had a hypophysectomy must be given information and medications so that he can increase the dosage of corticoids in times of stress, which is discussed more fully later in this chapter (page 679).

Thyroid is usually replaced gradually, so that the dosage is increased until the desired maintenance dose is reached. Thyroid status is measured by evaluating the level of thyroid hormones as described in the section about the thyroid gland. Men require replacement of androgens and women in premenopausal age ranges require estrogens to enable them to maintain normal reproductive tissues. Although sterility results from hypophysectomy, ovulation can be induced in women with the use of medications containing FSH to stimulate the development of the follicle in the ovary, followed by use of human chorionic gonadotropin. While not as effective, the same medications can be given to reinstate male potency.

When **panhypopituitarism** results from pituitary disease, the signs and symptoms of deficiencies are variable in degrees from mild to severe. Symptoms include nausea, vomiting, and physical and emotional inertia. Hyperthermia is also noted. As with treatment following hypophysectomy, hormones must be given exogenously. Adrenal insufficiency becomes evident first, while hypothyroidism may not become overt for as long as 10 years. Atrophy of the sex organs is usually pronounced. In men and women, libido decreases. Amenorrhea occurs in women, while the semen of men contains no sperm.

Skin changes appear early, as the person does not tan well, if at all, when exposed to the sun because of the reduced melanin. Fine wrinkles appear around the mouth and eyes, and body hair decreases. Men have a very sparse beard and both men and women tend to lose their axillary and pubic hair. Other skin changes, such as development of a waxy appearance of the skin, suggest hypothyroidism.

Metabolic changes vary and are most pronounced in diabetes. Generally, the fasting blood glucose level is below normal and hypoglycemia occurs in situations that place stress on metabolic functions such as fasting, infections, or surgery. The requirements for insulin decrease in people who are diabetic. This mechanism probably explains the reason for lack of noticeable changes in carbohydrate metabolism in people who have had a hypophysectomy or who have pituitary insufficiency.

Another change noted is development of anemia. Pernicious anemia may occur as a complication of hypothyroidism. In addition to this, the pituitary effects on erythropoietin in bone marrow are diminished so that normocytic or normochromic anemia develops.

Diagnosis of panhypopituitarism usually includes determining the level of growth hormone by radioimmunoassay. Prolactin levels are usually increased when the hypothalamus is involved in this pathologic condition. Thyroid function evaluation and determination of adrenal function and ACTH reserve are also carried out. When hypothyroidism occurs from pituitary dysfunction, the plasma cortisol levels are also low, whereas plasma cortisol levels are usually normal if the hypothyroidism results from thyroid disease. Checking the medical history of women who have borne children may be helpful, as postpartum hemorrhage resulting in necrosis of pituitary tissue may not be evident for a period of 10 or 20 years following the hemorrhage.

Further examination of the pituitary is conducted if there is demonstrated hyposecretion of pituitary tropic hormones. If x-rays of the sella turcica demonstrate sella turcical enlargement, a pneumoencephalogram is performed. Examination of the visual fields is carried out because of the possibility that a pituitary tumor might have extended to the optic chiasm. Treatment is determined by the findings of these examinations and may include surgical removal of the tumor if one exists. In every form of treatment, replacement of cortisol and thyroid is essential if the person is to live an active life. Without treatment, the person with severe panhypopituitarism will die. The alternative is taking exogenous hormones.

While the necessity for lifelong dependency is obvious to the nurse and may be intellectually accepted by the patient, who must take the medications, the nurse must realize that the patient may perceive this lifelong dependency as a lack of control over his own life. If the patient can learn to take the medication habitually and can accommodate routines and schedules, taking into account the need for having a supply of medications available at all times and in all places, the adjustment can lead to a feeling of emotional and physiologic well-being. The capability of being productive results. On the other hand, the person's self-concept and the need for medications consistently as part of a life style may be perceived as hindrances to enjoyment of life. The patient may have been too ill prior to surgery to realize this long-term effect.

Helping the patient resolve these feelings is a challenge for the nurse. The patient often must reshape attitudes concerning himself or herself in relation to the treatment and life goals. Often the major problems associated with taking medications do not come into the patient's level of awareness until he or she experiences the regimen following hospital discharge. For this reason, providing for ongoing contacts for guidance, reinforcement of the requisites of medications, and support in the adjustment is vital. Along with this need for continued medication is the requirement for periodic physical examination and monitoring of the effectiveness of the treatment. As the person ages and as life events bring about changes, adjustments will have to be made in the dosages of hormones. This is most prudently done on the basis of data including how the person feels and what the levels of hormones are in the plasma and urine. The term **prudent prevention** applies to the long-term care of people with endocrine dysfunction.

Hypophysectomy is sometimes used as an ablative measure in treatment of those who have **metastatic carcinoma.** This procedure is predicated on the fact that certain tumors are considered dependent on hormones for their growth. These tumors have needs and characteristics similar to those of cells at the site of their growth. An example is the mammary gland tumor, which requires hormones for growth and function. Among the organs involved in cancer growth that respond to hypophysectomy are the breast and the prostate. Ablative surgery is controversial and data are continually being collected either to prove or to disprove its value.

Criteria for establishing evidence of the probable response to ablative surgery have not been unquestionably set forth. Previous response to oophorectomy and identification of an estrogen receptor in the tumor cells indicate a probability of effectiveness in persons with breast cancer. If used, ablative surgery tends to be most successful in those who have been postmenopausal for more than one year. The procedure is usually done for persons who have had recurrence of cancer following previous therapy which may have included oophorectomy or chemotherapy or both. Use of hypophysectomy as an ablative measure for recurrent cancer of the prostate is based on the consideration that hormones secreted by the pituitary may support the tumor growth. Usually prostate carcinoma is first treated with estrogens and orchiectomy. As with ablative surgery for treatment of advanced carcinoma of the breast, the response is variable in advanced carcinoma of the prostate.

Another indication for hypophysectomy as ablative surgery is the rapid advancement of **diabetic retinopathy.** Hypophysectomy is done because of the influence of growth hormone, thyroid, and cortisol in promoting gluconeogenesis. Hypophysectomy is done in an attempt to decrease the possibility of blindness in diabetics who have rapid changes in vision probably because of altered carbohydrate metabolism. There is no guarantee that the hypophysectomy will be successful.

These are a few examples of the relation of the endocrine system to growth of cells and metabolism of nutrients. Hypophysectomy is an extreme measure made possible by the ability to provide the hormones necessary for life. In many instances, hormonal therapy is used, not only in treatment of carcinoma, but also in attempts to treat metabolic and long-term systemic diseases. When studying the various types of manipulations that are possible in the attempt to allay disease or to provide palliation of terminal conditions, one develops great respect for the complexity of the endocrine system and for the intricacies of the relationships among hormones.

The Thyroid Gland

The function of the thyroid gland is probably familiar to most people. The thyroid gland produces three hormones: **thyroxine** (T_4), **triiodothyronine** (T_3), and **thyrocalcitonin.** The first two are important for somatic and intellectual growth and maturation, influencing both intellect and musculoskeletal structure. They are also important for central nervous system function, metabolism, and temperature regulation, having a vital role in the maintenance of homeostasis within the body in response to both internal and external changes. Thyrocalcitonin functions as an antagonist to parathyroid hormone and is therefore important in calcium metabolism. The function of thyrocalcitonin is more fully discussed in the later section on parathyroid gland function (page 665).

Homeostatic mechanisms take place at the level of the thyroid gland, in the production and secretion of the thyroid hormones T_4 and T_3. Both the thyrotropin-releasing hormone (TRH), secreted by the hypothalamus in response to metabolic needs and the thyroid-stimulating hormone (TSH), secreted by the anterior pituitary, influence thyroid function in its role in maintaining homeostasis. Factors such as increased exercise, exposure to either hot or cold temperatures, and increased demands for growth during certain phases of the life cycle normally place demands on the thyroid gland for increasing production of hormones to maintain homeostasis.

Dysfunction of the thyroid gland is evidenced by symptoms caused by either excessive or insufficient hormone production or by interference with surrounding structures caused by increases in the size of the thyroid gland without clinical alteration in hormone balance. Excessive thyroid hormone levels are termed **thyrotoxicosis** or **hyperthyroidism** (the two terms are often used interchangeably [6]); insufficient levels are referred to as **hypothyroidism.** Enlargement of the thyroid gland causes symptoms resulting from compression on the surrounding anatomic structures. Specific causes of thyroid dysfunction may stem from disease processes affecting the anterior pituitary, the thyroid gland itself, or as secondary effects of dysfunction of other organs, primarily the liver and the kidneys. Diseases that arise in the thyroid gland are **primary thyroid diseases;** those that arise in other organs with resultant changes in the thyroid function are **secondary thyroid diseases.**

THYROID FUNCTION

Thyroid hormone production is stimulated by TSH. Low serum levels of thyroid hormones increase the production of TRF (thyroid-releasing hormone) by the hypothalamus, which in turn increases the production of TSH by the anterior pituitary. High serum levels decrease TRF and TSH secretion (Fig. 8-3) in a negative feedback loop. The biosynthesis of thyroid hormones depends on the presence of sufficient quantities of iodine. Some iodides are recycled and reused by the thyroid gland; the largest amount is supplied exogenously via foods, fluids, and medications containing iodine. Iodides are primarily contained in extracellular fluid, from which they are absorbed by the thyroid gland; iodides are also stored in the fluid of erythrocytes, in gastric juice, and in saliva.

The excretion of iodides occurs primarily via the kidneys, usually in inorganic form. Some iodides are also excreted via the skin, in expired air, and in feces.

The nurse must recognize that thyroid function is influenced by many factors. There is a normal decrease in thyroid metabolism with age. Anything that suppresses anterior pituitary function and thus secretion of TSH also depresses thyroid function. Diseases

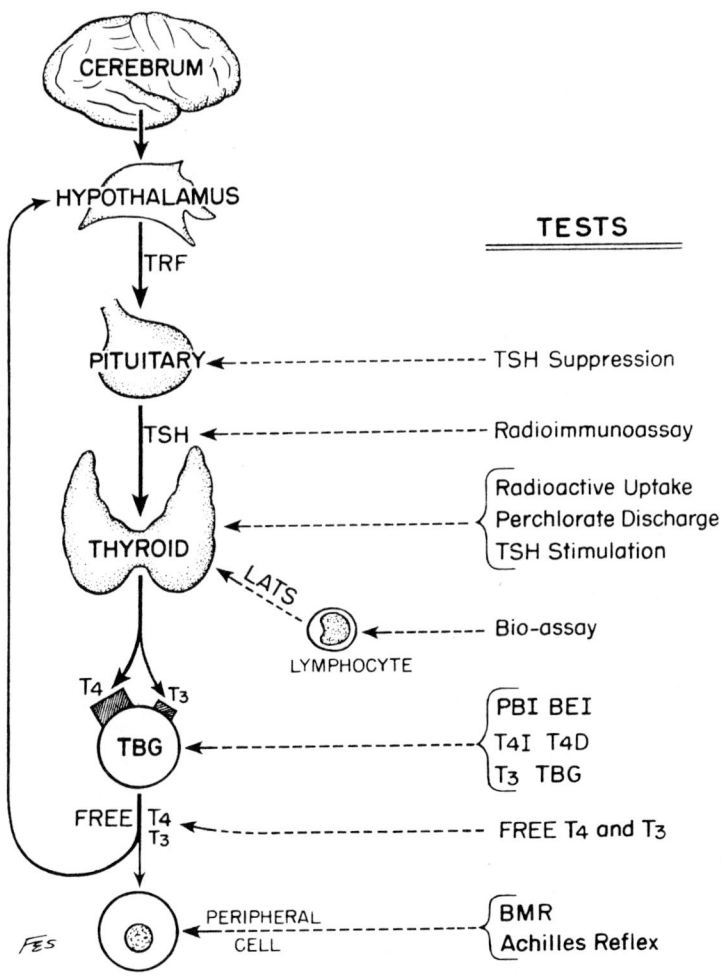

Figure 8-3
Physiological level of thyroid function tests. (From C. E. Sedgwick, *Surgery in the Thyroid Gland*. Philadelphia: W. B. Saunders Company, 1974. Reproduced by permission.)

suppressing the anterior pituitary production of TSH and administration of corticosteroids have this effect. Emotional and physical stress alter thyroid function. The exact mechanisms of the relation between stress and thyroid function, however, are not well understood. Some authorities feel that ACTH (adrenal cortical tropic hormone) is secreted in favor of TSH in the stress response. The increased demand for thyroid hormones during stress reactions may be more directly related to an increase in utilization of the thyroid hormones in peripheral cellular metabolism.

The thyroid gland is located at the level of the thyroid cartilage of the trachea with its upper margin below the cricoid cartilage. The two lobes of the thyroid are connected by a thin layer of tissue called the isthmus. The right lobe is slightly larger than the left and is more highly vascularized. Each lobe is approximately 2 to 2½ cm wide. The thyroid gland has the capability of greatly increasing in size. An abnormally large thyroid gland is referred to as a **goiter.**

The blood supply of the thyroid gland is provided by the superior thyroid arteries, which arise from the external carotids and the inferior thyroid arteries, which in turn arise from the subclavian arteries. The gland is highly vascular and also has an excellent lymph drainage. When the thyroid is enlarged, the blood supply increases so that a bruit or thrill can be heard by auscultation over the gland.

The major cells of the thyroid gland are the follicular and parafollicular cells. **Follicular cells** are filled with colloid and synthesize thyroglobulin, the matrix for forming and storing thyroxine and triiodothyronine. **Parafollicular cells** secrete calcitonin. Both the adrenergic and cholinergic nerves influence thyroid function, although the nervous system influences are not well understood. The adrenergic (sympathetic) nerves reach the thyroid from the cervical ganglia and the cholinergic (parasympathetic) nerves come from the vagus nerve. The known effect of nervous system control directly on the thyroid is that of increasing or decreasing the blood supply, which influences the rate at which iodide and TSH enter the thyroid gland. It is thought that thyroid function may also be influenced by adrenergic control at the level of the individual follicular cells.

NURSING ASSESSMENT

The nursing assessment of thyroid dysfunction, then, includes physical examination of the size, location, and position of the thyroid; observation of the patient's behavior; and careful interviewing to determine the types of problems the patient may be experiencing in terms of the effects of changes in metabolism and in cardiovascular and nervous system function. These effects are often noted in the specific signs and symptoms that are described in the following pages. In addition, there are many subjective symptoms that must be investigated through interviewing and observation. These include the patient's perception of changes in energy levels, emotional state, and general feeling of being able to cope with life events. The latter is often obscure because coping abilities are influenced by many different factors. Specific information about the function of the thyroid gland can be obtained through laboratory determinations of both iodine and hormone levels. These levels are also interpreted in terms of the patient's signs and symptoms.

The thyroid gland can be examined by palpation. In order to palpate the thyroid, the examiner usually stands behind the patient, who is in a sitting position. The examiner uses the fingertips of both hands for palpation to locate first the cricoid cartilage and then the thyroid just below. Palpation of the thyroid is done carefully. The gland should never be palpated if thyrotoxicosis (excessive thyroid hormone) exists. The thyroid gland normally feels slightly elastic and is movable; it tends to become firmer with increased age. The nurse should note the size, shape, and consistency of the gland. While the gland normally has the feel of an elastic substance, it becomes softer when there is diffuse enlargement. Certain disease processes such as Hashimoto's disease and carcinoma, to be discussed later, cause the gland to become firm. When palpating the gland, the nurse should be alert for the presence of nodules. If present, their size and position are noted. The consistency of the nodules is compared to the consistency of the surrounding tissues. As part of the palpation component of the examination, the lymph nodes in the region are also examined. Further observation of the gland is conducted by having the patient remain seated with the neck slightly extended.

The neck should be inspected from the front and side. Having the patient sip water allows observation of movement of the thyroid during swallowing. When goiters are present, they are usually freely movable when the patient swallows. Tumors, however, may not be movable, as they may be attached to surrounding tissues of the trachea or even to the base of the tongue.

While goiters are often indicative of hypothyroidism or hyperthyroidism, this is not always the case. Formation of a goiter is actually an adaptation of the thyroid in response to different factors. The hyperplasia of the thyroid tissue enables the gland to produce hormones for normal balance in metabolic functions when there is iodine deficiency, ingestion of goitrogenic substances, or inflammation of the thyroid. In these situations, low serum hormone levels increase TSH, which stimulates the thyroid and produces hyperplasia.

Pemberton's sign is elicited by having the patient raise his arms straight up along his head. If positive, raising the arms will cause congestion of the face and respiratory distress, indicating the presence of a retrosternal goiter. Lesions of the thyroid can displace the trachea by compression or they can impinge on the recurrent laryngeal nerve, located between the trachea and the lateral lobes of the thyroid. If the voice is whispery or hoarse, there may be compression on the recurrent laryngeal nerve. Any of these symptoms indicates the need for follow-up examination. In this case the physician will include esophageal x-rays or laryngoscopy in the more thorough examination.

While palpation of the thyroid gland may be conducted fairly easily, nursing assessment of the patient's total behavior and signs and symptoms of excessive or insufficient hormone production is much more difficult. Changes in behavior are characteristic of either excessive or deficient thyroid hormone production. If the nurse has not previously known the patient, behavioral changes may not be obvious. Because of the behavioral changes, the patient may not be able to give a clear history of the onset of the symptoms or of the significance of the symptoms to his life. For example, the emotional lability that occurs with excessive thyroid hormone production hinders the ability to carry on a conversation. Often very simple questions about disease elicit emotional responses out of proportion to the situation. Being aware of these behavioral changes is important, as the nurse may need to encourage the patient's family or friends to contribute information that will be helpful in ascertaining the patient's medical history.

Because many thyroid diseases are familial, a family history of thyroid disease is a cue to the nurse that questions related to thyroid function should be followed up more fully in the assessment interview. The onset of thyroid diseases may be either acute or may occur over a long period of time with vague symptoms that are difficult to distinguish from other general diseases. The nurse should try to piece together the information obtained to formulate a composite of the patient's history. Many cardiac, metabolic, and nervous system diseases influence thyroid function. In differentiating between primary and secondary thyroid dysfunction, the nurse should review the patient's history, if one is available, from previous medical records. Even if primary thyroid dysfunction is present, the existence of other diseases in the patient's history or current status may exaggerate the thyroid disease and often contributes to the nature of the specific symptoms he or she will develop.

The signs and symptoms of thyrotoxicosis and hypothyroidism are related to the effects of either excessive or insufficient thyroid hormones on metabolism, cardiovascular function, and nervous function. In many instances, the signs and symptoms of these two states are opposites. This is not true of all the signs and symptoms, however, as either excessive or insufficient thyroid hormone secretion can sometimes result in the same or similar signs and symptoms. Assessment of signs and symptoms is further complicated because not every person with hyperfunction or hypofunction has the typical or expected symptoms. There are degrees of excess or lack of the hormones.

A comparison of the effects of excessive thyroid hormone production seen in thyrotoxicosis and lack of thyroid hormone production seen in hypothyroidism helps the nurse to delineate the effects of the thyroid hormones in metabolism. In general, metabolism is increased in thyrotoxicosis and is decreased in hypothyroidism. Usually, thyrotoxicosis results in restlessness and nervousness or anxiety and loss of weight, while hypothyroidism tends to result in lethargy, apathy, and weight gain. The initial impression the nurse has of the patient during the assessment in terms of body weight and emotional affect can provide cues for further questioning and examination.

Tachycardia associated with hypermetabolic states is a classic symptom of thyrotoxicosis. The patient's pulse remains high (usually above 90) even at rest. For this reason, the nurse should take the hospitalized patient's pulse during sleep as a significant diagnostic measure in differentiating between thyrotoxicosis and other conditions that cause increased pulse only with exertion, diminishing with rest. The increased pulse represents the cardiac response to hypermetabolism. In addition to tachycardia, there may be palpitations and, frequently, anginal pain. In thyrotoxicosis, peripheral metabolism is increased and there is dilatation of the peripheral vascular bed, with concomitant increase in cardiac output. The heart muscle itself is influenced by thyroid hormones, and thyroid stimulation causes increased adrenergic activity. The resulting increased cardiac contractility and excitability noted in arrythmias is typical of thyrotoxicosis. Atrial fibrillation often results. In addition, the pulse pressure is widened so that the systolic pressure increases, while diastolic pressure decreases. In thyrotoxic people, digitalis is not usually effective. If the patient has underlying heart disease, he may not be able to compensate for the increased metabolic requirements and may develop congestive heart failure. This knowledge is very important to the nurse in planning activity and in assessing progress.

In hypothyroidism (called myxedema in adults and cretinism in children) the opposite cardiovascular effects occur. The person with hypothyroidism usually has bradycardia. Peripheral metabolism is decreased and there is vasoconstriction of the peripheral vascular beds with decreased cardiac output. The changes in the ECG represent a hypometabolic state. The term **myxedema heart** refers to cardiac muscle changes in which the heart becomes enlarged because of tissue changes. The myocardium becomes flabby and less efficient, so that persons with hypothyroidism may also develop congestive heart failure.

These cardiac changes are related to the metabolic state because thyroid hormones are important in carbohydrate, protein, and fat metabolism. Excessive thyroid hormone stimulates catabolism by increasing gluconeogenesis by increasing precursors in the metabolic pathways and gastrointestinal absorption of glucose and galactose. Glucose uptake by adipose tissue and insulin degradation are enhanced by thyroid hormones. There is a relation between the occurrence of diabetes and thyroid disease. (Diabetic patients with thyrotoxicosis have increased sensitivity to exogenous insulin and require less insulin, whereas diabetics with hypothyroidism have diminished sensitivity to exogenous insulin and require more insulin.)

Hypothyroidism results in hypometabolism. In this state there is a positive nitrogen balance and slower degradation of insulin. Mobilization of fat from tissue stores is impaired. In thyrotoxicosis there is usually an inadequacy of calories to support the hypermetabolism. This inadequacy results in catabolism of protein with a negative nitrogen balance, increased levels of free fatty acids, and increased mobilization of fat from tissue stores. The relationships between glucose and fat metabolism are somewhat similar to those that occur in diabetes with decreased insulin secretion.

In many persons the serum cholesterol values are abnormal because of the influence of thyroid hormones on lipid metabolism. An excess of thyroid hormones increases cholesterol synthesis; ATP (adenosine triphosphate, which contains chemical energy produced by glucose metabolism) is necessary for this reaction. The lipolytic response to growth hormones is increased in hyperthyroidism, decreased in hypothyroidism.

Persons in a hypermetabolic state have increased need for both water-soluble and fat-soluble vitamins and for calories. As caloric requirements are increased in the hypermetabolic states, the person tends to lose weight even though he eats increasing amounts of food. The person with thyrotoxicosis usually has an increased appetite. This is not always the case, however, for a few persons with thyrotoxicosis who are in younger and older age groups tend to have anorexia and weight gain. Persons with hypothyroidism tend to gain weight and are usually anorexic. This gain is caused by retention of fluid by hydrophilic mucinous deposits in the tissues rather than from increases in adipose tissue. Variations in patterns of weight gain in hypothyroidism are also seen in a few persons with hypothyroidism and in younger and older persons who tend to lose weight.

Gastrointestinal functions are also changed in thyrotoxicosis, with an increased gastric motility and a tendency for stools to become less well formed. There is decreased peristalsis and a tendency to gaseous distention, constipation, and even fecal impaction in hypothyroidism. If the gastrointestinal symptoms are severe, nausea and vomiting may occur. In both thyrotoxicosis and hypothyroidism there are circulating antibodies against gastric parietal cells. This often results in achlorhydria, and some persons, although very few, develop pernicious anemia. Vitamin B_{12} is absorbed poorly. The liver may be involved in severe cases with increased serum alkaline phosphatase in thyrotoxicosis and in some few situations, hepatomegaly and jaundice.

A number of signs in hyperthyroidism result from the synergistic effect of the thyroid hormones and catecholamines, thereby enhancing activity. Some of these signs are fine tremor in the outstretched hand, excessive sweating, and retraction of the upper eyelids, observed in thyrotoxicosis. People who are hyperthyroid have an intolerance to heat; those who are hypothyroid have an intolerance to cold. Comparison of the skin changes in both conditions again reveals the opposites. In thyrotoxicosis, the texture of the skin in protected body areas is smooth and the skin is pink and moist. The person's hair is fine, silky, and straight. Hypothyroidism causes the opposite; coarse dry skin and coarse brittle hair. Loss of scalp hair is common in hypothyroidism. The skin is usually flushed in thyrotoxicosis, and in hypothyroidism the skin may have yellowish discoloration or flushed patches typical of anemia.

Effects of thyroid hormones on the nervous system are evidenced by changes in behavior. Excessive hormones cause restlessness that is associated with a short attention span. People with thyrotoxicosis feel that they always must be doing something and they have a restless urge to be active. They are frustrated, however, because constant fatigue prevents them from doing the things they feel they need to do. Deficient hormone causes lethargy and mental apathy. People with hypothyroidism tend to have poor memories and may be depressed or even paranoid. When hypothyroidism occurs in infancy, irreversible brain damage may occur if treatment is not initiated promptly. In adults with acquired hypothyroidism, the decreased cerebral blood flow is thought to cause the slowing of all intellectual functions. Speech becomes slow and they suffer from headache and syncope. Trauma or infectious processes may precipitate the development of comas. Myxedema coma, while occurring infrequently, may be morbid.

In both states, previous emotional makeup is an important determinant of the emotional states accompanying the thyroid dysfunction. Symptoms of psychoses are frequently the reasons thyrotoxic individuals seek treatment. Irritability, flares of temper, and unprecipitated crying are common symptoms. While the person with hypothyroidism is usually lethargic, he may develop myxedema madness (emotional changes related to severe hypothyroidism) with great agitation. These emotional changes make the nurse's role in assessment challenging because there is a natural tendency to react to the overt behavior. Often the true diagnosis is missed by everyone involved because of the emotional changes, which distract attention from underlying physiologic causes of the behavior. The relation between emotional trauma and development of thyrotoxicosis is not clearly understood. Some authorities believe the excessive hormone precipitates emotional symptoms. Others feel that episodes of emotional trauma may precipitate the thyrotoxicosis in susceptible individuals.

The nurse may note the presence of muscle weakness and fatigue, which are symptoms common to both hyperthyroid and hypothyroid states. The hyperthyroid person has typical and often purposeless quick and jerky movements that use excessive energy. In hypothyroidism, there may be slow and clumsy movements and cerebellar ataxia, numbness, and tingling of the extremities. In thyrotoxicosis, the proximal muscles of the legs are affected so that activities requiring extension of the legs, such as climbing stairs, are difficult to accomplish. It is thought that this problem may result from infiltration of muscle tissue by fat cells. Muscle changes also occur with decreased muscle contraction and relaxation rates. The muscular dysfunction is similar to that experienced in muscle atrophy and tends to affect men more than women. There is an increase of creatine in urine in thyrotoxic people. Urine creatine is decreased in hypothyroidism. Many persons have symptoms similar to myasthenia gravis. The relation between myasthenia gravis and thyroid dysfunction has been demonstrated in thymic gland enlargement in persons with myasthenia. In myxedema, mucinous deposits may affect nerve function. For example, carpal tunnel syndrome may occur because of compression (by the mucinous deposits) on the median nerve.

There is a direct relation between increased hormone production and calcium and phosphorus excretion rates, so that hypercalcemia may occur in thyrotoxic states. The relation between thyrocalcitonin and calcium metabolism in hyperthyroid states is not well defined. Children who have excessive thyroid production have a higher than average height. Deficient thyroid production causes delay in bone development, and bone age is retarded. If the onset of hypothyroidism occurs during infancy and the condition remains untreated, the individual will have characteristically short legs while the trunk is of more normal size.

In thyrotoxicosis the person may have polyuria, with increased renal blood flow and glomerular filtration rates. Urine flow is reduced in hypothyroidism. Although the total body water is increased in hypothyroid individuals, the majority of the excess water is retained in interstitial tissues. This gives the face a puffy appearance. The mucinous deposits referred to as myxedematous infiltration may occur in the tongue and larynx also, contributing to development of slurred and thick speech or hoarseness. The extremities may be puffy as well.

Sexual maturity is also affected by deficiencies in thyroid hormone. If the dysfunction occurs prior to puberty, there will be a delay in the onset of puberty. In women, there is failure to ovulate and excessive or irregular menstrual bleeding, because of failure to secrete the luteinizing hormone. If the disease is of long duration or secondary in nature, however, there may be ovarian atrophy with amenorrhea. Both hypothyroid and hyperthyroid individuals have decreased fertility and the tendency to abort when they do become pregnant. In thyrotoxicosis that occurs early in life, sexual maturation will also be delayed, although the person's physical development may be normal or even accelerated. In older persons, there is increased libido and disturbed menstrual function which may vary from excessive to decreased or absent menses.

Because of the decreased oxygen consumption in hypothyroidism, there is a concomitant decrease in erythrocyte mass. Normocytic or normochromic anemia may result. The opposite is true in thyrotoxicosis with an increase in erythrocyte mass because of the increased oxygen requirement. Vitamin B_{12} and folic acid requirements are increased in persons with thyrotoxicosis. A small percentage tend to develop pernicious anemia.

DIAGNOSTIC TESTS

It should be noted that nursing care for patients with overt thyroid dysfunction is often difficult, particularly when behavioral changes are present. The nurse must devise creative techniques for helping the patient accept and follow through with diagnosis and therapy until the time at which the symptoms begin to diminish and the patient becomes a more willing participant in the care regimen. The nurse must be cognizant of the physiologic and psychological symptoms caused by thyroid hormone imbalance.

During the diagnostic phase, the nurse must determine the patient's needs for explanations of procedures and correct preparation for specific tests. The nurse may have to be directive and provide assistance for patients who are unable to carry out the necessary measures independently. Many of the tests of thyroid function are conducted periodically following initial diagnosis to monitor the patient's progress. The nurse must therefore understand the purposes of the tests and must be able to interpret the results.

Diagnostic tests of thyroid dysfunction are predicated on current knowledge of the negative feedback mechanism and biosynthesis of the thyroid hormones (Fig. 8-3). Since there is considerable variation in testing procedures and laboratory methods, test results and values differ from one institution to another. The nurse must be familiar with the laboratory methodology and values in each given setting. The basal metabolic rate, formerly used in diagnosis of thyroid dysfunction, is an indirect measure of greater value for evaluating the effects of therapy than for diagnosis. Only minute amounts of free thyroid hormones are present in circulating blood. These free or unbound hormones are physiologically active. The remainder (about 99 percent of the thyroid hormone in the blood) is bound to plasma proteins [4]; thyroxine-binding globulin, also called inter alpha globulin or TBG, binds with T_4 and T_3, thyroxine-binding prealbumin (TBPA) binds with T_4 and albumin binds with T_4 and T_3. T_3 is metabolically more active than T_4 as it is not as tightly bound to the plasma proteins. This binding provides a media for storing the hormones in circulation until they are needed or deactivated. In addition, the binding prolongs the life of the hormones to protect the body reserve and prevents the hormones from influencing metabolism indiscriminately. In maintaining homeostasis, there is an equilibrium between the amount of proteins that bind thyroid hormones and the hormone levels. Adaptation is made to accommodate either increased or decreased hormone levels by increasing or decreasing amounts of binding proteins so that the appropriate levels of free hormones can be maintained.

Normally, T_4 and T_3 remain in the serum for several days. The half-life of thyroxine is about 5 days in children and 6 to 7 days in adults. The half-life of T_3 is about 1 day in both children and adults. This half-life decreases in hyperthyroidism and increases in hypothyroidism.

T_3 is known to be more physiologically active than T_4 but is present in lesser amounts in circulation. The thyroid gland releases twenty molecules of T_4 for every one molecule of T_3 [4]. T_4, however, can be deiodinated at the peripheral level to form T_3 when T_3 levels become low or depleted. The hormones are deactivated in the liver. Unbound thyroxine in the serum is known as free thyroxine concentration. (It is the free thyroxine that influences metabolism.) Bound thyroxine is released in specific tissues of the body, as needed, in response to metabolic demands. The Murphy Pattee test provides for measurement of T_4 with levels of 4 to 11 μg per 100 ml being normal. The Murphy Pattee test measures T_4 by comparing displacement of labeled T_4 from TBG in dried residue of the patient's serum that has been added to a solution of serum proteins and labeled T_4. Other tests using similar procedures are available to measure both the T_4 and T_3 levels. Increases in unbound T_3 and T_4 imply hyperthyroidism either from primary causes or from secondary causes such as TSH-producing tumors located in the pituitary. Choriocarcinoma in the uterus or testes may also increase the T_4 and T_3 values, indicating the relation between the reproductive system and the thyroid hormones.

Usually T_4 and T_3 levels increase or decrease in the same direction, but this is not always the case. There is no direct relation in the ratio of the T_4 and T_3 values when dysfunction occurs. One may be present in relatively greater amounts than the other in disease states. The proportion of free T_3 to T_4 is normally 10 to 1. As previously mentioned, there is a tendency for the amount of plasma proteins and hormones to become equilibrated as differences occur in the amounts of either hormone. For example, if there are increases in the amounts of T_4, the available binding proteins will be used up. Conversely, if there are decreased amounts of hormone available, there will be free spaces in the available binding proteins. Gradually, as the dysfunction progresses, an equilibrium is reached and the amount of binding proteins and hormones reach relatively normal proportions. Therefore interpretation of tests for either free proteins or free or bound hormones is dependent on knowledge of the duration of the dysfunction.

There are many variations in the levels of binding proteins and hormones. Some of these variations are related to physiologic causes; others are related to external factors. Among the physiologic causes are increased estrogen levels in women who are pregnant or in those taking estrogens; this results in an increased capacity for binding thyroxine as well as increased levels of binding proteins even when thyroid function is normal. In pregnancy, T_4 increases at a greater rate than T_3. Some people have genetic variations in the normal capacity for binding thyroxine and may have either elevated or lowered levels of hormones or proteins with normal thyroid function. Age affects T_3 levels by decreasing them, while it does not seem to affect T_4 levels.

Among the external factors are the ingestion of medications or foods that have high iodine content. Many medications such as phenytoin sodium (Dilantin) or salicylates can displace thyroxine from binding with plasma proteins. Resorcinol and salicylic acid derivatives inhibit binding. The uptake of iodine is also suppressed if exogenous thyroid hormones are given. People who have had diagnostic x-rays that utilize dyes containing iodine may also have decreased uptake because the thyroid has accumulated iodine from the dyes. The dye used for intravenous pyelograms (IVPs) affects thyroid uptake for several days, while that used for cholecystography and bronchography affects thyroid uptake for several weeks; myelography affects it for several years. Other medications that affect iodine uptake by the thyroid are expectorants containing iodine, some suppositories, and some skin lotions.

Some disease states have a great effect on thyroid uptake tests because they cause abnormal increases in thyroid hormone excretion. These include chronic diarrhea and nephrosis. In the latter, there is excessive excretion of plasma-binding proteins so that T_4 is excreted in the feces in abnormally great amounts.

It should also be noted that there is an expected rebound increase in iodine uptake following cessation of antithyroid therapy or resolution of thyroiditis. Administration of exogenous hormones for a long period of time suppresses the uptake, as does cessation of administration of iodides over a period of time. The degree of influence of these factors is variable among individuals.

All these factors must be considered by the nurse in interpreting the various thyroid function tests, because the values of the measurements obtained with the various tests do not have absolute indications for a specific state of thyroid hormone balance. It is very important, therefore, that the patient's total status be evaluated.

In addition to measurements of T_3 and T_4, there are a number of different thyroid function tests. These include thyroid uptake, clearance, suppression, and stimulation tests. A description of these tests follows.

The **PBI** (protein-bound iodine) test can be used to measure the level of bound thyroxine. The normal value for PBI is 3.5 to 8.0 μg per 100 ml. In current practice, the T_4 and T_3 measurement tests are done more frequently than the PBI. A PBI test indirectly measures the amount of bound thyroxine, which is estimated from the amount of both organic and inorganic iodine available. Therefore, results of the PBI test are influenced by the ingestion of exogenous iodine in foods, medications, or from accumulated iodine from contrast media used in x-rays.

Butanol extractable iodine (BEI) is another test used to measure the amount of iodine so that the T_4 concentrations in the serum can be measured. The BEI test does not measure inorganic iodide and iodoproteins; therefore a comparison of the BEI with the PBI can reveal the types of substances being released by the thyroid. In certain disease processes, for example, iodoproteins are abnormally released from the thyroid because of dysfunction in biosynthesis of the hormones.

Radioiodine is used in several types of studies of thyroid function. ^{131}I is the most commonly used, as it has a physical half-life of 8 days. ^{125}I, with a 60-day half-life, is also used, as well as Tc^{99m}-pertechnetate, with a physical half-life of 6 hours. When radioiodine is used, studies can be done on the uptake of iodine by the thyroid, clearance of iodine from the gland, and absolute uptake.

In order to understand these tests, the biosynthesis of hormones will be reviewed. Normally the thyroid traps inorganic iodide from extracellular fluid following its ingestion and absorption by the gastrointestinal tract. This ability to trap iodide depends on an "iodide pump" mechanism for active transport into the follicular cells of the thyroid gland. Trapping is inhibited by anions such as perchlorate and thiocyanate. Iodide is oxidized within the thyroid by the enzyme peroxidase so that it can be incorporated into organic molecules of iodotyrosines. These are monoiodotyrosine (MIT) with one iodine molecule and diiodotyrosine (DIT) with two iodine molecules, plus tyrosine. A coupling of the iodotyrosine molecules occurs within the thyroglobulin to form the iodothyronines thyroxine and triiodothyronine. T_4 has four atoms of iodine and is formed by the coupling of two DIT molecules plus tyrosine. T_3 is formed by the coupling of one MIT and one DIT molecule and tyrosine and has three atoms of iodine. Anoxia inhibits iodine transport, as do inhibitors of metabolic phosphorylation (Fig. 8-4).

The thyroglobulin in the thyroid follicle holds the hormones within the gland until their release into circulation is required. Thyroglobulin (TBG) is contained in the colloid cells of the thyroid and has tyrosine residues. The antithyroid drugs, including propylthiouracil and methimazole, block the organic binding of iodine. Protease, another enzyme, acts to free the hormones from thyroglobulin. The thyroglobulin is proteolyzed to release the hormones for secretion into circulation, also liberating some MIT and DIT, which is retained by the thyroid and further broken down into its components so that the iodides can be recycled. The enzyme deiodinase releases the iodides from the MIT and DIT so that they can be reused in iodinization. This recycling is important in the conservation of iodine. Iodinization is mediated by NADPH (dependent microsomal dehalogenating enzyme).

By giving tracer doses of radioiodine, orally or intravenously, the uptake of iodine by the thyroid gland can be measured. This test is convenient for the patient because it requires no restrictions on diet or activity. The uptake reaches a plateau in 24 hours; the normal uptake range 24 hours after administration is 15 to 45 percent. (Uptake of iodine is usually increased in hyperthyroidism unless the body stores of iodine have been substantially increased by such factors as increased ingestion of exogenous iodine.) The time of measurement for determining thyroid uptake varies in different places. This is possible because increases in uptake are evident at any time the measurement is taken. Two or three sequential measurements may be taken to determine the time variables in uptake increase. For example, in severe thyrotoxicosis the thyroid hormones are released at a consistently high rate so that the thyroid content of iodine may be normal by the end of the 24-hour period even though the uptake is increased initially.

The nurse should recognize that several adaptive processes take place within the thyroid in the event of dysfunction so that the thyroid uptake test may not reveal dysfunction. In some cases the iodine cannot be used appropriately in the biosynthesis of the hormones so that there are low serum levels of hormones. As a consequence, there is an increased secretion of TSH or there is an increased sensitivity to TSH. Stimulation of the increased levels of TSH or sensitivity of the thyroid to TSH causes the gland to enlarge, forming a goiter. This hyperplasia enables the thyroid to produce enough hormone again to

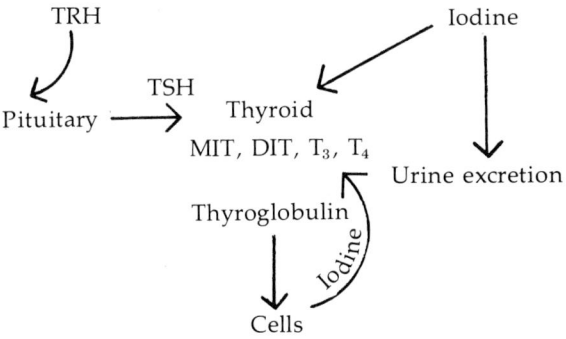

Figure 8-4
Formation of T_3 and T_4.

support metabolism, and the uptake of iodine will be in equilibrium and will appear normal in the radioactive uptake studies.

In other situations there may be hyperplasia of the thyroid without adequate biosynthesis of the hormones. This may occur as a result of a defect either in formation of MIT and DIT or in the coupling mechanisms. In some diseases there is a defect in the structure of thyroglobulin. In other diseases the thyroid releases iodotyrosines or iodoproteins abnormally, so that the iodine uptake test will show decreases.

When a person has hypothyroidism, the iodine uptake is decreased. There are two main categories of causes of hypothyroidism; the first is ineffective functioning of the thyroid, in which goiters usually form. This is termed **thyroprival hypothyroidism.** In the second, there is not enough TSH to stimulate the thyroid, and this is called **trophoprival hypothyroidism.** Thyroprival hypothyroidism is reflected in normal iodine uptake values that do not increase after administration of endogenous TSH. Since the thyroid does not respond to increased TSH, the thyroid uptake is not increased and there is increased TSH in the serum [10].

The clearance of iodine is measured by giving radioiodine intravenously. The serum is analyzed and serial counting of iodine is performed. Measurements of the plasma radioactive ^{131}PBI can be done 24 hours after giving the tracer dose. Values from 0.1% to 0.4% are considered normal. Values below this imply hypothyroidism and increased values imply hyperthyroidism.

Further evaluation of thyroid activity can be done by measuring the plasma ratio of ^{13}PBI to ^{131}I in 24, 48, or 72 hours after administration of the isotope. Increases in the clearance rate may be caused by iodine deficiency, low urinary excretion of iodides, or pregnancy. Use of ^{131}I is contraindicated in pregnancy. Iodine deficiency is most often related to insufficient dietary intake of iodine. Use of iodized salt has decreased the occurrence of iodide deficiency that was prevalent in the Great Lakes area, the thyroid belt. Now this deficiency is seen most frequently in persons who are on very strict salt-free diets. The turnover rate of iodide, if increased, causes a concomitant increase in the PBI. The amount of thyroid released in a given time period indicates turnover but does not indicate whether this is a normal or abnormal rate for the person. Urinary excretion can also be measured. If less than 40 percent of the urinary excretion of iodine occurs, uptake is increased, and if more than 80 percent is excreted, the thyroid uptake is decreased [8]. Values for the absolute uptake of iodine are determined by measuring both thyroid uptake and urinary excretion.

Resin and erythrocyte uptake of T_3 and T_4 is measured by adding ^{131}I-labeled T_3 to the blood sample, to test the reserve-binding capacity. In hyperthyroidism, the reserve-binding capacity is almost saturated and the T_3 is bound by erythrocytes at higher than normal rates. Placing a resin along with the hormones in a specially prepared blood sample indicates the reserve-binding capacity as the resin takes up the hormones that would have been taken up by the erythrocytes in the patient's serum. The reserve-binding capacity is decreased in hyperthyroidism and the resin takes up more labeled T_3. Hypothyroidism causes the opposite effect; there is a reduced concentration of serum thyroxine so that more than normal amounts of labeled T_3 are bound by proteins available to bind thyroxine. Consequently, the resin uptake is less. Anticoagulants and acid-base imbalances increase the binding capability.

Stimulation or suppression tests help differentiate among causes of dysfunction at different points in the negative feedback mechanism. The radioiodine suppression test is conducted by first giving the person sodium T_3 (liothyronine) for 3 to 5 days prior to the administration of the radioiodine. In persons with normal thyroid function sodium T_3 liothyronine suppresses uptake of the radioiodine. Those with hyperthyroidism will not respond to the suppression by administration of T_3. Persons with iodide deficiency will have an increased uptake despite the suppression dose. The concentration of the tracer dose of radioiodine is less when there is a larger extrathyroid pool of iodide. Suppression tests should not be done in the elderly or in those with heart disease, because these patients may already have reduced function.

The **TSH stimulation** test is performed by administration of bovine TSH and measuring the ^{131}I uptake and the PBI. Both should increase if the TSH stimulation is effective in activating the thyroid. Primary thyroid disease is indicated if the ^{131}I intake does not increase in response to exogenous TSH. This test may be done as a 1-day or 2-day test. In the 1-day test the iodine uptake, PBI, and TSH levels are measured 3 hours after ^{131}I has been administered. Five or ten units of TSH are given intramuscularly at this time; 24 hours after the isotope has been given, the PBI is again measured and another isotope dose is given with measurement of accumulation 3 hours thereafter. An increase of about 2.9 μg in the PBI is expected. This test distinguishes between those with true primary hypothyroidism and those with hypothyroidism because of factors external to the thyroid, and it gives an indication of the thyroid reserve. People with decreased thyroid reserves do not respond to TSH given exogenously, nor do those who have had pituitary dysfunction over a long period of time. Urinary excretion of iodine may also be measured. The thyroid hormones in the serum are conjugated with glucuronic acid in the liver. The inactivated hormones release iodides that are either recycled in the serum for trapping by the thyroid and liver or are transported, along with some free thyroxine and triiodothyronine, with bile into the intestine. Some of the thyroid hormone is returned to the liver; the remainder is excreted in the feces. The iodine removed may be excreted in the urine or may become part of the extrathyroid pool of iodine to be reused by the thyroid. The kidneys conserve iodide through tubular reabsorption. When radioiodine is given, it is taken up most quickly by the thyroid and the kidneys for excretion. For this reason, 24-hour urine samples may be collected for these tests.

In addition to thyroid function tests, biopsy of thyroid tissue may be obtained to confirm diagnosis. Needle biopsies may be performed, but some authorities believe that this method only serves to seed the carcinoma if it is present. Since the thyroid is highly vascular, bleeding may be a complication of needle biopsy. Biopsy by open method, requiring only local anesthesia and a small incision, is preferred by many. It is felt that this method provides for a more accurate biopsy because the tissues can be visualized. Complications are also fewer.

Other tests measure thyroid function indirectly. The basal metabolic rate (BMR) indicates the metabolic activity, which in turn gives an indication of thyroid function. The BMR, however, is changed by factors other than thyroid hormones, such as stress, disease processes, temperature changes, and activity. It is also very difficult to obtain a true basal metabolic rate because of difficulties in achieving a basal state.

Serum cholesterol is usually decreased and alkaline phosphatase is elevated in hyperthyroidism. Serum cholesterol is mainly used to differentiate between primary hypothyroidism and pituitary dysfunction. A normal serum cholesterol in a person with hypothyroidism indicates the possibility of pituitary dysfunction, rather than primary hypothyroidism.

The **Achilles reflex** time is measured when hypothyroidism or hyperthyroidism is suspected. There are many different ways to measure this reflex. Generally these measurements give specific information about the contraction and relaxation of muscles as observed in changes in the duration of the reflex. The reflex is shortened in hyperthyroidism and prolonged in hypothyroidism. In some instances, the Achilles reflex is measured to determine the patient's response to therapy, rather than as a specific diagnostic measurement.

Long-acting thyroid stimulator (LATS) has been found in the serum of some persons with hyperthyroidism or hypothyroidism. LATS is an immunoglobulin that simulates TSH in its function, except that its action is prolonged, with a peak effect after 8 hours, compared to the 1- to 2-hour peak effect of TSH. Initially, it was thought that LATS might be an important causative factor in the pathophysiology of hyperthyroidism; however, it has also been found in hypothyroidism. Tests for thyroid antibodies are becoming more common. Autoantibodies that are gamma globulins specific to the thyroid have been isolated. Antithyroglobulin antibody and an antibody against the microsomal component of the thyroid cells are two of the antibodies specific for the thyroid gland and are used diagnostically. Other antibodies have also been identified, giving support to the theory that many thyroid diseases may be autoimmune disorders.

Scintiscans following the administration of radioiodine can be taken to delineate **hot areas,** the areas of increased function, and **cold areas,** the areas of decreased function. The results of the scan are compared to the physical findings to determine the probable malignancy of nodules. For example, nodules that show up on the scan as cold are probably nonfunctioning and should be further investigated for malignancy.

Tests that measure thyroid function or its effects in the body must be evaluated in terms of the individual's history and symptoms. A clear-cut picture of the patient's disease is possible only through this type of total evaluation because of the adaptive mechanisms that take place in the thyroid and because the signs and symptoms may be vague and often are similar to those of many other types of disease processes. The results of diagnostic tests are expected to vary considerably among individuals and may be influenced by other disease processes. Liver dysfunction is particularly important for its influence on thyroid function, because the plasma proteins that bind T_3 and T_4 are synthesized in the liver. Such disease processes as liver cirrhosis may cause a decrease in the plasma proteins and result in lowering the values in tests such as the PBI. Hepatitis has the opposite effect, causing an increased binding capacity and an increased PBI. A number of other factors influencing the results of diagnostic tests for thyroid function have already been mentioned.

Thyroid function also changes according to body needs. For example, the thyroid function in temperature control is influenced by increased liver excretion of thyroid hormones and decreased binding capability by the plasma proteins in the serum when a person is exposed to cold. Long-term exposure to heat increases thyroid function. The calorigenic effect of thyroid hormones is stimulated by increased TSH. There is concomitant increase in the hormone production that causes an increased metabolic rate and increased heat production. This in turn also increases oxygen consumption. The levels of thyroid hormone, TSH, and plasma proteins, therefore, vary from one time to another in any given individual.

Other substances (goitrogens) ingested in food can affect thyroid function. **Goitrogens,** which are antithyroids, are present in many raw foods including cabbage, turnips, brussel sprouts, kale, and broccoli. Cooking reduces their goitrogenic activity. More important goitrogens are the antithyroid drugs used in treatment. These goitrogens can inhibit one or more phases of the biosynthesis of thyroid hormones. A result of ingesting large quantities of goitrogens is decreased synthesis and secretion of the thyroid hormones with resultant increased production of TSH. Since the thyroid cannot produce the hormones, the stimulated thyroid activity increases formation of thyroglobulin and increases the growth of thyroid cells, forming an enlarged gland or goiter.

THYROID DYSFUNCTION

Having discussed the broad scope of assessment factors, specific types of dysfunction will now be discussed. The nurse with a good understanding of these types of dysfunction can plan care that will be most beneficial to the people involved.

Among the disorders of the thyroid are **Graves' disease** (also called diffuse toxic goiter), exophthalmos, toxic multinodular goiter, and toxic adenoma, all of which can cause symptoms of thyrotoxicosis (hyperthyroidism). Goiter is considered an adaptive change in the thyroid gland and may or may not be associated with increased production of hormones. Carcinoma of the thyroid and thyroiditis occur less commonly and may render the person hyperthyroid or hypothyroid.

In general, nursing care for patients with thyrotoxicosis includes a number of factors, depending on the levels of the thyroid hormones and the individual's signs and symptoms. Intolerance to warmth requires that the nurse maintain a cool ambient temperature. In the hospital setting, this may be difficult, particularly if the patient's roommate prefers warmth. Placing the patient near a window that opens or in an air-conditioned room is important for the patient with thyrotoxicosis. In addition, the emotional atmosphere should be calm to reduce the patient's nervousness, anxiety, and irritability. Because of muscle weakness, the patient requires protection from falls and assistance when ambulating. Safety is promoted by placing the bed in low position, by the use of siderails, and by placing his or her belongings nearby. Appropriate measures for comfort and safety must also be taken in the patient's home environment. Caloric intake must be sufficient to meet the patient's increased metabolic needs. Frequent meals with snacks in between enable the patient to consume greater amounts of food. Finally, if gastrointestinal, cardiovascular, and other symptoms are present, the patient must receive specific care (Chaps. 4 and 7).

There are many causes of thyrotoxicosis. In the following section, nursing care of people with Graves' disease will be discussed followed by a discussion of other causes of thyrotoxicosis.

Graves' Disease

Diffuse toxic goiter (Graves' disease) occurs more frequently in females than in males. Its onset is often abrupt, but symptoms may develop gradually over a period of time. Frequently the person has experienced an emotional shock or trauma prior to the onset of Graves' disease. For example, death of someone close to the person and with whom she or he had a dependent relationship, major disappointments, or a personal crisis of any nature may precede the onset of Graves' disease. The disease often affects several members of the same family and can be traced through generations in families, giving credibility to the theory that it may be a familial disorder.

The symptoms of Graves' disease may be vague, resembling those of a nervous or emotional disorder, particularly if thyrotoxicosis is present. The patient is therefore often treated on the assumption that she or he is undergoing a reaction to the crisis and is in the depression stage of grief. Consequently, the physiologic symptoms may be overlooked while everyone—medical personnel and family—concentrates on the emotional changes in an effort to help the person adapt. Psychiatric counseling, participation in groups, and other forms of activity therapy are often recommended. The patient has difficulty coping with increased activity because of the fatigue that accompanies the thyrotoxicosis, and she or he becomes increasingly unable to manage the requisites of self-maintenance so that physical appearance deteriorates. This too, substantiates the belief that the person is depressed. Withdrawal from the usual activities the person previously enjoyed can also be interpreted as a symptom of emotional illness. The nurse should recognize that the patient's inability to participate in many activities may be a result of the muscle weakness and exertional dyspnea that sometimes occurs in Graves' disease. Weight loss, anxiety or restlessness, and increased gastrointestinal mobility are symptoms of nervous states as well as of thyrotoxicosis.

The irritability and emotional lability recognized as aspects of thyrotoxicosis may alienate family and friends who have made seemingly futile efforts to help the patient. The nurse may interpret this frustration as noncaring. It should be recognized, however, that the continual association with a person who seems to refuse help is stressful for the family and friends. They tend to react to the person's behavior on a very personal level and may have feelings of rejection or insecurity that are accentuated by the person's response to them. The nurse may then be placed in the role of mediator while helping the family members recognize the basis for these reactions and understand the nature of thyrotoxicosis.

Once the cause of the physical and emotional changes has been identified as a treatable physical illness, the family may be relieved. In some instances, however, the crises created by the illness may uncover underlying emotional problems that can be dealt with in psychological counseling or therapy. The emotional symptoms demonstrated by thyrotoxicosis may be preillness propensities or latent problems that require therapy even after treatment of thyroid dysfunction has rendered the patient euthyroid (having normal thyroid function). The family concerns and problems uncovered by the crises may require continuing therapy for successful resolution.

There are many forms of Graves' disease. The thyrotoxicosis is only one of three classic symptoms. The other two are **enlargement of the thyroid** (or goiter) and **ophthalmic changes**. The cause of Graves' disease is unknown. Among theories about the cause is that the disease may be an autonomous hyperfunction of the thyroid gland. LATS, which is considered either an autoantibody or an antibody, may cause abnormal stimulation of the gland. Other theories about the source of abnormal stimulation are related to the negative feedback mechanism, with TSH playing a major role. None of these theories has been proved.

A given individual with Graves' disease may have all three or any one of the three classic symptoms, singly without the others, or combinations of any two. Depending on the physical status certain symptoms may be accentuated while others are not present. This is particularly true in thyrotoxicosis, in which any one of the major body systems may seemingly be more affected than others. Cardiovascular signs and symptoms may be predominant in some patients while gastrointestinal signs and symptoms may be predominant in others.

There is also no direct relation between the size of the thyroid gland and the severity of the thyrotoxicosis or even the occurrence of thyrotoxicosis. Enlargement of the thyroid tends to be fairly evenly distributed throughout the gland, but the total increase in size may be of varying degrees. Diffuse toxic goiter implies that there is some degree of enlargement. When eye changes are present, there tends to be lid retraction and ophthalmologic symptoms of the infiltrative type.

Exophthalmos

Ophthalmic changes are characteristic of thyroid dysfunction. These changes are referred to as either **endocrine exophthalmos** or **malignant exophthalmos.** The former is associated with thyrotoxicosis while the latter may occur independently of overt thyroid hormone imbalances. Endocrine exophthalmos usually recedes with therapy, while the malignant exophthalmos does not respond to therapy specific for hyperthyroidism. Its progression is seemingly independent of this therapy. For this reason, this type of exophthalmos is referred to as malignant or **infiltrative exophthalmos.**

Signs and symptoms of exophthalmos vary considerably and may develop rapidly or gradually in varying degrees of severity. In mild exophthalmos, in addition to lid retraction, the person has a staring gaze. The staring is referred to as Dalrymple's sign, and dilated pupils may augment the effect of the staring gaze. Initially, the person may notice symptoms of eye irritation, with a feeling of having sand or dirt in his eyes. Excessive tearing occurs, especially during exposure to wind or cold air. It is thought that these symptoms are a result of increased sympathetic nerve activity. Blinking is infrequent and tremor of the eyelids may be noted. When the person looks upward, his forehead does not wrinkle but remains smooth. This is called Joffroy's sign. Lid lag may also be noted.

The prominence of the eyes may not be equal on both sides but rarely occurs unilaterally. When exophthalmos is present to a greater degree, the eyes tire easily, and there is a feeling of pressure behind the globe. Lids are often reddened and edema of the orbital and extraocular eye tissues mask the exophthalmos. The eyes then have a puffy appearance. This edema is caused by cellular infiltration, which is characteristic of immune disease. Chemosis (conjunctival edema) may also be present, and the conjunctiva may be enlarged. Vision may be blurred with frequent experiences of diplopia when looking upward or to the side. Visual acuity is often affected.

When exophthalmos is severe, lid retraction may be present to such a degree that the person cannot close his eyes, even during sleep. This loss of protection makes him susceptible to the development of corneal ulceration because of drying. Weakness of the extraocular muscles results in dysfunction as well. The person may not be able to converge his eyes and may find it difficult to gaze upward or to the side. In some instances, paralysis of the muscles occurs so that it is necessary to extend the neck in order to be able to see above the horizontal field of vision.

In assessing the presence and degree of exophthalmos, one can stand above the seated person and look downward to gauge the degree that the eyes protrude from the forehead. The nurse can test for resiliency of the eyeball by placing the thumb over closed lids and applying light pressure to move the eyeball back. In exophthalmos, the intraorbital tension is great and the eyeball does not move easily, if at all. Examination of the eyes with an ophthalmoscope may reveal venous congestion and papilledema.

The exophthalmometer is used to measure the degree of exophthalmos. This instrument measures the distance between the anterior section of the cornea and the lateral angle of the orbit. A distance of greater than 20 mm is considered abnormal. Since there is normally great variance in the size and shape of the eyes and their orbits, this test does not always establish the presence of exophthalmos. Instead, it is used primarily to determine the progress of the exophthalmos.

There are varying theories about the treatment of exophthalmos. It seems to run a natural course of an acute stage followed by some degree of remission. To what extent remission occurs and how long it takes is highly individual and cannot be predicted on the basis of signs and symptoms. As prognosis is a concern, this information is important in the nurse's counseling role. When exophthalmos occurs without changes in thyroid hormone levels, the patient's progress is monitored carefully, as a certain percentage of persons with this type of exophthalmos do eventually develop thyroid dysfunction. If, however, the exophthalmos occurs in conjunction with thyroid hormone imbalances, treatment for the imbalance will result in remission of exophthalmos as well. In other instances, the exophthalmos progresses independently of thyroid imbalances and does not always respond to treatment.

Nursing functions include conservative treatment measures such as having the person sleep with his head elevated. Limiting fluid and salt intake has some effect on decreasing the edema. Diuretics may be given. Administration of glucocorticoids reduces the inflammatory reaction. Some physicians prescribe low doses of thyroid hormones to achieve regression in the absence of thyroid dysfunction while others prefer to let the exophthalmos run its course. The nurse can advise the patient that wearing dark glasses may reduce eye strain and irritability. If the person's eyelids do not close, wearing protective shields over the eyes at night is helpful. Eye lubricants are necessary to prevent excessive drying. Special prism eyeglasses may improve upward and lateral vision, thereby reducing some of the discomfort and visual limitations. Complications of exophthalmos are caused by pressure on surrounding structures. Optic nerve disease may develop, and in rare instances result in blindness. Orbital decompression may be necessary to save the eyeball. Supervoltage radiation of the retro-orbital space is currently being used. Sectioning of the hypophyseal stalk has been tried in therapy, but is not always successful.

Other Signs and Symptoms

Pretibial myxedema, although not a frequent occurrence in hyperthyroidism, tends to be present along with infiltrative exophthalmos when it does occur. The skin of the anterior aspects of the lower legs and the dorsum of the feet is indurated. This edema may be distributed fairly evenly or may be nodular. The skin has a coarse appearance and there may be brownish or pink discoloration. Hair does not tend to grow in the indurated areas. When hair is present, it is usually coarse. Use of steroid creams applied topically or administration of systemic steroids usually relieves the symptoms. The nodules are filled with mucopolysaccharide deposits, again typical of an immune disorder.

Other signs of thyroid disease occur with great variance. Onycholysis (or Plummer's nails) may be present. The nails have the appearance of a fungus infection with abnormal separation of the nail from the nailbed. Thyroid acropachy, or clubbing of the fingers, may occur. The clubbing is caused by diaphyseal new bone that forms beneath the periosteum. While occurring most frequently in the phalanges, it may also be present in the long bones. The affected areas may be painful, with signs of an inflammatory response in that there is increased local heat along with edema. Thyroid acropachy rarely occurs and tends to be most frequent in males. Loss of skin pigmentation is another sign that, although occurring infrequently, tends to be associated with exophthalmia.

Of major concern in nursing care is the patient's feeling and response to changed body image. All the symptoms and signs previously described bring about changes in appearance that can prove distressful and may complicate the patient's total emotional response to the disease process. The nurse should explain the reasons for the changes, the prognosis, and the helpful activities that can reduce discomfort while also providing for protection and prevention of complications. When exophthalmos exists, for example, the bulging eyes may cause other people to either stare or try to avoid looking at the patient. It is difficult for the thyrotoxic patient to deal with such changes in other people's responses to him or her. The nurse must be aware of the meaning of the symptoms and signs of thyrotoxicosis for the individual and must establish trusting relationships with the patient and family in order to provide counseling and support.

Diagnostic tests used in differentiating Graves' disease include all the thyroid function tests. When the patient has all three of the classic symptoms (goiter, exophthalmos, and thyrotoxicosis), the diagnosis is obvious. Some persons do not have all these clear-cut symptoms, and it is necessary to complete extensive diagnostic tests. The iodine clearance rate is increased and ^{131}I uptake is increased with concomitant increase in the ^{131}PBI. In Graves' disease, there is decreased binding capacity of TBG with increased amounts of free T_4 and T_3. There is a greater increase in T_3 than in T_4. Two-thirds of the population with thyrotoxicosis have LATS in their serum while 40 percent have high titers of thyroid antibodies [10]. The thyroid suppression test may be done for diagnosis of borderline cases. A baseline thyroid uptake is done prior to and following administration of thyroid given to test suppression. If hyperthyroidism is present, the thyroid will not be suppressed by administration of thyroid for several weeks prior to the test. Suppression normally occurs as a result of administration of thyroid.

Therapy for Graves' disease is based on efforts to reduce the rate of hormone synthesis and secretion. Since there is no specific cure, therapeutic measures to facilitate adaptation of the thyroid gland are selected so that an euthyroid state can be achieved. This is accomplished by several methods: administration of iodine, administration of antithyroid drugs, surgical removal of all or part of the thyroid gland, or therapeutic administration of radioiodine. The disease tends to run a course with exacerbations and latent periods and may eventually end in hypothyroidism.

Iodine was formerly used in treatment of Graves' disease but in current practice is rarely used singly. Iodine inhibits the release of hormones and lessens secretion of T_4. If the patient has a high level of iodine stores in the thyroid, as do persons with hyperthyroidism, administration of exogenous iodine may precipitate severe thyrotoxicosis. Iodine also becomes ineffective as a therapeutic agent if used over a period of time; however, it does have a more immediate effect than antithyroid drugs. For this reason, iodine is administered when the patient is in danger of a thyroid crisis.

Administration of iodine inhibits the response to antithyroid therapy and precludes therapeutic use of ^{131}I. Only a small amount of iodine is required for therapy. When administering iodine, usually in the form of SSKI (saturated solution of potassium-iodide) or Lugol's solution, the dosage should be carefully measured, because one drop of either contains sufficient iodine for therapy (6 mg daily is considered sufficient by some authorities [10]. One drop of SSKI contains 48 mg of iodine and one drop of Lugol's solution contains approximately 8 mg of iodine. SSKI is administered by placing the dosage in fruit juice to dilute the iodine, to mask its unpleasant metallic taste, and to prevent gum soreness. Because SSKI evaporates readily, it should be prepared just prior to administration.

Thioamide drugs are given for their antithyroid effects. The most commonly used drugs in this class are propylthiouracil (PRU) and methimazole (Tapazole). These drugs inhibit the coupling of iodotyrosines. Large doses are used initially because the person may have a large supply of thyroid hormone stored and a large accumulation of iodine in the thyroid. Until these stores are reduced by use of the antithyroid drugs, the thyroid gland is to some degree resistant to the drugs. Therefore, the patient's symptoms do not abate rapidly with the initiation of drug administration. In general, the response of individuals to antithyroid drugs varies according to the amount of synthesis of hormones taking place within the glands, the amount of release of hormones, and the degree of inhibition the drugs bring about. As the stores are depleted, the dosage of the thioamide drugs is reduced to maintenance levels. Normal metabolism (an euthyroid state) is usually not achieved until about 6 weeks following initiation of drug administration. Initially, PTU is given in divided doses totaling 200 to 300 mg daily. If necessary, increased amounts are given by increasing the number of doses rather than the amount taken at any one time. Methimazol is about ten times as potent as PTU; the usual dosage is 10 to 15 mg q8h for moderately severe hyperthyroidism.

Mothers taking antithyroid drugs should not breast-feed their infants because the drugs are transmitted in the breast milk causing hypothyroidism in the infants. The expected effect of the thioamide drugs is reduction in the synthesis and release of hormones. The thyroid gland should decrease in size and be followed by a decrease in the symptoms of thyrotoxicosis. If too large a dosage is given, the person begins to demonstrate signs and symptoms of hypothyroidism: weight gain, fatigue, and perhaps enlargement of the thyroid gland. While trying to achieve adaptation of the thyroid toward an euthyroid state, some physicians give supplemental hormones routinely along with the antithyroid drugs, to prevent the occurrence of hypothyroidism. The nurse should assess the patient's signs and symptoms to determine the effectiveness of the drug therapy and should inform the physician of significant changes so that dosage can be adjusted.

Another effect of the antithyroid drugs in some persons is the development of iodine deficiency. Supplemental iodine may be given to counteract this effect. A significant measure of the effect of the antithyroid drugs is the thyroid suppression test. This is usually done about every 6 months to guide therapy. If the thyroid suppression test is normal, a schedule of reducing the dosage of the drugs gradually is followed; however, if the thyroid suppression test remains abnormal, the therapy is continued.

The nurse should advise the patient of the potential side effects of the antithyroid drugs. Skin rashes may occur along with fever. Agranulocytosis may develop during the first month of therapy. For this reason, leukocyte counts are monitored. The symptoms of agranulocytosis include sore throat and increased temperature. The patient should be aware of these symptoms and if they occur should be instructed to notify the physician. The drugs are usually discontinued when agranulocytosis develops. Other symptoms rarely occur, but may be serious. These include myalgia, arthralgia, neuritis, or even hepatitis or abnormal hair pigmentation. In the event the patient develops any of these symptoms, the drugs are discontinued and should not be prescribed again. When these symptoms occur, the nurse should understand that the patient may become discouraged about therapy.

It should be understood that antithyroid drugs do not cure Graves' disease. There is actually no cure for the disease. The anticipated effect of antithyroid drugs is the achievement of a prolonged stage of remission. Some 50 to 60 percent of the people with Graves' disease who take antithyroid drugs for periods of a year or so do go into a stage of remission. The remainder tend to have recurrences and the disease tends to become more active in the exacerbations following administration of antithyroid drugs. The type of response elicited by antithyroid drugs is somewhat dependent on the stage of Graves' disease the patient is experiencing. The disease has both latent and active stages and the active stages vary in severity. The periods of remission are also of varying length. Remissions may last for a period of only a month or so following the antithyroid treatment. Most exacerbations, therefore, do occur within the first few months after therapy has been discontinued. Others do not occur for several months or even years. Because of this, it is important that the nurse inform the patient of the need for follow-up care.

It should be noted that, when antithyroid drugs are given during pregnancy, the fetus will be affected. The drugs can cross the placenta, rendering the fetus hypothyroid during the first few weeks of life. Thereafter, as the effect of the antithyroid drugs diminishes, the infant becomes euthyroid.

In severe thyrotoxicosis, adrenergic antagonists have been used effectively to reduce the symptoms. These drugs function by depleting the tissues of catecholamines. Drugs usually given are propranolol (Inderal), reserpine (Serpasil), and guanethidine (Ismelin). Reserpine is given if nervousness is a predominant symptom. Although these drugs help to alleviate the symptoms of thyrotoxicosis, they cannot be used exclusively in treatment. In general, they are used as adjunctive therapy when the thyrotoxicosis is severe and when the symptoms are not relieved by antithyroid drugs. It is particularly important to monitor the patient's cardiovascular status when these drugs are being used. Postural hypotension may be expected if guanethidine is used. When the patient has underlying heart disease or if cardiac symptoms are predominant, one should be observant of signs and symptoms of cardiac insufficiency, such as tachycardia, shortness of breath, and weakness, that may develop as an effect of these drugs.

Because of the hypermetabolic state in Graves' disease, it is important that the patient have an adequate diet. A high-protein high-calorie diet with high vitamin content is advised. This diet provides for metabolic needs and helps allay catabolism of body stores of proteins and fats. Caffeine-containing beverages should be eliminated from the diet because they increase the metabolic rate. As it is often difficult to accommodate the great amount of calories required, the nurse must provide dietary counseling so that the patient selects appropriate foods and learns to space meals with frequent snacks in between main meals. It is helpful to have the patient keep a record of total caloric intake to ensure that the intake pattern can be evaluated.

Another important aspect of therapy in Graves' disease is the provision of a calm, quiet environment. The patient may be restless and hyperactive, nervous and irritable. Because of these changes the patient's interactions with friends and family may become distressful. Small problems that the patient formerly handled with little difficulty, such as reacting to loud music or laughing, may become monumental and normally insignificant events become important sources of stress. The patient and family must be involved in efforts to relieve this type of stress. Through the counseling process, the nurse must help the patient and family determine the sources of stress in the patient's environment and explore ways to reduce or remove the stress. The family and friends may tend to protect the patient from stress by not including him or her in events that have a potential for eliciting a strong reaction. This protection may be sensed by the patient as exclusion, causing him to be distrustful or suspicious. These issues must be resolved by the patient and family according to coping mechanisms normally used by the persons involved and in ways that they can handle. In general, dealing openly and honestly and with tactful diplomacy has better results than covering or hiding information or excluding the person from involvement in matters that are important to him or her. These are important considerations for the nurse in giving care.

A common focal point in stress situations is the interpersonal relationships one has developed. If a person closely interacts with others in a family unit, the position he holds in the family is important in determining his probable stressors. For example, if a mother with children becomes thyrotoxic, she will probably be less able to provide nurturing and care for the children. Depending on the stage of development of the children and the tasks they are working through, this loss of nurturing and understanding may contribute to exaggeration of the crisis and may delay or interfere with resolution. The type of relationship the children have with the father, or the presence or absence of the father figure, will also influence this crisis. If there is a father who can be supportive during the mother's illness, the crisis may be lessened. In addition, the relationship between the father and mother is significant. In situations in which there is understanding and a trusting relationship, the crisis of the mother's illness may be handled with less disruption of the family. In families in which the mother and father did not have a good relationship prior to the onset of illness, the crisis may be greater or the children may have already established coping mechanisms to deal with the family crisis.

If the person with Graves' disease does not live in a family unit, the problems may be different, but they usually revolve around the activities of daily living. For the single person who shares living arrangements with another, dealing with the environment to relieve stressors is very similar to the steps taken if the person lives in a primary family unit. Inevitably, persons who share living arrangements have an effect on one another and may develop dependent relationships not unlike those found in a primary family unit. A patient's illness may bring about a change in his or her ability to take care of his or her share of the daily routines and to participate in the relationship in a satisfying way for all persons involved. The reaction elicited from this change may vary from understanding and support from others to antagonism.

The person who lives alone may have fewer

stresses involving interdependent relationships with others. The very lack of this type of relationship may, however, be the source of stress. In some instances the person may have recently lost the support of someone on whom he or she depended. Accomplishing tasks for daily living may be more of a problem for the person who lives alone because there is no one in the home environment who can take care of cooking, cleaning, and maintenance activities. In this instance, the nurse may be of assistance by arranging for help in carrying out these activities. As an alternative, the person may be cared for in another setting such as the hospital or extended care facility until the illness is resolved sufficiently so that he or she can resume self-care at home. Counseling may also be necessary in an effort to bring this person into contact with others so that meaningful relationships can occur. This is sometimes an important long-term nursing care goal.

There are probably two alternatives for providing a calm and quiet environment; these are (1) remove the patient from a stressful environment or (2) change the environment so that stressors are reduced. In reality, neither solves the problem totally, but one is probably better for a given person than the other. It is necessary to ascertain what the patient considers the main source of stress and then to take measures to provide external assistance to accomplish the tasks necessary to reduce this stress. In certain situations it may not be possible for the person to leave the stressful environment, because of financial restraints or personal feelings. Therefore, the total condition and real and perceived restraints for accepting alternatives must be considered. Whatever is decided, the insight developed among the individuals involved in the problem-solving process can, in and of itself, prove to be very supportive of the person with thyrotoxicosis.

In the event that antithyroid drugs fail to produce a remission, radioiodine and surgery are alternative forms of treatment. There is controversy about the use of either of these treatment methods, however. As with antithyroid drugs, they do not cure the condition but are, instead, efforts to facilitate adaptation of the gland so that the patient becomes euthyroid. Radioiodine is the less expensive of the two and is a more simply accomplished form of therapy from the aspect of time and immediate risk; its use is controversial, however, because of the uncertainty about the long-term effects of radiation. Some authorities believe that radiation of the thyroid may make the patient more susceptible to the development of carcinoma or leukemia. This belief stems from the incidence of carcinoma of the thyroid in persons who were previously treated by external radiation for conditions involving the chest and neck. There is no evidence that the use of radioiodine results in an increase in the development of carcinoma. There is the possibility that radiation may result in genetic damage to children born to a woman who has had this therapy, limiting its use in women under the age of 40 years.

Initial effects of radiation on the thyroid are swelling of the epithelium and necrosis. The follicular cells of the thyroid are disrupted and leukocytes infiltrate the area. This process is followed by fibrosis and decreased vascularization of the thyroid tissue. The dosage of radiation used varies and is usually computed according to the estimated weight of the thyroid gland. The minimum amount of radioiodine that will produce relief of symptoms of thyrotoxicosis is used so that the gland remains sufficiently viable to produce adequate amounts of hormones. Hypothyroidism does result following radioiodine administration. Some physicians prescribe thyroid hormones to diminish the possibility of the occurrence of hypothyroidism following radioiodine therapy. The occurrence of hypothyroidism is greatest in the first year or two following radiation, and continues to develop in subsequent years at a rate of about 3 percent [10]. The proponents of radioiodine therapy generally believe that hypothyroidism is less of a threat to the patient than is continued thyrotoxicosis, as hormones can be given exogenously.

Thyroidectomy, the surgical excision of all or part of the thyroid gland, is carried out in persistent hyperthyroidism. Again, surgical removal of part of the gland does not cure but reduces the amount of functioning tissue, thereby reducing hormone production. Hyperthyroidism may occur again following surgery if sufficient tissue remains, and if conditions are such that the disease process continues. Hypothyroidism is the result of complete removal of the thyroid; the patient then requires administration of exogenous thyroid hormones. Subtotal thyroidectomy (removal of a part of the thyroid) allows the remaining thyroid tissue to be stimulated by TSH so that the adaptive functions of the thyroid in hormone production continue. Hypothyroidism does occur at a rate that increases with time during the years following surgery; the mechanism for this is not fully explained. One theory is that removal of part of the thyroid interferes with the blood supply sufficiently to cause eventual hypothyroidism. If hypothyroidism does develop, thyroid hormones are given exogenously and the person must accept that he is dependent on this thyroid.

Thyroid surgery requires careful preparation of the thyroid status in order to prevent postoperative complications. Very specific drug therapy schedules are prescribed prior to surgery. Antithyroid drugs are given for a period of time so that the stores of iodine and hormones within the gland are depleted. When this occurs, the patient will be in a normal or euthyroid state metabolically. Iodine is then given to produce decreased vascularity and increase in the size of the follicular cells. This process is referred to as **involution** of the thyroid gland. This regimen for administering antithyroid drugs until the person is euthyroid and then giving iodine for 5 to 7 days prior to surgery reduces the postoperative complications of thyrotoxicosis. These complications occur if the gland is in a highly vascular state and if it contains large stores of iodine and hormones. Other preoperative measures are the same as for persons having other types of surgery.

Following thyroid surgery, the patient is placed in a semi-Fowler's position, which prevents hyperextension of the neck and protects the suture line and the underlying surgical repair. There may or may not be drains in the wound, depending on the pathologic findings and the surgical procedure.

Thyroid surgery is associated with risks. Of these are interference with the blood supply to the thyroid, disruption or damage to the recurrent laryngeal nerve, and destruction of the parathyroid glands. Because of the location of the thyroid, postoperative bleeding may lead to symptoms of pressure and even asphyxiation. The nurse should monitor the patient's vital signs; tachycardia and hypotension imply hemorrhage. In addition, the wound is observed for hematoma formation. Edema is a significant postoperative sign. If postoperative bleeding is noted, the nurse immediately notifies the surgeon, as the patient will be returned to surgery for evacuation of the hematoma and ligation of the bleeding vessels.

The nurse also observes for signs and symptoms of damage to the recurrent laryngeal nerve. This damage may cause vocal cord paralysis and may be either bilateral or unilateral. Symptoms of respiratory obstruction that are severe enough to require tracheostomy may be noted in bilateral nerve damage. Stridor will be noted. Any indication of respiratory obstruction also presents an immediate need for intervention. When the damage is unilateral, the patient will experience dysphonia. His voice may be high-pitched, a state that may become a permanent condition, or it may gradually recede, depending on the extent of nerve damage.

It is wise to prepare for both an emergency tracheostomy and for suctioning, so that respiratory obstruction can be dealt with quickly if it occurs. Equipment for immediate intervention always should be at hand. The nurse should notify the surgeon if there is indication that respiratory obstruction is developing. This will be noted by tachycardia, dysphagia, and if the person is alert enough, by a feeling of being smothered. Restlessness and anxiety develop if intervention does not take place early. In the event of dysphonia, the nurse must be realistic in explaining the uncertainty of the prognosis concerning return of vocal cord function. Permanent damage may require a long-term adjustment, particularly if the pitch and quality of the voice are significant for the person. Complete loss of voice is very difficult to adjust to and is discussed more fully in Chapter 13.

If the parathyroid glands are destroyed, hypoparathyroidism results. Depending on the amount of disruption of parathyroid gland tissue, this condition may be transient or permanent. Hypocalcemia, the prominent feature of hypoparathyroidism, may be noted at any time during the week following surgery. To detect whether hypoparathyroidism has occurred as a result of thyroid surgery, the nurse observes the person for signs and symptoms of tetany. In this condition, the hypocalcemia causes increased neuromuscular irritability. The nurse observes for motor signs of twitching, muscle cramps, or dysphagia. Earlier symptoms are paresthesia and numbness; Chvostek's sign and Trousseau's sign are important in assessment (see Fig. 8-5 on page 670). Treatment involves intravenous administration of calcium gluconate to supply needed calcium.

Thyroid crisis was formerly a major complication following thyroid surgery. It does not occur as frequently now because patients are given antithyroid drugs and iodine prior to surgery to achieve an euthyroid state. In addition to surgery, however, thyroid storm or thyroid crisis may be precipitated by a variety of stressors in thyrotoxic people. Infections, abrupt withdrawal of iodine and antithyroid medications, metabolic causes, emotional stress, and pulmonary embolism are the most common precipitating factors. The condition is called thyroid storm because the signs and symptoms reflect exaggerated thyrotoxicosis. The basic cause of thyroid storm is not known. Its occurrence is greatest in persons who have hyperthyroid disease that is either not treated or is ineffectively treated so that the presence of excessive thyroid hormones results in the acute and life-threatening crisis. The onset of thyroid storm is usually abrupt, with an increased temperature of over 100° F (30° C) and diaphoresis. Cardiopulmonary symptoms include tachycardia of 120 beats per minute or more, arrythmias, congestive heart failure, and pulmonary edema. Embolism may be a serious complication. Gastrointestinal symptoms include abdominal pain that is severe and accompanied by nausea and vomiting, not unlike symptoms of an acute abdomen. Diarrhea and jaundice may occur. Central nervous system symptoms range from a feeling of tremulousness to severe agitation or psychosis with developing apathy and coma. There is an increase in free T_4 and T_3, and it is theorized that this may be of significance in bringing about the crisis.

Treatment consists in symptomatic and specific therapy. Adrenergic blocking agents, previously mentioned, are given to decrease the activity of the heart. Glucocorticoids may be given to help the person cope with the stress effects, and iodine is given depending on the person's tolerance. Sodium iodide 0.5 to 1.0 or 2.0 gm is given slowly in an intravenous infusion, or saturated solution of SSKI is given orally. The antithyroid drugs are given to prevent storage of hormones. Although their action in reducing hormone storage takes some time and they have no immediate effect on the thyroid storm, they do serve to initiate long-term therapy.

Nursing measures are extremely important for the patient in thyroid storm. It is essential to reduce the temperature by using aspirin or by applying external cold, or both, via a water mattress, ice packs, or whatever method is used in that particular hospital setting. The patient must be protected from infections, as the incidence of an infection may be the factor that proves fatal. Patients in thyroid storm are susceptible to the development of pneumonia.

Maintenance of fluid and electrolyte balance is also essential. The patient in thyroid storm quickly becomes dehydrated as a result of excessive diaphoresis and increased temperature, and he or she requires fluids to maintain an adequate urinary output. It is important that fluid and electrolyte balance be carefully monitored because the patient is in a precarious balance between underhydration and overhydration, with associated electrolyte shifts. Overhydration is a concern particularly if the patient has cardiac or respiratory problems. Serum electrolytes are monitored carefully and deficiencies are replaced accordingly. The occurrence of either vomiting or diarrhea, or both, contributes to sodium or potassium imbalances. The patient usually is monitored for changes in the ECG patterns, particularly if arrythmias are present and if adrenergic-blocking drugs are being given. Diuretics and other medications specific for the patient's cardiovascular-respiratory status are given according to his needs, and they may also affect his electrolyte balance.

Another area of importance in nursing care is provision for nutrients which may be complicated by the person's gastrointestinal status. Glucose is given intravenously along with large doses of vitamin B complex.

The person in thyroid storm is acutely ill and is usually cared for in an intensive care unit for continuous monitoring. In giving care, the nurse must be cognizant of comfort measures. If the person is agitated or psychotic, it is necessary to provide for protection and safety. Family members may be extremely upset, requiring both support and information about the patient's status. If appropriate in a given situation and if family members are able to be supportive, it may be helpful to involve them in caring for the patient and in assuming a role of providing for the patient's safety and protection as well as of giving comfort.

It is very important that the thyroid gland not be palpated in a thyrotoxic patient. This external stimulation of the thyroid may initiate increased symptoms, it may be sufficient to initiate thyroid storm, or it may increase the symptoms if storm is in progress.

The prognosis for patients in thyroid storm is good if treatment is initiated quickly and if they respond to the treatment. Cardiovascular-respiratory complications with the incidence of pulmonary embolism may be the cause of death.

Thyrotoxicosis may be caused by other factors in addition to Graves' disease. Toxic multinodular goiter, toxic adenoma of the thyroid, and taking excessive thyroid hormone which creates a condition known as **thyrotoxicosis factita** may result in symptoms of thyrotoxicosis. Other conditions that may cause thyrotoxicosis include tumors that secrete a thyroid stimulator which functions in a manner similar to TSH. Of these, hydatidiform mole, teratomas of the ovary, and carcinoma of the testes are the most common in occurrence.

Toxic-Nodular Goiter

Toxic multinodular goiter and toxic adenoma of the thyroid are grouped together in the classification, **toxic-nodular goiter.** Usually persons with toxic multinodular goiter have a formation of nodules with euthyroid states for some time prior to the onset of thyrotoxicosis. While the pathogenesis of toxic multinodular goiter is not fully understood, it has been found that the nodules comprise the functioning tissue of the thyroid for hormone production. For some reason, the nodular tissue functions autonomously without stimulation of TSH. Tissue surrounding the nodules may either be completely inactive or may respond to TSH stimulation by increasing iodine uptake.

The incidence of toxic multinodular goiter is greatest in persons over 50 years of age. The thyrotoxicosis that may develop is usually mild and cardiovascular symptoms tend to predominate. The person may experience some muscle-wasting and emotional lability.

Exophthalmos is uncommon in toxic multinodular goiter. Diagnosis is difficult, and when thyrotoxicosis is mild, thyroid function tests may not indicate dysfunction to any great degree. If results are borderline, one also has to consider that the tests of thyroid function are influenced by many factors.

Treatment is usually symptomatic. The patient is given antithyroid drugs until he becomes euthyroid and then radioiodine to suppress the overactive thyroid nodules. Antithyroid drugs are resumed several days following administration of the radioiodine, and are continued until the patient becomes euthyroid from the effects of the radiation. This takes about 2 weeks. Nodules that grow toward the sternum (retrosternal) may compress the esophagus and trachea if they are not treated.

Toxic Adenoma

Toxic adenoma may occur singly or in multiples. The nodules tend to occur more frequently in younger people and are slow-growing. As with toxic multinodular goiter, the adenomas do not respond to TSH but function autonomously. The remaining thyroid tissue is usually capable of functioning if TSH is supplied exogenously.

Treatment comprises either surgical removal of the adenoma, which cures the condition, or administration of radioiodine, which may reduce the size of the adenoma but does not ensure its complete removal. Prior to surgical removal of adenomas, exogenous TSH is given for about 3 days and a scintiscan is usually done to determine if the thyroid tissue surrounding the adenoma is capable of functioning. Usually the person responds well after surgery and the remaining thyroid tissue again becomes active. If the adenoma is long-standing, there may be suppression of the function of the surrounding tissue, as the adenoma has secreted increased amounts of thyroid hormones, increasing the serum thyroid hormone levels and decreasing TSH secretion. The thyroid no longer responds to TSH. In this case, the person requires exogenous thyroid hormone.

Thyrotoxicosis Factita

Thyrotoxicosis factita is a condition that develops as a result of taking exogenous hormones. In some instances, the individual has gradually needed to increase the dosage of thyroid hormones to achieve the desired effects. Eventually, the thyroid has adapted to extremely high levels of exogenous thyroid and decreased severely its own endogenous production. These people may develop mild thyrotoxicosis or may be susceptible to thyroid crisis in times of stress because they have minimal remaining adaptive capabilities. In this respect, teaching the person preventive measures is an important nursing function.

The general needs of the person with hypothyroidism are related to the many different types of signs and symptoms the person presents. These people have an intolerance for cold, requiring that the nurse provide for warmth. It is generally better to keep the ambient temperature in normal ranges and to provide warmth by having the patient wear warm clothing. The other needs related to hypothyroidism are protection and safety in ambulation, as the patient is often weak and lethargic because of muscular and nervous system involvement. The environment should be free of stressors, yet should provide stimuli to which the patient can relate. Caloric intake must be nutritious and provide for weight loss if the patient is overweight.

Signs and symptoms of other diseases should be treated accordingly. The over-all appearance of the person with hypothyroidism may be distressful and the nurse must make sure that excellent personal hygiene measures are carried out to minimize the effects of skin, hair, and weight changes. Every effort should be made to help the person develop a sense of self-satisfaction about personal appearance, which improves as he becomes increasingly euthyroid.

Juvenile Hypothyroidism and Myxedema

When hypothyroidism, the opposite of hyperthyroidism, begins in infancy it is termed **cretinism**. When it occurs in children, it is termed **juvenile hypothyroidism** and when it occurs in adults, it is termed **myxedema**. The age of onset of hypothyroidism is variable among children and probably depends to some extent on the degree of existing dysfunction. Congenital hypothyroidism may occur as a result of genetic defects in which there may be a developmental defect in formation of the thyroid resulting in absence of thyroid tissue. In other cases, there may be formation of ectopic thyroid tissue. **Lingual thyroid** is the occurrence of thyroid tissue between the anterior and posterior portions of the tongue. Endemic cretinism occurs in areas in which there is deficiency of iodine in the soil and water, usually in mountainous regions and previously in the thyroid belt of the Great Lakes area prior to use of iodized salt.

Children born of goitrous parents may have insufficient TSH from the mother during formative stages and may develop hypothyroidism later in life. Other genetic defects include impairment of the ability to synthesize thyroid hormones and defects in iodide-trapping. When thyroid hormones are not synthesized, there is a corresponding increase in TSH production and subsequent goiter formation. (This adaptive response may be adequate to provide sufficient hormones or it may be inadequate, resulting in hypothyroidism.) Iodide-trapping defects rarely occur. Finally, pituitary dysfunction also can cause thyroid dysfunction. When this occurs, the child may have adrenal insufficiency as well.

Severe hypothyroidism beginning in infancy is usually diagnosed through assessment of the infant's total behavior. Physiologic jaundice in the newborn may be the first sign of hypothyroidism. Other early symptoms include feeding problems, the presence of a hoarse cry, and somnolence. Treatment must be initiated prior to the age of 4 months or the infant will have stunted intellectual growth and will be mentally retarded. Thyroid hormone is essential for mental development. Treatment initiated after the age of 4 months may improve the mental development to some slight degree, depending on the child's age when therapy is instituted, whereas physiologic growth usually can be improved.

If the hypothyroidism is not diagnosed early in infancy, the symptoms and signs become more obvious. The infant develops a protruding abdomen and demonstrates failure to thrive. Hypothyroid infants do not develop motor skills at the expected age, with delayed sitting, standing, and walking skills. The untreated child does not grow. The extremities are short and the head and trunk tend to be of more normal size. The child's growth is permanently dwarfed if he or she is not treated. There is delayed closure of the fontanelles and maldeveloped femoral epiphyses, causing the child to walk with a waddling gait. Eruption of deciduous teeth is delayed and the teeth, when they do erupt, easily become carious. Bone age is generally retarded in accordance with the child's chronologic age. Protein synthesis is decreased in hypothyroidism and nitrogen excretion may be increased, also influencing failure to grow.

Children with juvenile hypothyroidism do not usually have as severe symptoms as cretins, whose growth and sexual development are retarded. Usually these children have decreased levels of both T_3 and T_4 and a decreased BMR. Both the serum cholesterol and creatine phosphokinase (CPK) is elevated.

Hypothyroidism in the adult commonly develops over a period of time. Tiredness is usually the initial symptom, along with increasing sensitivity to cold, constipation, and, in women, menstrual disturbances. Gradually the person becomes increasingly apathetic with slowing of both motor and intellectual functioning. As the disease progresses, there is a notable change in the person's appearance, as the skin becomes thick and coarse, the nails brittle, and hair tends to fall out. The facial features tend to flatten out and the face appears wider. The voice becomes husky, the eyes are matted together with mucus upon awakening, and there is increasing stiffness and muscular aching. Numbness and tingling of the extremities are common symptoms. The tongue may thicken, and speech becomes increasingly slow and halting. Progressive deafness and vestibular dysfunction sometimes occur. Eventually the eyes become puffy and the eyelids are particularly edematous and tend to lag. Eventually, the person has the appearance of a sedentary individual: slightly or moderately overweight with flabby muscles, nonpitting edema, and with slowness in all actions and movements. Males with hypothyroidism may also develop gynecomastia, which regresses after therapy. Persons with hypothyroidism should not be given medications that have antithyroid effects.

Treatment of hypothyroidism comprises administration of either synthetic or animal derivatives of thyroid hormone. The synthetic preparations are sodium levothyroxine (Synthroid) and sodium liothyronine (Cytomel). The thyroprotein derived from animal thyroid glands is called thyroid extract USP. Various methods of therapy are used. Some physicians prefer the synthetic hormone because of its uniform potency with identifiable hormone content. Thyroid extract varies considerably in potency and the composition of the extract is not exact for either T_3 or T_4, so that the effects of medications measured at different times may be variable. The dosage depends on the individual's condition and response.

Unless there is some reason to bring about a normal metabolic state quickly, such as need for surgery, the dose given is selected to provide for a gradual return to an euthyroid state. Usually a small dose is given and the response is carefully assessed. The dose is increased weekly until a maintenance dose has been reached. The amount required varies considerably for each individual, and excessive thyroid dosages result in hyperthyroid states. In the elderly, it is very important not to give excessive doses of thyroid extract, as it may activate underlying cardiac problems. The goal is to induce a balance between hypothyroidism and hyperthyroidism. The nurse must teach the patient self-care, keeping in mind that in hypothyroidism the person may have slowed mental alertness and cannot learn easily. The nurse and the patient must carefully observe for signs and symptoms of excessive thyroid.

As with the person who has thyrotoxicosis, the person with hypothyroidism often has emotional symptoms and may develop psychoses. Careful attention and support from the nurse during the early stages of treatment to ensure that the medication is being taken is required. Treatment usually brings about dramatic results, with improvement in all the signs and symptoms of hypothyroidism. Physiologic indications of the effectiveness of the thyroid drug that occur early in treatment are diuresis, weight loss, and decreased edema. Gradually, the skin becomes more normal in appearance and the hoarseness recedes with the voice becoming more normal. The person not only feels better but also begins to be more active. It is important that the patient be taught the importance of taking the thyroid consistently, for without this exogenous hormone, the condition will revert to the hypothyroid state. Frequently the patient does not consider medications necessary if he or she feels well and therefore discontinues taking the necessary, prescribed dose. The nurse will find then that the patient must be consistently "re-taught" as his or her learning capabilities improve.

The teaching role of the nurse also includes giving the patient the correct information concerning the complications that can occur following therapy. Angina and other cardiovascular effects are important complications that require treatment. Psychic disturbances may occur following therapy and may represent the person's preillness potential for emotional problems. These also require appropriate therapy. Signs and symptoms of thyrotoxicosis should also be recognizable to the patient. If the patient receives too much thyroid hormone, the metabolic balance can be disrupted toward the hyperthyroid state. For some reason, persons taking thyroid hormone for hypothyroidism are particularly sensitive to increased levels of thyroid hormone and require less hormone to induce thyrotoxicosis than do people with Graves' disease.

Monitoring the response to therapy with thyroid hormones may be done by measuring T_3 or T_4 levels or by measuring the BMR and serum cholesterol. The latter measures the metabolic effects of the hormone. The nurse must keep the person actively involved in the therapy, as relapse occurs in persons who do not continue to take their medication after they begin to feel better. Working with these persons often requires patience and persistence on the part of the nurse, particularly if they do not seem to take the initiative in their own care.

The nurse should know that, in many instances, patients with very mild hypothyroidism may not be treated with exogenous thyroid. This is controversial, as some authorities prefer to treat persons who demonstrate mild clinical signs and symptoms of hypothyroidism. Because of the adaptive nature of the thyroid gland, it is often difficult to discern from thyroid tests if a deficiency in hormone production actually exists. This is particularly the case if a person has been given thyroid hormone, because the exogenous hormone suppresses the thyroid function. A true picture of this person's thyroid capabilities is possible only after withdrawing the thyroid hormone for several weeks so that testing can be accomplished.

When true hypothyroidism exists the use of thyroid hormone is very effective in achieving weight loss and in providing more energy as the patient becomes euthyroid. The nurse should be aware that people who are responding to therapy have definitive needs for nutrition counseling in the selection of foods to accommodate their increased appetite and energy demands without adding unnecessary or empty calories. Principles of good nutrition therefore are applicable to people who are being treated for hypothyroidism as well as to those who are overweight for other reasons.

The administration of thyroid hormone for achieving weight loss is inappropriate if hypothyroidism has not been fully established. Some people take thyroid inappropriately because they are convinced that they need the hormone, or they have heard from others about the "magical cure" experiences as a result of taking thyroid hormones. The nurse should counsel the person toward developing positive health practices including proper diet and exercise when he or she is seeking a "cure" for weight gain. Formerly, thyroid hormone was used to augment establishment of menses in young girls who seemed to have difficulty beginning menstruation or who had irregular menstrual periods. By the time these girls reach womanhood they have often become dependent on the thyroid hormone and sometimes have never had an extensive examination of endocrine function, so that their need for thyroid hormone remains questionable. Giving exogenous thyroid interrupts the negative feedback mechanism so that after receiving exogenous thyroid the stimulation to secrete thyroid is suppressed and the overall effect is no change in thyroid hormone levels. If, however, the person has hypothyroidism and discontinues taking thyroid, overt dysfunction will develop and may progressively worsen.

Myxedema coma is the culmination of hypothyroidism and rarely occurs. The elderly are most susceptible and myxedema coma occurs most frequently in the winter months in persons with long-term hypothyroidism. Subnormal temperature is the initial outstanding sign of myxedema coma along with bradycardia, hypotension, and hypoventilation. Hyponatremia and hypoglycemia are present in some persons. Lactic acidosis can develop as a result of poor oxygenation. The coma may be precipitated by infections, trauma, or other illnesses which place a strain on the cardiovascular or respiratory systems. Exposure to cold can also trigger myxedema coma. Although the pathogenesis of myxedema coma is not fully understood, it is theorized that lack of adrenal hormones may be a major contributing factor.

The patient in myxedema coma is acutely ill and may have severe vascular collapse and respiratory insufficiency. Both problems must be treated definitively. Specific therapy is given to replenish the thyroid hormone in sufficient quantities to reestablish some thyroid function without placing the patient's cardiovascular status in jeopardy. Because of the hypotensive state, the patient does not have the ability to compensate for stimulation in cardiac activity. Thyroid hormone is generally administered intravenously at first. As the patient's condition improves, oral medications for replacing thyroid hormones may be given. Hydrocortisone is given to improve the adrenal function. Sedatives, particularly opiates, are never given, as they cannot be tolerated by the patient in myxedema coma because of the decreased adrenergic stimulation resulting from hypothyroidism and because of the patient's respiratory insufficiency.

Nursing measures focus on keeping the patient as warm as possible by application of external heat, taking care not to injure the skin. Mechanical ventilation may be required to treat the hypoventilation. Carbon dioxide narcosis may develop as a result of hypoventilation, and therefore blood gases must be monitored carefully as a guide to therapy. Oxygen may be required, but must be given with caution in accordance with the blood gas levels. Intravenous glucose can be given if hypoglycemia exists, and hyponatremia and lactic acidosis are treated according to the patient's condition. Myxedema coma occurs infrequently; however, there is about a 50 percent mortality rate in those who do develop myxedema coma. When the coma ensues, prompt initiation of therapy and constant attention to monitoring the person's physiologic and psychological status, with immediate intervention as indicated, may prevent death.

Nontoxic Goiter

Nontoxic goiter may result from iodine deficiency or from dysfunction in the biosynthesis of thyroid hormones. It is not certain why the goiter develops. A number of theories have been presented, but none has been proved. Nontoxic goiter tends to occur most frequently in females during adolescence, pregnancy, and menopause. The symptoms are related to the size of the goiter and range from discomfort when wearing garments that fit tightly around the neck to dysphagia and respiratory stridor, if the goiter impinges on the esophagus or trachea. The nontoxic goiter has the potential for becoming toxic and may precede development of Graves' disease or toxic multinodular goiter. The goiter progresses from a diffuse phase to a multinodular phase. In the latter stage, it is difficult to differentiate from carcinoma of the thyroid.

The nurse should know that treatment for goiter is controversial. Because iodine deficiency is rare in the United States, iodine is rarely given. If the person has been ingesting goitrogens (substances that produce goiters) in foods or medications, these are eliminated. The function of the thyroid gland may be suppressed in an effort to diminish the hyperplasia and to reduce the vascularity. Hemorrhage of the goiter may occur, further increasing its size. Suppression is accomplished by giving thyroid hormone. The ^{131}I uptake is measured to evaluate the effectiveness of the therapy. Suppression is accomplished gradually so that the person does not become thyrotoxic from taking exogenous thyroid hormone. This suppression essentially rests the gland and is continued for about 6 to 12 months. Reduction in the size of the thyroid relieves the symptoms. It is thought that the new state of adaptation in the thyroid prevents extension of growth rather than remission of the disease process. If suppression does not reduce the size of the thyroid, further treatment is indicated. Continued TSH stimulation may be a factor in the development of carcinoma.

If the goiter is in the multinodular phase, suppression may not be effective. In this case, surgery may be necessary, particularly if the thyroid size is so great that there is compression on surrounding structures. A scintiscan will determine whether the goiter is diffuse or if there are nodules present. The appearance of hot nodules, those that accumulate radioiodine, usually indicates that the nodules are benign. Cold nodules, which do not accumulate radioiodine, are usually malignant. Cold spots may also indicate a local inflammatory or degenerative process. Carcinoma of the thyroid occurs in many persons who have previously been treated with x-ray therapy in childhood, for lymphadenitis or for other conditions in the neck and chest. The most commonly occurring type is papillary carcinoma, which is found in children and in adults below the age of 40. Follicular carcinoma usually affects people over the age of 40. Other types are anaplastic and medullary carcinoma.

Carcinoma

Papillary carcinoma may be present for years without causing symptoms and tends to become more malignant with increasing age. The papillary tumors tend to be locally invasive and may involve regional lymph nodes. They do not take up radioiodine very well. **Follicular carcinoma** tends to spread to the bone, brain, and liver through the blood vessels. It can be differentiated to some degree from papillary carcinoma because it takes up radioiodine. **Anaplastic carcinoma** is a rapidly growing tumor that tends to change the size of the thyroid irregularly. This is a rapidly growing tumor that does not accumulate radioiodine very well. Anaplastic carcinoma occurs most frequently in persons over the age of 50. **Medullary carcinoma** is highly malignant and invades the lymphatics. This type of tumor secretes calcitonin, comprising parafollicular cells. It is associated with other endocrine pathology such as Cushing's syndrome, because it has the capability of secreting ACTH and serotonin. Medullary carcinoma is thought to be familial, being autosomal dominant.

Treatment of carcinoma of the thyroid depends on the type of tumor, the age and sex of the person, and the rapidity of growth. In persons who are under 40, single nodules are usually removed if they are functioning, because of the increased incidence of metastasis in young persons. Functioning tumors, those that secrete or accumulate iodine, may be treated with suppression therapy by thyroid hormone administration. If the tumor does not respond to suppression, use of radioiodine or surgical removal is usually indicated. When surgery is performed, the total thyroid and pericapsular lymph nodes are removed if the tumor is invasive and has involved the lymph nodes. A frozen section is done to confirm carcinoma. If the tumor tends to be encapsulated, removal is somewhat limited to the involved tissue. In many instances, a combination of surgery and radioiodine therapy is used to achieve a cure. Suppression therapy may also be added to subtotal thyroidectomy for removal of carcinoma to reduce the functioning of the thyroid and to allay tumor growth.

Thyroiditis

Thyroiditis occurs primarily in women. The major types identified are acute pyogenic thyroiditis, Riedel's thyroiditis, de Quervain's thyroiditis, and Hashimoto's disease. **Acute pyogenic thyroiditis** causes pain and tenderness of the thyroid with dysphagia and increased temperature. It is treated with antibiotics. **Riedel's thyroiditis** occurs in middle age and is associated with fibrosis of the thyroid. The gland is hard and may enlarge, causing compression of surrounding structures. Hypothyroidism may also result. Treatment consists in giving thyroid hormone for hypothyroidism and performing surgery if the compression symptoms are grave enough. **de Quervain's thyroiditis** is caused by a virus and usually follows an upper respiratory infection. Its occurrence is rare but when it does occur, it causes discomfort from pain, increased temperature, palpitations, nervousness, and extreme fatigue. Treatment is symptomatic and, if necessary, glucocorticoids are given to relieve the symptoms.

Hashimoto's disease is the most commonly occurring form of thyroiditis. It is an autoimmune disorder that often is present in persons with other autoimmune diseases such as pernicious anemia. People with Hashimoto's disease have a high titer of circulating antibodies. Women between the ages of 30 and 50 have the highest incidence of Hashimoto's disease. The thyroid dysfunction in this disease is defective biosynthesis of thyroid hormones with a defect in the organic binding of iodide, increased iodine turnover, and abnormal release of iodoproteins. The PBI and the T_4 ratio is widened because of the abnormal release of the iodoproteins which indicate higher iodine content than is demonstrated by the amount of hormone synthesized. The abnormal release of the iodoproteins prevents synthesis of hormones that would be possible if the iodine were available, rather than being abnormally released from the thyroid gland. TSH secretion is increased because of the decrease in production of thyroid hormones.

In Hashimoto's disease, goiters may be present, usually developing slowly until they become noticeable. There may be thyrotoxicosis initially but the person soon becomes hypothyroid as the disease progresses. Treatment is based on the symptoms. Thyroid hormone is given if the goiter is large. Glucocorticoids may reduce the symptoms and make the person more comfortable, but long-term use is contraindicated because of the many side effects that can ensue and because the symptoms tend to recur when the corticoids are discontinued. Hypothyroidism, if present, is treated by giving the person thyroid hormone. Surgery is carried out only if the goiter becomes large enough to impinge on surrounding structures. As with any goiter, it is necessary to determine whether carcinoma is present.

The Parathyroids

The parathyroid glands produce parathyroid hormone, which has three major target organs in the body: the kidneys, bones, and the gastrointestinal tract. The major function of parathyroid hormone is regulation of calcium metabolism in the body. Although there are usually four parathyroid glands, some individuals have fewer than four or more than four. Normally, the parathyroid glands are located on the surface of the thyroid gland. The two superior parathyroids are located on the posterior surface of the upper thyroid glands, one on each side. The two inferior parathyroid glands are located on the anterolateral surface of the thyroid, nearer the lower poles. Sometimes the parathyroid glands can be found in other locations, usually in the mediastinum. In this situation, the parathyroid glands tend to be located near the thoracic inlet.

PARATHYROID FUNCTION

Three major types of cells comprise the parathyroid glands: the **light and dark chief cells,** the **oxyphil cells,** and **water-clear cells.** The light chief cells seem to have no active function, whereas the dark chief cells synthesize the hormone. Oxyphil cells first appear at puberty and increase in number with increasing age. Adults also have a number of fat cells in their parathyroid glands.

Parathyroid hormone is synthesized by the chief cells in response to plasma calcium levels below 10 mg per 100 ml [5]. The hormone is not stored, but is secreted on demand. There seems to be no trophic control of parathyroid gland function. Plasma calcium levels determine parathyroid hormone release, decreased levels of plasma calcium trigger synthesis of parathyroid hormone, while increased levels of plasma calcium reduce the secretion of parathyroid hormone [6].

Because of its function in regulating calcium balance, parathyroid hormone is essential to many body processes. It should be noted that parathyroid hormone is closely related to vitamin D and thyrocalcitonin (a thyroid hormone) in the processes that maintain calcium balance. In addition, calcium is closely related to phosphorus in the metabolic processes of bone, gastrointestinal, and kidney control of calcium levels.

Calcium comprises about 2 percent of the adult's body weight. The major portion of calcium is found in the skeleton. That found in the plasma may be ionized, attached to organic anions or bound to proteins, primarily to serum albumin. Ionized calcium levels in the plasma cannot be measured easily and are estimated from the total calcium plasma levels in relation to the total protein. The levels of plasma calcium and phosphate vary inversely. Phosphate is primarily located in the bones and teeth, and unlike calcium, variable amounts are available in the plasma. A number of factors influence the plasma levels of phosphorus. These are the person's age, diet, and hormonal balance. In the plasma, phosphorus is mostly bound to proteins. Some phosphate may be combined with cations.

Calcium is required for activation of many enzymes, regulation of hormone release, the secretory functions of exocrine glands, and synaptic transmission of nerve endings. Calcium is important for maintaining skeletal integrity as well [4]. In addition, calcium is essential in blood clotting, milk production, and cellular membrane permeability; when extracellular calcium concentrations are low, membrane permeability is high [5]. Low levels of circulating ionized calcium increase the excitability of nerve and muscle tissue. Calcium and phosphorus are closely interrelated in body mechanisms.

Phosphorus is important in cellular physiology also. Although the mechanisms of its action in cellular metabolism are unknown, many important constituents of the cells contain phosphorus. For example, ribonucleic acids are polyphosphate polymers: phospholipids are a major component of the lipids of cellular membranes. Both adenine and guanine nucleotides are phosphorylated and provide an important source of chemical energy at the intracellular level. Glycolysis and energy metabolism are dependent on inorganic phosphate. Phosphorus is important in acid-base buffer systems.

When calcium is ingested, it is absorbed in the duodenum and upper jejunum. Parathyroid hormone increases absorption but is not essential, when both calcium intake and vitamin D are sufficient. Vitamin D is essential for parathyroid hormone activity in both bone and the gastrointestinal tract. Absorption is mediated by enzymes. Decreased absorption is influenced by corticosteroids, by the presence of excessive unabsorbed fatty acids in the intestine, and by excesses of inorganic phosphate or ingestion of alkali. From the site of absorption in the gastrointestinal tract, calcium enters the extracellular pool and is exchanged with intracellular fluids.

Phosphorus is also absorbed from the gastrointestinal tract. Absorption of phosphorus is increased by parathyroid hormone, growth hormone, and vitamin D. Acids and low-calcium diets also increase absorption, and ingestion of aluminum hydroxide decreases phosphorus absorption as well.

Parathyroid hormone acts directly on the kidney to increase the reabsorption of calcium. When serum calcium levels exceed 10 mg per 100 ml, parathyroid hormone synthesis is decreased and urinary excretion of calcium is increased. Acidity of tubular fluid limits calcium excretion. Calcium competes with saline and glucose and magnesium in reabsorption by the kidney tubules in acid-base balance mechanisms.

Renal excretion of calcium is increased by high plasma calcium levels; however, the kidney does not usually excrete calcium in excess of 500 mg per day. Therefore, when plasma calcium levels are excessively high, the kidneys cannot accommodate excretion beyond 500 mg per day and the amount in excess then remains in the serum so that hypercalcemia exists.

Parathyroid hormone inhibits tubular resorption of phosphate, thereby increasing its rate of excretion. Phosphate excretion is normally decreased when plasma calcium levels are high. The renal excretion of phosphorus is decreased by phosphate deficiencies in the diet by growth hormone, and in many normal and abnormal conditions such as during lactation, in osteoporosis, Addison's disease, and in metastatic neoplasia of the bone.

Parathyroid hormone, vitamin D, and thyrocalcitonin interact in maintenance of calcium balance. An antagonist to parathyroid hormone, thyrocalcitonin also participates in the regulation of calcium metabolism. Its action is more directly related to bone metabolism and it seems to have no effect on either gastrointestinal absorption or renal absorption or excretion. The effect of parathyroid hormone on bones is stimulation of bone resorption to release calcium and phosphorus to extracellular fluid. In this process, parathyroid hormone stimulates increased production of lactic and citric acid (organic acids) that decrease the pH so that calcium phosphate salts can dissolve. The osteoclasts in the bone are found in greater quantity at the site of bone resorption and secrete both lactic and citric acids. They also function to increase the breakdown of the bone matrix so that minerals can be released to extracellular fluid.

Thyrocalcitonin (TCT) antagonizes the action of parathyroid hormone (PTH) by inhibiting the action of PTH on osteocytes and osteoclasts and by increasing the rate of bone formation. It is thought that thyrocalcitonin inhibits resorption of phosphate directly while its inhibitory effect on calcium resorption is a result of the effect it has on inhibiting parathyroid hormone.

Vitamin D is also important in calcium metabolism. Some authorities consider vitamin D a hormone. It is an active sterol that promotes absorption of calcium and phosphate from the gastrointestinal tract. Vitamin D also promotes bone resorption and has a growth-promoting function.

PARATHYROID DYSFUNCTION

There are many causes of imbalances in calcium metabolism which may not be directly related to parathyroid hormone production. Parathyroid dysfunction is not frequent but can be serious. The two main types of dysfunction are hyperparathyroidism and hypoparathyroidism. There are varieties of each, depending on whether the cause is primary or secondary.

Hyperparathyroidism

Primary **hyperparathyroidism,** a rare occurrence, is the excessive secretion of the hormone by the parathyroid glands. The major cause of primary hyperparathyroidism is a single adenoma, usually involving the chief cells of the parathyroid. This type of tumor occurs most frequently in women between the ages of 35 to 65, being most common after menopause. Multiple adenomas may occur but much less frequently than single adenomas.

Other causes of primary hyperparathyroidism (5 to 10 percent) include (1) chief-cell hyperplasia, which is often related to corresponding hyperplasia of the pituitary, thyroid, or pancreas, and to the incidence of gastric ulcers and (2) clear-cell hyperplasia, which affects all the glands. Chief-cell hyperplasia is an autosomal dominant trait type of genetic disorder. Carcinoma of the parathyroids is the least frequent cause of hyperparathyroidism.

The predominant symptoms and signs of hyperparathyroidism may vary greatly. Hypercalcemia, hypophosphatemia, and hypercalciuria are usually present, along with an elevated alkaline phosphatase. There is a high incidence of nephrolithiasis and skeletal disease with adenomas. The formation of kidney stones is thought to be a result of the effect of parathyroid hormone on the kidney, as well as a result of impaired renal concentration and high excretion rates of both calcium and phosphates. Skeletal disease is related to increased rate of bone destruction with generalized demineralization. There is subperiosteal resorption of the bone which can be observed on x-ray. The changes are most evident in the hand, as the phalanges are readily affected. A ground glass or motheaten appearance on x-ray of the skull is typical of the bone changes found in hyperparathyroidism, as is absence of the lamina dura around the teeth. There is increased flexibility of the limbs and bone deformities are common. Pain and tenderness may be present and people with skeletal symptoms are prone to developing pathologic fractures. Cystic formations may also occur. Sometimes brown tumors appear as vascular masses containing osteoblasts and osteoclasts. Von Recklinghausen's disease (Osteitis fibrosa) may occur in about one-fourth of the cases.

Bone changes in the mandible and the maxilla are particularly characteristic of hyperparathyroidism. Hyperparathyroidism can be present with no symptoms for a long period of time. On the other hand, hyperparathyroidism may begin acutely and may be fatal in a short time. Generalized symptoms include anorexia, vomiting, abdominal pain, and constipation. Peptic ulcer occurs in about 10 or 20 percent of the people with primary hyperparathyroidism. Pancreatitis is another associated finding and may be confused with hyperparathyroidism in the sense that some of the symptoms are similar. Polyuria and polydipsia may also be symptoms of hyperparathyroidism, resulting from renal dysfunction with impaired concentration as well as from pancreatitis with resultant changes in insulin secretion. Generalized muscle weakness may be noticed by the person with hyperparathyroidism. The muscles and ligaments of the eye are particularly affected and there is characteristic band keratopathy of the cornea and conjunctival deposits of calcium that can be observed with a slit lamp. Cardiac function is affected, with resulting bradycardia and a shortened Q-T interval found on the ECG requiring cardiac monitoring when present. The person may experience fatigue and lethargy and may be depressed or confused. In the acute stages, coma may develop and the person may go into shock.

Some persons tend to have a predominance of the skeletal symptoms while others have a predominance of metabolic symptoms. About 50 percent of the affected people have both. The reason for the variance in symptoms is not clear. It is theorized that there may be different effects from different forms of parathyroid hormones. Three different forms of PTH have been identified. Another theory is that the symptoms are related to the quantity of excessive parathyroid hormone present and that the kidney is first affected as it is more sensitive to the hormone. Later, and in more severe cases, the skeletal symptoms occur. This is substantiated by the relation that seems to exist between higher calcium levels and the incidence of skeletal signs and symptoms. Another theory is that in some persons there is a compensatory increase in the secretion of calcitonin, which inhibits the skeletal effects of the excessive PTH. It is also postulated that the skeletal effects can be somewhat minimized if the person ingests a high-phosphate diet, so that the bone destruction is allayed.

TESTING AND TREATMENT OF HYPERPARATHYROIDISM

Hyperparathyroidism tends to go through periods of exacerbations and remissions. The tumors can rarely be felt on palpation. If they are large enough, they may displace the esophagus. A number of diagnostic tests can be done. First, hypercalcemia is usually present but may be less in those who have had the disease for a long time. Because the levels of calcium in the urine normally vary from time to time, it is important to measure the serum calcium levels three different times in extended time frames to ensure that levels are consistently high. While hypercalciuria is usually present, it is also important to evaluate kidney function, because people with renal insufficiency may have hypercalciuria without hypercalcemia.

The alkaline phosphatase is usually elevated in the people who have skeletal symptoms. In addition, an x-ray of the skeleton is also diagnostic for these bone changes. The hands are usually x-rayed routinely if hyperparathyroidism is suspected. Phosphate clearance studies may be done, but values are increased in people who eat diets high in phosphate. Giving calcium intravenously normally decreases phosphate excretion; in those with hyperparathyroidism, there is often no effect on phosphate excretion as a result of administration of intravenous calcium. Another test includes giving cortisone to observe its effect. In those with hypercalcemia from other causes, the condition is improved, but cortisone has no effect if hypercalcemia is caused by hyperparathyroidism.

The phosphate deprivation test may be done for differential diagnosis. By restricting a person's phosphate intake, it is possible to evaluate the results in terms of plasma phosphate and plasma calcium levels. Normally, phosphate reduction in the diet results in a decrease of plasma phosphate and an increase in plasma calcium. A low-phosphate diet with less than 350 mg of phosphate daily is given for 3 consecutive days. The dietary intake of calories or calcium is not restricted. Aluminum hydroxide gel or a similar substance may be given to decrease the absorption of phosphate from the gastrointestinal tract. On each of the three consecutive days during which the person has a restricted phosphate intake, fasting blood samples are taken for measurement of total calcium, inorganic phosphate and for total proteins. The blood sample is again drawn for these tests on the fourth day, after dietary restriction has ceased. If metabolism is normal, the person should have an increase in plasma calcium levels.

In addition to determining serum calcium and phosphorus levels (calcium is elevated, phosphorus decreased in hyperparathyroidism), kidney function is also evaluated to determine phosphorus and calcium clearance. Many tests can be done to determine the effects of PTH on both calcium and phosphorus clearance. Giving calcium (usually in the form of calcium gluconate) tests the effects of high calcium serum levels on PTH secretion, which will not be affected if adenomas secrete PTH autonomously. The phosphate excretion test (PEI) also indicates parathyroid function by determining the clearance of phosphate in relation to creatinine. (Creatinine clearance is more stable than phosphate and is used as a base for determining kidney function by determination of the efficiency of phosphorus excretion in the ratio to creatinine excretion.) Cortisone challenge tests are also done to determine the cause of increased calcium levels. In many conditions (vitamin D overdose, immobilization, milk-alkali syndrome, multiple myeloma, sarcoidosis, and hyperthyroidism), calcium levels are increased even though parathyroid function is normal. Cortisone causes a decrease in serum calcium in these conditions but does not affect serum calcium in hyperparathyroidism.

In some specialized laboratories, radioimmunoassay can be done to locate the site of parathyroid adenomas. Venous catheters are placed into the femoral vein and are passed to the innominate and jugular veins to obtain blood samples from both sides of the neck. Radioimmunoassay is then done to determine the levels of PTH in the samples. The venous samples should contain 10 to 15 times as much PTH as is present at the peripheral level. The samples from each side of the neck are compared to determine the size of the adenoma. There is a fairly positive correlation between the amount of PTH products in the venous sample and the size of the tumor.

Surgery is performed for treatment of hyperparathyroidism if the person's condition warrants and if the symptoms are severe enough. Parathyroidectomy is a major surgical procedure with serious implications because the location of the parathyroid glands is so variable in individuals. Radical neck surgery is usually required to explore possible sites of the glands in the mediastinal area. As diagnostic tests improve, and as the ability to determine the location of the adenomas and to differentiate between hyperplasia of parathyroid tissue and adenomas improves, the surgical risk may decrease.

The nurse should carefully plan care to include specific preoperative requisites. Prior to surgery, the patient will have had a chest x-ray, an esophagogram, and an angiogram. The neck is also scanned following administration of radioactive selenomethionine. Fluids are given prior to surgery in accordance with the patient's level of dehydration. In severely hypercalcemic persons, inorganic phosphate is given to reduce the plasma calcium levels. The phosphate must be administered carefully, particularly in those who are prone to hypotension. EDTA (calcium disodium edetate, a chelating agent) may also be used to reduce serum calcium when severe hypercalcemia is present. All these measures must be included in the preoperative nursing care to facilitate a positive response to surgery.

Following surgery, careful monitoring of the patient's vital signs is required, as well as other aspects of care similar to those following thyroidectomy. The major postoperative complications are tetany, which may develop within hours or days following the surgery, and fluid and electrolyte imbalances. Depending on the amount of parathyroid tissue remaining and the tissue trauma during surgery, the tetany may be mild and transient. If all parathyroid tissue has been removed or if the remaining tissue is permanently damaged or is incapable of secretion of hormones, the tetany is permanent and requires lifetime treatment. Tetany is further discussed later in the chapter in relation to hypoparathyroidism. The nurse must observe for signs and symptoms of tetany. As mentioned previously, the initial emergency treatment for overt tetany is administration of intravenous calcium gluconate. For mild or recurrent tetany, calcium is given orally along with vitamin D. Urinary hourly output is monitored by the nurse, and sodium and potassium levels are analyzed frequently. Diuresis is expected and electrolytes may have to be replaced. If the patient is in a state of adrenal insufficiency, steroids may be given. All these therapies are effective only if the nurse carefully monitors the patient's condition so that therapy may be initiated early.

Secondary hyperparathyroidism may be caused by hyperplasia of the parathyroid glands often because of hypocalcemia resulting from other diseases, the most important being malignant carcinoma. Secondary hyperparathyroidism resulting from any condition that causes hypocalcemia is an adaptive response in which hypocalcemia stimulates excessive secretion of parathyroid hormone and eventually causes hyperplasia of the parathyroid glands. Among the causes of hypocalcemia are malabsorption syndrome, renal insufficiency, vitamin D deficiency, and renal diseases. In secondary hyperparathyroidism, the serum calcium may be low or normal, but is usually not elevated. The serum phosphate and alkaline phosphatase are usually normal, and acidosis is common. Osteomalacia is predominant in conditions causing long-term hypocalcemia.

Usually treatment is focused on administration of calcium or agents such as aluminum hydroxide gel, or both, to decrease phosphate absorption from the gastrointestinal tract. In some instances, vitamin D is also given. In extreme cases, a subtotal parathyroidectomy may be performed.

Carcinoma that has metastasized is the most frequent cause of hypercalcemia, occurring with greater frequency than parathyroid adenomas. Usually the bones are involved in the metastatic process, with loss of bone mineralization so that extracellular levels of calcium are increased. Myeloma, leukemia, and lymphoma all cause increases in resorption of bone through invasion of the bone by the abnormal cells. It is therefore important to evaluate skeletal x-rays carefully to differentiate between primary hyperparathyroidism and these diseases, as the effects on metabolism may be similar.

Pseudohyperparathyroidism may be caused by carcinoma of the kidney or lungs. These tumors have the capability of producing a product that simulates parathyroid hormone and causes resulting hypercalcemia and increased alkaline phosphatase levels. Inorganic phosphates or corticoids may be given for treatment of this condition.

A number of other diseases may also cause hypercalcemia. These include the milk-alkali syndrome, hyperthyroidism, and diseases that result in immobilization with subsequent resorption of bone. Hypercalcemia is also a common occurrence following renal transplants. Vitamin D intoxication may cause hypercalcemia but with either hyperphosphatemia or hypophosphatemia and can result in acute renal failure and death if untreated. Treatment for vitamin D intoxication includes restricting vitamin D, calcium (and, if indicated, phosphorus) and giving fluids and adrenal steroids.

Hypoparathyroidism

Hypoparathyroidism is more often secondary to other conditions than a primary dysfunction of the parathyroid glands. The most common cause of hypoparathyroidism is damage to or removal of the parathyroid glands during surgery for removal of thyroid tissue, in which case calcium is required to prevent parathyroid crisis or storm. Damage to the vessels supplying the parathyroids may decrease the blood supply sufficiently to interfere with function. The parathyroid glands receive their blood supply from the inferior thyroid arteries or from the superior thyroid artery. They may also be supplied by arteries from the esophagus, trachea, or larynx. Hypoparathyroidism following thyroidectomy may be transient or permanent. If the parathyroids have been damaged, the tissue may regenerate and the symptoms of hypoparathyroidism may recede so that there may be a complete return of parathyroid function or minimal hypoparathyroidism; however, if all the parathyroid glands have been permanently damaged or removed, parathyroid hormone deficiency will be permanent.

Idiopathic hypoparathyroidism is rare and occurs most frequently in female children. In some instances, this condition is considered to be a familial disorder and it may be an autoimmune disease. The Di George's syndrome is a condition in which there is cellular immunity and hypoparathyroidism. A child born of a hyperparathyroid mother may be hypoparathyroid as a function of the prenatal compensation for the mother's excessive parathyroid hormone.

The early indications of hypoparathyroidism include decreased levels of plasma calcium and, later, increased plasma phosphate levels. The urinary excretion of calcium is initially greater and then falls along with reduced urinary excretion of phosphate. When there is insufficient parathyroid hormone, the normal compensatory function of parathyroid hormone for retention of calcium and excretion of phosphorus by the kidney does not take place. In hypoparathyroidism, there is also decreased absorption of calcium and phosphate from the intestine. Because of the low levels of parathyroid hormone, bone resorption also decreases so that eventually the bones may be more dense than usual.

Neuromuscular signs and symptoms are predominant when there is a decreased level of ionized calcium. The decreased levels of ionized calcium cause a concomitant increased excitability of the neuromuscular cells. Calcium is an important component in the transport of potassium and sodium and in the coupling of the phases of excitation and contraction in skeletal muscles. This increased neuromuscular excitation is called tetany, which occurs in over two-thirds of persons with hypocalcemia. Tetany may be latent or overt.

In latent tetany, there may be longstanding muscle weakness and fatigue, numbness and tingling of the extremities, and palpitation. Overt tetany is demonstrated by paresthesia of the fingers, toes, and the upper lip. There may be stiffness, and carpopedal spasm is common. This may be followed by laryngeal stridor in which dyspnea and cyanosis may occur. Spasms may involve the major organs of the body, occurring in the muscles of the eyes, bronchus, gastrointestinal tract, and the bladder. In severe cases there may be grand mal seizures. The emotional and mental effects of hypoparathyroidism may vary from irritability and anxiety to depression and psychoneurotic states. When the condition occurs in children, mental retardation may result.

Several diagnostic signs may be useful to the nurse in testing for tetany. One is the accoucheur's position, which is typical of carpopedal spasm in hypoparathyroidism. In this position, the person has flexion of the wrist and elbow and in the metacarpophalangeal joints. The thumb is adducted and the phalangeal joints are extended (Fig. 8-5). This position may occur spontaneously or it may be stimulated by applying a blood pressure cuff. Trousseau's sign is elicited by applying a blood pressure cuff and inflating the cuff beyond the systolic pressure for about 3 minutes. This initiates the carpopedal spasm, if Trousseau's sign is positive. Another commonly used diagnostic measure is testing for Chvostek's sign. In this sign, the facial nerve (seventh cranial nerve) is tapped briskly, near the middle of the masseter muscle, adjacent to the ear. If positive, there will be facial muscle contraction with a twitch that includes the upper lip. Greater contractions may include twitching of the entire side of the face. The peroneal sign is elicited by percussing the upper fibula to cause abduction and dorsiflexion of the foot.

People who have had hypoparathyroidism for a long period of time develop a number of epidermal lesions. The nurse should observe a patient for these lesions, which include coarse rough skin that tends to scale, and thinning of body hair, particularly on the scalp, axilla, and pubic areas, and on the eyebrows. The fingernails become brittle and deformed with horizontal ridges. The eyes are also affected. Lenticular cataracts form and with use of a slit lamp calcium deposits can be found in the lens. Papilledema may occur. Teeth formed after the onset of hypoparathyroidism are poorly developed and there are defects in the enamel; formation of yellow spots or grooves occurs. Cardiovascular function is affected with changes in the ECG. The Q-T interval is prolonged and the T wave is inverted. Calcium deposits may be found in the basal ganglia on x-rays.

The symptoms of hypoparathyroidism become increasingly generalized as the disease progresses. In overt hypoparathyroidism, laboratory findings reveal hypocalcemia and hyperphosphatemia; the alkaline phosphatase is either normal or low. The Ellsworth-Howard test, in which parathyroid extract is infused intravenously, or the Calcium Tolerance test, is done to determine the patient's response to changes in the feedback cycle of calcium and parathyroid hormones.

Goals of therapy for hypoparathyroidism include restoring the calcium balance to normal. The severity of the tetany is somewhat dependent on the amount of time it has taken for the calcium level to decrease. When the

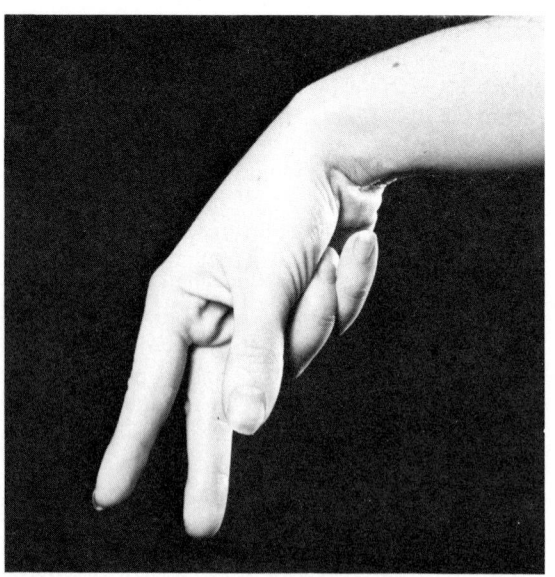

A

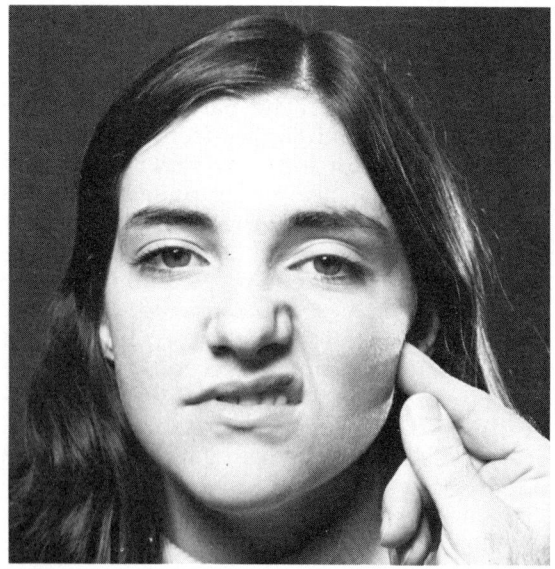

B

Figure 8-5
Carpopedal spasm in Trousseau's sign and facial muscle contraction in Chvosteck's sign.

ionized calcium concentration falls rapidly, tetany occurs at higher levels than when the ionized calcium level decreases more slowly. It is thought that the tetany may be a response to changes in the cellular pH, as it can also result from alkalosis. Treatment comprises giving calcium. If the situation is acute, calcium is given intravenously. Calcium gluconate is usually given or ionic calcium may be administered. There are different methods and doses used in current practice; however, calcium, when given intravenously, is administered slowly and carefully. If the tetany is not as acute, calcium is given orally in the form of calcium lactate, calcium gluconate, or calcium chloride. Calcium chloride is better absorbed in the intestine and is used if metabolic acidosis is present. If the person does not respond to oral calcium, magnesium may be given.

Calcium is supplemented with vitamin D. Dihydrotachysterol (DHT or Hytakerol) is more expensive, but may prove better than vitamin D. When vitamin D is being given, thyroid function should be evaluated as vitamin D is more effective when the person is euthyroid. Aluminum hydroxide gel or similar substances are given to bind the phosphate and to decrease its absorption in the intestine.

In addition to observing for signs and symptoms, the nurse must also assess the patient's response to calcium. Initially, plasma calcium levels may be measured every week or two. After the patient's condition has stabilized, measurements of calcium plasma levels are taken about every 3 months. The medications are withdrawn intermittently to test the patient's response. If necessary, calcium may have to be taken indefinitely. Both urinary and plasma calcium levels are measured routinely if this is the case. The nurse must also monitor the patient's response to vitamin D to avoid hypervitaminosis D. Symptoms and signs include hypercalcemia, calcification in soft tissue, anorexia, nausea, vomiting, diarrhea, polyuria, polydipsia, and headache. As the body slowly begins to build up its reserves, the excess vitamin D is stored and the patient may eventually accumulate excessive amounts of vitamin D. If this occurs, the vitamin D and calcium are stopped. The patient is then given large amounts of fluids and a diuretic such as furosemide (Lasix). Calcitonin may be given if necessary.

It should be remembered that while parathyroid hormone inhibits the urinary excretion of calcium, vitamin D does not.

Tetany is not limited to hypoparathyroidism; it also occurs in many other conditions that may result in metabolic acidosis. Potassium depletion, magnesium depletion, and vitamin D deficiency plus pancreatitis and renal insufficiency are among the conditions that can also cause tetany. The nurse should monitor all people with these conditions for fluid and electrolyte disturbances (Chap. 2).

Pseudohypoparathyroidism is a rare inherited disease in which skeletal abnormalities occur. The parathyroid glands may either be normal or they may be hyperplastic. The person with pseudohypoparathyroidism has a typical short stature and a round face. Strabismus may be present along with mental retardation. In addition, there are often areas of calcification in the soft tissues. The metacarpals and metatarsals and phalanges are usually short, and when the person makes a fist, dimpling may be noticed as the knuckles are often not apparent. Eye changes do not occur in pseudohypoparathyroidism.

This disease may be evident in either the skeletal symptoms or in biochemical symptoms alone, or both may occur. The metabolic symptoms are similar to those of hypoparathyroidism along with an abnormal glucose tolerance resulting from hypometabolism. It is necessary to differentiate pseudohypoparathyroidism from hypoparathyroidism. The plasma levels of parathyroid hormone are generally high in pseudohypoparathyroidism and they can be suppressed by giving calcium infusions. In hypoparathyroidism, calcium infusions do not affect the plasma parathyroid hormone levels. In the more traditional test, the Ellsworth-Howard test, parathyroid extract is given intravenously, to test phosphate excretion. In pseudohypoparathyroidism, there is less than normal urinary phosphate excretion. There are also few changes in the plasma calcium or phosphate levels after injection of parathyroid extract intramuscularly for 1 or 2 weeks.

Another rare condition, **pseudopseudohypoparathyroidism,** bears mention. The symptoms in this inherited disease are less severe than those in pseudohypoparathyroidism. Many of the symptoms and signs are similar to those in hypoparathyroidism with the exception of hypocalcemia or hyperphosphatemia. Tetany does not occur in pseudopseudohypoparathyroidism.

The Pineal Gland

That the endocrine system is closely aligned with the nervous system is exemplified by the presence of neuroendocrine transducers. The locations of some of these neuroendocrine transducers are the median eminence of the hypothalamus, which secretes tropic releasing factors; the beta cells of the pancreas, which secrete insulin; the juxtaglomerular cells of the kidney, which secrete renin; the adrenal medullary cells, which secrete epinephrine; and the pineal gland, which secretes melatonin. These transducers provide a mechanism by which the electrical nervous system impulses are relayed to the chemical endocrine system hormones. Neurotransmitters aid in this conversion. Some of these include serotonin, norepinephrine, and acetylcholine.

FUNCTION OF THE PINEAL GLAND

The pineal gland contains both norepinephrine and serotonin, and secretion of its identified hormone melatonin is cyclic, with peak secretion during darkness. Light inhibits secretion. The majority of pineal disorders are associated with either local symptoms from extensive tumor growth in the pineal gland or with development of precocious puberty, a condition in which pineal tumors are often found.

Not a great deal is known about the pineal gland. It is known to calcify normally. Experiments of pineal gland activities have demonstrated influence of melatonin to be important in adrenal, thyroid, and gonadal functions in mammals. The nature of pineal gland activity is as yet not identified in man. It is known that absence of pineal hormone results in accelerated gonadal function and that its presence inhibits gonadal function.

It is speculated that the pineal gland may have regulatory functions for other hormones. The gland is surrounded by cerebrospinal fluid, has neural input from postganglionic sympathetic nerve fibers from the superior cervical ganglia, and a segment of the optic tract from the retina to the pineal gland provides input of the exposure to light. All these findings have led to great interest in the pineal gland as being important for integrating input from man's external environment with input from his internal environment.

The Adrenal Glands

The adrenal glands secrete hormones important to maintenance of body homeostasis through their roles in metabolism, electrolyte balance, and support of nervous system function. There are two **adrenal glands;** one is positioned on the superior surface of each kidney, being imbedded in perirenal fat. Blood supply to these highly vascular glands arises from the aorta, from the inferior phrenic artery, and the renal artery. In some persons, the glands are also supplied by branches of the intercostal arteries and from the ovarian or spermatic arteries.

Each adrenal gland is divided into the **cortex** and the **medulla.** The outer area, or cortex, has the ability to synthesize cholesterol, which is converted into steroid hormones. The adrenals are also able to accumulate cholesterol from the circulation for hormone synthesis. ACTH stimulates the synthesis and the accumulation of cholesterol. Catecholamines, epinephrine, norepinephrine, and dopamine are secreted by the neurons located in the adrenal medulla, the inner division of the gland.

FUNCTION OF THE ADRENALS

Hormones secreted by the adrenal cortex are glucocorticoids, mineralocorticoids, androgens, and estrogens. There are three zones in the adrenal cortex: the zona glomerulosa, the zona fasciculata, and the zona reticularis. Aldosterone, the primary mineralocorticoid, is secreted in the zona glomerulosa while glucocorticoids, of which cortisol is the primary hormone, are secreted in the zona fasciculata. Androgens are secreted in the zona reticularis. The outer zone, the zona glomerulosa, is not as dependent on ACTH for its function as are the other two zones. Formation of the adrenal hormones takes place in a series of steps that are regulated by enzymes. Acetate is used to synthesize cholesterol, which then is converted to 20α-hydroxycholesterol. The latter is then converted in a number of steps to pregnenolone. This undergoes further conversions to form progesterone, which is further converted to cortisol in the 11β-hydroxylase system, in the zona fasciculata. Aldosterone synthesis follows the same pathways as cortisol to the point at which progesterone is formed. In the zona glomerulosa, progesterone is converted in several steps to form corticosterone, which is then converted through 18-hydroxylation to aldosterone. Knowledge of these metabolic pathways is important in the diagnosis of hormone formation abnormalities.

Glucocorticoids function primarily in metabolism to increase blood glucose levels, especially in the fasting state. This function protects body cells dependent on high levels of glucose for life when carbohydrates are not being ingested. The glucocorticoids stimulate the breakdown of proteins and the formation of substrates necessary for energy metabolism from deamination of amino acids by their action in stimulating or inhibiting enzymes. By stimulating gluconeogenesis, they maintain glycogen stores in the liver and in muscles. Glucocorticoids then stimulate protein catabolism in body cells, thereby increasing the uptake of amino acids by the liver, where they are converted to carbohydrate precursors. In this process, the enzymes necessary to stimulate transaminases are increased by glucocorticoids. Glucocorticoids also support mobilization of fatty acids and interfere with the utilization of glucose at the peripheral level [4].

Another important effect of glucocorticoids is their anti-inflammatory action. They impede diapedesis of leukocytes through the capillaries and stabilize lysosomes so that proteolytic enzymes are not released from the lysosomal membranes into damaged tissues. This stabilization reduces the destructive effects of proteolytic enzymes on surrounding tissues. Glucocorticoids have an effect on bacterial activity, probably from their influence on the body's response to the bacteria through interfering with histamine release and other activities that are not fully discovered. In addition, glucocorticoids can suppress delayed hypersensitivity reactions and are often used therapeutically for this effect. They decrease the blood lymphocytes and eosinophils as well as plasma cells and inhibit the formation of antibody-producing plasma cells.

Yet another function of glucocorticoids is their action in supporting the effects of catecholamine hormones in vasoconstriction. This is important in maintenance of blood pressure.

The glucocorticoids include cortisol, corticosterone, and compound A (11-dehydrocorticosterone). Of these, cortisol, an 11β-hydroxysteroid, is the most active and therefore is the most important in medical therapy. Normally, about 20 mg of cortisol is produced daily. Large quantities of cortisol not only produce anti-inflammatory effects and depression of hypersensitivity reactions, but also cause depression of the synthesis and secretion of ACTH. Cortisol in sufficient quantity inhibits the growth hormone and can therefore inhibit somatic growth. Stimulation of appetite and of hematopoiesis are two other effects of excessive glucocorticoids. Of the steroids produced for medical therapeutics, the glucocorticoid preparations used generally for inflammatory and allergic conditions include dexamathasone (Decadron), triamcinolone (Aristocort) and prednisone (Meticorton).

Mineralocorticoids function in regulation of electrolyte balance. Aldosterone is the most important mineralocorticoid and is produced in quantities of about 0.2 mg daily. The other major hormone in this classification is 11-deoxycorticosterone (DOC). Secretion of aldosterone by the adrenals is one of a number of complex mechanisms through which electrolyte balance is maintained. Many factors influence secretion of aldosterone, including blood volume, plasma levels of sodium and potassium, posture, and kidney function. Aldosterone affects transport of electrolytes in the gastrointestinal tract and in sweat glands and salivary glands, in addition to its action in the kidneys.

The **renin-angiotensin system** regulates secretion of aldosterone in a feedback loop. The enzyme renin is released to circulation by the juxtaglomerular cells in the kidney in response to low blood volume, low levels of potassium, and perhaps by sympathetic nervous system mediation. The macula densa cells in the distal tubules are thought to be sensitive to levels of potassium and sodium, transmitting messages to the juxtaglomerular cells. In the circulation, renin stimulates release of angiotensin I, which is hydrolyzed by another enzyme to form angiotensin II. This then stimulates the chain of conversions in the adrenal gland in which cholesterol is converted to aldosterone. Angiotensin II is a potent vasoconstrictor and stimulates the adrenals for synthesis of aldosterone. Intermediate substances in the order of formation in this chain of reactions are pregnenolone, 11-deoxycorticosterone, corticosterone, and 18-hydroxycorticosterone.

Androgens secreted by the adrenal glands are minimal in quantity compared to those produced by the gonads. Unless secreted in abnormally large amounts, they are not important in causing or affecting disease processes, except for their support of the growth of mammary and prostatic tumors. Estrogens are secreted in minute quantities by the adrenals and therefore adrenal estrogen products are normally not medically significant.

Adrenocortical function is controlled to a large extent by ACTH, which is secreted by the anterior pituitary. The corticotropin-releasing factor (CRF), secreted by the hypothalamus, influences anterior pituitary function and consequently adrenal function through a feedback system. Among the factors that directly influence the anterior pituitary secretion of ACTH are the plasma levels of cortisol, the diurnal body rhythms, and stress.

Levels of cortisol in the plasma influence the anterior pituitary secretion of ACTH through a negative feedback system. Low levels of cortisol stimulate secretion of ACTH, whereas high cortisol levels depress secretion of ACTH. This secretion is subject to the control of diurnal body rhythms. There is a definite pattern of cycles of increased and decreased ACTH secretion related to an individual's sleeping-waking habits and the light-darkness phases in a 24-hour period. This rhythm is also referred to as circadian rhythm or daily body rhythm. ACTH secretion is highest in the third to the fifth hours of sleep, reaching a maximum high within the first hour after wakening. The ACTH levels then decrease, reaching low levels about the eighth hour after wakening, being lowest during the hours just preceding and during the beginning of sleep. The diurnal rhythm is not constant or fixed, but instead is dependent on the person's routine or lightness and darkness. If, for example, the person changes his schedule, the diurnal pattern varies accordingly. When a person travels to another time zone, he or she requires about a week to adapt to the new phase relationship of the new time zone. Usually the variables of the person's routine and light and darkness are in phase, but these variables are separate and affect the diurnal rhythm independently.

Stress increases ACTH secretion. The type of stress that influences ACTH secretion can be either physiologic or psychological. Trauma to the body, infections, or surgical procedures are examples of physiologic stresses that increase secretion of ACTH. Psychological stresses are more difficult to define. What constitutes an emotional stress for an individual is unique to that individual's perception of or interpretation of the event. Emotions such as fright, grief, fear, and competitiveness may stimulate increased secretion of ACTH. In stress, ACTH is secreted independently of the negative feedback loop. Even when there is sufficient cortisol, ACTH is secreted. It is also thought that ACTH secretion in stress may be somewhat independent of the usual diurnal rhythm.

In addition to the diurnal or circadian rhythm, each person has an ultradian rhythm. In this rhythm of adrenal function, there are four to eight bursts of adrenal glucocorticoid production within a 24-hour period. These releases of glucocorticoids are closer together during the periods of high glucocorticoid secretion in the circadian rhythm and occur less frequently in periods of low glucocorticoid secretion in the circadian rhythm.

The steroid hormones diffuse readily into the cells, and different steroids have specific target receptor sites so that their activity is selective within the body. They are soluble in lipids and can activate or depress specific genes, thereby causing reactions in formation of RNA. Control of cell structure and cell growth can then be exerted by steroids that stimulate or inhibit RNA. Certain steroids compete for the same receptor sites. When this occurs, the steroids may be called biologic antagonists.

About 75 percent of the cortisol in the plasma combines with a glycoprotein called transcortin. The remainder is bound to albumin or is unbound. The free unbound cortisol actively functions to achieve the metabolic effects. Any disease process that affects the amount of transcortin or albumin available for binding cortisol also affects the amount of available free cortisol. Transcortin levels are increased in normal states; for example, in pregnancy because of the increased estrogen levels. Some people have genetically inherited low levels of these substances. It is possible to isolate the amount of cortisol in plasma for diagnosis by laboratory procedures that provide for freeing up the cortisol from the binding agents or by estimating the values by measuring the amount of binding substances available. Similar methods are used to determine cortisol levels in the urine. Tetrahydrocortisol glucuronide and tetrahydrocortisone glucuronide are the major metabolites of steroids that are excreted in the urine. Inactivation of the cortisol occurs primarily through metabolism in the liver. The cortisol is metabolized to form dihydrocortisol, which is further metabolized to form tetrahydrocortisol. A lesser quantity of cortisol is converted to cortisone, which is metabolized to form tetrahydrocortisone glucuronide. An enzyme, glucuronidase, is important in the reduction of cortisol. The metabolite of aldosterone derivation is tetrahydroaldosterone glucuronide.

About 40 to 50 percent of the metabolites of cortisol at the side chain of carbon 17 are not altered and can be measured in the urine as 17-hydroxycorticosteroids (17-OHCS). The 17-OHCS can be fractioned into two groups, the cortisol metabolites and 11-deoxycortisol metabolites. Only about 5 percent of the cortisol, however, is excreted in the urine as 17-ketosteroid (17-KS). The 17-ketosteroids are primarily made up of androgens, three-fourths of which come from the adrenal cortex. This is significant in tests to determine abnormal androgen secretion in disease states. Dehydroepiandrosterone (DHEA) is the principal precursor of ketosteroids and is the precursor of a weak androgen. DHEA appears in sufficient quantities to be measured and contributes to the total amount of ketosteroids found in the urine.

Methods for measuring the plasma and urine end products of steroid metabolism vary considerably. The Porter-Silber chromagen method measures the equivalent of plasma cortisols by identifying the presence of its metabolites in either blood or urine. Other methods for measuring cortisols include fluorometric methods in which cortisol is incubated in ethanolic sulfuric acid and radioimmunoassays which use tagged or labeled steroids.

TESTS FOR ADRENAL DYSFUNCTION

When dysfunction of the adrenal glands or pituitary gland occurs, adrenocortical function is affected with resultant changes in the levels of adrenal hormones. Several tests are conducted to differentiate pituitary dysfunction from adrenal dysfunction to determine the cause of the changes in hormone levels. These tests may be performed in different ways, but all depend on preciseness in carrying out the method being used so that the test results will be accurate. Both the adrenal glands' response to exogenous ACTH and the pituitary reserve for secretion of ACTH can be measured. In the first test, corticotropin (ACTH) is given either intramuscularly or intravenously. Usually, hourly doses are given for an 8-hour period, because a small quantity of ACTH stimulates more cortisol secretion if given slowly than is secreted if a large quantity or the same quantity is given rapidly. The ACTH may be given for a period of 2 or 3 days, and a 24-hour urine specimen is collected on the day prior to administration of ACTH and each day thereafter during the days ACTH is given. Plasma samples are drawn prior to administration of ACTH to determine the plasma level of cortisol, and another blood sample is drawn usually within the first hour during the administration of ACTH. In some instances, both plasma and 24-hour urine samples are collected on the day following the last day of administration of ACTH. This test measures the reserve capacity of the adrenal cortex. Normally, the adrenal secretes increased cortisol in response to the exogenous ACTH. If the person has adrenal insufficiency, the increase may be very small, indicating that the adrenal cortex reserve is minimal.

The metyrapone test measures pituitary reserves of ACTH. In this test metyrapone is administered either intramuscularly, intravenously, or orally, with the dosage determined by body weight. Metyrapone, an enzyme, suppresses cortisol synthesis by inhibiting 11β-hydroxylase, an immediate precursor to cortisol. If metyrapone suppresses cortisol synthesis, the resulting lowered plasma cortisol level should stimulate the anterior pituitary to secrete ACTH. Usually, metyrapone is given orally, every 6 hours for a 48-hour period. Normally, there is a twofold increase in urinary 17-OHCS if ACTH secretion has been increased as expected. This increase may occur on either the day of, or the day following, the test so that 24-hour urine samples are collected both days. If the pituitary reserve is low, the pituitary cannot respond to the lowered cortisol levels and there will be no resulting increase in ACTH production or in the subsequent production of 17-OHCS.

The metyrapone test may precipitate adrenal crisis and is contraindicated in adrenal insufficiency. Nursing observations during this test include monitoring of vital signs, as hypotension may result. Other effects are vertigo and vomiting. Giving metyrapone with milk, if the oral route is used for its administration, helps reduce the occurrence of vomiting. The test will not be accurate if the person is taking medications that depress ACTH secretion or stimulate the metabolism of metyrapone. In some instances, the dimension of purposefully induced physiologic stress is added to the metyrapone test for a precise evaluation of the pituitary reserve. Giving exogenous insulin to induce hypoglycemia is an example of an added physiologic stressor which causes identifiable symptoms of tremulousness, excessive perspiration, and mental confusion. In persons with borderline function, the added stress more realistically demonstrates pituitary reserve. When stress tests are added to the metyrapone test, nursing observations are critical both to protect the person from side effects and to determine the effects of the stress as demonstrated in signs and symptoms.

Another way of testing adrenal function is administering glucocorticoids to depress the secretion of ACTH. Dexamethasone is usually given in this test because it does not break down into the metabolites of cortisol and does not influence plasma and urine 17-OHCS levels. Dexamethasone is a glucocorticoid that normally causes a decreased secretion of cortisol and its subsequent metabolites. Both plasma cortisol and 17-OHCS levels in the urine should decrease on the day of, or the day following, administration of dexamethasone if the adrenal glands are functioning normally. The plasma cortisol levels may fall below 5 μg per 100 ml, and the 17-OHCS decrease to 2.5 mg per day or thereabouts with normal function.

It is important to note that because urinary excretion of 17-OHCS is variable, depending on body size, the values for excretion of 17-OHCS are measured in relation to a constant. Creatinine excretion remains stable and is not affected by diet or similar variables and can therefore be used to determine relative increases of 17-OHCS. Normally, a person excretes 3 to 7 mg of 17-OHCS per gram of creatinine. This increases to 12 to 25 mg of 17-OHCS per gram of creatinine following administration of ACTH.

Adrenal Dysfunction

Cortisol and aldosterone have been identified as the hormones that most affect the body homeostasis. Little is known about the function of the majority of the 48 or so hormones secreted by the adrenal glands. Dysfunction of the adrenal glands causes either **hyposecretion** or **hypersecretion** of the hormones. **Addison's disease,** also called primary adrenal insufficiency, is a form of dysfunction caused by "insufficient" adrenocortical hormones. **Cushing's syndrome** is the opposite, being caused by excess or hypersecretion of adrenocortical hormones. **Hyperaldosteronism** is a condition in which there is an excess of aldosterone. Adrenocortical dysfunction is also demonstrated by excessive quantities of androgens, or more infrequently estrogens, with resultant abnormal virilization or feminization.

Addison's Disease

Addison's disease can be caused by any process that destroys or interferes with adrenocortical function. Surgical removal, tumors, and autoimmune disorders are the most common causes. In adrenal gland atrophy from autoimmune disorders, Addison's disease may be only one aspect in a complex of dysfunction of other glands or organs susceptible to autoimmune disorders. These include the thyroid, the parathyroids, the parietal cells of the gastrointestinal tract, and the ovaries or testes. The resulting disease processes include hypothyroidism, hypoparathyroidism, and pernicious anemia. Infections of the adrenal gland can also cause dysfunction. Control of tuberculosis has reduced the incidence of adrenal atrophy from tuberculous infection.

Another cause of adrenal destruction is anticoagulant therapy in persons who are undergoing stress reactions. The anticoagulants may cause hemorrhage in the adrenal glands, resulting in destruction of tissue and loss of function. Women over the age of 50 years are most susceptible to hemorrhage from anticoagulant therapy. It is thought that factors such as enlargement of the adrenal gland with increased blood flow, which occurs normally in periods of stress with increased ACTH secretion, contribute to the incidence of hemorrhage.

Addison's disease may also occur in persons who have been receiving steroids for a long period of time if the steroids are abruptly discontinued. The lack of steroids causes the symptoms of Addison's disease.

Adrenal gland dysfunction may be secondary to changes in pituitary function. For example, insufficient secretion of ACTH resulting from pituitary dysfunction causes a concomitant hyposecretion of cortisol. Conversely, changes in adrenocortical function bring about changes in pituitary function. Low plasma levels of cortisol stimulate production of ACTH and therefore a demand for continuously increased anterior pituitary function. Increased secretion of anterior pituitary hormones often affects other body processes. The increased incidence of diabetes in those with Cushing's disease, perhaps due to increased GH or cortisol, demonstrates the relation between adrenal and pituitary function.

Addison's disease, or adrenal insufficiency, occurs more frequently in women. The symptoms are usually vague at first, becoming increasingly obvious as the adrenal cortex function gradually diminishes. As the reserve capacity of the adrenal cortex for synthesis of hormones lessens, the symptoms become more acute because the adrenal cortex eventually cannot produce sufficient quantities of hormones to meet the body's requisites. **Adrenal crisis** is the term used to describe the acute episode resulting from any form of stress that taxes the adrenal cortical function beyond its capabilities. Adrenal crisis is an acute form of adrenal insufficiency and is a possible complication for any person who has Addison's disease.

The mechanisms of the signs and symptoms of Addison's disease are the effects of insufficient cortisol and aldosterone. Lack of cortisol causes gastrointestinal symptoms, which may include anorexia, nausea, vomiting, abnormal stools similar to sprue, and abdominal pain. Hypoglycemia is common and is evidenced by apathy or drowsiness. Gluconeogenesis is decreased when there is a lack of cortisol, thereby decreasing the blood glucose levels. Changes in the glucose tolerance test in Addison's disease include both a low blood glucose level and a flattened curve. Hypoglycemia is precipitated by fasting or by missing a meal.

Hyposecretion of cortisol also affects cardiac function, as does hyposecretion of aldosterone. Without sufficient aldosterone, salt is lost in large quantities. The person with Addison's disease sometimes craves salt, probably because of the sodium deficiency. Another effect of salt loss is the inability to tolerate hot climates. Without sufficient aldosterone, the sweat gland ducts are unable to reabsorb sodium so that salt is lost in sweat. This contributes to loss of extracellular fluid volume, just as does loss of sodium from the kidneys without aldosterone. Water is lost along with the sodium so that the circulating blood volume is decreased. This in turn reduces the cardiac output so that the person has postural hypotension. The heart decreases in size, a sign that can be observed on x-ray.

Hypoaldosteronism results in signs and symptoms of electrolyte imbalance that may be exacerbated by loss of fluids and electrolytes from vomiting or diarrhea. Increased renin secretion somewhat compensates for the decreased aldosterone levels. Hyponatremia is the predominant form of electrolyte imbalance in Addison's disease. Potassium clearance decreases, as the normal exchange of potassium for sodium ions in the distal tubules does not occur when there is insufficient aldosterone.

Nervous system signs and symptoms may occur, particularly if hyperkalemia is present. The nurse should observe for these symptoms, which may include weakness, paresthesia or paresis, or even paralysis if the condition is severe. People with Addison's disease often have an exaggerated sense of taste or smell and may perceive auditory stimuli more acutely than normal.

Because the plasma cortisol levels are low, the anterior pituitary is stimulated to increase production of its hormones. ACTH is secreted in greater quantities as the anterior pituitary adapts to the lowered cortisol levels. MSH (melanin-stimulating hormone) is also secreted in greater quantities by the anterior pituitary causing changes in skin pigmentation. Characteristic skin pigmentation in Addison's disease is a yellowish-brown discoloration noted especially in the hands and in body creases, and around the nipples and the genitalia. Sometimes the buccal mucosa is affected. Because the body creases often form in areas where clothes fit more tightly, such as around the waist, the changes in pigmentation may not be easily observed.

Weight loss is a common sign of Addison's disease. This is related to the metabolic effects of insufficient cortisol as well as to the loss of body water resulting from hypoaldosteronism. Lipid metabolism is influenced by cortisol and without this influence, fat deposits decrease. Other changes include decreased libido resulting from hyposecretion of the androgens, and changes in hair distribution with loss of pubic and axillary hair.

Adrenal or **Addisonian crisis** is always a potential threat for the person with Addison's disease. The crisis may occur in persons who do not have overt symptoms, or from added stress in those known to have chronic adrenal insufficiency. Anorexia, nausea, vomiting, abdominal pain, persistent tachycardia, and azotemia are frequently precursors of crises. Among the other events that precipitate crises are infections, trauma, exposure to very high temperatures, or emotional upsets or critical life events. Giving anticoagulants, particularly heparin, may result in hemorrhage of the adrenal glands, which causes crises. Adrenal necrosis and hemorrhage are also seen in the Waterhouse-Friderichsen syndrome, a malignant form of meningitis with high fever, development of coma, and hemorrhage from the mucous membranes, skin, and adrenals. Addisonian crisis is life-threatening and must be immediately treated. The crisis is brought about by extreme deficiency of cortisol and aldosterone. Changes in the adrenal gland during stress include loss of demarcation in the zones, with ensuing necrosis of adrenal tissue in some instances.

Most predominant are the signs and symptoms of shock related to hypotension, fluid loss, and hyponatremia. Shock may occur in people who have latent Addison's disease so that the diagnosis of adrenal crisis must be made by ruling out other causes of the shock. In this instance, it is essential that the nurse carefully observe the signs and symptoms in relation to the person's previous history. As there is no single measure to detect Addison's disease, the composite of the person's present condition and previous history provides the best indication of the diagnosis, which is then confirmed by testing adrenal reserve. The history may reveal that the patient has had vague symptoms and lethargy with no apparent cause. In some instances, these patients sought medical attention and were not found to have any overt form of dysfunction.

Prior to initiating emergency therapy, blood samples are drawn for electrolytes, leukocyte count, cortisol levels, CBC, and glucose levels. The person in shock requires immediate therapy to replace sodium, fluid, and cortisol. Physiologic saline is usually started intravenously and a glucocorticoid is given. The specific preparation used is dependent on the physician's preference. The person in shock requires continual monitoring of blood gases, electrolytes, urine output, and vital signs, along with precise administration of electrolytes, fluid, and cortisol. The patient should be protected from unnecessary stimuli, and the nurse must conserve the patient's energy throughout the intensive care period. If the patient has a high temperature, the nurse must take measures for its reduction (water mattress, alcohol sponges). Observation must be made for any signs of infection. The infusion of glucocorticoid is continued for 24 to 36 hours. After the patient's condition has stabilized, oral glucocorticoids are given.

People with undiagnosed Addison's disease who have not previously received glucocorticoids often have more severe crises if their hearts are small and cannot adapt by increasing the stroke volume. In Addisonian crisis, the cause for the stress must be identified and treated simultaneously with the shock state.

As the patient's condition is stabilized, and normal sodium and cortisol levels are achieved, maintenance doses of glucocorticoids are given with fludrocortisone (Florinef) since it has mineralocorticoid activity. Diagnosis of Addison's disease is made by testing the adrenal reserve. In Addison's disease, the levels of adrenocortical hormones and 17-OHCS are low in response to stimulation by increased amounts of exogenous ACTH.

Because Addison's disease is chronic, there is a continued and essential need to replace the patient's adrenocortical hormones. These do not cure the condition but provide the patient with sufficient hormones to carry out normal activities. An individual cannot function effectively without these hormones. The person with Addison's disease must be acutely attuned to the events that cause stress for him or her because there is no automatic feedback cycle for increasing hormone levels during stress. Instead, the additional hormones must be supplied exogenously. This is also a requisite for persons who have had a bilateral adrenalectomy.

The amount of hormone secreted during stress varies with individuals and ranges from 100 to 300 mg daily. People who require exogenous hormones must increase their maintenance doses accordingly. It is generally advised that if doubt exists as to how much cortisol is required, more rather than less should be given to prevent the occurrence of a crisis. If stressors are known in advance—for example, elective surgery for any reason or participation in an event such as public speaking or a competitive event that produces stress—the dosage of glucocorticoid is increased gradually. If hydrocortisone is being used, the increments are usually made in 50-mg doses, until the desired dose, no more than 300 mg, is reached on the day of the stressful event. After the event, the dose is then gradually reduced by the same amounts as used in the daily increments until maintenance levels are reached. The nurse has an essential role in teaching the patient to use medications correctly for adaptation, as well as assisting him or her in developing life habits that will reduce stressful events.

Many stressors are not planned, and the patient must have a ready supply of hormone available for emergency injection. An emergency supply of dexamethasone should be carried at all times, usually 4 mg of dexamethasone sodium phosphate and a sterile syringe for the injection. Identification indicating that the person has adrenal insufficiency should also be carried at all times. A Medic Alert bracelet or pendant is quickly found in the event of an accident, whereas an identification card placed in a wallet might be missed by those giving emergency care.

The maintenance dose of glucocorticoids and mineralocorticoids may vary. The daily dose is generally divided with the maximum amount of cortisol given on awakening and the minimum amount prior to sleep, to correspond with normal body rhythms. Fludrocortisone (Florinef acetate) or a similar medication is given daily to supply mineralocorticoid needs. The need for mineralocorticoid replacement is variable among people and is somewhat dependent on preexisting medical conditions. People with hypertension may not require as much if any mineralocorticoid. The person is aware of the symptoms of hypoaldosterone secretion if he has experienced these symptoms prior to diagnosis of Addison's disease. He can then determine if these symptoms recur. Otherwise, the nurse should teach the patient about the possible symptoms. These include hypotension (low sodium and high potassium levels), weight loss, and weakness. The opposite symptoms occur if the person is overtreated; hypertension (high sodium, low potassium), and formation of edema, with perhaps weight gain. The dosage of mineralocorticoid is usually established by trial and error until the person achieves the proper balance in function.

Because of the loss of sodium resulting from decreased aldosterone, it is necessary that the diet be high in sodium, the amount determined by the total condition of the person. There is need for observation of signs and symptoms of fluid and electrolyte imbalances and the nurse should teach the patient how to monitor his or her own condition and when to seek medical assistance. Any event that alters electrolyte levels, the most obvious being diarrhea or vomiting, may require additional therapy. Excessive exercise accompanied by sweating may also alter the electrolyte balance through loss of sodium. The nurse should advise the person to ingest additional amounts of sodium chloride to cope with these events.

Infections pose a particular problem for the person with adrenal insufficiency because the infection is a stressor that places a demand on the body for an increased level of cortisol. Because of the anti-inflammatory effects of glucocorticoids, however, it is not always advisable to increase their dosage to cope with the stress. Usually the person will require the physician's guidance in determining the appropriate dosage. People with adrenal insufficiency may require hospitalization for infections that would normally be managed at home quite effectively. It is important not to cover the signs and symptoms of the infection with glucocorticoids, yet it is necessary to have adequate amounts of the hormone to cope with the stress. Intravenous saline may also be necessary if the individual is unable to eat a normal diet.

The nurse must emphasize the importance of regular physical examinations in Addison's disease so that the condition can be monitored and therapy evaluated for its effectiveness. In addition, autoimmune disorders in a complex of organ and gland involvement should be treated as early as possible. In Addison's disease as a result of an infectious process, it is important that the patients be taught to observe for signs and symptoms of the infection that might become overt following treatment for adrenal insufficiency. Preventive measures, especially physical examinations by the physician, provide for early detection and early treatment before long-term irreversible effects result.

When adrenal insufficiency results from pituitary dysfunction, it is called **secondary adrenal insufficiency,** as opposed to **primary adrenal insufficiency,** which is caused by lack of hormones because of disease processes directly affecting the adrenals. Often secondary adrenal insufficiency is only one of a number of disorders that are related to hyposecretion of pituitary hormones. Diagnosis of the adrenal insufficiency should differentiate between primary and secondary causes, as the treatment, to be effective, should deal with the cause of the dysfunction.

Hyposecretion of ACTH causes secondary adrenal insufficiency and may be related to deficiencies in corticotropin-releasing hormone (CRF) from the hypothalamus, from pituitary disease such as panhypopituitarism, or from long-term corticosteroid therapy, which suppresses CRF and ACTH secretion. In secondary adrenal insufficiency from pituitary dysfunction, ACTH is secreted in subnormal quantities, but MSH secretion is often normal; therefore, the patient will not have the skin pigmentation changes. Since aldosterone is primarily secreted in the feedback loop involving the renin-angiotensin system, it is usually not affected by hyposecretion of ACTH and the symptoms of fluid and electrolyte imbalances do not occur. Mineralocorticoid therapy then is not required. Unless the adrenal glands have been suppressed, stimulation by exogenous ACTH should increase cortisol secretion in the adrenal reserve test if the cause of insufficiency is of pituitary origin.

CRF or ACTH insufficiency may be brought about by steroid therapy. This may occur sometime after the glucocorticoids have been discontinued and may be evidenced by cardiovascular changes with postural hypotension. Secondary adrenal insufficiency can be expected if the person is abruptly withdrawn from steroid therapy. This is why steroid dosages must be gradually reduced.

Treatment for secondary adrenal insufficiency is based on replacement of glucocorticoids. If there is other endocrine gland involvement, as in panhypopituitarism, adrenal function is stabilized prior to administration of exogenous thyroid. This is done to prevent stimulation of adrenal crises from accelerated thyroid function. It is necessary in secondary adrenal insufficiency to follow the same therapeutic measures required by primary adrenal insufficiency, including provision for unforeseen stress by carrying dexamethasone and identification. Smaller replacement doses of glucocorticoids than are necessary in treating the primary form of adrenal insufficiency are often adequate in treating secondary adrenal insufficiency.

Cushing's Disease and Cushing's Syndrome
Cushing's disease, the opposite of adrenal insufficiency, results from hypersecretion of ACTH. The increased quantities of corticotropin-releasing factor, or ACTH, or both, stimulate the adrenal cortex causing hyperplasia of the cortical tissues and subsequent increase in the secretion of cortical hormones. This is differentiated from Cushing's syndrome, which is the result of increased secretion of cortisol by autonomously functioning adrenal glands or of production of ACTH-like peptides by carcinomas in other body organs. Another cause of Cushing's syndrome is excessive exogenous administration of glucocorticoids.

Certain tumors of the adrenal gland secrete hormones independently and are not responsive to diurnal rhythms. These tumors may increase hormone production when they are stimulated by exogenous ACTH. Oat cell carcinoma of the lung and tumors of the pancreas and thymus glands have the capability of secreting ACTH-like substances that function like ACTH in their ability to stimulate the adrenal cortex for adrenal hormone synthesis.

Glucocorticoids are often used in treatment of a number of immune diseases as well as for systemic diseases that respond poorly to other modes of therapy. Long-term administration of glucocorticoids, given for their anti-inflammatory effects, may result in Cushing's syndrome.

Cushing's disease affects women more frequently than men. It occurs most frequently between the ages of 30 and 40 years, and following childbirth; however, Cushing's disease can occur at any age, but usually in the age range of 20 to 60 years. The symptoms of Cushing's disease and of Cushing's syndrome are similar; however, the nurse should recognize that these symptoms do vary considerably among individuals. Not every person with Cushing's disease has all of the possible symptoms. Usually, the metabolic effects of the disease are the most prevalent with the muscles, bones, skin, and the deposition of body fat being affected. People with Cushing's disease have easily identifiable body changes that can make them unrecognizable to persons who have not seen them during the period of gradual changes in appearance. The nurse may have to rely on family members to describe these changes.

A typical sign is development of a "moon face" which is an accumulation of adipose tissue giving the face a round, filled-out appearance. Collection of adipose tissue in the area of the neck causes the typical "buffalo hump," and collection in the trunk area causes centripetal obesity. Along with this accumulation of adipose tissue, the person gains weight in varying amounts. At the same time there is protein-wasting with resultant muscle-wasting. The extremities become thin, appearing even thinner because of the centripetal obesity. Fat deposits in the retrobulbar tissues may cause ptosis of the upper eyelids, adding to the changed body appearance. These changes take place gradually and the person may exhibit symptoms of emotional instability as well, so that the diagnosis of Cushing's disease may be delayed in favor of emotional counseling. With experience the nurse may learn to identify these changes through observation. The protein breakdown affects connective tissue throughout the body. The nurse will note that there is a tendency to bruise easily, and the skin becomes extremely fragile as the disease progresses. Healing is delayed as the skin loses its tensile strength and becomes thinner and less resistant to trauma. Insignificant bumps against objects may cause debridement of the skin. Red or purple striae form on the abdomen, buttocks, thighs, and breasts. Plethora, an increase in the amount of blood in an area, makes the complexion florid. Acne is common. The plethora and acne are effects of increased androgen secretion. In women, amenorrhea is common and they may also have increased body hair, including an increase in facial hair; however, alopecia, to some degree, may be present.

There are also disturbances in metabolism of carbohydrates, fats, and proteins. These include a decreased tolerance for carbohydrates, increased gluconeogenesis, and increased glycogen breakdown. Pancreatic secretions are decreased and there may be fat necrosis of the pancreatic tissues. An increased resistance to insulin occurs in many persons with Cushing's disease. The glucose tolerance curve is often delayed and glycosuria may be present. About 20 percent of those with Cushing's disease develop overt diabetes.

In addition to the disturbances in carbohydrate metabolism, increased protein breakdown causes a negative nitrogen balance, which leads to changes in both muscle and bone. There are varying degrees of muscle weakness, disturbed calcium balance, and osteoporosis. Muscle weakness can be severe enough to interfere with the ability to perform daily routines and may add to the impression of an emotional disturbance. The vertebral bodies become susceptible to fracture because of bulging of the intervertebral disks. Kyphosis (increased convexity in the thoracic spine) with backache develops with fractures. Pathologic fractures may also occur in the lower extremities if osteoporosis from loss of bone matrix is severe enough. This has important implications for nursing care as the person must be protected from situations that may cause fractures. Growth is impaired when Cushing's syndrome occurs in children prior to epiphyseal closure.

Metabolic alterations are also evidenced in electrolyte imbalances. Sodium and chloride levels are increased with a concomitant decrease in the potassium level. The hypokalemia that results in some people causes changes in cardiac function. As loss of bone matrix develops, there is increased excretion of calcium and phosphorus with hypophosphatemia. With protein-wasting, albumin and globulin plasma levels decrease and there is increased excretion of proteins in the urine. Metabolic acidosis may result.

Other symptoms include hypertension, which may lead to congestive heart failure, changes in kidney function, and arteriosclerotic disease. These symptoms are associated with the susceptibility to arterial occlusions. Lymphoid tissue decreases, as does the eosinophil count, rendering persons with Cushing's disease susceptible to infections.

Personality changes develop in about 30 percent of people with Cushing's disease. Emotional lability, emotional overreaction to minor events, and mood swings with anxiety and overriding depression are frequently described by friends and relatives of people with Cushing's disease. A few develop psychoses and may have auditory hallucinations or paranoid delusions. Insomnia and a general irritability are not uncommon. There is also an increased incidence of peptic ulcers with the tendency to perforation.

Diagnosis of Cushing's syndrome or disease is made through assessment of the signs and symptoms and by laboratory and x-ray examinations. Because the range of signs and symptoms affecting body homeostasis is so great and because not everyone with Cushing's disease has all of the signs and symptoms, diagnosis cannot be made by assessment of the manifestations of the dysfunction without supporting evidence from laboratory and x-ray tests. In many instances, the symptoms may be of mild degree and are seemingly vague. Many signs and symptoms of Cushing's disease are typical of those observed in a variety of disease processes, so that evidence of their presence is not conclusive. Nursing observation is invaluable in piecing together a composite picture of the patient's history and present physiologic and psychological behavior.

Through the use of laboratory tests it is also possible to differentiate among the causes of the syndrome and the disease. In Cushing's disease, the plasma cortisol levels do not follow normal diurnal rhythms, but remain higher than normal all the time. Drawing plasma cortisol levels in the morning and evening to compare levels is therefore diagnostic. If the evening plasma cortisol level is high (above 7 μg per 100 mg), the person probably has Cushing's syndrome because with normally functioning adrenal glands cortisol levels are lowered prior to sleep. (This conclusion is based on the assumption that the sleep-wake habits are in phase with daylight and darkness.) Cortisol levels in plasma are also high if there is an adrenal tumor or if there is abnormal secretion of ACTH-like substances from carcinoma elsewhere in the body. In both of these instances, the secretion of cortisol does not follow normal body diurnal rhythms.

Collection of a 24-hour urine sample for testing the level of 17-OHCS is done to determine if further testing is necessary when Cushing's syndrome is suspected. The normal value of 24-hour urine 17-OHCS is relative to each individual and is therefore given in relation to creatinine. If the 24-hour urinary 17-OHCS is elevated, Cushing's syndrome is suspected.

A dexamethasone test is then conducted to suppress pituitary function. Normally, plasma cortisol levels decrease with dexamethasone suppression. In Cushing's syndrome, the urinary 17-OHCS remains elevated, indicating that cortisol secretion has not been affected by suppression of ACTH by dexamethasone. The dexamethasone test is performed differently in various hospitals. Different dosages and different time spans are used. In some instances, the test is conducted as a two-consecutive-day test. Therefore, the nurse must know the procedure used institutionally, so that the test can be conducted with precision to ensure reliable results from the standpoint of administration of the dexamethasone and collection of 24-hour urine samples, as well as collection of plasma samples for determining cortisol levels.

Tumors of the adrenal gland may be either benign or malignant, and in most persons are unilateral. They produce symptoms of Cushing's syndrome because of their ability to autonomously secrete cortisol and androgens independently of normal diurnal rhythm. Adrenal tissue not involved in the tumor growth atrophies because the high plasma cortisol levels arising from tumor cell secretion of hormones by the tumor cells depress ACTH stimulation. The remaining normal adrenal tissue then does not receive the necessary stimulation from ACTH. Without ACTH stimulation, the normal tissue atrophies. The dexamethasone test does not affect cortisol secretion by tumors that function independently of ACTH because dexamethasone does not affect the level of cortisol produced by the adrenal tumor.

The adrenal tumors also do not respond to the administration of metyrapone, which inhibits cortisol synthesis in its final phase. Results of this test are compared with the normal expected responses. Normally, the total urinary 17-OHCS are increased following metyrapone administration. Adrenal tumors do not respond to metyrapone and there is no increase in 17-OHCS following its administration. The pretest level of 17-OHCS is usually above normal, however, while plasma ACTH levels are lower than normal when adrenal tumors are present.

Tumors of the adrenal, then, are associated with low levels of ACTH and do not respond to dexamethasone or metyrapone. Diagnosis of adrenal tumors is assisted by x-rays. An IVP and an angiogram of the adrenals are used in diagnosis. Because adrenal tumors can grow very large by the time that dysfunction is diagnosed, they often impinge on surrounding structures such as the kidney and the abdominal wall.

The tumor may be unilateral, in which case it is removed. If the tumor is invasive and has involved the entire adrenal gland, the entire gland must be removed. If possible, however, the unaffected tissues are left intact. If the tumors are bilateral, both adrenal glands are removed. The cure rate for adrenal carcinoma is low—only about 25 percent. Chemotherapy is used palliatively if the adrenal tumor is so advanced that it cannot be resected. Adrenal tumors metastasize to the liver and lungs most frequently and also may involve other surrounding organs. Symptoms of progressive tumors include abdominal symptoms with distention and ascites, nausea, vomiting, and diarrhea, all requiring nursing care geared to comfort and support measures described in Chapter 7. There is also edema of the lower extremities and the patient progressively becomes debilitated. Metyrapone can be used to decrease cortisol levels in palliative therapy because of its action of interfering with production of 11β-hydroxysteroids of which cortisol is an example. The nurse is then challenged to work with the family and the person who is experiencing the problems related to terminal illness.

In contrast to adrenal tumors, Cushing's disease is associated with higher than normal levels of plasma ACTH. The 17-OHCS are generally found to decrease after administration of dexamethasone, although plasma cortisol levels remain high despite the point in the patient's diurnal rhythm. There is also an increase in total 17-OHCS following administration of metyrapone.

Cushing's disease is associated with dependency on pituitary ACTH. This is demonstrated by the dexamethasone test, in which the urinary 17-OHCS decrease if Cushing's is present. The metyrapone test results in an increase in total 17-OHCS and there is a high level of plasma ACTH. The primary cause for the initial increase in ACTH causing the disease can be dysfunction of the pituitary or disease processes in surrounding structures which affect the pituitary. Metyrapone enhances the dysfunction, through increased secretion of ACTH. A small percentage of those with Cushing's disease have a chromophobe pituitary tumor as the underlying cause of the disease. Skull x-rays are taken to determine changes in the sella turcica. If a tumor is present, the sella turcica will be expanded and there may be destruction of the clinoids posteriorly. If the tumor is impinging on the visual pathways, changes in vision occur. These are prevented by removal of the tumor.

Treatment for Cushing's disease or syndrome depends on the diagnosis. Surgical removal of the pituitary (hypophysectomy), removal of one or both of the adrenals (adrenalectomy), radiation of the pituitary, and use of adrenocorticolytic medications are the alternatives. Symptomatic treatment can be selected if the disease has not progressed. This is frequently followed by one of the more permanent forms of therapy.

When Cushing's syndrome is caused by abnormal secretion of ACTH-like hormones by tumors in other body sites, it is necessary to determine if the tumor exists and to find its location. Chest x-rays may reveal lung tumors or thymic tumors. The diagnosis for carcinoma of the lung is conducted by means of appropriate techniques for cytologic studies to determine the presence of carcinoma if x-ray changes are present. Depending on the site of the pulmonary tumor and its prognosis, treatment may involve either surgical removal or palliative therapy. The most commonly found tumor with capabilities for secreting ACTH-like substances is oat cell carcinoma of the lung, which is highly malignant and not curable. An adrenalectomy may be performed if the condition warrants, or chemotherapy may be used as a palliative measure.

Treatment in Cushing's disease or syndrome may include removal of either the hypophysis (pituitary) or the adrenal glands or radiation of the pituitary. The former removes all sources of the hormones secreted by the glands (tropic hormones if the pituitary is removed, and all the adrenal hormones if both adrenal glands are removed). Radiation of the pituitary has variable results, and the patient may or may not require exogenous hormones. The dosage of radiation is determined for each person individually. Treatment methods used include partial hypophysectomy or implantation of radioactive gold or yttrium in the pituitary. Chemotherapy is also used by some physicians: o,p'-DDD (mitotane) may be given over a period of several months for its adrenocorticolytic effects. When chemotherapy is used, small doses of the adrenocorticolytic agent are given over a period of several months, and plasma cortisol levels are monitored to evaluate the effectiveness of the treatment. Following reduction of excessive cortisol levels to normal (by therapy with adrenocorticolytic agents), some people have complications of excessive ACTH or MSH production by the pituitary. Many times pituitary adenomas are found following bilateral adrenalectomy and loss of the suppression by the high cortisol levels. The high levels of MSH, particularly β-MSH, may produce pigmentation as seen in Addison's disease.

Conservative treatment for Cushing's disease includes treating any existing disease such as diabetes, and giving a high-protein, low-sodium, high-calcium, and high-potassium diet. If the person has symptoms of emotional problems, these are treated by psychiatric counseling. The importance of recognizing the emotional instability that occurs in some persons as a part of the disease or syndrome must be emphasized. It is necessary to treat both the physiologic and the psychological manifestations of the dysfunction. Nursing care should be based on the premise that correction of the physiologic manifestations may or may not correct the emotional instability. Ongoing care may be required even after the physiologic manifestations have been corrected. Some theorists believe that the emotional problems and behavior exhibited may be preillness propensities that are exaggerated by the illness while others believe that there may be no relationship. At any rate, the types of behavior demonstrated are usually unique to the individual and should be managed with concern for long-term care.

There is really no "cure" for Cushing's disease or syndrome. Instead, the processes of hormone synthesis are manipulated. If the pituitary or adrenal glands are completely removed, the person is dependent on exogenous hormones for his lifetime. When the glands are partially removed in an attempt to preserve some function, the results are variable and the person may or may not be dependent on exogenous hormones, or may require smaller doses than if the glands had been completely removed. Some people respond well to radiation and retain function of the gland, whereas others may require further treatment including manipulation of hormones or surgical removal. Symptomatic treatment serves to make the person more comfortable, but does not allay the progress of the disease.

The nurse has an important role in both the diagnostic and treatment phases, and care given during diagnosis is important in preparing the patient for treatment. Preparation for adrenalectomy is similar to that for other surgery, with the added measure of providing exogenous glucocorticoids. The glucocorticoids are given intramuscularly or intravenously, beginning on the operative day. A maximum dose (300 to 400 mg of hydrocortisone) is given on the day of surgery and the dose is decreased gradually until a maintenance dose is reached. If subtotal adrenalectomy has been performed, the dose is regulated so that the adrenal-pituitary feedback system can be reestablished. This involves giving the glucocorticoid at the time of wakening and not prior to sleep, as is the procedure usually followed if the person is dependent on exogenous glucocorticoids. The nurse must arrange the person's schedule carefully so that the glucocorticoids are given precisely.

Prolonged administration of exogenous ACTH or hypersecretion of ACTH results in atrophy of the adrenal cortex. Return of adrenal cortical function following removal or reduction of the ACTH levels may take several months. The adrenal response to removal of excess ACTH generally is thought to take longer than the pituitary response recovery following removal or reduction of hypercortisol levels. The nurse must prepare the person being treated for the required long-term care, through both teaching and support, for the duration of the recovery, which may be extended.

Maintenance doses of both glucocorticoids and mineralocorticoids are given if the adrenals have been totally removed. The nurse should teach the patient how to adjust the dosage of glucocorticoids according to stress levels, as is required in Addison's disease. The maintenance dose is adjusted according to the person's requirements. A high-sodium diet is required in addition to mineralocorticoids, because of the absence of aldosterone.

The nurse should also teach people who are receiving chemotherapy for treatment of adrenal hyperplasia or tumors that they may develop side effects from the chemotherapy, in addition to being susceptible to development of adrenal insufficiency. The effects of chemotherapy may include lethargy, nausea and vomiting, diarrhea, and anorexia. If these effects occur, the dosage of the chemotherapeutic agent is decreased.

Since there is no cure for Cushing's disease and Cushing's syndrome, the patient requires continued evaluation periodically throughout his lifetime. Essentially, the patient has a chronic disease and must be reevaluated as body requirements change in the process of aging and living. The nurse should be aware of the patient's need for reinforcement of therapy requirements in those with disease of longstanding.

Aldosteronism

Aldosterone, important in fluid and electrolyte balance maintenance, is another important adrenal hormone that can occur in excess. **Aldosteronism** may be either primary or secondary. If primary, it is usually caused by hyperplasia of the zona glomerulosa or by an encapsulated adenoma that is usually single, but may be multiple. Women are affected more than men, and the disease occurs most often in the age range of 30 to 50 years. Secondary aldosteronism can be a complication of any disease that affects fluid and electrolyte metabolism. Secretion of aldosterone is predominantly determined by the renin-angiotensin system; factors that cause increases in the activity of the renin-angiotensin system also cause increases in the secretion of aldosterone. Viewed in this way, hypersecretion of aldosterone is an adaptive response that is important to the body's ability to compensate for such events as dehydration, reduced blood volume, fluid shifts, decreased renal blood flow, or other events that directly or indirectly influence fluid and electrolyte imbalances. Therefore, secondary aldosteronism can be a complication of cardiovascular diseases, renal diseases, liver diseases, or dehydration. The mechanism through which secondary aldosteronism occurs is through increases in the renin-angiotensin component of the feedback loop of renin-angiotensin and aldosterone. Only in rare instances is ACTH known to influence aldosterone secretion to any great degree.

The signs and symptoms of **primary aldosteronism** are typically similar to those of cardiovascular disease with hypertension. Increased levels of aldosterone cause the retention of sodium and the excretion of potassium. As a result, extracellular water is retained, the arterial blood pressure increases, and eventually, as potassium excretion increases, alkalosis secondary to hypokalemia ensues. The person then has increased systolic and diastolic blood pressure and may have frequent severe headaches from the hypertension. Muscle weakness, tetany, or paresthesia results from hypokalemia, and there are ECG changes with the development of arrhythmias. The urine specific gravity is usually low, as the kidneys have decreased concentration capabilities, with prolonged hypokalemia. Symptoms of polyuria with concomitant polydipsia occur along with nocturia. Protein is lost in the urine and the person cannot effectively metabolize carbohydrates because of the hypokalemia. A meal with high carbohydrate value can cause further decreases in the potassium level. In addition to potassium and sodium imbalances, some people with aldosteronism also have a negative magnesium balance.

Evaluation of aldosterone secretion rates is a diagnostic measure to differentiate between primary and secondary aldosteronism. For several days prior to this test, the patient is given a diet that has 100 mEq of sodium, while any medications, such as thiazide diuretics, that affect the aldosterone levels are withheld. In some procedures, potassium is given prior to the test. If the aldosterone excretion rate is above 20 μg per day, primary aldosteronism is suspected. Another test is measurement of renin production. Sodium ingestion is limited several days prior to this test. Since the upright position increases renin activity and bed rest decreases renin activity, the nurse asks the patient to stand or walk or sit in an upright position for several hours immediately preceding the taking of the blood sample. Furosemide (Lasix), a diuretic, is sometimes given prior to drawing blood for aldosterone level evaluation instead of withholding sodium. In this procedure, the person is also asked to remain in an upright position for 3 hours or so prior to the time the blood sample is drawn. In primary aldosteronism, renin levels remain low despite giving the diuretic or limiting sodium intake. In contrast, renin levels are elevated following these measures in most, but not all, instances of secondary aldosteronism.

The spironolactone suppression test is also used for diagnosis. In the spironolactone suppression test, spironolactone (Aldactone), an aldosterone antagonist, is usually given for 3 consecutive days. On the fourth day, the serum potassium should be increased. About 1 week after the administration of spironolactone, plasma electrolytes are again drawn and the potassium levels will again be reduced, which is diagnostic of primary aldosteronism.

Treatment for aldosteronism may involve surgical removal of the adenoma (if one is present) or giving spironolactone along with potassium. A combination of spironolactone therapy and surgery is sometimes preferred. In this method, spironolactone is given for a period of 3 to 5 weeks prior to surgery. This effects an increase in the potassium levels and also tests the response of the adrenal. In primary aldosteronism, the symptoms of hypertension and hypokalemia are reversed by giving spironolactone. When the renin-angiotensin feedback system has been suppressed by high aldosterone levels, spironolactone reverses the suppression so that, postoperatively, function may return to normal following removal of the adenoma. If spironolactone is not given preoperatively, the person may experience postoperative deficiency of aldosterone because of the suppression of the renin-angiotensin feedback system. Spironolactone is an aldosterone antagonist which is given in doses sufficiently high to reduce aldosterone levels to normal.

Depending on the stage to which the aldosteronism has progressed, the therapy may result in reversal of the symptoms. If the disease has progressed sufficiently to bring about changes in the renal and cardiovascular systems, these changes may be irreversible. Nursing care then changes according to the prognosis, as the person may require support and care for his chronic illness.

Some people with essential hypertension also have low renin levels. The association between the mineralocorticoid hormone secretion and the essential hypertension is not thoroughly understood. People with this relationship do have reduced blood pressure in response to spironolactone.

Secondary aldosteronism may be a complication of numerous disease processes that cause an increased secretion of renin. Sclerosis of the renal artery, extracellular fluid depletion, loss of protein with decreased blood volume, malignant hypertension, and vascular changes such as those that occur in cirrhosis of the liver can all affect the blood flow to the kidney. When a person stands or sits in an upright position, blood pools in dependent areas of the body so that the circulating blood volume is reduced. For this reason, renin secretion is increased with the upright position and is decreased when the person lies down, with resulting changes in distribution of blood.

Renin secretion is increased in response to the decreased blood volume. This is an adaptive response which generates the renin-angiotensin feedback system to increase aldosterone secretion. Both sodium and water are retained through the effects of increased aldosterone so that the extracellular fluid volume expands and thereby improves blood flow to vital organs.

Less frequent causes of secondary aldosteronism are Bartter's syndrome and renin-secreting tumors of the kidney. Bartter's syndrome is associated with hyperplasia of the juxtaglomerular cells of the kidneys; this increases renin secretion and subsequently increases aldosterone secretion. The cause and mechanism of Bartter's syndrome is not fully understood but is postulated to be a result of either changes in the refractory abilities of the blood vessels or loss of sodium. Blood pressure is typically low and the person with Bartter's syndrome may have edema if the extracellular volume expands to a great degree.

Diagnosis of secondary aldosteronism is made if the person has high levels of both renin and aldosterone. This is differentiated from primary aldosteronism, in which there is an increase in aldosterone and a decrease in renin levels. Treatment is dependent on the cause of the secondary aldosteronism. If the cause can be identified and treated effectively, the aldosterone secretion levels become more normal, as the adaptation requiring increased aldosterone is no longer necessary. Certain tests such as an intravenous pyelogram or an arteriogram are performed to determine the presence of stenosis of the renal artery, which increases renin levels in response to impaired blood flow. Tests are also conducted to determine both the amount of circulating renin and aldosterone secretion rates. Suppression of renin activity is accomplished by giving deoxycorticosterone acetate (DOCA), usually in doses of 10 mg, every 12 hours for 3 days.

In the renin-suppression test, the person with primary aldosteronism does not have a decreased aldosterone secretion rate, while the opposite is true in persons with secondary aldosteronism, who do have decreased secretion rates. Secretion of aldosterone can be evaluated by the salt-loading test, previously mentioned, or by administration of exogenous mineralocorticoid for 3 or 4 days. The urinary aldosterone levels are measured on the last day of the test from a 24-hour urine collection. With secondary aldosteronism, aldosterone levels are usually decreased.

Treatment for secondary aldosteronism includes treatment of the hyperaldosteronism and of the underlying cause. In chronic or terminal disorders such as cirrhosis, treatment of hyperaldosteronism is part of the palliative measures since the underlying cause cannot be cured. In curable conditions, treatment of hyperaldosteronism is necessary only as long as the symptoms persist. Spironolactone, an aldosterone antagonist, is usually the drug of choice for treating hyperaldosteronism. In persons who have symptoms associated with extracellular fluid volume increases, such as edema or congestive heart failure, reduction of extracellular volume is achieved by decreasing sodium intake and restricting fluids. It is very important that the nurse carefully monitor the person's response to therapy. The goal is to prevent fluid loss to a degree that causes aldosterone levels to increase further because of a decreased blood volume. Diuretics that alter the electrolyte balance are given only when necessary, because they may result in hypokalemia and decreased fluid volume.

Pseudoaldosteronism is a condition in which hypertension, loss of potassium, and decreased renin activity occur because of a familial disorder. In this condition, the abnormal potassium excretion is associated with renal tubular reabsorption of sodium. Hypokalemia may be severe enough to cause alkalosis. Treatment consists in giving medication to interfere with the exchange of sodium and potassium in the distal tubules. Triamterene (Dyrenium) is an example of a medication that achieves this effect.

In addition to the conditions mentioned, there are a number of abnormalities in sexual development that are caused by dysfunction of the adrenal. Excessive androgen secretion causes few changes in the male except for enlargement of the phallus. Females with excessive androgen secretion have an enlarged clitoris and may also have formation of a urogenital sinus into which both the urethra and vagina open. Generally, these abnormalities in sexual development are classified as those caused by enzymatic defects which lead to hyperplasia of the adrenal cortex.

Most often, the enzymatic defects are autosomal recessive. At least six identified types of enzymatic defects cause symptoms in early infancy or childhood. They differ in the point at which the specific enzyme involved affects the synthesis of the hormones. In all these defects, there is increased secretion of ACTH which causes adrenal cortex hyperplasia typical of the enzymatic defects. The symptoms produced in each type are related to the hormone synthesis that is inhibited by the particular enzymatic defect.

When there is interference with synthesis of cortisol in the last phase of its synthesis, cortisol secretion is decreased. The 17-KS levels in urine are increased and the 17-OHCS levels are decreased. DHEA levels increase. Symptoms include those caused by excessive androgen and 11-deoxycorticosterone (DOC). Females demonstrate virilization from the androgens and, in some females, pseudohermaphroditism occurs. Feminine characteristics such as development of mammary glands and menstruation are inhibited. Growth is accelerated and the epiphyses close earlier than normal. Hypertension derived from increased levels of DOC may eventually cause cardiovascular disease.

Glucocorticoids are given to suppress the ACTH secretion. This usually causes reversal of the symptoms. The sex of the child is determined by buccal smear and analysis of karyotype. Treatment is monitored by recording the child's weight and height and determination of bone age. An important component of treatment is counseling in regard to the genetic implications of the disorder, and support of the family while they are undergoing the counseling is one of the nurse's major functions.

Another condition, interference with the last step of aldosterone synthesis, is called 18-hydroxysteroid deficiency. The symptoms are those of hypoaldosteronism with loss of sodium and excessive potassium leading to water loss and hypotension. Renin levels are increased. Treatment is the same as given for Addison's disease: high-sodium diets or sodium supplements and administration of mineralocorticoids.

The most frequently occurring enzymatic deficiency is lack of 21-hydroxylase, which affects synthesis of both glucocorticoids and mineralocorticoids. The symptoms can be of varying degrees from mild to severe. They include virilization from excessive amounts of androgens and hypoaldosteronism. 17-KS levels are elevated. While the disorder can more readily be detected in females, the symptoms in males may not become obvious until childhood. In mild cases, the symptoms sometimes do not appear until growth is clearly abnormal. Females develop masculine characteristics: voice changes, and growth of pubic and axillary hair. They do not develop feminine characteristics. Males develop secondary sexual characteristics at an earlier age than normal. Treatment consists in giving glucocorticoids, and if they are given early enough the symptoms can be reversed.

Other enzymatic deficiencies include lack of 20-hydroxylase, of 3β-hydroxysteroid dehydrogenase, and of 17α-hydroxylase. In the first, a rare occurrence, male infants develop female genitalia. The infants affected usually have a very short life. In the second, there are deficiencies of both cortisol and aldosterone, and the child has ambiguous external genitalia. The last causes deficiency of cortisol with associated increases in ACTH. This in turn causes increased secretion of DOC and corticosterone. Children affected have low cortisol levels and do not develop secondary sex characteristics at the normal age. Treatment includes administration of glucocorticoids and estrogens.

The **adrenal medulla** is a target of much research. Following complete removal of the adrenals, there are no symptoms related to insufficiency as the amount of catecholamines produced by the adrenal medulla are minimal. There is no known dysfunction associated with insufficiency of the adrenal medulla. Tumors of the adrenal medulla, however, can cause symptoms. The three major tumors are pheochromocytoma, ganglioneuroma, and neuroblastoma.

Pheochromocytomas arise from chromaffin cells and are often associated with other disease processes. Predominant among these are autosomal dominant familial disorders including Lindau's disease, medullary carcinoma of the thyroid, Sturge-Weber disease, and Von Recklinghausen's neurofibromatosis. There is also a higher incidence of pheochromocytomas among diabetics. People with pheochromocytomas have a high incidence of gallbladder disease.

Pheochromocytomas occur in both males and females and most commonly occur in the age range of 40 to 60 years. The majority are unilateral, while they can occur bilaterally or in body tissues other than the adrenal. Extra-adrenal sites include the neck, chest, abdomen, and kidneys. They are usually encapsulated and also arise from chromaffin cells. While the greatest number are benign, a small percentage are malignant. The symptoms are caused by increased production of catecholamines which are thought to be related to impaired control of synthesis and release of norepinephrine and epinephrine.

The effects of increased catecholamine secretion are seen in increased peripheral vascular resistance. People with pheochromocytomas generally have hypertension either of the paroxysmal or consistent type. In addition, they have increased sweating, so that their hair is matted and damp. Periodic blanching or flushing of the skin may be noted. Often they describe periods of tachycardia and palpitations, tremulousness, and postural hypotension. The reason for the postural hypotension is not fully understood, but it may be caused by decreased blood volume or from ganglionic blocking activity from excessive quantities of catecholamines [10]. Headache, pallor, and weight loss may occur. Some people have predominant symptoms of nervousness and even develop psychoses.

While the most consistent sign of pheochromocytoma is hypertension, this can be variable. The hypertension may be mild or severe, constant or paroxysmal. It is usually labile. Some people also have a reflex bradycardia. When paroxysmal blood pressure elevations occur, both the systolic and diastolic levels are elevated. Usually the person has a pounding headache during the attack which can last for varying periods of time. Following the attack, the person experiences fatigue. In reconstructing the events that led up to the attack, the person may describe some form of stressful event or merely a change in posture.

People with constant labile hypertension may develop signs and symptoms of cardiovascular disease such as myocardial infarcts and heart failure. They often develop left cardiac enlargement and associated signs and symptoms. Complications of hypertension also include a susceptibility to cerebral vascular accidents and renal insufficiency.

Some people have signs and symptoms of increased metabolism. Among these are high blood glucose levels related to increased glyconeogenesis in the liver. There is a decreased ability to metabolize carbohydrates and a high level of free fatty acids. These metabolic changes augment the cardiovascular changes. The person with metabolic symptoms loses weight and has abnormally high fasting glucose levels.

The mechanism for the central nervous system symptoms is not well understood. It is theorized that when catecholamine levels are consistently increased, some catecholamines may pass the blood-brain barrier. Normally the blood-brain barrier is resistant to catecholamines. Among the nervous system symptoms are hyperventilation, tremulousness, and development of psychoses. In some people, the central nervous system symptoms predominate and diagnosis is sometimes missed because they are considered to have emotional problems.

Diagnosis comprises determination of the presence of the tumor. X-rays of the neck, chest, and abdomen, and an intravenous pyelogram and a tomogram are taken to locate tumors. Urinary excretion of free catecholamines and of their metabolites is measured. The catecholamine metabolites are vanillylmandelic acid (VMA), normetanephrine, and metanephrine. For measuring these, 24-hour urine specimens are usually obtained. For accuracy in measurements of VMA, it is important that foods containing phenolic acid are withheld as well as drugs that contain catecholamines. The foods containing phenolic acid, a stimulant, include coffee, vanilla and vanilla extracts or flavoring, chocolate, bananas, citrus fruits, and certain vegetables. Normally, VMA excretion levels are higher when one is active than during sleep. For this reason, the urine sample may be collected in two consecutive 12-hour periods. In pheochromocytoma both samples usually contain high levels of VMA, instead of the normal result which would be a higher level during active hours. The upright posture increases catecholamine excretion and it normally decreases during sleep when one is reclining.

The diagnostic value of the 24-hour urine test for VMA, normetanephrine, and metanephrine is great. The ratio of metabolites to VMA to normetanephrine and metanephrine is also of diagnostic value in determining the probable size of the tumor. When low VMA levels are found in relation to normetanephrine and metanephrine, the tumor is usually small. The converse is true if high levels of VMA in relation to normetanephrine and metanephrine are found.

Catecholamine levels in venous circulation can also be measured by obtaining blood samples during cardiac catheterization.

The Histamine Test may be performed to determine if an attack of hypertension can be stimulated by histamine because of the higher than normal levels of catecholamines. When the test is done, the nurse should have an alpha-blocking agent available in the event that the person responds to the histamine with extremely high blood pressure. A 2-hour urine sample is collected following administration of the histamine.

Formerly, the Regitine test was frequently performed to diagnose pheochromocytoma. Regitine is an alpha-blocking agent that causes a decrease in blood pressure in people with pheochromocytoma. The test is not currently used very often because it may induce prolonged hypotension and also is not considered reliable. The measurement of urinary excretion of the metabolites of catecholamines is more accurate in the diagnosis of pheochromocytomas [10].

If a tumor is found, the treatment is surgical removal. The exception to this is a far advanced malignant tumor. In this case, symptomatic treatment is initiated. Preparation for surgery includes administering alpha-adrenergic blocking agents to stabilize the blood pressure and the vascular reactivity. This is important to prevent complications during and following surgery. The blood volume is measured to gauge fluid replacement prior to and during surgery. It is necessary to take every precaution to prevent cardiovascular complications, and the nurse should carefully monitor the patient's signs and symptoms resulting from these preoperative measures. Nursing assessment is important for determination of the patient's status prior to surgery. Usually alpha-blocking agents are given for the week prior to surgery. Some authorities use beta-adrenergic blocking agents, and the selection of specific drugs and the route of administration varies. The nurse should protect the person from events that may stimulate hypertension. For example, enemas are contraindicated because they can precipitate a hypertensive crisis.

Following surgery, the patient is carefully monitored for the occurrence of hypotension or hypertension in addition to the normal postoperative care and monitoring for postanesthetic complications. During the recovery from anesthesia particularly, the blood pressure may fluctuate excessively, requiring the nurse's accurate assessment and intervention. There may be refractory hypotension following surgery which may be treated with norepinephrine or cortisol.

If surgery is contraindicated, as during the third trimester of pregnancy or in far advanced tumors, medications that inhibit the synthesis of catecholamines are given. These patients require careful instruction in recognizing signs and symptoms of the side effects of the medications being used and in determining the effectiveness of the medications. Routine visits to the physician or to the clinic are necessary to monitor the treatment.

The other two types of tumors occurring in the adrenal medulla mentioned previously are neuroblastomas and ganglioneuromas. Neuroblastomas are tumors that arise from neural crests and may occur in neural tissue in the brain or spinal cord. There is a familial tendency toward their development and they are highly metastatic through extension to surrounding tissues or through lymph channels. Neuroblastomas tend to occur in children, whereas ganglioneuromas occur in children or adults. Treatment includes surgical removal followed by radiation or chemotherapy or both.

In summary, the adrenal glands are important to body homeostasis. They have a broad range of influence on body processes including metabolism, electrolyte balance, and support of nervous system function. Because of the ability of steroids to support body functions, exogenous steroids are frequently given in the treatment of a wide variety of disease processes. Glucocorticoids are important in supporting body homeostasis during periods of stress as well as for their anti-inflammatory and immunosuppressive effects. The nurse must be aware of the implications of steroid therapy when explaining the dosage and possible side effects that may occur.

Essentially, steroids, whether given exogenously or secreted endogenously, have similar effects. When exogenous steroids are given to a person who has an adequate secretion of endogenous steroids, the additional steroids will increase steroid levels so that the effects of hypersecretion occur. These effects are relative to the dosage of exogenous steroids, the potency of the steroid being administered, its rate of absorption, and the person's health status.

Continuous steroid therapy suppresses ACTH secretion and causes the gland that normally produces the steroid being given to be depressed as well. Excessive amounts of glucocorticoids cause the same metabolic effects whether from an endogenous or exogenous source. Therefore, people who are receiving large quantities of exogenous steroids are subject to increased gluconeogenesis with protein-wasting and centripetal obesity. They can develop the characteristic moon face and buffalo hump of Cushing's syndrome. In addition, the increased glucose levels resulting from steroid therapy may be sufficient to bring about overt diabetes in latent diabetics.

When given for anti-inflammatory effects, the steroids can mask or suppress the signs and symptoms of infection or inflammation. Dosages are usually given to achieve a balance between the desired anti-inflammatory response and the normal adaptive response of the body to combat the infection. Steroids do not "cure" infections and if they are withdrawn the infectious process can become acutely overt after having been masked by steroids. To prevent this, steroids are gradually discontinued.

Steroids are often given for treatment of localized inflammatory processes such as bursitis. Usually they are given locally, being injected directly into the area of inflammation or applied directly to the skin, in the event of a skin dysfunction. Given this way, the steroids have a higher potency in the area injected or to which the steroid has been applied and do not cause the systemic increases in steroid levels that they would if administered systemically. Many times a single dose, applied locally or injected locally, is sufficient to relieve the inflammation and promote healing.

When given for systemic diseases such as rheumatoid arthritis, lupus erythematosus, or sarcoidosis, to name a few, the steroids are given systemically. To prevent the complications of excess hormone levels or to reduce these effects, a procedure of giving the steroids intermittently is often followed. Different procedures are used; for example, the steroid might be given every other day or on several consecutive days and then discontinued for several consecutive days. These intermittent patterns of administration decrease the suppression of ACTH that would occur if steroids were given continuously. When steroids are discontinued, the dosage is reduced gradually to reestablish the ACTH-adrenal feedback system so that the person may be given minimal doses for a period of months.

Some people who have chronic diseases that cause continuous pain and discomfort experience such great relief from symptoms following institution of steroid therapy that they become euphoric. This "steroid high" is now well recognized and has led to more discriminate use of steroids in chronic conditions because the symptoms do return after the steroids are discontinued. This return of symptoms may result in depression and in some people, a reduced ability to tolerate the discomfort or pain. Other methods that provide some measure of relief are more desirable for continuous therapy, particularly if the side effects of steroid therapy will be further debilitating in the long run.

Essentially, the concept of balance is applied to giving steroids in either acute or chronic diseases. Steroids are not given unless they can achieve a state that is more desirable than the person's condition will be if steroids are not given. The minimal dose necessary to achieve the desired effect without masking or covering other symptoms is given.

Steroids have untoward effects in people with certain types of dysfunction. Their effect in creating overt diabetes has already been mentioned. They are contraindicated in those with peptic ulcers as they can result in hemorrhage and perforation. Women in the postmenopausal age are susceptible to developing osteoporosis when taking steroids. People who are nutritionally debilitated may not be able to withstand the protein-wasting that occurs with steroid therapy.

Steroids are frequently used in treatment during acute episodes of shock, respiratory insufficiency, status asthmaticus, and similar conditions. When given for short periods of time, the disturbing side effects do not occur and the steroids augment recovery. In many instances, administration of steroids keeps the person alive so that treatment of the underlying disease can be maintained. Used in this way, the steroids are life-saving and supportive of other treatment modalities. Even when given for short periods of time for acute conditions, the steroids are withdrawn gradually by decreasing the dosage in daily increments. The length of time during which the steroids are withdrawn usually depends on the amount of dosage that has been given and the length of time the patient has been taking steroids.

The nurse has an active role in monitoring the effects of steroid therapy and in teaching people the correct methods for planning their daily regimens when they are taking the steroids at home. The nurse also must teach the importance of taking the correctly prescribed dosage; the patient is taught to respect the potency of the medication. It should be impressed on the patient that either too much or too little medication will interfere with the desired therapeutic effects, and that dosages other than those prescribed may be harmful.

When caring for persons with dysfunction of the adrenal glands, the nurse should be aware of the impact that changes in physiologic and psychological behavior have on the patient's life. An important aspect of nursing care is helping the patient and family resolve their conflicts about these changes, involving them in the treatment regimen, and following up to ensure that the patient continues treatment in the long run. In addition, nurses in various health care agencies should be aware of the early signs and symptoms of adrenal diseases. It is not uncommon for a person with adrenal dysfunction to be mistakenly considered emotionally unstable, and to be referred for treatment by a psychiatrist. In many instances, however, treatment for emotional instability is necessary for the person with adrenal dysfunction. When the dysfunction is mild, or when the symptoms are not clearly those of the typical adrenal dysfunction, diagnosis may be missed.

It is accepted that behavioral changes are a part of the dysfunction in both Addison's and Cushing's diseases. In experience, it is found that these changes are highly individual and do not follow a definite pattern. Some people have marked changes whereas others have few changes. This phenomenon further emphasizes the importance of developing individualized approaches to care.

The Pancreas

FUNCTION OF THE PANCREAS

The endocrine function of the pancreas focuses on the effects of two major hormones, insulin and glucagon. In contrast to the other endocrine glands, the pancreas has both endocrine and exocrine functions. The former are related to the islet cells of the pancreas, which are distributed throughout the gland, being most predominant in the tail. There are approximately 2 million islet cells, and they comprise different cell types: the alpha cells produce glucagon, the beta cells are the source of insulin, the delta cells are thought to contain gastrin, and the products of the F or fourth cells are yet to be identified. Beta cells occur with the greatest frequency; about 75 percent of the islet cells are beta cells, while about 20 percent are alpha cells and these are larger than the beta cells. Islet cells have a rich supply of blood and nerves. The nerve fibers are unmyelinated, with both sympathetic and parasympathetic nerve endings closely approximated to the plasma membrane.

DYSFUNCTION OF THE PANCREAS

Diabetes mellitus is the disorder most predominant in pancreatic hormonal dysfunction. The relationship between insulin and glucagon in the occurrence of diabetes mellitus is not clearly delineated. Current theories suggest that both pancreatic hormones may have a role in the pathophysiology of diabetes mellitus. Both hormones are associated with states of hypoglycemia and hyperglycemia. **Hypoglycemia,** the other common disorder in dysfunction of the pancreas related to hormone imbalances, is usually associated with increased levels of glucagon. Hyperglycemia associated with diabetes mellitus is caused by insulin imbalances. As more is discovered about the physiology of glucagon, it is postulated that the activity of this hormone may be found to have a more major role in the occurrence and treatment of diabetes mellitus [1].

Even though the syndrome of diabetes mellitus has been known for years, the pathophysiology remains obscure. Since the basic cause is unknown, there is much controversy about treatment; no cure is available and the syndrome is treated symptomatically by manipulating the metabolic factors of insulin, food intake, exercise, and other aspects of the syndrome.

The nurse must be familiar with the various theories of treatment and their application to individualized treatment and care regimens for people with diabetes mellitus. As with most disease syndromes, there is great variability in the signs and symptoms of diabetes mellitus among individuals. The point should be made early in the discussion that advancing research in the areas of islet cell function, in metabolism, and in the physiology of insulin and glucagon may eventually change current concepts in the treatment of diabetes mellitus as data about the course of the disease are collected and the treatment responses of people with diabetes mellitus are evaluated. Even these data may be controversial, however, because the treatment plans vary and the responses to treatment are highly dependent on uncontrollable variables within the individuals who have the disease syndrome. The nurse should be aware of the nature of the differences in treatment of diabetes mellitus. These differences reflect not only the varying theories of treatment, but also the different requirements of individuals with diabetes mellitus.

The nurse may encounter people in varying phases of diabetes mellitus—at the time of the initial discovery of a propensity for diabetes mellitus or of the initial overt presentation of symptoms; in follow-up care for known diabetics who are healthy as a result of positive responses to management; in caring for those who have uncontrolled diabetes mellitus and require hospitalization; and finally, in attending those who have developed serious complications or manifestations of the disease.

The primary problem resulting from diabetes mellitus is abnormal metabolism. There is some degree of carbohydrate intolerance associated with adaptive acceleration in catabolism of fats and proteins. Along with the metabolic abnormalities, people with diabetes mellitus may also have vascular disease that affects the small or large vessels or both. Diabetic neuropathies may also be present. The relationships among the metabolic abnormalities and the vascular and nerve dysfunction are not clearly understood. Some theorists believe that the vascular and nerve dysfunction are effects of or complications of the metabolic dysfunction, while others feel that these processes occur simultaneously as part of the syndrome of diabetes mellitus. A cause and effect relationship is not always substantiated, because an individual may first have symptoms related to vascular changes before demonstrating the metabolic alterations. It is more usual, however, for the metabolic alterations to become evident first.

Diabetes Mellitus

There are several theories concerning the causation of diabetes mellitus. It may be caused by viruses or it may be familial; however, the exact mode of genetic transmission of diabetes mellitus remains elusive. Theories presently considered include the following: Diabetes mellitus is transmitted as a recessive trait; or it is transmitted by multifactors; or it is an evolutionary gene stemming from man's biologic needs in prehistoric times [7]. Since the genetic transmission of diabetes mellitus remains unclear, a system of risk factors has been developed to identify the population susceptible to the syndrome. The risk factors include obesity, taking drugs that cause decreased tolerance for carbohydrates, stress, increasing age, and a family history of diabetes. The nurse should be alert for signs and symptoms of diabetes mellitus in people who are assessed to be within this population of risk.

In addition to the above risk factors, persons who have had pancreatectomies in which 80 percent or more of the pancreas has been removed will probably develop diabetes mellitus. Total removal of the pancreas results in diabetes mellitus.

The current knowledge of diabetes is undergoing continuous review as metabolic processes and the precise role of insulin and glucagon as well as other metabolic factors are further elucidated. It is known that diabetics do not have sufficient effective insulin. Why they do not have normal effective insulin function is not understood. There may be different types of dysfunction; for example, it is thought that some people do not secrete enough insulin, while others may secrete sufficient insulin, but its potency is low so it is ineffective. Yet others may have dysfunction in metabolism that is caused by factors that increase the body's resistance to insulin, or that create an antagonism to insulin so that the insulin secreted is ineffective. Insulin is required for transfer of glucose across cell membranes in muscle and adipose tissue.

Both assessment and nursing care are based on theories of insulin secretion and its effects, which are discussed in the following pages. Insulin is first secreted as proinsulin. Conversion of proinsulin to insulin through proteolytic cleavage is thought to take place in the granules located in the beta cells. The insulin is then stored in the granules along with C-peptide. When the beta cells are stimulated, granules are ejected and release insulin in a process called emiocytosis. The process of emiocytosis is dependent on the presence of calcium. Calcium uptake by the beta cells is directly related to the rate at which the granules are released from the islet beta cells. This dependency on calcium indicates that insulin release is supported by the action potentials of ionic exchanges. The uptake of calcium by the beta cells is thought to be depressed by the presence of sodium in extracellular spaces.

Insulin remains stored in the granules of the beta cells until there is a stimulus for insulin release. The number of beta cell granules present in the pancreas at any one time is an indication of the amount of stored insulin present. Glucose and glucagon both stimulate insulin release. When released, the insulin circulates in the plasma. Immunoassay techniques are used to measure the levels of insulin in plasma. It is thought that insulin secretion takes place in two phases. The first is an immediate response to the stimulus, which may be glucose or other stimulating substances. The immediate response takes place, and a peak of insulin secretion is attained in a few minutes. This is followed by a slower increase, related primarily to the glucose metabolism. The first phase of peak and drop in secretion rates is considered a function of the "islet set," which varies among individuals. The islet set functions in basal states as insulin secretion occurs in a pattern independent of stimulation in accordance with biologic rhythms. The release of insulin is stimulated by many factors. Glucose, the most important carbohydrate stimulator, has been mentioned. Glucagon stimulates insulin release by directly acting on the beta cells. Amino acids stimulate insulin secretion, and many of the hormones secreted in the gastrointestinal tract, including gastrin and secretin, augment insulin secretion. Glucosteroids, estrogen, progesterone, and growth hormone affect insulin secretion by causing increased resistance to insulin at the peripheral level. The increased resistance in turn causes an increase in insulin secretion to compensate for the resistance. There is much speculation about the neural control of insulin secretion. The basal secretion of insulin in a rhythmic pattern suggests that there is neural control, perhaps by the hypothalamus. Alpha blocking substances can effect an increase in insulin secretion. It is known that stress of varying forms increases insulin requirements in diabetics. Because stress is related to the activity of the adrenergic nervous system, alpha blocking agents are sometimes given to improve the insulin response. Some forms of well-identified stress include surgical procedures requiring anesthesia, myocardial infarction, and burns.

Insulin is largely degraded by the liver and kidney and can also be degraded by all body cells. In fact, all body cells are affected by insulin in some way. Cell structure, cell function, and energy production are dependent on the anabolic functions of insulin. At any given time, the effect of insulin is a composite of many factors: the amount of insulin secreted by the beta cells, the distribution of insulin to body cells through circulation, the types of tissue (for example, liver, kidney, and muscle tissue), and the concentration of nutrients, ions, and hormones present in the cells and surrounding the cells. It is not known whether insulin is bound by specific transport proteins in the blood [4]. Insulin is delivered to the body cells via the circulation. When the amount of effective insulin is insufficient to metabolize carbohydrates, lypolysis increases, because the cells then use fats for energy. Protein catabolism also increases without sufficient insulin. Therefore, insufficient effective insulin produces catabolic effects on metabolism. Insulin increases the threshold at which cells take up glucose. Once the glucose crosses the cell membrane, it is retained by phosphorylation. The glucose may then undergo several types of changes. These can be thought of as various roads that may be taken from one control point. Among these pathways are the Embden-Meyerhof pathway, also called glycolysis, the phosphogluconate-oxidative pathway, the glucuronic acid pathway, and glycogenesis.

Glucagon, the other pancreatic hormone, is secreted by the alpha cells. Its secretion is thought to follow a pattern similar to that of insulin so that glucagon is stored in the alpha cells for release. There is considerable interest in glucagon in current studies concerning metabolism. Generally, glucagon and insulin seem to function in reciprocal relationships so that both insulin and glucagon affect metabolism by regulating one another. Insulin secretion is stimulated by glucose and glucagon secretion is inhibited by glucose. Low glucose levels stimulate glucagon secretion and inhibit insulin secretion. The relationship between insulin and glucose in stimulating or inhibiting glucagon secretion is not defined. It is possible that glucagon responses are directly related to glucose levels, independent of insulin secretion. Certain amino acids stimulate glucagon secretion and it is postulated that fatty acids may also be related to glucagon secretion in their metabolic pathways. Sympathetic nervous stimulation increases glucagon secretion. Glucagon may then have metabolic functions independent of insulin, or it may be closely involved in regulation of insulin in the broad spectrum of metabolic activity.

Insulin is an anabolic hormone in terms of metabolism. After its release to circulation, insulin is distributed to body cells; the liver, the kidney, the skeletal muscle, and plasma have the greatest concentration. From the pancreas, insulin travels to the liver, where 40 to 50 percent is removed. The remaining insulin is distributed to body cells with the exception of the brain and erythrocytes, which have relatively little or no insulin. The kidney takes up as much as 40 percent of the insulin from that circulated to the kidney. The cortex and proximal convoluted tubules take up the insulin from the circulation.

When there is insufficient effective insulin for anabolism, alternative metabolic pathways are used for energy production. About 50 percent of the average diet of people in the United States comprises carbohydrates, and glucose is the major source of energy in people with normal metabolism. Nerve tissues and the brain are dependent on glucose, whereas most other cells can use other nutrients for energy production. (As previously mentioned, insulin is required for transfer of glucose across cell membranes in muscle tissue and adipose tissue.) When glucose is not able to enter cells because of lack of effective insulin, glycogen and fatty acids are utilized for energy. Certain adaptive processes occur when the glucose in the cells is insufficient. One of the most important processes is the stimulation of secretion of other hormones that aid the mobilization of fatty acids and the process of gluconeogenesis. These hormones include the growth hormone, cortisol, ACTH, glucagon, and epinephrine. The level of glucose in the blood rises because the glucose cannot gain entry to the cells without insulin. This in turn causes hyperosmolarity. As a result of fatty acid metabolism, ketone bodies are produced. As fatty acids are increasingly used for energy in the absence of usable glucose in the cells, increasing numbers of ketone bodies are produced so that acidosis occurs. Because of the hyperosmolarity and the acidosis, dehydration occurs along with fluid and electrolyte imbalances within the body. The extent of these changes and the duration of the metabolic adaptation are related to the severity of diabetes mellitus. For example, a person with minimal available effective insulin will demonstrate more severe metabolic symptoms than a person who has some but not enough insulin for metabolism.

Stages of diabetes have been classified as prediabetes (or potential diabetes), suspected diabetes, chemical diabetes, and overt diabetes. The first classification, **prediabetes** (or potential diabetes) is defined as the time period from conception to the evidence of glucose metabolism alteration. **Suspected** diabetes is also called subclinical or latent diabetes, which becomes overt only during times of unusual stress, such as during acute illness, in normal pregnancy, or when the person takes drugs that decrease carbohydrate tolerance. Psychological stress may also precipitate overt diabetes in those who are classified as suspected diabetic individuals. **Chemical** diabetes is defined in the same way as suspected diabetes but differs from suspected diabetes in that the standard glucose tolerance test is abnormal with borderline or low abnormal values. Clinical or **overt** diabetes is defined as demonstration of elevated fasting blood glucose as well as presence of the signs and symptoms of metabolic alterations, vascular changes, or neural changes. These classifications have been developed by the American Diabetes Association in an attempt to standardize the language used to describe diabetes mellitus.

Another commonly used classification is one developed according to the time in the person's life span in which diabetes mellitus first becomes overt. This classification uses **youth-onset** diabetes (or juvenile diabetes) and **adult-onset** diabetes (or maturity diabetes). Generally, juvenile diabetes occurs prior to the age of forty years; adult diabetes occurs after the age of forty. This differentiation has implications for the type of diabetes the person usually develops. For example, juvenile diabetic patients are more often "brittle diabetics," which means that the metabolic alterations are more difficult to control by diet, insulin, and exercise. People with youth-onset diabetes tend to be more prone to the development of ketoacidosis, a metabolic complication of diabetes mellitus. In general, the juvenile diabetic patient has no effective insulin, necessitating the provision of exogenous insulin by subcutaneous injection. These people are called insulin-dependent diabetics, and their carbohydrate intolerance is more severe and difficult to control.

In contrast, the person with adult-onset diabetes tends to have a milder form of the disease with less severe carbohydrate intolerance. This form of diabetes occurs when the amount of effective insulin present in the body is insufficient for metabolism of carbohydrates either because of decreased potency of the insulin produced or because of increased resistance to insulin. People with adult-onset diabetes are not usually insulin-dependent and do not tend to be prone to the development of ketoacidosis. Adult-onset diabetes is usually associated with a milder form of carbohydrate intolerance than is juvenile diabetes; however, adult-onset diabetes is often discovered because of the vascular or nervous system symptoms the person has developed, which can be life-threatening.

Diagnostic testing and screening programs Large-scale screening programs are often conducted for detection of diabetes mellitus. These screening programs frequently use **urine tests** for glycosuria and sometimes urine tests for ketone bodies. The nurse should recognize that use of urine tests cannot be definitive for detection of diabetes. Instead, these tests may identify those people who should be given further and more discriminative tests to determine the presence of diabetes. There are three major reasons for this. First, glycosuria may be transient, reflecting the person's metabolism of glucose for the specific time of the test, which is dependent on food intake, metabolic processes, and glomerular filtration. Second, urine tests are not specific enough for diagnosis. They are dependent on many variables, including the type of substances used for testing as well as other metabolites that may be present in the urine. Third, significant hyperglycemia must be present for glycosuria to occur. The plasma glucose must exceed 180 mg per 100 ml for loss of glucose in the urine to occur if the person has normal kidney function. Levels of glycosuria are variable at different times and the presence or absence of glycosuria is not definitive in diagnosis of diabetes mellitus. An example is that people receiving total parenteral nutrition excrete large quantities of glucose in urine so that glycosuria in these people is not evidence of diabetes.

Several types of testing materials are available to determine the presence of glucose: Clinistix, Clinitest tablets, Tes-Tape, and Diastix. Clinistix is the least specific of these, as it indicates the presence or absence of glucose in the urine without measurement of the amount. Clinitest tablets, which are poisonous, contain a copper-reduction indicator which is responsive to many substances. A consequence of this is that Clinitest tablets may give false positive results. They do measure the amount of glucose by comparison of color changes with the charts provided in the Clinitest tablet package. When using Clinitest tablets to test urine glucose levels, the nurse should watch the reaction both during the reaction phase and the waiting phase of fifteen seconds that follows the active reaction. This observation is necessary because of the pass-through phenomenon of rapid color changes that may occur during the reaction. The orange color, indicating 4+, may appear briefly at any time during the active reaction phase. In this event, the test results should be interpreted as 4+, rather than according to the color present after completion of the waiting phase. Tes-Tape and Diastix also measure the amount of glucose by changing colors, which can then be compared with color charts supplied in the package. They contain an enzyme specific for glucose oxidation which makes them more reliable indicators. A disadvantage of Tes-Tape is that it is very sensitive and may give meaningless positive results. Diastix is affected by ketones which delay the color changes. Color changes correspond with readings such as 1+, 2+, 3+, and 4+ for each color change. Percentages are also used from 1 to 4 percent, describing the amount of urine glucose present. Ketostix tests for the presence of ketones in urine and is used in both diagnosis and monitoring therapy.

When testing urine with any of these products, it is important for the nurse to follow the directions provided in the package for accurate timing and for comparison of color changes to evaluate the results. Since the first voiding contains urine accumulated in the bladder overnight, the second voiding after awakening is used to obtain a sample that represents the person's current status. Sometimes it is necessary for the patient to drink some water to obtain a second urine specimen. Obtaining a screening test may be difficult for those who have trouble producing a second voiding. Usually this is not a problem for the person with diabetes mellitus, who is polyuric.

It is also necessary to make certain that the testing substances have not deteriorated. Clinistix, Clinitest tablets, Tes-Tape, and Diastix are all subject to deterioration when exposed to moisture and air. Clinitest tablets become mottled and dark blue when they deteriorate. A convenient method for ensuring the potency of Clinistix, Tes-Tape, and Diastix is to place them in a solution with high glucose concentration, which normally causes a maximum, or 4+, reaction. The appearance of Tes-Tape and Diastix may not indicate deterioration, so it is necessary to determine their potency by some method such as this.

For those found to have glycosuria through urine screening tests, more specific measures such as fasting plasma glucose are used. A **fasting blood glucose** test is often done routinely as part of a physical examination to detect hyperglycemia. Normal values of fasting plasma glucose are 60 to 100 mg per 100 ml. Values above 120 mg per 100 ml are usually considered significant for diabetes mellitus. The term **fasting blood sugar** is frequently used instead of fasting blood glucose. This usage is misleading, however, as other sugars such as fructose and galactose, as well as glucose, are blood sugars. Since plasma glucose levels are variable in any one individual from time to time, one plasma glucose level is not sufficient to diagnose the presence or absence of diabetes mellitus. Oral or intravenous **glucose tolerance tests** are even more significant than urine tests or fasting blood glucose in the diagnosis of diabetes mellitus. Test results are most accurate when certain conditions are observed prior to and during the test. These include control of factors which influence glucose metabolism, such as intake of glucose, stimulants, exercise, or taking drugs that influence carbohydrate intolerance. In many instances, preparation for a glucose tolerance test begins 3 days prior to the test. Any drugs the person may be taking that influence carbohydrate tolerance, such as birth control pills and glucocorticoids, are discontinued and the person observes a regular diet during the 3-day preparatory period. In order to control the intake of carbohydrate, the person then fasts for 12 hours or so prior to the test. Stimulation is also avoided prior to the test. The nurse must advise the person not to smoke or drink coffee or tea. Exercise is also minimized. Both stimulants and exercise affect the uptake of glucose by the body tissues and therefore influence the test. The presence of stress, either from an illness such as an infection or psychological stress, including anxiety about the test, may also influence the results. When the person exhibits stress, the test is often postponed until optimum test conditions can be achieved. The nurse should make certain that the person is as relaxed as possible for the glucose tolerance test. Relaxation is often difficult, however, because the person is deprived of so many activities (such as smoking or chewing gum) that he may normally engage in during periods of stress. The restrictions listed above should be explained so that the person understands why they are important for test results.

The actual glucose tolerance test begins by obtaining fasting samples of venous blood and urine. Again, to obtain meaningful results, a second specimen is used rather than the stored urine from the first voiding. Glucose is then given; the amount varies in different testing regimens. Some use a standard 100-gm of glucose while others calculate the glucose load according to ideal body weight. The usual formula is 1.75 gm per kilogram of ideal body weight. In some places, Glucola is given. Glucola is made of corn syrup, carbonated water, and flavoring such as cherry or cola. Although Glucola is more palatable than glucose, false negative results may be obtained with its use. For this reason, many authorities prefer the use of the standard glucose. Another way to give glucose is in a meal which has been calculated to provide 100 gm of carbohydrate. This method is also not as desirable as giving a standard glucose load because of the variability in the rate of absorption of ingested carbohydrate in different foods. The glucose tolerance tests are dependent on evaluating the metabolism of glucose. Therefore, the tests are not valid if the person vomits after ingesting the glucose load, or if the prescribed amount is not taken, however it is given. If the person vomits, the test is discontinued and repeated at another time.

Both blood and urine specimens are collected at intervals, usually every hour or every half-hour, following administration of the glucose. The collection times vary with differing test regimens. It is important that the specific test regimen used be followed precisely to obtain meaningful test results. Specimens may be obtained up to 3 hours or may include a 4- or 5-hour collection. Each glucose tolerance test is designated by the span of time during which specimens are collected; a 3-hour glucose tolerance test, a 4-hour glucose tolerance test, or a 5-hour glucose tolerance test.

Interpretation of the standard glucose tolerance test depends on evaluation of the plasma and urine levels of glucose obtained as a total response pattern. There is a normal peak of plasma glucose 1 hour following ingestion of glucose with declining values to normal fasting levels thereafter. The person with diabetes mellitus demonstrates higher than normal blood glucose levels with each specimen, although the curve of the values often follows the normal pattern of peaking at 1 hour and declining thereafter.

Diabetes mellitus is confirmed if the blood glucose levels for the collected blood specimens significantly exceed the normal values along the curve formed by values for each time a specimen is obtained. A number of variations may occur in the glucose tolerance curve. In some instances, the blood glucose level does not peak at 1 hour as expected—in other instances the return to normal levels is delayed beyond 2 hours. Interpretation depends on evaluation of the total curve. One criterion for determining the presence of diabetes mellitus is elevation of three out of four values obtained from each of the sample collections. The amount of elevation above the normal or baseline curve is significant, and different levels are considered diagnostic by different authorities. In general, a 1-hour elevation above 160 mg per 100 ml indicates glucose intolerance.

There are many reasons for the differences in evaluation of the glucose tolerance curve. Individuals have differing baseline tolerances for glucose, so that a normal value for one person may be abnormal in another. This variation may be a result of genetic variations in normal levels. A number of factors influence the normal or expected curve. Pregnancy, with elevated hormonal levels, causes some amount of glucose intolerance. Aging is associated with gradual normal increases in glucose intolerance so that a 1-hour level of 180 mg per 100 ml may be "normal" in an elderly person. Both obesity and malnutrition are associated with glucose intolerance and higher than normal levels in the glucose tolerance curve.

A number of endocrine diseases, carcinoma, and stress also cause glucose intolerance. Another factor which contributes to the difficulty in interpreting glucose tolerance curves is that any one person only rarely demonstrates consistent levels of blood glucose with repeated glucose tolerance tests. A study conducted by West [8] reported that American specialists varied by 20 mg per 100 ml between the normal and abnormal values they considered in making a diagnosis of diabetes mellitus.

When a person is unable to ingest oral glucose, an intravenous glucose tolerance test is done. The presence of gastrointestinal dysfunction is one major indication for use of intravenous glucose tolerance tests. Usually 0.5 gm of glucose per kilogram of body weight is given intravenously. The test is then conducted according to the same regimen used for the oral glucose tolerance test.

Variations of the glucose tolerance test include measurement of creatinine clearance along with collection of specimens as an evaluation of kidney function. Another type of glucose tolerance test is the cortisone oral glucose tolerance test. Giving cortisone challenges the body's ability to metabolize and utilize glucose, and this test is most often used when results of the standard glucose tolerance test are borderline.

The **postprandial blood sugar test** is sometimes used for screening purposes. Generally, the test is done by collecting blood specimens 1 or 1 and 2 hours following a meal. Some authorities feel that this test is more useful in following progress of the identified diabetic patient than in screening, because the values are generally higher than those obtained with the standard glucose tolerance test. Postprandial blood sugar tests are less expensive than the standard oral glucose tolerance tests and are less stressful for the patient.

Early diagnosis and treatment of diabetes mellitus are desirable and warrant screening programs. Because of the uncertainty about the relationship in regard to the time of diagnosis and treatment and the occurrence of vascular and nerve changes, it is postulated that early treatment may allay the more severe manifestations of diabetes mellitus. Undiagnosed, diabetes mellitus may first become overtly apparent in a life-threatening situation resulting from severe hyperglycemia. Therefore, the general health of the person is better supported if diagnosis is made under optimum conditions.

Very frequently, diagnosis is made when the person begins to have symptoms of the metabolic alterations of diabetes mellitus. These include weight loss and a general decrease in energy as well as the classic triad of polyuria, polydipsia, and polyphagia. Some women are first suspected of having diabetes when they have repeated occurrences of vulvitis. Skin infections may also be indicative of diabetes when they recur with frequency. Other symptoms include headache, blurred vision, drowsiness, and loss of appetite. Awareness of these presenting symptoms should alert the nurse to the need for follow-up diagnostic tests.

When interpreting tests, the nurse should remember that the metabolic alterations underlying the symptoms of diabetes mellitus vary in degree according to the amount of effective insulin the person has. When the blood glucose levels exceed the renal threshold for glucose, the excess glucose is eliminated in the urine. This is called **glycosuria.** The glucose increases the osmolarity of the urine, causing water to be excreted in greater amounts. The result is **polyuria,** in which the diabetic patient excretes excess water as well as calories in the urine through glycosuria. **Polydipsia** is related to dehydration and the loss of calories in the urine contributes to weight loss. **Polyphagia** is related to the body's need for energy. Reduction in energy occurs as the calories that ordinarily would be used for energy are actually being wasted. The body cells, particularly of muscles and adipose tissue, cannot use the glucose because insulin, which is necessary for transfer of glucose across the cell membrane, is either not present or is not effective. As the cells then rely more on oxidation of fatty acids for energy, the body stores of energy are depleted. Triglycerides primarily from adipose tissue are the major source of fatty acids which are oxidized for energy when glucose cannot be utilized. Ketone bodies can also be used for energy by body cells. Gluconeogenesis and ketogenesis take place primarily in the liver, so that fatty acids are available to the body cells.

Increased blood plasma levels of free fatty acids and ketone bodies accelerate the problems of glucose utilization at the peripheral level. Both reduce the amount of glucose oxidation that is possible. Therefore, people who have minimal effective insulin eventually develop less ability to utilize glucose because fatty acids must be utilized; as the levels of free fatty acids increase along with increases in ketone bodies, glucose oxidation that is already minimal is further hindered.

Ketone bodies formed by the liver are important in development of acidosis in diabetic individuals. The ketone bodies include beta hydroxybutyric acid, acetoacetic acid, and acetone. Although ketone bodies are useful in that they can be used for energy through oxidation in body tissues such as muscle cells, they can increase to the extent that the amount of circulating ketones exceeds the amount that can be utilized for energy. As a result, the level of ketones in the blood plasma increases and ketones are excreted in the urine. As the level of ketones in blood plasma increases, however, a state of acidosis ensues; ketosis is then associated with the fluid and electrolyte changes of metabolic acidosis. This further complicates metabolism and also leads to symptoms such as drowsiness and confusion. Ketoacidosis may be an emergency condition requiring hospitalization.

Protein anabolism is also influenced by insulin. When there is depleted effective insulin, anabolism of proteins is depressed. The resulting increased protein catabolism leads to many of the overt symptoms of diabetes mellitus. The transport of amino acids across cell membranes as well as the building of amino acids into protein is insulin-dependent. With lack of effective insulin, many important cellular structures are influenced. Formation of RNA is decreased with a lack of insulin, and proteins generally used in cellular synthesis are degraded. Growth is then delayed in diabetic children who are not treated; it is also thought that delays in healing, which are characteristic of diabetics, are related to the changes in protein metabolism.

Vascular and neural changes in diabetes mellitus As previously mentioned, the first indications of diabetes mellitus may be vascular or neural changes. When the vascular changes are predominant, diagnosis of diabetes mellitus may be suspected from the presence of microaneurysms in the eyes, in renal insufficiency from vascular origin, or from myocardial or peripheral vascular disease. Pain and numbness in the extremities may be initial symptoms in those with predominantly neural involvement. Other neural changes indicative of diabetic neuropathy vary from localized or isolated neuritis to loss of motor function. Autonomic nerve involvement is characterized by such symptoms as diarrhea (usually at night), development of a neurogenic bladder, urinary incontinence, or in nausea or orthostatic hypotension or impotence. The symptoms any one person has may be different from those demonstrated by another person.

CARDIOVASCULAR CHANGES IN DIABETES MELLITUS In those people with cardiovascular symptoms, there can be extreme variability in the nature of the symptoms related to the vessels affected. Cardiovascular diseases in diabetic patients actually account for as much as 70 percent or more of the deaths. The large-vessel changes are those of arteriosclerosis and atherosclerosis. Plaques fill the arteries or form atheromas as a result of the accumulation of lipids in the subintimal tissues. These fatty plaques may undergo calcification or ulceration typical of cardiovascular diseases of other origins. Thrombosis and occlusion of major vessels may result from the changes. For some diabetic persons, these vascular changes may precede overt symptoms of carbohydrate intolerance. In fact, the severity of the vascular disease is related to the duration of the diabetes and the person's age, rather than to the severity of the carbohydrate intolerance. The specific symptoms the person will have from the vascular changes depend on the location of the changes. The changes can take place anywhere in the body. The brain, the kidneys, and the mesentery are most commonly affected. The complications of vascular disease for the diabetic patient occur because of disturbance in the function of the organ involved. Nursing care and treatment depend on the signs and symptoms.

Arteriosclerosis is common among diabetic individuals, and their signs and symptoms resulting from arteriosclerosis are the same as those found in any person with arteriosclerosis. Sometimes people who are thought to have essential hypertension are found to have diabetes also. Diabetics with the juvenile type of diabetes mellitus may have Mönckeberg's calcific medial sclerosis, in which there are deposits of calcium in the wall of the muscles, which makes the person susceptible to development of arteriosclerosis. This disease is not specific to diabetes, but when it occurs in people under age 40, they are usually diabetic.

Microangiopathy is common in diabetic individuals. This capillary disease may affect arterioles and venules, and the capillary basement membranes are thickened. The eye and the kidney are most commonly affected. Microangiopathies are the cause of both blindness and chronic renal disease in diabetics, and they decrease the adaptation abilities of the individual both physiologically and in carrying out the treatment plan. Diabetic retinopathy has been staged in four degrees of severity with stage I being the least severe. The stages include: stage I, in which the retinal veins are distended. These are called microaneurysms and may be found during a physical examination, alerting the examiner to the need for more definitive diagnosis for diabetes. Stage II is associated with punctuate hemorrhages. A waxy exudate is found as well. In stage III, the capillary networks are dilated; there is neovascularization and there may be hemorrhage of the retinal tissues along with fibrosis of the superficial retinal tissues. Stage IV is sometimes called proliferating retinopathy or rubeosis iridis diabetica. In this stage, there is vitreous hemorrhage and the individual may have retinal detachments or glaucoma. Blindness may result.

The eye changes associated with diabetes may also be classified as microaneurysms, exudates and hemorrhages, and retinitis proliferans. This classification follows the same progressive nature as that of staging; microaneurysms are the early lesions that progress to formation of sacs that fill with lipids. These sacs eventually leak and rupture. The **microaneurysms** appear as red dots that are very small and round in appearance. They tend to be most frequent in the perimacular region but occur along the course of the retinal capillaries. **Exudates** usually begin on the vitreous side of the retina and are often located in proximity to the microaneurysms. As the exudates and **hemorrhages** occur, the microaneurysms tend to regress or become obscure. When retinitis first occurs, it tends to go through periods of exacerbations and remissions. The cause of these eye changes is unknown and it is not certain why the periods of remission occur. When **retinitis proliferans** occurs in diabetes, it is associated with the duration of the disease process, being more frequent in those who have had overt diabetes for a period of time. Hemorrhagic glaucoma may result in proliferative retinopathy when there is depigmentation of the iris from deposition of glycogen on the surface of the iris. This often occurs in conjunction with central vein occlusion.

Cataracts of the eyes also tend to be related to carbohydrate intolerance. Metabolic cataracts often occur in people who are insulin-dependent and occur more frequently when the carbohydrate intolerance is not well controlled. Elderly diabetic individuals who develop cataracts are found to have a type that matures more rapidly. It is thought that increased production of sorbitol, a sugar alcohol, contributes to the more rapid maturity of such cataracts.

Insulin-dependent diabetic individuals may notice changes in vision that are thought to be related to changes in the lens or the ciliary body. It is not uncommon for the diabetic patient to develop myopia. This can be of great concern for the diabetic who knows that **retinopathy** is the fourth leading cause of blindness. These changes in accommodation and refraction may improve with treatment of the diabetes. Many authorities feel that retinopathy is related to control of the carbohydrate intolerance, whereas others feel that the retinopathies may occur independent of the carbohydrate intolerance, becoming overt prior to the occurrence of symptoms of altered metabolism. Many do feel that very careful management of metabolic alterations should be followed, however, since there is a possibility that good control or better control will decrease the severity of the retinopathy.

Many different types of treatment have been tried in efforts to reduce the occurrence of blindness among diabetics. Among these measures are hypophysectomy, vitrectomy (to treat vitreous hemorrhage), and photocoagulation using lasers. None is curative. The goal of treatment is to retain for the patient as much vision as possible.

The **kidney** is the other organ frequently affected with microvascular disease in diabetic patients. Kimmelstiel-Wilson syndrome is associated with diabetes. This syndrome includes the nephrotic syndrome resulting from glomerular sclerosis and hypertension. The kidney changes that take place in association with diabetes include both nodular glomerulosclerosis and tubular nephrosis. In order to determine kidney changes early in their development, creatinine clearance tests are performed routinely on a yearly basis or less frequently. The urine is also analyzed for the presence of leukocytes, casts, and protein.

When patients with diabetes mellitus develop the nephrotic syndrome, they are treated symptomatically. Management of the diabetic syndrome becomes more complicated in persons with the nephrotic syndrome, as they have symptoms of nitrogen retention, hypertension, and all the other consequences of the disease. When kidney function is impaired, the kidney cannot filter the excess glucose, and glycosuria decreases even in the presence of hyperglycemia in excess of the normal renal threshold. There is also decreased ability of the kidney to degrade insulin. It is not unusual for pyelonephritis to occur in persons with renal involvement, as diabetic patients are prone to infection. In progressive renal disease, uremia may be the cause of death. Microangiopathy as a cause of the nephrotic syndrome in diabetic individuals is not directly related to the severity of carbohydrate intolerance. Renal changes have been found to occur prior to overt symptoms of metabolic alterations. When the renal changes have progressed to the point of the nephrotic syndrome, they tend to be permanent. Tubular nephrosis, in which vacuoles of the epithelial cells of the tubules contain glycogen, is, however, related to the level of hyperglycemia.

This condition does usually respond to correction of metabolic alterations.

People with diabetes mellitus are particularly susceptible to **peripheral vascular disease in the lower extremities.** The reason for this phenomenon is unknown, but the incidence of vascular disease causing intermittent claudication, cool temperature of the feet and lower legs, and paresthesias is high. Gangrene may develop when circulation is greatly impaired and may affect large areas of tissue (when the large arteries are diseased) or small patches in various locations (when the small arteries and capillaries are involved) (see color insert Figure 6 on page 1078B). If arterial insufficiency is present, there will be **dependent rubor,** a characteristic reddening of the lower extremities. Assessment of peripheral pulse differences between the pulses in the tibia and those in the foot is an important nursing measure. If there is a great variation in pulses, the nurse can assume that arterial insufficiency is present. Other changes include a shiny appearance of the skin and atrophy of tissues. When the extremity is elevated, the color changes from the redness noted in the dependent position to a waxy paleness. Peripheral vascular deficiency is discussed in Chapter 4.

Gangrene may be of two types, wet or dry. Wet gangrene is a combination of poorly nourished tissue and infection. Usually surgical drainage of the infected gangrenous areas followed by antibiotic therapy and intermittent moist dressings is used to treat wet gangrene. If the infection does not clear and if the tissue necrosis continues, amputation is required. Dry gangrene is defined as tissue necrosis. It is caused by lack of blood supply because of atherosclerosis or occlusion of major arteries supplying the extremity. The initial event may be trauma to a small spot on the lower leg or foot. The inflammatory process may be hindered because of the already compromised circulation and may in turn further compromise circulation because of local swelling. When this occurs, the person is placed on bed rest or on limited activity, and the area of gangrene is exposed to the environment. It is important to avoid pressure on the area and to prevent further tissue damage. Since heat increases the demand for oxygen, it is not used. When possible, the gangrenous area is localized and excised after healing has advanced as far as possible. When the extremity does not respond to treatment, amputation is usually necessary. The care of people with amputations is described in Chapter 10.

NEURAL CHANGES IN DIABETES MELLITUS
Nursing care is essential in estimating the degree of neurologic involvement and teaching the diabetic self-protection in view of the increased vulnerability to trauma.

Many different forms of neural involvement are found in diabetic individuals. Among them are autonomic neuropathy, mononeuropathy, polyneuropathy, amyotrophy, and radiculopathy. **Autonomic neuropathy** generally is related to the time span of the disease and may involve any area of the body. When the bladder is involved, the symptoms are associated with urinary retention with a propensity to development of infections. Sexual impotence in the male is a common form of diabetic neuropathy. Gastrointestinal involvement leads to slowing of peristalsis and dilatation of the stomach. People with this form of neuropathy often have diarrhea at night. Sweating and orthostatic hypotension are also frequent types of neuropathies. **Mononeuropathy** is involvement of a major nerve trunk causing sensory loss, pain, and motor weakness. The onset may be acute and the person may demonstrate loss of reflexes in the involved area as well as tenderness of the nerve when it is palpated. This type of neuropathy may involve the extremities, or may be located in the cranial nerves.

Polyneuropathy is one of the more frequently occurring forms of the neuropathies. This type of neuropathy tends to involve the long nerves supplying the feet. There is loss of sensation to the part involved and skin changes typical of this type of neuropathy include thinning of the skin, a shiny appearance with loss of hair, and decreased sensation. **Amyotrophy** is associated with muscle weakness and muscle wasting, weight loss, and myalgia. There are typically dysesthesias of the reflexes, especially of the thigh and foot. Amyotrophy is most frequent in elderly men with adult-onset diabetes who are not insulin-dependent. **Radiculopathy** occurs with less frequency and may be difficult to distinguish from a ruptured nucleus pulposus (Chap. 10). In this condition, the roots of the nerves at the site of the dorsal root ganglion may be affected, as well as the nerves in the spinal columns of the spinal cord. Typical symptoms include loss of position sense and loss of deep tendon reflexes. Romberg's sign is usually positive. (Romberg's sign is elicited by having the person stand with feet together and with eyes closed; loss of position sense is indicated if the person sways.)

Treatment and nursing care in diabetes mellitus When symptoms of diabetes first present in the vascular or neural changes, the localized symptoms are treated according to the dysfunction that has resulted in the body organs and/or tissues involved. The diagnosis of diabetes mellitus is confirmed through glucose tolerance tests, and treatment is initiated according to the level of hyperglycemia found, in addition to specific treatment for vascular or neural dysfunction. Treatment and nursing care may vary considerably from one individual to another, depending on the individual requisites and on the types of symptoms the person presents.

In comparison, youth-onset diabetic individuals tend to have a more sudden onset of symptoms of carbohydrate intolerance while adult-onset diabetics may develop symptoms gradually. Adult-onset diabetics may demonstrate vascular changes and neuropathies before having symptoms of carbohydrate intolerance. Some adult-onset diabetics may be asymptomatic for a number of years and may be identified as having chemical diabetes or as being prediabetic.

Youth-onset diabetic individuals tend to be insulin-dependent because they usually do not produce insulin or produce very small amounts of it. The pathologic changes that take place in the pancreas are not fully understood. One process known to occur is hyalinization of the beta cells. This process, however, may occur in nondiabetic patients and it increases with age. There is speculation that diabetes mellitus may be an autoimmune disease. Some youth-onset diabetic individuals have demonstrated insulitis, which is characterized by lymphatic infiltration of beta cells. Destruction of beta cells (associated with chronic pancreatitis) may also cause diabetes mellitus. Whatever the cause, the person who does not produce sufficient effective insulin, whether of youth-onset type or adult-onset type diabetes, requires exogenous insulin, and treatment must include both dietary control and administration of exogenous insulin.

The treatment for diabetes mellitus is symptomatic rather than curative, because the cause is not known. From the previous discussion, it is obvious that there are many variations in the types of dysfunction that any given diabetic may present; therefore nursing care, as well as treatment regimens, must be very individualized. There is, however, one central symptom that all diabetic individuals share—that of hyperglycemia. For this reason, people often think of diabetes as a hyperglycemic state. Treatment for hyperglycemia is primarily accomplished through dietary reduction of carbohydrates, and if required, oral hypoglycemic medications to increase the amount of endogenous insulin or replacement of insulin by giving exogenous insulin, and nursing care focuses on teaching patients self-care. The patient must manage self-care in a precise manner in order to achieve reduction of hyperglycemia. The central common symptom, hyperglycemia, is often used as a measure of the effectiveness of self-care.

There are several different types or degrees of diabetes mellitus. When a person has sufficient effective insulin to metabolize the reduced carbohydrate load, this treatment alone may be sufficient; however, when the person's effective insulin is still not enough to anabolize the reduced carbohydrate load, he or she may be given oral hypoglycemic agents. These agents fall into two categories, the sulfonylureas and the biguanides. Both of these types of oral hypoglycemic agents depend on having sufficient insulin to be effective. The sulfonylureas are thought to increase the sensitivity of peripheral cells to insulin while the biguanides increase the uptake of glucose by the peripheral cells and decrease the rate at which glucose is absorbed from the small intestine.

For people who have insufficient effective insulin, it is necessary to replace insulin. This is accomplished by administering exogenous insulin. When insulin is administered, it is very important to control all the other aspects of metabolism that affect insulin's action or that are affected by the action of insulin. The types and methods used for control are variable and dependent both on the person's response to the treatment and to the physician's preferences.

Patient teaching by the nurse should emphasize the interrelationships among diet, insulin, exercise, and stress levels in metabolism. Since treatment for hyperglycemia centers on control of carbohydrate metabolism, it is easy to forget that the treatment actually affects the person's total metabolic processes. This then includes all ingested nutrients, the amount of energy utilized by the person, and the amount of insulin available to metabolize the nutrients so that energy is available. An essential nursing function is teaching the diabetic how to coordinate all these aspects of care: diet, exercise, stress, and medications.

Normally the body adapts to changes brought about by variations in any of these factors. The diabetic individual, however, does not have the capacity for internal adaptation to these factors and must learn to control the diet, exercise, stress, and medications in a coordinated way. A keynote for diabetic teaching for self-care is development of regularity in daily living habits. This means that the diabetic must eat well-balanced meals at regular intervals, develop regular sleep-waking habits, and follow a routine pattern of consistent activity and exercise, reducing stressors as much as possible.

The nurse, from personal experience, knows that it is not practical to assume that any person can establish precise regularity in daily living. Change can realistically be controlled only to a degree. Normal or usual variations, such as periods of more than usual activity, different sleeping patterns, and differences in food intake are expected in diabetic patients as well as in those who have normal adaptation capabilities. The difference is that the diabetic must develop patterns or habits to control these variations whereas the nondiabetic, who has normal metabolic function, will experience these variations automatically. Because of this difference, the nurse's teaching plan must include all the components of care important for the diabetic since effective life depends on effective control. The teaching must be individualized and, to be successful, must take into account the person's perceptions of his condition. The requisite to control metabolic processes externally, previously considered automatic by the diabetic, may be perceived as a severe limitation. The nurse may expect that responses to this limitation may include denial, frustration, anger, and any of the mechanisms that people normally use when confronted with a major illness. The goal of teaching is that the patients effectively control the disease so that they can live out their lives in good health. The nurse cannot deny the fact, however, that life-threatening neural and vascular involvement in diabetes mellitus cannot be predicted and may occur even when the patient follows the prescribed care plan exactly. When neural and vascular involvement are presenting symptoms, the disability they cause may hinder the person's ability to learn and to adapt to the treatment regimen.

Another important aspect of teaching is that all diabetic individuals should know that they are subject to hyperglycemic crisis (which will be discussed later) during periods of unusual stress. During these times, the diabetic may require exogenous insulin, even if it is not part of the ordinary treatment plan. In addition, the dietary management must be adjusted in certain situations. Therefore, when diabetic patients undergo some form of extraordinary stress such as a surgical procedure, a pregnancy, or psychological stress, their management and treatment must be evaluated to provide for their current metabolic needs. Diabetic individuals who routinely require insulin for treatment may require additional insulin and different dietary regimens during stress. Those who do not take insulin may require insulin during the stress.

Finally, since metabolism is adaptive as the body grows and changes, and in accordance with varying demands for energy requirements, the diabetic patient's treatment plan must be evaluated periodically throughout life. It is expected that requirements for management will change as the person ages and experiences different life stressors.

DIET Since dietary control is essential in the nurse's teaching plan for all diabetic individuals despite the type, stage, or age of onset, it will be discussed first. As with other aspects of treatment, there is controversy about the "best" form of diet control. Among the methods used to manage dietary control are the free diet and quantitative diets in which food exchanges or weighed diets or a combination of both is used. The purpose of dietary control in all these methods is to provide the body with adequate and appropriate nutrients for cell growth and function and for energy production. In general, it is agreed that the more consistent the dietary intake, the better the control of hyperglycemia.

The insulin-dependent diabetic patient cannot store nutrients for use when body requirements change, as during exercise or stress or when intake decreases; therefore consistent and regular intake of nutrients is essential. Diets for diabetic individuals provide for regularly spaced meals, often three main meals with in-between meal snacks. The amount of calories ingested is prescribed and should be the same each day; the intake of the daily quota of calories should also be divided into meals on a consistent basis. Many authorities believe that the consistency in intake in terms of both the total amount of carbohydrates, fats, and proteins and the distribution of the nutrients in each meal is more important than the total amount of carbohydrates allotted in the diabetic's diet for purposes of control. For example, a person who eats a consistent amount of carbohydrate calories regularly may be in better control than one who, although eating fewer total carbohydrate calories, does not consistently follow a pattern of regular meals with consistent distribution of calories among the meals on a day-to-day basis. There is considered to be a direct relationship between better control of hyperglycemia and the regularity of eating habits.

A goal of diet therapy for the diabetic person in all types of dietary control is maintenance of ideal weight. If the person is overweight (as many diabetics are at the time of initial discovery of diabetes mellitus of the adult-onset type), the diet is calculated for weight reduction. After weight reduction has been achieved, the diet is then calculated for maintenance of ideal body weight. It has been found that people who are obese and have hyperglycemia have increased insulin levels. The increase is proportional to the amount of obesity. These people are considered to have a higher basal insulin level because their basal islet set has accommodated; they have consistent requirements for more insulin. Those who are obese do not demonstrate the first phase or initial acute insulin secretion peak on glucose stimulus. Obesity causes resistance to insulin at the peripheral cellular level, so that more insulin is required for the metabolism of glucose, specifically in providing for transfer of glucose across the cell membrane. Consequently, more insulin is required to overcome the peripheral cellular resistance to glucose and the basal islet set is higher. The peripheral resistance to insulin is a determinant of the islet set.

Reduction of obesity or weight loss decreases the peripheral resistance to insulin and allows the islet set to be readjusted to lower levels. Less insulin is required as peripheral resistance is decreased, as the cells then become more sensitive to insulin. Therefore, people with adult-onset diabetes who are obese may control their diabetes mellitus to some degree by diet alone, if they can reduce their weight to ideal body weight. After losing the excess weight and thereby decreasing insulin resistance at the peripheral level, these people may have enough insulin to manage a controlled carbohydrate load. These people, to control metabolic symptoms successfully, must be taught to establish a regular pattern of nutrient intake. If they divert from the regular pattern by eating large quantities of food on a given day, such as one is prone to do on holidays or at picnics, they will not have enough insulin to cover the increased carbohydrate load and their symptoms of carbohydrate intolerance will become overt. Attempts to make up for excessive intake by not eating the next day or by severely restricting food intake also disturbs the pattern of insulin secretion. Essentially, these people cannot adjust to variances in carbohydrate load.

Teaching and counseling for weight reduction employ many techniques of nursing care described in Chapter 7. These people often find it difficult to form new dietary habits, particularly as the symptoms do not dramatically occur in direct relationship to intake of food. The nurse should teach the person to recognize cumulative signs and symptoms of carbohydrate overload such as lethargy, increased blood pressure if hypertension is a problem, and other manifestations of carbohydrate overload.

There are various opinions about the most appropriate distribution of carbohydrates, fats, and proteins in the diabetic diet. A free diet of 45 to 50 percent carbohydrate, 15 percent protein, and the remainder of calories from fats is commonly prescribed. Within the limits of this distribution, the person may select the foods he or she likes and is accustomed to eating. Selection of foods requires knowledge of food values. Several methods may be selected to help the person use correct food values, one of the most widely used being food exchange lists.

The **exchange diet** is one method of dietary control in which six food exchange lists are available for meal planning. The six exchange lists are milk, vegetable, fruit, bread, meat, and fat. The exchange lists were recently revised and include differentiation of polyunsaturated and saturated fats, important because many diabetics have cardiovascular problems. Each list contains foods that in the designated portions contain approximately equal amounts of calories and equal values of carbohydrate, protein, and fat, thereby allowing exchange of foods on a given list without the necessity for calculating food values. *Exchange Lists for Meal Planning* can be obtained from the American Diabetes Association, Inc., 600 Fifth Avenue, New York, N.Y. 10020 for a nominal fee. The portion amounts control the amount of calories as well as the amount of carbohydrate, fat, and protein. The lists can be compiled according to an individual's food likes by calculating the amount of carbohydrate, protein, and fat in each food and the total amount of calories in each portion. For example, the bread exchange list includes amounts of foods containing 15 gm of carbohydrates, 2 gm of protein, and 68 calories. The list contains a variety of foods and their approximate carbohydrate, protein, and caloric content in the size of the portions specified. Portion sizes may be estimated such as one large or one small slice; they may be measured or weighed.

Among foods included on the bread list are bread, flour, cereals, rice, crackers, noodles, spaghetti, and vegetables such as potatoes and dried beans. All the items on the bread list have about-equal values. If the prescribed diet specifies that a person may have three bread exchanges in one meal, the person may select three different foods or may use three portions of one food. The person who loves spaghetti may, for example, wish to use all three bread exchanges for spaghetti, adding meat from the meat exchange, butter or cooking oil from the fat exchange, tomatoes from the vegetable exchange. To balance the meal, a serving of milk from the milk exchange and fruit from the fruit exchange is added.

The exchange lists enable the person to compile a variety of meals, using exact exchanges so that the distribution of carbohydrate, fat, and protein values as well as the total amount of calories is consistent. The prepared lists can be used as the basis for helping the diabetic patient compile his or her own exchange list which contains the foods preferred. The dietitian can compute the food values for the person's preferential foods so that they can be added to the appropriate exchange list. Many diabetics or the persons who cook for a diabetic have, over a period of time, compiled highly individual yet accurate exchange lists of foods that are not included on published exchange lists. The flexibility and variety of foods allowed by use of exchange lists is limited only by the cook's ingenuity.

When the **weighted diet** method is used, the patient must weigh foods to calculate their nutritive value. All foods must be weighed rather than measured. While this method provides for very accurate calculations, it is time-consuming. A list of foods for the food groups is given and the person must quantitatively evaluate food intake according to the list of foods allowed. Weighed diets are not frequently used because exchange lists have proved to be more convenient and flexible and inclusive of greater varieties of foods. People using the exchange list method have achieved good results. When weighed diets are used, the nurse must provide for return demonstrations to ensure that the person knows how to determine portions.

The number of calories allotted for the diabetic depends on the person's body weight and the amount of physical activity the person performs in daily activities. As previously mentioned, a reduction diet is maintained for obese persons until ideal body weight is achieved. There are many charts that list ideal body weight. Among those frequently used are those published by insurance companies. Ideal body weight is approximated according to age, sex, and frame (small, medium, and large).

To calculate body weight for use in determining diets, kilograms are used. The weight in pounds is converted to kilograms by dividing the pound weight by 2.2 as follows: lb ÷ 2.2 = kilograms. Allowances for additional calories are made for growing children and physically active men and women for maintenance of ideal body weight. The number of calories allotted per kilogram is a matter of opinion and may vary from as little as 20 calories per kilogram for obese minimally active adults to a maximum of 50 calories per kilogram. Frequently, charts or formulas are used in initial calorie determinations, and these amounts are changed as necessary through evaluation of the person's response to the calories prescribed, using ideal body weight as the standard or basis for comparison.

Equally difficult is the decision about distribution of calories among fat, protein, and carbohydrates. The trend is currently to allow a more average percentage of calories in carbohydrates (45 to 50 percent). Previous diets have limited carbohydrate intake and have increased fat intake. Because diabetic patients are prone to the development of atherosclerosis, the fat allowances are controversial, just as the question of the contribution of diet and cholesterol levels in development of atherosclerosis in the general population is controversial. There is no succinct evidence that ingestion of diets lower in fat reduces the occurrence of atherosclerosis in diabetics. In an attempt to reduce complications as well as vascular manifestations of diabetes mellitus, however, many authorities prescribe diets lower in fat with compensatory increases in carbohydrate for provision of calories.

Of importance in determining the distribution of calories among carbohydrates, fats, and proteins is evaluation of the person's total health status. Those with known cardiovascular disease with high cholesterol levels are given a lower percentage of fats. Sodium may also be restricted in diets of those with cardiovascular or certain types of endocrine or renal diseases. People with renal disease (renal insufficiency with proteinuria) also require restriction of proteins. Those requiring special diets for treatment of gastrointestinal diseases may need to select foods that do not aggravate symptoms.

Other basic information needed to calculate diets is the caloric value of nutrients: 1 gm of carbohydrate provides 4 calories, 1 gm of protein provides 4 calories, and 1 gm of fat provides nine calories. Therefore, if one knows the total calories allotted and the distribution of calories according to carbohydrate, fat, and protein, the diet can be calculated. For example, if the person is given a prescription for a 2200-calorie diet, 45 percent carbohydrate, 15 percent protein, and 40 percent fat, the distribution is computed as follows:

Carbohydrate: 45 percent × 2200 = 990 calories ÷ 4 = 242.50 gm carbohydrate
Protein: 15 percent × 2200 = 330 calories ÷ 4 = 82.5 gm protein
Fat: 40 percent × 2200 = 880 calories ÷ 9 = 97.7 gm fat

Calories would then be distributed into the number of meals prescribed. If the prescription called for three major meals and two small feedings, the calories would be distributed so that each meal is balanced in carbohydrate, protein, and fat values. In this instance, 250 gm of carbohydrate, 85 gm of protein, and 100 gm of fat are distributed in the number of prescribed feedings. (The figures are rounded off to the nearest 5 gm.) The total distribution of nutrients is usually done by using a formula. An example is the Lilly formula, which distributes 2/7 at each of three meals and 1/7 for an evening snack.

Preparation of food is also of importance in provision of diets for diabetic individuals. Food values are calculated for the nutrients used in preparation as well as in the value of the foods being prepared. For example, fat used to fry eggs is calculated as part of the total calories used in the meal. For this reason, the diabetic patient is advised to prepare foods using items from the food exchange lists in preparation. Cooking techniques may be varied to minimize use of additional foods from the exchange lists. Baking, broiling, roasting, or boiling meats eliminates the need for adding a fat exchange that might otherwise be needed for frying. The fat may then be used for augmenting the flavor of other foods such as using fat for buttering bread or for potatoes or other vegetables. Creams or sauces may be used, but the ingredients must be taken from the appropriate food exchange lists.

The advantage of using the exchange diet is that foods are measured rather than weighed. In this way, the customary measuring tools can be used. Raw foods can be measured prior to eating; fruits are estimated in size according to small, medium, or large. Some foods, such as eggs, are measured in quantity, one or two. Cooked foods are measured after cooking.

Many diabetic persons as well as those who cook for them become adept at approximating measurements. This is useful when eating out and food cannot easily be measured. If full plates are served, the person should eat only the estimated required or allowed amount of food, leaving the remainder or adding other foods if portions are too large or too small, respectively. If the meal is served family style, the person can select foods according to the exchange lists and can serve himself or herself the estimated correct amount of foods needed. The nurse, in discussing these techniques with the patient, must base teaching on evaluation of his or her feelings about the dietary restrictions to find appropriate techniques that will help that patient be more comfortable in saying no or in developing ways to cope with the limitations.

Use of dietetic foods is also controversial. The major point of importance in regard to canned foods is that the diabetic or the person who purchases food for the diabetic should read food labels carefully to determine the nutritive value of the foods contained in the can or package. For the most part, there are few restrictions in the selection of foods for the diabetic patient. Prepackaged or canned foods with no sugar added should be selected. Water-packed canned goods should be used rather than those packed with sugar; water-packed fruits should be used rather than those packed in syrup. Fresh fruits, vegetables, milk and milk products, flour, and breads may be selected freely. Dried fruits may be used. Cereals with no sugar added should be used. Meats selected should be lean and of good quality. Polyunsaturated fats should be selected. Many authorities believe that highly refined sugar in any form should be avoided. This includes such items as jams, jellies, pies, cakes, and many types of cookies. Other authorities allow these foods if correct quantities from the food exchange lists are used in their preparation. In general, these foods provide more calories with less nutrient value than is required by the diabetic patient.

The diabetic individual should establish a routine of eating at approximately the same time each day and of eating about the same amount of calories according to the prescribed distribution for each corresponding meal on a daily basis. (Breakfasts should correspond to other breakfasts on a day-to-day basis; lunches with lunches, dinners with dinners, and snacks with snacks.) This is important to establish a body set for the routine amount of food that must be metabolized.

If the person is not hungry or is for any reason unable to eat a meal, liquids may be substituted to provide carbohydrates for calories. Fruit juices or milk are frequently substituted. For those diabetics requiring more rigid control, the portion of uneaten food is replaced for carbohydrate values. If, for example, a person does not eat a serving of fruit which supplies 10 gm of carbohydrate, one-half cup of orange or grapefruit juice may be substituted. The concept of replacement with foods of like value is an important one for those who have symptoms from dietary irregularities. It is especially important for insulin-dependent diabetic individuals as well as for those who are taking oral hypoglycemic agents.

Alcoholic beverages may be consumed in moderation; however, some authorities do not allow its consumption because it potentiates the action of both insulin and oral hypoglycemic reactions, and because it has a high caloric value. For those who wish to use alcohol, the nurse should clarify that 1 ounce of alcohol equals two fat exchanges. Therefore, alcohol should be used in minimal amounts because it does not provide nutrients available from other foods in the fat exchange. The use of alcohol as part of the dietary exchange provided actually depends on the importance of drinking alcohol for the individual. If having a cocktail is important to the person, the adaptation can be made. The social value of foods and their meaning and implications for socialization with others is probably the most important factor in the diabetic individual's decisions about drinking alcoholic beverages.

Some authorities believe that diabetic people should take supplemental vitamins and minerals, while others believe that if the person is eating a well-balanced diet, the use of supplemental vitamins and minerals is unnecessary.

Special alterations in the diet may be necessary during periods of illness. Generally, this is managed by providing small but frequent meals, using foods the person can tolerate such as soup, juice, soda crackers, jello, and even lifesaver candies. The carbohydrate values of foods prescribed are used to determine the amounts of fluids or to determine the foods to be included in the small feedings. In the event that the person is unable to tolerate this limited diet, glucose in high concentration is given. Those individuals who are unable to ingest foods or fluids will require intravenous glucose administration, according to the general plan for management of their total condition.

MEDICATION The next aspect of the nurse's teaching plan to be discussed is medication. Some diabetic patients are given medication to provide enough insulin for normal body processes, e.g., to support anabolism of carbohydrates, fats, and proteins. (Without insulin, catabolic processes provide for energy, with subsequent loss of body nutrient stores.) People who are able to secrete insulin may be treated with oral hypoglycemic agents. Oral hypoglycemic agents are often prescribed for adult-onset type of diabetes, as these people usually have enough insulin for stimulus of its release or secretion to be effective. A usual criterion is that oral hypoglycemic agents are indicated if the person requires less than forty units of exogenous insulin per day, when diet control has not reduced hyperglycemia.

The two types of oral hypoglycemic agents are the sulfonylureas and the biguanides. How the oral hypoglycemic agents (Table 8-1) actually work is unknown. In addition to stimulating the secretion of insulin, the sulfonylureas are thought to increase the sensitivity of peripheral cells to insulin. Sulfonylureas, to be effective, require that the person have enough beta cell function so that insulin can be secreted. There are both long-acting and short-acting sulfonylurea drugs. Tolbutamide (Orinase) has a duration of 6 to 12 hours, while chlorpropamide (Diabinese) has a duration of action of up to 36 hours. Side effects are more common with use of chlorpropamide. Tolazamide U.S.P. (Tolinase) has a duration of approximately 10 hours. Acetohexamide (Dymelor) is another of the sulfonylurea drugs. The short-acting sulfonylureas are metabolized in the liver and may cause hypoglycemia if given to people with liver damage. They are excreted in the urine; thus, kidney disease may also contribute to hypoglycemia from sulfonylureas. The long-acting sulfonylureas are not metabolized in the liver as well as are the short-acting ones and the long-acting sulfonylureas are excreted in the urine [10].

Side effects of the sulfonylureas include primarily gastrointestinal symptoms: an-

Table 8-1
Oral hypoglycemic agents

Generic name	Trade name	Dosage forms (mg)	Usual daily dose (gm)	Duration of action (hr)
Sulfonylureas				
Tolbutamide	Orinase	500	0.5–3	6–12
Tolazamide	Tolinase	100; 250	0.1–1	12–24
Acetohexamide	Dymelor	250; 500	0.25–1.5	12–24
Chlorpropramide	Diabinese	100; 250	0.1–0.5	24–36
Biguanides				
Phenformin	DBI, Meltrol,	25	0.025–0.15	4–6
	DBI-TD, Meltrol	50; 100	0.05–0.15	12–14

From G. B. Askew and K. I. Letcher, Oral hypoglycemic agents. *Nursing 75* 75:45, 1975.

orexia, nausea, and vomiting; abdominal pain; and diarrhea. These side effects are not common. The nurse must advise the diabetic patient that the drugs may cause a reaction to alcohol. Chlorpropamide, with a duration of up to 36 hours, is particularly associated with a reaction to alcohol. The symptoms and signs of the response to alcohol include headache, flushing, palpitation and tachycardia, and dyspnea. For those who want to drink alcoholic beverages, taking an antihistamine an hour before drinking alcohol minimizes this reaction. A few people who take sulfonylureas develop mild-to-moderate jaundice. The degree of jaundice is related to the dosage given. There is also an increased response to the sulfonylureas in those who are poorly nourished, so that hypoglycemia may result. In fact, actions of the sulfonylureas for causing hypoglycemia were first noted in malnourished persons who were taking the drugs. This discovery led to the later application of sulfonylureas in the treatment of diabetes mellitus. Sulfonylureas do reduce the fasting blood glucose, but do not cure the intolerance to carbohydrates.

The biguanides do not stimulate insulin secretion, but increase the uptake of glucose by the peripheral cells and decrease the rate at which glucose is absorbed from the small intestine. Side effects of biguanides include anorexia, nausea, vomiting, and, infrequently, diarrhea. Development of a metallic taste in the mouth is also a characteristic side effect of the biguanides.

There are two forms of biguanides; phenformin hydrochloride (DBI), the short-acting form, has a duration of 4 to 6 hours and phenformin hydrochloride (DBI-TD), a long-acting form, has a duration of 12 to 24 hours. The side effects are more common with the short-acting form.

The early enthusiasm for oral hypoglycemic agents has recently been dampened considerably as a result of longitudinal studies of people taking them. The National Institutes of Health study showed that 200 diabetics treated with a fixed dose of tolbutamide and followed for a period of 8 years had a high incidence of deaths from cardiovascular disease. In another study conducted by the University Group Diabetes Program, it was shown that phenformin increased the blood pressure and heart rate of people who were adult-onset diabetics taking the drug. The conclusion of the study at this point is that the mortality rate is greater for those taking phenformin than for people treated by diet alone or by diet and insulin [3]. While both of these studies have created controversy and speculation concerning the methodology of evaluation used, they have greatly influenced current practice, to the extent that many diabetic patients are unwilling to take the drugs and many physicians are more discriminating in selection of people for whom the drugs are prescribed. Research continues to be done in this area, and attitudes and opinions about use of the oral hypoglycemic agents may change in the future as results of current studies become known.

Many authorities believe that diet alone is the treatment most preferable for adult-onset type diabetics who do not develop ketoacidotic crises. The development of ketoacidosis from increased catabolism of fatty acids is discussed later in this chapter. If the person does not respond to diet control as measured by hyperglycemia, insulin is prescribed. As with most aspects of therapy for diabetes mellitus, this viewpoint is also controversial.

Various combinations of oral hypoglycemic agents, as well as combinations of oral hypoglycemic agents and insulin, have been prescribed in attempts to control the symptoms of diabetes mellitus. An example is the use of phenformin with insulin for treatment of the person who has brittle diabetes mellitus that is difficult to control, Sulfonylureas and biguanides are combined if one or the other given alone does not produce a satisfactory response. People who are taking sulfonylureas are often given prescriptions for taking them intermittently rather than consistently. Intermittent administration of the sulfonylureas is thought to achieve a better effect than consistent administration because the side effects and the occurrence of cardiovascular complications are thought to be reduced by intermittent administration. People who consistently have side effects from taking oral hypoglycemic agents, even after the dosage has been lowered, are usually placed on insulin therapy instead.

The use of insulin is a major mode of therapy for diabetics who do not respond to diet alone or to diet and the use of oral hypoglycemic agents. Insulin therapy may be required for long-term care on a consistent basis by diabetics who have need for more than forty units of insulin daily. Some people require insulin temporarily during periods of stress.

Insulin as an anabolic hormone is essential for the creation of nutrient stores in the body. For the insulin-dependent diabetic patient, the functions of insulin are the same as for the person who is able to secrete and release his or her own insulin in terms of anabolism. When these functions are lacking, symptoms of insulin deficiency are present. The diabetic individual has special problems because the types of insulin available for exogenous administration do not provide for the continuous adaptation to variations in body needs and ingestion of foods. Therefore, the dietary intake and exercise must be coordinated with the functioning capability of the insulins administered in terms of the time of onset and the duration of the different types of exogenous insulins.

The functions of insulin (that are known) include anabolism of carbohydrates, fats, and proteins as well as influencing the enzyme activity important to metabolism and the cellular exchange of ions. The effects of hormones on metabolism are shown in Figure 8-6. To review, insulin provides for the transfer of glucose across cell membranes. The cells of the nerves, renal tubules, and intestinal mucosa, as well as erythrocytes, are, however, not insulin-dependent for their uptake of glucose. Insulin supports esterification of fatty acids to form triglycerides as well as decreases lipolysis through decreasing the action of lipase (an enzyme) and decreasing cyclic AMP, both of which support lipolysis. In addition to being required for lipogenesis, insulin is also required for synthesis of proteins and for ribosomal development of RNA. Potassium enters the liver and muscle cells along with glucose, and is necessary for increasing the resting potential of the membranes of muscles and adipose tissue.

Insulin increases the permeability of cells to glucose. In the absence of insulin, glucose is unable to cross the cell membranes, particularly of adipose and muscle tissue. As a result, lipolysis increases and triglycerides are converted to free fatty acids. The liver, which is predominant in the control of blood glucose levels, takes up the free fatty acids and oxidizes them, forming ketone bodies in the process. The effect of insufficient effective insulin then on adipose tissue is loss of the action of insulin for synthesis of fatty acids to the storage form triglycerides. The fatty acids are released instead to the plasma, to be taken up by the liver, muscles, and kidney, to be used as a source of energy.

The plasma levels of glucose are increased in diabetes mellitus. When the plasma levels of free fatty acids increase, because they cannot be synthesized by adipose tissue without insulin, the liver responds by increasing gluconeogenesis. In normal states, the liver stores glucose when plasma glucose levels are high. The storage form is glycogen. These stores are utilized by the liver to form glucose in times when the plasma levels of free fatty acids increase. (The increased levels of free fatty acids signal the liver as to the need for glucose at the cellular level.) This normal adaptive mechanism of the liver (gluconeogenesis), however, is not effective in diabetic individuals because the cells cannot utilize the glucose supplied through gluconeogenesis, as insulin is either lacking or insufficient. The result then is further increase in plasma glucose levels.

Exogenous insulin administration, then, not only influences the uptake of glucose by adipose tissue, thereby promoting the storage of nutrients as triglycerides, but also reduces the liver's ability to produce glucose from the nutrient substrates of fatty acids and amino acids. It should be noted that insulin has an effect on enzyme levels, which contribute to the normal adaptive metabolic processes. For example, the enzymes that are important in gluconeogenesis (which include glucose 6-phosphatase, fructose 1,6-diphosphatase, and pyruvate carboxylase and pyruvate carboxykinase) are not present in as great quantities when insulin is present. They increase when insulin is either lacking or is not effective.

Muscle tissue is also affected by lack of effective insulin. Muscle cells utilize fatty acids and ketone bodies for energy. When insulin is not available for protein synthesis in the muscles, amino acids are released to the liver. The primary form for delivery is alanine formed by amino acids, and pyruvate. The alanine is utilized by the liver as a substrate for the process of gluconeogenesis to produce glucose, and actually provides a stimulus for glucose production by the liver. Urea is a by-product of gluconeogenesis from amino acids. The blood levels of urea are then in-

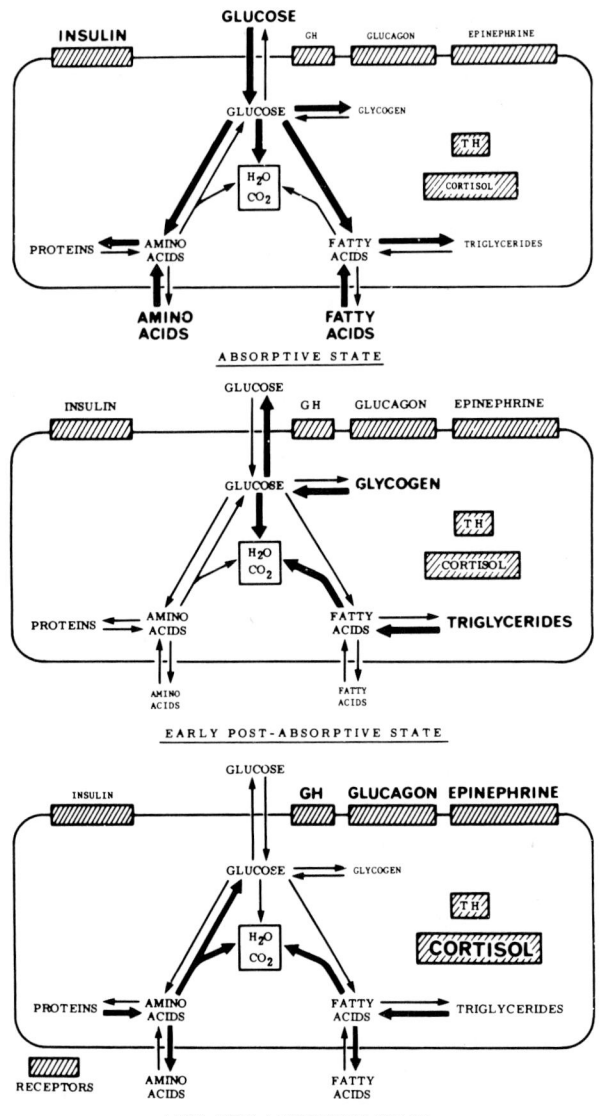

Figure 8-6
Effects of hormones on metabolism during the absorptive, early post-absorptive, and late postabsorptive states. Large lettering indicates high circulating or intracellular levels; medium lettering, medium concentrations; and small lettering, low concentrations. Pathways predominating in each state are indicated by heavy arrows. Cell membrane and intracellular hormone receptors are indicated. (Adapted from E. Selkurt, *Basic Physiology for the Health Sciences.* Boston: Little, Brown and Company, 1975. Reproduced by permission.)

creased so that there is also loss of nitrogen from urinary excretion.

In summary, insulin is needed by people with diabetes mellitus to promote the synthesis of fatty acids to triglycerides and to prevent utilization of fatty acids for energy. Muscle tissue requires insulin to prevent breakdown of protein stores and subsequent muscle-wasting so that the diabetic patient requires insulin for growth, as well as for energy. Children with diabetes mellitus who do not receive insulin therapy have stunted growth, a problem that was prevalent prior to discovery of insulin for therapy. The entire metabolic sequence of anabolism and catabolism that is normally going on within the body depends on insulin for stimulating or decreasing the amounts of enzymes that are available for metabolic processes. Without insulin, waste products of metabolism accumulate so that the blood plasma becomes acidic from increased urea and ketone bodies. Potassium, which normally enters the cell with glucose in the presence of insulin, does not enter the intracellular space, decreasing the membrane potential of the affected cells.

Finally, when body stores of glucose are depleted, cells of the body that are dependent on glucose for energy (in fact, as an exclusive source of energy) are deprived. This includes the nerve cells as well as erythrocytes, the cells of the gastrointestinal mucosa, and of the renal tubules.

Exogenous insulin is currently supplied from purified extracts from the pancreas glands of animals. Beef and pork are the most commonly used in insulin preparations for commercial distribution. Several different types of insulin are available and these can be broadly classified as fast-acting, intermediate, and long-acting insulins. These classifications are determined by the rate of onset and duration of action of each insulin preparation.

There are several different types of insulin: regular insulin, which has a rapid action; protamine zinc insulin, prolonged action; globin insulin, intermediate action; NPH insulin, intermediate; and lente insulin preparations, semilente (rapid), lente (intermediate), and ultralente (prolonged). Regular insulin is available in two forms: neutral regular insulin (NRI) and acid regular insulin (ARI). The neutral regular insulin is so called because it has a neutral pH. NRI is more stable than ARI and retains its potency longer than ARI. In many instances, insulin prescriptions require use of more than one type of insulin. The nurse should be familiar with each type and should know which insulins can be mixed.

Complexing of regular insulin with proteins allows for a gradual release of insulin, thus prolonging the onset, the peak, and the duration of the action of insulin. Both NPH and PZI have a phosphate buffer to maintain the pH of the insulins at about 7.2. This pH decreases the solubility of the insulin. Acid regular insulin, with a pH of 3.2, is more soluble. The differences in the onset of action, peak of action, and duration among insulins is achieved by complexing the insulin with proteins to vary the size of the insulin particles. Protamine is complexed with insulin extract in preparing protamine zinc insulin and neutral protamine Hagedorn insulin. For simplicity, these insulins are referred to as PZI and NPH. Globin is the protein included in globin zinc insulin. A combination of insulin extract and zinc results in an insulin with prolonged action and increased stability. The solubility of insulin is determined somewhat by the pH, as well as by the additives such as zinc. A phosphate buffer is added to PZI insulin to decrease the solubility.

The lente insulins are a mixture of crystalline and amorphous particles in a ratio of 3:7. The crystalline particles dissolve more gradually, prolonging the duration. Acetate buffers are used in lente insulins to delay breakdown of particles. Lente is dissolved by phosphate buffers and therefore cannot be mixed with either NPH or PZI insulins. Semilente and lente insulins can be mixed. Since the mixture of the two is stable, the lente insulins can be mixed in advance of use. Ultralente can be mixed with either semilente or lente insulins. Regular insulin can be mixed with lente insulin in a ratio of 1:1, and the mixing of these two insulins must be done immediately prior to use.

When mixing insulin, the nurse should be aware that the complexing of insulin affects the timing of the action of the mixed insulins. NPH insulin is a combination of protamine and insulin so that the insulin is completely bound or complexed to protamine. PZI insulin is a combination of protamine and insulin extract with free protamine; that is, there is more protamine in the combination than necessary to bind all the available insulin so that there is an excess of protamine. Regular insulin, in contrast, is not complexed. When neutral regular insulin is mixed with NPH insulin, both insulins remain stable, while if equal amounts of regular insulin and PZI are mixed, the excess protamine combines with the uncomplexed regular insulin, and the duration of action is not affected. Adding twice as much regular insulin to an amount of PZI, however, causes binding of the excess protamine and the excess regular insulin then decreases the time of action. This mixture results in an insulin mixture with a duration of action similar to that of NPH. It should again be mentioned that the pH of the insulins to be mixed influences the stability of the mixture. For example, since acid regular insulin has a different pH from NPH insulin, the two should be mixed immediately prior to being administered.

There are many regimens for establishing the dose of insulin required by a diabetic. Body weight is an important factor, as is the response to the glucose tolerance test and the amount of glycosuria. The initial insulin dosage is established beginning with an estimated dosage and measuring the response to that dosage in blood glucose values and glycosuria. Ketone in the urine is also measured in many instances. The measurements indicate whether the initial dosage of insulin is adequate according to the person's response. Several days or weeks are required to establish the desired dosage of insulin. Initiation of insulin therapy may be done on an outpatient basis if the level of hyperglycemia is considered mild. The person with moderate or severe hyperglycemia is often hospitalized for the evaluation and determination of an appropriate regimen of treatment. During the time of hospitalization, the person has an opportunity to learn how to care for himself by managing correct dietary intake, insulin administration, and testing of urine. The nurse must use this time with the person and his family or friends and relatives effectively. Often the initial experiences in managing the diabetes mellitus affect the patient's ability to be self-sufficient as well as attitudes about being a diabetic.

Various management programs are carried out for determining the appropriate therapy for an individual. Most frequently, a dosage of insulin is given prior to breakfast and urine is tested before breakfast and at intervals, usually prior to each meal and at bedtime. The level of glycosuria indicates whether there is a need for additional insulin. Usually, additional insulin is not given unless glycosuria is in the upper ranges. The amount of insulin prescribed is considered one component of the total therapy plan which includes ingestion of a controlled amount and distribution of calories and nutrients for each meal. This procedure of giving insulin, controlling the diet, and measuring glucose in the blood and urine is followed until the patient's condition stabilizes, that is, when the insulin dosage is adequate to prevent the occurrence of hypoglycemia or hyperglycemia. It is important that all aspects of the therapy—insulin administration, diet prescription, and all tests—be completed by the nurse on a regular time schedule, with the use of correct technique. The regularity of diet, insulin administration, and blood and urine testing in the evaluation procedure is essential for determining the patient's response to insulin therapy.

For the moderate or severe diabetic condition, many physicians begin the initial insulin administration with an intermediate-acting insulin and may or may not give regular insulin throughout the day to cover the amount of glucose estimated as being in excess as indicated by the urine glucose tests. Measurement of urine ketones is also important and is included in the evaluation for determining need for more insulin. A combination of fast-acting and intermediate-acting insulin is sometimes used if the initial dosage is not sufficient to prevent glycosuria. In many instances, people with youth-onset type diabetes mellitus have a temporary increase of endogenous insulin production. This remission of diabetes mellitus in the early phase of the disease is temporary, however, and is followed by a permanent decrease or lack of effective insulin.

The maintenance dosage of insulin is determined by the dosage at which the person stabilizes in terms of blood glucose levels as a result of dietary control correlated with exercise and drug therapy. This also applies to the care of people who are given oral hypoglycemic medications. During this period, the importance of the nurse's accurate monitoring of the person's reaction to therapy cannot be overemphasized. Youth-onset type diabetes is usually associated with dependency on insulin, and some adult-onset type diabetics are also insulin-dependent. The response to insulin therapy is variable among individuals, despite the type of onset of diabetes mellitus that they have. Some persons, particularly those with the youth-onset type, tend to be brittle diabetics; that is, they have great fluctuations in blood glucose and in glycosuria. As a result, it is more difficult to establish the adequate insulin dosage for these persons. Many times these people require a method called 6-hour management, or some similar method, in which a program of controlled diet, exercise, and insulin is established. In 6-hour management, one of the intermediate- or long-acting insulins is usually given in the early morning dosage and regular insulin is given as required, determined by the level of glycosuria every 6 hours.

It is also important that the nurse understand and carefully follow the management regimen used in a particular institution or by a particular physician for adjusting the insulin dosage. In some instances, regular insulin is given to "cover" glycosuria in the upper ranges at the time of the urine test such as before lunch or dinner. These plans utilize a scale for giving regular insulin in specific dosages for a 3+ or 4+ reaction in urine tests. Other plans vary the dietary intake as well as the insulin administration. In yet other plans, the next day's dosage is increased. One plan is to give five additional units of insulin the next day if all the urine tests demonstrated glycosuria on the previous day.

Glycosuria occurs at the times that the action of insulin is ebbing, and hypoglycemia at times of peak insulin action. The signs and symptoms of each of these states are discussed later in this section. It is essential that the diabetic patient understand the possible reactions to insulin and that the family be taught how to cope with these reactions. In addition, the diabetic should wear a Medic-Alert identification bracelet or pendant. This cues people to the fact that the person is a diabetic in the event of an emergency of any type, whether the person has an accident or is experiencing the onset of a different illness or a reaction to insulin.

Reactions of hypoglycemia occur at different times for each of the insulins, depending on the peak of action (Table 8-2). It is necessary to give the person a snack or meal at times of hypoglycemia. Given at 7:00 A.M., semilente insulin is most likely to cause a hypoglycemic reaction about 12 noon. Lente insulin, given at 7 A.M., will cause a hypoglycemic reaction at about 10 to 11 P.M., ultralente insulin at about 2:00 A.M. or 3:00 A.M. Figure 8-7 indicates the peak actions of these insulins. The nurse must teach the patient how to cover for these reactions by arranging meals accordingly. A small snack may be required at 10:00 P.M. for the person who is taking lente insulin to increase the blood sugar levels at the time of the peak action of the insulin. The management of a given person's insulin and diet is highly individual and must be determined according to his response to the insulin. For this reason, the nurse must carefully observe the person in evaluating the person's response and learning ability. If the patient is not able to learn how to cope with management, the nurse must find other resources to help the person carry out the management after discharge from the hospital. The nurse should also realize that treatment to correct imbalances while the patient is hospitalized serves as a model and is actually a demonstration of what must be done in self-care. Therefore, every nursing function—testing urine for glucose and ketones, giving insulin, demonstrating and asking the patient to give return demonstrations for insulin administration, and selection of diet as well as replacement of foods not eaten—are all examples of what the person must learn in order to manage his diabetes.

It should be understood that the insulin dosage established at the initiation of insulin therapy will not remain constant for the remainder of the person's life. In fact, the dosage often needs readjustment soon after dis-

Table 8-2
American preparations of insulin*

Type of insulin	Buffer	pH	Suspension	Zinc mg/100 U	Interval of maximum action (hr)	Total Duration of Action (hr)
Lente series						
Semilente	Acetate	7.1–7.5	Amorphous	0.2–0.25	4–6	12–16
Lente	Acetate	7.1–7.5	(30% amorphous 70% crystalline)	0.2–0.25	8–12	18–24
Ultralente	Acetate	7.1–7.5	Crystalline	0.2–0.25	16–18	30–36
Crystalline zinc	None	2.5–3.5	(Solution)	0.01–0.04	4–6	6–8
NPH (isophane)	Phosphate	7.1–7.4	Crystalline	0.01–0.04	8–12	18–24
Protamine zinc	Phosphate	7.1–7.4	Amorphous	0.2–0.25	14–20	24–36
Globin	None	3.4–3.8	(Solution)	0.25–0.35	6–10	12–18

*From Robert H. Williams (ed.), *Textbook of Endocrinology* (5th ed.). Philadelphia: W. B. Saunders Company, 1974. Reproduced by permission.

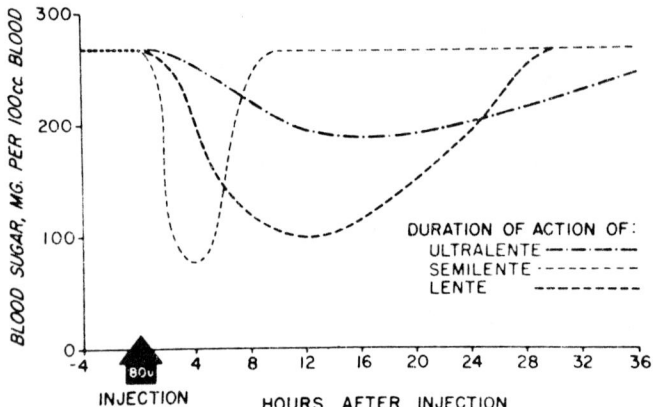

Figure 8-7
The duration of action of ultralente, semilente, and lente insulins. (From R. H. Williams (ed.), *Textbook of Endocrinology* (5th ed.). Philadelphia: W. B. Saunders Company, 1974. Reproduced by permission.)

charge, when the person returns to the usual pattern of exercise and activity. The maintenance dosage should be evaluated periodically and the evaluation may indicate a need either to decrease or increase the dosage. Many physicians believe that the diabetic person should be able to control his or her own dosage, given guidelines for increasing or decreasing the dosage according to different exercise and caloric requirements. This adaptive mode of therapy requires that the person thoroughly understand the therapeutic plan and know the rationale for changing any of the parameters—insulin, dietary intake, or exercise—so that the three can be coordinated. All diabetics, whether insulin-dependent or not, may require different therapy from the usual maintenance plan in the event of major stresses such as illness.

Responses to insulin vary considerably. Some people develop an allergic response to the insulin being given. The protein in the insulin or the animal type of insulin may cause allergies. When insulin allergies occur, there are two modes of intervention. One is to prescribe another type of insulin; the other is to give antihistamines to reduce the allergic response. Some persons may have localized skin reactions with hives or stinging or itching at the site of injection. This type of allergic response is different from the generalized body response to allergy, which is more similar to a hypersensitivity reaction. When a localized skin reaction occurs, the site may be indurated, and increased temperature of the area may be noted along with erythema at the site. The localized reactions occur 20 to 40 minutes after injection. Itching may continue for 2 to 6 hours, and the entire reaction may require a week to several months to subside. These local skin reactions are usually not serious and generally disappear.

Another problem encountered by some persons taking insulin is development of resistance to insulin. This is probably caused by insulin antibody formation. Insulins from beef derivatives are more likely to cause resistance than those from pork derivatives. Corticosteroids are usually given to treat insulin resistance.

In summary, the dosage of insulin, then, is regulated on a daily basis until stabilization is achieved. When the person attains normal blood glucose levels and "ideal weight" as a result of dietary control, the long-term therapy plan may become more stable if the exercise pattern is consistent. Exact control to normal ranges is difficult to evaluate because "normal" blood glucose and weight are variable and differ among individuals even when they do not have diabetes mellitus. People who are learning to manage their own schedule of diet, exercise, and insulin need to experience what is meant by minimal, moderate, or maximum exercise so that they can adapt accordingly. When exercise is minimal, additional insulin may be required. When exercise increases temporarily, the person should learn to increase food intake. Insulin-dependent patients are unable to release glucose from the liver as occurs normally during exercise, and they do not have decreased insulin secretion as a result of sympathetic nervous system activity; therefore, the diabetic patient has decreased blood glucose levels during exercise that require additional glucose to "cover" the exercise. This phenomenon is pertinent in the treatment of insulin-dependent diabetics because they must learn to manage their diet, insulin therapy, and exercise to accommodate changes.

The nurse should teach the diabetic patient the symptoms of hypoglycemia so that dietary management or insulin dosages, or both, can be adapted to prevent its occurrence. The signs and symptoms include increased perspiration, a feeling of nervousness, and hunger. Many physicians plan to have the newly identified diabetic patient experience these symptoms so that they can be recognized when they begin to occur. If dietary management does not rectify their occurrence through such measures as dividing meals so that snacks are provided when hypoglycemia occurs, the insulin dosage is reduced. It is most desirable to manage diet, insulin, and exercise so that hypoglycemia does not occur; however, in unusual circumstances, as when a meal is omitted or exercise increases, hypoglycemia may result as a one-time occurrence. In this instance, the person should pay attention to early symptoms of hypoglycemia: a nervous feeling, shakiness, irritability, followed by hunger, weakness, pale skin, and sweating, especially on the palms and forehead. The hypoglycemia is treated by ingesting sugar in the form of hard candy or fruit juice or another source of food with high carbohydrate value. Some candy, such as chocolates, has a high fat value and should not be used unless no other source of glucose is available.

Hypoglycemia by definition is a low level of blood glucose. This is an important point, as the degree of hypoglycemia can be evaluated only through blood tests. Usually a value of 60 mg per 100 ml of blood is considered borderline between hypoglycemia and normal ranges of blood glucose. A sudden drop in the blood glucose, even if the blood glucose level is not 60 or below, is also called hypoglycemia. Urine glucose is not always indicative of hypoglycemia because urine contains the glucose filtered by the kidneys and stored in the bladder, rather than corresponding directly to blood glucose levels at any given time.

If hypoglycemia is not treated in the early stages, symptoms increase in severity. The person may become dizzy, confused, and may exhibit uncoordinated movements. Swallowing is difficult, inhibiting the ability to take oral glucose. Reactose, a glucose gel, is useful because it may be swallowed by reflex action if the swallowing through voluntary action is not possible. If hypoglycemia continues beyond this stage without treatment, coma may ensue, requiring emergency care. This problem is discussed more fully later in this chapter.

In most instances, every person known to be diabetic is taught how to administer insulin, whether he is insulin-dependent or not, as a protective measure; the diabetic is then prepared for any contingency. In the course of one's lifetime, a number of stressful events may occur and one may become insulin-dependent temporarily. Among factors known to increase insulin resistance are glucocorticoids, estrogen, progesterone, alcohol ingestion, infections, major illnesses, and other forms of stress. The person should be able to give the injection to himself if necessary, and learning the technique of self-administration of insulin is easier when one is feeling well than when one is undergoing stress.

Several important points the nurse should stress in teaching the patient about insulin are: Regular insulin and globin zinc insulin are clear solutions. NPH, PZI, and lente insulins are normally cloudy suspensions. It is important to mix the suspensions by gently rotating the vial before withdrawing insulin. Gentle motions should be used, because shaking the insulin vial can reduce the potency of the insulin by disrupting the suspension. Insulins are stored in the refrigerator because they are heat-labile, losing their potency when they are exposed to high temperatures. Regular insulin is the least stable, retaining its stability and potency for about 6 months at room temperature of approximately 72 degrees. Lente, semilente, and ultralente insulin remain stable at room temperature for a 24-month period. PZI and NPH may remain stable for 36 months; however, they may be difficult to draw up and mix after this time because an aggregate tends to form. Insulins should not be placed in the freezer, as freezing disrupts the insulin particles. Usually, the patient is advised to store insulin in the refrigerator and to keep the vial presently being used for daily insulin injection at room temperature. Injection of insulin kept at room temperature reduces skin reactions. Insulins do lose their potency when they remain at room temperatures above 98 degrees, however. In warm weather, when room temperature exceeds 75 degrees, insulins being used should be refrigerated. When traveling, the diabetic should place the insulin within luggage so that it is protected from exposure to high temperatures. Some people use thermos bottles, and there are special insulin storage kits with refrigerator units for those who travel frequently. When it is necessary to check luggage, the person should keep the insulin in hand luggage, in the event that the checked luggage is lost or temporarily misplaced.

People who travel continuously or frequently usually find that insulin is available wherever they travel, and they can plan to purchase the supply needed when they are in cities and towns with such provisions. Those who visit outlying areas where insulin might be in short supply or difficult to obtain must make arrangements to have an adequate supply. Insulins are available in foreign countries. Usually, the diabetic person can inquire about the different forms of insulin available and the place where insulin may be obtained in the particular country or countries to be visited prior to leaving home.

Insulin is supplied in different concentrations, expressed as units. These concentrations are U40, U80, U100, and U500. U500 is not used clinically. Insulin syringes are also available with calibrations for U40, U80, and U100. One milliliter of U40 insulin contains forty units of insulin while 1 ml of U80 insulin contains eighty units of insulin per milliliter and U100 contains 100 units per milliliter. Through cooperative efforts, color-coding of labels and of syringes has been standardized. Markings on the syringes and on the vials are consistent in color: U40 is red, U80 is green, and the syringes of U100 are black while the vials have orange tops. U500 insulin vials are marked with white and brown stripes.

It is necessary to use the correctly matched syringe with the corresponding unit dosage of insulin: U40 syringes are used with U40 insulins, U80 insulins with U80 syringes, and U100 insulins with U100 syringes to ensure that the correct dosage prescribed is drawn. The nurse can adapt syringes and unit dosages when absolutely necessary. For example, when only U40 insulin is available and the dosage is prescribed in U80 insulin, the correct amount of insulin can be calculated as follows: 1 ml of U40 insulin equals 40 units of insulin; 1 ml of U80 insulin equals 80 units of insulin. Therefore, ½ ml of U80 insulin equals 40 units. People who have poor vision often have difficulty seeing the markings on the syringes. U40 syringes are easier to see than either the U80 or U100. Prescriptions of insulin take these special needs into account as well as the consideration of the dosage so that the syringe used is appropriate.

Syringes are available in glass or disposable plastic. Glass syringes may be sterilized and reused. They should be cleaned about once a week by first soaking them in an acid solution such as vinegar to remove deposits that accumulate on the insides of the barrel. They are then boiled for 5 to 10 minutes and stored in 70% isopropyl alcohol in between use on a daily basis. Disposable syringes are limited to an individual use, but they are convenient to use.

Selection of syringes is usually determined by cost and preference. The disposable syringes are equipped with needles. Some people prefer the disposables because the needles are always sharp and they do not have to be sterilized. One-half or five-eighths-inch needles are used for subcutaneous administration. The needle gauge should be appropriate for subcutaneous injection: 25-, 26-, or 27-gauge needles may be used. PZI insulin requires the largest gauge needle because the particles are larger. Long-barrel syringes are marked for each unit while short-barrel syringes are marked for only the even-numbered units.

Automatic injectors are available for use with either glass or plastic syringes. The Busher Automatic is one example of an automatic injector. This injector allows for automatic injection of the needle for administration of the insulin. For persons with impaired vision, specially adapted syringes are available from the American Foundation for the Blind. Another type of injector is the Medi-jector, which uses pressure to administer insulin subcutaneously, through a nozzle opening of 0.006 of an inch in diameter. U40, U80, and U100 insulins can be administered, and dosages can be set so that the Medi-jector measures the set dose from the vial placed in the apparatus. Others are the Insul gage (Meditec) and the syringe magnifier. Insulin administered with a syringe and needle is given subcutaneously. The area to be injected is carefully selected. The method used depends on the amount of subcutaneous tissue the person has. Those with minimal subcutaneous tissue find that pinching the area to be injected by placing the fingers about 3 inches apart and pushing the fingers close together creates an elevation of the skin so that the needle can be inserted easily into the subcutaneous tissue. Those with ample subcutaneous tissue may not require this technique. The angle of needle entry should be comfortable for the person giving the injection and should ensure that the needle does in fact enter the subcutaneous tissue. The angle of insertion should be at least 45 degrees, ranging to 90 degrees, to ensure that the injection is given subcutaneously. Insulin should never be given intramuscularly, as it is absorbed into the bloodstream too rapidly when this route is used. When given subcutaneously, the insulin is absorbed more slowly, rates of absorption differing with the area selected even in the same individual (Fig. 8-8).

When required, as for administration of insulin during periods of stress, regular insulin is administered intravenously and is stable in glucose and water. Electrolytes may be added to the same IV fluid bottle as insulin. It should be noted that only regular insulin can be given intravenously. When administered intravenously, regular insulin is delivered to the circulation at a rate constant with the delivery of glucose in the IV. When antibodies to insulin are present, the insulin may be bound to antibodies causing a delayed action of the insulin. Both IgG and IgM antibodies are produced in those who take insulin regularly. Insulin also binds to plastic and glass containers, so that the dosage added to the IV is not totally delivered to the person. As much as 20 percent of the dosage can be bound to the container so that when smaller doses are given intravenously a significant portion of the dosage is bound. With larger doses, less insulin is bound, proportional to the dose.

It is essential that the nurse emphasize that subcutaneously administered insulin be given in a different site at each injection. Failure to rotate sites may result in lipodystrophy, which is either hypertrophy or atrophy of adipose tissues. Hypertrophy results from the synthesis of lipids in fat cells. The cause of atrophy is thought to be related to inflammation or trauma from the injection, but the exact cause is not known. It is thought

Figure 8-8
Commonly used injection sites for insulin.

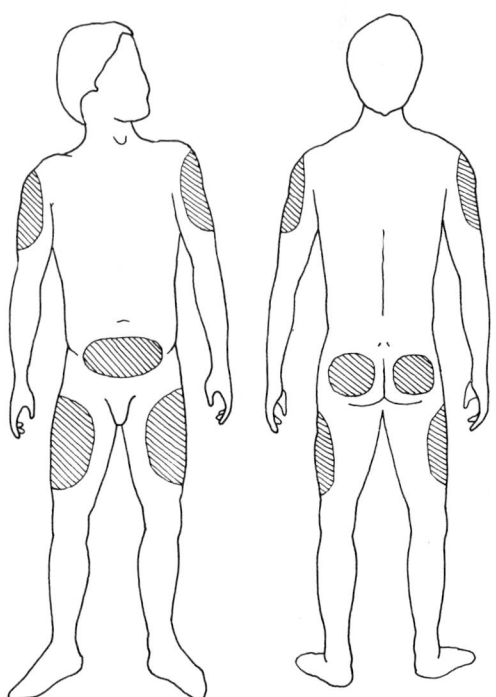

that injection of cold insulin taken directly from the refrigerator may also contribute to the occurrence of lipodystrophy. The condition is reversible if the site is not used for a while. Rotation of sites, then, is most important to prevent lipodystrophy. The formation of fibrous tissue changes the appearance of the site, and the hypertrophy leads to uneven absorption of insulin and loss of pain sensation. Injecting single-peak insulin into the atrophic site may fill the site, but usually insulin is not injected into fibrous or atrophic tissue.

When teaching people how to rotate sites for insulin injection, it is important to inform them about the most convenient and reachable sites for self-administration. The upper arms (avoiding the deltoid area), the thighs, the buttocks, the lumbar area, and the upper abdomen may all be used. The person should develop a routine for rotating sites. Many people keep a record of the site used each day. Others assign a certain site to each day of the week. A single site should not be reused (some authorities advise within each 10-day period) to prevent the occurrence of tissue damage.

It is necessary for the insulin-dependent diabetic patient to administer insulin regularly, at approximately the same time each day, according to his or her living pattern. When the dosage is excessive, hypoglycemia may result. When insulin is omitted for a day, or when the dosage is inadequate, the metabolic coordination achieved by insulin, diet, and other factors is disrupted. If glucose intake continues without sufficient insulin to "cover" the glucose usage, a number of events occur, leading to increased ketone body production. When the patient omits both insulin and dietary intake, gluconeogenesis may be stimulated within the liver. Hyperglycemia and increased production of ketone bodies may result. The presence of ketone bodies in the blood and in the urine is a good indicator of these metabolic processes and indicates the need for insulin.

Rebound hyperglycemia may occur following the administration of increased insulin dosages during periods of stress. Michael Somogyi discovered that rebound hyperglycemia is an aftereffect of insulin-induced hypoglycemia. This phenomenon, the **Somogyi effect,** has implications for stabilizing the diabetic's insulin dosage following stressful events such as surgery. The increased insulin dosage should therefore be sufficient to cover the stress, but not so great as to cause rebound hyperglycemia. Rebound hyperglycemia is difficult to correct as there is a tendency for the patient to go in cycles from states of hypoglycemia in response to insulin back to hyperglycemia as the rebound effect. Each patient's response to insulin is, however, highly individual.

When hyperglycemia occurs, some physicians advise increasing the daily insulin dosage by adding 10 percent of the dosage in regular insulin if ketonuria is measured in two consecutive urine tests. Other physicians prefer to have the diabetic patient continue with the prescribed dosage of insulin and to seek medical assistance if hyperglycemia continues. If hyperglycemia does continue without treatment, or with continued disruption of the treatment pattern, ketoacidosis may result. In addition to insufficient insulin, other factors that can contribute to the development of ketoacidosis are stress, infections, and emotional upsets. Any of the other previously mentioned substances that increase insulin resistance may also lead to hyperglycemia and catabolism of body nutrients, resulting in ketoacidosis.

Persons taking exogenous insulin develop antibodies to insulin. Some persons, in fact, develop antibodies to such an extent that the insulin administered becomes less effective. Attempts to reduce antibody formation from exogenous insulin have not been very effective to date. Insulins prepared from beef or pork are purified and contain about 95% insulin. Therefore, there is a 5 percent remainder which consists of proinsulin, degraded insulin products, and insulin polymers. Single-peak insulin, which is 99 percent pure has been prepared for commercial use. Some studies have shown that even with use of single-peak insulin, antibodies still may develop. Another preparation called single-component insulin, which is 100 percent pure, is being developed and tested.

Acute complications in diabetes The diabetic is subject to development of acute complications, particularly hypoglycemia, ketoacidosis, hyperosmolar coma, and lactic acidosis. While all these complications lead to coma, different physiologic changes take place in each person. Differential diagnosis is necessary to define the appropriate treatment for the specific disorder the diabetic is experiencing. Essentially, **hypoglycemia** occurs when the amount of insulin is in excess of available carbohydrates. Another name for hypoglycemia is insulin shock, and, in the susceptible diabetic, hypoglycemia may precipitate a myocardial infarction. **Ketoacidosis** is the opposite of hypoglycemia; in this condition, the patient has an excess of glucose which cannot be utilized because there is little or no effective insulin for its metabolism. Then excessive fat breakdown occurs. **Hyperosmolar coma** is similar to ketoacidosis in that there is excessive glucose in relation to the amount of effective insulin available for its metabolism. In hyperosmolar coma, there is an accumulation of glucose without the changes in fat and protein metabolism that contribute to ketoacidosis. Increased blood glucose levels result in fluid compartment shifts. **Lactic acidosis** most often occurs as a result of insufficient oxygen delivery to the cells. This type of coma may be caused by many disease processes in the diabetic; for example, the diabetic may have cardiovascular disease, a stroke, or a coronary occlusion, or any of the other conditions that compromise blood supply and subsequently result in coma or shock. Lactic acidosis, then, is not specific to diabetes, but can occur in anyone who suffers anoxia.

Hypoglycemia, the first of the complications to be discussed, occurs when the diabetic has an excess of exogenous insulin. This excess may result from an "overdose" of insulin, that is, administration of more insulin than the diabetic requires. It may also result when the person has decreased dietary intake so that the amount of exogenous insulin administered is more than is required according to the dietary intake. The condition also results when there are changes in the amount of insulin required because of resolution of problems that have led to increased resistance to insulin. This may include resolution of an illness or a stressor or even discontinuing drugs that have caused increased resistance to insulin. These events may all reduce the amount of insulin required because the cellular sensitivity to insulin is improved by resolution of the stressor. Discontinuing the use of drugs such as estrogen or glucocorticoids and termination of a pregnancy are examples of specific factors that lead to improvement of cellular sensitivity to insulin so that the person requires less insulin, even though his carbohydrate intake is maintained. Other causes of hypoglycemia include weight loss, which results in improved diabetic control by reducing the amount of insulin required; increased exercise levels; and satisfactory treatment of diseases such as hyperthyroidism or Cushing's syndrome, both of which are associated with insulin resistance. When the person experiences changes through resolution of an illness, discontinuing drugs that increase insulin resistance, or termination of a pregnancy, it is important that the condition be reevaluated for the purposes of redefining the correct insulin and dietary therapy.

In addition to insulin-dependent diabetic patients, those who are taking sulfonylureas may also develop hypoglycemia. Excessive dosage of sulfonylureas may cause hypoglycemia through their action of increasing the secretion of insulin. Similarly, diabetic patients who develop liver disease may become hypoglycemic if they are taking sulfonylureas, because these drugs are normally deraded in the liver. When degradation does not take place because of liver damage, the effect of the sulfonylureas is increased. In addition, the diseased liver cannot provide glucose through mobilization of glycogen stores through gluconeogenesis. This inability to provide for glucose augments the development of hypoglycemia in diabetics with liver disease who are taking sulfonylureas.

Renal disease in persons who are taking the sulfonylureas also contributes to the development of hypoglycemia. The action of sulfonylureas is increased when the drugs are not excreted in the urine. In renal disease, renal excretion is impaired, so that the drugs become more active.

Alcoholic diabetics being treated with sulfonylureas are also susceptible to hypoglycemia because of the states of malnutrition and starvation resulting from alcoholism. The alcoholic has inhibited substrate flow which reduces the liver's ability for gluconeogenesis. The alcohol is oxidized to acetate. As a result, the coenzyme molecule nicotinamide-adenine dinucleotide (NAD) is diverted from oxidation of substrates that are essential for gluconeogenesis.

Still other factors that contribute to development of hypoglycemia in diabetics who are taking sulfonylureas are antimicrobial sulfa drugs that potentiate the action of sulfonylurea drugs in some people and which may cause exaggerated sulfonylurea activity. The elderly are sometimes noted to have an exaggerated response to sulfonylureas. It is thought that hyperglycemia in the elderly may not always be indicative of diabetes mellitus but that it may be a function of the aging process. For this reason, the status of the elderly person is carefully evaluated prior to beginning therapy for diabetes.

Hypoglycemic coma, also termed **insulin reaction** or **insulin shock,** is the most frequently occurring acute complication of diabetes. Fortunately, hypoglycemic coma can be identified easily and early treatment instituted, thus preventing further complications. Many physicians allow diabetic patients, particularly those requiring exogenous insulin, to experience mild hypoglycemia in controlled situations so that the patient can learn to recognize the signs and symptoms and can institute appropriate treatment before coma ensues.

The individual response to hypoglycemia varies from one instance to another and there is also a wide variation among the signs and symptoms experienced. Although the signs and symptoms often do not occur in definite stages, some authorities refer to four phases of hypoglycemic reaction resulting from insulin shock in an effort to classify the stages of coma. In this classification the first phase, the **parasympathetic phase,** includes signs and symptoms of hunger and nausea; hypotension and bradycardia may be present. The second phase, termed **diminished cerebral function,** is characterized by generalized lethargy and slowed mental responses; speech is slowed and the ability to think and communicate is decreased. In the third, or **sympathetic phase,** there is increased sweating, tachycardia, and increased systolic blood pressure. The fourth phase is **coma,** and **convulsions** may occur [7]. The signs and symptoms of hypoglycemia are even more variable in children than in adults. Not every person has the warning signs and symptoms of hypoglycemia before developing coma; some people are in the third or fourth stage before having an opportunity to recognize and treat mild hypoglycemia.

If the person is aware of the signs and symptoms of hypoglycemia in the early phases, temporary measures can be taken to correct the condition by ingesting a readily accessible form of glucose. It should be noted, however, that not everyone goes through the four phases in the order outlined, but may instead go through all of them so rapidly that the signs and symptoms become severe without the person's awareness. This rapidity accounts for the occurrence of emergency situations in which the diabetic is found in a coma and then is brought to an emergency treatment center. In this instance, glucose is administered intravenously or other measures such as administration of glucagon are initiated. Because the person is often unable to relate the events that may have caused the coma, identification stating that the person is a diabetic is very helpful to the personnel in the emergency treatment center. This identification, in the form of a Medic-Alert bracelet or pendant, often facilitates diagnosis and treatment.

The development of hypoglycemia in diabetics who take insulin usually occurs at the time of the peak insulin effect. Factors such as increased exercise or decreased carbohydrate intake may change the time frame. People who take sulfonylurea drugs may develop hypoglycemia at any time after 30 minutes following their administration. Reactions tend to occur more frequently with the long-acting forms of the sulfonylureas. While it is generally thought that insulin shock or hypoglycemia occurs less frequently in those taking sulfonylureas than in those who are insulin-dependent, it should be recognized that insulin shock can and does occur in diabetic individuals who are treated with sulfonylureas.

When hypoglycemia ensues, blood glucose levels fall below 55 or 60 ml. Blood glucose is diagnostic and a blood specimen is drawn immediately. Some institutions utilize Dextrostix to obtain a rough measure of blood glucose, followed by laboratory evaluation of the blood glucose levels, as Dextrostix is only an indicator and is not always correct. The reaction of Dextrostix is based on an enzyme reaction that can be influenced by moisture, warmth, and light sensitivity. If hypoglycemia is established as the diagnosis, glucose is administered. If the person responds to intravenous administration of glucose, this action may also be considered diagnostic of hypoglycemia.

There are three major methods of treating hypoglycemia: administration of glucose, administration of glucagon, or administration of epinephrine. In the event that hypoglycemia is the established diagnosis, it is important to assess the person's level of consciousness to determine the route of administration of glucose. If the person is conscious and can swallow, oral glucose is given. Otherwise, glucose is administered intravenously, usually in 50% concentrations. The provacative test, mentioned above, includes administration of 50 ml of 50% glucose intravenously. If the person is hypoglycemic, the administration of glucose elicits a positive response. The provocative test provides for diagnosis as well as for treatment if hypoglycemia exists.

In severe hypoglycemia the diabetic may not have sufficient stores of glycogen in the liver. In that event, glucagon may be used to increase glycogenolysis so that liver glycogen can be broken down into glucose. Glucagon can be administered intravenously, intramuscularly, or subcutaneously. If hypoglycemia is mild, 0.5 to 2 mg of glucagon is given. If there is no response to the first injection, a second injection is given in 20 minutes. Oral glucose is given as soon as the person is able to swallow, because the effect of glucagon is of short duration. If the person does not respond to glucagon, 50 ml of 50% glucose is given. Usually the signs and symptoms of hypoglycemia begin to abate within 15 minutes after injection of glucose. When appropriate, the nurse should teach the family to give the glucagon and advise them to keep glucagon on hand in the event that an emergency onset of hypoglycemia occurs.

When neither glucose nor glucagon is available, epinephrine is given subcutaneously (0.5 ml of 1:1,000 solution is given to adults and no more than 0.3 mg of 1:1,000 solution to children). Epinephrine also increases gluconeogenesis and lipolysis. Epinephrine is used to treat the symptoms, but does not rectify the condition.

In some instances of severe coma, glucocorticoids are given in addition to intravenous injection of glucose because of their anti-insulin effects. Their use is adjunctive and is usually confined to situations in which the patient does not respond to therapy or when the shock is severe.

Stabilization is usually readily achieved when the hypoglycemia is not complicated by the presence of diseases such as cardiovascular, renal, or liver diseases. Following stabilization, it is important that the nurse obtain the history of events that precipitated the hypoglycemia in order to evaluate its cause further so that actions can be taken to prevent episodes of hypoglycemia. In some instances, the diabetic who frequently develops hypoglycemia requires teaching to promote better understanding of the treatment regimen so that he can better manage his diabetes, thereby preventing hypoglycemia. In other instances the physiologic status requires evaluation. Some people have poor control, despite their careful following of the treatment regimen. These people are brittle diabetics, and they often find the lack of control frustrating and demoralizing. The nurse should recognize that the brittle diabetic may be frustrated and therefore the teaching plans must focus on meeting the specific needs of this patient for emotional support and informative guidance. The person achieves the maximum possible control when the nurse is supportive rather than punitive or judgmental in discussing the cause and effect of the complications of diabetes mellitus in relation to control through diet, insulin or drugs, and exercise.

The second complication of diabetes mellitus to be discussed is **diabetic ketoacidosis,** an acute and critical complication. The events that occur in diabetic ketoacidosis are similar to those that occur when diabetes is first diagnosed. The development of diabetic ketoacidosis is a gradual process in which the person first notices polyuria, polydipsia, and polyphagia. There may be visual changes as well as constipation and exertional dyspnea. Eventually, the signs and symptoms include nausea, vomiting, and abdominal pain. The person may think that he has influenza or a minor infection when actually the early signs and symptoms of diabetic ketoacidosis are being experienced. Frequently, because the patient is not hungry or thinks that loss of appetite and malaise are caused by influenza, the diabetic neither eats nor takes the usual dose of insulin, thereby increasing the severity of the signs and symptoms of ketoacidosis because of depleted carbohydrate stores and little or no effective insulin for metabolism.

As ketoacidosis progresses, dehydration along with a flushed face and dry mucous membranes develops. The pulse becomes rapid and weak and there may be hypotension. Glycosuria and acetonuria are present as a result of hyperglycemia and ketonemia. Kussmaul's respirations and a distinctive acetone breath with a fruity odor are typical of diabetic ketoacidosis. Insulin levels in the blood are negligible. Stupor and coma are late signs and are not always indicative of the severity of ketoacidosis, being a function of individual response patterns.

Many factors affect the response to therapy in ketoacidosis. Among these are the patient's physical condition prior to the treatment, the duration of the coma, and the degree of the metabolic alterations that have taken place over a period of time. The mechanics of these metabolic alterations are those of adaptive processes utilized by the body when insufficient carbohydrate is available to the body cells because of lack of effective insulin. Essentially, the person in diabetic ketoacidosis is suffering from starvation. Along with the lack of insulin, there is an increase of glucagon, growth hormone, and glucocorticoids, and increased catecholamine levels. These substances are increased as the body attempts to provide for glucose. Fatty acids are mobilized from adipose tissue, because without insulin to keep them stored in the form of triglycerides, lypolysis increases. The lypolytic hormones, mainly glucagon; growth hormones T_3 and T_4; epinephrine and norepinephrine; and ACTH become more active in the absence of effective insulin. This freeing of fatty acids increases the precursors for gluconeogenesis as well as the production of ketone bodies (Fig. 8-9).

The liver takes up the liberated free fatty acids and activates them to the long-chain acetyl CoA. In addition to increased free fatty acids, muscle tissues release amino acids as part of the adaptive response to low glucose levels. The muscle tissues normally release the substrates for gluconeogenesis when insulin levels are low. These substrates include lactate, pyruvate, and amino acids. In the liver, acetyl CoA, the common intermediary among glucose, fatty acid, and amino acid metabolism, is formed from the substrates. Metabolic pathways of ketogenesis and gluconeogenesis are favored when there is a deficiency of insulin. Lipogenesis is decreased, and gluconeogenesis in the liver is the end result and is accompanied by the increased release of both glucose and ketones into the blood.

The ketones that are released are utilized for energy by muscle tissues, and the excess ketones are eliminated in the urine in the form of acetoacetate and beta hydroxybutyrate. When these anions are eliminated in the urine, they are coupled with the cations sodium and potassium, causing loss of these electrolytes. This loss of electrolytes, in addition to the loss of glucose, results in diuresis with symptoms of polyuria and signs and symptoms of dehydration. If the person can ingest fluids and sodium orally, dehydration is delayed; however, when nausea and

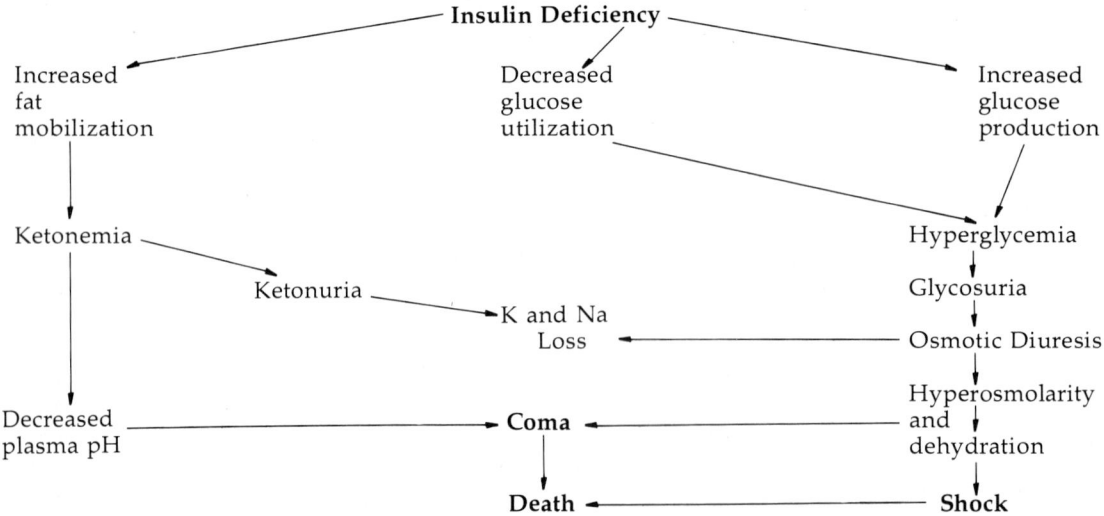

Figure 8-9
The pathogenesis of diabetic ketoacidosis. (Adapted from W. Sodeman, Jr., and W. Sodeman, *Pathologic Physiology*. Philadelphia: W. B. Saunders Company, 1974. Reproduced by permission.)

vomiting occur, loss of sodium increases and the dehydration increases.

The kidneys have a major role in delaying the onset of acute ketoacidosis. In addition to their function of producing glucose in ketoacidosis, the kidneys increase ammonia production and provide for buffering of the ketones. The acetoacetic acid is combined with sodium bicarbonate to form carbonic acid and sodium acetoacetate. The carbon dioxide formed from this buffering is excreted by the lungs while the sodium acetoacetate is eliminated in the urine. Disodium acid phosphate also combines with sodium acetoacetate to be excreted in the urine.

As ketoacidosis progresses, the adaptive mechanisms begin to fail. Even though the liver is functioning to provide for additional glucose, this glucose accumulates in the intravascular spaces, as it cannot be utilized by the cells without insulin. As a result, the plasma becomes hyperosmolar, causing diuresis of water and major electrolytes. If there is no intervention, hypovolemia results and the blood glucose levels continue to increase. Glucose levels may be as high as 1,000 or 1,500 mg per 100 ml.

As the levels of ketone bodies in the blood increase, the person is in a state of metabolic acidosis. In this state, the arterial carbon dioxide levels decrease and bicarbonate increases in greater proportion than the carbon dioxide. The pH falls, so that respirations increase in both rate and depth through the activity of the excess hydrogen ions in the respiratory center. Kussmaul's respirations result. These are deep and rapid respirations alternated with periods of apnea in regular cycles, which usually occur when the pH drops to a level of 7.2. Further complicating the respiratory ventilation difficulties is the development of muscle weakness which compromises the patient's ability to ventilate. The ketoacidosis becomes gradually more severe as the kidneys are increasingly unable to eliminate hydrogen ions through the buffering systems. The decreasing blood volume further decreases the kidney's function and impedes elimination of the hydrogen ions. The occurrence of the signs and symptoms of ketoacidosis is related to all these metabolic processes. Development of coma or impaired cerebral function, or both, is thought to be caused by increased levels of acetoacetate and hydrogen ions, and by the dehydration.

The diagnosis of diabetic ketoacidosis is made by careful evaluation of the patient's signs and symptoms, the history of diabetes mellitus, and laboratory findings. In some instances, the development of diabetic ketoacidosis is the first indication that the person has diabetes mellitus, so that prior diagnosis of the condition is not necessary to confirm diabetic ketoacidosis.

Laboratory values found in diabetic ketoacidosis include elevation of blood glucose levels, elevation of urine glucose and ketone levels, particularly of beta-hydroxybutyrate, decreased blood pH, and decreased arterial carbon dioxide levels. The blood osmolality is increased and various types of electrolyte imbalances, particularly involving sodium and potassium, are present. Intracellular potassium is depleted as the increased hydrogen levels cause potassium to leave the cells. It should be remembered that, without insulin, potassium does not enter the cell as it normally does in conjunction with glucose. For these reasons, the extracellular levels of potassium, which may be normal or elevated, are not indicative of intracellular potassium levels. Sodium levels are usually low, but they may also be normal or high.

Most frequently, emergency treatment is required. Administration of insulin is given priority in this emergency treatment. The initial insulin dose is given intravenously when the person is in coma or when ketoacidosis has progressed. The reason for intravenous administration of insulin is that circulatory impairment is usually present, and because of this circulatory impairment, insulin which has been given subcutaneously may be poorly perfused. The nurse can expect that the patient will not respond until about 6 hours after the initial insulin dosage has been administered. Unlike treatment of hypoglycemia, which is usually associated with a rapid response, the person with ketoacidosis requires a longer period of time before demonstrating a positive response. The metabolic processes that have led to the development of ketoacidosis develop over a long period of time and cannot be reversed immediately with the administration of insulin. Correction of the fluid and electrolyte imbalances as well as the nutritional deprivation associated with diabetic ketoacidosis may require up to 2 weeks for stabilization.

In the initial emergency treatment, the usual dosage of insulin given is 100 units. The dosage of insulin is repeated in lesser amounts on an hourly schedule until the blood glucose level decreases to 300 mg per 100 ml. The usual hourly dosage of insulin is 50 units or more. As much as 300 to 500 units of insulin may be given within the first 24-hour period. If the patient has high insulin resistance or if insulin antibodies are present, even greater dosages of insulin may be required. Glucocorticoids may be given to decrease severe antibody reactions (even though they increase insulin resistance). Reducing the antibody reaction outweighs the insulin resistance caused by glucocorticoids in making insulin more effective. Giving insulin via slow drip infusion is also effective in restoring normoglycemia in some patients.

When the blood glucose levels are decreased sufficiently by administration of insulin, further insulin therapy is calculated on the basis of blood glucose and ketone body levels, as well as by the levels of glycosuria and ketonuria. Essentially, management of the person's condition following resolution of acute ketoacidosis is similar to establishing the initial insulin dosage for newly diagnosed diabetic patients. The insulin dosage is prescribed in relation to dietary intake, and a regimen for long-term care is established.

Insulin therapy in ketoacidosis augments stabilization of both fluid and electrolyte balance. It is necessary, however, to treat the fluid and electrolyte imbalances according to the person's status, as there is great variability in each person's response. Even if ketosis is reduced to more stable levels, the fluid and electrolyte imbalances may cause death if not treated appropriately. Alkali solutions are administered intravenously to treat the acidosis. The nurse must maintain an exact record of intake and output, which serves as a guide to evaluation of kidney function, because kidney function determines, to a great degree, the effectiveness of treatment. In addition to monitoring fluid intake and output, the nurse also carefully monitors the effects of replacement of both sodium and potassium, observes for signs and symptoms of hypokalemia, and carefully monitors the ECG tracings. It is important to remember that intracellular potassium has been depleted and that merely giving additional potassium does not replace intracellular potassium. Instead, the intracellular potassium is replaced along with correction of the metabolic alterations that have occurred in ketoacidosis. When insulin is given, and when glucose is transported to the cells through the action of insulin, potassium can also be transported to the cells. The extracellular potassium levels may be depleted as potassium is transported to the intracellular spaces. Hypokalemia, therefore, continues to be a potential problem until the intracellular levels of potassium as well as the extracellular levels are restored to normal.

Since the person who is in ketoacidosis is suffering from starvation, it is necessary to give glucose when the blood glucose levels are reduced to about 300 mg per 100 ml [2]. This glucose can be given orally when the person's condition permits, but it may be given intravenously if necessary. In some settings, Dextrostix is used to measure blood glucose changes quickly. The nurse must remember that Dextrostix does not give an accurate measurement, but is used instead to determine trends of change. Stabilization from this point includes evaluation of both insulin and diet therapy if further increases in ketoacidosis are to be avoided. Throughout treatment the nurse must continually monitor the patient's condition to maintain the desired progression to normal blood glucose levels as the patient may easily shift from hyperglycemia to hypoglycemia.

The third complication of diabetes mellitus to be discussed is **hyperosmolar coma.** This condition results from elevated concentrations of the blood glucose level, which increases the osmolality of the blood. Intracellular sodium and potassium are generally depleted and the urinary excretion of urea increases. Serum insulin levels are lower than normal. Usually hyperosmolar coma occurs in older diabetic patients, who generally have some cardiovascular or renal disease. In comparison with the incidence of ketoacidosis, hyperosmolar coma occurs more frequently in diabetics with the adult-onset type, while ketoacidosis occurs more frequently in diabetics with the youth-onset type. While all diabetics tend to develop cardiovascular or renal disease, youth-onset type diabetics are more vulnerable to severe degrees of metabolic alterations because they have little or no effective insulin. Hyperosmolar coma occurs more frequently in diabetics who have sufficient insulin to prevent development of ketoacidosis in hyperglycemic states.

In hyperosmolar coma, central nervous system signs and symptoms predominate in the occurrence of seizures or coma. Usually an infection or stressful event precedes the hyperosmolar coma, and the person has enough reserve insulin to prevent development of ketoacidosis even though the blood glucose levels are elevated. In some ways, the development of hyperosmolar coma is similar to the development of diabetic ketoacidosis. The difference between the two is largely in the degree of metabolic alteration.

Elevated blood glucose levels increase the osmolality of the blood so that diuresis and subsequent dehydration occur. With diuresis, both sodium and potassium are excreted and the volume of blood is decreased. Hypovolemia is associated with increased blood viscosity and susceptibility to the development of thrombosis. Renal complications may ensue from hypovolemia so that fluid and electrolyte imbalances occur. There is also an increased incidence of cerebrovascular accidents. It is thought that coma in the hyperosmolar state results from dehydration of cerebral tissues.

Signs and symptoms of hyperosmolar coma develop rapidly. Warning signs include polyuria and polydipsia. The person may disregard these symptoms, thinking that they are not important. Coma occurs suddenly and the person may be found in a comatose state. If coma occurs, the person has all of the signs and symptoms of cellular hypoxia.

Treatment of hyperosmolar coma is similar to the treatment of ketoacidosis. Insulin is given, but in smaller amounts. The intent is to reduce the blood glucose levels gradually; they may have increased to very high levels of 250 to 2,000 mg per 100 ml. It is necessary to treat fluid and electrolyte imbalances, with particular attention to restoring potassium levels to normal. Serum electrolyte values are used as a guide to therapy.

When the person has impaired renal function, dialysis may be necessary. Peritoneal dialysis is selected because of the coexistence of circulatory problems in many persons with hyperosmolar coma. In both ketoacidosis and hyperosmolar coma, there is a possibility of cerebral edema following initial treatment. It is theorized that this cerebral edema occurs either as a result of increased glucose levels in the brain or as a result of the high acidity of the spinal fluid. It is believed that an accumulation of sorbitol (glucose is oxidized to sorbitol and fructose) in the brain may contribute to the incidence of cerebral edema. Treatment includes diuresis. Mannitol or dexamethasone (Decadron) is generally used to achieve this diuresis.

The fourth complication of diabetes mellitus is **lactic acidosis,** resulting from an interference with metabolism at the level of conversion of pyruvate to lactate such as occurs in muscle cells. When shock with anoxia occurs, the reconversion of lactate to pyruvate is hindered, and lactic acid levels increase as anaerobic glycolysis increases. The level of lactate considered normal is 1.0 to 1.5 mM per liter, while the normal pyruvate level is 0.08 to 0.16 mM per liter. The lactate-pyruvate ratio is normally 10:1.

Causes of lactic acidosis include both idiopathic and secondary factors. Idiopathic lactic acidosis has no defined cause at this time. Secondary causes include shock arising from any condition, overdose of drugs, carbon monoxide poisoning, excessive use of ethanol, and barbiturates. Any factor that interferes with oxidative phosphorylation may cause lactic acidosis; insufficient hemoglobin, impaired tissue perfusion, as well as previously mentioned substances such as carbon monoxide or cyanide interfere with oxidative phosphorylation. Ethanol and phenformin (DBI) inhibit gluconeogenesis in the liver and in this way contribute to increased lactic acid levels.

When formed, lactic acid is transferred directly to the brain, where the hydrogen ions of lactic acid stimulate the respiratory center, causing respiratory alkalosis. This adaptive mechanism, however, contributes to the continued formation of lactate, which in turn increases the level of lactic acidosis.

The diagnosis of lactic acidosis in the diabetic is made when lactate levels in the plasma are over 7 mM per liter. The serum bicarbonate is usually low, as are both the pH and the carbon dioxide levels. There are slight or no ketone increases in blood or urine. Sodium may be increased or decreased; potassium may be normal or increased. Often the BUN (blood urea nitrogen) and creatinine levels are increased. Lactic dehydrogenase, transaminases, and amylase levels are sometimes increased. Sodium bicarbonate is given to treat the acidosis, and all drugs are discontinued. The lactic acidosis occurs suddenly and is associated with a high mortality rate. Treatment includes administration of insulin along with fluids and sodium bicarbonate, the alkali of choice in the treatment of lactic acidosis. The amount of insulin required for glucose utilization is usually less than required in ketoacidosis. Fluid and electrolyte therapy is guided by blood levels.

Although the four types of acute complications have been discussed as separate entities, it is important to note that the last three discussed, ketoacidosis, hyperosmolar coma, and lactic acidosis, may occur together. It is more usual to find a combination of these conditions, or that one of these conditions progresses to the other as fluid and electrolyte imbalances and metabolic alterations progress. More specifically, hyperosmolar coma may develop with features of ketoacidosis. Anyone with anoxia from any cause may develop lactic acidosis. Therefore the nurse must be familiar with all the possible complications and must be prepared to initiate appropriate treatment.

Other long-term or more chronic complications of diabetes mellitus include emotional disturbances, a higher than normal incidence of gastrointestinal disturbances, and frequent infections. The emotional disturbances associated with diabetes mellitus are not well understood. Diabetic individuals, particularly those with the youth-onset type, who have poor control, as indicated by frequent incidences of hypoglycemia or ketoacidosis, or both, may eventually have cerebral damage. This may vary from mild to more severe degrees as a result of repeated insults to brain tissue. Diabetic encephalopathy, which refers to degenerative cerebral changes in the diabetic patient, is associated with diabetes mellitus of the youth-onset type because these persons tend to have more severe fluctuations in metabolism. It is thought that this degeneration of brain tissues may be associated with the vascular changes known to accompany diabetes mellitus. Just as emotional changes occur as a result of diabetes, some diabetic individuals may have behavioral patterns that tend toward instability. The ones who have unstable behavior patterns may have difficulty accepting treatment regimens and may be rebellious or refuse to participate in the treatment plan. The frequency of acute complications is usually greater in this group of diabetic patients, who also present a very difficult challenge to the nurse who tries to help them learn to control their diabetes mellitus.

Gastrointestinal disturbances that occur in diabetics as chronic complications of the condition are thought to be related to neuropathy. Diarrhea is the most common effect of neuropathy affecting the gastrointestinal tract. Usually, the diarrhea occurs at night. Treatment is usually symptomatic.

Liver enlargement and dental abscesses are problems which are more common in the diabetic population, as are increased tartar formation and the incidence of pyorrhea. In some diabetic patients, the liver is enlarged because of increased fat deposits. This does not necessarily cause liver dysfunction. Both the dental problems and the liver enlargement may, however, be considered gastrointestinal complications.

Diabetic individuals are more susceptible to development of infections than are healthy persons who are nondiabetics. Urinary tract and skin infections are the most commonly occurring types of infections in diabetics. Skin infections, which are often difficult to control in ordinary circumstances, are even more difficult to control in the diabetic, and present a challenge for expert and precise nursing care. Fungal and staphylococcal infections tend to be predominant in diabetics. For this reason, diabetics must take exceptionally good care of their skin. It is imperative that the nurse teach the person to seek treatment immediately in the event an infection occurs. Recovery from bacterial or mycotic infections is generally slower in diabetics than in nondiabetics who are healthy.

Diabetics who are underweight and who are insulin-dependent tend to have a high incidence of tuberculosis. Of all the illnesses that the diabetic is susceptible to, however, vascular diseases account for the most common cause of death. Youth-onset type diabetes is associated with neuropathy as a common cause of death. The life expectancy for youth-onset type diabetics is decreased in relation to the age of onset; the earlier the age of onset, the shorter the life expectancy.

In addition to the chronic complications that occur with diabetes, the disease itself progresses in some people to include the vascular and neurologic changes described earlier as part of the diabetes mellitus disease syndrome. The rapidity and the degree of severity of these symptoms and signs of neural and vascular dysfunction vary considerably.

The health practices important to maintaining good circulation (see Chap. 4) must be observed by the diabetic. This care includes protection of the extremities from trauma or injury, excellent foot care, and positive measures for prevention of circulatory distress. The diabetic must always seek prompt treatment for any wounds.

Loss of vision is a serious occurrence in the diabetic, who will require individualized care while learning to adapt to the loss. (Care of the visually handicapped person is described in Chap. 12.) The diabetic who is generally debilitated requires very gentle and realistic care, with emphasis on participation in life events within his or her capabilities.

Despite complications, it is possible for many diabetics to live a happy and productive life if they have learned to cope with their disorder. The nurse has a very important role in teaching the patient from the time diagnosis is established. To be successful in adapting to the disease, the diabetic must incorporate the therapeutic principles of medication, diet, and exercise into his or her life style, as well as the preventive measures for good skin care and avoidance of infections or trauma. When all these aspects of care become as customary as brushing one's teeth, the diabetic can feel less restricted or limited by the diabetes mellitus. The nurse should remain aware that the diabetic requires ongoing evaluation of physical status and corresponding treatment and emotional support as well as reinforcement of information important to the continuing adaptation to the disorder. As in the case of other chronic diseases, the treatment for diabetes changes over time, because of new findings in research and experimentation. As yet, there is no conclusive evidence that diabetes is caused by either viruses or by a combination of autoimmune factors or genetic susceptibility.

A number of aids are available for teaching patients and their families about diabetes and its management. Information and materials can be obtained from the

American Diabetes Association, Inc.
600 Fifth Avenue
New York, New York 10020

Periodicals to which the diabetic can subscribe to include

ADA Forecast
(American Diabetes Association; a bimonthly publication)

Diabetes in the News
Ames Company, Elkhart, Indiana 46514
(A quarterly publication)

The Diabetic Journal
Education for Health, Inc.
205 Deerwood Lane
Minneapolis, Minnesota 55427
(A quarterly publication)

Hypoglycemia in Nondiabetics

Hypoglycemia in nondiabetics is usually caused by metabolic derangements due to factors other than treatment for diabetes mellitus. The glucose level in hypoglycemia falls below 65 mg per 100 ml and may be a precursor of diabetes, the hypoglycemia being followed by hyperglycemia after a period of time elapses. Any factor that interferes with glucose metabolism may lead to hypoglycemia. Among these factors are genetic disorders; liver disease; pituitary, thyroid, or adrenal dysfunction; and tumors of the pancreas.

The genetic disorders include impaired reactions to galactose, fructose, leucine, and glucose. Leucine-related disorders are most common in children whereas glucose-related disorders are more common in adults. The genetic type of hypoglycemia is usually called reactive hypoglycemia, and in this type the blood glucose level falls approximately 5 hours after a meal but rises again in 15 to 20 minutes. During the hypoglycemic period, the person may have a number of symptoms that are related to the low level of blood glucose. The signs and symptoms range from sweaty palms, tremors, and nervousness to complete loss of consciousness. The pathologic factor may be within the pancreas (causing hypersecretion of insulin) or at the cellular level (due to factors that increase the resistance to insulin), or at any point in the metabolism of glucose.

Hypoglycemia following gastric surgery usually occurs 1½ to 3 hours after meals. One theory about the reason for its occurrence is that hypertonic glucose reaches the small intestine more rapidly than normal because the action of the pyloric sphincter is impaired. A second theory is that the normal delay of delivery of food to the small bowel does not occur following the removal of a large portion of the stomach.

The largest population with hypoglycemia are those persons with functional hypoglycemia. This form is not considered to be related to genetic impairment of glucose metabolism or to a specific event such as gastric surgery. The affected are generally tense and compulsive people and they tend to have gastric hypermotility or irritable colon, or both. One theory as to cause is that there is a greater than normal secretion of catecholamines which increases sympathetic activity.

In general, a person with hypoglycemia has exaggerated insulin responses. When the hypoglycemia occurs as a precursor to diabetes mellitus, it is thought that the beta cell function is impaired and that insulin reserves are being diminished. When insulin reserves are sufficiently low, the signs and symptoms of diabetes mellitus become evident.

Treatment in nondiabetic hypoglycemia consists mainly in dietary therapy. Carbohydrate intake is restricted and a high protein diet is mandatory because the amino acids yielded by proteins do not stimulate the release of insulin at as high a rate as do carbohydrates.

When gastric motility may be related to hypoglycemia, anticholinergic drugs are given to inhibit vagal action and to delay gastric emptying. Stimulants such as coffee and cigarettes, as well as phenobarbital, are avoided. Following dietary therapy, the person usually feels better. Some authorities believe that adherence to a carbohydrate-restricted diet and avoidance of stimulants and phenobarbital improve the patient's health because improved health practices are being followed.

Other Metabolic Disorders

Although rare, genetic disorders in the metabolism of galactose, fructose, and leucine should be mentioned. **Galactosemia** is the inability to metabolize galactose, which is found in milk lactose; the disorder is transmitted as an autosomal recessive gene. Treatment is simply the elimination of galactose from the diet. People who have galactosemia may also have liver disease and a tendency to develop cataracts. Galactosemia may be the cause of mental retardation in some infants. **Fructose intolerance** is also transmitted by an autosomal recessive gene and is related to deficiency of hepatic fructose 1-phosphate aldolase. Symptoms include severe hypoglycemia accompanied by vomiting. **Leucine hypersensitivity** usually becomes apparent in the first 2 years of life; it causes hypoglycemia because the leucine augments the release of insulin.

Other hereditary disorders of glucose metabolism include **inborn errors of gluconeogenesis,** usually a result of enzyme defects inherited as autosomal recessive genes. Patients with this disorder have decreased glycogen stores and cannot produce glucose during fasting states. Treatment consists in frequent feedings with high-protein diets.

Insulinoma is an uncommon condition in which there is abnormal storage and release of insulin caused by tumors of the islet cells of the pancreas. The condition occurs in both sexes and most frequently between the ages of 30 and 60 years. The person affected has high levels of insulin in circulation. This high level of circulating insulin impedes liver gluconeogenesis. The signs and symptoms of insulinoma include hunger, nausea, sweating, headache, diplopia, dilated pupils, and pale moist skin. Abnormal behavior and disturbances in consciousness may be exhibited. Often the symptoms are not consistent and they come and go without an established pattern.

Treatment usually involves surgical resection of the pancreas. Dietary management or infusions of glucose may be necessary.

References

1. Eaton, R. P. Evolving role of glucagon in human diabetes mellitus. *Diabetes* 24:523, 1975.
2. Guthrie, D. W., and Guthrie, R. A. Coping with diabetic ketoacidosis. *Nursing 73* 3:15, 1973.
3. Knatterud, G. L., Klint, C. R., Osborne, R. K., Meinter, C. L., Martin, D. B., and Hawkins, B. S. A study of the effects of hypoglycemic agents on vascular complications with adult onset diabetes. V. Evaluation of phenformin therapy. *Diabetes* 24:65, 1975.
4. Mountcastle, V. B. *Medical Physiology*, Vol. 2 (13th ed.). St. Louis: Mosby, 1974.
5. Selkurt, E. *Basic Physiology for the Health Sciences.* Boston: Little, Brown, 1975.
6. Sodeman, W., Jr., and Sodeman, W. *Pathologic Physiology*. Philadelphia: Saunders, 1974.
7. Waife, S. O. *Diabetes Mellitus.* Indianapolis: Lilly Research Laboratories, Eli Lilly and Company, 1973.

8. West, K. M. Substantial differences in the diagnostic criteria used by diabetes experts. *Diabetes* 24:641, 1975.
9. Walker, S. Sugar doctors push hypoglycemia. *Psychol. Today* 9:68, 1975.
10. Williams, R. *Textbook of Endocrinology* (5th ed.). Philadelphia: Saunders, 1974.

Bibliography

Azaroff, D. L. *Steroid Therapy*. Philadelphia: Saunders, 1975.

Bondy, P. K., and Rosenberg, L. E. *Duncan's Diseases of Metabolism: The Genetic and Biochemical Basis of Disease* (7th ed.). Vol. 1, *Genetics and Metabolism*. Philadelphia: Saunders, 1974.

Danowski, T. S. *Diabetes Is a Way of Life*. New York: Coward-McCann & Geoghegan, 1974.

Hall, R., Anderson, J., Smart, G. A., and Besser, G. M. *Clinical Endocrinology* (2nd ed.). Philadelphia: Lippincott, 1974.

Kramer, C. H., and Kramer, J. R. *Basic Principles of Long-Term Patient Care*. Springfield, Ill.: Thomas, 1976.

Paloyan, E., Lawrence, A. M., and Straus, F. H. *Hypoparathyroidism*. New York: Grune & Stratton, 1973.

Salzer, J. E. Classes to improve diabetic self-care. *Am. J. Nurs.* 75:1324, 1975.

Schwartz, T. B., and Ryan, W. G. (eds.). *The Yearbook of Endocrinology*. Chicago: Year Book, 1976.

Spencer, R. *Patient Care in Endocrine Problems*. Monographs in Clinical Nursing, No. 4. Philadelphia: Saunders, 1973.

Wiley, L. Diabetic out of control. *Nursing 73* 3:10, 1973.

chapter 9
Patients with Reproductive System Dysfunction

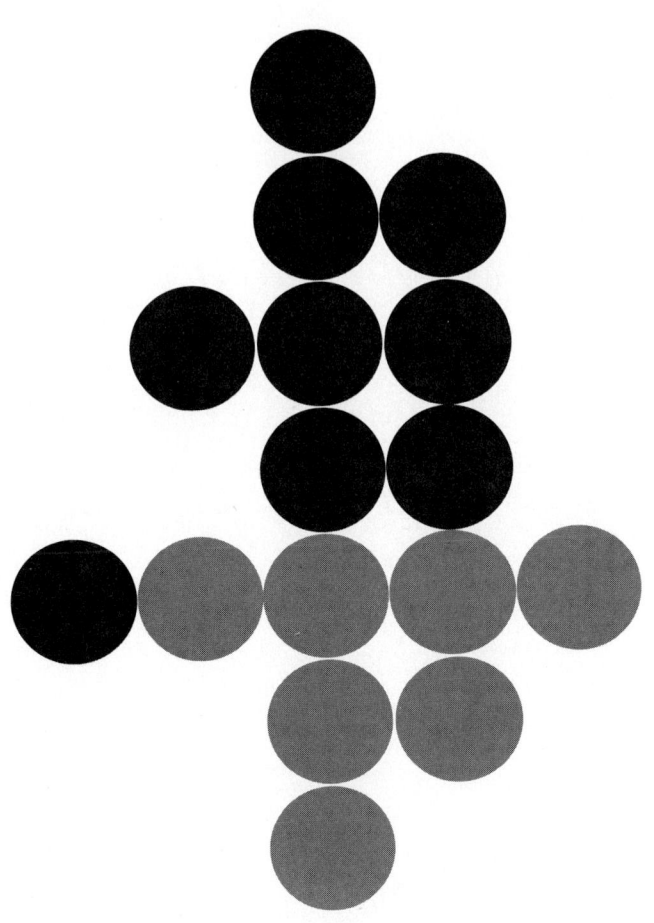

The primary function of the male and female reproductive systems is procreation, a requisite for continuation of human life. Because this primary function is essential, the impact of reproductive system dysfunction is a complex aggregate of physiologic discomfort and imbalance, psychological stress conditioned by cultural and personal values, and individual experiences. From a physiologic view the reproductive system, although primarily endocrinic in nature, is interdependent with the nervous, circulatory, and metabolic functions in the body. Psychologically the functions of the reproductive system are necessary for the development of a sense of self as determined by the individual genetic makeup (male or female) and the individual social and cultural implications of sexuality for the development of body image, self-concept, and personal well-being.

Procreation, requiring a male and female, also has significance in interpersonal relationships. The entire spectrum of developing male and female relationships, mating, marriage, and both single or family life are influenced by a person's sexuality. In and of itself procreation is an awe-inspiring phenomenon. Human concern with procreation is imbued with its essential nature and the personal and social implications of having children that are unique for individuals. Both individual family planning and world population control measures are current concerns related to personal values and beliefs and to the broader concern for support of the populations.

Human sexuality is a basic component of life, and sexual needs are intertwined with human needs for companionship. Some people enter into heterosexual relationships whereas others form homosexual relationships in their desire to meet these basic needs. In both types of relationships there is human interaction. Coitus is the most common means for sexual gratification in heterosexual relationships whereas male homosexuals use fellatio and anal intercourse; female homosexuals (lesbians) achieve sexual gratification through mutual masturbation and oral-genital contacts [27]. Some people achieve sexual gratification in both homosexual and heterosexual relationships. There is a great deal of variation in the types of activities people use to achieve sexual gratification, and sexual behaviors are highly individual. The nurse is therefore cognizant that sexuality and means of attaining sexual gratification are influenced by cultural and personal values and, as with other aspects of human relationships, respects each person's individual attitudes, beliefs, and practices as a part of that person's behavioral pattern. The nurse also recognizes that some people (including some nurses) are in conflict about their sexual roles and preferences. Nurses may normally feel threatened when dealing with individuals whose sexual values and attitudes are different from their own. It is therefore important that the nurse recognize his or her personal coping mechanisms and that these mechanisms should not compromise the professional care given.

Some sexually active persons tend to be vulnerable to certain types of dysfunction such as reproductive tract infections and genital lesions. Some of these infections and lesions are related to exposure of the genitals. There are many other types of reproductive tract dysfunction; some are related to infertility, others to changes in cell growth, and still others to the influences of the aging process.

When caring for persons with reproductive system dysfunction, the nurse deals not only with the dysfunction but also with the implications of that dysfunction in terms of personal and social values. As with many essential aspects of human life, problems arise when there is an inability to carry out function or the products of function are in excess, or when there is a wish to control function. The nurse encounters people who have too many children, people who are unable to have children, people who have carefully controlled the size of their families, and people who do not wish to have children. Human desires and wants are not always in keeping with actual status in this regard, causing conflict in relation to reproductive system dysfunction.

The essential function of procreation is associated with basic pleasurable experiences considered necessary to the sense of well-being. The ability to participate in sexual intercourse is a basic human need. When there is dysfunction of the reproductive system, this relationship is affected. Homosexual relationships can also be affected by reproductive tract dysfunction. Some of the types of reproductive system dysfunction discussed in this chapter result from sexual activity, others result from either primary or secondary disorders and often disrupt sexual activities. The nurse must therefore not only provide care directed toward alleviating the physiologic signs and symptoms of dysfunction but must also relate to the meaning of the dysfunction in terms of the affected person's needs and emotions.

Hormonal Factors in Reproductive Tract Function

Sexual maturity (puberty) is usually reached between the ages of 10 and 14. Females have a defined period of life during which they are capable of reproductive function beginning with **menarche,** the onset of menstruation, and ending with **menopause,** the cessation of menstruation. Males are capable of reproduction from the onset of puberty until old age. The **gonads** (ovaries in females and testes in males) are the primary reproductive organs. In females, the ovaries contain ova; in males, the testes form sperm. In both sexes the gonads secrete sex hormones. These sex hormones—estrogens and progesterone in females, and testosterone in males—are secreted in response to both positive and negative feedback systems. Releasing hormones secreted by the hypothalamus influence the secretion of gonadotropins by the anterior pituitary. The gonadotropins in turn influence secretion of hormones by the gonads.

There are about 1 million germ cells (ova) present in the female at birth and these cells both mature and regress throughout life. In the male, sperm are formed continuously along the length of the seminiferous tubules contained in the testes. Hundreds of millions of sperm are formed each day, and the maturation of a sperm takes about 60 days. Hormone production in the female ovary takes place in the theca interna and granular cells of the ovarian follicle, which secrete 17β-estradiol and estrone (the major estrogens); progesterone is secreted by the corpus luteum. The corpus luteum is formed from the collapsed ovarian follicle following ovulation (release of the ovum). The corpus luteum lasts for about 12 days. Testosterone, the major male sex hormone, is secreted in the Leydig cells (the interstitial cells) of the testes. Androgens are secreted in the adrenal cortex in both sexes. All these hormones are steroids.

The anterior pituitary secretes the gonadotropins **follicle-stimulating hormone** (FSH), which stimulates the growth and development of the ovarian follicle in females and spermatogenesis in the seminiferous tubules in males, and **luteinizing hormone** (LH), which contributes to the production and secretion of follicular hormones, increases the blood flow to the ovary, has a synergistic action with FSH for follicular development in females, and stimulates the Leydig cells of the testes to secrete testosterone in males. Both FSH and LH secretions by the anterior pituitary are stimulated by gonadotropin-regulating hormone (GnRH), which is secreted by the hypothalamus.

17β-Estradiol and estrone levels are highest in the preovulatory period in females; very small amounts of estrogens are stored. Estrogens are inactivated by the liver and excreted mainly by the kidney. The estrogens are necessary for the development and maintenance of the female reproductive tract including the fallopian tubes, uterus, vagina, and external genitalia (Fig. 9-1). The fallopian tubes transport ovum to the uterus via the cilia in the mucosal lining and by peristalsis, that is, the rhythmic contraction of both longitudinal and circular smooth muscles. Estrogen increases the activity of cilia and the contractility of the smooth muscles of the fallopian tubes. It also increases the thickness of the uterine walls, the height and number of endometrial cells, the number and length of endometrial glands, and the blood flow and water content. In addition, estrogen stimulates the growth of the spiral coiled vessels in the uterine wall and the muscular activity of the uterus by increasing the amount of the contractile proteins actin and myosin.

Estrogen affects the cervix by stimulating secretion of thin, watery mucus; the vaginal mucosa becomes thickened and there is cornification of vaginal epithelium from the action of estrogen. There are glycogen deposits in the intermediate and superficial layers of the vaginal epithelium. Glycogen breakdown produces lactic acid, which contributes to maintaining vaginal acidity, thereby diminishing the potential of infection. The pH of the vaginal secretions is normally 3.8 to 4.2. Estrogen also is necessary for the growth and development of mammary glands, including the development of the areola and nipples. Systemically, estrogens accelerate maturation of bone, contribute to the fusion of epiphyseal plates in long bones, and are responsi-

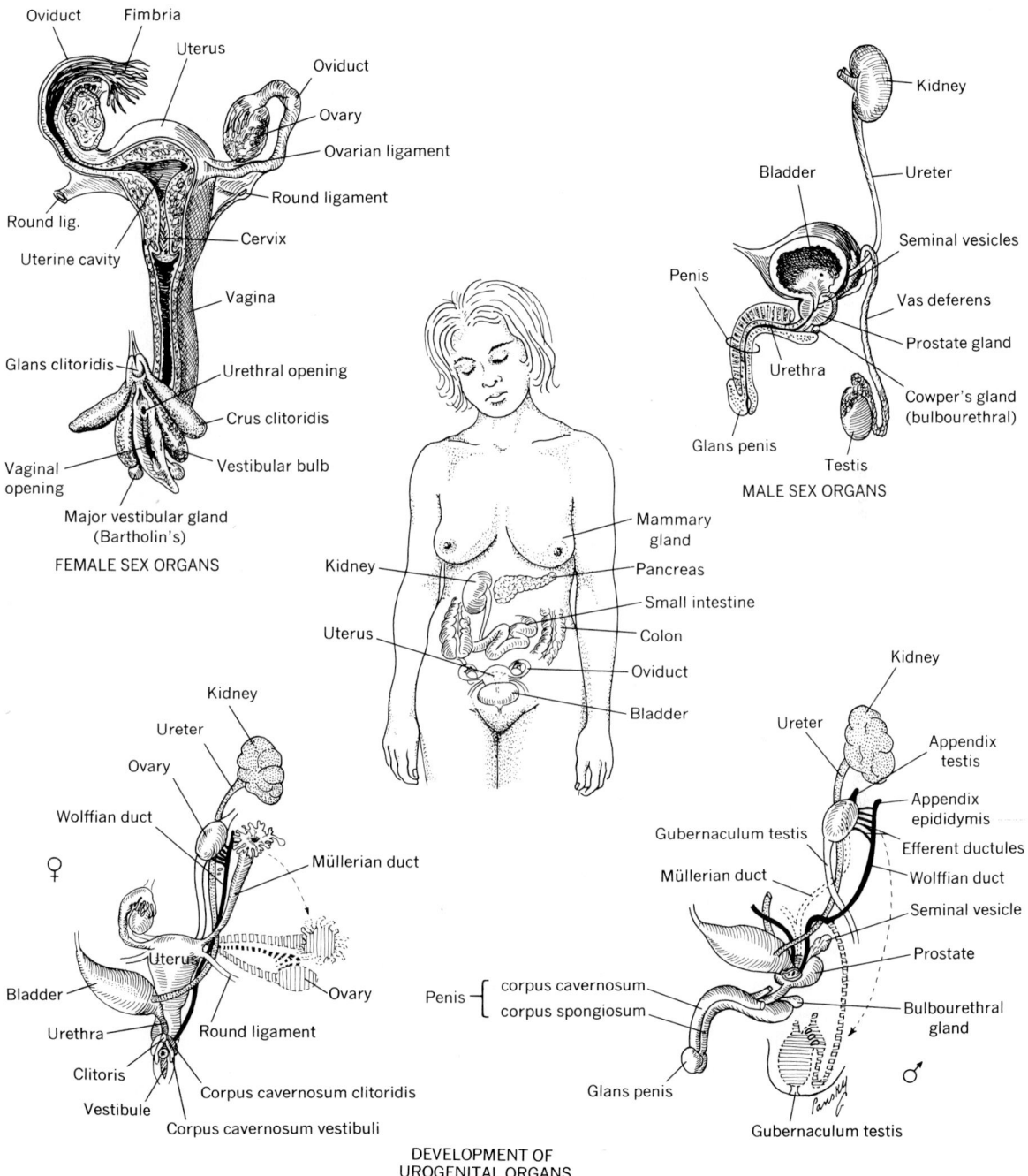

Figure 9-1
Female and male pelvic visceral embryology. The mature male and female reproductive tracts are also seen. (From B. Pansky, *Dynamic Anatomy and Physiology*. New York: Macmillan Publishing Company, 1975. Reproduced by permission.)

ble for fat deposits and changes in bone structure in the pelvis and shoulder associated with female characteristics.

Progesterone is the hormone of pregnancy and prepares the uterus for implantation of the fertilized ovum as well as maintains the ovum following implantation.

Testosterone, the major male hormone, supports the growth and development of masculine characteristics and is required for maintenance of these characteristics throughout life. Testosterone promotes protein anabolism, thereby contributing to tissue growth and influencing the nervous system by promoting muscular activity and aggressiveness [20].

The effects of the sex hormones are visible in body characteristics including hair growth, skin texture, bone structure, deposition of fat, voice, and in the development of the secondary sex organs (mammary glands and testes). As with other hormones, the sex hormones have general systemic functions and are influenced by and capable of influencing other hormones in the body in general regulation of body function. For example, estrogens antagonize the action of growth hormone.

Green cites several studies conducted to establish a biologic basis for homosexuality or heterosexuality [6]. In one study it was determined that testosterone levels and the sperm count are reduced in male homosexuals; the findings of this study are not definitive, however, because stress is known to reduce testosterone levels. This stress factor was evidenced by males who were in military combat in World War II and who demonstrated lower urinary excretion rates of testosterone and lower levels of plasma testosterone [6]. In another study the ratio of urinary etiocholanalone to androsterone, the metabolites of testosterone, was found to differ between homosexual and heterosexual males. It is questioned whether this ratio is the effect of other metabolic processes rather than an indication of biologic sexual preference; subsequent studies of urinary excretion of the metabolites of testosterone have not consistently confirmed the finding that the ratio differs between homosexual and heterosexual males. Some female homosexuals have been found to have lower levels of estrogen and higher than normal levels of testosterone [6].

Dysfunction of the reproductive system is complex because of its emotional impact and because the system is subject to influences of other body organs and systems. The reproductive system is influenced by emotions via the nervous system, by endocrine imbalances, and by both positive and negative feedback within the endocrine system. Metabolic function is also influenced by and influences endocrine function, and the nutritional status and endocrine function are closely aligned. It is therefore difficult to differentiate between primary and secondary causes of reproductive system dysfunction of endocrine origin. The anatomic locations of the male and female reproductive tracts subject the tract to pressure from surrounding abdominal organs. In addition, the proximity of the reproductive tract to the urinary tract makes it susceptible to secondary infection. The vaginal orifice is close to the urinary meatus in females, and the vas deferens in males opens into the prostatic urethra. The reproductive tract is also subject to bacterial invasion from external sources entering the tract through the vagina or the glans penis. Finally, the reproductive tract is affected by congenital abnormalities, acquired cellular changes, aging and degeneration, infectious or inflammatory processes, or abnormal cell growth. The discussion of reproductive dysfunction is limited to the more common conditions that occur in an adult's life cycle and does not include many of the endocrine or congenital classifications of dysfunction.

Nursing Assessment

THE PATIENT'S HISTORY

The patient's history is meaningful in the evaluation of reproductive system dysfunction and in determining appropriate nursing care. The nurse first creates trust by treating the patient with respect and conveying a sense of caring, thereby establishing a rapport which will enable the patient to share feelings and concerns in an atmosphere of confidence. Some patients, however, may be reluctant or embarrassed about discussing their signs and symptoms, and the nurse therefore must tactfully direct the interview to the patient's specific problems. The nurse must demonstrate an objective and nonjudgmental attitude to the information given by the patient. The problems presented by the patient with dysfunction of the reproductive system encompass the distress caused by the physical signs and symptoms, the perceptions of the causes of dysfunction, and the concern for the implications of the dysfunction in terms of self-concept and relationships with others. The nurse must realize that patients often associate these signs and symptoms with the concept of self. In the course of the history-taking interview, the astute nurse is alert for expressions of feelings, values, fears, and worries about the problems being discussed. The nurse directs the interview toward exploration of the patient's perception of the problems, obtaining specific information about the nature of the past and present signs and symptoms (onset, duration, precipitating causes), previous medications or treatments, and the results of their use.

Male patients are asked to describe abnormal drainage from the glans penis, changes in urination (particularly hesitancy or frequency); female patients are asked for the date of the last menstrual period, the frequency, duration, and usual rate of menstrual flow, and whether they experience pain or discomfort such as cramping and premenstrual signs and symptoms. In addition, information on irregular or unusual bleeding or vaginal discharge, the use of contraceptive devices or birth control pills, and past pregnancies, deliveries, abortions, or miscarriages is elicited. The presence of pain, tenderness, or other discomfort should be described by both male and female patients in relation to site, onset, precipitating factors, duration, methods used to alleviate the pain, and the effects of these methods. At the same time, the nurse observes the patient's affect and encourages free expression to convey assurance that he or she is understood, that the feelings being expressed are important, and that the physical examination and subsequent diagnostic tests, if any are required, will be beneficial although somewhat uncomfortable at times.

EXAMINATION OF THE REPRODUCTIVE SYSTEM

Physical examination of the reproductive system includes examination of the abdomen, the external genitalia, the rectum, and, in females, the pelvis and the breasts. Patients may be embarrassed by examination of the reproductive tract, and the nurse helps to minimize this embarrassment by the tone set in the history-taking interview and by conducting the examination in an orderly manner that conveys competence, purpose, understanding, and respect. Recognition of the patient's feelings helps to encourage the patient to discuss embarrassing aspects of the examination. It is necessary to have the patient as relaxed as possible to prevent tensing of muscles, which interferes with the examination.

Prior to physical examination the patient is asked to empty the urinary bladder so that the pelvic organs can be palpated easily. (A distended urinary bladder can be mistaken for a lower abdominal mass.) Assessment begins with examination of the abdomen, as discussed in Chapter 7. Normally the ovaries and uterus cannot be palpated in an abdominal examination. Tumors in either of these organs may appear as an asymmetrical mass below the umbilicus and can sometimes be found on abdominal palpation. An ovarian cyst may be felt as a mass near the midline of the suprapubic area, and tumors of either ovarian or uterine origin are dull on percussion. Large pelvic tumors may displace air toward the upper abdomen so that tympany may be heard. Abdominal tenderness may indicate the presence of either an infectious or an inflammatory process in the reproductive tract. The exact location of tenderness or pain is defined in terms of whether maximum tenderness occurs on light or deep palpation and whether there is rebound tenderness.

A good light source is necessary for examination of the external genitalia. Examination of the external genitalia in males includes inspection and light palpation. The pubic hair varies in distribution and amount and generally is not significant. The penis and scrotum are observed. If circumcized, the male has no foreskin (prepuce). When present, the foreskin is retracted from the head of the glans penis. Normally **smegma,** a thick whitish secretion, collects beneath the foreskin. **Phimosis** is a narrowing of the opening of the foreskin and is detected when the foreskin is not easily retracted from the head of the glans penis. The penis is observed for the presence of lesions, inflammation, or edema. The urethral meatus normally opens when slight pressure is placed near the end of the penis; failure to open easily indicates the presence of scars. Light palpation is used to determine the presence of either edema or tenderness of the shaft of the penis.

The scrotum, testes, epididymis, and spermatic cord are examined by palpation. Normally the skin of the scrotal sac is wrinkled in appearance. Both the scrotal sac and perineal areas are inspected. Skin lesions or reddened areas are noted in terms of distribution, size, and type of lesion and these areas are lightly palpated for swelling or edema. The color, consistency, and odor of discharge, if any, is noted. The scrotal sac is palpated gently to locate the testes, epididymis, and spermatic cord. With the index and middle fingers the examiner separates the testes and examines each testis bimanually by holding the testis in one hand and lightly palpating with the other hand in order to determine the presence of masses or inconsistency. The size of each testis is noted. The epididymis and spermatic cord are normally palpable from the lower pole of the testis along its passage to the spermatic cord, which continues to pass upward and which can be felt in the inguinal canal through the scrotal sac. The vas deferens is felt as a thin, wire-like line within the spermatic cord. Masses or areas of tenderness are noted according to size and consistency or extent.

Rectal examination is also discussed in Chapter 7. Specific findings in rectal examination in the male pertinent to the reproductive tract are swelling, masses, and tenderness of the prostate gland (Fig. 9-2). Firm masses indicate tumors whereas softer, more resilient enlargement indicates hypertrophy of the prostate gland; a boggy resilient enlargement may indicate inflammation.

Examination of the female external genitalia includes inspection and light palpation. The labia majora are inspected for swelling, masses, lesions, varicosities, or hematomas. Separating the labia majora, the nurse inspects the labia minora, the clitoris, and the urethral meatus. Any drainage or signs of inflammation or infection are noted. Vaginal examination requires a speculum warmed to body temperature and moistened with water prior to insertion. Speculums are available in different sizes, and smaller speculums are used for patients with smaller vaginas. The patient is asked to assume a

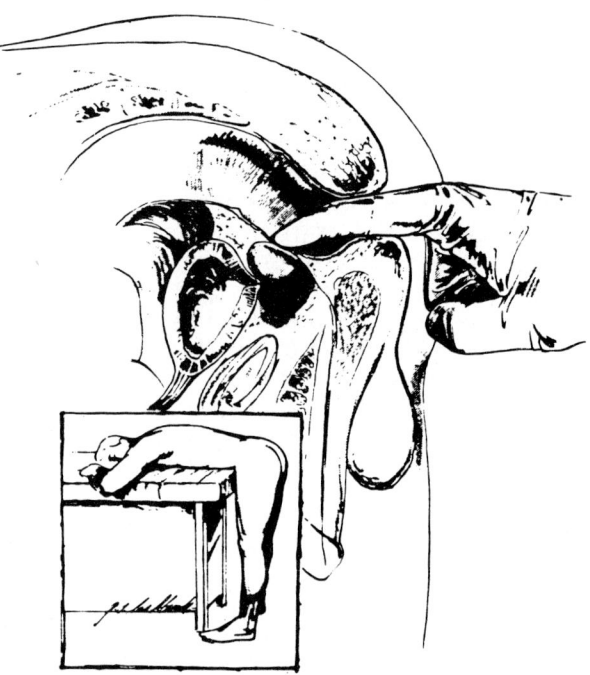

Figure 9-2
Examination of the prostate gland. (From J. M. Sana and R. D. Judge, *Physical Appraisal Methods in Nursing Practice*. Boston: Little, Brown and Company, 1975. Reproduced by permission.)

dorsal lithotomy position and is carefully draped. After the external genitalia are inspected and the vagina is examined with the fingers to note the consistency and smoothness of the vaginal mucosa and to locate the opening of the cervix (which, in the nonpregnant woman, is said to feel like the tip of a nose), the speculum is inserted into the vagina with gentle pressure and is rotated to follow the contours of the vaginal canal. To prevent contamination, lubrication other than water is not used if a specimen is to be obtained for cytologic study. Female patients should have a Papanicolaou (Pap) examination at least yearly or more frequently if the signs and symptoms of potential malignancy such as bleeding between menstrual periods occur. Therefore the Papanicolaou smear test is carried out routinely during pelvic examination if the patient has not had one within the year. Papanicolaou smears, discussed in Chapter 1, are a major preventive screening measure for detection of malignancy in the early stages.

The speculum is inserted and the cervix is

exposed by separating the blades of the speculum. It may be necessary to manipulate the speculum to locate the cervix. The cervix can be identified by its bright red color, which is clearly demarcated from the light pink of the vaginal mucosa. The specimen for the Papanicolaou smear is obtained by using a sterile cotton-tipped applicator, a wooden tongue blade, or a cytologic spatula firmly rolled around the walls of the cervical os (opening). The specimen thus collected is placed on a slide, made readily available prior to inserting the speculum. A specimen is also collected from the pool of vaginal secretions and may be collected by aspiration. Specimens of vaginal secretions or drainage are sent to the laboratory for culture tests to determine the presence of infection. Observation of the cervix exposed by the speculum includes notation of the color, such as abnormal redness, and the presence of lesions, erosions, polyps, or bleeding. The cervical os may be lacerated from trauma or everted (ectropion). The cervical os is dilated in females who have borne a child (parous). The vaginal wall is also observed for color, ulceration, polyps, or other lesions, and texture. Vaginal discharge may indicate inflammation or infection. Leukorrhea is often normal but may indicate dysfunction. Whitish, yellowish, or brownish discharge may indicate inflammation or infection.

A bimanual examination is conducted with the index and middle fingers of one hand placed in the vagina and the opposite hand placed on the abdominal wall (Fig. 9-3). When the patient is asked to bear down, the ligaments supporting the uterus are felt. The examining hand on the abdomen is used to gently palpate in the direction of the symphysis pubis from the iliac crest, so that the pelvic structures are placed in contact with the palpating fingers in the vagina. Areas of tenderness or pain elicited by this manipulation are noted. The cervix, normally freely movable, is moved from side to side by the intravaginal fingers held close to the posterior vaginal wall, which is longer than the anterior wall, to detect the size and firmness of the uterus. This part of the examination can be

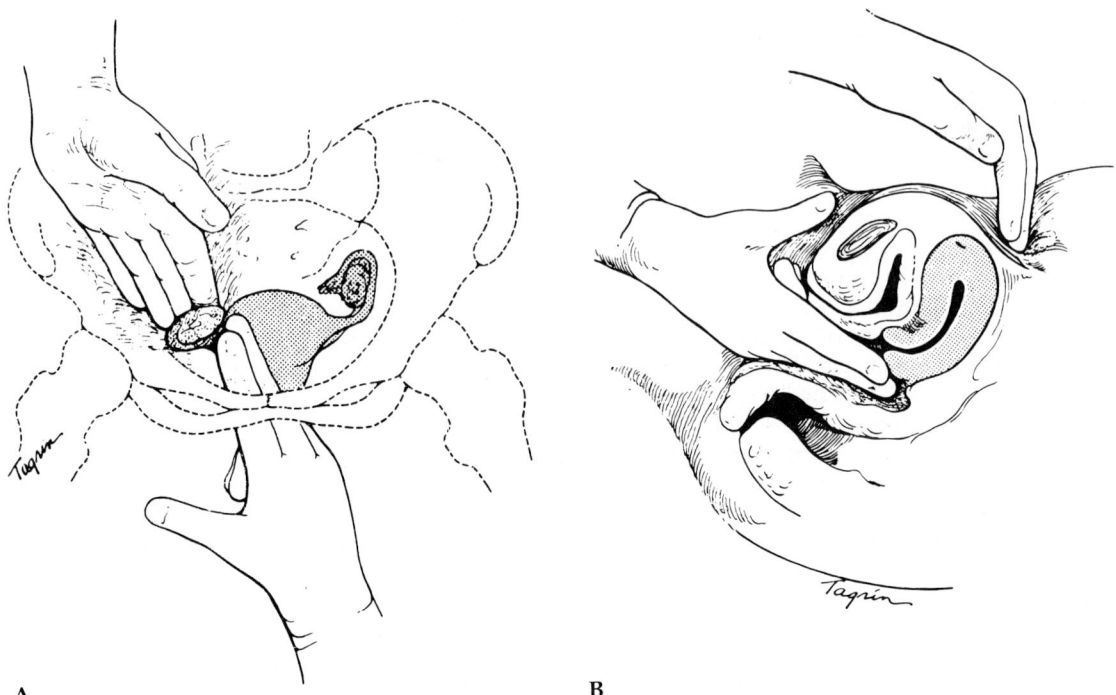

A B

Figure 9-3
A. Bimanual abdominovaginal palpation of the adnexa. **B.** Bimanual abdominovaginal palpation of the uterus. (From T. H. Green, Jr., *Gynecology: Essentials of Clinical Practice* [3rd ed.]. Boston: Little, Brown and Company, 1977. Reproduced by permission.)

uncomfortable and is painful if pelvic inflammatory disease is present. The size, contour, position, and mobility of the uterus are estimated. The ovaries and fallopian tubes are palpated. The intravaginal fingers are pushed upward and backward to better feel the ovary with the fingertips. The ovaries are firm and movable, but sensitive to palpation, and first must be located and held in position for examining by the fingers in the vagina and supported by the hand on the abdomen. The fallopian tubes are not normally felt. Following bimanual examination, the rectum and vagina are examined by inserting one lubricated finger in the vagina and the second finger of the same hand into the rectum, using the other hand to palpate the abdomen for the strength of supporting structures or the presence of abnormal bulges, nodes, or masses. The digital examination may cause bleeding if the vaginal or cervical mucosa is thin or its function is impaired. A rectal examination as described in Chapter 7 is then conducted.

BREAST EXAMINATION

Breast examination is carried out in both males and females. In females the breasts (mammary glands) provide for lactation as influenced by prolactin, adrenal glucocorticoids, and probably insulin. Normal growth of mammary tissue is dependent on estrogen, and progesterone in synergistic action with estrogen provides for development of the glandular components of breasts. Because changes in the structure of breasts can be identified by examination, self-examination of the breast is an assessment that every woman should carry out on a routine monthly basis. In the menstruating woman breast tissue is best examined about 5 days following cessation of menstruation because there is less swelling or engorgement and tenderness at that time and lesions may be more easily felt.

Breasts undergo normal changes with aging and during and following lactation. Breast tissue undergoes involution with the aging process. Youthful breasts are soft and of even consistency whereas aging breasts tend to become pendulous; the consistency may be nodular and stringy, especially following lactation. Breast size and tenderness increase during the early months of pregnancy, and gradually during the premenstrual period, reaching maximum monthly size just prior to the onset of menstruation. There is no normal size or shape of breasts because of normal variations among women.

The breasts are examined first with the patient seated, arms relaxed at the sides. The breasts are then examined for size, position, symmetry, presence of bulges, observable masses, retraction of skin, and dimpling. The contour of both breasts is noted. Differences in the sizes of the breasts may be attributable to congenital anomalies, inflammatory processes, or the presence of cysts or tumors. Following examination of both breasts with the patient's arms at the sides, the patient is then asked to raise her arms above her head. During this movement the breasts are observed for retraction or dimpling that may be observable only when the patient raises her arms, since the tumors or cysts may cause the ligaments to retract. The breasts are palpated with the fingertips or with the palmar aspects of the fingers. Pendulous breasts are better examined by supporting the breast from below with one hand while gently palpating breast tissue between two fingers of the other hand. Palpation takes place in an orderly fashion, by separating the breast into four quadrants: upper-inner, upper-outer, lower-inner, and lower-outer. The upper-outer quadrant extends to the anterior axillary fold (Fig. 9-4).

Following examination of the breasts with the patient seated, the patient is asked to assume a supine position to flatten the breasts. Palpation is then conducted. In thin persons, the pectoralis major muscle and the underlying ribs may be felt. Again, the breast tissue is examined in an orderly fashion, beginning in one quadrant and ending in the last of the four quadrants. The fingers and thumb are used to gently compress the breast tissue so that nodes, nodules, areas of tenderness, or cysts may be located. The fingers are moved in a rotary motion until the entire breast has been examined. Gentle compression of the areola and nipple reveals the presence of any drainage. The areola and nipple are also examined for mobility, crusting, color and pigment, and retraction. Some women have inverted nipples; this inversion may be normal if the nipples have not undergone any change. The patient should be asked whether her nipples have always been inverted, or, if a change has occurred, when it occurred. Drain-

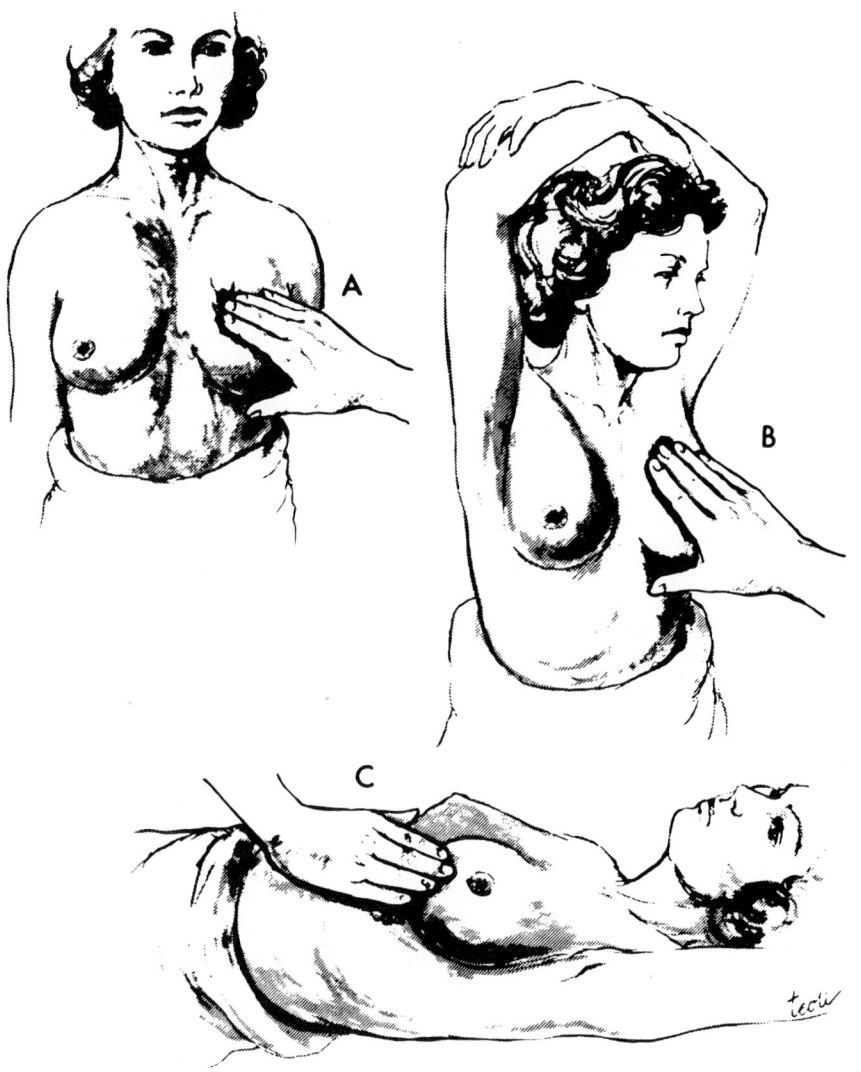

Figure 9-4
Positions used for palpation of the breast. **A.** Erect with arms at sides. **B.** Erect with arms raised overhead. **C.** Supine. (Modified from R. D. Judge and G. D. Zuidema, *Methods of Clinical Examination: A Physiological Approach* [3rd ed.]. Boston: Little, Brown and Company, 1974. Reproduced by permission.)

age from the nipples is described in terms of color, consistency, and amount. Crusting or scaling of the nipples or areola should be noted.

Breast tissue changes include cyst formation, the presence of nodes, masses, or inflammation. In an infection the skin appears red, is warm to touch, and may be tender or painful. Normal nodules in the breast are small, firm, and shaped like beans. If infected, the nodules may be tender to touch. Masses or nodes are described in terms of location, size, shape, consistency (whether they are firm, hard, or soft), and mobility (whether they are fixed to underlying or surrounding tissue or movable). The presence of cysts is noted in terms of extent and location. Cysts tend to increase in size during the premenstrual period. Any mass in the breast or a change in contour, and dimpling or retraction, may indicate malignancy and the patient is referred for further examination. In addition, peau d' orange thickening of the skin, resembling an orange peel, occurs when there is lymphatic obstruction and indicates a malignant process.

Part of the breast examination is inspection and palpation of both the axillary and supraclavicular lymph nodes. To examine the axillary nodes, the patient's arm is supported by one hand and the other hand is used to gently palpate for nodes, which are normally flat, movable, and soft. Enlargement of the nodes may be visible or may be felt. Enlarged nodes are described in terms of location, size, mobility, and consistency.

Examination of the male breast is similar to that of the female breast. The size of the male breast varies according to the amount of adipose tissue. As with the female breast, the male breast tissue is palpated to determine the presence of nodes, masses, tenderness, inflammation, or nipple discharge. The palpation required is not as extensive as in the female because the male breast is flatter and much smaller than the female breast.

The nurse uses the time of breast examination to determine whether the patient understands how to examine her own breasts. If appropriate, the nurse teaches the patient how to palpate the breasts in the positions described, the difference being that the patient uses one hand to examine her own breast while placing the opposite arm at the side or above the head for the different parts of the examination. Some patients feel more secure in their ability to conduct self-examination of the breast if given an opportunity to demonstrate the technique for the nurse. Patients should be encouraged in understanding that routine practice soon makes them expert in the technique and that familiarity with one's own breasts is the best method for evaluating changes that take place. The patients are also advised to seek medical examination without delay if any changes are noted, because there is a high cure rate for breast malignancies detected and treated in the early stages.

DIAGNOSTIC TESTS

The diagnostic tests used to determine reproductive system dysfunction include radioimmunoassay of hormone concentrations in serum and in urine, examination of the reproductive tract in males and females, and laboratory examination of drainage, secretions, and tissue. Because the reproductive tract in both males and females is associated with the urinary system, diagnosis of reproductive system dysfunction often includes evaluation of the urinary tract (see Chap. 6), such as by means of the intravenous pyelogram. The metabolic influences of the reproductive system are evaluated in terms of the suspected disease processes and are discussed in subsequent sections of this chapter.

There are variations in the methods of radioimmunoassay tests available in hospitals, and values considered normal are dependent on laboratory methods. It is more pertinent here to consider the hormones specific to reproductive function. In both males and females the hypothalamus is responsible for control of reproductive function. The pineal gland is thought to integrate neural stimuli from environmental and physiologic factors affecting reproductive hormone secretion rhythms and to exert inhibitory control from the brain on the hypothalamus [21]. In the hypothalamus, gonadotropin-regulating hormone (GnRH), sometimes called gonadotropin-releasing hormone, is secreted in response to gonadal hormones (estrogen, progesterone, and testosterone) in long feedback loops and in response to anterior pituitary hormones (FSH and LH) in ultrashort feedback loops. The anterior pituitary secretion of FSH and LH is responsive to gonadal hormones in a short feedback loop. It is thought that the anterior pituitary is more sensitive to hypothalamic GnRH when gonadal hormone levels are low and less sensitive to GnRH when the levels are high [9]. In general, GnRH stimulates anterior pituitary secretion of FSH and LH, as mediated by cyclic AMP. The test involves giving GnRH to evaluate pituitary response. If there is gonadal hormone insufficiency, GnRH increases pituitary secretion of FSH and LH. Failure of GnRH to increase pituitary secretion of FSH and LH indicates anterior pituitary disease [9].

The hypothalamus is considered to be the control center for the cyclic pattern of gonadal hormone secretion in women and the consistent secretion of gonadal hormone in males. Within the hypothalamus two centers have been identified: the **tonic center,** located in the ventromedial nucleus, and the **cyclic center,** located in the suprachiasmatic area. The tonic center is dominant in males and the cyclic center is dominant in females [9]. In males, testosterone is secreted fairly consistently (Fig. 9-5). The cyclic secretion of female

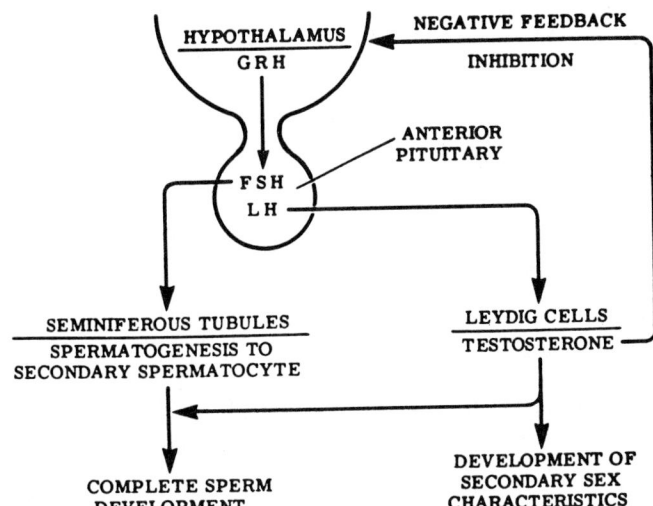

Figure 9-5
Regulation of testicular function. (From E. E. Selkurt, *Basic Physiology for the Health Sciences.* Boston: Little, Brown and Company, 1975. Reproduced by permission.)

gonadal hormones is evidenced by the menstrual cycle, which normally averages 28 days. This cycle takes place in three phases: the follicular phase, the ovulation phase, and the luteal phase. In the **follicular phase** an increase in FSH stimulates follicular growth. Usually one follicle in the ovary matures each month, although the reason any given follicle matures in preference to others is not known. The duration of the follicular phase of the menstrual cycle averages 14 days, but is variable among females and in the same female and accounts for the differences or normal irregularities in each menstrual cycle. As the follicle develops, it secretes increasing amounts of estrogen and small amounts of progesterone, but the FSH levels gradually decrease. As estrogen levels increase, LH levels consistently but slowly increase until a surge of LH secretion occurs 1 to 2 days prior to ovulation. This LH peak lasts only 2 or 3 days. **Ovulation** is the rupture of the follicle with the release of the ovum from the ovary. It should be noted that levels of LH remain fairly constant prior to and following the surge of LH secretion at midpoint in the menstrual cycle. The **luteal phase** begins after ovulation takes place and it lasts for 14 days. In this phase the follicle, now ruptured, takes on a new appearance and becomes the corpus luteum, with an accumulation of yellow pigment and enlargement of vascularized granulosa cells that secrete progesterone and estrogen. The corpus luteum gradually regresses in a process termed **involution** if pregnancy does not occur. (If pregnancy does occur, human chorionic gonadotropin [HCG] stimulates the viability of the corpus luteum until the ninth or tenth week of gestation, at which time the placenta secretes its own hormones and is no longer dependent on the corpus luteum.) With the involution of the corpus luteum there is a rapid decrease in progesterone secretion (Fig. 9-6).

While changes in the follicle are taking place, corresponding changes are also occurring in the endometrium of the uterus. During the follicular, or proliferative, phase, endometrial cells influenced by estrogen grow and vascularize. The coiled or spiral arterial vessels in the endometrium increase in length. During the secretory or luteal phase of menstruation, these coiled vessels undergo cyclic dilatation and constriction but the progesterone causes the endometrial cell size to decrease so that eventually there is vasoconstriction of the coiled arterial vessels with stasis in the endometrial circulation. Prior to the onset of menstrual flow, the vasoconstriction increases and the kinking of the coiled vessels is thought to result in menstrual bleeding.

The mechanisms of endometrial changes preceding and during menstrual flow are not understood. It is thought that progesterone stimulates the secretion of prostaglandin, which in turn influences vasoconstriction. In addition, as endometrial cell membranes break down, acid hydrolases are released from cell lysosomes to further disrupt the endometrial cells [15]. The endometrium sheds as a result of ischemia and is eliminated in menstrual flow.

Hormone levels may be evaluated by

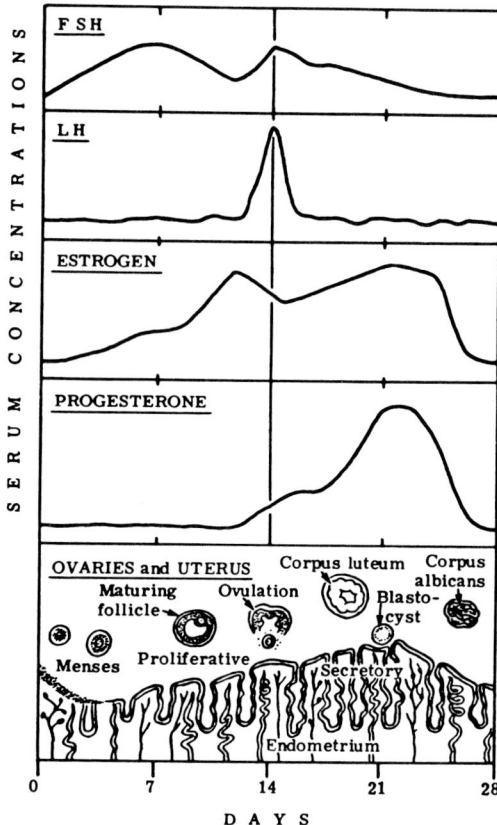

Figure 9-6
Hormonal, ovarian, and uterine changes during one menstrual cycle. (From E. E. Selkurt, *Basic Physiology for the Health Sciences*. Boston: Little, Brown and Company, 1975. Reproduced by permission.)

radioimmunoassay during different phases of the menstrual cycle and the levels, by nature of hormonal changes in the cycle, are different on any given day. Without knowledge of the pattern or cycle in the female whose function is being evaluated, single evaluation of hormone levels by radioimmunoassay techniques have little meaning. Usually, repeated evaluation is required, and thus radioimmunoassay evaluation of gonadal hormone function can be expensive.

Hormone excretion can be measured in urine studies. The total amount of estrogen excreted in urine indicates the secretion of estradiol and estrone by the ovaries plus the estrogens formed by precursors. Pregnanediol is the metabolite of progesterone that can be measured in urinary excretion. Measurement of 17-ketosteroids as discussed in Chapter 8 includes androgens excreted from adrenal secretion and testicular secretions but does not necessarily directly reflect the total amount of testosterone secreted.

An inexpensive method of evaluating the phases of the menstrual cycle and one that requires the patient's participation is determination of the pattern of the **basal body temperature** (BBT). Progesterone, when secreted by the corpus luteum in sufficient amounts, increases the BBT. Following ovulation, the rapid increase in levels of progesterone increases body temperature during the luteal phase of the cycle. While not as accurate as radioimmunoassay, the BBT can indicate the phases of the menstrual cycle, and the BBT pattern for nine months to a year provides a means for estimating the date of ovulation. Estimation of the date of ovulation is useful for females who wish to know when they are fertile. The BBT pattern can also be used in birth control to determine the period of fertility. Immediately preceding ovulation the BBT drops; 1 to 3 days after ovulation it increases. Birth control is accomplished by abstaining from intercourse or by using contraceptives from the few days prior to ovulation until the temperature has been elevated for at least 3 days.

When teaching patients the correct method for taking and recording the BBT either for diagnostic purposes or for birth control, the nurse explains what is meant by the word **basal,** that is, minimal metabolic functioning. It is important that the patient take her temperature in the morning on wakening and before performing any activity that would increase metabolic needs such as voiding, walking around, smoking, eating, or drinking fluids. Each person's basal temperature is different, and the patient who routinely takes her temperature each morning for months learns to recognize patterns. Recording the temperature on a graph better illustrates the changes in temperature for evaluation by the nurse and physician; the nurse can provide the patient with graph forms for recording temperatures. The actual dates of menstrual flow and coitus are recorded. Illnesses may affect the body temperature and therefore make the record invalid for that cycle. The normal span of menstrual flow varies and averages from 3 to 5 days. Information concerning the duration, amount, and pattern of menstrual flow is important in the diagnosis of dysfunction related to abnormal menstrual periods.

Another method of indirectly evaluating hormone levels is examination of secretions from the cervix. Estrogen stimulates secretion of thin, watery mucus in the cervical glands. This mucus, when placed on a clean glass slide, dries and forms crystals in a fern pattern; thus the name **fern test** has been given to this procedure. A positive fern test indicates the presence of estrogen. Vaginal epithelial cells demonstrate maturation in response to estrogen, and crystallization therefore indicates the high estrogen levels normally found in the follicular phase of the menstrual cycle. Progesterone decreases the amount of mucus secreted by cervical glands; when levels of progesterone are high, as in the luteal phase of the menstrual cycle, the fern test is negative. Cervical mucus secreted during the luteal phase also contains epithelial cells and is cloudy whereas mucus secreted in the follicular phase has few cells and is clear. The watery clear mucus secreted in the follicular phase also has characteristic spinnbarkeit qualities; the mucus forms or spins a thread that can be 5 cm or longer. Spinnbarkeit is an indication of cervical mucus of good quality.

In the evaluation of male reproductive function, semen is evaluated via microscopical examination for the quality of sperm including the density, motility, and morphology. Because the content of seminal fluid varies from day to day, comparison of two or three samples of seminal fluid is necessary for diagnosis. The fluid is collected by the male either by interrupting coitus or by inducing ejaculation. The sample is collected following a 4 to 6 day period of abstinence from sexual intercourse and the volume is measured. The entire ejaculate is collected in a clean, wide-mouthed container and the sample is examined within an hour following ejaculation; a glass jar is used because plastic affects motility. The normal volume of ejaculate ranges from 1 to 5 ml, the average being 2.5 ml. The seminal fluid normally coagulates quickly but then liquefies in 5 to 20 minutes. Evaluation of the density (count of sperm), motility (movement), and morphology (shape and size) under microscope is arbitrary and subjective. Sperm are difficult to count, motility is variable, but abnormal shapes may more or less be easily identified. Fifty percent of the sperm should be progressively mobile 2 hours after ejaculation.

The seminal fluid is also examined for epithelial cells, leukocytes, bacteria, and fructose. The amount of fructose indicates the function of the secretory epithelium in seminal vesicles. Both citric acid and fructose are contained in normal seminal fluid, and metabolism of fructose is a source of energy for sperm motility [12]. Absence or low levels of fructose in seminal fluid indicate dysfunction of the seminal vesicles or of the ductus deferens. Sperm in seminal fluid also are tested for agglutination. In some instances, dysfunction is related to antigen-antibody reactions. If the antibody titer in seminal fluid is high, the immune response in epididymal epithelium to infiltration of sperm or seminal plasma thus indicated can interfere with the motility and migration of sperm into the cervical mucus.

Another method of diagnosing reproductive tract dysfunction is examination of tissue by biopsy. A specimen can be obtained from any organ and be examined under the microscope for abnormal cell shapes indicative of malignancy or other changes in cell structure. The Schiller test is used when changes in the female cervical epithelium suggest cancer. The cervical squamous epithelium is stained with iodine and, if normal, the cells take up the stain and become deep brown. Abnormal cells do not take up the stain because the abnormal epithelial areas do not have the rich glycogen content found in normal cervical epithelium. Potentially cancerous areas then appear pale brown because they do not take up the stain as well.

A vaginal smear can be examined for the maturation index of its cells, which is a measurement of the relative percentage of parabasal, intermediate, and superficial cells. There are more superficial (karyopyknotic) and fewer parabasal cells in vaginal secretions during periods of high estrogen levels. The Pap test provides for identification of malignant cells that appear on the slide with cervical mucus (Fig. 9-7). Malignant cells have a different appearance when compared to normal cells, and finding these malignant cells in a Pap smear indicates the need for further investigation.

A cul-de-sac aspiration is carried out via culdocentesis (colpostomy). For this procedure the patient is placed in either the

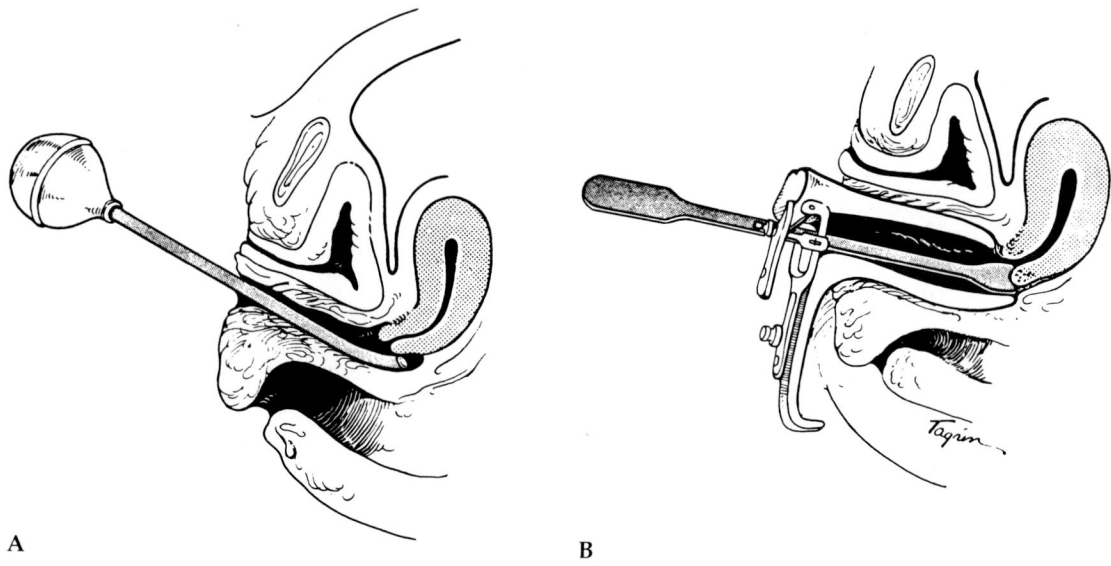

Figure 9-7
Technique for obtaining cytologic smears. **A.** Vaginal pool smear from the posterior fornix. **B.** Cervical scraping smear. (From T. H. Green, Jr., *Gynecology: Essentials of Clinical Practice* [3rd ed.]. Boston: Little, Brown and Company, 1977. Reproduced by permission.)

lithotomy or knee-chest position for insertion of the aspirating needle and is then placed in the dorsal recumbent position for the aspiration. The color of the fluid aspirated indicates the type of pathology present. In ectopic pregnancy, bloody drainage indicates rupture and in an infectious process, the drainage can be purulent. The specimen obtained in cul-de-sac aspiration is sent to the laboratory for cytologic studies.

A cone biopsy of the cervix is performed when changes in the cervical mucosa occur. To perform the biopsy, the physician excises a cone of tissue from the cervical os, using a scalpel blade, for cytologic studies. The cone biopsy can also be used for removal of localized lesions.

Dilatation and curettage (D and C) is a method of both examination and treatment and simply means that the cervix is dilated and the uterus is scraped. This procedure requires an operative permit, anesthesia, and thus preoperative preparation with premedication. The D and C may not require hospitalization but can be done on an outpatient basis provided the patient has adequate time to recover in an appropriate recovery room with nursing surveillance. Both the patient's stomach and bladder must be empty for the D and C. The uterus can be examined, and uterine size is measured by inserting a sound (probe) into the uterine cavity. The measurement is a guideline for both size and shape for the scraping part of the procedure. D and C may be complicated by perforation of the uterus or bleeding. The procedure is used for treatment when polyps are removed or lesions are cauterized. It should be noted that the nurse monitors vital signs and checks for vaginal bleeding during the patient's recovery from anesthesia and thereafter until the patient's condition has stabilized. Females with a retroflexed uterus or those who have just had an abortion are particularly susceptible to complications. The uterine walls are soft following abortion and are therefore more subject to trauma in the D and C.

The reproductive tract can also be evaluated by visualization of the tract. As may be the case with other diagnostic procedures in which contrast medium or dye is used, the patient may have an allergic or toxic reaction to the medium or the dye. A history of previous allergies should be obtained prior to tests for visualization. It is important to note that, because of the negative effect of radiation on gonadal tissue and on the fetus, if a fetus is present, the patient is not exposed to radiation unless absolutely necessary. Therefore, use of x-ray for diagnosis of reproductive system dysfunction is limited and is done with discrimination.

The male reproductive tract can be visualized by inserting a contrast medium via a catheter inserted into the urethra or via percutaneous injection of the contrast medium through the scrotal sac skin into the epididymis. A complication of the percutaneous route is formation of a stricture of the epididymis. In females, contrast medium is injected into the uterus and passes to the fallopian tubes and into the peritoneal cavity. This procedure, hysterosalpingography, does not give definitive information about pathologic conditions but it does outline the shape of the uterus and enables determination of the patency of the fallopian tubes. In some instances the contrast medium passes through only one fallopian tube because it follows the path of least resistance, and failure to visualize the other fallopian tube does not necessarily indicate an occlusion in that tube. There is controversy about selection of the appropriate contrast medium for a hysterosalpingogram. Many authorities believe that a water-soluble contrast medium should be used, on the premise that oil-based contrast media may cause oil emboli or granulomatous formation in the fallopian tubes. Speroff, Glass, and Kase report better results with the use of an oil-based contrast medium [21].

Another method used to visualize the reproductive organs is insertion of a Foley catheter in the uterus with inflation of the balloon to only 2 ml for insertion of a dye and examination of the pelvic organs via either culdoscopy or laparoscopy. In culdoscopy (colposcopy), the scope is inserted through the posterior vaginal fornix under local anesthesia and the uterus is visualized from below. The patient must be placed in an uncomfortable knee-chest position for this examination. In laparoscopy, a fiberscope is inserted through a small incision in the abdominal wall at the umbilicus, with the patient in lithotomy position, using general or local anesthesia. The laparoscopy allows direct visualization of the pelvic organs and viscera; adhesions can be detected, and the patency of the fallopian tubes can be determined by observing the dye as it passes from the uterine infundibulum, through the tubal fimbriae. Laparoscopy is also performed without use of a dye or contrast medium. The insertion of carbon dioxide or of nitrous oxide gas into the peritoneal cavity is used to separate the bowel from the reproductive tract organs in the pelvic area. A trocar on the laparoscope has a valve that prevents loss of the air from the peritoneal cavity. During the laparoscopy the patient's position can be changed so that the pelvic organs can be better viewed from different angles. In addition, a cannula inserted into the uterus is used to move the uterus so that the posterior of the uterus and underlying structures can be visualized. The fiberscope also provides for biopsy of endometrial tissue under direct visualization or for electric cautery to coagulate the fallopian tubes and achieve sterilization. Postcauterization bleeding requires recauterization. Perforation of the bowel with the potential for development of subsequent peritonitis and flare-up of a latent pelvic infection is another complication that may occur. Nursing care prior to these tests involves teaching the patient what to expect, ensuring that her bladder is empty (by catheterization if necessary), giving premedication, supporting her during the procedure, and assessing her status following the examination to detect signs and symptoms indicating the onset of complications. Immediate action must be taken if the patient's blood pressure decreases or pulse increases, or if bleeding occurs. The patient is returned to the examining room or the operating room for treatment of bleeding via cauterization or other appropriate methods as determined by the physician.

In the Rubin test for tubal patency gas is inserted via a cannula into the uterus to insufflate the fallopian tubes. If the tubes are patent, the presence of gas in the lower abdomen is detected by auscultation, and the patient will experience referred shoulder pain when sitting up. The insufflation test is normal if gas passes through the fallopian tubes at pressures below 180 mm Hg. If over 200 mm Hg pressure is required to insufflate the fallopian tubes, tubal occlusion is suspected.

Reproductive System Problems

Reproductive system dysfunction causes patients both emotional and physiologic distress. In this section the various types of dysfunction discussed are infertility, commonly occurring problems that result from congenital disorders, the effects of diseases, hormonal imbalances, normal deterioration in aging, abnormal cell growth, and mammary gland dysfunction. Also discussed are patient teaching in contraception and following abortion, rape, the menopause, and hysterectomy.

INFERTILITY

Infertility is defined as the inability to achieve pregnancy within a given period of time, usually arbitrarily designated as one year [15]. Approximately 12 percent of the marriages in the United States are involuntarily barren [15]. There are multiple causes of infertility, and unless a specific pathologic condition or dysfunction is found, the reason for a couple's infertility may be unknown and untreatable. While fertility of females is highest during young adult years and declines after the age of 35 years, some women become pregnant up to the age of 45 years. Pregnancy in women over the age of 45 is rare. Males, on the other hand, continue to be fertile throughout life, with fertility decreasing gradually after the young adult years.

Couples who seek treatment for infertility are initially interviewed to determine the motivation of each person for treatment and their attitudes toward sexuality, childbearing and childrearing, their marital relationship, and personal concerns about diagnosis and treatment. In some instances a physiologic cause can be determined and may or may not be treatable. In other instances no physiologic cause is evident and the couple may be referred for counseling selected according to the couple's preferences from among the available resources. This discussion of infertility includes physiologic causes and treatment. It must be stated, however, that the problems in infertility are complex and that this discussion is limited in scope in terms of the total array of interrelated problems the couple has.

Physiologically, infertility may result from congenital anomalies, hormonal imbalances, systemic diseases associated with metabolic imbalances and debilitated states, or from acquired pathology within the reproductive tract in the male or female or in both. In the male or female, impairment of the quality of sperm or ova may be of a genetic nature. The reader is referred to a genetics text to further explore this problem. If the genetic quality of the sperm or ova hinders or prevents fertility, counseling and genetic evaluation are required if the couple wishes to pursue diagnosis and treatment or receive guidance in alternate ways of having a family such as adoption or artificial insemination if no treatment is feasible.

Infertility in the Male

A number of factors contribute to infertility in males. These include mumps orchitis, previous herniorrhaphy in which the testicles were damaged, venereal disease, undescended testis or long-term exposure to excessive heat (both of which increase intratesticular temperature), exposure to industrial hazards such as x-ray (which can irreversibly damage the testes if dosages are sufficiently high), congenital anomalies or pathology in the reproductive tract, neurologic dysfunction causing impotence, and problems in coitus such as failure to penetrate the vagina.

Diagnosis of male reproductive function requires a history of the male's marriage(s), children, life-style (long periods of absence from home have been implicated as a cause of infertility), nutritional state, excessive use of alcohol, occupation to determine potential hazards, attitudes and emotions concerning his relationship with his wife, parenting, and infertility. A complete physical examination may reveal the presence of underlying dysfunction in other body systems that may influence infertility. Other endocrine dysfunction, particularly of the pituitary, adrenal, and thyroid glands, may be interrelated in causing infertility. Klinefelter's syndrome is a combination of anterior pituitary, adrenal, and thyroid dysfunction causing aspermatogenesis. The seminal fluid and sperm are evaluated, as is the reproductive tract. A testicular biopsy to determine whether trauma or inflammatory processes have caused fibrosis or aplasia of tissue is carried out and hormonal levels of FSH, LH, and testosterone are measured. The presence of varicocele (varicosity in the testicular vein resulting in increased temperature in the testes), phimosis, hydrocele, or undescended testes is ruled out. Medications being taken are also evaluated because certain medications, such as cyclophosphamide (Cytoxin), busulfan (Myleran), and the nitrofurans, interfere with spermatogenesis [18].

Treatment can be instituted in some types of defined dysfunction and is not feasible in other types of dysfunction. Treatable conditions include hormonal imbalances and general physical debilitation that responds to therapy. Repair of the varicocele by ligating the internal spermatic vein or carrying out a bypass procedure to correct an occluded ductus deferens may correct infertility. Testosterone may be given until the sperm count reaches 0 to cause a rebound increase in spermatogenesis when testosterone is abruptly withdrawn. Clomiphene (Clomid) may be given over a period ranging from 3 months to 1 year to treat oligospermia. Clomiphene is thought to act by stimulating secretion of FSH by the anterior pituitary. If the male's dysfunction is not treatable and if the female has no dysfunction, the male and female are given an opportunity to discuss the implications of the male's infertility in terms of their relationship, and the possibility of artificial insemination or adoption is presented as an alternative. The couple is a unit and as such must deal with the male's infertility together. Decisions made by consensus are more likely to have effective outcomes.

The male can also be counseled in ways to increase the quality of sperm. Good health practices including ingestion of a well-balanced diet, obtaining adequate rest and exercise, and emotional relaxation are advised. This effort is thought to have a positive benefit both for the male's health and the couple's relationship. The male is advised to avoid excessive heat because spermatogenesis requires temperatures a few degrees below normal body temperature. The scrotal sac provides insulation and mechanisms for regulation of scrotal temperature. The smooth muscle of the scrotal wall contracts in cold temperatures, thereby thickening the scrotal wall and holding the testes closer to the body, and relaxes in warm temperatures to thin the scrotal wall and to lower the testes from the body. Nerve endings and sweat glands abound in the testes and contribute to maintenance of optimum scrotal temperatures, and the high degree of vascularization provides for circulatory regulation of temperature [12]. Avoiding long hot baths, constricting undergarments and clothes, and exercise that increases body temperature for long periods of time augments spermatogenesis.

Other factors that are implicated as causes of decreased spermatogenesis include high alcohol intake, smoking, and high intake of caffeine. Van Thiel [25] reports that alcoholic patients have a decrease in plasma gonadotropins and loss of gonadotropin reserves resulting from a combination of gonadal and hepatic disease and alcohol toxicity. In alcoholic males, androgens are removed from circulation and are converted to estrogens at a more rapid rate as compared to nonalcoholics. It is thought that the metabolism of ethanol in the testes may reduce the level of nicotinamide adenine dinucleotide (NAD), which is an essential cofactor for enzymes necessary in testosterone secretion, or that ethanol may be toxic to the Leydig cells in the testes. In hepatic dysfunction, conjugation of estrogens is impaired and consequently plasma estrogen levels are elevated. Eventually the endocrine feedback loops including hypothalamic stimulation are irreversibly impaired in long-standing alcoholism [25].

Infertility in the Female

Evaluation of the female reproductive function is undertaken concurrently with that of the male reproductive function. The couple is informed at the onset that this evaluation takes many months, particularly because female gonadal endocrine balance patterns change within monthly cycles. The nurse attempts to establish a positive trusting relationship with the couple from the outset so that ongoing communication is maintained. The couple may become frustrated as the evaluation proceeds, and openly discussing this potential frustration in the beginning of the evaluation makes it easier for the nurse to help the couple deal with the frustration later on.

Evaluation of the female reproductive function begins with a detailed history of the patient's menstrual periods (menarche, irregularities, amenorrhea, dysmenorrhea), pregnancies, childbirth, previous marriages, coital history, medications being taken, and previous or present illnesses.

A complete physical examination is performed, and specific evaluation of reproductive hormones in relation to total hormonal balance is conducted along with evaluation of reproductive tract function. The female is asked to begin a basal body temperature chart in order to establish a baseline for evaluation of hormonal changes. For example, changes in cervical secretions should accompany the different phases of the menstrual cycle. The fern test can be performed on a daily basis by the patient and should indicate high levels of estrogen during the follicular phase of menstruation and high levels of progesterone during the luteal phase of the menstrual cycle. These changes in the cervical mucus are meaningful in determining whether ovulation has taken place. If progesterone levels increase as measured indirectly by the fern test, it can be assumed that ovulation has taken place and that the corpus luteum has developed.

The quality of cervical secretions is also evaluated 2 to 3 days prior to ovulation and within 6 to 24 hours following intercourse (The best evaluation of cervical mucus takes place within 6 or 7 hours following intercourse.) If the patient is unable to visit the physician's office or clinic within 6 or 7 hours following intercourse, testing may be delayed up to 24 hours following intercourse. In addition to testing for the quality of cervical mucus, the reaction of the male's fresh sperm placed in the female's cervical mucus is observed to test potential fertility.

Hostile cervical mucus is descriptive of sperm immobilization in cervical mucus and may result from immune reactions of sperm agglutination antibodies or sperm-immobilizing antibodies in cervical mucus to sperm antigens or from infections of the cervix. (Cervical mucus stores sperm and aids transport of sperm into the uterus.) The male's use of condoms for several months in intercourse is helpful in decreasing antibody formation in cervical mucus. Antibiotic therapy is given for infections, and diethylstilbestrol (stilbestrol) in low enough doses to prevent interference with the menstrual cycle is given during the ovulatory phase to increase the secretion of cervical mucus by estrogen. Different dosages and patterns of stilbestrol administration are followed. In some regimens the stilbestrol is discontinued 2 to 3 days prior to ovulation; in others, a low dose of stilbestrol is given continuously.

Sperm acquire their fertilizing ability in the female reproductive tract and survive in the tract for varying periods of time, averaging 2 to 3 days. Fertilization of the sperm takes place in the fallopian tube, usually in the ampullar portion. The ovum is fertile for only 6 to 12 hours following ovulation, and the fertile sperm must penetrate the ovum during the fertile period. The ability of the female reproductive tract to sustain the fertility of the sperm is determined through a variety of tests. The Sims-Huhner test includes evaluation of the effectiveness of coitus, the adequacy of male fertility, the quality of cervical mucus, and normal female gonadal production.

Evaluation of the reproductive tract includes examination of the uterus to ascertain the presence of any tumors that can interfere with sperm transport (or implantation of the conceptus in the uterus) and examination of the fallopian tubes to determine patency. Fallopian tubes not only transport the sperm and the ovum, but also the conceptus to the uterus for implantation. The fallopian tubes may be obstructed by adhesions resulting from previous infection or peritonitis (a complication of many types of abdominal organ dysfunction; see Chapter 7), endometriosis, pelvic inflammatory disease, previous abortion(s) or ectopic pregnancy, or any other condition that results in free blood in the peritoneal cavity. Diagnosis of tubal patency by insufflation or hysterosalpingography may also have the beneficial effect of releasing adhesions and may be curative. Complications include total rupture and activation of latent infections, and with the use of contrast medium or dyes, toxic or chemical reactions may occur. If indicated, fallopian tubes are repaired in tuboplasty procedures. If a stricture in the fallopian tube causes infertility, the stricture can be excised and the tube reanastomosed. This procedure gives early results as the patient may become pregnant within several months to a year. Peritubal adhesions may form close to the uterine wall, requiring reimplantation, or the fimbriae may be obstructed by adhesions. When the fallopian tubes must be reimplanted into the uterus (salpingolysis), or when the fallopian tubes' fimbriae require repair (fimbrioplasty), the patient may have to wait as long as 5 years for evidence of the positive effect of the repair, that is, pregnancy.

Another part of the examination in fertility evaluation is to determine whether the endometrium is capable of responding to progesterone, or whether there is a lack of progesterone or an imbalance in progesterone and estrogen levels. Patients who have a history of frequent spontaneous abortion and failure to maintain pregnancy often have dysfunction in progesterone secretion or endometrial cell function. The endometrium can be evaluated by biopsy 7 days following the estimated date of ovulation, when the corpus luteum is active and the endometrial secretory response to progesterone can be determined. Insufficient levels of progesterone sometimes cause the lack of endometrial secretory function during the luteal phase of the menstrual cycle. Therefore radioimmunoassay tests to determine progesterone levels in plasma obtained during the luteal phase of the menstrual cycle indicate whether there is failure to secrete progesterone. The progesterone secretion may be insufficient because of lack of LH secretion by the anterior pituitary. For this reason radioimmunoassay tests for LH are performed on daily blood samples for determination of LH prior to ovulation when the LH levels normally surge.

Another cause of infertility in the female is failure to ovulate. This failure may be induced by oral contraceptives, by any factor that interferes with ovarian function such as formation of scars or tumors, by premature ovarian failure, or by a number of systemic diseases. Primary anterior pituitary dysfunction may cause ovarian failure, and any of the endocrine diseases that interrupt anterior pituitary dysfunction may lead to failure to ovulate. Nervous system diseases that interfere with the function of the hypothalamus may interfere with ovulation, as can systemic, metabolic, or autoimmune diseases. Following evaluation of ovarian function, the patient may be found to have normal pituitary and ovarian function. It is recognized that failure to ovulate may be based in psychogenic causes that are difficult to identify and treat. Psychological counseling is then indicated, and changes in the patient's self-esteem or self-concept may be curative of failure to ovulate. When there is defined disease, such as ovarian tumor, a wedge resection of the tumor may be curative. Extensive disease requiring removal of the ovaries results in permanent infertility. Therefore conservative surgical procedures are carried out if the patient's condition permits and if she is of childbearing age. Various results have been achieved with hormone-induced ovulation, and the administration of clomiphene has proved helpful. If general endocrine imbalance exists, involving the adrenal or thyroid glands, treatment of the imbalance may correct the infertility. General measures of care including a well-balanced diet, adequate rest and exercise, and periods of relaxation may be helpful.

Treatment of endocrine imbalances of estrogen or progesterone or of FSH or LH includes giving the appropriate hormone. Clomiphene (Clomid) is sometimes given for failure to ovulate; its use, however, is associated with the risk that the drug may overstimulate the ovaries sufficiently to result in ovarian rupture. To induce ovulation, the patient is given gonadotropin, either HMG (human menopausal gonadotropin) (Pergonol) or HCG (human chorionic gonadotropin). Both HMG and HCG are expensive. A combination of FSH and HCG may be used to stimulate ovulation [7]. The dosages to induce ovulation and the specific hormone or combinations of hormones used vary according to the physician's preference, the patient's condition, and the patient's response.

General Considerations in Treatment of Infertility

Not every couple that undergoes extensive evaluation for definition of the cause of infertility is successful in achieving treatment. The nurse recognizes that failure to become pregnant may be disconcerting to both the male and female, and that couples who are upset with lack of positive results following their efforts and the expense of the evaluation may not wish to pursue the matter further. Other couples, however, continue to seek assistance from a variety of resources, and the nurse should discuss these resources with the couple. There are many clinics for people with sexual problems of varying nature, and not every clinic offers credible help for distressed couples. The nurse who is informed about the clinics in the area of practice can better counsel patients in the use of these clinics. Adoption is an alternative that often takes a long time and requires extensive social and financial evaluation by the adoption agency. Some couples select artificial insemination as an alternative.

Artificial insemination uses semen from either the husband's ejaculate when there is impaired coitus or from another male and may be obtained by the physician from semen banks. The procedure requires at least 3 to 6 months or longer, and there is the possibility that the female will develop antibodies to the semen. Prior to artificial insemination, the couple is interviewed to determine the motivation for the procedure and to explore their feelings about artificial insemination. Essentially insemination using semen from a male other than the husband is similar to adoption and must be accepted as such by the couple. To be effective artificial insemination requires that the female be fertile. The procedure is not carried out unless the male has proved to be infertile for a minimum period of 1 year.

INFLAMMATORY AND INFECTIOUS PROCESSES

Inflammatory and infectious processes in the reproductive tract are related; inflamed tissue is subject to infection, and inflammation accompanies the infectious process. Inflammation results from mechanical or chemical irritation of the mucous membranes and can be caused by trauma, use of preparations such as douches or antiseptics with high concentrations of chemicals that are irritating to the mucous membranes, or by irritating toxic secretions resulting from infectious processes within the reproductive or urinary tract or chemical toxins used to induce abortion. Trauma from external blows or from foreign objects placed in the tract, such as pessaries to reposition displaced pelvic organs in females, can cause mechanical injury to the mucosa. The reproductive tract can also be traumatized by bone fragments from orthopedic injuries in the pelvic area.

The reproductive tract is subject to infection by any number of organisms either singly or in combination. Gonorrheal infections occur frequently, as do trichomonal and monilial infections. Infections can also be caused by *Escherichia coli,* staphylococci or streptococci, or any other pathogenic organism. The degree or extent of the infection and its severity depend on the virulence and strain of the organism, the person's resistance to the infection, and the effectiveness of the treatment given. Mild infections cause few symptoms and can be overlooked by the affected person whereas moderate or severe infections cause discomfort that motivates the patient to seek treatment. Other conditions cause such discomfort and pain that the patient is motivated to seek medical assistance for relief. An example is Bartholin's cyst, which develops following inflammation. This cyst is associated with swelling and tenderness and causes discomfort when the patient sits and walks. Treatment is surgical excision of the cyst. When obtaining a history from a person suspected of having a reproductive tract infection, the nurse ascertains the events that precipitated the infection, the time of onset of the first signs and symptoms, and the history of previous infections. The patient is asked to describe the signs and symptoms including the presence of pain (its location, character, intensity, and duration), local signs of redness, edema or lesions, and any unusual drainage. Localized infection or inflammation is verified by examination when possible. It is necessary to differentiate reproductive tract infection from other causes of lower abdominal discomfort such as appendicitis, urinary tract infection, or nephritis. In venereal infections, sexual contacts are identified for follow-up treatment.

Inflammation or infection of the reproductive tract can be localized or general, involving more than one organ. The name given the localized infection implies the organ involved; for example, vaginitis, cervicitis, salpingitis, prostatitis, epididymitis, and orchitis. In females, pelvic inflammatory disease is generalized infection involving the fallopian tubes, the uterus, the ovaries, and the peritoneal structures. When an infection or inflammatory process is limited to one part of the reproductive tract, the inflammatory process includes induration of tissue with hyperemia, edema, redness, and pain or discomfort related to pressure. The amount of discomfort the patient has can be extensive if this inflammatory process extends to other reproductive tract structures. Inflammation or infection throughout a large portion of the reproductive tract, lower abdominal distress such as pain in the lower abdomen and abdominal distention, rebound abdominal tenderness, and referred pain to the inguinal area and groin are noted. The patient can also have generalized symptoms of malaise with nausea, vomiting, and increased temperature. Certain infections cause specific effects from the invasion of the organism on the involved tissue; formation of vesicles or erosions and typical drainage caused by an infectious agent are helpful in identifying the type of infection present. The infectious agent is diagnosed in laboratory examination of specimens of drainage by culture tests.

Nursing care is based on the type of infection and the extent of the signs and symptoms of the inflammation or infection. In both inflammation and infection, the cause is determined and treated. The patient is given supportive care to relieve generalized pain, discomfort, and malaise, as well as information about how to prevent or eliminate (if possible) the causes to prevent reinfection.

The external genitalia, the penis and the scrotum in males and the labia majora, the labia minora, the area surrounding the vestibule of the vagina, the urinary meatus, and the vagina in females, are susceptible to mechanical trauma. Wearing tight underclothing, participating in contact sports that subject the external genitalia to mechanical injury, and sexual exposure are some of the sources of mechanical trauma. The skin in the groin area and the external genitalia in males and females is subject to irritation from exposure that can lead to a variety of superficial lesions. The scrotum is vulnerable to dermatitis and psoriasis, and both the male and female genitalia are subject to herpesvirus infection (see Chap. 14). Sexual activity can lead to trauma to both the glans penis and the vagina, and in many instances pathogenic organisms are transmitted in sexual intercourse. Some of the specific organisms that cause reproductive tract infections are *Neisseria gonorrhoeae*, *Trichomonas*, *Candida albicans*, and *Treponema pallidum*.

INFECTIONS

Gonorrheal organisms cause infections that are initially acute, but may be so mild that the person does not know that he or she has been infected. If the acute infection is not cleared by treatment with chemotherapy, it often becomes chronic. The toxins produced by the gonorrheal organisms cause inflammation. In males, gonorrheal infection is usually evidenced in urethritis and there is a varying amount of purulent discharge. The infection spreads via the spermatic cord to the epididymis and is then difficult to treat. The prostate gland may also be infected, and symptoms of obstructed urinary flow can result if prostatic edema is great enough to impinge on the urethra. In females the initial gonorrheal infection can be limited to the vulva, and symptoms occur within 1 day to several days following the contact. These symptoms include itching, burning, frequency of urination, and leukorrhea. The gonorrheal infection can readily spread upward in the female reproductive tract and involve the vagina and the cervix. A thick viscous mucopurulent discharge then occurs. The infection usually remains in the external genitalia, in the paraurethral ducts (Skene's ducts) located on the posterolateral aspect of the urinary meatus, or in the vestibular gland at the vaginal introitus (Bartholin's duct) located between the hymen and the labia minora. The vaginal environment is not conducive to the growth of *Neisseria gonorrhoeae* organisms; however, if the cervix is invaded and if the condition is not adequately treated in the acute stages, the infection spreads via the uterus to the fallopian tubes. This spread takes place during the woman's first menstrual period following infection. The gonorrheal infection can be self-limiting, but without treatment the woman can then become a carrier of the disease and the gonorrheal infection can remain latent, only to flare up at a later time. For example, salpingitis caused by gonorrhea can be evidenced months following the initial infection, causing edema of the fallopian tubes and formation of a toxic exudate. This exudate can escape from the fallopian tubes and cause a pelvic abscess. It should be noted that the gonococcal infection predominates in mucosal surfaces. Determining the sexual contacts of infected persons is important in controlling the spread of gonorrhea to other people.

Trichomonas may also infect both males and females. It can be diagnosed by isolating the organism in the first portion of the male urine specimen (see Chap. 6) and causes urethritis with burning and itching on urination, and urgency or nocturia. In the female, trichomonal infections form a typical yellowish-green discharge that is frothy and foul smelling. The female also has burning and itching of the external genitalia as a result of the irritating discharge. The infected mucous membranes have a characteristic strawberry-like appearance with red spots and petechial hemorrhages. Because trichomonads live well in an acid medium, they flourish in the vagina where the normal pH, although variable, is 3.8 to 4.2. Trichomonads can also spread to the cervix or to the urethra, and affected persons often tend to be reinfected by sexual contact. For this reason the sexual partner is also treated in efforts to cure the infection.

Since this protozoan parasite resists treatment, trichomonal infections require medication, metronidazole (Flagyl), for a period of several weeks. Thereafter, Flagyl is taken during each period of menstrual flow for several months.

Candida albicans infections are characterized by ulcerations of mucous membranes with formation of white cheesy exudate that forms in patches. Candidiasis is a monilial infection that is also difficult to cure because the organisms proliferate in an acid pH. The monilial infections occur most frequently in women and can follow long-term antibiotic therapy or use of antibiotic suppositories. Treatment is local application of an antifungal agent such as nystatin (Mycostatin) or candicidin (Candeptin). In males *Candida albicans* can cause prostatitis and treatment involves acidification of the urine.

The spirochete *Treponema pallidum* first infects the external genitalia locally, but soon is disseminated systemically. The primary lesion, chancre, forms on the penis or on the vaginal mucosa near the vestibule of the vagina, or sometimes in the cervix. The lesion has a raised, indurated border with a central ulceration. Eventually a grayish-yellow hemorrhagic crust forms. Serologic tests are not positive until days or weeks following initial infection. Treatment with antibiotics is essential in the primary stages.

Tuberculosis can spread to the reproductive tract via the bloodstream, causing secondary infection. The primary infection is usually found in the lungs, and the secondary reproductive tract infection tends to occur in the fallopian tubes in females and in the prostate in males. Treatment includes the same medications that are used to treat primary tuberculosis (see Chap. 3).

The reproductive tract is susceptible to infection from the gastrointestinal tract, and *E. coli* is a frequent cause of reproductive tract infections. Staphylococci and streptococci are also frequent causes of reproductive tract infections. In each case of infection, it is necessary to identify the causative organism(s) via appropriate smear, culture, and staining techniques as well as tests for sensitivity to determine drug therapy. The nurse collects specimens of drainage or secretions for these laboratory studies and is careful to obtain the specimens from the localized site of infection to avoid contamination from other organisms that might be present at the site. Chemotherapy selected according to the sensitivity of the organism is instituted as early as possible to treat the infection. In health teaching, the nurse emphasizes the importance of early recognition and treatment of all reproductive tract infections. These infections can easily become chronic and, if infections occur repeatedly, the reproductive tract can be irreversibly damaged by the infectious process. For example, chronic infection in the fallopian tubes causes scarring and fibrosis of tissue so that the normal peristaltic movement of the tubes is impaired. Adhesions may form as a result of the fibrosis and can obstruct the fallopian tube. The same process may result in the epididymis causing obstruction in the transport of sperm.

SECONDARY INFECTIONS

In addition to infection by microorganisms, the reproductive tract can be traumatized by iatrogenic causes such as instrumentation for examination of the bladder in men or from procedures used in pelvic examination, or during delivery or induced abortion in women. Lacerations or mechanical trauma to the cervix or vagina during delivery or abortion make the woman particularly vulnerable to inflammation and infection at the site of the trauma. It is important that care be taken to protect the patient from injury when carrying out any type of procedure.

Many diseases also cause secondary inflammation or infection of the reproductive tract. An example is inflammation of the prepuce of the penis or of the vulva in diabetic patients with glycosuria. The viral disease mumps can be complicated by mumps orchitis, an inflammation of the testes that can result in chronic atrophy and fibrosis. Tuberculosis has been mentioned as a secondary reproductive tract infection. The prostate may be the focus of infection from another body part such as infected sinuses or infected teeth. Reiter's syndrome is a triad of conjunctivitis, arthritis, and urethritis and occurs in males. While Reiter's syndrome is self-limiting, it lasts for 1 to 5 months and the patient experiences great discomfort with diarrhea, chills, urinary tract symptoms of burning and frequency, and generalized malaise. The prostate is also a focal point in arthritis or myositis, and the patient may develop chronic perineal and low back pain.

Prostatitis

Prostatitis has serious implications for the male in that he not only experiences discomfort but also has impaired sexual ability in many instances. Granulomatous prostatitis is a nonspecific form of prostatitis that represents an inflammatory process caused by the granulomatous reaction. Other causes of prostatitis not previously mentioned are septicemia, or diffuse systemic pyemia. When the patient has acute prostatitis, the prostate gland becomes congested and stasis of fluid supports bacterial growth so that infections and abscesses may result. There may be blood in the seminal fluid in acute inflammation, and the patient has generalized symptoms of increased temperature, nausea, vomiting, premature ejaculation, decreased libido, and painful ejaculation. Pain in the perineal area and the rectum makes sexual activity difficult for some patients. For care and treatment, it is necessary to define the cause of the prostatitis. In some instances, the condition has a nonspecific cause; no organism can be identified and no source of inflammation can be found. Sometimes the patient has drainage containing bacteria and leukocytes. In other instances it is necessary to gently massage the prostate to obtain secretions; however, this is contraindicated in acute prostatitis because the massage causes exacerbation of the inflammation. Treatment is complicated because the prostate does not excrete antibiotics, and a lipid-soluble antibiotic is required to pass through barriers to the epithelial cell wall. Prostatitis can become chronic and may follow infections in the testis. Eventually, in chronic conditions, the patient suffers from the cumulative effects of the condition in emotional frustration as well as physiologic impairment.

Pelvic Inflammatory Disease

Pelvic inflammatory disease (PID) is a condition that results from the cumulative effects of chronic conditions. It occurs most frequently in females who have a history of being sexually active and who have had repeated reproductive tract infections such as gonorrhea or pyogenic bacterial infections (Fig. 9-8). It can also follow trauma to the reproductive tract following delivery or abortion or instrumentation, or systemic infections and sepsis. The use of an IUD can also contribute to increased risk for development of PID in susceptible individuals. The ovaries and fallopian tubes are usually most severely involved, and the patient is usually uncomfortable with abdominal distention, rebound abdominal tenderness, fever, lower abdominal pain, low back pain, perineal pain, nausea and vomiting, an increased sedimentation rate, an increased leukocyte count, and general malaise. If all the pelvic organs are involved, peritonitis may result or a pelvic abscess may form. Diagnosis is confirmed by laparoscopy, and by culture and sensitivity testing of a specimen obtained during laparoscopy. Antibiotics are given in treatment, and efforts are made to clear the condition as soon as possible. The patient may have long-term effects of adhesion formation from the serous or fibrinous exudates

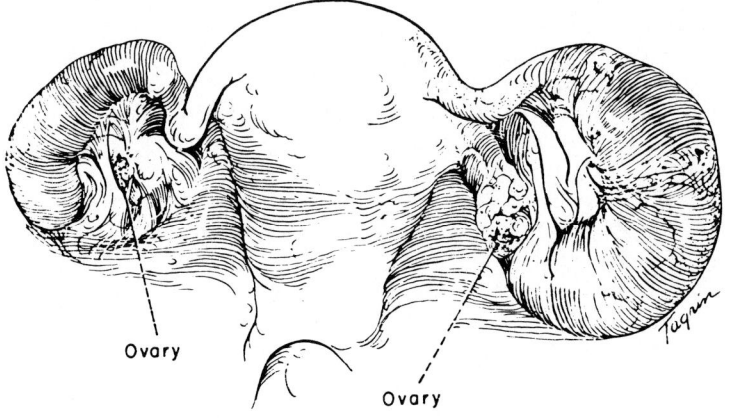

Figure 9-8
Typical gross pathology encountered in the chronic phase of gonorrheal pelvic inflammatory disease. (From T. H. Green, Jr., *Gynecology: Essentials of Clinical Practice* [3rd ed.]. Boston: Little, Brown and Company, 1977. Reproduced by permission.)

resulting from infectious processes, particularly if the infectious or inflammatory process is focused within the fallopian tubes. The adhesions may form between any of the pelvic organs including the fallopian tubes, the ovaries, the uterus, the bowel, the supporting structures of the uterus, and the peritoneum. Therefore early treatment (including laparotomy if necessary) of abscess formation is essential. Other complications from delayed treatment or failure to respond to treatment include septic emboli and pelvic thrombophlebitis. Sterility may result if the fallopian tubes become occluded or if their function is impaired by fibrosis and scarring. In impaired function, transport of sperm and of the conceptus is hindered, thereby increasing the potential for ectopic pregnancy.

In the overall nursing care and treatment for chronic prostatitis and pelvic inflammatory disease, the patient is advised to observe bedrest until the acute symptoms abate. Hospitalization may be necessary for treatment of abscess formation and sepsis or peritonitis that can result from ruptured abscesses. The severely ill patient may develop fluid and electrolyte imbalances and shock. Renal failure may result, requiring dialysis. Care of the patient in shock is discussed in Chapter 16. In both prostatitis and PID the patient is advised to avoid sexual intercourse until the condition has cleared. Males with prostatitis are counseled to avoid alcohol, spices, and coffee. When there are muscle rigidity and low back pain, warm baths may help relax muscles and relieve pain.

MALE REPRODUCTIVE TRACT DYSFUNCTION

Imperfect descent of the testis (cryptorchidism) may be diagnosed at birth or may be found during repair of an inguinal hernia. The testis can be **ectopic** (located in a position other than in the scrotum such as in the perineum or inguinal region); **retractile** (incompletely descended but capable of being manipulated into the scrotal sac); or **incompletely descended** (fixed in position because of a shorter than normal ductus deferens or abnormalities in the cremaster muscle). Either one testis or both may fail to descend into the scrotum. The reason for the imperfect descent is not known, but it is thought that hormonal imbalance may be causative. Usually, the incompletely descended testes are small and do not function well in the production of sperm, whereas ectopic testes are of normal size and function.

Treatment for ectopic testis includes gonadotropin therapy or surgery. Without treatment the ectopic testis may not function well because of the effect of body temperature on spermatogenesis. **Orchiopexy** is the surgical procedure in which the undescended testis is replaced into the scrotum. Incompletely descended testes of the retractile type often do descend during the growth period when the testes increase in size and weight. Incompletely descended testes that are fixed in position are often placed into the scrotum surgically because they are subject to trauma in their abnormal position. The imperfectly descended testis is also more susceptible to abnormal cell growth.

Torsion of the testis (Fig. 9-9) is another complication of imperfectly descended testes. Torsion often occurs in males who also have inguinal hernias and in those with absence of the scrotal ligament. The torsion can occur suddenly, causing pain that is similar to acute appendicitis. The scrotum swells, and there may be nausea and vomiting. Blood vessels in the twisted testis may become infarcted when the testis has been twisted for 6 hours or longer, and surgery for correction of the infarction is required immediately otherwise necrosis will occur. After 8 hours no treatment is necessary because the infarcted area has become necrotic, the pain has been relieved, and the tissue damage has become irreversible [18]. The surgical procedure for treatment of torsion of the testis involves untwisting the testis.

The development of a hydrocele is associated with the descent of the testes. Two layers of the peritoneum are normally carried down into the scrotal sac as the testes descend and the two peritoneal layers form the tunica vaginalis and are separated from the peritoneum by closure of the tunica vaginalis. A **hydrocele** is collection of fluid within the two layers of the tunica vaginalis. An acute hydrocele can occur following trauma or may develop more slowly following infection of the testes or epididymis. In some males the tunica vaginalis does not close and there is then communication between the peritoneal cavity and the tunica vaginalis, so that fluid from the peritoneal cavity can fill the layers

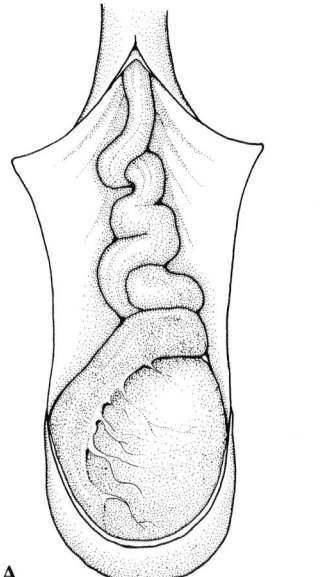
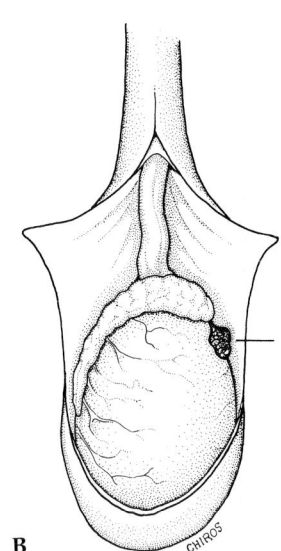

Figure 9-9
A. Torsion of the testicle.
B. Torsion of appendix testis.

and result in a hydrocele. This fluid flows back into the peritoneal area when the scrotum is elevated. Hydroceles are treated by aspiration of the fluid; this may have to be repeated several times. In some instances a sclerosing agent is injected.

Hydroceles may become chronic and are also subject to infection. If infected, the fluid in the hydrocele is cloudy and contains polymorphonuclear leukocytes. Usually, the fluid in the hydrocele is clear and pale yellow and varies in amount, ranging from about 100 ml to as much as 300 ml. When the hydrocele becomes chronic, both fibrosis and calcification can occur. In some instances the development of fibrous adhesions causes the hydrocele to become divided into a series of sacs separated by adhesions. Large chronic hydroceles compress the normal testicular tissue and can eventually result in atrophy of the testes with loss of normal function. If aspiration does not alleviate the condition, surgical excision (Fig. 9-10) of the sac containing the hydrocele is necessary. The major complication of this type of surgery is bleeding.

Hematocele is similar to hydrocele except that the tunica vaginalis is filled with blood. The hematocele is usually the result of trauma such as in torsion of the testes, following a surgical procedure in the abdomen or for repair of an inguinal hernia, or when there is an abnormal process such as tumor growth or systemic disease. The hematocele can also develop without any apparent cause, gradually filling with blood. If the hematocele is present for a long enough time, the blood becomes clotted and the wall of the hematocele thickens. Eventually, the hematocele may appear as a tumor in its consistency.

Cysts may also form, usually from remnants of embryologic development that degenerate. The cysts may be located on the spermatic cord or in the epididymis, and hydroceles can develop in the cysts. Treatment involves aspiration or surgical incision or excision of the cyst.

Another condition that occurs in males, particularly young men, is varicocele. A **varicocele** is a dilated vein of the spermatic cord. Because the left internal spermatic vein joins the left renal vein at an angle, the left side is more susceptible to dilatation. When a varicocele develops, blood flow in the internal spermatic vein is obstructed and corollary venous drainage from the testes must be established. The exact cause of varicocele is not known, but the condition is often associated with large retroperitoneal tumors in the abdominal cavity. Because varicoceles tend to occur more frequently in young, sexually active males, it is thought that the increased vasodilatation during sexual arousal may be a factor in susceptible males. Varicocele causes

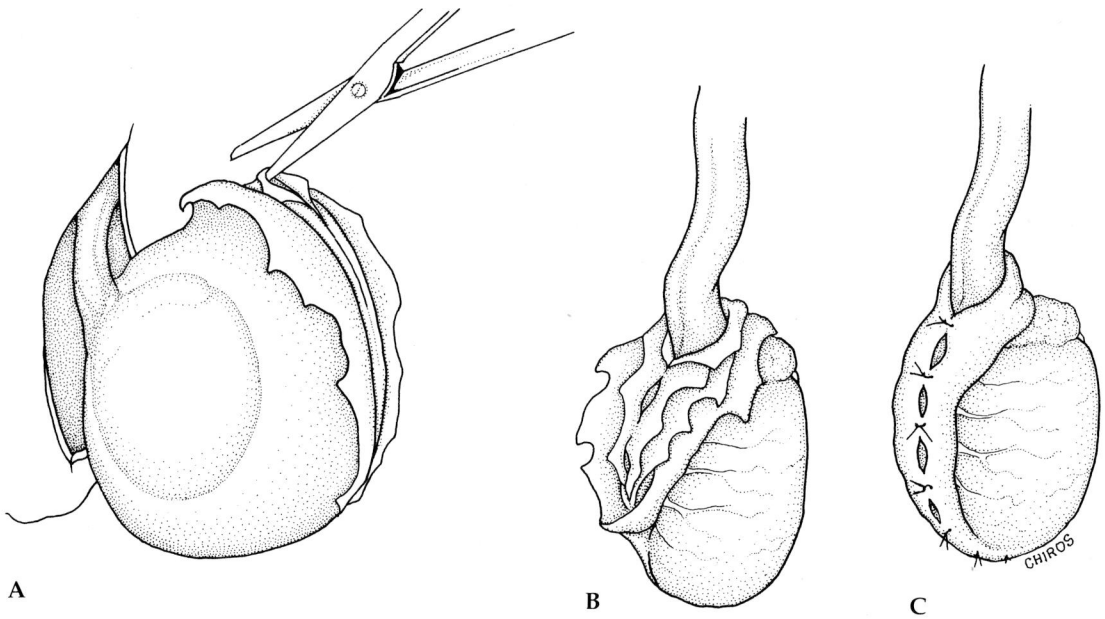

Figure 9-10
Repair of hydrocele. **A.** Layers of hydrocele are divided and peeled back. **B.** Excess sac tissue is trimmed and, **C,** sutured back around the epididymis and spermatic cord.

a vague but constant pain often described as a pulling sensation. Because the patient's complaints are often vague, the diagnosis of varicocele may be missed and the patient may be thought to have psychogenic complaints. Treatment involves ligation of the spermatic vein.

Simple removal of the spermatic cord, testes, and epididymis can be performed via an inguinal incision. Radical surgery includes removal of the retroperitoneal lymph nodes; this procedure requires general anesthesia and an abdominal incision. Postoperatively the patient has drains in the wound, and the amount, color, and character of the drainage are noted and recorded. The patient requires all the postoperative care essential for anyone who has an abdominal laparotomy, as described in Chapter 1.

When there is trauma to the testes the major complication is bleeding. An ice pack or cold compresses are applied to reduce swelling and to decrease bleeding. The testes are immobilized by placing a scrotal bridge formed by applying tape from one thigh to the other to support the scrotum. When lacerations occur in trauma, repair is performed in surgery. Again, bleeding is a major complication and the nurse examines the dressings for drainage. The dressings are held in place by a scrotal support. Drains are usually placed during the surgical procedure to promote drainage and to reduce edema. In every surgical procedure involving the sex organs, the nurse is cognizant that the patient has highly individual feelings about the meaning of the surgery and that the patient can be distressed about the impact of the surgery more than by the physical discomfort if the testes are permanently impaired.

Two other conditions that may occur involve the penis. These conditions are Peyronie's disease and priapism. **Peyronie's disease** is a slowly progressing condition in which irregular nodules form on the penis, usually near the glans penis. Fibrous plaques eventually form and cause the tissue to become inelastic so that, on erection, the penis curves abnormally. The condition causes edema and painful erection, and therefore interferes with intercourse. Peyronie's disease can be self-limiting and is treated by administration of cortisone. The plaques may be limited to localized patches or can occur more extensively. If the plaques are localized, they can be excised.

Priapism is the sudden onset of erection that persists, sometimes for days or weeks. This type of erection can be caused by systemic diseases such as leukemia or sickle cell anemia, or by inflammatory or neoplastic diseases involving the nervous system, or by spinal cord tumors. The male genital organs are innervated by parasympathetic fibers arising from the second, third, and fourth segments of the sacral cord. The muscles of erection (the compressor urethrae, the ischiocavernosus, and the bulbocavernosus muscles) can be controlled by reflex activity of the spinal nerves or by stimulation or inhibition from the parasympathetic impulses arising from the cerebrum. It is in the cerebrum where the afferent impulses for auditory, olfactory, visual, and touch receptors, all of which contribute to sexual arousal, are integrated. Parasympathetic stimulation increases secretion of mucus in the genital glands, such as the prostate, and dilatation of arterioles in the penis. The resulting increased blood flow to the penis causes venous flow to be shut off and the penis to become engorged, hard, and distended. In priapism, erection is not stimulated by sexual arousal, and the penis is somewhat soft although indurated. The continued distention can lead to both thrombosis and fibrosis in the corpora cavernosum (one of the columns of erectile tissue in the penis). The result can be loss of the capability for erection. Priapism can be transitory, and in this instance is often due to the reflex sacral spinal innervation for erection, as occurs in spinal cord injuries.

One of the more common conditions that affect aging men and that usually occur after the age of 50 years is **benign prostatic hypertrophy.** The reason for benign hypertrophy is unknown, but it is thought that changes in the ratio of androgens to estrogens may be a factor. The secretion of testosterone normally decreases in aging, thereby changing the relative amount of androgens and estrogens. The changes in this ratio with increasing estrogen levels in relation to androgen levels become greater at middle age and thereafter. Hypertrophy of the prostate may take place in either the muscular or the glandular structures of the prostate or both, and the resulting signs and symptoms depend on the effects of the enlargement on surrounding structures rather than on the size of the enlarged prostate.

The prostate gland surrounds the urethra and is located immediately below the bladder and just above the opening of the ejaculatory ducts into the urethra. (The ejaculatory ducts are formed by fusion of the seminal vesicles and the distal vas deferens, which passes through the posterior prostate and empties into the posterior urethra.) The ejaculatory ducts pass through the prostate gland posteriorly. Anteriorly the prostate lies behind the symphysis pubis and posteriorly it lies on the rectum. The prostate gland is contained in a fibrous capsule and consists of muscular fibers encircling the urethra and under the outer capsule and glandular portion of the prostate, in which small lobules (acini) are connected to tubules (ducts) that empty into the urethra. The prostate gland produces clear alkaline fluid that makes up about 20 percent of the seminal fluid volume [20]. The fibrous muscular portion provides support for the glands that contain this fluid, and the blood vessels enmeshed in the muscular portion of the prostate provide nutrients for the glandular portion. The prostate is normally about the size of a chestnut, and the glandular portion is arranged in three lobes, the two lateral lobes and the middle lobe. The anterior and posterior lobes are usually not present in adults.

When the glandular portion of the prostate hypertrophies, the outer fibrous structure is compressed and eventually forms a false capsule just inside the true capsule. When there is hypertrophy of the middle lobe, the enlarged prostate then impinges on either the urethra, the bladder, or both. The urethra becomes distorted and displaced as a result of the enlargement, and urine flow is impeded. The middle lobe enlargement can also encroach on the bladder wall so that the normal contour of the bladder is changed and, instead, dependent areas within the bladder are created around the encroaching prostate. Urine stasis can occur in these dependent areas because the bladder cannot be emptied completely.

The changes that take place within the prostate gland can vary from the formation of irregularly shaped nodules, the development of hemorrhagic areas, fibrosis or hyperplasia of the columnar epithelium that lines the ducts, to the formation of cysts that contain lymphocytes and the debris of necrotic tissue. A complication of these changes is the development of inflammation or infection in the complex glandular structures of the prostate

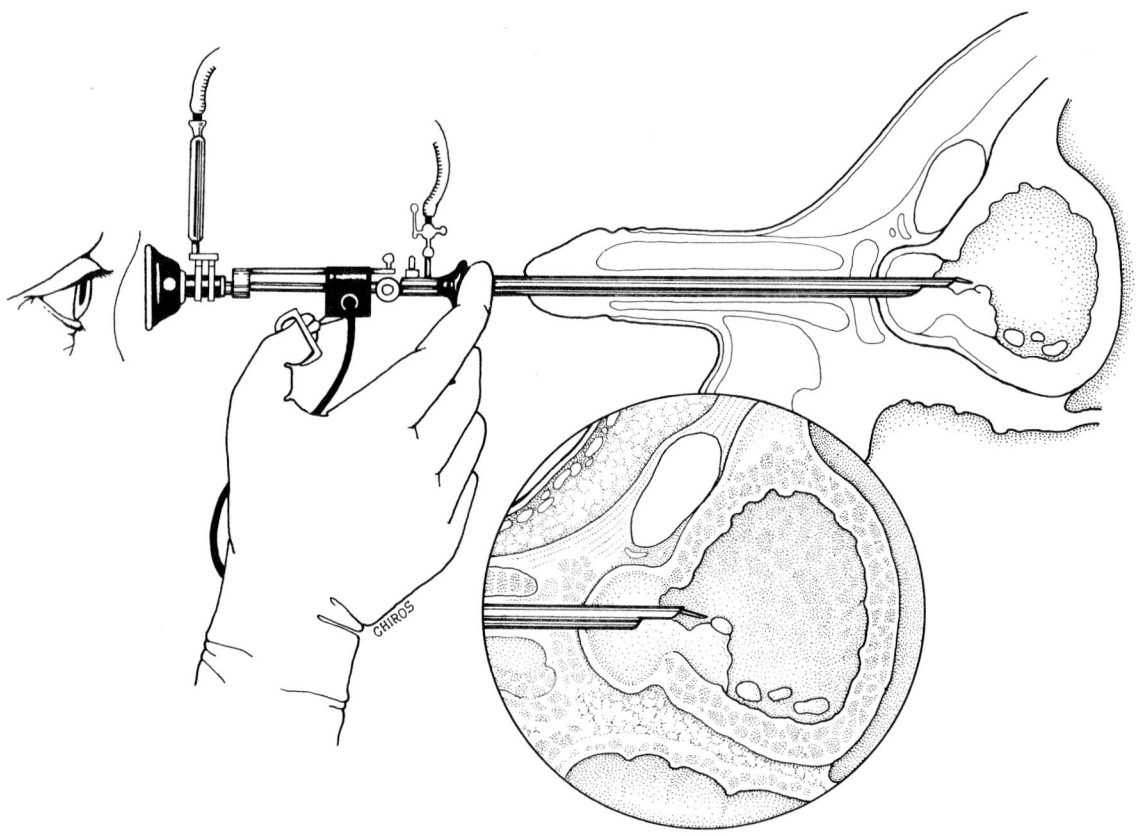

Figure 9-11
Transurethral resection of the prostate.

gland. Chronic prostatitis is a complication of prostate hypertrophy and may be the initial cause of obvious or visible signs and symptoms.

The patient with benign prostatic hypertrophy may have no symptoms because the processes of change take place gradually and because the prostate and surrounding structures can adapt to the gradual changes until urine flow is obstructed or infection occurs and does not respond to treatment. It is then necessary to treat the hypertrophy of the prostate to clear the infection. In some patients, obstruction of urine flow causes the initial obvious symptoms. Because the urethra is compressed, the patient may have difficulty in starting, maintaining, and terminating the stream of urine. He may experience intermittency in micturition in which the urine flow starts and stops, and he may also experience dribbling after termination of the stream.

Pressure of the enlarged prostate on the trigone of the bladder can cause increased frequency of urination and nocturia as well. It should be noted that the elderly normally experience nocturia because the ability of the kidneys to concentrate urine decreases with age. Patients with enlarged prostates that encroach on the bladder have more than normal incidences of nocturia. In addition to the changes in the urinary stream and in the frequency of urination, the patient may also experience pain and burning on urination.

Still other patients may not notice any of the signs and symptoms of obstruction of urine flow until kidney function is impaired as a result of urine stasis or until urine retention becomes acute. Urine retention results when the urethral structures are compressed sufficiently to preclude passage of urine. The patient is then susceptible to infection, has an urgent desire to micturate but cannot initiate the urinary stream and, if retention causes pressure on blood vessels in the bladder mucosa, the patient may develop hematuria. When the urinary bladder becomes full and overflows, the patient may be incontinent. Inability to empty the bladder also creates changes in the upper urinary tract and eventually the kidney. Ureteral dilatation, eventually leading to dilation of the kidney pelvis, may result from stasis of urine in the distended bladder. **Hydroureter,** distention of the ureter with urine, and **hydronephrosis,** distention of the kidney pelvis resulting from stasis of urine in the urinary tract, can lead to infection and urinary stone formation, and eventually to renal failure. These conditions are described in Chapter 6. In some patients with benign prostatic hypertrophy, renal failure is the first indication of pathology.

Diagnosis of benign prostatic hypertrophy consists in obtaining a complete history and physical examination. The abdomen is examined, and if the bladder is still distended after the patient has emptied his bladder, urinary retention is suspected. The amount of residual urine volume is checked by catheterizing the patient. With chronic retention of urine, the urinary bladder may contain as much as 1,500 ml of urine. In this event, the bladder is emptied slowly over a period of several days. A Foley catheter can be left in place for gradual decompression of the bladder or, if necessary, a suprapubic cystotomy tube through the abdominal wall and into the urinary bladder is used to decompress the bladder. In some patients this conservative treatment may alleviate the signs and symptoms for a time so that no further treatment is necessary. Decompression of the bladder, however, is also a necessary preparation for surgical removal of the diseased prostatic tissue.

Other components of the physical examination include examination of the urine to determine the presence of urinary tract infection, examination of the bladder by cystoscope (as described in Chap. 6), and a rectal examination. The prostatic enlargement may be felt on rectal examination unless only the middle lobe is involved. The prostate will feel small and firm if fibrotic changes predominate, and can be large, elastic, and rubbery in consistency if the outer areas of the prostate gland are hypertrophied. Crepitation may be felt if cysts are present. The patient may describe symptoms of constipation if the prostate protrudes on the rectum. If hematuria is present, the patient is carefully examined for the presence of tumors. The hematuria can be caused by pressure on blood vessels in the bladder mucosa when urine retention compresses the mucosa or by abnormal cell growth. It is also necessary to evaluate the patient's renal function through such tests as the blood urea nitrogen and serum creatinine tests and a creatinine clearance test. Other aspects of renal function evaluation are discussed in Chapter 6. The urinary tract is evaluated by intravenous pyelogram.

Treatment includes a number of different measures. As mentioned, catheterization relieves symptoms of urinary bladder retention. Complications that can occur when the bladder is decompressed too quickly include rupture of the blood vessels in the stretched bladder mucosa and postobstructive diuresis with secretion of up to 200 ml of urine per hour that can disrupt the patient's fluid and electrolyte balance. Prostatic massage can be used to relieve congestion from retained prostatic secretions if the prostate is not inflamed or infected. Urethral constriction can be alleviated in certain patients by passing urethral sounds. If frequency of urination and nocturia are the patient's major problems, anticholinergic drugs can be given to reduce the bladder tone, but these drugs also increase urinary retention by interfering with bladder contraction and therefore the patient's response to the anticholinergic drugs is monitored and the drugs are discontinued if urinary retention becomes too great. Infection is treated with antibiotics, but the patient may not respond to antibiotic therapy until the abnormal prostatic tissue is removed.

Prostatectomy is the surgical removal of abnormal portions of the prostate gland and can be an elective procedure (Fig. 9-11). Because many patients with benign prostatic hypertrophy are elderly, they may have a number of other medical problems such as cardiovascular disease or respiratory dysfunction. Some of these patients may prefer conservative treatment for their enlarged prostate instead of agreeing to have surgery since they are more likely to have complications from the anesthesia or from the stress of the surgical procedure. When the patient elects surgery, his physical status is carefully determined and the necessary precautions are taken to prevent complications that may occur in relation to other existing medical problems.

There are four surgical approaches to prostatectomy: transurethral resection, suprapubic prostatectomy, retropubic prostatectomy, and perineal prostatectomy. Each of these procedures can be used in specific situations, but transurethral resection is the procedure performed most frequently. All these procedures allow for removal of the abnormal prostatic gland by enucleation. Of major concern in these procedures are hemostasis and prevention of infection. When the gland is greatly enlarged or when there are bladder stones, suprapubic prostatectomy provides for more direct visualization and easier removal of prostatic tissue or bladder stones. A retropubic prostatectomy is indicated when the enlarged prostate is located high in the pelvic area. In the retropubic approach the patient has an incision in the pubic area but the bladder is not incised. When the gland lies lower in the pelvic cavity and it is desirable to provide for dependent drainage of urine and infectious materials away from the site of the surgery, the perineal approach is used. In the perineal approach, care to avoid damage to the external sphincter muscles and to the rectum requires meticulous surgical technique.

Transurethral resection is performed via a cystoscope that is passed through the urethra. The scope allows the surgeon to visualize the interior of the bladder and the operative site. An electric cutting loop and a cauterization loop are used to excise the abnormal prostatic tissue in pieces that are drained from the bladder by continuous irrigation throughout the procedure (see Fig. 9-11).

Following resection of the abnormal prostatic tissue in all these procedures, hemostasis is provided for by placing a Foley catheter with a 30-ml bag that is inflated in the prostatic urethral fossa. This catheter is left in place and provides sufficient pressure for hemostasis. During the procedure the prostatic tissue has been more or less shelled out of the capsule that surrounds the glandular tissue of the prostate. If the hypertrophy has compressed the outer layers of tissue to form a false capsule this false capsule, as well as the true capsule, is retained. The prostate gland function is thus maintained and the inner cavity fills in with epithelium in about 7 to 10 days. During the process of healing, however, bleeding can occur. Both a Foley catheter and a suprapubic cystotomy tube may be placed in surgery to provide for drainage, thereby preventing pressure on the bladder mucosa.

Nursing Care

Following surgery, the nurse monitors the patient's vital signs for signs of excessive blood loss (increased pulse, decreased blood pressure). The urine will be bloody initially, but this hematuria soon diminishes and the urine becomes pink and then returns to normal color. When the surgeon expects drainage of cellular debris and blood clots in great amounts, continuous irrigation is used to flush out the clots and debris. The nurse monitors this closed, continuous, sterile irrigation system, which can also be used for periodic flushing of the bladder. The type of equipment and procedure used for irrigation varies in different hospitals, but all formats and procedures mandate strict sterile technique to prevent infection. The bladder is flushed by allowing the irrigating fluid to run into the bladder slowly until the specified amount has been placed in the bladder. The irrigating fluid then passes from the bladder and is eliminated both from the Foley catheter and from the cystotomy tube if one is in place. When blood clots obstruct the elimination of urine or irrigating fluid, and if the ordinary irrigation measures have not loosened the clots, the surgeon should be notified. Because of the potential for bleeding, only gentle pressure should be applied in irrigating the bladder following prostatectomy.

The patient is also given fluids to tolerance and the nurse maintains an accurate record of intake and output, taking care to measure the irrigating solution as well as the oral and intravenous intake. Failure to subtract the irrigating solution from both intake and output records gives an inaccurate measure of the patient's renal function and of bladder retention. The nurse notes and records the color, consistency, and amount of output, including the presence of clots, cellular debris, and variations in color of the urine.

The patient who has had a suprapubic, retropubic, or perineal incision will have dressings that are checked for drainage or bleeding. In the suprapubic procedure the bladder wall has been incised, and urine leaks from the bladder can be irritating to the skin. Therefore meticulous care is taken to change the dressings as needed and to use a barrier to protect the skin from excoriation by the acid urine (see Table 7-1 for skin barriers described for ostomy care). The cystotomy tube is placed to reduce the pressure or urine retention in the bladder, and a Penrose drain may be placed to provide for drainage from the surgical site. The type of drainage and its color and consistency are noted.

The patient may experience chills postoperatively if the transurethral procedure has been performed since the continuous irrigation that is part of the procedure can reduce body temperature. Another distressing sensation to the patient is the feeling that he needs to void even though a catheter is in place. The Foley catheter in place and the pain and discomfort experienced from manipulation of tissue both contribute to the sensation of pressure. When the patient tries to void around the catheter, bladder spasms can occur and an antispasmodic medication such as propantheline bromide (Pro-Banthine) is given to relieve the bladder spasms. The antispasmodic medication is discontinued 1 or 2 days prior to removal of the catheter (which stays in place 4 to 7 days, depending on the patient's response) so that the bladder can contract normally. Following catheter removal the patient's output is measured with each voiding and if urinary retention is present, measures are taken to prevent bladder distention. Postoperative bladder spasms are less worrisome to the patient if he is told about their occurrence prior to surgery in the preoperative teaching phase of his care.

The patient often has concerns about what to expect in the months following prostatectomy. The nurse advises the patient to avoid lifting heavy objects and to prevent constipation so that undue stress is not placed on the healing prostate gland. The patient can expect to continue having some pus and cellular debris in his urine postoperatively; also urinary incontinence can occur following the procedure. The convalescence is shorter following a transurethral resection than following a suprapubic prostatectomy because the bladder is not incised in the transurethral procedure. Patients are advised to abstain from sexual activity for varying periods of time following the prostatectomy. Although two months is an average time, the surgeon advises the patient about when he can resume sexual activity; the type of procedure and the amount of manipulation that occurred in surgery determine the amount of time the patient should not place stress on the prostate gland. Finally, nursing care before, during, and after prostatectomy takes into account the patient's individual needs in relation to other medical problems, his age, and his concerns about the surgery. Unfortunately, prostatectomy is not always a permanent cure, but may have to be repeated in certain patients since the procedure provides for removal of abnormal prostatic tissue but does not remove the unknown cause of the hypertrophy.

FEMALE REPRODUCTIVE TRACT DYSFUNCTION

Some of the more commonly occurring conditions that affect the female reproductive tract as the result of congenital causes, hormonal imbalances, diseases, or the normal aging process include disorders in menstruation, endometriosis, and relaxation of the pelvic structures. Puberty normally begins at the age of about 14 years and may begin either earlier or as late as 17 or 18 years. The normal variations in the onset of puberty can be attributed to genetic influences, environmental factors such as climate and nutrition, and to the individual's make-up. Throughout life the female can have variations in menstrual periods. Some of these variations are normal, but others are indicative of disease or dysfunction. Both diagnosis and treatment of menstrual dysfunction are complicated by the complex central nervous system control of reproductive function in which emotional and physiologic aspects of the individual's experiences are integrated. While some of the conditions in reproductive tract dysfunction are congenital or genetic, others are acquired as a result of pregnancy, in the quality of relationships the woman experiences, or in the type of work she does.

The nurse is conversant with the terminology used in describing disturbances in menstruation. **Amenorrhea** is absence of menstrual flow. **Oligomenorrhea** is decreased frequency in menstrual bleeding in lengthened menstrual cycles. **Hypomenorrhea** is a decrease in the number of days of menstrual bleeding. **Hypermenorrhea** (menorrhagia) is increase in the number of days of menstrual bleeding, and **polymenorrhea** is increased frequency of menstrual bleeding in shortened menstrual cycles. **Metrorrhagia** is irregular menstrual bleeding that occurs between periods. **Dysmenorrhea** is discomfort and pain associated with menstrual bleeding, while the **premenstrual syndrome** is discomfort prior to menstrual bleeding. **Menopause** is the cessation of menstrual bleeding and occurs at varying ages. Delayed menopause rarely occurs as late as the seventh decade. **Climacteric** is another term that refers to cessation of menstrual bleeding. In summary, lengthened or shortened menstrual cycles, increased or decreased menstrual flow in regular cycles, irregular cycles, or the absence of menstrual flow are the types of menstrual dysfunction the woman can experience.

The pattern of menstrual cycles and the length and amount of menstrual bleeding are highly individual. When dysfunction in menstrual bleeding does occur, the change from the woman's usual pattern is significant in diagnosis. Many women normally experience infrequent changes from their usual menstrual patterns when they move to a different climate, undergo a stressful emotional experience such as participation in competitive events, begin a new job, undergo a traumatic experience, or have a temporary but serious illness. High fevers, for example, can interfere with follicular development. The menstrual history therefore is important in diagnosis, and this history becomes more meaningful when related to events in the woman's life. The nurse interviews the patient with the goal of establishing how the current situation differs from the woman's past experiences. In addition to determining the usual pattern of menstruation and the events that alter this usual pattern, the nurse also ascertains how much blood loss the patient has. It is difficult to estimate blood flow in menstruation; therefore the nurse asks specific questions such as: How many days does your period last? How often do you change your tampons or pads? The patient is also asked to estimate the amount of drainage that collects on the tampons or pads. Because menstrual flow is a normal function, many women do not keep track of their menstrual periods and are thus unable to give the nurse specific data about the history of duration of menses or the timing of their menstrual cycles. Other women are able to relate precise dates and times about their menstrual cycles and menstrual flow. Having the patient maintain a record of menstrual flow over a period of time is helpful in evaluating possible causes of dysfunction as well as the results of therapy.

In determining the possible causes of disturbances in menstrual flow the examiner first refers to the patient's history. When the disturbances were first noticed in relation to pregnancy and delivery, use of contraceptive medications, or the onset of symptoms such as weight gain, decreased energy, or other evidences of metabolic dysfunction are determined to evaluate possible systemic dysfunction that can influence menstrual cycles. Disorders in menstrual cycles can occur because of lack of pituitary hormones, a deficiency of ovarian hormones, or dysfunction of the uterus. Endocrine imbalances, particularly of thyroid and adrenal origin, are associated with changes in menstrual function. Diseases or dysfunction affecting the hypothalamus and the pituitary can result in altered menses. Therefore, evaluation of the patient's status often includes evaluation of thyroid, adrenal, pituitary, and pancreatic function in addition to function of the ovaries. Evaluation of dysfunction of the reproductive tract also requires a pelvic examination, tests of cervical mucus, biopsy of tissue from the vagina, cervix, and uterus, and laparoscopy if indicated.

This discussion of menstrual dysfunction is limited to amenorrhea, changes in the menopause, and dysfunctional uterine bleeding. Amenorrhea can be primary or secondary. **Primary amenorrhea** is associated with complicated endocrine imbalances or can be caused by congenital anomalies such as absence of the vagina or uterus or both, an imperforate hymen, or ovarian or pituitary dysfunction. In primary amenorrhea, the female has never had a menstrual period. **Secondary amenorrhea** is cessation of menses in females who have previously had normal menstrual cycles and menstrual flow. Pregnancy causes amenorrhea, as can contraceptive steroids, acquired hormonal imbalances, diseases affecting the pituitary, ovaries, uterus, or vagina, and systemic diseases. Figure 9-12 indicates the organs that can be involved in causing amenorrhea, along with etiologic fac-

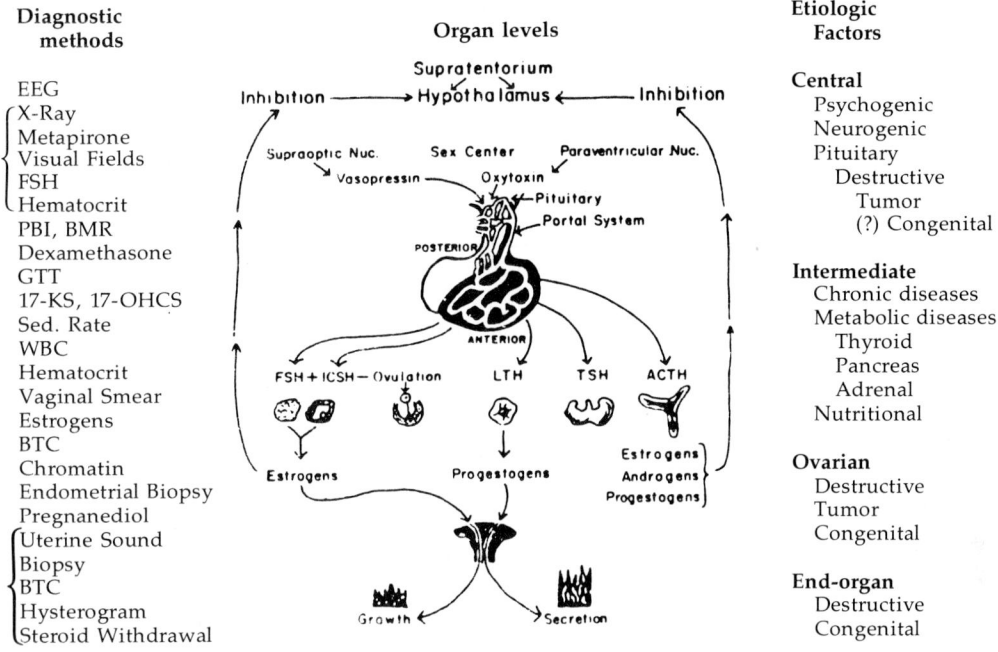

Figure 9-12
Diagnostic methods correlated with anatomic levels at which defects responsible for amenorrhea may occur. (From E. R. Novak, G. S. Jones, and H. W. Jones, *Textbook of Gynecology* [9th ed.]. Baltimore: Williams & Wilkins Co., 1975. Reproduced by permission.)

tors and diagnostic methods. (The reader is referred to Chapter 5 for details concerning blood tests such as hematocrit reading and to Chapter 8 for endocrine studies such as the metapirone, dexamethasone, 17-KS, and 17-OHCS tests.)

Treatment for amenorrhea differs according to the cause. In some cases, no treatment is given if the woman is otherwise healthy and no pathologic condition has been found. If, however, she wants to become pregnant or if she suffers psychological trauma because of the absence of menses, treatment may be given. Ovulation can be induced by giving gonadotropins. HMG (human menopausal gonadotropin) is often used for this purpose, as is clomiphene (Clomid). Because each person responds individually to these medications, dosages are individualized. The patient's response is carefully monitored by checking serum hormone levels and the menstrual cycles are evaluated by means of the BBT graph and examination of cervical mucus. Complications can occur from the use of steroids to induce ovulation, the major complications being excessive stimulation of the ovary with subsequent development of cysts that may rupture or even ovarian rupture. The serum levels of estrogen considered to be within a safe range in therapy range from as low as 150 pg per milliliter as the necessary level to induce ovulation to 700 pg per milliliter as the highest range that can be maintained without causing complications [15].

If the patient is found to have thyroid or adrenal hormone imbalances, treatment as described in Chapter 8 can result in menstrual flow. Improving the diet in malnourished females or the general state of health in debilitated females can also result in menstruation. Amenorrhea induced by steroid contraceptives usually occurs in females who had a pattern of irregular menses prior to taking the contraceptives. As long as 1 to 2 years may be required for return to usual function, and no treatment is given in ordinary circumstances. Amenorrhea following emotional stress can also be a temporary condition, and treatment is not given unless desired by the patient. When amenorrhea is associated with psychogenic causes, such as in anorexia nervosa, the treatment consists in psychiatric care (see Chap. 7).

Amenorrhea is normal in the menopause.

A few individuals can have a premature menopause in which ovarian follicles do not form either because of congenital factors or because of acquired pathology from inflammatory or infectious diseases that destroy ovarian tissue. Women who experience premature menopause have the same symptoms as are associated with normal menopause: cessation of menses and hot flushes.

Dysmenorrhea and the Premenstrual Syndrome

Many women experience difficulty with menstruation. Two types of problems are dysmenorrhea and the premenstrual syndrome. Dysmenorrhea (pain or discomfort associated with menstrual flow) can be either primary or secondary and its cause is unknown. One theory is that there is hypercontractility of the uterus. Finding evidence of prostaglandin in menstrual flow of these patients supports this theory since prostaglandin stimulates smooth muscle [10]. **Primary dysmenorrhea** is experienced with the onset of the menses at puberty. The female who experiences primary dysmenorrhea can have a variety of symptoms including colicky abdominal pain, nausea, vomiting, or lower abdominal pain extending to the back and to the thighs. Treatment for primary dysmenorrhea involves suppression of ovulation with steroids or dilatation of the cervix. Analgesics are given for pain. **Secondary dysmenorrhea** is acquired and begins during the adult years. It is thought that secondary dysmenorrhea might be caused by diminished progesterone levels. In some instances the discomfort can be caused by endometriosis, although not every woman with endometriosis experiences dysmenorrhea. The signs and symptoms of dysmenorrhea are indicative of nervous and vascular changes evidenced in increased irritability, gastrointestinal complaints, headache, and pain. The pain associated with dysmenorrhea is best relieved when analgesics are taken before the pain becomes severe.

Many assumptions have been made about why some women have dysmenorrhea while others have minimal discomfort with menstrual flow. It is thought that secondary dysmenorrhea might be related to immaturity, nonacceptance of the feminine role, initial traumatic sexual experiences, fear of childbirth, or emotional problems. Dysmenorrhea is usually accepted as valid by employers who allow time off when the woman experiences dysmenorrhea. Some persons believe that dysmenorrhea might be a functional disorder, but it is recognized that functional disorders cause real symptoms of discomfort and pain and that these symptoms need to be treated. Dysmenorrhea has been relieved in some women following marriage and pregnancy, and it is not known whether the positive effects of the woman's self-satisfaction or the hormonal changes in pregnancy have brought about the relief of symptoms. Some women do find that becoming actively involved in exercise or concentrating on interesting projects either relieves the symptoms of dysmenorrhea or decreases the awareness of the symptoms.

The premenstrual syndrome is associated with individualized symptoms that may include feeling depressed or irritable, weight gain with bloating or swelling, constipation, back pain, and soreness or tenderness of breasts. The symptoms of the premenstrual syndrome can begin as early as 10 or more days prior to the onset of menstrual flow and usually diminish 1 or 2 days after the flow has begun. It is thought that women who experience the premenstrual syndrome are affected by the hormonal and metabolic changes that take place in the menstrual cycle and that the swelling is related to changes in fluid and sodium retention. Some authorities prescribe diuretics to relieve fluid retention while others believe that no treatment should be given. When the premenstrual syndrome is associated with emotional disturbances, tranquilizers may be prescribed.

Mittelschmerz is pain and discomfort at midpoint in the menstrual cycle and is thought to be related to distention of the ovarian capsule. The pain in Mittelschmerz can be mild and transient or it can be a constant dull aching, with tenderness in the lower abdomen.

Abnormal Uterine Bleeding

Abnormal uterine bleeding can result from a number of different causes involving disorders of the uterus, hormone imbalance, or systemic disease. Young women who have abnormal menstrual bleeding often have blood dyscrasias that first become apparent when diagnostic tests are performed to determine the cause of the bleeding. In other instances bleeding is a symptom of cancer of the cervix or of the uterus. When no physical cause can be found, the bleeding is called dysfunctional uterine bleeding and is most often caused by **anovulation** (failure to ovulate). To determine the cause of bleeding, the patient is examined for the presence of abnormal cell growth, changes in structure resulting from inflammation or infection, and general systemic diseases. Occasional dysfunctional uterine bleeding may be a normal response to unusually great emotional tension.

Uterine bleeding occurs acutely but may be transitory, and blood loss can be minimal. The patient who has lost large amounts of blood in uterine bleeding can present in shock and must be treated immediately for hypovolemic shock as described in Chapter 16. Initial examination of the patient who presents with uterine bleeding includes not only emergency treatment to stabilize the patient's condition, but also examination to determine the source of the bleeding. The external genitalia and vagina are examined to determine the presence of lacerations, erosions, or foreign bodies. A pelvic examination is required to determine whether the source of bleeding is the upper vagina, the cervix, or the uterus. Bleeding can be caused by ectopic pregnancy that has ruptured, causing sudden and severe abdominal pain. In this situation, peritonitis can develop from the rupture into the peritoneal cavity. Pressure on the diaphragm also causes shoulder pain typically found in women who have ruptured ectopic pregnancies. Treatment for this condition involves emergency abdominal laparotomy for surgical removal of the products of the ruptured ectopic pregnancy and repair of strictures. Yet another cause of bleeding is incomplete abortion in which the patient has varying amounts of blood loss and cramping pain. Treatment for incomplete abortion is removal of the fetal remnants by suction or curettage. Uterine bleeding can also result from iatrogenic causes such as hemorrhage following surgery.

Although uterine bleeding begins without warning, the bleeding is not always life-threatening. Uterine bleeding can be of short duration, and the blood loss can be minimal or great. Therefore the patient's hemoglobin and hematocrit levels are monitored as a measure of blood loss. Not every episode of uterine bleeding is a medical emergency, but the patient who experiences the sudden onset of bleeding may be worried and anxious about the meaning of the bleeding, particularly if the patient is aware that uterine bleeding is a symptom of carcinoma. When the woman experiences prolonged menstrual periods (hypermenorrhea) or more frequent periods (polymenorrhea), she may adapt to the changes and often seeks medical assistance for signs and symptoms of anemia rather than for diagnosis and treatment of the uterine bleeding. These women often express their annoyance and frustration with having to cope with their seemingly constant menstrual flow. In polymenorrhea, intervals of less than 18 days between menstrual periods are considered abnormal and the patient should be evaluated to determine the cause of the uterine bleeding [4]. The diagnosis of uterine bleeding can involve long-term evaluation of the patient's menstrual cycle, and during this time the patient often becomes frustrated because she still has the inconvenience of excessive menstrual flow along with the added inconvenience of maintaining her BBT or having numerous diagnostic tests.

Abnormal uterine bleeding from endocrine causes can occur with ovulation or in the absence of ovulation. The presence of ovarian cysts or ovarian tumors that secrete hormones, or of corpus luteal cysts of the ovary, and uterine pathology can cause changes either in the secretion of progesterone or in the uterine response to progesterone following ovulation. It is necessary to determine therefore whether ovulation has taken place. If ovulation has occurred the patient's menstrual cycles are usually regular, but the duration and amount of bleeding are variable because the amount of progesterone secreted by the corpus luteum is inadequate to counteract the effects of the estrogen. Irregular ripening and shedding of the endometrium is evidenced by finding both secretory and proliferative endometrium when a D and C is performed 4 to 5 days after the onset of menstrual flow. The exact timing of the D and C is essential in the diagnosis. This irregular ripening and shedding can be caused by an abnormal endometrial response to hormones or to delayed regression of the corpus luteum.

In anovulatory bleeding the failure to ovulate is investigated. The primary cause of anovulatory bleeding may be found in the ovaries or in the pituitary. Secondary causes include systemic or endocrine diseases that influence ovarian and pituitary function. When the ovarian follicle does not mature, progesterone is not secreted in adequate amounts and the endometrium is in the proliferative phase, so that the patient's menstrual cycles are irregular and there is increased bleeding. Hemostasis is then necessary to stop the bleeding, and progesterone in oil is given intramuscularly for this purpose. If the bleeding ceases, a menstrual period is then induced by giving progesterone to cause normal shedding of the endometrium. If the patient does not respond to the progesterone, a D and C is necessary. Some patients resume normal menstrual cycles following the episode of bleeding and the treatment, but others require long-term therapy such as taking progestins during the last half of each menstrual cycle or progestins supplemented with estrogen. Many different drug therapy regimens are used to regulate menstrual cycles, and the selection of a specific regimen is made on the basis of the patient's response to the therapy and according to the physi-

cian's preference. The patient's response is evaluated periodically to monitor the effectiveness of therapy. Persistent abnormal uterine bleeding is an indication that the patient has a great potential for developing cancer of the uterus. Therefore, when other forms of treatment are not effective, the woman may have a hysterectomy to cure the condition. Hysterectomy is often the treatment of choice for an older woman who does not wish to become pregnant, but is deferred when the patient is a young woman who may wish to become pregnant; conservative treatment with progesterone or estrogen or both is continued.

Endometriosis

Endometriosis can also cause abnormal uterine bleeding. **Endometriosis** is the growth of endometrial tissue in abnormal sites, usually in the peritoneal cavity, and occurs most frequently in women between 30 and 50 years (Fig. 9-13). The ovaries and the peritoneum are the most common sites of endometriosis, but it has been found on the supporting structures in the pelvic floor, the rectum, and the posterior surface of the uterus; it can metas-

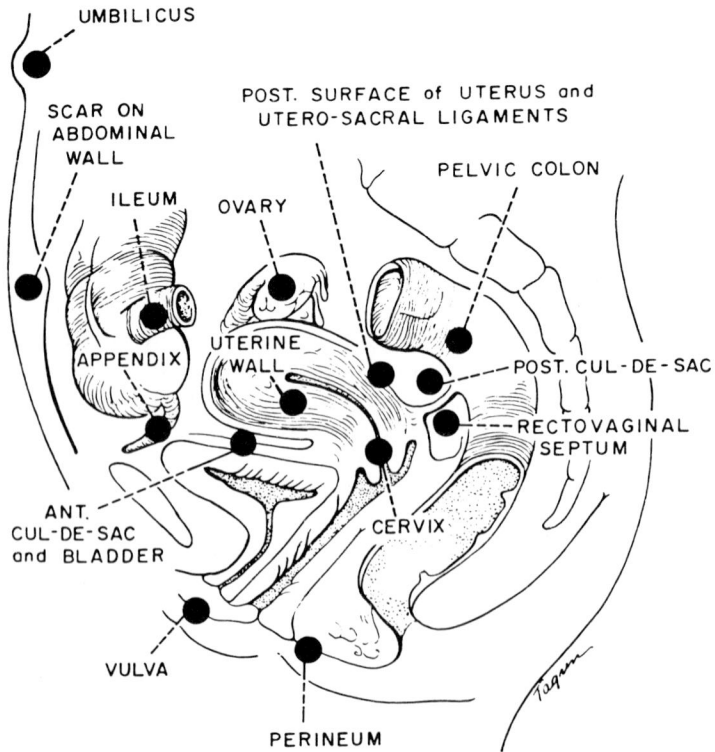

Figure 9-13
Sites of occurrence of endometriosis. (From T. H. Green, Jr., *Gynecology: Essentials of Clinical Practice* [3rd ed.]. Boston: Little, Brown and Company, 1977. Reproduced by permission.)

tasize to the kidneys, to scars in the vagina, and to the lungs.

The cause of endometriosis and the mechanism of metastasis are not known. There are several theories about endometriosis. One theory is that endometrial cells reach the peritoneal cavity from menstrual overflow via the fallopian tubes and that the endometrial cells in the menstrual flow are implanted in peritoneal or ovarian tissue, where they grow and differentiate. Another theory is that the peritoneal mesothelium, which has the same embryologic origin as the endometrium, undergoes metaplasia [17, 18]. Women who have been pregnant, thereby interrupting menstrual flow, are less vulnerable to developing endometriosis than are women who have had consistent menstrual cycles with no interruption [17].

In endometriosis, lesions can form as plaques or nodules of nonfunctioning tissue or can develop as functioning endometrial tissue capable of cyclic response to ovarian hormones. Endometriosis on the ovary that extends to the ovarian cortex is particularly likely to be the functioning type. The plaques in endometriosis are brown, and cysts can form and fill with blood. These cysts, called chocolate cysts because of their color, can either undergo atrophy and are then fibrous capsules filled with hemosiderin macrophages or they can rupture, releasing blood into the peritoneal cavity. This blood then causes an inflammatory response, and scarring and adhesion formation result. The adhesions can develop between any of the pelvic structures and cause numerous symptoms. Adhesions between the uterus and the peritoneum can cause retroversion of the uterus, holding the uterus fixed in place. When located on the ovaries, endometriosis can interfere with ovarian function and the cysts may rupture, causing acute abdominal pain and peritonitis.

The signs and symptoms associated with endometriosis are variable and range from mild discomfort to severe pain and interference with function. When the ovaries are involved there is increased frequency and irregularity of the menstrual cycle. If the uterus is retroverted, the patient may experience dyspareunia. Lower abdominal discomfort is caused by swelling and rupture of the endometriosis during the menstrual cycle. Adhesions can cause consistent discomfort.

Large lesions can be felt on abdominal palpation and cause discomfort from pressure. Endometriosis in the cul-de-sac causes premenstrual pain. Dysuria results from adhesions that form between the bladder and the peritoneum. Infertility will result when the adhesions obstruct the fimbriae of the fallopian tubes.

Treatment for endometriosis is variable. When the symptoms are mild, treatment may not be instituted. In some patients a normal pregnancy causes hormonal changes that result in atrophy of the lesions. Small localized areas of endometriosis can be cauterized or excised, or conservative therapy using progestins to bring about fibrosis and scarring of the nodules, thereby decreasing their function, relieves the symptoms while still allowing the patient to become pregnant later. Some patients are treated with testosterone such as methyltestosterone (Metandren) 5 mg daily for 6 months for relief of symptoms [17]. This dosage of methyltestosterone is low enough to avoid the masculinizing effect of higher doses and also does not interfere with ovulation. Other treatment measures require bilateral oophorectomy or lysis of adhesions, or both. The older patient may select hysterectomy for treatment. There is spontaneous remission of endometriosis with the menopause.

Adenomyosis is similar to endometriosis, but forms in the endometrial glands and in the myometrial stroma within the uterus. **Adenomyosis** occurs either as diffuse lesions or as a localized tumor, an adenomyoma. This condition is most common in women about 50 years of age who have delivered children. The symptoms include increased menstrual flow with subsequent increased blood loss, enlargement of the uterus causing back pain or other symptoms of pressure, and dysmenorrhea. The uterus becomes tender during menstrual flow. Diagnosis is made by endometrial biopsy.

Relaxation of Pelvic Structures

Another classification of dysfunction that occurs in women, particularly aging women, is relaxation of the female pelvic organs. This relaxation of the pelvic organs results from loss of muscle tone and atrophy associated with decreased estrogen levels. Contributing factors include weakening of the supporting pelvic structures from overstretching as occurs in delivery or from congenital weakness. Women who have delivered vaginally and those who have participated in long-term manual labor requiring lifting heavy objects are most vulnerable to relaxation of the pelvic organs. The major supporting structures in the female pelvis are the **cardinal ligaments** (Mackenrodt's) that support the upper vagina, cervix, and uterus; the **uterosacral ligaments** that maintain the position of the cervix near the sacrum; and the **pubocervical ligaments** that support the bladder. The muscles supporting the pelvic organs are shown in Figure 9-14. The bony pelvis in the female has a larger outlet than does the male's, to accommodate childbirth. This larger outlet makes the female more susceptible to prolapse of pelvic organs by gravity, as occurs in women who stand for long periods of time. The conditions commonly included in the classification relaxation of the pelvic organs are prolapsed uterus and herniations (cystocele, urethrocele, rectocele, and enterocele).

Prolapse of the uterus (Fig. 9-15) means that the uterus falls into the vaginal canal, causing the vagina to invert. In first-degree prolapse,

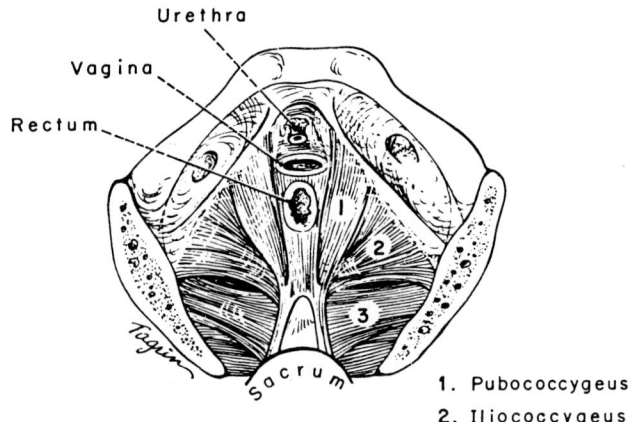

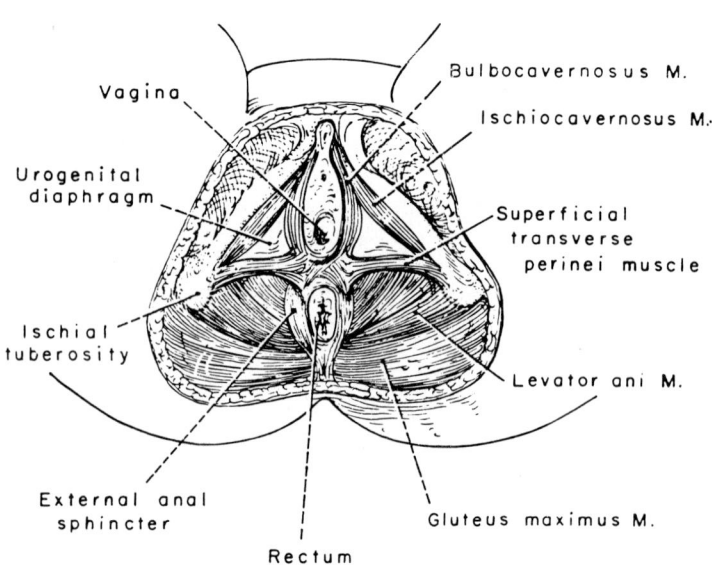

Figure 9-14
The muscular supports of the pelvic viscera. **A.** Muscles of the pelvic floor. **B.** Perineal muscle component. (From T. H. Green, Jr., *Gynecology: Essentials of Clinical Practice* [3rd ed.]. Boston: Little, Brown and Company, 1977. Reproduced by permission.)

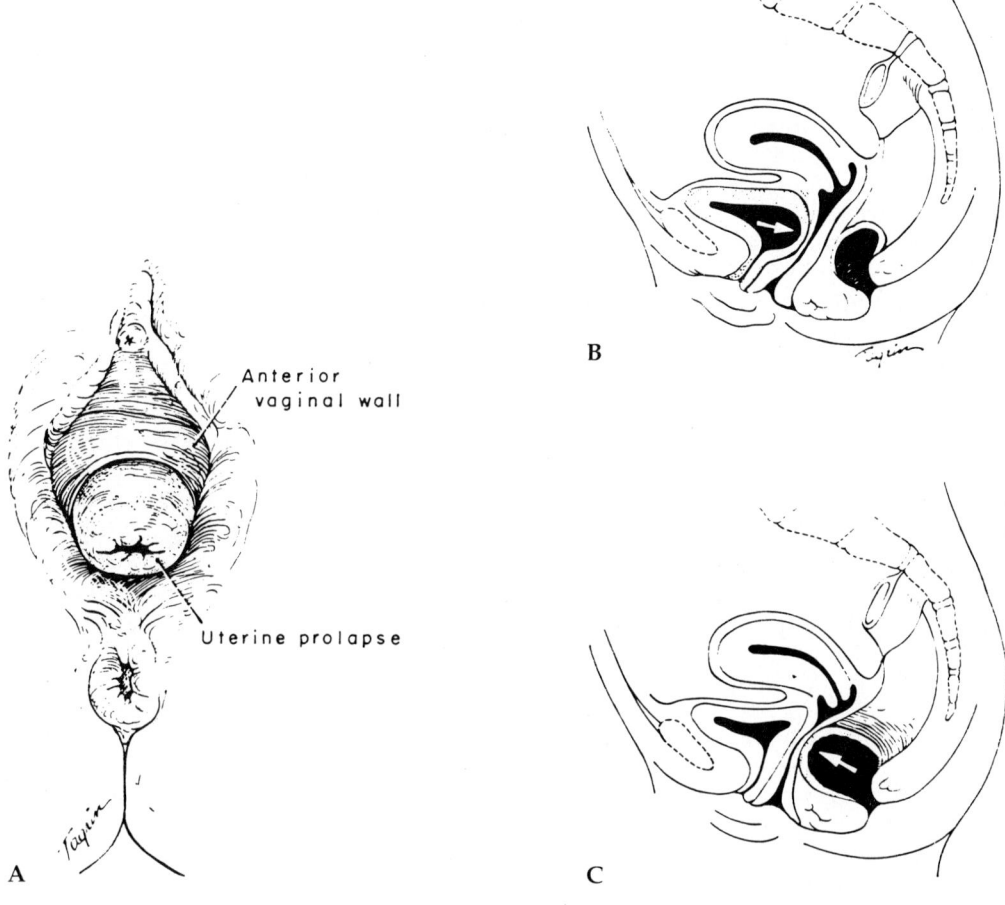

Figure 9-15
A. Uterine prolapse. **B.** Cystocele. **C.** Rectocele. The typical gross anatomic appearance of each of these common forms of pelvic relaxation is shown individually; actually they frequently coexist. (From T. H. Green, Jr., *Gynecology: Essentials of Clinical Practice* [3rd ed.]. Boston: Little, Brown and Company, 1977. Reproduced by permission.)

the cervix has fallen into the vaginal orifice; in second-degree prolapse the cervix protrudes from the vagina and the fundus of the uterus is at the level of the vaginal orifice (introitus); in third-degree prolapse the entire uterus has descended into the vagina and the vaginal wall, the urethra, and the base of the bladder can be pulled down with the uterus. When the entire anterior vaginal wall is prolapsed, the patient also has a cystourethrocele, and the cervix is usually stretched. Ureterocele can occur without cystocele and vice versa, depending on the area of laxity of the anterior vaginal wall. In rectocele, the posterior vaginal wall is pushed forward by the herniation of the rectum. When the upper portion of the posterior vaginal wall protrudes downward, the hernia involves the peritoneum and is called an enterocele.

The patient's symptoms vary according to the area of herniation and the degree of prolapse. Initially the patient has the sensation of something coming down or a dragging sensation, especially after standing or walking for a long period of time. This sensation is relieved when the patient either sits or lies down, enabling the organs to fall back into normal position. As the prolapse increases in degree, the symptoms become more consistent and the patient becomes increasingly uncomfortable. Some patients experience backache, but since backache is not necessarily a symptom of prolapse, other causes for its occurrence are investigated. Prolapse of the uterus is associated with congestion of the veins causing enlargement of the cervix and abnormal uterine bleeding. Cystocele causes urinary tract symptoms similar to those experienced by men with enlarged middle lobes of the prostate gland. The bladder contours can be encroached on by surrounding structures so that dependent areas form, causing retention of urine and difficulty emptying the bladder. There are increased frequency of micturition, hesitancy, and frequent infection resulting from stasis of urine in the bladder. When the bladder herniates, the ureters are obstructed and the patient can develop hydroureter and eventually hydronephrosis. The female is usually aware of the herniation and often learns to reduce the herniation of the bladder by pushing it back into place with her fingers in order to urinate. The patient with cysto-urethrocele may have loss of the urethro-vesical angle, thus impairing her ability to control micturition. Rectocele is associated with difficulty in fecal elimination or may cause no symptoms.

The symptoms of prolapse are aggravated by any activity that places downward pressure on the diaphragm or requires the use of abdominal and pelvic muscles. Symptoms tend to be worse in obese women, those who have a chronic cough or chronic constipation, or those who are debilitated. The diagnosis of prolapse is made by having the patient stand and bear down or cough to determine the degree of prolapse and to estimate the condition of the supporting structures. Hemorrhoids are often found in women who have rectocele. The patient is also evaluated to determine the presence of any other pathologic condition in the reproductive tract.

Pelvic floor exercises are prescribed for younger women who experience prolapse following delivery. In these exercises the woman alternately contracts and relaxes both the gluteal and the perineal floor muscles. Another helpful exercise is voluntarily interrupting the stream of urine during micturition. Some patients are unable to improve muscle tone, however, and may require surgical intervention if the signs and symptoms of prolapse are distressing. The specific surgical procedure to be performed is determined according to the patient's age, marital status, and severity of symptoms. A vaginal hysterectomy is performed in women who have other pathology in the vagina, cervix, or uterus. The Manchester procedure is amputation of the cervix along with curettage of the uterus and is used when the prolapse is mild or moderate. The Le Fort procedure consists in colpocleisis, which is approximation of the vaginal walls and is carried out in aged women with severe prolapse. The procedure can be modified to retain a portion of the patient's vagina. Anterior colporrhaphy is a surgical procedure in which the anterior vaginal wall is separated from the bladder and urethra; the bladder is then fixed into place by sutures and the vagina is reconstructed.

Nursing care for patients following repair procedures includes relief of swelling and pain, prevention of infection, and promoting elimination of feces. Ice packs can be used in the immediate postoperative period to relieve swelling and pain; analgesics are also given. Sitz baths are begun when the patient is ambulatory, and perineal care is performed following elimination of urine or feces. The nurse carries out the perineal care initially and teaches the patient how to carry out the procedure so that it can be done at home following discharge from the hospital. The patient is advised to avoid any activities that place strain on the surgical site. Stool softeners are given to promote elimination; rectal tubes or enemas are not used since they might cause disruption of the surgical site during the healing process.

A pessary can be used to relieve the prolapse. The pessary is placed into the upper end of the vagina so that the posterior fornix is distended, and, to be effective, it must fit correctly. If it is too large, the pessary causes erosion of tissue by friction and pressure, and if too small, it falls out. Pessaries are used in women with severe prolapse who are either not candidates for surgery or who do not elect to have the surgery. The patient with a pessary in place is taught that routine periodic changes of the pessary are necessary. Pessaries are removed and cleaned periodically, and the vaginal mucosa is checked to determine the presence of irritation or erosion that may have been caused by the pessary. There are a number of different types of pessaries (Fig. 9-16), and the physician selects the pessary that is most suitable for the patient. The Gellhorn pessary is a mushroom-shaped flat round plate and stem with a canal

Reproductive System Dysfunction

Stress Incontinence

Stress incontinence can be a symptom of prolapse but can also occur without prolapse. In stress incontinence, activities such as coughing, sneezing, lifting heavy objects, or laughing increase the intravesical pressure and can cause incontinence ranging from a few drops of urine to larger amounts. Certain women notice stress incontinence infrequently and it is often associated with infection, fistula formation, or prolapse. If stress incontinence is caused by loss of the urethrovesical angle, either the Marchetti test or the Bonney test prevents loss of urine when the patient strains. In the Marchetti test the vaginal wall is elevated with two clamps. In the Bonney test, two fingers are used to elevate the vaginal wall. The Marshall-Marchetti surgical procedure is performed to suspend the vesicourethral structures in stress incontinence. It is necessary to evaluate the patient's physical status to determine whether there is any other cause for the incontinence, such as kidney, urinary tract, or neurologic pathology prior to performing the Marshall-Marchetti procedure.

Fistulas and Retroversion of the Uterus

Other problems related to weakened or impaired structures are fistulas and changes in the position of the uterus. Fistulas can develop between any of the closely aligned pelvic organs and usually follow delivery or trauma in surgical procedures, or follow radiation therapy, accidents, or destruction of tissue by malignancy. Pessaries, because they are foreign bodies, can cause ulceration of the vagina and subsequent fistula formation. Fistulas between the bladder and vagina (vesicovaginal fistulas) are most common. Small fistulas often close spontaneously and require no treatment whereas intervention is required to augment healing of larger fistulas. Therapeutic measures such as the use of urinary antiseptics or a Foley catheter, bed rest, or limiting fluid intake reduce the irritation of urine on the fistula site in vesicovaginal, uterovaginal, or urethrovaginal fistula. If these measures are not effective, surgical repair is necessary when there is leakage since urine is irritating to the mucosa. Rectovaginal fistulas usually require surgical repair because it is difficult to protect the rectal mucosa from fecal material in efforts to promote healing.

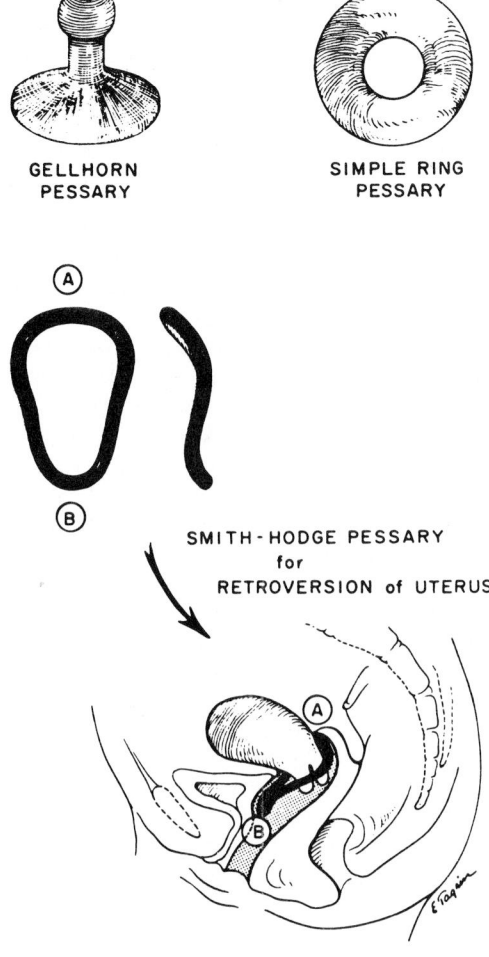

Figure 9-16
Types of vaginal pessary. The Gellhorn and the simple ring pessaries are employed in the conservative management of uterine prolapse. (From T. H. Green, Jr., Gynecology, Chapter 39. In G. L. Nardi and G. D. Zuidema [eds.], *Surgery: A Concise Guide to Clinical Practice* [3rd ed.]. Boston: Little, Brown and Company, 1972. Reproduced by permission.)

in the center for drainage. The Smith-Hodge pessary is a flexible ring that is easily inserted. A ring pessary is simply a rigid ring. The pessary does not cause pain if it fits correctly, but in some women it does cause pressure on the urethra with subsequent retention of urine. The patient is advised to notify the physician if she notices any unusual vaginal discharge or changes in her pattern of micturition following insertion of the pessary.

Changes from the normal position of the uterus can result in dyspareunia (painful coitus), vaginal discharge, dysmenorrhea, and backache. In **retroversion** of the uterus the uterus is tilted backward. Retroversion can be congenital or acquired. In endometriosis, adhesion formation can fix the uterus in a retroverted position. If the uterus is not fixed (it is normally movable) it can be manipulated into place bimanually. Retroversion can be classified according to degree; in first-degree retroversion the uterus is pointed to the sacral promontory; in second-degree retroversion the fundus of the uterus is in the hollow of the sacrum; in third-degree retroversion, the fundus of the uterus is below the level of the cervix. Evaluation of causes of retroversion by pelvic examination along with examination of the spine and of the patient's posture indicates the type of treatment that can be helpful for the particular patient.

To reduce retroflexion the patient with the potential for improving muscle tone can perform exercises. Having the patient assume a knee-chest position so that air distends the vagina changes the position of the uterus toward anteflexion. This exercise is performed for 5 minutes at least three times a day. If surgery is contemplated, a pessary is placed to determine whether surgery will be effective. If the pessary relieves the patient's symptoms, suspension of the uterus is performed surgically. If the pessary does not relieve the symptoms, it is assumed that the patient's symptoms will not be alleviated by surgical suspension of the uterus. Unless the retroflexion causes severe symptoms or interferes with fertility, surgical suspension is usually not performed.

Abnormal Cell Growth

The reproductive tract is subject to abnormal cell growth that can be either benign or malignant. Many of the benign growths are considered to be premalignant, and treatment is usually carried out with the potential for malignancy in mind. Basic consideration of abnormal cell growth and methods used for treatment are discussed in the section on oncology in Chapter 1 and are not repeated here. Early diagnosis and treatment improve the patient's prognosis and the Papanicolaou smear is a valuable screening measure for detection of epidermoid cervical carcinoma. The findings on physical examination and the patient's signs and symptoms of disturbed function indicate the need for further investigation by cytologic studies of secretions or of biopsied tissue. The nurse assures the patient that these studies are routine and preventive and not an indication that the patient does have cancer. Carcinoma in the reproductive tract does not always cause early symptoms, especially tumors in the prostate gland, the ovaries, or the cervix. Therefore any type of dysfunction is always investigated for the possibility of cancer. When abnormal cell growth is found, the tumors are graded to determine their activity or virulence or both, and grading gives an indication of the patient's prognosis. Staging of tumors is the method used in determining the extent of tumor growth and metastasis. Most staging procedures for tumors in the reproductive tract require surgical exploration of lymph nodes, blood vessels, and nerves in the peritoneal area. The surgical procedures used in treatment for reproductive tract tumors, however, do not always require surgical invasion of the peritoneal cavity, and alternative methods for staging are being explored, such as in testicular tumors. Bone marrow aspiration and lymphangiography are two procedures used in nonsurgical staging.

The routes of metastasis of tumors in the reproductive tract are not yet fully identified for each type of tumor, but lymphatic routes tend to predominate. The vascular, lymph, and nerve supplies to the reproductive structures follow common pathways and can all be involved in extensive tumor growth, giving rise to signs and symptoms of metastasis. The spinal cord segments two, three, and four give rise to the pudendal nerve plexus, which supplies the urogenital diaphragm, the levator and sphincter ani muscles, the urethra, the scrotum in males, the labia in females via its perineal nerve branch, the penis in males, and the clitoris in females via its dorsal nerve branch. The arterial and lymph vessels and the nerve plexus that supplies the reproductive organs stem from the area of the fifth lumbar vertebra. The hypogastric nerve plexus is the division of the autonomic nervous system that supplies the reproductive organs. The vesical plexus of the hypogastric nerve supplies the seminal vesicles and the ductus deferens; the prostatic plexus supplies the prostate, the seminal vesicles, and the penis. In females the vagina and the clitoris are supplied by the vaginal plexus while the uterine plexus supplies the uterus and the fallopian tubes.

The internal iliac artery supplies the pelvic organs and the pelvic wall, dividing into many smaller branches. The internal pudendal artery is one of these branches and supplies the external genitalia. In males the prostate is supplied by another branch, the inferior vesical artery. The perineal artery, a branch of the internal pudendal, supplies the urogenital diaphragm, the ischiocavernosus and bulbocavernosus muscles, and the scrotum. The testes are supplied by the internal spermatic artery, which arises from the aorta below the renal artery, and the vas deferens is supplied by a branch of the inferior or superior vesical artery. The cremasteric artery (external spermatic artery) supplies the tunica vaginalis. Venous drainage from the pampiniform plexus (which is made up of the internal spermatic vein, the external spermatic vein, and the veins from the vas deferens) empties into the epigastric and pudendal veins. Venous blood from the prostate also drains into the pudendal plexus. In the female the ovarian artery, the uterine artery, and the vaginal artery all arise from the internal iliac artery (the vaginal artery can also be found as a branch of the uterine artery in some females). The lymphatic vessels in the pelvic area are closely aligned with the blood vessels. The external and internal iliac nodes receive most of the pelvic lymph flow. This brief summary indicates the complexity of determining the route of metastasis from primary tumors in the reproductive organs and the complicated involvement of nerves, blood vessels, and lymphatics in extensive tumor growth.

There are many different cell types in tumors found in the reproductive tract. The following description of abnormal cell growth in the reproductive tract is limited to the most frequently occurring types. **Leukoplakia,** which appears as white patches, can be located on the penis (usually on the prepuce), the cervix, or the vulva and is considered to be a precursor to cancer. The lesions in leukoplakia can be edematous and associated with an inflammatory reaction. Fissures can form, and the involved areas are irritated by urine. These superficial epithelial patches of leukoplakia are surgically removed. If extensive, a vulvectomy can be performed in females, and amputation of the penis is performed in males with advanced leukoplakia that has caused the epithelium to become thickened and indurated. Carcinoma of the penis is rare and it is thought that circumcision is preventive. Any male who notices that the character of smegma is changed should contact his physician for examination. **Balanitis** (inflammation of the glans penis or the glans clitoridis) has many different causes and should be treated at the onset of signs and symptoms. Inappropriate treatment, including many self-treatment measures, can extend the lesions or inflammation and preclude correct diagnosis and treatment to prevent more serious consequences.

ABNORMAL CELL GROWTH IN MALES

The scrotum is usually affected by squamous or epidermoid cancer that is usually related to occupational hazards such as working with petroleum products or crude wool [13]. Tumors of the testes are infrequent and occur mostly in young men. Teratomas, which are epithelial cysts of embryonal origin, are benign but considered to be premalignant. Malignant tumors of the testes can be classified as either germinal or nongerminal in origin, and the germinal tumors occur more frequently. The germinal tumors usually arise from the unspecialized germ cells (spermatogonium) that line the seminiferous tubules. These germinal tumors include seminoma, teratoma, and choriocarcinoma and are highly radiosensitive and slow-growing, metastasizing via the lymphatics late in their course. If found early, the cure rate is high.

The Union International Center of Cancer staging system [22] for testicular tumors is as follows: **T1** refers to tumors that include less than one-half of the testis with the remainder of the testis being normal. **T2** indicates tumors including more than one-half of the testis, but the testis is of normal size. **T3** is a tumor that causes the testis to be enlarged or abnormally shaped. **T4** indicates that the tumor extends beyond the testis; **T4a** indicates extension to the epididymis; and **T4b** indicates extension to surrounding structures. Regional lymph node involvement is indicated by **N0** which refers to no involvement, **N1** referring to regional lymph node involvement, and **M1** to extensive metastases. In this classification **NX** refers to histologic evaluation, and efforts are currently being made to determine a valid histologic staging system through clinical research [22]. Diagnosis includes chest x-ray and lymphangiogram, venogram of the inferior vena cava, and a urogram in addition to physical examination. Since most malignant tumors of the testis produce hormones similar to pituitary hormones, the Aschheim-Zondek test for pregnancy is used in diagnosis. Treatment includes surgical excision or radiotherapy, or both, and chemotherapy. Orchiectomy is the procedure in which the testis and portions of the ductus deferens and spermatic vessels are excised. A retroperitoneal lymph node dissection is also included in many instances. Either a single chemotherapeutic agent or combinations of these agents are used for chemotherapy.

Adenocarcinoma of the prostate gland is the most commonly occurring prostatic tumor, and it affects men over 50 years of age. The adenocarcinoma is usually slow-growing, and when it occurs late in life the patient often dies of other diseases, such as cardiovascular or respiratory diseases. As with enlargement of the prostate, it is theorized that the development of malignancy in the prostate may be related to changes in the estrogen-androgen ratio. The tumors of the prostate have increased metabolism of zinc and acid phosphatase. Often there are no early symptoms, and the tumor can be present many years before the prostate becomes enlarged. Therefore presenting symptoms may be signs and symptoms of urinary tract infection, or, in late metastasis, bone pain or backache may be the initial symptom.

The Veterans Administration Cooperative Urological Research Group staging classification for prostatic tumors is commonly used. In this classification **stage I** includes tumors found in prostatic tissue, usually following surgery for an enlarged prostate. The patient has no other signs of tumor growth. In **stage II** the patient is found to have prostatic nodules on rectal examination, but there is no evidence of extension of the tumor. **Stage III** is tumor extension into the tissues around the prostate gland, but the patient has no other indication of tumor growth. In **stage IV** the patient has elevated serum prostatic acid phosphatase levels or metastasis, or both. Metastasis of prostatic tumors is determined by cytologic studies of bone marrow aspirations, lymphangiography, and bone scan. A needle biopsy is sometimes taken from the prostate for cytologic studies for diagnosis of a prostatic tumor.

Treatment for prostatic tumors has included hormonal chemotherapy, using estrogen to suppress the tumor. Tumors of the prostate are considered to be dependent on androgens and therefore, administration of estrogens or performing a bilateral orchiectomy to reduce secretion of testosterone helps in decreasing the androgen levels. Bilateral adrenalectomy to eliminate adrenal secretion of androgens, and hypophysectomy to eliminate pituitary hormone secretion, are sometimes performed for patients with extensive malignancy of the prostate as a palliative measure, with the goal of extending the patient's life. Another measure for suppressing the adrenal secretion of androgens is that of giving cortisone. Metastases of prostatic cancer occur via the lymphatic drainage and in order of greatest frequency involve bone, the lungs, the liver, and the brain. Since the lower urinary tract is frequently affected, treatment also includes measures to relieve urethral obstruction, such as transurethral resection.

Surgical excision of the prostate is carried out on patients who do not have extension of the tumor beyond the prostate gland. Singly, or in combination, chemotherapeutic agents are also used in treatment. Radical surgery can be performed, but because the consequence of radical perineal surgery is impotence, this method of treatment is often not selected since prostatic tumors are slow-growing and usually regress with hormonal or chemotherapeutic anticancer medications.

ABNORMAL CELL GROWTH IN FEMALES

A number of different types of abnormal cell growth can occur in the female reproductive tract. Ovarian cysts are the most frequent type of abnormal cell growth and can be benign or malignant. The ovarian cysts can arise from either the follicle or the corpus luteum, and become large in some cases before symptoms occur. Follicular cysts occur when the follicle fails to rupture and becomes overdistended by an accumulation of fluid as the ovum degenerates. These cysts can cause a dull aching or feeling of heaviness during menstrual flow and, if they rupture, the signs and symptoms are similar to those of ruptured ectopic pregnancy. Cysts arising from the corpus luteum cause delayed menstruation and are often mistaken for tubal pregnancy. The luteal cysts undergo spontaneous remission in many women. The Stein-Leventhal syndrome is associated with enlarged polycystic ovaries. The syndrome includes obesity, hirsutism, infertility, and disturbances in menstrual flow with amenorrhea or oligomenorrhea and some instances of menorrhagia. Treatment includes wedge resection of the ovary, in which one-half to one-third of the ovary is resected to reduce the ovarian mass to normal size. Another method is the administration of clomiphene (Clomid). The patient's total endocrine status is evaluated to determine pituitary and adrenal function imbalances that might be either associated with or causative of the Stein-Leventhal syndrome.

Dermoid cysts of the ovary are teratomas that probably arise from unfertilized ova. Teratomas may also be solid tumors and tend to occur in younger females. Teratomas, both cystic and solid, contain embryonal materials, as do those found in the testes. The symptoms include ascites and minimal bleeding; the tumors can usually be palpated. Since teratomas have a great potential for becoming malignant, surgical removal is indicated. The patient often has a hysterectomy and oophorectomy. The teratomas are radioresistant, though some respond to chemotherapy. Serous or mucinous cystadenomas occur more commonly than the dermoid cysts. The **serous cystadenomas** contain blood proteins, serum albumin, and serum globulin, can weigh several pounds, and usually are bilateral. **Mucinous cystadenomas** contain clear viscous fluid and can grow to huge proportions. The serous cystadenomas have great potential for becoming malignant and often form papillary growths on the external surface. The serous cysts contain psammoma bodies representative of calcium deposits in the papillary projections. The papillary growths can extend to the peritoneum, causing ascites. Serous cysts often recur following surgical removal. The signs and symptoms of these cysts are highly variable. If the cysts are large, they cause pressure with the feeling of heaviness in the abdomen, and interrupt either bowel or bladder function, or both, when they encroach on either of these organs. Complications include torsion and rupture of the cyst, and patients with these complications can present with the signs and symptoms of an acute abdomen as described in Chapter 7.

Brenner tumors occur infrequently and tend to be present in women over the age of 50. These tumors become large and can be malignant. In some cases the Brenner tumors are thought to be hormonally active and associated with carcinoma of the endometrium. Fibroid tumors of the ovary can also become large and are benign solid tumors. Comprised of fibrous tissue, the **fibroid tumors** begin as a small nodule and cause no symptoms unless they attain sufficient size to cause abdominal discomfort or pain. Fibromas are subject to torsion and subsequent infarction, as are the cystadenomas. When torsion occurs, the patient has venous obstruction and usually develops ascites. **Meigs' syndrome** is the occurrence of ascites along with hydrothorax in patients with ovarian fibroid tumors. The cause of hydrothorax in association with the ovarian fibroid tumor is unknown. It is thought that fluid either from the fibroid or from the ascites reaches the chest via the lymphatic drainage. The hydrothorax resolves following surgical removal of the ovarian fibroid tumor.

In general, treatment for benign ovarian tumors is resection of the tumor. A frozen section is performed at the time of operation, and if malignant cells are found, a panhystero-oophorectomy is performed. When only one ovary is involved and the patient is of childbearing age, conservative surgery (removal of the ovary and fallopian tube) is performed. This procedure is salpingo-oophorectomy. In women of menopausal age a complete hysterectomy is usually performed as preventive of further malignant growth.

Ovarian carcinoma is often insidious and far advanced before the patient experiences signs and symptoms. The patient may have vague symptoms that are mistaken for minor inflammatory or infectious processes in the gastrointestinal or urinary tract. Among the symptoms the patient experiences are gastrointestinal discomfort (nausea, vomiting, gallbladder colic, and abdominal distention), genitourinary symptoms of obstruction or infection or both, low abdominal discomfort or pain, backache, and the feeling of pressure in the pelvic area. Some patients have enlargement of the abdomen. The patient can have either an abdominal or pelvic mass and, sometimes, weight loss. Ascites is another sign of ovarian carcinoma and some patients have pleural effusion with chest pain and dyspnea. Unfortunately there are no screening tests for detection of ovarian malignancy, and diagnosis depends on investigation of the signs and symptoms. A complete physical examination along with a pelvic examination, upper and lower gastrointestinal x-rays, an intravenous pyelogram, and a flat plate x-ray of both the chest and abdomen is carried out. When the patient has ascites, paracentesis is performed; when the patient has pleural effusion, thoracentesis is performed. The fluid aspirated in these procedures is sent to the laboratory for cytologic studies. Laparoscopy is sometimes included in diagnosis.

Staging of carcinoma of the ovary by the International Federation of Gynecology and Obstetrics is as follows: **Stage Ia** is carcinoma limited to one ovary with no ascites. **Stage Ib** is growth limited to one or both ovaries with no ascites, and **stage Ic** is growth limited to one or both ovaries with ascites and malignant cells in the ascites fluid. **Stage IIa** is growth in one or both ovaries and extension or metastasis or both to the uterus or fallopian tubes or both. **Stage IIb** is extension or metastases or both to pelvic tissues. In **stage III** there is growth involving one or both ovaries with disseminated metastasis to the peritoneal spaces and to the abdomen that can involve the omentum, the intestine, the mesentery, the liver, and the retroperitoneal lymph glands. In **stage IV** there is distant metastasis beyond the peritoneal cavity.

Serous cystadenocarcinoma is the most frequently occurring type of ovarian malignancy followed by undifferentiated adenocarcinoma. **Serous cystadenocarcinoma** is the malignant form of the previously described serous cystadenoma. **Adenocarcinoma** is a solid tumor and the cell types present are variable, as is the size of the tumor. The adenocarcinoma frequently begins in one ovary and extends to the other ovary as the disease progresses. Adenocarcinoma can also be endometroid or mesonephroid. The mesonephromas of the ovary are thought to be of mesonephric origin and similar to renal tumors. The endometroid tumors are of endometrial origin.

As in the testes, ovarian malignancies can arise as germinal cell tumors. In the ovary these germinal cell tumors include dysgerminomas, granulosa cell tumors, arrhenoblastomas, and malignant teratomas. The dysgerminoma probably arises from embryonic germ cells and can be either encapsulated or infiltrative. The prognosis is better in encapsulated dysgerminomas. Granulosa and theca cell tumors have a common origin and since they secrete estrogen, granulosa and theca cell tumors are called functioning tumors. The arrhenoblastoma involves stromal cells and secretes androgens, causing amenorrhea, regression of secondary female sex characteristics, and the onset of masculinization that regresses following surgical removal of the tumor.

Treatment for patients with ovarian malignancy is immediate excision of the tumor. There is controversy about whether a unilateral oophorectomy or a bilateral oophorectomy along with panhysterectomy is the treatment of choice for patients with ovarian malignancy. Young and DeVita [28] found that the lack of data from controlled clinical trials leads to continued controversy about treatment of ovarian carcinoma [22]. As with other forms of malignancy, ovarian malignancy is treated via surgery, radiotherapy, and chemotherapy. It is thought that radiotherapy following surgical excision of the tumor improves the patient's prognosis when there is metastatic extension. Chemotherapy for treatment of ovarian carcinoma includes the use of single agents or combinations of agents. As one example, Kessinger et al. [11] cite the use of quadrichemotherapy for advanced ovarian carcinoma using cyclophosphamide, thio-tepa, chlorambucil, 5-fluorouracil, and methotrexate. Some ovarian tumors do recur, however, and some are resistant to therapy.

In preparing the patient for surgery the nurse includes all the preoperative measures indicated by the patient's needs for preoperative teaching and physiologic preparation. The patient is told that the findings in surgery determine the type of procedure that is performed. If the carcinoma has metastasized more extensive surgery is required and may include pelvic exenteration. A bowel preparation is included in preoperative care in the event there is metastasis to the bowel and a bowel resection is necessary. Total pelvic exenteration is removal of the distal sigmoid colon, rectum, perineum, and pelvic lymph nodes and muscles, and panhystero-oophorectomy. The exenteration can be anterior with cystectomy (creating a urinary stoma) or posterior (resulting in a colostomy), or both.

Carcinoma of the fallopian tubes is rare and usually is associated with chronic inflammation. The symptoms include watery vaginal discharge, and sometimes, irregularity in menstrual periods. Treatment is bilateral removal of the ovaries and fallopian tubes.

The Cervix, Vagina, and Vulva

The types of abnormal cell growth found in the cervix include changes associated with chronic cervicitis, polyps, and carcinoma. In **chronic cervicitis,** the cervical mucosa can undergo changes that are difficult to differentiate from carcinoma. The patient has vaginal discharge; usually there is leukorrhea with viscid mucopurulent or a whitish or yellowish discharge. The cervix undergoes metaplasia, and the involved areas are treated by cauterization. Following cauterization, the patient has vaginal drainage of the sloughing tissue during the first week or two and thereafter may have some bleeding in variable amounts until healing takes place. The patient is advised not to have coitus for 2 weeks postcauterization and is advised to see the physician if excessive bleeding or pain occurs. Healing takes about 2 months.

Cervical polyps occur either singly or in multiples and are usually pedunculated tumors of varying sizes. The major sign of polyps is bleeding following coitus or during straining for fecal elimination. The polyps are removed by cautery and are examined in cytologic studies as they can be malignant.

Carcinoma of the cervix, like that of the ovary, is often advanced before the condition is diagnosed. Women who have had intercourse at an early age have a high incidence of cervical carcinoma, as do women who have chronic inflammation or infections of the cervix, or who have had lacerations of the cervix such as during childbirth. The low incidence of cervical cancer in Jewish women suggests that circumcision of the male is preventive. In circumcised males there is less smegma, and it is theorized that smegma accumulations on the glans penis may be a factor in causing cervical carcinoma. Sexual activity seems to be a predominant factor associated with the occurrence of cervical carcinoma.

Epidermoid carcinoma is the most frequently occurring type; **squamous cell carcinoma** and **adenocarcinoma** of the cervix occur with less frequency. The lesions are usually rapid-growing and begin as a small erosion that bleeds easily on contact. In epidermoid carcinoma of the cervix, the lesions either develop into masses of papillary growths of tissue resembling a cauliflower or appear as nodular induration of the cervix. The cervix expands and assumes a barrel shape in some instances. The lesions are not always obvious and can extend into the structures of the cervix and vagina, the walls of the pelvis, the ureters, the bladder, and the rectum. When the ureters are involved the patient has symptoms of urinary tract obstruction and retention of urine, and when the rectum is involved the patient has symptoms related to difficulty in defecation. In extensive tumor growth, the patient can develop a bowel obstruction.

Involvement of surrounding structures can occur prior to the onset of other symptoms typical of cervical carcinoma, such as the thin watery vaginal discharge and bleeding between menstrual periods and following coitus. The patient's menstrual flow increases in duration and amount. A classic sign of carcinoma of the cervix in older women is postmenopausal bleeding. When the nerves are involved, the patient can have backache with pain radiating down the leg or flank. When lymphatic or venous flow or both are obstructed, the patient has edema of one or both lower extremities. Pain is a later symptom, and the patient can develop extensive disease, seeking treatment for urinary tract signs and symptoms before diagnosis of cervical carcinoma is made. Subsequent kidney failure can be the cause of death.

The International Federation of Gynecology and Obstetrics staging classification for carcinoma of the cervix includes **stage 0** for carcinoma in situ (intraepithelial), **stage I** for carcinoma confined to the cervix. In **stage Ia** the carcinoma is not found on clinical examination, and in **stage Ib** the carcinoma is clinically visible. **Stage II** includes carcinoma that has extended to the vagina; in **stage IIa** there is no perimetrial involvement, and in **stage IIb** there is perimetrial involvement. **Stage III** is carcinoma that extends to the pelvic wall, and in **stage IV** the carcinoma has extended to the bladder and rectum. The Shiller test is used in diagnosis as is colposcopy, a procedure in which the colposcope (a microscope with a high intensity light) is used to visualize the cervical epithelium. Using the colposcope allows for visualization of changes in the mucosa such as leukoplakia, changes in vascularization, mosaic patterns of tissue, and stippling of the capillaries.

Different methods are used in the treatment of cancer of the cervix, with surgery and radiation therapy being the most common. Excision of the tumor is often carried out prior to radiation therapy because radiation therapy is more effective if the tumor mass has been removed. As with carcinoma of the ovary, pelvic exenteration may be performed for advanced disease. The carcinoma of the cervix does not tend to metastasize beyond the pelvis. Cancer in situ is usually treated by excision of the localized intraepithelial lesion via conization, cauterization, or cryosurgery. A panhysterectomy is performed in some instances. (Previously, the stump of the cervix was retained and some patients then developed carcinoma in the cervical stump; therefore panhysterectomy is now the preferred procedure.)

In advanced carcinoma of the cervix a radical hysterectomy can be performed. The procedure used is the Wertheim operation or variations of it in which the internal, common, and external iliac and obturator lymph nodes are removed and the ovarian vessels and uterine arteries are ligated. In addition, parametrial and pericervical tissue and the upper third of the vagina are removed [6].

Radiation is also used extensively in treatment of carcinoma of the cervix. Basic principles of radiation therapy are described in Chapter 1. The patient with carcinoma of the cervix who is treated with radiation therapy is prepared with a douche and an enema as well as for general anesthesia for insertion of the applicators. The radioactive source, such as cesium 137, is placed following determination of the correct sites of applicator placement via x-ray. The radiation dosage is selected according to the tumor size and type and can be augmented by cobalt therapy. Nursing care of patients with radium implants requires attention to protection of the nurse and patient from radiation exposure as described in Chapter 1. Because radiation therapy is often selected for the elderly or obese patient, the nurse is aware of the special needs of these patients for safety, comfort, and care related to other medical problems they may have, as well as for monitoring the maintenance of applicators in correct placement, urine and fecal elimination, and measures to treat diarrhea that may occur with irradiation of the bowel, and pain relief. Most cervical carcinoma is radiosensitive, but a small percentage of tumors do not respond to radiation.

There is an increased incidence of vaginal and cervical carcinoma in young women whose mothers took diethylstilbestrol (DES) during pregnancy. Vaginal cancer occurs infrequently and is usually squamous cell carcinoma, but it can be of other types, such as adenocarcinoma or melanoma. The patient with carcinoma of the vagina can have discharge similar to that occurring in cervical carcinoma and eventually has pain. The carcinoma extends to the bladder, the rectum, and the cervix, and the growing lesion can eventually become a large mass that extends from the vagina. Radiation therapy is the most common form of treatment.

The vulva can also be the primary site of carcinoma. Leukoplakia is a precursor to cancer and the patient often notices persistent pruritus, an early symptom typical of vulvar carcinoma. Vulvar carcinoma grows slowly and tends to ulcerate, and urine irritates the eroded areas. Diagnosis is confirmed by biopsy, and treatment is by excision of the vulva. A **simple vulvectomy** is the removal of the vulva along with a margin of skin adjacent to the vulva. **Radical vulvectomy** is the excision of skin from the symphysis pubis to the anus. The excised areas are covered with a skin flap. The amount of skin remaining and the subsequent problems the patient has following the surgical procedure depend on the extent of the lesion and surgical repair.

Following vulvectomy, the patient's indwelling Foley catheter is left in place for 1 to 2 weeks to prevent constriction of the urethra. The patient remains on bed rest. The duration of the bed rest depends on the size of the surgical excision and the condition of the skin flaps, but the patient usually is allowed to ambulate after the first 24 to 48 hours. Use of elastic stockings prevents formation of leg edema, although patients who have had more radical surgery can have chronic lymphedema of the lower extremities following vulvectomy. The wound is usually dressed, and when changing these dressings the nurse should take care to maintain sterile technique; wound infection is a serious complication. Sitz baths are begun when the patient begins ambulation, and are continued following the patient's discharge from the hospital. Perineal care via irrigations is ordered to clean the wound, and the patient is taught to perform the irrigations in readiness for self-care at home.

Acceptance of and adjustment to her appearance following vulvectomy is often difficult for the woman, and the nurse tries to help her adjust to this change in body image. The patient may also require the nurse's support in helping her husband accept the change in her appearance. The patient is told about the possible complications of vulvectomy: bleeding, drainage, odor, and perineal pain. When these complications occur the patient should notify the physician. In addition, the patient can experience difficulty in coitus not only because of loss of tissue in the supporting structure of the labia and vagina, but also because of constriction of the vaginal orifice. The constriction may require dilation or surgical revision.

The Uterus

The types of abnormal cell growth in the uterus include polyps, myomas, carcinoma, and sarcoma. **Polyps** can vary in size and can be single or multiple growths. Often they cause no symptoms, but if they encroach on the cervix and vagina, there is bleeding. Polyps are removed and the tissue is examined in cytologic studies, since endometrial polyps can become malignant. Another type of abnormal growth is the hydatidiform mole, which can be benign or, rarely, malignant. This mole develops from placental tissue and is a formation of grape-like clusters of overdistended chorionic villi in the uterus. The major symptom is bleeding; the moles are surgically removed.

Myomas are smooth muscle fibers separated by connective tissue. Another name for myomas is fibroid tumors. The myomas can be **submucosal,** located in the endometrium; **interstitial,** located in the muscular wall; and **subserous,** projecting outward from the uterine wall. Symptoms associated with myomas are related to the location and size of the tumors. Endometrial myomas cause bleeding; the patient has longer menstrual periods and increased amounts of menstrual flow. The tumors can be located in the body of the uterus or near the cervical os. When the myomas are large, they cause pressure pains and can encroach on the bladder. The patient then has signs and symptoms of dysuria, retention, and subsequent frequency of micturition. Hydronephrosis can result from obstruction of the flow of urine. Other signs and symptoms experienced by patients with myomas include pelvic inflammatory disease, tenderness of the lower abdomen, and circulatory impairment. The patient may develop anemia with associated weakness and shortness of breath. The myomas regress with the menopause, and some patients are treated with radiation therapy to induce menopause. If the tumor can be removed without undue damage to the structure of the uterus, a myomectomy is performed when the patient is of childbearing age. Otherwise, total hysterectomy is performed and one ovary is retained so that the patient will not experience an abrupt menopause.

Patients who are of middle age and who also have other medical problems such as diabetes mellitus, hypertension, or obesity are at risk for developing **endometrial carcinoma.** Usually the endometrial carcinoma follows a long period of hyperplasia in those who have high levels of estrogen secretion and who frequently become infertile as a result of it. In diagnosis a D and C is performed, and an endometrial smear and biopsy are obtained for cytologic studies. In many instances the Gravlee jet wash is used to obtain samples of tissue for cytologic studies as an alternative to a D and C. The patient is also examined to determine the presence of ovarian carcinoma which, in some instances, accompanies endometrial tumors. Treatment includes total hysterectomy and removal of the ovaries via an abdominal incision. When the patient's disease has advanced to surrounding structures, radiation therapy is used. The use of progestins is also included in treatment, as are alkylating agents in chemotherapy. Pelvic exenteration is required in extensive disease.

The occurrence of **sarcoma** in the uterus is infrequent. Fibromyosarcoma arises from the connective tissue, and leiomyosarcoma is a complication of myoma. In some patients lymphosarcoma can be located in the uterus and extends rapidly via the bloodstream. **Chorioepithelioma** is a malignant tumor that arises from the same cells as do hydatidiform moles. The most common site for these tumors is at the placenta site in the uterus. These tumors grow rapidly, metastasizing to the pelvic organs and the lungs. The chorioepitheliomas usually follow pregnancy or abortion.

Because abnormal bleeding from the vagina, cervix, or uterus is an indication of carcinoma of the reproductive tract, its occurrence in women of postmenopausal age is considered a serious sign. Postmenopausal bleeding is any bleeding that takes place 1 year following the termination of the menses. When the woman is taking estrogen following menopause, she is advised to seek medical reevaluation of the dosage when bleeding occurs since the bleeding can be an indication that her metabolic needs for estrogen have changed or that she has carcinoma. If she abruptly stops taking estrogen, bleeding can occur. When postmenopausal bleeding occurs, a complete physical examination and cytologic studies of tissue obtained in the pelvic examination are recommended. The bleeding can be caused by ruptured endometrial cysts or by malignant lesions.

The Mammary Glands

This section deals with the female breast, or mammary glands. When caring for patients with dysfunction of the breast or with diseases that affect the breast, the nurse is cognizant that the breasts are accessory sex organs and that they are a visible sign of femininity as well as being a part of the body that can be stimulated in sexual arousal. For many females, the breasts are considered to be important for attracting males and for all females, the breast is part of their body and therefore its form contributes to body image. The breast is also the source of milk in nursing mothers. The breasts have a high level of emotional meaning for many women, and diseases of the breast can disrupt body image and self-concept in relation to the feminine role. When the breast is diseased, the woman often considers herself less of a woman or less able to attract male attention. For women of childbearing age, loss of breast function means the inability to nurse children. Amputation of a breast as is necessary in treatment of some breast diseases is therefore a stimulus for the grieving process.

The mammary glands are dependent on hormones. Estrogen stimulates the development of the ductal system in the breasts, and progesterone stimulates development of the lobular component of breasts. Breast development is also dependent on insulin, cortisol, thyroxine, prolactin, and growth hormones [12, 21]. The hormone prolactin is required for production of milk in nursing mothers. Estrogen and progesterone inhibit lactation by stimulating the hypothalamus to secrete prolactin-inhibiting hormone. The breasts respond to hormonal stimulation during the menstrual cycle and during pregnancy and lactation. The hypothalamus, the anterior pituitary, and the ovarian hormones all affect breast development and maintenance of breast structure and function through feedback loops of hormone regulation.

Anatomically the breasts vary in size and shape, depending on the amount of fatty and fibrous tissue present. The extensive ductal system in the breasts extends from the lobules comprising each of the lobes of the breast to the ampullae underlying the nipple. The ampulla is the reservoir for storing milk during lactation. There are 15 to 20 lobes in each breast. The nipple contains numerous tiny ducts in fibromuscular tissue, and the areola surrounds the nipple. The nipple is pigmented and is pink in caucasian women who have not borne children but becomes brownish in the first pregnancy, retaining the brownish pigmentation thereafter. The areola has tiny nodules that are formed by the underlying glands of Montgomery, which are modified sebaceous glands. The pectoralis major muscle lies beneath the mammary gland and is connected to the gland by a layer of fascia.

There is abundant overlapping vascular and lymph supply to the breast. The posterior intercostal arteries branch from the descending thoracic aorta, the internal mammary artery is a branch of the subclavian artery, and the lateral thoracic artery is a branch of the axillary artery. These major arteries form a plexus around the areola, and there is also a deeper plexus of the major arteries within the gland. Lymphatic vessels form a superficial plexus of lymph vessels around the areola, and there is also a deeper plexus of lymphatics. The superficial plexus drains to the central axillary nodes, which drain into the subclavian nodes. The deep plexus also drains to the subclavian nodes.

DIAGNOSTIC TESTS

There are several types of abnormal cell growth or changes in the breast structure. While not every breast change indicates that cancer is present, some of the benign lesions are precancerous and it is often difficult to differentiate between nonmalignant and malignant lesions. Therefore diagnostic procedures are indicated when breast lesions occur to ensure that early treatment is initiated if cancer is present. There are numerous diagnostic and screening procedures in current use: mammography, echography, thermography, xerography, and illumination of the breasts. None of these procedures is 100 percent accurate in diagnosing breast lesions.

Mammography is used for screening in women who are in the high-risk group for developing breast cancer. The soft tissue **mammography** is an x-ray of the breast in two planes, one from above and one from the lateral view. Malignancy is suspected when calcium deposits are seen on mammography. **Echography** uses ultrasonic waves that can reflect the difference between solid and cystic lesions. **Thermography** uses infrared emissions to detect lesions. The breast lesions, because of either increased vascularity or increased metabolism, have a higher temperature than normal breast tissue. The lesions with higher temperature appear as darkened or black areas on the thermogram. **Xerography** is an x-ray mammogram that charges a selenium plate, and the xerogram is transferred to special paper rather than to an x-ray film. Fibrous growths and distorted veins are demonstrated in xerography. **Illumination** is the use of a cold light in a dark room to illuminate the breast tissue. Cysts do illuminate whereas solid tumors are opaque.

Cytologic studies are the most accurate means of diagnosis of breast lesions. A biopsy can be performed by the needle aspiration method or by excision biopsy. The needle aspiration biopsy is more accurate when the tumor is large than when it is small since aspiration of small tumors may not be indicative of the growth of cancer cells if these cells do not predominate in the area being aspirated. Therefore excision biopsy is the most accurate of the diagnostic and screening tests because the total amount of tissue excised can be examined in the cytology studies. When the patient has nipple discharge, cytologic studies are also performed on the specimens of discharge. Failure to find cancer cells in the nipple discharge is not conclusive evidence that there is no malignant lesion.

RISK FACTORS

Risk factors for development of breast cancer have been delineated through clinical studies. Women who are in the high-risk group include those who have never borne a child, infertile women, women over the age of 35, women who have had one or two pregnancies, women who had their first child after the age of 25, women who were under 12 years of age at the onset of menarche, women whose mothers or sisters had breast cancer and, finally, women with a history of cystic breast disease [16]. Childbirth and prolonged nursing are considered protective in prevention of breast cancer. The incidence of breast cancer does increase as the woman grows older, and all women with one or more of these risk factors should be screened regularly to detect changes in the breasts.

CHANGES IN CELL STRUCTURE

Benign changes seen in the breast are fibrocystic disease, cyst formation, epitheliosis, mastitis, and papilloma. The malignant lesions include infiltrating carcinoma, fulminant carcinoma, adenocarcinoma, Paget's disease, and sarcoma. Each of these changes is briefly discussed in the following paragraphs.

Benign Tumors

The cause of fibrocystic disease is unknown and the disease can be either localized or diffuse. It is characterized by infiltration by lymphocytes and plasma cells. **Fibrocystic disease** (also called adenosis) is usually a freely movable mass that can be felt on palpation. Two types of changes can occur, either singly or in combination. One is proliferation of the ducts within the lobes; the other is fibrosis of the ducts. When there is proliferation, the ductile system expands and compresses the lobular cells. In fibrosis, there is compression of the ducts. Nodules form and are usually located in the upper outer quadrant of the breast. The patient experiences premenstrual pain and tenderness of the breasts and often has signs and symptoms of hypothyroidism or irregularities in estrogen and progesterone secretion.

Cystic disease is the formation of cysts in dilated ducts. Fibrosis of ducts or induration of ductile tissues can lead to kinking of the ducts so that there is obstruction and the ducts become filled with fluid. The cysts can rupture, and there is a granulomatous reaction. The cysts can be single or multiple and usually form in the upper outer quadrant of the breast. The patient usually experiences an abrupt onset of symptoms that include tingling or stinging sensations in the nipples. Patients who form cysts often have higher than normal levels of estrogen secretion at irregular intervals. There can also be nipple discharge with cysts; the discharge varies in color and can be yellowish, greenish, or brownish. Treatment of cysts is by aspiration of the fluid, but if the cysts recur, they are often excised. The aspiration procedure is done by having the patient in a supine position and under local anesthesia and injecting a needle for aspiration of the cyst. The fluid obtained is examined in cytologic studies. When cystic disease is chronic, the ducts may distend to cause hemorrhage from the vascular component of the cysts. **Mastitis,** which is a generalized inflammation of the breast, may be a chronic or an acute condition.

Epitheliosis, which is an apocrine-gland disease, is the conversion of ductules to apocrine-like sweat glands. In this condition the patient can develop papillomas. Epitheliosis is considered to be a precursor to malignancy. **Papillomas** are lobular tumors that can be single or multiple. They occur with increased estrogen levels and can be associated with cysts. There is a serosanguineous discharge from the nipples. The papillomas tend to form in the major ducts near the nipples. Changes in nipple discharge from serosanguineous to bloody indicate that malignant changes are taking place, although the occurrence of malignancy in intraductal papillomas is infrequent.

Malignant Tumors

Of the malignant tumors, **infiltrating ductal carcinoma** is the most commonly occurring type; the initial sign is usually a lump in the breast. The lump is usually hard or irregular and may be the only symptom. Some women have a transient sensation of pain in the nipple, and in others there is nipple retraction. An inflammatory type of carcinoma is **fulminant carcinoma,** which occurs most frequently in obese breasts. In this condition the lymph vessels are blocked and the inflammation can extend upward to the neck or to the axilla and arm. There is associated inflammation of the skin, which becomes edematous and discolored. When this reddish or purple discoloration occurs there is usually an underlying tumor. Nodules can be palpated, and usually there are enlarged axillary lymph nodes. Patients with the inflammatory type of carcinoma also tend to have a low grade fever and an elevated leukocyte count.

Adenocarcinoma occurs less frequently in the breast and usually is either a papillary or mucoid degenerative process within the ducts. Comedones form in the ducts, plugging them and causing the breast to bulge in the affected areas. On palpation, these lesions usually feel boggy and are somewhat movable. When the woman raises her arms, the lesions are demonstrated since they tend to remain in the dependent position and do not rise as normal breast tissue does when the arms are elevated.

Paget's disease of the nipple can either precede or follow the development of breast tumors. In this condition the nipples are crusted and red, and there is eczema. The crusted lesions gradually extend and ulcerate so that serum or blood oozes from them. The entire area around the nipple can be indurated, and this induration can extend into the deeper breast tissues to involve the connecting ducts. When this occurs, the larger ducts fill with blood.

Sarcoma of the breast is a rare condition and usually gives rise to a bulky fleshy tumor. Sarcoma of the breast is sometimes associated with fibroadenoma.

CHARACTERISTICS OF MALIGNANCY IN THE BREAST

There are some general observations about the occurrence and metastasis of breast tumors that are helpful to the nurse in caring for patients with possible breast cancer. The majority of breast cancers are detected by the woman herself, who notices the changes incidentally when taking a shower or dressing or who finds a lump or notices retraction of the skin during self-examination. Pain in the breast is a major symptom in about 20 percent of the cases. Breast lesions are most commonly found in the upper outer quadrant of the left breast and almost always occur unilaterally, although about 10 percent of the women who have cancer in one breast do develop cancer in the other breast. Nipple discharge is a less common initial symptom of cancer, as is the development of enlarged axillary nodes. Peau d'orange discoloration and skin edema are associated with cancer, and in some instances there is enlargement of supraclavicular lymph nodes, which usually indicates that the disease has become disseminated. Tumors become fixated as they extend, which means that the tumor is fixed or attached to the chest wall and cannot be moved.

Carcinoma can spread within the breast via the ductal system, and when the skin is involved the disease can spread to the pectoral muscle. Lymphatic spread to the axillary nodes occurs earlier than it does to the supraclavicular and cervical nodes. The pleural cavity is often invaded in advanced disease so that a chest x-ray is taken to determine extension of the tumor to the pleural cavity. In addition to intraductal and lymphatic spread, the cancer can also be disseminated to the bone via the bloodstream with subsequent development of painful osteolytic lesions. In these cases, patients have bone pain, hypercalcemia, and anemia. Spread via the bloodstream can also involve the lung, liver, brain, and adrenal glands. The dissemination via the bloodstream can occur prior to spread via lymphatic vessels. In order to detect metastasis, several tests are performed. Cytologic examination of the specimens via bone marrow aspiration is performed to detect the presence of malignant cells in the bone marrow. Lymphangiography, in which the lymph vessels in the dorsum of the hand are injected, is also used in diagnosis of metastasis. Other tests include evaluation of hormonal levels for estrogen, FSH, and prolactin, vaginal biopsy or smear, lymph node biopsy from axillary or supraclavicular lymph nodes, and liver function tests.

The American Joint Committee for Cancer Staging and the International Union Against Cancer Staging have agreed on a TNM (tumor, node, metastasis) classification of cancer of the breast in which TIS (tumor in situ) indicates carcinoma in situ of either noninfiltrating intraductal carcinoma or Paget's disease. **T0** is no tumor in the breast. **T1** is a tumor of 2 cm or less, **T1a** is no fixation to the pectoral fascia, and **T1b** is fixation to the pectoral fascia or muscle. **T2** indicates a tumor between 2 and 5 cm, **T3** is a tumor larger than 5 cm, and **T4** is a tumor with extension to the skin or chest wall, excluding the pectoral muscle. The **N** component of the TNM classification applies to lymph node involvement; **N0** is no lymph node involvement, **N1** is movable axillary nodes, **N2** is axillary nodes that are fixed and contain malignant cells, **N3** is involvement of the supraclavicular or infraclavicular nodes or arm edema. **M** refers to distant metastasis with **M0** referring to no evidence of metastasis and **M1** referring to distant metastasis with skin involvement extending beyond the breast. Staging is used to determine treatment, and grading of tumors is indicative of prognosis.

TREATMENT OF BREAST CANCER

There is controversy about the best method of treatment for carcinoma of the breast. The treatment can involve surgical resection, radiation therapy, or chemotherapy, often in combination. Hormonal therapy is used in treatment of advanced disease. Among the surgical procedures are wedge resection (lumpectomy), simple mastectomy, radical mastectomy, and supraradical mastectomy. The clinical studies concerning survival rates indicate that there is only moderate difference in the outcome of the radical and simple mastectomy procedures; however, there are proponents of both methods [1, 3]. When a lesion is confined to an area, a **wedge resection** can be performed. It is thought, however, that the procedure may not be effective since other areas of breast tissue that do not demonstrate disease may contain tumor cells. Therefore, some physicians prefer to perform either the simple or the radical mastectomy. The **simple mastectomy** is removal of the entire breast and is also called a total mastectomy. In this procedure the pectoralis muscle and the axillary lymph nodes are left intact. A **radical mastectomy** (Halstead radical mastectomy) is removal of the entire breast, the pectoralis major muscle, and the axillary lymph nodes. This procedure can be modified, in which case only part of the underlying chest muscles and the axillary nodes are removed or only selected axillary lymph nodes are removed. The **supraradical mastectomy** is removal of the breast, the underlying chest muscles, the axillary lymph nodes, and the chain of internal mammary lymph nodes [8].

The decision about whether the axillary lymph nodes should be removed is controversial [1]. In some cases it is thought that the axillary lymph nodes provide for the development of immunity to the tumor cells thereby preventing metastasis. In other cases the patient does not develop immunity and the disease disseminates rapidly. Unfortunately, there is no way to predict whether immunity will develop; therefore some physicians prefer a radical mastectomy since it offers protection against dissemination in the event immunity does not occur. It is possible, however, to closely observe the axillary lymph nodes and to later dissect the lymph nodes if the disease does spread.

In the past, radical mastectomy was considered the best method for treatment, and adjunctive radiation therapy was also included in treatment of many of the patients. Many physicians still prefer radical mastectomy with subsequent radiation therapy since the data about the relative cure rates with different procedures are inconclusive [1]. Lymph nodes in the axilla can be surgically removed or can be sterilized by radiation therapy. The radical mastectomy and lymph node removal or sterilization is considered appropriate when the patient has multifocal disease (located in different areas of the involved breast) or when the tumors are located in the medial or central portions of the breast. When the tumor is fixed to the chest wall, surgery is often not performed and radiation therapy is used instead as a palliative measure.

Following initial treatment for a primary breast cancer, the patient's response to treatment is monitored in frequent examinations to determine the presence of signs and symptoms of recurrence of the cancer or of dissemination of the cancer to other parts of the body. The woman of childbearing age usually is advised not to become pregnant for a period of 2 or 3 years since latent disease has been found to become activated during pregnancy. Although an infrequent occurrence, some women first become aware of cancer when they notice that their suckling infants reject their breast milk. It is not known how or why the infant determines that the breast milk should be rejected. When milk rejection is noted, the nursing mother should be advised to seek examination for early diagnosis and treatment if a malignancy is found.

Treatment for Advanced Breast Tumors

Treatment for advanced or recurring tumors usually involves chemotherapy. Some breast tumors are hormone-dependent although the dependency is not predictable. The type of hormonal therapy required depends on the age of the patient. When the patient is either premenopausal or is within 10 years of the menopause, tests are performed to determine levels of estrogen secretion. If estrogen secretion is demonstrated, either an oophorectomy or radiation ablation of the ovaries is carried out. If the patient responds positively to this treatment, as evidenced by reduction in tumor size in the breast or in areas of metastasis, androgens are given. The side effects of the androgens are masculinization and hypercalcemia. In women who have a positive response to oophorectomy, further treatment for inducing another remission to prolong life or to provide palliation is adrenalectomy or hypophysectomy. This surgical treatment is usually used for women who have slow-growing tumors and in whom the free interval is prolonged. The **free interval** is the period between diagnosis or treatment of the primary tumor and diagnosis or treatment of relapse [19]. While adrenalectomy and hypophysectomy are used in treatment of women with recurrence of bone metastases, they are not as effective when there is metastasis to the liver, lung, or brain. Corticosteroids are used for palliation to reduce the dyspnea caused by pleural metastasis and to relieve pain. The corticosteroids are also helpful in relieving the confusion related to cerebral metastasis, the hypercalcemia related to bone metastasis, and the anemia that occurs in advanced cancer.

In women who are 10 years beyond the menopause, estrogen therapy is used. The side effects of estrogen therapy can include nausea and vomiting as well as relaxation of the pelvic muscles and associated stress incontinence, and phlebitis. Androgens are given following the estrogen regimen, and following androgen therapy an adrenalectomy and a hypophysectomy can be performed in the women who responded to the estrogen therapy.

Another method of therapy is the use of alkylating agents, antimetabolites, and antibiotics in systemic chemotherapy. These agents are used alone or in varying combinations. Local chemotherapy such as nitrogen mustard is also used in some instances. For further detail about these chemotherapeutic agents, the reader is referred to the section on oncology in Chapter 1.

Radiation therapy is sometimes used along with chemotherapy. The patient's condition is evaluated for the status of the bone structure since pathologic fractures often occur following radiation therapy.

NURSING CARE

Nursing care of patients with breast cancer is complex since the patient must adapt to a new body image, and in so doing goes through the grief process. Many patients have reported having frightening dreams that leave them fearful and unsettled. Such patients require supportive nursing care. Recognition that these fears exist and helping the patient express them are important facets of preparing the patient for the surgical procedure and its aftermath. In many instances the diagnosis of cancer via frozen section and the surgical procedure for removal of the breast take place in one operation. The positive consequence is that the tumor cells are not seeded in biopsy performed separately, but of concern is the patient's lack of advance knowledge of the diagnosis and opportunity to become reconciled to having cancer. Essentially, the patient does not take part in a decision-making process about whether to have the radical surgery with full knowledge of the diagnosis when the biopsy and operation are carried out in the same procedure. Instead the patient, although knowing the possible outcomes of either benign or malignant findings, goes to surgery with some hope that the lesion is not cancerous and with some dread that it is. The nurse is cognizant of this ambiguity and helps the patient discuss her feelings in regard to the possible outcomes of the surgery.

The patient is prepared for the operation as for other surgical procedures requiring general anesthesia. Following the mastectomy, there will be drains in the wound. A vacuum drainage (Hemovac) is used to prevent accumulation of fluid in the wound. When a simple mastectomy or a radical mastectomy is performed, there will be skin flaps covering the wound. If serum is allowed to collect beneath these flaps the resulting pressure can cause sloughing of the flaps. Skin grafting is sometimes necessary when the patient does not have sufficient healthy skin to cover the wound or if sloughing occurs. The wound site is observed for drainage, and the amount and color of the drainage are noted. The drainage from the Hemovac is also checked to determine the amount and color of the drainage. Initially, the drainage is bloody and gradually becomes serosanguineous. The patient's vital signs are monitored, and intake and output are measured and recorded. The patient may require intravenous fluids.

Following the immediate postoperative period and after the patient's condition has stabilized, the nurse assists the patient with passive exercises. These exercises are necessary following breast surgery whether the surgery is a lumpectomy, a simple mastectomy, or a radical mastectomy. The initial passive exercises include flexion and extension of the elbow, pronation and supination of the wrist, and clenching and extending of the fingers, all of which are done to prevent muscle contracture and to preserve range of motion and muscle tone. At first the patient has pain and may reject the passive exercises, but the nurse must be careful to explain their importance and to continue the exercises within the patient's tolerance for range of motion. Since edema and trauma to the brachial plexus are postoperative complications that can occur, gentleness in carrying out the passive exercises is essential.

The patient is ambulated on the day of surgery or on the first postoperative day; ambulation is increased thereafter. More extensive exercise is gradually added to the patient's regimen by having her perform such activities as brushing her hair or reaching for things. The patient is helped to participate in an active exercise program while still hospitalized and to plan for a continuing program of full range of motion within her abilities following discharge from the hospital. One of the typical exercises the patient can perform postoperatively is the hand-wall exercise in which she places her palms on the wall at shoulder height and, using her fingertips in a walking motion, raises both arms to the height of tolerance and "walks" the fingertips back down to shoulder level. Many daily activities the patient usually performs at home can be adapted to the necessary range of motion exercises. Activities requiring flexion and extension of the shoulder and the wrist, adduction and abduction of the shoulder, internal and external rotation of the shoulder in addition to flexion and extension of the elbow, and pronation and supination of the lower arm provide the necessary exercises.

The American Cancer Society sponsors a Reach to Recovery program in which women who have experienced a mastectomy help those with new mastectomies adjust to the effects of breast surgery. The American Cancer Society, 219 E. 42nd Street, New York, New York 10017, also publishes booklets for informing patients about the exercises used following mastectomy.

Many patients who have had axillary lymph node resection develop lymphedema in the involved arm. Edema in the wound following surgery, infection in the wound, and tissue changes following radiation therapy as well as trauma to the vessels in the axillary region during surgery all contribute to development of lymphedema, a result of blockage of lymph flow. The patient with lymphedema has special care needs for protection of the arm that has impaired lymphatic and vascular circulation. The patient is advised to avoid infection and to protect the hand and arm from trauma such as cuts, lacerations, burns, or bruises. Wearing gloves to protect the hands, avoiding use of scissors or sharp instruments in giving nail care, avoiding carrying or holding heavy objects in the involved hand or with the involved arm, and placing the arm in an elevated position as often as possible are important preventive measures. Patients with lymphedema can wear elastic sleeves, and in some instances mechanical reduction of edema is achieved with compression devices.

The patient who has had a simple or a radical mastectomy also requires assistance in selecting a prosthesis. Initially the patient is advised to wear her regular brassiere padded with a soft material that will not adhere to the wound. Following healing, the patient is counseled about the various types of commercially available prostheses and of the places where they can be purchased. The patient is fitted for the prosthesis to ensure that she selects one that is comfortable and of the same size and contour of the opposite breast, all of which are important factors in helping the patient retain balance. Patients who have had radical or supraradical surgery may not wish to wear low-cut clothes since the depressions are visible. Otherwise, patients find that their clothing selections are often not altered by the mastectomy.

The patient who has advanced or disseminated disease requires special care for maintaining the maximum amount of energy and feeling of well-being within her capabilities. Many of the treatment regimens described in this section provide for remission and therefore for some relief of the signs and symptoms of metastatic disease. These treatment regimens do not cure the condition, however, and the patient is faced with accepting death. The major sites for metastasis are bone, soft tissue, visceral organs, and the brain. When there is bone metastasis the patient has bone pain, difficulty in ambulation, and frustration from the effects of decreased activity levels. Radiation therapy and narcotics or analgesics are used to relieve pain, and in some instances tranquilizers are also given. Following radiation the patient is vulnerable to pathologic fractures and is taught to protect herself from fracture-provoking motions such as lifting heavy objects, turning quickly or twisting, climbing stairs, reaching for items, and falling. The patient must become conscious of movement and instead of moving automatically at will she must learn to measure movements and to proceed slowly. When pathologic fractures occur, immobilization of the fracture is required, usually via a surgical procedure, as described in Chapter 10.

Patients with metastasis to the soft tissues also have pain and discomfort and require attention to positioning for relief from discomfort. The type of lesion the patient has determines special care needs. Patients with pleural effusion experience dyspnea and may require thoracentesis for removal of fluid. The thoracentesis provides temporary relief and may have to be repeated periodically. Patients with ulcerated lesions require dressings, cleaning of the lesions, and in some instances application of soaks or medications, or both. When the patient has metastasis to the viscera the signs and symptoms include ascites, nausea, vomiting, abdominal pain, and anorexia. Paracentesis is performed to remove fluid, thereby relieving pressure from ascites. Attention is given to maintenance of fluid and electrolyte balance; diuretics are sometimes prescribed. These patients also require either small feedings of foods they can tolerate, or if they are not able to eat, alternative methods such as gastrostomy feedings or total parenteral nutrition are required.

Patients who have metastasis to the brain can have different types of signs and symptoms ranging from confusion to inability to maintain balance, seizures, and paralysis. These women require comfort measures and must be protected from harm that could occur from falling or from trauma during seizures. Some patients experience visual disturbances. All of these patients require attention to intake and output and general nutrition, as well as comfort and body hygiene measures.

Patients with disseminated disease can have involvement of only bone, soft tissue, viscera, or of the brain whereas others can have multiple site involvement. The current reference to dominant site involvement indicates that disseminated disease is predominant in one site. When the metastasis is limited, it is considered that patients with metastasis to the soft tissues have a better prognosis in terms of length of life than those with involvement of the viscera [19]. Patients with metastasis respond differently to their treatment and their death is inevitable even though some of them have longer periods of remission than do others.

It is thus evident that patients with advanced breast cancer experience all the effects of a long-term chronic disease with exacerbations and remissions. The therapy given for palliation also causes discomfort. The nurse helps the patient by providing ways that the patient can conserve her energy for those activities she most enjoys or wants to participate in. In addition, nursing measures are essential for providing comfort or for teaching family members how to provide the maximum comfort for the patient. Throughout the period of terminal illness, the patient and her family must make adjustments and strive toward acceptance of the patient's eventual death.

MAMMAPLASTY

Mammaplasty is reconstruction of the breast either to reduce or to enlarge breast size. Reconstruction of small breasts is an elective surgical procedure requiring general anesthesia. In this procedure a space is created between the capsule of the breast and the pectoral fascia and a breast prosthesis is inserted into this space. Bleeding is controlled by electrocoagulation. Antibiotics are injected into the breast prosthesis as a prophylactic measure to prevent infection. The incision, which is made about 1 inch below the mammary fold, is then sutured.

Reconstruction of large breasts is also an elective surgical procedure and can be accomplished in several different types of operations. The areola can be excised similar to a full-thickness skin graft; usually some of the smooth muscle tissue is retained with the graft. This areolar graft is placed in gauze impregnated with isotonic saline for later placement in the desired location. The skin overlying the breast is then peeled back and wedge resections are performed, usually from the upper and lower quadrant of the breast. The skin is then placed over the reconstructed breast and sutured in place. Excess skin is excised. Following replacement of the skin, the areolar graft is then placed in the desired location by excising an area of skin the same size as the graft and leaving a thin layer of dermis since the dermis provides for better healing for the areolar graft than does subcutaneous fat. In other procedures, the areola is not excised as a free graft, but is resected so that the internal mammary artery attachment is retained. The internal mammary artery is the major source of blood supply for the areola along with the blood supply from the surrounding skin. When the ductile system and the blood supply are retained, the patient retains glandular function. Excess breast tissue is excised by wedge resections; the skin is replaced and the areola is sutured in the desired location.

Subcutaneous mastectomy is a procedure used when the patient has dysplasia of breast tissue from tumors or cysts or when the patient has scarring or tenderness of breast tissue. The subcutaneous mastectomy can be performed in either a single operation or in two stages. The breast tissue is excised by removal of the mammary gland and the axillary projection. If a one-stage procedure is used, a breast prosthesis is then placed and is covered with the skin flap. In this procedure the areola is removed as a separate graft and is replaced following placement of the skin flap. When the procedure is performed in two stages, the patient first has the mastectomy and then returns for placement of the prosthesis after a period of about 6 months.

Other reconstructive procedures include replacement of the areola when it is damaged, such as in burns or when there has been an infection with necrosis of tissue. The graft is taken from the labia minora, which have tissue similar to areolar tissue both in color and texture. Another type of procedure is repair of inverted nipples that are imbedded in muscle tissue. In this procedure the areola is resected from the muscle tissue, and triangular sections of the areola are also excised to create smaller areolar circumference so that there is some areolar constriction to hold the nipple in place.

Nursing care prior to mammaplasty includes preparation for general anesthesia. Following the procedure the patient has large pressure dressings in place. When the areola has been grafted, the graft dressings remain in place for about a week to 10 days and are removed only if there are signs of infection. Otherwise, the breast dressings are routinely changed and the wound is cleaned to remove drainage. Hematomas can form in the reconstructed breast tissue and are aspirated by the physician if necessary. Drains are placed in the wound in surgery and are usually removed 2 or 3 days postoperatively. The nurse checks the dressings and records the amount of drainage and its color and odor. Postoperative infection can be a complication and can interfere with healing. For this reason the patient's temperature is monitored postoperatively. Other complications include failure of the areolar graft to take and loss of some sensation in the nipple. A later painful complication can be venous thrombosis in the breast tissue. The patient is advised to buy a padded brassiere prior to surgery and use it to support the breasts 2 to 3 days after the mammaplasty has been completed. Dressings are placed within the brassiere and are changed as necessary.

Because the patient may have the complication of failure of the areola to grow or an infection, mammaplasty causes some concern during the immediate postoperative days while the wound is being observed to determine the effectiveness of healing. The nurse supports the patient by discussing these fears and by following strict sterile technique in all dressing changes to prevent infection. The patient may initially be disappointed by the sight of the breast with its suture lines but should be reassured that these sutures are removed and that the suture lines recede during healing. As the breast begins to look more normal, the patient can begin to appreciate the positive effects of the procedure.

Patient Teaching

Throughout the diagnostic phase of care the nurse has many opportunities for patient teaching. Many important factors pertinent to patient teaching are included in subsequent sections of this chapter. One area of general interest to many patients is birth control. Many couples or single males or females seek methods to control birth. A number of different methods are used for contraception and nurses are often asked for guidance and counsel in contraceptive use. The nurse is aware that patients can control birth without medical guidance or intervention (prescriptions or devices) and that the many control methods in current use require careful evaluation of the patient's status prior to determining the most appropriate methods of birth control for a particular patient. A general overview of various methods used for birth control is included in this section.

When the nurse is asked for advice about birth control, the patient's purpose in seeking contraception is ascertained prior to giving counsel or advice or to referring the patient for further care. Many persons seek information about family planning and require counseling different from that sought by those who wish to terminate the possibility of ever being fertile. Because world-wide attention has been given to birth control on the basis of reducing populations to ensure adequate food supplies as well as for other reasons, some patients have a broad but vague idea about birth control methods and do not realize that there are contraindications or difficulties associated with certain contraceptive methods such as steroid medications or contraceptive devices. As with any drug or foreign object used, there is a potential for untoward metabolic effects or injury resulting from indiscriminate use of these medications and devices, and preuse evaluation and follow-up care are recommended.

METHODS USED FOR CONTRACEPTION

Contraception may be accomplished in several ways. The use of rhythm or basal body temperature methods along with examination of cervical mucus, taking birth control pills, and using an intrauterine device (IUD) or a diaphragm are methods available to females. Males have the option of using condoms or interruptus coitus. Both males and females can use a number of spermatogenic medications or select to be permanently sterilized.

The rhythm method of birth control is practiced by females whose religious beliefs preclude the use of other types of contraception or whose physiologic conditions contraindicate the use of some of the other methods of birth control. In the 28-day cycle, the estimated day of ovulation is 14 days prior to the next menstrual period. Fertile days are from 2 to 3 days before and after the day of ovulation. In the rhythm method the woman's fertile period is calculated from a record of her menstrual cycles kept for 8 months to a year. The longest menstrual cycle and the shortest menstrual cycle within this time are noted; 11 days are subtracted from the longest cycle, and 18 days are subtracted from the shortest cycle, to determine the estimated fertile period. For example, if the shortest cycle is 24 days, the first fertile day is 24 minus 18, or the sixth day of the cycle. If the longest cycle is 30 days, the last day of the fertile period is 30 minus 11, or the nineteenth day of the cycle. These figures are based on the viability of the sperm for 48 hours in the reproductive tract of the female and the viability of the ovum for 24 hours. The period of viability of germ cells is, however, variable. In addition to charting the menstrual cycles according to menstrual flow, females using the rhythm method can also maintain a record of basal body temperature and evaluate cervical mucus to obtain further information about the date of ovulation.

Diaphragms and intrauterine devices are two methods of birth control that interfere with transport of the sperm. A diaphragm provides a mechanical barrier and must fit correctly to be effective. The female is fitted for a diaphragm following a gynecologic examination and is given complete instructions on how to insert the diaphragm. The gynecologic examination is important for determining the presence of any existing pathologic condition as well as for obtaining a Papanicolaou smear and evaluating the patient's needs for follow-up examinations. The patient is given an opportunity to practice insertion of the diaphragm since it is difficult to learn a motor skill from pictures or from either verbal or written instructions. The diaphragm is inserted a half hour prior to intercourse and is left in place for 6 to 8 hours following intercourse. A spermicidal cream or jelly is applied to the rim and either the inside or the outside of the diaphragm before insertion. Application to the outside is repeated every 2 hours, according to the particular product used, to ensure the spermicidal effect if intercourse is to be repeated. The diaphragm should be evaluated periodically and is replaced if it no longer fits correctly. Use of the diaphragm has few if any risks to the female's reproductive tract.

Intrauterine devices are thought to impede the transport of germ cells in the fallopian tubes and to prevent implantation of the conceptus into the uterus. Their action is not understood, but the use of an IUD is associated with an inflammatory reaction in the uterus. The IUD must be flexible and conform to the particular shape and size of the female's uterus since there is a potential for perforating the uterus or causing pain or bleeding or both if the IUD is too large. At the same time, the IUD must be large enough to prevent its spontaneous expulsion from the uterus. As with the fitting of a diaphragm, the female first has a complete gynecologic examination to rule out the presence of any pathologic condition and to determine the appropriateness of using an IUD. The gynecologist inserts the IUD carefully, using a uterine sound to evaluate the size of the uterus so that the IUD selected fits the uterus. The IUD is then inserted in the uterus, and threads from the

IUD remain in the vagina to facilitate removal if necessary. The patient is advised that the IUD may initially cause cramping and vaginal spotting or bleeding and that the menstrual periods may be both more painful and heavier in flow than normal. The IUD cannot be used in patients with chronic infection of the reproductive tract, but in noninfected women infection is a rare complication of IUD insertion. Following insertion, periodic follow-up examinations are important in order to evaluate the degree of inflammation or the onset of infection, if any, that may or may not be related to the presence of the IUD.

CONTRACEPTIVE MEDICATIONS

Birth control pills are synthetic steroids that change the hormonal balance, but have metabolic activity different from that of the natural steroids. The three major active components of the birth control pills are the estrogens, ethinyl estradiol and mestranol, and a progestin, norethindrone; these components are used singly or in combination. There are numerous combinations available, and the prescription for their use is based on individual needs and the physician's preferences for management. The pills act by interfering with normal hormonal balance; the progestins act on the hypothalamus to inhibit secretion of gonadotropin-releasing hormone and also cause atrophy of the endometrial glands. The progestins also affect cervical mucus, making it less effective in supporting sperm motility. The estrogens are given in combination with the progestins to prevent bleeding and undue atrophy of the endometrium since estrogens stimulate the growth of endometrial cells. Estrogens also stimulate FSH secretion. The combination oral contraceptives contain low doses of estrogen and are considered better for use if there is the potential for developing complications related to high estrogen levels. It should be noted that oral contraceptives have not been in use for a long enough period of time to evaluate their long-term results, and while their use is considered safe, some authorities believe that caution should be taken not only in carefully evaluating each female's physical status before prescribing the oral contraceptive, but also in conducting long-term studies to determine the occurrence of complications related to the use of oral contraceptives. The British Medical Research Council Survey conducted in 1967 included study of the incidence of venous thrombophlebitis or thromboembolism in women using oral contraceptives as compared with a matched control group of women who did not use oral contraceptives. The findings of this survey indicated that there is a relation between the use of oral contraceptives and the incidence of deep venous thrombosis, pulmonary embolism, and less frequently of cerebral thrombosis and embolism, but not with the incidence of coronary thrombosis [18]. These findings have led to the development of oral contraceptives with lower estrogen content to reduce the incidence of complications. The lowest dose that can be used to achieve birth control while also preventing complications is 50 μg of estrogen. Sequential pills, containing estrogen without progestins, have higher estrogen content than combination pills.

The incidence of complications resulting from oral contraceptives, while not frequent among the total population of oral contraceptive users, can be decreased by identifying women who are at risk for developing complications prior to prescribing the pills. Women who may be at risk are identified by physical examination prior to the use of these contraceptives and those who are taking oral contraceptives are examined periodically to determine their response to the drugs. One possible complication that can occur, although rarely, is cerebrovascular disease. There is usually a persistent headache for several months prior to the cerebrovascular accident. Women taking oral contraceptives therefore are cautioned to discontinue the medication when a persistent headache occurs. The effect of estrogen on regulatory and adaptive mechanisms in the body may lead to complications in susceptible women. Healthy women can adapt to these changes whereas women with dysfunctions such as adrenal or thyroid imbalance, diabetes, obesity, or vascular disease or hypertension may not be able to effectively accommodate the changes, and taking oral contraceptives may exacerbate an existing condition or induce a borderline condition previously not obvious. Some of the changes caused by estrogens include elevated cortisol levels, which lead to decreased ability to respond to stress;* impaired glucose tolerance requiring increased insulin secretion that may be diabetogenic in susceptible individuals; elevated serum lipid and lipoprotein levels that may eventually influence the development of atherosclerosis; interference with the active transport of biliary components that can lead to jaundice and pruritus in certain women; and increase in plasma angiotensinogen that may affect fluid and electrolyte balance through changes in the renin-angiotensin mechanism, thereby producing hypertension in susceptible women [21]. Nissen et al. [14] report an increased incidence of liver tumors in women taking oral contraceptives. Their report of eighteen young women who have developed nodular hyperplasia and hepatic adenoma with subsequent rupture and hemorrhagic shock indicates that certain susceptible young women may be unable to tolerate the hepatotoxic effects of oral contraceptives [14]. This finding further supports the theory that every woman who decides to take birth control pills should do so only after seeking consultation and a thorough physical examination, and that periodic physical examinations be conducted while the pill is being used to determine its effects. If this practice is followed, the incidence of complications can be better controlled.

Another important concept in relation to the use of oral steroid contraceptives is that the endocrine system requires a period of time to accommodate to changes. Therefore withdrawal of the oral contraceptives does not immediately result in potential for pregnancy. Rather, a period of time is required, perhaps a year, depending on the individual, for the endocrine balance to accommodate to loss of the oral contraceptive steroids. Some physicians prefer that female patients discontinue taking oral contraceptives approximately 3 months prior to major surgical procedures to give the endocrine system time to accommodate prior to the stress of surgery.

Side effects associated with the oral contraceptives vary in degree and in combinations. These include weight gain, nausea, breast tenderness, breakthrough bleeding, decreased libido, vaginitis, depression, and skin pigmentation. The skin pigmentation is now a less frequent occurrence because of the lower estrogen content in the oral contraceptives. All these side effects do not occur in every oral contraceptive user.

For birth control, the male can use a condom (disposable and often prelubricated and with spermicidal agents) to mechanically prevent passage of sperm into the female reproductive tract. The condom is inflated to test patency prior to use and is removed carefully following intercourse to prevent loss of sperm in the vagina. Spermicidal creams are used on the topical surface of the condom.

The spermicidal creams are available in a number of different preparations; creams, pastes, or jellies, and in suppositories or foams for use by the female. The components of the spermicidal medications include resorcinol, phenyl mercuric acetate, lactic acid, or ricinoleic acid, and some users may be allergic to certain of the components. Spermicidal agents also include a base that holds the agent and also provides a mechanical barrier to sperm. All spermicidal agents must be applied correctly to ensure effectiveness. For example, suppositories require about 15 minutes to become effective and then are only effective for about 1 hour. Foams are easy to apply and penetrate the vaginal and cervical mucosa more easily than can be accomplished by applying cream with an applicator. The duration of action of the spermicidal agents is usually short, and for repeated intercourse a new application is required.

Sterilization is another means of birth control and carries little risk physiologically except for that of the initial procedure. The decision to be sterilized is a grave one that has a different meaning for each individual as well as for each married couple. The psychological implications of sterilization must be explored with patients prior to the procedure. Therefore, sterilization procedures are carried out only after careful evaluation of the individual's motivation, particularly in younger persons, who may later change their life goals. Female sterilization is achieved by ligation of the fallopian tubes during the follicular phase of the menstrual cycle or removal

---

*Estrogens decrease metabolism of cortisol in the liver so that cortisol levels increase. The increased cortisol levels in turn decrease the stimulus for ACTH production in the anterior pituitary. With decreased ACTH production, the woman is less able to accommodate to stress since endocrine adaptations require a variable and individual period of time to achieve new balances in the feedback loops such as the cortisol, ACTH feedback loop (Chap. 8).

of the uterus. Tubal ligation can be performed with laparoscopy and may not completely terminate the potential for pregnancy since the tubes can recanalize. Hysterectomy is most often performed when there is a pathologic condition requiring removal of the uterus. Abdominal pregnancies have been known to occur even following hysterectomy. Vasectomy is the procedure used for male sterilization. In this procedure the ductus deferens is divided and the spermatic cord is incised. The male becomes infertile following use of the stored sperm (which usually takes about 3 months). Spermatogenesis continues, but the formed sperm undergo phagocytosis in the epididymis.

TERMINATION OF PREGNANCY

Abortion is the expulsion of a fetus. A **therapeutic abortion** is termination of pregnancy when the woman has health problems such as cardiovascular disease or diabetes that make pregnancy life-threatening or when she has been exposed to rubella during the first trimester and there is a possibility that the fetus has been damaged. Induced abortion is also indicated when there is evidence of genetic traits that are not compatible with the development of a healthy fetus or baby. Finally, abortion can be induced when the woman does not wish to continue the pregnancy. Abortion can also occur spontaneously. **Spontaneous abortion** can result from defects in the conceptus, uterine dysfunction, or endocrine imbalance, or occur in women with systemic illnesses that interfere with the ability to retain the fetus. Partial separation of the placenta is often the cause of threatened abortions. When abortion is induced, it is referred to as early abortion, first trimester abortion, or second trimester abortion. The 1973 United States Supreme Court decisions made termination of early pregnancy legal if the abortion is agreed to by the pregnant woman. Since the Supreme Court decisions in 1973, numerous state laws have been passed to legalize abortion. The terms of these laws vary from state to state. Prior to legalization of abortion in the various states, inducing abortion for the sole reason of being rid of an unwanted pregnancy was considered a criminal abortion. Abortion is a controversial issue.

When a woman has a spontaneous or induced incomplete abortion it is necessary to remove the remaining products of the pregnancy from the uterus to prevent bleeding and possible infection. A suction curettage or a D and C is performed, and the products obtained in this procedure are evaluated to determine whether a hydatidiform mole or other pathology might be present.

Statistics from clinical studies have indicated that early induced abortion, within the first 8 weeks following the last menstrual period, is to be preferred since there are fewer complications with early abortions. The number of complications that can occur increases according to the duration of the pregnancy. **First trimester abortion** is abortion within the first 13 weeks following the last menstrual period and **second trimester abortion** is abortion within 14 to 26 weeks following the last menstrual period.

Abortion can be induced through several methods. One method is to give the patient diethylstilbestrol (DES). This estrogen prevents the implantation of the fertilized ovum by inhibiting the function of the corpus luteum. Another technique is surgical intervention by dilatation and evacuation (D and E). For abortions at the sixteenth week of pregnancy, by which time the uterus is larger, either hypertonic saline or prostaglandins can be used to induce abortion. Other methods include hysterotomy and hysterectomy; these methods are used when the patient has reproductive tract pathology or when sterilization by ligation of the fallopian tubes is to be accomplished in the same procedure. Prior to abortion by any of these methods the patient should have a complete physical examination, confirmation of the pregnancy, and a pelvic examination to ensure that there is no pathology present that could complicate the abortion procedure. A complete blood count, urinalysis, blood typing and cross matching, and RH type are also obtained. It is important that preparations be made in the event the patient hemorrhages during the abortion procedure. In some instances cervical polyps or uterine tumors or other types of pathology are discovered during the evacuation procedure.

Early or first trimester abortion can be performed by a D and E, in which either a curet blade or a suction curet is used. In some instances physicians limit these procedures to termination of abortion in the first 10 weeks following the last menstrual period. A general anesthesia is usually used for a D and E, and following the D and E the patient has some postoperative pain or discomfort. Suction curettage by means of a vacuum aspirator causes less postoperative pain or discomfort and can be performed with local anesthesia via a paracervical block. In all these surgical procedures the patient is required to fast after midnight and to empty her bladder prior to the procedure. The physician first examines the cervix and uterus by means of a speculum and dilates the cervix. The uterine contents are then removed either with the suction curet or with the blade curet, depending on which procedure is being used. In some instances suction curettage is followed with blade curettage to ensure that all the products of conception have been removed from the uterus. All products removed are sent to the laboratory for examination.

The use of amniocentesis for injection of hypertonic saline or prostaglandin-induced abortion is indicated when the patient is in the sixteenth week of pregnancy. **Saline-induced abortion** is performed by inserting a spinal needle (usually 18 gauge) into the intrauterine cavity. Amnionic fluid is withdrawn to test for correct placement of the needle. Clear amnionic fluid verifies correct placement of the needle. Amniotic fluid is removed usually by gravity drip, and the amount of fluid is measured. Hypertonic saline equal to the amount of amniotic fluid removed is then instilled into the intrauterine cavity. The patient may abort in 2 to 3 hours to 2 to 3 days. Intravenous oxytocin can be given to augment the saline injection. The patient is observed carefully during this procedure; a test dose of hypertonic saline is usually infused slowly to evaluate the patient's response, and the infusion is stopped immediately if the patient has a headache, flushing, intense thirst, or other signs of hypernatremia. Severe abdominal pain may be an indication that the intestines have been perforated by the needle.

The use of prostaglandins to induce abortion is experimental and expensive. Prostaglandin compounds are considered beneficial because their action is effective at all stages of pregnancy. Dinoprostone and dinoprost are two of these experimental prostaglandin compounds. The oxytoxic prostaglandins (Pitocin or Syntocinon) can also be used to induce uterine contractions; these drugs are usually administered intravenously.

Both hysterotomy and hysterectomy require general anesthesia and abdominal incisions and therefore cause more postoperative discomfort and pain and a longer period of convalescence than do other methods of abortion. These procedures are used only when the patient has a condition that interferes with reproductive tract function. They are not commonly performed for routine abortion.

Following abortion, the patient requires care according to the type of procedure that was performed. Postsurgical care for a laparotomy is required when an abdominal hysterectomy or hysterotomy is performed. Following a D and E, the patient has vaginal flow similar to menstrual flow in amount. Antibiotics are sometimes given prophylactically, as infection can be a complication. It is important that the patient who wishes to have an abortion seek care and treatment from a qualified physician because there are many complications that can occur. For example, the cervix or the uterus can be perforated by the curet. As the contents of the uterus are emptied, the uterus reduces in size and the physician must be skillful in adjusting placement of the curet to the changing size of the uterus. In a few instances the uterus perforates very easily, but in such cases perforation is not a result of poor technique but indicates that the patient's uterus is fragile and tender. Serious complications of inappropriate technique can include chronic pelvic infections and infertility. When the abortion is incomplete and products are retained in the uterus, bleeding and sepsis can occur. Therefore post-D and E care includes observation for bright red vaginal bleeding, which indicates either a perforated uterus or a tear in the uterus or cervix. Bleeding in excess of normal menstrual bleeding can indicate that some of the products of the pregnancy have been retained in the uterus. Large perforations or tears are repaired by suturing whereas small tears often heal spontaneously. When it is suspected that there are retained products, a D and C is performed.

Despite liberalized concepts about abortion, some women who wish to have an abortion do not seek medical care. Some of these women use quinine or quinidine to induce abortion. These drugs have been used for years for induction of abortion and have oxytoxic action, that is, they stimulate uterine contractions. It should be noted that the effects of these drugs are not predictable, however, and some women may require such large dosages that the medications are unsafe. Women who have abortions performed by unqualified persons or who attempt self-abortion such as by trying to rupture the amniotic sac to induce abortion can develop sepsis. In these cases the term **septic abortion** is used. Septic abortion can be life-threatening because the infection can spread from the uterus via the lymph vessels or via the veins. The patient can develop signs and symptoms of sepsis in many body organs.

Streptococcus is a common causative organism in sepsis and can be aerobic or anaerobic, hemolytic or nonhemolytic. When the infection spreads to other body parts the patient can develop pneumonia, pleural effusion or empyema, endocarditis, nephritis, peritonitis, or thrombophlebitis. Septic shock can result, and the patient then requires emergency care and treatment. The patient can also develop focal abscesses in any part of the body, such as in the kidney or in the pelvic area. When the signs and symptoms of septic abortion are present, a complete physical examination is required to determine the extent of the sepsis. A pelvic examination is performed to determine if there are retained products of the conceptus. The patient is also asked to describe the technique that was used to induce abortion and to recall whether any foreign substances such as soap solutions were inserted into the uterus. The uterus can be perforated if sharp instruments have been used, or there may be intravascular clotting and hemolysis in the uterus if toxic products have been inserted into the uterus. Care of the patient in septic shock is described in Chapter 16.

RAPE

Trauma to the reproductive tract such as occurs in rape can also lead to the development of infection. Rape is a traumatizing experience both physiologically and psychologically. The rape victim can be male or female; young boys and particularly women of all ages are most commonly assaulted in rape. This discussion of rape is limited to immediate care and does not include the long-term counseling care needs of the rape victim. Burgess and Holmstrom of Boston City Hospital [24] have defined a **rape trauma syndrome.** They found that sexual assault included forced rape (against the victim's will), sexual encounters in which the victim was abused because of the inability to perceive what was happening, and sexual encounters that began with consent to intercourse but which turned out to be distressful because of violence or perversity. The victims of forcible rape are frequently seen in the hospital emergency room and sometimes have multiple assault injuries such as beating or knifing, or environmental exposure following the incident. Victims of sexual abuse may not seek medical treatment since they are often under pressure of fear to keep the sexual assault secret.

Initial treatment for the rape victim includes providing for physical examination and for the patient's comfort. Injuries are detected and treated in the order of priority; bleeding is treated before attention is given to fractures, bruises, or comfort measures. The woman may require hospitalization for treatment of injuries. The woman who has been raped outdoors is often dirty and may have torn clothing. When she is able, the patient is given the necessary equipment or facilities to bathe and to repair her appearance. The nurse provides this care if the patient is too upset for self-care. The woman may need time to discuss the encounter or to overcome the immediate feelings of anger, disbelief, or other emotional responses. Burgess and Holmstrom found that women either have a strong emotional reaction to the incident of rape or are controlled and composed in the initial reaction phase.

The patient is prepared for pelvic examination by cleaning the external genitalia to remove dirt that may be imbedded. It is important that the procedure be explained to the patient and that the patient understand the purpose of the examination. A specimen from the vaginal pool or from the vulva is collected for laboratory analysis for acid phosphatase, blood group antigen of semen, and for precipitin tests against human sperm and blood. A slide is prepared to determine the presence of motile sperm in secretions from the cervix or vagina and specimens are taken for culture and sensitivity tests. The patient is examined to determine whether there are any lacerations or other trauma to the vaginal walls and is given an antiseptic douche. Pregnancy is prevented by giving the patient a prescription for diethylstilbestrol. Antibiotics may be given prophylactically in some instances, and a follow-up examination is scheduled to determine the presence of venereal disease.

Since the rape victim may bring charges against the assaulter(s) and since there is need for a police report, the emergency room notes are carefully written to describe the patient's status at the time of admission, the findings of examination, and the treatment given. Hospital policy usually prescribes how the diagnosis is to be written. Since hospital personnel cannot evaluate whether physical assault did occur without the patient's consent in some cases of rape, the diagnosis may be written as alleged or suspected rape. The nurse may be able to help the patient prepare herself to discuss the incident with the police or can refer the patient to proper sources for legal assistance. These resources are different in each community.

In addition to caring for the patient's physical needs, the nurse is also aware of the needs for long-term care, which include a follow-up pelvic examination and counseling to help the rape victim cope with the physical and emotional aftereffects of the rape. These aftereffects can include physical symptoms of soreness or tenseness, gastrointestinal symptoms, vaginal discomfort, and often the development of infections that can become chronic. The patient may also experience nightmares, and fearful dreams and thoughts, and may be subjected to varying responses from family and friends. The nurse can help the patient by providing referrals to appropriate counselors and by informing the patient that these aftereffects are expected and that assistance is available. The nurse also makes certain that the patient has appropriate resources for transportation home and, when possible, that the family or friend of the patient is prepared to be supportive of the patient following discharge from the emergency room.

MENOPAUSE

Menopause is part of the normal aging process. As the menopause approaches, the woman secretes less estrogen and increasing amounts of luteinizing and follicle-stimulating hormones. The secretion of estrogen by the adrenal cortex continues. Changes in estrogen levels occur gradually, and the effects of diminished estrogen production also occur gradually. As aging progresses there is gradual atrophy of the genital organs and the breasts. The menses become increasingly irregular and finally cease. The hot flushes that typify the menopause are a result of vasomotor instability, but the cause of this instability is not known. In some women the hot flushes are distressing, particularly if they occur with frequency. The hot flushes generally involve the head and neck, and the sensation experienced is much like that in blushing. Some women also experience sweating, particularly at night. It is not known whether estrogen directly affects the blood vessels or whether it influences the autonomic nervous system in some way. Women of menopausal age are at risk for developing cardiovascular disease because there is an increase in cholesterol associated with decreased estrogen levels.

As with all behavior influenced by hormonal balance, the response of a woman to menopause is individual and varies from little discomfort or distress to serious emotional disturbances. The reason for this variation among women is not understood, but it is thought that menopausal behavior is to some extent influenced by social and cultural expectations. The woman of menopausal age is often experiencing many changes in her life at the time of menopause in addition to adapting to the changes in hormone balance. At this stage in life, for example, the woman may be adjusting to the effects of children leaving home and to accepting aging. The acceptance of the inevitable onset of old age is distressful to some women, and many women review their accomplishments at this time with a view toward determining future life goals. The woman's self-concept, the availability of supporting family and friends, and the degree of the woman's involvement in various activities all may influence how she copes with the changes associated with menopause.

A wide variety of signs and symptoms related to menopause can occur. The woman can experience arthritic-like aches and pains with paresthesia of the limbs. Some women gain weight at this time, and most women experience irregular menses. Sleep patterns may change, and some women develop insomnia. There is controversy about giving estrogens to women of menopausal age.

While estrogens decrease the symptoms of menopause, there is some evidence that long-term use of estrogen increases the incidence of tumor growth in postmenopausal women. Impaired glucose tolerance resulting from estrogen use can lead to the development of overt diabetes in women who have a borderline glucose tolerance. Therefore, if estrogen is given to alleviate the symptoms of menopause, low maintenance doses are given. Some of the benefits of estrogen therapy are reduction of cholesterol levels, relief of varied symptoms such as headache, insomnia, and irritability, and decreased bone pain. Osteoporosis can develop in postmenopausal women and is thought to be caused by estrogen deficiency, although the exact effects of estrogen on aging bone are not known (osteoporosis is discussed in Chap. 10). In addition, the use of estrogen also decreases the rate of genital atrophy and the woman feels better. Decreased estrogen is associated with senile vaginitis, which causes discomfort from itching, burning, and vaginal discharge along with dyspareunia (difficult coitus). Estrogen decreases these symptoms.

The nurse can support the patient and her family during the menopause first by listening to ascertain the implications that menopause has for the patient or family, and then by providing correct information about the menopause. Viewed as a normal occurrence and as an event that is adapted to in the patient's own manner, the menopause can be presented as a positive and expected change. The patient may require additional psychological support and the assurance that she is capable of adapting to this change. The nurse and patient can explore possible coping behaviors that the patient can use for adaptation. In some instances, recognizing that she has value and worth in the ability to contribute to the family's economic resources through employment or to contribute to the community through involvement in activities of her choice helps the woman overcome feelings of depression about aging. Support for the patient at this time is most effective if it relates to the patient's actual needs and circumstances. While the nurse knows that some women experience the menopause with little evidence that it has diminished the ability to be effective in employment, family, or community relationships, using these women as examples of successful adaptation can be frustrating to the patient who perceives that these other women do not have her own problems or limitations. Therefore the nurse relates to each patient with an understanding that the individual patient's perceptions, feelings, and symptoms are real and that the ability to cope with her situation must come from her, although supported by family, friends, and the nurse. The climacteric can be induced abruptly by removal of the ovaries, which is often accompanied by a hysterectomy.

Hysterectomy

A **panhysterectomy** is removal of the uterus and cervix; **panhystero-oophorectomy** is removal of the uterus, cervix, and ovaries; **salpingectomy** is removal of fallopian tubes. The operative permit signed by the patient includes the exact structures to be removed. In the event of removal of the uterus, cervix, fallopian tubes, and the ovaries, the operative permit reads panhysterosalpingo-oophorectomy (or total hysterectomy, salpingectomy, and oophorectomy), according to the terminology used in a given institution.

A hysterectomy can be total (panhysterectomy) with removal of the cervix and uterus or it can be subtotal with removal of the uterus and retention of the cervix. The subtotal hysterectomy is rarely performed because patients can develop leukorrhea and carcinoma of the cervical stump. Two surgical approaches can be used: the abdominal and the vaginal approach. The abdominal approach is used when the patient has large tumors, when it is necessary to explore the abdominal contents, when ovarian lesions are suspected, or when the uterus is in a fixed position. The patient has a longer convalescence following abdominal hysterectomy because of the abdominal incision and is subject to all the complications that can follow abdominal surgery of any type. The vaginal hysterectomy is performed to repair relaxations of the pelvic structures, when tumors are small, or when the condition precludes abdominal surgery.

Complications following abdominal or vaginal hysterectomy include development of hematoma in the operative site, bleeding, and formation of fistulas (especially if there is malignant disease or weakening of the tissues from the disease process or if the patient has had radiation therapy of the pelvic area). Patients can develop urinary retention and cystitis following procedures such as repair of prolapse. If postoperative bleeding is excessive, it may be necessary to return the patient to surgery for hemostasis. The patient is monitored carefully since the hemorrhage can be self-limited and may not require surgical intervention.

During convalescence patients are advised to avoid lifting heavy objects or taking part in activities such as driving a car or walking up the stairs to prevent straining at the surgical site. The patient is advised that exercise is important and that sitting for long periods of time causes pooling of blood in the pelvic area that can lead to the development of thromboemboli in susceptible patients. The patient normally has vaginal discharge that is usually of a brownish color following hysterectomy and the amount of discharge gradually diminishes and eventually ceases. The physician may prescribe douches or use of creams or suppositories to decrease the incidence of infection that can be a complication. The patient has no menstrual flow following hysterectomy and is infertile. Patients are advised to refrain from intercourse for a 6 to 8 week period following the hysterectomy. In the study entitled Comparative Study of Post Surgical Convalescence Among Women of Two Ethnic Groups: Anglo and Mexican-American it was found that women of premenopausal or perimenopausal age who had either a vaginal or abdominal hysterectomy for nonmalignant pathology had variable recovery periods ranging from 2 weeks to 6 months [26]. This study supports the concept that recovery from hysterectomy is highly individual and therefore must be managed according to the patient's needs. Patients who have had their ovaries removed do experience hot flushes like those that occur in the natural menopause.

When the patient has an oophorectomy with removal of both ovaries, changes from diminished estrogen secretion are noted; the patient has some atrophy of the breasts and the breasts can become pendulous, and the patient also has less pubic hair. When possible, the surgeon may elect to retain one ovary so that the patient will not experience the symptoms of abrupt menopause. In many instances removal of both ovaries is indicated.

The psychological impact of removal of the ovaries or uterus, or both, is variable and is influenced by the patient's attitudes and feelings about the loss of these organs. The nurse is sensitive to the patient's concerns about the removal of these organs and listens carefully for nuances of meaning in the patient's conversation and is supportive of the patient during the time of emotional adjustment to loss of the sex organs. Some patients may welcome the hysterectomy and may know that loss of the uterus or ovaries does not interfere with or change their femininity. Some patients are ambivalent about the loss, and their preoperative and postoperative experiences are important determinants in their perception of the impact of hysterectomy or oophorectomy. Other patients may be emotionally distressed and some require referral for counseling if their adaptation to the change is difficult. In addition to responding to the surgical removal of these organs, the patient who has malignant disease is also coping with the potential of death if therapy is not effective in curing the disease. This patient requires care as described in Chapter 1 for dealing with the fear of unknown outcomes of therapy and of death.

References

1. Anglem, T. J., and Leber, R. E. Operable breast cancer: The case against conservative surgery. *CA–A Cancer J. Clin.* 23:330, 1973.
2. Burgess, A. W., and Holmstrom, L. L. *Rape: Victims of Crisis*. Bowie, Md.: Robert J. Brady, 1974.
3. Crile, G. Operable breast cancer: In defense of conservative surgery. *CA–A Cancer J. Clin.* 23:334, 1973.
4. Danforth, D. N. *Textbook of Obstetrics and Gynecology* (2nd ed.). New York: Harper & Row, 1971.
5. Green, R. *Sexual Identity Conflict in Children and Adults*. New York: Basic Books, 1974.
6. Green, T. H., Jr. *Gynecology: Essentials of Clinical Practice* 3rd ed.). Boston: Little, Brown, 1977.
7. Hall, R., Anderson, J., Smart, G. A., and Besser, G. M. *Clinical Endocrinology* (2nd ed.). Philadelphia: Lippincott, 1974.
8. Holleb, A. I. (ed.). American Cancer Society policy statement on surgical treatment of breast cancer. *CA–A Cancer J. Clin.* 23:341, 1973.
9. Homburg, R., Potashnik, G., Lunenfeld, B., and Insler, V. The hypothalamus as a regulator of reproductive function. *Obstet. Gynecol. Surv.* 31:455, 1966.
10. Jacobs, T. J. Sexual aspects of dysmenorrhea. *Med. J. Hum. Sex.* 10(5):58, 1976.
11. Kessinger, A., Foley, J., and Lemon, H. Quadrichemotherapy for advanced ovarian carcinoma. *J. Obstet. Gynecol.* 48:134, 1976.

12. Mountcastle, V. B. *Medical Physiology* (13th ed.), vol. 11. St. Louis: Mosby, 1974.
13. Netter, F. In Oppenheimer, E. (ed.), *The Reproductive System*. Ciba Collection of Medical Illustrations, vol. 2. Summit, N.J.: Ciba, Ciba Medical Education Division, 1965.
14. Nissen, E. D., Kent, D. R., Nissen, S. E., and McRae, D. M. Association of liver tumors with oral contraceptives. *J. Obstet. Gynecol.* 48:49, 1976.
15. Novak, E. R., Jones, G. S., and Jones, H. W. *Textbook of Gynecology* (9th ed.). Baltimore: Williams & Wilkins, 1975.
16. Ochsner, A. Diseases of the breast. *Nurs. Dig.* 4:5, 1976.
17. Parmley, T. H. Endometriosis. *Hosp. Med.* 11:23, 1975.
18. Passmore, R., and Robson, J. S. (eds.). *A Companion to Medical Studies*, vol. 3, part 1. London: Blackwell Scientific Publications, William Clowes, 1974.
19. Rozencweig, M., and Heuson, J. Breast Cancer: Prognostic Factors and Clinical Evaluation. In Staquet, M. J. (ed.), *Cancer Therapy: Prognosis Factors and Criteria of Response*. New York: Raven Press, 1975. P. 139.
20. Selkurt, E. E. *Basic Physiology for the Health Sciences*. Boston: Little, Brown, 1975.
21. Speroff, L., Glass, R. H., and Kase, N. G. *Clinical Gynecologic Endocrinology and Infertility*. Baltimore: Williams & Wilkins, 1974.
22. Staquet, M. J. (ed.). *Cancer Therapy: Prognosis Factors and Criteria of Response*. New York: Raven Press, 1975.
23. Stoll, B. A. (ed.) *Mammary Cancer and Neuroendocrine Therapy*. London: Butterworth, 1974.
24. Treatment for rape: The listening ear. *Emergency Med.* 7:240, 1975.
25. Van Thiel, D. Testicular atrophy and other endocrine changes in alcoholic men. *Med. Asp. Hum. Sex.* 10:153, 1976.
26. Williams, M. A. Easier convalescence. *Am. J. Nurs.* 76:438, 1976.
27. Woods, N. F. *Human Sexuality in Health and Illness*. St. Louis: Mosby, 1975.
28. Young, R. C., and DeVita, V. T. Ovarian Carcinoma: Clinical Trials, Prognostic Factors and Criteria for Response. In Staquet, M. J. (ed.), *Cancer Therapy: Prognosis Factors and Criteria of Response*. New York: Raven Press, 1975.

Bibliography

Altcheck, A. The art of abortion. *Emerg. Med.* 5:144, 1973.
Avery, W., Gardner, C., and Palmer, S. Vulvectomy. *Am. J. Nurs.* 74:453, 1974.
Benton, B. Stilbestrol and vaginal cancer. *Am. J. Nurs.* 74:900, 1974.
Bloom, M. L., and Van Dongen, L. *Clinical Gynecology*. Philadelphia: Lippincott, 1972.
Byrd, B. *Standard Breast Examination*. New York: American Cancer Society Professional Education Publication, 1974.
Cali, R. W. Postmenopausal vaginal bleeding. *Hosp. Med.* 11:21, 1975.
Calvert, A. H. Chemotherapy in the treatment of breast cancer. *Nurs. Mirror* 141:63, 1975.
Coburn, D. Anticipating breast surgery. *Am. J. Nurs.* 75:1483, 1975.
Davis, J. E., and Minnberg, D. T. Prostatitis and sexual function. *Med. Asp. Hum. Sex.* 10:32, 1976.
Foss, G. Postmastectomy exercises: How to make them painless, more effective. *Nursing 74*, 4:23, 1974.
Goldsmith, H. S. Milk-rejection sign of breast cancer. *Nurs. Dig.* 4:37, 1976.
Goldstein, D. P., Goldstein, P. R., Bottomley, P., Osathanondh, R., and Marean, A. R. Methotrexate with citrovorum fador rescue for nonmetastatic gestational trophoblastic neoplasms. *J. Obstet. Gynecol.* 48:321, 1976.
Hamilton, M. S., and Schlapper, N. B. Pelvic Exenteration. *Am. J. Nurs.* 76:266, 1976.
Hatcher, R. A., Stewart, G. K., Guest, F., Finkelstein, R., and Goodwin, C. *Contraceptive Technology, 1976–1977* (8th ed.). New York: Irvington, 1976.
Hettlinger, R. *Sex Isn't That Simple*. New York: Seabury Press, 1974.
Hilkemeyer, R. Nursing care in radium therapy. *Nurs. Clin. North Am.* 2:83, 1967.
Holstrom, L. L., and Burgess, A. W. Assessing trauma in the rape victim. *Am. J. Nurs.* 75:1288, 1975.
Klinger, H. P., Glasser, M., and Kava, H. W. Contraceptives and the conceptus. I: Chromosome abnormalities of the fetus and neonate related to maternal contraceptive history. *J. Obstet. Gynecol.* 48:40, 1976.
Legans, J. Artificial insemination: Hope for childless couples. *J. Obstet. Gynecol. Neonat. Nurs.* 3:25, 1974.
Louka, M. H., and Lewis, G. C. Obstetric and gynecologic bleeding. *Hosp. Med.* 12:44, 1976.
May, H. *Plastic and Reconstructive Surgery* (3rd ed.). Philadelphia: Davis, 1971.
McCorkle, M. R. Coping with physical symptoms in metastatic breast cancer. *Am. J. Nurs.* 73:1043, 1973.
Milligan, C., Cummings, D., and Williamson, V. Screening for cervical cancer. *Am. J. Nurs.* 75:1343, 1975.
Mims, F. H. Symposium on human sexuality. *Nurs. Clin. North Am.* 10:517, 1975.
Novak, E. Uterine bleeding. *Hosp. Med.* 10:7, 1974.

Perras, C., and Camirand, A. Subcutaneous mastectomy. *Am. J. Nurs.* 73:1568, 1973.

Piver, M. S., Lele, S., and Barlow, J. Preoperative and intraoperative evaluation in ovarian malignancy. *J. Obstet. Gynecol.* 48:312, 1976.

Price, V. Rape victims: The invisible patients. *Can. Nurse* 71:29, 1975.

Rosenblum, R. Practical guide to the diagnosis of carcinoma of the prostate. *Hosp. Med.* 12:31, 1976.

Schaefer, G. (ed.). Legal abortions in New York State. *Mod. Treat.* 8:1, 1971.

Schwartz, W. H. Fever: When infection follows hysterectomy. *Contemp. Obstet. Gynecol.* 8:21, 1976.

Soika, C. V. Gynecologic cytology. *Am. J. Nurs.* 73:2092, 1973.

Stokes, W. Hysterectomy. *Nurs. Times,* 7:100, 1976.

The course of carcinoma and how to change it. *Emerg. Med.* 8:193, 1976.

The feminine condition. *Emerg. Med.* 7:144, 1975.

Thorn, G. W. (ed.). *Clinician: Medical Gynecology.* New York: Medcom Learning Systems, Searle & Co., 1972.

Vernon, A. Explaining hysterectomy. *Nursing 73* 3:36, 1973.

Wieke, V. R. Psychological reactions to infertility: Implications for nursing in resolving feelings of disappointment and inadequacy. *J. Obstet. Gynecol. Neonat. Nurs.* 5:28, 1976.

Wright, R. A. Pelvic inflammatory disease. *Med. Asp. Hum. Sex.* 10:139, 1976.

Yeadon, D. Uterine inversion. *Nurs. Mirror* 139:88, 1974.

Yussman, M. A. Principles and procedures of artificial insemination. *Contemp. Obstet. Gynecol.* 5:107, 1975.

chapter 10 Patients with Musculoskeletal System Dysfunction

Irene Schreck

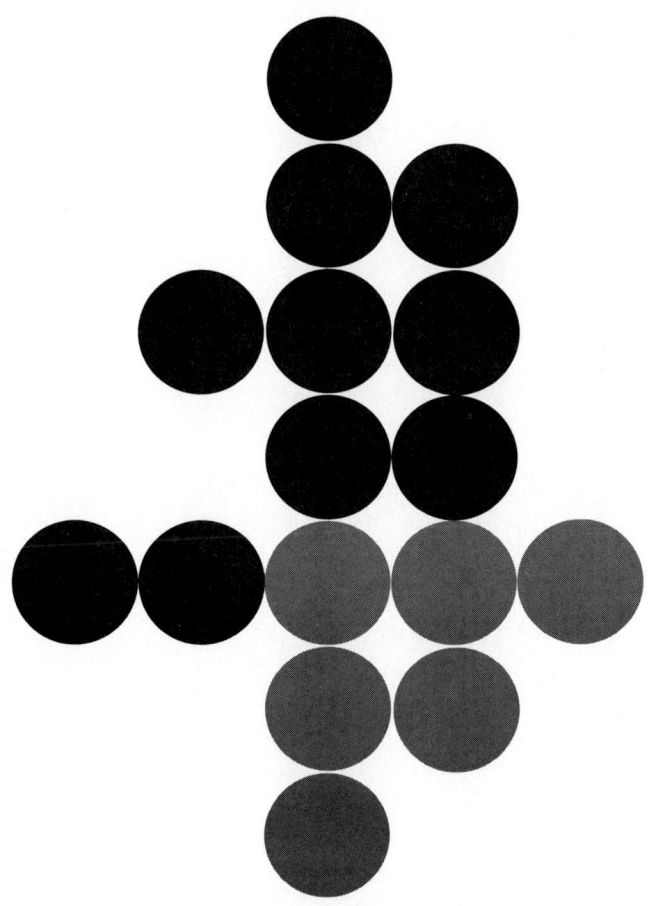

Alterations in the bones, joints, muscles, and connective tissue can affect any age group and occur primarily in well persons. Few musculoskeletal problems are terminal, and many of the patients with such problems are never hospitalized but are treated in clinics. Children comprise about one-third of these patients.

There are recognized periods in the life span when individuals are more vulnerable to musculoskeletal alterations. These periods are during accelerated growth and development, that is, ages 1 to 4, and during adolescence; during the later years of aging; and during any illness that involves long periods of immobility.

Musculoskeletal alterations can be short-term or long-term. A simple, closed fracture treated with cast application that heals without complications can be short-term in that the patient may be ambulant, although inconvenienced by the cumbersome cast. Methods used to correct deformities may continue for months or years, with the treatment involving a combination of surgery, casts, and traction. The greatest long-term alterations appear with spinal cord injury, amputations, and congenital problems. Long-term musculoskeletal problems may involve a change in self-image, role changes, and vocational and economic changes, and these patients may experience periods of discouragement and depression.

Of equal importance to any part of the treatment is the restoration of function to the part. Atrophy from disuse and stiff joints may take longer to correct than the initial trauma or disease. Function is not restored until all soft tissues are free of contractures and have regained their flexibility and strength. Well-planned treatment and avoidance of any complications give the patient a head start toward regaining function.

The nursing care of patients with musculoskeletal problems first involves assessment of the patient's needs and then all the basic measures aimed at maintaining the physical and psychological integrity of the person. Of special concern are care of the skin and routine exercises to maintain functional muscles and joints. Patient teaching is imperative, as the patient must understand the condition and assume increasing responsibility in the treatment plan. Orthopedic nursing involves all the basic principles of body mechanics for the patient as well as for the nurse giving care. In addition to care of the patient, the nurse is involved in the management of a variety of assistive devices and special equipment. Traction and casts must be maintained to be effective. Walkers, crutches, braces, and so forth must be used safely and correctly by the patient. Care of the orthopedic patient, whether hospitalized or in the community, involves the united effort of many health personnel: physicians, nurses, physical therapists, prosthetists, orthotists, and social workers. The more effective the communication and coordination, the greater the benefits for the patient.

Assessment of the Musculoskeletal System

Assessment and evaluation of the musculoskeletal system involve the use of some of the same tools used in assessment of other body systems. These are history-taking, inspection, palpation, blood tests, measuring, and x-ray.

The examination of a patient with acute injury of the musculoskeletal system is very different from the examination of a patient with no injury. With an acute trauma to the musculoskeletal system, diagnostic and therapeutic measures often occur in rapid sequence, frequently overlapping. Attention is directed to maintaining a patent airway, detecting and arresting hemorrhage, examination for coexisting brain or spinal cord injury, fracture, chest injury, intra-abdominal and urinary tract injury, and peripheral nerve injury [20].

When there is no acute trauma to the musculoskeletal system, the examination centers on evaluation of structure and function. The starting point is always careful history-taking to elicit the onset and course of the chief complaint.

Inspection is directed toward an assessment of body alignment, deformities, abnormal postures, gait, and skin color. Skin color may represent a change in pigmentation over an area, cyanosis, ecchymosis, or signs of ischemia. It is possible to note soft tissue swelling, muscle wasting, or nodules. Range of motion of all joints should be evaluated. Any scars that are present are noted.

Palpation involves feeling with the hands on external body surfaces to detect skin temperature, thickening, abnormal bony prominences, swelling, bogginess, or fluid where there usually is none. Tenderness can also be detected. Peripheral pulses should be palpated and compared on both extremities.

Blood tests including serology, bacteriology, and hematology are made to support or disprove other findings. Measurement of circumference, length, and angles will add important data about structural and functional changes and serves as baseline data to note improvements as therapy progresses. X-ray studies are usually the final but very important measure in the process of establishing a diagnosis.

Pain, deformity, and limitation of function are usually part of the presenting symptoms. Limited function may stem from pain resulting from previously normal body motion, from a stiff joint, or from joint instability. Joint restriction may in turn be caused by neurologic disease or trauma; muscle contraction resulting from disease or injury; fusion of bone or a mechanical block by bone fragments or torn cartilage within a joint [20].

Any complaint of pain must be evaluated in terms of its characteristics, location, and relation to activity. Deep, constant, boring pain is often associated with erosion of bone by tumor or an aneurysm. This pain is often not relieved by rest or position changes and may intensify at night. Aching pain that is accentuated by activity, by certain positions, and that is relieved by rest is usually associated with degenerative arthritis and muscle disorders. The pain of a fracture or bone infection is usually described as severe and throbbing. This pain is intensified by motion of the affected part. Compression of a nerve causes a sharp pain that radiates along the distribution of the nerve involved. Pain in an anatomic region remote from the site of the lesion is called referred pain and it occurs in diseases affecting the shoulder, hip, and lower cervical spine.

Following is a general overview of nursing assessment of structure and function of the musculoskeletal system. The patient is asked to walk, stand, sit, rise from a sitting position, run, and to jump if possible; any awkwardness, limp, or change in rhythm is noted. Much about posture and gait can be noted in just observing the patient's ability to perform certain activities of daily living such as getting in and out of bed or walking to the bathroom.

Good posture means maintaining body alignment that most favors function, requires the least muscular work to maintain, and puts the least strain on muscles, ligaments, and bones. It means keeping the body's center of gravity over its base. Posture is the result of continued partial contraction of many skeletal muscles, which makes standing, sitting, and position changes possible. All body systems being interdependent, posture cannot be maintained if muscles lack nerve and blood supply, or if the skeletal system is unstable.

Joints are inspected and palpated for any deformities, swelling, tenderness, and redness. Range of motion should be determined and always compared to the opposite side. As the joint is going through its range of motion, it is possible to detect crepitation manually. Any contracture of muscle near a joint will restrict its motion.

In observing the spine, it is possible to detect gross deformities or visible muscle spasm. **Scoliosis** is an abnormal lateral deviation of the spine. **Lordosis**, or "sway back," is an abnormal concavity of the lumbar spine. **Kyphosis**, or "hump back," is an abnormally increased convexity of the thoracic spine (Fig. 10-1). One should also note the flexion, extension, lateral bending, and rotation possibilities of the spine. The ribs should be observed for symmetry. Pain from the lower cervical spine may be referred to regions of the scapula, shoulder, and arm.

Assessment of the upper extremity includes examination of the shoulder, elbow, wrist, hand, and supporting structures and notation of any swelling, abnormal contours, nodules, changes in range of motion, or change in skin coloring. The carrying angle of the elbow, flexion, and extension possibilities are observed. The shoulder, being a ball and socket joint, is capable of many observable ranges of motion.

The lower extremity is first examined by observing gait. Gait is affected by leg-length, inequality, muscle weakness, habit patterns, fusion, contractures, pain-producing lesions of the hip, knee, ankle, and foot. Normally, the pelvis rises on the side opposite the leg bearing weight when one is walking. This is a result of contraction of the gluteus medius muscle on the weight-bearing side. The hip normally is capable of flexion, extension, abduction, adduction, and rotation. Pain in the hip can be referred to the anterior and lateral thigh muscle. The knee should be examined for any swelling or deformities and limita-

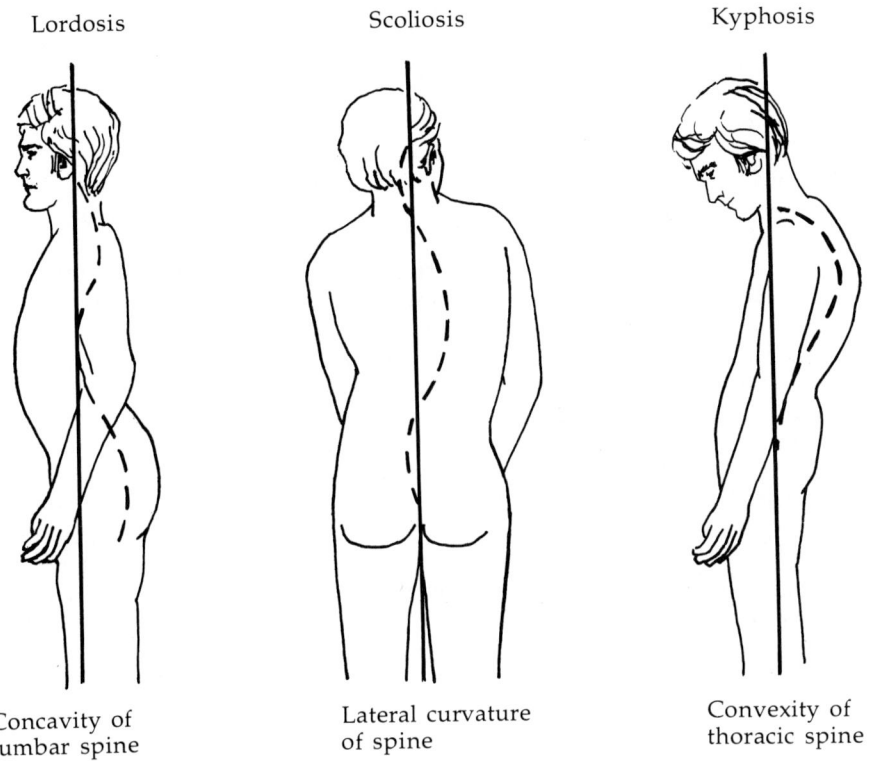

Figure 10-1
Curvatures of the spine. In lordosis, there is concavity of the lumbar spine; in scoliosis, there is lateral curvature of the spine; and in kyphosis, there is convexity of the thoracic spine.

tions in motion. Normally, the knee joint contains about 30 ml of synovial fluid. Increases in joint fluid can be felt as boggy, soft, and fluctuant swelling about the area. The ankles and feet should also be checked for any swelling or deformities and limitation in normal motion. Bunions, calluses, or hammer toe should be noted. Lower-extremity muscle strength can be tested by having the individual stand and first support weight on the heel, then on the ball of the foot, or push against resistance in a supine position. Joint stability means that a joint moves the way it is supposed to move. When assessing the structure and function of body extremities, the two extremities are always compared in terms of size, shape, and function.

Muscle tone is best evaluated when the person is warm, relaxed, and comfortable. The muscles are inspected and palpated for gross hypertrophy or atrophy. Fasciculation (isolated contraction of a portion of the fibers) may be noted. Muscle circumference of an extremity is measured at a given point above or below a joint and compared with the opposite side.

During examination of the muscles, the nurse should recall that the flexors are stronger than extensors, abductors are stronger than adductors, and flaccid muscles are easily stretched, and that for a muscle to function, it must be innervated and attached to either a bone, tendon, or ligament. In handling muscles, the nurse should remember that any time the body of a muscle is squeezed, pain can be produced. Therefore, extremities should be supported at the joints. Any bowing, angulation, or enlargement of bones is noted. Bones are palpated to detect areas of tenderness and masses.

X-ray diagnostic procedures related to the musculoskeletal system include roentgenography, tomography, cinefluorography, and polyphosphate bone scans.

Anteroposterior, lateral, posteroanterior, and oblique x-ray views may be taken. An **x-ray** is indispensable to diagnosis of musculoskeletal problems, for it demonstrates bone density, erosion, breaks, new growth, irregularity, deformity, and altered texture. Soft tissue abscesses or calcification or loose bodies in joints can also be detected. **Tomography** is body section roentgenography that can focus on certain tissue, blurring or eliminating surrounding tissue. **Cinefluorography** is a technique whereby motion of the skeleton is recorded on a movie film for more detailed study at a later date. This is accomplished with relatively small amounts of radiation exposure.

Contrast radiography includes arthrography, myelography, discography, and arteriography. **Arthrography** is introduction of air or a radiopaque material into a joint space, making it possible to outline radiolucent structures and to view joint surface detail on an x-ray. **Myelography** is the introduction of air or a radiopaque material into the subarachnoid space for the purpose of viewing filling defects that may indicate a tumor or herniated disk in the spinal column. **Discography** is a technique in which a radiopaque material is injected into the nucleus pulposus of an intervertebral disk so that the internal architecture of the disk may be studied. **Arteriography** is the injection of a radiopaque material into the arterial supply to an anatomic region and taking a series of x-ray films. This technique is helpful in studying vascular supply to bone, joint, or bone lesions. **Arthroscopy** is the inspection of internal structures of a joint with a lighted instrument inserted via a small incision. The internal structure can also be photographed with this instrument.

Bone-scanning uses an intravenous injection of radioisotope materials that have a special affinity for bone and emit penetrating gamma rays. The materials help detect, localize, and outline lesions of bone. Polyphosphates, ^{85}strontium, and radioactive gallium have been used. Radioactive estrone is used if the endosteum of bone is to be studied, and certain radioactive amino acids have an affinity for bone matrix. Usually the symmetrical uninvolved body part serves as the control in the comparison of data.

The musculoskeletal system is composed of bones, joints, muscles, tendons, ligaments, and cartilage. The system necessarily includes the associated blood vessels and nerves. These structures, working together, provide for voluntary motion, support body structures, and protect soft-tissue cavities. Essentially the bones and muscles give people their individual size, shape, strength, and coordinated graceful movement. Tendons, ligaments, bursae, and fascia hold the bones and muscles together and allow for the articulation of joints and motion. In addition, bones are reservoirs of essential minerals such as calcium and phosphorus. Bone marrow, which occupies the marrow cavity of all bones, also has a role in erythrocyte production (hemopoiesis).

The term **skeleton** (Fig. 10-2) means all the bones of the body, plus the joints formed by their attachment to each other, that permit movement. Bones and cartilage are the two predominant types of connective tissue of the skeleton. The two major divisions of the skeleton are (1) **axial**—skull, vertebrae, ribs, sternum, and (2) **appendicular**—shoulder, limbs, and pelvic girdle.

The skeleton is composed of 206 separate bones that are morphologically classified as flat, long, short, and irregular. The **flat bones** tend to be in positions that protect delicate organs or allow for attachment of large muscles (skull, sternum, scapula, ribs, pelvis). **Long bones** (humerus, ulna, radius, femur, fibula, tibia, phalanges) act as levers in movement. **Short bones** (carpals, tarsals) confer strength. **Irregular bones** (vertebrae, facial bones) permit movement. Vertebrae protect the spinal cord. The vertebral column is shown in Figure 10-3.

Long bones have the following parts: diaphysis, epiphysis, metaphysis, articular cartilage, periosteum, medullary (marrow) cavity, and endosteum. The blood supply of long bones comes from three sources: the nutrient artery, the periosteal arteries, and the epiphyseal arteries. The diaphysis is the shaft-like portion of thick compact bone with a medullary canal. It provides strength for strong support, yet is lightweight, since it has a hollow canal. The epiphysis is the end of long bones that is made up of spongy or cancellous bone. Epiphyseal ends have a somewhat bulbous shape, which provides for muscle attachment and gives stability to

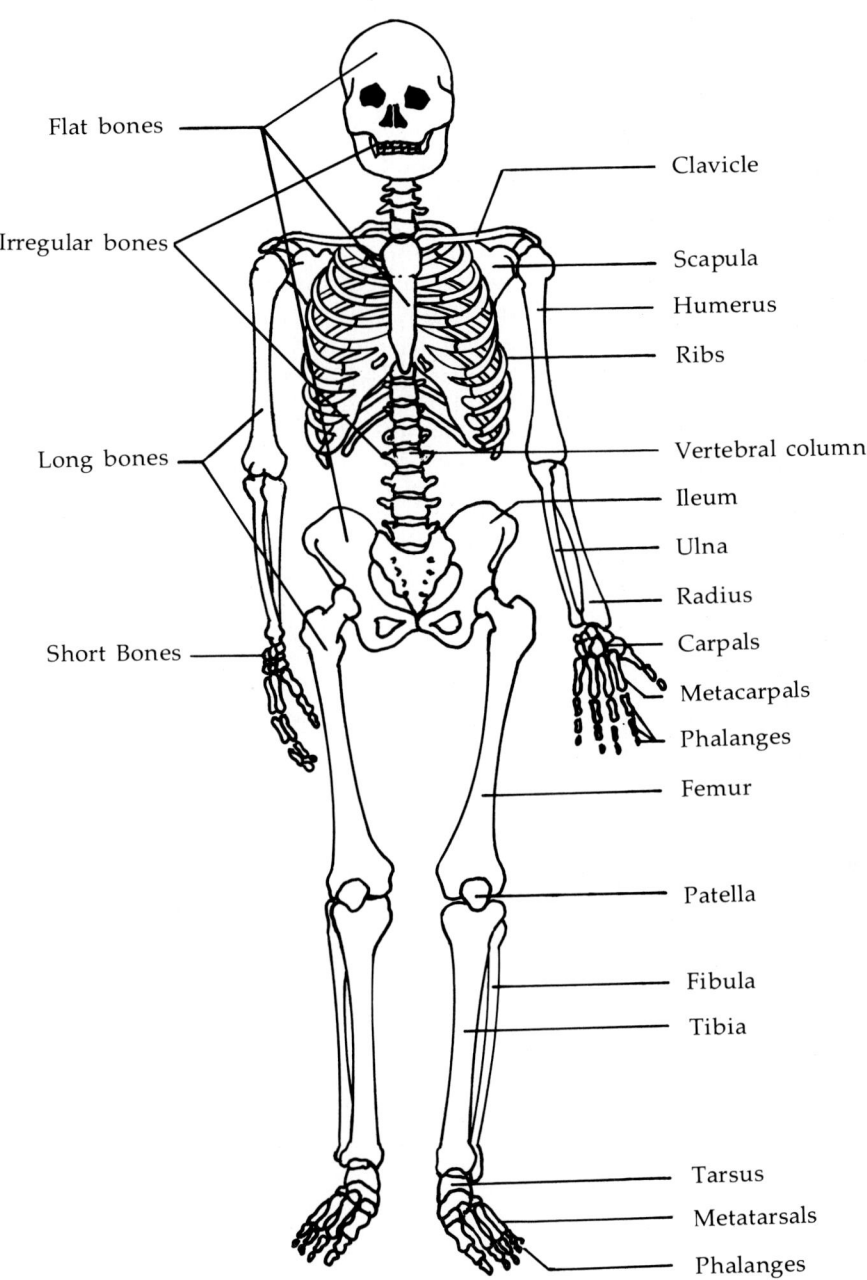

Figure 10-2
The skeleton gives shape and support to the body and is jointed to permit movement. Bones and muscles are concerned with movement of the body. All bones are attached to muscles and are classified according to their shape when growth is complete. There are four types of bones: (1) **flat** bones protect delicate organs; (2) **long** bones act as levers, (3) **short** bones confer strength, and (4) **irregular** bones, which are facial and vertebral, permit movement.

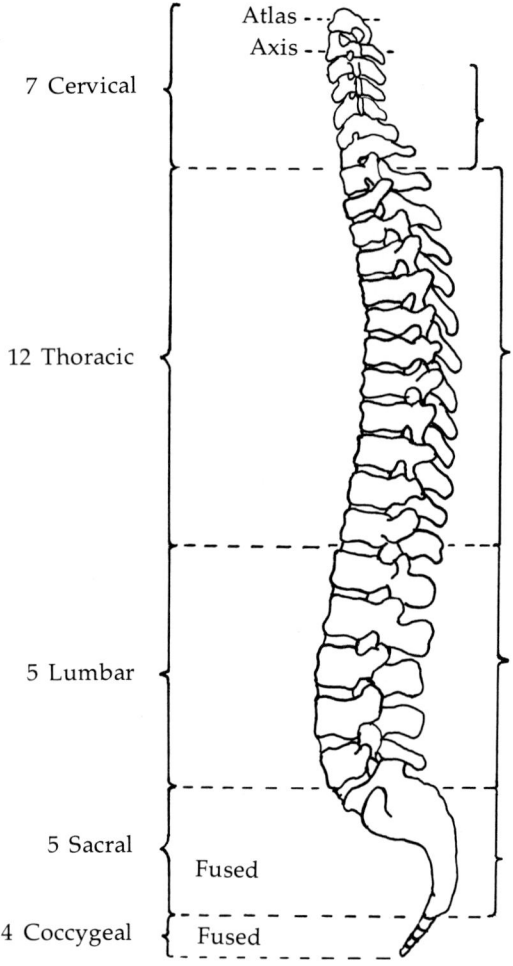

joints. The metaphysis is the flared portion of the bone lying at the junction of the diaphysis and epiphysis, which is a highly vascular area most often affected by bone infection. It arises out of the growth process at the physis. A cartilagenous disk, the physis, lies between the diaphysis and each epiphysis of long bones and is considered to be the growth zone. During maturation, a point is reached at which the epiphysis and diaphysis unite and further longitudinal growth ceases. Ossification is complete when the cartilage cells cease to divide and bone entirely replaces the disk. Epiphyseal closure occurs at about age 14 in girls and age 16 in boys, but it varies in different bones. Thus, complete ossification in all bones may not be achieved until age 25 (Fig. 10-4).

The articular cartilage is a thin layer of hyaline connective tissue covering the articular surface of each epiphysis. It is white, relatively hard, has no direct blood supply, but

Figure 10-3
The vertebral column. There are 33 vertebrae. The adult has 26 vertebral segments because the sacral and coccygeal vertebrae fuse. Vertebrae are united by intervertebral disks of cartilage and enclose and protect the spinal cord. The 7 cervical vertebrae are involved in movements of the neck; the 12 thoracic vertebrae attach to the ribs and allow rotation, forward flexion, and some lateral movement of the trunk; the 5 lumbar vertebrae allow dorsiflexion, lateral movement, and some rotation of the trunk; the 5 sacral and 4 coccygeal vertebrae transmit the weight of the body to the pelvic girdle and legs.

Figure 10-4
Structure of a long bone.

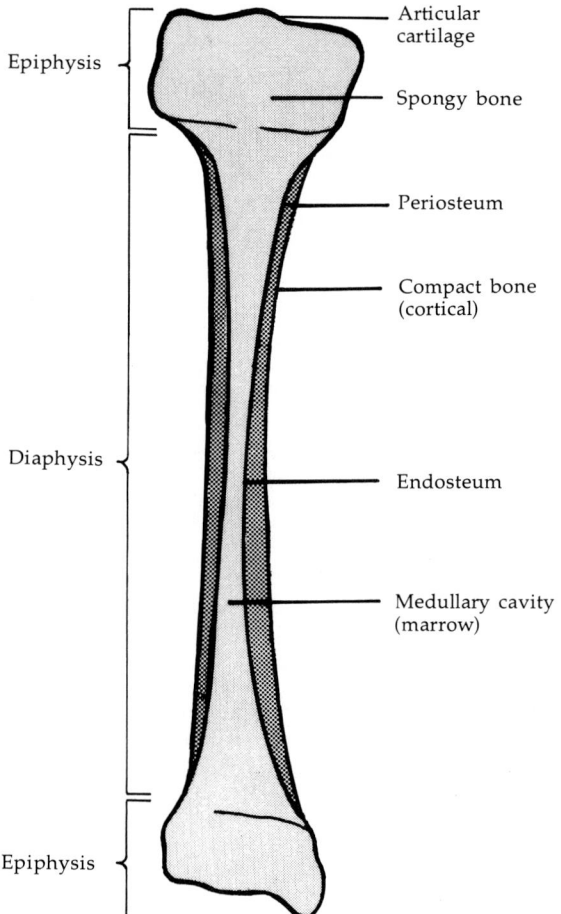

receives its nutrients from joint fluid. Cartilage is compressible tissue with a very smooth surface that cushions jolts and shock in many parts of the musculoskeletal system.

The **periosteum** is a dense white fibrous membrane that covers all bone except at joint surfaces. Periosteum is lined with osteoblasts; thus it is osteogenic and can form osteoid tissue directly when the necessity arises. Many fibers of the periosteum (Sharpey's fibers) penetrate the underlying bone to unite the two structures and allow blood vessels and nerves to enter bone. The periosteum has a rich blood and nerve supply. Periosteum serves to attach muscles and tendons to the bone and it is also necessary for bone growth, repair, and nutrition. The muscle tendon fibers interlace with the periosteal fibers to anchor muscles firmly to bone [2]. The **endosteum** is the thin layer of reticular cells that line the medullary cavity and haversian canals. It is the peripheral layer of bone marrow and has both osteogenic and hematopoietic functions. The endosteum, like the periosteum, is very active in fracture healing.

Bone arises from the embryonic layer of the mesoderm and it is a connective tissue, just as are fibrous tissue and cartilage. The connective tissues differ from one another in the types of cells and the chemical composition of the ground substance in each. Common to all connective tissue is collagen, which is protein made up of chains of organic molecules arranged longitudinally to form fibrils. The cell types for primitive fibrous tissue are the fibroblast, chrondroblast, and osteoblast which, as these tissues mature, become fibrocytes, chrondrocytes, and osteocytes [29].

Tendons, ligaments, and fascia are fibrous tissue with little ground or intracellular substance. Cartilage has fewer collagen strands, more ground substance, and more cells. Bone can be described as dense connective tissue in which osteocytes are immersed in the intracellular ground substance with the collagen fibrils. The hardness and rigidity of bone are attributed to the deposition of inorganic crystals in the ground substance or organic matrix. These inorganic salts are principally calcium and phosphorus, with some sodium, magnesium, potassium, and fluoride. The latticework arrangement of the inorganic salts with the matrix allows for continual exchange of these inorganic substances. The calcium in bone is of two types: a readily exchangeable reservoir and a larger pool of stable calcium that is only slowly exchangeable. Plasma calcium levels are in equilibrium with the readily exchangeable bone calcium [14].

The organic matrix of bone is about 95 percent collagen fibers, which extend in all directions and give bone its tensile strength. Inorganic calcium and phosphorus deposited in the matrix give bone its compressional strength. Calcium salt has physical properties similar to marble. Thus bone can be compared to reinforced concrete; the "steel" is the collagen matrix and the "cement" is the inorganic calcium and phosphorus.

Bones are not, however, static structures, but are dynamic in that they constantly undergo change: they remodel, metabolize, adapt, and respond. Bone is well vascularized. It is estimated that the total bone blood flow in man is 200 to 400 ml per minute [14].

Microscopically, bone cells are of three types: osteocytes, osteoblasts, and osteoclasts. **Osteocytes** are the bone cells that are surrounded by calcified matrix and whose function is to maintain bone as living tissue. **Osteoblasts** are the bone cells that are constantly producing the basic osteoid substance of bone. Osteoid is composed of collagen, which is protein, and a ground substance, "glue," which is made up of polysaccharides. Thus, osteoblasts are bone-forming cells that line the surface of actively growing bone in great numbers. In addition to forming the osteoid organic matrix of bone, osteoblasts also assist in the deposition of the inorganic salt that mineralizes and crystalizes the bone. This process is balanced by the activity of **osteoclasts,** multinucleated bone cells that erode and resorb previously formed bone. It is generally thought that these three types of bone cells are three phases of a single cell type. These cells are capable of reversible morphologic changes and are examples of cell modulation, as opposed to cell differentiation, which is an irreversible morphologic change [14, 23].

The process of constant bone production is called **accretion,** whereas the simultaneous absorption of both bone mineral and bone matrix is called **resorption.** When accretion and resorption are in balance, the normal toughness, size, and shape of bone are maintained. Both processes, however, decrease with age, that is, accretion and resorption are slower at age 60 than at age 20, resulting in the decreased bone mass associated with aging. When both accretion and resorption are abnormally increased, bone becomes thick, soft, and of poor quality. This abnormal bone remodeling is called Paget's disease [23].

The arrangement of the intercellular substance of bone consists of units of concentric cylindrical layers of calcified matrix called lamellae, enclosing a central longitudinal haversian canal containing blood vessels. The unit of lamellae surrounding the haversian canal is called the haversian system. Osteocytes of bone cells are located between the lamellae in minute spaces called lacunae. Microscopic channels (canaliculi) radiate in all directions from lacunae, connecting them with haversian canals and providing a means for tissue fluid to reach the bone cells [2]. The arrangement of the lamellae determines whether bone is compact or dense such as in cortical bone, or if bone is cancellous or spongy. The latter type has more open spaces, and is more vascular.

The haversian canals connect to the Volkmann's canals from the periosteal blood supply that penetrates bone. There are additional nutrient arteries in the marrow cavities of long bones.

The bone marrow forms erythrocytes, granulocytes, monocytes, and platelets. In fetal life and early infancy, all marrow cavities contain hematopoietic marrow. After the first few years of life, the distribution of hematopoietic (red) marrow changes. In adulthood, red marrow is found principally in the vertebral bodies, the sternum, and the bones of the pelvic girdle. All other bones contain adipose yellow marrow; however, in conditions of physiologic or pathologic stress, the yellow marrow can become active in hemopoiesis [2, 34].

FACTORS THAT AFFECT OSTEOGENESIS

Normal bone growth requires a diet with adequate minerals, vitamins, and protein. Normal calcium metabolism is dependent on a normal functioning gastrointestinal tract, kidneys, and parathyroid gland. Collagen and cartilage formation involves multiple biochemical processes [25].

When bone is not under stress, decalcification occurs. Forces exerted on bone lead not only to alterations in internal structure but also to changes in external form and functions. Wolff's law of bone growth states that when stresses are applied to a bone, the trabeculae within that bone develop and align themselves to adapt to these lines of stress. Bone thickens when subject to heavy loads. Thus, a football player, a person very athletically inclined, or a person whose occupation requires heavy lifting has heavier bone structure than a person whose life is more sedentary. Normal remolding and repair of bone as well as repair after injury depend on stress. This is the underlying rationale for early ambulation and weight-bearing following any type of skeletal injury.

Pressure forces exerted perpendicular to the axis of long bones, as in prolonged bed rest, cause resorption of bone, whereas pressure forces acting in the line of the long axis promote osteogenesis [32].

It is beyond the scope of this text to discuss in depth all the biochemical forces that affect osteogenesis. There is much interplay between vitamins, minerals, and hormones and their effects on the musculoskeletal system.

Calcium has a role in many physiologic processes: in cell permeability, cell adhesion, muscle contraction, synaptic transmission, blood clotting, and, in the skeleton, as a major inorganic salt. Calcium, a bivalent ion, is only absorbed from the gastrointestinal tract as a free ion, whereas phosphorus is readily absorbed. Absorption of calcium is decreased by phosphates and oxalates in the gastrointestinal tract, as these substances form insoluble salts with calcium.

The active transport of calcium from the intestinal tract is increased by the presence of vitamin D. Promoting the mineralization of bone, mobilizing calcium from bone, and elevation of serum phosphate levels are other roles of vitamin D. Deficiency of vitamin D can be a result of environmental factors (lack of sunshine), insufficient dietary intake, or absorption problems in the gastrointestinal tract. Most calcium is absorbed in the duodenum and jejunum.

Recent evidence suggests that vitamin D requires metabolic alterations within the body, first by the liver and then the kidney, to prepare it to function. Vitamin D is converted to an active metabolite, 1,25-dihydroxycholecalciferal (1,25 DHCC), by an enzyme in the kidney. This metabolite, 1,25 DHCC, is considered by some to be a hormone. In hypocalcemia, the parathyroid glands are stimulated to secrete parathyroid hormone, which then stimulates the conversion of vitamin D to 1,25 DHCC. Parathyroid hormone, along with 1,25 DHCC, then mobilizes calcium from bone. In addition, the 1,25 DHCC stimulates intestinal calcium absorption independently of the influence of parathyroid hormone. These two phenomena thus reverse the hypocalcemia and, when serum calcium levels return to normal, synthesis of 1,25 DHCC and secretion of parathyroid hormone are suppressed [8].

When there is a lack of vitamin D (or 1, 25-DHCC), bone becomes soft and bends abnormally. This condition is called rickets in a child and osteomalacia in an adult.

Parathyroid hormone excess occurs in hyperparathyroidism, resulting in overstimulation of bone resorption, which leads to bone demineralization and hypercalcemia. Idiopathic or spontaneous hypoparathyroidism is rare, but the parathyroid glands can accidentally be removed with a thyroidectomy. Lack of parathyroid hormone results in decreased removal of calcium from bone, decreased deposits of calcium in bone, and decreased intestinal absorption of calcium, all of which combine to cause deformed bone and hypocalcemia. There is also a pseudohypoparathyroidism in which blood plasma levels of parathyroid hormone are normal, but bone does not respond to it. Hypocalcemia and bone deformities result. Parathyroid hormone also influences the renal excretion of phosphate.

Calcitonin, secreted by the thyroid glands, lowers plasma levels of calcium and phosphates and inhibits bone resorption. Calcitonin has proved of value in treating Paget's disease. The enzyme, alkaline phosphatase, plays an active role in the mineralization of bone matrix.

The glucocorticoids from the adrenal glands are thought to lower plasma calcium levels and inhibit the action of vitamin D in the intestinal tract. Glucocorticoids, because they are catabolic, can decrease the protein matrix of bone leading to decreased bone mass.

Hyposecretion of growth hormone by the anterior pituitary leads to uniform dwarfism with failure of sexual and skeletal maturation. Hypersecretion of the growth hormone results in gigantism, a disharmonious enlargement of the skeleton. If excess growth hormone occurs past maturity, acromegaly results. It is believed that the pituitary growth hormone influences urinary excretion of calcium and increases intestinal absorption of calcium. Absorption is greater than excretion, leading to a positive calcium balance.

The estrogen and androgen hormones of puberty influence closure of the epiphyseal plate of long bones, which indicates when bone growth is complete in adolescence. Later in life, when these hormones diminish naturally, it is felt that decreased bone mass results. Senile and postmenopausal osteoporosis result.

Another vitamin that affects bone is vitamin C. Ascorbic acid is needed for osteoid production and to maintain intact capillaries. Chronic lack of ascorbic acid leads to a tendency to hemorrhage which, when occuring subperiostially, causes pain in the affected bones. This is one aspect of the syndrome called scurvy.

JOINTS

The tissues that join bones at their articulating surface make up a joint. These tissues are the joint capsule, ligament, muscle, and tendons. Articular cartilage is subjected to wear and tear unequaled by any other body tissue except the skin. The primary purpose of joints is to bear weight and provide motion.

Classification of articulation of joints is based on the presence or absence of joint cavities. Joints without cavities are called synarthroid or fibrous joints. There is a continuation of the two bone surfaces with fibrous tissue or cartilage which allows for little or no movement. The fibrous tissue cushions the two bone surfaces where they join. Examples of synarthroid joints are the suture lines of the skull, intervertebral disks, junction of the ribs at the point of their connection to the vertebrae and sternum, and the symphysis pubis joining the two pubic bones.

Diarthroses are joints in which a small space or cavity exists between the articulating surfaces of the two bones that form the joint. These joints move freely and are further classified according to their planes of motion as **ball and socket, hinge,** and **pivot** joints. The majority of joints in the body are diarthroid: ball and socket joints are the femoral and humeral heads; hinge joints are the knee, elbow, fingers; the skull on its axis is a pivot joint. Movements in diarthroid joints are described in such terms as **flexion, extension, abduction, adduction, pronation, supination, inversion, eversion, rotation,** and **circumduction.**

Structurally, each joint consists of two molded, contoured ends of bone shaped to permit motion of one bone upon the other. The bones are connected through a sleeve of dense, collagenous connective tissue, the joint capsule. The capsule is further supported by ligaments and tendons. **Ligaments** are fibrous tissue bands that reinforce specific anatomic areas around joints to provide greater strength. **Tendons** are strong fibrous cords of connective tissue in which muscle fibers terminate. Tendons attach muscles to bones.

The **joint capsule** is a specialized connective tissue that has a collagen matrix richly supplied with blood vessels, lymphatics, nerves, and a few elastic cells. The joint capsule is lined with thin, glistening epithelium called the **synovial membrane,** which secretes a viscous synovial fluid. This fluid lubricates the joint and prevents friction.

The **hyaline articular cartilage,** which covers the ends of bones within the joint, has elastic properties that help buffer the blows and jolts to the skeleton. Articular cartilage fibrils flatten and widen when subjected to pressure, changing in size and shape, but not in volume. When the pressure is relieved, the fibrils quickly regain their high, arched, resting shape. The subchondral surface of articular cartilage is irregular and is firmly attached to the bone surface, preventing separation during ordinary function. The joint side of the articular cartilage also has a somewhat irregular surface that prevents adhesion of the two opposing surfaces and, when lubricated by synovial fluid, provides a smooth gliding surface.

Articular cartilage has no blood supply, but is nourished by synovial fluid. This cartilage is capable of anaerobic glycolysis, but its metabolic rate is about one-tenth that of soft connective tissue. When injured, cartilage has negligible ability to regenerate, but is replaced by nonelastic fibrous tissue.

In addition to the joint capsule, synovial membrane, and articular cartilage, a joint also necessarily includes the associated ligaments, muscles, and tendons that provide the stability and motion. Some diarthroid joints have an additional crescent-shaped piece of cartilage called a meniscus, interposed between the articulating ends of two bones. Examples of a meniscus are the semilunar cartilage of the knee joint and the glenoid cartilage of the shoulder joint.

The synovial fluid within a joint is maintained by two opposing factors: capillary pressure and the osmotic pressure gradient between synovial fluid and plasma. Normal joint motion also assists movement of fluid in and out of a joint. Synovial membrane has greater permeability than true membranes. Normal joint fluid is about 95% water, 1 to 2% protein, and has a relative viscosity of about 124, pH of 7.3 to 7.4, and an average specific gravity of 1.010. Normally, the nonnitrogenous substance and uric acid in synovial fluid are slightly below those of normal blood plasma. Normally, synovial fluid is clear and straw-colored [12].

Synovial fluid shows characteristic changes in many types of joint disease. It changes in appearance, viscosity, mucin clot, and cell count. Increase in protein concentration occurs in inflammatory joint diseases. Physiologic alterations result from changing permeability of synovial and capsular tissue and from intra-articular metabolism disturbances.

Trauma is one of the most common causes of joint problems. Injury to the supporting structures of joints results in swelling about the joint causing stiffness and pain. Healing is usually rapid and complete, since these supporting structures have a good blood supply. Traumatic synovitis results in changes of dynamics and metabolism. Injury to articular cartilage results in more severe changes. Osteogenic proliferation may be stimulated, resulting in bone spurs or lipping, which is probably an attempt by the body to stabilize the joint. Degenerative changes can also occur. The nature and location of trauma to a joint determine the degree of dysfunction that results.

MUSCLES

Bones and joints must be moved by muscles, which have specialized properties of **contractility, extensibility,** and **elasticity.** It is only by the use of our muscles that we are able to act on our environment, to exert forces, and to move objects and ourselves around. Muscles are the movers of the body, and their action is dependent on an intact nerve supply.

The **skeletal** or **striated muscles** number more than 400 and comprise more than 40 percent of the body weight. Skeletal muscles are also called voluntary, as they are under the conscious control of the cerebral cortex. A decision originating in the cerebral cortex travels via a peripheral motor nerve and a contraction is set in motion. A contraction involves the conversion of chemical energy to kinetic energy. The three major functions of skeletal muscle are **movement, posture,** and **heat production** [5].

Microscopically, muscle cells are thin and long, and are called muscle fibers. The cell membrane is called sarcolemma; its cytoplasm is called sarcoplasm. Muscle fibers (cells) contain a network of tubules and sacs, known as sarcoplasmic reticulum, which store calcium. Each muscle fiber contains many **myofibrils,** which in turn are made up of thousands of **myofilaments.** The myofilaments are composed of molecules of myosin, actin, and other proteins. It is these proteins that give muscle its alternating light (A) and dark (I) bands, referred to as striated [2].

A sliding action between the actin and myosin allows the segment of muscle to shorten. Current theory holds that muscle contraction is triggered by release of small amounts of calcium from the sarcoplasmic reticulum into the fluid around the myofibrils, and that as calcium is withdrawn, the muscle relaxes.

Development and maintenance of muscle bulk depend on many factors, including inheritance, and stimulation of development by motor nerves and hormones. Adequate nutrition and optimal exercise also contribute to muscle mass [13].

Each skeletal muscle has a body and two attachments. Muscle body consists of the fleshy muscle tissue. The origin is proximal and is the more stationary attachment of a muscle. The insertion is distal and is the attachment that affects movement [5].

Muscles are attached to bone in one of three ways: directly, by a tendon, or by an aponeurosis. **Direct attachment** occurs when the fibrous white connective tissue of muscle is fused with the fibrous layer of bone periosteum. A **tendon** is a band or cord of white fibrous connective tissue that connects a muscle to bone. A tendon may slide over a joint like a rope on a pulley. Some tendons are protected by a tendon synovial sheath and the presence of fluid reduces friction. An **aponeurosis** is a heavy flat sheet of fibrous connective tissue that attaches muscle to bone.

The area of contact between a nerve and a muscle fiber is the **motor end plate,** or myoneural junction. When a nerve impulse reaches the end of an axon fiber in a skeletal muscle a chemical, acetylcholine, is released. This chemical contacts the end plate and causes an action potential to spread over the sarcolemma. This results in release of calcium from the sarcoplasmic reticulum and the fiber contracts [2].

A single motor nerve plus the muscle fibers in which its axon terminates constitute a motor unit. The number of muscle fibers in a motor unit varies according to the detail, the fineness of function of that muscle. For example, the muscles that move the eye have a ratio of almost one neuron to one fiber, whereas the ratio of neuron to fiber in the biceps muscle is considerably greater (one neuron to several hundred muscle fibers).

In addition to motor nerves, muscles have a generous supply of sensory nerves that provide information to the central nervous system. Sensory nerves convey sensations of pain and position sense.

Muscles need energy to contract and do mechanical work. This energy source is **adenosine triphosphate** (ATP). Resting muscle produces more ATP than it needs. Thus, some ATP combines with creatine to form creatine phosphate. This substance acts as a reserve supply for future energy needs. Muscle also stores glycogen and is capable of anaerobic gylcolysis. Working muscle also has a considerable oxygen demand. These constant biochemical processes serve to maintain and supply body heat.

The names of muscles usually describe one or more of the following features: **action** (abductor magnus); **direction** of fibers (transversus); **location** (intercostal); **number of origins** (biceps, triceps); **shape** (trapezius); and **point of attachment** (sternocleidomastoid). Other descriptive terms of muscles relate to their function, such as flexor, extensor, abductor, adductor, rotator.

Skeletal muscle and its motor nerve, along with its associated bone and joint, can be described as the physiologic unit for movement as a neuromusculoskeletal unit. Disease or injury to any part of the unit can cause dysfunction of the total unit. Figure 10-5 illustrates anterior skeletal muscles; Figure 10-6 illustrates posterior skeletal muscles. Multiple sclerosis and cerebrovascular accident are examples of insult to the neural component. Muscular dystrophy affects the muscular component, and arthritis is an example of skeletal involvement.

Muscles atrophy when they are deprived of their nerve supply. It is felt that this atrophy is caused mainly by loss of sarcoplasmic protein and energy-producing enzymes. In myositis, muscle fibers undergo necrosis and phagocytosis, and the muscle fibers are replaced with fibrous tissue. Muscle fiber regeneration is possible, but if the destructive process outstrips regeneration, atrophy ensues. Disuse atrophy occurs when muscles are prevented from contracting because of immobilization. If prolonged, there is an increase in collagenous protein in muscle, and fibrosis ensues. Other disease states result in either hypotonic or hypertonic muscle conditions. Neuromuscular irritability is influenced by serum calcium ion concentration and by the concentration of intracellular and plasma potassium [25].

Conditions That Alter the Musculoskeletal System

Bones are particularly subject to trauma because of their active motion and relatively exposed position. The joints have frictional surfaces; thus they are subject to the forces of wear and tear. Muscles may become ineffective as a result of diseases of the nervous system, or they may atrophy with disuse and malnutrition. Primary muscle disease occurs infrequently.

Accidents and trauma are the most frequent causes of injury to the musculoskeletal system. These are classified as mechanical injury and are the result of industrial, traffic, or home accidents. The injury may result in contusions or fractures of one or more bones, or in tearing of structures closely related to bones such as joints, tendons, and ligaments.

Congenital problems are structural or chemical imperfections present at birth. One example of a hereditary defect in ossification of bone is **osteogenesis imperfecta,** a condition in which the cortex of bone remains thin and fragile, resulting in frequent fractures.

Club foot, dislocated hip, torticollis, and scoliosis are defects in normal alignment of parts of the skeleton. The suffix **melia** refers to an extremity. **Amelia** refers to absence of a limb. **Hemimelia** refers to absence of the distal half of a limb. **Apodia** means absence of a foot. **Adactylia** refers to the absence of more than one finger or toe. **Polydactylia** means the presence of extra fingers or toes. When fingers or toes are webbed or joined, the condition is termed **syndactylia.** Many of the structural deformities present at birth lend themselves to correction; however, the defects in ossification may not always respond to treatment.

Figure 10-5
The anterior skeletal muscles. Bones move at joints by the contraction and relaxation of the muscles attached to them. The **facial** muscles are involved in expression, speech, and mastication (some muscles attach skin to bones). The **pectoral** muscles enable one to adduct the arms to the side and across the chest. The **biceps** enable one to flex the elbow, and the **flexors** enable one to flex the wrist and fingers. The **intercostal** muscles link the ribs; these muscles contract and relax during respiration. The **abdominal** muscles are arranged in sheets and protect delicate abdominal organs; they also contract to compress abdominal contents and aid in micturition, defecation, and vomiting. Abdominal muscles also assist in the childbirth process.

The most powerful muscles of the body are found in the legs: the **adductors** of the thigh; the **rectus femoris,** which enables one to flex the hip joint and extend the knee; the **sartorius** muscle, which is also involved in flexing the hip joint and the knee; and the **extensors,** which enable dorsiflexion of the foot and toes.

Figure 10-6
The posterior skeletal muscles. Some muscles work together to rotate a limb or other part of the body. The muscles of the back play a large part in maintaining erect posture. The **deltoid** enables one to abduct the arm. The **triceps** enable one to extend the elbow, and the **extensors** enable one to extend the wrist and fingers. The **hamstrings** enable one to flex the knee and extend the hip joint, and the **gastrocnemius** muscle enables one to flex the knee also; the **plantar** aids in flexing the foot. The **trapezius** muscle enables one to raise the shoulders and pull the head back. The **latissimus dorsi** muscles enable one to extend the arm. The **gluteal** muscles (maximum, medius, and minimus) enable one to extend the hip joint and abduct the leg. The **plantar flexors** enable one to flex the foot and toes.

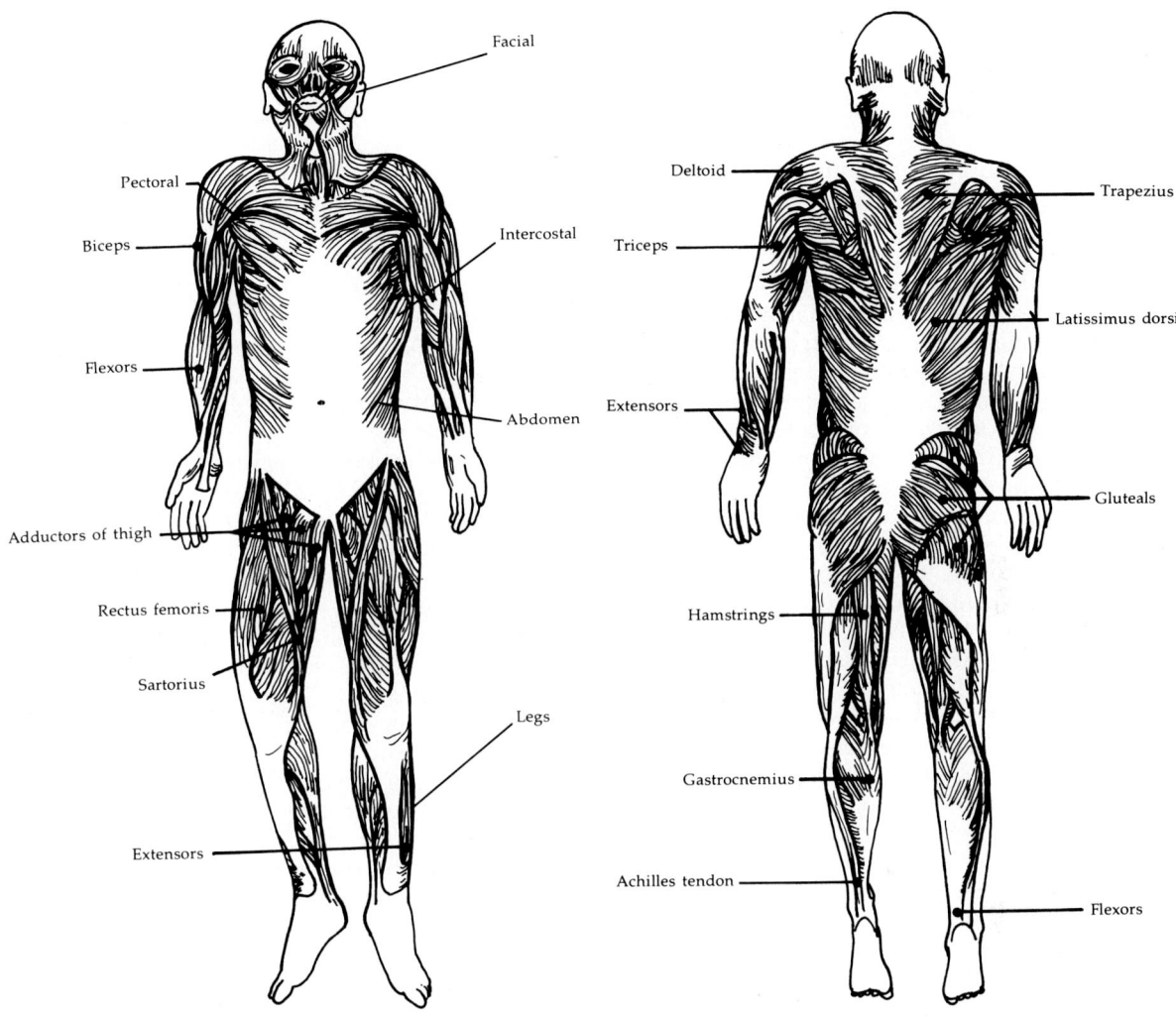

Figure 10-5

Figure 10-6

The principle of interdependence of all body parts is supported by the known fact that many generalized disease states or dysfunctions can also alter the musculoskeletal system.

Proteins, minerals, and vitamins A, C, and D are essential for normal bone and muscle growth, repair, and function. Problems can arise from inadequate intake or from faulty absorption or metabolism of these nutrients. Scurvy, rickets, and osteomalacia are considered to be related to nutritional insufficiency, although renal disease that alters calcium and phosphorus balance can also contribute to the development of rickets and osteomalacia.

Any condition that alters normal muscle tone, resulting in paralysis, affects locomotion. Cerebrovascular accidents, spinal cord injury, neurologic degenerative diseases such as parkinsonism, myasthenia gravis, and multiple sclerosis result in interrupted neural control of muscle activity. The various congenital or acquired dystrophies also interfere with musculoskeletal function.

The regulatory processes of bone—growth, mineralization, turnover, and maintenance—are influenced by metabolic processes. Hormones known to influence bone growth include the androgens, estrogens, adrenocortical hormones, thyroid and parathyroid, insulin, and growth hormone. Of all of these, it is the growth hormone of the anterior lobe of the pituitary gland that exhibits a specific effect on skeletal growth. Dwarfism, gigantism, acromegaly, and osteoporosis are classified as metabolic disorders of the skeleton.

Peripheral vascular disease is the most common factor involved in events that lead to lower extremity amputation. Ischemic vascular disease not only affects the tissues surrounding bone, but also has a physiologic effect on bone itself. The lacunae of bone become filled with minerals, the osteocytes die, and microscopically identifiable areas of necrosis are present. Impaired circulation to muscle or bone will eventually alter the conditions that provide optimum repair and function. Diminished vascular supply has been implicated as one factor leading to the development of osteoarthritis.

Abnormal proliferation of cells can be primary or metastatic, benign or malignant. Local overgrowth of bone may follow bone injury or fracture, which may not resolve for a long period of time. Of the various forms of primary malignant tumors in bone, the most important is osteogenic sarcoma, which occurs infrequently. Metastatic tumors of bone are much more common than primary malignancies, especially after middle age.

Infection in bone can result from direct implantation, from extension from an adjacent soft-tissue infection, or from hematogenous spread. Osteomyelitis (bone infection) can be acute or chronic, and is caused by such organisms as staphylococci and tubercle bacilli. Some forms of arthritis are related to the inflammatory process.

The skeletal system is resilient to mechanical forces such as a blow, twist, fall, or crush. When the external force is greater than the strength of bone and supporting structures, however, the musculoskeletal system yields in varying degrees.

A **strain** is the result of acute or chronic overstretching of muscles or tendons or use of a structure beyond its capacity to function. There usually is not a specific injury, but pain, stiffness, and swelling are present. Passive stretching of the involved muscle causes pain. Rest and application of cold relieve soft-tissue swelling. After a few days, application of heat helps promote comfort. Splinting the part, using a sling, or walking with crutches may be indicated in order to allow the damaged muscle to heal. It may require from 4 to 6 weeks for mature scar tissue to form in a damaged muscle. During the recovery period, the muscle activity in the affected part should never be increased to the point to cause symptoms. Resuming excessive activity of the affected part too soon delays recovery. Strain can also be caused by a long hike or result from strenuous physical activity undertaken by an individual who normally leads a more sedentary life. In this case, muscle joint capsule and ligament tissue tolerance are temporarily exceeded. Reduced activity and rest will reverse the symptoms.

A **sprain** results from forcible wrenching or hyperextension of a joint with injury to the ligament structures surrounding the joint. The synovial lining of the joint may also be injured with some hemorrhage into the joint (hemarthrosis). The joint is usually not rendered unstable. Any joint can be sprained, but the ankle is most commonly involved. At the ankle, the lateral ligament is attached to the tip of the fibula and the other end is attached to the astragalus bone. Forceful inversion (twisting) of the foot will tear the ligament. A sprain of the cervical vertebral joints and supporting tissues resulting from acute hyperextension and flexion is commonly called a whiplash injury.

Following sprain, the development of symptoms of pain, swelling, discoloration, and decreased motion may be delayed because it is a stable joint injury. The individual may continue to use the part. A few hours later there may be severe pain, swelling, and inability to use the part. Complete diagnosis of the extent of the injury requires taking a very careful history related to the injury, inspection, palpation, and x-ray studies.

Immediate treatment includes elevation of the part to reduce swelling, immobilization or splinting to prevent further tissue damage, and application of ice. Later treatment includes a compression dressing of Elastoplast or adhesive to provide support, elevation, and continued application of cold. The extent and duration of treatment depend on the extent of the injury. In moderate to severe injury, a cast may be applied. If ligaments have been torn, surgical repair may be indicated. Connective fibrous tissue heals by mature scar formation in 4 to 6 weeks.

A force of injury greater than that which would cause a strain or a sprain will result in a subluxation or a dislocation. A **subluxation** is an incomplete separation of the joint surface. The articulation remains in partial opposition, but the normal configuration of the joint is not maintained. A **dislocation** is a displacement or a complete separation of the articulating surfaces of the bones at the joint. There may be associated damage such as torn ligaments, rupture of muscle attachments, and ruptured blood vessels. The shoulder, elbow, hip, and fingers are the joints most commonly affected. A dislocation is usually described in terms of the direction in which the acting force displaced the distal portion of the joint. A posterior dislocation of the hip means that the head of the femur lies posterior to the acetabulum. The involved leg assumes an attitude of shortening, internal rotation, and adduction. If the internal rotation is severe, it tends to place extreme pressure on both the capsule and the arterial and venous supply to the hip. The sciatic nerve may also be injured when the hip is internally rotated.

With an anterior dislocation of the hip, the head of the femur lies anterior to the acetabulum. The involved leg is in abduction and external rotation.

A common cause of dislocated hips is a knee striking the dashboard in a motor vehicle accident. Keeping legs in extension rather than flexed at the knee while riding in an automobile will decrease the possibility of knees hitting the dashboard. Increasing numbers of motor vehicle accidents and failure to use seat belts contribute to the incidence of hip dislocations.

Pain, deformity, and loss of motion are the presenting symptoms. In order that the joint may function properly again, the dislocated portion of the joint must be relocated to its original anatomic relation with its articulating surface. The dislocation will usually cause muscle spasm in the surrounding area. Thus an anesthetic may be needed to relax the muscle sufficiently while the joint is relocated by simple manual manipulation. If soft tissue has become interposed between the dislocated parts, or if a fracture-dislocation has occurred, surgical intervention (open-reduction) will be needed to reduce the dislocation. After the bones are relocated in the joint, it is immobilized for 3 or more weeks to allow the torn ligament and capsule tissue to heal.

A **fracture** is a disruption or break in the continuity of a bone. Regardless of the size or extent of the break, all are called fractures. Depending on the force of stress or strain, there will be varying degrees of tissue disruption, disturbed blood supply, and muscle spasm. Bones will fracture as a result of **trauma,** direct force at point of contact such as occurs in accidents, violence, or falls. Another cause of fracture is indirect trauma such as stress, tension or twisting applied at a point remote from the fracture, as occurs when a tibia or fibula fractures following twisting of the foot. A violent muscle contraction can also result in fracture of underlying bone, as when an object is thrown with great force, causing the humerus to fracture. In electroshock therapy, severe muscle contraction can also result in bone fracture.

Pathologic fractures occur as a result of disease states accompanied by weakened bone.

No trauma has been involved. Severe osteoporosis or metastatic tumors may result in bone decalcification, making the individual more vulnerable to fractures.

Fractures of all types have the highest incidence in males up to age 45 and in females after age 45. Certain types of fractures are associated with certain age groups. Children have the highest incidence of fractures of the clavicle and supracondylar fractures of the humerus. Colles fractures at the wrist and fractures of the neck of the humerus are more common to females. The aged generally have the highest incidence of hip fractures and compression fractures of the vertebrae.

Signs and Symptoms of a Fracture

A fracture should be suspected if there is a history of a fall or trauma and increased complaints of localized pain and inability to use an injured part. The symptoms vary with the type of the fracture, the location, the normal function of the involved bone, and the amount of related tissue damage.

Upon examination of the patient, the presenting symptoms usually include pain at the time of injury and continuing severe pain. The periosteum of bone has a rich nerve supply; thus periostial injury occurring with the fracture results in pain. Palpation reveals acute tenderness localized at the fracture site. Loss of function is a result of the pain and muscle spasm and instability of the bone. With fractures, the muscle spasm that occurs pulls the fragments out of alignment, and may shorten the limb. This results in deformity because of the change in alignment and contour of the bone. Soft-tissue swelling also changes the contour of a limb. **Crepitus** is false motion or motion where there normally is none. It results in an audible grating sound or it can be felt as the fracture fragments rub against each other.

Ecchymosis is present if there has been subcutaneous hemorrhage. Extravasation of blood into the soft tissues around a fracture site can be considerable. A young adult can have as much as 500 to 1,000 ml of blood seepage into the thigh tissue following a fracture of the femur.

X-ray is the method of choice for diagnosis. Effective and definite treatment is usually based on accurate and precise x-ray findings. The final diagnosis of a fracture is a culmination of visual inspection, palpation, and x-ray findings. Concurrently, the injured part is inspected for any signs of circulatory or nerve impairment. Absent or diminished peripheral pulses distal to the fracture must be carefully evaluated by the nurse, as undetected arterial injury can lead to irreversible damage and eventual loss of the limb. Fractures around joints can lead to nerve damage. Nerve function is also impaired as a result of ischemia or pressure from swelling of the soft tissue.

Emergency Care

Following an accident or trauma, the individual should be examined in the position in which he or she is found. If this is not possible, he or she is moved only as much as is necessary to facilitate examination. The nurse should keep the patient at rest and promote comfort until the full extent of the injury can be determined. Improper handling or weight-bearing can cause more complications than the initial trauma, by injury to muscles, nerves, or blood supply. Inept handling can increase the deformity or convert a simple fracture to a compound fracture.

In a severe injury, the guideline usually followed is: save a life first, save a limb second. Priorities relate to the airway, breathing, and circulatory status of the injured individual. The mouth is checked for any foreign object such as gum, loose teeth, or displaced dentures. Repositioning the head may relieve an obstruction in the airway. An important exception is an individual with a suspected cervical vertebral injury who should not have the head flexed, hyperextended, or rotated. Checking the pulse and for any signs of bleeding, hemorrhage, lacerations, abrasions, or contusions reveals information essential to circulatory status. The use of a tourniquet to control bleeding is controversial, since it is often misused in the hands of inexperienced persons. When the examiner is satisfied that airway, breathing, and circulation are not impaired, attention is directed to the injury itself. If the fracture is open, it is covered with as clean a cloth as can be found. A sterile dressing is preferred as covering; however, one may not be available. If there is bleeding, a pressure dressing is applied.

The splinting of a fracture is both a method of emergency treatment and a method of definitive therapy. "A splint is a temporary nondefinitive method of immobilizing fractures so that pain is reduced, injury to soft tissue and neurovascular structures is minimized and, most important but seldom stressed, *edema is controlled and held to a minimum*" (italics ours) [1]. Basic principles of splinting are:

1. When splinting any fracture of a long bone, both the joint above and below the fracture are included in the splint if complete immobility is to be obtained.
2. The joint above and the joint below the fracture are immobilized in a position of maximum relaxation and comfort.
3. The part being splinted is amply padded to avoid pressure over bony prominences.
4. The splint is applied with sufficient overlying pressure to retard or prohibit excessive swelling in the extremity.
5. The splint and its manner of application should in no way impair the circulation in the extremity.
6. The splint is so designed and applied that it can be left on for hours or days if need be [1].

Briefly, a splint has these characteristics:
    It controls **S**welling, minimizes edema.
        Provides **P**osition that promotes relaxation of joints.
Has sufficient **L**ength to include joints above and below.
        Allows **I**ndefinite duration of use.
        Does **N**ot impair circulation.
        Has **T**hick and evenly applied padding [1].

Two general guidelines apply to the application of splint material. "When in doubt, splint" and "splint them where they lie." The goals are to reduce motion, friction, and edema. Splints properly applied minimize the amount of muscle spasm and the angulation and overriding that result from severe muscle spasm. An upper extremity can be splinted to the chest wall. The injured leg can be splinted to the uninjured leg if no other material is available. Cardboard cartons, several magazines together, a pillow, or a small piece of board could be improvised to splint the injured part. The principles of splinting are incorporated into whatever materials or method is used.

Various commercial splints are available and are readily used by rescue squads, police, and fire departments. The commercial pneumatic inflatable splint for use on extremities provides excellent support; however, it is nonporous. If left on a limb for an extended period of time, the limb may tend to become "hot" from the increased vasodilatation, causing the limb to perspire, and possibly precipitating skin breakdown.

To transport the injured individual, when possible, the stretcher is taken to the patient, rather than the patient to the stretcher. While waiting for adequate help to arrive, measures are taken to relieve anxiety and calm the individual.

On reaching the hospital or treatment center, further examination and assessment of the patient are conducted. It is essential to obtain data related to how the injury occurred: for example, was it a fall? impact? crushing? Important data include information about any preexisting diseases, such as epilepsy, cardiac disorders, diabetes, or prescription medications the person is taking. The physical examination reveals information related to the type and extent of the injury and the presence of any contaminants that might complicate or extend the injury. A skin wound may communicate directly or indirectly with the fracture. Crushing-type injuries that result in extensive soft-tissue damage are more serious than the fracture itself. There may be injuries remote from the known fracture site. Industrial accidents may involve wound contamination with strong acids or alkalis. Injuries resulting from automobile or farm accidents are often contaminated with dirt, grass, or glass.

Massive hemorrhage accompanying a fracture in an extremity constitutes a surgical emergency. In most other cases, definitive therapy follows thorough examination. Vascular or nerve impairment may accompany fractures directly involving the knee, hip, elbow, or shoulder. The physician usually manipulates the fracture to restore peripheral pulses distal to the fracture and to reduce abnormal compression or stretch on nerves. Throughout examination and treatment, the fracture should be kept splinted to prevent motion of the fracture fragments that could cause further soft-tissue injury.

The nurse in an emergency room should assess **pain, pulses, paralysis, paresthesias, and pallor.** These five "p's" are guidelines to the neurovascular status of the involved body area, and are checked every 15 minutes the first few hours after admission.

To assess pain, the nurse should check for overly constricting pressure dressings or splints that may have been applied prior to admission. Lack of splinting may lead to motion of fracture fragments causing pain. The patient should be asked to describe the pain and to help pinpoint the location of the pain. Any patient who has no relief from pain following administration of an analgesic should be closely observed. Pain associated with ischemia is not always relieved by analgesic medication.

All areas of peripheral pulses are checked on the involved extremity, especially distal to the fracture site. The pulses of the involved extremity are compared to those of the noninvolved limb.

Abnormal sensation, tingling, or numbness should be noted. The examiner can use a pointed object such as a sterile needle to check sensory changes that can occur in nerve injury or impending ischemia. The patient is asked to flex, extend, abduct, and adduct fingers and toes to detect any paralysis.

The color and temperature of the extremity are observed by the blanching test, which is done by applying pressure to the nail bed, releasing pressure, and noting the rapidity of blood return to the nail bed to determine adequate blood perfusion.

Gross inspection of the part reveals any shortening, angulation, muscle spasm, or swelling. Elevation of the part and continued splinting help reduce edema and safeguard the fracture site from undue motion.

A displaced fracture may involve damage to large blood vessels, and a hematoma may develop in the soft tissue. Blood loss may be considerable, and the vital signs should be monitored. Shock may ensue. If shock is present, medication should not be given intramuscularly, as the medication will not be absorbed from the tissue. As shock is reversed, the patient may have an overload of the medication as it is absorbed, especially if narcotics are given for relief from pain. A patient in shock frequently is very thirsty, because of fluid loss. The patient should have no oral intake if there is any possibility of shock or impending surgery.

Grossly contaminated wounds and compound fractures are examined and debrided under aseptic conditions by the physician. The patient is prepared for a surgical procedure, and tetanus prophylaxis, as well as antibiotic therapy, is usually instituted.

In summary, emergency care of an orthopedic injury is directed first to evaluation of and correction of life-threatening hemorrhage, impaired respiration, vascular or nerve impairment, and reduction of dislocation. Definitive reduction of the fracture is usually deferred until the life-threatening situations are attended to. Gentle, careful handling to promote comfort is important in the care of the injured person.

Classification of Fractures

As the diagnosis of fracture is established, the fracture is usually described in five ways regarding location, degree, communication with exterior of body described as open or closed, direction of the fracture line, and angulation or position of the bone fragments [7].

Describing the **location of the fracture** includes naming the bone that has been fractured; dividing the bone into thirds and stating which third is involved (proximal, medial, distal; or upper, middle, lower); relating the fracture to prominences or processes that serve as landmarks (trochanters, tuberosities, condyles, malleoli); indicating areas of the bone such as head, neck, shaft that may be involved; indicating if an articulating surface has been involved.

The **degree of the fracture** is indicated by stating whether it is complete, involving the entire diameter of the bone, or incomplete, in which case the diameter of the bone is partially interrupted.

Open versus closed fracture indicates if the skin overlying the fracture remains intact. A simple or closed fracture does not communicate with the external environment. Open fractures can result from severe angulation of a fracture fragment penetrating the skin from within or they can result from a penetrating wound from without, such as a bullet that breaks through the skin and bone as well. Open fractures (compound fractures) are much more likely to become contaminated and infected than are closed fractures.

Direction of the fracture line incorporates many descriptive terms. Fracture lines may be transverse, oblique, or spiral to the long axis of a bone. A transverse fracture runs in a

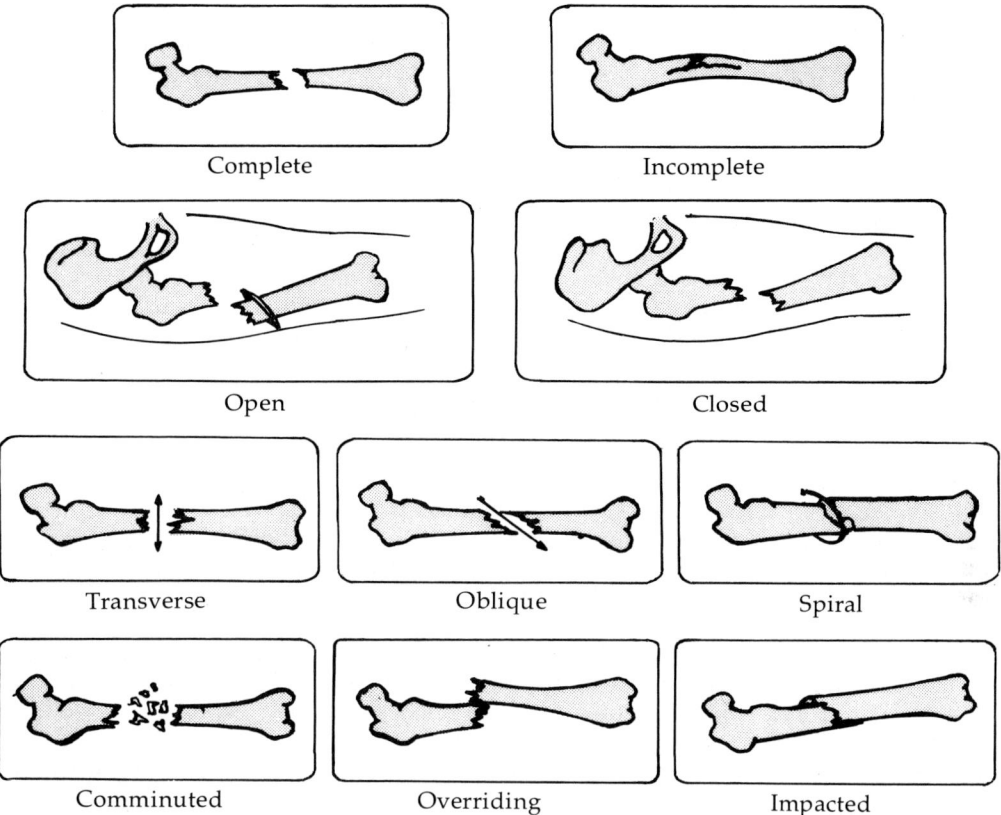

Figure 10-7
Some common types of fractures.

straight line across the bone. An oblique fracture slants at an angle across the bone. A spiral fracture encircles the bone in a slanting fashion. Spiral fractures often follow twisting types of trauma and the fracture follows the stress lines in the bone. A "greenstick" fracture disrupts the periosteum on one cortical surface and leaves the bone intact on the opposite side. These fractures are common to children whose bones are more pliable than those of adults. Some fractures may resemble a Y, T, or V; if this is the case, these letters are used to describe the direction.

The fifth aspect of classification of fractures describes the **angulation or position of the bone fragments.** A comminuted fracture is one that has more than two fragments. Overriding fragments are a result of muscle spasm or contraction that pulls the fragments over each other. A displaced fracture indicates that the fracture fragments are lateral, medial, posterior, or anterior to normal alignment. Impacted fracture indicates that the bone fragments are jammed together or into a joint space, which can result in a stable fracture. A compressed fragment is one that has been crushed or squeezed. The term **depressed fracture** usually refers to the skull in which a bone fragment is depressed below the surface. The terms **basilar, linear,** and **stellate** are also used to describe skull fractures.

Examples of this classification terminology found in patients' charts are: "Closed, complete transverse fracture of the M/3 left femur," or "Open, complete, oblique fracture of the D/3 of the right tibia and fibula," or "impacted, comminuted fracture of T/10 vertebrae." Figure 10-7 illustrates some of the common types of fractures.

Fracture Healing

Interruption in the continuity of bone, whether traumatic or surgical, is followed by a definite histologic sequence aimed at bridging the gap. Fracture healing is a unique process, as new bone is formed. Most other tissues of the body heal by scar formation. For example, following a myocardial infarct, the heart does not regenerate new myocardial muscle, but scar tissue replaces the injured area.

In a fracture, the bone is broken, soft tissues are damaged, periosteum is torn, and a hematoma surrounds the area within 24 hours. The coagulation of this blood gives rise to a loose fibrin mesh which helps seal off the fracture site and serves as the framework for ingrowth of fibroblasts and capillary buds. A reactive inflammatory process ensues and the area becomes swollen and friable. There is increased vascular congestion with the invasion of leukocytes. Phagocytosis of the debris occurs and the fibrin meshwork is then replaced by granulation tissue. Then the fibroblasts from the surrounding connective tissue, periosteum, and endosteum proliferate and invade the area. The periosteum and endosteum then stimulate osteoblast cell activity and new bone begins to replace the fibrocartilage bridge. By the end of the first week, the inflammatory process has subsided and procallus is apparent. The ground substance and matrix (osteoid) are laid down by their respective cells and then the inorganic salts are deposited. **Callus** is the name given to this newly formed bone and it is evident on x-ray as an overgrowth of bone on both the internal and external aspects of the fracture site. As the periosteum is actively building bony callus that encircles the external aspects of the fracture site, the endosteum is building callus on the marrow side of the fracture. As healing progresses, the excess bone within the marrow space as well as on the exterior aspect of the fracture is slowly remodeled. Stress or weight-bearing guides the remodeling of the bone. Eventually, the marrow cavity is rebuilt to its original size and shape, the bone marrow regrows in the space, and the exterior of the bone resumes its prefracture contour (if the bone has been kept in alignment).

The shape of the callus and the volume of tissue required to bridge the fracture depend on the amount of bone damage and displacement. The healing time is directly proportional to the total volume of damaged bone and the breadth of fracture defect. Age of the patient and site of the fracture also influence healing time. Solid callus may be present in the fracture of a child within 3 weeks; in a young adult it is 6 to 8 weeks, and 3 to 4 months in an elderly person. In general, bones of the upper extremity heal more rapidly (3 months) than a fracture of the lower extremity (6 months). Impacted fractures and spiral fractures heal more rapidly than transverse, displaced, or compound fractures.

Callus formation indicates that bony union has occurred but it is still incomplete and cannot withstand unprotected stress. This immature bone is gradually replaced by mature bone and the remodeling process is directed by muscle and weight-bearing stresses. If a fracture has been reduced to good anatomic alignment, the reduction has been retained by proper immobilization, and bone repair is uninterrupted, virtually perfect reconstruction of bone is accomplished. At some later date, the fracture line may not even be demonstrated on x-ray. Clinical union of bone follows the remodeling process and it is at this point that the bone may be used unprotected.

Blood serum levels of calcium and inorganic phosphorus are not altered during bone repair. The serum levels of the enzyme alkaline phosphatase are usually elevated secondary to new bone formation. The administration of minerals, vitamins, or hormones does not stimulate or hasten bone repair. The patient does need a good balanced diet to meet normal metabolic needs.

Fracture Complications

Perfect bone repair may be impeded or blocked by a variety of complications.

Delayed union is an arbitrary term implying that union is taking place over a longer period of time than is customary. Delayed union may proceed to complete union without active treatment [29].

In **non-union,** the reparative process ceases prior to bony union. Some factors present in non-union may be present in delayed union but to a lesser degree. Non-union of a fracture is characterized by bone deficit (lack of callus formation); false motion; sclerosing of bone ends; rounding or molding of the fracture surfaces; and sealing of the medullary canal with compact bone. Non-union requires treatment to reactivate the bone repair process. Some causes of fracture non-union include the following: soft-tissue interposition between fracture fragments, inadequate reduction, inadequate immobilization, infection secondary to compound fractures or open reduction, and extensive surgical dissection causing loss of vital soft-tissue attachments. Metallic fixation devices may cause bone necrosis and excessive traction may prohibit callus from spanning the gap. Preexisting metabolic or nutritional disturbances and inadequate circulation as a result of trauma, the immobilizing cast, or traction may also contribute to non-union. Certain bones of the body have a predilection to poor healing because of an anatomic deficit in vascular supply. These bones are the head and neck of the femur, the lower third of the tibia, the middle third of the humerus, and bones of the hand and ankle. In addition, nerve damage with resultant muscle dysfunction and post-traumatic arthritis, especially in fractures involving a joint, interfere with bone repair [33].

Non-union of fractures is usually treated with further surgical intervention to remove the cause if possible, to revitalize bone tissue, to remove necrotic bone, and to realign fragments. Inlay, onlay, and intramedullary bone grafts produce union in the majority of cases [23].

Needless to say, non-union of a fracture can be very distressing to the patient and those caring for him. Repeated surgery risks infection. Prolonged immobilization brings with it all the hazards of immobility. The psychological support of the patient is essential, as he is susceptible to periods of discouragement.

Fat embolism is another complication of crushing injuries, multiple fractures, or fractures of long bones. It is the release of fat droplets from the bone marrow into the venous-arterial channels. These fat droplets act as emboli and mechanically block pulmonary capillaries. The emboli are unique in that they become an impacted globule that conforms to the contour of the vessels in sausage-like fashion. It is possible for intact bone marrow emboli to pass through the vascular bed of the lung and cause cerebral embolization.

The mechanical obstruction of the vascular bed can result in perivascular hemorrhage and edema that can be foci of temporary metabolic changes or permanent structural damage.

In addition to causing mechanical blockage, neutral fat emboli are hydrolyzed by pulmonary lipase to free fatty acid, which disrupts alveolar capillary endothelium, producing hemorrhagic pulmonary edema. Free fatty acid is considered to be toxic to the lung. In addition, free fatty acids are thought to aggregate platelets and activate some of the clotting factors. There is much speculation about the pathophysiologic processes.

Pulmonary fat emboli occur within the first 12 to 72 hours after injury or surgery on long bones. The initial symptoms do not appear beyond 1 week after injury.

Dyspnea, tachypnea, cyanosis, and hyperpyrexia are major symptoms. A cough with foamy or blood-tinged sputum may occur. Altered states of consciousness are the most common cerebral effect of fat embolism. A classic finding in fat embolism syndrome is the appearance of petechial rash on the anterior aspects of the neck, shoulders, and chest. These petechiae are flat and do not blanch when pressure is applied to them. The presence of petechiae is not related to prognosis.

Treatment is directed to the underlying disorder and to complications. Proper management of the respiratory failure and hypoxemia is imperative. Arterial blood gases are monitored, and volume-controlled ventilators and oxygen therapy are used. Measures to clear respiratory secretions are essential. The patient is usually kept absolutely quiet; turning is not allowed.

Other supportive measures include the use of heparin for its anticoagulant effect as well as its effect in activating serum lipase to help reduce the circulating triglycerides. Intravenous glucose with alcohol may also be given for its lipolytic effect. Low-molecular-weight dextran may be used, since it decreases platelet cohesiveness. Intravenous corticosteroids are used to minimize the local inflammation and edema at the emboli site. Rapid-acting diuretics may be used if fluid overload occurs as a result of other therapy. Cardiotonic drugs and antibiotics may be needed. If there are associated thoracic injuries that cause pain with breathing, analgesics may be needed.

Nursing care is directed to ongoing assessment and observation of the presenting signs and symptoms, providing comfort measures, maintaining fluid balance, and achieving maximal respiratory function. Hypostatic pneumonia and secondary respiratory tract infection must be prevented. Allaying apprehension in both the patient and family is another important nursing function. The nurse is also involved in administration of the multiple therapies. Pulmonary fat embolism syndrome is a complication of initial trauma which is also being treated simultaneously.

Treatment of Fractures

The treatment of fractures involves four steps: recognition, reduction, retention, and rehabilitation. The objectives of treatment are to restore bone anatomically to its former length, alignment, and shape, and physiologically to restore joints, muscles, blood vessels, and nerves to their former function. The three major approaches to treatment of a fracture are closed reduction or external fixation, open reduction or internal fixation, and skin traction or skeletal traction. More than one method may be used in the treatment of the same fracture. A simple closed fracture may not need to be reduced if there is no alteration in the position, length, or alignment of the bone fragment. These fractures are immobilized by a cast or splint until healing occurs. Thus, the amount of reduction time and effort relates to the site and type of fracture, the degree of related soft-tissue damage, and the age of the patient.

CLOSED REDUCTION (EXTERNAL FIXATION)

Closed reduction is achieved by manually manipulating the fracture fragments into anatomic alignment and functional position. Three basic maneuvers are employed in the manipulation process: **traction** and associated countertraction, **angulation,** and **rotation.** Usually two sets of hands are needed to accomplish this because the proximal fragment must be stabilized by one person while the distal fragment (with muscle forces also acting on it) is manipulated into place by the second person. Following reduction, the realignment is checked by x-ray and then the part is immobilized in a cast.

Since closed reduction is usually done under general anesthesia, the patient is prepared for the anesthetic, that is, premedicated and fluid-restricted. There are many times when a true emergency exists, however. If the patient has recently eaten, gastric lavage may be necessary. The procedure is explained to the patient to allay any apprehension. If muscles are contracted during cast application, the cast does not fit snugly when the muscles relax.

A cast is a rigid dressing used to immobilize the fracture fragments and support the injured parts. Injured parts are held in the reduced position while the casting material is applied to include joints above and below the fracture. The cast then becomes a fixed type of traction adjusted to a specific distance or pull, which prevents displacement or overriding that could result from muscle spasm. A cast thus provides immobility, traction, and protection. It also allows for weight-bearing which, following Wolff's law, provides the stress needed to facilitate bone repair.

In addition to the utilization of casts to immobilize fractures, casts are also used to immobilize sprains, to support diseased joints, and to prevent or correct deformities.

Currently, two types of materials are being used as casts: plaster of Paris and plastic materials, such as Lightcast II (Table 10-1). In either case, the body part to be casted must be prepared for the cast. Tubular stockinette is applied over the skin in the correct size so there are no wrinkles in the stockinette. It is cut longer than the anticipated cast length; then, before the cast has been completed, the stockinette is turned over and incorporated into the last application of casting material to provide a smooth edge (Fig. 10-8).

All bony prominences are padded with sheet wadding or felt to protect these areas from undue pressure, which can cause ischemia. These paddings can be cut to specific sizes needed and they are applied over the stockinette. The casting material is then applied. The reduced fracture must be manually stabilized during application of the stockinette, padding, and cast. Postcast application x-rays are usually taken to assure that fracture alignment was maintained during the application of the cast.

During application of either plaster of Paris or plastic casts, only the palms of the hands are used in handling the wet casting materials. Use of fingers leaves indentations through the materials onto the skin below and can result in a pressure area under the dried cast.

The uncured Lightcast II tape and cast

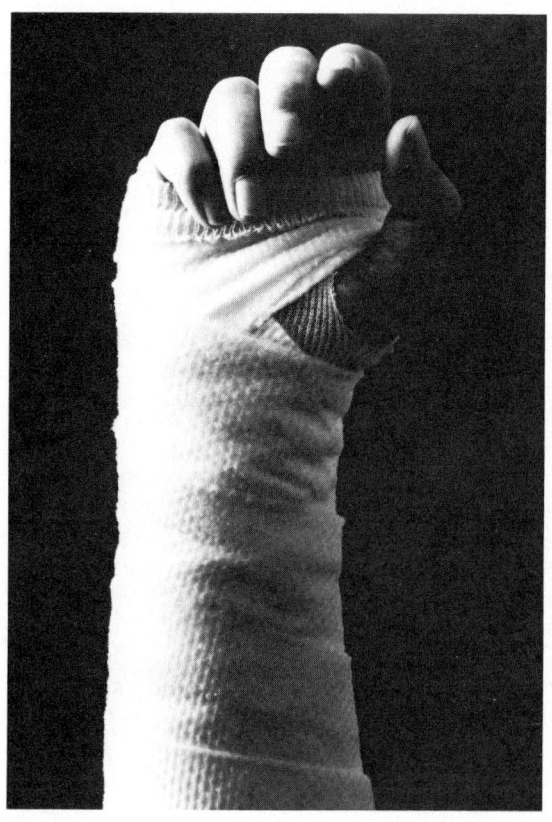 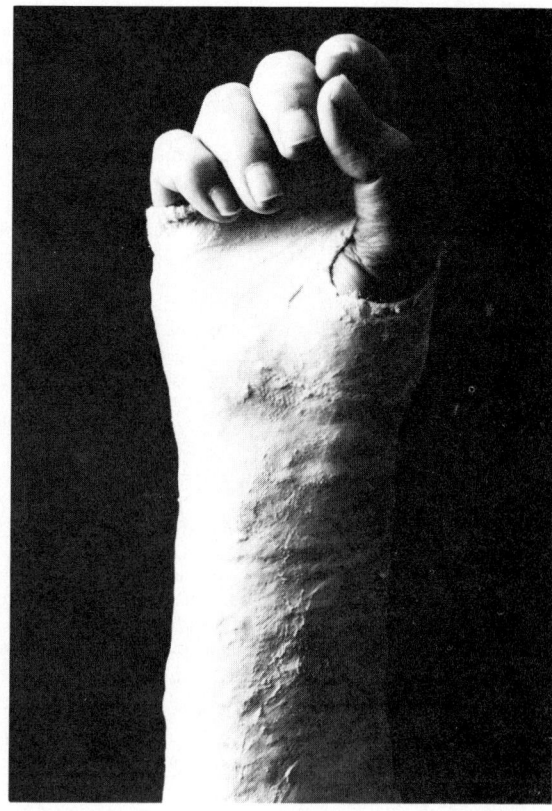

A   B

Figure 10-8
A. Tubular stockinette and sheer wadding applied to skin prior to cast application. **B.** Completed plaster of Paris cast. (Courtesy of Johnson and Johnson Company.)

burn over an open flame, but under normal circumstances the finished cast will not support combustion. It can be used in almost all types of situations that require a cast; however, if the cast will need to be changed frequently Lightcast II is not the material of choice. Lightcast II costs about twice as much as plaster of Paris. Both Lightcast II and plaster of Paris casts are removed with a cast saw, although Lightcast II requires a different type of blade.

Lightcast II does not disintegrate in water; thus a patient may have Whirlpool treatments, bathe, or shower while wearing this cast. Prolonged or too frequent wetting, however, can result in skin maceration. It takes about 3 hours for the stockinette and padding to dry. It is recommended that all excess water be removed by wrapping the cast in a towel and using a blower-type hair dryer to hasten drying. The wet cast gives the sensation of being in wet clothes until the stockinette and padding dry. Lightcast II is a very hard material when cured; it can scratch furniture if the casted part rests on a table or chair; however, rough edges can be smoothed with sandpaper or an emery board. The lightness, strength, and immersibility of Lightcast II impose fewer restrictions on the patients' activities than does a plaster cast, but immersibility of the cast is not an essential for most patients. No activity should be undertaken that will disrupt the fracture alignment or the integrity of the cast.

Plaster of Paris is still the most widely used cast when frequent cast changes are required. Cost and personal preference of the orthopedic surgeon may be other factors in the

Table 10-1
Comparison of the two types of casting material

Plaster of Paris	Lightcast II
Composition	
Crinoline impregnated with gypsum-dehydrated calcium sulfate dihydrate	Open-weave fiberglass tape impregnated with a photosensitive resin
Preparation	
Available in various size rolls that are dipped in water; the solid state returns to a fluid state to facilitate application	The soft, pliable tape in various sizes, prepackaged in airtight wrappers, ready for application
Stockinette and Padding	
Cotton stockinette and sheet wadding or felt	Stockinette and Web Wrap made of polypropylene that sheds water; dries in 2 to 3 hours
Application	
Moistened roll of plaster is unrolled onto the body surface without lifting it off the surface; it must not be pulled as it could become too constricting; molding and shaping to contours during application	Same technique in application of the Lightcast II (tape as is used in the application of the moistened plaster of Paris rolls)
Drying	
Plaster of Paris sets in about 8 minutes; 24 hours to dry depending on size and thickness of cast; recrystallization involves an exothermic reaction–gives off heat; weight-bearing in 48 hours; chemical reaction is reversible; cannot get it wet	Lightcast II tape is cured in about 3 minutes in a Lightcast II–controlled, near-ultraviolet lamp; the cast can be worked and shaped in the lamp for 10 seconds; when cured, immediate weight-bearing
Finished Cast	
Chemical reaction is reversible; cannot get it wet. Dried cast is white, shiny, hard, and radiolucent	Thin, porous open-weave; immersible, patient can bathe, shower; whirlpool; cast is radiolucent
Odor	
Plaster, until it is dry	Medicinal, until it is cured
Weight	
Arm cast about 3 to 4 lb	Arm cast about 17 oz

selection of plaster of Paris. When the plaster bandage is applied, it must be completely saturated to ensure that all the plaster of Paris undergoes the chemical change. The roll of plaster must be placed in water with one end up so that free air between the layers of the bandage rise to the surface and water can contact all areas of the plaster. When air bubbles stop rising to the surface, the roll is saturated. Excess water is then squeezed from the bandage prior to its application. Water temperature of about 65 to 75° F; 18 to 29° C is recommended because warmer water along with the exothermic heat given off may add to patient discomfort. Cold water causes plaster to set too slowly.

Types of Casts

There are numerous types of casts. Some of the more frequently used for the treatment of fractures are described. Casts to the upper extremity can be short-arm, long-arm, or hanging-arm. A **short-arm cast** completely covers the forearm, except the fingers and thumb, but does not restrict elbow joint motion. A **long-arm cast** extends from just below the axilla to include the palm and dorsum of the hand in either pronation or supination. The elbow, when included in a cast, is flexed at 90 degrees, since this is the most functional position. Finger, thumb, and shoulder motion are free. A **hanging-arm cast** is similar to a long-arm cast; however, its purpose is to provide traction to a proximal fracture of the humerus. The positioning of a neck sling attached to the cast provides the traction, as the shoulder joint is not immobilized. A patient with a hanging-arm cast must remain erect or semi-erect at all times, even when sleeping. The patient's head should be elevated to at least 45 degrees or higher during sleep.

Lower-extremity casts can be short-leg or long-leg and weight-bearing or nonweight-bearing. A **weight-bearing cast** has a walking heel incorporated into the cast. In application of a long-leg cast, the knee is usually flexed 15 to 20 degrees to provide relaxation of the ligaments that join the femur to the tibia. In either **long- or short-leg casts,** the toes remain exposed. Fractures of the foot, ankle, tibia, fibula, knee, and distal femur may be treated with either long- or short-leg casts, depending on the location and severity of the fracture. Fractures of the middle or proximal femur and fractures about the hip are usually not casted, as the immobilization would be of considerable duration.

Fractures of the cervical, thoracic, and lumbar spine can be treated with a body cast. A Minerva jacket is an ambulatory plaster cast that extends above the torso to include the neck and head and is used for cervical fractures. Shoulders and arms are free. A body jacket cast is utilized for immobilizing fractures of the thoracic or lumbar vertebrae.

A spica cast immobilizes an extremity to the torso. A shoulder spica cast includes a long-arm cast and body jacket, applied as a unit. The shoulder, arm, and elbow are immobilized. A hip spica immobilizes one leg and the hip joint. Spica casts can be unilateral or bilateral and are more commonly used in children than in adults. Bilateral hip spica casts often incorporate a crossbar in the cast between the legs, usually below the knee. The crossbar adds strength and helps to maintain abduction of the legs as well. This crossbar must never be used as a handle in moving or positioning the patient.

Nursing Care of a Hospitalized Patient in a Cast

In addition to assisting the patient in the emotional adjustment to injury, nursing care is directed to care of the skin, observation of circulatory and neural status, maintaining the integrity of the cast, position changes, and patient instruction regarding cast care.

Immediate care after a cast has been applied begins with preparation of the bed. A firm mattress or bed boards should be on the bed. Plastic-covered pillows should be ready to support the wet cast. This applies most of all to plaster of Paris casts, which require up to 24 hours or longer to dry, depending on the extent and thickness of the cast. A wet cast should never be left to rest on a hard flat surface. As the cast dries, it flattens and causes pressure on underlying tissue. The flattened cast can bend and crack. An air-pressure mattress on the bed may be helpful for the patient's total care as well as for supporting the cast appropriately. Supporting the wet cast on pillows serves a twofold purpose. The cast is supported in a manner to maintain its cylindrical shape, and elevation of the part serves to decrease edema and venous stasis.

Ice bags may be ordered for application to the elevated casted part. Cold serves to decrease edema and helps to diminish pain. Cold application has a local anesthetic effect.

As with Lightcast II, in handling a wet cast, only the palms of the hand should be used, rather than the fingers. Maximum cast strength requires that the water evaporate. In plaster of Paris casts, this chemical process is the recrystalization of gypsum; heat is produced in the recrystalization. Therefore the thicker the cast, the higher the temperature. The most effective way to reduce the temperature is to increase the circulation of air, which will hasten evaporation of water. This can be done with an ordinary circulating fan. The cast should be exposed to air; to cover it with blankets further insulates it. The use of heat lamps to hasten cast-drying only adds to the increased temperature; skin beneath the cast can be burned with careless use of heat lamps. Normally a cast cools in 15 to 30 minutes.

The patient is turned every few hours to allow the cast to dry on all sides. For the patient's comfort, plaster on the skin can easily be removed with a moist cloth. If the cast edges have not been finished by incorporating the stockinette into the last application of casting material they may be finished by applying petals of adhesive tape close together to cover the entire cast edge. All rough edges and irregularities of plaster are covered to avoid irritation to adjacent skin surfaces. Special measures are taken with spica-type casts of the lower extremity to protect the cast from urine and feces around the perineal area. Waterproof material can be tucked up under the cast at the buttocks, brought out over the cast, and taped to the cast. This material can be changed periodically. It is well to use a small-fracture bedpan for patients with lower body casts as a large bedpan can crack the cast when supporting the patient's weight and the buttocks.

A completely dry cast should be white, shiny, odorless, hard, firm, and resonant when tapped. Every effort should be made to keep the cast from becoming soiled, as washing off soil will lead to disintegration of the plaster.

In the immediate hours following cast application, the nurse must periodically assess the effects of the cast on the patient. The newer the cast, the more frequently the assessment must be done. Multisensory observation is an important function of the nurse; this means using the eyes to look, the nose to smell, the fingers to touch, the ears to listen, the mouth to question, and the hands to record the data. Instruction is begun immediately by informing the patient about the importance of reporting any unremitting pain or swelling. The involved extremity is compared with the noninvolved extremity.

Pain During the period of time immediately following the application of the cast, the patient may be concerned about the heat of the cast, and should be reassured that this is normal and will pass. Mild swelling of exposed fingers and toes is also an expected occurrence. Increasing edema may cause pain resulting from pressure. The exact location of the pain is determined by listening to the patient's description. Pain at the site of the fracture is probably a result of trauma. Pain remote from the injury may be a result of pressure over bony prominences under the cast. Pressure may be a result of insufficient padding or improper handling during cast application. The nurse must act promptly to relieve the pain according to the cause. The patient will stop complaining because the skin sensitivity diminishes within 12 to 24 hours. Without appropriate care tissue necrosis may occur: necrotic tissue has no sensation.

Circulatory impairment Very disruptive fractures, treatment by open reduction, and casts that maintain a limb in acute flexion may be more predisposing to vascular impairment than other types of injuries or casts. Arterial supply may be compromised as a result of the injury or surgery. Signs of arterial obstruction are pallor or blanching, numbness, coldness, and pain. Venous impairment usually results from mechanical constriction of soft tissue by the cast or from excessive swelling. The usual signs of venous impairment are cyanosis, warmth, edema, and pain. Three main factors in recognition that vascular impairment is in progress are that the patient's complaint of pain is out of proportion to that expected as normal for the type of fracture or surgical procedure; the pain is not relieved by narcotics; and it is excruciating on motion of the fingers or toes. This pain is caused by muscle ischemia. Irreversible muscle damage can occur within 4 hours. A cast can be applied a second time, when necessary, whereas, unrecognized and untreated vascular impairment leaves permanent disability in the affected part. The cast must be bivalved (split) or removed, and it may be necessary to explore the vascular supply surgically. Bivalving a cast at particular points does not alter its effectiveness in maintaining fracture alignment. Peripheral pulses may be unequal, but still present in vascular impairment; therefore, relying on the peripheral pulses for detection of vascular impairment can be misleading.

Nerve impairment Diminished sensation and sensations involving motion, tingling, or numbness of fingers and toes may be caused by edema or a poorly fitted or poorly padded cast. The patient should be asked to wiggle fingers or toes. Any inability of the patient to move previously functioning fingers and toes or to feel sensations from fingers or toes is indicative of decreased sensation. It is advisable to remove any rings from fingers prior to cast application. Swelling of a casted extremity is commonly relieved by elevation of the part, application of ice, and isometric exercises.

Odor Odor emitting from a cast can have several possible causes. It may indicate necrotic tissue, drainage from the underlying incision if the cast was applied following open reduction, or infection. Odor caused by infection has a "musty" character. Any drainage on a cast should be noted and accurately described. It is important to inspect the underside of the cast also, since drainage tends to follow gravitational flow. The site of the drainage can be circled on the cast with a pencil or pen, thus noting increase over a period of hours. In order to prevent the patient from becoming overly apprehensive, the nurse should explain that following open reduction with cast application, both the drainage and the nurse's act of circling the drainage site on the cast are routine.

The importance of astute, careful assessment of a casted body part cannot be overemphasized. It is equally important to record the detailed observations carefully. Legal literature is documented with cases where casted patients' complaints went unheeded and unnecessary disability resulted.

Skin care All the visible skin in areas which are adjacent to the cast is inspected on a daily basis for signs of irritation or abrasion. The nurse should explore under the cast as far as it is possible to reach using fingers moistened with alcohol which aids in toughening the skin and is drying as well. When cast edge covering becomes frayed or does not remain intact, it is repetaled.

Patient Teaching

The outpatient who has a cast is instructed to keep the cast uncovered until it is dry and should also be informed about how to support the cast properly. A casted leg is elevated when the patient is sitting, to minimize soft-tissue swelling. An arm cast can be supported on pillows when the patient is lying down. To relieve edema, the casted extremity is positioned so that it is even with or higher than the heart. Application of ice bags may be ordered. When the patient is ambulatory, a sling is worn to support an arm cast and crutches are used to prevent undue weight-bearing on a leg cast.

The patient is also instructed that some swelling will occur, but if swelling is excessive or if there is any pain, the physician should be notified. Any drainage on the cast or elevation in body temperature is also reported. The patient should know how to check for color, warmth, motion, and sensation. The cast should be protected, which means it should not be used as a weapon or to hit and kick objects. A plaster of Paris cast must be kept clean and dry. In some cases, several weeks postapplication, a short-arm cast may be tightly covered with a plastic bag and the patient allowed a short shower or tub bath. With more extensive casts or any lower-extremity cast, the patient is advised to sponge-bathe only. With the Lightcast II materials, a shower or tub bath is permissible, if the activity is permitted by the physician.

The patient is instructed in how to care for the exposed fingers or toes. These should not be neglected. Cotton applicators moistened with alcohol can be used to reach under cast edges, but under no circumstances should any objects such as a wire coat hanger, a toothbrush, or a table knife be used to scratch under a cast. Skin under a cast is tender and easily abraded. Also, objects can be lost inside a cast, with resultant abrasion and irritation more severe than the initial itching.

The patient is also instructed in the method of doing isometric exercises with the casted part and to do active range of motion with joints not enclosed in the cast. When the patient is ambulatory, all other joints of the body should be receiving adequate exercise; if not, an exercise program should be started. Neither an outpatient nor a hospitalized patient should be discharged without proper instruction and practice in the use of crutches, if they are to be used at home.

It is very helpful if written instructions are prepared and available to all discharged patients who have a cast. Verbal instruction and guidelines can be misunderstood or easily forgotten in the confusion of the cast application.

Cast Removal

The decision to remove a cast is made when x-ray evidence reveals adequate callus formation and good functional alignment. The rate of fracture repair is altered by age, site, and extent of the fracture. The cast may be removed and reapplied when it becomes too loose or a surgical incision beneath the cast needs inspection. Casts applied to correct deformities are usually changed at periodic intervals.

Casts are removed by means of a cast-cutter, an electric saw with a circular oscillating blade. The subcast padding and stockinette protect the skin during cast-cutting, and an experienced person can "feel" when the cast is cut through. Once the cast is cut, a cast spreader is employed to pry the cast apart and away from the limb or torso. The patient should be prepared for the experience in that the cast-cutter is noisy (like a vacuum cleaner), it makes dust, and the blade has dull teeth [29]. Most patients fear the blade will cut the skin.

Once the cast is removed, the limb feels light and unstable. There should be a gradual return to function and use. Excessive stretching, forced movements, and weight-bearing may result in further limitations of motion. A stiff joint should never be passively forced. Voluntary muscular contraction gradually stretches stiff joints; thus joint rehabilitation is best achieved with active motion.

Support is continued as directed with a sling, elastic bandages, and/or crutches. Elevating the uncasted limb reduces swelling. Graduated exercises and hydrotherapy may be ordered.

The skin under a cast is covered with exudate and crusty material that is best removed by oil or lotion. Excessive rubbing and soaking in water is to be avoided, as the skin is tender. Normal texture returns as the skin becomes accustomed to air and use.

OPEN REDUCTION (INTERNAL FIXATION)

Another approach to fracture treatment is open reduction with internal fixation. With the patient anesthetized, a surgical incision is made through the skin and soft tissue, and the muscle is spread to expose the fracture fragments. Under direct visualization, the fracture fragments are realigned and immobilized with a metallic device. While the metallic device is being attached to or inserted into the bone, the fracture fragments are held in alignment by manual traction. With the exception of prosthetic implants, metal devices are intended solely for use as internal splints to hold fractured bones in alignment during the normal healing process. Open reduction does not accelerate fracture-healing.

The type and location of the fracture dictate the type of metallic device that is used. A metal pin, nail, or rod may be driven into the medullary canal of the shaft of a long bone that has been fractured. This type of fracture can also be immobilized by fastening a metal plate to the surface of the bone with screws. Comminuted fractures can be immobilized by encircling the bone with heavy-gauge wire or a metal Parham band. The metallic devices used are nontoxic, inert, nonpyrogenic, nonporous, and nondegradable in the body. Vitallium (a cobalt-chromium alloy) and stainless steel are the two metals most commonly used. To avoid metal reactions, all parts of the metallic device must be of the same material; however, in joint arthroplasty, metals and plastics are combined in the prosthetic devices. This combination has lubrication advantages, a lower coefficient of friction, and, therefore, a slower wear rate. More than one type of metallic device can be applied to the same fracture. The periosteum is removed from the bone prior to the attachment of the metallic device. Since periosteum is rich in nerves, its removal reduces postoperative pain.

Metal devices are also used in bone reconstructive surgery and to correct deformities. The advantages of internal fixation are that the alignment is visualized, there is metallic immobilization, and early weight-bearing and mobility are promoted. The fracture does require some external support and protection until bone union is apparent and depending on the bone affected, casts, splints, a sling, or crutches are used for a period of time following the surgery.

The principle that bones respond to stress by becoming thicker and stronger is the underlying rationale for using a compression plate for internal fixation. With compression plate fixation, first the plate is securely attached to one fracture fragment with screws; second, a compression clamp is fixed to the plate on the opposite fragment; third, the clamp is closed or tightened, drawing the fragments together in a manner that impacts the fragments against one another. The plate is then fixed to the clamp side of the fracture, the clamp is removed, and the incision closed. Compression fixation adds stress and fosters the fracture-healing [27].

The two greatest hazards of open reduction are infection and delayed union. An open or compound fracture, whether a result of trauma or surgical reduction of a closed fracture, is potentially contaminated, but not necessarily infected. During the open-reduction procedure, the probing, debridement, and manipulation of tissue do disrupt the hematoma and can delay the development of callus. Additional trauma to soft tissue, nerves, and blood supply may also occur.

Open reduction is done when there is a compound fracture, when soft tissue is interposed between the fragments, when there is evidence of nerve and circulatory impairment, and when closed reduction has been unsuccessful. Internal fixation may be preceded by a period of skin or skeletal traction to reduce muscle spasm or severe angulation of fracture fragments. Internal fixation can be difficult in a comminuted fracture in which there are too many pieces of bone to be held together by the metallic device. It is desirable to leave all bone fragments in place, as they do stimulate new bone growth. Another difficulty with internal fixation occurs in the elderly who have osteoporosis. The bone may be too porous to hold the implanted metallic parts.

When a compound fracture occurs, especially of a long bone, it is generally felt that the incidence of fat emboli is reduced if the fracture is fixed internally within 6 hours after injury. This time span relates to less fluid loss from the wound. Any fracture with accompanying evidence of vascular or nerve impairment needs early surgical attention, as irreversible damage occurs within 4 to 6 hours in ischemic muscle [7, 21, 31].

Open reduction is not always the treatment method of choice, however. Some orthopedic surgeons feel that closed fractures should be left closed and contaminated open fractures should be left open.

Since open reduction is not without risks and repeated attempts at reduction and retention of a fracture are not advisable, the physician may decide to allow healing of a fracture that is not in perfect alignment. Minor angulation or shortening can result in a good functional extremity [29].

One of the classic examples of opening a closed fracture is the common and accepted practice of internal fixation for hip fracture. Orthopedic literature documents the benefits of this approach to treatment of hip fractures in the elderly. The primary rationale is that it affords early mobility, thus curtailing the development of all the hazards of immobility, and thereby reducing the mortality rate.

Open reduction is also done even when other methods of treatment would give satisfactory results, because internal metallic immobilization achieves early mobility, allows joints to remain active, and reduces hospital stay. Closed fractures at certain anatomic sites of the body are almost always treated with open reduction and internal fixation. These are fractures of the shaft, head, and neck of the femur; any intra-articular fracture; fractures of both bones of the forearm in an adult; and a fracture of the lateral condyle of the humerus in a child. As a rule, open reduction is not commonly used in children, because the epiphyses are open and there is a great potential for remodeling of bone structure following a fracture. In addition, hardware introduced into open epiphyses can make this bone vulnerable to infection.

There is always special concern when a fracture involves a joint. The ankle, knee, hip, elbow, and shoulder need to be kept active, and it is generally felt that if these joints are immobilized for more than 4 weeks, stiffness results. Blood in the joint provokes the formation of granulation tissue which can progress to a scar. These intra-articular adhesions plus contracture of the joint capsule often result in severe limitations of motion. Early active exercises to these joints are needed to improve the functional outcome. Internal fixation of fractures near or in a joint allows for more joint motion than retention of the fracture with a cast [27].

In an open fracture associated with massive trauma, the care of the fracture becomes secondary to the care of soft tissue. The healing of the fracture is dependent on the uncomplicated healing of surrounding tissues. Reduction, retention, and internal immobilization of the fracture are achieved along with exposure, inspection, and debridement of the wound. Any exposed fracture progresses to healing if circulation at the fracture site is good and the surrounding tissue is not infected. There must be some means of establishing drainage of the wound so that exudates and cellular debris can exit from the area. The wound heals with closure by secondary intention.

With this open treatment of compound fractures, the extremity may be placed either in traction or in a closed plaster cast that is changed every 2 to 3 weeks. Pins and wires used to stabilize the fracture are incorporated into the cast. Casts are applied if early ambulation is desired. With balanced suspension traction, joints can be kept active, but the person is confined to bed while the traction is in place.

Nursing Care in Open Reduction

Since open reduction involves a surgical procedure, usually with general anesthesia, the patient is prepared as for any surgical procedure; however, orthopedic surgery requires special preoperative skin preparation to curtail the incidence of infection. The patient may need to be assured that no probing or manipulation occurs until he or she is asleep.

The exposed bone, torn tissue, and abnormal angulation may be readily visible. Usually the wound is covered with a sterile dressing. Some patients request to see the wound; others do not want to view it, and they should not be forced to look at it. The patient may frequently ask, "Will I ever be the same again?" This may be an expression of concern about body image, because the patient's intact body has been disrupted. Every effort should be made to answer questions honestly, to keep the patient informed of the treatment plan and to keep the patient as comfortable as possible.

Open reduction may be emergency surgery and if the patient has had a full meal prior to injury, gastric lavage may be done, leaving the nasogastric tube in place during the surgery. Pain diminishes peristalsis, so to delay surgery for 4 to 6 hours does not result in an empty stomach. It is better practice to institute gastric lavage so that aspiration of food does not occur during the anesthetic. If surgery is not emergency, preoperative enemas may be ordered. These special procedures must be carried out with very careful handling of the injured part.

For medicolegal reasons, the wound may be photographed prior to, during, and after surgery; the patient must sign a consent form. Preoperative and postoperative photographs and x-rays serve as evidence in legal proceedings, especially in industrial accidents, or in decisions about compensation for lost work time.

Postoperatively the nursing care is the same as for any postoperative patient generally: assessment and relief of pain, adequate intake of fluids and food, elimination, coughing and deep breathing, and position changes to relieve stasis and pressure. The incision and dressing need to be assessed for drainage. A Hemovac-type drain may be in the incision. Therefore the type, amount, and other characteristics of the drainage need to be carefully observed. If a cast covers the surgical incision, the cast must be observed for drainage and any unusual odors. Nursing measures related to the care of a cast are the same as discussed previously. Support and elevation of the involved extremity are essential. There may be special orders related to position as well as to when to begin mobilizing the patient. Range of motion exercises to noninvolved parts can be started soon after surgery, with the patient progressing to independence in active range of motion in noninvolved joint areas. Physical therapists are often involved in the mobilization of the patient. It is then important that the nurse follow through and reinforce the efforts of physical therapy. At every step along the way to recovery, the patient's independence in self-care must be fostered.

Either skin or skeletal traction may also be used temporarily during the postoperative course following open reduction. Traction immobilizes the patient to a greater extent, and special nursing concerns are close observation for signs and symptoms related to pressure and stasis, as well as nursing measures to relieve sensory deprivation. The integrity of the traction must also be maintained so that the reduced fracture is retained in the desired position. Nursing care of the patient in traction is discussed in detail under the section on traction later in this chapter.

Open reduction almost always includes a course of prophylactic antibiotics given intravenously, intramuscularly or orally. It is common practice to use antibiotic solutions to irrigate the wound during the surgical open reduction procedure.

Hip Fracture

Hip fracture seldom occurs in the young. The incidence of hip fracture increases after age 60, the average age being 70, and is more common in females than males. The fracture is infrequently associated with severe trauma or an accident. More commonly, the elderly person, in the normal course of daily activities, may turn or twist his or her body, the bone breaks, and the patient falls. In the aged the strength of the bone decreases because of the osteoporotic and degenerative changes, and is no longer able to resist normal stresses. Other predisposing factors are the physiologic changes in balance and perception that occur with age [9].

Fractures involving the hip can be one of two types: (1) intracapsular, which involves the head and neck of the femur, and (2) extracapsular, which involves the trochanteric areas of the femur. These are trochanteric or intratrochanteric fractures occurring at the base of the neck through the trochanter of the proximal femur (Figs. 10-9; 10-10). Characteristically the leg assumes a postinjury position

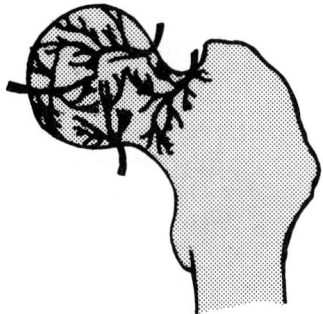

Blood supply to head of femur

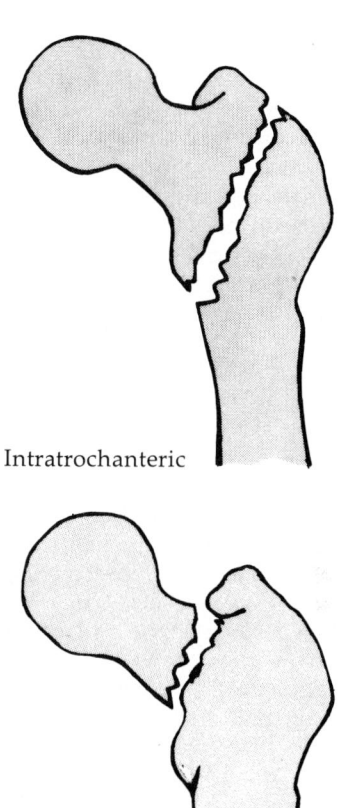

Intratrochanteric

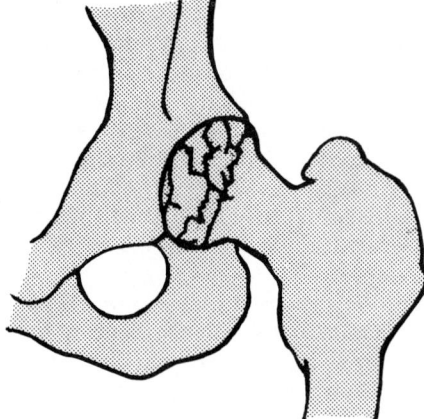

Intracapsular fracture of head of femur

Figure 10-9
Disruption of blood supply to head of femur with intracapsular fracture.

Base of neck

Figure 10-10
Extracapsular fractures.

of outward rotation because of the pull of the gluteus maximus muscle; the angle of the femoral neck is then decreased and the limb is shortened. The strong gluteus medius muscle pulls the distal portion of the fracture upward. There is associated pain and muscle spasm [9].

The hip, being a ball and socket joint, has a joint capsule that extends out along the neck to allow free range of motion. Blood vessels enter the head of the femur outside the point of attachment of the joint capsule. Most of the blood supply to the head of the femur enters the bone through the nutrient foramina at areas about the neck and travels to the femoral head inside the bone, and there is little or no blood supply to the femoral head and acetabulum from the ligaments in the area. Thus, fractures of the femoral head and neck easily disrupt the blood supply, which accounts for the number of persons who have non-union of these fractures even when perfect reduction has been achieved.

Following hip fracture, blood may accumulate in the area causing intracapsular pressure, which further compromises the blood supply. Some orthopedic surgeons routinely aspirate the hip as soon as possible after the admission of the patient with an intracapsular or extracapsular fracture. Aspiration of the hip to remove accumulating blood, along with definitive early internal fixation, is felt to decrease the possibility for development of avascular necrosis.

If the hip fracture is accompanied by severe muscle spasm and angulation of the fracture fragments, skin traction may be applied for a few days prior to surgery to reduce the abduction and muscle spasm. This traction is usually in the form of Buck's extension or Russell's skin traction with 5 to 10 pounds of weight. The amount of weight used is determined by the patient's general physical condition, size, and condition of the skin.

The prevailing approach to treatment of hip fracture is open reduction and internal fixation using metallic devices. Some of the metallic devices are Jewett nails, Austin Moore pins, Neufeld angled nails, Smith-Petersen nail with a McLaughlin attachment, Massie sliding nail, Ken nails, and Richard's compression plate or pin (Fig. 10-11).

Early mobilization and decreased mortality are the two major advantages of internal fixation of the hip. Closed reduction of a hip fracture utilizing a hip spica cast or some type of traction requires many weeks in bed. A hip spica cast includes both hip joints and the knee on the involved side. Thus, there is no motion of the hip and one knee joint. The elderly, with reduced circulation and other health problems, cannot tolerate these long periods of immobility.

The internal fixation device is always placed in bone using serial x-rays as a guide to placement throughout the surgical procedure. In this way, position of the reduced fracture can be checked prior to wound closure. Currently, compression plates and nails are becoming widely used for fractures of the head and neck of the femur. With compressing devices, the fracture fragments are impacted against one another, giving sufficient fixation to allow for immediate partial weight-bearing and ambulation. The fracture is overreduced from the anteroposterior view. These surgically impacted fractures enhance healing, as the added stress and muscle action facilitate better circulation to the fracture site; early ambulation also helps combat postoperative depression, thrombophlebitis, and pulmonary emboli. If the fracture is not impacted surgically, the impaction occurs within 3 to 4 months after surgery [9].

The surgically impacted hip fracture shows complete union in 5 to 8 months. When impaction is allowed to occur naturally, full weight-bearing is delayed for 3 to 5 months or until there is x-ray evidence of bone union. If, at the time of surgery, there is evidence of vascular insufficiency in the area of the fracture, bone graft can be used along with the metallic device.

Following the impacted technique, the patient begins partial weight-bearing aided by a walker or crutches by the first or second postoperative day. With the nonimpacted surgical technique, the patient is first allowed in the wheelchair, followed by a slower progression to walker and crutches.

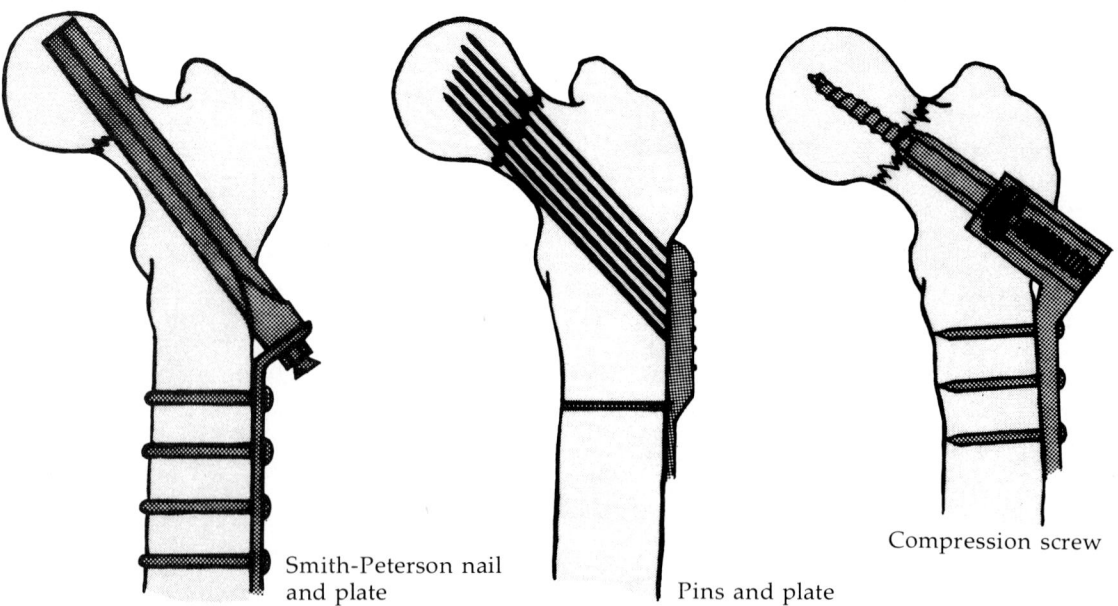

Figure 10-11
Metallic devices used in treatment of hip fractures.

Preoperative nursing care in hip fracture Because the patient with a hip fracture is usually elderly, he or she may be in poor physical condition and have coexisting chronic cardiac, vascular, renal, or respiratory disease or diabetes. These health problems increase the risk of surgery to the patient, and they must be treated so that the person is stabilized prior to the surgical intervention. Careful monitoring in the intraoperative and postoperative course is essential.

Patients with a hip fracture have pain both from the fracture itself and from the muscle spasm. The preoperative use of skin traction adds to the comfort of the patient, since it reduces muscle spasm. Any unnecessary movement is avoided, and manual traction is applied to the fractured limb when the patient moves, if skin traction is not used. Diagnostic x-rays are usually taken at the bedside, rather than moving the patient to the x-ray department.

The patient's pain is carefully assessed. Nursing measures useful for the relief of pain include maintaining good body alignment, giving backrubs, changing the patient's position, and providing individualized comfort measures. These measures are done before resorting to frequent administration of narcotics and barbiturates, which are physiologically depressing drugs in the elderly patient. These drugs may also be contraindicated if the patient has chronic respiratory dysfunction. Nonnarcotic analgesics such as propoxyphene hydrochloride (Darvon) and acetaminophen (Tylenol) can be very effective in the relief of pain. A firm mattress on the bed helps to splint the fracture, and the use of an alternating air-pressure mattress or synthetic sheepskin is helpful in relieving pressure on the body.

The patient's position is changed every 2 hours and requires two or more persons for proper management. The use of a turning sheet under the patient facilitates position changes. One person should stand on the side to which the patient is to be turned. Pillows are placed between the patient's leg from groin to ankle. One person places one hand on the patient's shoulder, the other on the patient's hip, and gently rolls the patient to his or her side. Prior to turning, the patient may need to be moved to the side of the bed away from the side to which he is to be turned. Thus, upon completion of the turning, the patient is centered on the bed and is not lying too close to the edge of the mattress. Another person must always support the affected leg. When turning the patient to the uninvolved side, it is possible to position him or her more fully on the side. The affected leg is supported at body level with pillows. The back is also supported by pillows. When turning to the fractured hip side, a partial turn of only 45 degrees may be possible. The mattress helps to splint the fracture, but placing full body weight on that hip may be uncomfortable.

When the patient is in a supine position, a small pillow or folded bath blanket can be placed under the affected limb from below the knee to the heel. Both the heel and Achilles tendon are kept free of pressure. The knee is more comfortable in slight flexion, rather than complete extension, and the heel is kept free of pressure from the bed. A trochanter roll or sandbag is placed against the hip-thigh area to prevent external rotation. Elderly patients often prefer to have the head of the bed slightly elevated; however, it may be necessary to keep the hip fully extended. Bed position is maintained in accordance with written orders.

A trapeze on the bed allows the patient to pull himself or herself up on the bed. If skin traction is used preoperatively, the patient may tend to slide to the foot of the bed. When the foot spreader of the traction touches the foot of the bed, the effectiveness of the traction is interrupted. With the use of the trapeze, the patient can be taught to shift his or her position periodically. Range of motion exercises are carried out by the nurse or physical therapist on all noninvolved extremities. Strengthening the upper extremities is especially necessary to the postoperative mobilization of the patient using crutches or a walker.

All bony prominences and potential pressure areas must be inspected and massaged at regular intervals. With the use of skin traction, the exposed toes are checked for signs of arterial, venous, or nerve impairment. Skin traction can also place undue pressure on the peroneal nerve resulting in plantar flexion (foot drop). The adhesive materials used to attach the skin traction may damage the thin, fragile skin of an elderly patient; thus, the nurse periodically checks all skin areas adjacent to the adhesive materials.

Coughing and deep-breathing exercises are part of preoperative care to prevent the development of hypostatic pneumonia and also to prepare the patient for what will be expected of him or her postoperatively. The patient may have difficulty voiding in this immobilized position. A small-fracture bedpan, offered at regular intervals, and adequate fluid intake are helpful measures. Intake and output are recorded. Placement of an indwelling catheter is avoided unless all other measures fail. A urinary drainage system may be established just prior to surgery and maintained for 2 or 3 days postoperatively, since in the early postsurgical days it is difficult for the patient to manage the movement needed to use a bedpan. Gas-forming foods are usually avoided, as they may produce abdominal discomfort and necessitate frequent use of the bedpan, which can be difficult for the patient.

Laboratory blood work, urinalysis, blood typing and cross matching, and other general preoperative preparation of the patient are required. The patient is usually transported to surgery in the bed to avoid unnecessary moving that might increase the extent of injury, because removal of the weights, which is necessary to move the patient from the bed to a surgical cart, can change alignment of the bone fragments. The bed-moving is done carefully, as jarring of the bed and swinging weights can cause pain to the patient. The surgical bed is then prepared in the surgical area so that it is ready for the patient's return following surgery.

Postoperative nursing care in hip fracture Following internal fixation of a hip fracture, nursing care is designed to provide general postoperative care, to prevent complications, to meet psychosocial needs, and to prepare the patient for mobilization.

If the hip appeared quite unstable during surgery, it may be immobilized for a few days postoperatively with the use of Buck's extension or a half-ring Thomas splint, which may have a Pearson attachment. The traction helps to overcome muscle spasm, allows soft-tissue healing, and increases the patient's comfort; the patient is restricted to bed, however, until the traction is discontinued. It is imperative to employ nursing measures that curtail the development of complications related to stasis and pressure.

Many factors can affect the postoperative course of internal fixation of hip fractures in the elderly. Chronologic age is not always an indication of biologic age. Thus patients' responses to surgery vary greatly. Barring complications of either surgery or fracture healing, bony union occurs in 4 to 6 months. Many individual variables are considered when initiating weight-bearing on the surgical side. These variables include the type of fracture, the type of metallic implant, the surgical technique, the postoperative course, the age and general condition of the patient, and the surgeon's judgment. Too much full weight-bearing too soon on the surgical side can result in dislodging of the metallic implant, or stress fractures of the metal device can occur. It is difficult to place the metal device a second time in the same site. Weight-bearing on the noninvolved leg begins the first or second postoperative day unless the patient is immobilized with traction. In the older age group, the metallic device usually is not removed after bony union. In younger persons who have internal fixation with plates, screws, or intramedullary rods, the metallic devices are often removed 1 to 2 years after fixation.

The involved limb must be handled gently and carefully, supporting all joints. Jerking movements or allowing the limb to flip off pillow supports can be very painful for the patient. Good body alignment is maintained at all times. Pressure points are relieved with both position changes and massage. After first trying out other comfort measures, analgesics are given as needed. It is important to assess the quality and type of pain as a basis for determining appropriate pain relief measures. Good skin care and a dry, wrinkle-free bed add much to patient comfort. A pain-free patient is better able to participate in turning, coughing and deep breathing, transfer activities, and other aspects of care. Pain can interfere with adequate rest necessary for tissue repair.

POSITION CHANGES Frequent position changes provide for some physiologic mobility, thus helping to curtail the development of postoperative complications. Usually, the patient may be turned to either side following internal fixation of a hip fracture unless the physician has ordered specific positions.

When turning the patient, at least two persons should be present to assist. Pillows are placed between the patient's legs from groin to ankles. The patient can assist in the turn, using the side-rail for support to pull himself or herself to the side. The patient should be turned as a unit. One nurse's hands are placed on the patient's shoulder and hip to assist in the turning and the other nurse supports the operative leg, ensuring that it is in good alignment, and not allowed to adduct over the other leg. Position is maintained by supporting the patient's upper leg with pillows and placing a pillow snugly against the patient's back. Both legs may be flexed when the patient is in the side-lying position. Some patients may not tolerate a full side-lying position on the operative hip the first few days postoperatively, as the mattress may cause too much pressure against the incision. The incision is painful and the large compression dressing is another source of pressure between the mattress and the incision. In these instances, a 45-degree turn may be substituted for a full side-lying position.

When the patient is lying supine, a sandbag or trochanter roll is placed against the surgical hip to prevent external rotation. The operative leg may be kept slightly abducted. A small pillow or folded bath blanket may be periodically placed under the operative leg from the knee to ankle to help relieve pressure on the heel. The patient is encouraged to exercise the uninvolved leg independently. The hip, knee, and ankle can be flexed and extended. Following repositioning the nurse should make certain that the call light is moved within the patient's easy reach.

NURSING MEASURES TO PREVENT COMPLICATIONS

Prevention of Respiratory Complications

Position changes, coughing and deep breathing, and adequate fluid intake help to raise secretions and prevent hypostatic pneumonia. The patient can be taught to cough and deep-breathe periodically without specific reminders from the nurse. Effectiveness of coughing is checked by auscultation of the chest before and after coughing. If secretions are raised, the nurse should observe the consistency, color, and amount. In some hospitals, intermittent positive-pressure breathing is employed to assist in respiratory expansion. The patient is protected from chilling or drafts and prophylactic antibiotic therapy is sometimes ordered. The nurse should be alert for signs of fat emboli or thromboemboli, both of which may complicate the patient's postoperative course.

Prevention of Cardiovascular Complications

Usually a large compression dressing covers the incision. Because of gravitational flow, bleeding may seep from the edges of the dressing and down under the patient's buttocks and thighs, rather than saturate the dressing. Frequently, a drain is placed in the wound during surgery. This drain may be attached to a Hemovac system. Vital signs are monitored at frequent intervals the first 24 to 48 hours after surgery and then every 4 to 6 hours, or as the patient's condition dictates. Pulse and blood pressure are compared with the preoperative and intraoperative data to determine the significance of changes. Intravenous feedings are closely monitored, particularly in the elderly, who tend to be susceptible to fluid overload and subsequent congestive heart failure.

Surgical trauma, stasis, and hypercoaguability of blood can result in thrombophlebitis postoperatively. The patient's legs therefore are assessed for edema, tenderness, and increased warmth. Lower-extremity peripheral pulses are checked, and measurement of the circumference of the lower extremities is made daily, comparing the two legs. Preventive measures to curtail the development of thrombophlebitis include antigravity measures such as elevating the leg, applying elastic stockings or bandages, leg exercises, and early mobilization. To decrease the cohesiveness of platelets, the patient may be given intravenous low-molecular-weight dextran (500 to 1,000 ml per 24 hours) or oral aspirin prophylactically. Patients who have had previous problems with phlebitis, or those who are considered high risks for other medical reasons, may be given anticoagulant drugs to keep prothrombin or bleeding time to one and one-half times normal.

Prevention of Gastrointestinal Complications

Immobilization and inactivity lead to the development of a sluggish bowel. Because of the physiologic changes of aging, the elderly are particularly vulnerable to constipation, but organic causes of constipation must be ruled out when it does occur. Generally, most patients respond positively to a well-balanced diet with adequate bulk, adequate fluid intake, and measures to establish bowel regularity. The nurse should help the patient reestablish the preinjury pattern of bowel evacuation as much as is feasible during the postoperative period.

Prevention of Genitourinary Complications

Indwelling catheters should not be placed unless necessary. Providing fluid intake of 2,500 to 3,000 ml per 24 hours and offering the bedpan at regular intervals are nursing measures important to prevention of urinary stasis. The color, odor, and amount of urinary output are noted. Ingestion of acid ash foods and fluids promotes urine acidity, which discourages bacterial growth and calculi formation.

Prevention of Integumentary Complications

Placing an air pressure mattress on the bed helps to alternate pressure on the body. Massage and the use of the synthetic sheepskin are helpful to reduce pressure on bony prominences. Sheepskin heel and elbow protectors are helpful in shielding the heels and elbows. Warm, moist body areas are inspected daily. A daily complete bath may not be necessary and it may even be contraindicated for elderly persons with dry skin.

Prevention of Musculoskeletal Complications

Either active or passive exercises of the extremities as well as position changes help to maintain the integrity and function of the musculoskeletal system. Transfer from the bed to the wheelchair, along with weight-bearing on the uninvolved leg, greatly assists all the muscles and joints. Use of an overbed trapeze helps to strengthen upper extremity muscles.

Prevention of Wound Infection

An elevated temperature may indicate the presence of infection of the incision, a dreaded complication. If the deep tissues become infected, fracture healing may be delayed or interrupted. The dressing is inspected for any unusual odor or drainage. After the dressing has been removed, the incision is inspected daily to note whether it is dry and intact.

Prevention of Depression

Depression is often part of the postoperative course and is related to the very real status of the patient's inactivity and helplessness. Other factors that contribute to the patient's depression and discomfort are dependency and loss of self-esteem; role changes; and concerns about financial burden. Another source of depression may be that following discharge, the patient, particularly one who lives alone, may not be able to return to previous living arrangements. Pain, a strange environment, sedatives, and analgesics may all contribute to the patient's confusion and disorientation.

The nurse must carefully assess the effects of medications on these patients. In addition, the nurse can manipulate their environments in any way that allows for more social contacts and increased sensory stimuli such as arranging for the patient to be out of bed and out of the hospital room. As soon as possible the patient is involved in activities of daily living: eating, bathing, oral hygiene, hair care, and position changes. The family is encouraged to bring hobby materials to the patient or, as an alternative, occupational therapy is suggested. A patient should be respectfully addressed by his or her proper name.

Prevention of Problems of Immobility

Early mobilization helps to prevent atelectasis, thrombosis, and embolism. It also serves as a morale booster. Mobilization involves weight-bearing on the noninvolved leg as ordered, and progression of activity increasing from bed to chair to wheelchair to walker, crutches, and cane.

Rather than lifting the patient out of bed physically it is better to enlist a patient's participation. When transferring the patient from bed to chair, the bed is placed in low position and the chair is placed parallel to the bed; the patient is assisted out of bed from the uninvolved side. The patient is first helped to a sitting position and allowed to sit for a few minutes to gain his or her balance and to allow the pulse to stabilize. The nurse supports the patient in an unhurried manner. The patient is then supported and assisted to a standing position, and by bearing weight on the unaffected leg, can pivot to the chair. Three shorter periods of 30 or 40 minutes in the chair are preferable to one long period per day. The nurse encourages the patient to maintain good posture when sitting and teaches the patient to grasp the arms of the chair and shift his or her weight in the chair periodically. This practice relieves pressure on bony prominences. When the patient is sitting up, the involved leg may need to be elevated.

Usually the patient is ready for discharge 2 to 4 weeks after surgery. The family should be involved in the discharge planning. The patient may go to an extended care facility until he or she achieves further strength and skill in ambulation. If the patient is going directly home, both the patient and the family need to be taught to remove potential hazards from the environment when possible or to minimize structural hazards in the home. The environment should be free from clutter, and scatter rugs should be removed. It may be wise to keep a small night light in the patient's bedroom and in the bathroom, if the patient has nocturia. Scatter rugs, a cluttered environment, and poor lighting may have precipitated the initial fall in which the patient fractured his hip.

ARTHROPLASTY OF THE HIP

Femoral Head Prosthesis

Intracapsular and extracapsular fractures of the femur may be treated initially with a prosthetic replacement of the head and neck. Among the types of femoral head prostheses are the Austin Moore, Matchette, Nadin Reith, and Thompson. These devices, as are other internal fixation devices, are made of Vitallium, which is inert and does not corrode (Fig. 10-12).

Insertion of a prosthesis is no more hazardous than internal fixation with nails, plates, and screws. Femoral head prosthetic replacement is done when avascularity of the head is apparent at surgery; when there is failure to obtain adequate reduction; when there are pathologic fractures; when there is spasticity such as in parkinsonism; and when the patient has generally poor health. The initial insertion of a prosthesis rather than internal

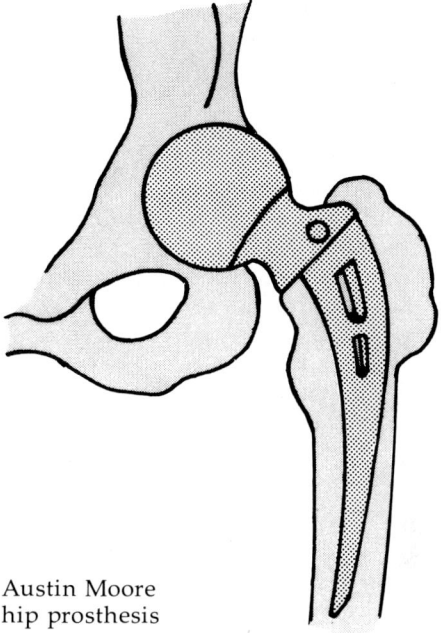
Austin Moore hip prosthesis

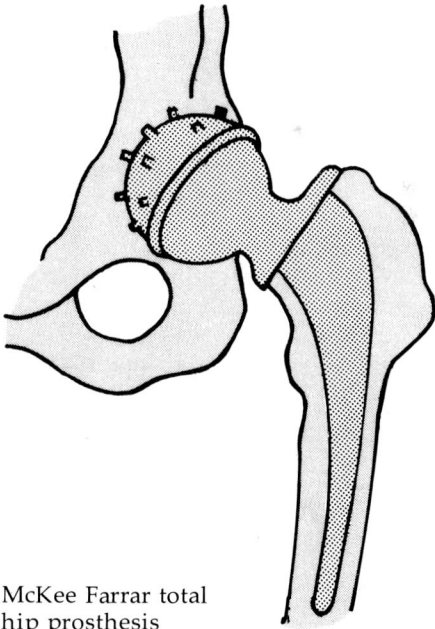
McKee Farrar total hip prosthesis

Figure 10-12
Femoral head prosthesis and total hip prosthesis.

fixation usually allows for more rapid weight-bearing and ambulation, shorter hospital stay, and less postoperative disability. When internal fixation is followed by avascular necrosis of the head of the femur or non-union, a second surgical procedure may be carried out to replace the head and neck of the femur with a prosthesis.

In this procedure the femoral head and neck are excised and the medullary canal of the femur is partially reamed out and the flange of the prosthesis inserted. The acetabulum may need to be reshaped to receive the head of the prosthesis. The Austin Moore femoral head prosthesis has openings in its stem intended for bone to grow through for additional stability.

These patients are subject to the same postoperative complications as are the patients with internal fixation. The most dreaded is infection. Infection around the prosthesis leads to instability of the prosthesis and it is almost impossible to place a prosthesis a second time. The infection must be cleared and there must be enough solid bone left to hold the second prosthesis.

Cup Arthroplasty–Hip Arthroplasty

In order to restore or improve joint function, the acetabulum may be replaced with a prosthetic metal cup. This procedure is done in fractures of the acetabulum, rheumatoid arthritis, degenerative joint disease, ankylosis, and complications of fractures of the head of the femur. Any of the conditions listed can interfere with a smooth joint surface. In this surgery, the hip joint is disarticulated, the acetabulum is reshaped to hold the metal cup, and the head of the femur is reshaped to glide smoothly within the metal acetabulum.

Postoperative care of these patients is similar to care following internal fixation. Special attention is given to keeping the involved leg in a position of abduction, which helps to keep the cup and head of the femur in the acetabulum to prevent dislocation. Russell's traction may be used along with sandbags. Postoperatively, a stationary bicycle may be used for flexion and extension exercises.

It has been found that the metal part induced fibrous changes in the exposed bone surface following the procedures in which bone is in constant contact with metal. For example, in a young active person, a metal femoral head prosthesis wears through the bony acetabulum. This problem has led to the development of the total hip replacement, the procedure now being used instead of cup arthroplasty.

Total Hip Replacement Arthroplasty

Currently, if either the acetabulum or the head of the femur is deteriorating because of trauma or disease, both are replaced with a prosthesis, fixed into place with an acrylic cement, polymethyl methacrylate. This is called total hip replacement or total hip arthroplasty. One type of total hip prosthesis is the McKee Farrar total hip prosthesis.

Dr. John Charnley, Professor of Orthopedics at the University of Manchester, England, is credited with much of the early work done in total hip replacement. The prosthetic femoral head was already in use, but the acetabulum component needed more development when he began to use these devices. Some of the early prosthetic pieces were made of glass, but these glass devices broke easily. Teflon also was used. Although Teflon has low friction properties, it did not wear well. In order to be successful, prosthetic joints must have a low coefficient of friction and be tolerated by body tissues. To meet these criteria, a high-density polyethylene plastic material was developed. This material is chemically inert in the body and has low friction properties. The sliding surface of a normal joint has a coefficient of friction of .02. By analogy, a skate sliding on ice has a coefficient of friction of .03. (The lower the coefficient of friction, the slower the wear rate.)

Synovial fluid is the product of activity of a joint; however, the fluid does not necessarily lubricate a prosthesis. The materials used in prosthetic joints must be compatible with each other and have no frictional resistance. Metal to plastic has these properties. Metal to metal, in which both components are made of either stainless steel or a cobalt chrome alloy, has higher friction between the parts which can lead to eventual loosening of the prosthesis. Stainless steel is not compatible with Vitallium.

The prosthetic joint components must also allow weight-bearing and range of motion without stress and without wear and tear to surrounding tissues. The impact of loading must also be tolerated. Normally, when one leg bears the body weight, such as in walking or standing on one leg, the force on the hip joint is 2½ times normal body weight. The femoral head can be loaded up to 12 to 15 times body weight before fracture of the neck occurs, assuming that the bone is healthy.

Dr. Charnley is also credited with the development of the self-curing cement (dental cement) now used to anchor the prosthesis in place. The cement serves two purposes: It holds the prosthetic components firmly in place so that the acetabulum prosthesis will not slip around in the socket, and the femoral head stem will not twist within the medullary canal, and it seals off the medullary canal guarding against infection. The cement powder (polymer) and a liquid (monomer) are mixed in surgery just prior to their use. An exothermic reaction occurs, and the temperature of the material may reach 100°C (boiling point of water). It is mixed to a doughy consistency and is then ready to be placed in the bone bed. Continuous wound irrigation is carried out with antibiotic solution to help cool the cement and prevent infection. The component parts are immediately positioned into place, as the cement solidifies within 10 minutes.

Some of the cement may diffuse into the bloodstream, resulting in a transient hypotension. Some anesthesiologists report that an odor is temporarily observed in the patient's breath. The cement does not adhere to bone, but acts as a filler or mechanical cement. The bone cement is opaque to x-ray. The long-term effects of this cement in the body are not yet known.

In the surgical procedure, a lateral incision is made. The hip is disarticulated and the head of the femur is removed. The greater trochanter is preserved; it needs to be cut away to facilitate approaching the head and acetabulum, but it is rewired into place later as it is needed for leverage of the abductor muscles. The acetabulum is then deepened and roughened with removal of all cartilage. Holes are drilled into the patient's bony acetabulum to match the studs on the plastic or metal acetabulum. The artificial plastic acetabulum is then cemented into place. The medullary canal of the femur is then reamed out and filled with the plastic cement, and the metal femoral head component is pushed or hammered into place.

These components come in various cup sizes, head sizes, neck lengths, and stem lengths. Thus, during surgery, various sizes are available so that the surgeon can more closely match the artificial pieces to the patient's bone parts being removed. Once the components are seated into place, the greater trochanter is reattached and the wound closed.

This is extensive surgery and the four major concerns in the early postoperative period are: (1) **hemorrhage** into the deep tissues which can initially go unnoticed; (2) **thrombophlebitis;** (3) **sepsis;** and (4) **dislocation** of the prosthesis.

Indications for total hip replacement are painful osteoarthritis of the hip in the aged; post-traumatic arthritis; rheumatoid arthritis; unreduced congenital dislocations of the hip; septic arthritis; necrosis of the head of the femur secondary to radium application for cancer of the cervix; and aseptic necrosis or non-union following the hip fracture. Repeated intra-articular injections of steroids can also lead to destruction of articular cartilage.

In general, total hip replacement is considered in any condition that results in a constantly painful hip; limited range of motion of the hip joint; or disturbed gait or deformity. Walking with an abnormal gait for any length of time not only weakens the muscles on the involved side, but also eventually jeopardizes the integrity of the contralateral hip joint.

The goals of total hip replacement are to alleviate a painful joint, to regain mobility, and provide stability. Criteria for patient selection are no history of osteomyelitis or wound infection; increasing severity of the arthritic pain; presence of good preoperative muscle tone and reflexes; and a patient highly motivated to undergo the surgery and maintain the prescribed exercise program. Since no prosthetic joint lasts forever and replacement is nearly impossible, age is a criterion as well. Fifty years of age is the usual lower age limit; however, age is becoming less of a criterion. The procedure is done on younger persons. Another concern in relation to age is that the long-term effects of the cement are not known; however, a person severely disabled from rheumatoid arthritis at age 30 is not denied surgery until reaching age 50.

Once the patient has made the decision to undergo surgery, preoperative preparation for total hip replacement begins with instructing the patient in the exercise regimen that will be carried out postoperatively. Usually the physical therapist conducts these teaching sessions. The patient must also be instructed in the special positioning needed postoperatively, and it is good to have practice sessions for teaching the patient to get in and out of bed without flexion of the thigh.

Systemic antibiotic therapy is initiated and anticoagulant measures with coumadin, heparin, or low-molecular dextran may be initiated as part of the preoperative preparation. The skin in the surgical area is prepared with hexachlorophene (pHisoHex) or povidone-iodine (Betadine) skin scrubs. The patient may have either a general or spinal anesthetic and is prepared accordingly. The patient is typed and crossmatched for blood replacement if needed during surgery. Other preoperative nursing measures are the same as for any surgery patient.

Postoperative care is directed toward prevention of any complications, maintaining the operative hip in abduction and slight internal rotation, and mobilization of the patient. The patient should be assessed for any signs of infection or thrombophlebitis. Vital signs must be monitored frequently to detect any signs of bleeding. A Hemovac drain may be in place. A certain amount of hemodilution occurs with the use of the low-molecular-weight dextran. This, along with blood loss, can result in decreasing hematocrit and hemoglobin, sometimes requiring blood replacement therapy. After the dextran has been discontinued, the hemoglobin returns to normal. This is referred to as self-correcting anemia.

Placement of an air-pressure mattress on the bed, use of sheepskin, and use of a single footboard for the unaffected leg are measures that add to patient comfort. Ace bandages may be wrapped on the lower extremity; removing and replacing elastic stockings on the affected leg in traction is difficult.

In addition to the special needs related to the specific surgical procedure, general nursing care is directed toward relief of incisional pain, checking all pressure points, maintaining fluid intake and elimination, pulmonary ventilation, dressing checks, isometric or active exercises, and maintaining the position as ordered by the physician.

Various approaches may be used for maintaining the operative leg in abduction. Russell's traction or Buck's extension may be used, bringing the patient's leg well to the side of the bed or extending beyond the mattress. Another approach is using a wedge-shaped foam rubber piece between the legs. Some surgeons prefer to keep the patient supine for 5 to 7 days postoperatively, with the leg in abduction and internal rotation. It is then necessary to have sufficient assistance to totally lift the patient for back care, linen change, and bedpan placement. Other surgeons allow the patient to be turned to the unaffected side for short periods, provided the operative leg is positioned in abduction and internal rotation. This requires good support with pillows.

The head of the bed can be elevated for meals, but never more than 90 degrees, as this places the femoral head in an unstable position. In the early postoperative period, the patient **cannot sit** for prolonged periods when ambulation is begun. The patient is usually mobilized out of bed within 5 to 7 days with the aid of a walker, crutches, or cane. The most characteristic outcome of this type of surgery is pain-free walking. Weight-bearing is allowed in 1 to 2 weeks; however, the supporting structures need up to 6 weeks to heal.

The major reason for maintaining abduction, internal rotation, and less than 90-degree flexion of the hip in the early postoperative period is to prevent dislocation of the artificial femoral head from the artificial acetabulum. Signs of a dislocated prosthesis are severe pain, a palpable bulge over the head of the femur, external rotation and shortening of the leg, and possible changes in circulation and nerve function in the extremity.

The patient is usually discharged in 2 weeks, on a graduated exercise program. The exercise program usually includes quadriceps and gluteal muscle setting exercises, active ankle exercises, straight leg raising, abduction, and adduction only to neutral position. Within 1 year after surgery, the patient can usually perform most activities as more and more flexion and extension of the hip are achieved.

TOTAL KNEE REPLACEMENT

Essentially, the knee is subject to the same deterioration as a result of disease or trauma as is the hip. The various forms of arthritis cause either inflammation or destruction of joint tissue, or post-trauma ankylosis can result in a nonfunctional knee. A failure in one structure in the knee joint often results in failure in other parts. Regardless of cause, eventually bone grates on bone and the result is a painful, useless joint.

Physiologically, the knee must transmit forces that support, accelerate, or decelerate body mass. When walking or climbing stairs, the knee is loaded up to three to four times body weight. The quadriceps, gastrocnemius, and hamstring muscles, and the cruciate and lateral ligaments assist in bearing the load and stabilizing the knee joint. The knee is a hinge-type joint where the concave superior surface of the tibia articulates with the convex inferior surfaces of the femoral condyles.

Usually, about 110 degrees of flexion are needed at the knee to stand up from a sitting position. A tall person may need more flexion. When descending stairs, the trailing leg needs about 90 degrees of flexion. For walking, the knee must be able to flex and extend, abduct and adduct, and rotate. Negotiating stairs, sitting, and lifting require flexion and extension. In rheumatoid arthritis and osteoarthritis, flexion-extension is severely limited and abduction-adduction and rotation are present in abnormal patterns. Rheumatoid arthritis tends to result in a tight, constricted knee, whereas osteoarthritis may result in a more loose, unstable knee. Successful knee arthroplasty that allows the person to return to activities of daily living and self-care should provide for at least 90 to 100 degrees of flexion-extension; about 10 degrees of abduction-adduction; and about 15 degrees of internal and external rotation after the surgery.

All knee prostheses replace the abnormal articular surfaces of both the tibia and femur. The diseased articular surface of the femoral condyles and tibial plateaus are resected surgically. There are a variety of knee prostheses on the market, but essentially they are either the single-unit, hinge type, or the polycentric type.

The hinge type usually consists of metal-to-metal, and it is either cemented into place or anchored with an intramedullary rod, nails, or screws. This process has been compared to "capping a tooth." These units have a more fixed center of rotation with limited anterior glide. The polycentric knee arthroplasty consists of two semicircular "runners" of stainless steel or Vitallium cemented into the articular surfaces of the femoral condyles. These runners articulate with two polyethylene plastic slots or grooves cemented into the tibial plateau. It is felt that the polycentric prosthesis allows a greater degree of flexion range and some axial rotation [19].

The same acrylic cement is used in knee arthroplasty as in the total hip replacement. During surgery, the wound is irrigated with antibiotic solution to guard against infection and to help cool the exothermic setting stage of the cement. Drains are placed in the wound and a pressure dressing is applied. During surgery, all effort is made to maintain the integrity of the joint ligaments so that postoperatively the stability of the joint will be assured.

Nursing Care in Knee Replacement

Preoperatively, the patient is evaluated for joint range of motion, muscle strength, and gaits to obtain baseline data for postoperative comparison. The patient is started on an exercise program and surgical scrubs prior to admission, and is instructed in what will be expected of him or her and what can be expected of others during the hospital stay. Prophylactic systemic antibiotic therapy is usually initiated and preoperative care proceeds as for any general surgery.

Postoperatively, quadriceps setting exercises, gentle knee flexion and extension, active ankle exercises, and straight leg raising exercises are started by the first postoperative day. The patient has considerable freedom to move about in bed; however, support and elevation of the operative leg are maintained. Ice packs may be applied to help curtail edema. Circulatory and neurologic function must be checked below the compression dressing. Intravenous therapy may be continued through the first 24 hours. Analgesics are given for pain; however, the presurgical joint pain is gone. Anticoagulant therapy may be initiated and used for 2 weeks to curtail development of thromboemboli.

By the fourth or fifth postoperative day, the compression dressing is removed and is replaced by elastic bandages or a light cylinder cast. Full ambulation is started the next day and discharge occurs in 8 to 10 days, or when the patient can ambulate safely with knee stability and motion. The exercise program includes body mechanics, muscle strengthening, range of motion exercises, and gait retraining. Transition from walker to crutches to cane progresses on an individual patient basis. The goal is to achieve 90 degrees of flexion of the operative knee by the time of discharge. This is possible if the patient is not sent home with the cast on.

Postdischarge, the pain-free joint allows for more function, a change in life style, and improved self-esteem. As their world widens, these patients experience new goals and new achievements. Depending on the degree of successful return of the planes of motion in the knee, these patients may no longer be housebound [30].

In all artificial joint replacement, perhaps the single most important gain is pain-free joints. Lower-extremity joint replacement has preceded arthroplasty of the upper extremity; however, artificial elbow and finger joints are being developed. If bilateral joints are to be replaced, the second joint is usually replaced 6 months after the first one.

TRACTION

Traction is the third method that can be used in the reduction and retention of a fracture. **Traction** is a steady pull on a part of the body. The application of the pulling force can be done by the hands (manual traction), or by a device attached to the body (skin and skeletal traction). The prescribed amount of traction is achieved by a system of ropes, pulleys, and weights connected to a metal frame on the bed.

Traction can be a temporary measure, as when either manual or skin traction is used to reduce a fracture. Some forms of skin and skeletal traction are of longer duration and are used to immobilize a reduced fracture, to relieve muscle spasm and pain, to treat an unstable fracture, to prevent or correct deformities, and to immobilize an inflamed joint or extremity to permit rest and healing.

When traction is used to treat a fracture, the goal is to exert sufficient force to keep the two bone fragments in alignment and just touching. The basic purpose is to produce a state of equilibrium with the resultant force applied to the fractured bone. In skin and skeletal traction, the forward force of the weights is balanced by the backward force of the muscle pull and the frictional force between the patient's body and the bed. Additional counterforce is supplied by the weight of the patient plus gravity [11].

Countertraction is the pulling force equal to and opposite (against) the traction weights. Countertraction is essential to keep the patient from being pulled against the pulleys, which will change the direction and magnitude of the traction. The body exerts countertraction by its gravitational pull. This gravitational pull can be increased by elevating the bed under the part of the body placed in traction. Elevating the bed is done by placing wooden blocks under the legs at the foot, the head, or the side of the bed. An additional 1½ pounds of countertraction is added for every inch that the foot of the bed is raised. Another method of providing countertraction is arranging the traction to pull against a fixed point. An example is the Thomas splint proximal ring, which presses against the ischial tuberosity. Thomas ring splints are used as an emergency measure or with a Pearson attachment in traction to treat fractures of the lower extremity.

Principles of physics are involved in the use of traction. One basic principle is Newton's third law, which states that *for every force there is an equal and opposite reacting force.* The acting force refers to the force that one body exerts on the second one, and the reacting force refers to the force that the second body exerts on the first one. For example, when a patient lies in bed, the weight of the body pushes against the mattress and in turn the mattress pushes against him. The heavier body parts receive a greater reacting force than do lighter body parts. A sagging mattress changes the direction of forces applied to the fracture treated with traction; a firm mattress and bed boards provide firm support and more equal distribution of body weight [11].

For traction to be effective, the forces of the traction and countertraction must be equal. Unequal opposing forces can result in too much pull, in which the bone fragments do not touch each other and cannot reunite, or too little pull, in which the fracture fragments override and deformity occurs with healing.

A force can be defined as a push or pull that tends to change the state of rest or motion of an object. The three characteristics of force are magnitude, direction, and point of application. Nurses encounter force daily as they care for patients. One type of force is scalar force, which has magnitude only. Examples of scalar force are a person's heart rate, height, or weight. The force of gravity keeps a person in bed. Friction is a force that opposes motion in two contacting surfaces. It is created when one surface moves over another. Continuous friction may produce abrasions. A vector force has both magnitude and direction. In skin and skeletal traction, the vector force is provided by free-hanging weights that pull in line with the long axis of the bone. Vector equilibrium is the simultaneous, equal amounts of pull in two opposing directions [11].

A pulley is used to transmit force and to change direction of force. A pulley is a simple machine containing a small grooved wheel around which a rope runs. The pulley transmits the exact force of the weight applied. A 10-pound free-hanging weight attached to an extremity by means of a rope going over a single pulley will apply 10 pounds of force in a straight line with the extremity in a distal direction. In some types of traction, more than one pulley, rope, and weight system are employed. When two concurrent forces act upon a given point but from different angles, the combined forces are called resultant force, a result of vector addition. When the forces are at right angles to each other, the resultant pull bisects the right angle. This principle is applied in Russell's skin or skeletal traction.

Traction can employ one or more of four basic systems: (1) the **traction** system, which is the pull applied to skin or bone; (2) the **countertraction** system, which helps to overcome unequal forces; (3) the **suspension** system, which elevates the limb in a supporting sling or splint and serves to hold the limb in constant alignment and also relieves pressure and edema; and (4) the **balancing** system, which supports the limb evenly and has a set of pulleys, ropes, and weights separate from the traction weights. The suspension and balancing systems allow some movement and facilitate care of the patient [3].

Manual traction is the pulling force exerted with the hands in the process of realigning a fracture. The fracture must then be held in alignment until the fixation or retention device is applied (that is, a cast, skin or skeletal traction) as well as during internal fixation. Manual traction is also used as a first-aid measure to prevent further displacement of the fracture fragments that could result in soft-tissue, blood vessel, or nerve injury. This is especially important if the fracture fragments have jagged edges. Nurses use manual traction when they guard the alignment of a fracture in an emergency room or in the preoperative and postoperative phases when the fractured limb must be supported during transfer or position changes.

Skin traction is the transmitting of a pulling force to the skin and indirectly to bone. Skin traction is also called straight or running traction, and it generally employs traction and countertraction. In the application of skin traction, an adherent material is applied to both sides of an extremity and the limb is then wrapped with an elastic bandage to help hold the adherent strips in place. The ends of the adhesive strips are then attached to a wood or metal spreader on which the pull is exerted by means of a rope, pulley, and weight.

The adherent material can be sponge rubber, Fas-Trac, Flex-Foam, or moleskin. Common adhesive tape does not have elastic properties and is therefore not recommended. Prior to application of skin traction, the extremity should be clean, dry, and clipped of hair. Shaving of the extremity is not recommended, because it denudes the skin. Application of benzoin to the skin improves adhesiveness. Padding can be applied proximal to bony prominences, but not directly over them. If moleskin is used as the adhesive material, it should be petaled to avoid wrinkles and ridges, which are potential pressure points. The adherent material should be applied over as wide an area as possible, since the skin cannot withstand shearing forces. The spreader must be as wide as the ankle to prevent pressure on bony prominences. If it is too wide, it will pull the adhesive away from the skin.

Skin traction is more readily tolerated in children than in adults, as a fracture of an extremity in children does not require large forces for alignment and immobilization. Their skin also tolerates the friction of the adhesive materials for longer periods of time than is possible in adults. Many orthopedic surgeons feel that if skin traction is used in fracture treatment of an adult, it should not be used for longer than 3 to 4 days. The use of

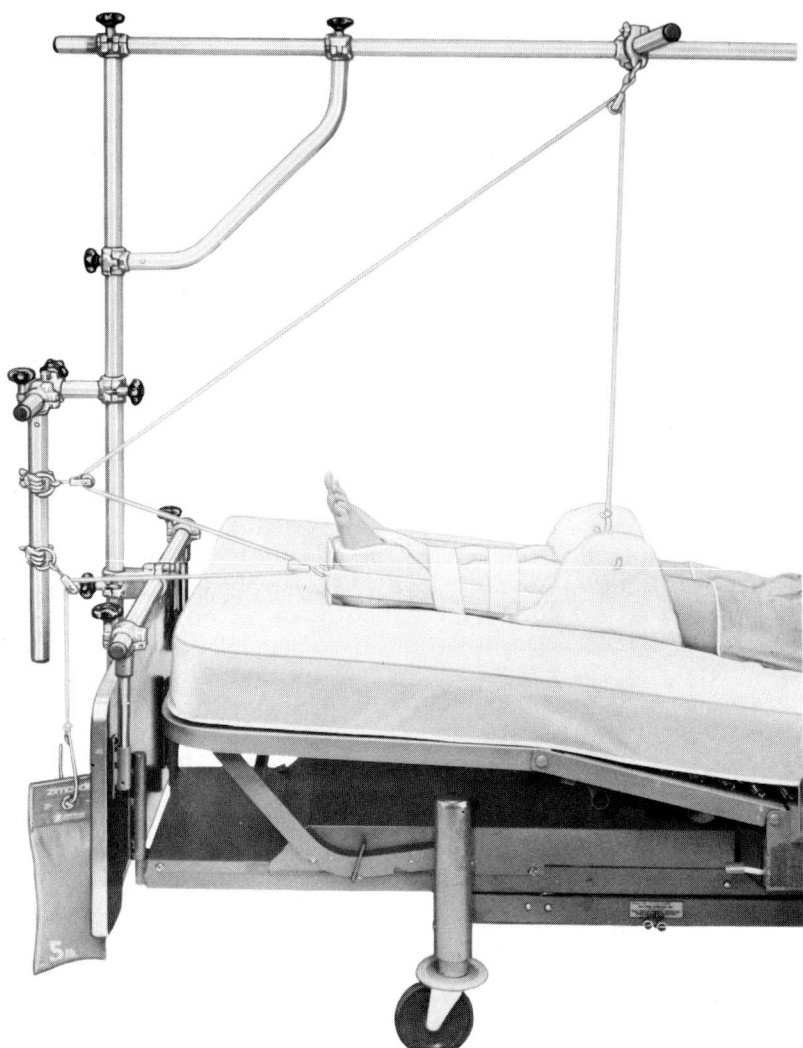

Figure 10-13
Russell's skin traction.
(Courtesy of Zimmer-USA.)

skin traction is restricted to the extremities, and a longitudinal force of 7 to 8 pounds is recommended.

One of the most frequent uses of skin traction in the adult is unilateral **Buck's extension,** which is used for temporary immobilization of a hip fracture prior to definitive therapy. The adhesive material is applied from the knee to the ankle and is attached to the pulley and weight at the foot of the bed. Special attention is given to the area just below the knee, where the peroneal nerve passes over the fibular head. The malleoli at the ankle, the heel, and instep are other potential pressure areas. Buck's extension traction usually requires elevation of the foot of the bed to provide appropriate countertraction. The traction force is in a straight line with the longitudinal axis of the femur, and it helps to overcome the external rotation and leg shortening that accompanies hip fracture.

Another form of skin traction is **Russell's skin traction** (Fig. 10-13), used to realign and immobilize femoral shaft fractures. Russell's traction employs Buck's extension and a sling under the knee attached to a separate system of pulleys and ropes. The underlying principle is the application of two vector forces at the knee. These two forces establish a single resultant force upon the long axis of the femur. The traction allows some flexion of the hip and knee. Russell's traction can also be used to treat certain types of knee injuries and fractures of the hip, and is often used for a few days following total hip replacement.

Skin traction utilizing adherent materials

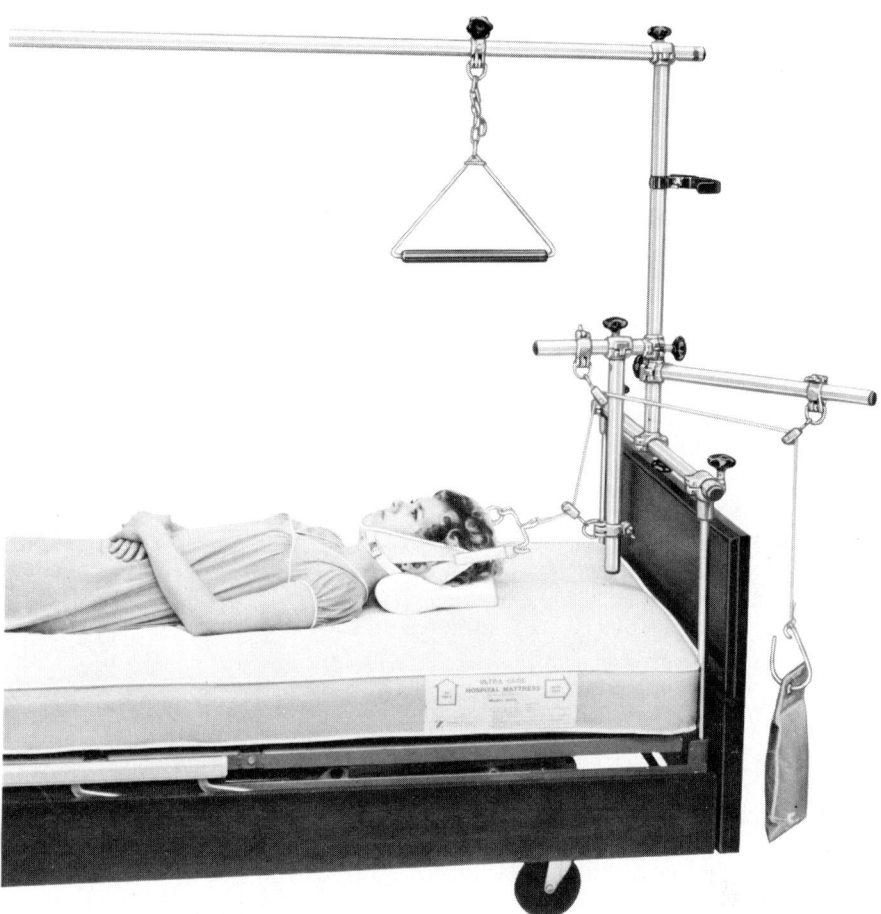

Figure 10-14
Cervical traction.
(Courtesy of Zimmer-USA.)

can also be applied to the forearm for the immobilization or stabilization of fractures, dislocations, and other pathology of the upper arm and shoulder. The traction system extends over the side of the bed.

Another type of skin traction is applied by encircling a part of the body with a belt or halter, as in **pelvic or cervical traction.** Weight is attached with force in a straight line. Both pelvic and cervical traction can be either continuous or intermittent, depending on the purpose for its use. Intermittent means that the halter or belt can be disconnected from the spreader bar and weights, allowing the patient to get out of bed for bathroom privileges or to go to physical therapy. Patients may discover how to get themselves out of the traction, however, and overuse the bathroom privilege; thus, patient instruction and supervision are essential.

Cervical traction is used to treat cervical myositis, subluxation, dislocation, minor fractures, and muscle spasm. Some physicians prefer to treat cervical dislocation and subluxation with skull tongs (skeletal traction) rather than with skin traction. A basic traction frame is attached to the bed. A canvas or leather head halter is applied to the patient's head, with special attention to pressure points on the ears, chin, and occipital area. These are the areas where the halter has contact with the skin. The halter then attaches to a spreader bar, which is above the patient's head. A rope tied to the spreader bar passes over a pulley and is attached to weights (Fig. 10-14). Countertraction can be provided by elevating the head of the bed on blocks or by elevating the backrest as prescribed by the physician. Hyperextension of the neck can be increased by placing a small rolled towel under the patient's neck. If the head is not to rotate, sandbags or rolled towels can be placed at either side of the head. The halter must be placed on the chin so that it does not

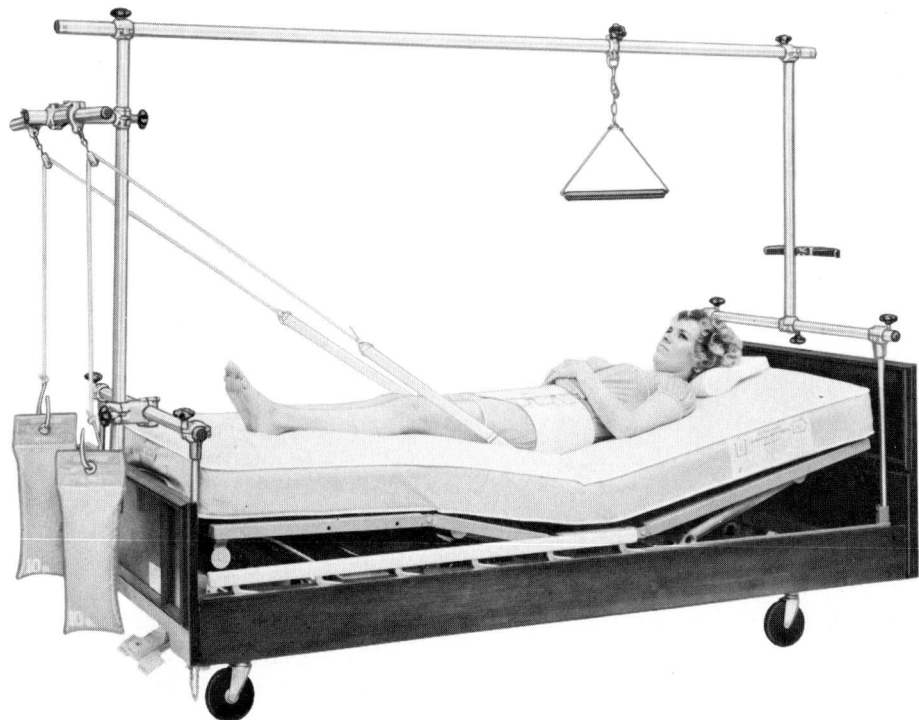

Figure 10-15
Pelvic traction.
(Courtesy of
Zimmer-USA.)

interfere with swallowing. If the patient is maintained completely flat in bed, he or she will need assistance with feeding.

Pelvic traction can be applied either with a pelvic sling or a pelvic belt, depending on the purpose of its use. A pelvic sling is used when a compression force is desired for pelvic fractures. The pelvic sling is attached to a pulley system directly above it on an overbed frame and then the ropes continue to weights at the foot of the bed. The use of a pelvic sling is usually continuous traction and is more restricting and immobilizing than a pelvic belt (Fig. 10-15).

Pelvic traction with a pelvic belt is also called Varco's traction, and is used to treat low back muscle spasm, nerve root disorders (herniated disk), sciatica, and minor fractures of the lower spine. Pelvic belts of the correct size should be selected following measurement of the patient's girth at the iliac crests. The belt must be applied directly to skin, snugly, above and on the iliac crests of the pelvis. Underwear worn under the belt causes slippage and interferes with the effectiveness of the traction. Lateral bands attached to the pelvic belt exert equal pull on the left and right sides. They must be placed posteriorly to "lift" the pelvis and apply a pulling force.

The lateral bands are then attached to a spreader bar that separates the bands enough to allow for leg movement. A rope tied to the spreader bar is attached to free-hanging weights at the foot of the bed. Usually 20 pounds of weight is used.

Pelvic traction is the most physiologic, most comfortable, and easiest method of traction to apply and maintain. In treating low back pain, pelvic traction assists in overcoming lumbar spasm and decreases lumbar lordosis; it also eliminates gravity by bedrest. In addition, the treatment includes medications to decrease pain and muscle spasm, as well as gentle exercises to prevent stasis and pressure point discomfort [6].

When in pelvic traction, the patient is usually placed in semi-Fowler's position, which is about a 45-degree elevation of the back rest along with elevation of the knee-gatch, to flex the hip and knee slightly. This is also referred to as the **Williams position.** The flexed position adds to patient comfort by flattening the lumbar spine and reducing muscle spasm. If additional countertraction is needed, the entire foot of the bed can be elevated on blocks.

Bilateral Buck's extension skin traction (Fig. 10-16) can be utilized to produce the

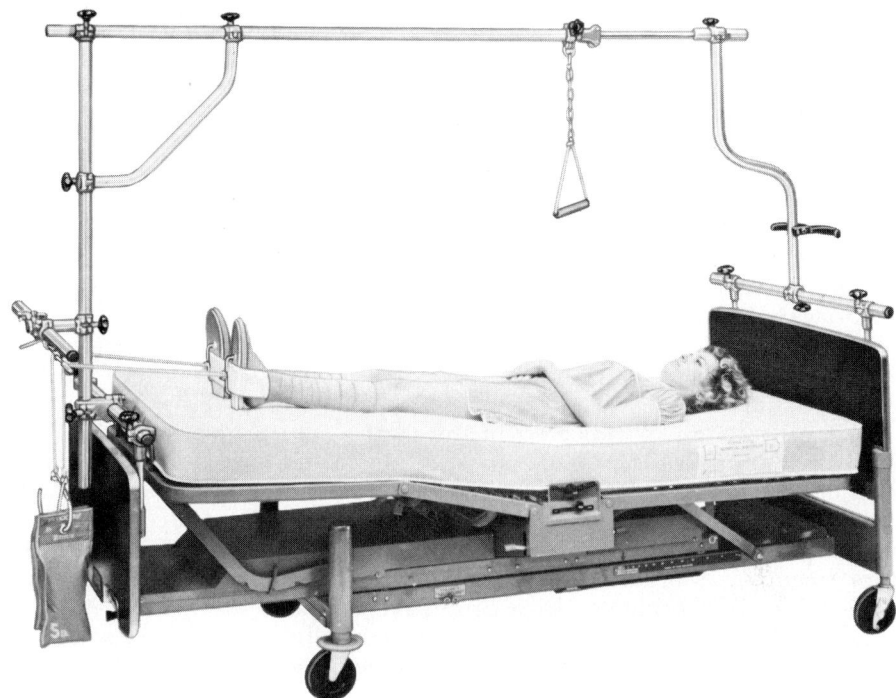

Figure 10-16
Bilateral Buck's extension skin traction. (Courtesy of Zimmer-USA.)

same effects as pelvic traction with the belt, lateral bands, and spreader. With the use of bilateral Buck's extension, the traction force tends to be dissipated at the knee and hip joints, with arching of the back rather than decreasing of the lordosis. Utilizing the Buck's extension is more restricting to the patient. There may be slippage of the adhesive materials causing skin irritation, and having the lower legs bandaged interferes with the ongoing sensory and motor assessment needed with low back problems [6].

In both cervical and pelvic skin traction, the patient must understand that eliminating the forces of gravity is as important as the traction. Thus the bedrest must be complete, correct, as continuous as possible, and of sufficient duration to allow for healing [6].

If bathroom privileges are allowed, the patient should be taught the proper sequence of getting in and out of bed. The following progressive stages provide the least discomfort to the patient and the body is moved as a unit. First, the patient should turn to one side and draw his or her knees up toward the abdomen in a semiflexed position. Then he or she pushes down on the mattress with the uppermost arm and simultaneously supports the partially elevated body on the dependent elbow. After gaining this position, the patient can then sit up by straightening the bent, dependent arm. While the arm is pushing the body away from the bed to a sitting position, the patient slowly lowers his or her flexed hips and knees over the edge of the bed as the body moves as a unit. When returning to bed, the sequence is reversed. Having the head of the bed elevated assists the patient in both getting up out of bed and returning to bed. The author suggests that each reader practice this procedure of getting in and out of bed. With practice and experience, one becomes more aware of each step in the process, and thus is able to teach patients more effectively.

Skeletal traction applies force directly to bone by the surgical placement of a pin or wire perpendicular to and completely through the bone. Insertion of tongs into the outer plate of the skull is another form of skeletal traction. The placement of the metallic device is usually done at the bedside, using surgical asepsis. Following placement of the pin or wire, a U-shaped metal yoke called a tractor bow is clamped to the pin and attached to a system of ropes, pulleys, and weights. The tractor bow must not impinge on the surrounding skin, as it can cause tissue breakdown. Traction directly to bone usually involves 20 to 30 pounds of weight, since the bone tolerates more pulling force than the skin. Skeletal traction can be maintained for weeks or several months; however, long-term use of traction is declining. The extremity is casted in the later stages of treatment and the patient can be mobilized [17].

Skeletal traction requires special measures to maintain countertraction, since more weight is used. If the Thomas ring splint is employed, it stabilizes against a fixed point. Skeletal traction to the upper extremity and skull usually does not provide for fixation against a fixed point.

Skeletal traction is indicated in the treatment of fractures of long bones that are surrounded by large muscle mass, as in the lower extremity. The contracting large muscles tend to cause considerable angulation of the fracture fragment. Markedly comminuted fractures of long bones that have concurrent overriding and displacement of the fragments are also treated with skeletal traction. Unstable fractures can be maintained in alignment with skeletal traction more effectively than in a plaster cast. Skeletal traction applies longitudinal pull to bone and in addition permits control of rotation of the fragments, which is not always achieved with a cast or skin traction.

Unstable fractures of the cervical vertebrae are always treated with tongs placed in the outer table of the cranial bones. The tongs are attached to a rope, pulley, and weights. Skull tongs can also be incorporated into a system called halo traction, which does not use ropes, pulleys, and weights, but the tongs encircle the head and are attached to a rigid brace system coming from the patient's shoulders and torso. The type of tong to be used determines the site of insertion. Some types of tongs are Crutchfield, Vincke, Barton, and Gardner Wells. Prior to placement of the tongs, hair is shaved and surgical preparation of the skin is carried out. A surgical field is established, the skin is infiltrated with local anesthetic, and the tongs are placed under aseptic conditions. Special drills are used that prevent penetration of the inner table of the skull. Skeletal traction applied for cervical fractures usually does not involve the use of a traction frame. These patients are often placed on a special turning frame such as a CircOlectric bed or Stryker frame, which provides the necessary physical immobility and some physiologic mobility as a result of the turning. These frames have a crossbar at the head for attachment of the pulley and weight. When turning the patient in the frame, one person must be assigned to watching the weight so that it does not dislodge or get caught.

When the decision is made to treat a fracture with skeletal traction, all needed equipment and supplies should be gathered and ready for use prior to placement of the pin or wire into bone, because the system must be set up as a unit to prevent displacement. The patient signs a permit and must understand the purpose of the traction: that it means staying in bed and in traction. The patient must know and understand the movements permitted and restricted. Sometimes the person is experiencing pain or has received medication, both of which prevent learning at the time. In this case, the nurse should reinforce these instructions at a time when the person can better concentrate.

The initial action is to attach the required overbed traction frame to the bed with the necessary cross, extension, and side bars that permit placement of pulleys in specific locations to direct traction forces. All clamps that hold the bars together must be functional and secure. Pulleys should be lubricated, and should turn and hang free prior to setting up the traction. Lubricating the pulley after the traction is operational reduces the degree of friction which in turn changes the balancing forces. Rope that is frayed or has weak spots should not be used, and the rope should be of sufficient length to allow knot tying at the proximal and distal ends. Knots should be wrapped with adhesive tape. The metal weight disks come in 1-, 2-, and 5-pound sizes and fit in a groove on the weight carrier, or weighted bags are used.

Skeletal traction to the lower extremity frequently involves the use of a Thomas splint. The Thomas splint was developed during World War I to transport persons with battle injuries involving fractures of the lower extremity. Its development and use greatly curtailed the mortality rate associated with leg fractures. The Thomas splint is still used in emergency treatment of leg fractures, since it allows traction against a fixed body part. Basically, the Thomas splint consists of two rods at each side of the limb joined together proximally by a ring and distally by a crossbar.

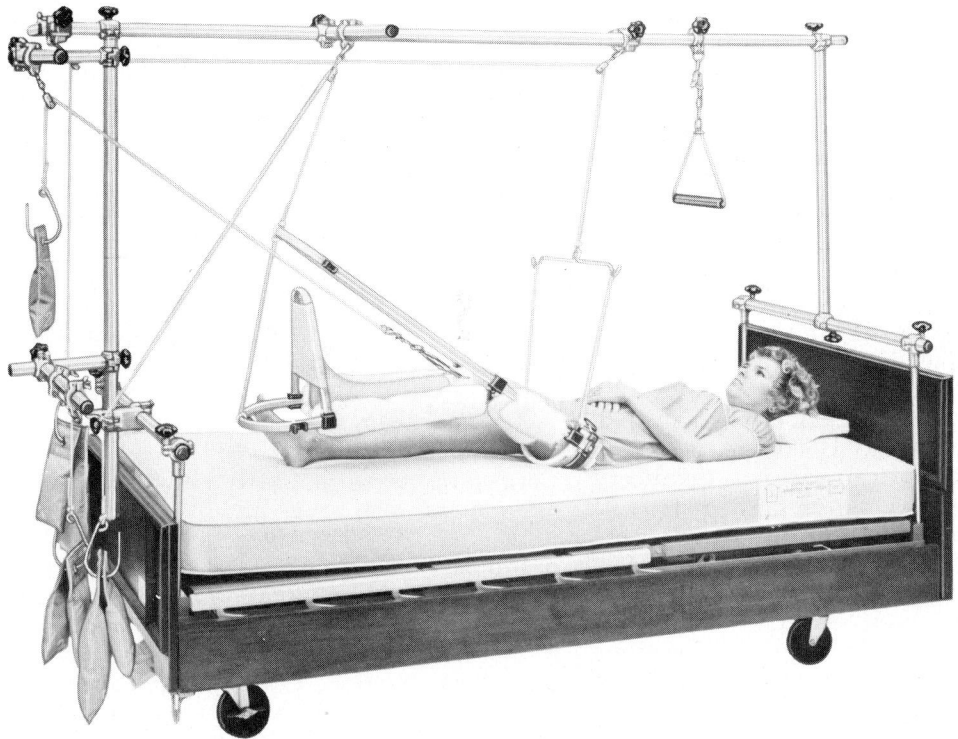

Figure 10-17
Balanced suspension traction. (Courtesy of Zimmer-USA.)

The two metal rods converge slightly toward the distal end so that it is wider at the thigh than at the ankle. The supporting splints are attached on the longer rod, which is placed on the lateral aspect of the leg. The right- or left-sided splints are also sized according to the transverse diameter of the proximal ring, so that a ring that fits the patient can be selected. A Pearson attachment is essentially a small Thomas splint without the proximal ring. It has clamps that attach to the rods of the Thomas splint at the level of the patient's knee.

Prior to placement of the Thomas splint with a Pearson attachment, the proximal ring is padded and sling materials are attached to the Thomas splint to support the thigh, and to the Pearson attachment to support the lower leg. The Pearson attachment is placed below the Thomas splint at about a 45-degree angle, so that the hip and knee are flexed when the leg is in the apparatus. The sling materials used must be smooth and nonstretchable.

The basic traction frame and the Thomas splint with Pearson attachment are used in balanced suspension traction that is either skin or skeletal (Fig. 10-17). The remaining discussion centers on balanced suspension skeletal traction that is applied for a femoral shaft fracture. When the traction frame and sling apparatus are prepared, the fractured leg is carefully placed into the Thomas splint with the knee in flexion, and the lower leg is supported by the Pearson attachment. After the leg is in place, the sling materials are adjusted so that the heel, popliteal space, tibial tuberosity, and malleoli are free of pressure. The proximal ring of the Thomas splint rests against the ischial tuberosity in the groin.

A Steinmann pin or Kirschner wire is then placed. Both Steinmann pins and Kirschner wires are round stainless steel rods with a point at one or both ends. They are available in smooth or threaded surfaces. The threaded surface has less tendency to slide around and thus is less likely to cause inflammation. A Steinmann pin has a larger diameter than a Kirschner wire, is stronger, and makes a larger tract through the bone.

The site of pin insertion is determined by

the type of injury and desired location to which the traction force is to be applied. Ideally, the pin should pass through only the skin, subcutaneous tissue, and bone. Muscle and tendons are avoided, as well as vital structures such as blood vessels and nerves. The pin or wire is placed in the distal fracture fragment in the metaphysis region of the bone. Although it is generally felt that a traction force should not pull across a joint, some orthopedic surgeons prefer to treat femoral shaft fractures by placing the pin in the proximal tibia. The traction force then does pull across the knee joint; however, a structurally sound knee that has no ligament damage will tolerate the traction. Distal femoral pin placement can cause scarring of the quadiceps muscle [17].

Prior to placement of the pin or wire, the skin must be clean, dry, and free from infection and abrasions. A local anesthetic is used and a small stab wound is made in the skin at the site of entry and exit of the pin. The pin is drilled through the bone perpendicular to the long axis. The drill is removed from the pin, sterile dressings are applied to the pin sites, and the tractor bow is attached. The excess pin or wire is clipped off and the sharp ends are covered with sterile corks, dressing, or adhesive tape. If left exposed, these pin ends can catch on linen or scratch the patient and personnel.

A rope is tied to the tractor bow and is attached to the pulley and weights at the foot of the bed. This exerts the traction force on the bone. The separate balancing system is provided by attaching a rope to the proximal ring of the Thomas splint. The rope leads to an overhead pulley system ending in weights at the head of the bed. Another rope, pulley, and weight system is attached to the distal crossbar of the Thomas splint. The distal crossbar of the Pearson attachment is usually tied to the distal crossbar of the Thomas splint. The weights at the foot and head of the bed are equal. This system then allows the patient to be lifted in bed without disrupting the traction force.

When skeletal traction is used to treat shoulder or humerus fractures, the pin or wire is placed in the olecranon through the elbow joint. There are many vital structures in the area of the distal humerus, making it inadvisable to use this area for pin placement. The arm is placed in flexion with the traction either to the side or to an overhead system of pulleys and weights. It is not possible to establish balanced suspension traction for the upper extremity.

In some settings, immediately following the application of traction, a Polaroid picture is taken and is posted next to the bed to remind those caring for the patient how the position and traction are to be maintained. Treatment of fractures with traction involves follow-up with serial x-rays taken at the bedside to ensure reduction and alignment of the fracture and to note the progress of callus formation.

Nursing Care of the Patient in Traction

Care of the patient in traction involves careful assessment, planning, and implementation to meet the physical and psychosocial needs of the patient. The body part held in traction requires special observations to detect early signs of arterial or venous impairment, nerve impairment, or bone infections at the pin site in skeletal traction. Other complications of traction are thrombophlebitis and foot drop. In addition to the care of the patient, the nurse has responsibility in maintaining the status and integrity of the traction equipment. The nurse must know why the patient is in traction, the type of traction employed, and the position to be maintained. The patient must also know the limitations of motion imposed by the traction.

General nursing measures related to maintaining respiratory function, normal bladder and bowel elimination, adequate fluid and nutritional intake, and relief of sensory deprivation have been discussed previously in this chapter and have equal importance in the care of the patient in traction. Sensory stimulation may need special emphasis, since traction is more confining than previously discussed types of fracture treatment. The patient may be extremely afraid of being held in the bed by the traction equipment. One patient described this fear: "My greatest concern was that there was no way I could get myself out of the skeletal traction in the event there was a fire on the ward. I felt so imprisoned." This fear was very real to this patient. Offering reassurance, being available and concerned, and listening and encouraging the patient to verbalize fears and concerns will foster the patient's psychological comfort.

The patient is usually maintained in a recumbent, supine position for the duration of the traction treatment. This constant position promotes many problems related to pressure and stasis. The coccyx, scapulae, elbows, and heels are constantly submitted to pressure. The use of an air-pressure mattress or synthetic sheepskin under the patient is helpful in relieving pressure but does not replace good skin care and massage. It is possible to turn the patient partially from side to side, carefully supporting the partial turn with pillows under the hip and shoulder to help relieve pressure. Bony prominences need lotion or alcohol massage every 2 to 3 hours. Prevention of skin breakdown is far easier than treating the breakdown after it has occurred.

The patient who is not in balanced-suspension traction poses more problems in management of back care and linen changes than does a patient who is in balanced-supension skin or skeletal traction. Suspension of the affected limb permits freedom of movement of the remainder of the body and facilitates nursing care while maintaining the desired alignment of the affected extremity. Back care and linen change are facilitated by having the patient grasp the trapeze, flex the unaffected leg, and firmly plant his foot on the mattress to assist in raising his body off the mattress. Several persons should assist in this maneuver to facilitate the process and to maintain the suspension system and weights. As the patient raises himself from the bed, the weight lowers and can catch on the bed or touch the floor. A long-handled mirror is helpful to inspect dependent body parts not easily visible. The posterior aspect of the Thomas splint ring as it rests in the gluteal fold needs daily inspection. Pushing down on the mattress with one hand, the nurse can slip the mirror under the patient to inspect areas. A dry, wrinkle-free bed is essential to protecting the skin of the patient in traction.

Any adherent materials applied to skin must be checked for slippage which can cause breakdown of adjacent skin areas. Elastic bandages must be checked frequently. Some experimental studies have been done in which tiny sensors are incorporated into elastic wraps of extremities. It has been found that pressure constriction can occur within 1 hour following their application [17]. Elastic bandages should be rewrapped daily.

In skeletal traction, the pin site is inspected daily for drainage, odor, redness, edema, or any sign that indicates pin tract infection. Usually pin site care and dressing change are performed each day. The entire extremity in skeletal traction is inspected daily using multisensory observation as described under cast care. The nurse should always investigate any complaint of the patient. Peripheral pulses and the temperature gradient between the two legs and feet and the blanching sign are checked frequently. Any numbness, paresthesia, or motor disturbance is reported. Femoral nerve injury can result from pressure to the groin by the Thomas splint. Pressure on the peroneal nerve under the knee, over the fibula head, and at the Achilles tendon can result in inability to flex the foot.

Early active exercises of all nontractioned body parts are imperative. Use of the overbed trapeze helps to maintain a functional upper extremity. The patient's independence in doing the active exercises should be fostered. Isometric exercises such as quadriceps setting can be done on the extremity in traction.

Proper body alignment is necessary to maintain the direction of the pulling force. Shoulders must be kept in straight alignment with the hips. Maintaining the prescribed position of the extremity in traction prevents deformity. Sandbags and pillows are used to hold an extremity in abduction, adduction, or some rotation if prescribed. The Thomas splint–Pearson attachment does have a footboard attachment that can be used to prevent plantar flexion. Elevation of the head of the bed interferes with the effectiveness of the traction, as it changes the direction of the pull. If the patient is in a bed that has a hand-controlled device and he tends to change his own position, the bed may need to be unplugged from the electrical wall outlet.

A traction frame should be attached with the bed in low position. Following application of the frame to the bed, the bed can then be raised to high position to facilitate care of the patient. If the traction frame is attached to the bed in the high position, at some later time someone may lower the bed without checking the placement of the vertical bars. As the bed lowers, the vertical bars may touch the floor before the low position is reached, causing the traction frame to dislodge from the bed. This causes total disruption of the traction forces and can be devastating to the patient.

The prescribed amount of weight is effective only when the weights are secure in the carrier, are hanging free, and are not in contact with the bed, floor, or equipment. Weights are never removed or changed without specific instructions. The countertraction that was initially established must be maintained.

All ropes should be secured with nonslip knots that are then taped. Ropes must be in the grooves of the pulleys and not touching each other, the patient, the bed, the linen, or the traction frame. The efficiency of the traction is reduced if the ropes are not free and if the spreader rests on the bed or against a pulley. Pulleys and all clamps on the frame must be checked periodically. A frozen pulley does not allow the rope to glide through it smoothly. Frayed rope or frozen pulleys must be replaced.

In summary, when traction is used to treat a fracture, the mechanical aspects must remain functional and the pull must be continuous to maintain the reduction. Anything that interferes with the rope, pulleys, and weights, or removal of the traction before bony union occurs, defeats the purpose of the treatment. The physician may adjust the direction of pull or the amount of weight based on the serial x-ray findings. When bony union occurs and the traction is discontinued, the patient progresses to an active rehabilitation program. Following 6 to 8 weeks in bed, the patient may have problems with orthostatic hypotension. Careful evaluation of the patient's transfer and mobility tolerance is imperative. The fractured limb needs protection for some time. Weight-bearing is delayed until more complete healing occurs.

Rheumatic Diseases

The Arthritis Foundation lists about one hundred diseases under the combined heading of arthritis and rheumatism. The term **arthritis** indicates inflammation and destruction of joints, specifically their lining. **Rheumatism,** a more general term, usually indicates symptoms that arise from tissue outside the joints, such as muscles, tendons, bones, and nerves. Most of these diseases stem from two major causes: (1) **degeneration,** which is the result of use and aging, and (2) **inflammation,** which can be exudative, proliferative, localized, or a manifestation of systemic disease.

Among the major categories of arthritis and rheumatism are arthritis of unknown causes, such as rheumatoid arthritis and ankylosing spondylitis; degenerative joint disease, osteoarthritis; connective tissue disorders, such as systemic lupus erythematosus; infectious arthritis; traumatic arthritis; and arthritis associated with errors in metabolism, such as gout. Each is a distinct disease entity not sharing common etiology or pathogenesis. All have one feature in common, however—joint dysfunction and disability. Differential diagnosis can be difficult in the early stages of some of the arthritic diseases. The two most common forms of arthritis are osteoarthritis and rheumatoid arthritis.

DEGENERATIVE JOINT DISEASE (OSTEOARTHRITIS)

Osteoarthritis is the most common of all forms of arthritis, afflicting about 40 million persons in the United States. Only about 10 percent of this group are significantly incapacitated by the joint changes. It occurs after age 50 and affects women more than men. Aging is perhaps the single most important factor in the development of osteoarthritis, which is almost as inevitable as wrinkling of the skin, greying of the hair, and other physiologic changes that occur with aging.

The two basic alterations in joints in osteoarthritis are degeneration of the articular cartilage and new bone formation. Currently the term **degenerative joint disease** is becoming more widely employed for osteoarthritis. It is also called hypertrophic osteoarthritis and degenerative arthritis.

There are two general theories about the causation of osteoarthritis. Mechanical stress to joints results from a combination of aging, chronic irritation, and normal wear and tear. Chronic irritation may come from excess weight, poor posture, previous trauma, or mechanical strain from one's occupation or recreation. Trauma to joints at an earlier age may lead to a period of joint edema, swelling, congestion, stiffness, and pain. If there has been no structural damage, healing is rapid and complete, as joints have a good blood supply, whereas early structural damage to joints can provoke osteoporosis in later years.

Biochemical factors implicated are heredity, metabolic factors, and endocrine factors. There appears to be an increased incidence of

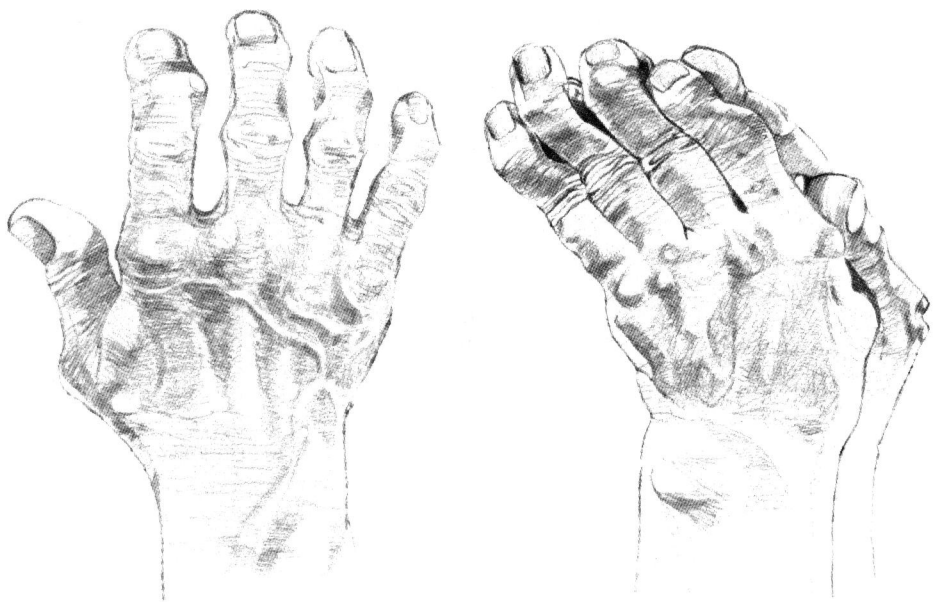

Figure 10-18
Comparing the hands in osteoarthritis and rheumatoid arthritis. In osteoarthritis, the distal interphalangeal joints are characteristically involved, with the bony enlargements called Heberden's nodes. In rheumatoid arthritis, there is ulnar deviation of the fingers and swelling of the knuckles; the proximal interphalangeal joints can be seen.

osteoarthritis in women as they reach menopause. Endocrine and metabolic alterations weaken joint cartilage. Persons with acromegaly have bony overgrowth which, when occurring in joints, interferes with function. It is believed that a combination of mechanical and biochemical factors contributes to the development of osteoarthritis.

Osteoarthritis is a disease of articular cartilage in contrast to rheumatoid arthritis, which attacks the synovial membrane of joints. It is a noninflammatory localized process and most often affects the weight-bearing joints of the lower extremity and lumbar spine, although other joints can be involved. There is asymmetrical joint involvement.

Osteoarthritis appears first in that part of the articular cartilage that receives the greatest wear and tear and has the poorest nutrition. Cartilage is a tissue that normally has limited ability to repair itself. With aging, cartilage loses its water content and its elasticity and softens. The fibers of the cartilage begin to separate, fissure, and fray. As the cartilage thins and wears away, the underlying bone is stimulated to grow. New bone forms on the articular surface causing bone spurs (osteophytes) and lipping, resulting in mechanical interference with joint function. In later stages, bone contacting bone is the source of much pain and limited motion. Synovitis is usually not present, unless late in the disease; the roughened cartilage and bone cause irritation that results in synovitis. The periarticular structures are not involved directly by the disease process, but the pain and restricted motion result in muscle spasm and contractures.

A classic manifestation of osteoarthritis is the development of bony nodules on the dorsolateral aspects of the distal finger joints. These are called Heberden's nodes and are considered to be familial. These nodes are permanent and can cause some flexion and deviation deformities. Figure 10-18 compares hand changes in rheumatoid arthritis and osteoarthritis.

Persons who present with osteoarthritis are usually in general good health. The most common clinical manifestation is joint pain and stiffness that is aggravated by use and relieved by rest. Temperature and humidity changes and weight-bearing also aggravate the symptoms. There may be tenderness on palpation and objectively the joints appear normal except for bony enlargement. There may be crepitus on motion resulting from bone spurs.

Synovial fluid aspiration and analysis reveal no pathology. Serologic tests are normal or negative. X-ray reveals narrowing of joint spaces surrounding bony sclerosis and the bone spur formation. When the vertebral column is involved, the spaces between the vertebrae narrow, causing painful and restricted motion. There may be pressure on nerve roots, resulting in motor weakness and paresthesia along the nerve segments involved.

The treatment for osteoarthritis is chiefly aimed at relief of symptoms and includes a combination of physical therapy, drug therapy, and surgery. Weight reduction, if indicated, reduces the strain on the weight-bearing joints. Joint replacement and reconstructive surgery in treatment of severe osteoarthritis were discussed earlier in the chapter.

The physical therapy is aimed at relief of joint and periarticular pain and stiffness and preserving the normal joint structure and function through exercise, application of heat, and massage. The Hubbard tank is useful for generalized symptoms. Short-wave diathermy to the knees, and ultrasound to the lumbar spine help to relieve pain and stiffness. Pain in the hands is relieved by paraffin or contrast baths. With contrast baths, the hands are placed in warm water for 4 minutes and in cold water for 1 minute, for a 15-minute period. Massage following the heat application helps to relax muscles and facilitates the exercise program [16].

Exercises are done to maintain range of motion and muscle strength. Stretching a joint capsule relieves an early contracture as well as pain. Isometric exercises help to strengthen muscles. The exercise program is individualized to each person's particular needs.

Both systemic and local drug therapy are used. Drugs bring about symptomatic relief and do not alter the course or outcome of the disease. Analgesics, sedatives, and muscle relaxants are part of the drug program. Acetylsalicylic acid (aspirin) is the most effective drug, since it has analgesic and anti-inflammatory properties. If the person cannot tolerate salicylates, indomethacin (Indocin) and phenylbutazone (Butazolidin) may be given. These drugs also have analgesic and anti-inflammatory properties. A short course of either of these latter two drugs is given for a week or 10 days. If ineffective after this period of time, they are most likely to remain ineffective. The adverse affects of indomethacin (Indocin) are nausea, vomiting, headache, and dizziness. Phenylbutazone (Butazolidin) has similar side effects and, in addition, can depress bone marrow.

Muscle relaxants used include such drugs as methocarbamol (Robaxin), diazepam (Valium), and meprobamate (Equanil). Reduction of muscle spasm also facilitates the exercise program. Local drug therapy includes the intra-articular injection of corticosteroids in selected joints such as the hip and knee. These injections help control symptoms of inflammation that may develop in a contracted joint. Local injection produces no systemic side effects.

Nursing care of the osteoarthritic patient may involve many aspects of geriatric nursing, since many of these patients are elderly. The patients' understanding and cooperation are needed in the weight reduction, modification of activity, and home exercise programs. The importance of taking the prescribed medications must be stressed. The patient should know the possible side effects of the drugs.

Canes, crutches, and special orthopedic shoes may be prescribed to relieve weight on joints. The patient may need to learn proper body mechanics and avoid heavy lifting or carrying heavy loads. Patient teaching becomes a very important aspect in the care of these patients. Nursing care following constructive surgery has already been discussed.

OSTEOPOROSIS

Osteoporosis is the most common systemic condition of the bony skeleton characterized by a reduction in bone mass. Bone resorption (mineral and matrix) outstrips bone accretion. One-fourth of all persons aged 50 to 70 are affected by the condition, which occurs in women four times more frequently than in men. The majority of patients of advancing age do not demonstrate underlying causes of osteoporosis; however, several causes have been identified: defects in osteoblasts result from the decreased stress and strain normally caused by physical activity and muscle contraction and loss of estrogens and androgens; defects in the bone matrix caused by excess (catabolic) glucocorticoids, which can be intrinsic (Cushing's disease), or a result of extrinsic administration; defects in metabolism of protein, calcium, and phosphorus. Bone marrow disorders, hyperparathyroidism, and hyperthyroidism are also associated with the development of osteoporosis. Disuse osteoporosis can develop with prolonged immobilization or bed rest. Osteoporosis that develops with advanced age is for the most part idiopathic and is termed **postmenopausal** and **senile osteoporosis** [23, 26].

Clinically, at least 30 percent of bone density is lost before changes are evident on x-ray. Osteoporotic bone appears moth-eaten and spongy, with a loss of cortical bone and enlarged medullary cavities on x-ray. Vertebrae appear concave. The bone cortex is brittle and lightweight. Serum calcium, phosphorus, and alkaline phosphatase levels are normal.

Patients with osteoporosis have pain and may feel insecure in walking. There is loss in body stature as a result of vertebral changes. The bone tissue loses its density; tensile strength leads to mechanical failure and very slight trauma can lead to fractures. Common sites of fractures are the proximal femur, the vertebrae, ribs, and distal radius.

The goal of treatment is to increase efforts to stimulate bone accretion and other factors needed for connective tissue synthesis. Physical activity and exercise provide the mechanical stimulus of stress needed for bone-building. Adequate nutrition with protein, minerals, and vitamins is essential. Replacement hormone therapy with estrogens and androgens has been of value.

RHEUMATOID ARTHRITIS

Rheumatoid arthritis is the most disabling of the various types of arthritis. It is a chronic diffuse connective tissue disease primarily affecting joint capsules and synovial membranes. Connective tissues of the body include membranes, tendons, ligaments, bone, and cartilage; thus systemically, there may be involvement of many other tissues in the blood vessels, heart, lungs, eyes, skin, muscle, and peripheral nerves. Rheumatoid arthritis causes a progressive disabling polyarthritis of the small peripheral joints of the hands and feet, advancing to the knees, wrists, elbows, shoulders, and hips in order of frequency. Typical joint involvement is bilaterally symmetrical. Rheumatoid arthritis affects about 3 percent of the general population, and about 10 percent of these persons are severely incapacitated. It affects women three times more than men, and occurs in all parts of the world. The onset usually occurs between ages 35 to 50; however, all ages are susceptible.

Diagnosing rheumatoid arthritis must be considered in the context of the many variants of rheumatoid arthritis and the many connective tissue disorders that can simulate it. Connective tissue diseases are characterized by a nonpurulent inflammatory process that primarily affects the soft connective tissue of joints and the periarticular connective tissues. In addition to rheumatoid arthritis, other connective tissue diseases are systemic lupus erythematosus, rheumatic fever, polyarteritis nodosa, scleroderma (progressive systemic sclerosis), and polymyositis/dermatomyositis. Although a common pathologic process is not clear, pathologic changes are similar in all these diffuse connective tissue diseases; however, the clinical features differ according to the organ systems affected. Because there may be overlapping symptoms, related conditions must be ruled out through objective and subjective findings, laboratory data, and x-rays.

The cause of rheumatoid arthritis is unknown. Currently, causation is ascribed to two related theories. One theory holds that rheumatoid arthritis is an autoimmune disease. The body, for unknown reasons, produces antibodies directed against its own tissues. The pathology of rheumatoid arthritis can be proliferative (synovitis, serositis, uveitis); necrotizing (nodules); or vascular (vascularitis). These are changes that occur in any known immunologic reaction and in connective tissue diseases [26].

Part of the supporting evidence of this concept is the abnormally high level of certain gamma globulins, resembling antibodies, that are present in the blood serum of about 80 to 95 percent of patients with rheumatoid arthritis. Rheumatoid factors are thought to be antibodies to self antigen-antibody complexes. The rheumatoid factor (RF) is detected by specific tests: latex fixation, the bentonite flocculation test, and sensitized sheep erythrocyte agglutination test. The serum titer of RF is most elevated in patients with severe disease and widespread involvement [26]. In the latex fixation test, the patient's serum will cause latex particles coated with human gamma globulin to clump together. There are times when the RF is present in joint fluid and tissue analysis before it is detected by serum serologic tests. RF has been identified in low titer in asymptomatic relatives of the patient. It is also found in other connective tissue disorders and in nonarthritic conditions [26].

The second theory supports an infectious process as the triggering mechanism. Streptococci, diphtheroids, mycoplasma, and viruses have been implicated. Experimental work done with mycoplasma has produced rheumatoid arthritis-like conditions in animals. The infectious theory may overlap with the autoimmune theory in that the infection could provoke the development of the autoantibodies [12].

Efforts to determine the cause of rheumatoid arthritis have also included investigation of nutritional excesses or deficiencies, metabolic abnormalities, and hormonal imbalance as possible sources of etiology. No conclusive evidence has been established from these investigations. Factors such as climate, heredity, and emotional stress have also been studied. Climate and heredity have been discredited as causative factors [12].

There has been some evidence that a series of stressful life events may precipitate the onset of rheumatoid arthritis. Some research studies have implied that such personality factors as inability to express anger, aggression, and lack of autonomy may be associated with the development of rheumatoid arthritis; however, these factors exist in persons who do not have rheumatoid arthritis. In order to identify personality and psychological factors as a cause-effect relationship to rheumatoid arthritis, one would need predictive studies that correlate psychological data to biologic variables such as the RF. These would need to be longitudinal studies. Most of the studies done in this area to date have been retrospective. It has been suggested that people with rheumatoid arthritis have high degrees of anxiety and depression; however, this is also true of other disabled persons. These factors could be secondary to development of the disease. To date there has been no psychological component identified that is specific to people with rheumatoid arthritis [18].

Although the cause remains obscure, the physiologic alterations are well understood. Rheumatoid arthritis joint pathology involves four stages that are in progress for months to years, and the symptoms are characterized by unpredictable spontaneous exacerbations and remissions. The four stages are synovitis, pannus formation, fibrous ankylosis, and bony ankylosis. There is accompanying osteoporosis of the bone.

The synovitis is chronic, proliferative, and nonpurulent. The synovial lining of the affected joints becomes inflamed, edematous, and invaded by polymorphonuclear leukocytes, lymphocytes, and plasma cells. The synovial membrane becomes greatly thickened, nodular, and hyperemic as a result of the invading granulation cells. This is called pannus, and it extends over the surface of the articular cartilage. In time, the pannus and inflammatory reaction produce lysosomal enzymes that erode articular cartilage and underlying bone. Joint motion can cause disruption of the pannus, and bleeding occurs into the joint space. Adhesions, which form between the layers of pannus, eventually progress to fibrous ankylosis and then to bony ankylosis. The joint is stiff and contracted most often in a nonfunctional position [22, 25].

The synovial fluid undergoes changes as the architecture of the joint changes. Synovial membrane permeability changes and synovial fluid volume increases, viscosity decreases, and the fluid is cloudy. The leukocytes (neutrophils) and gamma globulin are increased. Cells aspirated from the synovial cavities contain aggregates of rheumatoid factor.

Other body connective tissue is also invaded by the lymphocytes and plasma cells. Subcutaneous fibrous nodules occur near and around the joints. They can cause pressure and pain. Systemic muscle pain, stiffness, tenderness, and paresthesia result from other foci of inflammatory cells that develop throughout fibrous tissue. When these occur around periarticular structures, the joint capsule develops an elastic stiffness as opposed to a frictional stiffness. Sometimes this is termed **secondary fibrositis** and presents the same symptoms as primary fibrositis that is not related to arthritis. Fibrous tissue is stiff and achy when cold and after rest. This represents the common subjective symptom of "morning stiffness" that is relieved with gradual joint motion and warmth.

Fibrous tissue changes also account for the other systemic manifestations of rheumatoid arthritis such as vascularitis, which predisposes the patient to thrombosis and pericarditis. Fibrosis and nodules can develop in the lung. The eye can reveal uveitis and keratoconjunctivitis [25].

Laboratory tests show anemia, leukocytosis, elevated erythrocyte sedimentation rate (ESR), and positive rheumatoid factor. Blood cultures and cultures of synovial fluid are negative. X-ray early in the disease reveals periarticular osteoporosis and surface erosion in the joints. Later x-rays reveal loss of joint space, subluxation, and ankylosis [15].

Rheumatoid arthritis is usually insidious in onset with prodromal symptoms of fatigue, irritability, low-grade fever, malaise, weight loss, weakness, numbness and tingling of the hands and feet, and occasionally a period of physical and emotional stress. The patient appears chronically ill, and the symmetrically involved joints are tender, swollen, warm to touch, painful, and have limited motion. The hands are cold and clammy and the overlying skin is shiny, red, and atrophic in appearance. As the disease progresses, the fingers and wrists show ulnar deviation, flexion contractures, and muscle atrophy.

If the joints and surrounding tissue are inflamed, there is greater disability. Irritation and pain limit muscle strength and contraction, and may precipitate muscle spasm. The progressive joint destruction leads to muscle atrophy and much functional impairment. In the hands, this means the person loses small fine movement and cannot grasp things. In the wrists, flexion and extension are lost and the person cannot position his or her hands. In the elbows, motions used in feeding and grooming are impaired and the person cannot lift things. The person cannot dress himself or herself in addition to having the just-mentioned deficits. When the lower extremity is involved, the legs cannot serve as levers to lift the body and the person cannot rise from a seated position; he ambulates with great difficulty and has impaired ability to go up and down stairs [12].

The treatment of rheumatoid arthritis is directed toward the primary inflammatory process, with relief of pain as a goal. The treatment plan is directed toward preserving function and preventing and correcting deformities. The therapy includes drugs, rest, exercise, physical therapy, occupational therapy, and orthopedic devices and surgery. A coordinated team approach by the various disciplines is necessary to tailor the treatment plan for each patient.

Adequate rest is absolutely essential. Complete bed rest is needed during acute stages of the disease. At other times, it is recommended that the person have 10 hours of sleep at night and one or two daytime rest periods on a firm bed. Rest is therapy, as it helps to avoid excess fatigue, which can aggravate symptoms. A well-balanced diet is needed to maintain good nutrition and to combat weight loss. Being overweight adds excess stress to weight-bearing joints [24].

The physical therapy program includes heat applications, Hubbard tank, and whirlpool therapy to reduce pain and stiffness, thereby facilitating the exercise program. Exercising in a pool is helpful, as the buoyancy of water reduces stress on joints. The hydrotherapies are useful early in the morning to reduce the stiffness. The exercise program includes range-of-motion, strengthening, and endurance exercises. Some rheumatologists prefer complete rest with no exercise during acute exacerbations. Studies have shown that complete immobilization of joints for 2 or 3 weeks does not result in permanent stiffness [10, 24]. Others prescribe range-of-motion exercises to the point of pain during the acute episodes. Isometric and isotonic muscle-strengthening exercises are used on the lower extremities. Endurance exercises of the mild resistive type are used on the upper extremities. Strong resistive exercises can cause joint subluxation or other injury.

Paraffin baths and contrast baths are used on the hands. Some persons get more relief from pain and stiffness with the application of cold, and may hold some frozen item from the freezer in their hands for a few minutes to relieve stiffness. Cold acts as a local anesthetic and thus helps relieve pain.

A balanced program must be developed for each person, as rest helps to decrease pain, tenderness, swelling, and effusion of synovial membrane. All these are aggravated by activity, whereas guarded and progressive activity is needed to prevent disease phenomena from developing in the periarticular structures. Thus, rest helps to correct some problems and activity is needed to correct others.

Orthopedic devices such as splints, braces, serial casts, and cervical collars are used to increase the patient's independence and productivity while protecting affected joints. These devices are also used to correct existing flexion contractures and are prescribed to be worn during rest periods. Knee and hip flexion contractures can be helped by having the patient lie prone for certain periods of time. The patient should be taught to shift position periodically whether in bed or chair. Placing pillows under the knees fosters quadriceps wasting and flexion deformities. Fingers should be horizontal with the wrists while at rest. Knee and wrist splints may be worn at rest to maintain functional positioning. Shoes with metatarsal bars help to distribute weight-bearing stresses more equally over the foot.

Occupational therapy helps the patient with the necessary adaptations in activities of daily living. Various self-help devices such as long shoe horns, thick-handled eating utensils, raised toilet seats, grab bars, and shower seats can be utilized.

Orthopedic surgery is no longer considered a last resort. A **synovectomy** can be done to remove the synovial tissue. An **arthroplasty** removes enlarged and deformed bone. An **arthrodesis** may be done to fuse an unstable joint which is then stiff, but stable, pain-free, and usable.

Drug therapy includes the salicylates, analgesics, tranquilizers, muscle relaxants, cortisone, gold compounds, antimalarial agents, and immunosuppressive drugs.

Acetylsalicylic acid (aspirin) is the most widely used and most effective drug therapy. It has analgesic, anti-inflammatory, and antipyretic properties. It is relatively safe, nonaddictive, and inexpensive. Dosage is based on the patient's individual response and serum drug levels. A daily dosage to maintain a salicylate plasma level of 15 mg per 100 ml, or just below toxic level, is optimal. This may require up to twenty-five 5-grain tablets per day. Salicylates disappear from the plasma in 5 to 9 hours; thus dosage time must provide adequate coverage [24]. A late-night and early-morning dose is recommended. It must be impressed upon the patient that the aspirin must be taken during remissions as well as exacerbations of the disease. If tinnitus or hearing loss develop as side effects, dosage is usually decreased by 10 to 15 grains per day until those symptoms disappear. Gastric irritation from the aspirin can be reduced by taking the drug with milk or an antacid or right after meals. The patient should also be alerted to the bleeding complications that can occur with such high doses of aspirin. Acetaminophen (Tylenol), which also has analgesic and antipyretic properties, is not as desirable in the treatment plan, since it does not possess anti-inflammatory properties.

Propoxyphene hydrochloride (Darvon), Percodan, codeine, or other narcotics may be needed as analgesics during acute episodes; however, the use of narcotic drugs is discouraged in chronic conditions because of their addictive properties.

Phenylbutazone (Butazolidin and Tandearil) and indomethacin (Indocin) are also helpful as analgesics and anti-inflammatory agents. These drugs often bring about dramatic relief of the pain and stiffness, but they must be used under close supervision, as they have serious side effects.

Various tranquilizers and mood elevators may be employed to combat the anxiety and depression experienced by the patient. Many of these drugs also serve as skeletal muscle relaxants.

Usually the pain, range of motion, and muscle atrophy can be controlled by the conservative approach of salicylates and physical therapy. If these measures fail, cortisone drugs may be employed. Cortisone, its derivatives, or ACTH can be given systemically or via intra-articular injections. Its use brings about dramatic relief in symptoms; however, the use of cortisone is not without side effects. Some of the side effects are peptic ulcer development, moon face, and edema, and it can mask symptoms of infection.

Systemic cortisone can enhance osteoporosis, which may already be present, and predispose the patient to spontaneous fractures. Since cortisone does have such a dramatic effect on the relief of both local and systemic symptoms of rheumatoid arthritis, some investigators felt that adrenal disease or improper body utilization of adrenal hormones had a role in the development of rheumatoid arthritis. No supporting evidence was found, as when cortisone therapy is stopped, the disease progresses.

Gold compounds given by deep intramuscular injection and antimalarial drugs both have antirheumatic effects but take a number of weeks to develop results. The use of immunosuppressive drugs is thought to diminish production of antibodies at the cellular level.

The nursing care of the patient with rheumatoid arthritis involves several major goals: arrest of the disease process and control of pain through the administration of prescribed drugs; helping the patient and family adjust economically and emotionally to a chronic illness; assisting in the prevention and correction of deformities; and fostering the patient's physical and emotional involvement in the therapeutic plan.

Rheumatoid arthritis patients may not have a lot of faith in aspirin as the drug of choice. Much support and encouragement may be needed to gain the patient's cooperation in the drug program, to help him to recognize side effects, and to assume responsibility for proper self-medication. The patient must be alerted to the potential dangers of self-medication with over-the-counter drugs in addition to prescribed medications. Arthritic patients may fall prey to quackery promises of miracle drugs and total-cure devices. Patient education regarding activities, drug therapy, and exercise programs is imperative.

The psychological adaptation to a prolonged and recurring illness is not an easy task. Encouraging expressions of fear, hostility, and discouragement by the patient and family is necessary. Although cure is not possible, many patients can continue functional living with treatment. Allowing the patient to make decisions about his or her care schedule and fostering independence in activities of daily living can be morale-boosters.

General nursing measures to promote rest and comfort are important. The febrile patient needs good skin care and frequent linen changes. A firm mattress is necessary. A bed cradle will keep the weight of bed covers off the tender joints. The nurse should avoid hurried, jerky handling of extremities. All joints should be carefully supported and the patient should be advised of all movements before the nurse does them. Good body alignment is necessary to maintain functional position of all joints. This means judicious use of pillows: a small pillow under the head and none under the knees. The patient may have some previous habits with the use of pillows that need to be unlearned. When he or she is allowed up, a straight chair is better for joint function than a soft padded chair. It is also easier for the patient to sit down and to get up from a straight-back chair.

Application of splints and follow-through on the exercise program are also part of the nursing care. There should be three to four exercise periods a day with the goal in mind that the patient becomes independent in these by the time he or she is discharged. It is helpful if exercise periods are preceded and followed by periods of rest. Self-help devices are prescribed and should be at the bedside.

Teaching about proper nutrition and weight reduction may be necessary in individual cases. Dietary fads are part of the quackery approach to arthritis. No food has been known either to cause or cure rheumatoid arthritis.

Upon discharge, home visits by a visiting nurse, physical therapist, and occupational therapist are desirable for ongoing evaluation. There may be suggestions for alterations in the environment that would save energy for the patient; or different self-help devices may be beneficial. Since the patients with rheumatoid arthritis have difficulty in closing their hands to grasp and lift things, they should be taught to use the palms of their hands instead of their fingers. A variety of household activities can be analyzed and adaptations made in which larger and stronger muscle groups are utilized. The diet, medication, rest, and exercise programs can be reevaluated. In addition, the rheumatoid arthritic patient needs regular medical supervision and evaluation.

Rheumatic fever is a self-limiting local process that is characterized by acute inflammation of articular synovia, tendon sheaths, tendons, and other connective tissue about the joints. Rheumatic fever follows a streptococcal throat infection. It is a migratory polyarthritis that may simulate rheumatoid arthritis in initial intense joint symptoms of pain, warmth, swelling, and limited motion. These symptoms subside after a short period. Pannus does not form; cartilage and bone damage do not occur; and when the disease process subsides, there is no residual joint dysfunction.

Systemic lupus erythematosus (SLE) is a chronic diffuse connective tissue disease with joint pathology similar to rheumatoid arthritis, but less severe joint manifestations. It attacks body viscera more extensively, especially the kidneys. A butterfly skin rash can occur. SLE is a rare disease that predominantly affects young females. Serologic studies reveal the presence of lupus erythematosus cells, which aids in the differential diagnosis [12].

Bursitis is another condition that may need to be differentiated from rheumatoid arthritis. Bursae are sac-like cavities that are found between two soft-tissue layers which move upon each other. These bursae are filled with fluid that serves to pad and cushion joints. Bursitis results from repeated trauma, friction, and irritation. The joint is swollen, painful, and has restricted motion. When bursitis occurs at the shoulder joint, it is called "frozen shoulder." Other joints that can become involved are the elbow, hips, knees, and ankles. Rest of the affected part, heat application, and analgesics relieve the symptoms. If an occupational or recreational stress causes repeated bursitis, a change in life style may be indicated. A swelling and thickening of the walls of the bursae of the great toe result in a bunion.

GOUT

Gout is an inflammatory type of arthritis caused by the deposits of sodium urate crystals in and about joints, the cartilage, epiphyseal bone, and periarticular structures. Classic, primary gout results from errors in purine metabolism that lead to excessive uric acid levels. Normal uric acid concentration is less than 5 mg per 100 ml of serum. Acute gout is manifested by a rapid onset of severe, painful inflamed joints. It can be monoarticular or polyarticular. The joint most frequently affected is the great toe; however, the fingers, hands, toes, knees, and elbows may be involved. The disease has a familial tendency; it affects males 20 times more than females; and its onset usually occurs past age 30. If females are afflicted, it occurs postmenopause.

The hyperuricemia is caused by a combination of abnormal metabolic degradation of purines and decreased urinary excretion of urates. The excessive circulating urate crystals (uric acid) precipitate into the periarticular structures. A synovitis develops as phagocytes attempt to ingest the foreign crystals. This process is accompanied by an increased local anaerobic metabolism and the development of lactic acid, which causes the synovial cavity pH to drop. Because of the lowered pH, more urate crystals are deposited, more leukocytes enter, and the cycle continues. The inflammatory process results in a red, warm, swollen, and painful joint. Some of the crystals are so large that the phagocytes cannot engulf them; lysosomal enzymes are spilled into the joint cavity where they can attack joint surfaces.

Chronic, recurring gout is manifested by deforming joint changes, renal calculi, and subcutaneous urate crystal deposits called tophi.

The appearance of urate crystals in aspirated synovial fluid is a positive diagnostic criterion. The presence of the subcutaneous and osseous urate tophi is another diagnostic criterion. Other factors that aid in diagnosis are the very rapid onset of joint symptoms; a serum uric acid above 7 mg per 100 ml; and the complete relief of symptoms within 24 to 48 hours after the drug colchicine is initiated. Nongouty types of arthritis do not respond to colchicine. It is felt that colchicine acts by disrupting the leukocyte activity in the inflammatory cycle just described. When the acute onset subsides, the joint returns to normal anatomic and functional status.

An attack of gout can result from hyperuricemia related to recent surgery, leukemia, antineoplastic durgs, thiazide diuretics, recent ingestion of purine-rich foods (glandular and red meats), and excess alcohol intake. Acute infection and emotional trauma have also been linked to an acute onset of gout.

In addition to the elevated serum uric acid level, the erythrocyte sedimentation rate is also elevated. The complete blood count is normal, and RF and LE tests are negative. X-rays reveal soft-tissue swelling and a "punched-out" type of erosion near joints resulting from the soft-tissue swelling.

During an acute attack of gout, colchicine 0.5 or 0.6 mg can be given every hour until the attack subsides. Gastric irritation, nausea, vomiting, and diarrhea may develop. Since uninterrupted colchicine therapy is essential, the drug can be given intravenously every 3 to 6 hours instead of orally. Prophylactic colchicine is given on a daily basis to gout-prone persons. In addition to colchicine, a uricosuric agent such as probenecid (Benemid) is given. This drug facilitates excretion of uric acid by the proximal tubule of the kidney. Uric acid is more soluble in alkaline urine. If the uricosuric agent is not tolerated or is not effective, allopurinol (Zyloprim), which inhibits uric acid synthesis, can be used. These drugs are meant to sustain lower plasma urate concentration [4].

Salicylates, analgesics, phenylbutazone, and indomethacin may also be used for the same reasons they are used in other types of arthritis. It is felt that salicylates also help in the excretion of uric acid.

In addition to drug therapy, the patient is usually on bed rest to rest the inflamed part. Weight of the covers should be kept off the inflamed joint. Application of heat or cold may be helpful. A low-fat, low-purine diet is prescribed and abundant oral fluids are needed to flush the urate salts from the kidneys.

There is a condition similar to gout called pseudogout, in which calcium pyrophosphate crystals are found in the synovial fluid. Pseudogout, which presents with joint inflammation affecting larger joints, does not respond to colchicine [15].

INFECTIOUS ARTHRITIS

Infectious arthritis usually develops secondary to a bacteremia or adjacent osteomyelitis. It can be a primary infection resulting from a direct wound to a joint. Its onset and course resemble the other inflammatory types of arthritis; however, culture of joint fluid demonstrates the pathogenic organisms. Appropriate massive antibiotic therapy is then instituted according to sensitivity tests. An infectious process within a joint destroys articular cartilage and, if prolonged, can result in fibrous ankylosis of the affected joint. Other aspects of the treatment are aimed at the initial systemic infection, reducing joint pain and preserving joint function.

OSTEOMALACIA

Osteomalacia is a failure of bone matrix to calcify in the adult, and it involves the factors that affect osteogenesis previously discussed in this chapter. Bone matrix is adequate, but the mineralization process is abnormally prolonged. X-ray findings resemble those found in osteoporosis; however, bones affected by osteomalacia become soft, flattened, and deformed. There is usually a low serum calcium and low serum phosphorus and high serum alkaline phosphatase. The blood levels help to differentiate osteomalacia from osteoporosis [25].

In addition to the x-ray and laboratory findings, the patient has bone pain and tenderness. Spontaneous and pathologic fractures occur as in osteoporosis.

Several causes of osteomalacia have been identified. Deficient intake of vitamin D is a cause; in the adult it is most often caused by malabsorption problems such as seen in sprue. A second cause relates to chronic renal problems and chronic hypophosphatemia. A third cause can be fluoride or strontium intoxication. The skeletal changes in all three causes are not distinguishable from each other [25].

Treatment includes eliminating the cause, if possible, and prescribing a well-balanced diet, with calcium and phosphorus supplements. Currently, progress is also being made with the use of synthetic vitamin D.

OSTEOMYELITIS

Osteomyelitis is a bone infection caused by pyrogenic microorganisms. In the adult, *Staphylococcus aureus* is the most frequent causative organism, and it tends to remain intramedullary. The bone is involved secondary to this with spread to cancellous bone, and then cortical bone. When the suppuration reaches the periosteum, it erodes and a soft-tissue abscess appears. Osteomyelitis can be acute and localized or it can progress to a chronic state. If the infection progresses to the bone itself, the bone becomes necrotic and harbors the infection, retarding healing. Necrotic bone becomes a potential source of reinfection. This necrotic bone can be separated from sound bone, and the dead bone is called sequestrium. Bone has limited ability to resorb necrotic tissue and thus walls it off.

Osteomyelitis can result from direct bone infection which can occur with compound fractures; the infection can be blood-borne unrelated to trauma or it can be an extension from adjacent structures. Local symptoms include pain, tenderness over the bone, heat, redness, and restricted movement. Systemically, fever, chills, rapid pulse, leukocytosis, elevated erythrocyte sedimentation rate and, possibly, positive blood cultures are associated with osteomyelitis. Early recognition and treatment are very important if the chronic state is to be avoided.

Treatment includes bedrest, with immobilization of the involved part. Joints must be handled carefully and gently. A cast or splint can be used to immobilize a part, and a bed cradle will keep linen and pressure off the part. Surgery can be done for incision and drainage of the area or a sequestrectomy (removal of the sequestrum). Both local and systemic antibiotic therapy are used. Continuous-drip antibiotic instillation into the wound may be indicated. If drug-resistant organisms develop, the condition is very difficult to treat.

Amputations

An amputation is the removal of all or part of an extremity. When the extremity is removed by resection through a joint, the amputation is referred to as a **disarticulation.** The three major causes of amputation are those that result from trauma or the complications of trauma, a life-saving measure to arrest a disease process, and congenital defects.

Electrical, thermal, or chemical burns; freezing; and misuse of power tools can result in traumatic or accidental amputations. Accidents with automobiles, farm machinery, and firearms can also result in loss of a limb. Although newer surgical methods of blood vessel and nerve repair make it possible to save limbs injured by trauma, amputation is done when it is impossible to restore a blood supply sufficient for healing to occur. Following a severe fracture, there may be no union of bones or the nerve supply may be permanently disrupted. In these cases, amputation may be done to replace the nonfunctional extremity with a functional prosthesis.

Peripheral vascular disease, cancer, and infection are the disease processes that can result in amputation. Arteriosclerosis, diabetes mellitus, and Buerger's disease are implicated in the vascular diseases and account for the largest number of elective lower-extremity amputations.

In peripheral vascular disease, an inadequate blood supply prohibits the cells from meeting their nutritional needs. The leg, being farthest from the heart, has the lowest blood pressure of any part of the body; thus, blood flow can be easily compromised. One condition that absolutely demands amputation is the loss of blood supply to an extremity, with the resultant toxic products of tissue destruction causing systemic illness. Diminished blood supply to the lower extremity can result in infection, gangrene, and ischemia. The ischemic pain is unrelieved by rest, position, or medication. Vascular reconstructive surgery, and sometimes sympathectomy procedures, may be attempted prior to considering amputation. It is the elderly person who is most affected by occlusive vascular disease, which can be a generalized body process eventually affecting the total rehabilitation following amputation.

Both the upper and lower extremities can be involved in primary malignancies that affect the soft tissues, bone and periosteum, and skin. Primary cancer of the bone (osteogenic sarcoma) most commonly affects children, adolescents, and young adults. When it is reasonably certain that amputation will eradicate the disease, the current predominant mode of therapy is amputation of the involved extremity. Prognosis often has been poor even after amputation. A new mode of therapy is being utilized in some settings. High doses of methotrexate along with citrovorum factor are administered over a period of several months to destroy the malignant cells. The affected femur becomes necrotic and is then replaced with a metallic prosthesis. Femur replacement requires a long hospitalization during which a considerable length of time of complete bed rest is necessary. The effectiveness of this procedure is still being evaluated. In metastatic cancer of bone, a palliative amputation is done only if the cancer has resulted in a necrotic infected lesion and the patient's general condition is not too deteriorated. Removal of a large but benign bone tumor can create a defect that interferes with function, and amputation may be the eventual outcome.

Presence of uncontrolled infection in bone profoundly affects the general health of the patient; thus, amputation may be necessary. The onset of antibiotic therapy, however, has greatly reduced the incidence of amputation because of infection.

Congenital defects can result in the absence of all or part of a limb. Generally, the cause is unknown, with the exception of the

Thalidomide tragedy of 1959–1960. The left forearm is the extremity most affected, with a slightly higher incidence in females than in males. Reconstructive surgery is frequently done to convert the limb to a more cosmetic and functional extremity. If sensation is present in the affected limb, it is preserved as much as possible, so that the partial limb can help to control some part of the prosthesis.

There are about 320,000 amputees in the United States, about 1.5 per 1,000 population. There are six lower-extremity amputations to one upper-extremity amputation [35].

The anatomic and physiologic loss in amputation results in a loss of joints and surrounding tissue, loss of muscle power and balance, loss of ability to sense position (proprioception), and loss of the sense of touch. These physiologic factors relate very closely to a person's psychological components, such as sense of security, confidence, comfort, body image, and self-worth. Adjustment following amputation is more difficult than for any other type of orthopedic surgery. The patient must be physically, mentally, and emotionally prepared for amputation. Acceptance of amputation may be less difficult for a person who, prior to amputation, suffered from great pain in the affected limb or who required repeated surgery and hospitalization.

In traumatic or accidental amputation, there is no opportunity to prepare the patient. The person is healthy and active and within a matter of hours faces a drastic life change. Most amputees pass through the grieving process of denial, shock, anger, depression, and finally acceptance. The medical and paramedical teams assist the patient through the loss and grieving. Final acceptance to one individual may be spending the remainder of his or her life in a wheelchair, whereas to another acceptance is capitalizing on remaining strengths and abilities, working hard at the rehabilitation process, learning to use a prosthesis, and returning to a useful, independent life. A person has to want a prosthesis and be motivated to learn how to function with it. The prosthesis becomes incorporated into his or her body image.

Psychological preparation of the patient for elective amputation surgery ideally is done by a team that includes the surgeon, nurses, physical therapists, occupational therapists, the prosthetist, and social worker. This same team approach is needed with the traumatic amputee. Both the patient and family are prepared for the amputation and assisted in the coping process associated with loss and change in body image. Another amputee who has been successfully rehabilitated can be helpful in both preoperative and postoperative visits.

The team explains to the patient the usual course of events that occur with amputation. The expected level and type of amputation, the management of pain, dressings, activities, body positions, and exercises are discussed. Physical therapy is involved in teaching the patient isometric and isotonic exercises, demonstration of gait patterns, transfer techniques, and the use of crutches or cane. If an upper extremity is involved, occupational therapy begins training in conversion of activities of daily living such as feeding, shaving, etc., from right to left hand or vice versa. The prosthetist may brief the patient on types of prostheses available for limb replacement. If an immediate postsurgical pylon prosthesis is planned, the patient should know that this involves earlier ambulation than if conventional methods are used. The social worker can be of assistance in economic and vocational readjustments.

The patient and family must be given time to express their fears, concerns, and have their questions answered. The patient should know and understand that the total rehabilitation process with learning to use a prosthesis effectively will require much involvement and hard work on his part. It is very important that the patient make the decision to have a prosthesis or not have one. This should not be a decision imposed on him by others. For some patients, the use of a prosthesis is an unrealistic goal, if other health problems interfere with healing or mobility.

TYPES OF AMPUTATIONS

A **minor amputation** is one that is done at a level where no artificial limb will be worn, such as the removal of the metatarsals and metacarpals or parts distal to these bones in the foot and hands. The stump is planned so that as much of its original function is maintained or recreated. Following minor amputation of the foot, the remaining weight-bearing surface should be able to withstand the pressures of stance and gait, and its shape should not cause discomfort from any bony prominences within the shoe. Loss of all the toes does not alter slow walking, but hinders rapid walking or running. A minor amputation of the hand is reconstructed so that the remaining skin will not break down under the pressure of grasp, and function is not hampered by a painful scar. In the hand, the cosmetic appearance is a particularly important consideration.

A **major amputation** is the removal of any part or all of an extremity proximal to the metatarsals and metacarpals and is designed for the use of an artificial limb. In a major amputation, the stump at each level must conform to certain standards with regard to bone length, scar position, and general shape, if the best results are to be obtained with a prosthesis. The stump must be capable of activating a prosthesis and withstanding constant wear.

Amputations are further classified as open or closed. In an **open amputation,** the surface of the wound is not covered with skin, but is left open for drainage and control of actual or potential infection. Open amputation may be indicated in acute traumatic injuries until the viability of tissue is ascertained. Open amputation can be circular (guillotine) or with skin flaps done on the premise that final closure will be done early to avoid an open granulating wound. The open stump is covered with Vaseline gauze and an adherent type of dressing that allows for fixation of skin traction. Skin traction is used to prevent retraction of skin and muscle, especially in the circular flap type of amputation. Postoperative management includes dressing and wound care, maintaining the skin traction, and care of any problems associated with delayed closure. An open amputation is a temporary measure, followed by a final surgical repair and closure within 4 to 6 weeks. The initial open amputation is carried out at the lowest possible level to control the infection, so that maximal tissue is available for the final repair.

A **closed amputation** is usually an elective surgical procedure carried out for the purpose of creating a stump that permits effective use of a prosthesis. The procedure for doing an amputation usually involves initial wrapping of the extremity in an elastic bandage to compress blood flow. The extremity is elevated during application of the compression bandage, and it is applied starting distally and continuing to the proximal part of the limb. A pneumatic tourniquet is then applied above the area of expected amputation, usually the upper thigh or upper arm. The tourniquet is applied in these areas, as this allows for all soft tissue and blood vessels to be compressed against one large bone. The tourniquet minimizes blood loss and creates a somewhat "bloodless" surgical field, which makes it easier for the surgeon to identify vital structures. The pneumatic tourniquet is not used on patients who have occlusive vascular disease.

In general, the more length that can be preserved, the more functional the stump will be. An exception to this is a below-knee amputation through the distal third of the leg, where it is difficult to sustain adequate circulation and thus maintain healthy tissue in the stump.

The skin incision is made with the final skin flap in mind. Skin covering the end of the stump must have good blood supply, normal sensation, and subcutaneous fat. Some amputations utilize a long posterior flap, others have a longer anterior flap, and some have a midline incision. An amputation at the ankle is usually covered with heel tissue; and at the wrist, the palmar skin is used. These tissues are accustomed to pressure and thus make good stump covering to bear weight. The scar is placed where it is least subject to tension and pressure. A tight skin flap tends to break down because of tension and ischemia. Loose flaps result in skin folds within the prosthesis. Scars containing crevices are difficult to fit successfully and are hard to keep clean. Skin grafts on stumps rarely withstand the forces imposed on them.

Generally the deep tissues are handled in the following way. Large muscles are never placed over the end of the bone. In some cases, a **myodesis** is performed. In this procedure a hole is drilled in the cortex of the bone and a suture holding the muscle is knotted within the medullary canal of the bone end to reattach muscles just proximal to the bone end. **Myoplastic techniques** involve suturing muscles to each other. Reattached muscles can provide feedback, reflex information, and aid in proprioception. The muscles also contract isometrically, which prevents atrophy and fibrosis. The bone is cut so that it is parallel with the ground when the patient is standing. The bone ends are filed smooth, and rounded and projecting bony prominences are removed. Periosteum is usually removed to one-fourth of an inch above the bone end. Blood vessels are double ligated with catgut. Nerves are cut and allowed to retract above the end of the bone. Painful neuromas can develop at the end of the stump or in an area where the prosthetic socket exerts pressure if nerves do not retract. The skin is closed without tension sutures and there must be adequate subcutaneous tissue and fascia to cover the bone end for padding as well as to prevent adhesion of the scar or skin to bone. A drain is placed in the wound, and in conventional approaches, a soft dressing is applied, utilizing a sheet wadding pad and an elastic compression wrap. Vaseline gauze is usually used to cover the incision, as it prevents crusting, yet allows drainage.

Another approach used for below-knee amputations is the application of a rigid dressing of plaster of Paris over the soft dressing for the purpose of controlling edema and pain. If a pylon is to be attached, the commercially prepared unit is incorporated into the cast. It provides for easy attachment and detachment of a pylon and foot-ankle assembly intended for early partial weight-bearing and ambulation. The plaster of Paris socket, ideally, should be shaped in accordance with the basic patellar-tendon-bearing prosthesis design. If a rigid dressing and pylon assembly are utilized for an above-knee amputation, the plaster socket applied to the stump should conform to the quadrilateral design commonly used in above-knee amputation. This facilitates the process of adapting to the final prosthesis.

A variety of factors determine the site or level of amputation. These are the temperature of the skin, palpation of peripheral pulses, reactive hyperemia or color changes, venous filling time or tropic changes, and skin flushing following elevation of the extremity. Arteriogram studies, oscillometry tests, and tests for vasospasm may also be done before surgery. In the elderly, or any person with occlusive vascular disease, the absence of intermittent claudication in the remaining leg may also be a factor. The most reliable criterion in guiding the level of amputation is the amount of free bleeding that occurs from the skin at surgery. The end result must be a viable closed stump. Therefore the final decision regarding level of amputation frequently does not occur until the surgical procedure is under way.

Major lower-extremity amputations can be transmetatarsal, tarsal-metatarsal (Lisfranc), midtarsal (Chopart), ankle disarticulation (Syme's amputation), below-knee (B/K), knee disarticulation, above-knee (A/K), hip disarticulation, and hemipelvectomy. Optimum level for any lower-extremity amputation takes into account the extent of healthy tissue, length of stump sufficient for weight-bearing and function of the prosthesis, proper placement of the scar to avoid friction or to interfere with weight-bearing, and the cosmetic effect of the prosthesis.

In ankle disarticulation (Syme's amputation) the tibia and fibula are virtually intact, and tissues of the heel are preserved to cover the bone. Normal foot and ankle action is lost; however, the stump provides for full end weight-bearing. The severed muscles become bulbous about the stump, which helps to hold the prosthesis; however, a consideration in women is that this prosthetic leg does not match the shape of the other leg. The prosthesis most often used for this amputation consists of a snuggly fitting plastic socket extending to a point below the knee and a solid-ankle cushion-heel (SACH) foot. Another translation of SACH foot is single-axis cushion heel. A Syme's amputation and prosthesis must accommodate for loss of foot and ankle motion and length discrepancy, provide a firm base for standing, and provide a means of suspension. The SACH foot is solid rubber with a softer rubber heel. It is designed for compression of the material on heel stride, which simulates plantar flexion. During the heel-off to toe-off aspect of gait, dorsiflexion is prevented. The rubber also allows for some toe flexion in gait (Fig. 10-19).

Below the knee (B/K) amputations are most frequently done at the junction of the middle and upper third of the leg. This provides a 5- to 6-inch stump and avoids the circulatory problems that arise in distal-third amputations. Full knee action is retained as well as major leg flexors and extensors, which are inserted in the upper third of the leg. Two major types of prosthesis are used. The wooden prosthetic leg holds the stump in its socket and a good portion of the body weight is carried by a leather thigh corset or lacer attached to the prosthesis by means of steel hinges. Some wearers of these prostheses also

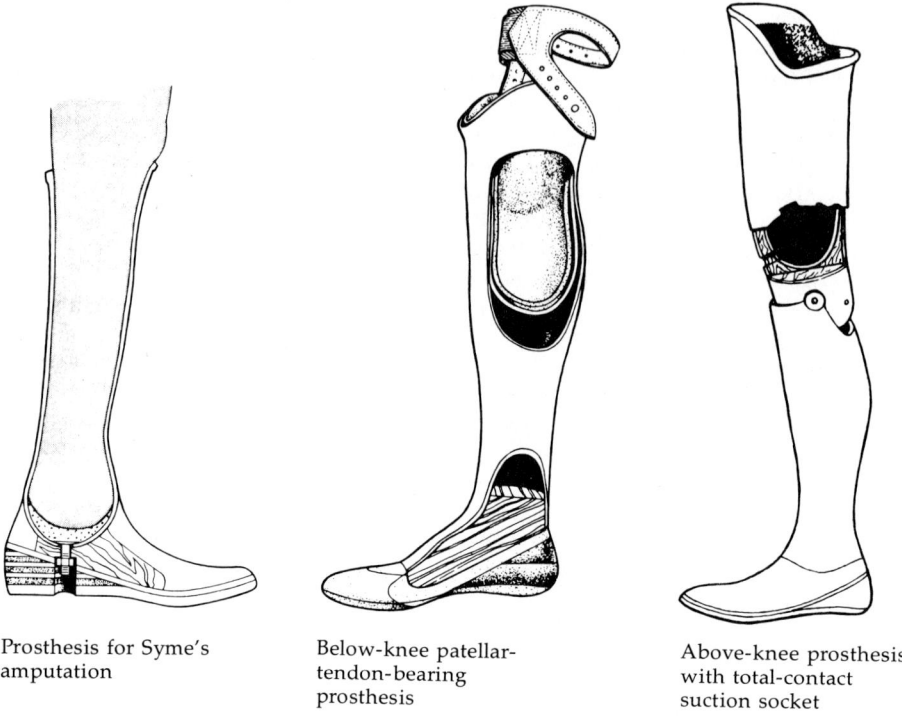

Prosthesis for Syme's amputation

Below-knee patellar-tendon-bearing prosthesis

Above-knee prosthesis with total-contact suction socket

Figure 10-19
Types of prostheses. (Courtesy of J. E. Hanger, Inc.)

prefer an additional suspension belt from the waist down to the prosthesis.

Currently, the patellar-tendon-bearing (PTB) total contact socket below-knee prosthesis is more commonly used. No thigh corset or hinges are used, and all the weight is taken through the stump by making the socket high enough to cover all the tendon below the patella. The patella tendon is an unusually inelastic tissue that is generally not adversely affected by pressure. The sides of the socket are also higher to provide stability against side loads. The PTB prosthesis is made of molded plastic laminate and may have a socket lining of sponge rubber and leather that is in total contact with the stump. The PTB prosthesis is suspended by means of a supracondylar cuff just above the knee or by a waist suspension belt if the wearer prefers. Some young amputees can suspend this prosthesis by the placement of medial and lateral wedges inside the higher socket sides (Fig. 10-19).

Below-knee amputations readily lend themselves to the immediate postsurgical fitting of prostheses, as previously discussed. With this approach, there is accelerated healing time, decreased postsurgical pain and edema, less contracture development, decreased stump shrinkage time, a better psychological adjustment, and an earlier return to employment, since mobility is achieved earlier.

In above-knee (A/K) amputations, it is important to preserve as much length as possible, since the adductor muscles of the hip are inserted low on the femur. Preserving adductor muscles helps counteract the strong hip abductor muscles. In short A/K stumps, muscle balance is lost and control of the stump is less efficient. The ischial tuberosity bears the weight in A/K amputations as high pressure is exerted on the soft tissues by the cut end of the femur. Total body weight cannot be taken by the soft tissues in an A/K amputation stump.

For most above-knee amputees, the prosthesis usually prescribed consists of a carved quadrilateral wooden socket, a single-axis knee unit (Back knee) with adjustable friction, a wooden shank, and a SACH foot. Various hydraulic knees are also available; however, they tend to respond to changes in humidity and temperature, so are not suited to all climates. The quadrilateral total contact socket is most common. It features four walls with the lateral and anterior sides higher, and lower posterior and medial walls. There is a bulge in the anterior medial section for Scarpa's triangle and a wide posterior medial brim called the ischia seat, which bears the body weight. The posterior outside wall has a soft rubber bumper for noiseless seating on wooden chairs and benches. The Bock knee provides more stability on heel strike for an elderly person. A constant-friction knee requires more control and is more suited to a younger amputee. Instead of a SACH foot, it is possible to have a single-axis ankle that allows for dorsiflexion and plantar flexion or a double-axis ankle that allows for dorsiplantar flexion as well as inversion and eversion.

Above-knee prostheses have several options in suspension systems. A pelvic belt attached to the prosthesis is most common. A young amputee may prefer a suction socket in which the quadrilateral socket is fitted to create negative pressure or suction between the stump and the bottom of the socket. No stump sock is worn, as the skin contacts the inside of the socket directly. No pelvic belt or suspender is worn with a suction socket.

A high, thigh amputation that preserves a few inches of the femoral shaft along with the head, neck, and trochanters of the femur is preferable to a hip disarticulation or hemipelvectomy. The presence of these tissues allows for a more stable hip socket on the prosthesis. The body weight is carried by the ischial tuberosity. Amputation is the only curative treatment for osteogenic sarcoma and chrondrosarcoma of the hip joint or pelvic bones. A prosthesis for these amputations must provide a hip unit that facilitates sitting in addition to the knee and ankle units needed for ambulation. Following hemipelvectomy, the lumbar spine must propel the prosthesis. This surgical amputation always has an anterior scar with a long posterior flap that utilizes the skin, fat, and superficial fascia of the buttocks to serve as padding within the socket shell.

Any upper-extremity amputation is considered carefully and in detail. Every effort is made to save any digit or hand tissue whenever possible, as the hand provides complex elements and functions unequaled in the body. To save some form of grasp is preferable to the best prosthesis. The hand has three basic functions: grasp (prehension), pinch, and hook. The length, strength, sensation, mobility, and power of every digit are evaluated prior to amputation.

The thumb is the single most important digit of the hand. The thumb is needed in both pinch and grasp, as well as being a principle tactile and pressure area of the hand. The index finger is the second most important digit, since it opposes the thumb in the pinching action. The other digits, middle, ring, and little finger, add span to grasp and serve the hook function of the hand. Each fractional loss of any digit of the hand carries with it a loss of function in direct proportion to the length lost. If sensation is present in any part of the hand, it is saved in lieu of disarticulation at the wrist.

Wrist disarticulation does preserve the important functions of pronation and supination of the forearm, which aids the functional use of the prosthetic hand. Amputations through the forearm are called below-elbow (B/E). When 60 percent of the forearm is removed, all supination and pronation are lost, and there is poor forearm flexion, with limited power and motion about the elbow. It is important to preserve length in a B/E amputation to save the long flexor and extensor muscles and tendons that power the wrist and hand. The shell of the prosthesis fits snugly over the stump in long B/E and wrist disarticulations. For shorter B/E amputations, either a figure-of-eight harness or chest strap harness connects to an upper arm cuff, which in turn has an elbow hinge unit connected to the B/E prosthesis.

Regardless of the level of upper-arm amputation, the hand replacement terminal device is essentially the same. The terminal device is any artificial grasping mechanism, a metal hook or cosmetic hand fitted to the end of the prosthesis. The plastic-covered hand has normal skin markings, color, and hair. It is capable of grasping, but otherwise is not a very useful device. The split-hook prosthetic hand substitute is more functional. The arm amputee must rely on his vision to handle objects and the hook provides more visibility. It also provides some prehension and can be used to retrieve items from pockets. Many arm amputees have a hook terminal device for manual skills and a plastic hand unit for social and cosmetic purposes. The terminal devices are exchangeable on the prosthesis.

Below-elbow amputees can also benefit from **biceps cineplasty,** which allows the biceps to move the prosthesis. The cineplasty procedure usually is not done until the stump has healed well and is freely moveable. A tunnel is made through the biceps muscle and the tunnel is lined with a pedicle skin flap. A skin graft is done over the area from which the pedicled graft is taken. A rod is then placed through the tunnel. This rod attaches to a control cable leading to the wrist and hand. The perforated biceps can then transmit its force externally to the prosthesis. The brachialis of the upper arm functions alone in flexing the forearm. A patient undergoing this procedure must be highly motivated, as he or she must learn the techniques used in operating the prosthesis as well as the daily care of the tunnel.

Above-elbow (A/E) amputation is any amputation of the upper arm. A stump that does not extend more than 2 inches below the axillary fold is of no functional value with or without a prosthesis; however, preserving the head of the humerus gives the shoulder a more normal rounded appearance. Loss of the upper arm tends to produce a deformity of the spine proportionate to the level of the amputation, because of loss of the weight of the limb, muscle atrophy, and overdevelopment of the opposite limb. Gait rhythm may also be disturbed because of loss of the arm swing.

Elbow disarticulation and long A/E amputations are fitted with similar prostheses that capitalize on the long biceps muscle. Elbow disarticulation provides a good bulbous end-bearing stump and allows for useful rotation in the upper arm. The elbow-locking mechanism is on the outside of the stump. In a long A/E amputation, the elbow mechanism is within the prosthesis. Both types of prosthesis have an identical chest or shoulder suspension harness. A/E amputees can have a pectoralis cineplasty procedure that helps to control the terminal device.

Short A/E amputations and shoulder disarticulations are fitted with similar prostheses. Any A/E prosthesis should have an elbow lock that does not require the other hand to activate the artificial joint. The action is accomplished by slightly depressing the shoulder as the arm is extended. The most popular harness used is the figure-of-eight, ring-type, dual-control design with a terminal control cable attached to a lever on the forearm. When the elbow is unlocked, tension in the control cable flexes the elbow. When the elbow is locked into position, the control force is diverted to the terminal device.

The prosthesis and the stump of an upper extremity bear no weight. The prosthesis must be capable of being propelled into desired position for gripping, lifting, and pushing by the stump, which acts as a lever.

A forequarter amputation involves removal of the entire arm, clavicle, and shoulder joint. It is done in malignant infiltrating tumors. It is very difficult to fit with a functional prosthesis.

PROSTHESES

A variety of artificial limbs are available for each type of amputation. The prescription for a prosthesis takes into account the site of the amputation, the type and condition of the stump and scar, the patient's age, physical and mental condition, motivation and interest, as well as the occupation and avocation of the amputee. The various components of prostheses are commercially produced; however, the prosthetist then selects and refashions the components to meet the individual requirements of the wearer. Appearance, weight, ease of application, probable amount of usage, and cost are factors that are considered. In the actual prosthesis, two very important aspects are the fit of the socket and the alignment of the various parts of the limb in relation to the stump and other parts of the body.

The total-contact socket has improved the functional performance of the amputee and reduced the local stump complications such as edema, irritation, and inflammation. Total contact of the stump with the socket increases proprioception and sensory feedback, as well as enhancing venous return, which reduces distal edema. Poor alignment of a socket will cause discomfort, which in turn can result in compensatory gait deviations with consequent increased energy expenditure. This may discourage the wearer from using it.

The artificial limb must be adjusted until its alignment is as close as possible to that of the remaining limb. In the lower extremity, a prosthesis that does not provide level support can lead to the development of scoliosis. An artificial arm should be the same length as the remaining arm. Knees and elbows should bend at the same level as the remaining extremity.

In addition to the total-contact socket, sockets that allow weight to be borne on the end of the stump are available. These are commonly used for joint disarticulations. Other sockets are designed so that the pressure of weight-bearing falls on bony support such as the metatarsal flare of the proximal tibia or the ischial tuberosity of a thigh stump. Even with the total-contact socket, some part of the skeleton bears body weight, rather than the soft tissues.

In addition to the socket fit and alignment considerations, the type of suspension is important. The suspension system varies with the age of the patient. It can be a suction socket, the wedge suspension system, or some type of belt or harness. Whichever type is selected, it must provide security to the wearer and prevent friction between the stump and socket. In an upper-extremity amputee, the suspension system incorporates the activity cable from the upper arm, shoulder, chest, or opposite shoulder that transmits power to the terminal hand device.

A variety of joints are available depending on the age and needs of the amputee. The Bock safety knee (variable friction) provides increased resistance as the knee flexes and reverses its action to provide increased resistance as the knee extends. Constant-friction knees do not have this feature, and the wearer must have more control. Hydraulic mechanisms for control of stability at joints are more costly, add more weight, and require more maintenance. They also respond to climate changes. With a hydraulic knee and ankle, the amputee can increase and decrease cadence (speed of walking) more readily.

Artificial limbs should be as light as possible and still withstand the loads placed on them. For years, wood has formed the basic construction material for prostheses; however, plastic laminates are now widely used, especially for upper-extremity prostheses. Plastic laminates are light in weight, durable, easy to keep clean, and do not absorb perspiration. They can be molded to any contour of stump and can be made extremely rigid or more flexible as the situation dictates.

The first step in making a prosthesis is to make an impression of the stump by wrapping it in plaster of Paris. When dry, the plaster cast is removed, and this plaster shell is then filled with liquid plaster to form an exact model of the stump. The model is then casted with plastic laminate, which becomes the socket that is then fastened to a temporary leg or arm for a trial period. Almost all amputees begin prosthesis training with a temporary, adjustable limb. When the amputee, prosthetist, and rehabilitation team are satisfied with all aspects of the prosthesis, the permanent one is made.

With use and wear, some parts of the prosthesis may need replacement. Leather, metal, and rubber parts wear with use. A SACH foot or the suspension system may need replacement every few years. A prosthesis requires maintenance and care for optimal function and the parts can easily be replaced by a qualified prosthetist. The prosthesis must be evaluated at regular intervals to assure proper fitting. For example, loss of weight in the amputee may affect socket-fitting.

To make and fit a prosthesis requires a complete understanding of anatomy, physiology, and the mechanics involved. In normal gait, the shoulders remain level; during weight transfer, the side sway of the body is minimal, the trunk is erect, arm swing is equal, there is symmetrical stride length, and there is a 2- to 4-inch walking base between consecutive heel contacts with the floor. The cycle of gait is the activity that occurs between heel strike on one side and the following heel strike on the same side. This cycle with the foot is: heel strike, foot flat, mid stance, heel off, and toe off. These actions are normally taken for granted. The goal of any prosthesis fitting and training is to restore lost function to as near normal as possible; thus, the prosthesis must allow for a complex sequence of actions that must be learned with the use of the prosthesis. Comfortable and cosmetic ambulation with a minimal expenditure of energy is important to the amputee.

The length of time required to master the use of a prosthesis depends on the complexity of the device and the physical condition and degree of coordination of the patient. For the lower-extremity amputee, achieving vertical balance is the first step in prosthesis training. Physical therapy is usually more involved in instruction for the use of a lower-extremity prosthesis, whereas occupational therapy is more involved in upper-extremity prosthetics. Although these appliances do not functionally or aesthetically replace the lost extremity, they are good substitutes and can be fitted for function and comfort.

POSTAMPUTATION CARE

The goals during the early postamputation period are to control edema and prevent flexion contractures. Complications during the preprosthetic period include bleeding, infection, wound separation, contracture formation, and mechanical skin lesions that may be caused by inadequate circulation. Later postprosthetic complications include the development of painful bone spurs, which may be caused by retained tags of periosteum, neuromas, and skin problems such as ulcerations, blisters, and edema resulting from a poorly fitted prosthesis. Many of the complications can be prevented by proper management of the dressing and proper positioning and exercises.

The stump requires a period of rest for tissue-healing. The stump is protected from contamination and injury by the elastic compression dressing, a well-padded plaster splint, or the rigid plaster dressing. Early, active motion of the stump can interfere with healing, increase edema, and provoke hemorrhage. The dressing helps to immobilize the stump. Elastic compression bandaging is needed for several days or weeks after a minor amputation and throughout healing and convalescence following a major amputation. When a rigid plaster dressing is used on a major amputation, the elastic compression dressing is not used.

Signs of active bleeding through the dressing are reported to the physician immediately, because of the danger of hemorrhage from the major blood vessels that are ligated in amputation. Some physicians request that a tourniquet be kept at the bedside at all times following amputation for immediate application if bleeding occurs. Vital signs are monitored frequently. The underside of the dressing is checked frequently because gravitational flow will cause drainage underneath the stump.

Signs of stump infection are increased temperature, pain, purulent discharge, edema, skin redness, leukocytosis, and possibly an odor from the dressing. If any of these signs is present, the physician is notified and the wound inspected. Frequently, the patient is on prophylactic antibiotics.

Wound separation may occur if there is excessive soft-tissue swelling or infection, or the sutures are too tight. The use of skin traction for a few days with a closed amputation will prevent wound separation. General good nutritional status promotes wound-closure. Hypoproteinemia, vascular problems, and diabetes predispose a patient to delayed wound-healing. Deep fingertip massage with cocoa butter may sometimes be prescribed to promote healing and to prevent the adherence of the skin flap to the bone end.

Contractures are easier to prevent than to cure. The most common contractures are hip flexion and abduction in the above-knee amputee, knee flexion contractures in the below-knee amputee, and shoulder adduction and elbow flexion in the arm amputee. A sagging mattress can promote hip flexion contractures. The use of an overbed trapeze encourages active use of the upper extremities and facilitates position changes. Positioning in correct body alignment is imperative. For lower-extremity amputees, hip flexion, abduction, external rotation, and knee flexion must be prevented. Sandbags or a trochanter roll should be used against the hip. No pillows are allowed under the stump or knee. As soon as possible, the patient is placed in a prone position for regular intervals daily to keep the hip in extension. Prolonged sitting is to be avoided. For the upper extremity, the stump is positioned so that the elbow is in extension for regular periods of time and the shoulder is abducted (Fig. 10-20).

For elective amputations, the patient has usually begun muscle-strengthening and range-of-motion exercises in the preoperative period. These are continued postoperatively by physical therapist and nurse. Early in the postoperative course, isometric exercises such as gluteal setting, quadriceps setting, adduction and internal rotation of the hip, and straight leg raising are initiated. Involved joints are given gentle partial assisted range-of-motion and passive resistive exercises. By the third postoperative day, the patient begins active exercises to the stump and gentle resistive exercises are also given. Within two weeks after surgery, healing should have occurred, and increased resistive exer-

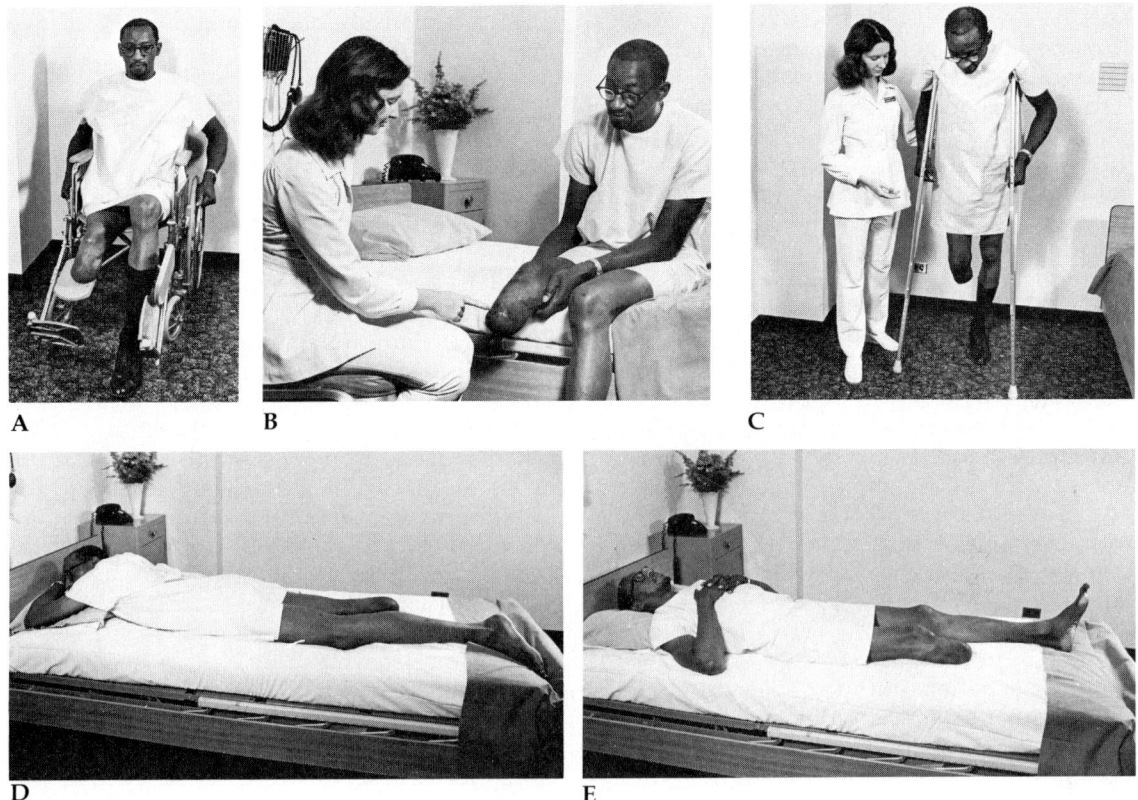

Figure 10-20
Patient with below the knee amputation (BK); beginning ambulatory efforts.

cises are done. Usually by this time the patient is mobilized in some manner, which also helps to decrease contracture formation. Being involved in self-care and activities of daily living encourages active use of extremities. Good stump hygiene promotes comfort, thus allowing the patient to be actively involved in all the exercises.

The closed-amputation stump is usually covered with one of two types of dressing: a soft dressing with or without tensor bandages or the rigid plaster of Paris dressing that is placed over the soft dressing covering the incision. The elastic tensor bandage, or a rigid dressing, is used to control edema and pain. Swelling is a normal physiologic response to the interruption of tissue and is anticipated in the stump. The degree of swelling that occurs can affect the rehabilitation and mobilization process.

A soft dressing without a tensor bandage may be used in an elderly debilitated patient. The soft dressing is converted to compression-wrapping with tensor elastic woven bandages a few days after surgery. A rigid dressing of plaster may be too heavy for an elderly amputee. In addition, the elderly amputee may have coexisting medical problems that guide the decision to a traditional approach to care. Such an approach includes the use of elastic compression bandages, teaching transfer techniques, and use of crutches or a walker, evaluating ambulation potential, and then deciding about the use of an artificial limb.

It is generally felt that stump swelling is best controlled by the use of a rigid dressing, which is applied immediately after surgery. It consists of a total-contact elastic plaster dressing and plaster of Paris outer covering. The rigid dressing conforms to the shape of the stump. A web belt suspension system is incorporated into the proximal end of the cast, which encases the knee at 10 to 15 degrees of flexion for below-knee amputations.

The rigid dressing can be a functional

socket to which the immediate postsurgical prosthesis is fitted at its distal end or intended for early prosthetic fitting, which occurs about 2 weeks after surgery. The original plaster stump socket is usually left in place for 10 to 14 days. If there is immediate postsurgical prosthesis fitting, the pylon and foot assembly are attached to the socket the first postoperative day and the patient is allowed to stand at the bedside. By the second or third postoperative day, a window is cut in the cast to remove the drain if there is one in the incision. The site is recasted. Ambulation progresses with a four-point gait and minimal weight-bearing on the amputated stump. In 10 to 14 days, the cast dressing is removed, the sutures are removed, and a new cast is applied immediately. The original prosthetic unit or an initial unit is incorporated into the cast socket and realigned as needed for ambulation.

Partial weight-bearing is continued for 4 to 6 weeks. The weight-bearing is protected by having the patient ambulate between parallel bars, with a cane or crutches. Some physical therapists prefer not to have the patient use crutches, as it is easy for the amputee to become dependent upon them. Full weight-bearing and plans for the final prosthesis begin when the stump has matured and the patient has balance, coordination, and sensation (usually four to six months depending on the individual patient's progress.)

The rigid plaster of Paris dressing requires the same nursing observations and care as a cast used in the treatment of a fracture. It must be kept intact, clean, and dry. If the rigid dressing slips off, elastic compression dressing must be applied immediately. When the patient is upright, the web suspension belt helps counteract the forces of gravity that may cause the cast to slip off. The pylon and foot assembly are always disconnected from the plaster socket when the patient is in bed.

Immediate postsurgical prosthesis is most widely used for below-knee amputations. Patients that require above-knee amputation frequently have more preexisting impairments that may interfere with the plaster dressing and pylon attachment. Above-knee and upper-extremity amputations may use the rigid dressing and terminal device as a temporary measure. The rigid dressing and temporary prosthesis curtail the development of joint contractures and muscle weakness, and diminish phantom sensation in all age groups.

Phantom Limb Sensation and Pain

Phantom limb sensation occurs in all amputees. Patients who have no phantom sensation may be denying the amputation. The amputee feels as if the lost limb is still present. This is a normal, expected reaction, and the patient should be alerted to its occurrence prior to amputation. Generally, the distal part of the limb such as toes or fingers are felt. As time progresses, phantom sensation progresses closer to the end of the stump. This is called telescoping. Phantom sensation diminishes as activity and weight-bearing increase; however, it may continue for 6 months to 2 years. It is less predominant in a child; its occurrence increases with age because "afterimages" in the cerebral cortex are increasingly fixed with age.

Phantom sensation is not a dermatome pain, and it occurs because of the neurophysiologic principle that no matter where a particular sensory pathway is stimulated along its course to the cerebral cortex, the conscious sensation produced is referred to the location of the receptor. Pressure on the stump can initiate an impulse in the nerve fibers that previously came from sense organs in the amputated limb. The cerebral cortex "reads" these as coming from the foot or hand even though they are now absent. These impulses may be sensations of pressure, touch, temperature, and pain [14].

When phantom limb sensations become painful they are called phantom pain. This pain occurs in less than 2 percent of all amputees. Phantom pain is described as constant burning, crushing, or stabbing. It may be caused by a painful neuroma. The axon of the cut nerve grows into the soft tissue at the end of a stump, and curls back on itself, producing a small bundle of nervous tissue. Pressure on the neuroma can cause an annoying pain that follows along the dermatome of that nerve root. Phantom pain tends to occur in the extremely anxious, easily depressed amputee who is having more than average problems with psychological adjustment to the amputation. It also occurs in the person whose amputation followed a long period of disability. Treatment includes increased use of prosthesis, novocaine or cortisone injections, whirlpool, massage, and heat to the stump. In some cases, a lumbar sympathectomy is done. Along with the medical treatment, appropriate psychologic care and support should be given to assist the patient in a more appropriate adjustment to the amputation.

Stump-wrapping and Stump Care

When the rigid plaster dressing is not used, proper *stump-wrapping* with elastic compression bandages is a vital part of the patient care. The purpose of stump-wrapping is to shrink and shape the stump. It is a compression dressing, not a pressure dressing, with the maximum compression at the distal end, minimal compression at the proximal end, and no circular bandaging. Smooth, even compression helps to decrease edema and eliminate dead space that may develop in the tissues, and helps to mold the stump. The ideal stump is cylindrical and is tapered to a rounded smooth end. Some authorities feel that an above-knee stump should be cone-shaped, whereas the ideal below-knee stump is cylindrical. Improper bandaging can lead to constriction of the stump, delayed healing, skin abrasions, and folds. Any skin or circulatory problems that develop, or a bulbous distal end on the stump, will cause difficulty getting into the prosthesis.

Proper width and length of woven elastic bandage must be used. It is best to use 6-inch width bandages for above-knee stumps and 4-inch width bandages for below-knee and upper-extremity amputations. Usually two to three bandages are needed, and they may be sewn together in one long continuous length, which helps to ensure a snug wrap.

The stump should be wrapped with a clean bandage each day and, regardless of how well the bandage stays on, the stump must be rewrapped at least four times a day to maintain proper compression. If the bandage slips off, it must be rewrapped as soon as possible. The bandage is worn day and night following a major amputation until the prosthesis is fitted and all edema subsides. Following adjustment to the prosthesis, stump-bandaging is continued at night. Nighttime bandaging may continue for years.

As soon as possible, the patient is taught stump-wrapping of a lower extremity. It is more difficult for a patient to self-wrap an upper-extremity stump effectively. A family member can also be taught stump-wrapping. The stump-bandaging can be done in the side-lying position; it can also be done while lying supine.

When bandaging the stump, the patient should be relaxed. It may not be possible to have joints extended during bandaging. For example, above-knee stump-bandaging is done with the hip flexed. In bandaging an above-knee stump, the bandaging is started medially at the groin with the 6-inch rolled elastic bandage. Recurrent vertical turns down the anterior surface of the stump, over the distal end of the stump posteriorly to the gluteal crease, are made. The patient can help hold the recurrent folds in place. Two additional recurrent turns are made, passing over the medial and lateral distal end of the stump. The recurrent turns are anchored with several figure-of-eight turns up over the iliac crest and around the hip in a spica. The spica turns are applied from the hip anteriorly down around the stump from medial to lateral to the distal end of the stump. This pattern is repeated a few times, pulling the stump into extension and adduction. Overlapping figure-of-eight patterns of turns from lateral to medial are done to bring the most compression on the distal end of the stump. The bandage is brought well up into the groin on some of the turns to eliminate bulges in this area; it is fastened with a safety pin on the anterior lateral aspect of the stump.

Below-knee stump-bandaging utilizes 4-inch rolled elastic bandage. Recurrent vertical turns on the posterior aspect of the stump inferior to the knee joint are made, followed by two additional recurrent turns, passing over the medial and lateral distal ends of the stump. The recurrent folds are anchored with several figure-of-eight turns. Figure-of-eight turns are continued until firm compression exists over the distal end of the stump. Both the medial and lateral aspects of the end of the stump are not included in one single turn because this causes creases in the skin. Some of the figure-of-eight turns should be spread above the knee. The bandage is anchored with adhesive tape or safety pins over the lateral or anterior aspect of the stump. If at any point semicircular turns are needed to bring the bandage into proper position, the turns should be made on the posterior aspect of the stump in order to compress soft tissue that will not interfere with circulation.

Instead of beginning the stump-bandaging with vertical recurrent folds, it is possible to begin bandaging and continue throughout with figure-of-eight turns. This approach may be easier for the patient to learn and manage, since it can be difficult for the amputee to hold on to the posterior and anterior folds of the recurrent bandaging. For above-knee amputees, the starting point, the hip spica turns, and medial-to-lateral turns remain the same. In below-knee amputees, bandaging is initiated at the anterior aspect of the stump, then down to the medial distal corner, back diagonally across the posterior aspect of the stump, and across the beginning of the bandage, to anchor it. Figure-of-eight turns above the knee and crossing the crest of the tibia are continued in an angular manner. Each figure-of-eight turn should overlap so that the whole stump is covered with the greatest compression at the distal end.

The goal of the preprosthetic care is to provide a stump that will bear weight, tolerate a socket, and give maximum control of a prosthesis. Adequate strength and endurance develop through muscle-strengthening and resistive exercises. The healed stump should have skin of good thickness and texture, adequate circulation, and scars away from the points of pressure. As soon as healing has occurred, measures are started to toughen the stump skin. General physical health and strength and psychological well-being are promoted during the period of interim ambulation. Periods of depression and feelings of guilt may occur, related to the precipitating cause for the amputation. For example, the amputee may feel that if he or she had stopped smoking or managed his or her diabetes more effectively he or she would still have the limb. The earlier the patient can be fitted with a temporary adjustable prosthesis, the fewer occurrences of depression and psychological maladjustments there will be.

Postprosthetic complications include skin breakdown resulting from friction, the development of sebaceous skin cysts from an excessively tight-fitting socket, bone spurs that grow at the end of the stump, and painful neuromas. If skin blisters or ulcerations develop, the patient may need to avoid wearing the prosthesis for a few days and return to stump-wrapping temporarily.

Many of the postprosthetic complications can be prevented by teaching the patient how to carry out daily stump inspection, care of the stump, care of the stump socket, and care of the stump sock and elastic bandages. The prosthesis must be maintained in good condition.

Abrasions, blisters, and infection can be prevented with proper care. Any time there is any evidence of stump skin problems, the patient should see his or her physician or prosthetist. Edema that leads to skin irritation can result from a poorly fitting prosthesis, or from having discontinued the practice of stump-wrapping at night. When an amputee complains that the prosthesis is getting too tight, it is wise to inquire about whether he or she has continued to stump-wrap when the prosthesis is not being worn.

Lack of ventilation within the socket can lead to an accumulation of perspiration and other skin secretions. This is a good medium for bacterial growth. Every evening the stump must be washed with warm water and mild soap, rinsed well, and dried thoroughly. At this time, the stump should be inspected. The posterior aspects of the stump can be visualized by using a hand mirror. Washing the stump in the morning may cause the damp skin to swell and stick to the prosthesis, resulting in irritation.

The inside of the socket must be washed every evening with water and mild soap, dried, and left open to air during the night. A single- or double-axis ankle unit on the prosthesis can be hard on foot socks, as the sock can get caught in the hinges. Wearing badly worn shoes should be avoided because they can alter alignment of the prosthesis.

A clean stump sock must be worn every day. It is important to make an initial purchase of five to six stump socks, as wool socks take longer to dry. The woolen stump sock should be washed in Woolite and cold water as soon as it is removed from the stump before perspiration dries into it. It should be laid flat to dry following rinsing in cool water. Stump socks are available in three- or five-ply wool, depending on the thickness desired. If the person is allergic to wool, cotton stump socks are available. A five-ply cotton stump sock equals a three-ply wool sock in thickness. Cotton stump socks can be washed with regular laundry, but both cotton and wool stump socks should be air-dried. Placing a rubber ball into the distal end of the sock while it is drying helps the sock retain a rounded shape.

As the stump shrinks, the amputee may wear two stump socks at the same time within the socket of the prosthesis; however, if more than two stump socks are required for the socket to fit snugly, it is an indication for a refitting by the prosthetist.

The elastic woven bandages must also be washed daily in warm water and mild soap, rinsed well, and laid flat to dry. Heat and sunlight damage elastic bandages. When dry, the bandages should be rerolled smoothly without stretching.

Additional patient teaching is required by the elderly amputee who has lost a limb because of vascular problems. The remaining extremity needs special care. The patient should be taught to make a daily inspection of the foot for any cracks in the skin, blisters, ingrowing nails, or calluses. Keeping the leg and foot warm promotes circulation. Daily washing and skin care are essential. No circular garters should be worn. The patient should stop smoking. Accelerated use of the remaining leg does not hasten the development of circulatory problems. The elderly patient also may find that the use of crutches requires more expenditure of energy than the use of the artificial limb. An elderly person requires a slower training program and more time to gain security and ease in managing the prosthesis.

It is well to recognize that not all persons are suited for prosthesis fitting and wearing. It may be beyond the physical capabilities of some elderly amputees to wear the prosthesis and expend the energy needed for ambulation. The rehabilitation goal in these amputees may be to become mobile in a wheelchair. Thus, learning independent transfer to and from a wheelchair, management of the environment from the wheelchair, and wheelchair safety become realistic goals. Special amputee wheelchairs are available for bilateral amputees who have an altered center of gravity. These special wheelchairs compensate for the missing lower extremities.

The rehabilitation program is tailored to each amputee. The amputee is not left to face the future unguided or without proper training. A multidisciplinary team of physicians, physiatrists, nurses, physiotherapists, occupational therapists, psychologists, and social workers should be available to the amputee as each respective service is needed.

For the lower-extremity amputee, the program begins initially by the patient learning to attach and remove the prosthesis. Then, various aspects of ambulation are mastered: straight walking, stepping sideways and backward, walking without an aid, going up and down stairs and curbs, and stepping over obstacles. Then the patient progresses to sitting and rising from a chair and the floor. The patient learns to kneel, and how to protect himself or herself during a fall. Later skills to be learned are walking outdoors on uneven surfaces and getting in and out of a car.

The arm amputee first needs to learn to put the prosthesis on and to manage the various controls, and then proceeds to learn all the necessary activities of daily living before beginning the special training needed for vocational and recreational pursuits.

Many amputees profit from sharing experiences with other amputees. In addition to the mutual learning that occurs, amputees may more readily express their fears and anxieties in a group setting. They may discuss such things as how bifocal or trifocal eyeglasses affect their ambulation. For some, amputee clinics may be the reentry into a social setting that gives them the needed encouragement to continue to widen their horizons.

Assisting in Mobility

Following any injury to the musculoskeletal system, restoration of function is as important as any part of treatment. Avoidance of complications provides a major step to regaining function of the injured part. Prolonged immobilization can result in disuse atrophy, and stiffening of joints. Proper positioning and bed exercises on a regular basis can deter the development of these conditions. Function is not restored until the muscles are free of contractures and have regained flexibility, strength, and endurance.

If a muscle has not been used for a time, it must be reconditioned to its normal strength and endurance. Muscle reeducation must be introduced gradually, since weak muscles are vulnerable to injury. Flaccid muscles are easily stretched. Muscle fatigue results from anoxia and an accumulation of waste products. Cramps can occur in muscles during the reconditioning process if excessive demands are made on them. Cramps and spasms are protective devices that immobilize the part and prevent further injury or strain.

When caring for patients with musculoskeletal injuries, it is well to remember that flexor muscles are stronger than extensor muscles, and abductors are stronger than adductor muscles. Thus, inappropriate positions are easily assumed by extremities. Any time a body of a muscle is squeezed, pain can result. For any muscle to function, it must have an intact nerve supply and be attached to either a bone, tendon, or ligament. Muscles that move a part usually do not lie over that part, but proximal to the part moved. For example, the lower leg is moved by thigh muscles and the forearm controls many movements of the hand.

Both the nurse and the patient must use principles of good body mechanics and good posture. The nurse must also observe good body mechanics. **Body mechanics** means the correlation of various systems of the body to produce motion and maintain equilibrium. **Good posture** is maintaining the most effective position of body segments, the relationship of body segments, and their adaptation to the laws of gravity. For the nurse lifting and moving patients, this means using large body muscles when possible, keeping feet apart to provide a broad base, and bending the knees, not the back. For the patient this means maintaining good body alignment and position when in bed, sitting, or standing. The nurse assists the patient maintain good body alignment and position by supporting extremities with sandbags, pillows, and a firm mattress, by teaching proper transfer techniques, and by providing exercises.

Passive range of motion involves movement of the muscle through its range of motion by the nurse or therapist. These are the limits of motion through which a joint can be moved without the use of muscles that cross a joint. There is no active muscle contraction, and these exercises do not build strength. Passive range of motion includes flexion, extension, abduction, adduction, and internal and external rotation of joints.

Active range-of-motion exercises use muscles that cross joints. There is contraction of muscle fibers and movement of extremities; muscle strength and function are facilitated.

Resistive exercises are those that are done against the forces of weight and gravity. They are used to increase muscle strength.

An **isotonic muscle contraction** is one in which the length of the muscle changes but muscle tension remains unchanged. These contractions produce movement and do work. Walking involves isotonic muscle contractions; muscles shorten and lengthen.

An **isometric muscle contraction** is one in which muscle tension increases but the length of the muscle does not change. These contractions "tighten" a muscle, but they do not produce movement or do work. Isometric or static muscle exercises are used to maintain strength of a particular group of muscles when joints cannot be moved. They help to strengthen the antigravity, or postural, muscles of the body. Quadriceps- and gluteal-setting exercises are examples of isometric exercises. The quadriceps muscle-setting exercises consist in having the patient in the supine recumbent position, pressing the back of the knee against the bed, and trying to lift the heel from the bed. The nurse can assist the patient to learn this exercise by placing his or her hand between the patient's knee and the mattress and asking the patient to press his hand against the mattress with the knee. Gluteal muscle-setting exercises consist in pinching the buttocks together and attempting to lift the hips when in the recumbent position. Muscle-setting for the foot consists in having the patient circle the foot in all directions and flex the foot toward and away from the knee.

The nurse will also be involved in assisting the patient in the use of crutches, canes, walkers, and wheelchairs. These assistive devices must be used correctly and safely. The patient should wear good supportive shoes, not soft slippers. Initially, when learning to use these devices, the patient may tend to watch the floor, his or her feet, and the device. This must be corrected, as accidents can happen if the patient does not look ahead to scan the environment for any hazards or obstacles. Posture should be erect with the head level. Crutches and walkers are adjusted to allow for 30-degree flexion of the elbow, whereas a cane allows for a 10- to 15-degree flexion of the elbow.

When getting in and out of bed or a chair, the patient should keep the affected extremity in the line of vision. The patient should push himself or herself to a standing position, then grasp the walker, cane, or crutches. When returning to bed or chair, the patient should feel the chair or bed against the back of his or her legs, grab onto the arm of the chair with one hand, and lower the body to a seated position. When using crutches, both crutches can be transferred to one hand prior to sitting and the handpieces of the crutches can be held while sitting down. A walking belt can be worn by the patient while the assistant stands close to the patient and helps stabilize the body by firmly grasping the belt. If no belt is worn, one hand on the shoulder and the other hand on the pelvis can help to stabilize the patient as he or she learns to use the assistive device. The crutches, cane, or walker of the patient with a faltering gait should never be grabbed by the person assisting in ambulation.

Correct fit of crutches is most important. The crutches should be 6 inches lateral to the foot when the patient stands. There should be a two-fingerbreadth width between the axillary bar of the crutch and the axilla. The hands should rest on the crutch handpiece with the elbows flexed 20 to 30 degrees. Most underarm crutches are made of wood and have adjustable height and armpieces, padding for the handpiece and axillary bar, and rubber tips on the end to prevent slippage. The hands bear the weight in crutch-walking. If there is prolonged pressure of the axillary bar into the axilla, nerve damage can result. Good upper-extremity strength is needed to manage crutch-walking.

The standard crutch gaits are the four-point alternate, the two-point alternate, the three-point, the swing-to, and swing-through gaits.

The **four-point gait** is slowest but safest, as there are always three points in contact with the floor. The four-point pattern is: right crutch, left foot, left crutch, and right foot. The **two-point gait** pattern is: right crutch and left foot advanced together followed by the left crutch and right leg. The two-point gait requires more balance than the four-point gait and it is a faster gait. Both the two- and four-point gaits allow some weight-bearing of both lower extremities.

The **three-point gait** is used when one leg cannot bear weight. This gait pattern is: both crutches and the nonweight-bearing leg are advanced, followed by the weight-bearing leg. When one leg bears all the body weight, it carries a load of two and one-half times body weight [28].

In the **swing-to gait,** both crutches are advanced and then both feet and body are swung up to the crutches. In the swing-through gait, both crutches are advanced and the feet and body are lifted and swung through and beyond the crutches. This is a rapid gait and is used when the lower extremities are braced. Both the swing-to and swing-through gaits require more space than the other crutch gaits.

When the patient goes up and down stairs or a curb, the crutches always stay with the affected leg. When going upstairs, the good leg is advanced up one step first, followed by the affected leg and crutches. To descend stairs, the crutches and affected leg are lowered first, followed by the good leg. When there is a hand rail on the stairs, both crutches may be transferred to one hand, and the other hand holds onto the rail. The pattern remains the same.

Normally, walking downstairs creates a load on the hip slightly less than level walking. Walking upstairs increases the load on the hip up to three times body weight; thus, when reduction of weight-bearing on the hip is needed, walking upstairs requires special care [28].

When the patient is using a walker, the patient is centered in the walker. The walker should be lifted with each step, not slid along the floor. The walker allows for a three-point gait. The walker should never be used to grasp onto to help raise the body from a sitting position, as it does not provide enough stability.

A cane is always used in the hand opposite the affected leg. This helps to reduce the forces acting on the affected hip. The cane and affected leg are advanced together, and then the unaffected leg is advanced up to or with a through step. In gait-training with a cane, the patient is sometimes asked to carry something in the opposite hand to help maintain balance; otherwise a limp can develop. Canes can be made of wood or aluminum, they are adjustable, and have a rubber tip.

There are many varieties of wheelchairs to meet the individual needs of patients. Removeable arms facilitate transfer of patients. Every wheelchair must have functional brakes that are locked during any transfer of the patient. Handrims on the wheels allow the patient to propel himself about his environment. These are used when the wheelchair is the only source of the patient's mobility. The front end attachments consist of a variety of footrests and legrests. They can be swung out of the way during transfer and elevated if the extremity should be kept in extension. The patient's feet should never be allowed to drag on the floor when he is in a wheelchair.

Training in the use of a wheelchair includes all factors related to safety, transfers, and mobility. Safety includes the proper use of brakes, how to lock and unlock them, use of the safety belt if required, and how to raise and lower the footrest. Transfer techniques include from the bed to the chair and back to bed, in and out of the bathroom, on and off the toilet, from the wheelchair to another chair, and in and out of an automobile. Mobility techniques include managing doorways, curbs, ramps, and backup maneuvers. A wheelchair-bound patient should be able to do the above independently and unassisted. The patient must also learn wheelchair maintenance and replacement of parts as needed.

Patients who have been immobilized for a period of time or who have had recent orthopedic surgery may be frightened and insecure about attempting ambulation. They must be given proper guidance, instructions, adequate demonstrations, emotional support, and appropriate supervision during the learning stages. Too often, patients are given assistive aids to use without provision for adequate practice under supervision so that they may often use the devices incorrectly or they limit their use. In contrast to such patients, other younger patients may be too eager to use the devices and abuse themselves or the devices, or both, in excessive and improper use.

Assessment of the patient's understanding and ability to use assistive devices is another important aspect of the nursing care involved in the rehabilitation of the patient with disorders of the musculoskeletal system.

References

1. Anast, G. The Splinting of Fractures. Paper read at AAOS course on Postgraduate Education in Orthopaedic Nursing. April 16, 1974, Richmond, Virginia. Unpublished data.
2. Anthony, C. P., and Kolthoff, N. J. *Textbook of Anatomy and Physiology* (8th ed.). St. Louis: Mosby, 1971.
3. Bailey, J. Tractions, suspensions and a ringless splint. *Am. J. Nurs.* 70:1724, 1970.
4. Ball, G. V., and Freeman, S. Management of chronic and recurrent gout. *Mod. Treat.* 8:829, 1971.
5. Beck, W. S. *Human Design: Molecular, Cellular and Systemic Physiology.* New York: Harcourt Brace Jovanovich, 1971.
6. Cailliet, R. *Low Back Pain Syndrome* (2nd ed.). Philadelphia: Davis, 1968.
7. Clissold, G. *The Body's Response to Trauma: Fractures.* New York: Springer, 1973.
8. DeLuca, H. F. Vitamin D: The vitamin and the hormone. *Fed. Proc.* 33:2211, 1974.
9. Deyerle, W. M. The Fractured Hip: From the Emergency Room to the Living Room. Paper read at AAOS course on Postgraduate Education in Orthopaedic Nursing. April 14, 1974, Richmond, Virginia. Unpublished data.
10. Ditunno, J., and Ehrlich, G. E. Care and training of elderly patients with rheumatoid arthritis. *Geriatrics* 25:164, 1970.
11. Flitter, H. H. *An Introduction to Physics in Nursing* (6th ed.). St. Louis: Mosby, 1972.
12. Freyberg, R. Musculoskeletal System. In Sodeman, W. A., and Sodeman, W. A., Jr. (eds.), *Pathologic Physiology Mechanisms of Disease* (4th ed.). Philadelphia: Saunders, 1970. Chap. 32.
13. Frohlich, E. D. (ed.). *Pathophysiology: Altered Regulatory Mechanism in Disease.* Philadelphia: Lippincott, 1972.
14. Ganong, W. F. *Review of Medical Physiology* (6th ed.). Los Altos, Calif.: Lange Medical Publications, 1973.
15. Goldenberg, D. L., and Cohen, A. S. Arthritis: A differential guide. *Hosp. Med.* 10:68, 1974.
16. Hardin, J. G. Approaches to the patient with degenerative joint disease. *Mod. Treat.* 8:840, 1971.
17. Harkess, J. W. Traction: When, where and why? Paper read at AAOS course on Postgraduate Education in Orthopaedic Nursing. April 16, 1974. Richmond, Virginia. Unpublished data.
18. Hoffman, A. L. Psychological factors associated with rheumatoid arthritis. *Nurs. Res.* 23:218, 1974.
19. Jackson, J. B., and Elson, R. A. Evaluation of the Walldius and other prostheses for knee arthroplasty. *Clin. Orthop.* 94:104, 1973.
20. Judge, R. D., and Zuidema, G. D. (eds.). *Physical Diagnosis: A Physiologic Approach to the Clinical Examination* (2nd ed.). Boston: Little, Brown, 1968.
21. Law, J. The fat embolism syndrome. *Nurs. Clin. North Am.* 8:191, 1973.
22. MacRae, I. Arthritis: Its nature and management. *Nurs. Clin. North Am.* 8:643, 1973.
23. McLean, F. C., and Urist, M. R. *Bone: Fundamentals of the Physiology of Skeletal Tissue*

24. Mills, J. A. The conservative management of rheumatoid arthritis. *Mod. Treat.* 8:753, 1971.
25. Robbins, S., and Angell, M. *Basic Pathology.* Philadelphia: Saunders, 1971.
26. Robbins, S. L. *Pathologic Basis of Disease.* Philadelphia: Saunders, 1971.
27. Roberts, J. New developments in orthopedic surgery. *Nurs. Clin. North Am.* 2:383, 1967.
28. Rydell, N. Biomechanics of the hip joint. *Clin. Orthop.* 92:6, 1973.
29. Schneider, R. F. *Handbook for the Orthopaedic Assistant.* St. Louis: Mosby, 1972.
30. Shoemaker, R. Total knee replacement, procedure and results. *Nurs. Clin. North Am.* 8:117, 1973.
31. Stein, A. M., Mandell, D., and Ferguson, J. Multiple fractures: Look out for those pulmonary complications. *Nurs. '74.* 4:26, 1974.
32. Thomas, B. J. Nursing care of patients with cancer of the bone. *Nurs. Clin. North Am.* 2:459, 1967.
33. Turek, S. L. *Orthopaedics: Principles and Their Application* (2nd ed.). Philadelphia: Lippincott, 1967.
34. Widmann, F. K. *Goodale's Clinical Interpretation of Laboratory Tests* (7th ed.). Philadelphia: Davis, 1973.
35. Wilson, B. A. *Limb Prosthetics-1972.* Huntington, N.Y.: Robert E. Krueger, 1972.

Bibliography

American College of Surgeons Committee on Trauma. *Early Care of the Injured Patient.* Philadelphia: Saunders, 1972.
Amstutz, H. C., and Finerman, G. A. M. Knee joint replacement: Development and evaluation. *Clin. Orthop.* 94:24, 1973.
Apley, A. G. Examination of the knee. *Hosp. Med.* 8:40, 1972.
Arnold, H. Elderly diabetic amputees. *Am. J. Nurs.* 69:2646, 1969.
Arthritis: The Basic Facts. New York: The Arthritis Foundation, 1970.
Arthritis Quackery. New York: The Arthritis Foundation, 1970.
Artificial Limbs: A Review of Current Developments. National Research Council Committee on Prosthetics Research and Development and Committee on Prosthetic Orthotic Education. Washington, D.C.: National Academy of Sciences, Autumn, 1971. Vol. 15, No. 2.
Aufranc, O. E., and Turner, R. H. Total replacement of the arthritic hip. *Hosp. Pract.* 6:66, 1971.
Bame, K. Halo traction. *Am. J. Nurs.* 69:1933, 1969.
Bates, B. *A Guide to Physical Examination.* Philadelphia: Lippincott, 1974.
Bayne, L. G. The emergency care and treatment of hand injuries. *Nurs. Clin. North Am.* 2:391. 1967.
Beaumont, E. (ed.). Nursing grand rounds: Ravages of rheumatoid arthritis. *Nurs. '75* 5:44, 1975.
Beaumont, E. Wheelchairs. *Nurs. '73* 3:48, 1973.
Bennage, B. A., and Cummings, M. E. Nursing the patient undergoing total hip arthroplasty. *Nurs. Clin. North Am.* 8:107, 1973.
Bertolinic, A. M. *Gerontologic Medicine.* Springfield, Ill.: Thomas, 1968.
Bilka, P. J. The painful shoulder. *Hosp. Med.* 9:6, 1973.
Blount, W. P., and Moe, J. H. *The Milwaukee Brace.* Baltimore: Williams & Wilkins, 1973.
Bonner, C. D. *Homburger and Bonner's Medical Care and Rehabilitation of the Aged and Chronically Ill* (3rd ed.). Boston: Little, Brown, 1974.
Bosanko, L. Immediate postoperative prosthesis. *Am. J. Nurs.* 71:280, 1971.
Brower, P., and Hicks, D. Maintaining muscle function in patients on bed rest. *Am. J. Nurs.* 72:1250, 1972.
Brown, P. W. The open fracture: Cause, effect and management. *Clin. Orthop.* 96:254, 1973.
Buck, B. I. Total hip replacement. *Supervisor Nurse* 3:74, 1972.
Burgess, E. M., and Romano, R. L. The management of lower extremity amputees using immediate post-surgical prosthesis. *Clin. Orthop.* 57:137, 1968.
Brunner, N. A. *Orthopedic Nursing: A Programmed Approach.* St. Louis: Mosby, 1970.
Cailliet, R. Shoulder pain. *Hosp. Med.* 9:48, 1973.
Calabro, J. J. The three faces of juvenile rheumatoid arthritis. *Hosp. Pract.* 9:61, 1974.
Cardea, J. A. Cast Complications: Prevention, Recognition and Treatment. Paper read at AAOS course on Postgraduate Education in Orthopaedic Nursing. April 16, 1974. Richmond, Virginia. Unpublished data.
Charnley, J. Arthroplasty of the hip: A new operation. *Lancet* 1:1129, 1961.
Christopherson, V. A., Coulter, P. P., and Wolanin, M. O. *Rehabilitation Nursing: Perspectives and Application.* New York: McGraw-Hill, 1974.
Clark, G. M. Infectious arthritis. *Hosp. Med.* 3:70, 1967.
Clawson, D. K., and Dunn, W. Management of common bacterial infections of bones and joints. *J. Bone Joint Surg.* 49-A:164, 1976.
Dodson, W. H. Immunosuppressive therapy in severe rheumatoid arthritis. *Mod. Treat.* 8:778, 1971.

Drain, C. B. The athletic knee injury. *Am. J. Nurs.* 71:536, 1971.

Dunn, A. W. Fractures and dislocations of the pelvis. *Am. Fam. Physician* 6:66, 1970.

Eaton, P., and Heller, F. Therapeutic nursing care of orthopedic patients. *Nurs. Clin. North Am.* 2:429, 1967.

Epstein, H. C. Traumatic dislocations of the hip. *Clin. Orthop.* 92:116, 1973.

Eyre, M. K. Total hip replacement. *Am. J. Nurs.* 71:1384, 1971.

Foss, G. Body mechanics: Use your head and save your back. *Nurs. '73* 3:25, 1973.

Foss, G. Breaking the architectural barrier with crutches, wheelchairs and walkers. *Nurs. '73* 3:17, 1973.

Foss, G. The "how to's" of bed positioning. *Nurs. '72* 2:14, 1972.

Francis, M., Sr. Nursing the patient with internal hip fixation. *Am. J. Nurs.* 64:111, 1964.

Galante, J. Total hip replacement. *AORN J.* 18:726, 1973.

Garner, J. H., and Peltier, L. F. Fat embolism: The significance of provoked petechiae. *J.A.M.A.* 200:226, 1967.

Golding, D. Diagnosis of rheumatoid disease. *Hosp. Med.* 8:21, 1972.

Gout: A Handbook for Patients. New York: The Arthritis Foundation, 1966.

Guyton, A. C. *Basic Human Physiology: Normal Function and Mechanisms of Disease*. Philadelphia: Saunders, 1971.

Harken, D. E., and Matloff, J. M. Initial management of rib fractures and their complications. *Hosp. Med.* 9:68, 1973.

Home Care Programs in Arthritis: A Manual for Patients. New York: The Arthritis Foundation, 1969.

Huxley, H. E. The mechanism of muscular contraction. *Sci. Am.* 213:18, 1965.

Jackson, R. W., and Abe, I. The role of arthroscopy in the management of disorders of the knee. *J. Bone Joint Surg.* 54-B:310, 1972.

Joint Motion: Method of Measuring and Recording. Chicago: American Academy of Orthopaedic Surgeons, 1965.

Keiser, R. P. Treatment of scoliosis. *Nurs. Clin. North Am.* 2:409, 1967.

Kerr, A. *Orthopedic Nursing Procedures* (2nd ed.). New York: Springer, 1969.

Kettlekamp, D. B., and Masca, R. Biomechanics and knee replacement arthroplasty. *Clin. Orthop.* 94:8, 1973.

Kurth, J. Correct application of the Thomas splint and Pearson attachment. *Nurs. '73* 3:20, 1973.

Larson, C. B., and Gould, M. *Orthopedic Nursing* (8th ed.). St. Louis: Mosby, 1974.

Levy, S. W., and Barnes, G. H. *Hygienic Problems of the Amputee*. Washington, D.C.: The American Orthotics and Prosthetics Association, 1961.

Licht, S., and Kamenetz, H. L. (eds.). *Rehabilitation and Medicine*. New Haven: Elizabeth Licht, 1968.

Manual of Orthopaedic Surgery. Chicago: American Orthopaedic Association, 1972.

Marmor, L., and Treace, J. A new balanced suspension. *Clin. Orthop.* 85:146, 1972.

Martin, N. Rehabilitation of the upper extremity amputee. *Nurs. Outlook* 18:49, 1970.

Massie, W. K. Treatment of femoral neck fractures emphasizing long term follow-up on aseptic necrosis. *Clin. Orthop.* 92:16, 1973.

McCollun, D. E., and Ogden, W. S. Surgery and its place in the therapy of chronic arthritis. *Mod. Treat.* 8:807, 1971.

McNaught, A. B., and Callander, R. *Illustrated Physiology* (2nd ed.). Edinburgh: Churchill Livingstone, 1973.

Meyer, P. R. Approach to long bone fractures. *Hosp. Med.* 6:36, 1970.

Michele, A. Principles of fracture care. *Am. J. Orthop.* 9:34, 1967.

Monteiro, L. A. Hip fracture: A sociologist's viewpoint. *Am. J. Nurs.* 67:1207, 1967.

Myers, A. Chrysotherapy in rheumatoid arthritis. *Mod. Treat.* 8:761, 1971.

Neufeld, A. J. Surgical treatment of hip injuries. *Am. J. Nurs.* 67:80, 1967.

Osteoarthritis: A Handbook for Patients. New York: The Arthritis Foundation, 1967.

Peltier, L. A brief history of traction. *J. Bone Joint Surg.* 50-A:1603, 1968.

Peltier, L. Complications of pelvic fractures. *Hosp. Med.* 3:88, 1967.

Perry, J., and Hislop, H. J. *Principles of Lower Extremity Bracing*. New York: American Physical Therapy Association, 1967.

Perry, T., and Miller, F. *Pathology: A Dynamic Introduction to Medicine and Surgery*. Boston: Little, Brown, 1961.

Phelps, P. Nongouty crystal deposit arthritis. *Mod. Treat.* 8:851, 1971.

Pinals, R. S. Salicylates in the management of rheumatoid arthritis. *Mod. Treat.* 8:796, 1971.

Ranalls, J. Crutches and walkers. *Nurs. '72* 2:21, 1972.

Rehabilitative Aspects of Nursing (A programmed instruction series). Part I. Physical Therapeutic Measure. Unit I. Concepts and goals. New York: National League for Nursing, 1966.

Rheumatoid Arthritis: A Handbook for Patients. New York: The Arthritis Foundation, 1966.

Rich, C. Changing concepts of osteoporosis. *Hosp. Med.* 3:24, 1967.

Riordon, F. H., and Holder, D. H. The painful back. *Hosp. Med.* 9:33, 1973.

Rosenbaum, E. Subdeltoid bursitis: The painful shoulder. *Hosp. Med.* 10:58, 1974.

Russek, A. S., Thompson, W. A. L., Clauss, R. H., and Truchly, G. *Investigation of Immediate Prosthetic Fittings and Early Ambulation Following Amputation in the Lower Extremity*. (Rehabilitation Monograph XLI). New York: Institute of Rehabilitation Medicine, New York University Medical Center, 1969.

Sarmiento, A. Recent trends in lower extremity amputation. *Nurs. Clin. North Am.* 2:398, 1967.

Sarmiento, A., et al. Lower extremity amputation: The impact of immediate post surgical prosthetic fitting. *Clin. Orthop.* 68:22, 1970.

Shepaed, R. C., and Holley, H. Role of physical therapy and rehabilitation medicine in the management of chronic arthritis. *Mod. Treat.* 8:787, 1971.

Soika, C. V. Combating osteoporosis. *Am. J. Nurs.* 73:1193, 1973.

Stein, I., and Beller, M. L. Therapeutic progress in osteoporosis. *Geriatrics* 25:159, 1970.

Tambakis, A. P., and Weinsaft, P. Fractures of the femoral neck: A ten-year review. *Geriatrics* 22:122, 1967.

The do's and don'ts of traction care. *Nurs. '74* 4:35, 1974.

The Traction Handbook. Warsaw, Indiana: Zimmer Manufacturing Company, 1971.

Townley, C., and Hill, L. Total knee replacement. *Am. J. Nurs.* 74:1612, 1974.

Walike, B. C. Rheumatoid arthritis: Personality factors. *Am. J. Nurs.* 67:1427, 1967.

Walike, B. C., Marmor, L., and Upshaw, M. J. Rheumatoid arthritis. *Am. J. Nurs.* 67:1420, 1967.

Webb, K. J. Early assessment of orthopedic injuries. *Am. J. Nurs.* 74:1048, 1974.

Whitehead, D. J. Emergency care in orthopedic injuries. *Nurs. Clin. North Am.* 8:435, 1973.

Wilkie, D. R. *Muscle.* London: William Clowes, 1968.

Young, C., Sr. Exercise: How to use it to decrease complications in immobilized patients. *Nurs. '75* 5:81, 1975.

Zvaifler, N. J. Antimalarials in the treatment of rheumatoid arthritis. *Mod. Treat.* 8:769, 1971.

chapter 11
Patients with Nervous System Dysfunction

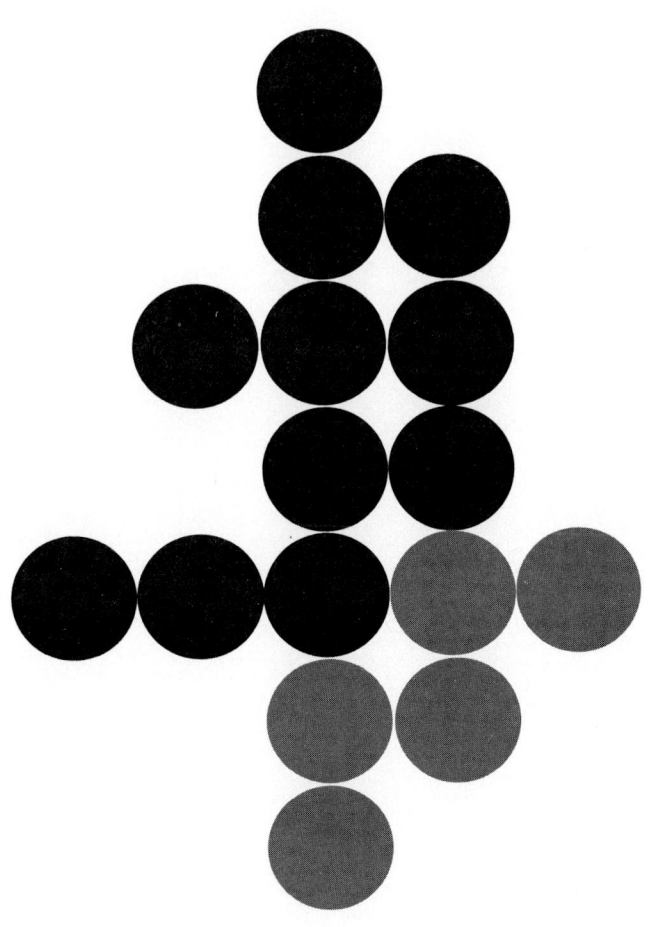

The nervous system has a dominant role in controlling and coordinating all body activities. It is a complex and highly organized system that affects all other systems in the body.

Neurology is the study of the nervous system and of the organic disorders and diseases that affect the system. To understand the changes that occur with dysfunctions of the system, the nurse must have some understanding of various parts of the system, their interdependence, and their normal function. Although the nervous system is susceptible to a great number of disorders and diseases of congenital, infectious, vascular, degenerative, neoplastic, or traumatic origin, the neurologic changes that result are related to the site of the pathology and the functions of the parts that are involved. Thus, knowledge of the anatomic and physiologic aspects of the nervous system enables the nurse to understand the changes that occur, regardless of the cause, and to determine the implications for nursing care.

Anatomy and Physiology of the Nervous System

The nervous system consists of two anatomic divisions: the **central nervous system** (CNS), which consists of the brain and spinal cord, which are contained within the skull and vertebral column; and the **peripheral nervous system** (PNS), which consists of the cranial and spinal nerves, their peripheral combinations, and the peripheral portions of the autonomic system. On a physiologic basis, the nervous system consists of two divisions: the **somatic nervous system,** also known as the cerebrospinal or voluntary nervous system, which transmits impulses to and from the nonvisceral parts of the body, and the **autonomic nervous system,** also known as the involuntary nervous system, which innervates the viscera and other smooth muscles, cardiac muscle, and glands.

THE NEURON AND NERVE IMPULSES

The **neuron,** or nerve cell, is the structural unit of the nervous system and is responsible for receiving and transmitting all stimuli and impulses in nervous system activities. The nerve cell is composed of a cell body with a nucleus and several processes of varying length. The short processes, the **dendrites,** receive and conduct impulses to the cell body; the long process, the **axon,** or nerve fiber, conducts impulses away from the cell body.

Nerve cell bodies are usually found in groups. Collections of nerve cell bodies outside the brain or spinal cord are referred to as **ganglia.** Within the brain and spinal cord, groups of nerve cell bodies, together with unmyelinated (unsheathed) fibers and supporting tissue, form the **gray matter.** The **white matter** of the brain and spinal cord consists mostly of nerve fibers that are covered with **myelin,** a white sheath. The gray matter of the brain forms the **cerebral cortex,** which is the surface layer of the cerebral hemispheres, the basal ganglia, various nuclei in the brainstem, and the central portion of the spinal cord. The characteristic appearance of the cross sections of the brain and spinal cord results from the contrast of the gray and white matter. The **neuroglia,** or glia, is the supporting tissue of nerves and consists of a network of glial cells and fibrils.

Nerve fibers that have a common origin and destination and a particular function tend to run together within the spinal cord forming tracts, or bundles. Fibers and tracts are usually named by using the site of origin followed by the site of termination. Thus the **spinothalamic tract** consists of fibers that go from the spinal cord to the thalamus.

Impulses are transmitted between neurons at the synapse (or synaptic junction), the junction between the axon of one neuron (the presynaptic neuron) and the cell body (or dendrites) of another neuron (the postsynaptic neuron). The **synapse** is an avenue for intercellular communication, primarily concerned with the transfer of electrophysiologic information between cells. Action potentials in the presynaptic neuron cause the release of neurotransmitters (chemical substances) that are stored in synaptic vesicles in the axon terminal. The neurotransmitters cross the synaptic cleft (the region of membrane separation) and either prevent (inhibit) or produce (excite) action potentials in the postsynaptic neuron [4, 11]. Synaptic transmission always takes place from the presynaptic to the postsynaptic element. Thus, impulses are conducted in only one direction, away from the region that receives the stimulation.

CENTRAL NERVOUS SYSTEM

The brain and spinal cord are protected by bony and membranous coverings, as well as by a cushion of cerebrospinal fluid. The skull, which covers the brain, is a rigid compartment of fused bone with a large opening in its base, the **foramen magnum,** where the cranial cavity and the vertebral canal meet. Other smaller openings in the skull provide passage for cranial nerves and blood vessels.

The vertebral column in the adult consists of 26 vertebrae: 7 cervical, 12 thoracic, 5 lumbar, 1 sacral, and 1 coccygeal. The vertebrae form a canal for the spinal cord, with the vertebral bodies in the front and an arch formed by the laminae and spinous processes in the back. The vertebral bodies are separated from each other by an **intervertebral disc,** which consists of a central cartilaginous portion, the **nucleus pulposus,** surrounded by a fibrous capsule, the **anulus fibrosis.** Spinal roots pass through an opening, the **intervertebral foramen,** which is located above and below each pedicle of the spinous process.

In addition to the bony coverings, the brain and spinal cord are protected by three membranes, the **meninges:** (1) the dura mater, (2) the arachnoid, and (3) the pia mater. The **dura mater,** the outer tough membrane of the nervous system, lines the skull and also extends through the foramen magnum and lines the vertebral column (although the spinal dura has no attachment to the vertebrae). The dura mater is separated from the arachnoid mater by the **subdural space,** through which fine blood vessels pass. The **arachnoid,** a delicate impermeable membrane, is separated by the subarachnoid space from the **pia mater,** the innermost membrane, which adheres to the brain and spinal cord. The subarachnoid space contains cerebrospinal fluid. The large subarachnoid spaces at the base of the brain are called cisternae (cisterns). The major cistern, the *cisterna cerebellomedullaris,* also known as the cisterna magna, is located over the dorsum of the medulla oblongata (page 896) and lies between it and the cerebellum. The cerebrospinal fluid circulates upward over the surface of the brain and downward, around the spinal cord, and serves as a cushion for these structures against trauma.

The folds of the meninges act as supporting structures both for the spinal cord and the brain. The dura folds vertically along the midsaggital line (medial longitudinal fissure) within the skull and forms the *falx cerebri,* the fold that separates the two cerebral hemispheres. At the superior and inferior boundaries, the layers of the falx cerebri separate and form the superior and inferior longitudinal sinuses, which function as cerebral veins.

At the posterior end of the falx cerebri, the dura projects laterally and forms the **tentorium cerebelli,** an important landmark within the brain that is used to describe the sites of lesions (supratentorial, infratentorial). The tentorium cerebelli supports the temporal and occipital lobes and separates the posterior cranial fossa from the remainder of the cranial cavity. The pia mater is closely attached to the surface of all the folds of the brain, the **gyri.** The **sulci** are the furrows of the brain.

The central nervous system can be divided into six major regions (Fig. 11-1). These regions are identified as the following: the telencephalon, the diencephalon, the mesencephalon or the midbrain, the metencephalon which is divided into the pons and cerebellum, the myelencephalon or medulla, and the spinal medulla or spinal cord. Within this chapter, however, disorders of the central nervous system will be discussed using specific structures, rather than using the regional terminology.

Cerebrum

The cerebrum occupies the anterior and middle fossae of the skull. It is incompletely divided by a longitudinal fissure into two cerebral hemispheres, which are joined at their base by a band of white matter, the **corpus callosum.** In each individual, one hemisphere appears to be more important functionally than the other and is called the dominant hemisphere. (In 90 percent of the population, the left hemisphere is dominant.) The concept of dominance in cerebral hemispheres is controversial. Mountcastle [22] cites that hemispheres differ with respect to the particular function for which they are specialized and that each performs its assigned role as a reciprocal specialization rather than as a hierarchy of importance.

Each hemisphere has a surface layer of gray matter, the cortex, and is divided into four lobes: (1) the frontal lobe, which is located most anteriorly; (2) the parietal lobe, in an upper central position; (3) the temporal lobe, in a lower lateral position; and (4) the occipital lobe, which is located posteriorly (Fig. 11-2). These lobes are bounded by deep fissures: The central fissure (**fissure of Rolando**) separates the frontal from the parietal lobe; the lateral fissure (**fissure of Sylvius**) separates the temporal from the frontal and parietal lobes;

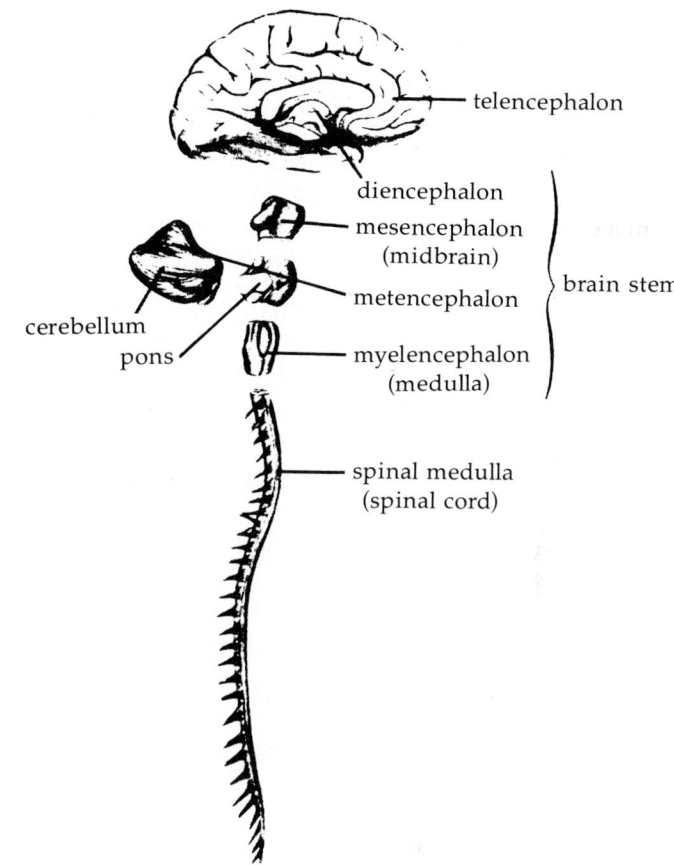

Figure 11-1
Six major regions of the central nervous system. (From G. B. Dunkerly, *A Basic Atlas of the Human Nervous System*. Philadelphia: F. A. Davis Company, 1975. Reproduced by permission.)

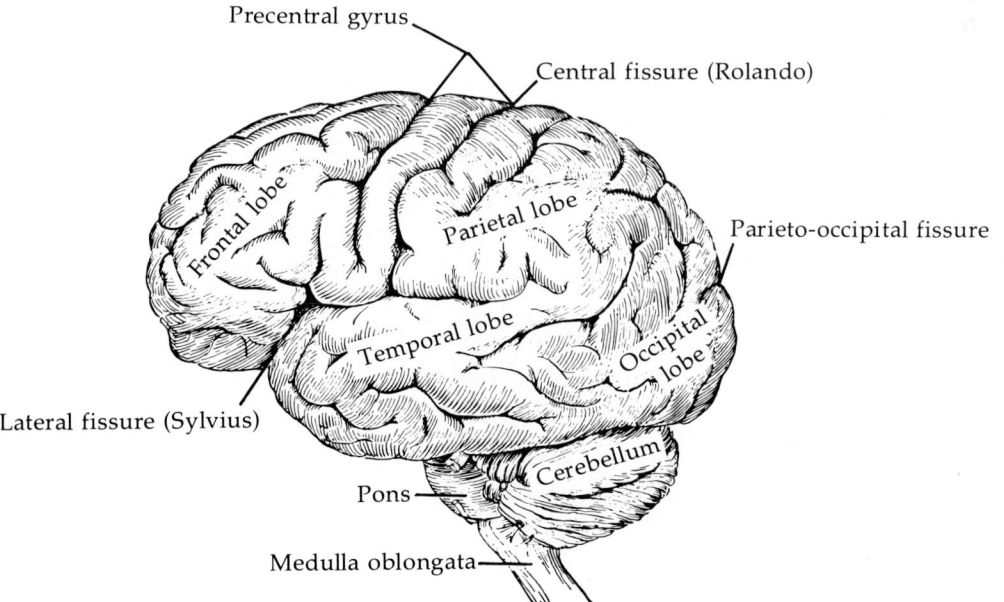

Figure 11-2
The four lobes of the cerebrum. (From E. Carini and G. Owens, *Neurological and Neurosurgical Nursing* [6th ed.]. St. Louis: Mosby, 1974. Reproduced by permission.)

and the **parieto-occipital fissure** separates the occipital from the parietal and temporal lobes.

The **frontal lobe** is primarily concerned with personality, behavior, and the cognitive processes: consciousness, learning, abstract and creative thinking, problem solving, judgment, memory, and social, moral, and ethical values. In the posterior part of the frontal lobe are the **pyramidal cells,** large cells that control motor activity throughout the body. This area, the **precentral gyrus,** or motor area, is the site of origin of motor nerves traveling to specific voluntary muscle groups throughout the body. If specific points in this area are electrically stimulated, movement is produced in specific areas on the opposite side of the body. The sites of these motor centers (Fig. 11-3) indicate the relation of these subdivisions to the consecutive parts of the body. (The diagram includes the motor speech center, but this center is found only in one hemisphere, usually the left.)

The **parietal lobe** is of major importance for interpretation of sensations, with the exception of smell, sight, hearing, and taste. It receives all the sensory impulses from the skin, mucosa, muscles, joints, and tendons from the opposite side of the body. The parietal lobe is also responsible for the **stereognostic sense,** the ability to recognize the size, shape, weight, texture, and consistency of objects, and the ability to differentiate between two skin contacts made simultaneously (known as two-point discrimination). It also provides for **proprioception,** the sense that gives information about the body's movements and position in space.

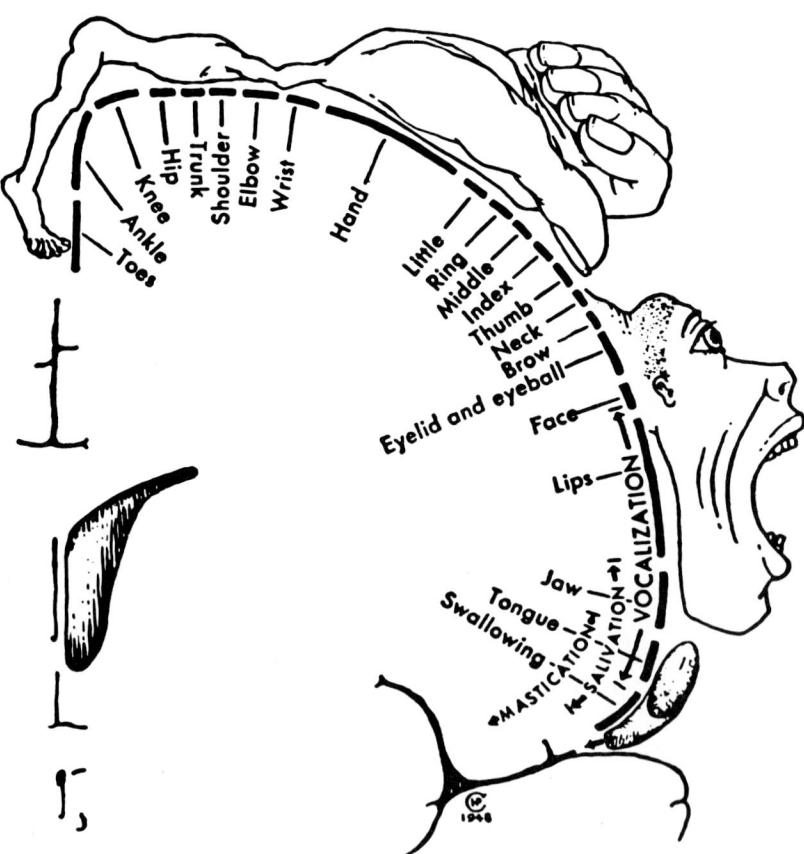

Figure 11-3
Relationship between sites of the motor centers and parts of the body. (From W. Penfield and T. Rasmussen, *The Cerebral Cortex of Man: A Clinical Study of Localization of Function.* New York: Macmillan, 1950. Reproduced by permission.)

The **temporal lobe,** located anteriorly to the occipital lobe but inferiorly to the parietal and frontal lobes, is the center for hearing, taste, and smell, three of the four special senses. In addition, the nerve fibers of the optic nerve travel through the temporal lobe to the occipital lobe. In the dominant hemisphere, the temporal lobe is also the center for understanding the spoken word [3].

The posterior lobe of the cerebrum is the **occipital lobe,** the end station for the optic nerve, receiving nervous impulses originating in the retina.

Other structures within the cerebrum are the hypothalamus, thalamus, basal ganglia, and internal capsule, as well as the third and lateral ventricles (Fig. 11-4). (The ventricles are described under Cerebrospinal Fluid on page 900.) The **hypothalamus,** located in the inferior part of the cerebrum in close proximity to the pituitary body, is the link between the neural and endocrine systems. By its regulatory effect on the pituitary gland and the autonomic system, the hypothalamus influences fat and carbohydrate metabolism, fluid and electrolyte balance, growth, sexual maturity, pulse rate, blood pressure, and sleep. It also affects the internal secretion of other endocrine glands and contains the temperature regulating center of the body. Thus the hypothalamus is the control center for a number of homeostatic mechanisms and for coordination of autonomic activity. The limbic system, in conjunction with the hypothalamus, controls visceral motor activity associated with emotional reactions. The limbic system comprises structures of the cortex, including certain gyri, that developed early in the brain's evolution and are common to all mammals.

The **thalamus,** which is either of two large masses of nerve cells adjacent to the third and on the floor of the lateral ventricle, is responsible for modifying and controlling the primitive emotions of pain, rage, fear, love, and hate, as well as serving as a relay station for all sensory information and other projections to the cerebral cortex. The thala-

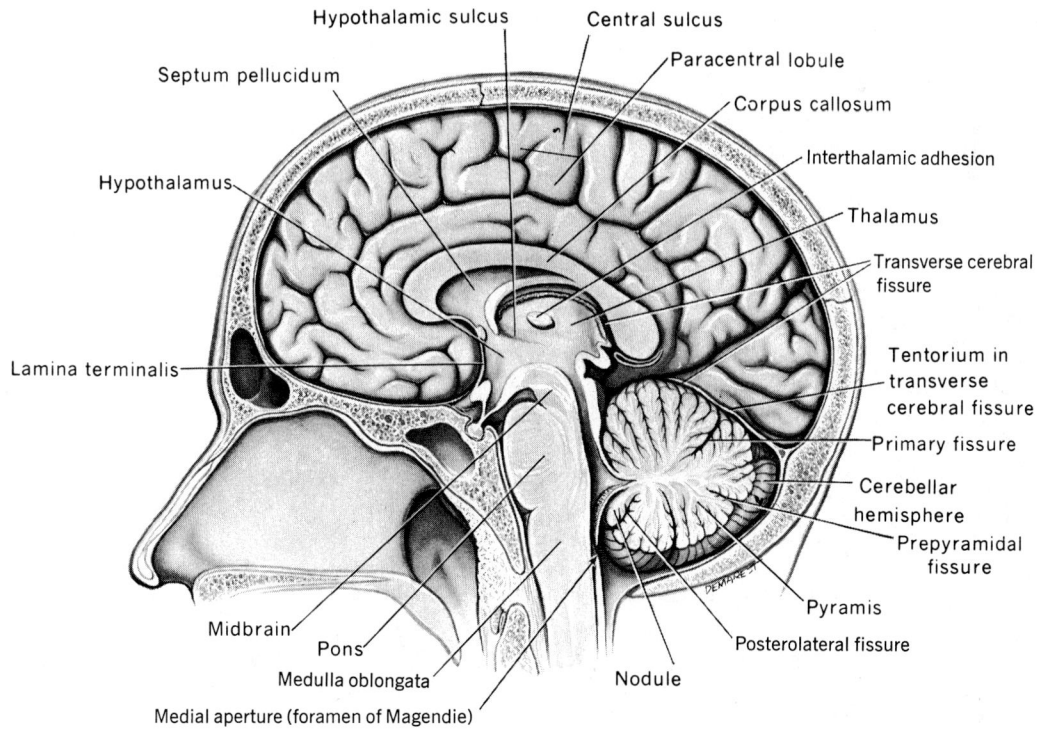

Figure 11-4
Other structures within the cerebrum. (From C. R. Noback and R. J. Demarest, *The Nervous System: Introduction and Review.* Copyright © 1972 by McGraw-Hill Book Company. Used with permission.)

mus contains many nuclei concerned with specific senses such as touch and temperature.

The **basal ganglia,** or basal nuclei, a group of cells that influence muscular activity, are located deep in the center of each hemisphere on either side of the midline and consist of 5 paired masses of nuclei: the caudate, putamen, the corpus striatum, the amygdaloid nucleus, or body, and the claustrum. The **corpus striatum** is composed of the caudate and lentiform nuclei. The basal ganglia are connected with the upper midbrain (page 903) via the red nuclei and substantia nigra, which also influence smooth and coordinated muscular activity. Diseases that affect the basal ganglia result in disruption of coordinated muscular activity, with loss of automatic movements of expression and walking and cause tremor and muscle rigidity.

Medial to the thalamus and lateral to the basal ganglia is the **internal capsule,** a large bundle of ascending and descending fiber tracts, or white matter. Lesions in the area of the internal capsule disrupt the flow of impulses through this area. This type of disruption is seen, for example, in cerebrovascular accidents.

Cerebellum

The cerebellum is located just below the occipital lobe, from which it is separated by the **tentorium,** the dura mater that supports it and the occipital lobes. It is attached to the brainstem by the cerebellar peduncles. The cerebellum has two hemispheres and a central section, the **vermis**. It contains many feedback circuits to the motor cortex and coordinates tone and movement of groups of muscles, including the skeletal muscles that maintain equilibrium and control posture. (Dysfunction of the cerebellum causes gait changes and hyporeflexia.)

Brainstem

The brainstem extends from the cerebral hemispheres to the foramen magnum at the base of the skull, where it merges with the spinal cord. All the nerve fibers passing between the cerebral hemispheres, cerebellum, and spinal cord are carried in the brainstem, which extends to the foramen magnum at the base of the skull, where it merges with the spinal cord. The components of the brainstem in descending order are the midbrain, pons, and medulla oblongata. As well as containing descending and ascending nerve pathways, the brainstem also contains the nuclei of 10 cranial nerves (III through XII) and the reticular formation.

The **medulla oblongata** is a cone-shaped structure that contains groups of neurons forming the vital centers for cardiac, respiratory, and vasomotor regulation and the reflex centers for coughing, salivation, sneezing, vomiting, and swallowing.

Within the brainstem is a central core of intertwining gray and white matter, the **reticular formation,** or reticular activating system, which receives sensory impulses from all over the body and plays an important role in the function of the cerebral cortex. Ascending nerve tracts from the reticular formation transmit impulses to the cerebral cortex that activate the cortical neurons and promote a state of alertness. An intact reticular formation is necessary to provide the arousal state of the cerebral cortex to receive and interpret incoming sensory impulses. Injury to this area produces loss of consciousness. Hypnotic drugs and anesthesia also selectively block transmission in the reticular activating system, and thus cause decreased wakefulness and reduced alertness.

Cranial Nerves

The cranial nerves provide for sensory and motor functions of muscles and autonomic functions as well as for the special senses of vision, hearing, smell, and taste. The 12 pairs of cranial nerves, each of which is designated by a Roman numeral, are as follows: olfactory (I), optic (II), oculomotor (III), trochlear (IV), trigeminal (V), abducens (VI), facial (VII), vestibulocochlear (acoustic) (VIII), glossopharyngeal (IX), vagus (X), accessory (XI), and hypoglossal (XII). The cranial nerve nuclei of the oculomotor and trochlear nerves are located in the midbrain, while those of the trigeminal, abducens, facial, and vestibulocochlear nerves are located in the pons, and those of the glossopharyngeal, vagus, accessory, and hypoglossal nerves, in the medulla oblongata. The latter cranial nerves in the medullar are "bulbar." The olfactory and optic nerves, which are two pairs of sensory tracts, originate in the nasal epithelium and retina respectively and do not have nuclei within the brainstem.

The **olfactory nerve** (I) is the special sense organ for smell. A small patch of olfactory mucosa in the upper rear portion of each nostril contains the receptors for smell. During normal breathing, little of the inspired air reaches the olfactory mucosa, but in sniffing, airflow is directed to this sensitive region and thus enhances the sensation of smell [11]. The fibers from the olfactory mucosa enter the skull through the midline portion of the anterior cranial fossa, where they join cells in the olfactory bulbs on the undersurface of the frontal lobes. The fibers then proceed along the base of the brain to each side of the optic chiasm where they enter the cerebrum and reach the thalamus and the temporal lobe.

The **optic nerve** (II) has the special sensory function of vision. Nerve fibers from the retina of the eye, which is the sensory receptor, come together as the optic nerve. The fibers pass posteriorly with approximately half (fibers from the temporal side of each eye) continuing on the same side to the brain and the other half (fibers from the medial half of the eye) crossing to the other side of the brain, creating the **optic chiasm,** which is located directly over the pituitary body. As shown in Figure 11-5, both the crossed and uncrossed fibers from the right side of the eye join together after the crossing and continue as the optic tract to the right lateral geniculate body, which is located adjacent to the thalamus; fibers from the left side of the eye join and pass to the left lateral geniculate body. The optic tract then continues around the tip of the temporal lobe posteriorly to the occipital lobe of the cerebrum.

Figure 11-5 is helpful in understanding

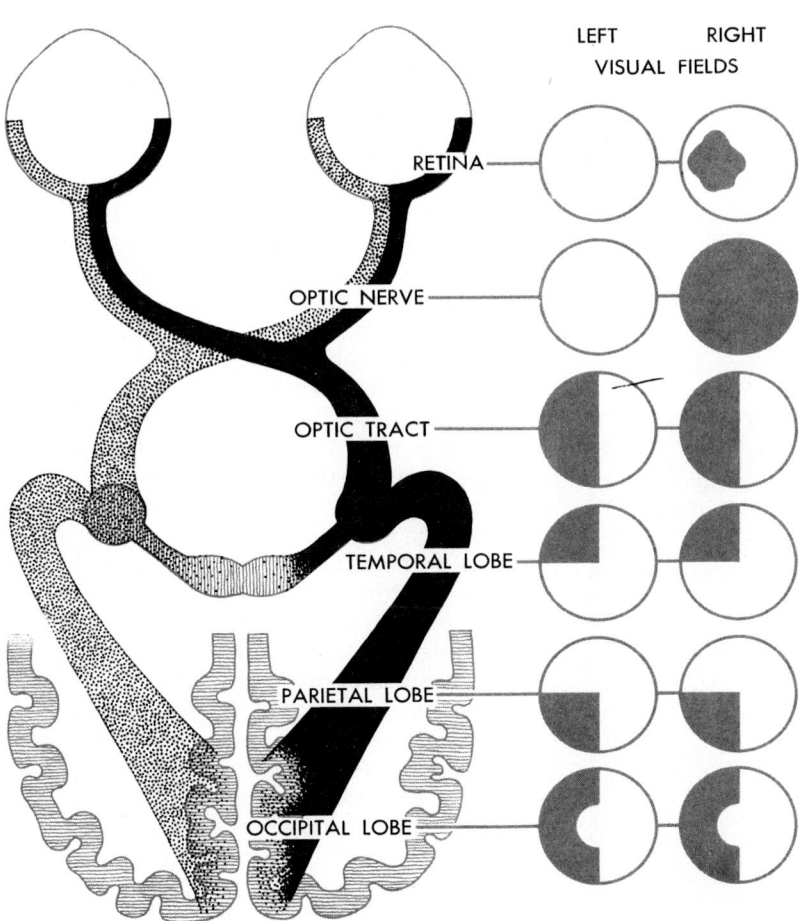

Figure 11-5
Visual pathways. (From *Essentials of the Neurological Examination*. Philadelphia: SmithKline Corporation, 1974. Reproduced by permission.)

why visual fields are disturbed when there is a lesion of the optic pathways. Thus, blindness in one eye results if one of the optic nerves is injured or diseased. If a tumor presses on the optic chiasm where the partial crossing of fibers occurs, the crossed fibers that come from the nasal side of the retina are interrupted, and **bitemporal hemianopia,** which is blindness in the temporal halves of each field of vision, results. If the compression on the visual pathway occurs behind the chiasm anywhere in the tract, the interference with both the crossed and uncrossed fibers causes **homonymous hemianopia,** which is blindness in the same halves of the visual field of both eyes. Thus, testing the field of vision is important in efforts to locate the site of a lesion.

Because the optic nerve is sheathed by a prolongation of the cranial meninges, increased pressure within the cranium causes stasis in the central retinal vein and pressure is transferred to the nerve, resulting in **papilledema,** or choked disc, which is swelling of the optic disc, the part of the optic nerve within the eye. This swelling can be observed with an ophthalmoscope (Fig. 11-6).

The **oculomotor nerve** (III) innervates the inferior oblique muscle and the superior, medial, and inferior rectus muscles, which control eyeball movements (up, down, and medially). It also innervates the muscle that raises the eyelid and constricts the pupil. Autonomic nerve fibers travel via the oculomotor nerve to the parasympathetic ciliary ganglion in the orbit, from which fibers go to the iris and control pupil constriction.

The **trochlear nerve** (IV) supplies the superior oblique muscle, which rotates the eyeball downward and outward. The **trigeminal nerve** (V), the largest cranial nerve, has both motor and sensory elements. The motor fibers innervate the muscles for mastication, the tensor tympani muscle of the eardrum, and the tensor veli palatini muscle, which tenses the soft palate and opens the eustachian tube. Damage to the motor root of the trigeminal nerve interferes with chewing and with opening the mouth. The sensory part of the trigeminal nerve originates in the trigeminal (gasserian, semilunar) ganglion, which has three branches: (1) The ophthalmic branch reaches the skin of the head, forehead, upper eyelid, and part of the nose as well as the mucous membrane of the nose and the cornea and conjunctiva; (2) The maxillary division goes to the skin of the cheek, the lower part of the nose, the lower eyelid, the upper lip, the mucous membrane, and the teeth of the upper jaw; and (3) The mandibular branch goes to the skin of the lower lip, chin, and ear, the teeth, and the mucous membrane of the lower jaw and the tongue.

The **abducens nerve** (VI) innervates the lateral rectus muscle, which regulates the movement of the eyeball outward. The **facial nerve** (VII), although primarily a motor nerve, also has sensory and autonomic components. It innervates the muscles of the forehead, eyelids, cheeks, and lips, ears, nose, and neck. The sensory portion of the nerve controls the perception of taste on the anterior two-thirds of the tongue.

The **vestibulocochlear (acoustic) nerve** (VIII) is a sensory nerve with two parts: a cochlear part and a vestibular part. The cochlear fibers represent nerve cells in the spiral ganglion in the cochlea and are concerned with hearing. The vestibular fibers, representing nerve cells in the vestibular ganglion, monitor and control equilibrium.

The **glossopharyngeal nerve** (IX) contains motor, sensory, and autonomic elements. The motor fibers innervate the constrictors of the pharynx and stylopharyngeus muscles to

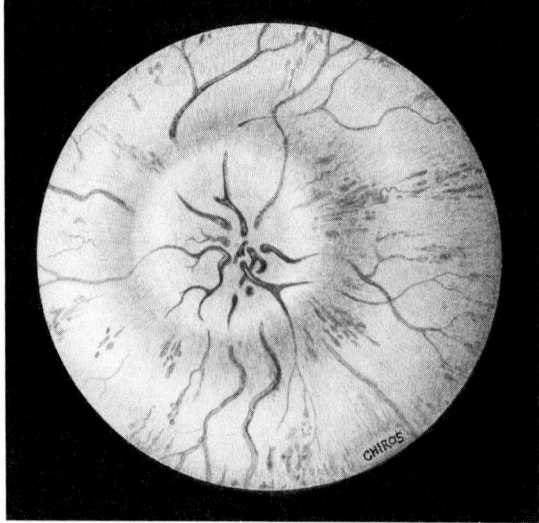

Figure 11-6
Papilledema.

facilitate swallowing. The sensory fibers transmit taste sensation from the posterior third of the tongue, sensation from the soft palate, fauces, and tonsils, and afferent impulses from the carotid body and sinus. Autonomic fibers are supplied to glands (mainly the parotid).

The **vagus nerve** (X) is also a mixed nerve, closely related to the glossopharyngeal in its position and function. It is the major segment of the parasympathetic nervous system. The motor fibers control the voluntary activity of the pharynx and larynx and the involuntary activity of the esophagus, bronchi, lungs, heart, stomach, small intestines, liver, pancreas, and kidneys. It also supplies sensory fibers to the tongue, pharynx, larynx, the back of the ear, and the posterior wall of the external acoustic meatus, as well as autonomic sensory fibers from most of the organs of the body.

The **accessory nerve** (XI) is a motor nerve that supplies the sternocleidomastoid and upper part of the trapezius muscles. The **hypoglossal nerve** (XII), also a motor nerve, supplies the muscles of the tongue. The functions of the cranial nerves are summarized in Table 11-1.

Vascular System of the Brain and Spinal Cord

The brain consumes 20 percent of the oxygen utilized by the body. This fact makes clear why the brain can withstand oxygen deficiency for only 3 to 5 minutes before irreparable damage occurs to the neurons. It is important for the nurse to remember that the more specialized a tissue is, the less likely it is able to survive a severe and sudden deficit in oxygen supply. These two physiologic characteristics of the brain have implications for the nursing care of the patient with intracranial disease with ypoxia.

The blood supply to the brain is derived from branches of the subclavian arteries, the two internal carotid arteries anteriorly and the two vertebral arteries posteriorly. These communicate at the base of the brain via the basilar artery (which is formed by the junction of the two vertebral arteries) and communicating arteries, forming the circle of Willis, an arterial circle (Fig. 11-7). This vascular structure provides continuity of the circulation if any one of the four main channels is disrupted. The circle of Willis surrounds the optic chiasm and the pituitary stalk.

The anterior and middle cerebral arteries branch from the carotid arteries at the base of the brain, and the posterior cerebral arteries branch from the basilar artery. Branches of the cerebral arteries extend throughout the cerebrum. The middle cerebral artery supplies most of the lateral surface of the cerebral hemispheres and the deep structures of the parietal, frontal, and temporal lobes. The anterior cerebral artery supplies the medial surface of the cerebrum and the superior border of the frontal and parietal lobes. The posterior cerebral artery supplies the entire occipital lobe and the inferior and medial portions of the temporal lobe. The cerebellum and brainstem are supplied primarily by other branches of the vertebral and basilar arteries.

The veins of the brain empty into sinuses of

Table 11-1
Functions of the cranial nerves

Number	Name	Function
I	Olfactory	Sense of smell
II	Optic	Sense of vision
III*	Oculomotor	Eye movements (autonomic to eye)
IV	Trochlear	Eye movements
V	Trigeminal	Chewing, facial sensations
VI	Abducens	Eye movements
VII*	Facial	Taste (autonomic to glands)
VIII	Acoustic	Hearing, equilibrium
IX*	Glossopharyngeal	Taste, swallowing (autonomic to glands)
X*	Vagus	Control of larynx, swallowing (autonomic to viscera)
XI	Spinal accessory	Control of neck muscles
XII	Hypoglossal	Movement of tongue

*Denotes involvement in the autonomic nervous system.
Source: E. E. Selkurt (ed.), *Basic Physiology for the Health Sciences.* Boston: Little, Brown and Company, 1975.

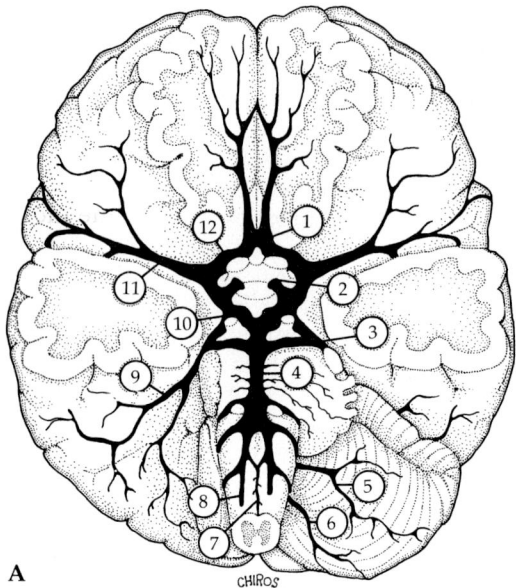
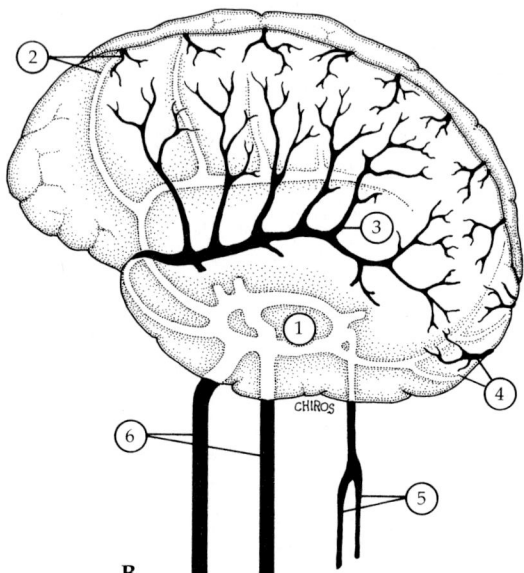

1. Anterior communicating artery
2. Internal carotid artery
3. Superior cerebellar artery
4. Basilar artery
5. Anterior inferior cerebellar artery
6. Posterior inferior cerebellar artery
7. Anterior spinal artery
8. Vertebral artery
9. Posterior cerebral artery
10. Posterior communicating artery
11. Middle cerebral artery
12. Anterior cerebral artery

1. Circle of Willis
2. Anterior cerebral artery
3. Middle cerebral artery
4. Posterior cerebral artery
5. Vertebral arteries
6. Carotid arteries

Figure 11-7
The blood supply to the brain.

the dura mater and then into the internal jugular veins to return venous blood to the heart. The cranial fossae (bony supports of the brain) and the dura mater are supplied by the anterior, middle, and posterior meningeal arteries, of which the middle meningeal is the most important. Laceration of this artery as a result of fracture of the temporal bone leads to increased intracranial pressure, brain displacement, and death.

The spinal cord receives its arterial supply from the anterior spinal artery and two posterior spinal arteries, which are branches of the vertebral arteries. In addition, these vessels receive blood at each segment of the cord via the lateral spinal arteries.

Blood-Brain Barrier

The blood-brain barrier prevents or delays the passage of certain substances into the brain tissue. Selective capillary permeability in the brain is different from that in other parts of the body. It is thought that the barrier in the walls of blood vessels of the central nervous system and the surrounding glial membranes has a protective function, since it helps to prevent the passage or the accumulation of chemical substances such as drugs within the brain. The existence of this barrier is an important factor in drug use. Drugs do not normally accumulate in the cerebrospinal fluid because protein is unavailable for binding. Substances used in brain scanning procedures are agents that readily cross the blood-brain barrier.

Cerebrospinal Fluid

Within the brain are four interconnected cavities: the right and left lateral ventricles, one in each hemisphere; the third ventricle, beneath the corpus callosum and between the two thalami; and the fourth ventricle, bounded by the pons and medulla in front and the cerebellum behind. The cerebrospinal fluid (CSF), often referred to as the third circulation, is formed (by secretion or dialysis) from the blood by the epithelial cells of the choroid plexuses, which are folds of pia mater in the ventricles. The CSF is formed especially in the lateral ventricles (Fig. 11-8).

The fluid flows from the lateral ventricles to the third ventricle via the interventricular foramina (of Monro), and then through the aqueduct of Sylvius to the fourth ventricle. It eventually flows via the foramina of Luschka and the foramen of Magendie to the cerebellomedullary cistern and finally to the other subarachnoid cisterns and throughout the subarachnoid space to surround the brain and spinal cord. It is reabsorbed into the bloodstream via venous channels primarily through the superior sagittal sinus. Any blockage within the circuit results in an excessive accumulation of fluid within the ventricles. If this blockage occurs before the bones of the skull are fused, the head becomes enlarged (hydrocephalus), with resulting brain atrophy and mental retardation. In the older child or adult the expanding volume of fluid in the rigid skull compresses the brain within the cranial cavity, causing increased intracranial pressure.

In addition to its role of serving as a protective cushion for the brain and spinal cord

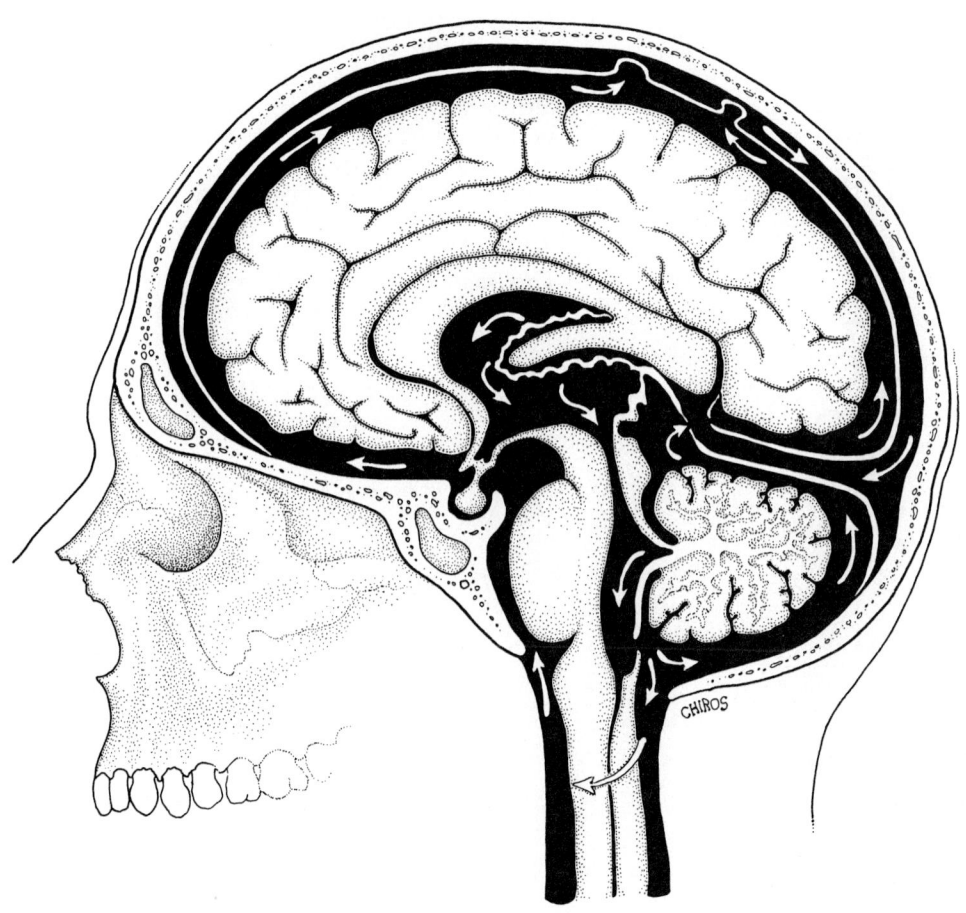

Figure 11-8
Circulation of the cerebrospinal fluid.

against trauma, CSF has a major role in regulating a balanced acid-base environment to maintain cerebral flow.

Spinal Cord

The spinal cord, continuous with the medulla oblongata, originates at the foramen magnum of the skull and extends down the vertebral canal approximately to the first or second lumbar vertebra. Thus, the spinal cord is shorter than the vertebral column. At this point it terminates in the **filum terminale,** a slender fibrous band that is attached to the coccyx. The cord contains long conducting fibers and serves as a link between the brain and the periphery.

The cord consists of 31 segments: 8 cervical, 12 thoracic, 5 lumbar, 5 sacral, and 7 coccygeal (Fig. 11-9). Each of these segments of the cord has a pair of spinal nerves. There are two areas of enlargement in the cord, one at the cervical region and the other at the lumbar region. The nerves from the cervical region supply the neck and upper extremities; the thoracic nerves supply the thoracic and abdominal muscles and the skin; and the lumbar nerves supply the lower extremities. The lumbar and sacral roots are grouped together as they exit from the cord, forming a pattern like a horse's tail, the **cauda equina.** The cord is composed of gray and white matter. In contrast to the cerebrum, however, the gray matter is concentrated in the interior, approximately in the form of an H, with the white matter completely surrounding the H on all sides. Afferent (sensory) information enters via the posterior column or horns and efferent (motor) information exits via the anterior horn. The efferent motor neuron cell bodies lie in the anterior horn, and the sensory neurons lie outside the spinal cord within the posterior root ganglia.

Reflex Arc

The basic defense mechanism and functional unit of the nervous system is the reflex arc

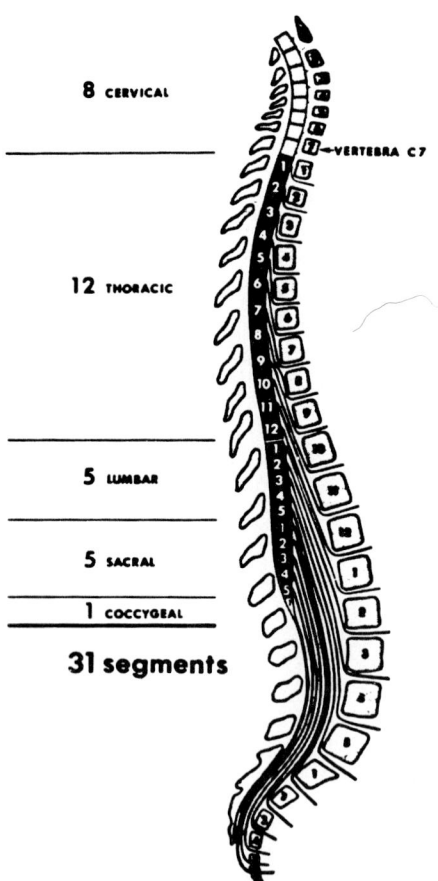

Figure 11-9
Relationship of spinal cord to vertebral column. (From Gary B. Dunkerley, *A Basic Atlas of the Human Nervous System.* Philadelphia: F. A. Davis Company, 1975. Reproduced by permission.)

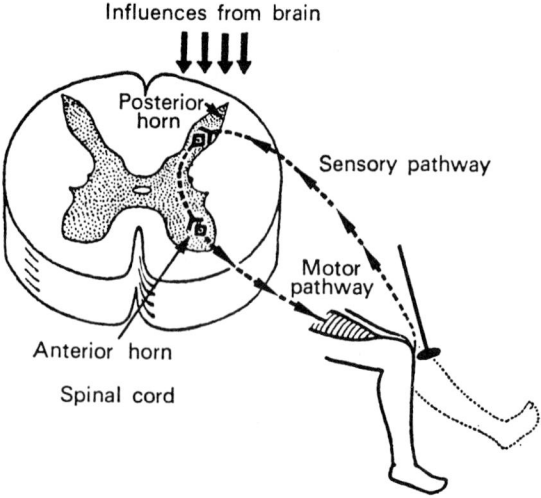

Figure 11-10
A reflex arc. The reflex illustrated is the knee jerk. (From E. R. Bickerstaff, *Neurology for Nurses* [2nd ed.]. London: English University Press, 1971. Reproduced by permission.)

(Fig. 11-10). It is the pathway for conducting the impulses of a receptor to an effector. The essential components of the reflex arc are as follows: a **receptor;** an **afferent neuron** to conduct the impulse arising from stimulation of the receptor; a **reflex center** in the central nervous system (an internuncial neuron, or interneuron, where a synapse occurs between the afferent neuron and an efferent neuron); an **efferent neuron;** and an **effector,** which consists of smooth or skeletal muscle or glands that respond to the nerve impulse. The simplest reflex arc is a synapse directly between a sensory neuron and an anterior motor neuron. An example of a spinal reflex is the knee jerk (Fig. 11-10).

An important function of the spinal cord is its role of reflex activity in association with peripheral nerves. These reflexes are stimulus-response mechanisms that have a regulatory and protective function. Spinal reflexes take place at the cord level by transmission of impulses from receptors via the sensory neurons to the central neurons within the cord, which send impulses directly to the motor neuron leading to glands and muscles.

Nerve Tracts

As mentioned previously, ascending and descending axons are grouped according to specific functions within distinct pathways or tracts. These pathways are located within the spinal cord. The **pyramidal motor tract** consists of the descending projectional tracts that arise from neurons in the cerebral motor cortex (precentral gyrus) and regulate voluntary control of muscle function. The term **pyramidal** is derived from the pyramid-shaped cells from which the corticospinal tract arises, an anatomic arrangement of the corticospinal tract within two triangular structures in the medulla. Below the medulla, most of the pyramidal tracts cross over to the other side, becoming the lateral corticospinal, or lateral pyramidal, tract; thus the cell bodies of the lateral corticospinal tract fibers lie in the precentral gyrus of the side opposite the side of the body they may innervate (Fig. 11-11).

Figure 11-11
The motor pathways. The pyramidal tract is responsible for fine control over voluntary muscle movements. Note the origin of the tract in the precentral gyrus of the cerebral cortex. In contrast to the pyramidal tract, the extrapyramidal tract originates in other gyri and is connected directly to the basal ganglia. The diagram illustrates the direct connection of the pyramidal cortex to the spinal motor neurons; the extrapyramidal cortex does not have such a direct connection. (From E. R. Bickerstaff, *Neurology for Nurses* [2nd ed.], London: English University Press, 1971. Reproduced by permission.)

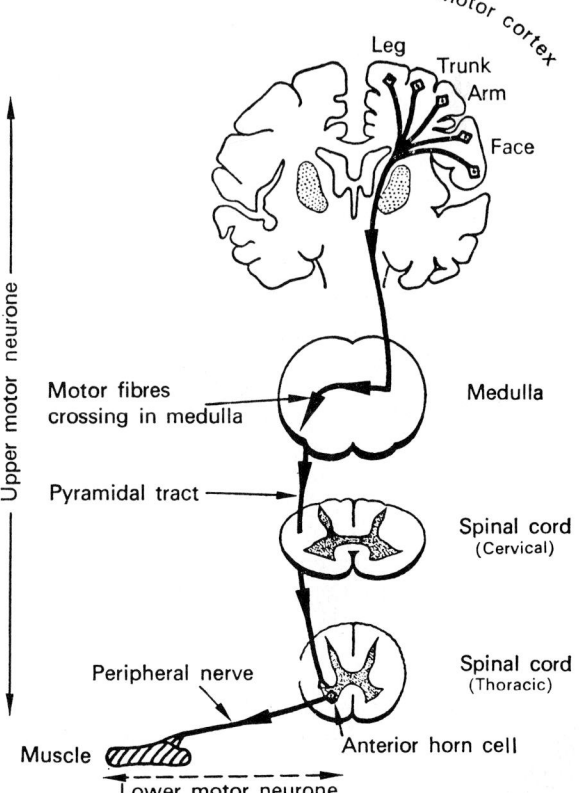

(The fibers that do not cross over are called the anterolateral, or ventral, corticospinal tract.) Therefore, if damage to the tract occurs above the pyramidal decussation, loss of voluntary function occurs on the opposite side as that of the lesion. If the injury takes place below the decussation site, paralysis occurs on the same side.

The extrapyramidal motor tracts facilitate the function of motor neurons to skeletal muscle (lateral reticulospinal tract) or have an inhibitory influence on muscle tone, automatic movements, and emotional expression (medial reticulospinal tract).

Sensory tracts include those for pain, temperature, touch, position, vibration, and recognition of shape, size, and texture, and are either spinothalamic or spinocerebellar tracts.

AUTONOMIC NERVOUS SYSTEM

The autonomic nervous system is that part of the central nervous system that regulates the activities of most organs of the body. Although these functions of the ANS are mainly on the unconscious reflex level, the ANS has neurons in the brain, spinal cord, and peripheral parts of the body.

By means of direct neurostimulation or by indirect hormonal stimulation, the autonomic nervous system controls the following body functions: (1) heart rate and the force of cardiac muscle contraction (via the cardiac pacemaker cells); (2) regional blood flow distribution, body temperature regulation, and blood pressure (by its effects on vascular smooth muscle); (3) gastrointestinal motility, secretion, digestion, urination, and defecation (by its effect on the smooth muscle of the intestine, and bladder); (4) sweating, salivation, and the texture of the body surfaces (by its actions on the exocrine glands); and (5) metabolism and endocrine function (by its indirect actions on the liver and on the pituitary and other glands [33].

The ANS is divided into two major parts: the **sympathetic system** (thoracolumbar) and the **parasympathetic system** (craniosacral). The efferent pathway arrangement consists of two kinds of fibers, preganglionic and postganglionic fibers, which connect at a ganglion, an isolated group of neuron cell bodies. The sympathetic system is also known as the thoracolumbar division because the preganglionic cell bodies of its neurons are located in gray matter of the lateral horn of the spinal cord and leave the cord from the thoracic and lumbar segments of the cord. The parasympathetic system is known also as the craniosacral division of the ANS because its cell bodies originate in autonomic nuclei of cranial nerves III, VII, IX, and X of the brainstem and from the sacral segments of the spinal cord. For example, the vagus nerve (cranial nerve X) supplies parasympathetic fibers to the heart, lungs, and almost all of the abdominal organs.

The sympathetic and parasympathetic divisions differ not only in the sites of the origin of their preganglionic fibers but also in the characteristics of their preganglionic and postganglionic fibers (Fig. 11-12). The sympathetic preganglionic fibers are short and enter a ganglion immediately upon leaving the cord; the postganglionic fibers usually are very long (and unmyelinated) compared with those of the parasympathetic division, and they terminate on or near the specific effector cells within the tissue that they innervate. The ganglia of the sympathetic system are linked together in a chain, the **sympathetic trunk,** which lies on either side of the vertebral column. The preganglionic neurons of the parasympathetic system are long and myelinated fibers and the postganglionic fibers are short and unmyelinated. The ganglia between the preganglionic and postganglionic parasympathetic neurons are located in or near the effector organ that they innervate [18].

Acetylcholine is the preganglionic transmitter for both the sympathetic and parasympathetic divisions and the postganglionic transmitter for the parasympathetic. The transmitter substance of the postganglionic fibers of the sympathetic system is a catecholamine, such as norepinephrine. (Acetylcholine is the transmitter for the sweat glands and blood vessels of skeletal muscles.)

The sympathetic and parasympathetic divisions also differ in their actions on specific tissues that they innervate. For example, the sympathetic nervous system dilates the pupils, constricts the blood vessels of the skin, increases the heart rate, decreases peristalsis, increases sweating, and raises blood sugar levels. These effects occur in periods of stress, in emergency situations, and in response to the injection of epinephrine (Adrenalin). These also reflect the actions of the

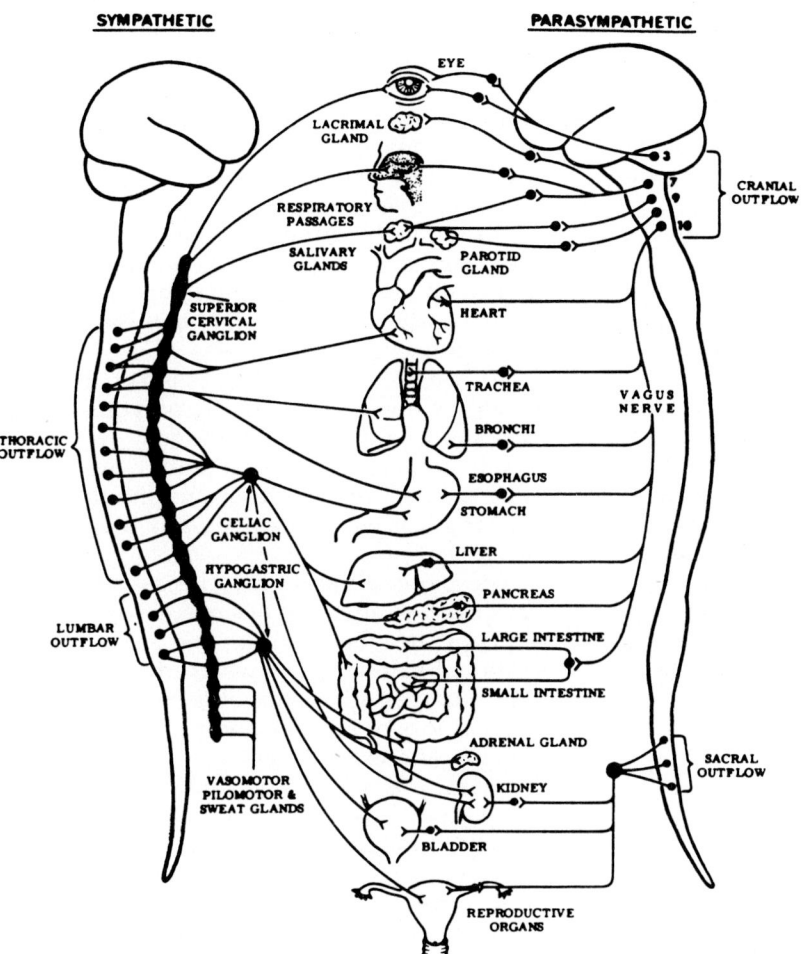

Figure 11-12
Sympathetic and parasympathetic neurons. (From E. E. Selkurt, *Basic Physiology for the Health Sciences*. Boston: Little, Brown and Company, 1975. Modified from B. S. Bergensen and E. E. Krug, *Pharmacology in Nursing* [12th ed.]. St. Louis, Mosby, 1973. Reproduced by permission.)

adrenal medulla, which is considered to be an extension of the sympathetic postganglionic system [18]. In contrast to these effects, the parasympathetic nervous system causes constriction of the pupil and dilation of the skin vessels, decreases the heart rate, increases salivation and peristalsis, and causes bladder contraction. The parasympathetic system plays a dominant role in nonstressful situations and tends to conserve bodily resources; it is thus restorative in nature.

The cerebral cortex, hypothalamus, pons, medulla, midbrain, and limbic system also have considerable influence on the functions controlled by the autonomic nervous system. The medulla and hypothalamus exert the greatest influence under normal circumstances, and in cases of stress the cortical areas exert particular influence [18].

The hypothalamus has a major influence on autonomic functions. The anterior portion has inhibitory effects on sympathetic function, and the posterior portion has excitatory effects. It is in this way that the hypothalamus has a great influence on homeostasis.

Neurologic Assessment

Responsibilities of the nurse for neurologic assessment will vary according to the setting in which a nurse functions, as well as according to the experience and knowledge of the individual practitioner. Certain aspects of the neurologic examination are essential components of any assessment made by a nurse in order to plan nursing care. These aspects will be considered, as well as some aspects that are regarded as the responsibility of physicians and neurologists (and, in some cases, nurse practitioners) in order to plan medical care. Even when not directly responsible for the various aspects of the neurologic examination, it is important for the nurse to understand their purposes and their relation to the patient's total assessment.

The major responsibilities of the nurse to the neurologic patient are to assess for normal and abnormal responses, develop baseline data, accurately monitor the patient for changes in his or her neurologic status, and report and record data accurately. The various aspects of the neurologic examination include a history, and assessment of the patient's mental status, cortical function, cranial nerve function, cerebellar, motor, and sensory functions, and evaluation of the reflexes and autonomic function.

HISTORY

A careful history is the first essential part of the assessment of the neurologic system. A general medical history is also necessary, because many other conditions are complicated by neurologic changes. During the history-taking procedure, the examiner is able to evaluate cerebral function by noting the patient's level of consciousness, alertness, contact with reality, appropriateness of responses to questions or directions, and the presence of drowsiness or periods of loss of contact. Orientation to person, place, and time should be carefully determined. The person's manner of dress and gestures and other behavior are also noted during this time. The person's ability to communicate impressions, thoughts, concerns, and symptoms and insight into his condition are important factors that the examiner should note in the patient's record. Any recent change in personality, behavior, and intellectual performance is particularly important, because lesions in the frontal areas of the cerebrum cause alterations in these functions. However, symptoms related to thought content, such as delusions, illusions, or hallucinations, may reflect psychiatric disorders as well as potential cerebral lesions. The person's emotional status should also be observed, noting any tension, hostility, depression, or euphoria. Both verbal and nonverbal observations should be recorded.

In many situations the family history is of considerable importance. Familial incidence, for example, is found in some cases of multiple sclerosis, amyotrophic lateral sclerosis, and brain tumor. A family history of epilepsy is also encountered in some histories of persons suffering from seizures.

A developmental history is particularly indicated when diseases of the nervous system occur in infancy and childhood.

When specific symptoms are evident, the time of onset of the symptoms should be ascertained, as well as progression or remission of the symptoms.

The patient should also be asked specific questions to elicit the occurrence of seizures, syncope, headache, diplopia, pain, and difficulty in bladder and bowel control, as well as any changes in motor or sensory function such as loss of balance and numbness or tingling in the extremities.

Symptoms should be carefully elicited in the patient's own terms. A careful description of pain should be elicited from the patient, and the factors that predispose to as well as relieve the pain should be recorded. When headache is described, the patient should be asked to identify its location (for example, frontal, focal, unilateral); its type (deep, superficial, severe or mild, throbbing or aching, constant or intermittent, periodic or irregular) and its frequency.

Terms such as **vertigo** or **numbness** are difficult for patients to understand and are thus often misinterpreted. The patient should be asked to describe the sensations; this should clarify for the nurse whether the patient means vertigo or dizziness. **Vertigo** is the sensation of movement or rotation felt by the patient; **dizziness** is the apparent movement of objects in the environment, but it is sometimes used for sensations of faintness or giddiness [1].

Although **numbness** means impairment or loss of sensation, persons often use the term when they are actually describing weakness of an extremity. When the patient describes a tingling sensation in the extremity, paresthesia is present.

Patients speak of "blurred vision" when

they mean double vision, the effects of visual field defects, or even reduced visual acuity.

When persons report that they have had seizures, information on the seizures should also be sought from members of the family or others who have actually observed the person during the seizure, since the patient is unaware of what occurs during these lapses of consciousness.

The head and neck should be examined, noting the scalp condition, any deformities, skull irregularities, mobility of the neck, and any bruits in the carotid bifurcation. The patient should also be checked for any nuchal rigidity, which indicates meningeal irritation. The patient may complain of neck stiffness, or stiffness may be noted when the examiner flexes the patient's head.

MENTAL STATUS AND CORTICAL FUNCTION

The patient's ease in communicating and vocabulary are important in the assessment of language ability; language impairment may be associated with various neurologic abnormalities. In assessing this aspect, however, the examiner should take into account the patient's visual and hearing acuity, level of education, and reading ability.

The presence of aphasia is noted. **Aphasia** is any deficiency in the ability to understand and communicate by means of the spoken and written word or communicatory signs. The examiner can detect deficiencies in language function by asking the patient to make different sounds, noting abnormal word usage in conversation, evaluating the coherence of the patient's conversation, and noting whether or not he comprehends what is said in his presence.

Factors used to evaluate the patient's intellectual abilities include the following: the manner in which the patient describes events and gives information about the illness; vocabulary, ease in communicating, and answers to direct questions; and level of education and occupation. However, social and cultural background, as well as level of education, are variables that affect testing results and must be taken into consideration.

Specific functions of the cerebral cortex may also be evaluated by testing the interpretation of sensory information (a cortical function), memory, ability to conceptualize, and cortical motor integration.

Agnosia is the term for the inability to recognize objects via any of the senses. The cerebral area that is affected may be identified by the type of agnosia present. For example, disturbances in tactile sensation suggest a lesion in the parietal lobe, while auditory agnosia implies a temporal lobe lesion.

Questions are asked to determine the recall ability of the patient, keeping in mind that in certain diseases remote memory is often intact, while memory for recent events may be lost. Other variations of testing for recall include giving the patient information to remember and then asking him to recall the information later in the interview. Normally, a person can repeat a series of six to seven digits in order and a series of four digits in reverse order [32]. Thus the patient may be given a series of digits and then asked to repeat them. The serial 7 test is often used, but the results must be evaluated in light of the patient's mathematical skills and education; in this test, the patient is asked to subtract 7 from 100 and then 7 from the remainder, and so forth [32].

Ability to conceptualize is evaluated by asking the patient to interpret proverbs or sayings (for example, "A stitch in time saves nine"). The patient who has impaired intellectual functioning will not have the ability to grasp the significance of a proverb and therefore will either repeat it or will interpret it literally.

Cortical motor integration can be evaluated by asking a patient to perform a specific task. **Apraxia** is the term applied to the inability to carry out purposeful, useful, or skilled acts in the absence of paralysis or motor or sensory nerve injury.

CRANIAL NERVE FUNCTION

The cranial nerves (except for nerves III, IV, VI, IX, and X), are tested to determine if there is any impairment of their specific functions.

The examiner should check the patient's nostrils for possible obstruction of the nasal passages (for example, fractures) before testing the **olfactory nerve.** With eyes closed (or blindfolded) and compressing one nostril at a time, the patient is asked to identify familiar odors such as coffee and tobacco. Inability to detect odors accurately may reflect conditions that affect either the primary olfactory receptors located in the nasal mucosa, or the neurons of the olfactory bulb and tract. **Anosmia** is loss of ability to smell.

To assess the status of the **optic nerve,** the patient's visual acuity (with or without corrective lenses, if worn) is evaluated by use of the Snellen chart. Visual fields are tested for gross defects, or perimetric testing is used for more accurate evaluation if indicated (see Chap. 12).

As described previously, disturbances in the function of the optic nerve may occur anywhere along the optic pathways—in the neurons in the retina, optic nerve fibers or tract, or occipital lobe. Figure 11-5 illustrates the types of visual field defects, or scotomas, associated with specific lesions along the pathway of the optic nerve. (A **scotoma** is an area of depressed vision within the visual field.) As Figure 11-5 shows, a retinal lesion may produce a blind spot in the affected eye, while an optic nerve lesion produces partial or complete blindness in the involved eye. A lesion involving one complete optic tract results in blindness in the opposite half of both visual fields. As noted previously, this is known as homonymous hemianopia and is characterized by a loss of half the visual field on the same side, either right or left, of each eye. A lesion in the temporal lobe may produce blindness in the upper quadrants of both visual fields on the side opposite the lesion. A lesion in the parietal lobe may produce blindness in the lower quadrants of both visual fields on the side opposite the lesion. An occipital lobe lesion characteristically causes contralateral blindness in the corresponding half of each visual field, but the central vision is intact [8].

Besides visual field testing, optic nerve assessment requires a thorough ophthalmoscopic examination to observe the optic discs, the vessels, and the retina and to detect the presence of papilledema. (These examinations are discussed in Chapter 12.)

The status of cranial nerves III, IV, and VI (the **oculomotor, trochlear,** and **abducens**) is determined by asking the patient to follow the movement of the examiner's fingers, or another object, through all directions of gaze. Disorders of the oculomotor nerve result in the patient's being unable to look up, down, or medially with the affected eye. Because the oculomotor nerve also supplies the muscles for pupillary constriction and elevation of the lids, dilatation of the pupil in the affected eye and ptosis (drooping) of the eyelid are observed in disorders of the oculomotor nerve.

The inability to look downward and outward reflects a disturbance of the trochlear nerve, while an inability to move the eye outward indicates involvement of the abducens nerve. **Nystagmus,** involuntary rhythmical movements of the eye, may occur on lateral or vertical gaze. The patient often complains of double vision (diplopia). Disturbances in the functions of these three cranial nerves reflect involvement of the nerves themselves or of their nuclei in the midbrain and pons.

To test the oculomotor nerve and its function in constricting the pupil, the pupils are examined in a darkened room. After the size, shape, and equality of the pupils have been noted, the patient is asked to focus first on a distant object and then on a close object. This enables the examiner to check for pupillary constriction (the pupillary accommodation reflex). Direct and consensual pupillary reflexes are observed by noting pupillary constriction in response to a light shown into each eye from the side; **consensual reaction** is contraction of the pupil of the nonstimulated eye. Differences in the equality and reactivity of the pupils is significant, because compression or stretching of the oculomotor nerve results in a dilated pupil on the side of pressure. Unilateral dilatation of the pupil occurring after head trauma or cranial surgery is a significant sign and must be reported to the neurosurgeon immediately. A unilateral dilated pupil usually indicates compression of the oculomotor nerve (or brainstem) by a herniation of the temporal lobe caused by a supratentorial mass (lesion above the tentorium) [34]. The patient's history, however, should indicate whether or not any medication causing pupil dilatation has been instilled in the eye.

To test the adequacy of the **trigeminal nerve** (V), several methods are used, because the nerve has both sensory and motor functions. The presence of several types of sensation are first evaluated, followed by tests to determine if both sides of the face are equally sensitive. The patient's eyes should be kept closed during the testing. The forehead, cheeks, and jaw are touched with a wisp of cotton; the inability to feel the cotton indicates anesthesia to light touch. Increased or decreased sensitivity to light touch may be detected by noting differences in response on opposite sides of the face. Pinpricks and warm and cold objects are also used to test for degrees of sensitivity. Neuralgia, tenderness, loss of sensation, and asymmetry of sensory responses are abnormal findings.

A wisp of cotton is also used to touch the cornea to determine whether or not blinking occurs as a protective mechanism when the cornea is touched (**corneal reflex**).

The motor portion of the trigeminal nerve supplies the muscles of mastication. The examiner should observe for any deviations of the jaw when the mouth is opened and should palpate the masseter and temporal muscles when the jaws are tightly clamped together in a bite. While the patient is asked to hold the mouth slightly opened, the examiner taps the middle of the chin with a reflex hammer to test the maxillary reflex, or jaw jerk. Normally, there is a sudden closing movement of the jaw.

The motor, sensory, and autonomic components of the **facial nerve** are evaluated. To detect any asymmetry of the face, the patient is asked to look at the ceiling, wrinkle his forehead, frown, whistle, smile, and raise his eyebrows. The patient is also asked to try to keep his eyes closed while the examiner attempts to open them, as a test to measure the strength of the eyelid muscles. When paresis is noted in the lower part of the face (as demonstrated by an inability to blow air into the cheeks or pull down the corners of the mouth), involvement of the supranuclear fibers supplying the face is suspected. Paralysis of the entire face indicates involvement of the motor nucleus or the peripheral portion of the nerve.

Because the facial nerve is responsible for the perception of taste on the anterior two-thirds of the tongue, the patient is asked to protrude the tongue and to identify the tastes of sugar and salt (or of sour or bitter substances) that are placed on this area of the tongue; the mouth must be rinsed carefully between each substance. The patient must be instructed not to retract the tongue or swallow prematurely, because the material will spread within the mouth, and the test will be inaccurate. A lesion in the sensory nucleus or the sensory fibers of the facial nerve is suspected when a basic taste sensation (sweet, salt, sour, or bitter) is disturbed.

The **vestibulocochlear (acoustic) nerve** (VIII) is tested for its cochlear and vestibular functions, although the latter is not always tested routinely unless the patient complains of vertigo, tinnitus, or disturbed balance. The tests should be done after the external ear is observed with an otoscope. The assessment of the two parts of the acoustic nerve is discussed in detail in Chapter 13 and is therefore not discussed in this section.

The **glossopharyngeal** (IX) and **vagus** (X) **nerves** are usually tested together because of their close anatomic and physiologic relationship. To test the pharyngeal gag reflex, each side of the pharynx is touched with a tongue depressor or applicator stick. The examiner then tests the palatal reflex by stroking each side of the mucous membrane of the uvula. As the side is touched, it should rise. The vagus nerve alone is tested by noting the patient's ability to swallow and speak clearly without hoarseness and by observing whether or not movements of the vocal cords and soft palate during phonation are symmetrical [8].

The **accessory nerve** (XI) is tested by noting the strength of the sternocleidomastoid and trapezius muscles during rotation of the head and shrugging of the shoulders. Weakness and atrophy are abnormal findings. The **hypoglossal nerve** (X) is tested by asking the patient to protrude the tongue and noting any lateral deviation of the tongue, asymmetry, atrophy, or tremor. The patient should then be asked to protrude the tongue and move it from side to side against a tongue depressor to determine its strength.

CEREBELLAR ASSESSMENT

To test the cerebellar control of balance and coordination, the patient is asked to touch a finger to the nose with each hand and then to repeat the test with the eyes closed. The patient should also be asked to make rapidly alternating movements, such as touching fingers to thumb in rapid succession. Tests for lower extremity coordination include asking the patient to run each heel down the shin, to point to the examiner's hand with each big toe, and make a figure eight in the air with each foot. The patient is instructed to stand erect with feet together, first with the eyes open and then with the eyes closed. The patient is also asked to walk naturally with the eyes open and then with the eyes closed and then is asked to walk on the heels and toes. The patient is also asked to provide a handwriting sample, which is also kept as part of the record.

During these tests, the patient's posture, ability to gauge distance, and swinging of the arms are all noted. Any **tremor** (rhythmic involuntary movement) or **ataxia** (incoordination of movement) is reported. These two symptoms are frequently present in cerebellar disease.

ASSESSMENT OF MOTOR FUNCTION

The status of the motor system is determined by inspecting and palpating the resting muscles for size and consistency and noting the presence or absence of atrophy, tremors, contractures, deformities, and abnormal movements. The examiner taps different muscle groups to test for mechanical irritability and myotonia (increased tone of muscle). The muscles are examined for abnormalities in tone, such as spasticity, rigidity, or flaccidity, and for muscle strength.

Any involuntary movements are important to note, because they generally indicate the presence of a disturbance of the extrapyramidal motor areas or pathways, although they may sometimes be caused by psychogenic disturbances. These movements include irregular and jerky choreiform movements, tremors, tics, or myoclonic contractions. Tremors should be described in terms of their relation to voluntary movement or rest. Intention tremors, for example, occur when voluntary movement is initiated.

To detect muscle weakness, the major joints are taken through their full range of motion without resistance and then with the examiner providing resistance. A disturbance or lesion along the pyramidal pathway is suspected when muscle weakness is detected.

SENSORY ASSESSMENT

The sensory examination is accomplished first by testing for superficial tactile sensation, superficial-pressure and deep-pressure pain, and sensations of temperature, vibration, motion, and position. The sensory tests are done with the patient's eyes closed. A wisp of cotton is used to test the patient's tactile sensory function, comparing one side of the body to the other, as well as comparing proximal to distal parts. A pin or other sharp object is used to determine sensitivity to superficial pain. The Achilles tendon and calf and forearm muscles are squeezed to determine sensitivity to deep pain. Test tubes containing hot and cold water are used to touch the various parts of the body, to determine the integrity of the patient's temperature receptors. A vibrating tuning fork is used over bony prominences to determine the patient's ability to feel when the vibration stops, also comparing reactions in different parts of the body and on opposite sides. Continuing the examination with the patient's eyes closed, the examiner, with light support of the digits, moves the fingers and toes passively while the patient is asked to identify the direction of the movement and the position of the digit.

A two-point discrimination test is used to evaluate the ability of the cortex to distinguish two stimuli applied in different locations. Disturbances suggest parietal lobe involvement. In this test, the examiner simultaneously touches various parts of the body with two sharp objects, asking the patient to state if he or she is being touched by one or two points. The patient is also asked to locate the site of the touch as a test of point localization. The function of stereognosis is tested by asking the patient, with eyes closed, to identify familiar objects that are placed in each hand. Texture discrimination is determined by having the patient identify materials that are placed in the hands. The sense of graphesthesia is tested by asking the patient to identify letters or numbers written on the palms with a blunt point.

ASSESSMENT OF REFLEXES AND AUTONOMIC FUNCTION

The last part of the neurologic assessment consists in testing the status of the reflexes and autonomic function. It is essential that the patient be relaxed during the testing of reflexes, although this is also important throughout the examination. Deep reflexes are tested by tapping briskly with a reflex hammer on a tendon or a bony prominence to cause a sudden stretching of certain muscles. Striking the biceps tendon, for example, results in the **biceps reflex,** a contraction of the biceps and flexion of the forearm. Tapping the triceps tendon above the olecranon causes the elbow to extend. The brachioradialis reflex is also tested, by striking the radius above the wrist, with the forearm placed on the lap. Normally, flexion and suppination of the forearm are observed. The patellar reflex is elicited by striking the patellar tendon and observing for extension of the leg at the knee. The Achilles reflex is tested by striking the Achilles tendon and observing for plantar flexion of the foot.

Superficial reflexes, such as the upper abdominal, lower abdominal, cremasteric, plantar, and gluteal, may be tested by stroking the skin with an object such as an applicator; the muscles in the area normally contract. In the upper abdominal reflex, the umbilicus moves up and toward the area being stroked, while stroking the lower abdomen normally causes the umbilicus to move down. Eliciting the cremasteric reflex causes elevation of the scrotum, and eliciting the plantar reflex normally causes flexion of the toes. When the gluteal reflex is elicited, the skin tenses in the gluteal area [8].

Certain reflexes that indicate the presence of a pathologic condition may be elicited. The most important of these is the Babinski reflex (Fig. 11-13), which is elicited by stroking the lateral aspect of the sole of the foot with a blunt object [8, 32]. Normally the patient flexes the toes and pulls the foot away by flexing the knee and hip. If there is disease within the pyramidal tract, the great toe is extended or dorsiflexed, and the other toes fan out. This reaction is recorded as a positive Babinski reflex. The examiner who tests for this reflex must be careful not to apply too much pressure, because the sudden reaction may be misinterpreted.

The autonomic nervous system is assessed by monitoring the vital signs, the color of the skin and mucous membrane, salivation, and perspiration patterns. Autonomic reflexes, such as pupil size and pupillary reaction, are also evaluated.

Diagnostic Tests

Abnormal findings in the physical and neurologic assessment may indicate a need for special procedures to determine the location and nature of lesions. Because usual palpation and auscultation tools have limited value in diagnosing intracranial lesions, various diagnostic procedures are used. These diagnostic procedures require that the nurse give the patient adequate physical and psychological preparation and that the patient be conscious during the procedures. Thus the patient must be given ongoing emotional support and appropriate explanations. Even if the particular examination is not a hazardous one, the patient is often fearful because of the implications that serious disease may be present. Calm reassurance is of paramount importance during the diagnostic phase of the patient's illness. A record of the procedure, as well as of any untoward effects and the patient's tolerance to the procedure, should be entered in the nurse's notes. The nurse is also responsible for observing the patient during and after the examination to detect complications.

The specific tests that are used for diagnosing neurologic disease may be divided into those that offer minimal or no risk to the patient and those that present risks. Each test detects different aspects; the tests are utilized from the simplest, nonrisk procedure to the risk procedures when a diagnosis seems elusive.

Skull and spine x-rays, electroencephalograms, electromyograms, and computer axial tomograms are generally considered nonrisk examinations. In some classifications, lumbar puncture and myelography are listed as procedures involving risks.

Tests that present risks to the patient include cisternal puncture, pneumoencephalography, ventriculography, and ateriography. However, most hospitals require that

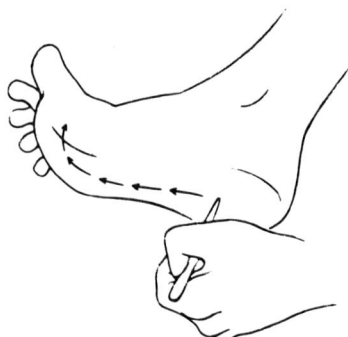

Figure 11-13
The Babinski reflex. (From J. F. Simpson and K. R. Magee, *Clinical Evaluation of the Nervous System.* Boston: Little, Brown and Company, 1973. Reproduced by permission.)

the patient sign an informed consent form prior to most of these procedures, except before skull and spine roentgenograms, which are frequently used to detect abnormalities such as fractures, deformities, and unusual calcified areas within the cranium.

LUMBAR PUNCTURE

A lumbar puncture is done both to measure CSF pressure and to obtain specimens for microscopical, chemical, microbiologic, and serologic examination. It is invaluable in differentiating neurologic disorders. The normal pressure of the CSF as measured by a manometer is 70 to 170 mm H_2O. The test must be done very cautiously (if at all) in the presence of increased intracranial pressure, since sudden reduction of pressure may cause herniation of the medulla oblongata into the foramen magnum [1, 26].

Increased CSF pressure is detected in meningeal inflammations, encephalitis, and poliomyelitis; in subarachnoid hemorrhage; in the presence of space-occupying intracranial lesions, such as brain abscess, subdural hematoma, cerebral hemorrhage, and brain tumor; and in cerebral edema associated with infection, head injury, hemorrhage, or craniotomy. The CSF pressure is decreased in patients with shock, dehydration, and following intravenous injections of hypertonic fluids [26].

For the spinal tap, the patient is placed on the side, with head and body in an acutely flexed position and knees drawn up onto the abdomen and clasped firmly by the patient's hands. (This position separates the spinous processes, which facilitates needle insertion.) The patient must lie still during the procedure; the nurse should provide both physical and emotional support. The puncture is performed aseptically; the back is prepared with an appropriate antiseptic, and surgical draping is utilized. A local anesthetic is injected at the site. The puncture is made with a very small and sharp needle and is usually made at a site between the third and fourth or fourth and fifth lumbar vertebrae.

During the lumbar puncture, a test for Queckenstedt's sign may be performed to determine the presence or absence of a spinal subarachnoid block to the flow of CSF. This is done as follows: The lumbar puncture is accomplished in the usual manner, and then baseline CSF pressure is established. The nurse then compresses the jugular veins for 10 seconds, which raises the intracranial venous pressure. If the circulation is unimpeded, the spinal fluid pressure is elevated 150 to 300 mm and returns to the original level within 10 seconds after release of the jugular pressure [26]. If a blockage is present in the subarachnoid space, no rise—or only an imperfect one—occurs with jugular compression. The test for this sign is contraindicated in the presence of increased intracranial pressure, particularly when a lesion above the foramen magnum is suspected.

After the lumbar puncture is completed, a sterile dressing or adhesive strip is applied to the puncture wound. The specimen of CSF should be taken to the laboratory promptly, because it deteriorates rapidly. The nurse should instruct the patient to lie flat, but not necessarily on the back, for several hours (varying from 3 to 24 hours in different protocols). This precaution is taken to avoid the occurrence of postlumbar puncture headache, which is attributed to the reduced volume of CSF. An icebag applied to the head and mild analgesics are used to control headache if it occurs. The patient should also be encouraged to inject an increased amount of fluids.

CISTERNAL PUNCTURE

Cisternal puncture is similar to lumbar puncture, but the needle used is shorter and is introduced below the occipital bone into the cisterna cerebellomedullaris. Before the procedure, the patient is shaved from the nape of the neck to the occipital protuberance. In this procedure, the patient is placed on the side, with the head sharply flexed and the chin on the chest. The head must be kept absolutely straight and still. The patient must be instructed to avoid rotating the neck. There is danger of injuring the medulla with the needle. Therefore, the patient is observed closely for any dyspnea or respiratory changes.

ANALYSIS OF CEREBROSPINAL FLUID

Routine examination of CSF specimens includes a cell count, protein and sugar count, colloidal gold reaction, and serologic tests for syphilis; special tests include smears, cultures, and estimation of the gamma globulin level.

Normally, CSF is a clear, colorless liquid, with a specific gravity of 1.005 to 1.009 and a pressure of 70 to 170 mm H_2O [26]. Normal constituents are: 1 to 5 lymphocytes per cubic millimeter, 15 to 45 mg per 100 ml of protein, 45 to 80 mg per 100 ml of glucose, and 119 to 128 mEq of chloride per liter [26]. The colloidal gold test is considered an indirect measure of gamma globulin. The level of gamma globulin is ordinarily below 12 percent [1].

The color of CSF changes in meningitis, with turbidity of the fluid being characteristic. It may be purulent in septic meningitis. Blood in the CSF (observed in test tubes other than the first one, blood in the latter merely indicating trauma during insertion of the needle) is diagnostic of hemorrhage in the subarachnoid space or hemorrhage of an intracerebral blood vessel into a ventricle or the subarachnoid space. Yellow (xanthochromic) CSF results from the breakdown of blood pigments from erythrocytes that have degenerated, which occurs a few days after bleeding into the subarachnoid space. It may also be noted in conditions in which the CSF has a very high protein content [1]; an increase in protein level and cell count is generally found in the presence of xanthochromic fluid.

In **pleocytosis**, an abnormal number of cells is present in the CSF. For example, in septic meningitis, the neutrophil count may rise as high as 1,000 to 10,000 neutrophils per cubic millimeter. An elevated cell count occurs in multiple sclerosis and brain tumors, and moderate rises occur in poliomyelitis, encephalitis, some types of meningitis, and neurosyphilis [26]. Acute bacterial infections are associated with an increase of polymorphonuclear leukocytes, and viral infections are associated with an increase in lymphocytes.

The CSF protein level is elevated in many organic diseases of the CNS, since the cells that produce CSF become abnormally permeable to serum proteins [26]. The protein level is particularly high in persons with septic meningitis and subarachnoid hemorrhage. The glucose level is normal or slightly increased in the presence of increased intracranial pressure but is reduced in acute bacterial meningitis and in meningeal metastases. The chloride level is reduced in septic and tubercular meningitis but remains normal in localized inflammatory conditions, encephalitis, and neurosyphilis [26]. Chloride levels appear to follow the blood levels of chlorides and thus are often low in cases of dehydration and vomiting. The colloidal gold curve of the CSF is found to be abnormal in neurosyphilis (especially in general paresis) and in many patients with multiple sclerosis.

It has only recently been determined that the CSF serves as an exchange medium for the products of both metabolism and catabolism and that its acid-base balance has an important role in the maintenance of cerebrovascular blood flow. Imbalances in this function are monitored by determining CSF carbon dioxide–oxygen tension, pH, and levels of lactate and bicarbonate.

MYELOGRAPHY

A myelogram involves the injection of isophendylate (Pantopaque) or another radiopaque substance into the subarachnoid space via a lumbar puncture (rarely, by a cisternal puncture) for the purpose of visualizing obstructions within the spinal canal. In some settings, air or a water-soluble material is now being used rather than the oil-base dye.

The procedure is done in the x-ray department, with the patient on a tilt table. After a conventional lumbar puncture, about 10 ml of spinal fluid is withdrawn, and 3 to 10 ml of the radiopaque substance is slowly injected. The oil is observed under the fluoroscope while the patient is positioned on a tilt table and manipulated into various positions to visualize possible defects. After the study is completed and to avoid meningeal irritation, the neurologist removes as much of the dye from the CSF as possible. To avoid some of the side effects associated with radiopaque substances, such as meningeal irritation, radicular pain, and arachnoiditis, air myelography is preferred by some neurosurgeons.

After the myelogram, the patient remains flat in bed for several hours. Persistent headache, pain, and neck stiffness (particularly when the head is flexed) are important symptoms to report because they indicate meningeal irritation.

ELECTROENCEPHALOGRAPHY

Electroencephalography is the amplification, recording, and analysis of the electric activity of the brain. An EEG is used primarily to differentiate organic disorders of the brain from functional disorders. The EEG may also be helpful in localizing cerebral lesions. However, the EEG is not an infallible test, for normal or nondiagnostic EEGs are sometimes recorded in patients with all types of seizures [1]. The EEG is also used to evaluate brain death, indicated by a persistent isoelectric tracing (one that shows no change in electric potential).

The person who is to have an EEG should be well prepared, because anxiety and tension may produce artifacts in the EEG tracing. The procedure is painless. It is helpful to have patients explain what they perceive the examination to be; often, the nurse may learn that patients think that it is a type of shock therapy or have some other misconception. The person should be informed that metal disks or small silver electrodes will be attached to the scalp in specific locations. In certain cases, nasopharyngeal leads are placed in each nostril to obtain information about electric activity at the base of the brain; this is done when temporal lobe seizures are suspected, or when previous EEG tracings have shown temporal region abnormalities [2].

The EEG tracing is made in a quiet room that is shielded from electric artifacts. The patient should be told to relax during the procedure and to lie still except when directed otherwise by the technician and that tracings may be taken for as long as an hour. The patient is also encouraged to keep the eyes closed to prevent any visual stimulation during the examination. The initial recording provides a baseline EEG for comparison with later recordings.

The EEG tracing is altered by drug therapy. The nurse preparing the patient should explicitly follow directions about drugs that are to be discontinued prior to the examination and those to be used for preparation of the patient. Usually, anticonvulsant drugs, tranquilizers, and stimulants, including coffee, tea, and cola drinks, are omitted for 24 to 48 hours prior to the test. Hypoglycemia may change normal brain wave patterns, and thus fasting is contraindicated prior to the test. Shampooing of the hair is required, in some protocols, to remove oils or hair spray that could prevent the electrodes from adhering to the scalp. In some settings, chloral hydrate is used for sedation of the patient. The time the prescribed dose is administered must be exact, so that the patient's EEG is not adversely affected. The chloral hydrate is usually given when a sleep recording is to be taken; this may be done when the patient has a seizure disorder, because sleep is a natural precipitator of abnormal EEG activity in susceptible persons, particularly those with temporal lobe seizures.

It is important that the patient be relaxed; if anxiety results in hyperventilation, the EEG tracing is affected because of response of the nervous system to alkalinity. However, hyperventilation may be instituted during the test as a specific evaluation measure. Since alkalinity increases the excitability of the nervous system and may stimulate abnormal waves, a seizure may result in a susceptible person. Resuscitation equipment and oral protective devices should be available if such provocative testing is done. In another type of provocative testing, photic stimulation consisting of flickering light of certain intensities is used to accentuate abnormal activity for diagnostic purposes [2].

The EEG tracings are examined for frequency, amplitude, voltage, rhythm, waveform, symmetry in the two hemisphere recordings, and uniformity as well as other aspects, as evaluated by the neurologist.

The patient returning from having an EEG is usually tired and wants to rest (the test may also be done on an outpatient basis). The collodion used to attach the electrodes should be removed, either with acetone or fingernail polish remover. Shampooing of the hair is usually required. If anticonvulsant drugs have been withheld for the test, they should be reinstated. The patient should also be observed for potential seizures, and precautionary measures should be taken.

ELECTROMYOGRAPHY

Electromyography involves the observation and recording of electric potentials within individual muscle fibers by means of needle electrodes placed in the muscle. The procedure is usually done by a physiatrist. The recording may be done on an oscilloscope or through an amplifying system, as well as by photographic methods. Normally, voluntary muscle is electrically inactive at rest but demonstrates a characteristic pattern when contracting. Electromyography is particularly valuable in diagnosing and evaluating the status of inflammatory muscle diseases, denervated muscles, and peripheral nerve injuries and other motor system diseases. For example, patients with myasthenia gravis demonstrate reduced amplitude of muscle potentials after successive stimulation, since the disease involves defects in transmission of neuromuscular impulses.

BRAIN SCANNING

Radioisotope (scintillation) scanning is a safe and painless screening procedure used to detect intracranial lesions. It is used before resorting to radiographic techniques requiring contrast medium. Various isotopes are used for the study, including ^{131}I-labeled serum albumin, ^{203}Hg-labeled chlormerodrin (Neohydrin), and ^{99M}Tc (technetium). The dye is injected intravenously 1 to 2 hours before scanning. The patient must be instructed to lie still during the procedure, which may take 35 to 50 minutes to complete.

ECHOENCEPHALOGRAPHY

Echoencephalography is a safe diagnostic procedure that involves the use of ultrasonic techniques and the recording of echoes derived from deep structures within the skull to visualize location of the midline structures of the brain and any displacement resulting from trauma, space-occupying lesions, or cerebrovascular disease. Echo pulsation patterns are significant for patients with subdural hematoma, arteriovenous aneurysm, carotid occlusion, and other cerebrovascular disorders. Echoencephalography is also used to determine lateral shifts of the pineal gland. It is not considered a substitute for other routine procedures but has been useful as an adjunct to the conventional diagnostic measures.

COMPUTERIZED TRANSVERSE AXIAL TOMOGRAPHY

Computerized transverse axial tomography with the EMI scanner (Electronics and Musical Instrumentation Ltd.) is one of the most recent developments in brain study. The machine uses a narrow moving beam of x-ray radiation in conjunction with a computer to produce anatomic and pathologic data about the brain, in order to diagnose both benign and malignant lesions. The procedure involves the use of a device that scans the patient's head with a narrow x-ray beam about 180 times and at different angles, so that various layers, or "slices," of tissue are visualized. Part of the machine rotates slowly around the patient's head as x-ray readings are taken. A computer is used to calculate the differences in tissue density in contiguous tissue slices; the machine is able to detect even minute alterations in absorption values and thus aids in detecting intracranial masses and associated ventricular shifts. The data appear on a computer printout (as well as on an oscilloscope), which corresponds to the density of the tissue. The density patterns can also be recorded on Polaroid film [29].

The major advantage of the method is that it is noninvasive, can be done on an outpatient basis, and takes only about 20 to 30 minutes to complete. The patient should be warned that he or she will be alone in a room during the procedure but will be able to communicate by intercom. The patient lies on a table in front of the scanner with the head in a rubber cap that projects into a water-filled Lucite tube [29]. The patient must be advised not to move whenever the machine is moving. Women should be instructed to wash their hair to remove hair spray and, since hairpins can produce artifacts in the test, they should be removed.

This new technique has proved to be more efficient than the conventional radiologic techniques that require the injection of contrast material (either radiopaque substances or air) to distinguish normal from abnormal intracranial tissue. Its increased use has resulted in less frequent use of pneumoencephalography.

CEREBRAL ARTERIOGRAPHY

Cerebral arteriography involves the injection of a radiopaque dye into the arterial blood vessels to study the cerebral circulation by x-ray. It is indicated to substantiate vascular lesions and anatomic changes in the brain and to detect vascular abnormalities, including malformations and aneurysms, and space-occupying lesions that distort the normal cerebrovascular pattern. The technique is especially hazardous for the patient with atherosclerosis and is not considered a screening technique.

A sedative, or a narcotic such as meperidine (Demerol), and atropine sulfate are usually given prior to the examination. Baseline data on vital and neurologic signs are obtained. The patient is prepared as if for surgery, with dentures, hairpins, and the like removed. A local anesthetic is usually given, but general anesthesia may be used in some patients.

The radiopaque material is injected directly into the carotid or vertebral arteries or indirectly through the aortic arch or brachial vessels. In some settings the femoral artery approach is considered a safer approach. In this approach, a long radiopaque catheter is threaded up the arterial vessels to the carotid or vertebral arteries or both. Serial x-ray films are taken to assess the arterial, capillary, and filling phases of the circulation.

The complications associated with the test are related to hemorrhage, emboli formation, and reactions to the dye. Test doses of the dye are usually given prior to the examination. This is of particular importance for patients with a history of allergies.

Following the examination, the patient remains on bed rest for periods ranging from 8 to 24 hours. A pressure dressing is maintained on the puncture site, and the site is observed for signs of hemorrhage or hematoma formation. An ice bag or collar may also be used at the site to prevent edema. Pressure from a hematoma may cause respiratory obstruction, requiring emergency measures. Vital signs and neurologic signs are assessed and recorded at frequent intervals. A delayed sensitivity reaction may occur with such symptoms as urticaria, pallor, pruritus, and respiratory difficulty. Vasospasm or embolism may occur within the cerebrovascular system, causing weakness or paralysis of the limbs, facial paralysis, dysphagia, speech difficulty, disorientation, or changes in level of consciousness. The nurse should observe closely for the onset of any of these symptoms, which should be reported promptly to the physician.

PNEUMOENCEPHALOGRAPHY

Pneumoencephalography is a contrast radiographic technique in which air or oxygen is introduced into the subarachnoid space and ventricular system via a lumbar puncture (or, less often, via a cisternal puncture). The technique is particularly used in studying atrophic and degenerative disorders and hydrocephalus. Although it has been used for detecting intracranial lesions, cerebral arteriography is usually preferred for this purpose today. (In some patients, both a pneumoencephalogram and arteriogram are taken if lesions are not clearly identified on the initial arteriogram.) When papilledema and other signs of increased intracranial pressure are present, a pneumoencephalogram is contraindicated. In these cases, ventriculography is used.

Preoperative preparation of the patient includes a thorough explanation of the procedure, which is anxiety-provoking for most patients. Baseline assessment data are obtained to allow for accurate monitoring during this potentially hazardous procedure. Food and fluids are restricted for 6 to 8 hours before the procedure, and a sedative and atropine sulfate are given about an hour before the examination. The patient is placed in a sitting position, strapped to a chair, with arms and chin resting on a pillow over a chair or overbed table. In some settings, a specially constructed revolving chair that is capable of rotating in any plane is utilized. A lumbar puncture is done, and about 4 to 10 ml of spinal fluid is withdrawn, and 10 ml or less of air is inserted. Serial x-ray films are then taken to visualize the ventricles, aqueducts, and cranial subarachnoid space.

After the pneumoencephalogram, the patient is required to remain at bed rest in a flat position for at least 12 to 24 hours and is kept as quiet and undisturbed as possible. Headache, nausea, and vomiting often occur and are relieved by mild analgesics, ice-bag applications to the head, and antiemetic medications. Ice applied to the head will cause contraction of the air that was introduced into the ventricles, thus helping to reduce headache. Vital signs are measured and neurologic assessments made at regular, frequent intervals to detect any untoward reactions, such as severe prolonged headache, fever, convulsions, continued vomiting, and signs of increased intracranial pressure (altering the pressure in the brain can cause displacement).

VENTRICULOGRAPHY

The ventriculogram is a variation of the pneumoencephalogram and involves the direct replacement of the CSF in the lateral ventricles with air as a contrast medium, followed by serial x-rays. The procedure is done in the operating room in the event brain displacement occurs and immediate craniotomy is required. This is done under local anesthesia by means of holes made in the skull with a perforator and a burr. A needle is passed into each lateral ventricle, and the air or contrast medium is introduced after some CSF has been removed. The size, shape, and filling of the ventricles are then observed by x-ray to localize lesions and cerebral anomalies.

The preparation for the ventriculogram is the same as that for the pneumoencephalogram, with the addition of shaving of the posterior third of the head and shampooing of the hair over the entire head.

Postexamination nursing care is similar to that described after the pneumoencephalogram, except that the nurse must also observe the scalp wounds. The sutures are usually removed within 4 to 5 days. Headache, nausea, and vomiting may occur but are generally less severe than following a pneumoencephalogram.

Manifestations of Neurologic Disorders

Neurologic disorders are caused by congenital deformities, vascular abnormalities, infections, trauma, neoplasms, and degenerative conditions, as well as by metabolic disorders. The neurologic system is a complex one, and the symptoms associated with a neurologic disorder are also complex, multiple, and varied. The types of disturbances depend on the area or areas of the nervous system that are affected, the extent of the lesion, and the nature of the pathologic condition. Normal responses may either diminish in quality or may be ablated, or the pathologic condition may result in defective or excessive activity.

Certain clinical manifestations of altered neurologic function are encountered with many different neurologic conditions regardless of the underlying cause. These common clinical manifestations include headache, vertigo, changes in level of consciousness, increased intracranial pressure, convulsive disorders, hyperpyrexia, and aphasia. A discussion of these common manifestations of altered neurologic function will precede the discussion of the specific neurologic disorders.

HEADACHE

Recurrent headache is a common symptom of an underlying problem. A headache may be a symptom of multiple causation including intracranial neoplasms, cerebral aneurysm, systemic disease, or psychological tension. Headaches particularly require investigation if they are sudden in onset, are associated with fever, confusion, and convulsions, or if they occur frequently. The brain itself has no pain endings; pain is caused by stretching of the dura mater, blood vessels, or muscle. Headaches, therefore, may be caused by tension or by displacement of pain-sensitive structures, dilatation of intracranial arteries, inflammation in a pain-sensitive structure of the head, and direct pressure on certain cranial nerves.

Diamond [9] classifies headaches into three types: (1) muscle contraction headaches, resulting from prolonged contraction of skeletal muscle; (2) vascular headaches; and (3) traction and inflammatory headaches. The latter are less common, more intense in the morning on awakening, and generally tend to involve the entire head.

Muscle contraction headaches, the most common type of headache, are generally considered to be of psychogenic origin and most often are associated with anxiety or depression. Usually the headache spreads over the entire head, most frequently in the occipital area, and is accentuated during stress. No nasal or ocular symptoms are associated with muscle contraction headaches, which usually respond to treatment with tranquilizers, analgesics, gentle massage, and hot applications to the head.

Migraines and cluster headaches are vascular in nature. Several factors, such as various allergies and food products containing tyramine and monosodium glutamate (found in wine and cheese), have been identified as precipitating vascular headaches; emotional stress, fatigue, vasodilating drugs, and a hereditary element have also been implicated.

Migraines are recurrent paroxysmal headaches that may last for hours to days;

they tend to occur more often in women than in men. They are characterized by severe, throbbing pain, are unilateral, and are often accompanied by nausea and vomiting. An aura, such as a visual phenomenon, often precedes the headache. Treatment consists in the administration of ergotamine tartrate (Gynergen), a vasoconstrictor, at the beginning of the attack. Ergotamine tartrate with caffeine (Cafergot) is also frequently used. Methysergide maleate (Sansert) is used to reduce the frequency and intensity of migraine attacks, but is ineffective once the headache has begun. Patients should watch for the side effects of ergotamine drugs, particularly peripheral arterial vasoconstriction, nausea, and vomiting. Ergotamine dependency often occurs, so that withdrawal symptoms become evident if dosages are decreased. The patient may also relieve the headache by applying ice packs to the head and lying in a quiet, darkened room until the headache subsides.

Cluster headaches, also called histamine headaches, are usually unilateral and are associated with lacrimation and nasal congestion. These occur more often in men than in women. The pain builds up quickly and then disappears rapidly; when it recurs, it is usually on the same side. Often, temporal vessels are prominent and ptosis and miosis are occasionally present.

A careful history and physical and neurologic examination are required to determine the underlying cause of recurrent headaches, whether they are functional or organic in nature. The nurse should determine the onset, site, intensity, duration, and precipitating factors of the headache. The presence of nausea, vomiting, or nasal stuffiness should also be determined. The nurse should also investigate what measures are helpful in relieving the discomfort of the headache.

Analgesics or tranquilizers may be used in the treatment of headaches, but symptomatic relief should follow an investigation into the underlying cause. Narcotics are contraindicated in the control of severe chronic headache, due to the danger of drug addiction. Control of precipitating factors in the environment is also necessary in treating headaches. If chronic headaches interfere with the activities of daily living, psychotherapy may also be indicated.

VERTIGO

Vertigo is a symptom often encountered in patients with neurologic disease, as well as in patients with otologic or cardiovascular disease. It may be of central origin, due to disease of the central nervous system, or of peripheral origin, primarily brought about by dysfunction of the vestibular mechanism. Vertigo is most often associated with multiple sclerosis, head trauma, epilepsy, migraine, intracranial neoplasms, increased intracranial pressure, vestibular disturbances, and cerebrovascular insufficiency.

Dizziness is a more general term to describe a sensation of movement within the head, including faintness and lightheadedness. Therefore the patient should be asked to explain what he or she means by being dizzy, to determine whether or not vertigo is actually present. **Vertigo** is a sensation that the environment is rotating or that one is moving within the surroundings [37]. Sensations of unsteadiness require the patient to sit, lie down, or hold onto something to keep from falling. The nurse should investigate the frequency and duration of vertigo and the prior activity and predisposing factors associated with it. Information should be elicited on additional symptoms, such as nausea and vomiting, an increase in vertigo with head movements, loss of balance, tinnitus, or hearing loss.

Nystagmus is an objective sign often associated with vertigo and can be either spontaneous or induced. **Nystagmus** is involuntary repetitive movement of the eyeball and may be horizontal, vertical, or rotary [10]. It is caused by impairment of the cerebellar system, as well as by drug toxicity and disorders of the labyrinth. Nystagmus can be induced via the optokinetic test, positional tests, or caloric tests (see Chap. 13). The presence or absence, direction, and rate of nystagmus are determined with these tests.

CHANGES IN LEVEL OF CONSCIOUSNESS

Consciousness is a state of awareness of oneself and one's environment. A conscious person is one who is awake, alert, able to carry on a rational conversation, and, if literate and without an organic speech or hearing defect, is able to comprehend the written or spoken word. Consciousness depends on the activation of a normal cerebral cortex by impulses from the reticular activating system.

Although sleep is a state of diminished awareness (or absolute unawareness) of the environment, a person who is sleeping can readily be aroused to a state of consciousness when stimulated (for example, by noise, pain, or touch).

A sleep state is different from a state of unconsciousness, such as coma, in which the person cannot readily be returned to the conscious state and is unresponsive to verbal or even painful stimuli. However, there are several stages in loss of consciousness; the characteristic behavior of a person at these various stages signifies a change in level of consciousness. A patient who is beginning to lose consciousness becomes less alert and less oriented to time, place, and eventually person. Restlessness and agitation, uncooperativeness, and excited confusion may also precede the state of unconsciousness. A sleep-like state (stuporous) then occurs, in which the patient is very lethargic and apathetic, difficult to arouse, and less responsive to questioning, as well as somewhat disoriented (again differing from normal sleep in the ability to be aroused readily). The sleep-like state progresses to a deeper state of stupor, until the patient no longer responds to verbal commands, only reacting to strong pain stimulation. When the patient progresses to a stage of profound unconsciousness and cannot be aroused, even with a strong stimulus, he or she is in a **coma.**

Initially responding to pain stimuli in an appropriate manner (for example, by withdrawing or grimacing), the patient losing consciousness then reacts inappropriately to pain and eventually does not respond to pain at all. From a stage of deep stupor, the person may then recede into a deeper stage of coma, in which he exhibits decerebrate or decorticate posturing and does not respond appropriately to any stimuli. However, deep tendon reflexes are present in this state. Absence of the cough, corneal, and gag reflexes is characteristic of the deepest stage of coma.

The decreased level of awareness can be graded on a continuum from a stage of drowsiness, lethargy, and indifference (in which uncooperativeness is also characteristic, and in which the person does not lapse into sleep but responds both to mild and deep pain stimuli and to his name being called) to the most severe stage, in which the patient does not respond to any stimuli. Such a patient also demonstrates flaccid extremities and the absence of deep tendon reflexes.

Assessing Level of Consciousness

The level of consciousness, the most reliable index of the neurologic state, evaluates the accuracy of the patient's answers to questions about person, place, and time; the nurse should also observe the speed with which the person answers. Ability to obey simple commands, such as "Touch your nose with your right hand," is also assessed.

If the person does not respond to verbal stimuli, the response to painful stimuli is then assessed. The minimal stimulation needed to promote a response to pain should be applied, such as pressing on the patient's fingertip between the examiner's thumb and index finger or pressing the Achilles tendon or tip of the little toe. The response should be noted as appropriate when the patient grimaces, withdraws, or makes noises; or as inappropriate when the patient makes nonpurposeful movements. It is important to record the type of response the patient makes, or the absence of any response.

When the patient does not respond either to verbal or to painful stimuli, the corneal reflex is used to determine the level of consciousness. The cornea is lightly stroked with a wisp of cotton. The normal response is immediate closure of the eyelid. If the corneal reflex is absent, the cough and gag reflexes are also likely to be absent.

Causes of Loss of Consciousness

Loss of consciousness occurs in the presence of any systemic or intracranial condition that depresses or destroys the brainstem activating mechanism or its pathways. Such conditions include diabetic acidosis, anoxia, drug or carbon monoxide poisoning, hypoglycemia, uremia, and epileptic convulsions. All these conditions interfere with the metabolic activities of the cerebral cortex. Cerebral conditions effecting a loss of consciousness are those that result in destruction of the brain cells: intracranial lesions such as a tumor or abscess, hemorrhage, and direct trauma. Elevated intracranial pressure due to an increased volume of CSF or to cerebral edema is another factor in changes of level of consciousness. Therefore, when a patient is admitted to the hospital, the nurse should investigate with the family possible factors related to these predisposing conditions.

Caring for the Unconscious Patient
With loss of consciousness, the awareness and responses essential for the patient's security, self-preservation, and comfort no longer are operational. Therefore, these functions become the responsibility of the nurse and others caring for the patient. The side rails of the bed, for example, must be continuously raised when the patient is not being directly cared for. In addition, the patient's environment must be controlled in terms of temperature, noise level, and safety factors.

The major aspect of the care of the comatose patient is to ensure that oxygenation and circulation are adequate. Maintenance of a patent airway has priority. If the underlying cause of the coma is known, the cause is treated. The nurse's role is oriented to protective measures and assessment of neurologic changes.

The comatose patient should be placed in a lateral or semiprone position to facilitate drainage of oropharyngeal secretions and to prevent obstruction of the airway by the relaxed tongue. An oral airway (endotracheal tube) and tracheostomy may be necessary to maintain a patent airway; a suction machine should be available to remove secretions. If increased intracranial pressure is present, suctioning is avoided except when it is absolutely necessary. A nasogastric tube may be inserted to empty gastric contents and prevent vomiting and aspiration as well as to provide a means for nutrition.

Observation of the vital and neurologic signs is an essential component of the care of the comatose patient. Increased intracranial pressure, trauma to the cerebral centers and brainstem, and an inadequate airway all affect the vital signs. In increased intracranial pressure, the systolic blood pressure rises, but the diastolic pressure often remains the same, resulting in an increased pulse pressure, and there is a decrease in the pulse rate. The respirations may be altered in rate and quality, from depressed respirations to respirations of the Cheyne-Stokes type, with periods of apnea. Elevated temperatures may result from a variety of factors, including pulmonary infections from aspiration and pulmonary stasis. However, elevated temperatures may reflect pressure or trauma to the thermoregulatory center in the hypothalamus. Regardless of the cause, elevated temperatures increase the metabolic needs of the brain and other body systems. Therefore, nursing measures are indicated (page 929).

Monitoring of the level of consciousness continues, and any changes in response to external stimuli or spontaneous movements are reported. Pupillary reactions and muscle strength are also assessed at regular intervals.

When the patient is placed in the lateral or semiprone position, proper body alignment must be maintained and measures taken to prevent the complications of contractures, drop foot and wristdrop, muscle strain, and joint injury. When positioning the patient, care is taken that there is no interference with circulation or chest expansion.

Immobility and loss of skin sensation may lead to pressure sores. Sheepskin pads or an alternating air pressure mattress may be used. The integrity of the skin is assessed at regular intervals, and the patient's position is changed every 2 hours. The skin must be kept clean, dry, and free from wrinkles (the care of decubiti is discussed on page 977). Immobility causes loss of skeletal muscle tone and predisposes to circulatory stasis and contractures. The nurse must therefore ensure that the joints are taken through full range of motion at least four times daily.

Loss of the corneal reflex and depression of lacrimal secretion may result in prolonged exposure of the eyeball, with drying and injury of the cornea. The threat of corneal ulceration and blindness is ever present in this situation unless eye shields are applied to protect the cornea from possible injury. (Eye patches may be contraindicated if the eyelid is able to move partially.) Ocular irrigations with sterile normal saline and the instillation of artificial tears (such as methylcellulose) are helpful in providing moisture and further protection.

Because the comatose patient is unable to eat or drink, fluids and nutrition must be provided by other means. No attempt should be made to give the comatose patient food or fluids by mouth. Aspiration into the respiratory tract will occur in the absence of the swallowing reflex. Intravenous fluids are usually started when the patient is in a comatose state, but other methods of providing longer-term nutritional intake are necessary if the comatose state is prolonged. Generally, this is accomplished by nasogastric tube feedings. (Nutritional intake by nasogastric tube feedings is discussed in Chapter 7.) A careful record of the amount and type of fluid and nutritional intake and an output record are necessary to monitor fluid and electrolyte balance and ensure an adequate nutritional state. Vomiting should be reported. After the patient begins to regain consciousness, the gag reflex should be tested periodically; oral feedings are gradually and carefully begun when gag and swallowing reflexes have returned.

Hygiene needs must be met by nursing personnel. Particular attention should be given to the nasal and oral orifices. Bleeding or dripping of CSF from the nose, particularly after a head injury, requires that sterile cotton be gently placed on, not in, the nares and changed when soiled. Cleaning of the nares or of the ears should be avoided in the presence of CSF rhinorrhea or CSF otorrhea because of the danger of transmitting an infection from the sinuses or the ears to the brain itself.

Oral hygiene is absolutely essential. Dentures or bridges should be removed from the mouths of patients who are unconscious. Brushing of the teeth and cleaning of the mucous membranes should be done at least four times a day and preferably every 4 hours to prevent odors, infections, and parotitis. Attention to other aspects of hygiene, such as hair care, nail care, and shaving, is important in the comatose patient.

To monitor elimination, as well as to control incontinence, an indwelling catheter is placed (or an external catheter may be preferred for a male patient). In some settings a catheter is not used, but rather the patient's urinary elimination pattern is monitored and the patient is placed on the bedpan at appropriately timed intervals. The approach used will depend on the patient's status and the ability of the staff to prevent complications from incontinence by proper and prompt skin cleaning after an accidental voiding. When an indwelling catheter is used for a male patient who is comatose, measures must be taken to prevent the formation of a fistula from the continuous pressure at the penoscrotal junction. The catheter should be taped to the abdomen as illustrated in Figure 11-14. (Refer to page 482 for the management of external catheters.)

Bowel elimination must also be monitored, because of the lack of bowel control in the comatose patient and the predisposition to fecal impaction, which results from limited intake of roughage, as well as from minimal exercise. Stool softeners or laxatives may be administered through the feeding tubes, or suppositories may be given at regular intervals. Enemas or manual removal of feces may be necessary in some situations, but they interfere with normal reflexes (see page 976 for measures used in bowel management).

In the care of the comatose patient, the nurse should remember, and remind other personnel, that hearing is the last sense the patient loses. The patient should be treated with dignity, and conversation in the presence of the patient should always be appropriate and professional.

The needs of the family and friends should also be considered in the care of the comatose patient. Often, they wish to help in the care of the patient, because their sense of hopelessness and insecurity render them distraught and anxious. For example, the family members often like to assist with the patient's

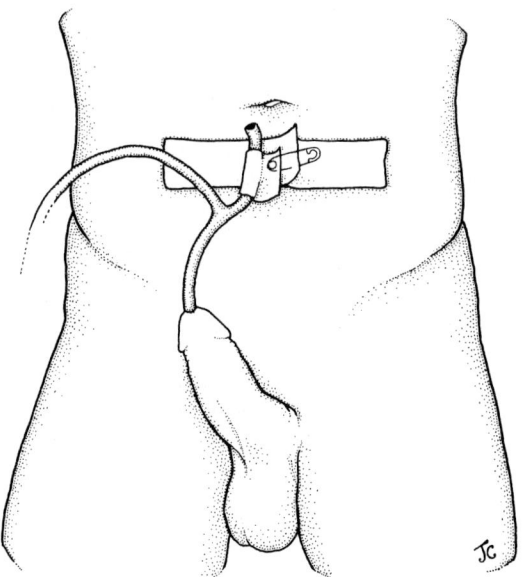

Figure 11-14
Male catheter taped to abdomen.

turning and positioning, shaving, or nail care. The many questions that the family members have for the nurse and physician should be answered as honestly as possible. Often, neither the outcome nor the length of time the comatose state may last can be predicted. In such cases, the nurse should consider the psychological and socioeconomic problems that may result in the family. Referrals to a social worker and appropriate agencies are often necessary.

If and when the patient recovers consciousness, he or she is usually initially confused and bewildered. The nurse must be calm and reassuring. Often, a familiar face and voice will be of significant support to the patient and, therefore, the family's presence at this time is important. Depending on the cause and length of the coma, as well as the severity of the coma, residual neurologic disabilities may be present, requiring appropriate rehabilitative and supportive services.

INCREASED INTRACRANIAL PRESSURE

The rigid skull that encases the brain allows only minimal room for expansion of its contents: the nervous tissue, cerebrospinal fluid, and blood volume. If there is an increase in the size of any one of these elements, the other elements are compromised. Brain tissue cannot expand without having serious effects on the flow and amount of CSF and cerebral circulation. The hazards of increased intracranial pressure are related to decreased cerebral perfusion and cerebral hypoxia, which can produce irreversible neurologic damage.

Increased intracranial pressure results from a variety of causes, including cerebral edema, hemorrhage, inflammation, and increased formation or decreased absorption of CSF. Space-occupying lesions such as neoplasms, abscesses, and hematomas compromise central nervous system functioning by their volume, pressure on vessels with decreased cerebral perfusion, and obstruction of CSF absorption. Ultimately, unless removed, space-occupying lesions lead to brain displacement and death.

Signs and Symptoms of Increased Intracranial Pressure

Although intracranial pressure monitoring is an important development in the care of the neurologic patient, it is not universally available, and it cannot substitute for careful assessment by the nurse caring for such a patient. The importance of precise assessment to detect subtle alterations and the accurate recording and reporting of these changes cannot be overemphasized. Baseline data must be established to enable detection of subtle changes. Neurologic assessment may be necessary as often as every 5 to 15 minutes or every half-hour to hour, depending on the severity of the patient's condition. The variables to assess include the level of conscious-vital signs. It is also essential to observe for seizures, vomiting, and CSF leakage from the nose and ear. Classic signs of increased intracranial pressure are headache, papilledema, bradycardia, defects in mentation, and deterioration in consciousness.

As noted previously, the level of consciousness is the earliest and most sensitive indicator of the onset of increased intracranial pressure, usually preceding changes in vital signs. A decrease in the level of consciousness reflects hypoxia of the reticular activating system and of specific brainstem nuclei and nerve tracts. This change in consciousness may be a subtle decrease in the patient's orientation, subtle changes in behavior with increased irritability or restlessness, drowsiness, or difficulty of arousal of the patient. The patient's response to stimuli should be described precisely rather than categorized as being a specific stage of consciousness (such as stuporous or comatose).

Evaluation of the motor and sensory function of the extremities is another important aspect of neurologic assessment for the detection of increased intracranial pressure. The nurse should observe for spontaneous movements of the arms and legs and evaluate the patient's voluntary movements by asking the patient to squeeze the nurse's fingers and hand and to move the extremity. Muscle tone is described as "spastic," "flaccid," or "apparently normal." Inequality of motor strength is a very important finding in detecting a focal neurologic deficit. Comparisons are made of the strength of each extremity: for example, bilateral hand grasps should be strong and equal. Facial symmetry is noted to determine cranial nerve involvement. Pressure on the motor cortex can result in paresis, paralysis, seizures, or purposeless movement.

When the patient does not respond to simple commands to enable evaluation of motor functioning, sensory stimuli are then used to elicit motor responses. The minimal stimulation necessary to cause a response is used; only if touch or pressure do not elicit a response is a painful stimulus used. Light stroking of the medial aspects of the patient's arms and legs or light digital pressure to the patient's fingertips or toes are examples of nonpainful stimuli. The normal response to pain is withdrawal of the part stimulated.

Inappropriate motor responses are decorticate or decerebrate posture. **Decorticate posture** occurs when the corticospinal tract is interrupted in its action through the motor segment of the cerebral cortex. It is characterized by the following: adduction of the arms; flexion of the arms, wrists, and fingers; and extension, internal rotation, and plantar flexion of the lower extremity. The **decerebrate position** indicates involvement of the midbrain and upper pons. Both the decorticate and decerebrate postures are ominous signs. The decerebrate posture is characterized by rigid extension of the extremities, with abducted arms and pronated hands and forearms. These characteristic movements may be associated with the opisthotonos position, with arching of the back, stiffness of the neck, and toes that are pointed inward. These abnormal postures may occur spontaneously or in response to a stimulus. When these assessments are made, the nurse must be careful not to pinch the skin or to cause trauma, especially when assessment is made frequently.

Pupillary signs are also important in evaluating the status of intracranial pressure. Normally, the pupils are equal in size and react readily to light. Deviations of pupillary size, equality, and reaction to light are therefore regularly assessed. The reaction to light is described as "brisk," "moderate," "sluggish," "fixed," or "nonreactive." The nurse should remember, however, that in addition to impairment of the oculomotor cranial nerve, certain ocular medications and opiates affect pupillary size and reaction. Although they are not always present, papilledema (choked disc), decreased visual acuity, and blurred vision are other ocular signs that are important in detecting elevated intracranial pressure. Any cause of increased intracranial pressure results in pupillary changes, which are important in locating the site of an expanding lesion or edema. Pupillary irregularity and hemiparesis on the same side, for example, indicates a shift of the brain and brain stem across the midline. In this situation, the motor fibers in the cerebral peduncle on the contralateral side become compressed against the tentorium cerebelli and cause ipsilateral paralysis and hemiparesis [34]. The side of a fixed and dilated pupil is usually considered the side of the expanding lesion. Deviations of gaze and nystagmus are also significant findings.

The nurse must immediately report a decreased level of consciousness and the presence of a dilated pupil. These signs indicate increased pressure to the brainstem and herniation into the foramen magnum. Respiratory failure and death occur rapidly unless medical and surgical intervention is obtained.

Vital-sign alterations develop as intracranial pressure rises, resulting in venous stasis and accumulation of CO_2 in the vasomotor center of the medulla. Initially, vital signs change to compensate and to preserve brain function, demonstrated by a slowly falling pulse rate, usually of a bounding quality, alterations in the respiratory rate, and an increase in the systolic and pulse pressures. When the compensatory mechanisms fail, the pulse may become rapid, thready, and irregular. Hyperpyrexia may or may not be present. Cerebral infection and pressure on the thermoregulation center located in the hypothalamus are associated with temperature elevations, but rapid hyperthermia is likely to be present in the decompensated stage of increased intracranial pressure.

Changes in respirations depend on the site of pressure. Initially, the respiratory rate may be increased or decreased, with ventilatory problems. The several different types of abnormal respiratory patterns that may occur include **Cheyne-Stokes respirations,** which are characterized by a rhythmic pattern of hyperpnea alternating with periods of apnea. This pattern results from hyperventilation due to raised carbon dioxide levels and then cessation of breathing (apneic period) when the carbon dioxide level drops. The cycle is repeated when carbon dioxide levels accumulate. This pattern of breathing is associated with deep cerebral lesions and lesions in the basal ganglia and diencephalon.

Other abnormal breathing patterns associated with neurologic disease are central neurogenic hyperventilation, apneustic breathing, and ataxic breathing. **Central neurogenic breathing** is sustained and regular hyperpnea, or abnormally rapid and deep breathing. **Apneustic breathing** is an irregular type of breathing with sustained pauses in both inspiration and expiration, while **ataxic breathing** is a completely irregular pattern, with random deep and shallow breaths and irregular pauses. Ataxic breathing requires immediate respiratory assistance.

To ensure adequate perfusion of the microcirculation, maintenance of respiratory function is of paramount importance. The nurse must make sure the airway is patent and provide adequate assisted ventilation as necessary. Arterial blood gases are drawn at regular intervals to evaluate the respiratory status of the patient. Suctioning must be done efficiently and quickly to prevent hypoxia during the procedure; usually, hyperinflation prior to suctioning is indicated. Chest auscultation is also performed to evaluate the effectiveness of suctioning and assisted ventilation.

Treatment and Nursing Care

To prevent even transient increases in intracranial pressure, the patient is positioned carefully and smoothly. The head is usually elevated 15 to 30 degrees, and neck flexion is avoided. Efforts are made to prevent the patient from performing the Valsalva maneuver, which increases intrathoracic and intracranial pressure. Stool softeners are indicated to prevent constipation, which causes straining (and the Valsalva maneuver) during evacuation of the stool. Patients also tend to perform the Valsalva maneuver spontaneously while turning or moving in bed, and they should be encouraged to exhale during these activities. The patient is also encouraged to prevent isometric muscular contraction during movements; these are contraindicated in a patient with increased intracranial pressure. Muscular contractions are likely to occur when patients try to push themselves up in bed by pressing the elbows into the bed or by pushing against the footboard; both of these movements should be avoided. The patient's tolerance for activities should be evaluated, and excessive movement or a cluster of activities during a short time should be prevented.

Fluid and electrolyte replacement is provided, but patients are kept somewhat dehydrated to prevent cerebral edema. Osmotic diuretics such as mannitol are given to increase cerebral blood flow by decreasing cerebral edema, which compromises the microcirculation [28]. All patients receiving osmotic diuretics should have an indwelling catheter, and a urimeter should be used for measurement of hourly urine output. These diuretics are given on a temporary basis by rapid intravenous infusion. Patients must be monitored closely for their neurologic status and kidney functioning. Pulmonary edema is a potential complication when osmotic diuretics are administered rapidly. There is also a danger of sloughing of the tissues from osmotic diuretics; proper administration and prevention of extravasation are essential.

Corticosteroid therapy is also used to decrease cerebral edema and reduce intracranial pressure. Dexamethasone (Decadron) is the most commonly used agent, because it produces less sodium-retaining effects than other steroids. Because of the danger of gastric hemorrhage associated with prolonged use of corticosteroid therapy, antacids are generally indicated; administration by nasogastric tube is necessary if the patient is unconscious.

The patient is observed for the onset of convulsions, and the necessary protective measures are taken. The patient is kept in a quiet room, and excessive noise or jarring of the bed is avoided. Phenytoin (Dilantin) may be used prophylactically; diazepam (Valium) is used if convulsions occur. Narcotics or other medications that cause respiratory depression are avoided. Restlessness is treated with mild sedation if necessary; restraints are avoided if possible, because they tend to excite the patient and thus increase intracranial pressure.

Intracranial pressure may be measured via a cannula in the lateral ventricle. The normal intraventricular pressure is within the range of 10 to 15 mm Hg when it is measured with the patient lying in a horizontal position. Intracranial pressure monitoring can be done on an intermittent or continuous basis. An intraventricular catheter in the lateral ventricle is attached to a pressure transducer.

Continuous ventricular pressure monitoring has provided data on the nonstatic nature of intracranial pressure; the pressure has transient fluctuations associated with activity, straining (the Valsalva maneuver), and isometric exercises. For the patient with neurologic disease, even these transient fluctuations are important, as are signs of transient worsening of neurologic status, and the physician must be notified of any changes in the status of either.

When intracranial pressure increases further, with enlargement of the ventricle and progressive neurologic deterioration, CSF may be withdrawn via the ventricular cannula. Continuous ventricular drainage may also be used to decrease intracranial pressure. This procedure involves the automatic withdrawal of ventricular fluid via a special device that maintains the intracranial pressure at a predetermined level. Another approach is via an indwelling catheter within the ventricular system and an external reservoir. In either technique, maintenance of an aseptic system is absolutely essential. In some situations, penicillin may also be introduced into the ventricular drainage system simultaneously with withdrawal of CSF.

Hypothermia may also be used when the patient is hyperpyrexic, because the metabolic rate of oxygen in the brain is increased in hyperpyrexia. Hypothermia reduces the cerebral and systemic metabolic need for oxygen and glucose [28].

During these critical stages of increasing intracranial pressure, the nurse must always be cognizant of the patient's emotional status and the family's concern and welfare.

CONVULSIVE DISORDERS

Convulsive disorders are caused by sudden brain dysfunction in which there is an uncontrolled, rapid, and excessive release of impulses by a group of neurons. Depending on the origin and pattern of spread of the abnormal neural activity, manifestations of the disorder vary from momentary suspension of activity and awareness to complete motor, sensory, autonomic, and psychic disturbances and loss of consciousness. The dysfunction may be localized or may spread to involve extensive areas of normal neurons. It is generally believed that the uncontrolled discharge of impulses results from the lowering of a normal seizure threshold or from an increased excitation within the neurons to minimal stimuli.

Convulsive disorders may occur both in intracranial and systemic disease. Seizures may be a symptom of increased intracranial pressure or brain damage associated with head injuries, cerebral edema, hemorrhage, infection, or intracranial space-occupying lesions. Hypoglycemia, hypocalcemia, renal insufficiency, hypoxia, fever (especially in children), and chemical poisoning (including alcohol, lead, and amphetamine poisoning), are examples of systemic conditions that may cause convulsions. Seizures associated with these conditions do not tend to recur after the systemic disease is corrected.

Epilepsy is a term used to identify chronic episodic brain dysfunction manifested by recurrent seizures. It is estimated that there are about 2 to 4 million epileptic persons in the United States [22a]. In the majority of patients, the specific cause of epilepsy is unknown (**idiopathic epilepsy**). An inherited predisposition is thought to have a role in idiopathic epilepsy. Rodin and Gonzales [31], in their studies of families with epileptic members, have determined that persons who start having seizures between the ages of 6 and 15 are likely to have a genetic component to their illness. These investigators stressed however that the genetic component is not necessarily the cause of the patient's illness, but that the immediate cause of the seizure relates to mechanisms that allow excessive electrical activity. It has also been found that relatives of epileptic persons often have abnormal EEGs even though they do not have seizures.

After seizures have occurred, an extensive physical and neurologic examination is necessary to rule out the presence of organic disease, particularly when a person over the age of 21 has a seizure for the first time. An accurate description of the seizure and an EEG are important in making the diagnosis. For example, EEG changes are characteristic for different types of epilepsy. A brain scan, lumbar puncture, skull x-ray films, CSF analysis, and a cerebral arteriogram may be indicated, before a specific cause can be ruled out.

Seizures may be generalized or local and they vary in form and length (from a brief transitory phase of a few seconds to several minutes) and in symptoms, depending on the origin and extent, as well as the course of the spread within the brain. Although there are various classifications of epilepsy and seizures, only the four major types (grand mal, petit mal, psychomotor, and Jacksonian [or focal]) will be discussed. Mixed forms of seizures may occur; for example, a psychomotor seizure may precede a grand mal convulsion.

Grand Mal Seizures

Grand mal seizures are generalized convulsions with a loss of consciousness that occurs suddenly, with or without an aura. An **aura** is a warning signal that usually consists of an unusual odor, tingling sensations, or a change in mood, as well as auditory or visual sensations. Spasm of the body is observed, and an audible cry is often heard as air is forced out of the lungs. Usually, the person falls and lies rigid for several seconds in tonic contraction, characterized by stiff arching of the body and causing a temporary cessation of breathing and transient cyanosis. Breathing is reinitiated when tonic contractions change to clonic movements, which are rhythmic muscular contractions. Spasms involving all body muscles begin to occur. During this time, the tongue may be accidentally bitten, and involuntary urination or defecation may occur. Within a minute or two the person relaxes and breathes normally, and normal color returns. On awakening the person remembers nothing about the seizure but becomes aware of it through the response of others around him, as well as by residual effects, such as a bitten tongue, injury, or accidental urination. Drowsiness often follows the seizure, and the person may fall into a deep sleep that may last only a few minutes or for an hour or longer. On awakening, the person often complains of achiness, fatigue, and a severe headache. The grand mal seizure varies in severity, frequency, and intensity among different persons but tends not to vary in these respects on recurrence in the same person.

Petit Mal Seizures

Petit mal seizures are the most common type of seizure in children and adolescents. They are characterized by a brief lapse of consciousness, a flickering of the eyelids, or simply a faltering in speech, usually lasting only 3 to 4 seconds. The person appears to pause in whatever he is doing and to stare into space, as if daydreaming, in a trance-like state. Although some persons experience a loss of balance and a transient loss of consciousness, the person having a petit mal seizure usually does not fall. Petit mal seizures are often referred to as absence seizures.

Psychomotor Epilepsy

Psychomotor epilepsy, also known as temporal lobe epilepsy, is most common in children 11 to 15 years of age. In this type of epilepsy, the patient remains conscious, but involuntary motor activities occur. These are often observed as chewing movements, mumbled speech, and other actions that may seemingly be purposeful but are inappropriate at the time (for example, removing clothes). At times, antisocial behavior may occur during these events. The person may appear angry, fearful, or irritable but later has no recollection of the seizure or the unusual behavior.

Focal Motor Seizures

Focal motor or **sensory seizures,** also known as Jacksonian seizures, indicate a structural cortical or subcortical lesion. Most commonly, they are associated with intracranial trauma. The seizure may start with clonic movements in the fingers and wrists, then involves the elbow, shoulder, and face, and then proceeds down the body or localizes at any point on the pathway. The seizure may also begin with a twitching of the lips that spreads across the face down into the neck and along the arm and leg of the same side. In some cases, the focal seizure may lead to a generalized convulsion.

Status Epilepticus

Status epilepticus is a condition in which a series of seizures occur in rapid succession without recovery of consciousness between seizures. The condition most often occurs when an epileptic suddenly withdraws his or her anticonvulsant medications but it may also be associated with infection and with cerebral edema. Status epilepticus with repeated grand mal seizures may have a fatal outcome, due to the decreased oxygenation that occurs with each seizure. Intervention is directed toward maintaining a patent airway and controlling seizures by medication. Currently, diazepam (Valium) is the drug of choice in most cases of status epilepticus. It is given intravenously for prompt effects. Phenobarbital and phenytoin sodium (Dilantin) are also used. If these medications are not effective, an anesthetic such as sodium thiopental (Pentothal sodium) may be administered intravenously, or tribromoethanol (Avertin) may be given rectally.

Status epilepticus may also occur with focal seizures. Although these are difficult to control, the condition in this case is not life-threatening.

Nursing Care

When a grand mal seizure occurs, the nurse should stay with the patient. The nurse's major responsibilities are to protect the patient from injury and to observe the pattern of the seizure.

If possible, a pad is placed under the patient's head to protect it from injury if the patient should fall. If the mouth has not become clenched, a padded tongue blade or other soft article is placed between the patient's teeth to prevent biting the tongue. However, if the jaws are clenched in spasm, no attempt is made to insert a tongue blade; this will cause more injury. Constrictive clothing should be loosened. If possible, the patient should be placed in a lateral position to facilitate drainage of mucus and saliva. It is important to observe the patient's respiratory status; transient apnea, however, is an expected effect during a generalized or grand mal convulsion. If the seizure occurs when the patient is in a wheelchair, he or she should be removed from the chair and eased to the floor with his head protected by supporting it in the nurse's lap. Any nearby objects should be removed if they are potentially injurious.

The patient should not be moved until the convulsion has ceased, unless there is danger of injury (the patient has fallen near a hot radiator or stove, for example). The patient should be screened as much as possible and privacy maintained. Other patients should be protected from observing the seizure, because it can be a very frightening event to watch. An explanation of what has happened is usually warranted, however, to reassure the observers. On awakening from the convulsion, the patient will usually be somewhat confused and should be allowed to rest quietly.

There are many important factors that the nurse observes and records during a seizure. First, the exact time of the seizure and its characteristics are noted and recorded. Other observations include the preceding activities of the patient and a general description of the seizure. The latter includes whether or not consciousness was lost, the duration of unconsciousness, type of onset, position at onset, types of body movements, and site of initiation of the movements if initially localized, as well as the pattern of spread. Any deviation of the eyes or any pupillary changes are recorded, as are any injury to the tongue, cheek, or other parts of the body, incontinence, postictal state, and the presence of confusion, speech difficulty, or drowsiness after the convulsion has ceased and the patient has awakened. It is important that the nurse remain calm during the event and that excessive noise and stimulation be eliminated when the patient recovers consciousness. When petit mal and psychomotor seizures are observed, the nurse notes precipitating behavior and factors and the length, frequency, and pattern of the seizures.

Treatment

The most effective method of treating patients with epilepsy is the regular administration of **anticonvulsant medications.** It is thought that they raise the seizure threshold, thus preventing the abnormal foci from discharging in response to minimal stimuli. Although a cure is not accomplished with drug therapy, control can be attained, so that the majority of patients can lead normal and active lives. The reader is referred to pharmacology textbooks for detailed information on these medications.

The most common anticonvulsants used for maintenance therapy are the following: phenytoin sodium (Dilantin) for the treatment of grand mal and psychomotor seizures; paramethadione (Paradione) for petit mal seizures; primidone (Mysoline) for grand mal seizures, psychomotor epilepsy, and focal seizures; and phenobarbital, which is used for both grand mal and psychomotor seizures. In 1974, the drug carbamazepine (Tegretol) was approved by the Federal Drug Administration for the treatment of epilepsy. Other anticonvulsant drugs include ethosuximide (Zarontin), mephenytoin (Mesantoin), and trimethadione (Tridione). These drugs may be used singly or in combination for synergistic effects while lessening the likelihood of toxic side effects.

The nurse must be alert for early signs of side effects of anticonvulsant drugs. Phenytoin sodium, for example, often causes gingival hypertrophy, blurred vision, nausea, vomiting, and skin eruptions. Ataxia, dizziness, and mental confusion may occur. Less often, but even more serious, are those effects resulting in sore throat and fever and associated with agranulocytosis. Megaloblastic anemia and bleeding tendencies have also been reported.

Proper oral hygiene is essential to prevent oral infections. Taking the medication with meals will usually control the side effects of nausea and vomiting. The sedative effects of phenobarbital may cause difficulties, although the initial lethargy associated with the drug usually decreases in time. Primidone may cause lethargy, light-headedness, and mental detachment, particularly if larger doses are used. Ataxia, nausea, vertigo, and a measles-like rash have been associated with the drug. Carbamazepine has caused hematologic and skin reactions. Blood counts and hemoglobin levels are monitored every 6 months to detect early signs of blood dyscrasias. Gas-liquid chromatography is used to determine blood levels of the drugs, facilitating adequate control and monitoring patient adherence to the regimen.

Anticonvulsant medications are continued for at least 3 years after the last seizure. If and when the medications are to be discontinued, dosages are gradually decreased and the patient is observed for recurrence of seizures. Strict adherence to the medication regimen is mandatory.

Surgery is used to treat a small number of epileptic patients whose disease is characterized by well-defined foci of abnormal activity in the brain and inadequate control with anticonvulsant drug therapy. The procedure consists of careful excision of the specific site of origin of the seizures in the cerebral cortex (usually in the temporal lobe), so that no serious neurologic deficit results. Postoperative care is similar to that following other types of intracranial surgery (see page 947). There is a potential for seizures postoperatively, and anticonvulsant drugs are usually continued for at least a year.

Another surgical procedure for seizure control that has been developed recently is implantation of electric stimulators to activate inhibitory mechanisms of the cerebellar cortex on skeletal muscle activity [19]. This procedure is used for control of intractable seizures secondary to stroke, cerebral palsy, brain injury, and epilepsy.

Patient Education
The epileptic patient needs a thorough orientation to the nature of the disorder and to the specific medication regimen, potential side effects, and the dangers of not taking medications as prescribed. Patients should be advised that the medications will be given for an indefinite period of time, and that recurrence of convulsions results from alterations in or omissions of the prescribed dosages. Often, patients who do not have a convulsion for a year or so after being started on medications begin to feel secure that the seizures have been controlled and discontinue taking their medications, only to have a rapid recurrence.

Precautions should be taken in the home to keep anticonvulsant medications out of the reach of children, for whom the drugs may be fatal. The epileptic patient should be advised to carry an identification card or a Medic-Alert tag to identify himself or herself as an epileptic and to ensure that proper treatment is given in case of a convulsion or accident.

It is important for the nurse to emphasize the necessity of adequate rest, regular meals, a well-balanced diet, and the avoidance of extreme physical exertion, fatigue, infection, fever, and emotional stress as measures to prevent recurrence of convulsions. For some persons, certain types of sensory stimulation tend to precipitate seizures. Such stimuli are sudden loud noises, some kinds of music, prolonged television viewing, and flickering lights. These should be avoided if known to precipitate seizures. Alcohol is generally contraindicated, although some physicians permit an occasional social drink. Only a moderate intake of coffee, tea, or cola beverages is advised; stimulant drugs such as amphetamines are contraindicated.

Epileptic persons must always advise their physicians and dentists of the medications they are taking, because some may interact with other drugs. For example, phenytoin augments the effect of coumarin, thus increasing bleeding tendencies. Isoniazid (INH) and chloramphenicol (Chloromycetin) increase the effect of phenytoin. Certain drugs interact with phenobarbital and cause an increase in the phenobarbital effects; these drugs include alcohol, meprobamate, and isoniazid. Phenobarbital, however, counteracts the effects of coumarin and cortisone.

Patients with epilepsy must be advised about the dangers of participating in certain activities in which a seizure would endanger the patient's life as well as the lives of others. These activities include driving an automobile (unless seizures are under control and legal requirements are met), working near dangerous machinery, working on scaffolds or ladders, and swimming alone.

Socioeconomic and Psychological Aspects of Epilepsy

The nurse caring for the epileptic patient is concerned with the socioeconomic and the psychological aspects of this chronic condition, as well as with the teaching aspects related to prevention of seizures. The patient should be advised of the available community resources and agencies that might be of assistance. Four national voluntary organizations are concerned with the problem of epilepsy and concentrate their efforts on changing the attitudes of the public toward persons with epilepsy. Besides providing literature about epilepsy for both professionals and lay persons, these organizations work toward the improvement of the social and economic conditions of epileptics and their families. (For example, members of the National Epilepsy League may purchase prescribed anticonvulsant medications by mail at reduced rates.) The agencies are

American Epilepsy Foundation
77 Reservoir Road
Quincy, Mass. 02169

National Epilepsy League
203 N. Wabash Ave.
Chicago, Ill. 60604

Epilepsy Foundation of America
1828 L St., N.W.
Washington, D.C. 20036

United Epilepsy Association
113 W. 57th St.
New York, N.Y. 10019

Often, patients try to conceal that they are epileptic because they fear negative attitudes, pity, or rejection. Although the stigma of epilepsy has lessened over the years, there are still many persons with misconceptions about and fear of the disease. Such misconceptions and fears have been institutionalized in various state laws concerning epilepsy, relating to drivers' licenses, sterilization, workmen's compensation, and reportability to a state agency. Only since 1972 has there been no statute prohibiting the marriage of epileptic persons in the United States. The last three states to have such laws repealed them in the years 1965 to 1971.

Periodically the Epilepsy Foundation of America does surveys to determine the status of laws related to epilepsy in the different states [9a]. The reader is referred to the reference list for the resource for current information in this area. The fourth edition of the survey reports that ten states still require that epilepsy be reported to a state agency. The Foundation is active in trying to have this type of statute revoked in all states.

The most common state licensing statutes for drivers prohibit the licensing of applicants whose driving, in the opinion of the commissioner or administrator, would be inimical to public safety or welfare. This type of requirement is considered inappropriate by the Epilepsy Foundation of America, which has taken the position that a permanent license should be granted after 2 seizure-free years. Their publication, *Legal Rights of Persons with Epilepsy* [9a], also includes a section that clarifies the meaning of workmen's compensation and second injury funds as they apply to persons with epilepsy. It is hoped that changes in these regulations will further lessen acts of discrimination against epileptic persons.

It is important that the nurse play a role in changing the public's attitudes and misconceptions about epilepsy, emphasizing that approximately 80 to 85 percent of persons with epilepsy whose seizures are controlled by medication can lead essentially normal lives.

HYPERPYREXIA

Hyperpyrexia, which is an excessively high body temperature (39.5°C; 103.1°F), often occurs in patients with intracranial diseases or injury or following intracranial surgery. It results from disturbances of the temperature control center in the hypothalamus or from associated infections. Because fever increases oxygen demand and glucose metabolism, the reduction of fever is an important component of care of the patient with neurologic problems.

Various approaches are used to reduce fever, depending on its cause and severity. Light covers are used, and excess clothing is removed. Room temperature is controlled with air conditioning or fans. Tepid or cold sponges, using ice water or alcohol, are given. Ice bags may be applied to the axillae, groin, and trunk. **Hypopyrexia,** using electronic cooling blankets, may be necessary if these other methods do not reduce the temperature. Aspirin may be given by rectal suppository. If not contraindicated, fluid intake is increased.

The patient's vital signs, including rectal temperature, should be measured frequently during attempts to reduce fever. The patient should be observed for the onset of chilling, shock, or emotional reactions, which may require discontinuing the treatment temporarily while providing supportive measures. Attention to the skin, with frequent massages and assessment for ischemic changes, is important to prevent injury when external cooling methods are used. If shivering occurs, the physician should be notified; ataractic drugs may be prescribed. When the temperature is changing rapidly, the patient should be observed carefully for changes in heart rate and rhythm. There is a danger of cardiac arrest with excessive or sudden cooling or rewarming; cooling increases the irritability of the myocardium. Urinary output should also be measured carefully, because hypopyrexia causes a decrease in the filtration rate and a lower specific gravity due to hemoconcentration.

APHASIA

The various types of language disorders that occur with neurologic deficits associated with cerebrovascular disease, brain tumors, and trauma represent varying degrees of disability. **Aphasia** (or dysphasia) is a general term used to describe organic disturbances in language, resulting from cortical tissue damage rather than from defective innervation of the muscles used in speech or from mental deficiency. Aphasia involves all areas of language, affecting speech, reading, writing, and understanding the spoken or written word. The pattern and severity of impairment depend on the location and extent of neurologic damage. The term **dysphasia** is used to reflect a degree of communication disability rather than a complete inability to communicate. However, in this discusssion, the conventional term aphasia will be used.

Any type of aphasia is overwhelming and frustrating to both patient and family, with devastating effects on the patient's psychological status and self-image.

TYPES OF APHASIA

Global aphasia is the inability to communicate and to understand communication and reflects severe, generalized brain dysfunction. **Receptive aphasia** is the inability to understand the spoken or written word (or, in some cases, even gestures) and reflects problems in perceiving and comprehending language. **Expressive aphasia** is the inability to communicate through speech or the written word or with gestures and reflects difficulty in using symbols in speech rather than difficulty in using muscles for speech. A neurologic deficit usually results in both receptive and expressive aphasia, but one function may be more impaired than the other. **Jargon aphasia** is the use of recognizable words but in a meaningless manner, with the patient apparently unaware that the words make no sense. Brief phrases with meaning may be interspersed with other meaningless phrases.

Other examples of language disorders are automatic speech and word-finding problems. **Automatic speech** is completely uncontrolled verbalization. Its use by the patient does not indicate whether or not language retraining will be successful. Patients may sing songs, count, or recite the alphabet and often do so correctly. It is generally felt that patients should not be discouraged from continuing these activities. **Word-finding problems** are difficulties in remembering words the patient wants to use; a similar word or an inappropriate one may be substituted.

These language problems may be associated with motor speech problems such as apraxia and dysarthria. **Apraxia** is impaired ability to make speech sounds voluntarily, with difficulty in carrying out the oral movements required in speaking. The patient substitutes sounds, so that, for example, the word *foot* may be called poot, toot, or foop. Although apraxia may make speech sound like jargon, the patient's message may be deciphered by careful listening and observation.

Dysarthria is an articulation defect due to physical weakness, paralysis, or incoordination of the muscles of the lips, tongue, pharynx, or larynx caused by either central or peripheral nerve damage. Slurring of words and monotonous speech are examples.

NURSING CARE OF APHASIC PATIENTS

Assessment requires early evaluation of the patient's understanding and use of speech. This assessment is only possible by speaking and listening to the patient and observing the patient's behavior. If the patient responds best to gestures alone, gestures should be used for communication. The nurse should convey this information to other nursing personnel working with the patient. Simple requests such as "Raise your arm" or "Touch your nose" are made to determine the ability of the patient to understand and carry out simple tasks. The patient can be asked to shake his head or nod in answer to questions if unable to say "no" or "yes." Simple questions such as "Is the light on?" can be used to assess understanding.

Information about the patient's background relevant to language should be obtained from family members; for example, information on the patient's education and interests and other languages spoken. Information about any visual problems, such as hemianopia or the need for eyeglasses, or hearing problems and the use of a hearing aid, should be obtained because such problems can interfere with understanding communications. If the patient wears dentures, they should be checked for proper fit to ensure that they do not cause slurring or problems in pronunciation. The patient should be asked to move the tongue up, down, and to the front and back. If able to do so, the patient probably does not have oral paralysis, and dysarthria should not be a problem.

People often tend to talk loudly to the aphasic patient, as though the patient were deaf or mentally incompetent. Raising the voice does not contribute to understanding but only succeeds in further frustrating the patient. Often, aphasic adults are spoken to as if they were children, or others tend to talk for them and thus inhibit their attempts at communication. All these habits are annoying and frustrating for the patient.

Skelly [33a], in studying the rehabilitation of aphasic patients, reported 12 areas of serious concern to aphasic patients who had recovered with a useful level of speech; for example, the tendency of people to talk about them rather than to them, even when their comprehension returned, and for people to talk too fast and ask too many questions at once without allowing enough time for an answer. These patients also were aware of behavioral cues that indicated impatience and frustration with their impaired communication. Further, they considered the level of many evaluation tests and exercises to be inappropriate. This study also showed that 6 to 12 weeks immediately after a stroke is the "optimum treatment period," but that additional improvement can take place for two or more years after a stroke (most spontaneous recovery of speech generally takes place within the first few weeks). This study has many implications for the nurse working with aphasic patients.

Formal speech therapy with a speech pathologist or speech therapist is generally started after the acute phase. The speech pathologist can suggest to the nursing personnel approaches and methods that will reinforce the speech therapy program. Even before a specific program is started, the nurse and family can follow certain basic guidelines in communicating with the patient.

It is important not to isolate the patient socially but rather to provide verbal stimulation and find some manner of communication if impairment is severe. Even if the patient does not understand speech, the tone of the nurse's voice may be reassuring. Fortunately, speech is not the only way of communicating; body language, facial expressions, the tone of voice, and gestures all convey messages to the patient. Sitting by the patient so that there is eye-level contact, rather than standing over the patient, helps to create a natural atmosphere for communication. Patience in allowing the aphasic patient time to speak and patience in trying to decipher the patient's meaning will encourage communication and the patient's participation in speech rehabilitation.

Guidelines for communicating with aphasic patients include the following: talking slowly and in a natural tone of voice;

using simple words and phrases and short sentences, allowing sufficient time for the patient to answer questions; and eliminating loud noises or distracting stimuli during communications. Listening carefully and patiently to the patient's labored efforts, avoiding excessive demands for near-perfect pronunciation, and preventing fatigue, which interferes with comprehension and tolerance, are equally essential. The nurse should also keep in mind that the patient with cerebral damage will have a short attention span and probably labile emotions, both of which will affect the patient's tolerance of learning and practice sessions. Short, frequent sessions are more effective than long ones.

It is also important for the nurse to avoid the use of abstract words, since the aphasic patient relearns speech in a sequence of nouns and verbs, then adjectives, then pronouns and articles. Using specific nouns (rather than collective or abstract nouns) and pointing to the article, or naming the article the patient is using, help to reinforce comprehension. When trying to teach the patient to use new words, the emphasis should be on words that are essential during hospitalization, such as *water, soap, hand, comb, doctor, nurse, toilet,* and *bedpan*. Patients who have problems with word finding should be given time to try to think of the word or to describe or explain the word. If the patient becomes frustrated, the nurse can suggest a few words and let the patient indicate which one is meant. Approaches to improve communication include the use of word cards, pictures, slate boards, audiotapes, and other audiovisual aids.

Dyslexia and dysgraphia are additional communication problems. **Dyslexia** is difficulty in comprehending the written word, while **dysgraphia** refers to the inability to write. Here again, the speech pathologist is best able to determine the extent of the problem and appropriate corrective methods.

Although few aphasic patients regain normal reading, writing, or speaking ability, some recover sufficiently to be considered almost normal. Probably the most important factor in communication rehabilitation (in addition to the extent of cerebral damage) is the attitude of those coming in contact with the patient. The patient responds positively when the nurse conveys the attitude that the patient is an important and communicating individual.

Specific Disorders of the Nervous System

DEVELOPMENTAL DEFECTS

The cranium, the vertebrae, and the nervous system may show evidence of a variety of developmental defects. The cause of many of these defects is often unknown. Many infants born with developmental defects do not live to adulthood. This discussion is therefore limited to the developmental defects the nurse may encounter in caring for adults.

Spina Bifida

Spina bifida, which occurs once in every 1000 births and is therefore not uncommon [26], is a failure of the dorsal arches of one or more vertebrae to develop, usually in the lumbosacral region. Spina bifida is often associated with hydrocephalus and talipes (clubfoot). In **spina bifida occulta** the defect is covered by skin and a patch of hair resembling a tail, or by a subcutaneous lipoma; there is no spinal protrusion in this type. Spina bifida in which there is a protrusion through the defect is known as **spina bifida aperta** and may be one of four types: meningocele, myelocele, meningomyelocele, or syringomyelocele. A **meningocele** is a protrusion of meninges through a bony and dural defect in the skull or vertebral column, usually at the sacral level. **Myelocele** is the absence of a dural covering but full exposure of the spinal cord. **Meningomyelocele** is a protrusion of both the leptomeninges and the spinal cord through a bony and dural defect in the vertebrae. **Syringomyelocele** is a rare defect characterized by distention of the central canal of the spinal cord in the myelocele, causing pressure atrophy.

The degree of motor deficit depends on the level and type of spinal cord lesion. The child with spina bifida or myelomeningocele can develop into a normal adult intellectually but have paralysis (paraplegia) and the loss of bowel and bladder control. Although the lesion in spina bifida occulta requires no treatment, back lesions can be repaired by dissection of the sac and repair of the skin and protruding meninges. Until this is done, the thin sac covering must be inspected regularly for signs of irritation, abrasion, rupture, and leakage. Meningitis may result from rupture or infection of the sac. Some persons with spina bifida are able to ambulate with crutches, whereas others are totally dependent on the wheelchair.

Hydrocephalus

Hydrocephalus is characterized by excessive amounts of cerebrospinal fluid (CSF) within ventricles, resulting in dilatation of the ventricles, subsequent compression of surrounding cerebral tissue, and atrophy. Infants with hydrocephalus have enlarged heads, with widely separated cranial bones and prominent scalp veins. In some infants, the head may be of normal size with bulging fontanelles. The condition is caused by excessive production or inadequate absorption of CSF in the brain. It may also be caused by an obstruction that interferes with the circulation of CSF in the ventricular system. Hydrocephalus may be noncommunicating or communicating. In the noncommunicating type there is ventricular block; in the communicating type, there is no obstruction in the ventricular system and the CSF readily passes out of the ventricles and into the subarachnoid space but is not absorbed.

Cerebrospinal fluid flow may become obstructed at three points: (1) the aqueduct of Sylvius; (2) the roof of the fourth ventricle; and (3) around the midbrain, where it passes through the narrow opening in the tentorium. The first two locations are the ones likely to be involved in infants and children. Although hydrocephalus is sometimes idiopathic, it is often secondary to congenital malformations, infections, skull damage, or intracranial neoplasms, such as choroidal papillomas that produce excessive CSF.

Surgical treatment of hydrocephalus involves removal of obstructive lesions affecting CSF circulation. Ventriculostomy (providing an opening into the lateral ventricle) may be performed to allow the CSF to escape into the subarachnoid space. Another approach is to insert a tube into the lateral ventricle and the other end into the cerebellomedullary cistern to bypass the site of obstruction. Auricular ventriculostomy (or ventriculoatrial shunt) involves the insertion of a silicone catheter from a lateral ventricle to the right atrium of the heart via the external jugular vein. A valve is included in the system to permit only a one-way flow. The last procedure promotes normal ventricular pressure by channeling excess CSF into the general circulation, from which it can be excreted. Yet another shunting procedure is the ventriculoperitoneal route.

Compensatory hydrocephalus (adult hydrocephalus) is not associated with a rise in CSF pressure but is secondary to general or local atrophy of the brain. It occurs in senile dementia, diffuse atherosclerosis, or localized brain atrophy due to trauma.

Down's Syndrome

Another relatively common developmental defect, Down's syndrome (mongolism), is a gross congenital defect involving mental retardation and a characteristic physical appearance and is thought to develop during the eighth week of gestation. Although many children with Down's syndrome used to die at early ages because of associated anomalies and susceptibility to infection, more adults with Down's syndrome are now being encountered by the nurse. Most persons with Down's syndrome have 47 chromosomes in their body cells due to an additional short, acrocentric chromosome 21. A smaller proportion have 46 chromosomes, with translocation of a small autosome on chromosome 15.

As attitudes toward the mentally retarded have changed somewhat over the years, more mongoloid children (and other retarded persons) are being kept at home rather than being institutionalized, so that the nurse in the general hospital often cares for the adult retarded person. The degree of retardation varies, and an accurate assessment of mental status is essential to planning care that is meaningful and anxiety-free for these patients. If retardation is severe and the person unmanageable in the stressful hospital atmosphere, the presence of a family member is often necessary to assist with the care. Assumptions should not be made about the abilities of a retarded person unless they have been verified with family members or by testing the person in specific situations. It is as inappropriate to do too much for a retarded person on the assumption that he or she is totally incapable of performing as it is to make excessive demands that the retarded person cannot fulfill.

Communicating with the adult retarded person may be difficult; it is wise to obtain specific information from the family as to the best ways to communicate and the specific words to use. The professional nurse often finds that nonprofessional personnel need orientation to the care of retarded persons.

Often, they do not recognize that there are varying degrees of retardation. The nurse must ensure that care is adapted to the abilities and needs of the individual retarded patient.

Cerebral Palsy

Cerebral palsy is a neurologic disorder resulting from lesions that develop during embryonic or fetal life or early infancy, primarily in the pyramidal tracts but also in the extrapyramidal tracts. It is the most common single cause of crippling in children. Symptoms, which vary from patient to patient, result from the loss or impairment of control over voluntary muscles. The three most common types of cerebral palsy are those characterized by spasticity, athetosis, or ataxia. Spasticity of one or more extremities due to involvement of the pyramidal tract is more common than athetoid movements, which reflect extrapyramidal tract involvement. Ataxic gaits are associated with cerebellar damage. Contrary to popular opinion, all persons with cerebral palsy are not mentally retarded; severe mental retardation occurs in about 30 percent [26]. Involvement of the motor cortex may result in convulsions, and speech defects, visual disorders, and hearing difficulties are often present. Emotional and social problems may result from motor, sensory, and intellectual impairment.

Cerebral palsy may be a developmental defect due to lesions that are hereditary, or it may result from systemic causes such as anoxia neonatorum, prematurity, erythroblastosis fetalis, encephalitis, or local causes such as mechanical birth injuries. Although some infants with cerebral palsy die at an early age, others live to adulthood. The amount of independence attained depends on the severity of the defects and the general health status of the individual patient, as well as on the patient's motivation, education, and family support. The drug dimethothiazine is being used experimentally in the management of spasticity. The goal of long-term care is to provide physical therapy and education to attain and maintain as much independence as is realistic in terms of the individual patient's abilities.

Infections of the Nervous System

Infections of the brain and spinal cord are most often viral in origin whereas infections in the meninges are most often caused by pyogenic organisms, tuberculosis bacilli, and fungi. The most frequently encountered infectious processes are meningitis, encephalitis, and brain abscess. Common to all of these infectious processes is the treatment required: antibiotic therapy for the specific causative organism, control of fever and increased intracranial pressure, and provision of symptomatic care, including fluid and electrolyte balance and control of seizures.

MENINGITIS

Meningitis is the inflammation of the meninges. The most common type is **leptomeningitis,** which is the infection of the pia mater and the arachnoid with accumulation of the exudate in the subarachnoid space. **Pachymeningitis** is the inflammation of the dura mater. Meningitis occurs following bacteremia from infectious agents traveling via the bloodstream and choroid plexus, or by direct invasion from contiguous tissues such as in acute otitis media, osteomyelitis, mastoiditis, or orbital cellulitis. Meningitis may also develop from accidental contamination during administration of anesthesia, lumbar puncture, or surgical procedures involving the central nervous system.

Clinical Symptoms

Meningitis is characterized by a classic triad of symptoms: nuchal rigidity, headache, and vomiting. Other associated symptoms are fever, photophobia, irritability, confusion, lethargy, changes in personality and behavior, and convulsions. The presence of Brudzinski's sign (flexion of both thighs and legs when the head has been subjected to passive flexion) and Kernig's sign (resistance or pain when the patient's thigh is flexed at the hip in an effort to completely extend the leg at the knee) is characteristic of meningeal irritation. A history of a recent upper respiratory tract infection is usually reported. Any type of motion becomes painful; irritability increases, and the patient may alternate from periods of delirium to drowsiness.

The onset of symptoms varies according to the type of causative organism. Clinical symptoms develop in most patients within 48 hours of onset. Meningococcal meningitis, however, may be very rapid in its onset, with death occurring within 8 to 12 hours. The onset of *Hemophilus influenzae* meningitis may be insidious, with the patient's condition becoming worse over a period of 4 to 5 days before the disease is even recognized. Meningococcal disease often begins with a petechial rash, which may proceed into generalized purpura and severe subcutaneous bleeding.

Diagnosis

The diagnosis is confirmed by analysis of the CSF. A specimen of CSF is obtained for smear and culture, chemical analysis, and cytologic examination. The CSF in meningitis is cloudy and under increased pressure and demonstrates an elevated cell count. The protein level is usually elevated in bacterial, tubercular, and fungal meningitis [16b]. The three most common causative organisms are the meningococcus, pneumococcus, and *H. influenzae*. The causative organisms must be identified promptly, so that appropriate antibiotic therapy can be initiated; inadequately treated meningitis is associated with a high mortality. In most cases, penicillin is administered as soon as the CSF specimen is obtained, because it is effective against the most common types of meningitis.

Neisseria is the causative organism in meningococcal meningitis and is introduced into the bloodstream via the nasopharynx. It occurs predominantly in children and young adults. Fulminating infections may occur, with peripheral vascular collapse, shock, and death. Hyperemia is usually present in the meninges, and serous or purulent exudate collects in the subarachnoid space.

Tubercular meningitis is usually associated with generalized miliary tuberculosis, especially in infants and small children. Treatment involves the use of two or three of the antituberculosis drugs, usually for at least a year.

Viral meningitis is usually a brief illness and requires no specific therapy. Classic symptoms of meningitis are present, but serious alteration in the sensorium is not a usual finding.

Treatment and Nursing Care

Treatment of patients with meningitis requires prompt and specific antibiotic therapy (which may be administered intrathecally as well as parenterally), bed rest, supportive therapy, and fluid and electrolyte replacement. Accurate intake and output records are mandatory; fluid replacement must be supervised closely to prevent rapid infusion, with the hazard of cerebral edema. Ice bags to the head and analgesics for pain are indicated; measures to control fever are important. Isolation precautions are instituted in meningococcal meningitis. Persons who have intimate respiratory contact (such as in mouth-to-mouth resuscitation) may require antimicrobial prophylactic therapy. The nurse should anticipate the onset of seizures and be prepared to observe and protect the patient in the event one occurs.

The nurse should observe the patient for complications associated with meningitis, such as coma, increased intracranial pressure with brainstem compression, brain abscess, disseminated intravascular coagulation, and shock. Death or permanent neurologic disabilities may result from meningitis. Cranial nerve damage, especially deafness, often occurs.

ENCEPHALITIS

Encephalitis, or inflammation of the brain, is usually caused by a viral infection but occasionally it is of bacterial origin. Encephalitis lethargica (sleeping sickness) is thought to be caused by a filterable virus. Although it occurred in epidemics in the early 1900s, it occurs only sporadically today.

Encephalitis is characterized by marked congestion of the meninges and brain tissue, particularly affecting the brainstem. The flow of the fourth ventricle characteristically shows evidence of small hemorrhages. The onset is usually abrupt, with fever, headache, and nuchal rigidity as the predominant symptoms, associated with mental deterioration. The patient may be somnolent (as a result of hypothalamic lesions) or hyperkinetic (indicating involvement of the basal ganglia) [26]. Damage to the substantia nigra results in postencephalitic parkinson syndrome. Findings in the CSF include an elevated white cell count, predominantly polymorphonuclear leukocytes in the early stage and lymphocytes in later stages, a normal glucose level, and a normal or slightly elevated protein level.

St. Louis encephalitis is caused by a filterable virus and is transmitted by mosquitoes that are prevalent in swampy areas, particularly in stagnant pools. The symptoms include high fever, headache, vertigo, signs of meningeal irritation, ataxia, tremors, and often lethargy and spastic paralysis. This type of encephalitis occurs periodically in small epidemics.

Treatment of encephalitis is supportive and symptomatic. Isolation during the acute infectious stage is dependent on the specific type of encephalitis. If respiratory difficulties occur, tracheostomy or assisted mechanical ventilation is necessary. Convalescence is usually prolonged. Residual disability may be present, requiring educational programs and physical therapy over a long period.

BRAIN ABSCESS

A brain abscess is a collection of purulent exudate within the brain. Usually, it results from one of three sources: (1) from direct extension from infections within the cranial cavity, particularly the nasal sinuses and mastoids, from sinus infections, or from osteomyelitis of the skull; (2) from infections secondary to skull fracture; (3) from infections outside the cranial cavity, particularly the lungs in adults. The location of the brain abscess may indicate the underlying source of the infection; abscesses in the frontal lobe, for example, are associated with infections of the frontal and ethmoidal sinuses [21].

Local clinical manifestations and local neurologic defects depend on the site and size of the abscess; usually, generalized symptoms such as fever and chills are also present.

Brain abscess is suspected when signs and symptoms of increased intracranial pressure are associated with chronic ear infections, sinus infections, or suppurative lung disease [21]. Diagnostic procedures include EEG, arteriography, and brain scans to differentiate brain abscess from a brain tumor or encephalitis. The causative organisms most often involved in brain abscess formation are *Staphylococcus aureus,* streptococci of the viridans group, and pneumococci.

Treatment consists in determining the source of infection, correcting the underlying disease, and treating the abscess with antibiotic therapy. In addition, drainage or excision of the abscess is indicated. If the abscess is not drained, it may rupture into the subarachnoid space or ventricular system, causing a purulent bacterial meningitis, which is often fatal. Aspiration and excision of the abscess may be done through a burr hole made over the site of the abscess. A cannula is inserted into the cavity for aspiration of the pus, and antibiotics are often instilled into the abscess cavity. Even when the abscess is treated with antibiotics and drained, neurologic deficits may be permanent.

Intraspinal abscesses may also occur and cause back pain and flaccid paralysis of the extremities, with bowel and bladder disabilities.

MYELITIS

Myelitis, a general term for inflammation of the spinal cord, may be diffuse and may include inflammation of the brain **(encephalomyelitis),** or it may be selective in its involvement, affecting specific structures of the spinal cord and brainstem **(anterior poliomyelitis)**. Myelitis may be a primary infectious process or a complication of an acute infectious disease such as measles or influenza. In **transverse myelitis,** there is sensory and motor involvement across the spinal cord at a specific level. Treatment of myelitis is supportive and symptomatic and includes bed rest and prevention of complications. Residual disabilities are common. The extent and severity of the lesion and the prevention of complications are the major factors affecting prognosis.

Poliomyelitis, or infantile paralysis, is an acute infectious disease that affects the motor neurons of the spinal cord and brainstem and may affect the motor cortex, but it primarily involves the anterior horns of the lumbar segments of the spinal cord. The three types of poliomyelitis are bulbar, involving the medulla oblongata and pons; encephalitic, in which there is diffuse brain involvement; and spinal (anterior poliomyelitis). The causative organism, poliovirus, which is a neurotropic filterable enterovirus, can be recovered from the pharynx of a patient or carrier, from feces of an acutely ill or convalescent patient, and from the intestinal wall and mesenteric lymph nodes at autopsy [26]. The most communicable period is during the latter part of the 7- to 14-day incubation period.

Poliomyelitis has occurred in endemic and epidemic patterns in the past, affecting both children and adults. There has been a sharp decline in its incidence since 1955, when widespread use of the poliovirus vaccine was initiated. Two types of vaccine are available. The Salk vaccine is an intramuscular injection of a solution of killed viruses, while the Sabin vaccine is an oral preparation of attenuated living viruses. There is concern, currently, that the public has become nonchalant about poliomyelitis and that laxity in using the available immunizations may result in an increased incidence of poliomyelitis.

A prodromal period of 1 to 3 days with fever, headache, irritability, sore throat, stiff neck, nausea, and vomiting is typical of acute poliomyelitis. The initial symptoms, which closely resemble those of a common cold, are followed by a paralytic stage, characterized by rapidly developing flaccid paralysis. Neurologic symptoms vary according to the level of involvement and degree of damage to the motor neurons. Weakness of the lower abdominal and back muscles may also be present. Paralysis is often unilateral, but this depends on the particular motor neurons that are affected. Since bulbar poliomyelitis involves the brainstem and various cranial nerve nuclei and thus may interfere with circulatory and respiratory mechanisms, it is more often fatal than are the other types. Mechanical respiratory support is usually necessary in bulbar poliomyelitis. If neurons are irreversibly damaged, permanent disability results. Affected muscles atrophy, resulting in restricted growth of the involved extremity.

The care of patients with poliomyelitis is primarily symptomatic and directed toward relief of pain, prevention of deformities, and maintenance of function. Pain due to muscle spasms is often intense; hot moist packs or dry heat are used to relieve it. Isolation precautions with particular attention to oral and nasal secretions and intestinal excreta are necessary in the early stage. Exercises with passive range of motion are initiated as soon as the acute pain and muscle tenderness subside; physical therapy is a major aspect of the rehabilitation program. Residual disability, such as drop foot, may require surgical intervention. Bracing is often required to provide support for ambulation, and crutches may be necessary for persons with extensive residual disability.

NEURITIS

Infections of the nerves and nerve roots (radiculitis) do not occur frequently. However, polyneuritis and herpes zoster are among the more common ones the nurse is likely to encounter.

The **Guillain-Barré syndrome,** also known as acute idiopathic polyneuritis, is a relatively rare disease. Although the specific cause is unknown, the disease may occur within 2 weeks after a febrile illness. It is thought to be of viral origin or the result of an immunologic disturbance.

Guillain-Barré syndrome is characterized by the rapid development of symmetrical weakness or flaccid paralysis, particularly in the lower extremities but sometimes spreading to the upper extremities and face. Paresthesia and other sensory disorders are also characteristic. The cranial nerves, particularly the seventh, are often involved. A lumbar puncture and CSF analysis frequently show normal cell counts, but protein is elevated. This finding is referred to as albuminocytologic dissociation. The greatest threat associated with the Guillain-Barré syndrome is respiratory failure, due to weakness or paralysis of the intercostal muscles and diaphragm. Occasionally, respiratory failure in the early stages has resulted in death. Close observation of the patient's respiratory status and alertness to signs of cerebral hypoxia are mandatory. Assisted mechanical ventilation and oxygen therapy are often necessary, and a tracheostomy may be indicated. Suctioning to maintain a patent airway is a major nursing responsibility.

Nursing measures are focused on maintaining respiratory function, ensuring proper body alignment, and maintaining good nutrition and fluid and electrolyte balance. If dysphagia is present, nasogastric feedings are given. Passive range of motion exercises are necessary to prevent postural deformities, and position changes at regular intervals are of paramount importance in the prevention of pneumonia, thromboembolic phenomena, and decubiti formation. The nurse should observe for urine retention, which often occurs as a result of loss of bladder tone and weakness of the abdominal muscles. Intestinal ileus may develop in patients with the Guillain-Barré syndrome; constipation and fecal impaction should be prevented.

The rapid onset of symptoms, the critical nature of the syndrome, and the patient's total dependence in the acute stage on those caring for him are anxiety-provoking for patient and family. Both require clear explanations of the nature of the disease and the assurance that the patient will receive appropriate care during the critical state. The usually transient nature of the disease and the high probability of complete recovery without residual neurologic deficit are emphasized. Improvement usually begins before the third week, and complete functional recovery generally occurs within six months. Corticosteroids have been used to hasten recovery in some patients.

Herpes zoster, or shingles, is a viral disease characterized by clusters of blister-like lesions on the skin or mucous membranes in a pattern that follows the course of either a cranial or peripheral sensory nerve. Typically, the skin lesions do not cross the midline of the body but are unilateral like the peripheral nerve that is involved. The vesicles usually crust and dry up within a few days, but the pain remains longer. The causative organism is the chickenpox (varicella) virus. Fatigue, stress, and malnutrition appear to be predisposing factors. A neuritis of the sensory neurons occurs, primarily affecting the sensory neurons of the dorsal root ganglia of the spinal nerves and the ganglia of the sensory portions of the cranial nerves. Hypersensitivity, malaise, fever, and pain are characteristic of the disease.

There is no special treatment, but care is directed primarily toward the relief of pain and prevention of secondary infection of the vesicles. Scratching of the lesions is to be avoided. Various medications are used on the lesions, including calamine lotion, wet dressings, topical ether, and corticosteroids. Rest and nutritious meals are encouraged. The disease tends to recur in susceptible persons. Postherpetic neuralgia may persist for several years and may require surgical division of the involved posterior root.

NEUROSYPHILIS

Prevention and control of syphilis as a communicable disease has been effective to some degree, and neurosyphilis is relatively uncommon, although it may develop if treatment of early syphilis has been inadequate. The clinical picture varies, depending on the type and extent of the lesions. Acute neurosyphilis has symptoms like those found in acute meningitis, such as nuchal rigidity and headache. In the chronic form, hemiplegia may be present. Cranial nerve involvement may occur, such as optic neuritis and infection of the oculomotor, trochlear, and abducens nerves.

Diagnostic measures include the complement-fixation and agglutination tests, which are typically strongly positive. Lumbar puncture and CSF analysis usually show elevations in the colloidal gold curve and protein level, and pleocytosis.

General paresis, or dementia paralytica, is a type of neurosyphilis that primarily involves the cerebrum. It usually occurs as a late manifestation, 10 to 15 years after the initial infection. In this condition, the brain is atrophic; other pathologic changes include a thickened pia mater, dilated ventricles, and severe degenerative changes of the cerebral cortex. These pathologic changes result in varied mental symptoms, ranging from slight memory loss to megalomania and marked euphoria [26]. Tremors and generalized muscle weakness are common findings.

Tabes dorsalis is a type of neurosyphilis principally involving the spinal cord, with degeneration of the dorsal roots and posterior tract. Like general paresis, it is a late manifestation of syphilis, occurring 10 to 15 years after the primary infection. The patient typically complains of having the feeling of walking on a rug, with varied sensations of the legs that are the result of irritation of posterior nerve roots. Loss of pain, position, and vibration sensations occur later. Cranial nerve involvement may result in blindness, ptosis, diplopia, and facial paresthesia.

The use of procaine penicillin is the principle method of treatment, but it does not reverse the existing neurologic deficits. Care is focused on protecting the patient from injury caused by unsteady gaits, poor balance, irrational behavior, and lack of judgment. Institutionalization may be necessary for long-term care when the condition is incapacitating.

TETANUS

Tetanus, or lockjaw, is caused by invasion of the central nervous system by the anaerobic bacterium *Clostridium tetani*. It may occur as a complication in either large or small wounds. The *C. tetani* organism, which is commonly found in soil and manure, enters the body through open wounds and releases a virulent substance containing tetanospasmin, a neurotoxin, and tetanolysin, a homolytic toxin. These substances produce hemorrhage, edema, and inflammatory changes in the brain, particularly the brainstem, and spinal cord. The disease is characterized by hypertonicity of the skeletal muscles and repeated attacks of intense tonic spasms. The jaws are initially involved; hypertonicity of the muscles causes difficulty in opening the mouth and chewing. Headache, back pain, leg stiffness, fever, and apathy are common symptoms. As spasms increasingly affect the back muscles, the head becomes retracted, producing the opisthotonos position. Signs of tetanus include a typical facial appearance characterized by tense and immobile muscles and a fixed smile called risus sardonicus.

Tetanus can be prevented by routine immunizations and administration of a booster injection after injuries. Meticulous cleaning and surgical debridement of wounds and the administration of antibiotics in the presence of contaminated wounds are other preventive measures.

Specific treatment depends on whether the patient has previously been actively immunized with tetanus toxoid, and also on the extent and type of wound. Only a booster injection of tetanus toxoid is required at the time of injury if the patient has been previously immunized, unless he has received a booster or has completed an initial immunization series within the past 5 years [6]. Homologous (human) tetanus immune globulin (Hypertet) by intramuscular injection is the treatment of choice for passive protection against tetanus, when indicated. Tetanus antitoxin is now considered an obsolete treatment in the management of tetanus, because the antitoxin frequently has caused allergic reactions and delayed serum sickness.

Any kind of stimulus may trigger spasms; therefore a quiet semidark room is essential to minimize external stimuli. Nursing care must be given carefully, with gentle and smooth movements, in order to prevent spasms. The patient should not be moved unnecessarily. Sedatives, anticonvulsant therapy, and antispasmodic agents are usual medications; penicillin is also usually required. Fluid and electrolyte management is of paramount importance; nasogastric feedings are used only after spasms have been controlled, since aspiration of the feeding may occur during a spasm that dislodges the nasogastric tube.

Respiratory complications, nephritis, and pneumonia frequently occur, and the disease often results in a fatal outcome. In other patients the paroxysmal muscle spasms gradually decrease after 7 to 10 days, and normal muscle tone may return within several months.

RABIES

Rabies, also known as hydrophobia, is a disease caused by the transmission of a filterable neurotropic virus transmitted to man by the saliva of a rabid animal. Although the disease is usually associated with bites by an infected animal (such as dogs, cats, skunks, foxes, and bats), skin contact with rabid saliva is also a possible cause [6]. Rabies is almost always fatal.

Laboratory diagnosis is made by testing the serum of the patient to detect neutralizing antibodies to rabies. Local treatment of the bite includes cleaning, irrigation with betadine solution or hydrogen peroxide, and debridement, if necessary. Strong antiseptic solutions are contraindicated because they destroy vital structures within the wound [6]. Antibiotics and tetanus immune globulin or toxoid are administered.

All animal bites should be reported to a hospital, physician, or local Board of Health. The domesticated animal that bites a person is isolated, confined, and observed for 10 days. If abnormal symptoms develop in the animal, it is sacrificed and the brain is examined for distinguishing lesions. A classic finding in rabies is the appearance of Negri bodies, which are viral inclusion bodies in the cytoplasm of cerebral ganglion cells.

The Center for Disease Control recommends both active and passive immunization for persons exposed to rabies. Active immunization is provided via 21 daily doses (plus a booster dose on the 31st and 41st days) of 1 ml of 10% tissue emulsion duck embryo vaccine (DEV). The vaccine is given subcutaneously by injections in the abdomen, lower back, and lateral thighs, rotating the sites. Besides causing pain, injections of rabies vaccine may cause encephalitis; the injections should be discontinued if any neurologic signs appear. Passive immunization for immediate protection is provided via a single dose of human rabies immunoglobulin (HRIG) or antirabies serum of equine origin.

There may be a delay in the onset of symptoms after the incriminating bite or contact has occurred. Initial symptoms are irritability, malaise, headache, fever, anorexia, insomnia, restlessness, and local sensory changes at the wound site. Vomiting, dysphagia, convulsions, personality changes, choking due to pharyngeal spasms, and hypotension are later symptoms.

The major factor in preventing human rabies is the maintenance of immunity in pets via the enforcement of laws pertaining to rabies vaccination of domestic animals. People should also be advised to avoid handling sick or wild animals, which might be affected by rabies.

BOTULISM

Botulism is a relatively rare, but often fatal, toxic disease, caused by the *Clostridium botulinum* organism. The spores of this organism germinate in an airtight, low acid environment and produce a toxin called *botulin*. Because the bacillus is heat resistant, it is found in improperly processed food that is stored in jars or cans.

Symptoms appear 12 to 36 hours after ingestion of the contaminated food. Nausea, vomiting, sore throat, voice changes, dysarthyria, dysphagia, a decreased gag reflex, and weakness of the facial, lingual, and arm muscles are the presenting symptoms. Weakness, dizziness, headache, and paralysis are other symptoms associated with the disease. Death is often due to respiratory failure.

The botulin toxin may be detected in a specimen of serum. Trivalent (ABE) botulin antitoxin is used to combat the toxin. Immediate treatment is stomach lavage and supportive ventilation. The major method of controlling botulism, however, is through public education about the proper processing of home-canned foods. It is important that people understand the need for boiling food to specific temperatures before use in order to destroy spores. Storage of canned food is most appropriate in a cool, dark environment. People should also be cautioned not to use food in cans that are swollen or bent and not to eat canned foods that look or smell different than usual. Suspect cans or foods should be reported to the local health department. If it is a commercial product, the can and its number should be given, so that other cans with the same number can be examined for the presence of the organism.

CRANIOCEREBRAL INJURIES

The brain is normally protected from trauma by the cushion of the cerebrospinal fluid, the meningeal covering, and the rigid, bony skull. However, the high incidence of automobile and motorcycle accidents and violent assaults has made head injuries the second most common cause of major neurologic deficits after stroke. Head injuries also result from accidents at work, at play, and in athletic activities. Head injury is the major cause of death in persons between the ages of 1 and 44 and is the cause of death in two-thirds of all fatal accidents. Initial irreversible cerebral and brainstem damage from cerebral contusion or laceration, secondary compression effects on the brainstem and cerebrum by expanding intracranial lesions, and cerebral edema are the major factors responsible for the mortality and morbidity associated with head injuries.

Head injuries may result in lacerations of the scalp, skull fracture, penetration of the skull, or injury to the brain itself. Injuries are classified as **closed** if the skull remains intact without obvious external damage and **open** if the wound is confined to the scalp and skull or penetrates the dura and brain tissue. Closed head injuries result from sudden acceleration or deceleration of the head; open injuries result from sharp instruments or projectiles [25].

Scalp Lacerations

Because of the vascularity of the scalp, scalp lacerations may cause significant blood loss, with resultant hypovolemia. If bleeding is excessive, a sterile dressing with direct compression of the wound edges is used to control it. Or pressure can be applied over the superior temporal artery in front of the ear until severed vessels can be ligated. The wound is cleaned thoroughly after bleeding is controlled and it is debrided before suturing. Tetanus toxoid immunizations and antibiotics are administered to protect against infection.

Skull Fractures

A skull fracture is suspected when an area of the scalp is swollen, tender, and ecchymotic; the fracture is confirmed by a series of skull x-ray films. Skull fractures may be linear, comminuted, depressed, or compound. A **linear fracture** is a simple break in the continuity of the bone with no change in its contour. In a **comminuted fracture,** multiple fragments from multiple linear fractures are present in the skull. A **depressed fracture** is the displacement of comminuted fragments; displacement of the fragments inward compresses the meninges and brain. A **compound fracture** is any of these types combined with an external opening through the scalp, paranasal sinuses, or eardrum. A compound depressed skull fracture requires debridement of the scalp laceration, elevation of the skull fragments, and repair of the dural laceration [34]. Basal fractures (fractures at the base of the skull) are particularly hazardous because they open into paranasal sinuses or the middle ear, often leading to infection.

It is important for the nurse to remember that the presence or absence of a skull fracture does not indicate the seriousness of the patient's condition. Fractures may occur with little or no brain injury, while serious and lethal brain damage may occur without a fracture. Any patient with a skull fracture, however, should be observed for abnormal neurologic signs because of the danger of subsequent intracranial hemorrhage. If a patient is discharged from an emergency room after a head injury, the nurse should instruct the family to contact the physician if the patient is hard to arouse or complains of persistent headache, vomiting, and weakness. While a linear fracture requires no special treatment, one that crosses a meningeal artery is likely to cause serious intracranial hemorrhages [17a].

Cerebral Injuries

Cerebral injuries range from cerebral concussion, which is generally considered a minor injury,to epidural and subdural hematomas, which are life-threatening.

Concussion A cerebral concussion is characterized by the absence of abnormal neurologic signs except for a momentary loss of consciousness or transient loss of neurologic function, such as a brief focal neurologic deficit with disturbances in vision or equilibrium. Alterations in nerve cells and fibers occur due to jarring of the brain against the skull but do not cause significant changes.

There is a complete recovery of all neurologic function. Some patients who have suffered a cerebral concussion may later complain of recurrent headaches, dizziness, vertigo, anxiety, and fatigue. These symptoms are termed the **postconcussion syndrome,** which is considered to be a psychoneurotic disorder [39].

Cerebral contusion Cerebral contusion results in bruising or hemorrhage of the brain surface; consciousness is generally not lost with cerebral contusions, but other signs of neurologic dysfunction persist for more than 12 hours. These signs may be weakness of the extremities, sensory or speech disturbances, or visual changes. When cerebral contusion is suspected, the patient is hospitalized and observed for progression of the neurologic deficits. There is a danger of secondary hemorrhage or cerebral edema developing at the site of contusion. Surgical decompression via lobectomy or subtemporal craniectomy may be indicated in a cerebral contusion that threatens the life of the patient [34].

Hematomas Small hemorrhages and brain congestion in addition to alterations in the nerve cells and fibers may occur with contusion (bruising) of the brain, resulting in a longer period of unconsciousness than in concussion and often associated with abnormal neurologic signs and permanent tissue damage and scarring. Severe head injuries are generally characterized by prolonged unconsciousness and various abnormal neurologic signs due to compression of the brain, caused by a depressed fracture, edema, and hemorrhage. Hemorrhage may be subdural, epidural, subarachnoid, or intracerebral.

A subdural hematoma is caused by venous bleeding beneath the dura and may be classified as acute, subacute, or chronic, depending on the rapidity and volume of bleeding and the severity of the accompanying symptoms. Patients with acute or subacute subdural hematoma become unconscious almost immediately after the head injury [39]. The classic picture of chronic subdural hematoma is a lucid period immediately after the head injury, followed by a gradual loss of consciousness over a period of several weeks or months. Headache and confusion are common findings in chronic subdural hematoma.

Extradural (epidural) hematoma is usually

due to arterial hemorrhage. The most frequent location of epidural hematoma is the parietotemporal region, and it is associated with a tear in the middle meningeal artery. In epidural hematoma there is a momentary loss of consciousness, which is followed by an initial lucid interval, but within minutes to hours, there are increasing signs of intracranial compression and focal neurologic signs of a progressively deteriorating state. The expanding hematoma causes unconsciousness, dilatation and fixation of the ipsilateral pupil, contralateral hemiparesis or hemiplegia, and increased deep tendon reflexes, including the Babinski reflex. Prompt surgical aspiration and removal of the clot is indicated.

Emergency Care of Patients with Cerebral Injury
Treatment of patients with lesions such as intracranial hematomas, contusions, and cerebral edema associated with injury is directed toward reducing the effects of compression of these lesions on brain tissue and preventing interference with adequate cerebral oxygenation. Therefore, when a person's head is injured in an accident, provision of a patent airway and control of hemorrhage are priority emergency measures. An adequate oxygen level must be maintained to prevent affected brain cells from being further compromised by hypoxia. If hypovolemic shock is present, sites of bleeding other than intracranial lesions should be considered; except for excessive blood loss from scalp wounds, hypovolemic shock in the adult with head trauma is not likely to be caused by intracranial bleeding [39].

Evaluation of vital signs and neurologic signs, particularly the level of consciousness, is a major responsibility in case of head injury. Any patient with a head injury that causes loss of consciousness or other neurologic signs should be treated as having a potential cervical spinal cord injury as well and should be moved in a manner that will prevent further cord damage.

Assessment of Cerebral Injury
History A description of the type of accident, the direction and force of any blow that was received, and the site of injury, such as the forehead, occiput, or temporal regions, should be obtained even when the findings of the initial neurologic examination are negative. This information is necessary to determine the potential hazards of the injury. Knowledge of the velocity of the object causing the injury is also important. In assessment of the traumatized patient, information on the level of consciousness since the injury occurred should be obtained. If the patient lost consciousness, the time this occurred and the duration of unconsciousness should be noted. The patient or the person who observed the accident should be asked if there was any paralysis, seizure, bleeding, or flow of clear fluid from the nose or ears, vomiting, headache, or confusion during the interval before the patient was seen by professional staff. It is also important to determine whether or not the patient had been using drugs or alcohol prior to the accident. These agents affect the neurologic findings and also may cause respiratory depression or cerebral confusion.

Neurologic examination A neurologic examination is done to assess the patient's present neurologic status, thus providing baseline data that will enable detection of even slight subsequent changes. The level of consciousness, comprehension, and orientation is described carefully, so that alterations in consciousness can be readily recognized. Pupillary size and reaction, headache, recurrent vomiting, and focal neurologic signs such as hemiparesis, hemiplegia, and the presence of the Babinski reflex are also noted. The eyes should be examined for the presence of contact lenses, which should be removed to prevent corneal damage (see Chap. 11). The ears and nose should be examined for CSF rhinorrhea or otorrhea (CSF flowing from the nose or ears). The nature of the fluid may be readily determined by testing for glucose content, which is lower in nasal discharge than in CSF. Often, the patient will complain of a sweet-tasting liquid trickling down the oropharynx [39].

Diagnosis After hemorrhage is controlled, cardiovascular and respiratory problems are corrected via endotracheal intubation, suctioning, and assisted ventilation, and the neurologic examination is completed, the nature and extent of neurologic involvement are determined. Diagnostic procedures may include skull roentgenograms, cerebral angiograms, brain scans, electroencephalograms, echoencephalograms, and computerized transverse axial tomograms, but the selection of tests to be used depends on the clinical status of the patient. Skull roentgenograms are indicated to detect skull fractures, foreign bodies, and shifts in the pineal body and other midline structures. Cerebral angiography is done to determine the presence of supratentorial, extracerebral, and intracerebral hematomas, cerebral contusion, or cerebral edema. Although brain scans are controversial in acute head injuries because of their lack of specificity, they are particularly useful in determining the extent of chronic subdural hematomas. As stated previously, lumbar puncture and pneumoencephalography are not used routinely in patients with acute head injuries because of the danger of causing transtentorial herniation and further deterioration. For the patient in a critical condition, burr holes are usually made in the skull to permit immediate exploration.

Treatment of Cerebral Injury

Reduction of intracranial pressure Patients whose condition necessitates reduction of cerebral edema are given mannitol and dexamethasone (Decadron) intravenously to reduce increased intracranial pressure. The effect of these osmotic dehydrating agents is monitored by measurement of urine output and improvement in neurologic signs. Mannitol, however, is generally used only temporarily, while the patient is prepared for definitive surgery. A Scott cannula is usually inserted through a burr hole into a lateral ventricle to measure intracranial pressure [28].

Surgical treatment Immediate surgical intervention to prevent intracranial compression is indicated for depressed skull fractures, intracranial hemorrhages, and subdural and epidural hematomas. Hematomas may be removed through burr holes or a craniotomy flap. In lieu of multiple burr holes, a pneumatic craniotomy technique may be used to permit removal of an entire clot. Penrose drains or silicone rubber drains connected to a sterile reservoir are often placed in the subdural space to remove residual subdural fluid.

Nursing Care in Cerebral Injury

Nursing care of the patient with a head injury requires measures to maintain adequate respiratory and cardiovascular function and to prevent complications. The care of the patient is directed toward supporting cerebral metabolism and preventing cerebral hypoxia, which is the primary cause of brain damage. Cerebral edema and increased intracranial pressure increase hypoxia and impair the microcirculation of the brain. Arterial gases should be monitored for oxygen, carbon dioxide, and pH levels, so that hypoxemia will be recognized and prompt treatment provided. The nurse should observe for hyperventilation, hypoventilation, and signs of impaired cellular respiration [25]. Recent advances in the diagnosis and treatment of neurosurgical conditions are measurements of cerebral blood flow, the metabolic rate of oxygen in the brain, cerebral perfusion pressure, intracranial pressure, and CSF acid-base balance. These measures are used to determine pathophysiologic and metabolic alterations in the brain and to evaluate the patient's response to various kinds of therapy.

Regular and thorough neurologic assessment is essential to prevent complications and to detect signs of an expanding intracranial mass. Changes in the level of consciousness are the major index of the patient's neurologic status. The patient should be aroused every hour to determine the level of consciousness, and the nurse should immediately report any decrease. Any increase in focal or generalized neurologic deficit should also be reported at once. Increased difficulty in arousing the patient is an important sign to report to the physician. It is important for the nurse to remember that pupillary dilatation, bradycardia, systemic arterial hypertension, and respiratory depression are late signs associated with significant irreversible neuronal damage [39].

The nurse should assess the vital signs, pupillary reactions, the size and equality of the pupils, and motor function, the latter by evaluation of motor strength of the extremities. Pupillary irregularity and hemiparesis on the same side indicate a shift of the brain and brainstem across the midline by an expanding lesion. In this situation, the cerebral peduncle on the contralateral side becomes compressed against the tentorium cerebelli and causes ipsilateral hemiparesis [34]; the side of a fixed and dilated pupil is usually considered the side of the expanding lesion [39]. The onset of headache, convulsions, or unusual behavior, and signs of cranial nerve impairment are important to report to the neurosurgeon promptly.

The nurse should observe for any drainage (and note the amount and characteristics) from the nose or ear. A dry sterile cotton placed loosely into the ear, or a sterile gauze over the ear, is used to manage the ear drainage. The external ear should not be cleaned or irrigated because of the danger of introducing bacteria. The patient with rhinorrhea should be allowed to wipe drainage from the nose but be warned not to blow the nose. Attention is also necessary to the patient's safety and to temperature control, maintenance of bladder and bowel function, and prevention of skin breakdown. Opiates are contraindicated in the first 24 to 36 hours after a head injury because they cause respiratory depression and mask important neurologic signs by altering pupillary reactions.

The care of the comatose patient and the patient who has convulsions has been discussed previously. The care of the patient requiring cranial surgery is described in the last section of this chapter.

The nurse should be prepared to maintain accurate intake and output records of the patient to assist in accurate fluid and electrolyte replacement. Generally, fluids are restricted to approximately 1,500 ml in a 24-hour period to decrease or control cerebral edema. Oral fluids are not given to the patient after a head injury in the event that diagnostic procedures or surgical intervention are necessary; intravenous infusions or nasogastric feedings are used.

As previously mentioned, either osmotic diuretics such as mannitol are given intravenously as a temporary measure to reduce cerebral edema, or corticosteroids such as dexamethasone are given. Corticosteroids and mannitol may both be utilized in some situations. The effect of these drugs is monitored by the measurement of urine output, via an indwelling catheter, and by changes in neurologic signs. Prolonged corticosteroid therapy may precipitate gastric bleeding, and the nurse should observe for signs that it has occurred. Often, antacids are administered orally or by a nasogastric tube. Diazepam (Valium) or phenytoin sodium is used to prevent and control convulsions that may occur with severe head injuries. A focal seizure that occurs soon after injury implies cerebral contusion or depressed fracture; seizures occurring within a few hours after trauma and associated with changes in level of consciousness or other neurologic signs are usually indicative of an intracranial hematoma. In some patients, seizures may be delayed until weeks later. Hyperthermia may develop after head injury due to disturbances of the temperature control center of the hypothalamus (measures to control hyperthermia in the neurologic patient have been discussed earlier).

Rehabilitation of the patient who has suffered a head injury focuses on helping the patient and the family to adjust to any residual disabilities. This is often a very difficult task, particularly when the neurologic deficits are severe. Diversional and occupational therapy activities are helpful during prolonged rehabilitation. Emphasis is placed on the full utilization of remaining faculties and abilities to provide as normal a life as possible.

Intracranial Neoplasms

Vital cerebral function is threatened by all types of intracranial neoplasms, whether they are benign or malignant. Symptoms of intracranial tumors result either from increased intracranial pressure or from neurologic dysfunction of a focal or generalized nature due to tissue destruction, irritation, or compression by the space-occupying lesion. The type of symptoms and their progression in a given patient depend on the location of the brain tumor and its histologic type. Unless the progression of the tumor is interrupted, cerebral function is increasingly compromised, and a fatal outcome results.

Clinical symptoms Focal symptoms of intracranial tumors are caused by localized destruction, irritation, or compression of brain tissue and cerebral vessels in specific areas. Thus, symptoms vary, depending upon the area of the brain affected. For this reason, accurate observation of focal symptoms is important in determining the presence and location of the lesion. These focal symptoms include muscular weakness, olfactory phenomena, language disturbances, hearing difficulties, visual disturbances, such as hemianopia or diplopia, dizziness, particularly with position changes, paresthesia, and focal or generalized convulsions. Seizures are often associated with tumors and are important signs, particularly if the onset of seizures occurs after the age of 25. The presence of preconvulsion visual phenomena such as (flashing lights) indicates that the lesion is in the occipital lobe.

Personality disturbances are associated with tumor involvement of the frontal lobes. These personality changes range from subtle personality disturbances to psychotic behavior or intellectual impairment. Apathy, lack of concern, and indifference to urinary control are examples of these inappropriate responses. These symptoms usually appear insidiously and increase in severity, although they are occasionally abrupt in onset. The nurse needs to be vigilant to detect subtle changes in the symptom complex; often it is the family who recognize these subtle changes.

Gradual changes in mental status, in the absence of focal neurologic signs, are often attributed to emotional stress, depression, agitation, or other nonorganic mental illness. Consequently, intracranial neoplasms may be misdiagnosed initially and improper treatment provided. For example, sedatives, tranquilizing, or stimulant drugs may be prescribed to provide symptomatic relief and thus often obscure the underlying organic problem.

Brain tumors of any type or in any location eventually cause generalized symptoms of increased intracranial pressure and cerebral edema. Although symptoms of increased intracranial pressure are usually a late development, after other neurologic signs become evident, certain tumors, such as those located in the frontal lobe, third ventricle, fourth ventricle, or in and around the aqueduct of Sylvius, are manifested initially by symptoms of increased intracranial pressure.

The classic generalized symptoms of brain tumors are those mentioned previously as important symptoms of intracranial pressure, namely, papilledema, headache, nausea and vomiting, drowsiness, and, later, changes in the level of consciousness. The headache is frequently located in the frontal and suboccipital region but the site varies widely. Usually, headaches initially occur in the morning and are transient but later become persistent and increasingly intense, particularly when the patient coughs, strains, or stoops. As intracranial pressure increases, headaches become more generalized, increasing in severity, and becoming refractory to the ordinary medications.

Diagnosis of intracranial tumors In addition to a detailed history and a physical examination for abnormal neurologic signs, various diagnostic procedures are used in detecting intracranial tumors and delineating the site and nature of the lesion. These diagnostic tests include skull x-rays, echoencephalograms, electroencephalograms, brain scanning, angiography, ventriculograms, and pneumoencephalograms. As mentioned previously, because of the increased use of the EMI scanner for computerized transverse axial tomography, pneumonencephalograms and even ventriculograms are often bypassed today.

Skull roentgenograms may demonstrate shifting of intracranial contents, abnormal calcifications, and bone erosion. Echoencephalography is useful in defining the exact location of the pineal gland and in outlining the size and position of the ventricular system. Displacement of the pineal gland may indicate the presence of a mass. Dislocation of normal cerebral vessels near the tumor may be demonstrated by angiography. Lumbar puncture may be utilized to obtain specimens for analysis of CSF. An elevated protein content in the CSF, for example, is often associated with brain tumors. Lumbar puncture is generally used only in the early stages of the disease, before signs of increased intracranial pressure are evident. It is contraindicated in the presence of increased intracranial pressure because there is a danger of causing a shift of intracranial contents, adversely affecting the brainstem. If the lesion is supratentorial, buckling of the midbrain may occur during a lumbar puncture. If the lesion is infratentorial, medullary compression occurs.

Types of tumors Intracranial tumors occur at all ages but predominantly in the fifth decade of life. The lesions are generally described by their location, as either supratentorial (cerebrum or anterior two-thirds of the brain) or infratentorial (cerebellum or brainstem). The tumors may involve the brain substance, supporting structures, the vascular structure, the meninges, or the cranial nerves. The most common type of intracranial neoplasm is the glioma. About half of all intracranial tumors are gliomas. **Gliomas** are derived from the neuroglia, the supporting cells of the central nervous system, and may infiltrate any portion of the brain. Gliomas are subclassified according to the predominant cells: astrocytoma; glioblastoma multiforme; oligodendroglioma; ependymoma; and medulloblastoma. **Astrocytoma,** the most common of the gliomas, is composed of astrocytes, which are neuroglial cells, and varies in degree of malignancy. In adults, it is found most often in the cerebrum, especially the temporal lobe, but in children it is most often found in the cerebellum. **Glioblastoma multiforme,** which is a highly malignant astrocytoma, and **medulloblastoma,** which originates from undifferentiated nerve tissues, are the most malignant and rapidly growing of all neoplasms in the brain. Most glioblastoma multiforme tumors occur in the cerebrum, usually affecting persons of 45 to 55 years of age and rapidly causing death, usually within a year after the onset of symptoms. **Oligodendrogliomas** are slow-growing and often benign neoplasms. **Ependymomas** originate in the linings of the ventricles, especially the fourth ventricle, and are also frequently benign. Medulloblastomas are the most common type of intracranial tumor in children, usually occurring at about age 12 and causing rapid deterioration and death within about 18 months.

Meningiomas are tumors of the meninges. They are found most often in middle-aged adults, primarily in women. Meningiomas are generally benign but occasionally undergo sarcomatous changes. Some may be massive, causing bone destruction and proliferation, whereas others are small. **Hemangiomas** and **hemangioblastomas** are benign tumors of the blood vessels.

Tumors may also develop in any of the cranial nerves. The most common is the **acoustic neuroma,** a benign tumor that initially involves the sheath of the vestibulocochlear nerve, but also involves the nerve fibers as it grows. Vestibulocochlear nerve involvement causes unilateral tinnitus and loss of hearing and vestibular function. As the tumor grows, it compresses other cranial nerves and the cerebellum, leading to the following: disturbances of the facial nerve, with weakness of facial muscles; trigeminal nerve involvement, with paresthesia of the face; loss of the corneal reflex; and diminished touch and pain sensations. Cerebellar compression leads to ataxia of the limbs. Vertigo and nystagmus are other associated symptoms. Characteristically, an acoustic neuroma is a slow-growing tumor, most often occurring after the age of 40.

Tumors may also develop in the pituitary and pineal glands (pinealomas). Pituitary adenomas are diagnosed by symptoms associated with hormonal disturbances, as well as by visual disturbances and blindness resulting from compression on the optic chiasm. Changes in the sella turcica (the bony structure containing the pituitary gland) also may be detected by skull x-ray. Hormonal disturbances vary from acromegaly to pituitary deficiency, according to the type of pituitary adenoma present.

Metastatic neoplasms of the brain are common and most often arise from primary sites in the lung, breast, or kidneys. In some patients, the metastatic cerebral lesions produce neurologic symptoms even before symptoms become evident from the primary lesion.

Pseudotumor cerebri is a syndrome that simulates a brain tumor, causing increased intracranial pressure and symptoms of headache, papilledema, and blindness. The syndrome occurs most often in young adult females and overweight adolescents. Hypervitaminosis A and prolonged corticosteroid therapy have been cited as causes; remission of symptoms results when these underlying causes are corrected [26].

Treatment It is estimated that more than half of brain tumors are malignant and infiltrate the brain substance. This fact explains why it is frequently not possible to remove intracranial tumors completely if severe neurologic deficits would result from extensive resection. When possible, early treatment consists in surgical resection of the tumor, often followed by radiation therapy. Metastatic tumors (unless solitary lesions are amenable to surgical excision) are generally treated only by irradiation. Complete removal of meningiomas is often possible by surgery, irradiation, or both. Acoustic neuromas are completely excised, with care taken not to injure the facial and other cranial nerves.

When gliomas are located in an area that does not compromise vital functions, they are treated by surgical excision, followed by radiation therapy and chemotherapy. When the tumor is located in critical areas, irradiation and chemotherapy are the treatment modalities used.

Chemotherapy for intracranial lesions is limited, because many of the commonly used agents cannot pass the blood-brain barrier in large enough quantities to be effective. Bis-beta-chloroethyl-nitrosurea (BCNU) is an agent that does cross the blood-brain barrier and is frequently used in the treatment of malignant brain disease; 1,2, chlorethyl-3-cyclohexyl-1-nitrosurea (CCNU) is another agent that is used. Corticosteroid therapy, such as with dexamethasone (Decadron), is often used as adjunctive therapy to control cerebral edema.

Hypophysectomy (removal of the pituitary gland) may be done for primary pituitary disease or as a palliative measure in cancer therapy for patients who have metastases that are dependent on sex hormones. In the latter situation, the operation in some patients appears to control metastasis and to provide pain relief. Hypophysectomy via a conventional craniotomy or by a transphenoidal approach is discussed in Chapter 8.

Nursing Care

Nursing care of the patient with an intracranial tumor requires the provision of extensive psychological support for patient and family during all stages of the illness. Many crisis periods occur from the time of initial onset of symptoms and diagnosis to either recovery or a fatal outcome. The variety of symptoms leading to definite changes in motor and sensory function are confusing and frightening for both patient and family. The fear of cancer and the fear of severe neurologic deficits are ever present. The patient and family need careful explanations to help understand the neurologic changes and how to cope with them.

Careful assessment of the patient, with early recognition of neurologic changes, is an essential component of care. Prevention of complications from sensory and motor deficits also is a major focus of care. The nurse must provide the nursing measures that are indicated by the patient's specific symptoms. For example, the person with gait disturbances requires assistance in ambulation, precautions for safety, and possibly assistive devices. Patients with seizures require appropriate precautionary measures to prevent trauma. Most patients with brain tumors tend to tolerate an upright position better than a supine position. The upright position appears to decrease venous congestion and often relieves headache.

All patients with intracranial tumors need attention to their nutrition and elimination. Straining at stool, for example, is to be avoided, because it results in increased intracranial pressure. The patient should be kept as independent as possible, and diversional therapy should be provided. It is important for the patient's family to have time to discuss the patient and his previous capabilities and personality. This need is particularly evident when the intracranial tumor has caused severe mental changes and behavioral disturbances. Narcotics are avoided because of their effect on respiratory depression. The nurse must observe the patient closely for signs of increasing intracranial pressure and neurologic changes during both the preoperative and postoperative period.

Intracranial Surgery

Intracranial surgery is performed for exploratory purposes and to obtain biopsy specimens, remove intracranial neoplasms, relieve intracranial pressure, and evacuate hematomas or fluid. Intracranial surgery is also done to control hemorrhage, repair a decompressed or compound fracture, remove scar tissue to relieve tremors, repair aneurysms or vascular anomalies, and drain an intracranial abscess. The goal of intracranial surgery is to treat the disease with minimal neurologic deficits.

Craniectomy is excision of a part of the skull, varying in size from that of a small burr hole to several centimeters in diameter. In the latter incision, a rongeur (bone forceps) is used to enlarge the original hole. Craniotomy involves freeing a portion of the skull via a large opening in the cranium to form a bone flap. The flap remains attached to muscular tissue and is resutured after the operation is completed. Cranioplasty is the repair of a cranial defect by inserting a substitute bone graft, tantalum, or Vitallium plate. Cranioplasty is indicated to protect the brain and to improve cosmetic appearance, particularly in supratentorial defects. Other specific neurosurgical operations are discussed with their related diseases or conditions elsewhere in this chapter.

GENERAL PROCEDURES

General anesthesia is usually used for extensive intracranial operations, as well as for many operations on the spinal column. The skull and the brain itself, however, are insensitive to pain; the scalp, extracranial arteries, and portions of the dura mater are the only structures that are sensitive to pain. Local anesthesia is used for most diagnostic and some neurosurgical procedures. To supplement general anesthesia, to reduce bleeding, and to decrease oxygen requirements, hypothermia is often used, particularly when cerebral aneurysms are being repaired or when vascular tumors are being removed.

The position of the patient for intracranial surgery is determined by the operative site. Usually, the supine position is used, but an upright, sitting position is generally preferred to the conventional prone position when suboccipital craniectomy is to be done. Special headrest attachments are used to hold the head in the desired fixed position. The incision is made through the cranial bone over the site of the pathologic condition; its size and direction depend on the area to be exposed. The bone is either completely removed at the incision, elevated, or turned back to expose the operative site; it is put back in position during the closure. In some cases, the bone is not replaced in order to provide temporary cerebral decompression. However, these skull defects are eventually repaired with autogenous bone grafts or synthetic plates.

Whereas in most operations the lesion is fully exposed, only limited access and visualization are possible in most neurosurgical procedures. Neurosurgery is also prolonged because lesions often cannot be removed intact but rather in a piecemeal fashion.

Bleeding requires careful control and is managed with pressure, forceps, or metal clips specifically designed for cranial surgery. Bone wax rubbed into the incised cranial bones is used to prevent oozing. Electrocautery is used to control bleeding from intracranial cerebral vessels, or metal clips may be used. In contrast to the coarse mesh gauze sponges usually used in operations, compressed absorbent rayon and cotton strips are used to absorb blood and fluids because of the fragile nature of brain tissue. Thromboplastin materials, such as Gelfoam sponges saturated with thrombin solution, control oozing where ligatures are not usable. Microneurosurgical techniques utilizing a microscope and very fine instruments have been developed and have facilitated new procedures for establishing collateral blood flow in patients with occlusive cerebrovascular disease, for the removal of neoplasms, and for the repair of aneurysms and severed nerves.

PREOPERATIVE PREPARATION

Preoperative preparation requires a thorough explanation of the operation by the neurosurgeon with a clear statement as to the anticipated findings and results. The patient and family should be advised that any neurologic defect present preoperatively may persist postoperatively. The patient should be told the reasons for required preparation, including the head shave. Some patients are particularly apprehensive because of the fear of a permanent change in appearance and neurologic deficits that may cause dependency or death. Psychological support of the patient and family is of paramount importance. If, because of presenting symptoms, the patient is not considered competent, relatives must sign the informed consent document.

Routine preoperative measures are carried out, including preparation of the site itself. The hair of the patient with long hair is braided and cut close to the scalp; it is labeled and saved. The scalp is shampooed, and any signs of lesions or abrasions are reported. The head is shaved cautiously to prevent cutting the scalp and then is covered with a clean towel. The time of preparation varies in different hospitals; sometimes it is done the night before, sometimes on the morning of the operation, and sometimes in a two-step process. An indwelling catheter is inserted preoperatively for postoperative monitoring of urine output. A spinal catheter may be inserted to decrease cerebral edema if indicated. Enemas, if ordered preoperatively, should be given slowly to avoid straining and increased intracranial pressure.

A detailed assessment should be carried out preoperatively for baseline data with which to evaluate the patient's physiologic status postoperatively. These data include the vital signs, level of consciousness, status of mental functioning, motion and strength of the extremities, facial muscle mobility and symmetry, and the status of pupillary reaction.

POSTOPERATIVE CARE

Postoperatively the patient's position will vary, depending on the site of surgery. Any restrictions in position should be clearly understood by all personnel and the patient's family, so that the patient is not accidentally positioned improperly. Lesions in the cerebrum are supratentorial. (Intracranial lesions are described as supratentorial or infratentorial, that is, above or below the tentorium, the fold of dura mater between the cerebellum and occipital lobes.) After supratentorial surgery, the patient is not allowed to lie on the operative site, and the head is generally elevated to 45 degrees. Lesions in the cerebellum or brainstem are infratentorial; the incision is usually in the occipital region of the skull. After infratentorial operations, the patient is generally kept flat, on either side but not on the back. Position changes are necessary every 1 to 2 hours to prevent skin breakdown and pneumonia. Patients should be observed closely for respiratory difficulty.

Patients who have had an infratentorial operation are usually given nothing by mouth for 24 to 48 hours. Such an operation may cause trauma or edema, affecting the functioning of the glossopharyngeal and vagus nerves and resulting in the loss of the gag reflex and the onset of dysphagia. Such a patient must be evaluated carefully before oral food or fluids are given. Vomiting should be prevented, because straining may increase the intracranial pressure. If increased intracranial pressure or cerebral edema is present, osmotic diuretics, corticosteroids, or both are administered.

Confusion and restlessness often occur after intracranial operations. Repeated but calm efforts to orient the patient to the surroundings and ongoing events, and constant attendance by staff or family are preferred methods to reduce restlessness and manage confused states. The use of restraints tends to agitate the patient, who then tends to strain against them, leading to increased intracranial pressure. Side rails should be raised at all times. The side rails may require padding to prevent injury to the confused patient or the patient in whom seizures are likely to develop.

Ice bags are applied to the head and often help relieve headache. Headache is generally present for 24 to 48 hours postoperatively. Pain is relieved with mild analgesics. Sedatives and opiates are used cautiously, if at all, because they cause respiratory depression and mask neurologic signs of increased intracranial pressure.

The wound dressing should be checked frequently for drainage. If drains have been placed, reinforcement of dressings with sterile dressings is often necessary. The drainage should be described precisely; if leakage of CSF is detected, it should be reported immediately. Asepsis is of paramount importance in handling dressings; the danger of meningitis is great. After an infratentorial operation (in the suboccipital region), lateral and forward flexion of the head is avoided to prevent tension on the incision. The time of removal of the dressing varies, depending on the surgeon. When the dressing is removed, the scalp is cleaned with hydrogen peroxide to remove crust formations. Wigs or kerchiefs may be used to cover the head.

Periocular edema with swelling of the eyelids and surrounding tissues may occur after intracranial surgery as well as after head injuries. Light compresses of cracked ice are placed within Pliofilm ice bags and are placed on a patch covering the eye. Petrolatum jelly is used to lubricate and protect the eyelid and surrounding ocular tissue. At regular intervals, the patch should be removed to replace melted ice and to check the condition of the eye. Collections of mucus or crusts on the eyelids should be removed. Care must be taken to avoid trauma to the eye, particularly if there is a loss of the corneal reflex. If the facial nerve (seventh cranial nerve) is damaged during surgery, the cornea must be protected with an eye shield or a protective transparent covering, such as Saran wrap. Artificial tears are instilled to prevent corneal drying and scarring. A tarsorrhaphy (suturing of the eyelid) may be done to treat permanent facial nerve paralysis.

Vital and neurologic signs are evaluated at

regular, frequent intervals. The patient should be observed for complications and immediate measures taken to prevent the following: respiratory failure and airway obstruction (primarily due to compression of the respiratory center of the medulla); shock; increased intracranial pressure from bleeding or cerebral edema; and hyperthermia (related to disturbances of the heat-regulating mechanism or other systemic disease). Meningitis, wound infection, respiratory infections, thrombophlebitis, seizures, and deformities related to motor dysfunction are other potential complications. Arterial blood gas studies are done regularly to determine the adequacy of respiratory function and the need for ventilatory assistance. The patient is observed for any disturbance in motor function or in orientation, visual disturbances, alterations in pupillary reactions, and changes in personality and behavior.

Activity is governed by the patient's condition and whether or not increased intracranial pressure is present. Supervision in ambulation is required; dizziness and disorientation frequently recur after intracranial surgery. Any neurologic disability resulting from the operation must be dealt with realistically to facilitate acceptance and adjustment by both patient and family. For those whose lesions proved inoperable or who have serious neurologic deficits, care continues to focus on making the patient as comfortable as possible and independent for as long as possible.

Cerebrovascular Disease

Cerebrovascular disease is used here to refer to any functional abnormality of the central nervous system resulting from a primary disorder of blood vessels supplying the brain tissue. The magnitude of the problem of cerebrovascular disease is demonstrated by the fact that stroke is the third most common cause of death in the United States and is the major cause of chronic disability. Stroke, or cerebrovascular accident (CVA), is identified as an abrupt onset of neural deficits resulting from interference with the blood supply to the brain. The major causes of stroke are hemorrhage, thrombosis, and embolism. Embolism is often associated with cardiovascular disease. Less often, subarachnoid hemorrhage occurs as a result of a ruptured aneurysm.

It has been estimated that in the United States there are about 25 million survivors of stroke with varying levels of disability. Although about 30 percent of these stroke survivors return to normal activity or employment, 15 percent require total nursing care because of severe disability, and 55 percent, though incapable of working, can carry on the activities of daily living [22b].

STROKE SYNDROME

The rehabilitative aspects of stroke have been emphasized in the past, but the current emphasis is on prevention. The signs and symptoms of impending stroke should be recognized, so that medical intervention can be obtained before a stroke occurs. Some of these symptoms are vertigo, recurrent lightheadedness, syncope, intermittent unilateral temporal or occipital headache, blurred vision and transient monocular blindness, and transient loss of muscle tone of all extremities, resulting in falls. Transient episodes of ataxia, dysphasia, disorientation, and paresthesia are also important signs. Behavioral changes and convulsions in persons over 45 years of age are other important symptoms that require further investigation.

The types of stroke may be divided into transient ischemic attacks, lacunar strokes, and the completed stroke.

Transient Ischemic Attacks

A transient ischemic attack (TIA) is a temporary or reversible focal cerebral ischemia that does not result in an infarction or tissue damage. It is sometimes called "cerebral angina." Symptoms develop suddenly but last less than 24 hours. These attacks should be recognized as warnings of impending stroke, because about 15 to 20 percent of patients who have transient ischemic attacks ultimately have cerebral thrombosis.

Transient ischemic attacks are the result of a temporary reduction of blood supply to a focal area of the brain and are frequently caused by partial or total obstruction of an extracranial artery in the carotid or vertebrobasilar system or narrowing of intracranial vessels in the circle of Willis and its branches (page 899). Symptoms in a TIA vary, depending on whether the carotid or vertebrobasilar arteries are involved. Predisposing factors leading to a transient ischemic attack include vertebral artery compression, microemboli, decreased arterial blood pressure (causing a fall in regional cerebral perfusion pressure), cardiac arrhythmias, cerebral vasospasm, and hypoglycemia.

Symptoms associated with a TIA include unilateral weakness or numbness, ipsilateral visual disturbances, diplopia, confusion, slurred speech, dizziness, ataxia, and sudden falls. Symptoms may last for only a few seconds or a few hours, and complete recovery occurs within 24 hours. If these symptoms last longer than 24 hours, it is likely that a lacunar stroke, rather than a TIA, has occurred.

Cerebrovascular disease almost always is accompanied by one or more other medical problems, such as hypertension, cardiac disease, an elevated blood cholesterol level, diabetes mellitus, and peripheral vascular disease. (Typically, the patient with cerebrovascular disease is a 50- to 60-year-old man with a history of hypertension, is overweight, and is a smoker.) Therefore, persons who have symptoms of TIAs should be assessed for hypertension and obesity and should stop smoking; controlling these factors may prevent a stroke from progressing. Anticoagulants may be started, although there is some controversy over the use of anticoagulants as prophylactic therapy in this syndrome. The use of anticoagulants for the patient with hypertension is hazardous because they may cause a cerebral hemorrhage. Some physicians use low doses of aspirin as a type of anticoagulant therapy. Vascular surgery is often indicated when TIAs occur frequently and when an area of vascular occlusion can be identified and is accessible for surgical repair.

Lacunar Strokes

Lacunar strokes are very tiny infarcts caused by occlusion of the smaller vessels. They tend to be multiple and most often occur in the basal ganglia and the pons. Associated with hypertension, they can be prevented when hypertension is controlled. Four types of clinical syndromes are associated with lacunar strokes, which also can be asymptomatic. The syndromes are: (1) the clumsy hand syndrome with dysarthria, which is associated with slurred speech, weakness, clumsiness, and ataxia of the involved arm; (2) pure motor hemiparesis, with unilateral paralysis of the face, arm, and leg but without significant sensory loss; (3) crural paresis and ataxia, with slight weakness and clumsiness in one leg; and (4) the pure sensory stroke, in which there is unilateral loss of sensation without weakness or other motor deficits [31a]. These symptoms may last from hours to days.

Completed Stroke

A completed stroke may result from cerebral thrombosis, hemorrhage, or embolism, thrombosis being the most frequent cause. The majority of patients with cerebral thrombosis or embolism survive acute episodes whereas mortality is increased in cerebral hemorrhage. Interference with tissue perfusion causes ischemia or infarction, and hemorrhage destroys nerve cells by clot formation (causing increased intracranial pressure) or by disrupting blood flow (causing infarction), or both. Bleeding may be either intracerebral or in the subarachnoid space. Intracerebral hemorrhage is commonly caused by spontaneous bleeding in a patient with hypertension whereas subarachnoid hemorrhage is most often caused by rupture of an aneurysm into the meningeal space.

Signs and symptoms vary according to the site and extent of nervous tissue affected by altered blood flow and also by the availability of collateral flow when obstruction in the vessels occurs. Damage to a minute area of the brain tissue may result in significant impairment or death. For example, if an infarct occurs at the internal capsule, where many nerve fibers are located in proximity, a very tiny lesion may cause a very severe permanent hemiparesis. Intracerebral hemorrhage is characterized by a rapid onset and a progressive pattern of a focal deficit over a short period. Usually there are no focal warning signs and the patient is typically awake and active when the hemorrhage occurs.

In contrast to the sudden development of neurologic deficits associated with cerebral hemorrhage, there is generally a slower step-by-step development of neurologic deficits in cerebral thrombosis. Atherosclerotic degeneration tends to occur at sites of vascular bifurcations or curves and involves both extracranial and intracranial vessels.

NURSING CARE OF STROKE PATIENTS

General Nursing Measures

During the acute phase of the stroke, the medical and nursing goals are oriented to meeting the survival needs of a critically ill patient and preventing extension of cerebral damage. If the patient is comatose, maintenance and protection of vital functions take priority. Ensuring a patent airway requires frequent suctioning and positioning of the patient to prevent aspiration of mucus; a tracheostomy may be necessary. The nurse must also provide oxygen therapy, adequate hydration, and medication to liquefy secretions. If the patient is alert, deep breathing and coughing are encouraged to prevent pneumonia, one of the most frequent complications after stroke.

Vital signs must be monitored accurately. Adequate blood pressure must be maintained to ensure adequate perfusion of vital organs. The patient who has had a hemorrhage and has suffered neurologic defects of the vasomotor center may be in a state of shock, and vasopressors may be necessary; however, the blood pressure of patients on vasopressors must be carefully monitored to prevent untoward effects from the therapy. Some patients who have suffered a stroke continue to have high blood pressure levels, which require treatment to prevent further complications. The patient who has suffered a stroke is also vulnerable to peripheral vascular complications such as thrombosis. Measures are taken to prevent venous stasis, and the extremities are placed in a position that does not precipitate venous obstruction. Antiembolic elastic stockings may also be applied.

Neurologic assessment is done at regular intervals to detect changes in the neurologic status and impending complications. Again, the patient's level of consciousness is a major indicator of increased intracranial pressure and must be evaluated frequently. If the patient is restless it must be determined whether hypoxia or pain is the precipitating factor. Sedatives or narcotics are avoided due to the hazards of respiratory depression. If convulsions occur, diazepam or phenytoin is administered, and precautions are taken to protect the patient while observing the pattern of the convulsion for diagnostic purposes.

Prevention of Complications Due to Immobility

The patient who is unable to move freely because of a stroke is vulnerable to all the hazards of immobilization. Even during the acute phase of the illness, the nurse should place particular stress on measures to prevent contractures, decubiti, hypercalciuria, negative nitrogen balance, vascular complications such as thrombosis, and disuse atrophy of muscles. The patient's position must be changed at least every 2 hours. However, the length of time on the affected side is limited because of the hazards of decreased blood flow in the involved extremities. (The paralyzed arm must be kept free of pressure from the patient's body.) The nurse who is aware of the types of contractures and deformities to which the stroke patient is susceptible takes special precautions to prevent their occurrence. Functional restoration will not be possible if contractures and muscle shortening due to prolonged nonphysiologic positioning result in deformities.

The potential deformities and contractures are in general of a flexor pattern. The shoulder becomes adducted and internally rotated, the elbow is flexed, the forearm pronated, and the wrist and hand totally flexed. In the lower extremity, the knee may become flexed, the hip flexed, the leg externally rotated, and the foot in an equinovarus position. Contracture of the gastrocnemius muscle causes heel-cord shortening. To prevent the leg from external rotation and the foot from resting in the flexed position while the patient is supine, a footboard and sandbags or a trochanter roll along the lateral aspect of the involved leg from the hip to the knee is absolutely essential. When the patient is positioned on the side, a pillow must be placed between the legs to prevent pressure and to promote proper positioning. In the upper extremity, a pillow should be placed in the axilla to keep the shoulder abducted and partly flexed at about a 45- to 50-degree angle. The forearm is placed on a pillow, so that the elbow and hand are higher than the shoulder; this position prevents edema in the upper extremity. The wrist is placed in a neutral or slightly extended position. Hand rolls are placed within the palm and the fingers and thumbs are placed in an opposed position to maintain the normal grasping position. Dayhoff [8a] recommends the application of hard hand-positioning devices rather than the traditional soft hand-positioning devices such as cloth or Kerlix rolls. It is important to stress that the patient is not constantly maintained in one position. If the patient is able to tolerate it, the prone position is effective in preventing decubiti and deformities. It promotes hyperextension of the hip joint, which is essential for a normal gait. The patient can be placed in a prone position for 15 to 30 minutes once daily or more often if tolerated, with folded bath towels or a small pillow placed under each shoulder to prevent inward rotation. A small flat pillow is placed under the ankles, and the feet are extended beyond the mattress to prevent plantar flexion. The affected arm is adducted and extended; the head should be turned to one side, and a pillow under the head should not be permitted. A flat support, such as a folded towel, may be placed under the patient's chest if this contributes to comfort.

The patient's position should be changed at intervals, and the joints of both the involved and noninvolved extremities should be put through their full range of motion by gentle passive movement. This early activity of gentle passive movement should begin the first day after the stroke occurs and should be done three to four times daily. (As soon as possible, the patient is taught to use the unaffected hand to exercise the weak hand.) In fact, if hemorrhage is not the cause of the stroke, the patient is usually allowed up in a chair the next day, assuming vital signs are stabilized. Ambulation is generally delayed when the patient has had a cerebral hemorrhage.

In some situations, splinting may be indicated to prevent deformities. However, if the splint is kept in place too long without removing it to exercise the extremity, other types of contractures may occur. When used correctly, a half-cast with the foot at right angles is effective in preventing drop foot, a frequent complication after stroke. Cock-up splints for the upper extremity to keep the wrist and fingers extended may also be used. Again, it is important to emphasize that these devices must be combined with changes of position and exercise to be beneficial.

Fluid, Electrolytes, and Nutrition

Providing for adequate fluid and electrolyte balance is another major responsibility in the care of the stroke patient. Depending on the patient's neurologic status and level of consciousness and the presence or absence of the gag and swallowing reflex, food and fluids are provided by intravenous infusion, nasogastric tube, or oral intake. Often, intravenous infusions are used for at least the first 24 hours. Mouth care must be given at frequent intervals and always after every feeding; often, food particles will accumulate on the paralyzed side of the mouth.

The swallowing reflex must be tested before giving any fluids orally. The stroke may cause compression of the cranial nerves in the medulla and particularly the glossopharyngeal and vagus nerves, affecting the gag and swallowing reflex. When eating is permitted, the food should be placed on the unaffected side, and the patient should be encouraged to eat slowly and concentrate on coordinating chewing, breathing, and swallowing. Gaffney [12] recommends stroking the back of the neck near the occiput with a washcloth or icing the sternal notch to stimulate swallowing if necessary. Some utensils that facilitate swallowing have been designed; for example, a long spoon with a bladelike plunger that allows the patient to put food in the back of the mouth.

Bladder and Bowel Care

The comatose patient requires an indwelling catheter to assure proper urinary elimination and to facilitate accurate output records. Adequate hydration and early removal of the catheter are important in preventing urinary tract infection. Patients should be placed on a bladder training program; the bedpan is offered, or the patient is taken to a commode at regular, frequent intervals to establish a voiding schedule. These intervals gradually decrease in frequency as control is reestablished. Records are kept to determine the appropriate time to offer the patient the bedpan.

Constipation and fecal impaction must be avoided because of the danger of straining and distention. Straining with defecation may increase intracranial pressure. An appropriate bowel-training program is initiated when the patient's physiologic status permits (see page 976).

Psychological Aspects of Care

The patient is likely to be confused on regaining consciousness. Orientation to time, place, and person should be provided slowly and calmly. Familiar persons and objects should be provided to assist in reorientation. If the patient is aphasic, measures are taken to establish some means of communication. (The presence of aphasia is determined by various approaches, as described on page 931.) During this time, both the patient and family require emotional support as the realities of the neurologic deficits become evident.

Mancell [20b] identifies the first several days or weeks after the stroke as the period of the greatest degree of functional restitution.

(Functional recovery occurs as cerebral pressure and edema subside.) Therefore, the nurse should capitalize on any spontaneous recovery and provide reinforcement as the patient begins to communicate verbally. However, Mancell also notes that improvement may be observed for as long as 18 to 24 months after the onset of the stroke. These factors should be taken into consideration when patients and families seek reassurance from the nurse about the type of recovery to be anticipated.

Depression is a normal reaction as the patient intellectually and emotionally reacts to the bodily changes in stroke and the need to depend on others for even basic needs and body functioning. It is important that the nurse communicate with the patient as a normal person. Too often, emotional changes in the patient that result in labile emotions and crying, for example, influence nursing personnel to talk to the patient in a condescending manner or as though to a child, and this must be avoided. When the patient cries inappropriately, the nurse should intervene by distracting the patient, asking a question, or engaging the patient in another activity. The patient's emotional and intellectual status should be carefully evaluated to determine appropriate methods of giving directions and what can realistically be expected of the patient during rehabilitation.

Depending on the site of the lesion, certain types of problems can be anticipated. The patient with right hemiplegia, for example, will usually have associated aphasia. The patient with left hemiplegia generally has spatial-perceptual difficulties and thus cannot accurately judge body position, distance, and movement, or correctly perceive the body in relation to the environment. All these factors influence the ability to ambulate safely.

It is important to remember that the patient may have difficulty in mentally processing directions and has a short attention span. Stroke patients often find it hard to concentrate, are apathetic or euphoric, and have poor judgment, difficulty in estimating time, lapses of memory, and a low frustration threshold. They may be irritable, impulsive, and sexually uninhibited, and may have problems making decisions.

All these characteristics are manifestations of the neurologic effects of the stroke and they affect the following: the length of time needed for activities; the type of instructions given in teaching the patient self-care; fatigability and physical endurance; and the type of supervision required as the patient begins to regain function. New tasks should be initiated slowly and step by step. Directions should be given one at a time, and the patient should be praised for any success, however small.

Although it may be simpler and less time-consuming for the nurse to perform various tasks, the most therapeutic approach is to allow the patient to take over when he or she can. However, it is also important to prevent frustration if the patient has great difficulty doing a task. The patient is not rushed and is encouraged but not forced to perform. Frustration may lead to feelings of failure and cause the patient to lose heart. It is helpful for the nurse to observe the patient closely to determine the times during the day when the patient appears to function best and is least fatigued. The nurse should schedule planned therapies and new experiences and tasks for these peak periods.

Ambulation, Eating, and Dressing

Vasomotor tone is facilitated by early ambulation, which also has positive psychological effects on the patient and family. Ambulation is generally started in the physical therapy department between parallel bars to help the patient adjust to an erect position; a tilt table may be necessary for some patients who tend to faint on adjusting to an erect position. The nurse who assists the patient in transfers from the bed and in ambulation must keep several principles in mind to help the patient ambulate safely. Generally, the hemiplegic patient should transfer toward the strong side of the body. In walking, the nurse should stand on the patient's weak side, since the patient tends to fall toward the weak side. To prevent knee flexion, a posterior knee splint may be used if the patient has weakened or absent quadriceps muscle function. A sling may be used to hold the affected arm during ambulation in order to prevent subluxation of the shoulder joint, because the weight of the affected arm tends to pull on the shoulder, but it should not be used while the patient is in bed because continuous use of the sling promotes deformities. As balance is learned, the patient gradually progresses to independent ambulation with the use of a cane. (Leg braces or a foot-drop splint may be necessary for patients with flexor spasms.) The cane should be the right height for the patient and provide for bending at the elbow at a 30-degree angle with the patient's hand resting on the handle of the cane. If indicated, a tripod or quadruple cane is prescribed for additional stability. It is important that the patient wear good walking shoes rather than slippers during ambulation to prevent slips and falls. The tip of the cane is covered with a rubber safety grip. The patient holds the cane in the unaffected hand, placing it about 6 to 8 inches in front on the unaffected side.

To facilitate independence in eating, the patient may be taught one-handed techniques and may use assistive devices such as a food guard, rubber suction cups, and forks with one semisharp curved edge for one-handed eating and cutting. Many other assistive devices are available for eating, homemaking, and self-care activities.

Dressing is facilitated by using loose-fitting clothes, preferably with fastenings in the front. Velcro fasteners are preferred to buttons. Long-handled shoehorns are useful; laced shoes are avoided. The patient should be instructed to start with the involved extremity when dressing, and with the unaffected extremity when undressing.

Discharge Planning

Long-range goals for the stroke patient are related to the restoration of function, education in the use of restored function, and adaptations for carrying out activities of daily living. Both patient and family should be involved in planning for the care of the patient after hospitalization. Continuity of care after discharge is essential to prevent regression, and long-term follow-up is necessary. Referral for home health care is frequently warranted. The home situation and the family's ability to care for the patient should be carefully appraised. Physical changes in the home may be required for the patient's safety (such as eliminating throw rugs, widening doorways, and installing handrails and grab bars in strategic locations). The family is encouraged to emphasize the abilities that the patient has retained rather than those that have been lost and is advised to observe the patient's energy pattern to determine the periods of greatest effectiveness and to capitalize on these periods. All these efforts are aimed at enabling the stroke patient to function at the maximal level possible.

SUBARACHNOID HEMORRHAGE

The most common causes of spontaneous subarachnoid hemorrhage, another cause of stroke, are ruptured intracranial aneurysm, vascular malformations, trauma, and hypertensive vascular disease with intracranial hemorrhage. Blood dyscrasias and vascular tumors (angiomas) also may cause spontaneous subarachnoid hemorrhage.

Cerebral aneurysms are usually developmental defects in the tunica media (middle coat) of the arteries, causing an outpouching and weakening of the vessel. The most common type is the berry aneurysm, a saccular congenital type that occurs at or near bifurcations, most often in the anterior portion of the circle of Willis. These aneurysms are distinguished from arteriosclerotic aneurysms, which are usually fusiform, tortuous, and associated with atherosclerotic degeneration. Subarachnoid hemorrhages associated with congenital aneurysms most often occur in patients between 30 and 50 years of age.

Physical Findings

Physical findings include a sudden, severe, and throbbing headache, usually occipital; nuchal rigidity; vomiting; neurologic signs such as visual defects, hemiparesis, cranial nerve paralysis (especially of the oculomotor nerve, causing pupil dilatation), convulsions, lethargy, delirium, or coma. In aneurysm of the carotid artery there is often a prodromal headache associated with ptosis and pupillary dilatation. The presence of a bruit over the ocular orbits or skull is associated with arteriovenous anomalies. A lumbar puncture is done and usually demonstrates an elevated pressure and the presence of blood in the CSF. The presence of an intracranial aneurysm is confirmed by angiography.

Treatment and Nursing Care

The patient is placed on a bed rest in a darkened and quiet room, remaining flat in bed but allowed to turn from side to side. The patient's activities are restricted during the first 2 weeks because there is a high incidence of recurrence of bleeding, particularly 7 to 14 days after the initial episode. Rebleeding is sudden and severe and often fatal. The patient is protected from any increase in intracranial pressure that might incite bleeding. Vomiting, sneezing, coughing, hiccoughing, and straining are to be avoided, because they may increase intracranial pressure. Total care is provided for the patient. Straining during bowel evacuation is particularly hazardous; constipation must be controlled with stool softeners and appropriate diet. Headache is treated with mild analgesics, and hypotensive agents may be used to treat underlying hypertension. Diuretic therapy may also be indicated to control hypertension and to reduce intracranial pressure. Monitoring of vital signs and the patient's neurologic status at regular, frequent intervals is essential to detect early signs of increased bleeding or increased intracranial pressure. The nurse should immediately report any alteration in the level of consciousness, an unexplained elevation in temperature or blood pressure, an increase in the intensity of headache, or an increase in neurologic deficits. An intracranial clot forming from the rupture of the aneurysm may cause an increase in intracranial pressure or an obstruction to the CSF pathways. Cerebral vasospasm is another complication associated with subarachnoid hemorrhage.

Early rebleeding is currently being controlled by the use of the antifibrinolytic agent, epsilon-aminocaproic acid (EACA; Amicar), which is used to prevent lysis of the clot sealing the bleeding site until surgical therapy can be provided. Hypotensive agents are also used to prevent the blood pressure elevations that usually preceed a bleeding episode. Measures are taken to control cerebral edema, vasospasm, and secondary hydrocephalus. Corticosteroid therapy is often used.

Surgery is indicated after the patient's condition has stabilized, usually within 2 to 6 weeks. A direct surgical approach is used for clipping or ligating the neck of the aneurysm. If the aneurysm has ruptured (rather than leaked), the clot is evacuated before the aneurysm is clipped. For aneurysms that cannot be repaired or clamped internally, an external carotid or Crutchfield clamp is used [20a]. The clamp is turned progressively each day to occlude the carotid artery completely and to block the blood supply to the aneurysm. Since it is essential that the clamp not be dislodged, jaw movement is restricted; the patient is asked to communicate by writing, and intravenous feedings are given temporarily. The recovery period is prolonged when the external clamping method is used.

Degenerative Disease

Degenerative diseases of the central nervous system include those in which parenchymal degeneration occurs, often for undetermined reasons, but possibly due to deficiencies, familial factors, or viral and immune mechanisms. The major degenerative conditions that will be considered here are multiple sclerosis, amytrophic lateral sclerosis, syringomyelia, Parkinson's disease and Huntington's disease. Although myasthenia gravis is not among the degenerative diseases, it will be discussed in this section, because of its many similarities to these conditions.

All these conditions entail problems with mobility, visible symptoms characteristic of progressive stages, periods of remissions and exacerbations, and the actual or potential threat of increasing disability and dependence on others for carrying out the activities of daily living. Since there is no cure for these conditions, control of the diseases is the goal of medical and nursing care. Because of the long-term care required and the expense of necessary therapy, these diseases impose an ever-present economic burden.

The psychological impact of a chronic, progressively disabling disease on the person and his family cannot be overestimated. Therefore, the nurse's role should be centered on assisting patients to maintain function and independence as long as possible and to provide them with the means of coping psychologically and physiologically with the manifestations of the disease process. Patients often react with pessimism when a diagnosis of degenerative neurologic disease is made, and providing psychological support for both the patient and the family is a major component of nursing care.

MULTIPLE SCLEROSIS

Multiple sclerosis is a chronic disease of the central nervous system that is characterized by remissions and relapses. The disease is called multiple sclerosis because its typical lesions, which are areas of demyelinization in the white matter of the spinal cord and brain, occur in multiple (disseminated) sites. Later, patches of scarred (sclerosed) nervous fibers develop at these sites.

It is estimated that approximately 250,000 persons in the United States have multiple sclerosis. Studies have shown a high incidence of the disease in certain geographical locations, especially in temperate zones (roughly 40 to 60 degrees north or south of the equator). A particularly interesting finding of these studies is that for those who move from a high-risk to a low-risk area before the age of 15, the risk that multiple sclerosis will develop becomes equivalent to that in the new location. Epidemiologic studies have also shown a higher incidence in persons from higher socioeconomic groups. Other factors are being studied in the Shetland and Orkney Islands, which are sites of abnormally high proportions of persons with multiple sclerosis.

Current research in multiple sclerosis is centered on virology and immunology, as well as on epidemiology. A slow, latent virus that lies dormant in the body for months or years before some other factor causes the onset of the disease itself is thought to be directly responsible for the disabling disease. Other evidence supports the theory that the disease results from an autoimmune process, or that an immune deficiency permits a viral process to produce the lesions associated with multiple sclerosis.

It is difficult to diagnose the disease in its early stages, since there are no specific diagnostic tests for the condition; rather, the pattern of the symptoms and ruling out other causes lead to the diagnosis. The CSF level of gamma globulin is often elevated in the majority of these patients, and an abnormal colloidal gold curve is also often detected.

Clinical Symptoms

The disease has an insidious onset, tragically affecting young adults in the prime of their lives, between the ages of 20 and 40. The disease occurs more often in women than in men. Vague symptoms may be present, such as diplopia, awkwardness in handling articles and frequent dropping of articles, and stumbling or falling for no apparent reason, but are forgotten when they spontaneously subside. Often, the initial symptom is temporary blindness or visual disturbances related to optic nerve involvement.

Three major symptoms, namely, nystagmus, intention tremors (those developing during volitional movements but absent at rest), and scanning speech, known as **Charcot's triad** after the physician who first noted their significance, are often seen in multiple sclerosis. In scanning, or staccato, speech, there are long pauses between syllables. Other symptoms vary, depending on the location of the lesions, and include spastic paraplegia, increased deep reflexes, a positive Babinski sign (due to pyramidal tract involvement), frequent mood swings, and often an inappropriate euphoric state.

Course

The course of the disease is unpredictable and the duration uncertain. It is sometimes rapidly progressive, with death occurring within a few years, usually from secondary complications. The majority of patients, however, suffer varying degrees of motor and sensory disability in a course of alternating remissions and exacerbations with progressive incapacitation over the years. Even for the person who recovers from an exacerbation with minimal residual effects, there remains the constant fear of another exacerbation. The long-term effects of the disease result in instability, spasticity, paraplegia, speech defects, eating difficulties, and extreme fatigue.

Management

Because there is no specific treatment or cure for multiple sclerosis, management centers on supportive care to treat symptoms and secondary complications. Corticosteroids have been used to lessen the intensity and duration of exacerbations. Maintenance of motor function by preserving the strength of muscles is extremely important, and physical and occupational therapy are indicated to facilitate this aspect of care. Activity within the patient's capacity should be encouraged. Physical exhaustion, however, should be avoided and adequate rest periods provided. Gait disturbances may precipitate falls, so safety factors must be considered. It is essential to maintain good nutrition to avoid infections, which tend to aggravate the condition and compromise the patient's functional ability. Self-help devices are indicated when there is considerable weakness, or deformity, or both.

The patient frequently has poor bladder tone and incontinence, and bladder infections are common. In some patients, neural prostheses (see the section on bladder control under Spinal Cord Injuries) are being utilized for activating bladder action. The spasms and pain that are often present are treated with muscle-relaxant therapy. The dorsal column stimulator (see under Peripheral nerve stimulation, page 48) has also been used to control spasms and pain in some patients.

When the patient is hospitalized during an exacerbation, the nurse has an important role in teaching the patient and family the techniques of proper hygiene, back care to prevent pressure areas, and ways to conserve energy for priority activities as incapacitation becomes increasingly severe. Provisions for follow-up care with referral to local health agencies is important for assistance in long-term management.

Many communities have chapters of the National Multiple Sclerosis Society, a voluntary nonprofit organization. These local chapters meet regularly and provide opportunities to discuss and solve common problems. Family participation in these programs is encouraged, because the spouse or a family member has the major responsibility for managing the patient's care and also requires emotional support and encouragement from others in similar situations.

In 1972, Congress established the National Advisory Commission on Multiple Sclerosis to devise plans for finding the cause, cure and optimal treatment of the disease.

AMYOTROPHIC LATERAL SCLEROSIS

Amyotrophic lateral sclerosis (ALS) is a motor neuron disease (affecting both upper and lower motor neurons) in which there is a degeneration of motor cells in the brain and spinal cord, leading to muscle weakness. About 8,000 to 10,000 persons in the United States are afflicted with the disease, and approximately two-thirds are men. Onset is most often between the ages of 40 and 60. The cause is unknown, although susceptibility is possibly genetically related. A slow virus infection has also been implicated.

Symptoms depend on which nerve cells are affected. Muscle weakness is a prevalent feature. The initial symptom, however, is often the occurrence of irregular muscle twitchings known as fasiculations. Muscle cramping also occurs. Muscles of the legs and hands become spastic and progressively weaker until flaccidity and atrophy occur. Brainstem involvement causes difficulties in speech, chewing, and swallowing. Damage to cortical centers results in mood swings, although mental faculties are generally not affected. There is no treatment for the disease, and care is directed toward relieving the symptoms. The condition is usually progressive, leading to helplessness and total dependency, with a fatal outcome usually within 3 to 4 years. However, some patients have remissions and are able to lead reasonably active lives. As in other degenerative conditions, the pattern of the disease varies in different individuals.

Nursing care measures are oriented toward meeting the physical and psychological needs of the patient, preventing complications, and providing intellectual stimulation. As mentioned previously, the patient remains mentally alert in this degenerative disorder. Death usually results from aspiration pneumonia or respiratory failure.

SYRINGOMYELIA

Syringomyelia is a chronic and slowly progressive disease of the spinal cord but may also involve the lower brainstem. The disease is characterized by the development of a cyst within the spinal cord or gliosis (scar tissue), with damage to the nerve fibers that cross within the cord [2]. Thus, disturbances in the perception of pain and temperature result, making the patient vulnerable to burns and other injuries. The condition is often associated with skeletal deformities, which appears to support the theory that syringomyelia is a developmental disease.

Although there is no specific treatment for this condition, laminectomy is done if a cerebrospinal fluid block occurs, and the spinal cord cyst is opened and drained [3]. Nursing care is directed toward the prevention of burns or other kinds of injury and monitoring the patient carefully because of the insensitivity to pressure or pain. When the brainstem is affected, nursing measures include the provision of nutritional intake via artificial methods, suctioning to prevent aspiration, and alternative means of communication. As in all other degenerative conditions, the importance of psychological support cannot be overemphasized.

PARKINSON'S DISEASE

Parkinson's disease, also known as paralysis agitans or shaking palsy, is a progressive neuromuscular disease involving degenerative changes and dysfunction of the basal ganglia. It is a progressively debilitating disease and often leads to total dependence on others for care. It is estimated that there are more than half a million persons with the disease in the United States. Onset is usually between the ages of 50 and 60.

It has been determined that patients with Parkinson's disease have deficient amounts of a naturally occurring biogenic amine, dopamine, which is required for normal functioning of the basal ganglia. Dopamine is essential for the regulation of synaptic transmission of nerve impulses within the basal ganglia; the deficiency particularly occurs in the substantia nigra of the midbrain and the corpus striatum (the caudate and lentiform nuclei; page 896). Parkinsonian syndrome is a variation of the disease that is often associated with a history of previous encephalitis. A pseudoparkinsonian syndrome is associated with adverse effects of certain drugs, including the phenothiazines and *Rauwolfia* alkaloids such as reserpine.

Clinical Symptoms

The extrapyramidal system is affected in Parkinson's disease, resulting in difficulty in carrying out smooth and coordinated muscular activity, particularly affecting gross and automatic movements. The classic symptoms include tremor, rigidity, and akinesia (difficulty in starting movement) or bradykinesia (slowness in movement). The rhythmic tremor in Parkinson's disease is characteristically regular and rapid. It may be limited to the digits of the hand, with a characteristic pill-rolling movement of the fingers and thumbs, or it may involve the entire hand or limb. The tremor occurs at rest, tends to disappear temporarily when the limb or hand is moved voluntarily, but returns with persistent effort. The tremor is aggravated by emotional stress and fatigue but tends to disappear during sleep.

Rigidity causes postural changes; the trunk and head are flexed forward, so that the center of gravity is changed. The patient's gait is characteristically shuffling, with short steps and dragging of the feet. The reflex arm swing in walking is absent; the arms are adducted and semiflexed. Changes in position are difficult, as are turning and moving. (Initially, the rigidity characteristically is not accompanied by muscle atrophy or weakness.) The ability to write deteriorates, and the handwriting becomes shaky, smaller (micrographia), and illegible.

The patient typically has a masked facies, due to facial muscle rigidity. Rigidity of the mouth muscles results in dysarthria. The voice is muffled, and the patient speaks in an inexpressive nasal monotone; the ends of sentences fade into unintelligible muttering. Later, difficulty in mastication and swallowing may be experienced. The patient is also susceptible to respiratory complications because muscular rigidity hinders respiratory excursion and the ability to cough.

Disturbances in autonomic nervous system functioning are demonstrated by increased salivation (sialorrhea) and lacrimation, constipation, incontinence, and decreased sexual activity. Drooling often occurs because of poor control of the muscles of the mouth.

All these symptoms are distressing and socially embarrassing to both the patient and the family. Because the lack of affect in speech and problems of articulation interfere with communication, the patient often feels alone and alienated. Depression is common, and family relationships may be adversely affected. The patient's appearance may deteriorate because of inability to attend to activities of daily living.

Treatment

Medical treatment The discovery of the therapeutic effects of levodopa, the synthetic form of L-dopa, has made an important impact on the welfare of patients with Parkinson's disease. The drug has proved effective in relieving the symptoms of parkinsonism, particularly tremor and rigidity. In contrast to dopamine, which does not pass the blood-brain barrier, L-dopa, its metabolic precursor, readily passes the barrier. Levodopa (Dopar, Larodopa, Bendopa) is an oral preparation that is readily converted into dopamine after passing the blood-brain barrier. The dose of levodopa is gradually increased until the maximal response with the fewest side effects is achieved.

The response to the drug is variable, and there is a high incidence of adverse reactions. Its long-term effects are still unknown. The adverse reactions include nausea, vomiting, cardiac arrhythmias, constipation, increased blood urea nitrogen levels, postural hypotension, and agranulocytosis. The most common symptom associated with the drug is dyskinesia (abnormal involuntary movements) of the musculature of the tongue, jaw, and anterior neck, so that grimacing, lip smacking, tongue clicking, tongue protrusion, and rotary movements of the neck and shoulder may occur. The adverse reactions are usually dose-related. Psychological symptoms (agitation, delusions, insomnia, nightmares), and overt psychosis with hallucinations have been observed. An increased libido is a well-publicized side effect.

To prevent the onset of nausea and vomiting, levodopa should be taken with food or after meals. Antacids are often prescribed, and antiemetic agents may be necessary. The drug should not be given concomitantly with monoamine oxide inhibitors, which block the metabolism of dopamine, nor should they be given with phenothiazines. Large amounts of chocolate, wine, and aged cheese tend to neutralize the activity of the drug. Pyridoxine hydrochloride (vitamin B_6) may reverse the effects of levodopa and has been used to control side effects of the drug in some instances. Excessive dietary supplements of pyridoxine (as found in large doses of multiple-vitamin preparations) should be avoided. When the patient receives levodopa combined with a decarboxylase inhibitor, low pyridoxine diets and pyridoxine-free vitamin preparations are not necessary [18a]. Certain agents, such as alcohol, can antagonize the effects of levodopa.

Patients who are obese tend to have difficulty in dosage regulation; apparently, levodopa is absorbed into the fat depots and is released sporadically. Monitoring of the blood pressure with the patient in the supine and standing position is important to detect signs of postural hypotension. The use of elastic stockings and teaching the patient about avoiding rapid postural changes are important measures to prevent fainting and accidental falls.

Carbidopa-levodopa (Sinemet) is a new preparation that provides levodopa in combination with an inhibitor of the enzyme dopa decarboxylase, which limits the peripheral metabolism of levodopa. This action reduces the incidence of cardiac arrhythmias, nausea, vomiting, dizziness, and fainting associated with higher dosages of levodopa. Carbidopa reduces the amount of levodopa required; it does not, however, reverse the adverse reactions of levodopa on the central nervous system.

Other adjuvant drugs used in symptomatic treatment of Parkinson's disease include anticholinergics such as trihexyphenidyl hydrochloride (Artane), benztropine mesylate (Cogentrin), and procyclidine hydrochloride (Kemadrin). Biperiden hydrochloride (Akineton) is a synthetic anticholinergic agent also used in the treatment of mild Parkinson's disease. All these anticholinergic agents may cause blurred vision, dizziness, mouth and skin dryness, nausea, tachycardia, urine retention, and constipation.

Surgical treatment Although surgical treatment of Parkinson's disease has diminished since the advent of levodopa therapy, stereotactic surgery (destruction of areas controlling specific functions) is still performed on some patients as a means of controlling tremor. In this procedure, done under local anesthesia, a burr hole is made into the skull, and a cannula is inserted into the thalamus. Destruction of a well-defined area of tissue is accomplished with alcohol or with a freezing technique using liquid nitrogen. This technique is also called cryothalamectomy.

Nursing Care

Nursing care of the patient with Parkinson's disease focuses on maintaining muscular and joint function, so that the patient may remain as independent as possible. Physical therapy is indicated to provide moderate exercise. Because muscle rigidity prevents prompt regaining of balance, these patients often fall. They need supervision in ambulation, the use of ambulatory aids such as handrails, particularly in the bathroom and bathtub, and instruction in walking slowly and carefully. Although exercise is encouraged, there should be an adequate balance of rest and activity in order to avoid fatigue. Assistive devices may be necessary for the activities of daily living, and clothes should be simple and easy to put on. Sufficient time should be allowed for eating, and assistance should be given as needed.

The patient with severe disease must avoid the supine position because of the danger of aspiration of food or excess saliva. Adequate fluids, diets with adequate fibrous content, stool softeners, and mild laxatives are indicated to prevent constipation and fecal impaction. When patients are receiving anticholinergic drugs, oral hygiene is particularly important to relieve dryness of the mouth. Skin care and personal hygiene are important because of the increased perspiration, seborrhea, and sialorrhea in Parkinson's disease. Urinals and bedpans should be readily available, because the patient may be unable to get to the bathroom in time.

Both the patient and family require clear explanations of the symptoms of the disease and the drug therapy. Psychological support is essential to counteract the depression, discouragement, and hopelessness that are often associated with the disease. Family members and patients must understand the effects of levodopa, particularly the "on-and-off" characteristics of the drug effect after long-term use. Otherwise, they will not understand why the patient's ability to carry out activities varies during a single day.

Encouragement to continue appropriate activity is of paramount importance. Exercises are prescribed according to the degree of disability and the patient's tolerance. Speech therapy may also be necessary for some patients to correct problems of dysarthria.

HUNTINGTON'S DISEASE

Huntington's disease (Huntington's chorea) is a hereditary disease (autosomal dominant) that is characterized by degeneration of the basal ganglia and cerebral cortex. Usually, the age at onset is usually between 30 and 45, with death occurring within 10 to 15 years and following progressive weakness, pneumonia, or heart failure.

Clinical Symptoms and Management

The disease affects the extrapyramidal tract, resulting in abnormal involuntary movements and tremors. Initially, these abnormal movements may be minor and limited to rapid twitches of the fingers, but later they become jerking, twisting, and severe spasms of the muscles of the face, tongue, neck, trunk, and legs. Sudden flinging movements of the patient's limbs may result in injuries to other persons. These abnormal movements are also associated with progressive mental deterioration. Personality changes may be the first sign of the disease in some patients; irritability, carelessness in personal habits, and apathy are some of the changes encountered. The deterioration may become so severe that patients endanger themselves or others. Institutionalization is usually required in the late stages of the disease.

There is no specific treatment for the disease, but tranquilizers and sedatives are used to treat symptoms. The effects of the enzyme glutamic acid decarboxylase on the progress of Huntington's disease is now being studied as a possible treatment modality. The basis of the treatment is that a deficiency of the neurotransmitter gamma-aminobutyric acid (GABA), which is thought to inhibit neural excitation, is due to a decreased activity of this enzyme, which is a precursor of GABA and passes through the blood-brain barrier. Stereotactic surgery has also been tried for some patients with Huntington's disease to control abnormal movements, although the effects have only been temporary. Various biochemical tests are being studied for possible use in the detection of Huntington's disease before symptoms appear. Such a test would be a valuable aid to genetic counseling and control of the transmission of the disease.

Nursing care measures are oriented toward safety and maintenance of independent functioning as long as it is realistically possible. These patients tend to fall often, and their illogical thought processess often result in unpredictable and often hazardous behavior. Progressive loss of sensation also leads to susceptibility to burns and skin trauma.

The psychological effects of the disease are devastating. Fear of inheriting or transmitting the disease and fear of ostracism are ever-present in the families of patients with Huntington's disease. Because of personal experience with these problems, the wife of Arlo Guthrie, the famous folk singer and composer, helped to establish the Committee to Combat Huntington's Disease, a national voluntary organization. The Commission for the Control of Huntington's Disease and Its Consequences was officially established under the Health Revenue Sharing Act of 1975. Its purpose is to develop a comprehensive national plan for the control of the disease.

MYASTHENIA GRAVIS

Myasthenia gravis is a neuromuscular disease characterized by varying degrees of weakness and fatigue of voluntary striated muscles. It usually affects people between the ages of 20 and 40 and most often occurs in females. Males are generally affected at an older age.

Although, as previously mentioned, myasthenia gravis is not actually a degenerative disease, it resembles degenerative disease in its frequently insidious onset, its pattern of exacerbations, its effects on mobility and the ability to carry out normal activities, and its chronicity.

The site of the functional disturbance in myasthenia gravis is the neuromuscular junction. In muscle contraction, acetylcholine is normally released on neural stimulation and causes repolarization of the muscle membrane. Acetylcholine is partly broken down by cholinesterase, which permits the muscle membrane to repolarize in preparation for subsequent chemical activation and contraction. The defect in myasthenia gravis has been postulated to be a result of (1) impaired synthesis or storage of acetylcholine, or of (2) an insufficient amount of acetylcholine being released at the nerve ending, or of (3) the presence of an antiacetylcholine substance in the extracellular fluid, or of (4) a blockade at the motor end-plate, even in the presence of normal amounts of acetylcholine. Recent studies appear to confirm that the defect is predominantly postsynaptic, occurring in the motor end-plate, and is attributable to an abnormal response to acetylcholine, probably due to an autoimmune disturbance. Although the disease is not considered hereditary, genetic factors are also implicated. Infants of myasthenic mothers may be born with a transient form of the disease, and anticholinesterase drugs may be temporarily required by the neonate.

Clinical Symptoms and Management

The onset of symptoms is often insidious and may include any single symptom or a combination of the following: unilateral or bilateral ptosis; diplopia; blurred vision; general fatigue; limited physical activity; difficulty in chewing and breathing; dysphagia; and fatigued, slurred speech (often with a nasal quality). The muscles are characteristically strongest in the morning but become exhausted with continued effort. Weakness may range from slight reduction of strength on repeated use of involved muscle groups to severe motor failure. Weakness in the arms and hands, with difficulty in raising the arms overhead, is a frequent finding, and the person may complain of tiring from just combing the hair. Prompt recovery of strength, however, may occur with rest. Early symptoms may be vague and diagnosis is often delayed. Unless the physician suspects myasthenia gravis and does specific tests to diagnose the disease, the person in these stages may often be considered as having a psychoneurotic problem.

Symptoms are often aggravated by emotional upsets, alcoholic intake, lack of adequate rest, onset of menstruation, and respiratory infections. When the diaphragm and intercostal muscles are affected, respiratory difficulties may be severe, and the patient may be admitted to the hospital in a critical state. (The symptoms of restricted lung disease are discussed in Chapter 3.)

The diagnosis is made on the basis of a history and physical examination and electromyography. Pharmacologic testing with cholinergic drugs is used to confirm the diagnosis. Administration of a test dose of neostigmine (Prostigmin) or edrophonium (Tensilon) results in revival of the function of exhausted muscles within a few minutes. These drugs prolong the action of acetylcholine at the neuromuscular junction and increase muscle strength in myasthenia gravis. Edrophonium is usually preferred in diagnostic testing because it can be given intravenously and has a rapid action of brief duration. An anteroposterior chest x-ray and a tomogram are done to detect the presence of thymus enlargement or tumor (thyoma), which is often encountered in patients with myasthenia gravis. (The thymus gland is a mass of lymphoid tissue located posterior to the sternum and normally atrophies with adulthood.) A majority of patients with myasthenia have demonstrable thymic abnormalities. Although its exact role is not known, the thymus appears to play an important part in myasthenia gravis. It is thought that a substance in the thymus, thymopoietin, is produced in excess, leading to a characteristic neuromuscular block [16a]. Thymic venography is a recently developed procedure that permit visualization of the thymus and detection of tumors.

Treatment

Treatment of the patient is determined by the severity and course of the disease. In some persons, spontaneous remissions have occurred. Traditionally, the anticholinesterase drugs such as neostigmine, pyridostigmine bromide (Mestinon), or ambenonium (Mytelase) have been used to counteract the symptoms of fatigue and weakness. These drugs prevent the breakdown of acetylcholine by cholinesterase. The optimal maintenance dose is individually determined to provide therapeutic effects without causing the adverse side effects that result from increased acetylcholine activity at the parasympathetic postganglionic nerve endings. These adverse effects include bradycardia, increased peristalsis, urgency and frequency of urination, abdominal cramping, diarrhea, sweating, nausea, vomiting, miotic pupils, increased salivation, and bronchial mucus production. Atropine sulfate is used as an antidote for these symptoms.

Dosage requirements of the cholinergic medications change periodically, requiring that the nurse closely observe the patient for effects of the drug. It is the nurse's responsibility to instruct the patient and the family about medications so that complications will be prevented and optimal relief obtained. Marked overdosages *cause* rather than relieve weakness and may result in cholinergic crises with respiratory distress (due to inability to expectorate secretions and to muscle weakness).

Corticosteroids have been utilized for treatment of myasthenia gravis as a means of controlling the autoimmune process; in fact, it is felt by some authorities that corticosteroids may become the preferred treatment. Hospitalization is generally prescribed when such therapy is initiated, because there may be an initial worsening of the disease before improvement occurs. Increasingly, oral prednisone therapy on a single dose daily or on an alternate-day basis is being evaluated in the treatment of these patients.

Another approach to therapy that is under investigation is the use of germine monoacetate (GMA), a potent skeletal-muscle stimulant, which appears to benefit the patient without causing the toxic side effects associated with anticholinesterase drugs.

A major development in the control of the effects of myasthenia gravis is surgical removal of the thymus gland (thymectomy). When performed in the early stages of the disease, thymectomy has proved effective in bringing about early remission in a significant number of persons, with marked improvement in electromyographic findings. The operation is performed through either a sternum-splitting incision or a transcervical approach; the latter generally is preferred because it is associated with less morbidity. In the majority of patients who have had thymectomies, the excised thymus gland demonstrates central clear areas, called germinal centers, within the densely packed cells of the cortex. Improvement after thymectomy generally occurs gradually over a period of years rather than immediately after the operation. Therefore, the results of the surgery are not immediately apparent. The patient who is hopeful of immediate benefits must be supported psychologically during the lengthy recovery period.

Nursing Care

The nurse must reinforce the importance of continued follow-up and monitoring of the effects of medications. The patient's status may change for a variety of reasons, requiring adjustment of dosages in order to prevent complications. The patient should carry a Medic-Alert identification card or wear a Medic-Alert bracelet to facilitate proper management in case of accidents or crisis states. Substances that act on the neuromuscular junction should not be taken by or administered to a person with myasthenia gravis. These substances include morphine, barbiturates, tranquilizers, ether, curare, strong cathartics, quinine (including tonic drinks), and antibiotics such as streptomycin and neomycin. Careful observation is necessary when quinidine sulfate or procainamide (Pronestyl) is required for cardiac disease because of the effects of these agents on the membrane potential and their possible accentuation of the symptoms of myasthenia gravis. If diuretics are required for other medical conditions, they must be given with caution. The potassium-depleting effect of diuretics may cause hypokalemia and increase muscle weakness.

The patient should be instructed to have adequate rest and avoid excessive physical activity and emotional stress, which predispose to exacerbations of the disease. Prevention of infections is important, since they also exacerbate symptoms.

When a crisis state arises, with exacerbation of respiratory insufficiency, the patient must have emergency care. Respiratory support, using a positive-pressure machine or a volume respirator, is required. Endotracheal intubation or a tracheostomy may be indicated for prevention of airway obstruction. During this time, cholinergic medications are usually reduced to diminish pulmonary secretions. Fatal outcomes in myasthenia gravis are usually due to pulmonary complications such as pneumonia and to respiratory failure.

It is important to remember that when a myasthenic patient is admitted to the hospital with respiratory difficulty, it may be hard to determine whether the problem is an exacerbation of the myasthenic state (myasthenic crisis) or the symptoms are related to an overdose of the cholinergic medication (cholinergic crisis). Administration of edrophonium may be necessary to differentiate the cause of the crisis; the patient improves if the crisis is myasthenic rather than cholinergic. Regardless of the cause, mechanical respiratory support and maintenance of a patent airway are priority measures. Once respiratory problems are controlled, the patient is slowly returned to increased activity.

Nursing care of the myasthenic patient requires monitoring vital capacity and the strength of affected muscles as a means of determining the schedule that will allow the patient to function maximally. Family members should be taught how to monitor the patient's strength and respiratory status and observe the patient's tolerance. They also should be informed about signs and symptoms of crisis states, and be involved in devising measures to avoid stressful situations for the patient.

If dysphagia is present, provisions for adequate fluid and nutritional intake may initially require the use of nasogastric feedings. When the patient begins eating, supervision and assistance are necessary. The patient is often reluctant to eat because of the fear of choking. Medications to control myasthenia gravis symptoms are usually given before meals to facilitate the muscular activity required for swallowing and chewing. Medications must be given precisely as ordered to ensure continuous effects and to prevent the recurrence of symptoms. Diet modifications, using soft, strained, or blenderized foods, may be necessary when dysphagia and chewing difficulties are present.

When the patient is discharged from the hospital, the family needs assistance in learning to manage his home care. Special equipment, such as a hand respirator (for example, an Ambu bag), a suction machine, and plastic oral airways, is often required to handle any potential respiratory emergencies that might occur in the home. The patient and family must be thoroughly prepared in how to use this equipment. Referral to public health agencies is indicated to assist patients and their families in adapting to home care. The medications may be extremely expensive, and some chapters of the Myasthenia Gravis Foundation and certain myasthenia gravis clinics provide them at a reduced rate. In addition, the Myasthenia Gravis Foundation, a national voluntary agency, supports research in myasthenia and provides educational materials for both professionals and lay persons.

Neuropathies

Although disorders of the cranial nerves are often secondary to other diseases, a few are primary disorders of specific nerves. Trigeminal neuralgia and Bell's palsy are two examples. Peripheral nerve dysfunction may result from neoplasms or direct local trauma (such as pressure, infection, and severance) or may be secondary to systemic conditions such as malnutrition, chemical poisoning, or alcoholism.

TRIGEMINAL NEURALGIA

Trigeminal neuralgia (tic douloureux) is characterized by excruciating, unpredictable, and paroxysmal pain along the distribution of one or more divisions of the trigeminal nerve (fifth cranial). This nerve has both sensory and motor fibers and has three main divisions: the ophthalmic, with fibers distributed to the anterior part of the scalp, the forehead, eye, and nose; the maxillary, which supplies the skin of the cheek, upper lip, upper jaw and teeth, and palate; and the mandibular division which has sensory fibers that carry impulses from the lower lip, chin, lower jaw, teeth, and the tongue. The mandibular division also has motor fibers which innervate the muscles of mastication. The mandibular branch is most often affected in trigeminal neuralgia.

Trigeminal neuralgia usually occurs in the fourth to sixth decade and occurs more often in women. The cause is unknown; sometimes infections of the sinuses, teeth, and mouth are aggravating factors. The pain may occur spontaneously or may be initiated (or aggravated) by facial movements, such as those involved in eating, talking, brushing the teeth, shaving, and washing the face. Emotional excitement or exposure to a draft may also be precipitating factors.

Clinical Symptoms

Twitching, grimacing, frequent blinking, and tearing are often observed during an attack of intense pain. The pain is described as a stabbing or burning pain and usually lasts only seconds to 2 or 3 minutes. However, the pain is so intolerable that the patients often try to avoid anything that may bring it on, even to the point of not washing and not eating properly. Social isolation is often preferred by the patient.

Treatment and Nursing Care

Medical therapy includes the use of phenytoin sodium (the anticonvulsant agent), tranquilizers, analgesics, and cyanocobalamin (vitamin B_{12}). Recently, carbamazepine has proved to be effective in the control of trigeminal neuralgia. However, serious side effects, such as aplastic anemia, agranulocytosis, thrombocytopenia, and leukemia, have occurred with carbamazepine administration. Alcohol blocks have also been used to provide temporary pain relief.

Surgical sectioning of the sensory nerve roots of the affected divisions of the nerve (retrogasserian rhizotomy) has also been done. Surgical sectioning of the nerve results in some permanent effects that must be clearly understood by the patient preoperatively. These effects are loss of sensation, numbness, stiffness, and heaviness along the distribution of the nerve. Problems with mastication may result due to trauma to the motor fibers of the mandibular nerve; trauma to the facial (seventh cranial) nerve may cause temporary facial paralysis. Care must be taken postoperatively when the patient begins to eat. The patient is advised to place the food in the unaffected side of the mouth and to avoid hot foods, because the affected area is not sensitive to heat. Oral hygiene is very important, particularly because food particles may accumulate on the desensitized size. Regular dental checkups should be emphasized, because the patient cannot feel the pain that indicates a dental problem. If the ophthalmic division of the trigeminal nerve is sectioned, the conjunctiva and cornea become insensitive to foreign particles and injury. Therefore, the eye must be examined regularly to detect any redness or irritation. Irrigations of the eyes are usually required, and the patient must remember to close the eyelid often to keep the surface lubricated. Glasses are worn to protect the eyes.

A recent development, which does not require major surgery, is radio-frequency retrogasserian rhizotomy. This procedure involves threading an electrode through the cheek into the foramen ovale and advancing it to the gasserian ganglion and the rootlets behind it, where a lesion is made with the radio-frequency current [24]. The procedure can be done under local anesthesia. The use of implanted electrodes to block pain impulses have also been investigated; radio-frequency impulses are initiated to block the pain impulses.

Patients who have recurrent trigeminal neuralgia must be advised to avoid the stimuli that are likely to precipitate an attack of severe pain, such as drafts and exposure to cold and hot or cold foods. Pureed food may be necessary if chewing solid food aggravates the pain. Mouth care must be encouraged, even though the patient is frequently tempted to avoid it for fear of precipitating pain. Personal hygiene and grooming are encouraged, and suggestions are made on ways to eliminate movements that might initiate pain. Above all, the patient needs consideration and understanding during the periods of intense pain and when limiting activity because of anxiety about the recurrence of pain.

BELL'S PALSY

Bell's palsy results from dysfunction of the facial (seventh cranial) nerve, which has both motor and sensory components. The condition is characterized by a loss of the ability to move the muscles on one side of the face. The cause is unknown, although viral infections, exposure to drafts, occlusion of the blood supply to the nerve, and compression of the nerve fibers by edema associated with inflammation have all been implicated.

Clinical Symptoms

Some patients experience pain posterior to the ear for a day or two before one side of the face becomes paralyzed. The affected side becomes flaccid, and the patient is unable to whistle, or drink through a straw, or eat on the affected side. The mouth is drawn to the unaffected side, and drooling occurs. The patient is unable to wrinkle the brow; the eyelid on the affected side does not close, and the eyeball rolls upward if the patient attempts to close the eyelid. Frequently, there is increased lacrimation. In addition to these motor changes, taste sensation is lost over the anterior two-thirds of the tongue on the affected side. The distorted facial expression and speech difficulties interfere with social relationships, and social isolation may result as the patient avoids awkward situations.

Treatment and Nursing Care

The patient is advised to protect the head from exposure to cold and drafts because these aggravate symptoms. Passive exercises of the facial muscles, moist cloths applied to the affected side of the face, and gentle massage are all measures to improve muscle tone and prevent facial muscle atrophy. The affected muscles usually begin to regain tone within a few weeks, and progressive improvement occurs over a period of months. Active exercises, such as forced closing of the eye, wrinkling of the forehead, pursing of lips, blowing out the cheeks, and attempting to whistle, are prescribed as recovery of muscle tone occurs. In some patients, there may be some residual deficit or even permanent paralysis if nerve degeneration has occurred.

The patient is advised to maintain good nutrition and to chew the food on the unaffected side of the mouth. Residual food may accumulate in the affected side of the mouth, resulting in sores and parotitis unless adequate oral hygiene measures are carried out.

Because the blinking reflex is lost in Bell's palsy, special efforts must be made to protect the cornea of the affected eye and prevent keratitis (corneal inflammation). The eye must be kept moist and free from dust and dirt. Sunglasses are indicated to protect the eye; an eyepatch may be worn at night on the affected eye. Artificial tear solution is instilled in the eye several times a day. The patient is also instructed to close the eyelid periodically to relieve eyestrain and promote ocular moisture.

Electrical stimulation to the face is often prescribed to stimulate return of function. Analgesics are given to relieve discomfort, and corticosteroids are sometimes prescribed to minimize nerve tissue inflammation and trauma. Spontaneous recovery may occur within three to five weeks, although some patients may not recover for 6 to 12 months. If complete facial paralysis results, the tone of the facial musculature may be restored via anastomosis of the peripheral end of the facial nerve with the accessory or hypoglossal nerve.

NEOPLASMS OF THE PERIPHERAL NERVES

Neurilemmoma, a common type of peripheral nerve tumor, is almost always benign and most often develops along the nerve roots and large peripheral nerves.

Neurofibroma is a benign neoplasm that occurs subcutaneously or along peripheral nerves. A variation of neurofibroma is multiple neurofibromatosis (Recklinghausen's disease), a rare familial disease in which hundreds of subcutaneous neurofibromas develop, along with lesions in the central nervous system and peripheral nerves. This disease presents with a variety of symptoms, depending on the sites of involvement.

POLYNEURITIS (PERIPHERAL NEURITIS)

Polyneuritis is the dysfunction of peripheral nerves, associated with pain but not with inflammation. Dysfunction is usually symmetrical and involves both sensory and motor disturbances. Vitamin B deficiencies, malnutrition, alcoholism (discussed previously), chemical poisoning, and prolonged gastrointestinal disease have all been implicated in polyneuritis. It is also associated with diabetes mellitus and peripheral vascular disease. Symptoms of pain, tingling, and weakness in the hands and feet and the inability to perform fine movements are frequently experienced by the patient. The involved areas are tender to light touch, and there may be a progressive loss of sensation, with diminished tendon reflexes.

Treatment focuses on controlling the underlying cause. Vitamin B complex is usually administered and a nutritious diet is provided. A cradle is often necessary to protect the feet and legs from the weight of the bedding. The patient generally tries not to move the affected extremities, but limbs are gently moved through range of motion to prevent contractures. Gentle massage may also be helpful. Analgesics are administered to control acute pain. Heat therapy may be prescribed but must be used carefully because of the danger of burns to desensitized areas of the body.

Alcoholic polyneuritis is caused by a nutritional deficiency which is secondary to prolonged and excessive alcoholic intake. It is a slowly progressive chronic disease and has an affinity for the extremities with pain, paresthesia, muscle tenderness, and sensory and motor loss. It is treated by controlling alcoholic intake and correcting any nutritional deficiency. Prevention of residual disabilities such as foot drop and wrist drop is a major aspect of nursing care in this type of peripheral neuritis.

SPINAL CORD INJURIES

Spinal cord damage, with its resultant motor and sensory neurologic deficits, is most often caused by trauma. Spinal injuries include injuries to the bones and joints with associated trauma to the spinal cord. The usual causes are vehicular and diving accidents, falls, and bullet wounds. Less often, spinal cord disease is caused by tumors within the spinal cord or tumors outside the cord that compress it, congenital defects such as spina bifida aperta, infectious and degenerative diseases, and ruptured intervertebral discs.

Spinal cord injuries are of four types: (1) concussion without direct trauma (mechanical compression) to the cord; (2) compression, contusion, or laceration of the cord substance by penetrating wounds or fracture dislocation; (3) hemorrhage into the cord substance; and (4) compression of the blood supply to the cord [22b]. Any interruption of the ascending tracts causes loss of sensation below the site of injury. Interruption of the descending tracts results in paralysis of the body parts that derive innervation from the cord below the level of the lesion. Consequently, the autonomic nervous system is also disrupted in spinal cord injuries. Transections of the spinal cord are described as either partial or complete.

The phases of care in spinal cord injury are usually described as follows: (1) the emergency phase; (2) the bed phase, or the period during which the patient's condition stabilizes; (3) the transfer and wheelchair phase; (4) the period for bracing, crutching, and ambulation for certain patients; (5) the vocational rehabilitation phase; and (6) the return to the community. The period from the emergency phase to the return to the community may take anywhere from 12 to 18 months or longer, depending on the patient's level of injury and remaining abilities and the presence of any complicating situations.

It is estimated that from 10,000 to 12,000 persons, most often in the younger age group, sustain spinal cord injuries annually. Most of the progress made in spinal cord injury management has been in rehabilitation rather than in correcting the defect. Currently, research efforts are focusing on reversing the effects of the spinal cord injury itself. It has been thought that the hemorrhagic destruction of tissue in the spinal cord is caused by bleeding that occurs immediately after the trauma. However, experimental studies have shown that hemorrhage may not occur for a number of hours after injury. This delay is now considered to be due to an increase in the concentration of norepinephrine (or a closely related substance) in the injured area of the cord, which results in constriction of blood vessels to the cord. Osterholm [23] has used injections of alpha-methyltyrosine in experimental animals to interfere with the synthesis of norepinephrine and to combat the loss of circulation and tissue destruction. The effects of catecholamines in the production of some of the functional and anatomic abnormalities from spinal cord trauma are now being studied in national spinal cord injury centers. This new focus of research efforts may ultimately provide new methods for the treatment of spinal cord injuries.

Emergency Care

A major aspect of the care of persons with spinal cord injuries relates to the prevention of complications. Even in the early period of injury, care is given that emphasizes maintenance of vital functions and prevention of respiratory and circulatory failure and further trauma to the spinal cord. Proper handling of the person who has had a spinal cord injury must start at the time of injury, before the person is moved for the first time.

When a person has been involved in an accident or has fallen, is unable to move the extremities, and complains of a loss of sensation in the limbs and trunk, a spinal cord injury should be suspected and precautions taken to prevent further damage to the cord.

Although maintenance of respiratory and cardiovascular function takes precedence, avoiding flexion or hyperextension of the neck and spinal column is essential; even lifting the patient's head is contraindicated unless it is absolutely necessary for establishing a patent airway. It is better not to move the patient than to move him hurriedly and possibly cause additional injury. The injured person should be on a firm, level surface such as a stretcher, wide, flat board, or even a door, and no pillow should be used under the head. Manual support to the head, or sandbags at the side of the head, is essential to prevent turning of the head or flexion of the neck. The patient is moved very carefully by at least three to four persons but preferably by six. When the patient is being moved, the head, neck, back, and legs should be supported to maintain good alignment at all times. There should be no bouncing or jostling of the patient during transport. A reversible spinal cord lesion may be changed to an irreversible lesion merely by a single twisting or flexion of the spine.

When possible, the patient should be transported to a special trauma unit. However, initial evaluation may have to be done in a general hospital setting, prior to air transportation to a special center. When the patient arrives at the hospital, he or she is moved as little as possible. If x-ray films are made precautions are taken not to bend the patient's back or neck, since loose fragments of the vertebrae might be dislodged and cause further injury to the cord.

In cervical cord injury, careful assessment of respiratory function takes precedence over other measures. The cord-injured patient is dependent on the diaphragm and accessory muscles for respiratory ventilation. Diminished vital capacity in the cervical cord injuries leads to susceptibility to pneumonia. Tracheostomy, endotracheal intubation, and suctioning are necessary; assisted mechanical ventilation is necessary for high cervical injuries.

If cervical fracture has occurred, skeletal traction with skull tongs (such as Crutchfield or Vinke tongs) (see Chap. 10) is used to reduce the fracture and prevent trauma to the cord. Although the patient may be cared for in a fracture bed, he is usually placed on a turning frame, such as the CircOlectric bed or else a Wedge turning frame may be used. The frame makes it possible to maintain traction and immobilization while adhering to the turning schedule; position changes are necessary to prevent skin breakdown. A laminectomy may be performed in the early post-trauma period to relieve compression of the cord, remove bony fragments from the injury site, and reduce the fracture.

Any motion is contraindicated in cervical cord injuries until skull tongs have been applied to the parietal or temporal bones. The patient is placed in a regular bed and skull tongs applied if cervical injury is present. In fractures below the cervical level, the patient may also be cared for in a regular bed, but the patient is limited to the supine position. When turned, the patient must be turned carefully by a log-rolling technique and using a turning sheet to prevent flexion and further damage. This technique requires at least two persons to perform it adequately to assure proper support and good alignment.

Spinal Shock

Immediately after acute spinal cord injury, the syndrome of spinal shock occurs; it does not occur in progressive spinal cord lesions. Spinal shock may last from several days to many weeks with an average of 2 to 3 months. It results in flaccid paralysis and complete loss of all sensation and of both somatic and visceral reflexes. (In lifting an extremity with flaccid paralysis, it falls quickly when released.) Most of the autonomic control over internal structures is lost as a result of the cessation of all sympathetic activity directed to the periphery. This results in vascular dilatation and hypotension as a result of the loss of the sympathetic influence on the blood vessels. In contrast to patients with other types of shock, the person in spinal shock has a slow, steady pulse and warm, dry skin. There is no vasomotor control or neurogenic sweating stimulus; the patient with a spinal cord injury does not perspire below the level of injury. This loss of the normal cooling mechanism results in an inadequate thermal regulation, the loss of ability to lose body heat, and frequent febrile episodes. The environment should therefore be kept cool and coverings minimal. Cool or tepid sponging is often necessary, and excessive exposure to cold must also be avoided.

Other reflex activities that are temporarily (and in some cases permanently) lost are those involved in bladder, bowel and sexual function. The patient should be observed for paralytic ileus and urine retention. An indwelling catheter is inserted to prevent bladder distention.

It is not possible to determine the extent of the spinal cord injury until spinal shock subsides. If the function of the spinal segmental reflexes is restored after the spinal shock period ceases, many of the reflex activities will return, at least partially.

Pain and Muscle Spasms

Pain associated with cord injuries can usually be controlled with mild analgesics, such as aspirin compounds and codeine. Analgesics such as morphine sulfate are contraindicated, especially in cervical lesions, because of their depressive effect on respiratory function. Often, pain is increased because of anxiety and fears related to the injury and its implications, and sedatives and tranquilizers may be indicated. Patients often suffer from constant burning pain or from muscle spasm, particularly those with incomplete severance of the cord. The spasms are aggravated by various factors such as bladder stones, jarring of the bed or wheelchair, sitting for long periods, tension, and anxiety. The nurse has a role in helping the patient identify those factors which promote spasms and in helping to control these factors. Muscle relaxants may be prescribed to control muscle spasm. When spasms are severe and interfere with performance of activities of daily living, control may be achieved by various procedures, such as selective nerve blocks or surgical sectioning of specific nerves.

Edema

The feet and ankles of the patient with spinal cord injuries often become edematous due to the lack of muscle action in the legs and poor vascular tone. Elastic stockings, body corsets, or abdominal binders may be necessary to prevent pooling of blood in the abdomen and legs. Elevation of the extremities at regular intervals also helps combat this problem.

Positioning

Correct positioning of the body is essential to prevent contractures or deformities. External rotation of the legs, for example, is prevented by placing rolls from the hip to the knees. Foot drop is prevented by use of a foot board. Passive range-of-motion exercises for all joints are important to prevent contractures, which limit independence, interfere with mobility, and cause pain.

Nutrition

A high-calorie, high-protein diet is essential; tube feedings are utilized if the patient is unable or unwilling to eat. If skin integrity is disrupted and decubiti are present, the need for protein increases. A high-protein diet will also combat the tendency for some patients with spinal cord injuries to gain weight because of decreased activity. Excessive weight creates difficulties in mobility later. Low-calcium and low-cholesterol diets are also often prescribed. Citrus fruits are avoided because they tend to produce alkaline urine, which makes the patient prone to calculi and infection.

Psychological Needs

The person who has suffered a cord injury requires extensive emotional support as the reality of the injury becomes evident. The assurance of prompt attention to all the patient's needs promotes emotional security. Regular and frequent measurement of vital signs, neurologic status, and motor and sensory function is necessary. Initially, care is centered on patient survival. But when the patient becomes aware of the paralysis and other symptoms that indicate the permanence and extent of the disability, the nurse must provide support in the grieving process. The threat to the patient's body image and integrity is exceedingly difficult to cope with, and the patient responds by denial, anger, hostility, and depression. For some persons, the period of adjustment is lengthy.

The importance of being truthful with the patient in the acute phases of adjustment cannot be overemphasized. However, as stated previously, the exact amount of disability that will result cannot be predicted immediately unless a laminectomy has been done, and surgical exploration confirms that the cord has been completely transected. Besides spinal shock, which masks the actual extent of the injury, edema at the injury site may temporarily cause symptoms suggesting complete transection of the cord.

Brown-Séquard syndrome The Brown-Séquard syndrome is a unique syndrome that occurs with transverse hemisection of the spinal cord, resulting in paralysis on the side of the lesion. Since the sensory fibers for pain and temperature cross in the spinal cord and travel on the opposite side in the spinothalamic tract, this kind of injury results in loss of pain and temperature sensation below the level of the lesion and contralateral to the transected side. Sensory fibers for light touch and position travel up the cord on the same side; thus, there is a loss of these sensations on the side of the lesion. There is also a loss of autonomic function on the ipsilateral side. These varied symptoms in different parts of the body confuse the patient and cause considerable anxiety. Therefore, the reasons for them should be carefully explained.

Autonomic Hyperreflexia

Autonomic hyperreflexia (or autonomic dysreflexia) is a unique complication in which there are exaggerated autonomic responses to stimuli. It occurs in patients with cervical or high thoracic spinal cord lesions (above the seventh thoracic level) and is a medical emergency that can lead to cerebral hemorrhage and death unless emergency measures are taken. Various precipitating factors are recognized, the most common ones being bladder and bowel distention or manipulation, pressure sores, digital stimulation, and enemas. Other causes are pressure on the penis or testis and stimulation of the pain receptors.

The symptoms of autonomic hyperreflexia include the following: pounding headache and blurred vision; severe hypertension, with a rapid rise in both systolic and diastolic pressure (systolic pressure may rise as high as 300 mm Hg in some patients); and severe diaphoresis above the level of the spinal injury. Restlessness, a flushed face, cutis anserina (gooseflesh), nausea, bradycardia, and nasal congestion are other symptoms. These symptoms reflect exaggerated autonomic reflexes to stimulation of the pelvic and presacral nerves to the spinal cord. These reflexes are uncontrolled by higher autonomic centers because of the level of the lesion in the spinal cord.

When these symptoms occur, the nurse should immediately elevate the head of the bed or place the patient in a sitting position to lower the blood pressure and prevent a cerebrovascular accident. (Quadriplegic patients usually have a lowered blood pressure in the sitting position.) The nurse should immediately check for bladder distention, a plugged catheter, or other precipitating stimulus, so that the problem can be corrected. If the catheter is plugged, it should be irrigated with a small amount of fluid (50 ml or less). The patient with a distended bladder should be catheterized, if no catheter is in place. If bladder distention is not the cause, the nurse should look for other sources of sympathetic stimulation, such as cold air, drafts, or sharp objects on the patient's skin, which should be corrected or removed. However, if the cause is fecal impaction, attempts to remove it may cause more sympathetic stimulation and further increase the blood pressure; thus, local anesthetic ointment is often inserted into the rectum prior to manual evacuation to prevent excessive sensory stimulation, and manual removal is delayed until symptoms have subsided.

If emergency nursing measures do not relieve symptoms, the physician is notified and ganglionic blocking agents are given intravenously or atropine sulfate is administered. Diazoxide (Hyperstat) or hydralazine (Apresoline) may be used in these emergencies. The use of these agents requires close monitoring of the blood pressure to prevent hypotensive reactions to the drugs. Antidotes to treat hypotension, such as metaraminol bitartrate (Aramine), should be available.

Measures are then taken to control the factors that precipitate episodes of autonomic hyperreflexia because, once such an episode occurs, it may be repeated. Patients and their families must be taught to recognize the symptoms and how to implement control and emergency measures. When these episodes are chronic, adrenergic blocking agents such as phenoxybenzamine (Dibenzyline) or an agent such as guanethidine sulfate (Ismelin) are used prophylactically. For some patients who have frequent episodes of autonomic hyperreflexia, surgical procedures such as pelvic or pudendal nerve sectioning or posterior rhizotomy (division of spinal nerve roots) may be necessary.

Effect of Level of Injury on Function

Because of the difference in the level of the vertebral bodies and the segments of the spinal cord, the vertebral level of injury does not coincide with the level of spinal cord injury. The spinal cord shortens, relative to the bony spinal canal; 31 spinal segments lie within 21 vertebrae. It is the level of the cord injury, not the level of the bone injury, that determines the extent of damage and the prognosis. (Paraplegia is paralysis of the legs and quadriplegia is paralysis of all four limbs.)

The most important factor in determining the eventual functional potential of the patient with a spinal cord injury is the distribution of muscle power remaining (assuming that there is an absence of other medical complications). This can be determined if the level of the lesion is known. However, regardless of the level of the lesion, complications such as spasm, decubiti, insufficient motivation, deformities, contractures, and urinary infection or incontinence will interfere with maximal use of remaining muscle power. In addition, age and degree of tolerance account for differences in abilities among different patients with lesions at the same level.

Spinal cord injuries at the C-4 level and above have usually been considered incompatible with life because of the resulting respiratory failure. However, emergency services that provide immediate respiratory support have saved the lives of patients with C-3 and C-4 lesions. However, these patients do not have any potential for self-care. Recently, electrophrenic stimulation, using two phrenic-nerve pacemakers implanted in the chest wall, have been developed to eliminate the need for prolonged use of respirators for patients with high cervical injuries.

The patient with a lesion just below the C-5 segment has full innervation of the trapezius, and sternocleidomastoid muscles and the upper cervical paraspinal musculature [20]. Thus, the patient is able to stabilize and rotate the neck and to elevate and rotate the scapulae. However, there is no muscular function in the wrist or hand, and the patient is thus unable to use the hands; some patients are able to use special hand devices to assist them in eating. A low respiratory reserve causes limited endurance, and the patient with an injury in this location cannot ambulate or push a wheelchair. No self-care activities are possible, and the patient must depend on others. However, some exceptional patients have learned to use their mouths and teeth for such activities as painting.

The patient with a C-6 level injury has fully innervated shoulder rotator muscles and partial innervation of the serratus, latisimus dorsi, and pectoralis major muscles. Wrist muscles have innervation, and the biceps are also innervated, allowing for elbow and wrist flexion. Although these patients can grasp some large but light objects, they need wrist devices to grasp most objects. They are also able to roll over in bed because the shoulder muscles are innervated. Although these patients have some partial lifting capacity, they cannot lift themselves into or out of a wheelchair without help. Sometimes it is possible for the C-6 quadriplegic to self-propel a lightweight wheelchair and to transfer it in and out of the car independently [35]. Assistance is also needed in toileting and dressing, although the patient may be able to feed himself with specific hand devices.

Some patients with lesions at the C-6 level have been successfully trained to gain independence with a minimum of adaptive devices other than a raised toilet seat, urinary collection equipment, automobile hand controls, and a lightweight wheelchair. Trigiano [35] states that an intact C-6 level is the division point between permanent dependence and the potential for independence. He has found that with an intact deltoid-rotator-pectoral mechanism, the patient with a C-6 lesion can use the biceps, brachioradialis, and radial extensors to assist in using the upper extremity for weight bearing, thus increasing the ability to transfer.

When the C-7 segment of the spinal cord is intact, the patient has function in three additional muscles, the triceps, the common finger extensors, and long finger extensors. The presence of triceps function facilitates the lifting of the body by enabling stabilization of the elbow in extension. Although the finger extensors and flexors are functional, they are not strong, and extension dexterity is not present. These patients can roll over, sit up in bed, and move about in the sitting position. They need some assistance in transferring to the wheelchair but do not have to be lifted into the chair. Although eating can be done independently without assistive devices, some assistance is still required for toileting and dressing. This patient, if trained, is able to do bookkeeping, mimeographing, and typing; use office machines; and perform telephone services. These must be done in the home situation, unless there is adequate transportation service to an office [20].

The patient with a T-1 injury has full innervation of the upper extremity musculature, including the essential intrinsic muscles of the hand. Therefore, this patient can be independent in bed and transfer activities. Except for lifting the body while recumbent (which is necessary for putting on trousers), the patient is generally independent in self-care activities. Such a patient, however, does not have trunk stability, so that full-body bracing is necessary. Ambulation is not functional but is often prescribed for exercise purposes [20]. Many sedentary jobs are possible for such a patient if transportation can be provided. Although the patient can readily transfer, help is needed to lift the wheelchair in and out of the car.

The patient with a T-6 injury has innervation of all the upper extremity and thoracic muscles, with respiratory reserve being enhanced by intercostal innervation. Such a patient therefore can be wheelchair-independent in all phases of self-care. Bilateral long-leg bracing permits ambulation, but ambulation is slow and taxing. Thus, except for those who have good balance and coordination and very strong upper extremities, patients with a T-6 injury are limited in their ability to ambulate. However, they are usually able to drive a hand-controlled car, and some can lift their wheelchairs in and out of the car.

Patients with T-12 lesions are increasingly independent, even in ambulation with bilateral long-leg braces and crutches. Such patients may not require a wheelchair for daytime activities if adequately braced but often use it for convenience [20].

The patient with a low lumbar or sacral lesion can, with minimal bracing, be completely independent in all activities, because full upper extremity and trunk strength, hip flexors and extensors, knee extensors, and ankle control are intact.

NURSING CARE IN SPINAL CORD INJURY

Nursing care during the early period after spinal cord injury involves the management of any life-threatening events and controlling symptoms of spinal shock. It also centers on prevention of such complications as further cord injury and pressure sores, provision of nutritional intake, the control of pain, bladder and bowel care, and meeting psychological needs. Some of these activities are facilitated by the use of the CircOlectric bed and other turning frames.

Positioning and Turning

The CircOlectric bed provides for vertical rather than lateral turning by means of electrical power that turns the entire frame on which the patient lies (Fig. 11-15). The patient can be turned into a variety of positions from the supine to the prone, as well as to an erect position later in the recovery phase, depending on his tolerance. The bed also facilitates bowel management, since a circular removable section in the mattress permits the patient to use the bedpan without being moved or lifted. The bed has a footboard, so that footdrop can be prevented. Changes in the patient's position are made by pressing a switch until the desired position is reached. Straps are attached, so that the patient feels and is secure and is maintained in good body alignment. It is recommended that the bed be unplugged from the wall except when being turned. Otherwise, personnel can accidentally bump into the switch, jolting the patient and causing further injury.

Before the patient is turned to the prone position, an anterior frame is placed over the

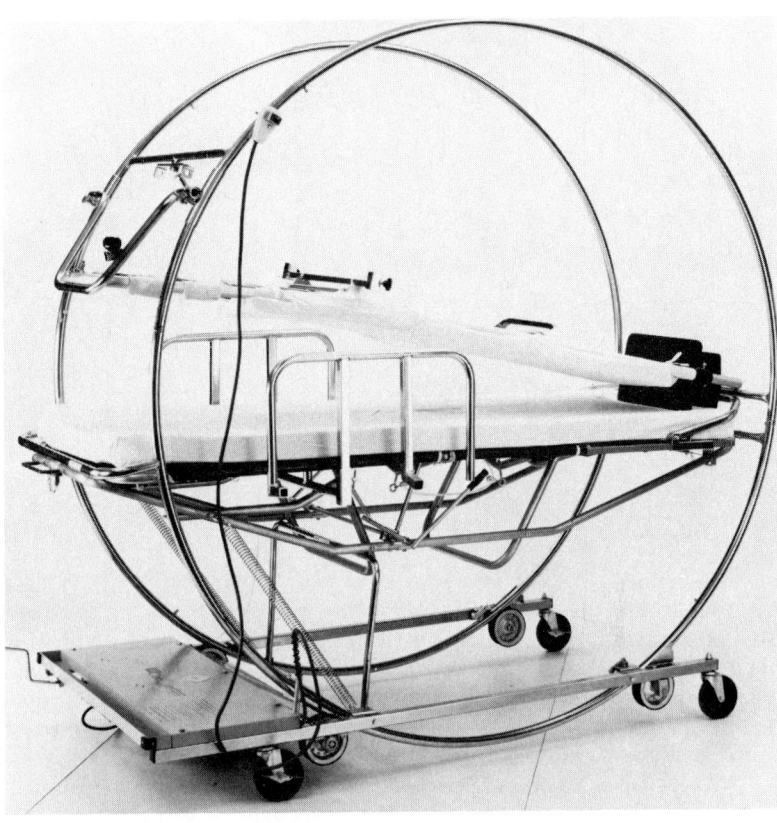

Figure 11-15
CircOlectric bed. (Courtesy Stryker Corporation, Kalamazoo, Michigan.)

patient and fastened securely by tightening the lock nuts at the head and foot of the frame. The forehead and chin straps are adjusted, and the patient's arms are slipped into slings, so that the patient literally hugs the anterior frame while being turned. When first turned into the prone position, the patient must be observed carefully. Initially, physiologic adjustments may not be made readily, and the patient may lose consciousness on being placed into an erect position. The procedure for turning should be explained to the patient before it is started, and the turning should be done in a confident and smooth manner; turning is frightening and the patient is usually apprehensive, until he or she becomes accustomed to the personnel and the equipment. The patient should also be forewarned about a possible light-headed feeling and tingling sensations in the legs and feet.

When the patient is placed in the prone position, the posterior frame is released and pushed upward. It is locked into position on an overhead metal bar over the patient, so that treatments and back care can be given. Bands of canvas are used to support the patient's forehead and chin. In the prone position, the patient can read, eat, write, and perform other activities (assuming that the muscles to carry out these functions are still intact). Another advantage of the CircOlectric bed is that the frame is on wheels, so that it can easily be moved anywhere within the hospital when necessary.

Other turning frames, such as the Stryker frame, the Wedge turning frame, or the Foster frame, function on the same basis as the CircOlectric bed, except that they are manually operated and permit only the supine or the prone position. The Wedge turning frame has the advantage of requiring only one nurse to turn the patient easily on the frame (Fig. 11-16). If possible, turning schedules with any of the turning frames should be planned with the patient. The nurse should take into consideration the patient's activities during the day. For example, the patient should be turned for correct positioning to coincide with the meals and with bowel, bladder, and therapy schedules. It is

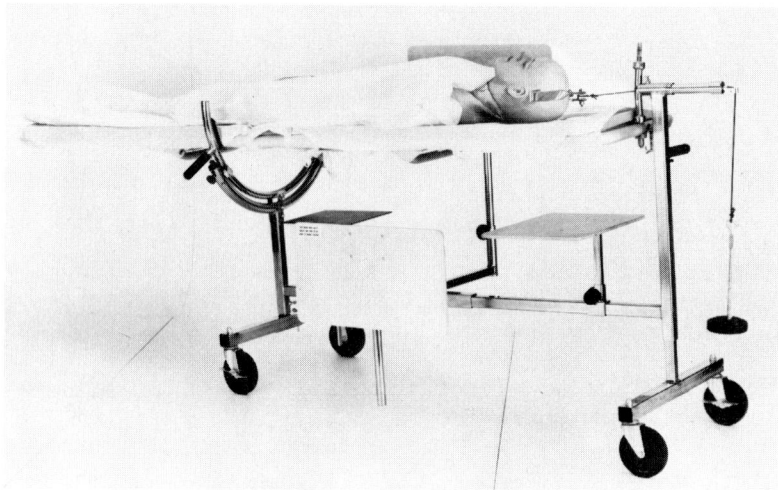

Figure 11-16
Wedge Turning Frame. (Courtesy of Stryker Corporation, Kalamazoo, Michigan.)

also helpful if the patient is not lying prone during visiting hours. Position changes are necessary around the clock.

For later stages in the rehabilitation process, a tilt table is used to help the patient to stand. For the paraplegic patient who has had a laminectomy and whose condition is stabilized, the tilt table may be used as early as 10 to 14 days after surgery. The patient stands on the foot end of the table and is strapped to it with soft leather-padded straps across the knees, above the knees, at the pelvis, and across the thoracic cage. Actually, the tilt table is not necessary if a CircOlectric bed is being used, because the patient can be turned into the standing position gradually on the frame. The patient should be observed for signs of discomfort, such as pallor, increased perspiration, and tachycardia. The time for standing is gradually increased to a minimum of 1 hour daily.

Bladder Care

Initially, during the spinal shock stage, the patient with a spinal cord injury needs an indwelling catheter because the bladder is atonic. However, usually after the spinal shock phase ceases, other methods are quickly substituted. These include indwelling catheters, external collection via a condom in the male patient, bladder control by the Credé (external reflex) method, or intermittent catheterization. In some patients with a neurogenic bladder with frequent infections, an ileal conduit or permanent urostomy is performed. Prevention of urinary tract infection is essential no matter what method is used, because these infections may lead to kidney damage, a leading cause of death in patients with spinal cord injuries. However, Price et al. [30] found in their study of renal function in spinal cord injuries that progressive renal deterioration rarely develops in patients who receive adequate medical supervision and who are meticulous in personal care. They found that (1) reflux renal calculi, calyceal blunting (denoting pyelonephritis), and recurrent decubitus ulcers were the factors most frequently associated with renal deterioration, and (2) all of these could be prevented by urinary dilution, acidification, and control of bladder hygiene.

When an indwelling catheter is in place, efforts must be made to keep it patent and to maintain the acidity of the urine; the latter is promoted by giving the patient cranberry juice, avoiding citrus fruits, which cause an alkaline urine, and administering supplemental ascorbic acid. The pH of the urine is tested regularly to determine the presence of asymptomatic urinary infections; cultures are taken when indicated. Antibacterial agents such as methenamine mandelate (Mandelamine) may be prescribed. Fluid intake of 3,000 to 4,000 ml daily is encouraged as a means of maintaining patency of the catheter in preference to bladder irrigations. However, some institutions continue to use bladder irrigation regimens. When a catheter is in place in the male patient, it is important to prevent fistula formation at the penoscrotal junction of the posterior urethra by taping the catheter to the abdomen. The catheter is taped to the thigh of the female patient. In some institutions, catheters are regularly irrigated with agents such as Renacidin, which keeps deposits from forming in catheters and thus prevents bladder calculi; usually, the catheter is irrigated twice daily, and the catheter is not changed except when necessary. When patients drink adequate fluids, and equipment is kept scrupulously clean at all times, it is possible to retain the catheter for as long as 3 months. Some protocols prescribe clamping the catheter on a regular schedule as a means of maintaining bladder tone. However, this approach can cause overdistention or reflux, and clamping is generally considered to be contraindicated. Maintaining perineal hygiene and a sterile collecting system is essential to prevent infection. Early mobilization is important, because inactivity predisposes to hypercalcemia and renal and bladder calculi formation.

When a male uses a condom, care should be taken that it does not cause excessive pressure, which would constrict the blood supply. The condom should be removed at least daily to clean the area, provide perineal care, and detect signs of pressure.

Following the resolution of spinal shock, the type of bladder functioning depends on whether the patient has an upper motor neuron or lower motor neuron lesion. Determining which type of lesion is present is essential for selecting the appropriate method of bladder management. The goal of bladder programs is for the patient to become catheter-free with adequate bladder emptying. A urologic examination, including cystometry, cystoscopy, and intravenous pyelography is carried out to determine the condition of the kidneys, ureters, and bladder. Cystometry is used to evaluate detrusor muscle function and bladder capacity.

The sacral segments of the spinal cord contain the reflex center for micturition. Reflex arcs through the pelvic nerves and internal pudendal nerves are intact if the S-2 through S-4 segments and their nerves are intact. But if the sacral segments or their nerves are damaged, the reflex arc through the pelvic and internal pudendal nerves is absent [38].

In an upper motor neuron lesion, the sacral segments of the cord are not damaged; the reflex arc is intact and the bladder is therefore a reflex type. The presence of an intact sacral segment can be verified by testing for the bulbocavernous reflex via a rectal digital examination. If this reflex is positive (indicated by contraction on the finger), an upper motor neuron lesion is present.

To cause reflex bladder action, various stimulating mechanisms are used, such as tapping the abdominal area at the site of the bladder, stroking the inner thigh, and pulling the penis. When these techniques are used, the patient is periodically catheterized to check for residual urine and to determine the effectiveness of the technique. The male patient usually wears an external catheter to serve as a receptacle for intermittent incontinence. Anticholinergic drugs such as propantheline bromide (Pro-Banthine) may be prescribed to control urinary incontinence caused by bladder spasms. For the female patient, there is no available method for external collection of the urine in case of spontaneous urination, so that an indwelling catheter may be necessary; some patients may prefer to wear plastic-lined briefs and absorbent pads, which are changed frequently. Urinary diversion procedures may be required.

The patient with a lower motor neuron lesion has an areflexic, or flaccid, bladder, because the reflex arc is interrupted. On rectal digital examination the sphincter muscle remains flaccid, and no contractions are felt over the inserted finger. The patient has no sensation of needing to void, and retention of urine is the major problem. Manual expression of urine, using the Credé method, is the approach to bladder control in these patients.

The Credé method is initially done by the nurse and later by the patient. The nurse strokes the abdomen in a downward movement from the level of the umbilicus to the bladder to remove urine from the ureters. Pressure is then applied suprapubically by moving the fists toward the pubis in a rolling fashion (usually six times). The nurse then places his or her hands, one on top of the other, slightly above the pubic arch and applies sufficient pressure to expel the urine manually [36]. The urine is measured and the amount recorded.

The patient who has sufficient hand control and can use the toilet learns to do the Credé method. In self-Credé, the patient can bend slightly forward to help expel the urine. Initially, the Credé method may be required every 1½ to 2 hours to maintain continence but later is used every 4 hours.

There is some controversy about the use of the Credé method; some professionals feel the technique may cause reflux of the urine, particularly if done incorrectly.

Intermittent catheterization is increasingly being used as a method of bladder control. The technique is contraindicated in the presence of outlet obstruction or active pyelitis.

On the first day of intermittent catheterization, stimulation and voiding techniques followed by catheterization to check the amount of residual urine are done on a prescribed schedule. Catheterization is done every 4 to 6 hours for 48 hours; however, it is done any time that symptoms of autonomic hyperreflexia occur. If the catheterizations demonstrate less than 100 ml of residual urine, the catheterization is only done every 8 hours and finally on a once-a-day schedule. Some patients are able to achieve a catheter-free status with a random catheterization done only weekly to check residual urine. Later, catheterization may be done only every 3 months to check residual urine and obtain a urine culture. The urine should be checked regularly for its pH level, however, and adjustments made in the diet to maintain a pH of 5 or lower. Some patients catheterize only at night to check for residual urine, leaving the catheter in place overnight, connected to gravity drainage. Male patients use the triggering mechanisms but have a urosheath or condom in place to collect the urine and control any accidental voiding or dribbling.

A recent approach to the management of bladder elimination in the presence of a neurogenic bladder is the use of electronic bladder stimulators. Selected patients in several centers throughout the country are being studied to evaluate this method. Under either general or spinal anesthesia, an electronic pacemaker is implanted through a vertical incision made about 2 cm above the pubis or 2 cm below the umbilicus. An external hand-held transmitter is used to activate the pacemaker whenever urination is desired. The transmitter is held close to the body (without touching) over the implanted pacemaker. The pacemaker then conducts electrical impulses through the detrusor muscle, producing bladder contraction and evacuation. Problems that can occur with the technique include intermittent incontinence, chronic urinary infection if the system does not function adequately, lead detachment or breakage, and, rarely, a lead erosion through the bladder wall. The long-term effect of the bladder electronic pacemaker has not yet been determined.

Bowel Management

Bowel incontinence is a major problem for patients with spinal cord injuries, affecting both the psychological and physiologic status of the patient and often interfering with therapy and delaying rehabilitation. Unless bowel continence is achieved, independence and socialization of the patient is hindered, even when the patient is mobile and functionally independent otherwise.

A major factor in the success of any bowel program is to facilitate a soft to unformed consistency of the stool, because many patients with cord injuries cannot do sufficient abdominal straining to try to expel hard stools. The preinjury pattern of bowel evacuation should also be considered in determining the appropriate schedule for bowel evacuation. Rigid adherence to a schedule for elimination is essential. A well-balanced diet with sufficient bulk to stimulate peristalsis, adequate fluid intake, avoidance of constipating drugs, and the use of prune juice and stool softeners such as dioctyl calcium sulfosuccinate (Surfak) are other essential elements of a successful bowel program.

Reflex or automatic bowel habits may be developed in the patient with spinal cord injuries. The technique depends on causing reflex activity in the bowel musculature by anal stimulation via insertion of a suppository or digital stimulation. Initially, suppositories are used, but digital stimulation is sufficient in many situations. In digital stimulation, the lubricated and gloved finger is inserted into the rectum about 1 to 2 cm and is rotated to stimulate rectal activity. Mild stretching and massage of the anal sphincter triggers reflex responses involved in evacuation (assuming the reflex arc is intact). The finger is removed to allow bowel evacuation, and the procedure is repeated one time if necessary. If able, the patient is instructed to inhale deeply, tighten the abdominal muscles, and push down. The patient can also stroke the abdomen with slight pressure from right to left and downward to stimulate peristalsis.

The patient should sit on the toilet to attempt bowel evacuation rather than using the bedpan. If defecation does not occur within 30 minutes, the patient should be transferred off the toilet. Otherwise, prolonged pressure from the hard toilet seat could initiate skin breakdown.

If the patient cannot use the toilet, a side-lying position in bed with collection of the feces into an incontinence pad is the technique that is used. Enemas tend to produce overdistention of the paralyzed bowel and are therefore not used routinely in most bowel programs. They may be necessary in some situations, however. On occasion, digital removal of the feces may be necessary if there is a fecal impaction or if peristalsis is inadequate.

A major consideration in the selection of the elements of a bowel program is to evaluate the individual patient's abilities, disabilities, and responses to different approaches. A regimen should be selected that is most effective and makes the patient feel most secure about bowel management. Methods for bowel control require further study and evaluation.

Cornell and others [7] compared three types of bowel management programs in 20 patients with recent spinal cord injuries to determine which was most effective; irritant-contact, stimulant, or mechanical programs. The irritant-contact approach used bisacodyl (Dulcolax) orally and rectally and diocytl calcium sulfosuccinate (Surfak) orally. The stimulant approach consisted of oral anthracene laxatives and senna rectal suppositories. The third approach was mechanical evacuation with a 500-ml tap-water enema using a rubber stopper to compress the flaccid anal sphincter to ensure retention of the solution. Bulk stool softeners such as psyllium hydrophilic mucilloid (Metamucil) were also used in this regimen.

The data showed that the mechanical method was more consistently effective than the others because less time was required for evacuation after stimulation, and more patients obtained results from the stimulation and had fewer accidental evacuations than with the other techniques. However, the investigators found that families often objected to the mechanical program after the patients were discharged and that impactions occasionally occurred. Again, it is important to stress that long-term management is to be considered in selecting an appropriate bowel program for the individual patient.

Skin Care

Rubbing and scraping the extremities or other parts of the body occur readily if special precautions are not taken during transfer activities or when moving the paralyzed legs or arms. The person with a spinal cord injury no longer has normal sensation in the affected body parts and is not aware when excessive pressure is being exerted. There is no substitute for this sensory loss. Early in the care of the patient, the nurse emphasizes the importance of proper skin care and regular, thorough assessment of the skin's integrity, demonstrating their importance by consistent adherence to frequent assessment.

The nurse should teach the patient that preventing pressure on vulnerable areas of the body is necessary to prevent skin breakdown and decubiti. The patient should be taught to use a long-handled mirror to examine the torso and sacral areas daily to detect skin abrasions or pressure areas. The reason for the pressure should be determined and corrected.

A thick foam-rubber cushion should be used on the wheelchair. The patient should be encouraged to raise himself at least four times every hour to relieve the pressure over the sacral area. If the patient is unable to do this, a staff person must shift the patient in the wheelchair at regular intervals. The patient in bed may use a sheepskin pad under the buttocks, as well as sheepskin boots to prevent breakdown at the heels. A footboard is applied to the bed to prevent drop foot.

It is important that the patient learn to transfer carefully to avoid bruising or abrasions of the buttocks, thighs, or legs. A wheelchair with removable arms and leg rests and a trapeze over the bed are important devices to assist in making smooth transfers. A sliding board may be needed for sitting transfers to bridge the space between two surfaces.

Exercise and Ambulation

Atrophy of the upper extremities may result unless active exercise of the unaffected parts of the body is promoted. Atrophy results from disuse, malnutrition, and general lowering of metabolism. For the paraplegic patient, strengthening of the triceps muscles is most important, because the triceps are used in transfer activities and in ambulation with crutches. Use of the overbed trapeze is an excellent measure for upper extremity strengthening.

Once the patient's physiologic status has stabilized, all joints of the affected extremities should be passively carried through a complete range of motion to prevent contractures. It is important for the paraplegic patients to develop the muscles of the upper extremities and the abdominal and trunk muscles to facilitate transfer and ambulation on crutches, when possible. The use of a Balkan frame with a trapeze over the bed facilitates the paraplegic's independence as well as strengthening the upper extremities. The patient is promoted to the wheelchair as soon as possible.

After a strenuous muscle-strengthening and trunk-balancing program, the paraplegic patient is fitted with long-leg braces and is taught to stand in an upright position between parallel bars. The patient learns to balance himself on the parallel bars then progresses to a swing-to gait and finally to a swing-through gait. When these are mastered, the use of crutches is taught, so that the patient can ambulate outside the parallel bars with supervision. Often, paraplegic patients are encouraged to stand in braces and crutches at least 1 hour a day. It has been determined that standing enhances calcium metabolism in the long bones and also helps prevent the formation of renal and bladder calculi. However, excessive energy may be required for standing and thus the patient prefers not to utilize this activity. In some spinal cord centers bracing and standing are not emphasized.

Education in Activities of Daily Living

The patient who is confined to a wheelchair requires instruction about mobility, safety, and methods of carrying out the activities of daily living from the chair. Proper upkeep of the wheelchair must also be learned. Lint and dust from the hubs and folding crossbars must be removed weekly, and the chair should be oiled monthly or as necessary. The pressure of the balloon tires of wheelchairs should be checked weekly.

Braces also require regular attention. All the locks should be opened weekly to permit removal of lint. A drop of machine oil in each lock is usually indicated at the time of cleaning. Saddle soap and lukewarm water are used to wash the leather parts of the braces. The brace should be propped against the wall or placed on the floor or table in good alignment when it is not being used. Proper handling will prolong the life of the brace. When assessing the patient on return visits to the clinic or hospital, the nurse should check for worn parts and loose or missing screws. Adjustments in the brace become necessary when the patient begins to gain weight. The joint alignment of the brace should be checked regularly, to make sure that it is appropriate for the individual patient.

A major part of the rehabilitation program is learning adaptation to the activities of daily living. The paraplegic patient must learn to put on and take off braces, transfer from bed to the wheelchair and vice versa, to start to ambulate with crutches, as well as learning how to dress, handle bladder and bowel programs, and carry on a job from the wheelchair. When the activities of daily living are mastered, the paraplegic patient who requires a new type of employment because of the spinal cord injury is given vocational tests.

While some quadriplegic patients are able to carry out certain activities by using various electronic devices and can return to work, others require attendants for their care and are unemployable. Pneumatic devices, activated by the tongue, breath, or even eye movements, are being used to increase independence for the quadriplegic patient. Breath-operated wheelchairs are also available to facilitate independent mobility.

Psychological Aspects of Care

The impact of spinal cord injury is overwhelming for both the patient and the family. When the implications of complete paralysis of portions of the body are realized, it is only natural that a severe depression ensues. However, the patient may use denial as an initial defense mechanism and continue to hope that neuromuscular function will return. For the patient who first has complete flaccidity of the extremities, even initial spastic movements are looked on as a positive sign that complete return of function is possible.

It is important to avoid implying to the patient and family that functional recovery is likely to occur when it is known that it is not possible. As the acute phase passes, the patient and family go through a period of depression. This is not to be viewed as a discouraging sign but as the first step in facing the reality of the injury. This depressed state is a necessary stage in the process of grief and adjustment to the disability. In fact, the nurse should be concerned about the patient who becomes detached and seemingly unconcerned, because such a patient is not able to deal realistically with the implications of the injury. However, when the depression becomes profound and interferes with the person's health, psychological consultation is indicated. Inappropriate reassurance about recovery and attainment of unrealistic goals only delays depression and also contributes to mistrust of the staff, when the patient finds out that they have not been honest with him or her.

The nurse should provide an accepting and open atmosphere for communication, allowing the patient to express anger and hostility. The importance of a trusting relationship and provision of emotional support for the patient with a spinal cord injury cannot be overemphasized. Perrine [27] has documented their importance in his account of his own reactions to spinal cord injury. He also described the phases of grief, protest, despair, and detachment that he passed through during his prolonged adjustment to his injury.

It is not only the patient who requires time to adjust to the permanent injury. The family and friends also must adjust, and they need opportunities to discuss their fears and concerns. Often, the family may negatively affect the patient's rehabilitation by overestimating the disability or denying its reality. Since family and friends may feel uncomfortable around the patient and insecure about how much assistance they should provide, they need specific guidelines as to how to deal with the patient.

Although patients require time to adjust psychologically to the injury, they should become active participants in their care as soon as possible. Only active participation will prepare a patient for becoming independent in self-care to the degree possible. The nurse should always consider, however, the patient's readiness to learn a new aspect of care before proceeding with the instruction. Teaching actually begins in the early stages, when the nurse stresses the paramount importance of regular changes in position and skin inspection and instructs the patient about the techniques of bladder and bowel control. If the nursing staff adheres to the principles of management that are taught, the patient will be prepared for taking over the responsibilities. Depending on the severity of the disability, family members and friends may have to be taught specific aspects of the patient's care. An attendant may be necessary for the more severely disabled patient.

A majority of patients with spinal cord injuries are in the adolescent or young adult group. For the adolescent, who is striving for independence and identity, the onset of a spinal cord injury augments the emotional stress and difficulties of this developmental period. It is not surprising that disciplinary problems often occur in a hospital or rehabilitation unit where groups of several adolescents with spinal cord injuries are cared for.

The relationship of the patient to other members of the family may suffer strains. The nurse should remember that the family also needs support in adjusting to the change in the role and image of the injured family member. Initial reactions of overprotection may alternate with feelings of complete rejection. Economic burdens brought on by the prolonged rehabilitation program may tax financial resources and further disturb family relationships. If the injury has been the result of an accident, guilt on the part of both patient and family members may also disrupt the family relationship. It is obvious, therefore, that in addition to being prepared psychologically for the posthospitalization period, the patient must also be prepared to adjust to living at home if continued progress is to be assured. Often, the spinal cord injured patient is psychologically ready to leave the hospital and reenter family life, only to find that relationships are changed and strained, that employment is difficult, and even that physical barriers in the home interfere with mobility. Frustration after hospitalization often results in neglect of measures that prevent complications, and the patient returns to the protective atmosphere of the hospital.

The many Vietnam veterans who suffered spinal cord injuries represent a different type of patient with different needs. This group has been more aggressive than other patients in seeking understanding of treatments and procedures and more demanding about having a voice in decisions about therapy programs. The veterans have also been found to be impatient about delays in receiving the services they feel they need. They are typically better educated than previous veterans and are also more interested in vocational activities and development. Studies of this group of veterans have shown that improved communication and increased opportunities for participation in decisions affecting their lives are necessary for their successful rehabilitation. Another distinctive need among this group is assistance with problems of drug abuse and addiction, which complicate the rehabilitation of these patients [38].

Sexual Aspects of Spinal Cord Inury

Immediately after a spinal cord injury has occurred, it is not possible to determine whether sexual function will be restored. However, important signs of potential sexual functioning are the ability to contract and relax the rectal sphincter voluntarily and the presence of sensations in the penile and scrotal skin of the male patient.

For too long, patients with spinal cord injuries have been deprived of sexual counseling or even diagnosis and treatment of sexual dysfunction and care oriented to meeting sexual needs. Often, disabled persons have been treated as if they were not expected to have sexual needs or desires, or as though they had excessive or perverted sexual needs [17]. As the importance of the sexual aspects of spinal cord injuries has become recognized, various approaches have been developed to assist professionals in carrying out their responsibilities in this area. In some settings, workshops have been held for both professionals and disabled persons to provide information on ways of meeting sexual needs. Most workshops are designed to "demythologize" sexual behavior, "desensationalize" sexual stimuli, and aid both the disabled person and the professional to accept their own sexuality as well as that of others [17].

The patient may feel that sexual drives are no longer appropriate for him or her and may thus repress them. It is important for the nurse to observe the patient for any signs of interest in discussing the sexual aspects of the injury, and the patient must be made to feel that it is appropriate to discuss these topics, or the subject may not be brought up. Often, the male patient tests his sexuality by making passes or crude remarks to the female nurse; it is important for the nurse to show acceptance of the patient at these times without degrading him.

No assumptions should be made about the patient's attitude toward sex; the patient should clarify what sexuality means to him or her. Then, an assessment is made to determine the patient's concern about sexual activities. The male patient is encouraged to try different stimuli to attempt to elicit an erection; such techniques include stroking or pulling the pubic hairs and rubbing the thighs. Studies have shown that 80 percent of male patients with spinal cord injuries can have an erection [16].

Comar and others [5] studied various groups of patients with spinal cord injuries and concluded that the chances of having psychogenic erections (produced by external stimulation) and the ability to ejaculate among the patients in the upper motor neuron–complete transection group become possible only as the lesions approach the distal thoracic and lumbar segments [38]. They also concluded that the lower the lesion segmentally, the better the chance for a psychogenic erection, and that most upper motor neuron lesions in patients with complete transection prevent psychogenic erections. This is in contrast to some patients who have complete lower motor neuron lesions but are able to achieve psychogenic erections. (It is thought that even if the pelvic nerve arc is damaged, the sympathetic nerves may take over the function of erection [38].) These investigators also reported that patients with incomplete upper motor neuron lesions may have both psychogenic and reflexogenic (produced by spontaneous reflex action) erections. However, reflexogenic erections do not ensure successful coitus, because erection may not occur at an appropriate time or may not last long enough.

It has been reported that ejaculation may occur in a patient with either upper motor neuron or lower motor neuron lesions, even though volitional control of the external sphincter is absent [38]. Thus, the patterns of sexual functioning will vary among patients with spinal cord injury, ranging from a smaller number who have essentially normal sexual functioning, to those who can have intercourse but do not experience orgasm or ejaculation, to those who are unable to participate in genital sex but are able to have sexual relationships by using digital stimulation, caressing, cunnilingus and other types of foreplay in the sexual activity.

The patient with a spinal cord injury should prepare for coitus by emptying the bladder. In the case of a patient with an upper motor neuron lesion, the bladder may empty reflexly. The person with a lower motor neuron lesion may urinate during intercourse because of vaginal pressure.

Women of childbearing age may be able to become pregnant and deliver infants, depending on the degree of disability as well as their desire for pregnancy. The pregnancy is not without complications in some cases. For the woman with a spinal cord injury the risks associated with pregnancy are urinary tract infection, premature or precipitous delivery, autonomic hyperreflexia during labor, and decubiti formation [13]. Even with the potential for these risks, however, the pregnancies usually result in vaginal deliveries of healthy infants [14]. The female patient has additional hygiene problems related to menstruation. Tampons or adhesive strip napkins are preferred to sanitary belts with plastic hooks, which may cause pressure ulcers.

Because the supine position is likely to have been the premorbid pattern of the woman's participation in the sexual act, women often do not appear to have the problems with sexual intercourse that male patients do. Although it is thought that orgasm is absent in females with complete lesions of the spinal cord, heightened arousal or orgasm by means of intense tactile sensation above the sensory level affected, especially about the breasts, is possible [14, 21a].

Although various resource materials and books [14, 21a] are now available on sexual approaches for the patient with a spinal cord injury, health workers should consider the religious and moral attitudes of both sex partners before discussing the couple's sexual relationships and alternate sexual techniques. If the nurse is uncomfortable about discussing sex, referrals should be made to a person skilled in this type of counseling.

Discharge Planning
Before the patient is discharged from the hospital, both patient and family must be thoroughly grounded in the details of care that are essential to maintain function and prevent complications. The patient must understand the importance of a high fluid intake and must develop a pattern for provision of this intake. The patient must also be aware of the importance of keeping the urine acid and know how to test the urine for acidity. Careful perineal hygiene and proper bladder care should be stressed so that the patient will understand the benefits to be derived from these activities. The patient should be reminded to inspect the skin daily and change body positions frequently, particularly when in the wheelchair for prolonged periods. A properly fitted wheelchair is prescribed, and the proper care of the wheelchair should be reviewed. A 3-inch foam rubber cushion should be provided for the wheelchair as further insurance against decubiti formation.

Before the patient is discharged from the hospital, the home should be evaluated for potential physical barriers that would interfere with mobility. For example, stairs may have to be replaced with a ramp to allow access to the home. The doorways may need to be widened to allow wheelchair entrance. These changes can be a heavy financial burden to some families.

Once the patient is discharged, follow-up care should be planned to evaluate adherence to the teaching and activity programs. This evaluation should also include a physical examination to determine the adequacy of skin care, nutritional habits, perineal care, bladder and bowel care, and transfer techniques. The patient's urine should be examined to determine the adequacy of fluid intake. The pH is tested, and a specimen for culture and sensitivity is obtained if indicated.

Factors in Successful Rehabilitation
The success of rehabilitation will depend on a variety of factors, the most important being the patient's personality and motivation. The level of the lesion, the presence and nature of any complications, and the patient's age, intelligence, and general health all are factors that influence rehabilitation. It is important that realistic goals be established by the patient and the professional staff and that planning and coordination be a team effort. The major role of the staff after the crisis period is to teach the patient to begin to take as much

responsibility for his or her own care as is possible within the limitations imposed by the injury. Diligence in adhering to the routines that have been prescribed is the patient's responsibility and guarantee for rehabilitation.

The paraplegic patient can acquire complete independence in personal care, assuming that no serious complication or other pathologic condition is present. The quadriplegic patient can attain varying degrees of independence. The higher the level of the lesion, however, the more time and effort are required to develop approaches to facilitate as much self-care as possible. Functional splints are often used to improve upper extremity mobility. An example is the flexor-hinge hand splint, which is used to enable a patient without hand function to write, dial a telephone, self-feed, and shave. Reconstructive surgery is often indicated for selected patients to facilitate increased mobility of the upper extremities. For the quadriplegic patient with high lesions, power-driven splints and wheelchairs are available.

The goal for the patient with a spinal cord injury is to be at home, trained, and rehabilitated to live successfully and productively within 6 to 12 months after injury, depending on the level of the lesion and the absence of complications. The ultimate goal is maximal independence [38]. To accomplish this goal, the talents of people from various disciplines must be coordinated, including the physician, neurologist, urologist, nurse, physical therapist, occupational therapist, social worker, psychologist, and vocational counselor. Self-care and training for functioning independently as much as is possible are essential for economic and social functioning as well as for psychological health.

If and when the patient is to return to employment, the setting should be evaluated in terms of physical barriers. The professional worker is most likely to be able to return to a former job, but this depends on the type of profession. The skilled worker probably is more handicapped by the physical limitations of the injury and may require training in alternate types of occupations. The unskilled worker will have the most difficult time obtaining training for some type of employment. Vocational assistance through the state Division of Vocational Rehabilitation or the Veteran's Administration (for eligible persons) is an important resource in the rehabilitation of persons who are disabled from spinal cord injuries and are unable to return to former employment. Counseling, medical services (such as purchasing necessary equipment and self-help devices), job training, and job placement are the types of services available.

The National Paraplegia Foundation (432 Park Avenue South, New York, N.Y. 10016), a national voluntary health agency, supports activities related to research and education, both public and professional, in all aspects of spinal cord injury. A publication, *Paraplegia News*, printed in conjunction with the Paralyzed Veterans of America, is financed partially by the National Paraplegia Foundation. The Foundation does not give direct aid to individuals but assists paraplegic persons in contacting cooperating agencies and other organizations. The local chapters that have been established in different parts of the country have varying programs.

Intravertebral Tumors

Although the pathologic types are similar, intravertebral tumors occur less frequently than do intracranial tumors. Also, metastasis occurs more frequently to the vertebrae than to the cranium whereas hematomas and abscesses are much less common in the vertebrae. The intravertebral tumors are either extradural (the majority type) or intradural. Some of the tumors can be excised surgically, but often they infiltrate and are not removable because of potential damage to the spinal cord.

Spinal tumors most often involve the thoracic region of the spine but may involve any part of the spinal column. They occur most frequently in young or middle-aged adults, but they are not as common as intracranial tumors. Although the spinal cord itself is rarely involved in metastatic lesions, metastatic tumors in the epidural space (space between the dura mater and walls of the vertebral canal) occur with some frequency. Metastasis to the vertebral column from various primary sites often occurs, causes compression on the cord, and may extend into the cord. Symptoms vary widely, depending on the level of cord involvement, but are similar to the symptoms of patients with spinal cord injuries who require similar nursing care (see

Spinal Cord Injuries for a detailed discussion).

Signs and symptoms associated with intravertebral tumors depend on the level and location of the tumor and the effects of the compression of the tumor on the meninges and spinal cord. Pain may be the first symptom and may be prolonged for months or years before symptoms of cord compression appear. In other patients, such as those with metastatic tumors in the thoracic spine, rapidly developing paraplegia is characteristic. A slowly developing paraplegia of a spastic type is associated with intramedullary tumors.

The diagnosis is confirmed by examination of the CSF, x-ray, and myelography if necessary. Laminectomy is indicated to decompress the spinal cord as a palliative procedure in the management of malignant and nonresectable lesions. Removal of the tumor is attempted if possible. Radiation therapy is used when tumors are nonresectable.

Nursing care before and after surgery is similar to the care of patients with spinal cord injuries (page 972). Even after surgery, the patient may have residual disability. The psychological impact of increasing dependency and permanent disability, along with the diagnosis of primary or metastatic cancer, is overwhelming for the patient and family. Provision for psychological support is of paramount importance.

Herniated Intervertebral Disk

The vertebral bodies are separated by fibrocartilaginous disks that serve as cushions and shock absorbers. The intervertebral disk consists of three parts: (1) the cartilaginous end-plate of the vertebral body; (2) the anulus fibrosis, which is a meshwork of dense collagenous fibers surrounding and enclosing the disk material; and (3) the nucleus pulposus, a thin meshwork of collagenous fibers with a mucoprotein gel [1a]. Degenerative changes cause a tear in the posterior rim of the anulus, allowing the nucleus pulposus to herniate into the neural canal. The herniated pulposus compresses the nerve roots and the fibers leaving the cord at that level. The most common locations for herniated intervertebral disks are the cervical and lumbar spine; the fourth and fifth lumbar disks are most frequently affected.

CLINICAL SYMPTOMS

Herniation of the lumbar disks causes severe low back pain and often occurs immediately or within several hours after heavy lifting or twisting of the body during the moving of a heavy object. Severe muscle spasm is usually present, and the patient finds that bending forward, sneezing, and straining aggravate the pain. When the herniated disk compresses one or more nerve roots, severe sciatica results. **Sciatica** is pain that radiates along the course of the sciatic nerve; the pain is centered in the lumbar area but radiates over the buttock, the posterior thigh, the calf, and even the foot. Paresthesia and numbness may also be present. When a herniation of a cervical disk occurs, pain, disturbed sensations in the arm and hand, and limitation of neck movement are usual findings. Weakness of the biceps and triceps muscles is also evident.

DIAGNOSIS

Disk herniation is diagnosed by the clinical history and a physical examination to determine muscle strength, the presence of reflexes, and the status of motor and sensory function in the involved extremity. Although roentgenograms are not always useful in detecting herniated disks, they may show a narrowing of the disk space. Electromyography and myelography are done to confirm the diagnosis.

When a herniation of a lumbar disk is suspected, the physical examination includes measurement of the calf circumference (the calf muscle is frequently flabby on the involved side) and the straight-leg-raising test. A positive straight-leg-raising test is associated with nerve root irritation from lumbar disk lesions. Straight leg raising with the hip flexed and the knee extended normally can be done to 70 or 90 degrees. In the presence of an acute disk lesion, however, the leg can only be raised to 30 or 40 degrees (or sometimes only to 10 degrees) because of the onset of leg and back pain. Diminished reflexes (for example, the Achilles reflex) also reflect nerve root involvement.

TREATMENT AND NURSING CARE
Medical Treatment

Disk herniation is treated conservatively by absolute bed rest on a firm mattress, analgesics (such as Empirin with codeine), diathermy, sedation, anti-inflammatory agents such as indomethacin (Indocin), and muscle relaxants such as diazepam or methocarbamol (Robaxin). Corsets may also be helpful in providing additional support. When herniation of a cervical disk occurs, a cervical collar is often used to keep the head in a neutral or slightly flexed position; the collar should never cause hyperextension. Traction with a cervical halter may also be prescribed for cervical disk herniation to relieve pressure on the nerve. The use of traction for herniated lumbar disks is controversial; however, it is used to help maintain the patient at bed rest. A flexed bed position with the knees and hips flexed helps relieve the tension on the lower lumbar and sacral nerve roots. The patient with a herniated lumbar disk is gradually started on progressive spinal exercises to strengthen the back. (The Williams exercise program is discussed in Chapter 10.)

Surgical Treatment
When conservative treatment is ineffective or when neurologic deficits increase, surgical intervention is indicated. Laminectomy is done to permit excision of the herniated disk material in order to permit surgery on the spinal cord and its nerve roots. In addition to the excision of intervertebral disks, laminectomy is done for the removal of neoplasms, abscesses, and in operations involving dissection of the anterolateral tracts for treatment of intractable pain (cordotomy). A midline incision is made in the back over the spinous processes of the vertebrae to be exposed. The spinous processes and laminae are excised with rongeurs, and the dura and pia-arachnoid are incised for definitive procedures. Spinal fusion may also be performed in conjunction with laminectomy to stabilize the spine by bridging over the defective disk. In this procedure, two or more vertebrae are fused together with a bone graft obtained from the posterior ileac crest.

Postoperative care Following laminectomy, the patient is placed in a flat position for at least 4 hours. The patient's vital signs and motor and sensory function in the extremities are monitored. After cervical laminectomy, the patient should be observed for respiratory distress. The patient should be asked to flex the toes and to dorsiflex the feet. Any complaints of numbness or tingling in the feet (or in the arms after a cervical laminectomy) should be reported to the surgeon. There is a danger of injury to the motor roots during the operation, and paralysis may occur.

After a lumbar laminectomy, the patient may be distressed to find that sciatica is still present and should be informed that this often occurs but will subside within a few days or weeks.

The patient is turned every 2 or 3 hours and is turned as a unit in log rolling fashion (a turning sheet will facilitate this procedure). The patient should not be allowed to twist or to move his hips separately from the rest of the body. Jerking, and angulation of the spine, must be prevented. When the patient is positioned on the side, a pillow should be placed between the legs, and knee flexion should be avoided. After cervical laminectomy, a pillow under the head is not permitted.

Urine retention is a frequent postoperative problem, particularly after lumbar laminectomy; temporarily a retention catheter may be necessary until the patient begins to ambulate. The patient should also be observed for abdominal distention, which is often associated with this type of surgery.

Ambulation Most patients ambulate within a day after lumbar laminectomy. When ambulation is initiated it must be supervised, and the patient must be told to walk erectly and not to bend forward or stoop. Prolonged sitting is discouraged; the patient should either be walking or lying in the bed. A brace or corset may be used by some patients, particularly if a spinal fusion has been done. Ambulation may be delayed slightly longer after a spinal fusion than after lumbar laminectomy alone.

Chemonucleolysis
Chemonucleolysis is a relatively new approach to the treatment of low back pain and herniated disks. It is used primarily when laminectomy has failed to control pain, but in some settings it is considered a primary mode of therapy.

Chymopapain, an enzyme that is isolated from the leaves of the papaya plant, is injected into the herniated disk. The enzyme apparently causes depolymerization of the mucoprotein when it comes in contact with the disk, but it does not appear to have any effect on the collagenous structures [1a]. The Food and Drug Administration, however, has not approved the use of this drug, and thus it is, at the time of writing, limited to experimental use only.

Chemonucleolysis is carried out either in an x-ray room or in the operating room. The medication is instilled preferably while the patient is under general anesthesia to facilitate proper positioning. The patient is placed on the left side with the left flank elevated, so that the pelvis tilts to the right. Spinal needles are inserted into the disk space under fluoroscopy. The chymopapain is injected into all abnormal disks after they have been identified on x-ray films. When the substance is injected, the patient should be observed closely for an anaphylactic reaction.

The major complication of chymopapain injection is anaphylactic reaction. In some protocols, corticosteroid therapy is used preoperatively to reduce any potential reaction. The reaction almost always occurs immediately; symptoms of urticaria, severe hypotension, tachycardia, and respiratory stridor occur. Epinephrine is given immediately, and corticosteroids are given. Maintenance of a patent airway to prevent anoxia and its resultant deficits is the major intervention necessary during this crisis. Sodium bicarbonate is utilized to combat the metabolic acidosis that often accompanies the anaphylactic reaction.

After the chemonucleolysis, the patient should be observed for delayed reactions to the enzyme. Patients are allowed to get up the same evening, although they are told to avoid sitting for prolonged periods. Thus, the patient is encouraged either to remain recumbent or to walk; stooping or bending should be avoided. After discharge, the patient should avoid lifting more than 10 pounds of weight for a period of time and should avoid driving or riding long distances. For 2 weeks, the patient should not participate in exercise or sports; gradual return to some sports is then permitted.

Patient Education

Patients who have had a herniated disk should be instructed in practicing good body mechanics. The nurse should also practice good body mechanics as an example for all patients and should emphasize the need to avoid strain on the back muscles and ligaments. When the patient is picking up objects from the floor or lifting heavy objects, the knees and hips should be flexed and the back kept straight, so that the muscles of the thighs and buttocks, rather than the back, sustain the strain. The nurse emphasizes the importance of avoiding bending at the waist with the knees straight, and twisting of the spine.

References

1. Alpers, B. J., and Mancall, E. L. *Essentials of the Neurological Examination.* Philadelphia: Davis, 1971.
1a. Apfelbach, H. W., et al. Chemonucleolysis in the treatment of low back pain and sciatica. *Surg. Clin. North Am.* 55:181, 1975.
2. Blount, M., and Kinney. A. B. What to remember about EEG. *Nursing 74* 4:36, 1974.
3. Carini, E., and Owens, G. *Neurological and Neurosurgical Nursing* (6th ed.). St. Louis: Mosby, 1974.
4. Clark, R. G. *Manter and Gatz's Essentials of Clinical Neuroanatomy and Neurophysiology* (5th ed.). Philadelphia: Davis, 1975.
5. Comarr, A. E. Sex among patients with spinal cord and/or cauda equina injuries. *Med. Asp. Hum. Sex.* 7:222, 1973.
6. Committee on Trauma, American College of Surgeons. *Early Care of the Injured Patient* (2nd ed.). Philadelphia: Saunders, 1976.
7. Cornell, S. A., et al. Comparison of three bowel management programs. *Nurs. Res.* 22:321, 1973.
8. DeJong, R. N., Sahs, A. L., Aldrich, C. K., and Milligan, J. O. *Essentials of the Neurological Examination.* Philadelphia: SmithKline Corporation, 1974.
8a. Dayhoff, N. Re-thinking stroke. Soft or hard devices to position hands. *Am. J. Nurs.* 75:1142, 1975.
9. Diamond, S., and Baltes, B. J. Clinical clues to different types of headache. *Hosp. Med.* 9(10):56, 1973.
9a. Epilepsy Foundation of America. *The Legal Rights of Persons with Epilepsy* (4th ed.). Washington, D.C.: Epilepsy Foundation of America, 1976.
10. Fields, W. S., Rubin, W., and Wolfson, R. J. *Essentials of the Examination and Evaluation of the Patient with Vertigo.* Philadelphia: Smith Kline Corp., 1967.
11. Freeman, A. R. Physiology of Intercellular Communication, Neuronal Interaction, and the Reflex. In Selkurt, E., *Basic Physiology for the Health Sciences.* Boston: Little, Brown, 1975.
12. Gaffney, T. W., and Campbell, R. P. Feed-

ing techniques for dysphagic patients. *Am. J. Nurs.* 74:2194, 1974.
13. Griffith, E., et al. Sexual dysfunctions associated with physical disabilities. *Arch. Phys. Med. Rehab.* 56:8, 1975.
14. Griffith, E. R., and Trieschmann, R. B. Sexual functioning in women with spinal cord injury. *Arch. Phys. Med. Rehab.* 56:18, 1975.
15. Guyton, A. C. *Textbook of Medical Physiology* (4th ed.). Philadelphia: Saunders, 1971.
16. Hanion, K. Maintaining sexuality after spinal cord injury. *Nursing 75* 5:58, 1975.
16a. Hadden, J. W. (ed.). Thymopoietin, ubiquitin and the differentiation of lymphocytes. *Clin. Bull.* 5:66, 1975.
16b. Harvey, A. M., Johns, R. J., Owens, A. H., and Ross, R. S. *The Principles and Practice of Medicine*. New York: Appleton-Century-Crofts, 1972.
17. Held, J. P., et al. Sexual attitude reassessment workshops: Effect on spinal cord injured adults, their partners and rehabilitation professionals. *Arch. Phys. Med. Rehab.* 56:14, 1975.
18. Judy, W. V., and Freeman, A. R. The Autonomic Nervous System, In Selkurt, E., *Basic Physiology for the Health Sciences*. Boston: Little, Brown, 1975.
18a. Langan, R. J., and Cotzias, G. C. Do's and don't's for the patient on levodopa therapy. *Am. J. Nurs.* 76:917, 1976.
19. Loetterle, B. C., et al. Cerebellar stimulation: Pacing the brain. *Am. J. Nurs.* 75:968, 1975.
20. Long, C., and Lawton, E. B. Functional significance of spinal cord lesion level. *Arch. Phys. Med. Rehab.* 36:249, 1955.
20a. Maddox, M. Subarachnoid hemorrhage. *Am. J. Nurs.* 74:2199, 1974.
20b. Mancell, E. L. The stroke: A review of current diagnostic and therapeutic considerations. Part I, *Hosp. Med.* 10:8, 1974; Part II, *Hosp. Med.* 11:38, 1975.
21. Miller, C. A., and Kindt, G. W. Brain abscess. *Hosp. Med.* 10:26, 1974.
21a. Mooney, T. O., Cole, T. M., and Chilgren, R. A. *Sexual Options for Paraplegics and Quadriplegics*. Boston: Little, Brown, 1975.
22. Mountcastle, V. B. *Medical Physiology* (13th ed.). St. Louis: Mosby, 1974.
23. National Institutes of Health. *Research Advances 1975*. Bethesda, Md.: DHEW Publ. 75-3, 1975.
23a. National Institute of Neurological and Communicative Disorders and Stroke. *The NINCDS Epilepsy Research Program*. Bethesda, Md.: NIH, 1974.
23b. National Institute of Neurological Diseases and Stroke. *The NINDS Spinal Cord Injury Research Program*. Bethesda, Md.: NIH, 1975.
24. Ostrow, L. S. New hope for patients with trigeminal neuralgia. *Am. J. Nurs.* 76:1301, 1976.
25. Parsons, L. C. Respiratory changes in head injury. *Am. J. Nurs.* 71:2187, 1971.
26. Peery, T. M., and Miller, F. N. *Pathology: A Dynamic Introduction to Medicine and Surgery* (2nd ed.). Boston: Little, Brown, 1971.
27. Perrine, G. Needs met and unmet. *Am. J. Nurs.* 71:2128, 1971.
28. Pizzi, F. J., Hector, J., Derek, B., and Longfitt, T. W. A protocol for the management of head trauma. *Am. Fam. Phys.* 10:163, 1974.
29. Pohutsky, L. C., and Pohutsky, K. R. Cancer update: Computerized axial tomography of the brain. A new diagnostic tool. *Am. J. Nurs.* 75:1341, 1975.
30. Price, M., Kotte, F. J., and Olson, M. E. Renal function in patients with spinal cord injury: The eighth year of a ten-year continuing study. *Arch. Phys. Med. Rehab.* 56:76, 1975.
31. Rodin, E., and Gonzales, S. Hereditary components in epileptic patients: Electroencephalogram family studies. *J.A.M.A.* 198:221, 1966.
31a. Ross, G. S., and Klasson, A. The stroke syndrome. Part 1, Pathogenesis. *Hosp. Med.* 9:8, 1973; Part 2, Cranial and Diagnostic Aspects. *Hosp. Med.* 9:58, 1973.
32. Sana, J. M., and Judge, R. D. *Physical Appraisal Methods in Nursing Practice*. Boston: Little, Brown, 1975.
33. Selkurt, E. E. *Basic Physiology for the Health Sciences*. Boston: Little, Brown, 1975.
33a. Skelly, M. Re-thinking stroke. Aphasia patients talk back. *Am. J. Nurs.* 75:1140, 1975.
34. Tinball, G. T., and Fleischer, A. S. Head injury. *Hosp. Med.* 12:89, 1976.
35. Trigiano, L. L. Independence is possible in quadriplegia. *Am. J. Nurs.* 70:2610, 1970.
36. Tudor, L. L. Bladder and bowel retraining. *Am. J. Nurs.* 70:2391, 1970.
37. Van Meter, M. J., and Diehl, E. A. Detection of Alterations in Neuromuscular Functioning. In Sana, J. M., and Judge, R. D., *Physical Appraisal Methods in Nursing Practice*. Boston: Little, Brown, 1975.
38. Veterans Administration. *A Source Book for Rehabilitating the Person with Spinal Cord Injury*. Washington, D.C.: Veterans Administration, Sept., 1972.
39. Weiss, M. H. Axioms on the management of head injury. *Hosp. Med.* 11:94, 1975.

Bibliography

Alexander, M. M., and Brown, M. S. Physical examination; part 17: Neurological examination. *Nursing 76* 6:38, 1976.

Alter, M., and Hauser, W. A. *The Epidemiology of Epilepsy: A Workshop* (DHEW Publ. 73-390).

Bethesda, Md.: National Institute of Neurological Diseases and Stroke (NINDS Monograph #14), 1972.

Alter, M., and Seltzer, A. P. What do taste and smell disturbances tell you? *Patient Care* 8:76, 1974.

AMA Department of Drugs. *AMA Drug Evaluation* (2nd ed.). Acton, Mass.: Publishing Sciences Group, 1973.

Aphasia and the Family. New York: American Heart Association, 1969.

Aurelia, J. C. *Aphasia Therapy Manual.* Danville, Ill.: Interstate Printers and Publishers, 1974.

Barr, A. Treatment of Huntington's chorea with L-glutamate. *Proc. Inst. Med. Chic.* 30:117, 1974.

Behrends, E. A. Revascularization for intracranial stroke. *AORN J.* 20:405, 1974.

Bergstrom, D. A. *Care of Patients with Bowel and Bladder Problems: A Nursing Guide.* Minneapolis, Minn.: American Rehabilitation Foundation, 1968.

Bernatz, P. E., Khonsari, S., Harrison, E. G., and Taylor, W. F. Thymoma: Factors influencing prognosis. *Surg. Clin. North Am.* 53:885, 1973.

Bickerstaff, E. R. *Neurology for Nurses* (2nd ed.). London: English University Press, 1971.

Blount, M., and Kinney, A. B. (eds.). Neurologic and neurosurgical nursing. *Nurs. Clin. North Am.* 9:591, 1974.

Boyle, M. A., and Ciuca, R. Amytrophic lateral sclerosis. *Am. J. Nurs.* 76:66, 1976.

Bruya, M. A., and Bolin, R. H. Epilepsy: A controllable disease. *Am. J. Nurs.* 76:388, 1976.

Burch, G. E., and DePasquale, N. P. Axioms on cerebrovascular disease. *Hosp. Med.* 11:8, 1975.

Burt, M. B. Perceptual deficits in hemiplegia. *Am. J. Nurs.* 70:1026, 1970.

Cailliet, R. *Low Back Pain Syndrome* (2nd ed.). Philadelphia: Davis, 1968.

Carr, C. J., and Fisher, K. D. *A Study of New Methods of Measuring Cerebral Circulation.* Bethesda, Md.: Life Sciences Research, 1970.

Cassidy, F. M. Adult hydrocephalus. *Am. J. Nurs.* 72:494, 1972.

Cohen, L. K. *Communication Problems After a Stroke.* (Rehabilitation Publication #709). Minneapolis, Minn.: Sister Kenny Institute, 1971.

Coleman, P. G., and Kittle, C. F. Aneurysms of the common carotid artery. *Surg. Clin. North Am.* 53:231, 1973.

Conn, J., Jr. Thoracic outlet syndromes. *Surg. Clin. North Am.* 54:155, 1974.

Cooper, C. R. Anticonvulsant drugs and the epileptic's dilemma. *Nursing 76* 6:45, 1976.

Davis, R., and Lentini, R. Transcutaneous nerve stimulation for treatment of pain in patients with spinal cord injury. *Surg. Neurol.* 4:100, 1975.

Delehanty, L., and Stravino, V. Achieving bladder control. *Am. J. Nurs.* 70:312, 1970.

Dillon, A. M. Nursing care of the patient with multiple sclerosis. *Nurs. Clin. North Am.* 8:653, 1973.

Drake, W. E., Dietrich, B. J., Hunt, G., and Moga, D. Community action in stroke management. *Am. J. Public Health* 62:522, 1972.

Drew, N. How to cope with speech defects in stroke patients. *Nursing 74* 4:21, 1974.

Dunkerley, G. B. *A Basic Atlas of the Human Nervous System.* Philadelphia: Davis, 1975.

Ehni, G. The surgical nurse and neurological surgery. *J. Neurosurg. Nurs.* 6:7, 1974.

Eliasson, S. G., Prensky, A. L., and Hardin, W. B., Jr. *Neurological Pathophysiology.* New York: Oxford University Press, 1974.

Feustel, D. Autonomic hyperreflexia. *Am. J. Nurs.* 76:228, 1976.

Fields, W. S. Aortocranial occlusive vascular disease (stroke). *Clin. Symp.* 26:3, 1974.

Flaherty, P. T., and Jurkovich, S. J. *Transfers for Patients with Acute and Chronic Conditions.* Minneapolis, Minn.: Sister Kenny Institute, 1970.

Ford, J. R., and Duckworth, B. *Physical Management for the Quadriplegic Patient.* Philadelphia: Davis, 1974.

Fowler, R. S., and Fordyce, W. E. Adapting care for the brain-damaged patient. *Am. J. Nurs.* 72:1832, 1972.

Fox, M. J. Talking with patients who can't answer. *Am. J. Nurs.* 71:1146, 1971.

Gaffney, T. W., and Campbell, R. P. Feeding techniques for dysphagic patients. *Am. J. Nurs.* 74:2194, 1974.

Graber, R. F. The minor head injury: a major dilemma. *Patient Care* 8:16, 1974.

Guth, L., and Clemente, C. D. *Experimental Neurology.* Part 2, vol. 48, no. 3 (Sept.), 1975.

Hafey, L. W., and Keane, B. A. Patients with acute insult to the central nervous system. An observational tool. *Nurs. Clin. North Am.* 8:743, 1973.

Hayter, J. Patients who have Alzheimer's disease. *Am. J. Nurs.* 74:1460, 1974.

Heilman, K. M. Neuropsychologic changes in the stroke patient. *Geriatrics* 29:153, 1974.

Hekmatpanah, J. The management of head trauma. *Surg. Clin. North Am.* 53:47, 1973.

Henderson, G. M. Teaching—learning for rehabilitation of the spinal cord-disabled individual. *Nurs. Clin. North Am.* 6:655, 1971.

Hewitt, W. *Functional Neuroanatomy.* London: Macmillan Journals Ltd., 1972.

Hinkhouse, A. Craniocerebral trauma. *Am. J. Nurs.* 73:1719, 1973.

Hrobsky. A. The patient on a CircOlectric^R bed. *Am. J. Nurs.* 71:2352, 1971.

Jackson, F. E. The Pathophysiology of Head Injuries (reprint from *Clinical Symposia*). Summit, N. J.: Ciba, 1966.

Jackson, F. E., Back, J. V., and Pratt, R. Current management of acute injuries of skull and brain. *Am. Fam. Phys.* 10:82, 1974.

Jimm, L. R. Nursing assessment of patients for increased intracranial pressure. *J. Neurosurg. Nurs.* 6:27, 1974.

Johnson, M. R. Emergency management of head and spinal injuries. *Nurs. Clin. North Am.* 8:389, 1973.

Johnson, I. Radiofrequency percutaneous rhizotomy. *J. Neurosurg. Nurs.* 6:92, 1974.

Judge, R. D., and Zuidema, G. D. *Methods of Clinical Examination: A Physiologic Approach* (3rd ed.). Boston, Little, Brown, 1974.

Kay, E., and Boone, E. Stereotactic surgery for Parkinson's disease. *Am. J. Nurs.* 72:2200, 1972.

Korte, M. L. Intensive care of the neurologic patient. Meeting the challenge. *Nurs. Clin. North Am.* 7:335, 1972.

Lehmann, J. F., et al. Wheelchair propulsion in the quadriplegic patient. *Arch. Phys. Med. Rehab.* 55:183, 1974.

Mack, E. W., and Dawson, W. N., Jr. Injury to the spine and spinal cord. *Hosp. Med.* 12:23, 1976.

Matzke, H. A., and Foltz, F. M. *Synopsis of Neuroanatomy* (2nd ed.). New York: Oxford University Press, 1972.

McCullough, E. C., et al. An evaluation of the quantitative and radiation features of a scanning x-ray transverse axial tomograph: The EMI scanner. *Radiology* 111:709, 1974.

McDonald, J., and Lapham, L. Central Nervous System Tumors. In Rubin, P. (ed.), *Clinical Oncology for Medical Students and Physicians* (4th ed.). New York: American Cancer Society, 1974.

Merrill, D. C., and Conway, C. J. Clinical experience with the Mentor bladder stimulator. Patients with upper motor neuron lesions. *J. Urol.* 112:52, 1974.

Michael, J. A. Physiology of the nervous system: From the molecular to the behavioral. *J. Am. Assoc. Nurse Anesth.* 43:140, 1975.

Moeller, E. Cervical common carotid to supraclinoid intracranial internal carotid artery saphenous vein bypass. *J. Neurosurg. Nurs.* 6:132, 1974.

Moeller, B. A., and Scheinberg, D. Autonomic dysreflexia in injuries below the sixth (6th) thoracic segment. *J.A.M.A.* 224:1295, 1973.

Monken, S. S. After assessment—what then. *Nurs. Clin. North Am.* 10:107, 1975.

Murphy, J. J., and Schoenberg, H. W. Principles of management of the neurogenic bladder. *Hosp. Med.* 3:83, 1967.

Murray, R. L. E. Principles of nursing intervention for the adult patient with body image changes. *Nurs. Clin. North Am.* 7:697, 1972.

National Advisory Commission on Multiple Sclerosis. *Report and Recommendations of the National Advisory Commission on Multiple Sclerosis* (Vol. I). Bethesda, Md.: DHEW Publ. 74-534, 1974.

Nelson, G. Current approaches in the treatment of malignant gliomas of the brain. *J. Neurosurg. Nurs.* 6:109, 1974.

Odachowski, S. Cerebrospinal fluid–acid base balance: Importance in neurosurgical nursing. *Am. J. Neurosurg. Nurs.* 6:117, 1974.

Patient Assessment: Neurological Examination (Parts I, II, III). *Am. J. Nurs.* 75:1, 1975; 76:1, 1976.

Passmore, R., and Robson, J. S. *A Companion to Medical Studies,* Vol. 3. London: Blackwell, 1974.

Ransoff, J. Treatment of ruptured supratentorial aneurysms. Current concepts of cerebrovascular disease. *Stroke* 8:21, 1975.

Robinson, M. B. Levodopa and Parkinsonism. *Am. J. Nurs.* 74:656, 1974.

Ruge, D. *Spinal Cord Injuries.* Springfield, Ill.: Thomas, 1969.

Schontz, F. C. *The Psychological Aspects of Physical Illness and Disability.* New York: Macmillan, 1975.

Seedor, M. M. *The Physical Assessment: A Programmed Unit of Study for Nurses.* New York: Teachers College Press, 1974.

Selkurt, E. E. *Basic Physiology for the Health Sciences.* Boston: Little, Brown, 1975.

Sodaro, E., and Perlick, J., Sr. Guillain-Barré: The syndrome, patient care and some case findings. *J. Neurosurg. Nurs.* 6:97, 1974.

Soll, D. B., and Schaffzin, L. Horner's syndrome. *Am. Fam. Phys.* 9:141, 1974.

Stackhouse, J. Myasthenia gravis. *Am. J. Nurs.* 73:1544, 1973.

Stayman, J. W. Thoracic outlet syndrome. *Surg. Clin. North Am.* 53:667, 1973.

Taylor, A. G. Autonomic dysreflexia in spinal cord injury. *Nurs. Clin. North Am.* 9:717, 1974.

Taylor, M. L. Understanding aphasia. *A Guide for Family and Friends* (Patient Publication No. 2) New York: Institute of Rehabilitation Medicine, N.Y.U. Medical Center, 1958.

Taylor, J. W. Measuring the outcomes of nursing care. *Nurs. Clin. North Am.* 9:337, 1974.

Valencius, J. C. Guidelines for neuroassessment. *AORN J.* 20:442, 1974.

Wells, R. W. Huntington's Chorea: Seeing beyond the disease. *Am. J. Nurs.* 72:954, 1972.

Whisnant, J. P. Epidemiology of cerebral infarction. Current concepts of cerebrovascular disease. *Stroke* 9:1, 1974.

Wright, G. N. (ed.). *Epilepsy Rehabilitation*. Boston: Little, Brown, 1975.

Yahr, M. D. Brain tumors. *Hosp. Med.* 9:8, 1973.

chapter 12 Patients with Eye Dysfunction

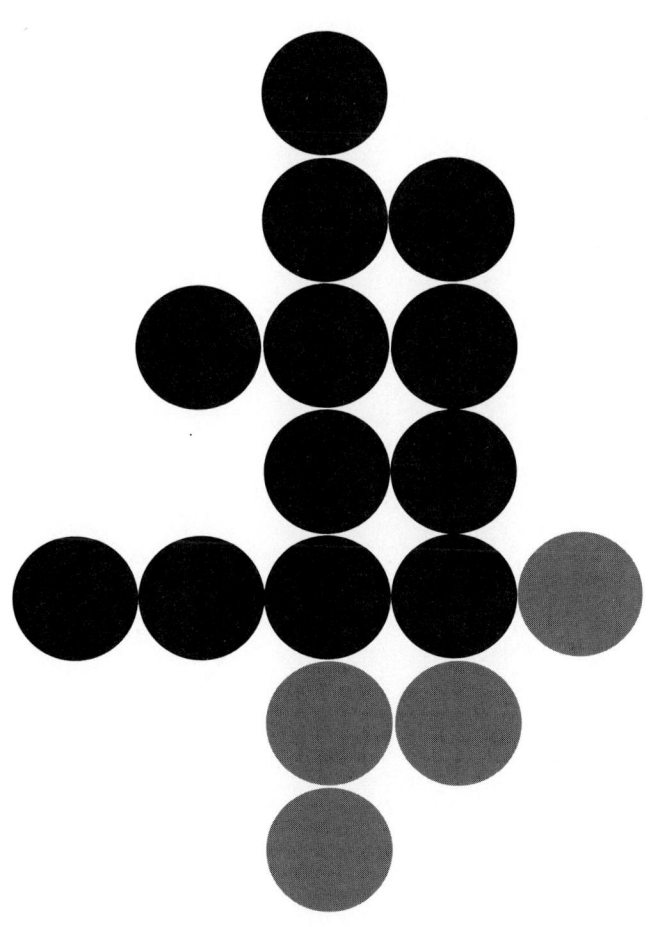

Vision is considered the body's most valued sensory function. The world is oriented to sighted people so that when visual impairment or blindness occurs functioning is hindered. Vision loss interferes with safe and free mobility and deprives a person of enjoying the beauty, sights, and colors around him. Not only is the blind person handicapped in the ability to function and move about freely, but his or her interpersonal relationships are also affected. The person who is blind loses the facility for interpreting nonverbal communication. In addition, verbal and written communication is also affected by visual impairment and blindness. Thus loss of vision results in reduced sensory input and stimulation.

The value of vision is felt most explicitly when a person is faced with the threat of visual impairment or blindness. It is understandable therefore that such a situation is a crisis for the person and the family, requiring that the nurse provide emotional support and assistance to cope with the crisis. The implications of vision loss are great, affecting the person's social, physical, emotional, and psychological state. The nurse should therefore be concerned with the prevention of both blindness and impairment of vision, the maintenance of eye health, measures to enhance healing in ocular disorders, and the rehabilitation of the patient with blindness or visual impairment.

Prevention of Blindness

Although some persons are blind from birth, a great number of people are blind as the result of preventable conditions. The major cause of blindness on a worldwide basis, for example, is the disease **trachoma,** which is prevalent in Africa, Asia, and parts of South America [14]. The disease is transmitted by the common fly as well as by direct contact with infected eyes. Trachoma is prevalent in areas of poverty, crowded living conditions, and poor hygiene. Effective education regarding hygiene and the transmission and treatment of this disease should have an impact on decreasing blindness caused by trachoma. Progress has been made in combating this disease through the efforts of the World Health Organization in conducting education programs and in treating trachoma with specific antibiotics.

The eyes are vulnerable to injury because they are exposed organs and thus are susceptible to infections and trauma. Protection of vision can be facilitated with the enforcement of safety regulations and standards regarding the use of shatterproof automobile glass and safety eyeglass lenses to prevent eye lacerations. Safety goggles or welding masks must be used in industrial and farm work, especially where caustic solutions are used or where particles of dust, wood chips, or metal may enter the eye, and in any other situation where potential eye injuries exist (e.g., in classroom laboratories). The potential danger of eye injuries from BB guns, pointed sticks, and similar objects should be emphasized. Outlawing the sale of dangerous toys and fireworks and requiring the use of protective sports equipment are additional measures to prevent blindness from trauma. Traumatic causes of blindness can also be reduced through proper education in first aid measures for eye injuries.

Health education for the public should emphasize early consultation and referral when ocular symptoms occur or when vision-screening programs detect abnormalities. Laws requiring the instillation of silver nitrate drops in the eyes of every newborn have controlled the incidence of blindness resulting from venereal disease in the mother. Improved prenatal care, including rubella inoculations to protect the fetus from maternal rubella, has made a positive impact on the incidence of congenital blindness in the United States.

In educating the public about eye health and the importance of positive habits in preventive eye care, the nurse should clarify the different types of specialists and their services so that patients are informed about the appropriate person to consult. The **ophthalmologist** or **oculist** is a physician specializing in the diagnosis and treatment of defects and diseases of the eye who is able to perform surgery and prescribe treatment, including eyeglasses. An **optometrist** should be distinguished as a nonmedical practitioner who is trained only to measure refractive errors and eye muscle disturbances. The optometrist's practice is limited to the examination of the eye for refractive errors and prescription eyeglasses, optical aids, and therapeutic exercises. An **optician** is a person who is trained to grind lenses, fit them into frames, and adjust the frames to the wearer.

Several agencies are involved in the various aspects of care of the blind and the prevention of blindness; these agencies are listed in the last section of this chapter. One of these agencies is the National Society for the Prevention of Blindness, Inc., a voluntary health agency with a single purpose, to save sight. The Society claims that half of all blindness is preventable, and it conducts a comprehensive program of community services, public and professional education, and support of research related to the prevention of blindness.

It is estimated that about 1.5 million persons in the United States are blind in one eye and more than 300,000 are legally blind. Although the United States has one of the lowest incidence rates of blindness among the nations of the world, efforts must be continued to prevent the approximately 30,000 new cases of blindness that occur annually [9]. The National Eye Institute, a division of the National Institutes of Health, is the national federal center for promoting research geared to the prevention of blindness and the management of visual disorders. Existing programs of the Institute are concerned with etiology, better screening methods, medical management, and new surgical procedures. For example, the National Eye Institute has been conducting an epidemiologic study to identify risk factors for the four leading causes of adult blindness in the United States—senile cataracts, senile macular degeneration, chronic simple glaucoma, and diabetic retinopathy. This study utilized the same population from Framingham, Massachusetts, that has been since 1950 a part of the well-known Framingham Heart Study. The presence of these four ocular conditions in the study population is being reviewed to determine if there is a relationship between their incidence and factors such as cigarette smoking, diet, and high blood pressure. The report is not available at the time of this writing.

Much information about a patient's physical and emotional status can be gained through careful observation of the eyes, which are good indicators of health or illness. It is a well-recognized fact that changes in the eyes can be indicative of systemic or localized disease. The importance of including an eye examination as part of the routine physical examination cannot be overemphasized as a major factor in the early detection of ocular disease and the prevention of blindness.

Anatomy and Physiology of the Eye

A review of the mechanism of vision and the structures involved in visual functioning is necessary as a basis for understanding ocular disorders, their prevention, and treatment.

Vision provides for sensory input. Figure

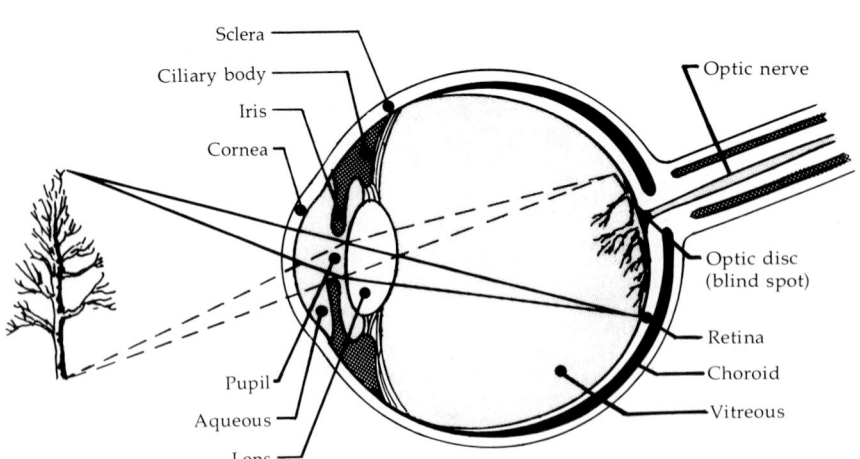

Figure 12-1
Structures of the eye and mechanisms of sight. Light rays enter the eye through the cornea, pass through the opening in the iris, the pupil, to the crystalline lens, which then directs the rays through the vitreous body and focuses them on the retina.

12-1 illustrates how an image is viewed by the eye with specific refracting media identified as the cornea, the aqueous humor, the lens, and the vitreous humor. This diagram can also be used to clarify the structural arrangement of the globe, or eyeball, and its components. The light rays that strike an object in a person's field of vision are first transmitted through the cornea, which is normally completely transparent. Blinking of the eyes spreads tears over the corneal surface, maintaining transparency and preventing scarring of the cornea. The cornea is the anterior portion of the outer layer of the eye and becomes the sclera posteriorly at the junction identified as the limbus. The sclera, the protective opaque outer layer, is observed as the white portion of the eye. (The sclera may become discolored in certain systemic diseases, such as in jaundice associated with liver disease.)

The light rays pass through the anterior chamber of the eye, which is filled with aqueous humor (the fluid behind the cornea), and then proceed through the pupil. The iris (the colored part of the eye) surrounds the pupil and regulates its size and the amount of light reaching the retina by enlarging the pupil in darkness and reducing it in bright light. The iris controls the pupil size through the reflex action of the iris sphincter muscle, which is supplied by the parasympathetic nervous system, and the action of the iris dilator muscle, which is innervated by the sympathetic nervous system. The iris is part of the uveal tract, which consists of the iris, the ciliary body, and the choroid. The ciliary body produces the aqueous fluid, which fills the anterior chamber of the eye and also has a muscular function of opening the trabecular spaces through which the aqueous fluid escapes from the eye. The ciliary muscle also controls the tension on the zonular fibers, which suspend the lens in proper position and change its shape to produce accommodation. The choroid, a very vascular layer, supplies the nutrition for the outer half of the retina, to which it is normally attached.

The light rays are transmitted through the transparent crystalline lens of the eye. The lens bends the light rays appropriately to focus on the retina, the innermost layer of the eye. The crystalline lens is normally biconvex in shape, but it deepens or becomes more shallow in order to accommodate for near or far vision. Although the image is received upside down on the retina (as shown in Fig. 12-1), it is transmitted via the optic nerve to the brain, where the image is perceived appropriately. Two types of visual receptors are located in the retina: the rods, which are used for vision in dim light, and the cones, which are used for daylight vision and for recognizing colors. The retina contains a depression, the fovea centralis, surrounded by the macula, which is the area of the fundus (the inner lining of the eyeball) with the greatest concentration of visual receptors. The macula therefore permits detailed central vision.

The optic nerve exits from the retina, creating a retinal defect known as the physiologic blind spot, which results from the absence of visual receptors at this point. The meningeal sheaths that encircle the optic nerve are continuous with the meninges of the brain, with the result that increased intracranial pressure is reflected in papilledema (swelling of the optic disc). The optic nerves join to form the optic chiasm just behind the orbits overlying the pituitary gland. At this point the medial or nasal fibers cross over so that the left optic tract contains fibers only from the left half of each retina and the right optic tract contains fibers from the right half of each retina. The visual pathway is an important factor in locating and understanding visual defects associated with intracranial disease. These defects are discussed in detail in Chapter 11. The visual pathways continue to the visual cortex in the occipital lobes of the brain.

The bony cavity surrounding the eye provides considerable protection for the eye through its sturdy orbital walls. The eyelids also serve as protective coverings; they close by the action of the orbicularis muscle of the eye, which is innervated by the facial (seventh cranial) nerve. The eyelids shield the eyes from excessive light and rays and provide for blinking to keep the corneal surface smooth and to keep a film of tears evenly distributed. The upper lid is pulled into the orbit by the action of the levator muscle, which is innervated by the third cranial nerve. The lacrimal gland, which is located in the upper lateral part of the orbit, produces the tears that lubricate the eye surface. The tears normally drain into the lacrimal puncta, located at the inner part of the upper and lower lids, and are carried by the canaliculi into the lacrimal sac, which is a small pouch located in the nasal corner of the orbit.

The nasolacrimal duct then drains fluid from the sac into the nose.

The shape of the eyeball is maintained primarily by a viscous, gel-like substance, the vitreous humor, which is located behind the lens in the posterior cavity of the eye. Each eye is suspended in the orbit by means of six extraocular muscles, ligaments, vessels, nerves, and a cushion of fat. The extraocular muscles, which are innervated by the third, fourth, and sixth cranial nerves, include the four rectus muscles, the superior oblique muscle, and the inferior oblique muscle. The extraocular muscles are responsible for aiming the two eyes at the same point in space.

Assessment of the Eye and Vision

Assessment of the eye includes obtaining an ophthalmic history; examination of the external eye, its orbit, and surrounding tissues; assessment of visual acuity through visual screening techniques; assessment of ocular movements, testing of pupillary reactions, determination of intraocular pressure, and examination of the internal eye with an ophthalmoscope and other special instruments to evaluate the ocular fundus; and specialized examinations done only by an ophthalmologist. The nurse's role in these various aspects of the ocular examination varies in different settings. All nurses, however, should be knowledgeable about the purpose of each part of the eye examination.

Eye examinations are especially important at birth to detect malformations, injuries, and infections, as well as during the preschool period and whenever ocular symptoms occur. They are also recommended in early adolesence and every five years during young adulthood. After the age of 35 to 40, when there is usually a beginning of reduction in vision, eye examinations are advised every two years. The more frequent eye examinations after age 40 are indicated by the fact that the highest incidence of blindness occurs in the older age group. However, the eyes should also be examined as part of the routine complete physical examination and especially when the patient complains of blurred vision or other symptoms of possible ocular origin. Some patients require more frequent eye examinations, particularly when there is a family history of diabetes or glaucoma.

A history of any systemic disease with possible implications for visual dysfunction, a history of familial ocular diseases, and the patient's own symptoms and description of visual changes are essential parts of the assessment of ocular function. The examiner should determine the presence of symptoms of pain, light sensitivity, itching, tearing, redness, and blurring or veiling of vision. The onset of these symptoms, precipitating factors, and measures that provide relief should also be determined.

Because the nurse, particularly the school nurse, is often involved in visual screening examinations, measurement of visual acuity will be considered first in the discussion of assessment of the eye and vision.

MEASUREMENT OF VISUAL ACUITY

Visual screening is most often done with the use of the Snellen wall chart, which has block letters in gradually decreasing sizes. The smallest line that the patient can read from a specific distance is determined. Measurement of visual acuity is done on each eye separately, with the other eye totally occluded with an opaque card. The visual acuity is recorded as a fraction but does not reflect a ratio; the numerator reflects the distance of the patient from the chart and the denominator is the distance at which a normal eye can read the specific line. For example, when a patient 20 feet from the chart cannot read beyond the line that a person with normal vision can read at 30 feet, the visual acuity is recorded as 20/30 vision. The largest letter on the Snellen chart can normally be seen at 400 feet. If the patient can read only this line at 20 feet, his visual acuity is recorded as 20/400. If the patient normally wears glasses, the eyes are then tested with the glasses in place and visual acuity is measured as corrected vision.

Variations of the Snellen chart are used in certain situations. For example, if the patient being examined is illiterate or cannot read English, the block E chart may be used; the patient reports the position of the legs of the E in the different lines. If the patient being tested is a young child, variations of the chart using animal figures, birthday cakes, or toys may be used. Any patient with vision less than 20/30 should be referred to an ophthalmologist for further testing and treatment. If the visual acuity is decreased, for example to 20/70, the ophthalmologist will usually assess vision with the use of the pinhole disc. This test provides a rough determination as to whether vision that is subnormal without glasses is caused by a refractive error or by other conditions. If the visual acuity score is not improved with the use of the pinhole, some cause other than a refractive error is suspected, such as opacities in the ocular media or disease of the retina or optic nerve.

Legal blindness is defined as visual acuity of 20/200 or less in both eyes with full correction or less than a 20° field of vision in each. This definition is used to determine eligibility for special services and income tax benefits. Blindness is defined medically, however, as the inability to perceive light.

To test near vision, the Jaeger chart is used. The Jaeger card contains print of varying sizes with scores beside each size; it is held 14 inches from the eye and as many lines as possible are read. If a Jaeger card is not available, regular newsprint can be used to evaluate near vision. This test is particularly important for patients more than 40 years old, in whom presbyopia is most likely to occur. (Presbyopia is impaired vision resulting from the aging process with loss of elasticity in the crystalline lens of the eye, causing defects in near vision.)

TESTING FOR OCULAR MOVEMENTS

The range of extraocular muscular control over eye movements is tested for normal version and direction. Movement of both eyes jointly is **version** and individual movement is **direction**. The patient is asked to focus on a moving finger or pencil held at a comfortable distance from his or her eyes. The object should then be moved through the six cardinal fields of gaze, which include the straight nasal, up and nasal, down and nasal, straight temporal, up and temporal, and down and temporal fields (Fig. 12-2). The muscles and cranial nerves involved in these positions are the medial rectus (oculomotor or third cranial nerve), inferior oblique (third cranial nerve), superior oblique (trochlear or fourth cranial nerve), lateral rectus (abducens or sixth cranial nerve), superior rectus (third cranial nerve), and inferior rectus (third cranial nerve), respectively. Any abnormal movements of the eye are reported.

Convergence of the eyes is tested by asking the patient to follow the examiner's finger or a pencil as it is moved toward the bridge of the patient's nose. Strabismus, commonly known as "crossed eyes," is a faulty alignment of the two eyes. It is usually caused by an abnormal extrinsic muscle resulting in diplopia or double vision. Strabismus may be convergent (estropia), divergent (exotropia), or vertical (hypertropia) and may be congenital or the result of disease or trauma. Convergent strabismus is the most common type seen in children.

VISUAL FIELD TESTING

Measurements of the visual field are indicated as part of a thorough eye examination. Disease of the retina and optic nerve, as well

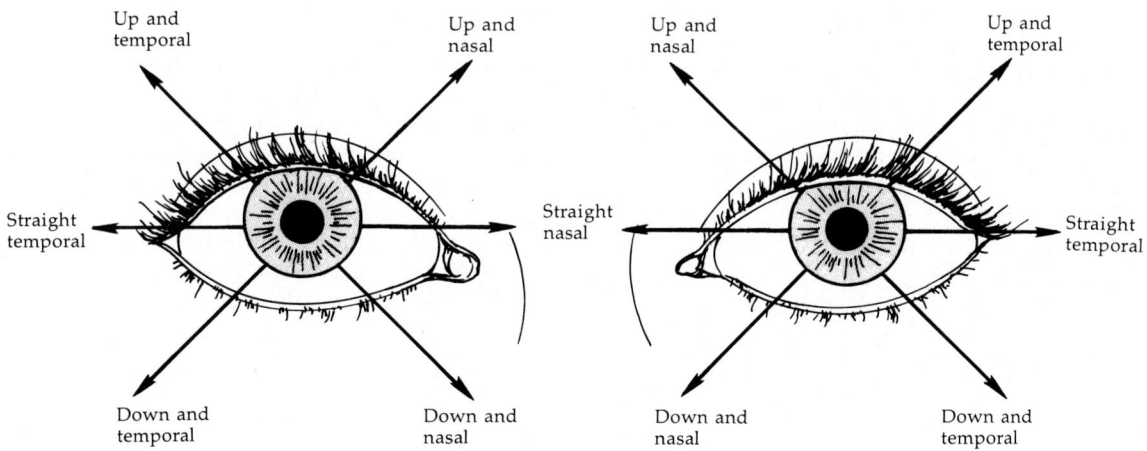

Figure 12-2
Testing for ocular movements; the six cardinal positions of gaze.

as glaucoma and intracranial lesions, can cause visual field defects. Normally, a person's visual field should be 60° nasally, 50° upward, 90° temporally, and 70° downward [8].

The perimeter, a semicircular instrument that is marked in degrees, is used to determine the extent of the patient's peripheral vision. In the absence of a perimeter, the examiner may obtain a rough estimate of field vision using his finger as a target. The examiner can bring his finger from behind the patient to determine the point at which it is first seen while the patient's gaze is fixed straight ahead. Assuming that the examiner's field vision is normal, a confrontation test may be used as a rough measurement of the visual field. In this test, the examiner and the patient are seated about three feet apart. One eye of the examiner is closed and the eye of the patient on the same side is patched, and each person fixes his open eye on the other person's open eye as a target. An object is moved inward from outside the visual field until seen by the patient who is being tested. The examiner and the patient should detect the object at the same time, if the patient's visual fields are normal. Another method for visual field measurement is the tangent screen. A large black felt cloth with a central mark for fixation is used to record the central visual fields.

ASSESSMENT OF THE EXTERNAL EYE

Inspection of the external eye includes observation for local infection or disease and systemic disease, and evaluation of the extent of injury following trauma to the face and eyes. In conversing with the patient, the nurse should note the overall appearance of the eyes and their movements. The lids, conjunctiva, cornea, anterior chamber, iris, pupils, and lacrimal ducts are examined.

The lids are examined first to determine the adequacy of closure and to check for the presence of **ptosis** or drooping of the eyelid. Normally the upper lid does not cover any part of the pupil when the eye is opened. Ptosis may be caused by congenital underdevelopment of the lid muscles or by heaviness of the lid resulting from edema or excess fatty material or by trauma. Ptosis is also a symptom of abnormal neuromuscular transmission as found in myasthenia gravis or with damage to the third cranial nerve. The blinking reflex of the eyelid is a mechanism by which the eye is protected from injuries. Absence of the blinking reflex may be the result of neurologic disease and requires further examination by an ophthalmologist and neurologist. (Eye shields are applied to the eye to protect it, when the blinking reflex is absent.)

Exophthalmos (abnormal protrusion of the eyeball) of only one eye may indicate a tumor and should definitely be reported as a significant finding. The eyelids consist of thin skin and thus collect excess fluid more readily than any other skin area in the body. Systemic fluid retention may therefore result in edematous eyelids. When the lids are chronically swollen, nephritis or nephrosis should be suspected. Allergic reactions that are nonocular in origin may also cause edematous eyelids. The skin of the eyelids should be examined for lesions, nodules, or ulcers, which may be symptoms of basal cell or squamous cell carcinoma. Basal cell carcinoma occurs more commonly on the lower lid in persons older than 50 years of age. The patient with a suspicious lesion should be referred to an ophthalmologist for surgical excision and biopsy.

Prior to examining the eye, the nurse should wash his or her hands. If there is any infection in one eye, the nurse should again take hand washing precautions prior to examining the opposite eye in order to prevent cross-contamination. Infection should be suspected if there is any redness or discharge from the eyelid. Infection of the small meibomian glands located along the lid margin, known as marginal blepharitis, is fairly common. The infection is usually of staphylococcal origin, with pus or pustules at the base of the lashes. It may also result from seborrheic dermatitis. Seborrheic dermatitis usually causes waxy and greasy scales that cling to the lids; when they are removed, they leave open lesions. Discussion of the management of infectious lesions of the eye is found in a subsequent section of this chapter.

The nurse should examine the position of the lashes, which normally curve outward from the eye. Progressive relaxation of the lid muscles caused by physiologic aging can result in **entropion** (inversion of the lid). The curling inward of the lashes causes the cilia to come in contact with the conjunctiva and the conjunctiva and cornea are frequently irritated by the lashes. Corneal scarring results and plastic surgery is often required to evert the lashes. Therefore, the presence of entropion is an important finding to report.

Another ocular change that can be observed in elderly patients is **ectropion,** in which the lid turns outward from the eyeball; this causes the lower lid to droop and exposes the cornea and conjunctiva. Drying and exposure of the conjunctival tissue can produce excessive tearing and redness of the conjunctiva. This finding also requires referral to an ophthalmologist, because surgery is often indicated to correct excessive tearing, exposure keratitis, or cosmetic problems.

Madarosis (loss of eyelashes) may be a local condition associated with inflammation of the lid margins, or it may be associated with generalized alopecia.

The lacrimal system is evaluated and examined for the presence of infection or blockage. Tearing, swelling over the area of the inner canthus, redness, pain, and purulent discharge are all associated with infection of the lacrimal sac, known as **dacryocystitis.** Chronic dacryocystitis with complete obstruction of the nasolacrimal duct causes an overflow of tears from the eye, which is termed **epiphora.**

The nurse should examine the eyes for localized swelling and inflammation. An acute inflammation at the lid margin around a hair follicle of the eyelashes may be recognized as a **hordeolum,** commonly known as a sty. Initially tender, swollen, red, and inflamed with the appearance of a boil or pimple, the hordeolum may progress to a pustular condition (usually of staphylococcal origin). If precautions are not taken, the infectious exudate may be transmitted to the other eye. Sties occur singly or in groups. People who have sties frequently should be suspected of lowered or altered states of health, particularly anemia or diabetes mellitus.

In contrast to the hordeolum, the **chalazion,** which is a granuloma of the internal sebaceous (meibomian) glands of the lid, is not usually inflamed or tender to the touch. The chalazion has the consistency of a firm nodule or swollen lump, and thus, when located inside the lid, it may cause irritation or subsequent infection of the underlying parts.

The conjunctiva, which is the mucous membrane lining the back surface of the eyelids (palpebral conjunctiva), is normally pink in color. The conjunctiva also covers the sclera (bulbar conjunctiva) but is transparent so that the white sclera is actually observed. Conjunctivitis may result from bacterial or viral infections or from mechanical, chemical, or allergic causes. Normally, many small blood vessels are visible in the conjunctiva; when they become dilated, the symptom of redness becomes quite evident. (A "red eye" indicates the presence of conjunctivitis, but may also be a sign of corneal abrasion, acute iritis, or acute glaucoma.) The conjunctiva covering the back surface of the eyelids cannot be seen until the lids are everted. By pulling the skin over the lower orbital rim downward and asking the patient to look upward, the nurse can examine the conjunctiva of the inferior lid. This procedure is also necessary for examining the conjunctiva for foreign bodies, since this is the most common location of superficial foreign bodies. To examine the conjunctiva of the upper lid, the patient should look down while the nurse grasps the lashes, pulls downward, and everts the lid over an applicator. This technique is illustrated in Figure 12-3.

A **pterygium,** an abnormal growth of the conjunctival tissue in a pyramidal shape containing blood vessels, may often be seen on the white of the eye and it may extend to the cornea. The patient with a pterygium should be referred to an ophthalmologist. Although a pterygium usually does not require removal, it may be cosmetically undesirable or may obstruct vision if growing over the cornea and require surgical treatment.

The cornea is examined with a penlight for smoothness, clearness, and reflective properties. Irregularities or dullness in any area are abnormal findings. The size and shape of both corneas should be compared. If the patient complains of **photophobia** (increased sensitivity to light) or blurred vision, or has irregularities or dullness of the cornea, he should be referred to an ophthalmologist for diagnosis and treatment. The corneal reflex may also be tested (this test is described as part of the neurologic examination in Chapter 11).

EXAMINATION OF THE IRIS, PUPILLARY REFLEXES, AND LENS

The iris should be examined for color, texture, and pattern, and for any unusual markings or

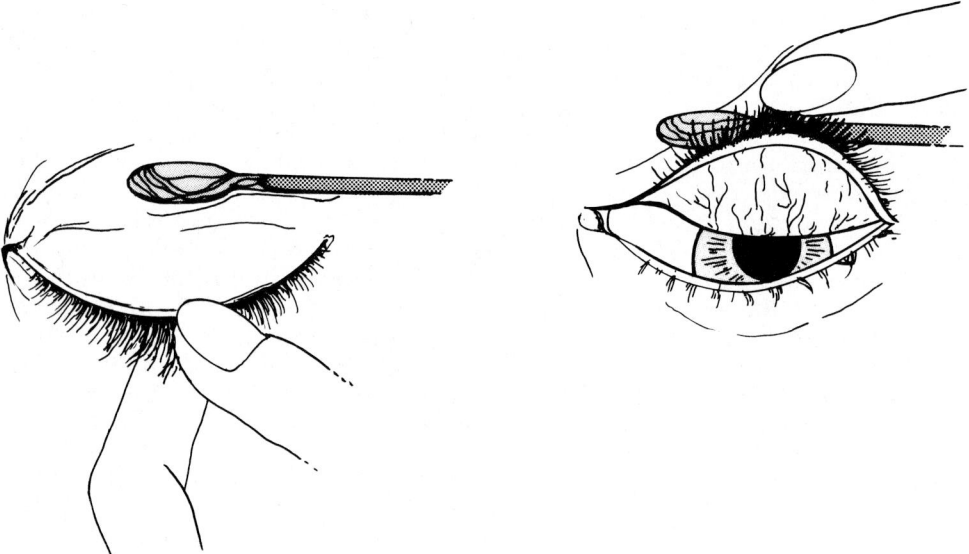

Figure 12-3
Examination of the conjunctiva of the upper lid by everting the eyelid. The eyelid is grasped with the fingers of one hand, and the upper lid is pulled outward and upward over the applicator. This technique is also used for removing a foreign body resting on the conjunctiva.

growths. The pupil of each eye should be checked for configuration, equality in size, and reflex reaction to light. Enlargement of the pupil may be caused by drugs, acute glaucoma, eye injury, or systemic poisoning by parasympatholytic drugs, so a careful history is required. When pupil inequality is detected, the nurse must investigate whether the patient has used mydriatic or miotic eye drops in either eye or if the patient has a past history of eye surgery or neurosurgery. It is important for the nurse to make this investigation before assuming that a serious neurologic or ocular disease is present. For example, constriction of the pupil may be present in the patient with glaucoma who has recently administered a miotic drug such as pilocarpine into the eye. Constricted pupils may also be present in patients who are taking narcotics or heroin and in patients with iritis.

To test pupil reaction, the nurse should use a penlight or a flashlight and approach the eye from the side (approaching the eye from straight ahead with a flashlight will cause the patient to accommodate to the light source, which can be misleading in evaluating the reaction). In physical assessment, the abbreviation **PERLA** is often used to indicate that "the pupils react equally to light and accommodation." Both eyes are checked for pupil reaction; direct reaction results in constriction of the pupil receiving the light but will also cause constriction of the opposite pupil through stimulation of either optic nerve (consensual reaction). This simultaneous constriction will occur even in an eye that is blind. However, if the light source is brought initially to the blind eye, there will be no constriction in either eye.

Since the pupil is normally round, any irregularity is reported as an abnormal finding. Opacity of the lens, as found in cataracts, may cause the normally black-appearing pupil to have a cloudy or discolored area. The size and shape of the pupil may deviate as a result of swelling of the iris, which may be discolored. When this symptom is detected, especially in conjunction with ocular pain, iritis is suspected and the patient should be referred to an ophthalmologist. **Iritis** is the most common inflammatory process of the uveal tract. Inflammation of the ciliary body and choroid may also occur and present similar symptoms. Iritis causes cells and protein materials to collect in the anterior chamber; this can be detected by the ophthalmologist using a special binocular microscope with a fine slit-light beam (the slit lamp) to visualize fine detail in the anterior segment of the eye.

EXAMINATION OF THE INTERNAL EYE

Ophthalmoscopic examination is a necessary part of the eye examination, and in some settings it may be the responsibility of the nurse who has been trained in its technique. Using the ophthalmoscope, the examiner can look through the pupil to examine the internal components of the eye (the chambers and ocular fundus). A darkened room is used for the examination. The ophthalmoscope is held 2 or 3 cm (1 inch) from the patient's eye and should not touch the eye. When the examiner observes the patient's left eye, the ophthalmoscope is held in the left hand and the left eye is used for the examination. The examiner's right eye is used to examine the patient's right eye, with the ophthalmoscope held in the right hand.

The location of opacities in the cornea, lens, or vitreous humor is determined by observing the way the opacity appears to move when the examiner moves his or her own eye. For example, an opacity that appears to move in the same direction as the examiner's eye is probably located behind the lens in the vitreous humor, whereas an opacity that does not seem to move at all identifies opacity in the lens. Corneal opacity usually causes movement in the opposite direction [12].

Fundoscopy consists in examination of the optic disc, the macula, and the blood vessels located in the posterior wall of the eye. The fundus is the only area of the body in which blood vessels can be directly examined; this fact establishes the importance of the ophthalmoscopic examination in diagnosing and evaluating systemic diseases that affect the vascular system throughout the body. The optic disc, which is normally red-orange in color, contains a small depression in its center called the physiologic cup. Although the cup is sometimes not visible, it usually appears as a whitish area near the middle of the disc. Normally the cup is less than half the diameter of the disc but may be larger in glaucoma. The optic disc is normally round or slightly oval with sharply defined margins. Papilledema is present when the entire disc is reddish and congested with swollen margins and scattered "cotton wool" patches. Excessive pallor of the disc indicates a decreased blood supply.

The ophthalmoscope permits direct visualization of the central retinal artery and vein, the largest blood vessels visible in the fundus. This examination facilitates the diagnosis of arterial occlusion, which is a medical emergency characterized by sudden visual loss due to retinal deprivation of oxygen. Permanent damage usually results. Occlusion of the central retinal vein can also cause gradual visual loss. The fundus is checked for abnormalities of pigmentation, hemorrhages, swelling, and production of exudates. Pigmentation of the fundus is similar to the patient's general pigmentation, so that a patient with dark skin would be expected to have a highly pigmented fundus [12]. Clumping of pigment, however, is considered abnormal and may be a sign of degenerative retinal disease. A nevus, the accumulation of pigment in the choroid layer, is another abnormal sign.

Hemorrhages can be seen as crescent-shaped, solid areas in front of the retina, as dots or blots in the deeper layers of the retina, or as small, thin lines radiating from the optic disc [12].

Arterioles and veins are distinguished from each other by color, size, and light reflex. The arterioles are light red in contrast to the dark red veins. Arterioles are smaller than veins and have a bright light reflection, while veins have inconspicuous or dull light reflection [1]. Occlusion of the terminal arterioles with swelling of the nerve fibers results in large, fluffy, white areas described as "cotton wool" patches. Exudates are generally visualized as abnormal, yellowish, small areas with sharp and clear margins; they are usually the result of vascular leakage. Because the macula of the retina is the area having the highest density of visual receptors, hemorrhages, exudates, or occlusions in this area are potentially more serious than in other areas of the retina.

Evaluation of retinal vessels is helpful in assessing the patient with arteriosclerosis or hypertensive disease. Hemorrhage and exudates occur in advanced hypertension, severe renal disease, certain collagen diseases, advanced diabetes, blood dyscrasias, and severe retinal venous occlusion.

Early signs of diabetic retinopathy include venous congestion, tortuosity of the vessels, the presence of microaneurysms, and minute, localized varicosities of the smaller veins. These vascular changes may occur even before any overt systemic symptoms are observed. When the changes are detected, a glucose tolerance test is indicated. Unfortunately, institution of treatment may not improve or arrest the course of diabetic retinopathy.

A patient who has any abnormalities on the fundoscopic examination should be referred to the ophthalmologist (or internist if systemic disease is suspected) for further diagnostic evaluation and treatment. One of the most recent diagnostic tests being utilized for retinal disease is fluorescein angiography. In this technique, a fluorescein dye is injected intravenously into an arm vein. The dye circulates in the bloodstream and permits direct visualization of the blood flow within the vessels of the retina and choroid. The technique facilitates locating the sites of leakage or blocking of blood flow and has proved to be a valuable adjunct to the diagnostic procedures of the ophthalmologist.

MEASUREMENT OF INTRAOCULAR PRESSURE

Every person over the age of 35 should be tested for glaucoma through the initial screening process of tonometry to determine the presence of excessive intraocular pressure, which is a significant finding in the detection of glaucoma. The only contraindication to the tonometry test is the presence of an ocular infection. Tonometry may be performed by a physician or nurse practitioner using a Schiøtz tonometer, which is considered a screening device. Ophthalmologists generally use the applanation tonometer, which is applied to the cornea during observation with the slit lamp and is considered more accurate than the Schiøtz tonometer. Nurses should be knowledgeable about the technique of tonometry, even if they only assist in the procedure, in order to prepare the patient better and to educate the public about the value of tonometry in detecting glaucoma.

The thought of having an instrument placed on the eye can be very frightening to the patient who has never experienced tonometry, unless he receives an explanation of the procedure, how he will feel, and what is expected of him. The patient should be assured that he or she will not experience any pain during or after the test. Each eye is first anesthetized with a drop of tetracaine hydrochloride or proparacaine hydrochloride (Ophthaine or Ophthetic) [18]. The patient is encouraged to relax during the procedure. Tight collars should be loosened to ensure that venous blood flow is not obstructed, since this would cause an artificial increase in intraocular pressure. The patient is directed to fix his or her gaze on an object above while the tonometer is placed to rest on the center of the cornea (Fig. 12-4). The patient is cautioned against rubbing the eyes for about one-half hour after the test while the topical anesthetic continues its effect, in order to prevent any accidental injury to the anesthetized eye. False-positive results may occur if the patient squeezes his or her eyes, if the examiner presses on the eye instead of holding the lids open against the bony orbits, or if the tonometer sticks.

The tonometer measures the indentation resistance of the globe by means of a central plunger fitted into a footplate. The scale should be pretested for accuracy on a testing block, where it should register zero. The footplate is rested gently on the cornea, and the movement of the plunger is transmitted to a lever scale. The reading is considered normal within the range of 12 to 22 mm Hg. The instrument must be held vertically so that the plunger is freely movable. The instrument is cleaned with alcohol or ether after each use, and the alcohol is allowed to evaporate before the tonometer is placed on the eye. Disposable membrane covers for the footplate made of sterile latex are now available for individual use.

Although a diagnosis is not made on the basis of one abnormal reading, the presence of increased intraocular pressure indicates the need for a complete evaluation by an ophthalmologist. When glaucoma is suspected, the ophthalmologist may test visual fields and use a gonioscope to view the angle of the anterior chamber. The gonioscope is a microscope that is held in the hands, and is used with a corneal contact lens, a prism, and a light source. Gonioscopy is used to determine the presence of either open-angle or closed-angle glaucoma (these disorders are discussed later in this chapter).

The ophthalmologist may also on some occasions request that a water provocative test be done to detect or specify the presence of

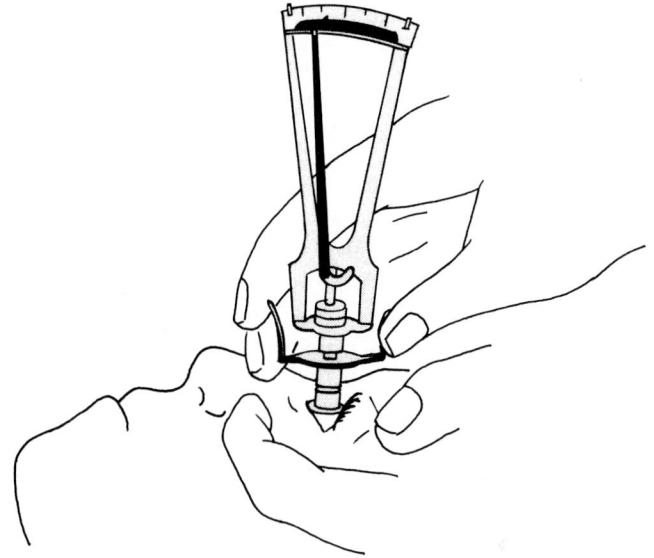

Figure 12-4
Use of the Schiøtz tonometer to measure intraocular pressure.

open-angle glaucoma. A baseline tonometer reading is recorded, and the patient then drinks 1 liter of water. The intraocular pressures are recorded at 30-, 45-, and 60-minute intervals after ingestion of the water to detect the presence of increased intraocular pressure.

MANAGEMENT OF COMMON VISUAL PROBLEMS

The patient who has eye dysfunction is often referred directly to the ophthalmologist for further examination, prescriptions, and continued management, which often takes place on an outpatient basis. The nurse augments the ophthalmologist's care by monitoring the patient's progress, evaluating the effectiveness of the treatment and the patient's understanding of care given, and teaching about potential problems requiring further assessment. The nurse must therefore know about the common visual problems that are treated on an outpatient basis and about management modalities. The nurse also has a responsibility to teach patients about the maintenance of eye health and appropriate methods of eye care.

Refractive Errors

Refraction is tested objectively by an ophthalmologist, using the technique of retinoscopy. In this procedure, movement of focused light merging from the patient's eye is observed. This procedure is performed by means of a refractor, an instrument containing varied lenses on a rotating wheel; the lenses are dialed into the refractor eyepiece. Interpreting the distortion of the light focus facilitates an objective and accurate evaluation of the refractive error. Retinoscopy permits accurate prescriptions for eyeglasses or contact lenses or both. Cycloplegic agents, such as atropine, homatropine, or cyclopentolate hydrochloride (Cyclogyl), are applied topically prior to the procedure to facilitate accuracy; these drugs block accommodation and dilate the pupil. When these drugs are used, the patient should be advised that his near vision may remain somewhat blurred for several hours and that dark glasses may be needed for several hours when outdoors to avoid discomfort caused by excessive light entering the dilated pupils.

The corneal curvature, the strength and flexibility of the lens, and the length of the eye all affect the proper focusing of images on the retina. Normally the ciliary muscles increase and decrease the curvature of the lens as needed for either far or near vision. However, accommodation decreases with age, resulting in presbyopia; after the age of 40, accommodation is often inadequate for close work due to the loss of elasticity of the crystalline lens. The person may then require eyeglasses for reading or close work or may require bifocal lenses, which have different strengths for the top and lower sections to facilitate both near and distant vision. Too often, however, other signs of ocular problems, such as blurred vision and decreased vision, are ignored by older people because they assume these symptoms are also part of the aging process. This attitude may be an important factor in causing delays in obtaining proper examinations and treatment.

Types of refractive errors **Emmetropia** refers to normal refraction of light rays, when the image is appropriately focused on the retina. The person with emmetropic vision adjusts to seeing clearly without effort for distant images and then is able to focus appropriately for close objects. (Emmetropia is illustrated in Figure 12-1.) Refractive errors are those in which there are disturbances in the focusing function of the eye; they include myopia, hyperopia, astigmatism, and anisometropia.

When the light rays are focused behind the retina the condition of **hyperopia** (farsightedness) occurs. The hyperopic eye is the result of insufficient refraction (of either the cornea or lens) so that the eye is unable to focus light upon the retina, particularly when the person is viewing objects at close range. The farsighted eye may also be shorter than the normal eye.

In **myopia** (nearsightedness), parallel rays of light come to focus in front of the retina, as a result of excessive refractive power of the cornea and lens or because the eye is too long for the amount of refractive power. Thus the person with myopia is unable to see distant objects clearly. When myopia is detected in early childhood, new glasses are prescribed every year or every two years as the condition progresses. The status of myopia tends to stabilize in adolescence. Often parents want to give their child extra vitamins, eye exercises, or varied types of treatment to prevent myopia from progressing. The nurse should advise the parent that none of these measures has been shown to prevent the progression of myopia.

Astigmatism, which may accompany myopia or hyperopia, is a fairly common condition caused by uneven curvature of the cornea. This uneven curvature results in distortion of the focus of light rays on the retina so that there is no clear point. Blurred vision and eye discomfort necessitate the use of eyeglasses that are ground to neutralize the unequal curvature of the cornea and thus to produce a clear image on the retina.

The person with **anisometropia** cannot see clearly with both eyes at the same time because there is a different focus in the two eyes. Eyeglasses are required since the person is unable to compensate for the different focusing.

Correction of refractive errors The prescription of **eyeglasses** or **contact lenses** is indicated to correct the various refractive errors. Some persons alternate between contact lenses and eyeglasses. Eyeglasses should be changed as needed when reduced visual acuity or discomfort of the eyes occurs; they do not have to be changed at regular intervals unless these changes occur. However, eyeglasses do require periodic replacement in children as the child outgrows the size of the eyeglasses. People who are required to wear eyeglasses should be oriented to proper care. They should be taught to wear the eyeglasses as prescribed and to prevent trauma or scratches resulting from careless handling. The glasses should be kept clean and properly aligned. When a person wears contact lenses, the nurse should assess his or her habits and management of use of the lenses. Although persons with contact lenses prefer them to the more cumbersome eyeglasses, there are precautions with which the wearer should be familiar. Contact lenses are generally more expensive than eyeglasses and are also lost more readily. The ability to adapt to contact lenses varies. Some persons never do learn how to insert and remove the lenses properly and thus are never free from minor discomfort on wearing them; in spite of the expense of the lenses, some persons discontinue their use. Others find the increased light sensitivity associated with contact lenses uncomfortable. Still others, in their eagerness to use the lenses, ignore the precaution to insert the contact lenses for only a short period of time initially and then gradually to wear them for longer periods until they are well tolerated. Gradual utilization will prevent the occurrence of irritation and corneal abrasion. Contact lenses should be removed during sleep and at periodic intervals to prevent scarring from overuse. Instructions for cleaning and storage must be followed carefully. Lenses should not be used in the presence of any ocular infection, inflammation, or allergic reaction.

Many wearers of contact lenses have the habit of using their saliva to moisten the lenses before insertion; they should be reminded of the danger of corneal infection since saliva is high in bacterial content. Bacterial contamination of any source can result in permanent corneal scarring.

When a patient is admitted to the hospital, the nurse should find out when taking the history whether or not the patient wears contact lenses or eyeglasses so that proper care is given to them. When a patient is comatose, his or her eyes should be checked for the presence of contact lenses, which should be removed. If the cornea of the patient's eye is not visible, the nurse should not attempt to remove the contact lens but should ask an ophthalmologist to remove it. Contact lenses are removed prior to general surgery, when the patient will be unconscious under general anesthesia, to prevent trauma to the eye as well as to prevent trauma or loss of the contact lenses. The lenses should be stored in individual containers and identified properly (i.e., right and left).

The nurse may on occasion have to remove contact lenses in emergency situations when the wearer is injured and unable to remove the lenses or when the patient is in a comatose condition. The nurse should therefore be familiar with the two types of contact lenses, because each is removed differently.

The **corneal (hard contact) lens** is smaller than a dime, is usually tinted, and covers most of the cornea when correctly positioned. This type of lens is held in place by the surface tension of the eye's natural tears. To remove the corneal lens manually, the edges of the lids are positioned on either side of the contact lens. Pressure is increased on one of the eyelids, which causes the lid to move under the contact lens (Fig. 12-5). The lens will slide out as it is tipped slightly outward and the eyelids are moved toward each other. (No force should be used to remove contact lenses, since corneal damage may result.) If this procedure does not work, the contact lens should be moved off the cornea onto the sclera. If the nurse is certain that a contact lens is in place and it cannot be removed manually, a suction cup can be used. The lids are opened wide and the end of a compressed suction cup is touched to the contact lens only. As pressure is released on the suction cup, the lens is lifted from the eye. The cup should not touch anything but the contact lens, since suction can damage the cornea.

Scleral contact lenses are larger than the corneal type (about the size of a quarter) and fit over a portion of the sclera as well as the cornea, which makes them harder to dislodge. Currently, they are less frequently prescribed by physicians. Scleral lenses are removed in a different manner from that used for corneal lenses. The patient, if responsive, is instructed to look downward when scleral lenses are removed to avoid abrasion of the cornea. In manual removal, the examiner's index finger is positioned near the edge of the lower lid. The lid is slowly and carefully slid back to reveal the edge of the lens. Moving the finger away from the patient's nose and pulling the lid taut causes the lid to slide under the lens, thus making the lens lift out so that it can be grasped and removed (Fig. 12-6).

In the suction cup method for removing scleral contact lenses, a larger suction cup is used. The lid is opened with the thumb and index finger of one hand and the suction cup is applied with the other hand. If the nurse

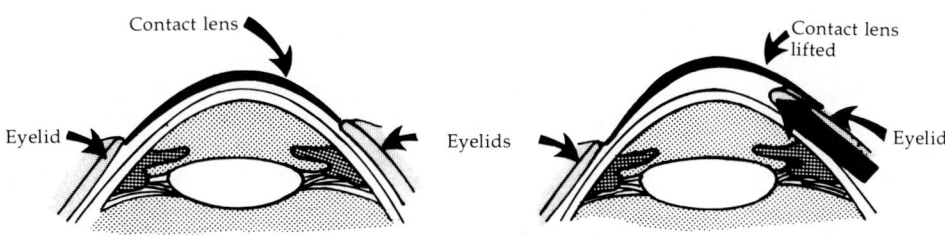

Figure 12-5
Removal of the corneal contact lens.

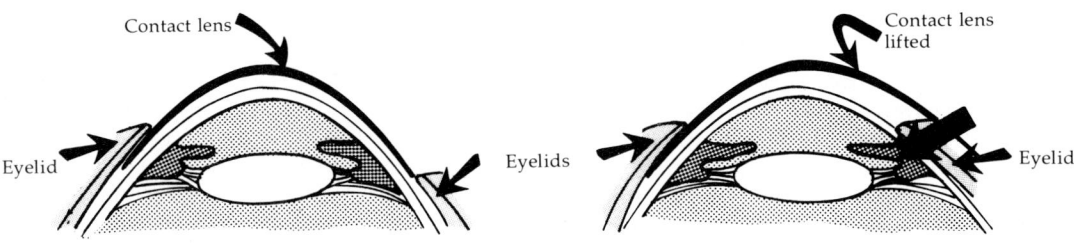

Figure 12-6
Removal of the scleral contact lens.

has difficulty in removing the contact lens, an ophthalmologist or optometrist should be consulted. The nurse should not attempt to remove a contact lens from an injured eye because of the danger of increasing the damage to the cornea.

Soft contact lenses (hydrophilic lenses) are a fairly recent development. Some patients prefer them to the hard lenses, stating that there is less discomfort. Soft contact lenses have been used with corneal disease because they appear to aid healing and are painless. To remove, the soft lens is grasped with thumb and forefinger. As they are tolerated for longer periods, there is less urgency to remove them from injured eyes. They may be difficult to manage and on occasion may cause edema and staining. Soft lenses also require more care; directions for care are supplied with the sterilization kits that come with the lenses.

Strabismus

There are two types of strabismus, paralytic and nonparalytic. **Paralytic strabismus** is caused by involvement of the extraocular muscle itself or by damage to the third, fourth, or sixth cranial nerve. The cranial nerve damage may be the result of a tumor, brain injury, or infection. The presence of diplopia, the usual visual symptom associated with paralytic strabismus, is therefore significant; when it is detected, the patient is referred to an ophthalmologist.

Nonparalytic strabismus is an inherited abnormality of the position of the two eyes without any paralysis of the muscles. Because the two eyes do not view the same object, vision in one eye is suppressed. This can result in suppression amblyopia, the loss of vision in the eye that is not utilized regularly. Occlusion therapy, which consists in covering the good eye and forcing the suppressed eye to function, can be successful in treating suppression amblyopia. If amblyopia is not treated by the age of 6, however, vision is usually lost in the suppressed eye. This is an important point to emphasize with parents who are reluctant to seek treatment because they feel their child will outgrow the condition. It is possible to treat nonparalytic strabismus with eyeglasses and topical medications. Orthoptics to train the patient in simultaneous use of the eyes to facilitate fusion is no longer accepted by most physicians as a useful method of treatment. Surgery may be indicated to transfer the muscle attachments of the eye.

Promotion of Eye Health

During the assessment of the eye and visual function, the nurse has opportunities to determine the patient's understanding of eye health and often discovers misconceptions about eye care. The nurse can immediately use this time for patient teaching or can determine goals to be included in the care plan for patient teaching.

The patient may state that he takes a lot of extra vitamins to keep his eyes in good condition. Patients should be advised that while vitamin A and vitamin B deficiencies may cause night blindness, corneal damage, and retinal changes, there is no evidence that excessive vitamins will promote eye health. In fact, an excess of vitamin A may cause increased intracranial pressure and papilledema with consequent decrease in vision [9]. A well-balanced diet with adequate vitamins A, B, and C is encouraged. Patients may also admit that they have used a relative's or friend's eye drops for an ocular irritation similar to the friend's problem. Self-dosing with another's medication may be dangerous. Medication prescribed for an eye with bacterial infection may be harmful for a condition of viral origin. The danger of spreading infection through contaminated medication should be stressed. Since ocular conditions may be similar in symptoms but different in etiology, the danger of using medications that may be contraindicated for an ocular condition should be emphasized. Patients should also be alerted to dangers in using outdated eye medications.

Some patients, particularly the elderly, may try to wear another person's eyeglasses to correct visual problems. The fact that prescriptions are individually made to correct specific refractive problems should be emphasized. Some people will use magnifying glasses rather than get a new prescription or will purchase used eyeglasses. The nurse should realize that the motive for this practice may be an economic one, rather than a lack of knowledge of proper care.

Prolonged exposure to sunlamps should be discouraged and eye covers should always be worn when sunlamps are used. Many patients ask questions about the use of sunglasses and whether or not they are beneficial and necessary. Sunglasses should be worn in bright light to reduce glare, especially by people who are sensitive to light. The use of sunglasses depends on the amount of comfort obtained when they are used in bright light. Sunglasses vary in the amount of light that is blocked, ranging from tinted glasses that block only 5 percent of the light to others that block as much as 90 percent. Reflected light causing discomfort from glare can be relieved by wearing polarized sunglasses. However, some people are tempted to wear these glasses while driving at night, because they block glare from the headlights of oncoming cars. People should be discouraged from wearing polarized glasses at night because they limit visual acuity in darkness.

Patients should be advised not to rub their eyes, because rubbing may introduce bacteria into the eyes or cause irritation. If there is a specific purpose in touching the eye, the hands should be washed prior to touching the eye. Habits of rubbing and picking at the face, hair, and eyes should be discouraged because of the danger of contamination. When aerosol spray products are used the nozzle should be pointed away from the eye before pressing the spray button. Patients should be advised about measures to reduce eyestrain by providing adequate lighting that does not cast shadows on the object being illuminated and by periodically resting the eyes when engaged in prolonged periods of close work, reading, or watching television. The eyes may be rested by closing them occasionally or by pausing to look at distant views.

Opportunities for health teaching should be utilized to teach patients about the warning symptoms of eye disease, about proper eye care and safety precautions, and first aid techniques to prevent blindness. Eye changes and symptoms that indicate the need for consultation with a physician include the following: persistent redness of the eye; persistent discomfort or pain in the eye, particularly after injury; disturbances of vision (such as loss of peripheral vision, seeing halos or fogginess around lights, double vision, or the sudden development of floating spots before the eyes); crossing of the eyes, especially in small children; growths on the eye or eyelids; continuing discharge, crusting, or tearing of the eye; and pupil irregularities. Persistent redness can be indicative of serious disease, especially when associated with vision loss, pain, opacities of normally transparent parts of the eye, pupil irregularities, redness encircling the cornea, pressure abnormality, history of previous serious eye disease, or failure to respond after three to four days of adequate treatment [9].

General Nursing Measures for Eye Care

Whatever the type of eye disease present or whatever the type of ocular surgery required, certain nursing procedures are likely to be included in the care of patients with visual dysfunction. These procedures should be carried out appropriately and safely in order to achieve the most therapeutic effect. Opportunities for teaching proper procedures to the patient should be utilized, because these procedures are often continued by the patient after hospitalization.

ADMINISTRATION OF EYE DROPS OR OINTMENT
Hand washing should be carried out diligently before and after the administration of any eye treatment or medication. Eye drops

may be used to relieve pain and discomfort, to dilate or contract pupils, to act as an antiseptic, or to treat infections. When eye drops are to be instilled, the patient should be in either a sitting or a lying position with his or her head tilted back; the patient is then asked to look upward and to fix his or her eyes at a point toward the top of the head. The nurse should open the lids with his or her fingers placed over the bony structure of the orbit and not by pressing over the eyeball itself. With the forefinger, the nurse should gently retract the lower lid until the conjunctiva is exposed and a small pocket is formed. With the other hand, the nurse instills a drop of medication directly on the conjunctival lining of the inverted lid (Fig. 12-7). During this procedure, the dropper (or squeeze bottle of medication) should not touch the eye. The eye drops should not run down into the lacrimal ducts leading to the nose, because the medication could be absorbed and cause systemic effects. Manual compression of the lacrimal passages is necessary to minimize systemic absorption. The patient then blinks his or her eyes and can blot them with a clean tissue to wipe off excess solution, but should not rub the eyes. One drop should be instilled at a time. Sterility of the eyedropper and the eye medication should be maintained during this procedure. If there is an infection in one of the eyes and the same medication is ordered for both eyes, a duplicate bottle should be used for each eye. In this situation the hands are washed before the medication is administered in the opposite eye. If either the eyedropper or the medication becomes contaminated, it is discarded. Eye medications should not be interchanged among different patients. If the patient is reliable and institutional policy permits, it is safer to leave individual eye medications at the patient's bedside rather than in a central location.

The same approach used in administering eye drops is used to administer eye ointments, except that a small amount of ointment is placed at the same point where the eye drop is placed (Fig. 12-8). The ointment will melt and be distributed over the eye surface by the mechanical blinking action of the eye and by the body temperature. For this reason it is not necessary to place an excessive amount of ointment along the entire length of the conjunctiva. The same precautions as are taken with the eyedropper should be taken to avoid touching the eye with the ointment container.

APPLICATION OF EYE PATCHES
When an eye patch is applied, the patient should close both eyes while the nurse gently

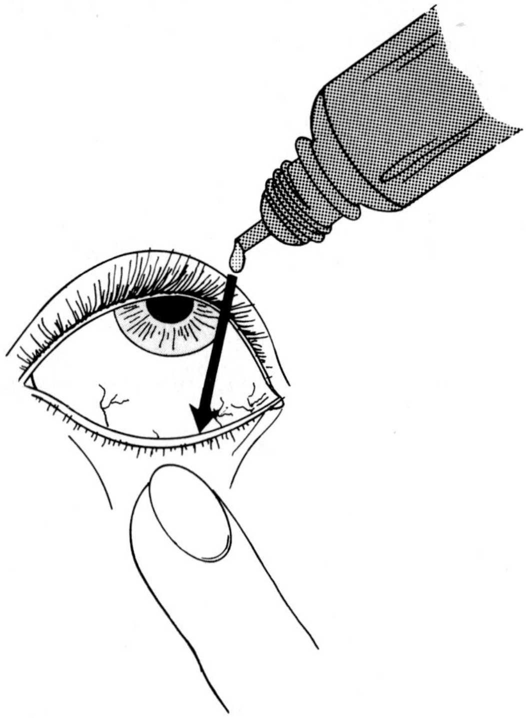

Figure 12-7
Administration of eye drops.

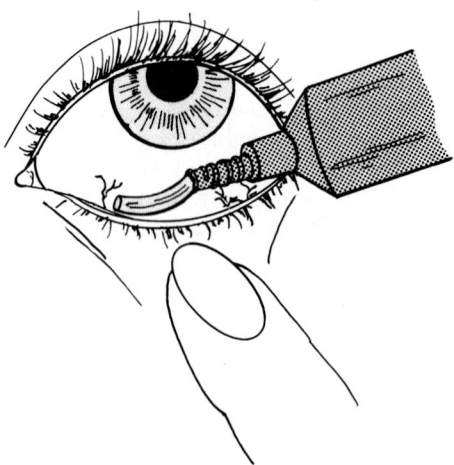

Figure 12-8
Application of ophthalmic ointment.

places the patch on the eye without touching the inner surface of the pad. Nonallergic paper tape or cellophane tape is preferred for applying the eye patch. Two diagonal strips of tape are stretched from the center of the forehead over the cheek near the earlobe or in the center of the cheek. Eye patches are usually used postoperatively to prevent excessive eye motion and to promote eye rest. They may also be used to absorb secretions or blood. They should be changed when soiled, or each time that medications are applied. Once removed, they should not be reused. Eye pads should not be used to cover infected eyes because of the likelihood of spreading the infection by creating an environment of warmth and darkness suitable for bacterial growth.

Sometimes pressure dressings are utilized to minimize edema. In this situation, two eye patches are usually placed over the affected eye, and several strips of adhesive tape are applied diagonally across the patch to the jawbones with firm pressure.

USE OF HOT OR COLD COMPRESSES

Hot compresses may be used for superficial infections of the cornea, conjunctiva, or eyelids. However, caution should be taken so that the water is not too hot. The hot compress may be either a sterile compress or a clean washcloth soaked in hot water and placed in a flat position over the *closed* eye after wringing out the excess water. The need for sterility is determined by the type of condition present and the purpose of the compresses. The compresses are reheated when they cool. This technique will soften crusts attached to the eyelids and facilitate their removal.

Cold compresses are applied in the same manner except that ice water is used instead of hot water. Cold compresses are used to control ocular itching, swelling, or pain. If an ice cube wrapped in a washcloth is used postoperatively to reduce ocular swelling, the ice should not be applied directly to the lid. Cold compresses should not be used in the presence of ocular infections.

IRRIGATION OF THE EYE

Contrary to the popular belief that the eye should be irrigated to relieve symptoms of irritation and fatigue, the cornea and conjunctiva do not need washing or irrigation except when tears are deficient or the lids do not close as a result of eye pathology. Ordinarily the tears and the blinking of the eyes provide sufficient lubrication. When the lids are damaged or paralyzed, or when the patient is unconscious, there is danger of damage to the cornea, which is sensitive to drying caused by the absence of the blinking mechanism. In such cases, eye ointments and methylcellulose eye drops or tear substitutes such as Adsorbotear may be used to protect the eye from permanent scarring. The nurse should ensure that the eyes of the unconscious patient are closed to prevent such scarring.

When eye irrigations are ordered, the patient should lie or sit with his head tilted backward and toward the side to be treated. A small basin is placed close to his head to collect excess fluid and drainage. The eyelids are opened with the thumb and forefinger of one hand while the eye is gently flushed with a stream of fluid (usually sterile water, sterile saline, or an antibiotic solution); the fluid should be directed away from the patient's nose. Either a plastic bottle, a small bulb syringe, or an eyedropper is used for the irrigation procedure. The procedure is repeated several times, depending on the amount of drainage and the purpose of the irrigation. The area is dried with a sterile gauze pad.

After some eye operations the patient's eyelids may be edematous, uncomfortable, and bruised and may stick together. There is often a serosanguineous discharge. The discharge and crusts may be wiped from the eyelids with a gently held gauze pad soaked in sterile saline or sterile water.

TOPICAL MEDICATIONS FOR THE EYE

A variety of topical medications are used for treating pathologic conditions of the eye. Table 12-1 lists some of the more commonly used eye medications, their indications, and the precautions associated with their use. Some of these are categorized as miotics, causing miosis or constriction of the pupil; mydriatics cause mydriasis or dilation of the pupil.

The nurse should be familiar with the abbreviations used by ophthalmologists to indicate which eye is to receive medication. The abbreviations are as follows: O.D. (oculus dexter), referring to the right eye; O.S. (oculus

Table 12-1
Selected drugs used in the treatment and diagnosis of ocular disorders

Medication	Action and Indications for Use	Precautions

Topical anesthetics
  Proparacaine hydrochloride (Ophthaine, Ophthetic) 0.5%
  Tetracaine hydrochloride (Pontocaine) 0.5%
  Benoxinate hydrochloride (Dorsacaine) 0.4%
  Cocaine hydrochloride 1.0–4.0%
	Produce relatively rapid anesthesia of short duration. Used to prevent pain in ocular procedures	Long-term use for pain control is contraindicated due to danger of ocular injury

Miotic drugs
  A. Cholinergic drugs
    Pilocarpine hydrochloride 0.5–6.0%
    Carbachol (Doryl) 0.75–3.0% solution and ointment
    Ocusert Pilo-20, Pilo-40
	Cholinergic drugs act directly on myoneural junction, causing contraction of iris and ciliary muscle. Used as miotics to control intraocular pressure in both open-angle and narrow-angle glaucoma. These drugs widen the angle of filtration and increase aqueous humor outflow	Safety precautions indicated relative to dimming of vision. Eye drops cause local irritation initially. Patients should not discontinue miotic therapy for any reason and should be encouraged to tolerate transient discomfort

B. Cholinesterase inhibitors
    Echothiophate iodide (Phospholine Iodide) 0.06–0.125%
    Physostigmine salicylate (Eserine) 0.25% ointment
    Demecarium bromide (Humorsol) 0.25%
	Cause accumulation of acetylcholine at myoneural junction, resulting in contraction of iris and ciliary muscles. Longer-acting than cholinergic drugs. Strong miotics	Action of these drugs is difficult to reverse due to long action. Systemic absorption may cause nausea and vomiting, diarrhea, cholinergic crisis. Advise anesthesiologist of use, since patients on these drugs are at higher risk

Mydriatic drugs
  A. Anticholinergic mydriatic-cycloplegic agents
    1. Long-acting
      Atropine 1.0%
    2. Intermediate-acting
      Cyclopentolate hydrochloride (Cyclogyl) 0.5–1.0%
      Homatropine methylbromide 1.0–2.0%
    3. Short-acting
      Tropicamide (Mydriacyl) 0.5–1.0% for refraction use
	Produce mydriasis and cycloplegia to facilitate examination of eye structures. Useful before cataract extraction to facilitate removal of the lens	Blurred vision results temporarily; safety precautions indicated. Caution required in all patients over 40 because of possibility of glaucoma. Patient should wear sunglasses in bright light when medication has been used. Systemic absorption can cause raised blood pressure and tachycardia

B. Adrenergic mydriatics
    Hydroxyamphetamine hydrobromide (Paredine) 1.0% solution
    Phenylephrine hydrochloride (Neo-Synephrine) 10% solution
	Used for mydriatic action	

Topical antiinflammatory drugs
  Hydrocortisone acetate (Cortef, Cortril) 0.5–2.5% suspension
  Dexamethasone (Decadron) 0.1% solution; 0.05% ointment
  Prednisolone (Hydeltrasol) 0.1 to 0.5% solution
	Used in treating inflammatory conditions that are nonpyogenic; also in allergic reactions and severe ocular injuries. Sometimes prescribed in combination with antibiotics for inflammatory conditions	Long-term use of topical steroids may raise intraocular pressure. Contraindicated in corneal infections caused by fungus or virus, such as herpes simplex

Table 12-1 (Continued)

Medication	Action and Indications for Use	Precautions
Topical antiinfective drugs		
Bacitracin ointment (Baciguent)	Used in treating infectious conditions of the eye and as prophylaxis in injuries	Contraindicated for specific allergic states
Chloramphenicol (Chloromycetin, Chloroptic) 0.16–0.5% solution; 1% ointment		
Gentamicin sulfate (Garamycin) 0.3% ointment or solution		
Neomycin sulfate 0.5% ointment; 0.1–0.5% solution		
Sulfacetamide sodium (Sodium Sulamyd) 10% ointment; 10–30% solution		
Idoxuridine (Herplex, IDU, Stoxil) 0.5% ointment; 0.1% solution		May be toxic to corneal tissue when used for prolonged periods
Lubricants		
Methylcellulose (Isopto-Tears) 0.5% solution	Artificial tears to provide moisture and lubrication in absence of normal tear production. Relieves conjunctival dryness and prevents corneal abrasion	
Polyvinyl alcohol (Liquifilm Tears) 1.4% solution		
Hydroxypropyl methylcellulose (Isopto-Alkaline) 1.0% solution		
Carbonic anhydrase inhibitors (systemic)		
Acetazolamide (Diamox)	Administered orally to decrease aqueous humor production in long-term treatment of chronic glaucoma. May be given intravenously in acute attacks	May cause electrolyte loss in diuresis. May also cause dermatitis, malaise
Osmotic agents		
Glycerin (Osmoglyn, Glyrol) 50–75% solution (oral)	Used preoperatively to decrease intraocular pressure and in acute glaucoma	Lemon added to glycerin makes it more palatable. May cause nausea after ingestion
Mannitol (intravenous)	Administered intravenously. May be used preoperatively or in acute attacks of glaucoma	Rapid administration can cause vascular overload in patients with poor cardiac reserve

sinister), referring to the left eye; and O.U. (oculus uterque) referring to both eyes.

The patient who is receiving eye medication should be observed for toxic reactions, which may be either local or systemic or both. Caution must be taken in teaching the patient about the medication, including timing, dosage, proper concentration, and proper administration. Patients should be taught to compress the lacrimal passages manually after drops are administered to minimize systemic absorption of the medication. For example, systemic toxicity from pilocarpine, the most frequently used drug for glaucoma, can cause nausea, emesis, diaphoresis, hypotension, muscle tremors, and sinus bradycardia.

Patients receiving eye medication should be taught how to use the eyedropper correctly to prevent trauma or the spread of infection. The patient should be cautioned against the use of outdated medications and also against using medications belonging to other people. Older patients, particularly, may tend to use eye drops belonging to a friend when their own medication is used up or when there is difficulty in getting the prescription refilled. This is dangerous not only because the medication may actually be contraindicated for such a patient but also because there is a danger of cross-contamination even if the medication happens to be exactly the same as his own.

Diffusional systems for controlled release of drugs to the eye have recently been developed and utilized. These miniature drug dispensers, which are slightly larger than a contact lens, are inserted into the conjunctival cul-de-sac. The complex system consists of a central reservoir of a drug enclosed between specially tailored membranes that allow the drug to diffuse from the reservoir to the eye; this device permits precise, programmed delivery of the medications for 24-hour control in glaucoma. The Ocusert Pilocarpine Delivery System* is an example of this type of system. It consists of two cross-linked polymer membranes between which is sandwiched another polymer impregnated with the drug. The convenience of once a week insertion of the system, which is a clear, wafer-like object, has obvious advantages over the multiple doses ordinarily required daily for traditional eye drop administration [15]. The system appears to be more successful with younger patients who have glaucoma than with older patients. Some patients develop irritations from the device and never learn to tolerate it; others have accidently lost the device from the eye without even realizing it. Some leaks of the medication have also been reported. Currently, the system is more expensive than the comparable doses in eye drop formation.

Care of the Visually Impaired Patient in the Hospital

Whether a person is completely blind from birth, has gradually lost his vision, or has some impaired vision, certain general principles of nursing care should be followed when such a person is admitted into the hospital setting. Approaches to these patients should be carefully handled in a calm manner, creating (as much as possible) a nonstressful atmosphere. Some patients may be completely adjusted to being totally blind and want to be as independent as possible even in the hospital setting after an initial orientation to new surroundings and an explanation of routines and expectations. Other visually impaired patients will need very specific directions, much companionship, and a great deal of support to counteract their fears in a strange new setting. The stage of adjustment and specific needs of the blind patient admitted to the hospital should be carefully assessed and recorded appropriately on the nursing care plan. If vision is better in one eye than the other, this should be indicated on the care plan so that the staff will approach the patient from the side of best vision.

Whether the patient is blind, has decreased vision, or is unable to see because of bilateral patching of the eyes, the nurse should approach the patient only after giving a verbal greeting and clarifying the nurse's name and role. It is important to address the patient by his name so that the patient will know that someone is talking to him or her and not to others in the room. Physical contact is good for the patient, but not prior to announcing one's presence, since this only increases the patient's anxiety and startles him or her. It is also important to tell the visually impaired patient when one is leaving.

People who are communicating with a blind patient often tend to talk very loudly or very slowly and distinctly, implying that the person is not only blind but deaf and has difficulty in reasoning. When blind people are accompanied by sighted family members or friends, others may not address the blind person directly but rather speak to the sighted person. Both of these habits are annoying to the blind patient, and the nurse should avoid doing either and caution others to avoid their use.

Verbal communication is one of the most important aspects of the care of patients with visual impairment. They need the security of knowing what is being done around them and to them, and what is expected of them. They also need the security of having someone to listen to their needs and expectations. These patients will be able to participate in their care if they are adequately oriented to their surroundings and to the procedures that will be performed for them.

The hospitalized blind patient should be given a tour of his or her room and should be oriented immediately to the furniture in the room, the bathroom, the location of important equipment, and especially the means for getting assistance when needed (the use of the call bell). If desired, the independent blind person should also be guided outside the room to the nurse's station and other strategic areas.

The patient who is blind or visually impaired should be guided in a manner that will prevent him or her from bumping into obsta-

---

*Manufactured by Alza Pharmaceuticals, Palo Alto, California.

cles. This is most appropriately done with the nurse placing the patient's hand in the crook of his or her elbow (or with the patient touching the nurse's elbow) and walking in an unhurried pace about one foot ahead of the blind patient (Fig. 12-9). In this way the nurse can describe the obstacles, such as doors, stairs, and obstructing furniture, and can warn the patient of hazards. When a blind patient is guided to a chair, he should be allowed to feel the front of the chair with his knee and the seat and arms with his hand to prepare him for the height of the chair. Excessive furniture and unnecessary equipment should be removed from the patient's area since they may precipitate accidents. Doors should be left either fully open or shut, but not half open, so that the visually impaired patient will not bump or injure himself. The location of articles that the patient will need, for example the water pitcher, telephone, and call bell, should be clarified. The patient should be allowed to feel each item as an explanation is given of its use. The patient's personal articles should be put in the drawer in the manner he or she prefers. These possessions should not be moved and furniture should not be moved without advising the patient of any necessary change.

At mealtime the nurse or assistant should be available to assist with the meal as necessary. The patient who has been blind for a long period of time will be able to feed himself satisfactorily if given specific guidelines about the arrangement of food trays. Most blind people are familiar with the "clock" arrangement of food, so that when the patient compares the meal tray to a clock, he or she can be oriented to finding food readily (Fig. 12-10). This technique facilitates the patient's knowing where specific articles and food are located. It is very important for the nurse to be available at initial meal periods to assess ways in which each new patient needs assistance. The patient's suggestions should be solicited as to the type of assistance needed or preferred. These observations and identified needs can then be included in the care plan so that appropriate follow-through is provided without creating anxiety for the patient. For the patient who is recently blinded or who has bilateral eye patches and cannot be independent, more assistance will be necessary. After certain eye operations, movement is ex-

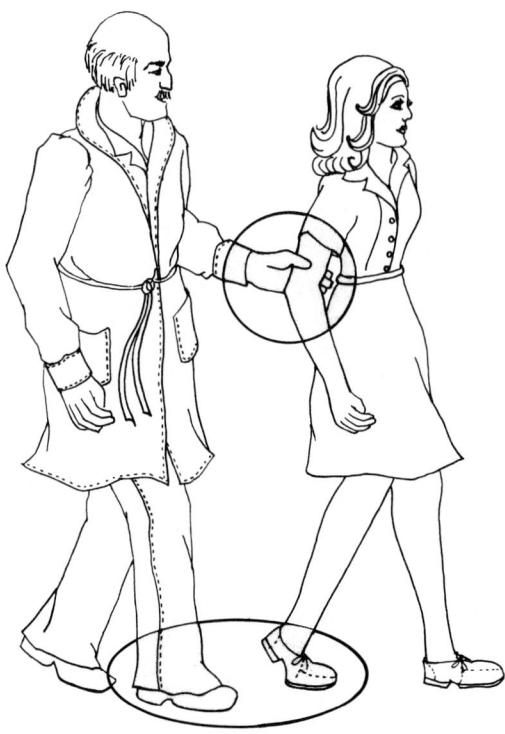

Figure 12-9
Guiding the blind or visually impaired patient.

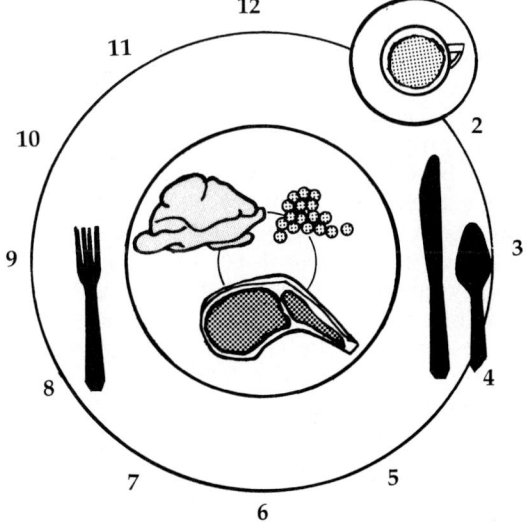

Figure 12-10
The clock guideline used for determining food arrangement.

tremely restricted so that totally assisted feeding is required. When feeding the patient, the nurse should act in an unhurried manner, advising the patient of what is on the tray and asking his preference for the order in which the food should be given.

When administering medications to the blind patient, the nurse should give thorough explanations. Efforts should be made to avoid awkwardness or accidents caused by inadequate preparation of the patient. If the patient is receiving new medication, it is helpful to allow him or her to handle the tablet to become familiar with its shape. Touching unfamiliar items (such as tablets or capsules) is essential for the blind patient's orientation. He or she should also be informed of the dosage and anticipated effect of the medication.

The need for verbal communication with the visually impaired patient cannot be overstressed. Hospitalization can be boring even for patients with good eyesight, who have ready access to books, television, and other diversions; boredom and even confusion and disorientation are more likely to occur in the visually impaired patient, who does not have access to appropriate diversional activities. Patients with recent visual impairment or those with bilateral eye patches will profit by the use of a radio, tape recorder, or phonograph and by frequent visits by the nursing staff to provide sensory stimulation. References to the time of day at frequent intervals will assist them in their orientation; the nurse can relate time to specific auditory cues that may be present in the environment. Frequent visits by the nursing staff can be utilized as periods to discover the patient's special assets or limitations, on which a teaching plan should be based. A calm, unrushed atmosphere at these times implies to the patient that he or she is important and valued and results in an increased sense of security.

Safety precautions are an important element of nursing care for all visually impaired patients and particularly for those who are newly blinded or have bilateral patches. For these patients, side rails should be constantly kept on the bed to avoid accidents or injuries. Supervision in ambulation should be provided by the nursing staff until the patient is ready for increased independence. Unless the visually impaired patient (particularly the elderly one) is stimulated sufficiently, disorientation and confusion may lead to restlessness and increased activity. Restraints should be avoided with such patients, since fighting the restraints only results in increasing anxiety and may cause increased intraocular pressure, which may be harmful.

PREPARATION FOR EYE SURGERY

There are certain aspects of eye surgery that differ from general surgery. Many patients who are scheduled for eye surgery have impaired vision; if this has developed gradually, as with cataracts, they may have made some adjustment to poor vision. Others may not have adapted and may fear that permanent blindness will result from the surgery. In addition to preparing the patient for preoperative and postoperative care, the nurse must also deal with the patient's fears related to the outcome of the surgery.

In preparing the patient for eye surgery, the nurse should be very thorough in explanations of procedures and routines. The room should be set up preoperatively according to anticipated postoperative restrictions. For example, the call bell and telephone should be placed on the side that will not be operated on. This is done to avoid the patient's turning on the operated side postoperatively, which would cause pressure on the surgical site. In some hospitals, the eyelashes are clipped routinely prior to ocular surgery. When this is ordered, the nurse should place a thin film of ophthalmic ointment or petrolatum on the blades of small, curved scissors with blunt tips; the cut lashes thus adhere to the scissors rather than falling into the eye. The patient should be assured that the eyelashes will grow back in 6 to 8 weeks.

One major difference in eye surgery is that local rather than general anesthesia is usually used. The patients, on learning that a local anesthesia will be used during eye surgery, often fear that they will have excess pain. However, they should understand that local anesthesia will permit them to be awake during the procedure but they will not have pain. The patient should be advised about the preoperative medication that will be given for sedation and about the preoperative preparation of the eye itself. The patient should be forewarned that eye drops will be given at fairly frequent intervals during the preoperative preparation. Unless advised of this, the patient may question the frequent administration of eye medications the morning of the operation or may become overly anxious about the preparation. Preoperative eye drops are given to dilate the pupil and to paralyze the accommodation muscle; for example, phenylephrine hydrochloride (Neo-Synephrine), a vasoconstrictor and mydriatic drug, and Cyclogyl, a cycloplegic drug, may be used. The ocular medications must be given at exactly the specified times in order to facilitate maximum dilation of the pupil at the time of surgery. The patient should not be exposed to bright sunlight, especially when mydriatics are being administered. (Many patients with various ocular diseases cannot tolerate bright sunlight even when mydriatic drugs are not used.)

Even when the patient receives only a local anesthetic, breakfast and fluids are usually restricted to prevent postoperative nausea and vomiting. Nausea and vomiting following surgery can cause increased intraocular pressure and result in damage to the suture line.

Osmotic agents such as mannitol may be given intravenously prior to surgery to reduce intraocular pressure. The nurse must observe the patient closely for cardiovascular complications, because the drug may be prescribed at a fairly rapid rate of administration over a 45-minute period, and should notify the physician if rapid urine output does not ensue.

POSTOPERATIVE CARE

Postoperative nursing care will vary depending on the underlying pathology, the type of surgery, and the preference of the surgeon. There is a wide variation in the approach of postoperative care regarding the amount of activity permitted. Usually the surgeon is very specific about the type and amount of activity allowed and about the positioning of the patient. These directions should be followed explicitly and the patient should be thoroughly instructed about specific restrictions.

The major concern of the nurse postoperatively is to provide for the physical and emotional safety and security of the patient. The patient frequently requires another orientation to the surroundings, particularly to the location of the call bell, and should be reassured of constant attention to his or her needs. Usually an aluminum shield covers the operative eye continuously during the first 24 hours postoperatively and also at night or during naps throughout the hospital stay. This shield is also used at night for at least one month following discharge from the hospital after cataract surgery. Some surgeons replace the metal shield with a simple eye patch during the day and allow the patient to wear his glasses. The shield is applied carefully on the operated eye at night to ensure protection during sleep. The patient is directed to avoid touching the eye. Safety aspects include preventing increased intraocular pressure and protecting the patient from injury or falling due to loss of vision or visual impairment imposed by the use of eye patches postoperatively. Attention should also be given to protecting the patient from intravenous poles, television equipment, drinking straws in glasses, and other hospital hazards. Because the eyes move simultaneously, both eyes may be patched postoperatively to maintain rest of the surgically repaired eye; surgeons vary in their preference for bilateral patching or patching of only the operated eye. Even if the unoperated eye is unpatched, the patient should be encouraged to close the eye voluntarily to rest the operated eye. Often the patient with only the operated eye patched will have diminished vision in the unoperated eye. It is essential that the nurse make a careful assessment of the patient's visual ability.

Depending on the type of surgery, total movement may be restricted, turning only on the unoperated side may be allowed, or complete freedom of movement may be permitted. For the patient who requires prolonged bed rest after surgery, provision for isometric exercises is needed. Leg exercises are usually indicated to prevent complications of thrombophlebitis. With most eye operations, early ambulation is being encouraged as long as it is supervised and not strenuous.

The nurse should be concerned about preventing increased intraocular pressure, which might traumatize the surgically repaired eye. The nurse should instruct the patient to avoid bending over, straining (especially during defecation), nausea, vomiting, coughing, and sneezing, all of which contribute to increased intraocular pressure. The patient should also avoid the use of sprays or dusting powder, which could enter and irritate the eye. Combing or washing the hair and shaving may be contraindicated also. The patient must understand that the eyes are not to be touched or rubbed. Proper instructions regarding the maximum type of activity allowed, the administration of antiemetics to prevent vomiting, the use of stool softeners early in the postoperative period, and the avoidance of upper respiratory infections preoperatively and postoperatively are all necessary precautions to prevent these problems from occurring. Questions about these factors should be investigated with the patient prior to surgery so that potential problems can be eliminated. For example, the operation would probably be postponed if the patient had a cold or if he seemed to sneeze excessively during the preoperative period. A history of constipation might necessitate a preoperative enema the night before surgery to avoid discomfort and straining in the early postoperative period. The patient's usual manner of handling constipation (e.g., the use of stool softeners) should probably be followed during the postoperative period to ensure effectiveness. Because smoke is irritating to the eye, the patient and visitors should not be allowed to smoke.

Patients do not usually complain of much postoperative pain and mild analgesics will control discomfort. For this reason, excessive pain should be reported to the surgeon immediately, since it may indicate that hemorrhage, increased intraocular pressure, or other complications have occurred. Usually the ophthalmologist prefers to do the dressing changes himself in order to use special equipment and measures to evaluate the condition and progress of the eye.

Posthospitalization plans should be investigated early to determine how the patient will be assisted with meals, eye treatments, and medications after discharge. For example, corrective refraction after cataract surgery is not possible for several weeks, so the patient initially may have a serious visual deficit that will prevent self-care and independence. If the patient cannot be taught to apply ointments, instill eye drops, and apply and tape the metal shield in place, some other family member or friend should be taught these procedures. However, many patients requiring eye surgery are elderly and may not have family or friends to care for them. Even when the patients do have family or friends, referrals to home health agencies may be necessary to ensure that postoperative management is appropriately arranged following discharge. The patient must avoid lifting heavy objects and will be restricted in activity for one to two months after most ocular operations.

Care of Patients with Specific Ocular Problems

The previous discussion of care of the visually impaired patient and nursing care measures for patients with ocular diseases or ocular surgery applies to many different situations. The following section is concerned with the care of patients with specific types of ocular problems: ocular infections, ocular injuries, cataracts, glaucoma, retinal diseases, corneal diseases, and enucleation.

INFECTIONS OF THE EYE

The source of eye infections is usually contamination by the hands rubbing the eyes, contamination from the nose or face, foreign bodies in the eyes, or contamination from equipment or solutions used in the treatment of ocular conditions. Cosmetics, particularly eye makeup and false eyelashes, are also a source of contamination.

Applications of antibiotic ointments are generally utilized for inflammatory conditions of the eyelids (blepharitis). Warm, moist compresses and antibiotic ointments are usually prescribed for hordeolums of the eyelid, which usually open spontaneously without surgical excision of the abscess. Surgical excision, however, is occasionally necessary. The patient with a hordeolum must be cautioned not to squeeze the "pimple" because of the danger of extending the infection and causing cellulitis. In all cases of infection, precautions must be taken to prevent transmission of the infection from one eye to the other. Cleaning the lid margins is necessary to remove the adherent crusts that tend to form with the infectious process.

Acute conjunctivitis ("pink eye") is a highly contagious viral infection that is fairly common among children. Conjunctivitis may also occur as the result of an allergic reaction or bacterial infection and is characterized by tearing, itching, and ocular redness. Topical antibiotic drops and procedures related to the prevention of recurrent infections generally eliminate most types of conjunctivitis without any residual scarring or abnormality of the eye. Corticosteroids are contraindicated in viral infections. Since redness of the eye can also be associated with corneal infection, the cornea should also be checked for opacity to determine whether or not there is a corneal infection.

Acute dacryocystitis with accumulation of pus in the lacrimal sac and swelling over the inner canthus of the eye is treated with systemic antibiotic therapy, irrigation of the lacrimal sac with penicillin, and surgical drainage of the abscess when necessary. Chronic inflammation with complete obstruction of the nasal lacrimal system may result from persistent dacryocystitis, and a surgical dacryocystorhinostomy may be required. In this procedure a new, large opening between the lacrimal sac and the nose is created for drainage.

Uveitis, the inflammation of the uveal tract (the iris, ciliary body, and choroid), requires prompt treatment with antibiotics or steroids or both to prevent secondary complications of adhesions leading to glaucoma, cataracts, or retinal detachment.

Inflammation of the cornea (keratitis) requires prompt medical treatment to prevent visual damage caused by scarring or ulceration from the inflammatory process. Keratitis is treated by bed rest, antimicrobial medications, and warm, moist compresses. Photophobia is a usual complaint; it is relieved by cycloplegics and dark glasses. Corneal infections are not patched, as this may tend to increase infection. A topical anesthetic may also be necessary to relieve the pain associated with infection. Herpes simplex keratitis is treated with idoxuridine. Corticosteroid treatment is contraindicated in herpes simplex because it can cause extension of the infection with corneal scarring.

Infections of the eye should not be treated lightly. Small, localized infections may spread, affecting internal structures and resulting in visual impairment. Sympathetic ophthalmia is a severe form of uveitis that may occur in the opposite eye after severe injury or infection of one eye; it is thought that this may be an allergic reaction to the pigment the damaged eye releases. Enucleation of the injured eye may be necessary in sympathetic ophthalmia and corticosteroids are used to treat the other eye.

OCULAR INJURIES

Whenever the nurse receives a patient who complains that something "hit" his eye, resulting in sudden impairment of vision or a sudden gush of tears, or when the nurse observes a pupil change, hemorrhage in the anterior chamber (hyphema), a conjunctival hemorrhage, or bleeding from the eye, a perforating wound or the penetration of the eye by a foreign body should be suspected. The eye should not be touched, and no medication should be instilled into the eye. Both eyes should be lightly patched and covered with a Fox shield (a metal shield with tiny perforations) to protect the eye against pressure. The patient must be seen immediately by an ophthalmologist.

A patient with a **perforating wound** may not have any pain and therefore may feel that the injury is not serious. The nurse should be knowledgeable about the fact that internal eye injuries frequently do not cause pain. Trying to wipe away blood, tears, or discharge from the eye can result in further damage; these actions should be avoided by both the nurse and the patient. During transfer of the patient to the ophthalmologist, the patient should avoid any exertion that would increase intraocular pressure. It is very important for the nurse to remain calm in this emergency situation, since it is an extremely frightening crisis for the patient.

A **foreign body** in the eye is one of the most common types of eye injury and is a frequent problem for the school nurse and the occupational health nurse as well as for nurses in a variety of other settings. If the foreign body is located on the conjunctiva, it may often be removed by blinking the eye. However, neither the patient nor the nurse should rub the eye or use pressure, because a superficial foreign body can then abrade the cornea and even penetrate it. If the foreign body is on the cornea, no attempt at removal should be made by the nurse. Foreign bodies tend to lodge in the inner surface of the upper tarsal plate, and the lids must be everted to examine the area for the location of the foreign body (see Fig. 12-3). A sterile cotton applicator is then moistened with sterile saline solution and the particle is gently removed. If the foreign body is not readily removed by irrigating the eye with either sterile water, sterile normal saline solution, or an irrigating solution such as Dacriose or Eye-stream, or by using a small sterile applicator moistened with sterile water, the nurse should not attempt any other means of removal. The eye should be covered and the patient referred to an ophthalmologist.

Severe pain or the sensation of a foreign body, especially when the lid is moved over the cornea, should make the examiner suspect corneal abrasion even if no foreign body is detected. If the abrasion cannot readily be seen, staining techniques using sterile fluorescein sodium are utilized to disclose the presence of corneal abrasions. Sterile single strips of porous paper impregnated with fluorescein are preferred to liquid fluorescein, which may support *Pseudomonas* or other pathogenic growth once the container is opened. The fluorescein strip is moistened with normal saline or Dacriose, touched to the lower conjunctiva, and then dispersed by the tears. Denuded corneal areas stain a green color, so that the examiner can detect where corneal epithelium has been lost.

Treatment of ocular injuries consists of antibiotics, tetanus prophylaxis, removal of the foreign body or particles (by the ophthalmologist, who uses special instruments such as an eye spud), suturing of any lacerations, and the use of analgesics for pain. Usually a local anesthetic is needed for the examination and removal procedures; however, prolonged use of anesthetic drops is discouraged because they retard healing and may cause corneal damage. The patient's blinking reflex is masked by the anesthetic, and the patient may not be aware of any foreign body in the eye. In the case of a penetrating ocular injury, an x-ray should be taken to rule out the possible presence of a retained intraocular foreign body. Foreign bodies often cannot be seen by the naked eye, especially small, high-speed particles caused by explosives, metal splinters, or hammering stones. Glass fragments or slivers from broken glasses or bottles can also result in lacerations of the eye.

The above examples indicate that the nurse should not be aggressive in the treatment of ocular injuries due to either perforation or foreign bodies, but rather should protect the eyes until prompt attention by an ophthalmologist is obtained. The eye can be destroyed if pressure is exerted on it. Most authorities recommend the approaches just outlined, although some even advise against irrigating the eye if a foreign body is suspected.

Chemical Injuries and Burns

The nurse's responsibility changes when chemical injuries or burns of the eye from acids, solvents, poisons, and other caustic agents occur. Immediate and aggressive first aid care is essential. Copious irrigations with plain water within seconds of the injury are absolutely necessary to prevent permanent scarring. The water may be poured gently on the eyeball with the eyelids separated. This irrigation procedure should be continued for at least 10 to 20 minutes prior to applying a sterile dressing to the eye and having the physician see the patient. The nurse should use a pH strip to determine acid or alkaline toxicity, and the eye should then be irrigated until the pH is at a neutral point. Even if the irrigation seems to relieve the trauma, the patient should be seen by a physician since some chemicals may cause a delayed reaction. Plain water should be used whether the toxic chemical is an acid or an alkali. The emphasis should be on eliminating contact of the toxic chemical with the cornea and conjunctiva. Neutralization of an acid burn with an alkaline substance (or vice versa) is contraindicated because the irrigating agent itself may cause additional damage.

If a **flash burn** of the eye has occurred, cold applications to the eye will provide relief. In some settings the nurse may have a standing order to then apply a topical anesthetic if the pain continues to be severe. Ultraviolet burns of the cornea may result from germicidal lamps, electric flashes, arc welding, and probably most commonly from exposure to sunlamp rays. In the concerted effort to obtain a quick tan, young people especially may forget to close the eyelids or wear protective goggles to protect the corneal epithelium, which is susceptible to ultraviolet burns. Severe pain is usually delayed in its initiation and can usually be relieved with aspirin, codeine, and cold compresses. Photophobia, pain, and blurred vision indicate the need to investigate for corneal ulceration. If the burn is severe, topical antibiotics are used to prevent infection.

If the patient has a **laceration** of the lid with active bleeding, it should be assumed that the globe may also be lacerated. The patient or the nurse may want to apply pressure to control the bleeding. However, pressure on the lid may control the bleeding but may damage the eye itself. A dressing is applied and the patient is seen by an ophthalmologist for repair of the laceration and determination of any other intraocular damage.

If a **black eye** occurs as a result of a blow or trauma, the eye is examined with an ophthalmoscope to determine whether or not internal damage has occurred. Hyphema (hemorrhage into the anterior chamber) may result from the ocular trauma. Black eyes are too often treated lightly and no investigation of internal injury is made even when the patient has blurred vision. If the injury was severe enough to cause a black eye, it may cause immediate complications such as fractures of facial or orbital bones, detached retina, lens dislocation, and intraocular hemorrhage, or it may cause delayed complications. Therefore, an ocular examination with an ophthalmoscope is indicated.

Sympathetic Ophthalmia

Following an eye injury, especially a deep and penetrating one, sympathetic ophthalmia is always a potential complication. In this condition uveitis (inflammation of the ciliary body, choroid, and iris) may develop in the noninjured eye. This inflammation is considered to be an antibody-antigen reaction to the foreign protein of the uveal tissue that is dispersed during the injury. The condition must be treated aggressively to prevent visual impairment. Corticoid preparations are generally used locally and systemically. Rarely, removal of the injured eye may be necessary to prevent sympathetic ophthalmia from developing.

CATARACTS

Visual impairment may be caused by **cataracts,** a partial or total opacity of the normally transparent crystalline lens. Opacity alters or blocks the passage of light rays. Although there are several types of cataracts, the most common is the senescent (senile) cataract, associated with aging and occurring after the age of 55. The specific etiology of cataracts is not known, although persons with senescent cataracts often have overt or occult diabetes mellitus or a history of prolonged topical therapy for glaucoma, intraocular surgery, or previous inflammation or trauma to the eyes. Congenital cataracts most often occur when the mother has a history of a viral infection such as rubella during the first trimester of the pregnancy. Cataracts may occur at any age secondary to trauma, acquired systemic disorders such as metabolic disease or dietary deficiency, or acquired ocular disease such as inflammatory or neoplastic conditions. Cataracts may also result in cancer patients who require radiation therapy to the head. Systemic and topical steroid therapy has been implicated in the development of some cataracts.

If some lens transparency remains, a cataract is identified as **immature;** if it is entirely opaque it is identified as **mature.** The mature senescent cataract is visualized as a diffusely opaque lens that is usually white. Normal refractive ability of the lens is lost as opacity of the lens prevents light rays from being focused on the retina. Typically, a slowly progressive and painless decrease in visual acuity occurs, although some persons report a rapid onset of visual distortion. They frequently complain of a "yellowing" of vision, which is caused by nuclear sclerosis and which also reduces and modifies the light reaching the retina. The lens is best examined by use of the slit-lamp after the pupil is dilated. The location, the density of the opacification, and the likelihood of progression can best be evaluated by this technique.

In adults, surgical removal of the lens is the treatment of choice when visual performance is reduced to a level that is unacceptable to the patient, but it is done only after the presence of other abnormalities that could impair vision have been ruled out. Cataract extraction is not indicated when there are other ocular diseases that would prevent improvement of vision even if the opaque lens were removed.

Cataract surgery is the most common type of eye surgery that is performed. There is a low incidence of complications, and usually the results of surgery are good. There are several surgical techniques for the removal of cataracts; the current standard method is the intracapsular extraction, in which the complete lens with its capsule is removed through an incision about 18 mm long at the corneoscleral junction. Local anesthesia is usually preferred for the procedure, especially since most cataract operations are done on elderly patients who usually have other systemic diseases that complicate the administration of general anesthesia. Preoperative sedation is generally used, and an eyelid block with lidocaine is followed by a retrobulbar block for local anesthesia. Many surgeons use a cryoextractor for removal of the lens. A control console connected to a carbon dioxide or nitrogen source is connected in turn to a cooled cryoprobe, which is used to grasp the lens to deliver it intact through the incision.

A new microsurgical technique called phacoemulsification is currently being used to remove cataracts in younger patients as well as in infants and children. It requires special instruments and special training. A smaller incision (about 3 mm) is required in this technique than is required in the conventional cataract extraction procedure. The tip of a phacoemulsification hollow probe is introduced into the lens material. At the same time that ultrasonic vibrations are used to break up the firm portions of the lens, an aspiration-irrigation system is used to remove the particles of the lens through the probe. Physiologic saline solution is used to replace the volume of the anterior chamber, so that the normal depth is maintained [7]. Thus all the lens material except for the posterior capsule is removed in this technique. The patient usually has fewer restrictions and a shorter hospitalization with this technique than with conventional cataract surgery. Not all patients, however, can be treated by this technique; it is limited to patients who have corneas free of disease, pupils that are able to dilate fully, anterior chambers that are of normal depth, and lenses that are not too hard [13].

A new approach to cataract surgery that is under investigation involves the use of intraocular lens implantation. The cataract is removed and a prosthetic lens is secured within the pupillary space by clips on the pupil or by plastic loops resting in the chamber angle [3]. Problems with intraocular intolerance, corneal damage, and proper sterilization appear to be overcome. This method of cataract correction may facilitate easier management of ocular function, especially in the aged.

In conventional cataract surgery the patient has a metal shield on his eye postoperatively; if he cannot voluntarily keep his other eye closed, he may require a patch on the unoperated eye also. Pain is usually minimal and is relieved by mild analgesics. Severe pain may indicate increased intraocular pressure or hemorrhage and should be reported immediately to the ophthalmologist. Precautions for postoperative management have already been described, with emphasis on the prevention of increased intraocular pressure (the avoidance of coughing, sneezing, bending, or pressure), which could disrupt the sutures. Complications of cataract surgery may be intraocular hemorrhage, infection, and vitreous loss with danger of subsequent retinal disease.

The loss of the lens (aphakia) requires the temporary use of thick eyeglasses that initially create discomfort for the patient because of distortion of image size and loss of panoramic vision. For the older patient, these eyeglasses may actually interfere with balance while he or she is learning to adjust to spatial changes. The magnification created by the eyeglasses results in distorted or enlarged images, so that the patient often reaches short of objects and also has difficulty walking or using stairs. For this reason patients must be thoroughly prepared for this period of adjustment to visual changes and must be supervised during the readjustment phase. Most patients accommodate to these eyeglasses, however, within a few days or weeks. The patient who has limited vision or difficulties with depth perception should be taught how to put on the eyeglasses correctly in order to prevent injury to the eyes. The patient should hold the ends of the earpieces and gently slide them up the side of the face and over the ears. This method of putting on eyeglasses also helps to maintain their alignment.

Some of the disadvantages of the thick eyeglasses are overcome by the use of contact lenses, which are often preferred even by the older cataract patients as long as their manual dexterity is still adequate to handle the care of the lenses. These contact lenses only magnify about 6 to 10 percent (in comparison to 35 percent magnification in eyeglasses) and provide a full, undistorted field of vision [3]. The use of a contact lens is especially beneficial when only one eye requires cataract surgery. A prescription for permanent eyeglasses is not usually made for 2 to 3 months; however, when soft hydrophilic contact lenses are used, the prescription is made earlier in the postoperative period.

If the patient has bilateral cataracts, the second operation may be done within 5 days of the first, or it may be delayed until full recovery from the previous operation occurs.

GLAUCOMA

Glaucoma, one of the leading causes of blindness and visual disability, is characterized by an abnormal increase in the intraocular pressure. This is often followed by progressive loss of vision in parts of the visual field caused by atrophy of the retinal ganglion cells and the optic nerve. Unless prompt, proper, and continuous treatment is initiated, blindness may result. Vision already lost at diagnosis cannot be restored. Therefore, emphasis on early detection remains the major factor in preventing blindness from glaucoma. As mentioned previously, regular eye examinations, including tonometry and peripheral vision testing every two years after the age of 35, could have an impact on preventing blindness by detecting the early stages of glaucoma. People with a family history of glaucoma should be examined even more frequently.

Normally the aqueous humor, which is produced by the ciliary body, passes from the posterior chamber through the pupillary aperture of the iris into the anterior chamber. It then passes through the trabecular meshwork located in the peripheral angle of the anterior chamber into the canal of Schlemm and ultimately into the venous circulation. When the intraocular pressure is within normal limits, there is a balance between aqueous production and aqueous outflow. However, when there is a blockage in the drainage of the aqueous humor through the canal of Schlemm, intraocular pressure is increased. The constant increased intraocular pressure causes atrophy and degeneration of the optic nerve. To prevent blindness from occurring, the intraocular pressure must be decreased by either decreasing the production of aqueous humor or by promoting its drainage.

Glaucoma may be congenital, occurring within the first six months of life. Primary glaucoma, either of the open-angle (chronic simple) type or the angle-closure (narrow or closed-angle) form, usually occurs after the age of 40. The terms **open-angle** and **angle-closure** refer to the angle of the anterior chamber where the cornea and iris meet (Fig. 12-11). Hereditary factors appear to be an important influence in the development of adult primary glaucoma, particularly in the open-angle type, which is the most common. Secondary glaucoma may result from trauma; from a preexisting, generalized eye disease such as a tumor or inflammation; from vascular disorders or diabetes; or from postoperative complications after ocular surgery (such as keratoplasty).

Chronic simple glaucoma (**open-angle glaucoma**) is usually asymptomatic with an insidious onset, but it progressively destroys peripheral vision over a span of years. The person may visit his physician when he becomes aware of peripheral vision loss,

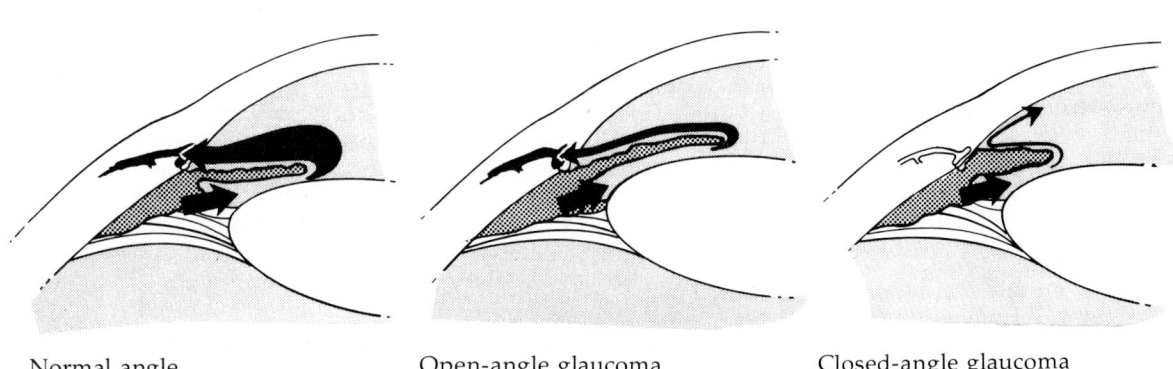

Normal angle   Open-angle glaucoma   Closed-angle glaucoma

Figure 12-11
Comparison of the normal angle with open-angle glaucoma and angle-closure glaucoma.

blurred or foggy vision, seeing halos around lights, difficulty in focusing on close work, or difficulty in adjusting to darkened rooms. In this type of glaucoma the anterior chamber angle is open and the trabecular meshwork is in communication with the anterior chamber, but there is some type of blockage to the outflow of aqueous humor through the meshwork. Although open-angle glaucoma can be controlled, vision that is already lost cannot be restored. This condition requires the use of topical miotic drugs to facilitate aqueous outflow by increasing the efficiency of the outflow channels. Pilocarpine, which is a direct-acting parasympathomimetic drug, is the usual drug of choice. Another miotic frequently used is carbachol (Carcholin). These miotic drugs produce pupillary constriction, stimulate the ciliary muscle, and facilitate increased outflow of aqueous humor. Carbonic anhydrase inhibitors such as acetazolamide (Diamox), which is administered orally, are used to decrease the rate of secretion of aqueous humor by the ciliary processes. Since this disease is chronic and progressive, the medication has to be carefully adjusted for each patient. The patient will require evaluation of the effectiveness of therapy at regular intervals by measurement of the intraocular pressure with tonometry, visual field examinations, and observation of the optic nerve with the ophthalmoscope. If visual field loss continues to progress in spite of therapy, surgery may be indicated to reduce intraocular pressure.

Angle-closure glaucoma occurs when the iris occludes the anterior chamber angle structures, the trabecular meshwork, and the canal of Schlemm, thereby preventing the aqueous humor from reaching its usual outflow channels [16]. This type of glaucoma often occurs in hyperopic eyes with shallow anterior chambers. Dilation of the pupil, trauma, emotional upsets, or any ocular change that pushes the iris forward may precipitate an acute attack of glaucoma as the angle is blocked by the iris [16]. Any patient complaining of ocular pain, headache, blurred vision, and halos around lights, and demonstrating a fixed pupil and a red, hard eye with a steamy (cloudy appearing) cornea should be seen by an ophthalmologist immediately. The intraocular tension may be so severe that it results in nausea and vomiting, which may even cause the examiner to suspect gastrointestinal disease. To prevent rapid damage to the optic nerve and permanent blindness, the intraocular pressure must be reduced immediately. Repeated administration of a miotic until the pupil is constricted and the oral or intravenous administration of a carbonic anhydrase inhibitor such as acetazolamide are initiated. Analgesics are also administered. If the intraocular pressure cannot be decreased, the use of intravenously administered hyperosmotic agents such as mannitol may be required. Oral glycerin, another hyperosmotic agent, is utilized in some situations. Immediate surgical intervention may be necessary when medical therapy is not effective. Even if the acute attack is controlled with medical therapy, surgical intervention may be indicated to prevent subsequent attacks.

A peripheral iridectomy is performed by excising a piece of the iris to allow aqueous humor to flow from the posterior to the anterior chamber; this prevents the iris from pushing forward into the angle and allows aqueous humor to pass freely through normal channels. Other types of surgical procedures include iridencleisis, which also provides for filtration of aqueous humor from the inner eye, and trephination, a procedure in which a small piece of sclera is removed to permit aqueous outflow through the artificial tunnel that is created. Cyclodialysis is a procedure in which the sclera is opened behind the limbus and the ciliary body is separated from its normal attachment to the sclera. This procedure creates a passage from the anterior chamber to the suprachoroidal space.

Cyclodiathermy, in which diathermy is applied from the outside of the eye through the sclera over the ciliary body, and cryosurgical (freezing) techniques are both utilized to reduce the formation of aqueous by partially destroying the ciliary body. For patients with intractable glaucoma a new microsurgical procedure, the aqueous-venous shunt, has recently been developed. This operation establishes aqueous drainage by the insertion of a tiny plastic or collagen tube between the anterior chamber and the lumen of an extraocular vein [11]. Postoperative care for patients having surgery for glaucoma is similar to that for other types of ocular surgery, with modifications indicated by the individual patient's needs.

In caring for the patient with glaucoma, the

nurse must place major emphasis on patient teaching to ensure complete understanding of the disease and compliance with the necessary treatment regimen [17]. Therapy to reduce and control intraocular pressure must be followed explicitly. Eye drops of miotic drugs must always be given at the specific times prescribed in order to lower intraocular pressure consistently by decreasing resistance to aqueous outflow. The patient with glaucoma will have to administer eye drops of miotics at specific intervals daily for the rest of his life. Since this can be a problem for the elderly patient who is either forgetful, confused, or generally unreliable, provision must be made for supervision of the regimen of these patients. Even the alert younger person may have difficulty fitting the time schedules for the administration of the eye drops into his or her daily pattern of activities. Eye drops tend to burn for the first few minutes after administration, and until the patient adjusts to this effect, he or she may want to omit the eye drops. Again, the emphasis on absolute follow-through of the prescribed regimen must be conveyed to the patient.

The patient with glaucoma is advised to carry a Medic-Alert card or some type of identification to verify the presence of glaucoma. This is especially important in case the patient is rendered unconscious by an accident, since a constricted pupil that was actually caused by medications for glaucoma might suggest pupil dilatation of the opposite eye, causing a misinterpretation during neurologic assessment.

Nurses should allow patients to continue taking their eye medications for glaucoma when admitted to the hospital for conditions other than ocular problems. The physician may neglect to include the eye drops in the medication orders when the patient is admitted for other conditions. Patients with angle-closure glaucoma should not use other drugs that may induce intraocular pressure by causing pupil dilation. Drugs such as atropine or propantheline bromide may be used for a variety of medical regimens but are contraindicated for the patient with glaucoma because of the pupil dilation associated with the drugs. Drugs used for coronary and peripheral vasodilatation are considered safe to use with glaucoma patients [6], but certain antihypertensive agents and some synthetic narcotics are contraindicated. This is only true in the case of angle-closure glaucoma, in which the patient is vulnerable to an acute attack when the pupil is dilated. Overuse of topical or systemic corticosteroids can also increase intraocular pressure. In fact, open-angle glaucoma has developed in susceptible patients who have had repeated instillation of corticosteroids [5]; in these cases, the glaucoma is generally reversible on cessation of the topical steroids.

Patients with glaucoma should be advised about activities and situations that predispose to increased intraocular pressure. Leading as tranquil a life as possible is important, to avoid emotional or stressful situations that increase intraocular pressure. The patient should avoid excessive exertion, such as shoveling snow or heavy lifting, and wearing constrictive clothing such as tight collars. Although ocular damage that has occurred prior to the initiation of treatment is not reversible, further visual impairment can be prevented by proper medical management and the patient's compliance with the prescribed regimen.

DISEASE OF THE RETINA

Detachment of the retina, which is the separation of the retina from the choroid, is usually spontaneous, although it may be secondary to trauma. It occurs most frequently in persons over the age of 50 and in persons with myopia. Aging and other types of damage may cause the vitreous body to shrink, causing a retinal tear where it is attached to the retina. The patient with a detached retina may complain of "floaters," heavy black spots or lines in his line of vision; these are caused by shadows cast on the retina by clumps of shrunken vitreous gel or by hemorrhage in the vitreous cavity. Vision is reduced wherever the retina is detached, but a person may not notice the visual loss if the other eye has good vision. Central vision may remain normal as long as the macula is not involved. However, once the macula is detached, visual loss is profound. Total detachment of the retina prevents light perception only.

There is usually no pain or redness of the eye. The patient generally complains of blurred vision in one eye and flashes of light, and he often describes the sensation of "a curtain coming down over my eye." When retinal detachment is suspected, the patient should be referred immediately to an ophthalmologist. If possible, the patient should be moved with both eyes patched. As soon as the retina is torn, a transudate from the choroidal vessels mixed with vitreous causes an abnormal vitreous traction on the retina so that the retina is stripped from the choroid, from which it normally receives nourishment (Fig. 12-12).

By using the binocular indirect ophthalmoscope and a scleral depressor, the ophthalmologist is able to obtain a three-dimensional view of the retina and can usually visualize a tear, most commonly found at the superior temporal area of the retina. Most retinal tears are about the size of the tip of a lead pencil but sometimes may be much larger and are known as giant retinal tears [4]. The patient is placed on complete bed rest, and both eyes are covered to prevent further detachment until surgery is accomplished. Since the eyes move simultaneously, binocular patches are needed to limit eye movements. If the macula has already been detached, reattachment may not totally restore vision.

There are two basic types of detachment of the retina. The most common is the **rhegmatogenous** type, which is usually caused by one or more holes in the retina. Degenerative changes in the vitreous causing shrinking of the vitreous with pulling on the retina are considered the cause of most retinal detachments. Although some people may associate the symptoms of detachment with those of a mild blow to the head, the trauma is not likely the direct cause but rather the culminating factor. Rhegmatogenous detachment can be treated by surgical correction and modern methods of attachment.

Secondary or **nonrhegmatogenous** detachment occurs as the result of another local or systemic condition, such as an intraocular tumor, and as the result of exudate accumulation from the choroid rather than from tears in the retina. Direct contusion injury to the retina, corneal scleral lacerations, and intraocular foreign bodies can also cause retinal detachments. Inflammatory disease of the eye involving the vitreous may cause contraction of the vitreous with pulling on the retina, resulting in retinal detachment. A relation between aphakia (absence of the lens after cataract extraction) and retinal detachment has also been recognized, especially when the vitreous is traumatized during the surgery. Treatment of the nonrhegmatogenous types of detachment usually involves the correction of the underlying cause.

The aim of treatment of retinal detachment is to seal the retinal break, reattach the retina, and prevent the retina from detaching again. The most common operation used for repair of the retina in the rhegmatogenous type of detachment is the **scleral buckling** procedure. An adhesive, exudative choroiditis is produced in the choroid at the site of the retinal hole by the application of diathermy or cryocauterization to the sclera overlying the choroid. A strip of silicone plastic is anchored to the sclera by Dacron sutures, and cinched up to make a buckle in the sclera and choroid,

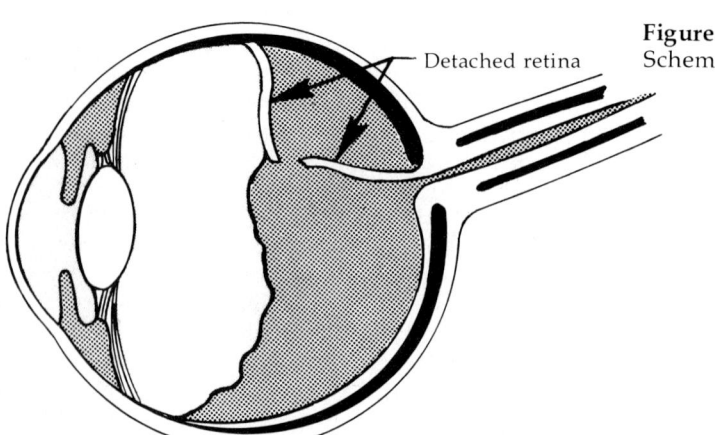

Figure 12-12
Schematic illustration of retinal detachment.

much like a belt or girdle [10]. The choroid is punctured with a small needle, allowing the subretinal fluid to be drained, which in turn allows the retina to settle back on the choroid. A chorioretinal scar forms and permanently seals the hole.

Maximum ocular rest is necessary while the chorioretinal scar is forming, requiring bed rest with bilateral eye bandaging (or unilateral patching in some protocols) for several days postoperatively. The uninvolved eye may then be uncovered, but the patient may wear a pinhole glass or patch over the operated eye for about 2 weeks longer. Progressive ambulation is usually initiated on the second or third postoperative day but is done very gradually. The patient must be cautioned against bumping his head and making rapid eye movements (such as in reading) or rapid jerking movements of the head. There is a gradual return to normal activity, but contact sports are usually not allowed for 3 months.

If retinal holes are discovered before actual detachment has occurred, the tear may be sealed nonsurgically by using the **laser** or xenon arc photocoagulator. Light of high intensity produces a localized burn and an inflammatory reaction, creating adhesion of the retina to the underlying choroid. Transconjunctival cryopexy has also been utilized to prevent further progression. The purpose of both techniques is to form an adhesive chorioretinal scar to seal the retinal hole. The laser works as a glue, so that the retina must be lying against the back of the eye for the laser to be effective. For this reason, the laser cannot work once the retina has become significantly detached [2].

Lasers have also proved to be useful in treating various vascular problems, including diabetic retinopathy, a progressive disorder of the blood vessels of the retina leading to impaired retinal circulation and impaired vision. Retinal hemorrhages and microaneurysms frequently occur in this condition. In proliferative retinopathy, new blood vessels sprout from existing vessels, erupting through the retinal surface and growing between the retina and vitreous, which leads to visual impairment. Lasers are used to produce clotting and to destroy vascular channels that would otherwise cause visual impairment or total blindness. The laser is also being utilized to treat tumors of the eye, such as retinoblastoma and melanoma.

In most cases, laser treatments are done on an outpatient basis, with no hospitalization required. The treatment takes approximately 30 minutes and is essentially painless. The number of treatment exposures varies according to the type of lesion to be treated.

Another less frequently used approach for treating diabetic retinopathy to halt progressive blindness is to perform a hypophysectomy (removal of the pituitary gland). This procedure is discussed in Chapters 8 and 11.

A leading cause of blindness and visual disability is **degeneration of the retina,** which occurs in people over the age of 60. The macula, which is a small indentation along the retina, is usually the site of involvement. The macula controls sharp vision, such as that required in reading, and therefore damage to the macula results in a gradual loss of central vision. There is no known treatment for the condition, although the use of special low-vision aids is helpful to allow continued activity.

Another retinal disease is **retinitis pigmentosa,** an inherited disease that usually produces its first symptom, night blindness, in children and adolescents. Another major symptom is "tunnel vision," or loss of peripheral vision. The disease derives its name from the characteristic black pigment deposits scattered throughout the retina, particularly around the edges. An abnormality in the biochemistry of the eye or in the body's metabolism is thought to be the precipitating factor. There is no known treatment to halt the progression of the disease, although complete blindness does not always occur. Reading vision may be retained, although it is limited to a small central part of the visual field.

Retrolental fibroplasia, an abnormal proliferation of the retinal vessels in premature infants, is decreasing in incidence since the cause has been found to be the use of excessive oxygen concentration in early incubator care. This knowledge has resulted in the improved management of oxygen control in the care of premature infants by careful monitoring of arterial oxygen concentration.

Retinoblastoma is a highly malignant cancer arising from the retina of one or both eyes in children. The symptoms, including secondary strabismus or glaucoma or a pupil that is whitened by the underlying tumor, occur so late that removal of the eye is usually necessary when the diagnosis is made. There is a tendency for the tumor to recur in the other eye, so frequent examinations of the second eye are carried out to detect a possible tumor in its early stages. Treatment is essential to prevent metastasis to the central nervous system. Radiation therapy, chemotherapy, and photocoagulation may be used to treat the tumor that is discovered in its early stages. The condition is often familial, occurring in more than one child; therefore funduscopic studies of siblings are indicated when there is a history of retinoblastoma.

DISEASE OF THE CORNEA

The cornea, which is the transparent membrane at the front of the eye, may be the site of infections, injury, and degenerative changes. When not treated promptly, corneal diseases cause scarring and opaqueness, resulting in impaired vision or blindness. Foreign bodies in the cornea cause visual impairment either from edematous reactions or from surface irregularities. Complete debridement of all foreign material is the primary treatment and is best done with topical anesthesia under the slit lamp. When the cornea is destroyed by disease, infection (keratitis), or injury or loses its transparency, corneal transplantation (keratoplasty) may be an effective treatment. A cornea from a cadaver is used to replace the central portion of the cornea, which is removed surgically. (People can arrange before death to donate their eyes to a state or national Eye Bank.) The cornea is removed from the donor's eye within 6 hours after death, and the sooner the cornea is transplanted, the better are the results. However, a technique called cryopreservation is now being utilized for freezing donated eyes to preserve the corneas for later use.

A full-thickness graft, also called penetrating keratoplasty, goes through the entire thickness of the cornea, although the size or width of the graft will depend on the extent of the area to be replaced. The lamellar keratoplasty, a partial-thickness graft, is primarily used to improve the structure of the cornea. In a penetrating keratoplasty, the cornea is removed from the donor eye and a disc of the required diameter is punched out. A disc corresponding in size is marked on the recipient eye, and sutures are inserted in the cornea around the disc for direct suturing of the graft. The disc is completely removed, and the graft is carefully laid on its bed and sutured in place. The procedure for the lamellar or nonpenetrating keratoplasty is similar except that this partial-thickness method does not involve perforating the deeper layers or entering the anterior chamber.

Postoperatively, complete bed rest with binocular patches for several days may be required for the graft to begin to heal. Since many delicate sutures are used, pressure or strain on the suture line must be prevented. The postoperative precautions for preventing intraocular pressure are similar to those described for cataract surgery, but the period of restricted activity is much longer. The major complication to be prevented is displacement of the graft, which must heal with its edges exactly flush with the surrounding cornea. Limiting activity and providing sensory stimulation for the patient who has prolonged bilateral patching after a corneal transplant can be a real challenge to the nurse. Often these patients feel fine and think that they should resume more activity unless the necessity for absolute bed rest and the dangers of excess activity are completely explained to them. Other complications that can occur after keratoplasty are ocular infections, uveitis, and secondary glaucoma.

Improved surgical techniques using the operating microscope and the use of newer and finer suture materials have contributed to success in maintaining clear grafts. Immune graft reactions and allograft rejections, however, can occur after transplantation. Through screening for HL-A antibodies (HL-A antigen system), donors and recipients can be matched more appropriately so that graft rejections occur less often. In some cases, the inflammatory response can be successfully treated with immunosuppressive therapy, but in other cases, endothelium may be destroyed in the rejection process. As surgical techniques are improved and homograft reactions decrease, the number of patients benefiting from corneal transplants will be increased.

ENUCLEATION OF THE EYEBALL

Enucleation of the eye (surgical removal of the eyeball from its orbit) is most often performed when severe injuries cause so much damage to the eye that no other alternative is possible. Enucleation may also be done to prevent the spread of a malignant tumor, such as retinoblastoma or malignant melanoma. Intraocular melanoma is the most common type of intraocular malignancy in the adult and is second to trauma as a cause for enucleation. If it is not controlled, metastasis (especially to the liver) readily occurs. Any part of the uveal tract, including the iris, may be involved in malignant melanoma. When the iris is involved, the tumor may be visualized even on direct inspection. If only the iris is involved, excision of the iris may control the disease; otherwise enucleation is indicated. Since malignant melanoma is generally radioresistant, radiation therapy is not indicated for intraocular melanoma.

Enucleation may be necessary after a severe ocular injury as a prophylactic measure to protect the unaffected eye from developing sympathetic ophthalmia. This process can occur in the unaffected eye when the diseased eye is extensively injured or infected. On rare occasions, enucleation may be necessary when intractable pain occurs in severe, uncontrolled glaucoma.

The patient having an enucleation requires much emotional support. The fears associated with the loss of a vital feature of the facial contour result in concerns about the postoperative cosmetic appearance. The fear of spread of the disease process and the definite loss of a vision source (even if the affected eye has only minimal vision) is a frightening experience. In a society that tends to be oriented toward visual contact, the patient fears that the nonmovable artificial eye will be very obvious to others. However, the patient should be reassured that the prosthesis is so artistically designed that it is usually very difficult to discern.

The surgical procedure for enucleation involves making an incision into the edge of the conjunctiva, severing the rectus muscles and the tendons, and sectioning the optic nerve before the globe is finally removed. Saline-soaked gauze and a plastic compressor are then compressed into the empty socket to control initial bleeding, and an implant similar to a white or clear ball is placed in the socket and sutured in place. A white plastic shield called a conformer is placed over the implant to give a normal contour to the eyelid.

Postoperatively there is danger of hemorrhage, but a pressure dressing is usually applied to the area to prevent hemorrhage or edema formation. As in other types of eye surgery, the patient should avoid stooping or bending postoperatively, which might increase the pressure on the suture line. Early ambulation is encouraged. Pain is generally minimal and can be controlled by mild analgesics, although headache is a frequent postoperative complaint. There is always the possibility that the implant may escape from its position; when this occurs, the implant must be replaced under general anesthesia.

The patient is taught how to irrigate the socket (a procedure similar to the technique of eye irrigation described previously, except that a rubber ear syringe is usually used) and to apply antibiotic eye solution, using the principles of asepsis to prevent infection. Patches are used to cover the surgical area. As noted previously, a temporary plastic conformer is placed in the socket to retain its shape. The patient should be warned that the conformer may fall out and should be instructed in the procedure for replacing the conformer in the event this occurs. The conformer is used until the ocular prosthesis is available. Fitting for the ocular prosthesis is not done until approximately 2 to 3 weeks after surgery, when swelling completely disappears. The patient is usually discharged several days after the operation.

Care of the Ocular Prosthesis

The patient will require instruction in the use and care of the ocular prosthesis. It is generally advantageous for the nurse to understand the care, removal, and insertion of an ocular prosthesis, because patients may be admitted to the hospital in a condition that prevents their caring for or removing the prosthesis. It may be necessary, for example, to remove the prosthesis in an emergency situation or prior to general surgery in order to prevent loss or trauma to the prosthesis.

The ocular prosthesis is designed to be worn day and night. It should not be removed daily, as some patients tend to think; rather it should be removed weekly or at least once a month for cleaning. When crusting occurs around the prosthesis, the crusts should be removed. The prosthesis should be irrigated externally every day with warm saline solution. An eye irrigation solution such as Eyestream may be used to clean the eye.

When the nurse is to remove the ocular prosthesis, the patient should preferably be in a flat position so that the prosthesis is not broken when it falls out. A suction cup is the preferred method for removal, but it can be done manually. The lower lid is depressed, which allows the prosthesis to slide up and out into the nurse's hand.

The prosthesis is scrubbed with mild detergent and water. No other chemicals should be used for cleaning since they can damage the prosthesis. The prosthesis is polished and dried and then stored in water or contact lens soaking solution until it is reinserted. Some authorities recommend the use of a drop of a bacteriostatic agent on the prosthesis. When the prosthesis is reinserted, it is dampened with water. The upper lid is lifted with one hand and the other hand is used to place the notched edge of the prosthesis toward the nose. The prosthesis is slid as far as possible under the upper lid, and the lower lid is then depressed so that the prosthesis will slip into place. When wiping of the eye is necessary, it should be done toward the nose, since wiping toward the ear is apt to dislodge the prosthesis.

The person with an ocular prosthesis will adjust to turning his head rather than his eyes. Many people learn to do this so expertly and gracefully that the prosthesis may not be noticed by others.

Rehabilitation of the Blind Patient

Aspects of caring for the visually impaired or blind patient primarily in relation to the hospital situation have already been discussed. In addition, the general rehabilitation of the newly blind patient and aspects of long-term management should be considered. One must also consider that the entire family is affected by a person's blindness; the family members as well as the patient require support in adjusting to the handicap and a different life-style. The effect of blindness on the total life pattern is overwhelming in most instances.

Each newly blind person will react to the problems imposed by his loss of vision in an individual way. The shock and grief associated with the onset of blindness require time for adjustment in the grief process before adaptation is possible. Even face-to-face communication with people is disrupted; normal reading and writing abilities are major losses. The problems encountered may seem insurmountable until the blind person is reconciled to learning to adapt to new techniques for carrying out essential and important activities. Contrary to popular opinion, the remaining senses do not automatically become more sensitive, but rather the newly blind person gradually learns to adapt by making greater use of the other senses. Hearing, for example, becomes more efficient because the blind person is not distracted by the sights around him and learns to sharpen his listening skills. If the blind person is elderly and has hearing difficulties, he is more seriously handicapped.

Even in familiar surroundings, the newly blind person feels confused and insecure because of an uncertain sense of balance and direction and awkward doing even ordinary activities such as eating, dressing, and walking. The newly blind person realistically feels insecure, dependent, and frightened. The danger of physical injury or the fear of embarrassment in moving about in the sighted world may physiologically and psychologically immobilize him. After gaining confidence and increased ability to move about comfortably, the newly blind person will want to expand his or her environment.

The blind person needs assistance in carrying out certain tasks. For example, grocery shopping requires that someone assist him or her in locating specific items in the store. At home, the blind person can organize cabinets and make braille markings to facilitate locating specific items. Certain appliances in the home may be adapted for the blind person; for example, braille dials may be applied to ovens. Telephones with touch-tone systems rather than conventional dials are more readily used by the blind person.

The newly blind person must learn to handle coins. He can usually identify most coins readily, except that distinguishing pennies from dimes may be difficult (however, pennies have a smooth edge as compared to the serrated edges of dimes). Braille watches are available. The newly blind person must also learn to arrange his or her hair without benefit of looking in a mirror. The woman must learn to put on makeup in new ways; the man must adjust to learning to shave without the use of a mirror. Until the blind person becomes agile with eating utensils, meal times are likely to be tension-producing and awkward.

It is often difficult initially for sighted people to determine how much assistance is needed by the blind person. This problem should be discussed with the blind person prior to attending social situations so that a system of smooth assistance can be provided. Even communication becomes awkward as sighted people try to avoid using words that imply vision. It takes time for both the blind person and his sighted family and friends to overcome these communication problems.

The blind person can benefit from using a cane to warn him of obstacles ahead of him. The white cane with a red tip is readily recognized by others, who may have to give assistance at strategic times. Some people learn to use a guide dog after proper training. The Seeing Eye, Inc. has specialists to train blind people in this technique. However, using a guide dog is a very technical process requiring much time and concentration, and not all blind people are able to learn the technique. Some people use both a guide dog and a cane.

Recent developments in the use of laser canes have facilitated increased independence for the blind person. Laser canes are specially designed long canes that emit beams of colorless light to detect objects up to 20 feet ahead of the blind person. The system is also able to detect and signal changes in the terrain. Other technologic aids have been developed to facilitate safer mobility, such as ultrasonic transmitter-receiver devices on eyeglasses to detect overhanging obstacles.

Learning the braille system, an arrangement of embossed or raised dots that are read with the fingers, is a valuable tool when the blind person has the motivation to learn the method. Braille is written with the aid of a metal slate or a specially constructed braille typewriter. Correspondence courses in braille are available, and talking books and long-playing discs or tapes are available from various libraries. The Library of Congress lends many of these talking books and recording machines on a free basis. Some magazines (such as *Newsweek*) and newspapers provide a talking magazine (or newspaper) service, placing the material on records or tapes.

The person with partial vision loss will usually benefit from optical aids such as telescopic and microscopic eyeglasses. Large-print books and newspapers are also helpful.

A variety of visual aids for magnification of visual materials are available both for direct observation and for projection, so that a person may use efficiently what remaining vision he has.

Recently a reading instrument has been developed to enable a blind person to read the same printed material any sighted person would read. Using advanced electronics, this device, known as the Optacon (OPtical-to-TActile-CONverter),* converts the visual images of letters into tactile forms that can be identified by the blind person. To read with the Optacon, the blind person moves a miniature camera across the line of print with one hand. The index finger of the other hand is placed on the Optacon's tactile screen, which is approximately one inch long and one-half inch wide. As the camera is moved across a letter, the image is simultaneously reproduced on the tactile screen by means of vibrating reeds. The person using the Optacon senses the outline of a regular letter conveyed through the raising and lowering of an array of tiny rods that fit onto a single finger. The Optacon weighs only four pounds, is battery operated, and can be easily transported. The current cost of the instrument is approximately $3,500. Optacon instruction is being integrated into some public education settings.

Another type of vision substitution device uses images captured by a television camera to activate a series of stimulators arranged on a grid and positioned over the abdominal skin. With training and practice, a sightless person learns to translate these impulses automatically into crude spatial images within his brain.

The blind person will find his adjustment facilitated by having appropriate support from his friends and family and appropriate understanding and guidance by professional people. After the newly blind person adapts to his environment and gains independence, he may be able to return to his former occupation, if vision is not absolutely essential to it. Adaptations may be possible to facilitate the return to a former position; for example, the use of tape recordings or Dictaphones may facilitate the carrying out of responsibilities in certain types of employment. If the person cannot return to his former employment, the

---

*Telesensory Systems Inc., Palo Alto, California.

blind person may seek assistance from the local or state Office of Vocational Rehabilitation. Vocational guidance, training, placement, and follow-up are available through these agencies.

Social activities such as dancing, swimming, or skating are encouraged for the blind person who has always been interested in such activities. The ultimate goal for the blind person is to adjust to the reality of the loss of vision while taking advantage of the assets and capabilities that remain to permit his leading a full and satisfying life.

Many agencies, some of which are listed below, serve the needs of blind persons. It is advantageous for the nurse to know about these agencies so that appropriate information and advice may be given to patients needing their services. Some of these agencies provide professional as well as lay publications and films to increase the understanding of those working with blind people.

1. American Foundation for the Blind
   15 W. 16th Street
   New York, NY 10011
   Publishes books, pamphlets, monographs, and professional reports; sells special appliances for the blind.
2. American Printing House for the Blind
   1839 Frankfort Avenue, South
   Louisville, KY 40206
   Prints books and magazines in braille; publishes the *Reader's Digest* in braille and talking book forms; produces *Newsweek* magazine in talking book form; publishes books in large print for visually handicapped children.
3. Braille Institute of America, Inc.
   741 N. Vermont Avenue
   Los Angeles, CA 90029
   Produces braille books.
4. Eye Bank Association of America
   3195 Maplewood Avenue
   Winston-Salem, NC 27103
   Furnishes corneas, scleras, and vitreous humor free of charge.
5. Hadley School for the Blind
   700 Elm Street
   Winnetka, IL 60093
   National school of tuition-free correspondence courses for the blind, including some university and vocational courses.
6. Library of Congress
   Division for the Blind and Physically Handicapped
   Washington, DC 20540
   Provides books in braille and talking book records; serves many geographic areas through 34 distributing libraries.
7. National Eye Institute
   National Institutes of Health
   Bethesda, MD 20014
8. National Society for the Prevention of Blindness, Inc.
   79 Madison Avenue
   New York, NY 10016
9. Recording for the Blind, Inc.
   215 E. 58th Street
   New York, NY 10022
   Provides records and tapes of textbooks and other educational material free of charge; will record books by specific requests.
10. The Seeing Eye, Inc.
    P.O. Box 375
    Morristown, NJ 07960
    Offers one-month courses for qualified blind people to learn to use and control guide dogs.

References

1. Bates, B. *A Guide to Physical Examination.* Philadelphia: Lippincott, 1974.
2. Berler, D. K. Lasers in ophthalmology. *Am. Fam. Physician* 9:118, 1974.
3. Emery, J. M. Cataract treatment and rehabilitation. *AORN J.* 20:992, 1974.
4. Freeman, H. M. Recent advances in retinal detachment and vitreous surgery. *AORN J.* 18:1896, 1973.
5. Friedman, E., and Lessell, S. Diseases of the Eye and Ocular Manifestations of Systemic Disease. In C. Keefer, and R. Wilkins (eds.), *Medicine: Essentials of Clinical Practice.* Boston: Little, Brown, 1970.
6. Grant, W. M. Ocular complications of drugs: Glaucoma. *J.A.M.A.* 207:2089, 1969.
7. Gutierrez, A. Nursing care during cataract removal by phacoemulsification. *AORN J.* 15:929, 1973.
8. Havener, W. H. *Synopsis of Ophthalmology* (3rd ed.). St. Louis: Mosby, 1971.
9. Havener, W. H., Saunders, W. H., Keith,

C. F., and Prescott, A. W. *Nursing Care in Eye, Ear, Nose and Throat Disorders.* St. Louis: Mosby, 1974.
10. Jarrett, W. H., and Hagler, W. S. Retinal detachment. *Hosp. Med.* 7:87, 1971.
11. Lee, P., and Wong, W. Aqueous-venous shunt for glaucoma. *Ann. Ophthalmol.* 6:1083, 1974.
12. Patient assessment: Examination of the eye: II. Programmed instruction. *Am. J. Nurs.* 75:1, 1975.
13. Paton, D., and Craig, J. A. Cataracts: Development, diagnosis and management. *Clin. Symp.* 26:2, 1974.
14. Roy, F. H. World blindness: Definition, incidence and major treatable causes. *Ann. Ophthalmol.* 6:1049, 1974.
15. Shell, J. W., and Baker, R. W. Diffusional systems for controlled release of drugs to the eye. *Ann. Ophthalmol.* 6:1037, 1974.
16. Soll, D. Glaucoma. *Am. Fam. Physician* 9:125, 1974.
17. Vincent, P. Factors influencing noncompliance: A theoretical approach. *Nurs. Res.* 20:509, 1971.
18. Weinstock, F. J. Tonometry screening. *Am. J. Nurs.* 73:656, 1973.

Bibliography

Abrahamson, I. A. Anterior segment eye disorders: I. *Hosp. Med.* 7:56, 1971.
Abrahamson, I. A. Anterior segment eye disorders: II. The red eye. *Hosp. Med.* 7:96, 1971.
Alexander, M. M., and Brown, M. S. Physical examination: V. Examining the eye. *Nursing '73* 3:41, 1973.
Allen, J. H. Disorders of the eyelids. *Hosp. Med.* 8:102, 1972.
Ammon, L. Surviving enucleation. *Am. J. Nurs.* 72:1817, 1972.
Appleton, B. Some aspects of ocular trauma. *Hosp. Med.* 7:96, 1971.
Armaly, M. F. Annual review: Glaucoma. *Arch. Ophthalmol.* 93:146, 1975.
Babel, J. Safeguarding your eyesight. *Bull. W.H.O.* 2, 1970.
Bean, M. A. Camp Lighthouse. *Am. J. Nurs.* 72:950, 1972.
Branson, H. K. The blind mother. *Am. J. Nurs.* 75:414, 1975.
Brueggen, S. L. Tonometry and the professional nurse. *Am. Assoc. Indust. Nurs. J.* 16:13, 1968.
Brust, A. A. The eyegrounds in hypertension and other disorders. *Hosp. Med.* 7:38, 1971.
Caring for the Visually Impaired Older Person. Minneapolis, Minn.: Minnesota Society for the Blind, Inc., 1970.
Casey, T. A. Examination of the eye. *Hosp. Med.* 7:20, 1971.
Condl, E. D., et al. Ophthalmic nursing. *Nurs. Clin. North Am.* 5:449, 1970.
Duane, T. D., ed. *Clinical Ophthalmology* (Series 5). Hagerstown, N.J.: Harper & Row, 1976.
Fernsbener, W. Etiology and treatment of glaucoma. *AORN J.* 20:996, 1974.
Fulton, M., Schweizer, D., Ruhland, F., Brownfield, J., and Etzwiler, D. Helping diabetics adapt to failing vision. *Am. J. Nurs.* 74:34, 1974.
Gordon, D. M. Diseases of the eye. *Clin. Symp.* 14:115, 1962.
Guyton, A. C. *Textbook of Medical Physiology* (4th ed.). Philadelphia: Saunders, 1971.
Hamilton, M. J. What the nurse should know about eye banks. *Nurs. Clin. North Am.* 5:483, 1970.
Harvey, A. M., Johns, R. J., Owens, A. H., and Ross, R. S. *The Principles and Practice of Medicine* (18th ed.). New York: Appleton-Century-Crofts, 1972. Pp. 1563–1571.
Hiles, D. A. Strabismus. *Am. J. Nurs.* 74:1082, 1974.
If Blindness Occurs. Morristown, N.J.: Seeing Eye, Inc.
Jordon, H. The use of the argon laser photocoagulator in retinal surgery. *AORN J.* 18:914, 1974.
Judge, R. D., and Zuidema, G. D. *Physical Diagnosis: A Physiologic Approach to the Clinical Examination* (2nd ed.). Boston: Little, Brown, 1968. Pp. 75–100.
Neu, C. Coping with newly diagnosed blindness. *Am. J. Nurs.* 75:2161, 1975.
Patient assessment: Examination of the eye: I. Programmed instruction. *Am. J. Nurs.* 74:1, 1974.
Rabb, M. F. The present status of corneal transplantation. *Nurs. Clin. North Am.* 5:477, 1970.
Reinhards, J. Flies, sand and trachoma. *Bull. W.H.O.* 9, 1970.
Rizzuti, A. Trauma to the anterior ocular segment. *Hosp. Med.* 10:26, 1974.
Rodman, N. J., and Smith, D. *Pharmacology and Drug Therapy in Nursing.* Philadelphia: Lippincott, 1968. Pp. 586–597.
Rosborough, J. F. Ocular emergencies. *Hosp. Med.* 7:46, 1971.
Roy, F. H. A practical approach to children's eye problems. *Am. Fam. Physician* 10:101, 1974.
Scheie, H. G., and Albert, D. M. *Adler's Textbook of Ophthalmology.* Philadelphia: Saunders, 1969.
Smith, J. F., and Nachazel, D. Retinal detachment. *Am. J. Nurs.* 73:1530, 1973.

Weinstock, F. J.   Emergency treatment of eye injuries. *Am. J. Nurs.* 71:1928, 1971.

Wells, P.   Use of ultrasonics in cataract surgery. *AORN J.* 18:922, 1973.

Zucnick, M.   Care of an artificial eye. *Am. J. Nurs.* 75:835, 1975.

Media Resources

Nursing Techniques for the Care of Patients with Impaired Vision (series of eight single-concept films). Available from The Ohio State University, Columbus, Ohio.

chapter 13
Patients with Ear, Nose, and Throat Dysfunction

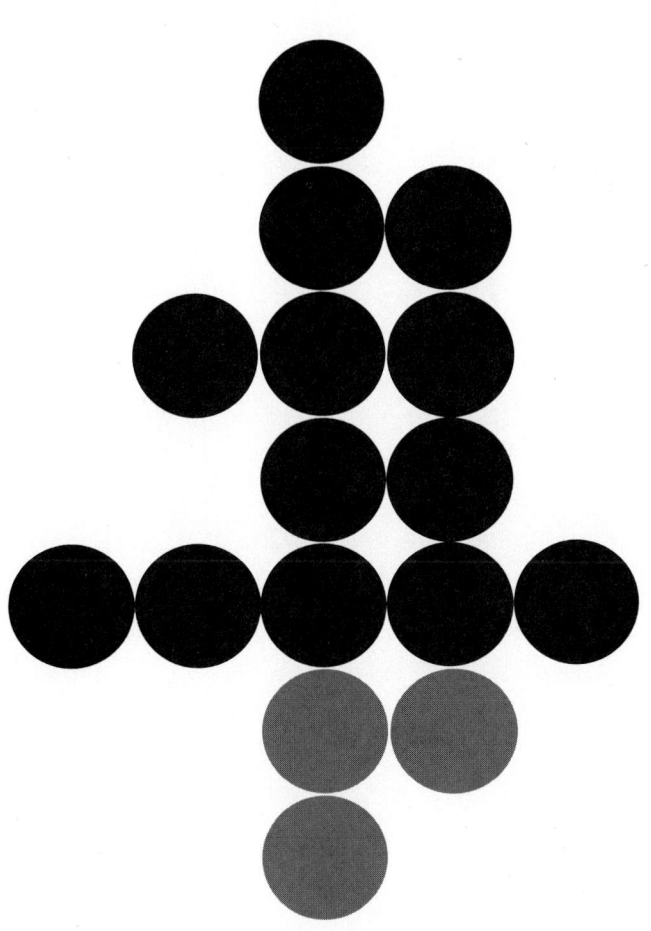

This chapter includes information about the most commonly occurring types of dysfunction in the ear, nose, and throat. Dysfunction of the ear, nose, and throat disrupts a person's normal activity and requires sensitive and perceptive nursing care. The ear is essential for both hearing and equilibrium; the nose and throat are important for respiration. In addition, the nose provides the essential sense of smell, while the vocal cords in the larynx are necessary for production of sound. The upper respiratory passages also contribute to the production of sound and influence the tone and quality of a person's voice. The functions of the ear, nose, and throat have multiple meanings for the individual since hearing, smelling, and speaking have both esthetic and protective implications. Smelling good food or hearing pleasant music or conversing with a friend is pleasurable, while smelling fire, hearing loud noises, and being able to call out in the event of danger are protective functions. When any of these functions are disrupted, patients must make adjustments in order to accurately perceive and relate to their environment. A basic element in nursing care for these patients is helping them to adapt to the basic changes in their lives required by the dysfunction.

The Ear

The ear is a sensory organ with two major functions: hearing and maintenance of equilibrium. Both of these functions are associated with complex neural mechanisms for perception and interpretation in the highest centers in the brain. The ear provides for sensory input and contains end-organ receptors that transmit impulses to and receive stimuli from the central nervous system. **Hearing** is one of the senses through which people become oriented to their environment as they move from place to place or when their environment changes, as when people and things move in and out of the range of hearing. Hearing is basic to a person's relating to others or to objects in his or her environment and it serves both for pleasure and for protection. Humans are constantly learning to discriminate among sounds and to define for themselves sounds that are pleasurable or disturbing. Responses to what is heard constantly change as attitudes and knowledge about what is heard change. For example, new experiences are often associated with new sounds. Familiar sounds often help one to adjust when adapting to new experiences and may take on new meanings.

The sense of hearing is finely developed, so that changes in the character of sounds are heard as cues to understanding or knowing about the events taking place in the environment. Hearing is also a major component in communication with other persons, being essential to both listening and speaking. Persons who are deaf or those who are hard of hearing are deprived of auditory sensory input. This deprivation requires adaptation, which never fully replaces the loss of pleasurable auditory sensations. Sound is a function of the environment and is produced by visible and invisible components. The sounds a person is able to "hear," that is, perceive, interpret, and respond to, vary from instant to instant. Emotional and physical well-being and the total array of sensory inputs received at any given time influence the person's ability to receive and interpret sounds. The nurse should be aware that a person does not and cannot always "hear" everything that is said; this concept is important to remember in teaching-learning situations and in analyzing responses to situations. The emotional impact of any situation and the amount of new and unfamiliar sensory stimuli may interfere with a person's usual ability to concentrate on and comprehend the spoken word, and the patient's values, attitudes, and emotions determine the perception of or the meaning of the sensory input he received.

The other major function of the ear, **equilibrium,** is an automatic function that enables a person to maintain balance and position sense in relation to gravity. Maintenance of equilibrium is important for both body balance and position in space. The vestibular functions of the ear enable a person to maintain orientation in relation to gravity as he moves his head. The function of equilibrium is not limited to the ear. Instead, it is accomplished by complex coordination of body movements through vestibular sensations, visual sensations, and proprioception. The integration of these stimuli occurs through complex neural mechanisms to initiate skeletal muscle and visual responses so that a person can remain in appropriate contact with his environment.

NURSING ASSESSMENT OF EAR FUNCTION

Assessment of ear function is part of the care the nurse gives to every patient. General observation of speech, hearing modes, balance, and coordination as demonstrated in body movements are important aspects of the assessment. As a person converses, the nurse should listen carefully for speech patterns. People with hearing loss often have concomitant impairment of speech. Reception of auditory stimuli is necessary for the correct production of vocal sounds. The nurse should be aware that certain relationships among hearing, speaking, and seeing are important in assessing the functions of the ear.

The nurse should observe for indications of hearing loss. These include the patient's asking for repetition of verbal communication, misunderstanding of words or phrases as evidenced by inappropriate answers or failure to follow simple directions, and expression and body posture indicating intense concentration as evidenced by leaning forward or by a tense or strained facial expression. People with hearing loss confined to one ear often form habits of positioning the head so that their good ear is toward the speaker.

Some of the vestibular functions can be observed as the patient walks or moves. A tendency to veer in one direction when walking and other indications of lack of coordination are meaningful signs in assessing balance.

When obtaining a patient's nursing history, the nurse should inquire about the history of hearing impairment in relatives. Many types of hearing dysfunction are either known or thought to be familial, and this information may serve as a cue that more careful assessment of the individual's hearing through examination techniques is indicated.

The nurse should also ascertain whether the person has noticed changes in his hearing or equilibrium and obtain a description of the changes. Information about the nature of the changes, their onset, the conditions present when the person noticed the changes, and the current signs and symptoms all are important considerations. The duration of the signs and symptoms (if transient), or the length of time they have been present (if permanent), are meaningful data. Tinnitus, vertigo, or occurrences of motion sickness should be further examined, as these are classic symptoms of ear vestibular dysfunction.

Most people normally experience tinnitus at some time or another. Infrequent occurrences may be considered normal if the tinnitus is transient and if it is related to exposure to loud noise or change in air pressure, as may be experienced in air travel. On the other hand, tinnitus may be the presenting symptom of ear disease or of neurologic diseases.

Tinnitus is a subjective symptom and is defined as noise in the ear. Infrequently, tinnitus is auditory, that is, it can be heard by an observer. Each person has a unique perception of the noise he hears. Most often tinnitus is thought to be a ringing or tinkling noise, but may actually include a wide variety of sounds. People are generally more aware of tinnitus when they are alone or in a quiet environment. It is usual to be most bothered by tinnitus at night, when trying to fall asleep, or at times when there are few other distractions. Tinnitus is often worse when the person tries to relax and has time to think about his symptoms. Tinnitus can be distracting and unsettling, as the person tends to worry about the cause of the unusual noises and often has grave fears about his health.

Certain types of tinnitus are associated with specific causes. For example, a blowing noise synchronized with respirations is related to blocked eustachian tubes or to blockage of the external meatus by cerumen (earwax). Inflammation of the inner ear is often associated with pulsatile tinnitus, which occurs in rhythm with blood flow through the vessels. Ménière's syndrome (a condition that impairs hearing or equilibrium or both) and middle ear diseases frequently produce tinnitus of lower frequencies. Gradual loss of hearing function as a result of the aging process and vestibulocochlear (acoustic) nerve trauma tend to produce tinnitus of higher frequencies. Persistent and continuous tinnitus is associated with inner ear dysfunction or acoustic nerve or central nervous system diseases. Transient tinnitus may be caused by a variety of factors including exposure to noise, changes in pressure experienced when swimming, or changes in altitude. Aspirin causes tinnitus in certain susceptible people, particularly when taking repeated doses as in arthritis. The tinnitus disappears when the aspirin is discontinued. Other ototoxic drugs are quinine, quinidine, and streptomycin, all toxic to the acoustic nerve.

Another classic vestibular symptom associated with ear diseases is **vertigo,** defined as hallucination of movement. The person with true vertigo sees objects moving in the line of vision, often tending to go around him in circles. Some people describe this as a sensation of objects whirling around. When he closes his eyes, the person feels that he is moving. Sometimes the sensation of body movement in vertigo is localized to the head, but it may encompass the entire body. It is important to ask the patient about the duration of the attack of vertigo and the specific times and circumstances that vertigo is noticed. For example, is the vertigo related to any special place or event? Positional vertigo may be experienced only when the head is in certain positions.

Vertigo is a subjective symptom, and the nurse should carefully define the patient's perceptions of vertigo. He or she may describe the feeling of being off balance as vertigo when in reality it is an instance of transient dizziness caused by cardiovascular insufficiency. Usually, movement of the head exaggerates vertigo. When trying to walk during attacks of vertigo, the patient veers to one side and describes sensations of unsteadiness because "the room is moving." It is important that the nurse provide adequate support for patients with severe vertigo to prevent trauma or injury. Usually bedrest is necessary, and assistance in ambulation will be required. Vertigo is often accompanied by nausea and vomiting. Other vagal nervous system symptoms associated with vertigo are perspiration, pallor, and bradycardia.

Motion sickness is another disturbance of vestibular function of the osseous labyrinth. (The semicircular canals, the utricle and saccule comprising the vestibular apparatus are the end-organ receptors in equilibrium.) In motion sickness, varying degrees of vertigo and usually nausea, a swimming sensation in the head, or dizziness may be experienced.

In addition to obtaining the patient's history, the nurse also examines the ear. This examination includes observation of the structure of the external ear and of the external auditory meatus. The examination is done gently because of the delicacy of the ear structures. The pinna and the preauricular and postauricular areas of the ear are observed and palpated. Each person's ear has a unique size and shape. The pinna, also called the auricle, is a cartilage flap that collects sound waves. Systematic examination of the preauricular and postauricular areas (the areas in front of and behind the pinna) requires the patient to open and close his mouth so that the examiner, by placing the tip of the index finger on the preauricular area, can feel the mandible slide anteriorly. Palpation for tenderness, fluctuations, depressions, or swelling of the preauricular and postauricular areas is done gently (Fig. 13-1).

Tenderness and swelling may denote infection or inflammation of the middle or outer ear. Normally the tragus, the small appendage located on the anterior margin of the external auditory canal, can be moved without discomfort. A number of changes related to different disease processes may be observed in the soft tissue about the ear. Tophi (pale, hard, nontender nodules) are often present in patients with gout. Calcifications, which are collections of urate crystals, may be noted in patients with Addison's disease. Pigmentation is noted in ochronosis, a discoloration of the body tissues that results from exposure to noxious substances or is due to a metabolic disorder. Rashes or redness of the soft tissue may be caused by either localized reactions or generalized dermatitis. Sebaceous cysts appear as red and swollen areas, usually on the ear lobe. These cysts are generally not related to other diseases.

An otoscope with an aural speculum is used to examine the external auditory meatus. Pneumatic otoscopes are preferred by many specialists, and they have a device that can be used to test the patency of the eardrum. A Zeiss operating microscope is often used by physicians for ear examinations since its magnifying power enables visualization of minute changes in the external ear canal and eardrum. It not only has an excellent light source, but also provides for binocular sterescopic vision. The size of the auricle and any observable deformities should be noted before inserting a speculum into the ear. Different-sized speculums can be attached to the otoscope. The speculum selected should fit the diameter of the auricle comfortably without causing damage to the sensitive ear structure. Holding the pinna slightly back and upward somewhat straightens the double curves of the external meatus so that the eardrum can be observed. Sometimes it is necessary to first remove cerumen or drainage that may have accumulated in the external meatus in order to visualize the drum.

Cerumen is secreted by glands located in the tissue of the external auditory meatus. Cerumen is conveyed to the exterior of the ear

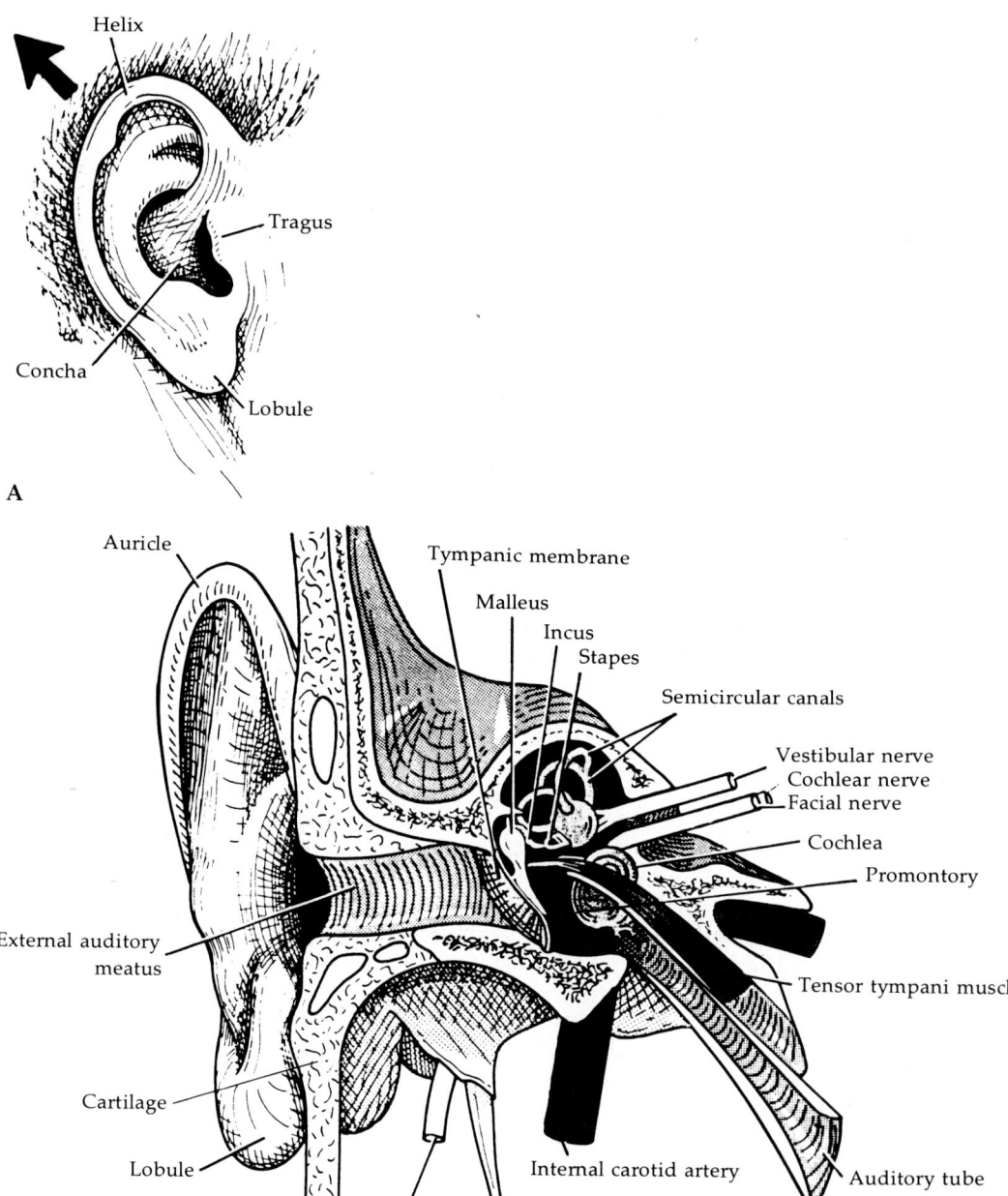

Figure 13-1
A. The external ear. Arrow indicates the direction the auricle should be pulled to straighten external auditory meatus prior to insertion of the otoscope. **B.** The external and middle portions of the right ear as viewed from the front. (From R. S. Snell, *Clinical Anatomy for Medical Students*. Boston: Little, Brown and Company, 1973. Reproduced by permission.)

by jaw movements and protects the ear by trapping dust and particulate matter and bacteria, thereby preventing contamination of the middle or inner ear. Cerumen has the protective functions of maintaining the humidity, temperature, and patency of the eardrum. The length (approximately 1 to 1½ inches) and shape of the outer meatus with its two curves also protect the middle and inner ears.

Excessive cerumen or drainage can be removed by irrigation with water or hydrogen peroxide warmed to body temperature. (Ear drops may be used prior to irrigating to soften cerumen.) Vertigo or nystagmus can result from caloric stimulation of the semicircular canals if the irrigating solution is either too hot or too cold. When irrigating the ear, insert the syringe just a short distance into the lumen and with gentle pressure direct it to the lateral surface of the ear. Irrigation is contraindicated if there is evidence of swelling or tenderness, as the sensitive ear tissues may be further irritated or damaged by irrigation. The eardrum, when inflamed, is vulnerable to rupture. Patency of the eardrum can be crudely tested by asking the patient if he feels changes in pressure when swallowing. If he cannot discern pressure changes, the drum may be ruptured.

If the drum is ruptured, cerumen is removed by means of a curet or a small ear loop. A thin, cotton-tipped applicator prepared for ear examination may be used; care must be taken to discard each applicator after use, to prevent contamination of the ear. However, it is sometimes difficult to avoid pushing wax further into the canal with the large cotton tip.

For purposes of description in assessment, the eardrum can be visually divided into four quadrants: anterosuperior, posterosuperior, anteroinferior, and posteroinferior. The drum, a thin oval membrane, is normally pink or gray and is semitransparent. Certain structures in the middle ear can normally be seen through the drum (the tympanic membrane). These structures are landmarks for evaluation of the drum and include the short process, the handle and umbo of the malleus, and the incudostapedal junction. Normally there is a core of light reflected on the eardrum that also serves as a landmark. The short process of the malleus appears as a knob. The umbo, which is a portion of the handle (or manubrium) of the malleus that is attached to the inner tympanic membrane, is normally visualized whereas the incudostapedal junction cannot always be seen. Schrapnell's membrane, also referred to as the attic area, is located in the upper part of the eardrum. This small triangular area is the weakest part of the drum. The lower part of the drum is the pars tensa (Fig. 13-2).

Fluid in the middle ear may be seen as tiny bubbles of air behind the tympanic membrane, absence of the core of light reflection, and reddening and dulling of the tympanic membrane. Reddening and dulling also occur when the eardrum is inflamed. In addition, the blood vessels become injected (congested) and more visible, particularly around the periphery, when inflammation is present. The landmarks also may be obscured. If the

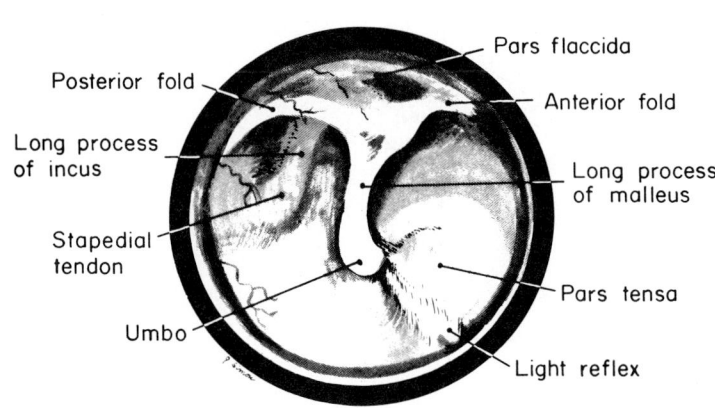

Figure 13-2
Landmarks of the tympanic membrane, right ear. (From J. Sana and R. Judge, *Physical Appraisal Methods in Nursing Practice*. Boston: Little, Brown and Company, 1975. Reproduced by permission.)

drum is ruptured, structures of the middle ear can be visualized. Healed perforations result in red and thickened membranes and scarring. The eardrum (tympanic membrane) separates the external ear from the middle ear and responds to changes in both passages. Normally the membrane is concave. Blockage in the eustachian tube causes the membrane to retract whereas inflammation with fluid collection in the middle ear causes the membrane to bulge. Mobility of the drum is tested by means of a pneumatic otoscope. Normally the drum is mobile. It is important to use as large a speculum as is comfortable for the patient to create a seal so that the pneumatic pressure is achieved when testing for mobility of the drum.

Except for the landmarks mentioned, the structures of the middle ear, which is located in the temporal bone, cannot be seen in ordinary circumstances. The auditory ossicles, the malleus, the incus, and the stapes, are held in place by the tensor tympani and the stapedium muscles, which contract with sounds of high frequency. As previously mentioned, the handle of the malleus is attached to the tympanic membrane. The head of the malleus is attached to the incus, the arm of the incus articulates with the stapes, and the base of the stapes is attached to the oval window membrane. The middle ear opens into the inner ear at the oval and round windows and into the eustachian tube, which is connected to the pharynx. Air pressure differences between the middle ear and the outer ear are equalized as the eustachian tube opens during swallowing. The ossicles are protected from intense vibrations by the tensor tympani muscle, which tightens the tympanic membrane and reduces the amplitude of vibrations by making the membrane less resilient. Changes in the vibratory patterns of the stapes also protect the ossicles from intense vibrations (Fig. 13-3).

The inner ear is protected by the petrous portion of the temporal bone and cannot be examined. This hard bone contains the labyrinth (the vestibule and semicircular canals), which is the end-organ receptors for maintaining equilibrium, and the cochlea, which is the end-organ receptor for hearing. Because the inner ear cannot be examined, a number of different tests are done to determine hearing and equilibrium dysfunction. In order to understand the methods used in these tests and the interpretation of results, a

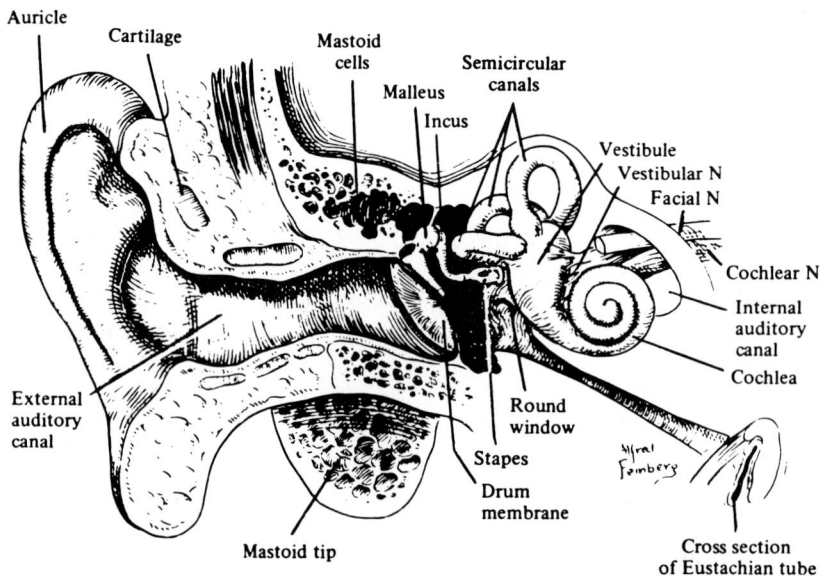

Figure 13-3
Anatomy of the human ear. (From H. Davis and S. R. Silverman, *Hearing and Deafness* [3rd ed.]. New York: Holt, Rinehart & Winston, 1970. Reproduced by permission.)

brief review of the physiology of these ear functions is presented prior to description of the specific tests.

EAR PHYSIOLOGY AND HEARING TESTS

Hearing is a complex function in which sound waves are transmitted from the tympanic membrane, which vibrates in direct relation to the frequency of the sound waves. Vibration of the tympanic membrane causes motion of the auditory ossicles. The stapes moves in the oval window to transmit vibrations to the inner ear fluid, and the round window bulges in response to sound waves. As the oval window vibrates, sound waves are passed to the perilymph contained in the bony labyrinth in the inner ear. The perilymph separates the membranous labyrinth from the bony labyrinth and is similar to cerebrospinal fluid. The aqueduct of the cochlea carries the perilymph into the subarachnoid spaces. The cochlea, the organ of hearing, is divided into the scala vestibuli, the cochlear duct, and the scala tympani. The scala tympani is the lower division and terminates at the round window; the scala vestibuli forms the upper division and terminates at the oval window. The cochlear duct (which contains the organ of Corti) divides the two and is filled with endolymph. Endolymph is similar to intracellular fluid. The areas for secretion of endolymph are the secreting epithelium and the area vascularis.

The basilar membrane separates the scala tympani from the cochlear duct; it is narrow and stiff at its base, and wider and softer at its apex. Sound waves transmitted through perilymph cause mechanical movement of the basilar membrane. Low frequency sounds cause waves of vibrations that extend to the apex whereas high frequency vibrations are limited to the base. The organ of Corti, the primary receptor for hearing, rests on the basilar membrane. Movement of the basilar membrane activates the cilia of the receptor hair cells in the organ of Corti and causes depolarization. This depolarization occurs as nerve impulses are generated at the top of the hair cells by vibrations. In this way the mechanical vibrations become electrical, initiating impulses in the nerve fibers located at the base of the hair cells. The intensity of sound is related to both the amplitude and the extent of the basilar membrane displacement. More intense sound activates more nerve fibers.

Fibers of the cochlear branch of the acoustic nerve (the eighth cranial nerve) terminate at the lower end of each hair cell. There are numerous neural pathways from the ear to the brain. The most direct sensory pathway from the ear begins with the spiral ganglion of the cochlea, passing to the cochlear nerve and synapsing with the cochlear nuclei in the brainstem. Synapses occur in several other locations before impulses reach the auditory cortex in the temporal lobe of the brain. Some of the impulses pass through more indirect and less defined routes by passing through the recticular formation and from there through more diffuse pathways, intercrossing with fibers from both ears so that sound in space can be localized. All the fibers terminate in the cortical hearing center in the superior temporal lobe. Because some of the impulses are transmitted on the same side and others cross to the opposite side, hearing loss does not occur if the temporal lobe on one side is impaired. Efferent impulses from the brain pass into the cochlea through the olivocochlear nerve bundle and synapse with hair cells and the afferent endings below the hair cells. The efferent impulses inhibit afferent activity. It is postulated that their function is for frequency discrimination.

Hearing tests are based on the principles of sound. Sound waves travel in air, liquids, and solids. The characteristics of sound are intensity, frequency, duration, and complexity. **Intensity** is defined as amplitude and is expressed in decibels (db). The intensity of a sound is referred to as loudness and is influenced by the frequency. Cycles per second (cps or Hertz [Hz]) describes the number of vibrations per second and is an expression of frequency. **Frequency** is defined as the rapidity of vibrations; **duration** is the length of endurance of the vibration; and **complexity** is the combination of sounds of varying frequencies. The pitch of a sound is determined by frequency, with sounds of higher frequency having higher pitch. A tuning fork produces a sound of single frequency and thus produces a pure tone. The tone varies with the frequency of the particular tuning fork used. The quality of a sound is produced by harmonic combinations of frequencies, and noise is complex in that many discordant frequencies are mixed.

Normally a person can discriminate among 1,000 or so different pitches of sound, a fantastic function that is not fully understood. Localization of sound is a function of discriminating between the sound intensity and the minute difference in the time that the sound reaches each ear. Hearing tests determine the acuity of hearing and are diagnostic of the type of hearing loss, differentiating between conduction hearing loss and sensorineural hearing loss. Conduction is a function of the middle ear; sensory reception is a function of the inner ear and neural pathways to the brain.

A simple hearing test that does not require complex equipment is the watch test. The watch test simply evaluates the estimated distance of the watch from one ear at the time the person first hears the ticking of the watch. By testing each ear separately, it is possible to estimate differences in hearing in each ear. During this test the opposite ear is covered, or sound is masked in the opposite ear when this test is being done.

The whispered voice test is similar. In this test one ear is plugged or sound is masked by locally applied noise such as vibrating a finger in the ear. The examiner stands 20 feet away from the person being examined. He then whispers and asks the person to repeat the words. Bisyllabic words such as airplane, fireplace, or baseball are used. The examiner covers his lips to prevent lip reading and is careful to mask his facial expression; people with hearing loss become astute at both lip reading and interpretation of facial expressions. This test can be done by using prerecorded words with controlled intensity, which provides for a more accurate measure of the person's hearing than does use of the examiner's voice, which is difficult to control with any exactitude. If the person cannot discern a soft whisper, he or she has a mild or moderate hearing loss. Inability to hear softly spoken words implies sensorineural hearing loss; inability to hear loudly spoken words indicates severe hearing loss.

A tuning fork is used for three hearing tests: the Weber, the Rinne, and the Schwabach. Usually a 512 cps tuning fork is preferred. The **Weber test** evaluates bone conduction. The tuning fork is activated and then is held by the stem to place the base of the fork against the person's forehead at the midline. Normally the person hears the sound equally well in both ears. Unilateral conduction deafness causes the sound to be lateralized (heard better) to the affected ear. In unilateral sensorineural hearing loss, the sound is heard in the better ear, and not in the affected ear.

The **Rinne test** compares air and bone conduction. The activated tuning fork is first held a short distance from the auricle to test air conduction for sound. The fork, still weakly vibrating, is then placed on the mastoid bone to test bone conduction of vibrations. If hearing is normal, the person can hear the tone of the tuning fork better by air than by bone conduction. However, if conduction deafness is present, the person will hear the tone of the fork better when it is placed on the mastoid bone. Persons with sensorineural hearing loss hear the sound better through air conduction than through bone conduction.

The **Schwabach test** compares the examiner's hearing through bone conduction with that of the person being examined. In this test the activated tuning fork is first placed on the mastoid bone of the person being examined and then on the examiner's mastoid bone. As with the Rinne test, the person with conduction loss will hear the sounds better through bone conduction than can the examiner. If sensorineural hearing loss is present, the person will not hear the tone as well through bone conduction as the examiner can.

Audiometry is indicated when these hearing tests show abnormal results as well as for routine hearing tests. Audiometry provides for more accurate testing of hearing. This method allows for evaluation of the ability to hear pure tones of known frequency in each ear individually. Pure tones of 250, 500, 1,000, 2,000, 4,000, and 8,000 Hz are transmitted to one ear at a time. The patient being examined indicates the level at which he or she can first barely hear the tones well. This level is recorded on an audiogram. The tones are first presented through air conduction and then by bone conduction. For the latter, a small bone conduction hearing receiver is placed over the mastoid process and pure tones are repeated in the same frequencies used to test air conduction.

Evaluation of the audiogram is based on comparison of the level of intensity with the baseline level of 0 db. This baseline has been determined as the lowest intensity at which a control population with healthy ears can hear the sounds [6]. The number of decibels of intensity above the baseline 0 db level indicates the hearing ability. For example, normally one hears within a range of 10 to 20 db; the person requiring intensity of 25 db above the norm is considered to have mild hearing loss. The person requiring 30 to 50 db of intensity for hearing usually has a mild or moderate hearing loss and has difficulty understanding normal conversation. Hearing thresholds vary and they differ at separate testing times in the same individual.

Speech discrimination is also tested as part of the audiometric examination. This testing is done by asking the patient to indicate when he hears monosyllabic words. Phonetically balanced words are presented with increasing intensity until they are heard. The responses are recorded as speech reception threshold (SRT). Hearing loss ranges from mild loss at 30 to 50 db to severe loss at 80 to 90 db. Audiometry tests are conducted in noise-controlled environments and earphones are used to minimize noise distraction as well as to control intensity measures.

The **vestibular receptors** in the ear are also located in the inner ear. The posterior portion of the cochlea opens to the vestibular apparatus in the inner ear. The three semicircular canals, arranged at right angles with each in a different plane, detect motion in three dimensions in space. Messages from the anterior, posterior, and horizontal semicircular canals are transmitted to a receptor organ, the *crista ampullaris*. The hair cells of the crista are stimulated by changes in velocity, and the otoliths transmit neural impulses to maintain the relationship of the body to gravity. The otoliths, utricle, and saccule in the crista ampullaris function for balance and position and are separated from one another and from surrounding structures by perilymph. The utricle and the saccule each have a receptor organ called the macula that has supporting cells and hair cells. The utricle's macula is horizontal to the head and the saccule's macula is vertical to the head when a person is standing. The cristae and maculae are innervated by the vestibular branch of the 8th cranial nerve. Sensory pathways for vestibular impulses from the cell bodies in the vestibular ganglion synapse in the brainstem at the vestibular nuclei. The impulses travel through the spinal cord to the reticular formation and to the motor nuclei of the extrinsic eye muscles, the cerebellum, and the cerebral cortex for the coordination of skeletal muscle movement. The vestibular portion of the labyrinth initiates vestibulo-ocular reflexes that influence eye movement to keep retinal images fixed and that contribute to orientation in space. Abnormal stimulation results in vertigo and motion sickness or both. Either acceleration or deceleration normally stimulates the semicircular canal on the side of the body to which the movement was made.

Nystagmus can be associated with vertigo in dysfunction of equilibrium. The nystagmus is rhythmic ocular movement from side to side or up and down that occurs normally only when the person's head is rapidly turned or moved in any direction. Vestibular impulses in the semicircular canal stimulate the reflex movement of the eyes in nystagmus. The reflex movement is the slow component of eye movement in the direction of the turn and there is a compensatory rapid movement or component in the opposite direction. Nystagmus is the rapid component of the eye movement. In vestibular disease nystagmus can be vertical, horizontal, or rotating [2]. When testing vestibular function, nystagmus can be induced by the Bárány test, in which the person is rapidly rotated. The person is turned ten times clockwise in a specified amount of time. In normal function the slow component or reflex eye movement is in the direction of the turn and this slow movement orients the person in space. There is then a rapid movement of the eyes in the opposite direction that helps fix the eyes in the new direction. The patient is then turned rapidly in the opposite direction to test the opposite labyrinth. It should be noted that head movements also cause movements of the otoliths, which transmit neural impulses to maintain the relationship of the body to gravity (Fig. 13-4).

The **caloric test** differentiates between labyrinths in the right and left ears. In this test, 1 ml of ice water is instilled into the external auditory meatus of one ear and is retained for 1 minute before allowing it to drain. The patient's head is tipped slightly backward and the eyes are examined for nystagmus. Normally there is biphasic nystagmus with the fast component to the opposite ear, lasting for approximately 1½ minutes. Graphic measurement of eye movements is accomplished by placement of leads around

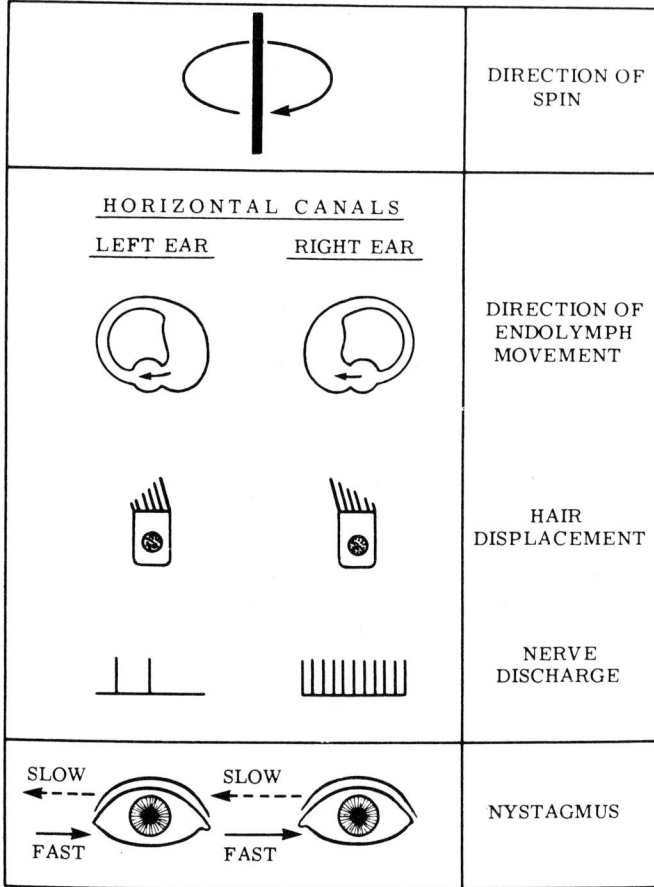

Figure 13-4
Effects of spinning a subject clockwise to the right. On acceleration, the endolymph in the horizontal canals will lag with respect to the movement of the canal wall. The hairs in the cristae will be displaced to the left. In the left canal, hair displacement is away from the kinocilium, leading to a decrease in nerve discharge below the resting level. On the right, hair displacement is toward the kinocilium, leading to an increase in nerve discharge above the resting level. A vestibular nystagmus to the right (slow component to the left) results. (From E. Selkurt, *Basic Physiology for the Health Sciences*. Boston: Little, Brown and Company, 1974. Reproduced by permission.)

the eyes; this test is called electronystagmography. Use of ice water in the caloric test is contraindicated if there are defects in the tympanic membrane or in the presence of external otitis or mastoid disease. Air may be used instead.

Following these tests, the patient is asked to stretch his arms outward and to close his eyes. The examiner places his index fingers under the patient's index fingers to establish a point of reference. The patient is then asked to raise his arms over his head and to lower his fingers in an attempt to again touch index fingers with the examiner's. Normally the patient can touch the examiner's fingers; a person with abnormal labyrinth function deviates to the right or left. This test is the **pass-touch test**.

X-ray examination of the mastoid bone and the temporal bone reveals abnormalities caused by factors that destroy normal bone tissue. The posterior wall of the middle ear space in the temporal bone opens to the tympanic antrum, which leads to the mastoid air cells; these air cells form during the growth process. The mastoid air cell space can be visualized on x-ray and cloudiness in the space is indicative of a disease process.

Neurologic examinations are used to determine involvement of the seventh and eighth cranial nerves in advanced ear diseases. The seventh cranial nerve branch innervates the tongue, passing between the malleus and incus near the lateral wall of the middle ear space, and the eighth cranial nerve is located near its medial wall. In addition to the proximity of these nerves to the middle ear, the jugular vein is located near the floor of the middle ear space and the carotid artery is located near the posterior wall. Both can be involved in middle ear diseases, especially those that cause erosion of surrounding structures.

Ear dysfunction can range from a temporary problem such as a foreign object in the ear to permanent and serious problems that result in deafness. Because a number of disorders or diseases of the ear are treated on an outpatient basis, the nurse's function often focuses on assessment and teaching about ear care. Dysfunction of the ear disrupts normal hearing and, sometimes, equilibrium. It is possible to have disruption of hearing without loss of equilibrium, and vice versa. In addition to taking care of those with active diseases of the ear, the nurse also meets many people who have hearing loss as an outcome of disease processes, as well as people who are congenitally deaf. Therefore the nurse should be able to detect and differentiate among the types of hearing loss and determine care accordingly.

NURSING CARE IN HEARING LOSS

Hearing loss is described in different ways. Types of hearing loss include congenital deafness and adventitious deafness. **Congenital deafness** means that the person has been born without the function of hearing. **Adventitious deafness** is hearing loss acquired through disease processes or trauma. **Hard of hearing** describes the person who has the ability to hear sufficiently well to communicate either with or without the use of a hearing aid. Another way to describe hearing loss is by using a system of grades. In this system grade I is the inability to hear long-distance speech. Grade II is the inability to hear in close conversation, and grade III is the inability to hear loud conversation. Hearing loss or deafness may be either unilateral or bilateral. The onset of hearing loss may be acute, or it may develop gradually over a long period.

Classifications of deafness according to the physiologic dysfunction include conduction deafness, sensorineural deafness, mixed deafness, central deafness, and functional deafness. Normally, sound waves are transmitted through the external auditory meatus to the eardrum. Vibrations that reach the eardrum are sequentially transmitted by the ossicles in the middle ear to the organ of hearing, the cochlea, located in the inner ear. Vibrations in the inner ear are converted to neural impulses, which are transmitted via neural pathways to the brain. Conduction deafness is caused by a disorder or disease in the middle ear that prevents the normal conduction of sound vibrations by the ossicles, the small bones that include the malleus, incus, and stapes. When a disorder affects the organ of hearing in the inner ear, or the eighth cranial nerve, the patient has loss of nerve function and is said to have sensorineural hearing loss. In many cases, the middle ear structures function normally. Mixed or combined deafness indicates a combination of both conductive and sensorineural hearing loss. Central hearing loss refers to a pathological condition at any level along the nervous pathways that transmit auditory impulses to the brain, including in the brain itself. Functional hearing loss is caused by psychological factors. Often this type of loss is difficult to identify, and treatment is primarily based on psychological evaluation and counseling.

Persons with ear diseases may experience transient hearing loss. For example, when the middle ear is inflamed and serous fluid collects, the fluid dulls sound and impairs the ability of the middle ear structures to convey vibrations. As the disease process regresses, hearing may return to normal. In some instances the cure may not be complete, and chronic ear disease may develop. The result may be loss of hearing in varying degrees, depending on the extent of the residual dysfunction.

The person who cannot hear lives in isolation from sound. One who is congenitally deaf or who has a permanent acquired hearing loss may adapt to this isolation by learning to respond to sensory stimuli in a different way. The success of adaptation to this permanent disability is individual and is relative to capabilities and goals. Persons with transient deafness and the newly deaf may have great difficulty adjusting to the loss of hearing. The inability to hear evokes anxiety and concern in one who is accustomed to hearing. The isolation from sound may cause a reciprocal tendency to isolate oneself from people. The permanently deaf person must learn new adaptations for developing communication skills, and must eventually establish a new pattern of communication. He has to adapt not only to his own feelings and attitudes, but also to the reactions of others to his deafness. The person with transient deafness or deafness of a sudden onset initially has no techniques or tools to use in communicating. As a result, the nurse must be empathetic to the impact of that initial loss of hearing and must be supportive of the patient's adjustment to either the temporary or permanent hearing loss.

Speech is affected by hearing loss and the person who has never heard sound has needs for learning speech that are different from the needs of the person who learned to speak before acquiring the permanent hearing loss. People with congenital deafness cannot speak and must be taught how to articulate words without the input of audible sensory stimuli. This learning requires the special skills of speech and hearing therapists. In contrast, people with acquired deafness have learned to articulate words but have lost auditory stimuli that are necessary to continually reinforce the ability to speak and that prevent lapse of correct sound production abilities. They cannot monitor their speech and this loss interferes with learning to pronounce new words. Without the sense of hearing, the person cannot tell if these words are being pronounced correctly. People with acquired deafness may feel very strange when talking when they cannot hear what they are saying. People who cannot hear themselves are not sure that others can hear them, have no gauge to use in controlling the volume of the speech, and sometimes tend to compensate by speaking too loudly.

The nurse must be aware of the varying needs of the hard of hearing or deaf person. It is also important that the nurse be aware of the stage of adjustment to hearing loss a person has reached. Care will be different for the person who has been deaf for some time, as compared to that required by the newly deaf person. Care for a person who knows that the hearing loss is to be permanent is different from that required in transient deafness. The nurse must be able to provide for the person's communication needs, from becoming familiar with the deaf person's established pattern for communicating to helping the newly or temporarily deaf person find appropriate resources for learning to communicate. The nurse can facilitate development of an effective individualized communication pattern for the patient's use in everyday living.

When deafness is transient, a temporary alternative means of communication must be established. If the recovery of hearing is uncertain, the nurse must recognize the patient's response to the possible loss and should encourage open expression of his or her uncertainty and fears so that appropriate information and support can be given.

The newly deaf can adjust to hearing loss by learning new or maximizing existing communication skills. A deaf person needs feedback to become aware of mispronounciations so that errors can be corrected. In addition, he needs to learn how to adjust the volume of his voice appropriately.

Lipreading is valuable for deaf persons with good vision. Many people with hearing loss become skilled in combining a number of stimuli in order to interpret communication. The use of sign language is controversial. Some authorities consider it a useful tool for communication whereas others feel that learning sign language may prevent the deaf or hard of hearing from learning oral communication and lipreading. Some deaf persons may become so adept at these skills, that an observer is unaware that they are deaf. Others may have difficulty in adapting to sign language because of visual disabilities that prevent maximum use of visual stimuli in communicating. Each person has individual needs and must learn to communicate according to his or her capabilities. Some deaf people learn both signing and oral communication.

Nonverbal communication figures predominantly in the ability of the deaf or the hard of hearing to interpret the nuances of communication. Observation of the speaker's facial features and body movements and observations of the activity in the milieu provide input for discerning what is being said and what is happening in the environment. With practice in improving perception of the visible aspects of speech through lip reading and interpreting nonverbal communication behaviors, it is possible for the deaf or the hard of hearing person to actively participate in conversations. For those persons who live alone, it is difficult to receive continuous feedback, which is important in correcting errors and preventing deterioration of speech. A cooperative and understanding friend or social group is helpful for these persons.

People with some hearing acuity must make good use of the auditory stimuli they do receive by improving their listening skills to become increasingly aware of sounds and to discriminate between what they hear and what persons with normal auditory function hear. One of the problems experienced by the deaf or the hard of hearing is that their disability is not easily recognized. Blind people can carry a cane marked for recognition, but deaf people find that people relate to them as though they can hear. Until others learn of the disability, both the deaf person and the one trying to communicate with him or her can become discouraged or frustrated in attempts at communication. The nurse should recognize that being deaf or having hearing loss presents unique stresses for persons with these disabilities.

There is a natural tendency to speak loudly to a person who cannot hear well. This loudness sometimes accentuates the noise that the person with impaired hearing perceives. This phenomenon is called recruitment, and is most common in persons with presbycusis (senile nerve hearing loss associated with aging). Several techniques can be used to improve communication with the person who has severe or complete hearing loss. First, it is important not to startle the person. Rather than touching the person to announce one's presence, it is usually better to place oneself in the line of vision. If the person has both vision and hearing disabilities, touch is effective in gaining the person's attention. Second, it is helpful to the person with impaired hearing if the speaker faces him and speaks directly to him. The speaker should articulate normally; spreading out words or exaggerating the enunciation of words interferes with lipreading. Speakers who cover their mouths or obscure speech movements by eating or drinking make lipreading difficult. Third, proximity enables the person to both lipread and hear the sounds better. Using a normal tone of voice is usually more effective than speaking loudly and it minimizes distortion of the sound. If a person has better hearing in one ear than in the other, the speaker should place himself in proximity to the good ear.

When verbal communication is not effective, the use of written words or phrases may be necessary. The writing should be large enough for the person to see. During initial or transient deafness, when the person has not learned to lipread or to respond to expressions, the use of a magic slate for writing messages is helpful. Other techniques include message cards on which commonly used directions are written or signals devised with the person's cooperation. The nurse should remember that vision determines the nature of the signals, touch being necessary for the blind person.

Hearing aids are available in different sizes and different formats. Often people are sensitive about wearing hearing aids and have difficulty accepting them. Present day hearing aids are small, however, and can be worn unobtrusively. They function either by air or bone conduction and are useful in conduction hearing loss. Hearing aids that function by air conduction amplify sound through transmission of air waves to the eardrum and through the middle ear to the hearing organ of the inner ear. Aids that function by bone conduction transmit the amplified vibrations through bone directly to the hearing organ in the inner ear.

Hearing aids are often rejected because they merely amplify all sound. The wearer may be disturbed by the loudness of amplified background noise. This noise may cause confusion and may disrupt the sounds the person wishes to hear, such as conversation. As a result, the hearing aid may not improve hearing of the sounds the person would prefer to select for hearing. Instead, he has to learn to use the hearing aid at times and in places when and where it is functional for improving hearing.

Hearing aids are more useful with middle ear hearing loss than with inner ear dysfunction. Conduction of vibrations to the inner ear either through air or bone does not improve the function of the inner ear if the hearing loss is caused by inner ear dysfunction. Hearing aids are often sold in noise-controlled rooms, and ear phones are sometimes used. The person who is buying the hearing aid does not initially realize that, while the hearing aid is useful in these quiet conditions, it may be distracting in noisy environments because all noise is amplified. The person who is considering buying a hearing aid should consult an otologist or an audiologist for advice prior to purchase. Hearing aids are expensive and often remain unused because the person finds he has purchased a device that is not helpful in improving his hearing.

There is no treatment for complete sensorineural hearing loss. In this type of loss, there is difficulty understanding what is said and sounds cannot be discriminated. Amplification of the sound does not improve understanding. Many people with a mild or moderate sensorineural hearing loss can hear better if only one person speaks at a time. In conditions of stress, the person tends to hear less well than when he is comfortable and relaxed. Hearing loss and inability to interpret what is being said may cause anxiety and confusion and contribute to the inability to understand what is being said. Persons with sensorineural hearing loss usually do not have an even pattern of loss for specific ranges of sound frequencies as do those with conduction loss. Modulation of voice sounds to frequencies at which the person hears best aids his hearing.

An electronic cochlea has been developed and is now being tested. This device increases sound awareness for persons with inner ear dysfunction and consequent sensorineural hearing loss. Implanted electrodes provide an electrical source for conduction of neural transmission. The experimental electronic cochleas now being tested produce sound wave signals in the 30 to 120 cps range. If successful, this electronic cochlea will be a major breakthrough for the person with inner ear dysfunction who has intact neural pathways for transmission of neural impulses to the higher centers of the brain.

Central deafness is often untreatable, particularly if the cause is a degenerative neurologic disease or a result of trauma that caused irreversible neural damage. Functional or psychological deafness is also difficult to treat. People with this type of deafness are examined very carefully to rule out the possibility of middle or inner ear dysfunction. Because the basic problem is psychogenic, hearing aids or other devices do not help. As with other psychogenic illnesses, treatment is aimed at counseling to help the person recognize and deal with the source of the dysfunction.

The Nurse's Teaching Role

Diseases that affect the ear directly, or systemic diseases that interrupt the function of the ear or the neural pathways for the transmission of auditory stimuli to the brain, have the potential for causing some degree of hearing loss. The nurse can often be instrumental in helping to prevent this hearing loss by assessing the function of the ear and then by taking measures to help the patient receive appropriate treatment as necessary. The nurse also has many opportunities to discuss proper ear care in the course of daily contacts with people. Because the ear is such a sensitive structure it is necessary that the nurse teach the importance of seeking professional examination and treatment. People should be discouraged from trying to treat themselves when they experience ear dysfunction. Screening of hearing acuity is now a routine part of most school health programs. Adults should follow through with this routine periodic screening as well as with routine ear care.

Many persons tend to "overclean" their ears, using cotton-tipped applicators following a bath or shower. Only small, thin applicators should be used in the ear. The usual size applicator is too large for the ear and often causes cerumen to be pushed further into the ear, rather than cleaning the ear. Ear care should be limited to cleaning with a washcloth and drying with a towel, with the cloth positioned over the little finger. Nothing should be inserted into the ear beyond the point the little finger reaches. The normal protective and cleaning function of cerumen is adequate for cleaning the external meatus. If, however, a person has an abnormal accumulation of cerumen, he should have his ears irrigated by either a nurse or a physician.

Another area in which nurses can teach about ear care is in methods for piercing ears. It is important that sterile technique be used when ears are pierced. A few states are now requiring that ears be pierced by a physician. One should first ascertain the safety of the type of technique used before having the piercing done by friends or in commercial establishments that offer the service of ear-piercing. Diseases such as viral hepatitis may result, as can ear infections. Ordinarily there is no long-term discomfort or trauma when the lobule of the ear is pierced. Some persons may develop keloid formations at the site of the piercing, but this is unusual.

Proper insertion of ear drops is another technique that should be explained. Ear drops are inserted as follows: The person is positioned with the head tilted to one side, with the affected ear upward. The pinna (or auricle) is drawn back and upward to straighten the ear canal, and the medication is dropped into the external meatus without touching the dropper to the ear. Mild pressure is then placed on the tragus to force the fluid inward. A cotton wisp is placed in the canal to keep the drops in place.

Ointments are applied with a cotton tip inserted deeply into the canal with a twirling motion so that the ointment reaches as deeply as possible along the surface of the meatus. The responsiveness to stimuli initiating the perception of itching is greater in the external ear canals, the nostrils, and the perineal area than in other areas of the body. Therefore, itching of the external auditory canal is a common symptom, particularly in chronic otitis. For this reason, another person should insert ear medication to avoid the natural tendency to scratch the epithelium with the cotton tip when the medication is inserted by the individual who is experiencing the itching.

There are several different types of ear medications and many proprietary medications. It is best for the person to have a medical ear examination, so that the appropriate medication can be prescribed for acute external otitis. Keeping the canal clean and dry to provide for contact of appropriately prescribed topical ear medications can often prevent chronic external otitis. If one does not know the appropriate medication, it is very easy to further damage affected ears by choosing the wrong form of treatment.

Because a number of the disorders or diseases of the ear are treated on an outpatient basis, the nurse's function often focuses on assessment and teaching about positive ear health practices and treatment for temporary conditions. Some types of diseases or dysfunction require hospitalization for treatment, and the nurse must then provide for care during the acute phase of the illness. In the following discussion, a number of different types of ear dysfunction and diseases are described in relation to assessment factors and the usual treatment.

Earache is one of the most common types of ear dysfunction and may be secondary to other diseases or the primary disorder. An earache is pain in and around the ear and is most often caused by inflammation of the external or middle ear or from dysfunction in the mouth or bones surrounding the ear structures. Excessive quantities of cerumen or the presence of foreign bodies in the ear may be a source of earache. Costen's syndrome, a disturbance of the temporomandibular joint caused by unequal bilateral bite of the dentures, infections of the teeth (particularly the posterior teeth), and diseases of the parotid and salivary glands as well as ulcerations of the pharynx are among the sources of earache related to dysfunction in the mouth or bones. Therefore when a person has an earache, it is important to examine the tongue, the nasopharynx, and the pharynx to determine whether there is any abnormality in these areas. The ear itself should be examined. The color, amount, character, and odor of drainage should be noted. Chronic earache is usually associated with foul-smelling discharge whereas an acute inflammation or infection of the outer ear is usually associated with a more watery discharge that smells like ear accumulations.

Cerumen (wax) accumulation is another common problem; accumulation in the ear in sufficient amounts can cause deafness by occluding the external meatus so that vibrations do not reach the drum. Hardened cerumen may stimulate inflammation of the epithelium of the meatus. Cerumen can be softened by placing olive oil, glycerin, or hydrogen peroxide in the ear 2 or 3 days prior to removal by syringing. Care must be taken to avoid irritating or damaging the meatal epithelium, which normally bleeds easily. External otitis media may develop following irrigation. Foreign bodies may be removed by syringing or by means of a curet or forceps. It is amazing that so many different kinds of foreign bodies can find their way into the ear; these may range from a piece of grain to an eraser or an insect. If an insect is lodged in the ear it should be drawn out if possible by placing a light near the auricle. If this light does not lure the insect from the ear, it should be smothered by placing a drop of mineral oil or olive oil in the ear [3] prior to removal by irrigation with a syringe. Because of the danger of irritation or trauma to the external meatus and drum, objects that fit the meatus but cannot be removed easily by syringing should be removed by the physician, who uses instrumentation, often with anesthesia.

Keratosis obturans is another cause of a mass in the ear that is differentiated from accumulation of cerumen. Normally the superficial layer of cells is constantly migrating from the surface of the tympanic membrane to the exterior through the external meatus. The skin that lines the cartilaginous aspects of the external meatus contains sebaceous and apocrine glands. The migration of the cerumen formed by these glands to the exterior of the ear facilitates removal of dead superficial cells. When this migration of the superficial epithelial cells does not occur, the desquamated epithelium accumulates in the meatus near the drum, causing pain or even deafness. A white debris may be noted on inspection of the meatus. It becomes necessary to remove keratosis obturans surgically, usually with general anesthesia.

EAR DYSFUNCTION

Trauma

Trauma to the ear may result in perforation of the tympanic membrane or dislocation or damage of the ossicles in the middle ear. A blow to the ear, loud noises such as explosions or gun blasts, piercing with a sharp object, or fractures of the facial bones may cause perforation of the tympanic membrane. These perforations usually heal spontaneously in approximately six weeks. Systemic antibiotics may be given prophylactically and the patient's condition is monitored to determine whether there is any hearing loss. Loss is not always evident at the time of injury. Hearing loss will result if the ossicles have been disrupted.

Blows to the mandible can be transmitted to the external auditory canal. If fragments of bone in the canal are not surgically removed, stenosis of the canal may result during the healing process. If the fracture involves the temporal bone, particularly the petrous portion, the inner ear can be traumatized and sensorineural hearing loss may result. There can also be facial nerve paralysis, particularly if the fracture is transverse. Bleeding is usually a symptom in this instance. The drum has a characteristic bluish black color, indicating hemorrhage behind the drum. There may also be leakage of cerebrospinal fluid (otorrhea) if there is a passage from the subarachnoid space as a result of the fracture. Whiplash injuries or fractures of the base of the skull can cause trauma to the ear. Cochlear function may then be impaired, resulting in hearing loss in the high frequencies.

Exposure to a loud blast may be followed by ringing in the ear and by deafness. In some persons this deafness may be permanent. The fact that noise levels, not just a sudden explosive blast, can be traumatic is recognized in the Federal Noise Abatement Program, which declares noise a pollutant. People have individual tolerances for noise, but the level for average human tolerance has been set at 140 db. For comparison, a low whisper produces 10 db and normal conversational speech ranges from 40 to 60 db (or 250 to 4,000 cps [or Hz]). Cycles per second are interchangeable with Hz, with 1 cps being equal to 1 Hz. Many everyday objects produce excessive noise. An alarm clock produces approximately 80 db, and a siren can be as much as 150 db.

Noise can affect a person's psychological and physical well-being. Communication is disrupted by increasing noise, particularly in industries in which people must shout or write notes to communicate. The quality of work is diminished in the presence of noise. Sleep is affected by noise. It has been postulated that noise more than 30 db affects sleep. Some studies have shown that noise as low as 50 db interrupts REM sleep. Physiologic responses to noise include vasoconstriction of the peripheral blood vessels, slow and deep breathing, skeletal muscle tension, and galvanic skin responses. It is also thought that there are endocrine and metabolic effects. Persons exposed to loud noises of long duration have an increase in urinary output, an increase in urinary catecholamines, and increased blood pressure. The startle effect of noise has long been known; there is a temporary physiologic and psychological loss of contact with environmental stimuli when one is startled. The startle effect is sometimes used in an effort to help a person stop continuous hiccoughing.

While noise pollution affects people differently, it is thought that there is no specific pathologic entity related to noise. Rather, susceptible individuals who cannot tolerate a noise annoyance level, often above 90 db, develop symptoms related to their individual propensities for behavior or disease. These people develop cochlear damage with a sensorineural hearing loss in many instances. Both the intensity and the duration of noise are factors in the development of this type of hearing loss, which begins with a perceptive hearing loss followed by loss in the high frequency ranges. People who live in urban environments, those who listen to loud music (the rock and roll syndrome), and those who work in a noisy industry are most frequently affected. Persons in the latter group are said to have occupational deafness. Hearing tests and ear examinations should be routinely performed for people about to begin employment in noise-polluted industries, to establish a baseline for further testing of susceptible individuals.

In the current law the standard is that anyone exposed to greater than 90 db during an 8-hour shift must wear personal protective equipment. The types of personal protective equipment most common are ear masks and ear plugs. If a company is not in compliance with the standard of the law, that company must institute engineering control for noise reduction and a program that may include wearing of personal protective equipment, reducing the time of exposure to noise, or rotating personnel in the high noise areas. This law has been tested in at least one case in which the employee was fired for not complying with the standard of wearing personal protective equipment. The employer's right to fire this employee was upheld in court [4]. It should be noted that ear masks or muffs are generally more effective than ear plugs for reducing the impact of the noise.

Trauma to the ear is experienced in different ways. A blow to the pinna can cause hematomas. A cauliflower ear results when the hematoma organizes and calcifies. To prevent cauliflower ear, the clot should be incised and aspirated. A packing or splint is applied to keep the cartilage in proximity to its blood supply and to promote healing so that the ear will remain normal-appearing.

Trauma to the pinna can result from sharp objects, bullets, or burns. Reconstructive surgery with pedicle grafts from the mastoid area is done to repair holes or to replace missing portions of the ear when sufficient cartilage remains to provide for the framework of the pinna. Cartilage from the costal area on the same side as the defect is commonly used to prepare grafts for replacing cartilage. If, as in the case of burns, the area surrounding the ear is also damaged, skin is used from other body areas and an effort is made to match the texture and color of the skin. In burns, scars and contractures are removed and the area is grafted. Cervical tube grafts are often used to reconstruct the ear and the postauricular areas.

Depending on the extent of the defect, surgery involves staged procedures for preparation of the pedicle flap or flaps, for replacement of cartilage between layers of skin grafts, and for gradual separation of the pedicle or tube graft as closure is achieved. To repair a small hole in the ear, for example, a single pedicle from the mastoid area may be sufficient. To be prepared for the graft, the ear is held back and the hole is traced on the mastoid area, leaving about one-third more skin in the pedicle than necessary to just close the hole. Skin is then sutured to the peripheral end of the pedicle and the pedicle is replaced. About two weeks later, the pedicle is mobilized at the peripheral end and is sutured into the hole, so that skin appears on the anterior and posterior sides of the pinna. The pedicle is left attached for about two more weeks, at which time it is severed and replaced to its original site. A separate graft may be needed to cover the mastoid area from which the graft used to cover the hole of the pinna was taken; the pedicle is then severed and replaced to its original site.

Congenital Deformities

Some people have congenital absence or deformities of the pinna. Surgical repair, reconstructive surgery, or both can be done to improve appearance and hearing. Reconstructive surgery to reconstruct ears demands patience and exacting and skillful surgery.

The external auditory canal is usually absent in congenital absence of the ear, but hearing by bone conduction is possible because the inner ear is usually intact. In addition to the ear deformity, the person often has other deformities of the facial structure, indicating the need for more extensive reconstructive surgery. Because surgical reconstruction is a painstaking procedure, the external auditory canal may not be reconstructed if hearing by bone conduction is good.

To repair the pinna of the ear, cartilage grafts from the costal cartilages are used along with grafts from the mastoid area. Reconstruction involves a gradual building up of the auricle in sequential procedures. The entire reconstruction may take several months to a year, depending on the amount of rudimentary ear present. The reader is referred to a text about reconstructive surgery for detail. A prosthetic graft may be used to provide the framework for the ear, giving a more normal contour and shape for overlying grafted skin.

Protrusion of the ear is another deformity that can be corrected surgically. This operation to construct a more normal-appearing pinna is done by folding the cartilages back on each other to form the anthelix ridge of the normal auricle; The anthelix is often missing in protrusion. Excessive cartilage is usually excised. Sterile dressings with a head bandage to hold the ear firmly in place are not disturbed for about a week or ten days. This bandage is then replaced by smaller dressings that are left in place for about another week. Following removal of the dressings, the patient wears a tight-fitting skull cap at night to hold the ears close to the head. This cap is worn for about 3 weeks.

Some people have overly large pinnas, and surgical repair is accomplished by preserving the normal landmarks and profiles of the ear while excising the extra cartilage. Prior to surgery, lines are drawn on the back of the pinna to provide a guide for the excision. Following surgery, which can be done under local anesthesia, the ear is taped back for about a week. Although this surgery is best done in children around the age of 5, adults may benefit from the surgery if they are very conscious of their large ears and wish to have them reduced in size.

Abnormal Cell Growth in the Ear

Several types of tumors may occur in the external ear. These include osteomas, benign tumors usually found in the external meatus and thought to be related to continued irritation from swimming. Surgical removal of these bony tumors is indicated only if the ear becomes occluded by a combination of the tumor and cerumen accumulation. Adenomas generally arise from the ceruminous glands and squamous or basal cell carcinoma may occur in the epidermis. Crusting lesions in the ear may be associated with deep boring pain, weeping, or drainage from the ear. Hearing loss and peripheral facial paralysis are late symptoms of tumor development. Excision of basal cell carcinoma is usually curative if the lesion is diagnosed early. Squamous cell carcinoma may be treated with preoperative radiation followed by surgical excision; the prognosis is usually not as good as with basal cell carcinoma as there is a propensity for spread to the lymph nodes and extension to adjacent tissues.

Squamous cell carcinoma may follow chronic otorrhea or chronic otitis media. The symptoms are pain and bleeding. The glomus tumor may occur at the dome of the jugular bulb in the middle ear and is referred to as glomus jugulare. If the tympanic branch of the glossopharyngeal nerve is affected, the tumor is a glomus tympanicus. The auricular branch of the vagus may be affected. Symptoms include tinnitus of the pulsating type, deafness, and bleeding from the ear. The tumors are highly vascular and slow growing, and symptoms arise after the tumor becomes large enough to impinge on vital structures. If the tumor involves the cranial nerves, symptoms may include diplopia, dysphagia, dysphonia, and unilateral atrophy of the tongue. X-ray may show mastoid bone erosion. If diagnosed early, the tumors can be excised locally. A mastoidectomy is done if the bone is involved. Radiotherapy is used in the treatment of large lesions unless the cartilage is involved; radiotherapy is then contraindicated and surgery is the treatment of choice. If the lesion is limited to the external ear, the facial nerve can be spared in the surgery. Radical resection of the temporal bone is required in advanced disease if the middle ear is involved; resection is a neurosurgical procedure.

Another type of tumor is a ceruminoma. This tumor usually occurs in the outer third of the external auditory canal and is excised because of its malignant-like invasive growth pattern.

Cholesteatoma, an abnormal squamous epithelial growth, may form in the middle ear extending from the external meatus. Normally epithelial tissue is sloughed to the exterior with the movement of cerumen, but in this case, the dead epithelial tissue forms a sac and produces keratin. The lesion grows in size and contains fibrous stroma, cholesterol crystals, and keratin and squamous epithelial tissue. The area bleeds easily so the examination is performed with care. In the absence of perforation, this lesion is thought to stem from rests left during developmental stages in the middle ear evolution. There is usually a conduction hearing loss and x-ray examination shows absence of mastoid cells and enlargement of the mastoid antrum.

Treatment includes control of infection; radical surgical excision is rarely performed since this procedure involves exenteration of the middle ear spaces with resulting conduction deafness. Less radical surgery can be performed if the patient's condition indicates, so that the ossicles are retained. Left untreated, the cholesteatoma can destroy the bone. People with cholesteatomas tend to have associated polyp formation.

Inflammation and Infection in the Ear

Perichondritis of the pinna is accumulation of pus between the perichondrium and cartilage, eventually causing septic necrosis of the cartilage. The area is incised and drained, and a pressure dressing or splint is applied to ensure correct positioning of the ear during the healing process. Culture and sensitivity of the drainage are done for determination of antibiotic therapy.

External otitis media, a general term for inflammation of the auricle and external meatus, can be caused by any irritation to the ear. Swimming, use of certain soaps or shampoos, placing objects like hairpins into the ear, application of heat, incorrect cleaning of the ear, and bacterial infections are the most common sources of irritation. Various organisms may cause otitis, and it is often related to dermatitis or to fungal infections. Patients who have been on long-term antibiotic therapy are likely to acquire fungal infections. External otitis media can be localized or it may involve the entire surface of the meatus.

Inflammation of the external meatus is demonstrated by reddened epithelial tissue. Swelling may be present to such a degree that the meatus is obstructed. There is usually a serous weeping or drainage that gradually becomes more purulent. The external ear may be swollen and tender, and the skin in the preauricular and postauricular areas may be reddened. Itching is a common symptom, and the regional lymph nodes may be enlarged. Generally the condition is treated with topical antibiotics or antiseptics. If there is extensive cellulitis, systemic antibiotics may be given. The ear drainage is cultured and sensitivity tests are done to determine specific bacteria and drug therapy. Often more than one organism is involved in the infectious process. Neomycin or hydrocortisone or both, in the form of an ear ointment or as drops, may be given along with systemic antibiotics.

Middle ear infections (middle ear otitis media) are common in children and are related to adenoiditis or tonsilitis, colds or sinusitis, allergies, or rapid pressure changes. Suppurative otitis is a pyogenic infection with systemic symptoms of chills, fever, and malaise. Streptococci, pneumococci, or staphylococci are commonly the causative organisms. A combination of symptoms includes pain, which may be severe; a feeling of stuffiness in the ear; dulled or impaired hearing; and a feeling that there is fluid in the ear. There may be hemorrhagic bullae on the drum or in the external meatus. The drainage may be sterile, or it may become purulent if the eardrum is perforated. The characteristic finding is injection of blood vessels in the periphery and over the handle of the malleus of the tympanic membrane; the tympanic membrane appears reddened and dull; initially it is retracted, but bulges as the infection progresses. Bulging of the tympanic membrane precedes rupture. The mastoid process and the preauricular and postauricular areas may be tender and swollen.

Treatment includes antihistamines for allergies, nasal decongestants if there is upper respiratory tract infection, and systemic antibiotics. Bed rest is ordered to promote healing, and analgesics may be required for pain relief. In some instances a tube may be inserted into the eustachian tube to provide for continuous ventilation. This tube is usually made of Teflon or another nonirritating substance and remains in place as long as necessary. A **myringotomy** is advised if there is evidence that the tympanic membrane might rupture. In this procedure a central curvilinear incision is made in the eardrum. Usually general anesthesia is used. Myringotomy facilitates better healing than occurs following perforation by rupture and allows for incision in the area of the membrane that heals best. The drainage from the ear is cultured following either a rupture or a myringotomy, and sensitivity studies are done for determination of antibiotic therapy. Following a myringotomy, the patient will have a sterile cotton wick drain in place. This drain is changed as necessary. The tympanic membrane usually heals within 24 hours, and hospitalization is not necessary. A small tube may be placed following myringotomy to facilitate drainage. This tube is similar to those used in the eustachian tube and remains in place as long as is necessary to promote healing.

Otitis may be so severe that the mastoid bone is involved in the infectious process with formation of an abscess in the mastoid. In this event the person has severe pain in the postauricular area. Tenderness is followed by swelling and increased temperature. An abscess in the mastoid bone, if severe, may cause swelling in the external meatus. **Bezold's mastoiditis** is an abscess in the zygomatic area, whereas **Gradenigo's syndrome** is mastoiditis that has extended to the temporal bone, sometimes involving the sixth cranial nerve.

Surgical drainage of the abscess is required. This procedure is done with extreme care to avoid damage to the facial nerve, the surrounding structures of the middle and inner ear, and the dura mater. Necrotic bone tissue is removed, and a drain is left in the wound to facilitate drainage until the abscess is resolved and healing begins. The area is then covered with a dressing held in place by a head bandage.

In applying the dressing, gauze is placed over the affected ear, forming a protective soft covering; several layers of gauze are used. The head dressing is wrapped in the fashion of a turban, using figure-of-eight wrapping around the head to keep the dressing in place. Gauze is wrapped above and below the ear on the affected side and in a similar fashion on the other side, leaving the unaffected ear unbandaged. The dressing may be tied or taped to fix the ends in place. Postoperatively there may be vertigo with nausea and vomiting, requiring antiemetics and assistance in ambulating until these vestibular symptoms subside. The mastoid bone heals by filling in with granulation tissue. Particular attention is given to oral hygiene and dietary management, with a soft diet being necessary in the postoperative phase. Observation for signs of facial nerve damage is accomplished by having the patient open and close his eyes, raise his eyebrows, and show his teeth. Impaired ability to perform these functions indicates facial nerve damage (Fig. 13-5).

Chronic otitis media may occur as tubotympanic disease or as atticoantral disease. The former usually follows acute otitis media with perforation of the tympanic membrane that does not heal. Infections of the upper respiratory tract may cause secondary infection in the middle ear, and the patient may experience a mild or moderate deafness. The upper respiratory infection is controlled and appropriate ear medications are used in treatment. It may also be necessary to repair the tympanic membrane by grafting. This procedure is called myringoplasty. It decreases the possibility of continuous infections from either external infection or from the respiratory passages. Perforations located centrally are easier to treat than those located marginally. The bony substance of the tympanum annulus may be destroyed or impaired in marginal perforations, and surgical repair is difficult.

When the bony portion of the ear is involved in chronic infection the disease is atticoantral. It is more serious than tubotympanic disease because of the possibility of spread to surrounding tissues and structures. In this condition there is a mucopurulent discharge and the tympanic membrane is perforated into the bony margin. A polyp of granulation tissue forms following the infection. This polyp may extend into the middle ear, and there may be ulceration of epithelial tissue and epithelial glands may become cystic. Bacteria most commonly found include *Pseudomonas aeruginosa, Escherichia coli, Klebsiella aerobacter, Proteus vulgaris,* or *Staphylococcus aureus.*

Many conditions result in damage to the tympanic membrane, requiring surgical repair. **Tympanoplasty** is the surgical procedure for repair of the tympanic membrane. There are several types. Type I provides for restoration of the tympanic membrane. A soft tissue graft is used. Type II includes repair of the tympanic membrane and relocation of the ossicles if their position has been dislocated. Type III is used when the malleus and incus have been destroyed but the stapes is in good condition. In this surgery, a graft is placed between the tympanic membrane and the stapes to reconnect the ossicular chain. All these procedures provide for protection of the round window and for transmission of sound waves.

Following these procedures the patient requires nursing care for comfort and protection. Vestibular symptoms of vertigo require the nurse to assist the patient when he or she is ambulating. Nausea and vomiting are treated with antiemetics. Maintenance of oral hygiene and hydration is important. Gener-

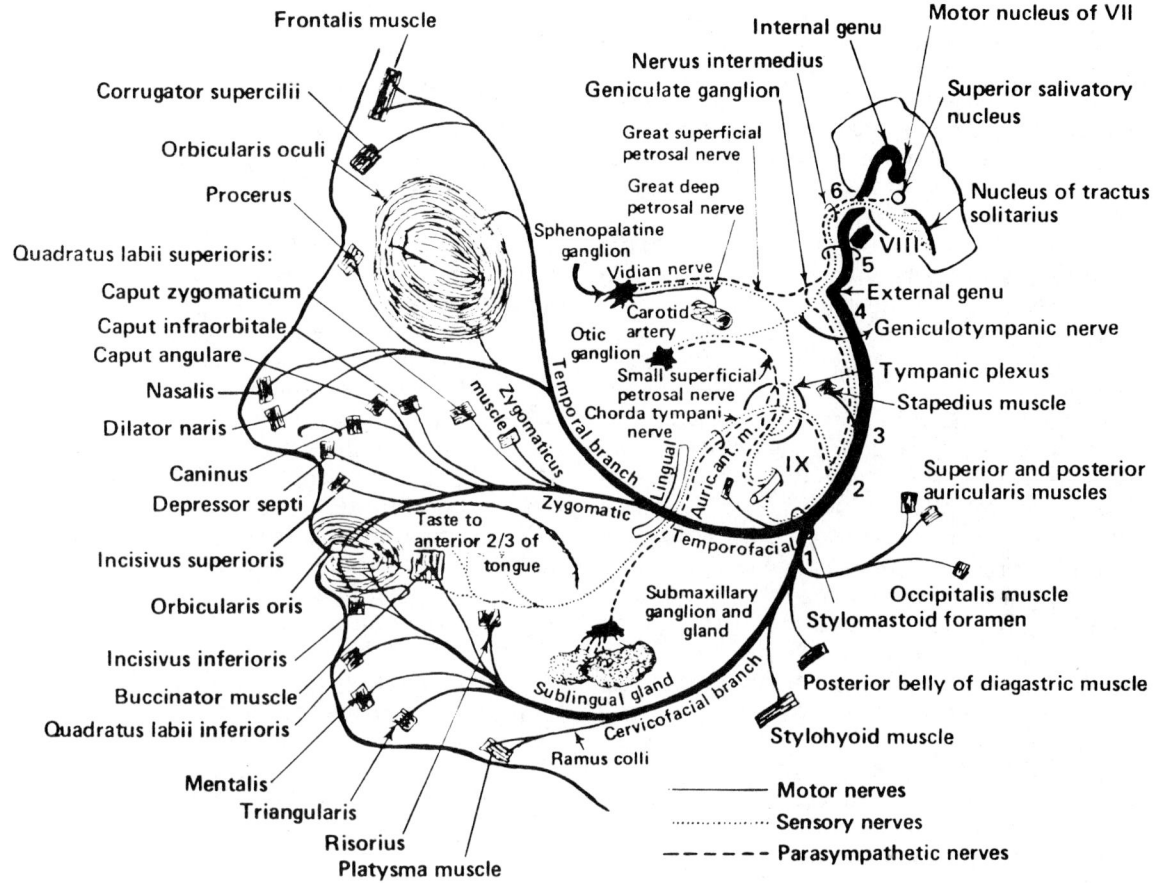

Figure 13-5
The facial nerves. (From J. G. Chusid, *Correlative Neuroanatomy and Functional Neurology* [16th ed.]. Los Altos, California: Lange Medical Publications, 1976. Reproduced by permission.)

ally, the inner ear packing is never touched. The outer dressing (if present) should be changed as necessary. The surgeon usually changes the inner ear dressing, using great care to prevent disturbance of the delicate structures that have been repaired in the surgical procedure. The patient usually experiences discomfort caused by swelling and tenderness in the operative area and may have a feeling of heaviness on the operative side. Analgesics may be required for pain. Systemic antibiotics are generally given, as infection is a major complication of ear surgery and should be avoided if possible. Follow-up care requires monitoring of hearing function and observation of healing and facial nerve function.

Otitis media can be complicated by thrombosis of the lateral sinus, labyrinthitis, facial nerve paralysis, and extension of the infection to the intracranial spaces. Abscess formation in the lateral sinus may cause growth of a mural clot that blocks the sinus. The neck is swollen with enlarged lymph nodes. Mastoidectomy is required if internal drainage is not adequate.

Labyrinthitis usually occurs from infection spread via the oval or round windows, the lateral sinus, or the vascular supply. Symptoms include vertigo, which is sometimes transient. Nausea and vomiting are common. Increasing pressure in the external auditory meatus produces nystagmus that is diagnostic. If the inner ear fluids are involved, there may also be perception deafness.

Diffuse serous labyrinthitis refers to labyrinthitis with mild or moderate hearing loss. **Diffuse purulent labyrinthitis** refers to total hearing loss. Bedrest, antibiotics, and, if necessary, mastoidectomy are the treatment modes.

Toxic labyrinthitis can result from ototoxic drugs; streptomycin, vancomycin, kanamycin, and neomycin are among the drugs known to have ototoxic effects when given intramuscularly. Streptomycin has been found to cause vestibular damage. People with kidney impairment are particularly sensitive to ototoxic drugs.

Infection in the middle ear may extend through the midcranial fossa or to the posterior fossa. Extradural or subdural abscesses or meningitis or both may result. When the bony canals are infected, the facial nerve may be involved at the site where it passes through the middle ear. Necrosis of bone may erode the nerve as well if the abscess is not treated or if it does not resolve.

Otitis media of secretory origin is a condition in which sterile fluid accumulates in the middle ear. The person hears his voice echo and has a feeling of fullness in the middle ear. Sometimes intermittent mild pain occurs and a sensation of fluid accumulation is felt only when the head is in certain positions. Conductive hearing loss is related to immobility of the tympanic membrane. A number of events including pressure changes during air flights, upper respiratory infections, and adenoiditis may precipitate secretory otitis media by causing the eustachian canal to be blocked. The middle ear is not ventilated if the eustachian tube is blocked. Oxygen is then absorbed by the blood vessels in the mucous membranes. Initially the drum is retracted, but returns to normal; as there is a transudate of fluid from the vessels, the drum bulges with the pressure of the collected fluid. On inspection, the tympanic membrane appears yellowish, and bubbles may be seen behind the drum. Glue ear is the name given to this condition when the fluid is mucoid.

Therapy consists in identifying and treating the precipitating cause. It may be necessary to drain the fluid by myringotomy. If the condition is not treated, adhesions may form and the ossicles become immobilized, resulting in deafness. A tympanostomy tube may be inserted to ventilate the middle ear until the eustachian tube returns to normal. This tube may be left in place for weeks or months. The tympanostomy tube is a small plastic tube that is placed in the tympanic membrane through the external auditory meatus. It cannot be seen externally and it is not uncomfortable for the patient.

Otosclerosis

Otosclerosis is replacement of the temporal bone with spongy vascular bone. It occurs twice as frequently in females as in males, and the symptoms are noticed when the footplate of the stapes is immobilized. Although the cause is unknown, the disease is familial in about one-half of the cases. Symptoms are first noticed in the late teens or early adulthood, and there are exacerbations during pregnancy. Conduction deafness results and tinnitus is a common symptom; vertigo may also be a symptom. The tympanic membrane is intact and cochlear function is often good. Otosclerotic bone appears as irregularly arranged bone with numerous vascular pathways embedded in the bone. These changes cause ankylosis of the footplate of the stapes and sometimes affect the area posterior to the oval window. The focus of the disease may also be in the scala media, in which case there is a sensorineural hearing loss.

Surgical treatment is stapedectomy in carefully selected candidates. This procedure involves removal of the stapes and insertion of a prosthesis that may be either a soft tissue graft or a tiny wire prosthesis, to complete the ossicle chain from the incus to the oval window. Hearing is improved in the majority of persons who have this surgery; however, deafness may result. If the otosclerosis is bilateral, the stapedectomy is first performed on the most involved ear. If surgery is not selected as an option for treatment, a hearing aid may be worn. Because hearing acuity is improved in the majority of people postoperatively, most persons do elect to have the surgery.

Stapedectomy is an elective surgical procedure requiring that the patient be advised of the expected outcomes and potential complications prior to making the decision to have surgery. Preoperatively, the patient should wash his hair because it is contraindicated in the postoperative phase. The ear must remain dry. On the night before the operation, the patient is given nothing by mouth after midnight. Local anesthesia is generally given to avert the postoperative effects of general anesthesia. In addition, local anesthesia enables monitoring of vestibular function.

The surgical site is usually prepared in the operating room. Hair around the auricle is shaved, and that in the auditory canal is cut with scissors. A skin preparation is done.

Following stapedectomy (a microsurgical procedure involving finely developed skill on the surgeon's part), the patient is usually kept in bed for 24 hours. Ambulation thereafter is increased slowly to the person's tolerance and with assistance, particularly if vestibular dysfunction is present. The patient should not blow his nose or sneeze. A liquid diet, gradually increased to soft foods, is given according to tolerance.

The patient is usually anxious about the status of his hearing postoperatively. He should be informed that hearing acuity does not immediately improve on the day of surgery.

The nurse monitors the patient's condition in the postoperative phase for early detection of complications that may occur following stapedectomy [5]. Facial nerve paralysis may occur immediately following surgery because of injection of anesthesia near the nerve. This paralysis is usually transient, with function returning in about 4 hours after surgery. Prophylactic antibiotic therapy is given to prevent another complication: otitis media. If otitis media occurs, sensitivity studies are done to determine appropriate antibiotic therapy. Injury to the chorda tympani nerve may occur during surgery and causes dryness of the mouth or decreased taste sensations or both. These symptoms are transient, but may last for several months, requiring oral hygiene and hydration. Vertigo may occur following stapedectomy because of surgical trauma, loss of perilymph, or labyrinthitis. This symptom requires protection of the patient's safety, particularly in ambulation. This is also usually transient, but if it persists, the surgeon may have to repair the prosthesis or its attachments. Hearing loss may occur; this may be either a fluctuating conductive hearing loss or sensorineural hearing loss of sudden onset. The latter is a rare occurrence. Fluctuating hearing loss indicates that there is intermittent loss of conduction because of loose fittings in the prosthesis and is corrected by replacing or tightening the prosthesis. Sensorineural hearing loss is often delayed, occurring months after the surgery, and is usually associated with changes in pressure experienced in changing altitudes. A revision of the surgery may be necessary to correct this loss.

The patient is advised to avoid, during the convalescent phase, situations in which he is subject to air pressure changes. Swimming is contraindicated.

The nurse may meet people who have had fenestration surgery. This operation was frequently performed for treatment of otosclerosis, but is rarely done in current practice. In this operation an artificial opening is made to provide for the passage of sound waves to the inner ear. The oval window, which is impaired by the otosclerosis, is bypassed. People who have had this surgery may later require a stapedectomy.

Vestibular Dysfunction

Ménière's disease is also known as labyrinthine hydrops and is usually unilateral, occurring before the age of 50. Although the cause is not known, the disease is thought to be due to autonomic nervous control impairment, which influences labyrinthine circulation, with dilatation of the membranous labyrinth. There is strong evidence that the disease may be a hypersensitivity disease. It is thought that there is a relationship between allergy and endocrine dysfunction as a primary factor in its incidence. Three types of Ménière's disease have been identified: endolymphatic hydrops of vestibular variety, true endolymphatic hydrops, and endolymphatic hydrops of the cochlear variety. In the first there is vertigo and no specific cochlear symptoms. True endolymphatic hydrops is characterized by ear stuffiness and hearing loss. Eventually persons with either the vestibular or the cochlear variety develop all the symptoms of true endolymphatic hydrops. Some persons also have migraines along with the symptoms of Ménière's disease. The vertigo attack may be preceded by discordant hearing. The tinnitus is noted to be more severe just before or following an episodic attack of vertigo. Hearing loss is noticed more after vertigo. The attacks of vertigo are of varying lengths and duration, lasting from 2 hours to as long as 24 hours. Nausea and vomiting may occur along with the vertigo as does spontaneous nystagmus. The hearing loss in Ménière's disease is generally in the low frequencies. It is related to caloric response, with the loss being greater when caloric response is weak.

Treatment includes use of vasodilators to relieve the vertigo. This treatment is effective in about one-half the cases. Low sodium diets and diuretics are also used for establishing a mild dehydration. Between attacks there may be no symptoms. If the cause is thought to be allergic, an elimination diet is given to determine food allergies. A Rinkel serial dilution antigen titration is helpful in determining allergies to inhaled substances. Some authorities prescribe hyposensitization.

In some cases there is no response to medical management and no hearing improvement. In other cases the response is good and there are few if any symptoms following treatment. In other instances radical surgery may be performed. The most radical procedure is destructive labyrinthectomy, which results in deafness.

Tinnitus, while often associated with specific and nonspecific disease processes, may occur singularly with no apparent cause. There is no specific treatment for tinnitus as its cause is not really known. Initially, efforts are made to trace the cause to diseases of the ear. If a disease is found, treatment may provide for relief from the tinnitus. In some people, however, tinnitus may prove to be untreatable. These persons should be helped to learn methods for relief from the sounds. The use of other sounds to counteract the tinnitus is helpful. Music from a clock radio or a record player or a television set connected to a timer during quiet periods and prior to sleep has been found useful. Preoccupation with handwork or reading may help to "tune out" the tinnitus. Persistent tinnitus with no identifiable or treatable cause may induce such grave psychological distraction that ligation of the acoustic nerve may be necessary. The loss of hearing in the affected ear is counterbalanced by relief from the psychological distraction of the tinnitus.

Presbycusis is associated with aging and is thought to be related to arteriosclerosis. The affected person first notices impaired hearing at higher frequencies with gradual progressive loss of speech frequencies. The hearing loss is neurosensory and there is no definitive treatment.

Numerous other conditions are associated with hearing loss. **Bell's palsy,** a unilateral facial paralysis, causes pain in the postauricular area. This condition begins acutely and if recovery is not spontaneous in about three weeks, surgery is often performed to relieve compression on the facial nerve. This condition is discussed more fully in Chapter 11.

Vestibular neuronitis is another acute illness in which there is impairment of vestibular function. It is thought that this disease is caused by demyelination following infections usually of viral origin. The predominant symptom is vertigo with nausea and ataxia. As the patient attempts to walk, he veers to the affected side. Treatment involves bedrest and limiting of head movements that exaggerate the vertigo. The symptoms usually disappear after about three weeks with great improvement within 2 or 3 days after the onset.

Allport's syndrome is characterized by sudden cochlear deafness. The disease usually occurs in males. Treatment is bedrest with the head of the bed elevated at a 20° to 30° angle. It is thought that the disease may be caused by a rupture in a labyrinthine window membrane or by perilymphatic fistulas. If a fistula is present a portion of the tragus is used as an autograft to repair the membrane. This graft is placed around the fistula to close the opening. Following this procedure, the patient remains on bed rest for 2 days and limited activity for about 2 weeks. Prophylactic antibiotics are given, and the patient is advised to avoid swimming for several months.

Ramsey Hunt syndrome is a herpes infection of the geniculate ganglion. The symptoms are tenderness, swelling, tinnitus, and hearing loss. There may also be facial palsy and symptoms of vestibular impairment. As with other types of neural involvement, treatment is symptomatic.

Persons with multiple sclerosis often have symptoms of inner ear lesions. These symptoms are usually subtle and transient and require diagnosis to rule out inner ear disease.

Many diseases, then, can affect hearing and vestibular senses. The nurse should constantly be aware of each person's need for communication and for position sense, and should observe and assess the function of the ears in this regard for every person. In many instances, the observant and understanding nurse can help a patient find the correct resources for diagnosis and treatment of specialized hearing problems. If treated, many of these problems can be resolved and the patient will be able to lead a fuller and more satisfying life. For people who have chronic health problems that cannot be treated, the nurse should adapt care to meet their special requirements.

As more is found out about the relationships among various disease processes, previously vague symptoms may take on greater meaning. For example, it has been found that the tympanic membrane may be a source of the coughing spells that some people experience. Because of the presence of afferent vagal nerve fibers in the pathway from the concha of the ear and the posterior portion of the external auditory canal, irritation can give rise to cough. One report cites three incidences in which a hair lying on the tympanic membrane caused chronic cough [7]. Ordinarily one would associate this chronic cough with chronic sinusitis or bronchitis. It is important to listen carefully and to follow up on patients' concerns in an effort to discover the primary source of dysfunctions. This principle is particularly true of the ears because the person who has ear discomfort but also has other types of dysfunction such as cardiovascular or respiratory disease may be treated for the more obvious and seemingly more crucial problem while the seemingly merely bothersome problem of earache is left undiagnosed and untreated. Nursing assessment should therefore be complete and should include hearing and vestibular functions. The nurse should also investigate the possible causes of the symptoms by checking the patient's medications for side effects, reviewing the relationships among diseases, and by making certain that the patient is provided appropriate diagnostic examinations.

Care and ongoing support is facilitated by cooperation with health personnel in many different types of health agencies. Information for the hard of hearing or deaf person may be obtained from several sources. Two of these are:

Alexander Graham Bell Association for the Deaf
1537 37th Street, N.W.
Washington, D.C. 20007

National Association of Hearing and Speech Agencies
919 18th Street, N.W.
Washington, D.C. 20006

The Nose

A person's nose, with its unique size and shape, is a predominant facial feature. The significance of a person's perception of his nose in terms of self-image and personality is as vital as the physiologic functions of the nose. Physiologically the nose has multiple functions. These functions include olfaction and the conditioning of inspired air. The sense of smell (olfaction) is one of the most important components of a person's ability to relate to and interpret his environment. The air-conditioning functions of the nose are the protective mechanisms of screening and preparing air for passage to the lower airways. The nose is also an accessory organ in the articulation of speech and it contributes to the quality of the voice.

Normally a person breathes through his nose, tending to breathe through the mouth only when the nasal passages are obstructed, during strenuous exercise, and when respiratory insufficiency is present. Mouth breathing reduces the total work of breathing. Although nasal breathing nearly doubles the work of breathing, it is more beneficial. The nose warms inspired air to body temperature and saturates the air with water vapor. About two quarts of water are added to inspired air within the nose every 24 hours. Warming and humidification of air in the nose are protective mechanisms, and air entering the lower airways normally reaches a body temperature of approximately 98.6° F (37° C) and a 75 to 80 percent humidity level.

Another protective function of the nose is removal of particulate matter, water-soluble gases and vapors from inspired air. Particulate matter in the air is deflected by the hairs near the opening of the nares and is impacted in the nose, being caught up by the mucous blanket. Several factors are important in the efficiency of this process. They include the size and density of the inhaled particles, the linear velocity of the airstream, the size of the nasal passages, and the surface area of mucous membrane in contact with the air. With normal nasal function most of the remaining particles that pass through the nose are small enough to be exhaled during normal ventilation or removed by protective mechanisms within the lower airways. Both sneezing and nose-blowing facilitate removal of irritants from the nose. The nose also is an outlet for some of the tears from the lacrimal duct and for drainage of sinuses surrounding the nose.

NURSING ASSESSMENT OF NASAL FUNCTION

Assessment of nasal function begins with visual observation of the shape and symmetry of the nose and notation of swelling, redness, or skin lesions on the soft tissues of its outer surface. A nasal speculum and a light are needed to examine the interior of the nose. The speculum is inserted just inside the naris for a distance of 1 cm so that the naris can be opened wide with the speculum. The lower two-thirds of the nose is supported by flexible cartilage; the upper third by bone. The patient holds his head upright so that the nasal mucosa in the anterior naris can be examined. Normally the nasal mucosa is pink to red. A pale gray color suggests allergic rhinitis. Reddened mucosa indicates an acute inflammation. The amount and color of mucus in the nose should be noted. The nose is lined with epithelium-containing and mucus-secreting cells and cilia. Mucus from the nose is passed to the pharynx by ciliary action, to be swallowed for clearance to the stomach.

Paranasal sinus secretions continually contribute to the secretions in the nose to aid in the clearance function. The nasal mucosa vaporizes inhaled air to remove water-soluble gases and vapors. The latter pass into solution in the serous covering of the mucosa. The narrow airstream and the low linear velocity of the air in the nares allow for maximum contact of air with the mucous membrane.

After the nasal mucosa in the anterior nares is examined, the patient is asked to tilt his head back so that the posterior aspects of the nose can be visualized. A light is needed for this part of the examination. The nasal septum (cartilage covered by mucoperiostium) is formed by the medial wall of each nostril. Three turbinates (also called conchae), the inferior, middle, and superior, are attached to the lateral wall of each nasal cavity. Of these, the superior turbinate usually cannot be visualized. The inferior turbinate, the largest of the three, can be visualized and the middle turbinate can usually be seen. A meatus lies below each turbinate. The turbinates are bony and curved, and are covered with a highly vascular mucous membrane and erectile tissue. The large surface area of the mucous membrane of the turbinates warms inspired air and the mucous membranes contain swell spaces that enlarge and become engorged with particulate matter, thereby trapping particles to prevent their passage into the airways. It is normal to find the inferior turbinate enlarged or swollen in appearance. This is particularly true if the inspired air contains a high level of pollutants. Spraying the mucosa with a vasoconstrictor such as ephedrine about five minutes prior to examination decongests the turbinates, allowing for better visualization of the posterior aspects of the nose that are obstructed from view by the swollen turbinates.

The vestibule of the nose is a widened area located posteriorly. The opening to the pharynx is a slit-like passage. This narrow portion of the air passage is smaller than the major airways of the lower respiratory passages. The narrowing contributes to removal of the particulate matter, as does the bend in the airways at the nasopharynx.

Paranasal sinuses are air-filled cavities within the skull bones. They are lined with mucous membrane and drain into the nose. Only the maxillary and frontal sinuses can be examined. The ethmoid and sphenoid sinuses can be visualized only by x-ray. The frontal, maxillary, and anterior ethmoid sinuses drain into the middle meatus, which lies below the middle turbinate. The posterior ethmoids and the sphenoid sinuses drain into the superior meatus. The nasolacrimal duct drains into the inferior meatus. These openings are not visible on examination. Pus in the cavity indicates that sinusitis or another type of inflammatory process is present.

The frontal sinuses can be palpated by applying firm pressure on the infraorbital areas above the supraorbital ridge. Tenderness or pain implies inflammation. The maxillary sinuses can be palpated just below the orbits and across the cheekbone. The maxillary sinuses should be palpated for swelling and tenderness. The frontal and maxillary sinuses can be visualized by transillumination in a dark room, although this procedure is used infrequently. X-ray visualization, using contrast medium if desired, gives more precise information about the sinuses.

Olfactory receptors are located in the posterior nasal cavity and are small areas containing olfactory epithelium. The mucosa in these areas has a characteristic dark yellow pigmentation, and there are no cilia. Bowman's glands, supporting cells, and olfactory cells make up the olfactory receptors. Olfactory cells contain bipolar sensory neurons with unmyelinated axons at the basal end. They project to the surface of the olfactory areas. The olfactory nerves enter the cranial cavity through the ethmoid bones and synapse to two tissue masses below the frontal lobe. Axons in the olfactory bulb and olfactory tract transmit impulses to the temporal lobe of the brain. Integration of sensory perceptions, including the perception of odors, takes place in the higher brain centers. This integration is significant in appetite and in many other aspects of behavior.

Little is known about olfaction. It is believed that the air molecules must have sufficient vapor pressure to reach the olfactory receptors and that to activate the neural receptors these air molecules must be soluble in both water and lipids contained in the mucous membrane secretions. The amount of vapor pressure required to stimulate receptor cells is not known, but it is considered to be minimal. It is possible for a person to distinguish odors from one another and to detect a specific odor from a mixture of smells. It is thought that the olfactory receptors do not have specific sensitivity for specific odors, but that the ability to discriminate odors is a higher nervous center function. The olfactory receptors are easily fatigued, losing their ability to detect odors after exposure of a few minutes thus allowing one to become accustomed to odors. For example, when one first enters a room one smells its odors most clearly, becoming less aware of them in a brief time.

DYSFUNCTION OF THE NOSE

Functions of the nose can be impaired by infection, trauma, or abnormal cell growth. Narrowing of the lumen of the nostril or nasal constriction interferes with passage of air and increases the resistance to airflow. Injury or infection of the mucous membranes impairs the protective mechanisms for humidification, temperature adjustment, and removal of particulate matter as well as interferes with the sense of smell. Anosmia (loss of smell) may result. Injury or trauma that involves the structure of the nose or the soft tissues of the nose may cause internal and external nasal deformity. Treatment of nasal dysfunction can include both medical and surgical intervention. In both it is important not to damage or impair the function of the delicate structures and membranes of the nose.

Rhinitis, an inflammation of the mucous membrane of the nose, is one of the most common causes of nasal dysfunction. It is usually associated with colds, but it can be acute or chronic and related to many other conditions. Bacteria, viruses, or irritation of the nasal mucosa by irritants including chemicals, air pollutants, and smoke, or chronic conditions such as allergies or chronic bronchitis, may be factors in the occurrence of rhinitis. The mucosa is congested and a nasal discharge is often present. Congestion may extend to the sinuses or to the nasopharynx and to the pharynx. Decongestants such as phenylephrine hydrochloride (Neosynephrine hydrochloride) and oxymetazoline hydrochloride (Afrin) and steam inhalation with analgesics to relieve the discomfort are the primary modes of treatment. The effect of nasal decongestants is vasoconstriction. The use of decongestants is contraindicated in hypertension; for example, ephedrine stimulates the heart, increasing cardiac rate and force. Blood pressure is then elevated.

Chronic rhinitis occurs with continuous exposure to pollutants (dust or dry air) and is frequently associated with chronic bronchitis. The nasal mucosa may be hypertrophied, requiring surgical intervention to reconstruct the nasal passages. This is done by trimming or removing a portion of the turbinates. If the passage is too large, atrophic rhinitis may occur causing thickened viscous mucus and dry nasal secretions with crust formation. Use of softening agents such as water-soluble oils to remove crusts and irrigating the nares with an alkaline solution such as sodium chloride are helpful in preventing discomfort.

Sinusitis may result from bacterial or viral infections, from diving and swimming, and from dental disease. Hypersensitivity reactions or obstruction of nasal passages that prevent draining of sinuses may also result in sinusitis. Symptoms of **sinusitis** are pain and tenderness of the affected sinus, fever, malaise, and headache. When the sinuses drain well, pain is lessened. Sinus drainage causes engorgement of the nasal mucosa, causing a "stuffed up" nose. Drainage passes from the nasopharynx to the pharynx and may cause a sore throat.

X-ray examination is done to detect which sinuses are affected. The inflamed sinuses appear opaque on x-ray. Normally the sinuses are filled with air and appear as clear cavities on x-ray. Nasal decongestants, which act by local vasoconstriction, are given to relieve the symptoms and reduce edema to promote drainage. If nose drops are used, the person should tilt his head backward to administer the nose drops. When administering a nasal spray, the head is held upright and the spray is directed into the nostril. Position changes allow passage of the medication to the sinuses. Sinusitis may be chronic and occurs with varying degrees of severity. Headache, pain, and tenderness in the sinus areas, fever, and malaise may be transient symptoms in chronic sinusitis.

Chronic maxillary sinusitis may be relieved by irrigating the sinus with isotonic sodium chloride to empty the purulent secretions and debris, allowing the cilia to become active and the mucous membrane to function better. Local anesthesia is used for this procedure and may be repeated as necessary. In severe cases, a **radical antrostomy** may be performed. This procedure involves creating an opening from the maxillary sinus to form a window to the inferior nasal meatus. The maxillary sinus is reached through the anterior surface of the maxilla in the mouth for drainage. An **intranasal antrostomy** provides drainage into the nose by opening the maxillary sinus through a resection of part of the anterior wall of the maxillary sinus. In either procedure, the sinus is cleared of debris. The former allows for better visualization of the interior of the maxillary sinus and for better clearing of cellular debris and secretions. Following surgery the patient experiences pain and discomfort from edema. The patient's face is swollen in the area of the nose and cheeks and this swelling gradually decreases but causes discomfort during eating or talking. Adequate nutrition and hydration must be provided despite lack of appetite, nausea from swallowing drainage, and discomfort. Nasal ice packs may be used along with analgesics to relieve pain and edema. As the edema is reduced, the patient begins to feel better, realizing the positive effects of the surgery in improved breathing and a sensation of openness or clearing of the sinuses.

Maxillary and frontal sinusitis are often related. Relieving mucosal engorgement of the middle nasal meatus to provide better drainage from the maxillary sinuses relieves the frontal sinuses. There is a reciprocal improvement in the frontal sinus drainage into the medial meatus when the maxillary sinus is draining well. Surgical drainage of the frontal sinus is done by making a small incision medial to the supraorbital notch. Excision of occluded areas can also be performed to create a drainage passageway at the bottom of the frontal sinus; ethmoid cells are removed to create a passage to the nasal septum.

Ethmoid sinusitis is associated with signs of orbital cellulitis: edema of the eyelids and proptosis (downward or forward displacement of the eye). Orbital cellulitis is relieved by treating the sinusitis. Treatment is essential because of the location, which threatens potential damage to the optic nerve. Orbital edema may cause loss of eye motion and, if pressure on the optic nerve is great enough, blindness can result. Ethmoid sinusitis may be associated with allergies and the formation of nasal polyps. If medical treatment does not provide relief, an ethmoidectomy is performed, either through the nose or externally. This procedure creates an opening between the ethmoid sinus and the nasal cavity through removal of the anterior portion of the middle turbinate. For draining procedures, the sphenoid sinuses may be reached through the ethmoid sinus. The operation is performed only after effective treatment of infections.

Complications of sinusitis are consequential as they involve adjacent or continuous structures. Rhinitis, pharyngitis, laryngitis, bronchitis, and bronchiectasis occur in association with sinusitis. Infection may travel through the venous supply to the brain and cause meningitis or a brain abscess. Abscesses may also form in the frontal sinuses. Osteomyelitis of the frontal bone may also occur, so that the infection extends through bone erosion.

Nasal allergies often occur in persons prone to hypersensitivity reactions. They may occur seasonally or year-round, depending on the allergen. Hay fever is typical of a seasonal allergy. In this condition the person is very uncomfortable with watery discharge from the eyes, irritation of the nose with sneezing, and copious secretions and general symptoms of headache, fever, and malaise. The eosinophil count may be high. Antihistamines are given to relieve symptoms, and the affected persons are advised to avoid the allergens if possible. Some authorities believe that persons suffering from hay fever should be desensitized. However the results are variable and the procedure is not always effective.

Polyps that originate in the sinuses or in the nares often occur in association with allergies or infections. **Nasal polyps** are edematous swellings of the mucosa. Secondary infection and obstruction of the nasal passages occur with polyps. Speech may be affected, becoming nasal in quality, and sometimes there is anosmia. The polyps appear pale gray or pink and are sometimes translucent. Polypectomy is performed with a snare either under local or general anesthesia, depending on the accessibility to the site of the polyps. Nasal packs may be used to prevent bleeding postoperatively, and it is important to observe for bleeding. Unfortunately the polyps tend to recur.

Epistaxis occurs often in relation to a systemic disease or from trauma. Little's area, located in the anteroinferior part of the nasal septum, is the most common site of nosebleeds (epistaxis). At this point branches of the internal and external maxillary arteries join. Because nasal mucosa is highly vascular, bleeding can occur at any point. In emergency care for epistaxis the patient is asked to sit up with his head bent slightly forward and breathe through his mouth. Bleeding in the anterior part of the nose can often be stopped by pinching the cartilaginous part of the nose firmly, applying consistent pressure for 5 minutes or more, depending on how long cessation of the bleeding takes. Apposition of the thumb and index finger provides the best control for firm consistent pressure. Efforts are made to prevent the swallowing of blood. A basin or other receptacle is placed below the patient's nose to catch the blood and protect him from swallowing the blood, which could cause gastrointestinal problems later. An estimate of how much blood the person is losing should be made. The person should have a thorough nasal examination following the nose bleed; even if bleeding is quickly controlled, he may require treatment for the vessel rupture.

Bleeding from the posterior aspect of the nose is more difficult to control and the site cannot be visualized well. Nasal packing or cauterization is required to stop posterior bleeding. Some authorities believe that cauterization has fewer complications than packing the nose. Following stabilization, the patient is given a physical examination as nosebleeds may be either an early or late sign of hypertensive disease. Other causes are anticoagulant therapy and vitamin C or K deficiency.

If cauterization is used, the site of bleeding is located and a topical anesthetic and vasoconstrictor are applied to the bleeding vessel with a cotton pledget to stop the bleeding. Cauterization may then be performed either with a chemical agent such as silver nitrate or by electrocautery. Bleeding that continues following cauterization requires the pressure of a nasal pack for control. Some authorities believe that the inferior or middle turbinate should be fractured to allow for visualization of the bleeding vessel if the bleeding site lies in the posterior aspect of the nose and cannot otherwise be seen.

Intranasal packing must be done correctly to be effective. A topical anesthetic is applied first. Then the recesses of the nose are lightly packed, followed by placement of packing gently but firmly into the remainder of the nostril. The packing should be placed tightly enough to produce sufficient pressure to stop the bleeding and to prevent the packing from displacing into the nasopharynx or the oropharynx. If the packing is displaced, the patient will have the feeling that he is suffocating and may panic. When this problem occurs, someone should quiet the patient, open his mouth, locate the string or the pack, and remove it. If available, a forceps can be used. If the patient goes home with a pack in place, he should be forewarned of the possibility of this problem occurring and how to handle it.

Postnasal packs are prepared by folding a 4 by 4 gauze square in half, rolled tightly. These rolls are secured with presterilized umbilical tape or #2 black silk. The two ends of the tie are left long enough to be used as a guide for inserting the pack and for its removal. The pack is placed by first inserting a French catheter through the nose to the mouth. The string at one end of the pack is tied to the catheter in the mouth; the catheter is withdrawn through the nose to place the pack at the posterior choana (the opening at the posterior nose; Fig. 13-6). The string pack is then held tightly while the remainder of the nose is packed with petroleum gauze or with gauze impregnated with antibiotic ointment. The antibiotic ointment is applied just prior to insertion of the pack. Three-inch wide fine mesh gauze is usually used for nasal packs.

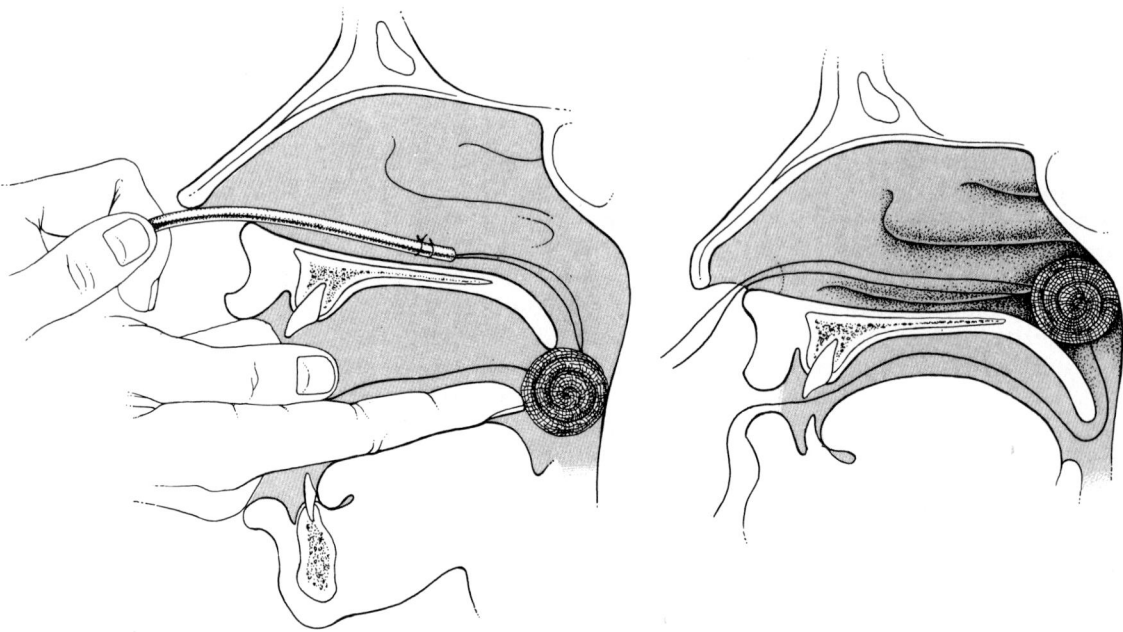

Figure 13-6
Placement of a posterior nasal pack. (From P. J. Donald, Leading with the nose. *Emergency Medicine* 11:29, 1975.)

Packs remain in place for 4 days. One string is trimmed and left in the nasopharynx. The other is taped to the cheek. Systemic antibiotics may be given, as infection is a complication of nasal packing. In addition, packing may cause ulceration of the mucous membrane and may cause synechiae (adhesions of the mucous membranes). The patient with a nasal pack usually is very uncomfortable. The pack distorts his appearance. In addition the pack may interfere with swallowing, so that the patient will require a soft or liquid diet. Often the combination of discomfort and foul taste in the mouth, caused by old, dried blood, causes nausea and lack of appetite. Both can be relieved by frequent oral hygiene and mouthwashes. The pack is observed for bleeding. Some bleeding continues following placement of the pack, making the appearance even more distressful to the person. Mouth breathing is necessitated and often results in dryness of the oral mucosa. This dryness can be reduced by taking ice chips and frequent sips of water. Temperatures must be taken rectally.

Bilateral packing is contraindicated because the pressure of packs on both sides of the nasal septum may cause necrosis. It is important that the basic cause of the hemorrhage be determined. Nasal fractures are most commonly the cause in young persons, and epistaxis is often not as serious in the healthy young adult as for older persons. Hypertension is the most common systemic cause of epistaxis. Persons with chronic lung disease who have low Pa_{O_2} levels may require supplemental oxygen while the pack is in place. When epistaxis is associated with liver disease, and if a large amount of blood has been swallowed, sterilization of the gastrointestinal tract may be required to prevent breakdown of blood with subsequent release of ammonia. Cathartics and enemas may be given to rid the tract of blood as soon as the patient's condition permits. Hemoglobin and hematocrit levels are obtained to determine the blood loss when excessive bleeding occurs, particularly because the patient with debilitating diseases may require replacement of lost blood.

Following removal of the pack, the nose is inspected to ascertain that the mucosa is intact. The inspection is again carried out 1 or 2 weeks after the pack has been removed to observe for indications of sinus infections, crusting, or purulent discharge, or for synechiae.

A **foreign body** may be inhaled or placed in

the nose (usually by small children). There may be no symptoms until a foul-smelling nasal discharge leads to the discovery of its presence. Foreign bodies tend to lodge between the inferior turbinate and the nasal septum. A blunt hook is used to remove the foreign body, taking care not to push it further into the nose. Local anesthesia and vasoconstrictors are first placed into the nose to provide for maximum visibility and to increase the area available to manipulate the foreign body. Using a forceps tends to push the foreign body deeper in the nose and should be avoided. A suction machine may be needed if the patient has large amounts of drainage, so that the nasal cavity can be better visualized.

In adults, **deviation** of the nasal septum may be normal. The septum is usually straight in children but becomes slightly deviated with age. A deviation is not serious unless it obstructs the nasal passages or interferes with sinus drainage. Surgical removal of part of the cartilages of the septum, of the perpendicular plate of the ethmoid, and of part of the maxillary crest, may be required for straightening the septum. This procedure is called submucosal resection. The amount of tissue resected depends on the particular type and degree of deviation any one individual has. Submucosal resections are usually delayed until full growth has been reached, because the teeth may not have erupted.

Splints or packing may be placed following resection, to hold the septum in alignment until healing occurs and to prevent bleeding. If a nasal pack is used, the patient has to breathe through his mouth and has difficulty swallowing and chewing. It is not unusual to have a sucking sensation when swallowing; the pack establishes a partial vacuum in the throat as air cannot pass through the nose. There may be some bleeding following a submucosal resection; in this case a drip pad is placed below the nose to catch the blood. If bleeding is continuous, additional nasal packing is usually inserted by the physician.

Perforations of the nasal septum can cause epistaxis and may follow submucosal resections. They can also result from trauma caused by putting objects in the nose or from picking the nose. Whistling sounds may be produced by the perforation when the person breathes through his nose. People with nasal dryness or crust formation are advised to use a bland ointment to promote healing of mucous membranes and to loosen crusts, which helps to prevent ulcer formation and subsequent perforation. Perforations that do not heal spontaneously are repaired by grafting.

Rhinoplasty is a surgical procedure performed for restructuring the nose. Structural deformities that obstruct the air passages and displeasure with the appearance of one's nose are the two major reasons for performing rhinoplasty. The procedure may also be performed to repair damage caused by trauma or in treatment of cancer. In this procedure the bony and cartilaginous structure of the nose is revised to achieve the desired shape. Overlying soft tissue takes the shape of the nasal structure. The nares are stabilized by placing a nasal pack and a protective nasal splint is applied by taping the outer skin and placing a hard metal or rubber shield over the nose for protection. Postoperatively, the patient is placed in Fowler's position to facilitate breathing through his mouth. Frequent sips of water and the use of mouthwashes keep the oral mucosa moist and the person more comfortable. An ice pack or an ice glove is applied gently to the nose to relieve pain and swelling from tissue trauma. The bag or glove should not be filled so full that it causes pressure on the nose. The patient is often nauseated from swallowing blood and requires antiemetics and supportive care to prevent vomiting.

During the first week or so after the rhinoplasty, the patient has difficulty in swallowing and chewing. Liquid diets or very soft foods are tolerated best and should be given according to the patient's preference and tolerance. Oral hygiene before and after eating is very important for comfort as well as for reducing the possibility of an infection. Soft tissues of the nose and surrounding areas become discolored. Ecchymosis appears within 24 to 48 hours after the operation, followed by a dark blue color that becomes yellow and dissipates in about two weeks. The discoloration is expected and the patient should know that it does not signify a complication. The nose and surrounding tissues are also edematous, with gradual reduction of the edema during the 2 to 3 week period following rhinoplasty. After this period, the patient can begin to appreciate the cosmetic result of the surgery.

Fractures of the nose occur commonly as

open fractures with tearing of the mucous membrane and may involve the ethmoid, sphenoid, and frontal bones that surround the nose. Deviation of the nasal septum may occur. Hematomas or frank bleeding or both may be present because of the tears in the mucous membranes. Swelling of the soft tissues of the nose with ecchymosis of the eyelids occurs rapidly following trauma, so treatment should be initiated as soon as possible. The internal nasal swelling can obscure the site of the fracture. The nose is usually abnormally mobile and tender, and crepitation of tissues may be felt. X-rays confirm the diagnosis. The paranasal sinuses and facial bones are x-rayed in addition to the nose to determine the extent of the fracture.

Drainage from the nose should be noted in extensive fractures because cerebrospinal fluid may drain through the nares. If rhinorrhea occurs, the patient should not blow his nose. A frontal craniotomy to preclude infection to the brain may be necessary if the rhinorrhea does not stop.

Nasal fractures are usually reduced under general anesthesia if they require repair of the bony structure and the septum. Splinting of the nose helps to stabilize the reduction until healing takes place. It is important to treat the nasal deformity caused by the fracture so that the air passages will not become obstructed. It is also important to repair the cosmetic deformity.

Hematomas may occur in conjunction with nasal fractures or with trauma. They are usually located between the mucoperichondrium and septal cartilages and appear as soft red swellings. Hematomas are incised and drained as they tend to become infected and can cause sepsis and necrosis. Either a drain or nasal packing is placed after drainage. If abscesses do form, they are also incised and drained. General anesthesia is often used, particularly if the hematoma is in a posterior location. Systemic antibiotics are given, and the patient may require analgesics, as the abscess causes throbbing pain. The patient may have an elevated temperature, a headache, and general malaise.

Papillomas, fibromas, or neurilemmomas may occur in the paranasal sinuses. Papillomas, which are usually benign tumors, also may occur in the nasal vestibule in the nasal cavity. Inverted papillomas may be invasive and involve surrounding tissues, tending to recur after removal. Viruses are thought to be the cause of papillomas.

Squamous cell carcinoma is the most commonly occurring type of malignant tumor of the nose. Adenocarcinomas, melanomas, lymphomas, or fibrosarcomas may also occur. The growth of tumors in these sites is infrequent, however. More commonly, carcinoma involves the soft tissues of the nose. Treatment for skin carcinoma of the nose includes cauterization and radiation whereas surgical excision is used for treating large lesions in the nasal cavity and in the paranasal sinuses. Radical resection along with radiation therapy may improve the cure rate.

Because of their location, tumors of the frontal and sphenoid sinuses cannot be treated easily. Radiation therapy is used to allay tumor growth in these areas and is sometimes effective. Lymphomas respond to radiation therapy or chemotherapy whereas melanomas are difficult to treat and their cure rate is low, despite therapy. The symptoms of tumors in the nasal cavity and paranasal sinuses vary according to the size and location of the tumor. They may cause obstruction of the lacrimal duct, loosening of the teeth, or swelling and obstruction of the nares. Pain is usually a late symptom.

Many times, a radical procedure is required in the treatment of invasive tumors of the paranasal sinuses or nasal cavity. Radical surgery is time-consuming and disfiguring. The exact procedure done depends on the amount of tissue to be removed. Often the initial surgery is followed by several sequential procedures for building up the nose. Efforts are made to create as normal an appearance as possible, because of the importance of the facial features in the person's maintenance of self-concept and body image.

The immediate effects of the operation are pain, a constant uncomfortable feeling of fullness and distortion of the facial structures and interference with normal nutrition. The diet must be adjusted to the patient's tolerance and limitations. Nasogastric tubes are often necessary for feeding following extensive surgical procedures. The patient experiences loss of appetite, depression, and anxiety about his condition. Concerns about death are real and must be considered by the nursing staff planning for the patient's support and maintenance of his well-being. A positive and trusting relationship with the nurse is essential to both the patient and his family. Family members must be helped to discern how they can best convey love and trust and acceptance to the person who feels "messy" and disfigured as a result of the surgery. All these measures are accomplished with regard for the patient's need for independence and acceptance. Rejection is not an uncommon feeling, because the patient knows and reacts strongly to his or her own disfigurement and expects to be rejected by others. Coping with the feeling of rejection is a basic focus of the nursing care. Creativity in restructuring the nose through use of bone and tissue grafts and adjunctive materials often results in a good cosmetic appearance although nasal and sinus functions may be permanently impaired.

The occurrence of nasal cancer is somewhat related to industrial pollutants. There is a high incidence of nasal cancer in persons who are exposed to wood dusts, such as furniture makers. Exposure to certain chemicals and metals such as nickel tend to be related to the incidence of nasal cancer.

There are many unanswered questions about the nasal functions and the relationships of nasal dysfunction to systemic diseases. The sense of smell is little understood, although it is known how the passage of air through the nose contributes to the articulation of words. It is postulated that some persons are particularly susceptible to respiratory diseases and that there may be a relation between the nasal and tracheobronchial clearance through the mucus and ciliary action. People with chronic respiratory conditions, including bronchitis and asthma, also have a tendency to have sinusitis or nasal allergies. Because of these relationships, people with nasal dysfunction are advised not to work in industries where they will be exposed to dusts or gases that may be harmful to the lower respiratory airways as well as to the nasal passages.

Some people affected with nasal discomfort become addicted to nose drops and steam inhalation. Overuse of nose drops should be avoided; **rhinitis medicamentosa** may occur with overuse. In this condition, there is rebound swelling after the initial effect of the nose drops has worn off. Treatment is simply stopping the use of the nose drops. It should be noted by nurses that water aerosols breathed through the nose are ineffective for humidifying the airways beyond the nose. Ultrasonic nebulizers provide finer vapor that reaches more deeply into the nasal passages. Because of their questionable effectiveness, the use of nebulization therapy and of water aerosols may not be beneficial since nebulizers can be a source of infection.

People with debilitating diseases may also have nasal discomfort related to dry indoor air or to medications they are taking. Certain medications dry all mucous membranes, including those in the nose. Hypertensive drugs in the rauwolfia group can cause nasal obstruction, as can hypothyroidism. The nurse should be aware of the patient's potential nasal discomfort, and should take measures to provide for appropriate intervention. Many people habitually use patent medications such as ointments containing menthol to moisten and soothe their nasal passages. As part of the total assessment of the patient's needs, the nurse should ascertain if the person does experience nasal discomfort and how he or she usually relieves this discomfort. If the person uses acceptable methods, these should become part of the hospitalized person's care. If, however, the methods the person has been using are potentially harmful, such as overuse of nose drops, the nurse should teach the person to use more appropriate methods.

Facial Injuries

Facial injuries can involve any aspect of the face, including the bony framework, the cartilaginous structures, and the soft tissues. These injuries are always life-threatening if they compromise the airways. Early assessment focuses on respiratory status, followed by assessment of the extent of the injury. Facial injuries are treated as early as possible to prevent deformity, to achieve maximum function of the involved parts, and to reduce the cosmetic defects.

Assessment of the respiratory status includes search for any foreign materials that might be present in the oropharynx; broken dentures or debris from external sources or vomitus must be removed. The tongue may be displaced if there is central nervous system impairment. The tongue may also be injured by blunt or sharp objects, causing edema and obstruction of the airways by the swollen tongue. The larynx or tracheal cartilages can be injured from either direct or indirect trauma, and suction and intubation are life-saving in occlusion of the air passages. Often the patient requires support of mechanical ventilation.

Hemorrhage is also treated immediately. Pressure applied externally controls bleeding from external lacerations. Application of packs or occlusive dressings may be necessary for hemostasis in bleeding in the nostrils, mouth, or sinuses. Efforts are made to prevent swallowing of blood to prevent later gastrointestinal distress and to provide for some measure of estimating blood loss. Laboratory analysis is essential to confirm blood loss (Chap. 16).

The nurse should remember that extensive pressure on the facial nerve can cause damage to the nerve; therefore pressure should be applied only with sufficient force and sufficient duration to stop the bleeding.

Pain associated with facial injuries is often mild. Narcotics are contraindicated if the patient has respiratory difficulty or if central nervous system damage is suspected.

Once the patient has been examined and priority needs have been cared for, the management of facial injuries that are not life-threatening is begun. A determination of the extent of the injuries is made by careful examination of the soft tissues of the face and neck and of the underlying bony framework. Facial wounds are carefully cleaned to remove all foreign debris and care is taken to prevent further damage to the tissues. Because facial injuries are usually not painful, the cleaning can usually be accomplished without anesthesia.

Special consideration is given to assessment of the facial nerve function and to lacerations of the ducts, including the lacrimal and parotid ducts. These require surgical treatment in the operating room. Superficial facial lacerations may be repaired in the emergency room. Following cleaning, debridement of nonviable tissue is done. All viable tissue is retained because the face has an excellent blood supply and healing usually progresses well. Repair of lacerations is easier if accomplished prior to the onset of swelling. Careful repair of lacerations is done to achieve the best cosmetic results possible.

Fractures of the facial bones can be difficult to assess, particularly in the presence of edema. The nurse should obtain x-rays of the facial bones if the patient's condition warrants. This facilitates diagnosis and treatment by the physician. Crushing injuries may cause damage to any of the structures of the face. An ophthalmologist should be called if there is damage to the eyes.

The face absorbs stress, thus protecting the cranium. Many small fractures of the facial bones may occur in various patterns, interfering with the sinuses, the eyes, the nasal septum, and the dental structures. Specific types of facial fractures are discussed briefly in terms of treatment and nursing care in the following paragraphs.

Fractures of the orbit may cause displacement of the eye. Diplopia is a frequent sign, as is limitation of eye motion. Mandibular fractures are assessed by noting preauricular pain when the bite is closed, malocclusion, or displacement of the mandible to one side. Maxillary fractures are determined by unusual motion of the maxilla, either segmental or total. Epistaxis, drainage of cerebrospinal fluid, crepitation, and obvious displacement indicate fractures of the nose. The nurse should observe for rhinorrhea of cerebrospinal fluid, indicated by clear drainage that can be differentiated from mucus by determining the mucin or glucose content of the drainage. Cerebrospinal fluid glucose is approximately half that of serum glucose levels [1].

Repair of facial fractures is often difficult because maintenance of reduction is impeded by lack of stable structures to which attachments can be made. Careful examination, cleaning of the wound, and approximation of all structures usually requires anesthesia. A variety of methods are used to stabilize the fractured part; wires, pins, packs, and special arch bars are all used. External splinting of the part is done to stabilize structures when appropriate.

Mandibular fractures can be stabilized with interdental wiring or with arch bars in **closed reduction methods.** Kirshner wires may be used in **open reduction** to stabilize bone fragments. In some instances both Kirshner wires and interdental wiring are necessary. Maxillary fractures also require stabilization with either open or closed reduction or both, depending on the extent of the fracture (Fig. 13-7). Both mandibular fractures and maxillary fractures require attention to the status of the teeth. It is necessary to place the teeth in proper approximation. Splints applied exter-

Ear, Nose, and Throat Dysfunction **1069**

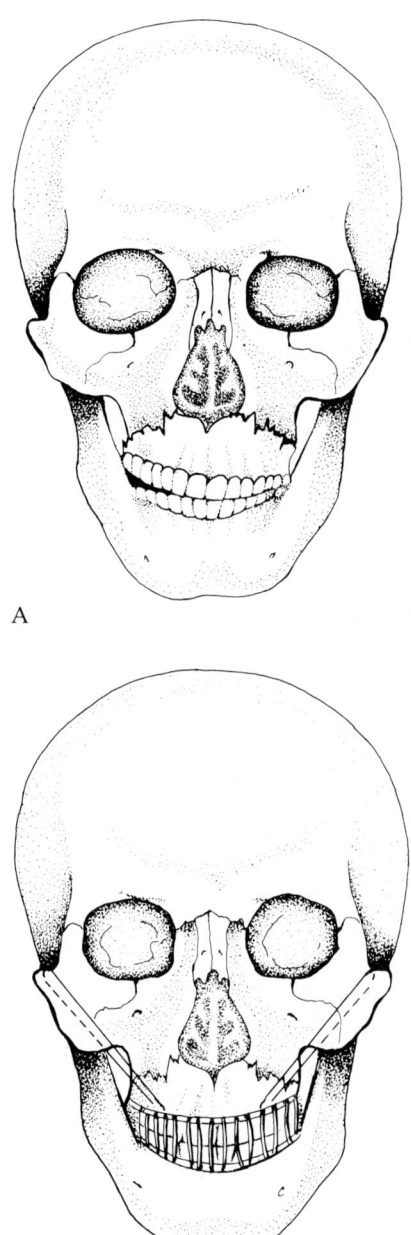

Figure 13-7
A. Transverse maxillary fracture. **B.** Transverse fracture stabilization with circumzygomatic wires to arch bar. (From C. W. Sproul and P. J. Mullanney, *Emergency Care, Assessment and Intervention.* St. Louis: Mosby, 1974. Reproduced by permission.)

nally are necessary to hold loose teeth in place. If the person wears dentures, these may be incorporated into the stabilization procedure with wiring and arches to hold them in place.

Nursing care for patients with maxillary or mandibular fractures includes provision of nutrition in liquid form and careful oral hygiene to provide comfort and the cleanliness necessary to prevent infection without disrupting the stabilization achieved by wiring. The nurse carefully inspects the mouth and teeth to make certain that there are no loose wires or that the wires do not protrude to cause irritation or damage to the mucous membranes of the mouth. A patient cannot communicate easily with "wired jaws" and communication methods must be found that are easily understood by the patient and the nurse as well as by others. Pain and discomfort also interfere with talking. When the pain and discomfort decrease the patient can articulate words more comfortably even though the teeth are wired together. Appearance is of great concern to many people with facial fractures. The nurse should give realistic explanations of the amount of damage that has been sustained and prepare the patient for ongoing treatment that may be required for dental repair, or further cosmetic surgery if appropriate, following consultation with the physician. The nurse can be instrumental in helping the patient develop the patience necessary during the healing period by providing for diversional activities and by listening to the patient's concerns. When the dental involvement is extensive, the repair may take weeks, months, or years. The time and effort expended by the person and the dentist are realized in the reconstruction of near normal or normal abilities for function and for appearance.

Fractures of the zygoma occur frequently and require repair with wires for fixation (Fig. 13-8). Facial contours may be impaired if there has been significant bone splintering. These contours are repaired with adjunctive materials such as Silastic or bone grafts, if there is insufficient tissue in the area for repair. Extraocular muscles may be involved and require reduction of the fracture as soon as possible to prevent muscle damage. Reduction of these fractures may require external incisions so that the patient has an incision line that must be observed following surgery. Healing of fractures is further discussed in Chapter 10.

Fractures of the nose may involve any of the

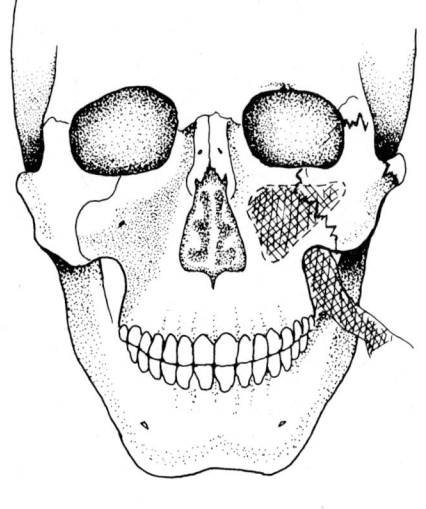

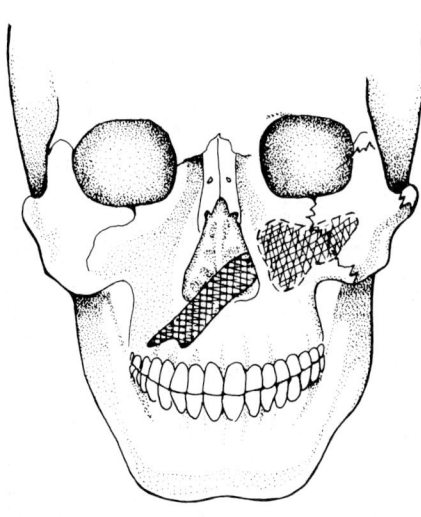

Figure 13-8
Intra-antral gauze stabilization for fractured zygomatic compound. **A.** Oral exit. **B.** Nasal antrostomy exit. (From C. W. Sproul and P. J. Mullanney, *Emergency Care, Assessment and Intervention*. St. Louis: Mosby, 1974. Reproduced by permission.)

aspects of the nasal structure. They are repaired via the techniques previously discussed for nasal reconstruction. Rhinoplasty involves reduction of the fractures, approximation of all of the fragments, repair of the cartilage or nasal lining, and fixation, using nasal packs and external splints.

Patients who undergo repair of nasal fractures have the same needs as those following any rhinoplasty. They require special attention to nutrition, to oral hygiene, and to observation for bleeding or disruption of the packs or splints. Edema may be severe and may hinder vision; thus the nurse must provide for the patient's safety in use of articles and in ambulation. Placement of personal articles within the patient's reach is helpful in preventing accidents and in encouraging the patient to feel more self-sufficient. Nausea is a common symptom and antiemetics and comfort measures are necessary to prevent vomiting that can disrupt the repair.

Depending on the type and extent of facial injury, further reconstructive surgery following initial healing for revision of scars or for building up facial structures may be required. Often these reconstructive procedures necessitate several sequential surgeries with both bone and skin grafting. Use of adjunctive materials for reconstructing the framework of the ears, the nose, and the orbits has greatly facilitated the surgeon's efforts in this extensive and very delicate series of operations. While the outcomes of the surgical procedures are gratifying for both the surgeon and the patient, there are times throughout the extensive waiting periods and healing phases when the patient may become discouraged and doubt the usefulness of the efforts involved. The nurse who recognizes these feelings can take measures to help the patient express his or her feelings and to acquaint him or her with others who have had similar experiences. Use of pictures and personal contact with others often restores the goal orientation. Continued support and understanding on the part of the nurse is invaluable to the patient.

Although the surgeon often uses preinjury pictures of the patient to reconstruct the features, exact replication of features is often not possible. Therefore the patient must adjust to a new appearance and cope with all the questions, curious looks, and comments directed to him from acquaintances. The facility with which the patient adjusts is highly individual, and the nurse should be aware that personality characteristics and pretrauma behavioral patterns are important factors in the patient's adjustment. The alert nurse recognizes the need for counseling and emotional therapy and provides the patient with adequate resources when possible and appropriate.

The Pharynx

The pharynx connects the nasal passages and the trachea and is a passageway for both air and nutrients. Dysfunction of the pharynx may occur as a result of infection or from irritation caused by foods and fluids that contain spices or are hot in temperature. Noxious gases also cause irritation of the pharynx. Changes in cell structure, such as cysts and benign or malignant tumors, can occur in the pharynx. Usually the pharynx is examined in conjunction with examination of the nose and mouth. The three major divisions of the pharynx are the nasopharynx, the oropharynx, and the hypopharynx. The oropharynx is most easily examined, while the nasopharynx, the soft palate, and the hypopharynx cannot be visualized without a mirror and a reflecting light.

When the pharynx is to be examined, a tongue blade is used to keep the tongue from obscuring the examiner's view of the pharynx. Correct placement of the tongue blade on the middle third of the tongue prevents gagging and curling of the tongue, both of which hinder visualization. The gag reflex is initiated if the tongue blade is placed on the posterior part of the tongue or on the tonsils. The tongue curls if the blade is placed on the anterior third of the tongue. People vary in their ability to tolerate the tongue blade without gagging. If the tongue or pharynx is inflamed, examination of the throat can be painful or uncomfortable.

Landmarks in the oropharynx include the uvula (the fleshy portion of the soft palate above the tongue), which is pink in color and variable in size. The anterior tonsillar pillar is the tissue connecting the tongue and palate; the posterior tonsillar pillar is located behind the anterior tonsillar pillar. Waldeyer's tonsillar ring is composed of lymphoid tissue forming the pharyngeal, palatine, and lingual tonsils and the lateral pharyngeal bands. The pharyngeal tonsil is more commonly referred to as the adenoid. When examining the walls of the pharynx and the tonsils the examiner proceeds systematically, first examining one side and then the other. The presence and character of mucus, pus, discoloration, or inflammation are noted. Having the patient say "ah" enables the examiner to better visualize the posterior pharynx. The uvula should be located in the midline and should not deviate to one side; the tonsils should appear equal on both sides.

Following examination of the pharynx, the cervical lymph nodes are palpated with the tips of the fingers of both hands. The locations of cervical lymph nodes vary, and the examiner must therefore systematically palpate the neck posteriorly, laterally, and anteriorly. The areas anterior and posterior to the pinna of the ear and along the junction of the mandible and the course of the jugular vein and carotid artery are usually examined with a smooth downward motion of the hands, using the fingertips to feel for enlarged nodes. The entire neck area is then lightly palpated, including the posterior neck. Normally the nodes are not palpable. The parotid glands may be palpable in the elderly and in disease states. These glands lie downward below the ear and into the upper neck at the angle of the jaw. The neck may be enlarged from the presence of a thyroid goiter or from abnormal cell growth in the pharynx, trachea, or larynx. The sternocleidomastoid and trapezius muscles should be equal on both sides of the neck. To check this aspect the examiner stands slightly away from the patient and observes for symmetry of the neck.

Infections are the most common cause of dysfunction of the pharynx and are often related to infections of the sinuses or of the respiratory tract. Sinusitis may cause inflammation as mucoid material drains postnasally into the pharynx to be swallowed. Infected teeth may cause sore throat, as can many infections or disorders of the oral cavity. A number of disease processes are associated with sore throat. For example, dehydration results in dryness of all mucous membranes. Breathing through the mouth in sleep may cause one to awaken with a sore throat that disappears after eating breakfast or brushing the teeth. Certain communicable diseases such as measles may be associated with a sore throat. Leukemia often causes soreness of the throat.

In general, children are more susceptible to the development of sore throats than are adults. Exceptions are adults who are continually exposed to dry air or to pollutants such as inhaled gases, cigarette smoke, or environmental pollutants in inspired air, and those with hypersensitivity reactions. Pharyngitis associated with respiratory dysfunction from bacteria or viruses is discussed in Chapter 3. Viral infections occur with greater frequency than do bacterial infections.

Tonsillitis most frequently occurs in the palatine tonsils, but may involve all the tonsils. Reddened, swollen tonsils with purulent debris in the crypts are indicative of tonsillitis. The condition may be either acute or chronic and is generally treated with antibiotics following throat culture and sensitivity tests. Gargles or throat irrigations are prescribed to reduce the inflammation (warm saline is usually prescribed). Fluids are given to prevent dehydration. A tonsillectomy may be performed when chronic tonsillitis does not respond to treatment or when the enlarged tonsils obstruct the eustachian tube openings or interfere with swallowing. It has been postulated that chronic tonsillitis is associated with the development of rheumatism and certain other systemic diseases. Tonsillectomies are performed only when necessary, however, as some authorities believe that the tonsils have immunologically protective functions. Following removal of the palatine tonsils, lingual tonsillitis may occur. The symptoms are similar to inflammation or infection of the palatine tonsils: low grade fever, soreness when swallowing or talking, and pain referred to the ear.

The adenoids may also become inflamed or enlarged. The latter may require removal if enlargement is great enough to consistently interfere with swallowing or if the eustachian tubes are blocked. Enlarged adenoids cause snoring, rhinitis, and a twangy monotone voice. The voice change is related to blockage of the posterior choanae, which connect the nasal passages with the nasopharynx. People with enlarged adenoids tend to breathe through their mouths because of the obstruction of the airways.

Adenoid facies is a condition in which there are characteristic changes in the nares, palate, and teeth. The nares are narrowed and have a pinched appearance. The palate is usually arched, and the teeth are crowded together. It is not known whether these changes precede or result from enlarged adenoids. In addition to these changes there is rhinitis; there also may be collection of fluid in the middle ear or otitis media. Diagnosis includes either posterior rhinoscopy or lateral x-ray of the nasopharynx.

The adenoids are usually removed along with the tonsils, a procedure referred to as T and A (tonsillectomy and adenoidectomy). Children have T and A's more frequently than adults because the adenoids normally atrophy about the time of adolescence; adults rarely have enlarged adenoids. Preparation for tonsillectomy or adenoidectomy or both includes blood tests for complete blood count, leukocyte count, hemoglobin and hematocrit, bleeding and clotting time, serologic tests, and a throat culture. Active infections and diseases that interfere with normal clotting, such as hemophilia, are contraindications. A general anesthetic is usually required, but some adults require only a local anesthetic.

Postoperatively, the patient may have a postnasal pack in place. The packing provides for hemostasis if there is considerable or uncontrollable bleeding. Bleeding vessels are often cauterized in surgery. Packing soaked in a hemostatic agent such as epinephrine is usually used. The patient recovering from general anesthesia is placed on his or her side with the head lowered to facilitate drainage by gravity and to prevent aspiration of drainage. Because hemorrhage is the most frequent postoperative complication following tonsillectomy, the vital signs are checked frequently. Signs and symptoms of bleeding are monitored and include paleness, tachycardia, decreased blood pressure, and frequent swallowing of drainage in the throat. The throat is inspected routinely by depressing the tongue with a tongue blade to visualize the tonsillar bed to note drainage and to observe for the presence of blood clots. The blood clots can indicate the source of bleeding. A flashlight provides a good light source for inspection of the throat. In some patients bleeding may not occur until about the fifth postoperative day so that the patient is taught how to inspect the throat as a self-care measure to be carried out at home. Bleeding beyond the first week after the tonsillectomy is infrequent. Whenever bleeding does occur, surgical intervention for ligation of the bleeding vessels is necessary. Another indication of bleeding is coffee-ground emesis or dark stools caused by swallowing blood. If the patient notes these signs, the physician should be notified.

Following tonsillectomy, a secondary infection can occur within a few days. Pain and soreness of the throat and sometimes earache are to be expected and may mask infection. Some physicians give antibiotics prophylactically. The patient is told that his postoperative pain will include earache because of referred pain to the tympanic membrane. A soft diet with soothing foods (e.g., ice cream) is prescribed according to the patient's tolerance. Postoperative nausea is a frequent occurrence, especially if the patient has swallowed a quantity of blood or if he or she has a reaction to the anesthetic. Ice chips are helpful for their soothing effect and for hydration when the patient is nauseous. Coughing and clearing the throat should be avoided in the early postoperative phase. There is considerable variation in the recovery time following tonsillectomy. An ice collar may be used to relieve discomfort.

A **peritonsillar abscess** is called **quinsy** and it usually occurs as a complication of tonsillitis. The throat is usually sore and edematous with resulting dysphagia and pain or soreness when speaking. Pus can collect under the tonsil and displace it toward the midline. The uvula is usually displaced also and is swollen. The soft palate appears reddened. Trismus (tonic spasm of the jaw muscles) and difficulty in opening the mouth may occur because of irritation of the pterygoid muscles. Sometimes the patient appears to have a stiff neck and holds his head toward the affected side.

Quinsy may occur with or without pus formation. When an abscess forms it may rupture spontaneously or, more often, it may require incision and drainage. The actual incision is usually painful, but the relief following the incision is considerable. Unless a tonsillectomy is done after the abscess has resolved, peritonsillar abscesses tend to recur.

Infections of the mouth may extend to the throat. These infections include thrush and trench mouth. **Thrush,** or **Ludwig's angina,** is caused by *Candida albicans*, a yeast-like organism normally found in the mouth. The infection usually occurs on the floor of the mouth in the spaces between muscles, with formation of white patches that can extend to the tissues of the pharynx and tonsils. This infection is most common in debilitated patients (because of lowered resistance), in those who have had extensive antibiotic therapy, and in diabetics. Treatment includes the use of nystatin (Mycostatin). Gentian violet may be used to paint the white patches. The nurse should be aware that gentian violet stains clothes and skin.

Trench mouth, or **Vincent's angina,** is caused by a combination of gram-negative anaerobic bacterium, *Fusobacterium mecrophorum*, and a spirochete, *Borrelia vincentii*. These organisms are normal in the mouth and do not cause infection unless the patient's resistance is lower due to injury or tissue damage, viral infection, malnutrition, or poor oral hygiene. The gums, pharynx, and tonsils may be affected with ulcerating lesions, which may appear gray and which have a tendency to bleed. Sore throat, low grade fever, and lymphadenitis occur. Mouthwashes and throat irrigation with oxygen-releasing preparations such as half-strength hydrogen peroxide are used in treatment.

Inflamed or obstructed salivary glands can affect the pharynx. Obstructions can be caused by formation of calculi, strictures, or trauma from rubbing of teeth along the duct or from biting the cheek. The ducts can be examined with a probe and by injecting contrast media and taking x-rays.

Types of abnormal cell growth include thyroglossal duct cysts, lingual thyroid, and tumors. The thyroglossal ducts usually form from an embryonic remnant generally found in the anterior midline of the neck. Treatment is excision of the cyst.

Lingual thyroids may occur as the only functioning thyroid tissue or in addition to a normally functioning thyroid. This feature is investigated prior to treatment by excision to determine whether the patient is dependent on the lingual thyroid for normal function. Symptoms of lingual thyroid include edema of the tongue posteriorly with dysphagia or voice changes. These symptoms may not occur until adulthood, even though the lingual thyroid has been present since birth.

Tumors most frequently occurring in the pharynx include angiofibroma, squamous cell carcinoma, lymphosarcoma, reticulum cell sarcoma, and pleomorphic adenoma. Angiofibromas are generally located on the lateral or anterior wall of the nasopharynx and are initially highly vascular. As they enlarge they may obstruct the nares and extend as far as the orbits of the eyes or back toward the base of the skull. Deafness may be a result.

Pleomorphic adenomas are usually located on the lateral wall of the nasopharynx and extend to the cervical lymph nodes. These adenomas also may invade the eustachian tubes or the base of the skull. Squamous cell carcinoma of the tonsil can be invasive or exophytic and extend to the base of the tongue, causing sore throat and pain radiating to the ear. These carcinomas may become very large and can then be observed as a mass in the neck. With all these tumors, diagnosis by biopsy followed by radiation is the treatment. A radical neck dissection may be performed when the tumors are large or extended, usually 6 weeks after completion of the x-ray therapy. As with radical surgery for lesions in the neck, the extent of the neck dissection is often based on the extent of cervical lymph node involvement in the pharynx, trachea, larynx, thyroid, or the oral cavity.

Nursing care in dysfunction of the pharynx begins with a thorough examination of the pharynx and the surrounding structures. Disease processes first occurring in the oral cavity, ears, sinuses, the nose, or the lower or upper respiratory tract may all affect the pharynx and cause similar symptoms. Most often these symptoms include soreness, pain, dysphagia, difficulty in speaking because of pain or soreness, trismus (tonic spasm of the law muscles), earache from referred pain, and irritation noticed when eating very sweet or very sour foods. Changes in the voice and otitis media may occur from edema or obstruction. The treatment, to be effective, must be based on the causes of the symptoms.

Sore throat or irritation of the throat is common, and there are many patent medications available for self-treatment. People often tend to treat themselves, using a number of different types of remedies. While some of these remedies are adequate for viral sore throats, none are adequate for treatment of a bacterial infection that requires antibiotics or for treatment of changes in cell growth. The nurse must teach principles of positive health care and preventive medicine by encouraging people to seek adequate medical examinations if they have recurring pharyngitis or persistent throat irritation. Lozenges, irrigations, and aspirin are usually effective for viral infections and following tonsillectomy to reduce irritation and soreness. The nurse should teach the person who requires irrigations how to correctly instill the irrigating solution so that it comes into contact with the irritated tissues. Finally, the nurse should always be alert to the possibility that the pharynx may be irritated because of other disease processes. Careful observation and recording of symptoms are important in following the progress of a person who tends to have a chronic throat condition.

The Larynx

The larynx functions as a guard to prevent aspiration of food and fluid into the lungs, as a passage for air in respiration, and as a vibrator to produce voice sounds in phonation. Extending from the pharynx to the trachea, the **larynx** is made up of cartilages, muscles, and ligaments. The **epiglottis,** which is a cartilage, and the aryepiglottic folds form the inlet of the vestibule of the larynx. The thyroid cartilage, forming the front and upper section of the larynx, is the largest of the laryngeal cartilages. Other cartilages include the arytenoid, corniculate, cuneiform, and cricoid and form the remainder of the structure of the larynx. As the only completely circular cartilage, the cricoid cartilage maintains the patency of the larynx.

Both the true and false vocal cords are located in the glottis. The true vocal cords are attached to the thyroid cartilage and the arytenoid cartilage. Contraction and relaxation of the laryngeal muscles stretch and relax the vocal cords. The transverse arytenoid muscle approximates the cords for sound production. Contraction of the posterior cricoarytenoid muscles stretches the vocal cords while the lateral cricoarytenoid muscles pull the arytenoid cartilages forward and apart to open the airways for respiration. The lumen of the larynx is smallest in the glottis; approximation of the vocal cords further narrows the diameter of the larynx. Both the intrinsic and extrinsic laryngeal muscles are innervated by the superior and inferior recurrent laryngeal nerves, which are branches of the vagus. The superior laryngeal nerve provides sensation to the mucous membranes and innervates the cricothyroid muscle. The inferior laryngeal branch of the vagus supplies motor innervation for the intrinsic muscles (Fig. 13-9).

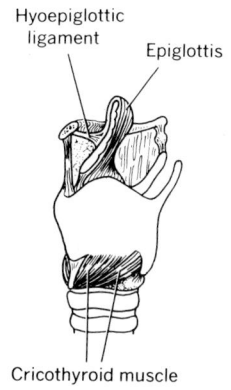
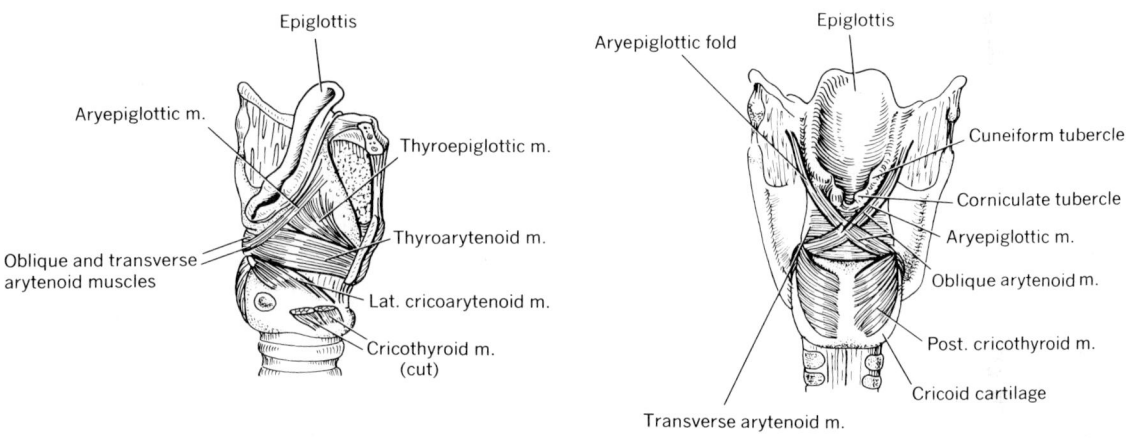
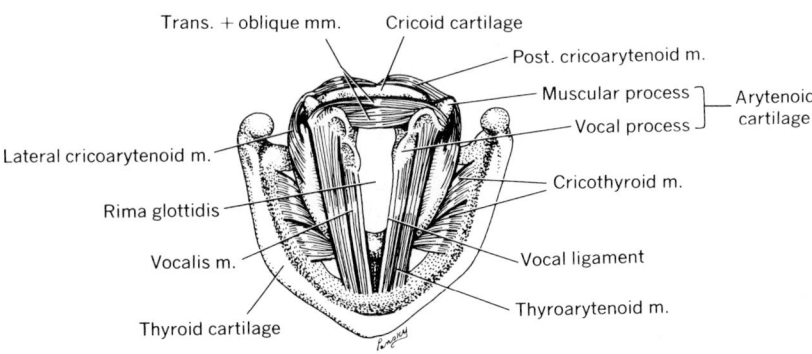

Figure 13-9
Intrinsic muscles of the larynx. (From B. Pansky, *Dynamic Anatomy and Physiology*. New York: Macmillan, 1975. Reproduced by permission.)

1075

The glottis functions as a valve or sphincter, changing shape by opening during inspiration and becoming triangular at rest and linear during phonation. Closing of the glottis helps to stabilize the thorax and the diaphragm when a person strains to lift a heavy object, to urinate, or to defecate. Any activity that pulls the shoulder muscles expands the thoracic cage, closing the glottis and limiting the passage of air from the thorax (Valsalva maneuver; see Chaps. 3 and 4). The glottis guards the entrance of the respiratory airways by closing when swallowing takes place. When the glottis closes, the epiglottis is drawn over the closed sphincters so that food and fluids pass into the pyriform sinuses and into the esophagus.

Phonation is produced by vibrations of the vocal cords as air passes through the glottis. Pitch is a function of the stretching and relaxing movements of the vocal cords. Changes in the frequency of vibrations are the source of the melodious quality of the voice. High frequency sounds are produced by upward movement of the entire larynx, which tenses and shortens the true vocal cords, whereas bass sounds are produced by downward movement or loosening of the entire larynx, with relaxation and lengthening of the true vocal cords. Frequency is also adjusted by changing the approximation of the vocal cord edges. High frequency occurs when the sharp edges of the cord are approximated while low frequency occurs when the broad edges are approximated. Tone is articulated in speech by the pharynx, palate, tongue, teeth, and lips.

Internally the larynx is covered with connective tissue and mucous membrane lined with ciliated epithelial cells and a few goblet cells. Squamous epithelial cells cover the portion of the larynx that comes in contact with food or fluids. Externally, there are two laryngeal landmarks. The first is known as the Adam's apple, or laryngeal prominence, which is formed by the fusion of thyroid cartilage laminae. The second is the anterior prominence of the cricoid cartilage.

Assessment of laryngeal function includes observation of movement of the external landmarks, inspection of the skin, palpation of the neck for determination of tenderness or swelling or loss of motion of the underlying structures, and laryngoscopic examination. There are two types of laryngoscopy, direct and indirect. **Indirect laryngoscopy** is a technique in which the throat is first sprayed with an anesthetic agent. A warmed mirror is then passed through the mouth into place against the soft palate so that a mirror image of the movements of respiration and phonation is seen as the person breathes normally and says "ee." **Direct laryngoscopy** provides direct visualization of the larynx. Either a rigid or a flexible fiberoptic laryngoscope is used. The rigid laryngoscope requires anesthesia and is somewhat limiting in the area of the interior of the larynx that can be visualized. The flexible fiberoptic laryngoscope can be inserted through the nose or mouth and does not require anesthesia. Visualization of the internal larynx is better with the flexible scope.

Prior to laryngoscopy, the patient is premedicated to induce relaxation; foods and fluids are withheld. After laryngoscopy, if anesthesia has been given, monitoring of vital signs and respiratory status is imperative. The patient cannot be given food or fluids until the swallowing reflex returns. Soreness of the throat is expected and is treated with soothing gargles and lozenges.

Dysfunction of the larynx can result from infection, inhalation of irritants, or impairment of the innervation of the larynx. Trauma or changes in cell growth can also cause dysfunction. Voice changes are usually an early symptom of laryngeal dysfunction from any cause. Because tone is produced by movement of the vocal cords, any changes in cord movement result in either asynchrony or aperiodicity of vibration so that harmony is disrupted. A monotone voice results from loss of flexibility of the cords. When the cords do not approximate, air is wasted and the voice has a breathy quality. Hoarseness and complete aphonia are caused by failure of the cords to approximate. Respiratory distress with dyspnea, stridor, or asphyxiation occurs if the larynx is occluded. Dysphagia may result from edema or changes in tissue mass.

Laryngitis occurs commonly with upper respiratory infections such as colds, tonsillitis, sinusitis, or respiratory influenza. The symptoms of laryngitis include hoarseness, sore throat, and dysphagia as the vocal cords become edematous and there is concomitant muscle paresis. Voice rest and inhalation of steam relieve the symptoms and allow for healing.

When laryngitis is associated with pharyngitis, the free edges of the epiglottis may be edematous. In this situation, Fowler's position (semireclining) facilitates breathing and swallowing. Antihistamines and epinephrine may be given to reduce the edema.

Laryngitis may become chronic in persons who use their voices excessively, or in association with chronic tonsillitis or sinusitis, or in infections of the teeth. Prolonged exposure to atmospheric pollutants, to fumes or irritants such as cigarette smoking and either very dry or very humid climates, may also cause chronic laryngitis. Usually the major symptom is hoarseness that is more noticeable in the morning. The person may have a constant feeling that he needs to clear his throat and often experiences a cough with production of mucous plugs. If hoarseness persists for more than 2 weeks, the person should have a thorough examination, including laryngoscopy. Dysphagia and dyspnea may occur. Treatment includes voice rest, lozenges and soothing gargles, frequent oral hygiene, and steam inhalation.

Impairment of innervation results in laryngeal paralysis and may occur in diseases that affect the motor neurons or with lesions involving either the medulla or the vagus nerve. Brainstem lesions, acoustic neuronomas, meningitis, or basal skull fractures may damage the vagus nerve as it passes to the jugular foramen in the neck. The recurrent laryngeal nerves are susceptible to trauma because of their position in the groove between the trachea and the esophagus. These nerves may be involved in disease processes affecting either the esophagus or the thyroid. The laryngeal nerves are subject to damage in thyroid surgery. The left recurrent laryngeal nerve may also be involved in tissue changes of structures in the mediastinum. Because this nerve is located in the lower part of the superior mediastinum, disease processes of the lung and mediastinal structures such as aortic aneurysms or carcinoma of the thoracic esophagus may involve the left recurrent laryngeal nerve.

Paralysis of the vocal cords may be incomplete, complete, unilateral, or bilateral. Function of the adductor muscles is retained when incomplete paralysis exists so that the cord lies adducted to the midline. In complete paralysis, the cord lies between full abduction and adduction. When there is incomplete paralysis, the normal cord can adduct to the paralyzed cord so that phonation is possible, and the hoarseness may be transient. In instances of complete unilateral paralysis, the normal cord does not meet the affected cord so that the person whispers and cannot cough normally. As a compensatory measure, the normal cord may move across the midline to meet the affected cord. This occludes the larynx and causes respiratory distress, requiring tracheostomy. If the respiratory distress is noticed only on exertion, a tracheostomy tube with a flap valve may be used to allow for inspiration during distress. If the respiratory distress is severe, however, a standard tracheostomy tube is used.

Another method of treatment is surgical intervention in which the more affected cord is fixed so that it does not occlude the larynx, allowing for passage of air. When this operation is done the patient cannot speak audibly because phonation cannot occur with an immobilized vocal cord.

When paralysis of the vocal cords is caused by brainstem lesions, the prognosis is grave. The paralysis is often bilateral and although the airways may be sufficient, the patient cannot cough effectively as the sphincter action does not function. There is also danger of aspiration of food and saliva; supplemental gavage feedings may be necessary to minimize aspiration in swallowing. As with paralysis of the vocal cords from other causes, airways may be blocked by the paralyzed cords and require tracheostomy.

Functional aphonia is a disorder in which there is paralysis of the adductors of both vocal cords. It usually results from emotional stress and can be differentiated from true paralysis if the cords do not adduct on phonation but do adduct for coughing. There is a sudden loss of voice; recovery is just as sudden. There is no specific treatment except for speech therapy and emotional counseling to deal with resolution of the emotional stress.

Trauma to the larynx may be caused by aspiration of a foreign body, with serious consequences. **Cafe coronary** is the term used to describe the symptoms experienced when a person has aspirated a bolus of food. When foreign bodies are aspirated, they may be retained in the larynx. If the foreign body is sharp, it may lodge in the mucous membrane. Large, soft foreign bodies may be caught between the vocal cords. Laryngospasm occurs in response to the foreign body so that the larynx may become completely occluded. Presence of a foreign body is diagnosed by observing passage of air. If the larynx is occluded, there will be no air passage and the patient will have suprasternal, intercostal, and subxiphoid retraction. Emergency care to establish an airway is important as the patient may suffocate if no action is taken. If the person has swallowed a bolus of food he may be helped in one of two ways. The first is to remove the bolus by pulling the tongue forward and by a tweezer or forcep action, with two fingers, grasping and removing the bolus. If this maneuver is not effective, pressure is used to remove the bolus by having someone stand behind the person who is choking and encircle him below the level of the diaphragm with arms clasped in front of him. The person standing behind applies pressure with the arms and hands. Changes in air pressure caused by compression of the rib cage may be sufficient to force the bolus of food outward. If this is not effective, it is necessary to establish an airway by performing an emergency cricothyroidotomy. This procedure is explained in Chapter 3.

Even though foreign bodies may not completely occlude the larynx, they may cause enough respiratory distress to require tracheostomy. Removal of foreign bodies from the larynx is accomplished by laryngoscopy and requires general anesthesia.

Among other types of trauma that affect the larynx are fractures, crushing injuries, and prolonged endotracheal intubation. People with long, thin necks are more susceptible to fractures of the larynx involving the hyoid bone. Those with short, thick necks are more susceptible to fractures of the cricoid cartilage. Usually trauma of the larynx causes hoarseness or aphonia. There may be hemoptysis; immediate care involves provision for an adequate airway by suctioning the blood and mucus. A tracheostomy may be required. Edema may form later, resulting in dyspnea or respiratory distress. Therefore, observation and monitoring of vital signs and respiratory status are important aspects of nursing care following trauma.

Examination of the larynx is carried out as soon as possible following trauma to determine whether there are lacerations of the mucous membranes, the cartilages are exposed, or the cords are paralyzed. If the cricoid cartilage is lacerated, it must be repaired immediately because it is the only complete circular cartilage, and when it is damaged, the larynx tends to close. Repair of these injuries is usually accomplished through a transverse incision of the neck and direct repair of the larynx. If the alignment of the larynx has been interrupted, a solid core mold is sometimes left in place following surgery to provide for healing with correct internal alignment of the larynx. A total laryngectomy may be necessary if the larynx cannot be repaired. Any trauma to the lining of the larynx should be repaired as soon as possible; laryngeal stenosis may occur if treatment is not initiated soon enough.

When the repair does not take place soon after injury, it may be necessary to perform surgical procedures to relieve stenosis or to repair tracheoesophageal fistulas to restore the function of the larynx. Among the procedures used for this purpose are arytenoidectomy, supraglottic partial laryngectomy, and subglottic excision of the area of stenosis. Healing of the larynx with these procedures may require a period of 4 to 6 weeks or more. Without repair, the patient may experience voice loss, obstruction of the airways, or dysphagia.

Changes in cell growth or structure result in varying degrees of laryngeal dysfunction. Among the types of cellular growths are laryngoceles, vocal nodules, laryngeal polyps, ulcers, papillomas, and keratoses.

Laryngoceles are diverticuli of the epithelial lining of the mucous membrane. Depending on their location, laryngoceles may either displace or cause enlargement of the false vocal cord. The symptoms are hoarseness, respiratory distress, and discomfort. External laryngoceles may be seen as a mass in the neck, which rises with the larynx when swallowing takes place. Formation of laryngoceles is most common in musicians who play wind instruments and persons who are glass blowers by trade. As air passes through the larynx, the laryngoceles may expand and fill with air or collapse, depending on changes in laryngeal pressure. Infected laryngoceles may become filled with mucoid fluid and are called laryngopyoceles. Treatment for laryngoceles includes dissecting the sac of the laryngocele and repairing the mucous membrane. External laryngoceles may be repaired

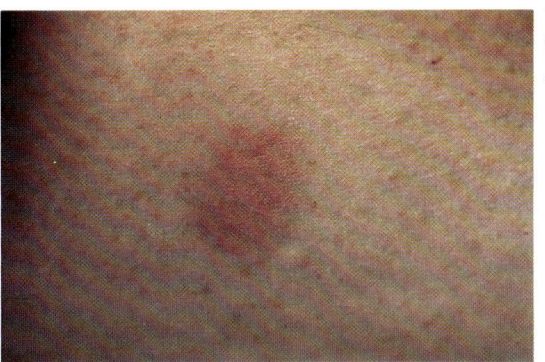

Figure 1
A positive tuberculin reaction.

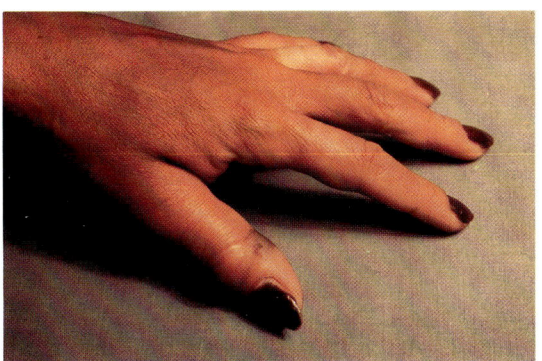

Figure 2
Inflammation of the hand following an insect bite.

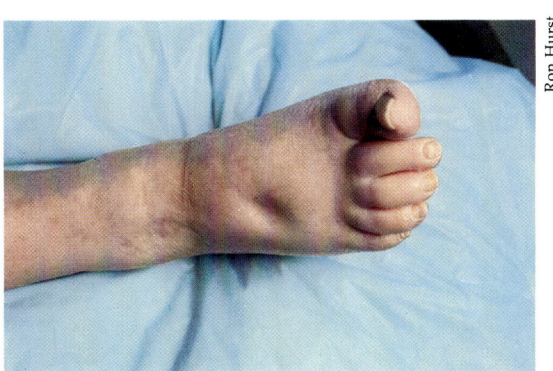

Figure 3
Pitting edema in a patient with cardiopulmonary disease.

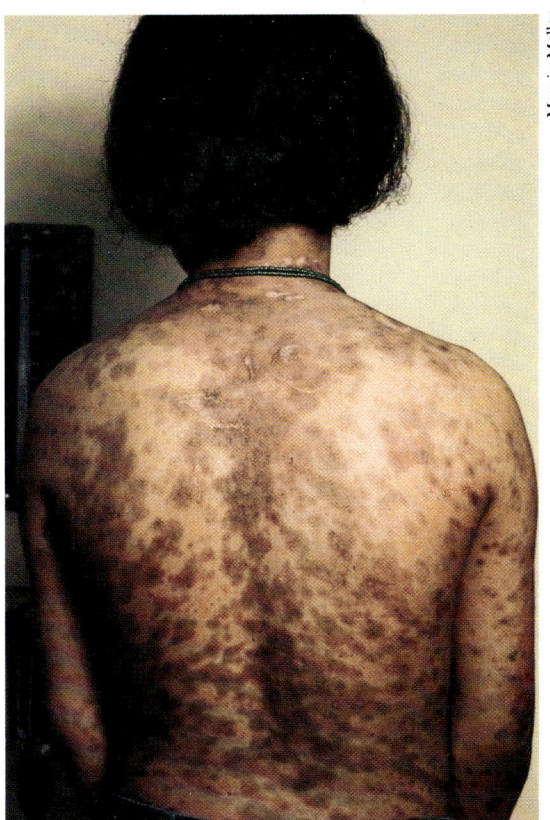

Figure 4
Loss of pigmentation in a black woman following a drug reaction.

Figures 1 to 12 courtesy of Evanston Hospital, Evanston, Illinois.

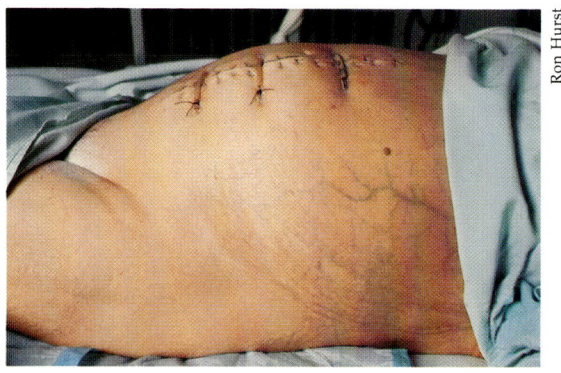

Figure 5
Ascites in a patient with liver disease.

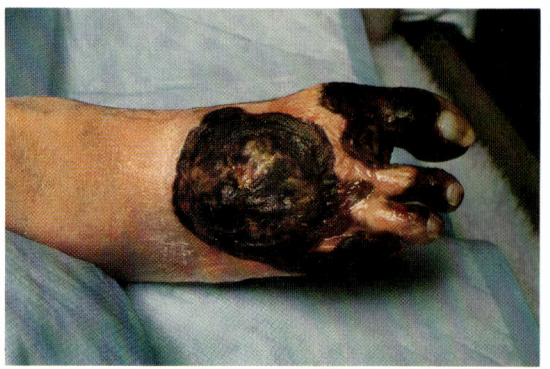

Figure 6
Gangrene of the foot in a patient with vascular disease.

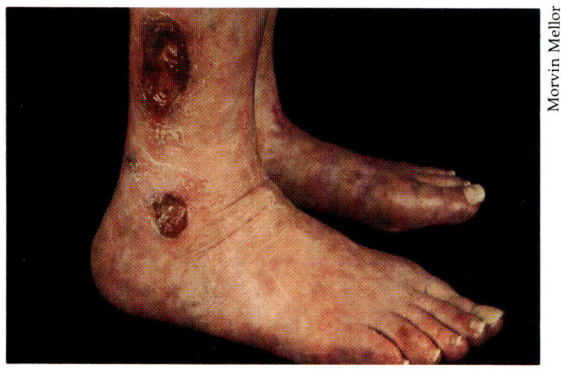

Figure 7
Ulcer formation in a patient with venous insufficiency.

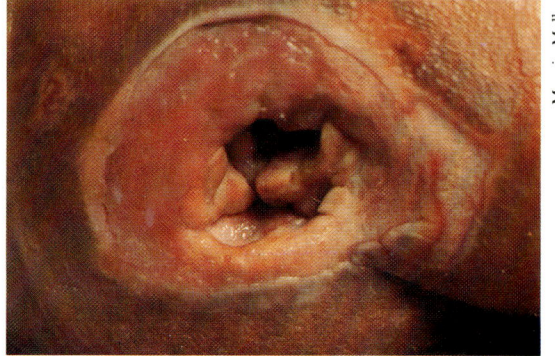

Figure 8
Decubitus ulcer formation in a debilitated patient.

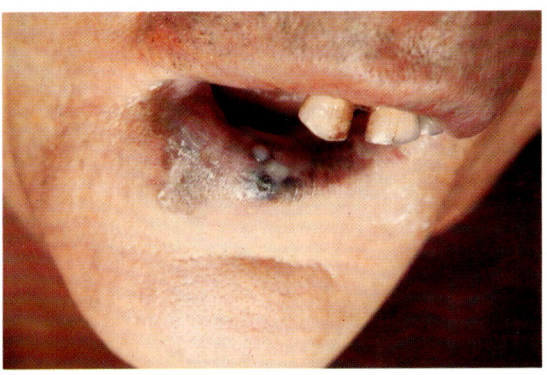

Figure 9
A patient with malignant melanoma of the lip.

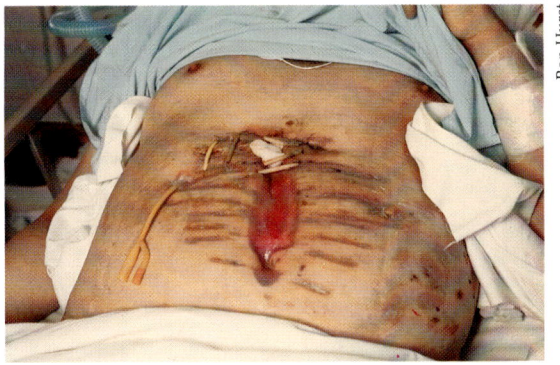

Figure 11
Wound dehiscence in a patient following surgery.

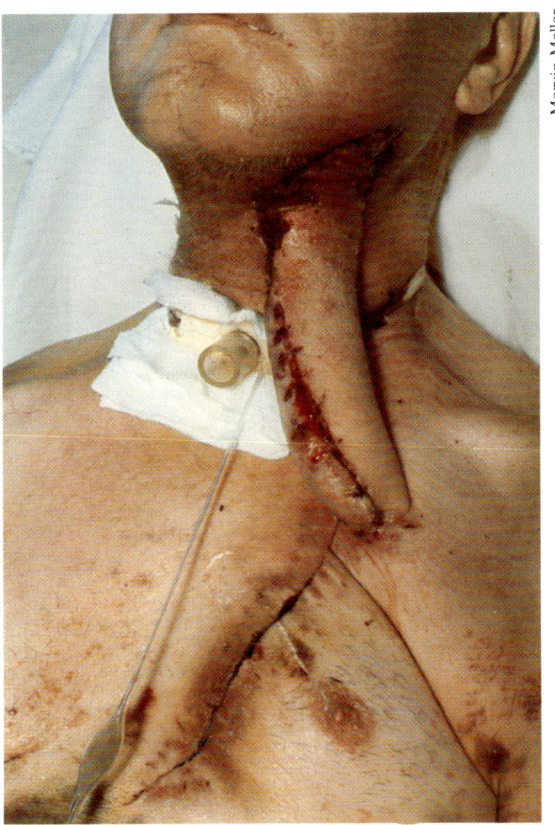

Figure 10
A patient with a pedicle skin graft following radical neck dissection.

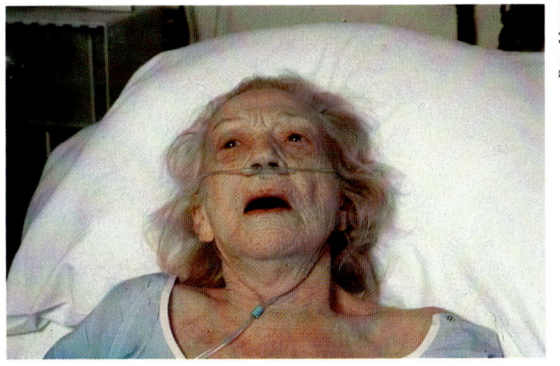

Figure 12
A patient with chronic obstructive lung disease.

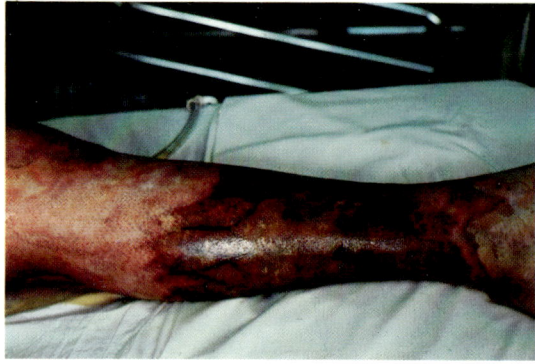

Figure 13
Thrombosed blood vessels within the eschar in a patient with a full-thickness burn.

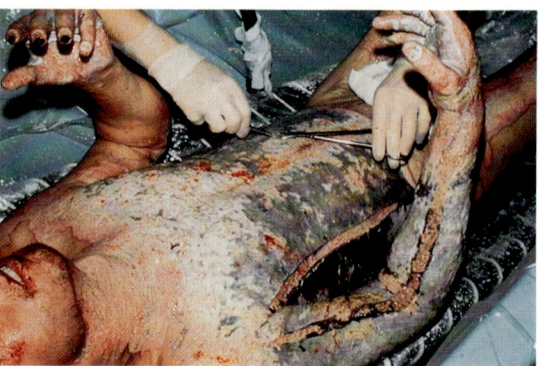

Figure 14
Debridement of a patient's burn wound.

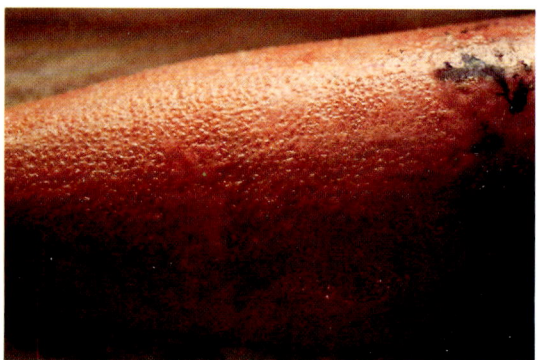

Figure 15
A patient with healing in the area of partial thickness injury.

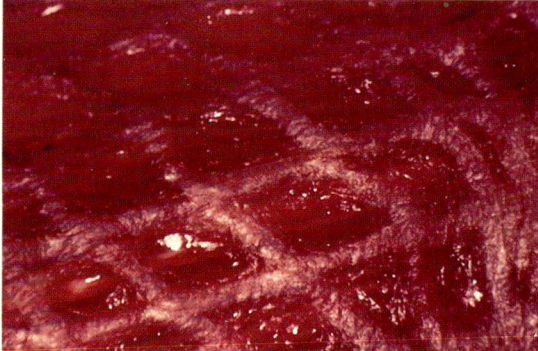

Figure 16
A patient with freshly meshed skin applied to the wound bed.

Figures 13 to 16 courtesy of The University of Texas Health Science Center at Dallas.

through a transverse cervical incision while a thyrotomy is required for repair of internal laryngoceles.

Vocal nodules are sometimes called singer's nodes as they occur frequently in people who consistently strain their voices. These nodules occur on the membranous vocal cord at the point of maximum vibration. They are more common in males under the age of 20 and in females, being related to production of high frequency sounds. They do not occur as frequently in people with bass or baritone voices. Vocal nodules are isolated masses of connective tissue covered with mucosa. They are soft and red at first, becoming small, firm, and pale in appearance as they progress. Nodules are usually located at the junction of the middle and anterior portions of the vocal cord and may affect one or both of the cords.

The symptoms of vocal nodules include hoarseness and the sensation that there is constantly something in the throat that must be cleared. Conservative treatment of prolonged voice rest may be effective. However, the nodules may have to be surgically removed through direct laryngoscopy. Vocal nodules do not tend to become malignant, but they recur if continued strain is placed on the vocal cords. Because vocal nodules are associated with voice strain, speech therapy in how to avoid voice strain may be necessary. It is also important to avoid voice abuse. Forcing a voice to a lower pitch than is natural places strain on the cords as do shouting and screaming and prolonged voice use. Voice fatigue with cracking of the voice at higher notes is indicative of voice abuse.

Laryngeal polyps are also associated with using the voice excessively or forcing the voice to loudness not normal for the individual. Polyps are formed from edema of the subepithelial tissue in the lamina propria of the anterior or middle third of the true vocal cords. They may originate from small hematomas that form as a result of voice strain or following laryngeal infection. Polyps cause hoarseness because they interfere with the approximation of the true vocal cords, and they are excised during direct laryngoscopy either with local or general anesthesia.

Ulcers of the larynx can also form as a result of voice abuse. They are associated with mild pain when speaking or swallowing. The pain may be referred to the ear. Hoarseness may be variable. These ulcers usually heal by voice rest.

Papillomas on the vocal cords or on the vestibular folds are benign tumors. They may extend upward to the epiglottis or downward to the trachea. The major symptom is hoarseness. Treatment is surgical removal through endoscopic techniques with care to preserve the integrity of the underlying structures.

Keratosis, or leukoplakia, appears as white raised patches on the vocal cords. These patches cause hoarseness. Leukoplakia may be premalignant and is considered an important signal requiring periodic follow-up examination. Persons with leukoplakia should have routine laryngoscopic examinations to determine any changes in cellular growth.

Carcinoma of the larynx, when diagnosed early, is highly curable. The early presenting symptom is hoarseness. Diagnosis is made by laryngoscopic examination with a biopsy, tomography, and contrast x-rays. Carcinomatous vocal cords usually appear irregular in size and are gray in color. Early diagnosis of carcinoma is possible; persistent hoarseness of two weeks' duration should be evaluated by laryngoscopic examination. In many cases, leukoplakia or laryngeal polyps may precede cancer. If either of these conditions is present, periodic examination of the larynx is essential so that tissue changes can be noted as soon as possible for early diagnosis. Swelling in the neck may also be indicative of carcinoma. There are, however, many causes of cervical lymph node enlargement, and it is necessary to conduct a laryngoscopic examination as well as a diagnostic physical examination to determine the actual cause.

Excessive alcohol intake, cigarette smoking, and voice abuse are thought to be directly related to the incidence of laryngeal carcinoma. The majority of people with diagnosed carcinoma of the larynx are men between 40 and 60 years of age. There is currently an increase in the incidence of laryngeal cancer in younger people and in women. The most frequently occurring type of carcinoma of the larynx is squamous cell carcinoma. Adenocarcinoma and basal cell carcinoma may also occur in the larynx.

Treatment for laryngeal cancer may include radiotherapy, surgical intervention, or a combination of radiation and surgery. When the lesions are small and localized to the cord and have not involved adjacent structures in the larynx, radiotherapy alone is often effective. More advanced lesions require surgical removal. The type of operation performed depends on the size of the tumor, the amount of fixation of the vocal cord, and the depth to which the lesion has extended into the laryngeal structures. The thyroid and cricoid cartilages are often involved in advanced lesions that have extended beyond the vocal cords. The patient's general physical condition is also an important consideration in determining what type of treatment is most suitable. Many people with laryngeal carcinoma are elderly and have multiple health problems that preclude successful surgery.

A **cordectomy** is done when the lesion is localized to one cord and if the mobility of the cord is not impaired. Cordectomy may also be performed following ineffective radiation. After a cordectomy the voice may be permanently hoarse, although some persons have a more normal voice than others following this procedure. Generally the metastasis is minimal in lesions localized to the middle third of the vocal cord because the lymph supply in this area of the larynx is negligible.

Lesions involving the laryngeal muscles and cartilage with impairment of the mobility of the vocal cords metastasize through the lymph and blood supply in the supraglottic and subglottic areas. If lesions are located on one side, a **partial vertical hemilaryngectomy** may be performed to remove only the lesion, thereby preserving the sphincter and phonation functions of the larynx. A **total laryngectomy** is done if the lesion has vertically invaded the supraglottic, glottic, and subglottic areas. In this procedure the entire larynx is removed, including the laryngeal cartilages, the hyoid bone, and the upper segment of the trachea. The end of the trachea is sewn to the skin to form a permanent stoma that serves as the airway. The pharynx is repaired to restore the integrity of the food passages as there is no longer a connection between the air and food passages. Techniques are being developed to restore the normal air passages by connecting the pharynx and the trachea so that a permanent laryngectomy may not be necessary.

When the lymph nodes are involved, a radical neck dissection is done on the same side as the lesion in conjunction with removal of the larynx. This procedure includes dissection of the sternocleidomastoid muscle at the clavicle. There is then paralysis of the trapezius muscle and the eleventh cranial nerve is interrupted (the spinal accessory nerve). Depending on the amount of tissue removed, radical neck dissection is obviously disfiguring in varying degrees. Not only is the capacity to speak normally removed, but there is also an outward and visible change in the body image. Both are extremely difficult to cope with for the patient and his family.

Radical surgery is usually done in several stages. Following dissection of tissue, there is additional staged surgical repair with skin grafting to close the wound. Various types of skin grafts are used, including pedicle grafts (see color insert Figure 10 on page 1078C). These grafts require long-term surgical processes, discomfort because of the nature of the repair, and restrictions of movement imposed by the pedicle graft in the interim stage when it is connected to both the site being repaired and the site of origin of the tissue. These procedures not only change appearances, but also precipitate concerns about whether the surgical procedure will be successful. Many times the long periods of isolation the hospitalized patient experiences make the adjustment to home, family, and friends difficult when he or she does again become part of the family group. The family often builds up fears about the patient's ability to speak, work, and live normally. These concerns influence the family's ability to support the patient when he or she returns home.

A total laryngectomy, most often performed for treatment of carcinoma or for repair of trauma, has serious implications. Following surgery the patient will not be able to produce sound, as the phonation function of the larynx has been removed. The air passage is also disrupted and the patient breathes through a stoma in the neck. These persons are called neck breathers as there is no continuity of the airway from the trachea to the pharynx. Treatment for carcinoma often involves total laryngectomy with a radical neck dissection and may result in physical limitations and disfiguring, causing even more disruption of the patient's body image. Because of these serious implications it is very important that the patient and his family be involved in making the decision to undergo the operation if there is a choice. It is also important that the preoperative care prepares the patient for the immediate postoperative period and for the adjustment to living as a neck breather. The patient requires a careful explanation of how he or she will breathe following surgery, the use of tube feedings, the presence of drains and dressings, the importance of frequent oral hygiene, and the loss of voice. The nurse should develop plans for alternate means of communication with the patient.

Laryngeal carcinoma is classified according to its anatomic location. The sites of the lesions are classified as supraglottic, glottic, transglottic, or hypopharyngeal. Carcinoma in the epiglottis is usually located in the pyriform sinus or in the postcricoid area. Women with the Plummer-Vinson syndrome (see Chap. 8) tend to have postcricoid carcinoma. The symptoms include cough, dysphagia, and pain that radiates to the ears when swallowing. Metastasis to both sides of the neck is common. Cervical nodes may be enlarged, and the cancer readily metastasizes through this abundant lymph supply. Laryngeal carcinoma in this location is often treated by a two-stage operation. A total laryngectomy and radical neck dissection are performed in the first stage, followed by a radical neck dissection on the other side after a month or so has elapsed. Radiation may be prescribed prior to and following surgery. Depending on the experiences with the first stage of the surgery the patient may be conditioned to a feeling of dread, fear, and anxiety for the second procedure, or if the first experience was positive and well managed, even though distressful, the patient may be better able to cope.

Supraglottic lesions may involve the epiglottis, the aryepiglottic folds, or the false vocal cords. Cough, pain that radiates to the ears, and hoarseness may be the presenting symptoms. Treatment may consist of a hemilaryngectomy, which leaves the person with some of his natural voice. This procedure leaves the airways intact so that the person may breathe normally through his mouth or nose.

Lesions confined to the glottis do not tend to metastasize because of the lack of lymph nodes in the glottic region. When the lesions are limited to the free edge of the cord and are diagnosed early, the prognosis is very favorable. However, if the lesion extends beyond the cord, either to the anterior commissure or to the arytenoid cartilage, the probability of metastasis through the cervical lymph nodes increases and the cure rate decreases. The anterior middle third of the true vocal cord is the most common site of glottic carcinoma, and hoarseness may be the only symptom. Treatment involves either a partial laryngectomy, also called laryngofissure, or a complete laryngectomy.

Subglottic carcinoma may originate in the true vocal cord or below its free edge and involve the cricoid cartilage. These lesions tend to metastasize because of the good lymph and blood supply to the area. Transglottic carcinoma extends vertically to include the supraglottic, glottic, and subglottic areas. Both the true and false vocal cords can be involved; extensive lesions may involve the thyroid as well as the cricoid cartilage with metastasis to the same side. Treatment includes total or complete laryngectomy and radical neck dissection on the same side.

Unless the surgery is emergent, as in cases of trauma, preoperative preparation for both the surgery and the postoperative period is important. The surgical procedure is explained so that the patient understands that following the operation he will have to adjust to breathing through the permanent stoma in the neck and will not be able to talk. In the immediate postoperative period the patient has several special needs that will not be permanent. Initially, there are one or two hemovacs connected to drains in the wound to provide for drainage from the operative site, and a nasogastric tube for gavage feedings. Both of these measures are temporary, but they add to the general discomfort and fear when the patient wakens from anesthesia and experiences the inability to speak for the first time.

Preoperative teaching for the person with carcinoma who is about to have a laryngectomy is complicated by the nature of the crisis he or she is undergoing. The patient not only has to accept the diagnosis of cancer but also must deal with the concept of not being able to communicate normally. Although different persons react to this crisis in different ways, it can be expected that fear, panic, and denial may be predominant in the patient's reactions. Many people feel that they are losing control when confronted with this crisis. They understand the consequences of not having the operation, but the implications of the surgery for normal interaction and for earning a living threaten their security. Underlying fear of the outcome of surgery is the fear of death. The nurse should openly discuss the patient's feelings and fears about death, the options for treatment and therapy, and the measures that will be taken to help in the adjustment to the changes imposed by the surgical procedure.

The essential element in the preoperative period is development of trust among the family and the patient and those who will care for the patient after the operation. The nurse should recognize that teaching is ongoing throughout the preoperative and postoperative periods. As the patient works through the crisis, the nurse provides counseling, information, and support and helps plan for postoperative needs. During this time the patient, family, and nurse should work together to formulate an appropriate means of communication. Communication will be important to the sense of security following the operation and must take into account any special problems the patient has in vision or hearing. For those with good vision and hearing, flash cards can be made and verbal responses are adequate. With the guidance of the nurse the patient can write cards for special likes, needs, and requests to be used postoperatively to ask for food, fluids, or information. Three-by-five cards work well; color coding can be used if the person's vision is poor. This process elicits the patient's cooperation and involvement in his or her care.

Another method for communication is that of using a magic slate for conversations following surgery when the patient begins to feel better and becomes more alert in the postanesthetic period. Some people are able to work out a system of signals and interpretations that can be used for communication in the postoperative period.

Nursing care in the immediate postoperative period includes providing for the patient's comfort needs, and monitoring for the occurrence of complications. Obstruction of the airway is one of the most serious complications. Symptoms of restlessness or dyspnea, tachycardia, and tachypnea indicate that the airway is obstructed. A laryngectomy tube is left in place for the first three or four days postoperatively until the amount of secretions from the larynx subsides. Usually the patient has copious secretions at first and must either be helped to cough up the secretions or be suctioned, depending on his condition and ability to remove the secretions by coughing.

Because the air passage has been interrupted and the normal protective mechanisms of the nasal passages are cut off from the lower airways, the patient is prone to the development of infections that may complicate his progress. Care should be taken to use correct technique in suctioning secretions in the laryngectomy tube. In the initial postoperative period frequent suctioning of secretions is essential to keep the laryngectomy tube patent; the initial copious secretions diminish by the third or fourth postoperative day and suctioning then is less frequent. Humidity should be provided to keep the secretions liquified. Antibiotics may be given prophylactically.

A number of different types of laryngectomy tubes may be used following surgery. A laryngectomy tube is shorter and has a slightly larger lumen than a tracheostomy tube. These tubes may be single or double with an inner and outer cannula, and may be made of either sterling silver or plastic. Depending on the site of the stoma, a tracheostomy tube may be used. Selection of the tube depends on the shape of the trachea remaining following surgery. Usually the upper portion of the trachea has been removed and the remaining trachea has less curvature than is normal. It is necessary that the laryngectomy tube fit correctly to prevent injury to the tracheal tissues.

The patient is placed in a semi-Fowler's position to facilitate ventilation of the lungs. Turning, coughing, and deep breathing are essential to prevent atelectasis and hypostatic pneumonia. In some hospitals, positive pressure treatments are prescribed. If symptoms of respiratory distress occur, the laryngectomy tube may have to be changed by the physician. Intensive respiratory care may be required if symptoms of respiratory insufficiency occur from such causes as infection of the lung or from postanesthetic lung changes. People with chronic lung disease are particularly likely to develop respiratory insufficiency following surgery. Many persons who have laryngectomies are heavy smokers and have lung dysfunction in addition to the laryngeal carcinoma. Respiratory distress may require oxygen therapy utilizing mechanical ventilation given according to arterial blood gas evaluations of pH, O_2, and CO_2.

Hemorrhage is the second serious postoperative complication that may occur. A carotid artery blowout may suddenly occur or may follow a slow steady leak with a sudden rupture. This complication often follows the formation of a fistula in the operative area. Any oozing of blood at the suture line should be noted, as this may indicate imminent hemorrhage. Direct pressure is immediately applied to the bleeding vessel if hemorrhage occurs and is maintained until the patient can be taken to surgery for repair of the rupture.

Other complications that may follow surgery are formation of fistulas and sloughing of the skin flap covering the operative area. These complications occur more frequently if the patient has had radiation therapy prior to surgery. Healing may also be delayed if the tissues have been exposed to radiation. If the suture line does not heal adequately, further surgery or skin grafting is required to repair the sites of inadequate healing. Delayed healing can be disconcerting and may cause depression. The patient may interpret delayed healing as a sign of poor prognosis and may become progressively more despondent, unless some positive sign of healing or recovery can be demonstrated. Poor healing prolongs the postoperative recovery period, increasing the patient's anxiety about returning home and concern about the increased cost of hospitalization and care. The nurse must deal realistically with the patient's feelings and responses.

Immediately following surgery, the patient has a nasogastric tube in place. Some authorities believe that a soft diet with no liquids is tolerated better than the nasogastric tube and that ingestion of food does not interfere with healing. Fluids are not given orally in this instance because of the danger of aspiration through the surgical suture lines. Others believe that the nasogastric tube should be left in place 3 or 4 days or until the wound has healed sufficiently to prevent the possibility of delayed healing. Gavage feedings are then given, beginning with clear liquids, according to the patient's tolerance. The swallowing and respiratory functions are separated from one another by the total laryngectomy, and patients often fear that swallowing will be painful and harmful. It is important that the nurse stress that food will not cause choking and that a normal diet can be eaten following healing. Increasingly, solid foods are introduced after the fourth postoperative day if gavage feedings are used. Frequent oral hygiene is imperative and is a necessary comfort measure.

One problem associated with a total laryngectomy from the standpoint of nutrition is an impaired sense of taste and smell. This loss is more noticeable when the patient begins to eat a normal diet. Some persons begin to eat increasing amounts of food as their appetites are not satisfied by the seemingly bland food; then follows a corresponding tendency to gain weight. If forewarned, a patient can anticipate this problem and can avoid weight gain from overeating.

Stenosis of the stoma may occur following surgery. Surgical insertion of the laryngectomy tube provides for initial healing and prevention of stenosis. Use of the laryngectomy tube after the first three or four postoperative days is controversial. The tube may be removed so that the patient can become accustomed to his permanent stoma while still in the hospital. Some persons, however, prefer to use the laryngectomy tube while they are sleeping. Others more readily become comfortable with the stoma and do not want to use the tube.

Two important factors determine whether the tube should be left in place: the amount of secretions the person has and the tendency of the stoma to close. Secretions may continue to be copious in the early postoperative period, especially if the patient has a respiratory infection or postoperative lung congestion. In some instances the stoma tends to close and the tube is replaced until healing is more advanced. People who are prone to stenosis are advised to keep the laryngectomy tube in place periodically to prevent stenosis.

Skin care and stoma care are ongoing needs in total laryngectomy. Initially the nurse provides this care, teaching the patient how to clean the stoma and helping him to perform this procedure for himself. Use of a mirror aids visualization of the stoma so that the patient can observe the nurse's technique and later so that he can see what he is doing as he performs stoma care. The nurse should encourage and expect the patient to begin self-care as soon as he is able to do so. Cleaning the stoma may be needed more frequently during the initial postoperative period because of the tendency to blow air forcefully from the stoma. Secretions are blown out with the air and collect around the tube. This forceful blowing is diminished as the person learns to control his breathing and as secretions diminish. When the blowing-out is accompanied by secretions, the ring of mucus that collects around the stoma gives rise to an odor that is characteristic of laryngectomies.

The laryngectomy stoma is different from a tracheostomy stoma in that the trachea is sutured to the skin. The tube can be easily removed and replaced and the laryngectomy stoma remains stable, whereas a tracheostomy stoma tends to close when the tube is removed. Initially the stoma may tend to close because of postoperative edema. The condition of the tissues in the surgical area also influences the integrity of the stoma.

Cleaning of the stoma reduces irritation from accumulated mucus and reduces stoma odor. Care of the stoma and of the laryngectomy tube, if one is used, is a clean procedure after healing has occurred. Up to that time, sterile procedures are most often followed. In the clean procedure, the patient should wash his or her hands before touching the stoma or tube. Soap is not used; instead a water-soluble cleaner such as hydrogen peroxide may be used. The stoma is cleaned by wiping the area around the stoma and the lip of the stoma carefully so that the solution does not enter the trachea. It is important to prevent aspiration. If the person is being treated with radiation therapy, the skin may be particularly sensitive and should be cleaned very carefully. Care of the laryngectomy tube with an inner cannula includes removal of the inner cannula. The inner cannula is scrubbed with a brush and an abrasive cleaner or hydrogen peroxide. A toothbrush serves nicely to clean the cannula; a pipe cleaner may be used, depending on its size. The tube is then washed. Silver tubes are boiled and cooled before being replaced. A thin layer of abolene cream or petroleum jelly may be placed on the skin around the stoma before replacing the tube, to keep the tube from sticking to the skin when mucus collects and dries around the stoma. An antibiotic ointment may be applied to the skin around the stoma until initial healing is complete.

Stoma size varies, but usually the stoma is one-half to three-fourths of an inch in diameter. It must be large enough to provide for an adequate airway. In addition to keeping the stoma clean, long-term care includes covering the stoma with a bib to filter dust particles that are normally removed by the nose when air is inspired. The bib also warms the air and increases the moisture content of the inspired air. The bib is worn with a string around the neck.

Crusts tend to form around the stoma because of drying secretions. These crusts around the stoma should be wiped off two or three times a day and medical assistance should be sought for removal of crusts that form inside the trachea. The patient should never place anything inside the stoma, as dry mucous membranes are very fragile and easily injured. The nurse may remove crusts that form inside the stoma, using a forceps or tweezers.

Humidity is very important to reduce this crusting, particularly during sleep. Usually 45 percent humidity is advised. People with laryngectomies may have difficulty providing adequate humidity at all times but must make adaptations so that there is proper humidification in the places where they spend the most time, at home or at work. In addition to the need for humidification, the person should not spend time in places that are extremely hot or cold, or in places that have atmospheric gases, dusts or fumes, because the stoma has no mechanism for filtering and warming or cooling the air. Going out for walks or shopping may expose the person to atmospheric air and pollutants. The neck bib helps to protect the lower airways for normal activities that take place outside the home. This precaution provides sufficient protection. Both powders and aerosol sprays should not be used.

The bib is also useful for absorbing secretions and for reducing the noise of stoma breathing. Initially the person who is learning to breathe through the neck has noisy, wheezing respirations. He sometimes exhales air under pressure, which increases the noise. It takes time to learn to breathe quietly through the neck stoma. The person should be aware of the sounds of his breathing, as more noisy than usual breathing may be indicative of infection.

Long-term care needs for the person who has had a total laryngectomy include adjustment to being a neck breather, learning to communicate, and resolving the crises of the surgical experience and its implications, all important for well-being. The patient's emotional stability and the quality of his or her relationships with others are significant determinants of the adjustment to the postoperative period. Even though the inability to speak following surgery has been anticipated, the impact of not being able to talk is not fully realized until the patient assumes a normal daily life and is then constantly reminded that he or she cannot express feelings in words, cannot speak on the telephone, cannot shout, laugh, cry, or scream, and cannot easily carry on a normal conversation. The continual frustration experienced may impede adjustment.

Because of these factors, speech training is begun as early as possible (when the mucous membrane and muscles are well healed). Each person must be approached according to his own needs. A useful idea is having a successful esophageal speaker visit the patient early in the postoperative period. Selecting someone that the patient can identify with is helpful, as it demonstrates that a successful recovery is possible. Another person with a laryngectomy can understand the fears and concerns that normally follow the surgey.

Some persons find use of an electrolarynx, a device that oscillates sound when placed on the submandibular area, helpful while learning esophageal speech. This device enables one to produce a monotone vibrating voice. Although this voice does not sound normal to the person, in that it is different from his presurgery voice, it does allow for verbal communication. Esophageal speech is quickly learned by some persons while others find the technique difficult and sometimes never learn its use. Many authorities feel that the person's motivation to learn esophageal speech is a singular component of the success rate.

Esophageal speech uses the eructation of swallowed air through the cricopharyngeal muscle to produce sound. The resulting voice is low volume and more monotone than a normal voice. It cannot be varied in inflection or tone as can a normal voice, but many persons master the technique so well that if one has not known them previously it is difficult to discern that they are using esophageal speech. In many instances, those with chronic laryngeal dysfunction may have already adapted to voice changes prior to surgery, having lost the normal range of tone, pitch, and voice flexibility.

In order to learn esophageal speech, a person must learn to draw air into the esophagus during inspiration. When learning to swallow and regurgitate air for speech, gastrointestinal distention may occur, making the person uncomfortable. This distention may be treated with antacid medications and is minimized when the person begins to learn how to contain the air in the upper portion of the esophagus. If the person has a hiatus hernia, learning esophageal speech may be difficult, since swallowing air may precipitate symptoms. Some people are bothered by regurgitation of stomach contents as they learn esophageal speech. This may cause pain similar to heartburn or may be as severe as cardiac pain.

Encouragement is given to help the laryngectomee overcome the depression experienced because of the inability to communicate in addition to the discomfort the effort to learn to swallow and regurgitate air causes. The amount of time required for learning esophageal speech varies with each individual. Some people learn quickly, seeming to catch on to the technique, whereas others may need 3 or 4 months to learn to speak adequately. Those who do learn (65 to 75 percent) are gratified with their success and are able to communicate very effectively as esophageal speech soon feels more normal to them.

A hearing test precedes the teaching of esophageal speech. Learning esophageal speech depends on being able to hear the sounds produced. If one cannot hear well, the sounds cannot be produced accurately as the mouth is shaped in accordance with the sounds one hears. Fifteen of the English language consonants require the vocal cords; the remaining ten can be formed by the shape of the mouth. If hearing is impaired, a hearing aid can be worn to improve hearing, but this also increases the background noises, hindering the hearing of specific sounds. Elderly people often have more difficulty learning esophageal speech because of their inability to hear well. Another problem sometimes experienced is the wheezing noise of breathing through the neck stoma. It may be so loud that it interferes with hearing the sounds well. Improvement of breathing technique diminishes this problem.

People who do learn esophageal speech derive corollary benefits from the improved tone of both respiratory and abdominal muscles. This improvement enables them to breathe more easily and often increases their ability to cough and raise secretions. Regurgitation of air through the esophagus also causes air to flow through the nasopharyngeal passages and somewhat increases the ability to smell and taste, both senses that are impaired following a laryngectomy.

The patient's family should be included in the process of learning esophageal speech. There is a natural tendency to help the person who has a disability. If that disability involves speaking, family and friends may speak for the person, rather than letting him or her take time to articulate thoughts. Family members may tend to interrupt or to answer questions before the person has time to reply, rather than waiting for a response. This habit leads to frustration and a feeling of nonacceptance. The family and friends can accommodate to the person's stage of learning by patiently giving him or her time to speak. Other supportive measures include forming habits of standing or sitting in proximity to the person so that his or her voice can be heard better. Learning to draw the person into the conversation, listening, and speaking more slowly help the person feel included and reduce feelings of being left out, unwanted, or unaccepted. It is sometimes difficult for families and friends to respond to the person with a laryngectomy. Occasionally the family members require help in accepting the disability as well as in overcoming the tendency to overhelp.

More appropriate assistance for the laryngectomee involves learning to encourage him or her by demonstrating acceptance and by giving positive reinforcement. People who do not learn esophageal speech usually get along without speaking and for some reason are not motivated to learn. They can communicate by whispering or by using an electrolarynx. An alternative that has limited use thus far is insertion of a VoiceBak prosthesis.

The VoiceBak prosthesis (LaBarge, Inc., St. Louis, Missouri) has been devised for people who are unable to learn esophageal speech. In addition, insertion of the voice prosthesis requires that the person be in good medical condition, that the skin in the area of the laryngectomy and neck has not been damaged or impaired either from radiation or from other causes of poor healing, and that the esophageal and cricopharyngeal muscles function normally. Another important consideration is the desire and motivation to use the voice prosthesis. The voice prosthesis uses the esophageal air flow through to the cricopharyngeal muscle to produce sound. The prosthesis is attached to the laryngectomy stoma, and the internal flange is placed into the esophagus through a surgically produced fistula. The portion of the prosthesis that communicates with the esophagus is attached by a short tubing to a valve that is then connected to the laryngectomy stoma tube. The valve allows passage of air from the lungs into the esophagus and provides for inspiration and exhalation of air through the laryngectomy stoma to and from the lungs. The valve can be adjusted for the proper balance of air flow. When the person is exercising and requires more air for respiration, the valve can be adjusted to allow passage of more air. The entire prosthesis is small enough to be covered easily by regular clothing. A nice feature of the prosthesis is that the voice sounds produced are more like normal speech than the sounds produced by the electrolarynx. Since the prosthesis uses the method of producing sound through the esophagus with air flow produced by normal increases in breathing during speaking, the person can learn to produce sound with little extra effort or new learning.

Prior to inserting the prosthesis, a fistula is made surgically by an external incision into the esophagus. Placement of the incision is determined by testing the person's ability to produce sound when a Foley rubber catheter is inserted through the nose and into the esophagus. Placement is usually slightly above the level of the stoma and must be below the cricopharyngeal muscle. If the person cannot produce sound with the Foley catheter test, the procedure is not done. Another preoperative measure is that of testing the integrity of the mucosa of the esophagus by x-ray examination with contrast media (a barium swallow). The person is prepared prior to surgery by insertion of a

Foley catheter into the esophagus. Following the surgical formation of the fistula, gavage feedings are given until healing has advanced. Usually the gavage feedings are discontinued on the fourth postoperative day and food and fluids can be given orally. Prophylactic antibiotics are given.

The voice prosthesis is then inserted approximately three weeks following surgery. In teaching the patient how to use the prosthesis, it is important that he or she understand that the system of air flow must be closed, with a good seal around the fistula opening where the internal esophageal flange is inserted. Passage of fluid and secretions from the esophagus is prevented by a valve external to the esophagus. As with any device that is used to assist respiration, the prosthesis must be kept free of contamination; the external valve provides this protection by preventing passage of fluids into the prosthesis.

Use of the voice prosthesis is a creative way of providing an important normal function. It has limitations because it cannot be used for those who have had radical neck dissection or for those who have had extensive radiation. However, the example of the possibility of use of a voice prosthesis is an important breakthrough that will hopefully be followed by other creative inventions that will make life more normal for people who have had laryngectomies.

Having a laryngectomy not only changes one's ability to speak, but may have effects on the rest of the person's life. The laryngectomy is noticeable, even though the stoma may be covered. For example, the normal neck movements and facial movements that are an almost imperceptible part of breathing are absent when the person has a laryngectomy stoma. There is a quietness about the person that can be noticed most when he or she is sitting still and not interacting with anyone or anything in the environment. If the person has had a radical neck dissection, the neck will be different in appearance; the neck may seem thin or the tissue of the neck appear taut. These differences can be covered effectively by facial movements, by movements of the neck, and by wearing clothes that cover the neck. Some of the changes, particularly those in breathing, cannot be covered as easily and may be disconcerting to those who live intimately with the person.

The nurse should recognize that one of the areas of major difficulty for the person may be the development of marital problems precipitated by the stoma. In some marriages the odor of the stoma, the noise of breathing, and the changes in physical appearance may be very disturbing to the laryngectomee's spouse. The stoma may become an overt barrier to interaction in the marriage, which may include not only general communication but also sexual recognition such as physical contact, kissing, or even intercourse. The nurse should anticipate these difficulties and should openly discuss them with the person who is having the laryngectomy and his or her spouse. Open discussion of these problems may be sufficient to enable the couple to work out their feelings. The variety of feelings is unlimited and may range from a fear of rejection by the person who has the laryngectomy to annoyance or distaste by the marital partner. If there are underlying problems with the marriage itself, couples are counseled to work out these problems with the assistance of a counselor, if necessary. In many instances, covering the stoma with a guard or with clothing, using deodorizers or perfumes to mask the stoma odor, and learning techniques to improve breathing may be sufficient.

Every person with a stoma must learn how to take care of the stoma on an ongoing daily basis. Careful attention to daily cleaning is important to reduce the odor. Actually, the stoma requires simple care that does not hinder or incapacitate the person in his daily routines. Teaching stoma care actually begins postoperatively, while the patient is still in the hospital. Care does not vary much from the procedures used in the hospital. If a laryngectomy tube is used, it must be cleaned. It is important to inform the patient that cotton or paper tissues should not be used in cleaning the stoma or tubes because of the possibility of aspirating fragments of cotton or tissue; this aspiration could cause a respiratory infection. Printed instructions, diagrams, and pictures are useful in teaching. The nurse should encourage active involvement through return demonstrations of procedures and should provide the patient with a guide to self-care that can later serve as a reference.

Many people fear that the stoma will cause difficulty or interfere with their normal activities. The patient can participate in all the activities enjoyed prior to surgery with the exception of water sports. Inhalation of water is avoided because the stoma opens more directly to the lungs than the oral or nasal passages and the protective mechanisms are limited. Showering or taking a bath can be adapted so that no water is inhaled. Stoma shields can be worn during the bath or even while brushing teeth to prevent aspiration. The humidity of a bath or shower is actually helpful in keeping secretions thin and in preventing crust formation. The steam from a shower or bath can also replace the water normally supplied by the nasal passages. Shaving is another activity that may require a stoma shield or guard to prevent aspiration of lather. Many persons with laryngectomies use electric razors to eliminate the need for lather, which might be aspirated.

Oral hygiene is important. The person with a laryngectomy needs to maintain excellent oral hygiene, brushing the insides of the mouth, the palate, and the tongue, as well as the teeth. The passage of mucus downward in the gastrointestinal tract from the pharynx is not lost with the laryngectomy. However, air does not pass through the nose and mouth in inspiration or expiration so that secretions and particles are retained. The nose cannot be "blown," as the upper airways are separated from the trachea and lungs. These differences will become acutely obvious in the immediate postoperative period when secretions are greater. Teaching good oral hygiene begins at this time when the nurse demonstrates proper oral hygiene. Use of mechanical water sprays that provide cleaning by pressure are very good for oral hygiene, particularly in the postoperative period. During this phase the patient needs routine oral hygiene to prevent discomfort and to facilitate removal of secretions. Water spray devices for oral hygiene are also available for home use.

Adaptations can be made in choice of clothing to cover the stoma. Blouses, shirts, sweaters, and scarves or ascots can be worn and still allow for passage of air. Clothing actually protects the stoma from atmospheric pollutants and also serves to cover the stoma bib, which can be worn over the stoma and under the clothing. Clothes can be selected to allow access to the stoma to remove mucus when coughing. Acrylic stoma buttons are available. These can be used if the person fears that the stoma will close; they are most frequently used during sleep. As previously mentioned, some people continue to use their laryngectomy tubes during sleep.

Respiratory distress is always a concern for the person with a laryngectomy. This is a major complication, and the person with a laryngectomy should carry a special identification card or Medic-Alert bracelet or pendant to call attention to his being a neck breather. Cards are available with directions for giving mouth to stoma resuscitation in the event of respiratory arrest. In this procedure, the neck stoma is uncovered and secretions are removed by wiping or sucking, using mechanical suction if available. The resuscitator's mouth and lips are placed tightly over the stoma so that air can be blown into the airways. This procedure should be repeated every 1 or 2 seconds for the first 5 seconds and then slowed to a pace of about 12 to 20 times per minute. The person may begin to breathe spontaneously or may require more sophisticated resuscitation. Some laryngectomees may have some normal respiratory passages; these persons are called partial neck breathers. In this case, the palm of one hand is placed firmly over the mouth and two fingers are used to pinch off the nasal airways so that air can be blown into the stoma. Dentures are removed if they are present. The cards with these directions are available from the International Association of Laryngectomees.

Some laryngectomees fear going to sleep as they think that the stoma may be occluded by linens or blankets or that it may close spontaneously during the night. Using pillows or elevating the head of the bed facilitates ventilation for persons who have difficulty breathing while sleeping. Warm compresses placed over the stoma are beneficial, as is steam inhalation. As previously mentioned, stoma buttons or laryngectomy tubes can be worn during sleep to keep the stoma open.

Because the trachea is shortened by the total laryngectomy procedure, only 3 inches or so of the trachea may remain, making the person susceptible to bronchitis. Avoiding exposure to extremes of temperature is important. Cold winter air and warm dry air are both irritating to the airways and stimulate coughing. Normal saline may be inserted into the stoma with an eye dropper, using care to avoid placing the tip of the dropper into the stoma. The saline loosens secretions and facilitates their removal by coughing. Persons susceptible to hypersensitivity reactions, sinusitis, or rhinitis may be able to use a suction tip syringe to remove secretions from the nares as secretions cannot be "blown" from the nose. Antihistamines are not usually prescribed for neck breathers because these medications dry the mucous membranes. Other drugs that cause drying of mucous membranes are also contraindicated.

Proper humidity in the air is also an important preventive measure in avoiding respiratory infections. When infections do occur, edema of the airways and increased secretions may cause respiratory insufficiency. Coughing must be learned so that secretions may be raised effectively. It is important that secretions be removed from the stoma, using a cloth handkerchief. Paper tissues should be used carefully *if at all* because of the danger of aspiration of tissue fragments. Some authorities advise against their use, particularly when one is sleepy, as it is difficult to be careful when one is sleepy.

Everyone with a neck stoma should have an emergency laryngectomy tube available for use in periods of respiratory distress, whether caused by infection or other types of pulmonary dysfunction. These tubes should be custom made following surgery and after the shape of the trachea is known. The tube should fit the curvature of the trachea to prevent injury to mucous membranes. Most laryngectomees keep two tubes on hand. Persons with short necks may need to use a laryngectomy tube more frequently or even all the time, particularly if the skin folds of the neck tend to cover the stoma. Those prone to stenosis also need to continue periodic use of the tube to keep the stoma open. For others, the tube represents security and they are afraid to go without it. Still others have no desire to use a laryngectomy tube. Some people continue to have copious secretions and may need to leave the tube in place all of the time to facilitate suctioning. In this case the family, as well as the person with the laryngectomy, must learn to use the suction effectively to clear the airways. Suction machines can be obtained for home use.

Following surgery, the patient should have routine periodic examinations for detection of any signs or symptoms of recurrence of the carcinoma and for examination of the stoma. Any tissue changes, bleeding from the stoma, enlargement of cervical lymph nodes, coughing, dysphagia, dyspnea, and hemoptysis are important signs and symptoms that should be further examined. Changes in the esophageal voice may also indicate changes in the tissue structures. The recurrence of carcinoma following laryngectomy usually occurs in the cervical neck nodes or, less frequently, along the suture lines on the skin. Lesions in the glottis do not tend to metastasize, as the true vocal cords have a very sparse supply of lymph. The recurrence of transglottic or subglottic lesions is more common.

The adjustment each person makes following a laryngectomy is highly individual. Those with radical neck dissections may be unable to resume former jobs, particularly if their job involves heavy lifting with arm raising. These persons may require vocational retraining, and physical therapy may be necessary if they have a drop shoulder following the radical neck dissection. The physical therapy is needed for retraining in use of the remaining neck and shoulder muscles. Those who work in environments with a high level of atmospheric pollution must also find new jobs and may need vocational retraining. Fortunately, the majority of persons who have their disease diagnosed early and who receive early treatment do not have these problems and most usually can resume their former work.

The most important adjustment every laryngectomee who is a neck breather has to face is self-acceptance and learning to relate to others with his or her new self-image. Some authorities have found that the laryngectomized person tends to be asocial. Personal counseling is helpful to increase socialization. Membership in an organization that has a purpose meaningful to the person may be helpful. There are also a number of clubs specifically for people with laryngectomies. Among them are the Lost Chord Club, the New Voice Club, and the Anamilo Club. Agencies such as speech and hearing clinics, rehabilitation institutes with speech and hearing services, and the American Speech and Hearing Association provide help for neck breathers. The International Association of Laryngectomees, 219 East 42nd Street, New York, New York, 10017, an affiliate of the American Cancer Society, offers many services. Vocational retraining is available through state and federal agencies. These groups provide valuable information about special phone devices and other supportive devices and techniques.

Membership in a Lost Chord Club or similar organization is very supportive for the laryngectomee and his family. In these clubs, members support one another and learn how others have managed to cope with the problems of esophageal speech training, cleaning stomas, reducing the stoma odor, adapting clothing to cover the stoma and allowing for wiping secretions when coughing, and for keeping the stoma open during sleep. Helpful information about how to avoid colds and respiratory infections, and the very important considerations of how to relate to others and to the environment, can be obtained from sharing with others who are in similar situations. The support and sharing that take place in these club meetings are invaluable adjuncts to adjusting to and coping with the laryngectomy. Even though it may be necessary to travel some distance to attend a meeting, the benefits derived from the experience are very worthwhile for learning to live more fully. It should be pointed out that the person who has a laryngectomy as a result of damage to tissues during trauma also has the same types of problems with the exception that he usually does not have the fear of recurrence of cancer. Therefore these people also benefit from participation in groups in which people share their experiences in learning to live with and cope with the laryngectomy. When no organized group is accessible, nurses can be instrumental in forming and supporting such a group.

References

1. American College of Surgeons Committee on Trauma. *Early Care of the Injured Patient*. Philadelphia: Saunders, 1972.
2. Chusid, J. G. *Correlative Neuroanatomy and Functional Neurology* (16th ed.). Los Altos, Cal.: Lange, 1976.
3. DeWeese, D., and Saunders, W. *Textbook of Otolaryngology* (4th ed.). St. Louis: Mosby, 1973.
4. *Federal Register* CFR 29, Parts 1910.95, OSH 2206, General Industry Standards.
5. Schuknecht, H. *Stapedectomy*. Boston: Little, Brown, 1971.
6. Selkurt, E. *Basic Physiology for the Health Sciences*. Boston: Little, Brown, 1975.
7. Wolff, A. P., May, M., and Nuelle, D. The tympanic membrane, a source of the cough reflex. *J.A.M.A.* 223:1269, 1973.

Bibliography

Ballantyne, J., and Groves, J. *Diseases of the Ear, Nose and Throat* (3rd ed.). London: Butterworth, 1971. Vols. 1–4.

Boyd, E. M. *Respiratory Tract Fluid*. Springfield, Ill.: Thomas, 1972.

Connor, L. E. *Speech for the Deaf Child: Knowledge and Use*. Washington: Alexander Graham Bell Association for the Deaf, 1975.

Davis, H., and Silverman, S. R. (eds.). *Hearing and Deafness* (3rd ed.). New York: Holt, Rinehart & Winston, 1970.

Dickson, S. (ed.). *Communication Disorders: Remedial Principles and Practices*. Glenview, Ill.: Scott, Foresman, 1974.

Donald, P. J. Leading with the nose. *Emerg. Med.* 7:26, 1975.

Donald, P. J. Guide to diagnosis and management of eustachian otitis. *Hosp. Med.* 12:44, 1976.

Fowkes, W., and Hunn, V. *Clinical Assessment for the Nurse Practitioner*. St. Louis: Mosby, 1973.

Gardner, W., and Taylor, P. *Health at Work*. New York: Wiley, 1975.

Glorig, A., and Gerwin, K. S. *Otitis Media: Proceedings of the National Conference, Collier Hearing and Speech Center, Dallas, Texas*. Springfield, Ill.: Thomas, 1972.

Havener, W., et al. *Nursing Care in Eye, Ear, Nose and Throat Disorders* (3rd ed.). St. Louis: Mosby, 1974.

Lawless, C. A. Helping patients with endotracheal and tracheostomy tubes communicate. *Am. J. Nurs.* 75:2151, 1975.

Martin, F. *Introduction to Audiology*. Englewood Cliffs, N.J.: Prentice Hall, 1975.

May, H. *Plastic and Reconstructive Surgery*. Philadelphia: Davis, 1971.

McCorkle, R. Effects of touch on seriously ill patients. *Nurs. Res.* 23:125, 1974.

Medic Alert Foundation. P.O. Box 1009, Turlock, California 95380.

Minifie, F. D. (ed.). *Normal Aspects of Speech, Hearing and Language*. Englewood Cliffs, N.J.: Prentice Hall, 1973.

Montgomery, W. *Surgery of the Upper Respiratory System*. Philadelphia: Lea & Febiger, 1973.

Mountcastle, V. *Medical Physiology* (13th ed.). St. Louis: Mosby, 1974. Vol. 1.

Myers, D. Tinnitus. *Hosp. Med.* 11:55, 1975.

Myers, D., et al. Otologic deafness and the treatment of deafness. *Clin. Symp.* 22:35, 1970.

Newby, H. A. *Audiology*. Englewood Cliffs, N.J.: Prentice Hall, 1972.

Paparella, M. M. (ed.). *Yearbook of Ear, Nose and Throat*. Chicago: Year Book, 1974.

Paparella, M. M., and Schumrick, D. *Basic Sciences and Related Disciplines,* vol. 1; *The Ear,* vol. 2; *Head and Neck,* vol. 3. Philadelphia: Saunders, 1973.

Paparella, M. M., and Strong, M. S. (eds.). *Yearbook of Ear, Nose and Throat.* Chicago: Year Book, 1975.

Pollack, M. C. *Amplification for the Hearing Impaired.* New York: Grune & Stratton, 1975.

Rose, D. E. (ed.). *Audiological Assessment.* Englewood Cliffs, N.J.: Prentice Hall, 1971.

Sabiston, D. C. *Davis-Christopher Textbook of Surgery.* Philadelphia: Saunders, 1972.

Sana, J., and Judge, R. D. *Physical Appraisal Methods in Nursing Practice.* Boston: Little, Brown, 1975.

Searcy, L. Nursing care of the laryngectomy patient. *R.N.* 35:35, 1972.

Serratius, D. Laryngectomy: Paving the way to successful treatment. *Nursing 74* 4:60, 1974.

Shah, N. Examination of the ear. *Hosp. Med.* 9:86, 1973.

Snidecor, J. C., et al. *Speech Rehabilitation of the Laryngectomized* (2nd ed.). Springfield, Ill.: Thomas, 1968.

Sproul, C. W., and Mullanney, P. J. *Emergency Care, Assessment and Intervention.* St. Louis: Mosby, 1974.

Taub, S. Air bypass voice prosthesis for vocal rehabilitation of laryngectomees. *Ann. Otol. Rhinol. Laryngol.* 84:45, 1975.

Taylor, R. *A Primer of Clinical Symptoms.* New York: Harper & Row, 1973.

Thomas, B. J. Coping with the devastation of head and neck cancer. *R.N.* 37:25, 1974.

Traver, G. *Nursing the Patient with Respiratory Insufficiency.* League Exchange no. 96. National League for Nursing, 1972.

Walsh, T. Rehabilitation: Sound the way for laryngectomies. *Patient Care* 6:58, 1972.

Wolstenholme, G. E. W., and Elliott, K. M. *Human Rights in Health.* New York: Assn. Scientific Publishers, 1974.

chapter 14
Patients with Integumentary System Dysfunction

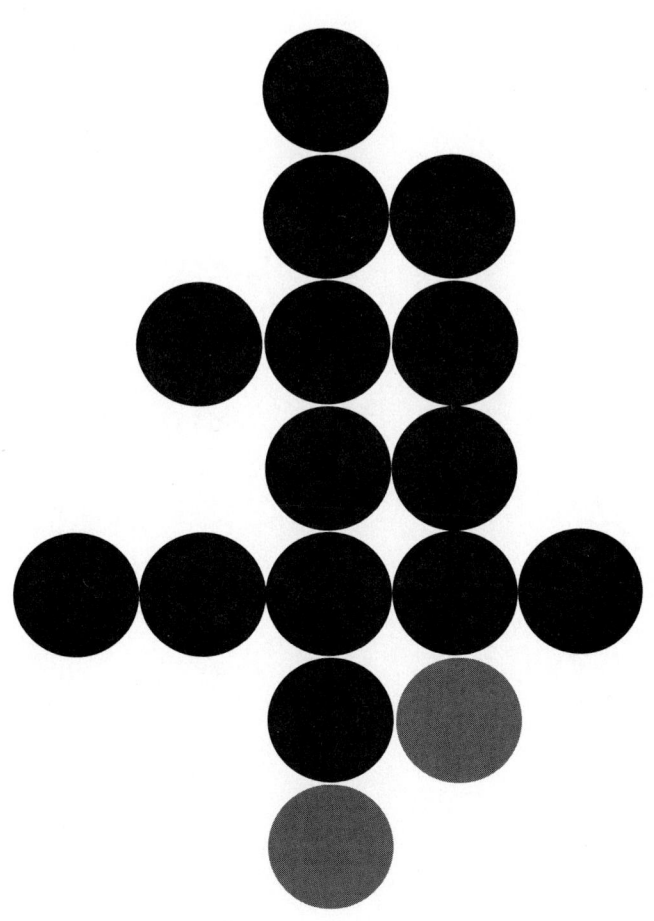

The integumentary system comprises 15 percent of the body weight and includes the skin, hair, and nails. As one of the largest and most visible of the body organs, the integument is important both to the body's function and to a person's appearance.

The cells of the skin are constantly growing and ever-changing; they respond to stimuli from within the body as well as from the external environment. The skin has properties that make it a pliable and tough body covering. It is resilient enough to adapt to the many positions assumed by the underlying structures that give the body and the skin covering its shape. The skin may be considered as a shield for the underlying body organs, protecting them from environmental forces such as heat, cold, pressure, friction, chemicals, electromagnetic forces and radiation, and bacterial invasion.

Anatomically the skin is made up of three layers (Fig. 14-1): the epidermis or outermost layer, the dermis, which is the thickest of the layers, and the subcutaneous or adipose layer. The epidermis varies in thickness from as thin as $1/50$ inch in areas over the eyelids and eardrums to as thick as $1/4$ inch over the soles of the feet. Cells in the epidermis grow from the inside to the outside. The majority of the epidermal cells are keratinocytes, the cells that produce keratin. These keratinocytes change in structure as they grow and move toward the outer layer of the epidermis and are given different names in each layer of the epidermis. In the bottom layer of the epidermis, called the stratum germinativum, the keratinocytes are tall columnar cells, called basal cells. These basal cells are germinative cells that divide into two daughter cells. Some of the daughter cells move up to the next epidermal layer to form the stratum spinosum, a layer of prickle cells that produce keratin. Gradually the prickle cells form granules and move up to form the next epidermal layer, the stratum granulosum. The granular cells gradually flatten out and begin to die in this epidermal layer, moving up to form the outermost epidermal layer, the stratum corneum. Keratin cells in this outermost layer, the horny layer of the epidermis, are dehydrated, but it is the keratin, a largely insoluble protein, which provides the protective coating of the outside layer of the skin, hair, and nails.

The outside layer of the **epidermis,** then, contains keratinocytes that have only cell walls and lipid residues remaining. These cells are essentially dead cells and form a semipermeable membrane that retains body fluid and electrolytes while at the same time preventing entry of substances from the environment. **Keratinization** is the process through which the outermost layer of skin is formed as epidermal cells lose their nuclei and flatten out to form the stratum corneum. The new cells require about 2 weeks for their development, and loss of viability of epidermal cells takes about 2 weeks. The nonviable cells are gradually sloughed off. As long as the delicate balance of the skin functions is maintained, the constant shedding of skin cells goes unnoticed. At times, however, when new cells form at a rate faster than the sloughing process, the horny layer may appear as scales or as thickened, irritated skin. Conversely, when new cells form at a rate slower than the sloughing of dead cells, the skin becomes thin and may appear eroded.

The **dermis** lies beneath the epidermis. This skin layer is comprised mainly of collagen fibers along with reticulum and elastin fibers, water, and a ground substance which is a gel. The collagen fibers give the skin its tensile strength whereas reticulum fibers link the collagen fibers together. Elastin fibers, as their name suggests, are elastic. The gel, or ground substance, is composed of mucopolysaccharides (elements of colloid and water) and serves as a medium for the fibers. The dermis provides substance and structural support for the epidermis and absorbs strain and stress. The dermis communicates with the epidermis through papillae, which are finger-like projections of dermal tissue extending into the dermis. These cells contain nerves, capillaries, and lymphatics; they supply the epidermis with its required nutrients.

The dermis communicates below with the subcutaneous tissue, which contains fatty cells. The subcutaneous layer varies in thickness in different areas of the body and is not present in areas such as the eyelids. The subcutaneous layer of skin provides insulation, a cushion for absorption of stress, and a deposit for nutrients in the fat cells.

Hair and nails are often referred to as appendages of the skin and are also made up of keratin. Hair is either terminal or vellus. Terminal hair is found on the scalp, arms, legs, and face, while vellus hairs are found all over the body. The vellus hairs are very short and fine and are often not readily visible.

Hair grows according to a mosaic pattern in

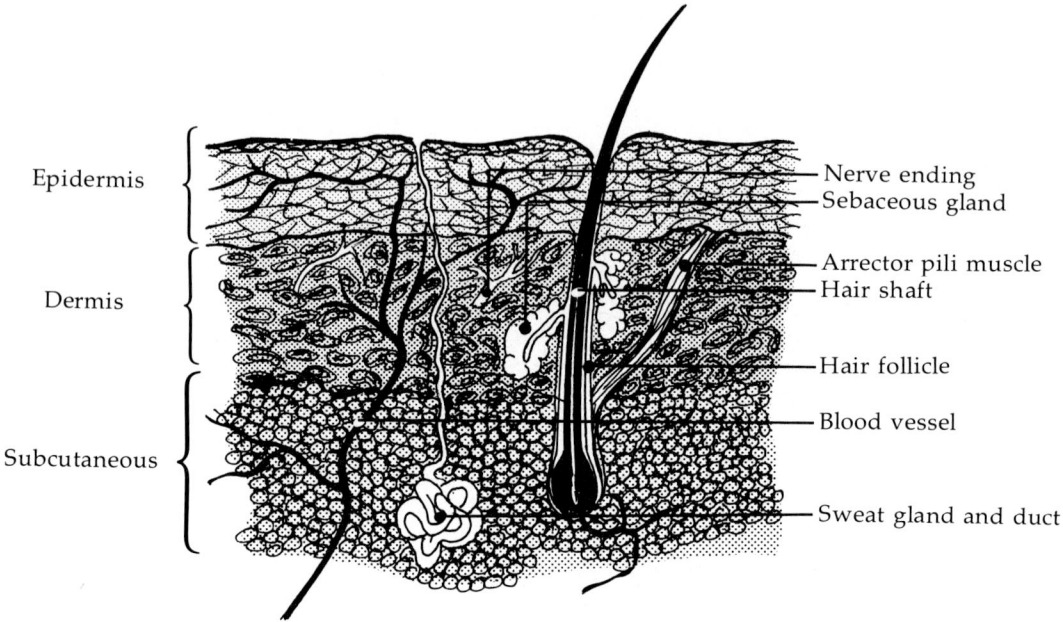

Figure 14-1
The layers and appendages of the skin.

which each hair follicle functions independently. The life phases of a hair include the anagen phase, or new growth; a period of atrophy which is the catagen phase; and finally a resting phase called the telogen phase. Hair follicles are always in different phases with some beginning the cycle of hair growth in the anagen phase and others in the other two phases. Thus, hair is constantly being formed and shed, at a rate of up to 100 hairs per day from the scalp in normal conditions. **Alopecia,** loss of scalp hair, is a normal occurrence that is part of the aging process. It results from changing cycles of the hair growth pattern. Abnormal loss may also be induced by mechanical trauma to the hair by pulling or twisting as well as by certain illnesses, including metabolic dysfunction, infections, or systemic diseases such as lupus erythematosus. Certain forms of therapy, such as x-ray, antimetabolite drugs, and some chemicals may also interfere with hair growth.

Both apocrine and sebaceous glands are associated with hair cells. The apocrine glands are found in the axilla, the areola, the genital areas, and the anal area. The **apocrine glands** secrete odorless secretions that promote bacterial growth with bacterial degradation of the secretions and cause body odor. **Sebaceous glands** are called oil glands and produce sebum. The function of sebum is really not known, but it is thought that sebum inhibits bacterial growth. Plugged sebaceous gland ducts cause acne.

Another type of skin gland is the **eccrine sweat gland.** This type of gland is present on the palms of the hands and the soles of the feet, and secretion is increased in times of emotional stress. The axillae also contain eccrine sweat glands that are responsive to emotions. Other eccrine glands are responsive to body temperature, functioning to retain or lose moisture in regulation of the body's heat balance. Maintenance of the heat balance within the body is one of the skin's regulatory functions.

Another regulatory function of the skin is that of cutaneous sensation. This function is most highly developed in the fingertips and on the lips. Among the cutaneous sensations are pain, itching, tingling, tickling, wetness, dryness, temperature, and pressure. Cutaneous sensations are described as cold, warmth, touch or pressure, and pain. One appreciates the functioning of the skin when one realizes that all four of these cutaneous sensations may be present in a small area of skin. The term **sensory field** describes the body area served by the branches of a sensory axon. The population of receptors for cutaneous sensation differs in various parts of the body. Each portion of the body that normally contains the axon branches usually contains overlapping branches. The sensory network of branches in the skin is actually dense and interwoven.

The electrophysiologic classification of nerve fibers is A, B, and C fibers. The A fibers are designated alpha, beta, gamma, and delta. The A and B fibers are myelinated and C fibers are nonmyelinated. A-beta fibers are receptors for touch and pressure; A-delta fibers receive pain and temperature sensations and may be thinly myelinated or have free nerve endings. C fibers serve as receptors for pain and temperature and are mechanoreceptors. In the skin, the Pacinian corpuscles located deep in the dermis and subcutaneous tissue receive pressure sensations. Meissner's corpuscles, located in the papillary dermis, detect movement. Ruffini's endings are receptors for heat and Krause's end bulbs are receptors for cold; both are located in the dermis. Merkel's disks, located in the lower layer of the stratum germinativum, detect transient and steady sensations for pressure. These receptors have been presented as having specific receptor functions. It should be noted, however, that the specificity of sensory receptors is currently being questioned; it may be that these receptors have overlapping functions.

The mechanoreceptors include those for pressure and touch. Receptors for pressure are located both in the subcutaneous tissue and dermis. It is thought that receptors in the papillary dermis detect movement while the deeper receptors detect indentations of pressure. Touch receptors are the most sensitive of the mechanoreceptors and can be stimulated by deflections of hair, their terminals being located around the lower part of follicles. Temperature receptors may be either specific for hot or cold or for both cold and pressure. It is interesting to note that some of the cold receptors are also stimulated by extreme warmth, causing a sensation of cold even though the person's skin is very warm. This is evidenced by chilling, which occurs in persons who have high fevers. Sensations of temperature are dependent on changes in the temperature rather than on detection of the actual temperature. For example, when the skin is very cool, exposure to warmer but still cool air causes the sensation of warmth. The receptors detect the change in temperature from very cool to less cool and cause the sensory interpretation of "warmer."

Pain receptors are free nerve terminals located in connective tissue and in between dermal cells up to the layer of the stratum corneum. Pain receptors are responsive to a variety of stimuli including mechanical, chemical, electrical, and thermal. The mechanics of pain sensation are not well understood. It is thought that pain elicited by a pinprick is produced by the A-delta fibers while burning pain, which has a slower onset and lasts longer, results from stimulation of the C fibers of peripheral nerves. When skin tissues are damaged, proteolytic enzymes released from the injured cutaneous tissue are thought to excite pain sensations. Itch and tickle sensations are also thought to be conducted by C fibers. Itching, a sensation that causes an urge to scratch, has a sensory afterimage; that is, the sensation continues after the source of stimuli has been removed. The tickle sensation is thought to be a component of the itch sensation and also has an afterimage. The itching sensation is inhibited by the pain sensation. Scratching must cause pain to be effective in relieving itch. The itch sensation is different from the pain sensation in that the stimulus for itch is localized in the skin, the conjunctiva, or mucous membrane of the nose whereas pain can be evoked from deep tissue stimuli. Proteinases injected into the skin may elicit the itch sensation, as is seen in allergic reactions. The chemical enzymes thought to be important stimuli for pain and itch sensations are not fully understood.

The previous overview of the integument has included the skin and hair. The remaining portion of the integument, the nails, is also made up of keratinized cells, modified to become the nail structure. Nails grow from their base in a continuous fashion.

Nails are either cut, filed, or broken or worn off at the ends. If they are not subjected to such alterations, they grow to indefinite lengths. The matrix of the nail can be seen at its distal end as the white moons of the fingernails. In the matrix, the process of keratinization takes place. The visible portion of the nail is made up of keratin; it derives its color not from the keratin, but rather from the vascular bed underlying the nail. Because the nails are metabolically active in their formation, changes in metabolism from any source, such as insufficient oxygen, inadequate nutrition, or other causes, bring about changes in the nails.

Factors Influencing Changes in the Integumentary System

Examination of the integumentary system provides the nurse with information about the patient. The texture and color of the hair and skin are clues to ethnic origin. The condition of the hair, nails, and skin indicates to some degree how the person takes care of his or her health as viewed by personal appearance. In addition, the condition of the hair, nails, and skin also indicates the presence of disease conditions associated with skin changes. The integument is affected by many different systemic diseases, and some of the changes in hair, skin, or nails are specific to certain disease processes. The integumentary system is also subject to exposure to environmental factors. This exposure causes normal skin changes of an adaptive nature. Finally, the integumentary system normally undergoes changes in the aging process.

In view of all the functions of the skin, it is amazing to consider that, in most parts of the body, the epidermis is only as thick as a page in this textbook. Light can be transmitted through the skin and can be demonstrated by holding a flashlight close to the palm of the hand and viewing the light from the upper surface.

While skin color is influenced by reflection of light, melanin in the epidermis is the primary basis for skin color. The amount of melanin (skin pigmentation) in the skin is genetically determined. In addition, the color of the skin is influenced by the volume of blood in the capillary circulation. Low blood volumes are associated with paleness and pallor, increased circulation with pinkness of the skin. Cyanosis results when the capillary venous plexus contains more than 5 gm of unsaturated oxygen. There are variations in the transparency of the skin among people as well as in different body parts. The changes in skin color are more readily observed in areas of transparent or thin skin; they are more difficult to observe in people whose skin is thicker and more opaque.

The integumentary system is influenced by exposure to environmental factors. In dry hot environments, the skin becomes dry and may crack if sufficient fluid is lost. Overexposure to sunlight causes skin to become erythematous. Soaking the skin causes it to become wrinkled and pale. Chemicals and toxic substances applied to the skin or in contact with the skin cause localized responses including erythema or allergic reactions or both in susceptible individuals.

The integument is metabolically active and is dependent on major body processes such as circulation, respiration, ingestion, assimilation and metabolism of nutrients, elimination, and nervous system function. An example of this interrelatedness of the integument with other body processes is skin turgor, which reflects the fluid balance of the body. When appropriately hydrated, the skin can be pinched and released and it quickly returns to its normal shape. In overhydrated states, when the fluid content of the skin is greater than normal, the pinched skin holds the shape of the finger indentations for a longer than normal period of time. Dehydrated skin becomes brittle and is subject to cracking and scaling. Skin color is another example of this interdependency—the presence of jaundice indicates liver or biliary tract dysfunction. The amount, texture, and distribution of hair on the skin is influenced by hormones. An obvious example is change occurring in thyroid dysfunction. Coarse hair is characteristic of hypothyroidism, whereas fine silky hair is characteristic of hyperthyroidism. Growth of genital and facial hair is influenced by androgens and estrogens.

Metabolic changes are also associated with nail changes. For example, clubbing of the fingernails is caused by decreased oxygen saturation in many diseases. Abnormalities that may be seen in addition to clubbing, in which the angle between the nail base and nail is lost, include **splinter hemorrhages,** which appear as streaks in the fingernails, usually in persons with subacute bacterial endocarditis; **Beau's lines,** which are horizontal depressed lines that occur in conjunction with severe illnesses of any type; and finally spoon nails or **koilonychia,** in which the nail is shaped in a concave fashion, generally associated with iron deficiency anemia and nutritional deficiency.

Certain people are susceptible to dysfunction of the integumentary system. Among them are persons who have long-standing and continuous exposure to the sun, chemicals, or toxins, and the aged. Exposure to sunlight, chemicals, and toxins may either cause diseases such as cancer or may accelerate aging of the skin.

EFFECTS OF AGING

As a person ages, resistance to trauma to the skin decreases because of generalized atrophy. With aging there are normal changes in both the consistency and the appearance of the skin. Wrinkles are associated with aging as is an increasing dryness of the epidermis. The dermis of an aged person contains fewer mucopolysaccharides, and the composition of the collagen changes so that there is more insoluble collagen. Just as the epidermis becomes thinner and irregularly pigmented, the dermis loses some of its normal elasticity and its capacity to remain hydrated. Growth of the integument is slowed, as evidenced in slower growth of hair and nails and in decreased sebaceous gland secretion. The nails become brittle and hard and sometimes crack as part of the aging process. The specific changes and their rate of occurrence vary according to genetic makeup and are not totally dependent on chronological age. An important implication of the aging process for care of skin dysfunction is that as a person ages, there is a gradual increase in the amount of time required for repair of wounds. This time may double between the ages of 20 and 40.

TERMINOLOGY USED IN ASSESSMENT

The nurse should become familiar with the terminology used to define the most commonly occurring types of skin dysfunction. The following paragraphs describe the lesions (Fig. 14-2) often referred to later in this chapter.

Macules are small areas of change in color of the skin. The skin does not change in consistency. The color change is due to changes in pigmentation or to the blood supply in the area. Macules are usually no larger than 1 cm in size and are smooth and flat. **Papules** are usually smaller than macules and are caused by a proliferation of cells or by the accumulation of metabolic or fluid products. The papule can be felt because it is an elevated lesion. **Nodules** are similar to papules but are somewhat larger and usually extend deeper into the skin layers than do papules. A nodule can be felt as a bump and is usually firmer in consistency than a papule. Like papules, nodules are formed from collections of metabolic substances, fluids, or proliferation of cells in the area of skin affected.

Plaques are sometimes formed by closely aligned papules. A plaque is an elevated portion of skin that has a flat surface. The areas of skin affected may vary from small areas to large portions of skin, as a result of thickening of the layers or of one of the underlying skin layers.

A **wheal,** sometimes called a hive when occurring spontaneously, is a rounded elevation of the skin that usually represents edema of the upper layer of the dermis. A wheal is usually superficial and may have irregular edges. **Vesicles** are also formed by edema or an accumulation of fluid and are called small blisters. A vesicle appears as a contained fluid area that assumes the status of a bubble. **Bullae** are large vesicles or blisters, also being filled with serous fluid. The major difference between vesicles and bullae is that the bullae are larger in size. When vesicles or bullae fill with blood they are called hemorrhagic vesicles or bullae.

Cysts are also similar to vesicles, but they have thicker walls and may have semisolid contents. Other differences between cysts and vesicles or bullae are that cysts are larger and deeper and are usually covered with normal-appearing epidermis.

Pustules are also similar to vesicles and bullae except that, instead of containing serous fluid, they contain white blood cells and necrotic debris and may appear as white or yellowish bubbles. The formation of pus gives the pustule both its name and appearance.

Scaling of the skin is associated with dryness or thickening of the uppermost layer of the epidermis, the stratum corneum. Scales are sometimes easily sloughed from the skin. In other instances scales are difficult to remove. **Crusts,** on the other hand, appear as a dried covering over a previous lesion and contain dehydrated serum that was formerly contained in the lesion. Crusts are usually composed of dried fluid which is mixed with keratin cells. A large, adherent crust is referred to as a **scab.**

Erosions of the skin are areas in which the epidermis has been destroyed. The eroded area of superficial epidermis leaves a moist surface. An **ulcer** is similar to an erosion but extends deeper into the skin layers. Ulcers

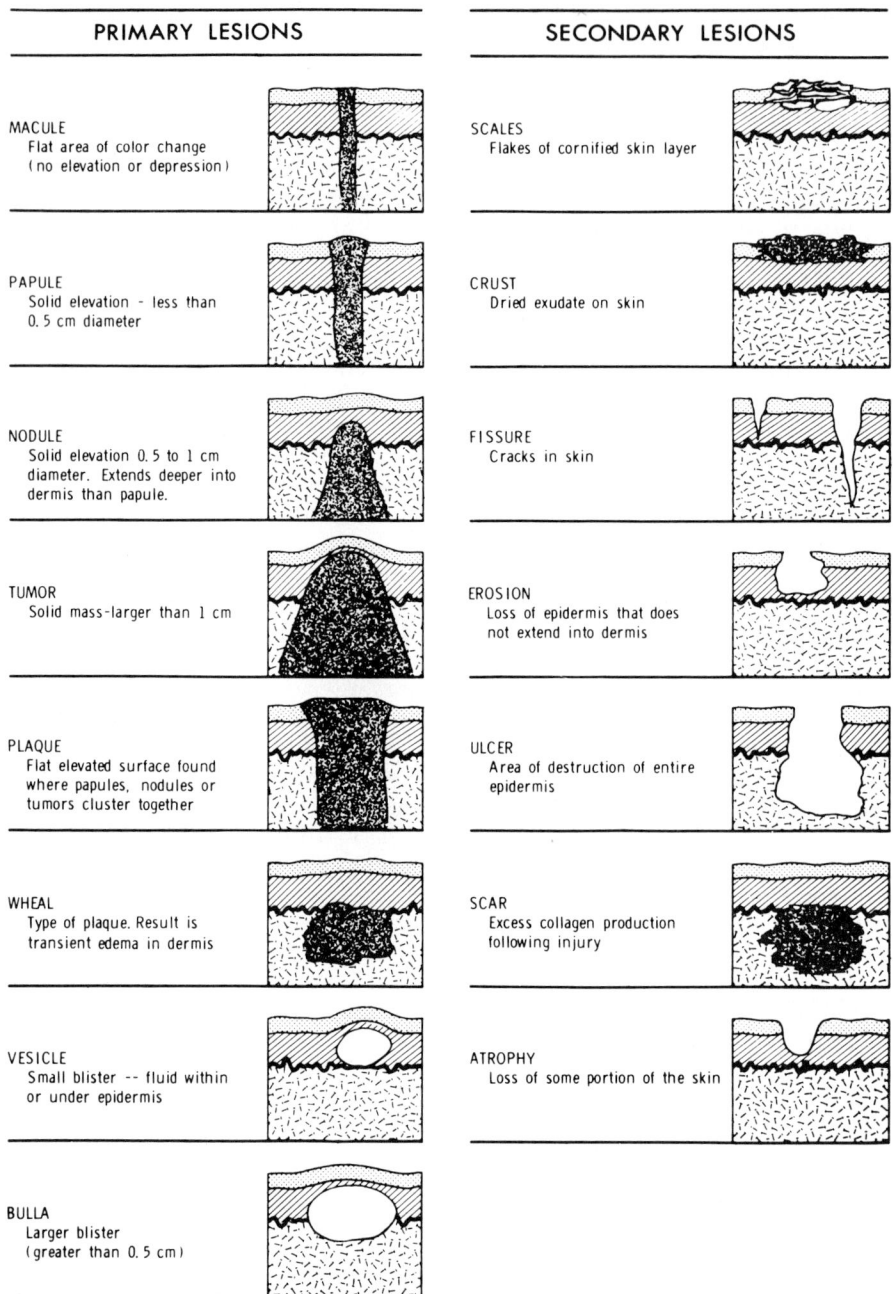

Figure 14-2
Characteristics of common skin lesions. (From J. Sana and R. D. Judge, *Physical Appraisal Methods in Nursing Practice*. Boston: Little, Brown and Company, 1973. Reproduced by permission.)

often bleed and may leave scars following the healing process. **Fissures** are lesions that interrupt the integrity of the skin surface. Fissures are recognized by their line-like appearance and tend to form in areas where the skin naturally folds or creases, such as at the sides of the mouth or in the gluteal folds.

Erythema is redness caused by capillary dilatation, commonly noted in sunburn or underlying areas in which skin has become scaled. Another type of skin discoloration is **hyperpigmentation,** which is usually related to increased melanin production. **Freckles** are examples of hyperpigmentation in an area with increased melanin. **Moles** are caused by increases in the number of melanin-producing cells. A bluish-gray color indicates that melanin is being formed in the dermis rather than in its normal placement in the epidermis [10].

Hypopigmentation may occur as a result of various traumatic substances either applied to the external surface of the skin or resulting from disease processes internal to the body. **Vitiligo** is a type of skin dysfunction of unknown cause that results in loss of pigmentation in an area of skin. Chemicals, radiation, or other substances that destroy melanocytes result in areas of hypopigmentation (see color insert Figure 4 on page 1078A).

Pruritus, also called itching, is a protective reflex mechanism. Stimulation of nonmyelinated peripheral nerve fibers in the deep epidermis evokes the sensation of itching, which serves as a warning that the skin is in contact with harmful substances. Factors that initiate pain stimuli also initiate itching stimuli, including enzyme release, vasodilatation, and mechanical or chemical stimuli. When one has pruritus, the urge to scratch is evoked to remove the harmful substance. When scratching interferes with the integrity of the skin, it becomes excoriated. (Another term for excoriations is scratches.) Pruritus results from stimulation of nonadaptive nerve receptors and therefore is continuous as long as the stimulus endures. Therefore, pruritus is extremely distressful to affected individuals and may cause tenseness or anxiety as demonstrated by body movements and an inability to concentrate. Pruritus may also interfere with sleep and relaxation, which in turn may cause the individual to be tired and cross. Management of severe pruritus is often a challenge to the nurse, because of the emotional response to the continuous discomfort.

Several systemic diseases, notably uremia, are associated with pruritus. Liver diseases, some types of vascular dysfunction with venous stasis, and diabetes mellitus are also associated with pruritus. In addition, pruritus may be caused by localized skin diseases or lesions. Atrophy of the cutaneous glands, which occurs normally in the aged or in persons with excessively dry skin, may cause pruritus.

Hyperkeratosis is thickening of the stratum corneum as a result of friction, rubbing, or continued pressure. Examples of causes of hyperkeratosis are the pressure on the fingers when writing with a pencil, wearing tight shoes that rub, or long-term playing of instruments that require the use of unprotected fingertips so that the fingertips become callused. A **callus,** then, is an area of hyperkeratosis. A corn **(clavus)** is a confined area of hyperkeratinization in which the skin layers lose their demarcation. A callus usually has a ball or a central core of keratin. **Lichenification** is increased thickness of the skin that results from repeated scratching. When this occurs, the skin appears furrowed and rough. Superficial skin markings become more prominent and there is increased pigmentation in lichenification.

Urticaria is a transient edema caused by leakage of plasma from the blood vessels into the skin; it appears as a white, itchy lesion with an erythematous halo. Urticaria usually results from factors that cause histamine release, such as chemical, thermal, or mechanical irritation. The histamine causes increased permeability of the blood vessels, which leads to the leakage of plasma. Usually urticaria is associated with hypersensitivity reactions and with allergies; it may be localized or appear in patches.

Erythema is also caused by dilatation of vessels with leakage of fluid that collects within the skin. In certain types of erythema, the fluid can collect between the dermis and the epidermis, which causes formation of a round lesion. Externally the appearance of the center of the lesion is different from its periphery. The center of the lesion may be either clear or redder than the outer margin. Erythema occurs in the inflammatory response and in allergic responses.

Erythema nodosum is a deep subcutaneous vasculitis that is also associated with the hypersensitivity response. In this response, there is an initial formation of nodules that may flatten out to appear as a bruise or ecchymosis. The nodules are filled with fluid that has leaked from the vessels; healing occurs as the fluid is reabsorbed.

Purpura is a reddish-purple discoloration of the skin caused by extravasation of blood from the vessels in the skin. Purpura is most frequently macular, without a raised lesion. When there is inflammatory vasculitis, in which the vessel walls are thickened and disrupted (as in infections or allergic responses), the purpura occurs as elevated skin discolorations.

Spongiosis is the formation of edema between the cells of the epidermis. The fluid eventually escapes from the intraepidermal areas to the outside so that there is weeping of fluid from the skin. This weeping may lead to scaling and may be associated with erythema followed by epidermal thickening.

In the healing process, the skin forms scales and scabs and crusts. **Eschar** is the name given to scabs that cover a large area of skin, such as occurs in burns.

A **scar** represents healing of an area in which fibrous tissue has replaced the destroyed epidermis or deeper layers of skin. **Keloids** are scars that have hypertrophied. **Striae** are streaks or lines that may appear paler than the surrounding skin usually as a result of mechanical stretching of the skin surfaces, as occurs in pregnancy. Purple striae result from increased corticosteroid levels.

The appearance of skin dysfunction is often described by the terms given above. The nurse should be able to identify skin lesions and communicate findings, using this terminology.

Nursing Care

Nursing care for patients with dysfunction of the integumentary system is predicated on the awareness that the dysfunction may have caused disruption of the patient's body image. Because skin dysfunction often results in visible lesions, the affected person is subject to reactions of persons who view the lesions with curiosity or distaste. These reactions may influence the patient's body image, which is partly formed by the responses of others. The nurse should be cognizant that initial impressions are formed by spontaneous and often unconscious assessment of appearance as evidenced by shape, size, and the condition of the skin, hair, and nails. In addition, impressions of personality and state of health are formed by observation of the shape of body structures and body movements. Because the integument is a body covering, it is difficult to separate that covering from underlying body structures. Facial features, for example, may not be perfect, but are enhanced by healthy skin. The nurse may react either to the patient's skin lesion or to the implications of the skin lesion. In some instances, skin dysfunction is related to poor health habits or sloppiness and the nurse may unconsciously make judgments about the patient because of his or her appearance. It is interesting to note that the skin also reflects emotions and feelings through reactions such as blushing, wrinkling of brows, smiling, perspiration, and tensing. All these reactions are visible elements of both the nurse's and the patient's state of feeling. Patients who are sensitive to negative reactions from the nurse may find it difficult to trust the nurse.

The public is generally conscious of appearance and the condition of the visible integument. Fashion often dictates which products one ought to use to achieve the current look in skin, hair, or nails. In an article published in the *Saturday Review* the statement was made that consumers spend $500 million for deodorants, shaving items, and perfume and another $1.5 billion for hair preparations [7]. A number of ingredients in some of these preparations have been found harmful to the body. The Food and Drug Administration continually reviews and improves existing controls and determines controls for new products in attempts to protect consumers from harmful products. Consumer interest in safety and protection from harmful products is an important impetus to the controls established by the Food and Drug Administration.

Changes in hair, skin, and nails are difficult for the affected person to deny or forget, because they are always visible. The affected person is often distressed about the dysfunction; people who value physical appearance and suffer a change in body image may consequently withdraw from social interaction because of visible dysfunction of the integument. A dramatic example of the impact of skin problems is the withdrawal from social activities by a person who has visible skin changes following a severe burn. The presence of skin lesions, patches of changes in pigmentation, or even minor bruises may prove to be just as distressful to a person as an extensive burn scar. The nurse should recognize that there is often no direct correlation between the size and extent of skin lesions and the distress they can cause the patient.

In addition, physical appearance and a healthy integument are often a requirement for certain types of employment. Dysfunction of the integument may preclude continuing employment in these types of positions. The nurse should be sensitive to the economic implications that skin lesions or dysfunction may have for affected individuals in terms of employment. Another important economic factor associated with dysfunction of the integument is the cost of treatment. For many persons, this cost is a financial burden.

PATIENT HISTORY AND PHYSICAL EXAMINATION

The patient's perception of dysfunction should be elicited, if feasible, through a history-taking interview. The nurse then describes the nature of the dysfunction, using appropriate terminology when writing up the history. Information obtained from the history is then used to guide the initial examination and follow-up assessment of treatment. When there is a skin lesion or an area of change in the character, consistency, or texture of the skin, the nurse should ascertain when the patient first noticed the change. If possible, events that may have caused the change should be explored. These are some examples: Is the onset associated with the use of certain medications? Related to certain experiences, such as travel to a foreign country? Related to a certain type of employment in which the patient is in contact with irritating or toxic substances? Related to any hobbies or projects that require the use of glue or chemicals? Related to new products used in the home?

Some skin dysfunction, because of its nature, is chronic, and there may be a long history of periods of remission followed by periods of exacerbations in the skin changes. Some of these changes are seasonal. For example, **ringworm** often appears in the warm summer months or in warm climates and disappears in cold weather. Sometimes skin lesions may be related to emotions. In times of stress, there may be an exacerbation of the problem, while in times of relative calm, there may be no skin changes. In other instances, skin changes may be the first clue to the presence of a systemic disease. People who notice jaundice of the sclera may become aware that symptoms they previously thought to be due to influenza might be related to liver dysfunction. Similarly, certain systemic diseases result in skin changes for which the patient seeks treatment.

Finally, certain types of skin dysfunction occur in relation to age. Diaper rash occurs in infants while acne is associated with puberty. Women notice the formation of striae following delivery of their babies or extreme loss of weight. Areas of hyperplasia are noted in the aged. These are but a few examples of the different types of skin dysfunction that may occur in concert with an age group. Knowledge of these relationships gives the examiner information about what is important and significant to look for in the patient being examined.

Examination of the integument is included in a general physical examination. The examiner observes and evaluates the condition of the integument throughout the physical examination when evaluating muscle tone and muscle strength, listening for chest sounds, or palpating a body area. Specific skin manifestations associated with various disease processes often alert the examiner to conduct more specific diagnostic tests.

It is important that the examination of the integument be done in a place where the light source is good. Some lesions and changes in skin color are not evident when lighting is poor. Inspection of the skin is made in a systematic manner. One can easily miss small lesions if a systematic approach is not used. Some examiners prefer to examine the skin of each body part separately before beginning further examination of the part through auscultation or palpation. In this way the body folds can be smoothed out and examined, body hair distribution noted, and changes in the skin texture, color, or presence of lesions noted. At some point in the examination, the skin is viewed in its totality to determine variations from one body part to another in color, texture, or pigmentation. Skin turgor, sensitivities to touch, and the amount of moisture on skin surfaces are also important observations.

Individual variations in normal skin are influenced by the genetic makeup, sex, age, and race. The external environment also influences the skin's texture and consistency, as does nutritional status. These variations make diagnosis of skin lesions complicated. The nurse must be able to define types of lesions, describe the lesions with some degree of specificity, and note the location, distribution, size, and nature of lesions. If the skin lesion appears as a mass, it is important to note the degree of elevation, mobility, and presence of pain or tenderness. Often, changes in skin lesions from one time to another are most significant in determining the type of lesion as well as the cause of the lesion.

Skin lesions are often viewed through a magnifying glass or hand lens to enable the observer to see the fine lines and markings of the lesion not visible to the naked eye. A lens is, then, an important tool for use in diagnosis. The Woods light, which is a high-pressure mercury lamp with a filter of nickel oxide and silica, transmits longwave ultraviolet wavelengths. Certain skin lesions fluoresce under this light so that a diagnosis can be made. For example, superficial fungus infections fluoresce a blue-green color. Vitiligo fluoresces white and *Pseudomonas* organisms fluoresce a yellowish-green color.

A **diascope** is an instrument made of clear plastic and is used to apply mild pressure to the skin to observe the effect. An example is applying pressure to the central body of telangiectasis to occlude the dilated vessel. If the lesion is not a permanently dilated vessel, the central body depression will not result in disappearance of the lesion.

A **patch test** is used to determine sensitivity to allergens or antigens, which are applied to the skin and occluded for 48 hours to determine the response of the skin. An erythematous response indicates sensitivity to the allergen or antigen being used to test for hypersensitivity.

Biopsy in the diagnosis of skin lesions can be carried out as a punch biopsy or through incision or excision of the lesion. A **punch biopsy** is performed with a special instrument (a punch) that has a terminal end about 4 to 6 mm in size. Following application of local anesthesia, the punch is applied with firm pressure and then rotated to obtain a round skin specimen for biopsy. The punch biopsy is used for lesions less than ½ cm in size. A **shave biopsy** is used to obtain a specimen from a raised or elevated skin lesion. The skin is first prepared with alcohol and the upper portion of the lesion is shaved off with a scalpel. Lesions may be incised to obtain tissue for laboratory study. Excised lesions are sent to the laboratory for cytologic study.

TREATMENT OF INTEGUMENTARY DYSFUNCTION

Nursing care of patients with skin diseases is complex. Not only are there many variations in normal skin, but there are also many different types of manifestations of skin diseases. Not every affected person has the same type of problem. There are differences in the location of lesions, in the response to therapy, and in the capability for self-care. Because many people take care of their skin lesions at home, visiting clinics or doctors' offices only for diagnosis, treatment procedures, and follow-up care, a primary aspect of the nurse's role becomes that of health teaching.

The broad topic of health teaching encompasses observation; counseling; giving information; helping the patient learn to apply topical medications, dressings, and other forms of treatment; and finally, advising about positive health practices to prevent recurrences of problems. Often the nurse notices skin lesions that should receive medical attention while giving care related to another health problem. The nurse must be aware of significant changes, must develop an ability to recognize skin lesions, and must be able to refer the patient to proper sources for treatment.

Skin dysfunction caused by systemic diseases is usually cured when the underlying systemic cause is treated effectively. In debilitated persons skin lesions may not respond to treatment until the general health status improves. Treatment for skin lesions includes systemic medications, topical medications, wet and dry dressings, and surgical techniques. There are numerous medications available for topical application to the skin. These medications can be classified as ointments, creams, lotions, gels, tinctures, solutions, pastes, and powders. An **ointment** is oil with water, whereas a **cream** is an emulsion of oil with water. **Lotions** are suspensions of insoluble powders in water (a shake lotion is a lotion that requires shaking to suspend the particles prior to use). A **gel** is a transparent colloid that liquefies on application, leaving a thin film following drying. **Pastes** contain powder and are used to hold therapeutic ingredients in place, usually being mixed with an ointment. Sprays and aerosols are similar to lotions.

Water may be used alone, on dressings, or in baths to soften and soothe the skin in mild inflammation. Solutions are also used for their soothing effects and contain ingredients that promote healing. The most commonly used include Burow's solution, saline, silver nitrate, and potassium permanganate solutions. Powders are used to dry the skin by absorbing moisture and fostering evaporation; they also have a cooling effect. Ointments, such as petroleum jelly, are applied to occlude the skin and to keep it moist; they may be used as a vehicle for holding therapeutic ingredients in place. Creams have variable ingredients and may be similar to ointments if they contain a high amount of grease. Some creams contain more water than grease and disappear through evaporation, leaving a powder on the skin. Others contain more grease and may be occlusive, protecting the skin.

Topical medications include steroids, such as triamcinolone diacetate (Aristocort) and triamcinolone acetonide (Kenalog); antibiotics, of which gentamicin (Garamycin) is frequently used, as is bacitracin; fungicides such as amphotericin B (Fungizone) and nystatin (Mycostatin), which are antifungal antibiotics, and antifungal agents as selenium disulfide suspension (Selsun), or salicylic acid; keratolytic agents include resorcinol (Resorcin), salicylic acid tar compounds and medications containing sulfur; and antipruritic agents such as menthol, phenol, and camphor, which soothe and reduce itching. The reader is referred to a pharmacology text for additional information about medications used in the treatment of skin lesions. There are many different trade names and types of preparations in common use, and different medications are preferred by different physicians. In addition to topical medications, systemic antibiotics, antifungal agents, antihistamines, tranquilizers, and pain medications are used in the treatment of skin dysfunction.

The nurse, however, should be knowledgeable about methods for applying medications to the skin. Lotions are usually applied with the hands, and their use is designed to protect the skin, to dry the skin, and to cool it. Some lotions contain alcohol or astringents to provide for additional cooling and drying. Ointments are used to lubricate the skin. Some are water-soluble whereas others are difficult to remove with water. Yet others, such as silicone ointments, are designed to protect the skin from water. Pastes are used to absorb and contain powder and ointment.

Application of lotions and emulsions (creams) for topical treatment of skin lesions is often facilitated by use of a soft-bristled paint brush. Pastes and ointments may be applied with a spatula or tongueblade. The amount of pressure used for application should be controlled to prevent further damage to the involved skin. Paint brushes are useful for spreading lotions and emulsions evenly. Thicker preparations such as ointments and pastes are often applied with a rubber spatula to enable even distribution of the medication with a light touch. Powders are applied by sprinkling on the skin surface. Puffs may be used to facilitate dusting with powders.

Dressings are used for a variety of purposes including protection, provision of moisture, and for keeping medication in contact with the desired skin surfaces. **Wet dressings** are either open or occluded. They can be used to apply solutions to the skin, to moisten the skin, and to absorb debris from the skin lesions. Wet dressings are applied by placing on the affected skin area gauze or cloth saturated with the solution being used to soothe and cool the skin. When there is no drainage, the dressings can be maintained with moisture applied with an Asepto syringe. When there is drainage, the dressings should be removed and fresh dressings applied.

When moist dressings are being applied, the nurse should make certain that the room temperature is warm enough to prevent chilling of the patient. Heat lamps are sometimes used to provide the necessary heat, particularly if a large portion of the body is dressed. Dressings are removed carefully to prevent irritation and trauma to the skin, and unless there is significant drainage, dressings are removed infrequently. It is important, however, to remove all dressings periodically to allow the skin to dry, to prevent maceration of the tissues, and to examine the skin.

Occluded wet dressings are similar to open wet dressings except that a covering is applied over the wet dressing to prevent the escape of heat and to facilitate increased blood flow to the part being dressed. It is important that the nurse observe the condition of the skin periodically, as maceration and tissue damage can result from occlusive dressings. The skin should be exposed periodically, examined, and allowed to dry in between dressings.

Another type of dressing is the **wet-to-dry dressing,** which means that a wet dressing is applied and then allowed to dry. This technique is useful in removal of eschar or debris from skin lesions, for the drying dressing retains the debris, which is then removed with the dressing. It is necessary to remove dry dressings carefully so that the lesion is not traumatized by this form of debridement.

Finally, **dry dressings** are used to keep medications or topical applications in contact with the skin. They can also protect skin lesions from friction or further trauma and keep the lesions clean. Dry dressings may be left in place for a period of days. When there is drainage from the lesion, the dressing is changed to prevent bacterial invasion. A plastic film wrap may be used to provide airtight occlusive dressings.

It is difficult to place dressings on some areas of the body so that they stay in place without requiring the use of large amounts of tape or tubular coverings that occlude nonaffected areas. It is important that dressings be applied so that they remain in the desired location; they must not interfere with the integrity of the lesion or surrounding skin by friction caused by slipping. Many people with skin diseases also have allergies, which preclude the use of conventional tapes. When possible, the nurse should apply the dressing with a minimum amount of tape, using tie-type binders or other devices to hold the dressing in place.

In some skin diseases, soaps that mechanically clean the skin or soothing baths are prescribed. Oatmeal baths are soothing. It is necessary that the patient be advised to fill the tub with sufficient water so that the major portion of his body is immersed in the bath to achieve maximum benefit for lesions covering the body. Usually, the patient is advised not to remain in the tub longer than 20 or 30 minutes.

The nurse must be aware that certain topical medications can be absorbed by the skin. While the dosage of topical applications cannot be measured precisely, the nurse should be aware of the concentration of the medication being used and should develop a technique of applying topical medications in thin, even coats.

People who have skin diseases are often very uncomfortable. They are not only physiologically uncomfortable, but also suffer from the distress of an altered and disconcerting body image. The affected person may express feelings of uncleanliness because of the presence of skin lesions, even though his or her personal hygiene is impeccable. This feeling permeates the person's whole being and often affects normal social patterns. For example, when one feels "unclean" one is reluctant to engage in conversation and to participate in contact with others. This feeling has far-reaching effects for the affected person in terms of daily social contacts.

One of the distressing aspects of having a skin disease that covers a large portion of the body is the feeling that one must isolate oneself from others. This feeling may be supported by feedback from others who are reluctant to touch the person who has visible lesions. Touching, or tactile sense, is one of the primary components in nonverbal communicative processes and is an integral part of one's relationships with others throughout life. Tactile sensations provide information about the environment. This information varies from notification of danger signals to intimate and meaningful communication. Skin diseases often interfere with these tactile sensations and, depending on the location of the lesions, may deprive the person of a valuable source of input as well as a needed source of physical contact. When providing nursing care to patients who have skin lesions, the nurse should be aware of the implications of touch. Many nursing actions may convey disapproval, distaste, and nonacceptance unless the nurse gives good explanations for the actions. The simple act of using a paint brush to apply medications may be interpreted by the patient as an indication that the nurse is unwilling to touch his or her skin. This interpretation may make the patient feel rejected. If, however, the patient is told that the paint brush provides for even application of the medication to the skin with the least amount of trauma, he or she will appreciate the method.

The person with skin lesions who is also confined to bed requires very special attention to comfort. Linens may be particularly uncomfortable. Some persons are allergic to soaps or rinses used in laundry and require specially laundered linens. When scaling lesions are present, the scales can collect in the bed linens, giving the patient the feeling that he has "cracker crumbs" in his bed. Frequent change of linens and removal of the scales are required. Consistent routine application of topical medications is also important to maintain the patient's level of comfort. Maintenance of a feeling of well-being is facilitated by constant attention to such details as carefully following routines for application of topical medications and comfort measures. Once the person becomes uncomfortable, the treatment is somewhat less effective compared to the results achieved from prompt and consistent applications designed to maintain the comfort level. The latter often serves to decrease the amount of systemic pain medication required to achieve comfort.

Often people with skin lesions are generally uncomfortable and are unable to determine a specific problem they are experiencing. The alert nurse, through observation and knowledge of the condition, can often discern the primary source of the patient's discomfort. If, for example, the patient has a painful lesion on his mucous membranes he or she may experience generalized discomfort if localized treatment is not applied. The nurse may tend to administer a systemic pain medication to provide relief in such instances when actually a localized topical application of medication would be more effective. With localized treatment, the patient may also remain more alert and better able to participate in activities that might facilitate distraction from the skin lesions. Administration of systemic pain medications may render the patient lethargic.

Involvement in activities that engage the patient's interest requires concentration and is useful in facilitating comfort. However, the patient who has prolonged and severe pruritus may be unable to concentrate on anything and it may be necessary to administer tranquilizers in addition to topical applications. Pruritus is often most bothersome at night or when the sufferer has fewer distractions.

Another important role of the nurse in caring for persons with skin lesions is determination of the effectiveness of the treatment. In many instances, treatment is nonspecific and trial and error methods of selecting measures to provide comfort and relief are used. The nurse should observe results of specific treatment to ascertain its effectiveness and should document the results. It is possible that the conditions or methods of self-treatment either hinder or augment the results. Therefore, teaching self-care and assessing the results may be an ongoing process with patients who have long-term problems. The affected person may feel that more of a medication is useful in expediting the healing process, or he may discontinue a treatment prematurely because he has begun to feel better. The nurse must be aware of all of these possibilities and must teach the person correct care habits to promote full recovery if this is possible.

Finally, skin lesions are variable and often it is difficult to define specific causes for some lesions. The rash that results from a drug reaction may resemble that of measles or eczema. The nurse must realize that this variability prevents an accurate diagnosis of a skin rash or lesion and must learn to associate events to determine possible sources for the cause of the skin lesions. Assessment of skin lesions is facilitated when the nurse learns to be inherently observant of not only the types of skin lesions but also of the nature of the lesion, its pattern of spread, its response to therapy, and its effect on the patient.

As in every disease process or type of dysfunction, the purpose of examination and treatment is to determine ways to help the patient return to a state of health. This help is complicated when the person has skin dysfunction because of the human tendency to be overzealous in self-treating dysfunctions of hair, skin, and nails. One obvious problem in this regard is the ready availability of patent medications and home remedies designed to "cure" minor skin problems. One has only to visit a community drug store, a grocery store, or a department store to view the multitude of preparations available. Yet another aspect of self-care is that many people consistently use cosmetics to beautify the skin. They find it difficult to accept the knowledge that some of these beautifying and "good" products may actually cause dysfunction of the integument.

Electrosurgery is often used in the treatment of skin lesions. This method utilizes the tip of an electrode with high-frequency current. Electrodesiccation refers to superficial destruction of the lesion through application of heat, which causes the cells to become dehydrated and disrupted. Electrocoagulation is deeper than electrodesiccation and provides for deeper destruction of the skin cells. Electrosurgery is contraindicated in those who have pacemakers.

Cryosurgery is the application of cold for the purpose of destroying lesions. A slush made of precipitated sulfur, powdered dry ice, and acetone, or of solid carbon dioxide and acetone, is an example of substances used to apply cold. Liquid nitrogen is also used and needs to be stored in a container that allows for evaporation to prevent explosion. Liquid nitrogen can be applied with cotton applicators, metal discs, or sprays.

Ultraviolet light is used to suppress the rate of mitosis of the basal cells. Following suppression, there is a rebound increase in the turnover rate of the cells. Sources of ultraviolet light are the natural sun, sun lamps, or ultraviolet lights available for hospital and treatment center use. When using ultraviolet light, one should wear goggles to protect the eyes. The black light is a longwave ultraviolet light that is used with photoactive dyes to destroy viruses such as the DNA virus of herpes simplex. In many special care units, germicidal lamps, which are shortwave ultraviolet lamps, are used to kill bacteria.

Skin Dysfunction

Skin dysfunction may be categorized in many different ways. One of the simpler categorizations includes arrangement of skin dysfunction according to mechanical, chemical, or thermal sources; infection; allergies or hypersensitivity reactions; abnormal metabolism; abnormal cell growth; and systemic causes. Among the types of dysfunction related to trauma are cuts and scrapes, callus formation, and ulceration. Burns result from thermal or chemical trauma. Trauma to the skin may be intended, as in a surgical procedure, or it may be caused by accidental injury to the skin. Wound healing is discussed more fully in Chapter 1. Burns are discussed in Chapter 15. The following paragraphs will describe the remaining categories of skin dysfunction that occur most commonly.

INFLAMMATORY AND ALLERGIC SKIN DYSFUNCTION

Acne is a condition associated with puberty or with middle age. Acne vulgaris, an inflammatory disease that involves the pilosebaceous follicle, is the form of acne that occurs most commonly at puberty. Acne rosacea, which is caused by permanent dilatation of vessels, usually occurs between the ages of 30 and 50 years, being more common in women but more severe in men. Taking certain drugs, particularly the bromides, iodides, and corticosteroids, may cause acne. Women notice that acne is more severe during the premenstrual period. Both conditions predominate in areas of the skin in which there are very large and active sebaceous glands, primarily on the face, the upper chest, and the upper back. Neither acne vulgaris nor acne rosacea has a clearly defined cause. For this reason, treatment is symptomatic.

Acne vulgaris is a physiologic response to the hormonal changes of puberty. It tends to be more severe in those with a familial tendency toward its occurrence. The condition is not physiologically harmful and is usually outgrown, even without treatment. It is, however, psychologically disconcerting to the affected individual. The appearance of the face is important to everyone to some degree and particularly to a person in the life stage of adolescence who is finding his or her identity in relation to others. One of the most significant aspects in the treatment of acne is the patient's attitude toward and feelings about the acne. These feelings must be dealt with actively because self-confidence may be marred by the presence of acne. While physiologic treatment may improve the appearance, the emotional overtones and the self-concept may not improve along with the appearance unless this aspect of care is also managed.

The primary lesions of acne vulgaris are blackheads and whiteheads. Almost everyone has blackheads and whiteheads, and their occurrence does not always develop into acne vulgaris. Blackheads, or comedones, are hair follicle canals that have been dilated by an accumulation of sebum and keratin that has obstructed the canal. The black color is caused by melanin pigments. Whiteheads are closed comedones that contain less compactly accumulated keratin and sebum. The opening of the follicle, which is a pore, is dilated and the blackheads and whiteheads can be seen visibly. Both blackheads and whiteheads may cause an inflammatory response, as seen in the incidence of pimples or papules. The papules may become pustules or nodules, and even cysts; in some instances abscesses may form.

The process that causes the inflammation is one of disruption of the hair follicle. When the hair follicle ruptures, the sebum and keratin enter the dermis where they cause inflammation. Bacteria are present with the accumulated sebum and keratin. Sebum is particularly irritating to the dermis. It contains free and esterified fatty acids, and the free fatty acids are the most irritating to the dermis. When the papules become suppurative, pustules or cysts form to wall off the debris.

Treatment consists in discontinuing any practice that may contribute to the development of acne and includes removal of the pressure that occludes the pores. The patient should be advised to avoid placing pressure on the face. The habit of leaning the chin on the hand is an action that applies pressure to the pores. If acne is present on the shoulders or upper chest, tight-fitting clothes or those that apply pressure can cause occlusion, particularly when worn in warm and humid climates. Another practice that can be discontinued is the use of oil-based cosmetics or hormonal creams or wearing the hair low on the forehead or over the cheeks.

Another factor that may contribute to acne is the ingestion of bromides. These drugs are discontinued if alternative medications are available for treatment. Irregular sleep patterns with loss of sleep, stress of any kind, or emotional crises may also contribute to acne. Regular sleep patterns and increased calmness in interactions with others and with the environment help to reduce acne.

In the treatment of acne much attention is given to the relation between dietary patterns and the occurrence of acne, especially the cycle in which overeating leads to obesity and subsequently to acne. The emotional stress of being obese, particularly for an adolescent, can contribute to the occurrence of acne.

There seems to be no relation between the ingestion of sweets (chocolates, cola, candy) or foods of high fat content and the occurrence of acne.

Unfortunately, many relationships between personal practices and acne are held to be true, even though a basis for the relationship does not actually exist, at least in a direct way. For example, some people think that acne is related to masturbation whereas others attribute its occurrence to eating chocolates. The stresses associated with being an adolescent probably do contribute to the development of acne, however. In managing the adolescent's behavior, adults often relate acne to a behavioral practice that is considered undesirable in attempts to have the adolescent conform or comply with the expected behavioral patterns. It should be mentioned that whenever there is no well-defined cause for a condition, people usually attempt to determine cause-and-effect relationships in order to make the condition more understandable and manageable.

Treatment goals in acne vulgaris include reducing the occurrence of acne or preventing the inflammatory response so that emotional or physiologic scars do not remain. First, the skin is freed of occlusion by use of abrasive soaps that remove sebum, keratin, or dirt. These soaps function by irritating the skin, causing increased vasodilatation and turnover of cells. Use of keratolytic agents enhance the removal of dead cells by causing them to slough off. The most commonly used keratolytic agents are sulfur, resorcinol, and salicylic acid. Comedones are sometimes removed, using a comedo extractor to prevent progression of the lesions to the inflammatory state.

A second treatment modality is the use of ultraviolet light or exposure to sunlight to increase vascularization of the skin and the rate of cell turnover. It also has a drying effect. Tetracycline is sometimes given to treat severe or cystic acne. Some authorities use oral vitamin A, although the basis for the effects of vitamin A has not been proved. Large cysts are sometimes responsive to intralesional injection of steroids. Antibiotics, according to culture and sensitivity, are given for treatment of abscesses. Cryosurgery may be employed by using a slush made up of sulfur, powdered dry ice, acetone, or solid carbon dioxide to cause involution of the lesions.

Along with these forms of therapy, a third aspect of treatment is counseling for the emotional component and use of positive health practices. Exercise, appropriate nutrition, and thorough cleaning of the skin are advised. The latter may be sufficient treatment for less severe acne. There is some controversy about the amount of treatment required in acne because the condition is usually outgrown and disappears with aging. In general, aggressive treatment is employed when the lesions are large and inflamed and have the potential for leaving scars following healing. Large keloids may result from deep cysts. When these scars form, treatment may consist in dermabrasion, which is removal of the superficial epidermis by mechanical means. This treatment is often indicated when keloids have formed in the healing of large cysts, and is done only when the acne has been inactive for several years.

Acne rosacea is a chronic condition that begins with vascular dilatation. Often the cheeks and nose are affected. Blotchy or diffuse erythema occurs transiently at first and gradually becomes more constantly present. Subsequently, lesions similar to those seen in acne vulgaris may develop and be followed by rhinophyma. **Rhinophyma** is a chronic inflammation in which the distal area of the nose becomes lobulated and bulbous because of thickening of the skin. The follicles are dilated and the affected areas appear discolored, often becoming deep red or purple.

The cause of acne rosacea is unknown. Suggested causes include vitamin deficiency, hormone imbalance, allergies, or excessive use of substances such as caffeine or alcohol. Unfortunately there is no specific treatment. The affected person is advised to avoid extremes in temperature and sunlight. Dietary restriction of spices, alcohol, and caffeine is also advised.

Several other benign but distressing conditions affect the skin. Among these are miliaria, pityriasis rosea, seborrheic dermatitis, psoriasis, and atopic dermatitis. Each of these conditions will be briefly described in relation to its effects and treatment.

Miliaria is a condition in which the flow of eccrine sweat to the superficial epithelium is hindered. It occurs most frequently in persons who sweat profusely and consistently and is more common in hot, humid climates. Keeping the skin covered so that it is occluded also contributes to the incidence of miliaria. There are many forms of miliaria: miliaria rubra, commonly known as heat rash; miliaria crystallina, or sudamina; and miliaria pustulosa. Any factor that injures the eccrine sweat pores such as inflammation, sunburn, or chemicals may cause this condition.

Miliaria rubra appears as tiny papules from vasodilatation and accumulated sweat in the dermis. The lesions may tingle, itch, or burn. In **miliaria crystallina,** the sweat cannot be excreted and forms bubbles on the skin that disappear without treatment. **Miliaria pustulosa** is simply a condition of miliaria in which the blisters become pustules. An extreme state of miliaria not previously mentioned is **miliaria profunda** and is related to anhydrosis; it interferes with the evaporation of heat from the body. Symptoms and signs may include severe headache, tachycardia, and increased temperature. If severe enough, the condition may lead to heat prostration or collapse.

Treatment for miliaria involves prevention of the condition by avoiding becoming overheated and by wearing loose and light clothing in hot, humid environments. When the condition occurs, the affected person should rest in a cool environment and should remove tight-fitting or loose clothing. Should miliaria profunda result in collapse, emergency treatment may be necessary, particularly if there is a fluid and electrolyte imbalance.

Pityriasis rosea is a harmless condition that tends to occur in young persons. It is evidenced by multiple scaly patches that can occur anywhere on the body. Although the cause is unknown, it is thought to be related to a viral infection. The lesions most commonly occur in the spring and in the fall. They begin with a herald patch, which is a small lesion, and spread as this patch is followed by the appearance of smaller lesions that are round, light red, and scaly. Sometimes the lesions itch, but often they are asymptomatic. Pityriasis rosea disappears spontaneously within about 2 months. Treatment is symptomatic with the administration of antihistamines if itching is present.

Lichen planus is an inflammation of the skin that often follows trauma. It appears as papules with flat tops that occur in the wrists, the inside of the knees, the ankles, the oral mucosa, and the penis. It may be associated with severe, persistent itching, and the lesions may become bullous. Topical steroids are usually given with good response.

Seborrheic dermatitis is another common and often chronic disorder involving the sebaceous glands. The affected skin—scalp, face, chest, and back—has a high population of sebaceous glands. While the cause is unknown, the condition is common in adolescents and may continue throughout life. Exacerbations frequently occur during periods of stress or crises.

The most common sites of seborrheic dermatitis are the areas of hair growth—the scalp and eyebrows—and in men, the bearded areas of the face. A mild form of seborrheic dermatitis is dandruff. Some people have a typical butterfly rash over the nose and cheeks. Severe seborrheic dermatitis is associated with the formation of red plaques with yellowish-red scales. The dermatitis may extend to the eyelids and the ears.

The treatment is similar to that used in acne. Use of sulfur, salicylic acid, resorcinol preparations, or other keratolytic agents applied topically is usually effective in reducing the symptoms, through promoting removal of the scales. Whatever topical preparation is used, it is important that an appropriate agent for the specific site be used, such as shampoo for the scalp, and that the agents be in contact with the skin for sufficient time.

Psoriasis involves the epidermis with demarcated erythematous lesions and flaky scales. The lesions may occur anywhere on the body and most frequently are seen on the skin overlying bony prominences such as the elbows and knees. Sometimes the lesions itch, but usually they are bothersome because of their appearance and tenderness rather than because of itching. There may also be pitting or ridging of the nails. Although the cause of psoriasis is unknown, it is considered to be genetically transmitted and is chronic, with periods of exacerbations and remissions. The disease is not contagious.

It is thought that the activity of psoriatic lesions stems from excessive multiplication of basal cells and a rapid acceleration of cell differentiation processes that lead to the formation of the stratum corneum. Imperfectly formed cells are reproduced every 3 to 4 days as opposed to the normal monthly reproduction rate of the epidermis. The process is enhanced by stress and by exposure to sunlight. The cells scale off rapidly, and there is then no protective skin layer in affected areas. Lesions that develop quickly and are mild tend to heal quickly with simple treatment: washing the areas with soap and water and applying a lubricant such as vaseline.

Depending on the severity, treatment may include topical application of medications. Well-established remedies include tar-based preparations to promote healing. Sulfur preparations also promote healing, and salicylic acid is used to augment scale removal. The combination of application of crude tar ointment, which has a photosensitizing action, followed by ultraviolet light exposure is called the Goeckerman technique and is used for extensive body lesions. The tar is applied and left on usually overnight; it is then removed prior to exposure to the ultraviolet light. Some patients require a sunscreen to protect the skin from burning from the ultraviolet light. Corticosteroid creams or injections into the lesions may be used in severe cases. Triamcinolone (Aristocort) is often used for injection directly into the lesion. Usually systemic steroids are not used because their side effects and the implications of long-term steroid therapy for hormonal balance are more harmful than the benefits of the short-term remission. Systemic steroids are also not used because following short-term administration the condition often flares up and becomes worse than it was prior to treatment.

Systemic therapy with chemotherapeutic drugs, usually methotrexate, is used only in very severe cases. Precautions and nursing care measures important in administration of chemotherapeutic agents is described in Chapter 1.

The scales in psoriasis are sometimes removed by the use of keratolytic agents. Baths and shampoos along with the keratolytic agents also may be used to facilitate removal of scales.

Because psoriasis is chronic and frequently affects small areas of the body, the treatment is usually carried out by the affected person in the home. The nurse should explain the basis for the treatment and how to conduct it so that the greatest effectiveness possible can be achieved. There are many patent medications available for the treatment of psoriasis. Some persons independently use a variety of these medications along with prescribed treatments without mentioning this fact to the doctor or nurse. This practice can be counterproductive. However, it is important to recognize that having a chronic condition such as psoriasis is often very frustrating for the individual involved. There is a tendency to overtreat oneself in an effort to cure the condition. One may feel that the accelerated efforts will be effective in overcoming the psoriasis. Sometimes, after considerable time and effort have been spent in carrying out the treatment regimen, the condition persists. The person may then lose hope and cease all efforts or may be haphazard about following a treatment plan. The nurse's verbal recognition of these problems and demonstration of concern may facilitate the patient's motivation to follow through with treatment.

Many other conditions are just as disconcerting. One of these is **dermatitis**. There are many forms of dermatitis that are classified as eczema. Among them are atopic eczema, nummular eczema, pompholyx, and hand eczema.

Atopic eczema is considered an allergic response that is familial. Some affected persons also have other atopic conditions such as asthma or hay fever. Vasoconstriction is characteristic of atopic eczema. Stroking the skin or applying light pressure to an area elicits blanching when vasoconstriction is present. The most predominant symptom is itching, which can be stimulated by wool clothing, certain irritating soaps and cosmetics, and extreme temperature changes. The itching occurs more frequently in dry climates with low humidity. The skin is erythematous and may be edematous. When there is weeping of vascular products into the skin from the vessels, crusts or scales may form on the stratum corneum. If the affected areas are scratched consistently, lichenification occurs.

Atopic dermatitis may appear at any age and frequently proceeds into stages of transitory or permanent remission without any obvious reason. Affected persons are susceptible to viral infections such as fever blisters (herpes simplex) or to bacterial infection.

Contact with certain medications and toxins, such as substances containing mercury, or contact with ragweed may exacerbate the dermatitis. Affected people are also hypersensitive to smallpox vaccinations and may have hypersensitive reactions following administration of penicillin.

Treatment includes avoidance of substances that bring about the dermatitis. Use of humidifiers during periods of dryness or low humidity is helpful, as is minimal bathing or exposure of the skin to temperatures or substances that reduce the skin's moisture. For severe dermatitis with weeping and itching, Burow's solution (aluminum acetate solution) or saline compresses may be used to relieve itching. Baths containing a preparation that either relieves itching, such as oatmeal, or moisturizes the skin, such as bath oil, are helpful. The dermatitis usually responds well to topical steroid creams applied as a thin coat and rubbed in thoroughly. Antihistamines may be given to provide rest from the itching.

The particular problem experienced by a person with atopic eczema is that of the effects of continual and bothersome itching that is relieved, if at all, only for a short period of time. The tension induced by this continual annoyance of itching may be very great. The affected person may become irritable, tense, nervous, or anxious. Many people with dermatitis are thought to be hyperactive and tense individuals. Nonetheless, a direct relation between the personality characteristics and the occurrence of dermatitis has not been demonstrated. The nurse should recognize that the psychogenic aspect of dermatitis is central in any treatment regimen. The nurse must be sensitive to the particular attitudes and behavior of the affected person.

The remaining types of eczema are briefly described in a general way, as each is similar to atopic eczema in some way and each can be precipitated by emotional stress.

Nummular eczema affects the arms, legs, buttocks, and the dorsum of the hand. **Pompholyx** is eczema of the soles of the feet and the palms of the hands with formation of reddened, weeping vesicles. **Hand eczema** is often localized on the dorsum of the hand and on the fingers. It is thought to be related to exposure of the hand to many different substances. People often develop hand eczema from excessive washing of hands in harsh soaps or from handling substances that dry or irritate the skin. Hand eczema may also be related to infectious processes including fungal and bacterial causes. Itching of the lesions leads to scratching with weeping and formation of fissures or crusts. Avoidance of irritating soaps is advised. Steroids applied topically are helpful.

INFECTIONS OF THE SKIN
Bacterial Infections

An entirely different classification of skin dysfunction, which can include both temporary and chronic conditions, is that of infection. The skin has many resident bacteria. Most of the dominant bacteria found on the skin are gram-positive organisms. The most prevalent are staphylococci, either albus or epidermis. *Staphylococcus aureus* predominates in the nostrils. Resident organisms normally found in the throat, the axilla, and the perineal areas are also potentially infectious to the skin. Gram-positive diphtheroids or bacilli are commonly found as is *Corynebacterium acnes,* an anaerobic bacillus dependent on lipids for nutrition.

Bacteria, while found all over the skin, tend to be more highly populated in the body folds or in the protected moist areas such as the axilla, scalp, vagina, anus, and ear canal. The face has significant bacteria because of the sebum that accumulates as a layer on its surface. Sweat and sebaceous gland secretions are generally thought to protect the skin from bacterial invasion. It should be noted that apocrine gland activity does not begin until puberty and that both sweat and sebum production are less in children than in young adults, decreasing again with aging. Therefore the child and the aged person are more susceptible to skin infections.

Among the factors that help protect the skin from infection are the dryness of normal skin, the presence of fatty acids on the skin surface, and the active sloughing off of old dead cells and their replacement with new cells. When the integrity of the stratum corneum or underlying epidermis and dermis is disrupted, bacteria can readily invade the skin. Bacteria thrive on the nutrients provided by the blood serum and the intracellular components.

Bacterial infections are common in the skin, the most common being impetigo, folliculitis, furuncles, and carbuncles.

Impetigo may be caused by either staphylococci or streptococci. Impetigo, most common in children, is usually caused by *Staphylococcus aureus* and is a superficial skin lesion. Staphylococcal impetigo is typically vesicopustular with thick crusts. Streptococcal impetigo tends to have bullous lesions with thin shiny crusts. Impetigo is limited to the epithelium.

Impetigo contagiosa, an epidemic form caused by group A beta hemolytic streptococci, also occurs most frequently in children and is more common in the months of August and September. One of the major factors leading to its incidence is considered to be uncleanliness. It is thought that the skin lesions stem from infected fecal material, from *Hippelates* (the eye fly), or from contamination by the organism from lesions elsewhere in the body. Acute glomerulonephritis may be a complication in a small percentage of cases.

The disease begins with an erythematous macule that develops into a vesicopustule, rupturing easily and releasing seropurulent drainage. Crusting of dried drainage is usually honey colored. Lesions spread to surrounding areas and to exposed body parts and are usually from 1 to 2 cm in size. The lesions may burn or itch and generally heal within a few days. Following healing, staphylococci may be found as the secondary invader. The lesions should be kept dry and open to air. Systemic antibiotics (usually penicillin or erythromycin) are given for large lesions, topical antibiotics for small lesions. Bacteriostatic soap is used to gently debride the lesions to remove crusts. The nurse should follow hand washing procedures before and after handling the lesions to avoid contamination of the lesions and to prevent spread by direct contact with the drainage. Dishes and towels and other items that come into contact with the lesions should be isolated and disinfected.

Ecthyma is a form of streptococcal impetigo in which the dermis and the epidermis are affected. The occurrence of ecthyma is related to poor body hygiene. Healing of the deeper (dermal) lesions is slower than that with epidermal lesions. Scarring may also result from the dermal lesions. In a small percentage of cases, glomerulonephritis may occur as a complication, particularly in small children. The glomerulonephritis usually occurs within 2 to 6 weeks following the skin infection. Streptococci M types 44, 2, 55, and 57 are the most commonly involved.

Treatment of ecthyma includes systemic

antibiotics, usually penicillin or erythromycin. Warm compresses, using tap water or saline, are applied to the lesions several times a day. Crusts are washed with soap and water. Neosporin or other topical ointments may be used.

Pemphigus, a skin condition of various types, is a condition similar to impetigo. Some forms of pemphigus are serious. Pemphigus neonatorium appears in the infant as impetigo lesions. The infant may have extensive lesions associated with increased temperature and lymphadenopathy in the affected regions. Pemphigus must be treated promptly, to prevent severe fluid and electrolyte imbalance. Moist compresses and tetracycline ointment are usually the treatment of choice.

Folliculitis, another condition caused by staphylococci, most frequently occurs on the scalp, on the extremities, or on the bearded areas of the face. **Sycosis barbae** is the term used to describe chronic folliculitis of the bearded areas of the face. Folliculitis may be either superficial or deep and is simply the infection of a hair follicle. Other organisms in addition to *S. aureus* may cause the infection. The folliculitis appears as a raised dome around the follicle. The infection may spread into the entire follicle and may extend into the dermis surrounding the follicle. If this happens, pain is felt.

The typical lesion is a pustule surrounded by erythema. The pustule weeps so that a crust forms. Often the hair seems to be growing from the center of the crust. Treatment includes removal of excess moisture, oil, or grease from the area and use of soaps to dry and clean the area. Antibacterial soaps are often prescribed. Treatment should begin early in the course of folliculitis. If the lesion extends deep into the hair follicle, there is a possibility that the follicle will be permanently damaged and a scar will form. Hair cannot grow from permanently damaged hair follicles.

Furuncles (boils), often caused by staphylococci, tend to be familial and recurrent. They may result from exposure to oils or chemicals and are often related to poor body hygiene. Furuncles are often preceded by folliculitis caused by friction or pressure on the skin, the presence of oil, or excess moisture of the skin surfaces. Furuncles frequently occur on the neck, face, axillae, buttocks, thighs, and perineum.

The furuncle is at first firm, tender, and reddened in the area around the hair follicle. The lesion then becomes enlarged, indurated and, finally, boggy and fluctuant. The top of the lesion becomes yellow prior to rupturing through a point or head. The head may also appear white. On spontaneous rupture, thick, creamy yellow pus comprised of white blood cells, fibrin, and necrotic debris usually forms as a core is released. Following rupture the furuncle begins to heal. During their progression to the rupture state, furuncles may be very painful and may have an associated increase in systemic temperature. Warm compresses aid in comfort and sometimes seem to hasten the progression to the rupture state.

Sometimes furuncles are incised and drained. It is important to wait until the center begins to become soft and boggy before incising a furuncle because incision prior to the soft state only extends the inflammation. When the center is soft, the furuncle can be incised. A culture is taken of the drainage and a dressing is applied. The dressings are changed frequently to reduce the possibility of reinfection or of spread to unaffected areas. Hand washing before and after touching the area or the dressings is an essential precaution. When a person has a draining furuncle, he should use separate personal hygiene items, including towels, washcloths, brushes, or other items that may come into contact with the infected area. Linens should be washed carefully; some authorities suggest boiling or using antibacterial soaps. The dressings are discarded with care to prevent infection of others as well as reinfection. In some instances antibacterial soaps are prescribed to prevent further occurrence.

Carbuncles are larger than furuncles and involve many hair follicles. They are often found in areas of thick skin. Multiple pustules appear around the hair follicle pores and the entire area becomes erythematous. Rupture and drainage precede healing. Scar formation often follows carbuncles that are deep. The patient may have an increased systemic temperature and leukocytosis, and may experience generalized malaise. Treatment includes use of warm compresses, comfort measures to reduce the effects of the malaise, reduction of temperature, and systemic antibiotics based on a culture of the drainage if possible.

Untreated carbuncles may continue to spread and may eventually cause bacteremia, metastasizing to other organs. Carbuncles can be septic foci for systemic infections. Nasal and throat cultures are sometimes taken in affected persons with recurrent furuncles and carbuncles, and topical antibiotics are given to reduce the population of bacteria in these areas. If the antibiotics are ineffective, further tests are often done to determine whether there is a systemic cause for these repeated infections.

Cellulitis is an inflammation of the cells. In cellulitis, there is erythema, edema, and ill-defined extension of the inflammation in the superficial skin cells. The affected area is warm and tender. There may be increased systemic temperature, lymphangitis, or lymphadenopathy in the affected areas. In some instances, vesicles and bullae occur because of the dilatation of both blood and lymph vessels. Another form of cellulitis is **erysipelas.** This condition is actually a more superficial cellulitis in which the erythematous area is warm and especially tender. Vesicles and bullae may also form in erysipelas.

The occurrence of cellulitis or erysipelas often follows trauma to the skin. The affected person may have generalized malaise, fever, and chills. Frequently, staphylococci or streptococci are the causative organisms. The specific bacteria involved may influence the degree of inflammation, with those that produce enzymes causing more cellular inflammation. Beta hemolytic streptococcus is an example of enzyme-producing bacterium. The treatment for cellulitis is application of warm soaks to the affected areas. Antibiotics, given orally or intramuscularly if necessary according to the patient's condition, are often prescribed. Bedrest is often advised to treat the fever and malaise. Erysipelas can contribute to the debilitation of individuals who are not physically strong. This primarily includes infants, children, and invalids, in whom the condition occurs with the greatest frequency. When it occurs, erysipelas should be treated promptly as the condition may spread, causing bacteremia.

Fungal Infections

Fungal infections make up another classification of infections commonly involving the skin. **Candidiasis** is caused by a yeastlike fungus, *Candida albicans*. This fungus is most prevalent among the normal flora of the mucous membranes, the gastrointestinal tract, and the vagina. *Candida albicans* thrives in warm, moist environments and becomes infective when the balance of the normal flora is upset by systemic antibiotics, corticosteroids, or birth control pills. Pregnancy, diabetes mellitus, and Cushing's disease are associated with excessive candidal growth. Persons with debilitating illnesses are also susceptible to infection by *Candida*.

A number of different conditions may be caused by *Candida*. These include paronychia, intertrigo, perleche, vulvovaginitis, and thrush. Evaluation of infection by fungi is usually made by applying potassium hydroxide or Swartz Medrick stain, which demonstrates the budding yeasts. *Candida* can also be grown on culture; its growth takes 2 or 3 days.

Paronychia is a fungal infection of the fingernail which causes rounding and lifting of the folds of the fingernail. Usually the infection causes erythema and swelling of the distal end of the finger. The nail may become yellowish, and ridges may form in the nail. This condition is very difficult to heal. Treatment involves avoidance of moisture. Gloves are worn to avoid contact with any liquid or moisture. An antifungal cream such as nystatin (Mycostatin or Nilstat) is applied to the nail folds. If the condition is painful, as it often is, a steroid or nystatin cream may be used. The nails often crumble and disintegrate as the condition progresses. Following healing, the nail will again grow out normally.

Another condition caused by *Candida* is **intertrigo,** characterized by itching. This fungal infection occurs most frequently in obese persons with large body folds, and in those who have debilitating diseases that require bedrest. It is often associated with diseases that are evidenced by high temperatures and excessive sweating. The infection is found in the body areas that are moist and protected and is decreased by keeping the areas as clean and dry as possible. Occlusive clothing also contributes to its incidence. The axilla, the groin, perineal areas, behind the ears, and in the folds of pendulous breasts are common areas for the incidence of intertrigo. The lesions may extend to surrounding areas—to the scrotum from the groin, to the hands from between the digits, and around the lobes of the ears from behind the ears. The lesions appear as moist red scales. Intertriginous areas deep in body folds often become macerated.

Intertrigo is treated by reducing the moisture in the body folds as much as possible and by avoiding clothing that occludes the skin. Wearing clothing that supports the body folds and holds them apart is helpful. In obese persons, losing weight is advised, but may not be feasible. Maintenance of a cool dry environment also helps to treat intertrigo. Air conditioning is advised if the climate is warm. Powders with antifungal effect are prescribed and their use is advised for a long term to prevent recurrence of the infection. Active lesions are often soaked with compresses, such as Burow's solution compresses. Soaking serves both to cool and soothe the affected skin and to remove the endotoxins of the fungus. Following the soaks, the treated areas are dried gently but thoroughly and an antifungal cream is applied. Further drying is achieved by exposure to a heat lamp so placed that drying occurs without further damaging the tissues through excess warmth. Fans may also be used to circulate air to the exposed areas to facilitate drying.

Perleche is a fungal infection in the cracks at the sides of the mouth. Other names for perleche are chelitis and angular stomatitis. This condition may be precipitated by any factor that increases the moisture at the sides of the mouth, such as drooling or licking the areas. Use of cosmetics that are irritating may predispose to perleche as can inappropriate dental occlusion. Treatment is geared to correcting the cause. Dental repair or improvement of dental occlusion, breaking the habit of licking, diminishing the incidence of drooling, if possible, or discontinuing the irritating cosmetics are all measures that can be taken to prevent perleche. In some instances perleche is thought to be related to vitamin deficiency. If this is the case, the nutritional status should be improved. The active lesion is treated with an antifungal topical cream and the area of the lesion is kept as dry as possible.

In **vulvovaginitis** the walls of the vagina become erythematous and edematous. There is usually a vaginal discharge. Treatment is by the use of antifungal vaginal suppositories. The incidence of vulvovaginitis is more frequent in women who have been taking systemic antibiotics for other conditions. It is frequently associated with diabetes mellitus.

Thrush affects the vaginal mucous membranes. It also affects the oral mucous membranes. Thrush may occur at any age; oral thrush may occur in children or under the dentures of older adults. The appearance of oral thrush begins with tiny white plaques with shiny red mucosa underneath. The plaques tend to run together, forming a cheesy appearance that is typical of thrush. If the plaques are removed, the mucous membranes underneath may appear eroded. The vaginal form of thrush is most prevalent among diabetics. Treatment involves the use of an antifungal agent as a mouthwash or oral medication for oral thrush and as a vaginal suppository for vaginal thrush. Methylrosaniline chloride (gentian violet) is the traditional treatment for thrush but is now more commonly used for oral thrush when it does not respond to other forms of therapy. While it is a very effective medication, gentian violet is difficult to use because it stains materials with which it comes in contact and gives a poor cosmetic appearance.

Onychomycosis, a fungal infection of the nails, often occurs along with fungal infections in other parts of the body. This infection causes the nails to become brittle and thick. The nails also become discolored and may be easily lifted from the nail bed. Treatment requires avoidance of moisture. The toenails are most frequently affected. For this condition antifungal powder is used twice a day and cotton socks are worn. Cotton is more absorbent than other materials. It is advisable to wash the socks and other clothing that come into contact with the fungal infection in hot water. Many authorities advise wearing leather shoes as opposed to wearing those of canvas or synthetic materials. When vesicles are present, they are treated by moist compresses, followed by drying and application of an antifungal cream. In many instances, this fungal infection of the toenails cannot be cured unless the toenails are removed. This may seem to be an aggressive form of treatment. However, the toenails affected become discolored and lose their healthy cosmetic appearance. The toenail does not grow back when the germinative cells have been removed; however, the appearance of the toe following removal of the nail involved in the fungal infection is much improved in comparison with the appearance of the affected nail. Most people adapt easily to loss of the toenail and other than experiencing increased sensitivity of the site for a time following removal, until the skin on the site thickens, they tend to have no further difficulties.

Treatment of onychomycosis on the nails of the fingers is the same: warm moist compresses on the vesicles, drying the areas, and applying an antifungal cream. If the infection is extensive, keratolytic agents may be used to soften the hands. It is also important to trim the fingernails carefully. Because they are brittle and thicker than normal nails, the affected nails tend to catch on linens and clothing. By trimming them short and removing rough edges, this problem can be somewhat lessened.

Another fungal organism, *Malassezia furfur,* causes **tinea versicolor,** an infection somewhat similar to those previously described. This condition affects young adults and is most prevalent in the temperate zones. The lesions appear as white, pink, or brown, hence the name "versicolor." There are fine scales on the affected skin but the fungus cannot be cultured. The scales can be seen with staining, using either potassium hydroxide or Swartz Medrick stain. This infection causes change in pigmentation that can be observed under a Wood's light (a light with long ultraviolet rays). The affected areas do not tan and the change in pigmentation is obvious when the area is exposed to sunlight.

Tinea versicolor causes no special discomfort, but it may be cosmetically annoying. Treatment includes use of antifungal medications, laundering clothing and linen in hot water, and using a brush with stiff bristles when taking a bath. Selenium disulfide (Selsun) is the most popular treatment for this condition; its use has to be continued over a long period of time to prevent reinfection.

Yet another group of fungal infections includes the dermatophyte class of fungi. Dermatophytes technically include all fungi infecting the skin, but the common usage refers to organisms that cause ringworm. Dermatophytes live on dead keratinized tissue and often secondarily infect skin that is already diseased.

Dermatophytes live in the superficial layers of the epidermis, the nails, and the hair. They thrive on a person who is poorly nourished or who uses poor hygienic practices. These infections are more common in hot humid climates and in debilitating diseases. The dermatophytes are found in the soil, on animals, and on human skin. It is therefore possible for a susceptible individual to become infected from contaminated soil or from animals. Usually the affected person develops an immune response to ringworm after the first incidence, which protects him or her from further incidences. The condition becomes chronic in about one-fifth of those affected—these people do not develop an immune response [1].

Ringworm can affect any portion of the body; it is often referred to as **tinea** plus the area affected or by the source of contamination. **Tinea capitis** refers to ringworm of the scalp; **tinea barbae** refers to ringworm of the beard and moustache. **Tinea corporis** is ringworm of the body; **tinea cruris** is ringworm of the groin. **Tinea manuum** is ringworm of the hand; **tinea pedis** is ringworm of the foot. Of all these conditions, tinea pedis is the most common.

Tinea capitis, ringworm of the scalp, usually follows minor trauma to the scalp. The condition is usually asymptomatic and is associated with scaling, inflammation, and broken hairs. The hairs are broken at a point close to the scalp. There may be patches of hair loss.

Tinea barbae, ringworm of the beard and moustache, appears as an inflammation of the hair follicle that develops into a kerion. A **kerion** is a deep boggy area of inflammation that is edematous and quite painful.

Tinea corporis is infection of the skin. It may be asymptomatic or it may be associated with itching. The lesions occur in hot and humid climates and begin as papules with flat surfaces that are red. The lesions spread outward from the papules so that there is a circular formation of papules surrounding a center of healing. The borders at the periphery of the lesions are usually well demarcated. The lesions tend to occur with greater frequency on the arms, shoulders, and the face.

Tinea cruris, commonly called jock itch, is ringworm of the groin. This condition is usually related to heat and is accelerated by friction of clothing. Obese men tend to be affected more than thinner men. Often, the lesion spreads to cover the entire groin, equally on both sides, forming a typical butterfly appearance. Itching is prevalent as is maceration of the insides of the folds of the skin.

Tinea manuum is ringworm that affects the hands; tinea pedis affects the feet. Tinea manuum tends to appear more as an erythematous area of hyperkeratosis. Tinea pedis is precipitated by wearing tight-fitting shoes. The organism may be found on floors, linens, or socks. Both tinea manuum and tinea pedis cause itching. The lesions may be vesicular and may form fissures. They can extend from the digits to the other areas of the hand or foot, whichever is affected. In both conditions there is scaling. Some persons develop both tinea manuum and tinea pedis at the same time.

Treatment for tinea capitis or any of the other forms of ringworm requires a dry, clean environment on the skin. If poor nutrition or poor hygiene is a causative factor, these conditions are rectified. In hot and humid climates, the patient is advised to keep as cool as possible to relieve itching and to wear nonocclusive clothing over the affected areas. As with other fungal infections of the foot, cotton socks are advocated to provide for absorption of moisture. Appropriate antifungal preparations are prescribed and are used following resolution of the infection in order to prevent recurrence. The time for continued use often depends on the duration of the infection and is extended if the infection has occurred repeatedly.

Viral Infections

Yet another classification of infections of the skin is caused by viruses. The major types of viral infections of the skin include warts and herpes.

Warts are benign growths that involve the intraepidermal areas of the skin. They are caused by a DNA virus, the human papilloma virus, which depends on living tissues for its function and spread. Warts can be spread from one area of the body to another by autoinoculation via a scratch or a broken area of skin. The virus that causes warts is normally present only in humans. The occurrence of warts caused by this virus is most common in children and in young adults. The warts have an incubation period of 1 to 6 months and often disappear spontaneously with no treatment.

There are many different types of warts. Common warts (**verruca vulgaris**) are small, pinhead-sized, flesh-colored papules. They appear most frequently on the dorsum of the hand and on the fingers. As they develop they become larger and elevated. Their surface becomes rough because of irregular papillary projections of keratin. Sometimes they contain black dots, which represent blood pigment in the capillary loops that have thrombosed. Flat warts (**verruca plana**) are simply multiple warts of about 1 to 3 mm in size. They occur in any area of the body, frequently appearing on the face or on the hands.

Filiform or juvenile warts (**verruca filiformis**) begin as papules and are flesh colored. They appear most commonly on the face, neck, shoulder, axilla, forearms, or hands. Filiform warts are slender projections as opposed to the flat warts.

Plantar or palmar warts (**verruca plantaris**) occur most frequently on the feet and are elevated or flat areas of hyperkeratotic tissue. Plantar warts are usually firm and cone-shaped. Because of the pressure on the feet, they tend to grow inward. The base of the cone-shaped plantar wart is on the surface of the skin and its point (or tip) grows into the deeper layers of the skin.

Condylomata acuminata warts grow in the intertriginous areas including the vaginal or penile areas around the urethra, and in the perianal area. These lesions are fleshy growths that often have a cauliflower-like appearance.

Treatment of warts is often controversial. Because they often have a life span of only 1 or 2 years and then tend to go away spontaneously, treatment is not always advised. When the wart interferes with function, as on the fingers or hand, or in the case of genital warts in which the virus can be transmitted through contact during sexual intercourse, the warts are generally removed. The size, placement, and appearance of the warts are basic considerations in the decision to remove them or not. In some instances warts have disappeared through the power of suggestion. It is not certain, however, if the wart would have disappeared spontaneously without the intervention of suggestion. It remains an interesting question.

Removal of warts is accomplished in several ways: electrosurgery, chemical applications, cryosurgery, or surgical removal with a blade. Some wart-like lesions are thought to be squamous papillomas that are premalignant and not caused by a virus. These are difficult to differentiate from warts of viral origin. Suspicious warts are examined in the laboratory to determine malignancy. Topical keratolytic preparations may also be used for removal of warts. The major goal in treatment is to remove the wart while not damaging the underlying cells of the surrounding skin. Sometimes the pain caused by some methods of removal is worse than the discomfort initially caused by the wart. In this instance, the psychological implications of removal may counterbalance the pain. Nonetheless, carefully removed warts leave no residual pain or scar.

The other type of viral skin infection is the herpes infection. Herpes infections include herpes simplex, herpes zoster, and varicella. Herpes simplex is also caused by a DNA virus. The **herpes simplex** virus affects man exclusively and is not present in animals. There are two types of this virus, type 1 and type 2. **Type 1** herpes infections are usually located on the face or neck. **Type 2** herpes infections involve the genital areas. Other names for type 1 infections around the lips are cold sores or fever blisters.

The precursor to the herpes simplex lesion is pain and tenderness in the area. Vesicles then erupt and are often associated with erosion of the surrounding area, particularly if the lesion is located in the buccal mucosa or in the vaginal mucosa. The affected areas are edematous, and the tenderness extends to the surrounding skin areas. The affected person has symptoms according to the location of the herpes. If located in the mouth, eating and drinking are difficult. When located in the urethral area, there may be painful voiding. There is usually discharge associated with lesions located in the urethra or the vagina. In men, the discharge is usually watery and associated with urethritis. There may also be systemic fever.

The lesions go through a progression that begins with the vesicle. The vesicles then become purulent and begin to dry. A crust forms over the lesion. The entire process takes from about 7 to 10 days. The underlying area remains erythematous and edematous during the healing process. It is possible for herpes simplex lesions to be secondarily infected by bacteria. In this case, the crust appears yellow.

Usually the primary infection is more severe and lasts longer than recurrent infections. The herpes virus goes into a latent stage after resolution of the primary infection. It is activated when there is physical trauma to the area, or when the host is subjected to emotional trauma. A number of other precipitating factors include menstruation in women, systemic infections, elevated systemic temperature from any cause, and exposure to sunlight.

There is no specific treatment for herpes simplex because a vaccine has not as yet been developed. Therefore treatment is symptomatic. Analgesics are given as necessary, and topical anesthetics are given when required. In some instances systemic antibiotics may be helpful. If the infection is debilitating, intravenous fluid may be required. Soothing mouthwashes or cool compresses, according to the area involved, may be used to relieve tenderness. Sitz baths are helpful in providing relief for genital lesions. Topical medications for drying and soothing are sometimes used. These medications may include topical antibiotics and steroid creams.

Some specific treatments for the DNA virus include the antiviral agent idoxuridine (Dendrid, Herplix, Stoxil), which inhibits the synthesis of DNA. Another treatment is the use of dyes that bind viral DNA and are also photoactive. The dyes are first applied and then either a fluorescent or a tungsten bulb light is directed on the area to activate the dye.

Herpes zoster is a viral infection commonly known as shingles. It is very similar to varicella. The lesions typical of herpes zoster appear in the cervical or thoracic region most frequently. They tend to follow the distribution of the peripheral nerve and usually cause symptoms involving the nerve's dermatome. The lesions are most commonly unilateral, but can appear bilaterally. Their appearance is preceded by erythema, followed by macules, papules, and plaques. Vesicles may appear later. In severe cases, the zoster lesions may become hemorrhagic and bullous. They can be infarctive and cause gangrene of the affected body part; the lesions heal slowly and sometimes there is scarring.

In herpes zoster there may be an itching sensation prior to eruption of the macules. There may also be tenderness and pain. The pain may be severe. Treatment includes cool compresses on the vesicles, if they are present, and systemic analgesics for pain. The lesions are sometimes painted with tincture of benzoin, or other drying powders are used. When the areas are painful and are located on the thorax, they can be splinted with occlusive dressings made of cotton and covered with an elastic bandage. Topical antibiotic creams are sometimes used, particularly in the crust stage. Topical corticosteroids are sometimes used if the patient is elderly. If treatment is begun early it somewhat lessens the complication of neuralgia that sometimes occurs. In this complication there may be a residual paresthesia in the dermatome affected. Paresthesia occurs as a complication less frequently in younger persons. Intralesional injection of steroids is sometimes helpful in the treatment of post-zoster pain.

The herpes zoster lesions usually erupt for a period of several days and then disappear within 3 to 4 weeks. The lesions are often limited to a localized area and do not tend to spread.

The other form of herpes is **varicella,** commonly known as chickenpox. It is caused by a virus, which is spread by respiratory droplets, and it has a 2-week incubation period (14 to 16 days). The disease is communicable from the day preceding the appearance of the lesion and continues to be communicable for 6 days. The lesions begin with erythematous macules that lead into papules. Vesicles containing the virus may form with crusting as they begin to dry, the moist crusts being infectious. The lesions are found most often on the scalp, mucous membranes, the face, and the thorax. The lesions erupt on different days and usually lesions in various stages of progression are present at one time. The crusts eventually fall off and are not infectious when dry. There is a general feeling of malaise, fever, and often a cough and dyspnea, prior to developing the rash. It is essential to prevent scratching the lesions. By scratching, the inflammatory process is furthered and scars form at the site of the lesion. Ways to prevent excoriation of the itching areas include trimming the patient's fingernails so that they are very short. Children are often given gloves that are carefully attached to prevent the child from scratching.

Because there is no known cure for varicella, medications are usually limited to symptomatic treatment. Calamine lotion may be applied to the lesions to reduce itching. Antihistamines may also be given for the same reason. If there are lesions in the mouth, a mouthwash is used. Saline or hydrogen peroxide is useful in this condition. Sometimes topical antibiotics are used. It is also important that a chest x-ray be taken because there may be nodular pulmonary infiltration, which may not cause symptoms. The extent of the lesions can vary considerably from a few clusters to many lesions. The discomfort and also the treatment required vary with each individual. Prevention of spread of infection via direct contact with infectious crusts and via respiratory droplets requires appropriate isolation control measures.

INFESTATION BY PARASITES

Another type of skin dysfunction is infestation by parasites. The two infestations of major importance are pediculosis and scabies. Both are caused by obligate parasites, so named because they must obtain their nutrients from another organism, in this case the human body. Parasites are spread from one person to another by close personal contact or from infested clothing or personal articles, linens, or other materials such as upholstered furniture. People who live in crowded conditions most commonly become infested. Poor hygiene or poor sanitation also contribute to infestation.

Two types of lice cause **pediculosis.** *Pediculosis humanus* is the louse that infests hair-producing and smooth areas of the body. The louse that affects the body has feeding habits different from those of the louse that affects the scalp and bearded face [10]. *Phthirus pubis* is the louse that infests the pubic areas. It is spread most frequently through sexual contact. This louse is smaller in size when compared to the body or hair lice. Lice have the appearance of crabs with claw-like legs and a rounded body. The largest are only about 4 cm in length and are a light gray color. Sometimes they can be seen, particularly if the infested person has a great number of lice. If fairly good personal hygiene is practiced and there are only a few lice, these few may not be easily found. The lice attach their eggs, which are called nits, to hair or clothing.

The female louse lays the eggs and deposits them on the surface of the hair (most commonly at the nape of the neck and behind the ears) if it is a head louse, or on clothing fibers if it is a body louse. The female first coats the area where the eggs will be placed with a cement-like substance that causes them to stick in place. The lice then tend to be found where the hair is the thickest and in the protected areas of clothing, particularly in the seams. The louse moves to the body for its nutrition gained from sucking blood. It then returns to its habitat in the clothing or in the hair. The life span of the louse is about 10 days whereas the egg requires 8 to 10 days to hatch and mature.

Itching is the primary complaint of people who are infested. The itching stems from the saliva and the excrement of the lice that are left on the skin and act as antigens. The site of feeding appears as a reddened pinpoint or in some cases as purpura where the blood was sucked. Because the itching is severe and scratching is unavoidable the infested areas become excoriated. Often these excoriated areas become subject to secondary infection by bacteria. The lesions are better seen with a magnifying glass, and patches of excrement, the pinpoint areas left from feeding sites, or the lice or nits may be found.

Treatment includes use of gamma benzene hexachloride (Kwell). This medication is available in many forms: creams, shampoos, or topical lotions. The hair is shampooed thoroughly with the prescribed shampoo if head lice are present. Following this, the nits are removed by combing. The shampoo may be repeated within a few days if necessary. Because the lice can be spread through use of combs and brushes or infested hats or linens, the best precaution is to treat these items carefully. It is advisable to throw away any combs and brushes that may be infested. Clothing can be dry-cleaned or washed carefully, using hot water. If clothing is stored and not worn for a period of a month, the lice will die because they are obligatory parasites and cannot live without a human organism as a source of nutrients. The period of a month is based on the knowledge that the nits require at least 3 weeks to become mature.

Treatment for body lice is similar to that used for head lice. The person is advised to bathe thoroughly and then to apply the cream or lotion on the affected areas. Clothing and linens are treated in the manner just described.

The incidence of head lice usually increases when people are crowded together and often becomes a problem in schools and camps where children are grouped together. Appropriate personal hygiene measures and being careful not to wear hats and garments belonging to infested persons are important preventive measures. Borrowing combs and brushes may also lead to infestation, if lice are present on these items. The use of modern medication has greatly facilitated removal of infesting lice. Formerly, treatment was long and rigorous and uncomfortable, and was followed by long sessions of nit picking. If the medications available today are used appropriately, the need for nit picking can be minimized.

Scabies, the other parasitic infection, is caused by *Sarcoptes scabiei*. The predominant symptom of scabies is severe itching. The parasite lives on the skin, with the female mite piercing the stratum corneum and burrowing into the skin. Warm, protected environments foster their growth and they are spread by prolonged personal contact. The female leaves about three or four eggs each day and the eggs hatch in 3 or 4 days. As with lice, the itching and edema that follow the burrowing are allergic reactions. Often, the infestation has taken place some time before these symptoms are noticed. The allergic reaction is also accompanied by formation of vesicles.

The burrowing trails left by scabies are either straight or S shaped. They are most frequently found between the fingers, on the flexor surfaces of the wrists, in the axillary folds, and on the penis, nipples, or buttocks. In addition to these channels, there may be pustules, papules, and edema from scratching and from secondary bacterial infection. The scabies can live for several months in the skin before they die. When burrowing occurs, the mites can be removed from their tunnels by means of a scalpel blade. Eggs and excrement, usually formed in small brown oval shapes, can also be removed. In some infested persons, the burrows are difficult to find, and the redness and edema of the area may lead one to the mite infestations.

Treatment for scabies is very similar to that used for pediculosis. Kwell is helpful and should be applied in its cream or lotion form after the person takes a bath; it is left on for 24 hours. While controversial, some authorities recommend applying medication in two stages: the first to destroy active mites and eggs and the second, 7 days later, to treat any eggs that may have hatched. Others suggest that a single application is sufficient. Some authorities advise bathing in a tubful of hot water, using a stiff bristle brush to scrub every area of the body. This bath is then followed by the application of medication and complete change of clothing. Other useful preparations are benzyl benzoate, benzocaine, and DDT emulsion prepared as Topocide.

Care is taken to treat the clothing by washing it in hot water or by having it dry cleaned. Often each person in the patient's living quarters must also follow the same treatment because the scabies can spread very easily from one person to another.

This discussion has summarized some of the more frequently occurring infections and infestations. Many others occur, however. Some are particular to a specific region or country in the world, while others are rarely found in the United States. The reader is referred to a definitive text about dermatology for information about conditions that may be encountered and are not included in this chapter.

LESIONS CAUSED BY ABNORMAL CELL GROWTH

There are many types of skin lesions that are the result of abnormal cell growth. Many of these lesions are benign. Others are benign with the potential for becoming malignant. Still others are malignant. Among the group of benign lesions are seborrheic keratosis, actinic keratosis, leukoplakia, molluscum sebaceum, and Bowen's disease. Each is described separately in the following paragraphs.

Seborrheic keratosis usually appears as a round, elevated growth. The lesions often occur in multiples and are distributed on the forehead, the chest, or the back. A greasy, flaking appearance is typical of these lesions, which are tan or black. They appear to be pasted on the skin rather than growing from the skin. If traumatized, the lesions are irritated and may bleed. In many instances, they slowly increase in size. The lesions represent cyst formations arising from the horny layer of the epidermis and are treated by surgical excision only if they are disturbed by friction from clothing or pressure, or if they create displeasing cosmetic appearance in the affected person's perception.

Actinic keratosis is also called senile keratosis and occurs most frequently in people over 60. These lesions usually occur on areas of the face and arms that are exposed to sunlight—on the cheeks, forehead, lips, and forearms. They are more likely to develop in fair-skinned people and in those who are consistently exposed to sunlight.

The lesions may have an irregular shape and are similar in appearance to warts. About 20 percent of the actinic keratotic lesions become malignant, proceeding to squamous cell cancer by invasion of the dermis. Usually, the lesion undergoes changes that signal the premalignant state. The obvious change is the formation of a halo, representing inflammation around the base of the lesion.

Treatment includes surgical removal. The lesions are excised to the level of subcutaneous tissue because of the potential for malignancy. If the lesions occur in multiples, surgical removal of that portion of the skin affected may be required, with skin grafts to cover the area.

Leukoplakia is the precancerous lesion that appears on the mucous membranes. This condition is related to actinic keratosis. Leukoplakia presents as white plaques that form on the mucous membranes of the mouth and lips. It is considered that the white plaques appear most frequently in smokers. Because of the constant irritation, hyperplasia of the epidermis may occur. Sources of constant irritation, such as irregularly shaped teeth or oral trauma, may contribute to the formation of leukoplakia. In some instances, there is no history of trauma or irritation, and the lesions appear spontaneously. When the lesions begin to change, as evidenced by erosion, ulcer formation, or the appearance of fissures, the leukoplakia is considered to be precancerous. When undergoing change, the lesions become thicker. The cancerous lesions may form in situ, which means localized to the site, or as squamous cell carcinoma.

Early treatment for leukoplakia includes

elimination of any factor that causes irritation to the mucous membranes. As previously mentioned, this may include discontinuing smoking cigarettes, cigars, or pipes or the use of chewing tobacco. Correction of dental problems and a regular plan of excellent dental hygiene are important preventive measures. Discontinuing the use of irritating substances such as toothpastes or mouthwashes, spicy or thermally hot foods, and chemicals is also useful. People with leukoplakia are advised to keep their lips moist by using one of the commercial sun filters for lips or by using lipstick.

When lesions demonstrate change, or when the diagnosis is uncertain, the lesions are removed. A biopsy may be done prior to removal to ascertain whether the lesions are cancerous. In some instances, the decision is made to remove the lesions as a preventive measure.

Molluscum sebaceum occurs more frequently in males who are exposed to tars. The lesion grows for 1 to 2 months in an active state and in this phase appears round and shiny with a depressed center. The lesions are usually located on the face. While the initial lesion is firm, it begins to change after the active growth phase, becoming softer in the inner portion. An ulceration begins to develop and is followed by the next phase, which is the phase of healing. A scar is usually left following the healing. The lesion itself is thought to stem from the hair follicles. Treatment is usually initiated after the lesion has ceased its active growth period. The level of excision varies.

Histologic examination of the tissue is important to differentiate the lesion from squamous cell carcinoma. If squamous cell carcinoma is present, a deep excision is made to eliminate the abnormal cells. If carcinoma is not present, a more superficial excision may be made.

Bowen's disease, in contrast to the other types of lesions mentioned in this section, occurs most frequently on body parts usually covered by clothing. Usually the lesions appear singly, but they may be multiple. They appear as a brownish red or dull red patch on the skin, with an irregularly formed border. The lesions slowly spread, and the surface of the lesion crusts over. When the crusts are removed, the center of the lesion is granular and oozing. The lesions never seem to heal, and sometimes they are mistaken for psoriasis when in the crusting stage. Treatment includes x-ray therapy or surgical excision. Squamous cell carcinoma develops in about 25 percent of the people with Bowen's disease.

Other lesions are classified as carcinoma. Usually, carcinoma is diagnosed by evidence of delayed healing of a pimple, sore, or an inflamed area. The presence of a lesion that persists and does not heal and examination of the tissue are two criteria used to determine whether lesions are cancerous. Skin cancer is the most commonly occurring malignancy.

A number of risk factors have been identified in the formation of skin cancer. There seems to be a familial predisposition to cancer. Blue-eyed, fair-skinned Nordics have a high rate of skin cancer. Prolonged exposure to sunlight or to chemicals (arsenic and tar being the most predominant) increases the risk of developing skin cancer. The incidence of skin cancer also increases with age. Other factors include increased risk of skin cancer in persons who have experienced previous damage to the skin from x-ray therapy or from burns. For example, the incidence of skin cancer is greater in those who have burn scars; the cancer occurs at the site of the scar. Exposure to x-ray or radiation therapy also predisposes to developing carcinoma of the skin. On the other hand, persons who have more melanin, such as dark-skinned people; those who tan quickly; and blacks, whose melanocytes produce melanin in greater amounts, are less susceptible to skin cancer because the melanin absorbs the harmful ultraviolet rays.

Because exposure to sunlight is such an important risk factor, susceptible persons who recognize the signs of overexposure should attempt to reduce the amount and duration of exposure. Formation of small white spots on the sun-exposed skin or the appearance of flaking areas are both signs of susceptibility. Not only should the total amount of sun exposure be reduced, but the time span of exposure should be distributed over a longer period of time, with periods of nonexposure in between. The use of sun-screening agents during exposure to the sun is advisable to reduce the possibility of development of skin cancer. Of the available topical agents, those containing para-aminobenzoic acid (PABA) and creams containing cinnamates and benzophenones are most effective in blocking the middle ultraviolet light that causes sunburn [8].

Sunlight exposure is related to the ultraviolet ray exposure; there is a direct correlation between the amount of ultraviolet exposure, the wave length of the ultraviolet rays, and the amount of skin cancer. Most harmful are middle ultraviolet rays of 2,900 to 3,200 angstroms. Noonday sun is the least filtered, and heat may augment the damage from ultraviolet light. Long-wave ultraviolet light can be harmful in photosensitive persons, particularly when drugs such as Declomycin are being used.

Sun-exposed skin demonstrates several changes as a result of the exposure. These changes include thinning of the dermis, more superficial location of sebaceous glands, and breakdown of collagen fibers in the skin. The areas most often exposed are the face, the skin covering the forehead, the nose, cheeks, ears, and the lower lip.

Basal cell carcinoma, squamous cell carcinoma, pigmented nevi, and malignant melanoma are the most commonly occurring types of skin cancer. The majority of skin cancers are **basal cell carcinoma,** which occurs most frequently on the head and neck. Variations of basal cell carcinoma are nodulo-ulcerative basal cell epithelioma, pigmented basal cell epithelioma, and superficial basal cell epithelioma.

The **nodulo-ulcerative epithelioma** is the most frequently occurring type of basal cell carcinoma. Initially, the lesions appear as pale nodules with a waxy appearance and with telangiectatic vessels on the surface. This stage is followed by formation of a raised lesion with a shiny edge. Gradually the lesion then develops a depressed center of ulceration with a pearly colored rounded edge. The basal cell carcinoma grows slowly. **Pigmented basal cell epithelioma** is very similar to nodulo-ulcerative epithelioma except that the lesions are pigmented and dark in color. **Superficial basal cell epithelioma** involves one or more plaques that tend to form crusts. The edges are also pearly in color, and ulcerations occur.

Treatment for basal cell carcinoma is far less traumatic if it is begun early and before the lesions have spread. Either x-ray therapy or surgical excision is used for treatment. Surgical excision is preferred if the underlying structures such as cartilage would be particularly subject to destruction by x-ray therapy. Basal cell carcinoma rarely metastasizes, but left untreated it may cause extensive tissue destruction extending to underlying structures. Surgery performed for removal of deep lesions may be a major surgical procedure involving reconstruction of the body part.

Squamous cell carcinoma is an invasive carcinoma that tends to extend deeply into underlying structures in an irregular fashion and that may metastasize. The squamous carcinoma appears anywhere on the body and most frequently on the face and hands. The lesions appear initially as ulcerated areas with wide borders. Crusts form over the granular tissue exposed by the ulcerations. The treatment includes surgical excision with removal of the underlying tissues involved in the tumor growth. It is even more important for squamous carcinoma to be diagnosed and treated early, because of the irregular and extensive growth that occurs.

A **nevus** is a benign growth of tissue which is usually present at birth but which may first become obvious in adulthood. Nevi can be vascular, arising from blood vessels; pigmented, arising from melanocytes; or they may arise from squamous epithelium. They appear as small flat areas, nodules, or warty growths. Pigmented nevi are precancerous, for a small percentage do develop into malignant melanoma. These nevi vary in color from blue to brown to black. The size also varies considerably. Some nevi are covered with scales. The nevi may be present anywhere about the body.

Nevi may undergo many changes. Some authorities refer to stages of nevi growth: lentigo stage, junctional change, compound nevus, and intradermal nevus. During the lentigo stage, the nevus appears as a freckle, with increased melanin pigmentation. In the junctional change, the nevus appears as a nodule because cells at the junction of the dermis and epidermis proliferate. When the growth enters the dermis, the epidermal areas of the nevus become detached and nevus cells appear in the dermis. This is called the stage of compound nevus. Finally, the nevus is localized in the dermis, and the nevus is then called an intradermal nevus.

If there is a suspicion that the nevus is

malignant, surgical excision is the preferred mode of therapy. The depth of the tumor is an important indication of prognosis. Rapidly growing nodular lesions are considered to be the most highly precancerous. Potential malignancy (development of melanoma) is also determined by increase in size of the nevus, an extension of a halo of pigmentation of the nevus, development of nodules around the original nodule, the appearance of ulcers or hemorrhage, or location of the nevus in areas of the body subject to friction or pressure. Any change in the appearance of a nevus is significant and should be brought to the physician's attention. Another reason for surgical removal of nevi is the affected person's feelings about the lesion. They are usually removed if the person finds them to be cosmetically stressful.

Malignant melanoma may arise from pigmented nevi. However, the tumors may also occur without the precursor nevi, arising from otherwise normal skin. Malignant melanoma is a tumor of the pigment cells, the melanocytes. These tumors most commonly occur in fair-skinned persons between the ages of 50 and 60. They are most common on the head and neck (see color insert Figure 9 on page 1078C) and also occur in the lower extremities. The lesions may occur as nevi that increase in size with ulcerated centers, or when they occur without the precursor nevi, they are irregularly shaped pigmented areas. The tumors enlarge peripherally and ulcerated areas form in the center. In many instances, the central tumor is surrounded by satellite tumors.

Melanoma spreads rapidly through invasion of the lymphatic system. The many lymph channels in the dermis of the skin connect to regional lymph nodes. From these regional lymph nodes, the melanoma spreads to the bloodstream, depositing tumor cells throughout the body. Because of the rapidity of spread, it is important to diagnose melanoma as early as possible so that treatment can be instituted before spread to the lymphatic system occurs.

Treatment for malignant melanoma consists mainly in wide, deep local excision of the lesions, and of the regional lymph nodes if they are involved. Melanomas are generally not responsive to radiation therapy; regional perfusion of the melanoma with an alkylating agent such as phenylalanine mustard (Alkeran) is sometimes used. Development of melanoma cell vaccines for use in immunotherapy is currently experimental.

Immunotherapy uses nonspecific prophylaxis with the vaccine BCG (bacillus-Calmette-Guérin), an attenuated organism which is a strain of *Mycobacterium bovis*. The BCG vaccine is being used in treatment of malignant melanoma. It acts by nonspecifically stimulating the reticuloendothelial system to bring about resistance to tumor growth. It may be injected directly into the nodules of melanoma in persons who are sensitive to tuberculin, and if effective, it causes the melanoma to regress [11]. This mode of therapy is discussed more fully in Chapter 1.

If treatment is given prior to metastasis via the lymph nodes, the prognosis is very good. When metastasis has occurred, the prognosis is poor.

In general, skin cancers make up the most common type of malignant disease. If early diagnosis is made and treatment is initiated promptly, the prognosis is very good with as much as a 90 percent cure rate (except for malignant melanoma). The staging of skin lesions has been established, with T_1 being lesions with a diameter of less than 2 cm and a depth of less than 1 cm. These lesions may be treated by excision. T_2 refers to lesions from 2 to 5 cm in surface area with a depth of 1 to 2 cm. Lesions in this staging do not involve the deeper structures. They are treated by excision. Large lesions may require grafts following excision if necessary for cosmetic benefits. T_3 includes lesions whose diameter is greater than 5 cm with a depth of 2 cm or greater. Lesions in this stage involve underlying bone or cartilage and must be surgically removed. Finally, stage T_4 lesions involve underlying structures.

Therapy for skin lesions is primarily excision. Radiation is effective in some instances but, as previously mentioned, it is not used when the underlying tissues are vulnerable to damage by radiation. Cartilage and bone may be adversely affected by radiation for skin lesions lying over these structures. Chemosurgery may be used, and often follows treatment by surgery with subsequent recurrence of the lesions. When chemosurgery is used, the area is first treated with a substance such as dichloroacetic acid, which makes it more permeable to treatment. Zinc chloride paste is then applied in a thin layer and is kept in place 24 hours by an occlusive dressing. This procedure fixes the tissue so that it can then be surgically excised. The excised tissue is examined by frozen section to determine the depth of the lesion. If the lower areas are involved in tumor growth, the excision is carried out to a greater depth. If the lower areas of the tissue are not demonstrative of tumor growth, however, no further excision is necessary. In situations in which tissue is removed deeply, grafting may be necessary to restore the integrity of the skin.

In many instances treatment for skin lesions is done on an outpatient basis. The nurse's involvement includes observing for the presence of lesions, assisting in early diagnosis, advising the patient to seek medical advice for diagnosis and treatment of the lesions, and finally caring for the patient during the treatment phase. The latter includes teaching the patient how to care for the lesion postoperatively. This care usually involves dressing changes, according to the method of treatment used in a particular treatment setting, observation of the healing process, and emotional support during the treatment.

SKIN LESIONS IN CONNECTIVE TISSUE DISORDERS

Four other skin diseases should be discussed in relation to chronic skin lesions. These diseases are sarcoidosis, mycosis fungoides, discoid lupus erythematosus, and scleroderma.

Sarcoidosis is a complex disease and is classified as granulomatous. This disease is discussed elsewhere in this book as it affects any organ or body system, such as the lungs. It is a chronic disease and it progresses slowly. Typical skin lesions occur in about one-fourth of the affected persons [10]. The lesions occur as plaques, papules, or nodules and, sometimes, existing scars become elevated and reddened because of the granulomatous growth. The lesions are most frequently found on the face, neck, and trunk. Treatment may involve systemic corticosteroids.

Mycosis fungoides is a disease of the lymphoreticular system which is localized to the skin for a long period. The disease begins with skin lesions that appear similar to eczema or psoriasis. The lesions respond slowly to treatment and are sometimes nonresponsive. Ulcers and eroded areas gradually form, and as the disease progresses, the lymph nodes and body organs are often invaded. Treatment consists in chemotherapy, radiation, or ultraviolet light. The disease may progress slowly and the affected person may die of other causes. When the disease has advanced, the prognosis is poor, with a life expectancy of only about 3 years. Many other malignant diseases of the reticuloendothelial system may either begin with skin lesions or may eventually involve the skin. These diseases, including lymphosarcoma, Hodgkin's disease, and leukemia, are discussed in Chapter 4.

Discoid lupus erythematosus is a collagen disease that occurs in two forms: discoid lupus or systemic lupus. DLE refers to the former, SLE to the latter. Discoid lupus appears as erythematous raised lesions with irregular borders. As the lesions progress, telangiectasia, changes in pigmentation, and atrophy may occur. Healed lesions often leave scars. The lesions occur most frequently on the face (the typical butterfly lesion that appears over the nose and cheeks), neck, and trunk. In some instances there is scaling or alopecia or both. It is not unusual for affected persons to be sensitive to cold; the skin lesions tend to be sensitive to sunlight.

Although the cause is not known, it is believed that lupus may be an autoimmune disease. The disease is variable and it causes different symptoms in different persons. Sometimes the symptoms are vague and, generally, discoid lupus is less serious than systemic lupus. The severity of systemic lupus erythematosus depends on the organ involved and on the extent of the disease. Specific diagnostic tests include the LE cell test. The LE cell is a blood cell that is typically found in the majority of persons with lupus erythematosus. The fluorescent antinuclear antibody test is usually positive in those with lupus. Skin biopsies are also done and often demonstrate abnormal cell reactions.

Treatment for lupus erythematosus depends on the symptoms. The patient is advised to avoid exposure to sunlight as this aggravates the lesions, causing them to worsen. Some authorities also advise counseling to help the patient learn to avoid stresses and events or experiences that cause nervousness in the individual. Because the disease tends to flare up at intervals, special care including rest and taking corticosteroids is advised during the periods of exacerbation. The nurse should inform the patient about management when taking corticosteroids, including gradual reduction of dosage as well as the side effects of maintenance doses (Chap. 8). Other aspects of treatment include avoiding drugs to which the patient may be sensitive, such as sulfa drugs or penicillin. Antimalarial drugs such as quinine are useful in treatment of the skin lesions. When there is aching or painful discomfort of the joints or other areas of the body, aspirin is given. The person with lupus is advised to follow consistent schedules of daily living in an effort to minimize exacerbations that might be caused by unusual events.

Scleroderma is another connective tissue disease that has no known cause and may occur at any age. The disease is typified by a hardening of the skin; the skin becomes leathery. As with lupus, there is one form of scleroderma that is particular to the skin, called morphea, and a form of systemic sclerosis that is progressive and involves the internal body organs.

The skin lesions of morphea scleroderma are plaques of erythematous and sometimes edematous areas. These plaques eventually become waxy and shiny, surrounded by a ring of erythema. Lesions may occur in a confined area or may be distributed all over the body. The disease progresses and may eventually disappear, leaving little residual effect. In some instances, however, there is atrophy of the subcutaneous tissue beneath the morphea. Healing in these instances occurs with a residual of atrophied skin in which there may be changes in pigmentation.

Skin changes are also apparent in the systemic form of scleroderma; edema, followed by smoothing and tightening of the skin, are typical skin changes. The skin seems to tighten over the underlying structures so that the person becomes immobile and subject to ulceration at pressure points, such as the tips of the fingers. A characteristic mask-like appearance is noted when the skin changes involve the face. There is no specific treatment for scleroderma. Corticosteroids are often used in an effort to reduce the size or occurrence of the lesions. Systemic scleroderma is discussed more fully in Chapter 10.

In all four of these diseases, the nurse is challenged to provide the patient with comfort, support, and health teaching to minimize the distressful effects of the lesions. Because they are all chronic conditions, the long-term effects of care include those related to the stresses common in any continued and unresolved problem. Medications are expensive; the price of not feeling well over a long period of time is also expensive in terms of the person's ability to tolerate frustrations. Simply having the condition is, in itself, a frustrating situation. Because there is no specific treatment and therefore no cure for these diseases, the person involved often develops an attitude of hopelessness. The nurse must deal with the patient's feelings and emotions, and with the family's response to him or her and to the disease. It is important that the nurse understand that a cosmetically distressful disease that is also somewhat physically disabling can have a serious effect on the patient's relationships with others.

SKIN DYSFUNCTION OF VASCULAR ORIGIN

A number of skin lesions arise from vascular sources. These include xanthomas, purpura, and hemangiomas. Vascular spiders, also called telangiectases, are actually permanently dilated small vessels. The lesion appears as a spider because it has a central body from which small vessels radiate. The central body can sometimes be observed to pulsate. These lesions may be hereditary, or they may occur in association with liver disease, pregnancy, or with taking birth control pills. The lesions are common in persons who have high alcoholic intake and often develop in the elderly. Sometimes telangiectasia occurs in healthy persons with no apparent reason for its development. This group of people is usually light skinned, and when telangiectasia occurs, it is predominantly located on the face. It is postulated that exposure to weather or to sunlight may contribute to the development of this condition. It may occur anywhere on the body, and there is considerable variation in the size and shape of the lesions. Treatment consists in injection of the body of the spider to occlude the dilated vessel.

Xanthomas are deposits of macrophages that are known to have a high lipid content. They occur in persons who have problems in lipid metabolism. The lesions appear as yellowish or brown plaques. They most frequently occur on the upper and lower eyelids. There is no specific treatment for these lesions. Often, observation of the presence of these lesions may lead to diagnosis of cardiovascular or nutritional diseases.

Diabetic xanthomatous tissue develops in people who have diabetes mellitus. Xanthomas may occur anywhere on the body as reddish or yellowish lesions; they are small and are often multiple. They generally occur as an acute outbreak and disappear when therapy for diabetes mellitus is instituted.

Purpura is a reddening of the skin in disseminated plaques. The lesions may occur in otherwise healthy persons, or they may be present along with diseases such as anemia or leukemia. The lesions are not treated, but their presence usually indicates the need for physical examination to rule out any possible underlying causes.

Hemangiomas are also called nevus flammeus. This lesion is sometimes called a port wine stain, known as a birthmark; it appears frequently at birth and lasts for the person's lifetime. The lesion may be flat or raised. One type of the latter, known as strawberry mark, is bright red. Hemangiomas often disappear spontaneously and therefore are not treated initially. They disappear by involution. In instances in which the hemangiomas involve the deep areas of the skin, there may be a residual indentation through which the underlying vessels may be observable. An infrequent type of hemangioma is the **racemose hemangioma** in which there is an outgrowth of veins, forming bluish spots.

When a hemangioma is present at birth or soon thereafter, the parents of the child are often eager to have the lesion removed, particularly if it is located in highly visible areas such as on the face. It is important that the parents be counseled that the lesion may regress spontaneously. Surgical removal of a hemangioma may result in scarring that leaves a more displeasing cosmetic appearance than the person would have if the lesion is left alone to disappear spontaneously. Involution of the hemangioma is seen as a gradual fading of the red areas. The redness is replaced by a gray or whitish color that is barely noticeable in white-skinned persons. The process of involution usually requires about 5 or 7 years. If the lesion appeared as an elevated mass, involution may leave a residual of loose skin which can be treated by plastic surgery. More frequently, the lesion completely disappears.

Some general guidelines are usually followed in determining treatment for hemangiomas. If the lesion interferes with the function of a body part or if it involves a vital body organ, it is excised. When hemangiomas become infected, they must be treated with warm compresses and antibiotic therapy; in some instances systemic corticosteroid therapy is used.

BLISTER FORMATION

Another type of pathology affecting the skin is blister formation. Blisters form by collections of fluid and are covered with epidermal tissue; they may vary considerably in size. Damage to the skin from heat, cold, or infectious agents may cause blistering. A particularly serious disorder characterized by blister formation, followed by denudation of the area, is **pemphigus,** which affects people in middle age. The cause is unknown. Initial blisters occur in the mouth, quickly eroding the skin so that the mouth is painful and eating is difficult. Lesions progress to cover the face and often become secondarily infected by bacteria. If untreated sepsis and death may follow. Methotrexate and systemic steroids are used in treatment, and meticulous nursing care of denuded areas and maintenance of nutritional, fluid, and electrolyte balance are required.

There are several forms of pemphigus. Familial benign pemphigus is a less severe genetically transmitted form. It is a chronic condition with exacerbations and remissions characterized by lesions in the folds of the neck and in the intertriginous areas that appear most commonly in warm weather. Treatment consists in the use of systemic and topical antibiotics.

ULCERS

Many patients with dermatologic conditions or with vascular insufficiency from any cause develop ulcers. The following paragraphs briefly describe ulcers and more specifically deal with decubitus ulcers.

An **ulcer** is defined as an area of skin in which the entire epidermis has been destroyed. This interruption in the skin is different from an **erosion,** in which part of the epidermis remains. Erosions may result from lesions that destroy the skin, from deep scratching, or from trauma. Erosions usually heal without scarring as long as the skin appendages are not damaged. If the skin appendages have been traumatized, scars will form in the healing process. Sometimes healing is evidenced by either hypopigmentation or hyperpigmentation in the eroded area. An ulcer, when healed, leaves a scar because the entire epidermis has been destroyed. Plastic surgery with grafting may be required to close an ulcer.

When ulcers result from vascular insufficiency there are usually differences in the temperature, color, and hair distribution of the surrounding skin. Coolness, paleness, or a bluish color and lack of hair in the area signify vascular insufficiency. People who fall in the high-risk group for skin ulcer formation include those with diabetes mellitus or with arteriosclerosis or hypertension, or with vasoconstriction to an area for any reason. They tend to have ulcer formation on pressure points such as the heels or toes, or in areas that are easily traumatized, such as the shin. Leg ulcer formation is common in persons with ischemia as a result of poor circulation.

Ulcers that form from ischemia usually begin as tender, painful areas that become reddened and then cyanotic. The area then appears to break down and the ulcer crater develops a scab, an **eschar.** Ulcers caused by arterial occlusion often appear on the medial aspects of the shins. They tend to be more painful than those caused by insufficient venous flow. In arterial ulcers, pain is aggravated by elevating the leg. Venous ulcers are usually associated with edema formation and become more tender with standing in an upright position (see color insert Figure 7 on page 1078B).

Treatment for ulcers is controversial. Most authorities prescribe bed rest to promote healing by increasing the blood supply to the affected part. The primary issue in treatment is to do no harm to the ulcer; excessive use of therapy including medications and application of heat to the area may actually extend the ulcer instead of facilitating healing. It is important to keep the ulcerated area clean by irrigating it to remove all debris and necrotic tissue. In many instances, treatment of the patient's cardiovascular disease is most beneficial in aiding ulcer healing. The amount of ambulation desired depends on the patient's capabilities for exercise, his or her need for movement to prevent venous stasis, and tolerance for exercise. It is necessary to prevent pressure on the area as well as overexertion, which may tire the patient. When the area does not heal, grafting may be necessary. If the circulation is poor, however, grafting may not be successful. In some instances arterial reconstruction prior to grafting improves the potential for graft healing.

Because ulcers are sometimes so difficult to heal, they are an enigma to nursing care. Both leg ulcers and decubitus ulcers can interfere with a person's return to normal activities, can prolong hospitalization, and may contribute to a feeling of hopelessness in those who have chronic diseases. The complications of ulcer formation are formidable, and nurses should therefore observe for early signs of pending ulcer formation. Treatment initiated as soon as these early signs are discovered may enable the patient to avoid the discomfort and the emotional and financial cost of ulcer care.

Decubitus ulcers are a frequent complication occurring most often in persons who are chairridden or bedridden, generally debilitated, and in a poor nutritional state (see color insert Figure 8 on page 1078B). The most appropriate solution to the problem is *prevention*. The nurse has the prime responsibility for prevention. Yet the occurrence of decubiti continues to complicate illnesses, cause pain and discomfort, increase costs of hospitalization, and delay rehabilitation.

The most important factor in the prevention of decubiti is the frequent and proper change of position to avoid long-term pressure on vulnerable areas of the body. The importance of this factor is reflected in the other names used for decubiti, such as bedsores and pressure sores. All the terms refer to localized areas of necrosis. Both intensity and duration of the pressure influence decubiti formation [3].

The weight of the body pressing over bony prominences compresses the capillaries and venules in the area and causes ischemia. An early stage of decubitus formation is reddening of the skin which disappears as pressure is relieved. Induration of the tissue occurs as superficial circulatory and tissue damage persist, leading to excoriation and blistering or superficial necrosis and ulcer formation. Decubitus ulcers may become large and deep, destroying subcutaneous tissues, fascia, muscles, and even bone. Such decubiti require months of treatment before healing is possible. Ulcerated areas may become infected, retarding healing, and in some cases leading to systemic infection (Fig. 14-3).

The most frequent sites of decubiti are those at or near bony prominences without padding of adipose tissue, such as the sacrum, coccyx, greater trochanters, and ischial tuberosities. Other sites include the heels, elbows, malleoli, and the knees. The incidence of decubiti tends to increase with age and is related to the loss of elasticity and subcutaneous fat as well as the decreased glandular secretions and general skin atrophy that occur with aging [6]. The presence of circulatory disorders is also a predisposing factor.

The prevention of decubiti requires the recognition of persons susceptible to decubiti and early initiation of preventive measures. Susceptible persons are those who are unable to freely change their positions, such as those paralyzed from a stroke or from a spinal cord injury. Persons who have sensory loss due to circulatory or neurologic conditions or both are particularly vulnerable since they are unaware of pain and pressure. Other susceptible persons are unconscious patients, weak and debilitated patients, or patients confined to bed and limited in movement due to equipment or therapeutic restriction, such as the patient in traction or in a cast.

In addition to continued pressure, shearing forces contribute to decubiti formation. Shearing forces are those that pull tissues rather than press on them and cause movement of one layer of tissue over another [9]. Shearing forces are encountered when patients try to move themselves in bed by digging their heels or elbows into the mattress. Improper positioning while sitting in a chair or in a sitting position in bed results in slumping, which also produces the effects of shearing forces.

Healthy tissues are less likely to develop decubiti than tissues that have had any type of abrasion. Abrasions may result from irritation from scratching, excessively dry skin that peels or cracks, or skin exposed to excessive moisture. The classic example of the latter is the incontinent patient or the patient who sweats excessively and lies for extended periods of time in wet linens. The importance of a dry, wrinkle-free bed cannot be overemphasized. Edematous patients also have a tendency to develop decubiti, because the superficial skin is stretched excessively over the underlying accumulation of fluid.

Persons who are malnourished, especially those in negative nitrogen balance and hypoproteinemia, are vulnerable to decubiti formation. In such persons, decubiti are resistant to healing unless the nutritional state is improved. A dietary intake high in calories and rich in protein, minerals, and vitamins is absolutely essential. Evaluation of dietary intake and instruction in dietary habits must be a part of any nursing plan for the patient susceptible to decubiti or who already has a decubitus ulcer.

Knowledge of the predisposing factors should guide nurses in preventive measures for susceptible patients. Any patient who is unable to move himself and change his position must be turned and have his position changed on a regular schedule that is adhered to by all. This schedule may vary from an hourly to 4-hour interval, depending on the tolerance and degree of susceptibility. Position changes should be accompanied by thorough drying of the skin and massage to stimulate blood flow. Hygienic care is essential, but excessive use of soap is discouraged because of its alkali content, which contributes to cracking and chapping of the skin [3].

When turning aids are required to facilitate the process a Foster frame, Stryker frame, or the CircOlectric bed may be used. Their

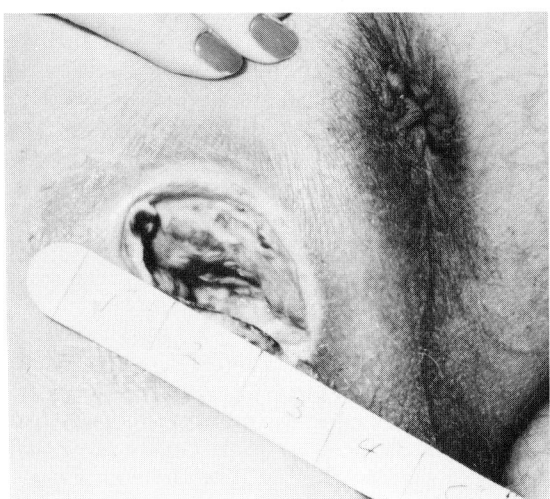

Figure 14-3
Decubitus ulcer.

use is described in detail in Chapter 11 in relation to the care of the spinal-cord-injured patient.

To reduce pressure under bony prominences, soft, form-fitting supporting surfaces are substituted for hard surfaces. Hard surfaces cause pressure concentration over small areas, whereas soft surfaces spread the weight over a large skin area. Soft, thick mattresses with a stretchable cover and a nonsagging bottom have been evaluated as the most appropriate to prevent decubiti formation [9]. Soft foam rubber or foam plastic pads may be added to hard mattresses. Soft, moisture-absorbing pads under the bottom sheets are substituted for hard, waterproof sheets or mattress covers.

Pillows are utilized to relieve pressure on vulnerable areas of the body. They are used to prevent two body parts from pressing on each other, such as the legs when the patient is positioned on his or her side. Sheepskin pads of various sizes may be used to protect either the entire back area or specific areas of the body. The softness and resilience of sheepskin padding under the patient provides for even distribution of pressure, absorption of moisture, and avoidance of friction. Soft pads may be applied to the heel or elbow, but should not be strapped tightly. They should also be removed at frequent intervals to allow for skin inspection and cleaning.

Providing a form-fitting supporting surface is the basis for the use of water beds and water-filled chair seats for selected patients. The weight of the water bed, the difficulty of changing the position of the patient with retention of flotation, spatial disorientation, seasickness, and difficulties in general nursing care often make the use of the water bed impractical [12]. Other flotation systems include the water mattress; gel flotation pads made of Silastic, silicone, or polyvinyl chloride; and even an ordinary camper's air mattress partially filled with water. All these devices help to disperse pressure over a larger surface rather than on specific vulnerable body areas.

Alternating pressure mattresses are used frequently as a means of equalizing pressure distribution. These polyvinyl or rubberized canvas air mattresses require a pumping system to inflate and deflate alternate series of cells that are arranged either vertically or horizontally. These mattresses, also referred to as a ripple-celled mattress, require proper maintenance to assure proper functioning. A frequent misuse of the mattress is the use of pillows or pads over the mattress. Only a thin sheet should be used over the mattress, or the purpose of the mattress is negated.

None of the devices available should be viewed as a single means of prevention of decubiti. Nor should the nurse mistakenly feel secure that preventive measures have been initiated simply because one of the devices is being used. Thorough assessment of all areas of the body is carried out regularly and systematically to determine any change in the integrity of the skin or to detect any area showing effects of compression. The patient is kept as active as possible to increase skin and vascular tone. Active and passive exercises are indicated if the patient has limited activity. The patient with a neuromuscular disorder should be taught to use a mirror to inspect posterior regions of the body for signs of decubiti formation. Patients who sit in wheelchairs for long periods should lift themselves and shift their positions frequently; if they are unable to do so, nursing staff should move the patients at regular intervals. Foam-padded seat boards that may be cut out posteriorly over ischial areas are useful for the chairridden patient.

Patients who are incontinent should be put on a schedule for bladder and bowel programming and should be checked often for any episodes of incontinence. A retention catheter may be indicated in some situations. Attention to proper hygiene is essential to prevent skin breakdown and infection. When patients are to be moved in bed, they should be lifted rather than pulled or slid across the bed to prevent the strong shearing forces that contribute to the development of decubiti. Nurses have the responsibility of teaching other staff personnel, the patient, and the family the importance of positioning and moving patients in the proper manner.

Another role for the nurse in the prevention of decubitus ulcers is that of conducting or participating in studies to determine the effectiveness and efficiency of various measures utilized in the prevention of decubiti. Berecek frequently refers to the lack of *controlled* studies with sufficient numbers of study and control subjects as the major problem in determining the most effective means of preventing decubiti [3]. She also cites the need to study the posttreatment effect of various measures and devices to determine if their use actually increases later susceptibility to decubiti development [3].

If a decubitus ulcer develops, or if the presence of one is detected on an initial assessment, care is focused on preventing extension of the lesion and on promoting healing. The decubitus should be described in detail and accurately to provide a baseline for determining the effectiveness of treatment. All the previously discussed preventive measures should be carried out even more rigorously in order to prevent pressure on the decubitus. Mechanical cleaning of the decubitus is necessary to promote healing and prevent infection; regeneration of epithelium is also stimulated by mechanical cleaning. Healing and epithelial regeneration are not possible, however, without regular and careful debridement of the ulcer. A culture and sensitivity test of any drainage from the ulcer is necessary to determine the use of appropriate topical or systemic antibiotics.

Various topical agents have been prescribed in the treatment of decubitus ulcers. Their use is determined most often by the personal preference of either the physician or the nurse and is usually based on past successful experiences. Again, this area of decubiti care is one that requires further investigation via controlled studies with adequate numbers of subjects to determine which agents are most effective and when their use is indicated.

The agents used include, but are not limited to, various ointments, tinctures, lotions, solutions, antacids, antiseptics, antibiotics, egg white mixtures, granulated sugar, gelatin sponge, scarlet red ointment, karaya, gold leaf, gentian violet, enzymatic preparations, corticosteroids, and oxygen under pressure. In addition, exposing the ulcer to air and sunlight or to heat lamps or infrared treatment provides drying effects.

Only a few of these topical agents will be considered individually. The reader is referred to pharmacology textbooks to obtain more specific information about actions of specific agents.

Zinc oxide cream and pHisoHex have been shown to offer some protection against decubiti formation [3]. Vitamin A and D ointment has often been utilized on decubiti, but this practice is questionable since the vitamin needs to be metabolized in order to be effective [4].

Granulated sugar is often used to fill decubiti cavities after thorough cleaning with hydrogen peroxide. The technique has been shown to stimulate granulation of tissue by substituting sugar as a medium for bacteria to feed on rather than on living tissue and by altering the pH of the tissue and influencing the toxicity of invading organisms [3, 4].

Gold leaf is applied in 2 to 4 layers at the base of ulcers after they have been cleaned with hydrogen peroxide and debrided. The gold leaf, which is absorbable, is thought to have an electrochemical effect [3, 4].

Absorbable gelatin sponge (Gelfoam) placed at the base of the ulcer may hasten granulation. Oxygen under pressure has been applied directly to ulcerations on schedules of three or four times daily for 15 minutes. Karaya, a substance obtained from the sap of the *Sterculia* tree, has been shown to have healing characteristics and has been used for treatment of decubiti when combined with aseptic cleaning with hydrogen peroxide [13].

Local enzymatic agents that have a debriding action include the following drugs: (1) collagenolytic-acting agents such as collagenase (Santyl), which apparently digest collagen as well as debris; (2) proteolytic agents such as Travase ointment; and (3) fibrinolytic agents such as Elase [2]. These agents are thought to "digest" the necrotic soft tissue and purulent exudate. The decubiti are cleaned with either normal saline, hydrogen peroxide, or Dakin's solution prior to fresh applications of the ointment, usually once or twice daily. Directions supplied with the medications must be followed specifically. Certain substances used for cleaning, such as detergents, antiseptics containing heavy metal ions, and acidic solutions that decrease the pH of the skin, tend to inactivate the enzymatic action of local agents used for debriding. The substances to be avoided when local agents are used include hexachlorophene, tincture of iodine, and Burow's solution.

Some authorities recommend that nothing be applied on decubiti while other authorities recommend the use of some of the agents previously listed. It is felt by some authorities that the specific agent used is not as important as the mechanical cleaning and debridement of the decubiti [4].

When conservative management is inadequate and not successful in healing a decubitus, surgical intervention is indicated. Debridement, combined with sterile saline soaks (or Dakin's solution in some settings), is used to provide a clean granulating wound, followed by a closure of the wound with skin grafts. Recurrence of decubiti is likely to occur, however, if special precautions to eliminate predisposing factors are not accomplished. Reconstructive surgery, utilizing pedicle flaps for grafting, may be necessary to prevent recurrence. Reconstructive surgery consists in wide excision of the ulcer, including the bursa and adjacent bone, and covering the defect with pedicle tissue. Either soft tissue adjacent to the ulcer, or tissue obtained via a tubed pedicle or regional rotation flap, is used for the graft. The pedicle tissue serves as a cushion of subcutaneous fat over the defect [4, 5].

The success of radical excision and reconstructive surgery for decubitus ulcers is dependent on nursing care that provides for relief of pressure to the site, proper positioning, good nutritional intake, and strict adherence to aseptic technique in the care of the wound.

As stated previously, the most appropriate solution to the problem of decubitus ulcers is prevention. A broadened view of the nurse's role in prevention of decubitus ulcers will include an emphasis on controlled studies to determine (1) specific predisposing factors, (2) the most effective preventive measures, and (3) the most effective treatment.

References

1. Arndt, K. *Manual of Dermatologic Therapeutics.* Boston: Little, Brown, 1974.
2. Barrett, D., Jr., and Klibanski, A. Collagenase debridement. *Am. J. Nurs.* 73:841, 1973.
3. Berecek, K. H. Etiology of decubitus ulcers. *Nurs. Clin. North Am.* 10:157, 1975.
4. Brandner, J. (ed.). Treating the open ischemic ulcer. *Patient Care* 8:231, 1974.
5. DiPirro, E. Surgery: Successful treatment for deep decubiti. *RN* 38:28, 1975.
6. Gosnell, D. J. An assessment tool to identify pressure sores. *Nurs. Res.* 22:55, 1973.
7. Houston, J. The great cosmetics safety debate. *Sat. Rev.* July 26, 1975.
8. Johnson, S. A. M. (ed.). Symposium: Coping with common skin conditions. Part 2. *Geriatrics* 30:44, 1975.
9. Miller, M. E., and Sachs, M. L. *About Bedsores.* Philadelphia: Lippincott, 1974.
10. Parrish, J. *Dermatology and Skin Care.* New York: McGraw-Hill, 1975.
11. Sell, S. *Immunology, Immunopathology and Immunity* (2nd ed.). New York: Harper & Row, 1975.
12. Tummes, J. J., et al. Treating and preventing decubitus ulcers with a new flotation unit. *Am. Fam. Physician* 10:150, 1974.
13. Verhonick, P. J. Decubitus ulcer observations measured objectively. *Nurs. Res.* 10:211, 1961.

Bibliography

Brown, M. S., and Alexander, M. Physical examination. Part 3. Examining the skin. *Nursing 73* 3:9, 1973.

Fisher, M., and Wittner, M. *Bacterial Infections of the Skin.* New York: Abbott Laboratories, 1973.

Fitzpatrick, T. B., Arndt, K. A., Clark, W. H., Jr., Eisen, A. Z., Van Scott, E. J., and Vaughn, J. H. (eds.). *Dermatology in General Medicine.* New York: McGraw-Hill, 1971.

Graham, J. M., Johnson, W. C., and Helwig, E. B. (eds.). *Dermal Pathology.* New York: Harper & Row, 1972.

Morley, M. H. Decubitus ulcer management: A teaching approach. *Can. Nurs.* 69:41, 1973.

Mountcastle, V. B. (ed.). *Medical Physiology* (13th ed.). St. Louis: Mosby, 1974.

North, C., and Weinstein, G. D. Treatment of psoriasis. *Am. J. Nurs.* 76:410, 1976.

Pillsbury, D. M. *A Manual of Dermatology.* Philadelphia: Saunders, 1971.

Rice, A. Common skin infections in school children. *Am. J. Nurs.* 73:1905, 1973.

Roach, L. B. Assessing skin changes. *Nursing 74* 3:64, 1974.

Roberts, S. L. Skin assessment for color and temperature. *Am. J. Nurs.* 75:610, 1975.

Rodman, M. J. Systemic and topical drugs for psoriasis and acne. *RN* 38:63, 1975.

Rogers, R. S., and Callaway, J. L. Contact dermatitis. Part I. *Hosp. Med.* 7:6, January 1971.

Rubin, P. (ed.). *Clinical Oncology for Medical Students and Physicians.* Rochester: American Cancer Society, 1974.

Sana, J., and Judge, R. D. *Physical Appraisal Methods in Nursing Practice.* Boston: Little, Brown, 1975.

Sauer, G. Skin diseases due to a virus. *Hosp. Med.* 7:82, August 1971.

Torelli, M. Topical hyperbaric oxygen for decubitus ulcers. *Am. J. Nurs.* 73:494, 1973.

Torrey, F. A., Morris, W. J., and Sulzberger, R. Z. Hemangiomas: Visible vascular birthmarks. *Hosp. Med.* 7:6, August 1971.

Wallace, G., and Hayter, J. Karaya for chronic skin ulcers. *Am. J. Nurs.* 74:1094, 1974.

Williams, A. Study of factors contributing to skin breakdown. *Nurs. Res.* 21:238, 1974.

Wilson, J. W., et al. Superficial fungous infections of the skin. *Hosp. Med.* 7:98, July 1971.

chapter 15

Patients with Thermal Injuries

Cornelia Kenner

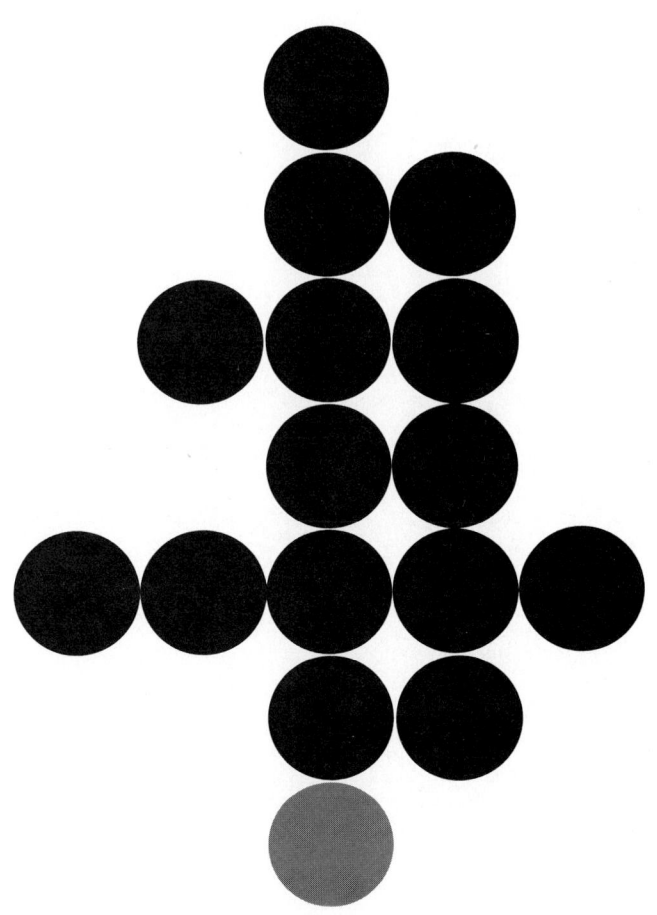

The patient who has undergone severe thermal injury is constantly confronted with severe illness, numerous complications, psychological alterations, and adjustments to lifelong physical disability. The nursing care administered must be comprehensive and detailed. The toll on a nurse is also great, not only in terms of physical strength but also in terms of emotional expenditure.

The nursing process is inherent in all phases of hospitalization and posthospitalization. The nurse must be capable of making a comprehensive assessment, planning nursing care, implementing the interventions, and evaluating the effectiveness of the care administered. The entire process is governed by the nurse's level of competence, the patient's individual response to injury, and the family and social structure of which the patient is a part.

It is well recognized that special burn units and burn teams have contributed to the decrease in mortality from burn injury. Although patients with severe burns are most appropriately treated in special burn centers, nurses may work in settings where such facilities are not immediately available. Nurses may also care for burn patients who do not require hospitalization in a special unit but who still require nursing care. It is therefore important for all nurses to understand the basic principles of first aid care in burn injuries and also to understand some of the basic terminology used in burn care.

Care of the thermally injured patient will be discussed in relation to initial care, fluid and electrolyte balance, respiratory status, metabolic status, gastrointestinal function, sepsis, psychological adjustment to stress, wound coverage, and decreased range of motion and contractures.

Initial Care

In any situation, whether in the first aid room at the industrial site, on the highway following an automobile accident, or in the emergency room, the medical team must systematically assess the patient's overall condition. Priorities are established and the principles of emergency management are followed. Thermally injured persons are approached first as individuals who have undergone trauma. Frequently, they have been in a motor vehicle accident or an explosion, and associated injuries are common. In essence, the burn itself will not cause death in the first few minutes after injury, but death will ensue from an obstructed airway or an open chest injury. Care thus includes the maintenance of an adequate airway, treatment of any associated life-threatening injuries, assessment of the injury (including history, physical examination, and laboratory studies), initial fluid therapy, attention to the details of asepsis to prevent infection, and relief of pain.

HISTORY

The details of the accident are of particular significance. Information concerning the depth of the burn may be ascertained by the type of injurious agent, be it hot water, flames, a hot object, or a flash explosion. Knowledge of the circumstances surrounding the injury provides much valuable information. A history of being burned in a closed space or of excessive smoke inhalation is important in the early determination of respiratory damage. The findings of a physical examination of respiratory status may be negative, but such a history would alert one to be particularly observant for the symptoms of respiratory distress that may develop several hours later. One can thereby prevent situations in which the patient is treated for a minor injury and discharged, only to return later in severe respiratory distress.

With respect to the circumstances surrounding the injury, it is particularly important to note whether the patient lost consciousness. For example, if the patient has been lying unconscious on top of a hot automobile engine, one should be alert for extensive involvement of underlying tissues. If the patient had an epileptic seizure while cooking and fell on a hot stove, one would also be alert for extensive tissue involvement as well as for another convulsive episode.

A known history of cardiovascular, pulmonary, renal, metabolic, or neurologic problems is of utmost importance in treating the patient and assessing his or her response to therapy. To increase the patient's chances for survival, one must be cognizant of all the potential complications, since early recognition and treatment can perhaps alter the clinical course. A knowledge of present and past drug usage, drug sensitivities, excessive alcohol intake, and narcotic usage or abuse is necessary. Tetanus immunizations are also recorded. An in-depth history, including family status and health history, sleep patterns, and dietary habits, can be obtained at a later time when the immediate emergency has passed.

ESTIMATE OF TOTAL BODY SURFACE AREA BURNED

Initial fluid resuscitation is based on the extent of total body surface area (TBSA) burned rather than on the depth of the burn. The simplest method of determining the extent TBSA burned is the Rule of Nines: The head (including the neck) and each arm represent 9 percent of the TBSA (total, 27 percent); the chest, back, and each leg represent 18 percent (total, 72 percent); and the perineal area represents 1 percent. These percentages are different for children. Although not entirely accurate, the method is particularly helpful in the triage of burn patients. The more accurate Berkow formula is shown in Figure 15-1 and is now available on prepared charts in most emergency rooms. Utilizing these body diagrams, the health team member can identify which parts of the body are burned. The percentages of the body parts are estimated according to the patient's age and then added together to give the TBSA burned. As a check, after the extent of the burn has been estimated, the same calculation is performed on the unburned area; the two percentages should add up to 100. Later, after the patient's wounds have been cleaned aseptically, the same calculations are repeated for a more accurate estimate of the TBSA burned.

FLUID RESUSCITATION AND MONITORING

Fluid resuscitation can be initiated according to several different formulas: crystalloid, Evans, Moore's burn budget, hypertonic, Brooke, or an alteration of any of these. (These formulas will be discussed in detail later in this chapter.) Any formula the physician chooses to administer serves only as a guideline, and the patient's response is closely monitored, so that the rate of fluid administered can be altered if necessary.

Many of the physiologic alterations that occur in the patient are a systemic response to injury, and several procedures are necessary to treat and monitor the patient's total condition. Intravenous fluid is administered via a large line(s). Cutdowns are often necessary and are preferably placed in an unburned area. Peripheral veins are initially used if possible, so that central veins are saved for later total parenteral nutrition. Central venous pressure readings are used in monitoring the response to fluid therapy and are mandatory in elderly patients with cardiovascular disease. Pulmonary artery and wedge pressures are often used. Blood is drawn for a complete blood count, serum electrolytes, blood urea nitrogen, and glucose. An arterial blood sample is obtained for Po_2, Pco_2, and pH. Since a paralytic ileus is likely to occur in all persons with injuries involving more than 20 percent of the TBSA, nasogastric intubation is performed. In all with injuries involving more than 15 percent of the TBSA, a Foley catheter is inserted and hourly output is measured. Urine sugar and acetone levels are determined every 4 hours, since a pseudodiabetes (high blood sugar levels, glycosuria, and high urine volumes) might be present.

ASSESSMENT OF DEPTH OF THE BURN

Clinical assessment of the depth of injury aids in observation and treatment of the patient's wounds and in selection of the appropriate type of hospitalization. It is helpful always to remember that injuries are not entirely partial-thickness or entirely full-thickness but are mixtures of different depths and that skin thickness varies with age and body site. The actual depth of the injury is very difficult to assess in the early stages. Accurate determination of depth cannot be made until several days after injury.

A **first-degree burn** is the most superficial and involves only the epidermis. It occurs after sun exposure or very brief contact with intense heat following flash explosions. The main characteristic is erythema. Pain and discomfort are present, but there is little systemic involvement other than vasodilation and chilling. Healing occurs within a week by a scaling process.

Superficial second-degree burns or **superficial partial-thickness burns** involve the entire thickness of epidermis and part of the dermis. They usually are caused by hot liquids or by a flash from an explosion. Blister formation is characteristic (Fig. 15-2), although blisters also occur in full-thickness injury from steam trapped in the dermis. The skin is usually mottled red or pink, moist, and very painful. Healing occurs in 10 to 14 days.

Deep second-degree burns or deep partial-thickness injuries are often clinically difficult to distinguish from full-thickness injuries.

DALLAS COUNTY HOSPITAL DISTRICT
DALLAS, TEXAS

BURN RECORD

To be completed upon admission:

Unit # _____
Name _____
Address _____
Birthdate _____
Classification _____
OP ☐ ER ☐ IP ☐ Admit # _____

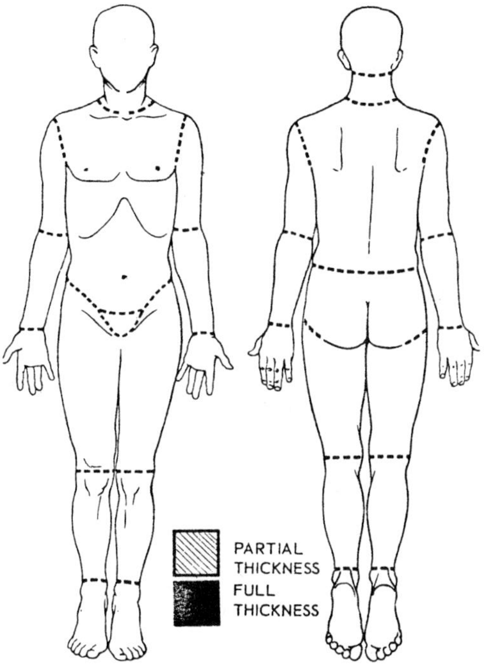

Date: _____

Height: _____ Weight: _____

2° _____ + 3° _____ = _____ %

PARTIAL THICKNESS
FULL THICKNESS

Percent Surface Area Burned
(Berkow Formula)

AREA	1 YR.	1–4 YRS.	5–9 YRS.	10–14 YRS.	15 YRS.	ADULT	2°	3°
Head	19	17	13	11	9	7		
Neck	2	2	2	2	2	2		
Ant. Trunk	13	13	13	13	13	13		
Post Trunk	13	13	13	13	13	13		
R. Buttock	2½	2½	2½	2½	2½	2½		
L. Buttock	2½	2½	2½	2½	2½	2½		
Genitalia	1	1	1	1	1	1		
R.U. Arm	4	4	4	4	4	4		
L.U. Arm	4	4	4	4	4	4		
R.L. Arm	3	3	3	3	3	3		
L.L. Arm	3	3	3	3	3	3		
R. Hand	2½	2½	2½	2½	2½	2½		
L. Hand	2½	2½	2½	2½	2½	2½		
R. Thigh	5½	6½	8	8½	9	9½		
L. Thigh	5½	6½	8	8½	9	9½		
R. Leg	5	5	5½	6	6½	7		
L. Leg	5	5	5½	6	6½	7		
R. Foot	3½	3½	3½	3½	3½	3½		
L. Foot	3½	3½	3½	3½	3½	3½		
TOTAL								

Figure 15-1
Burn record for estimation of total body surface area (TBSA) burned.

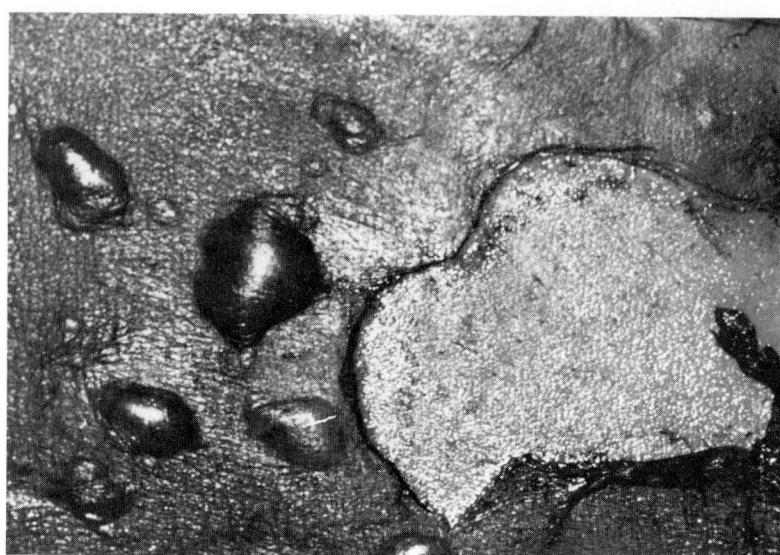

Figure 15-2
Blister formation in partial-thickness injury.

All the dermis except the basal layers are injured. The wounds are dryer than in lesser injuries, appear mottled, and may contain waxy white areas of injury. Healing occurs in 30 to 60 or more days by reepithelialization from epithelial elements in the hair follicles (see color insert Figure 15 on page 1078D). Infection, metabolic depletion, or rejection complications result in conversion to full-thickness injury.

Third-degree burns or **full-thickness injuries** involve the epidermis, dermis, and even subcutaneous tissue. The destroyed tissue is called eschar, and healing cannot occur since all dermal elements have been destroyed. Once the eschar has been removed, skin is taken from another area of the body and grafted to the wound site. Commonly, the cause of full-thickness burns is flame injury; however, burns resulting from contact with a hot object or hot water can be partial-thickness or full-thickness, depending on the temperature of the object or water and the duration of contact. Elasticity of the dermis is destroyed, and the wound appears dry, hard, and leathery. It is white, cherry red, or black in color, with or without bullae, and edema is marked. Thrombosed blood vessels within the eschar (see color insert Figure 13 on page 1078D) are characteristic of full-thickness injury. The nerve endings are destroyed, and the wound is painless to touch or pinprick.

In the older person, as in the young child, areas that at first appear to be partial-thickness injury actually are usually full-thickness injury; accurate depth assessment is difficult, but, as a rule of thumb, these burns are deeper than initially anticipated. Because the skin of these patients is thin and translucent, the red color of the vascular bed under the burn is visible and appears to be the color of the burn itself.

ESCHAROTOMY AND FASCIOTOMY

Once fluid therapy has been instituted, any circumferential burned area must be closely observed. The underlying tissues swell, but the area of a circumferential full-thickness burn is inelastic and remains contracted. The area acts like a tourniquet and impairs venous return and arterial flow. Elevation decreases the edema, but escharotomy is often necessary [51]. An **escharotomy** (Fig. 15-3) is an incision through the entire thickness of eschar, so that the underlying viable edematous tissues may expand. In the case of a deeper burn, the fascia is incised, a procedure called **fasciotomy.** Circulation is constantly evaluated to determine the need for escharotomy. Pulses are palpated and an ultrasonic Doppler flowmeter is used to hear the arterial flow. Clinical signs of impaired circulation are (1) numbness, decreased sensation, and decreased motor activity; (2) decreased capillary refill; (3) cyanosis; and (4) deep aching pain. After the incision is made, the eschar separates, and the edematous tissue bulges because of underlying pressure. Es-

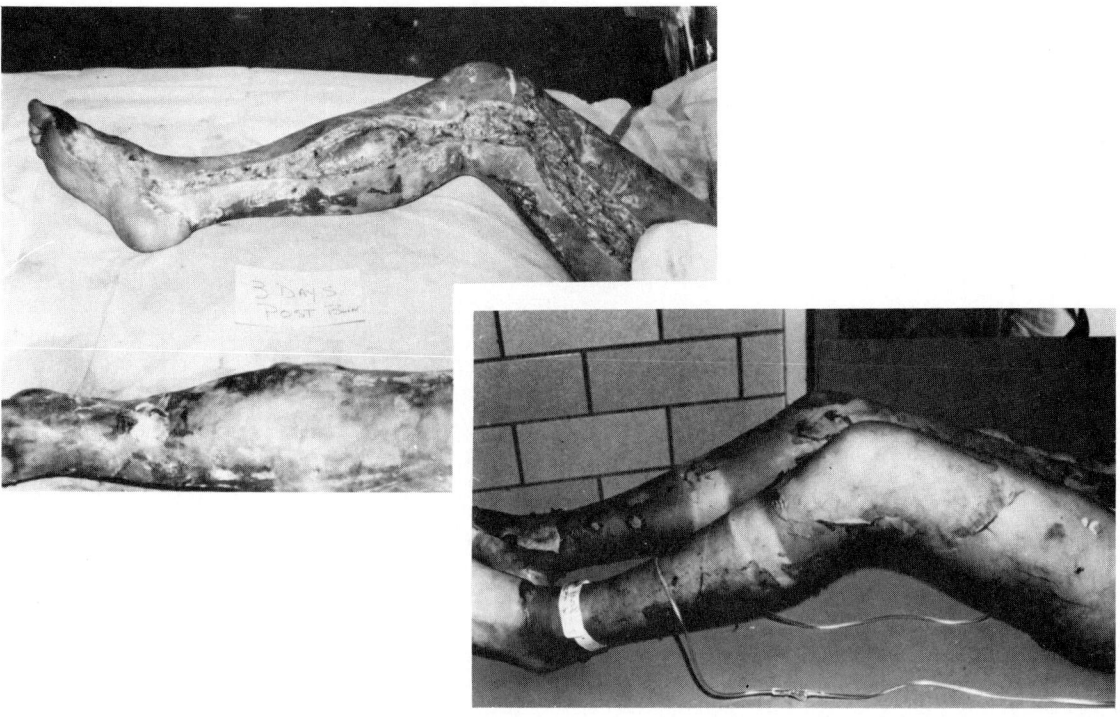

Figure 15-3
Circumferential full-thickness injury of both legs with escharotomy of left thigh and fasciotomy of left calf.

charotomies are carried from one end of the burn to the other to prevent constriction and distal damage. Any bleeding is controlled by direct pressure and the application of sterile microcrystalline collagen hemostat (Avitine).

OPTIMAL CRITERIA FOR HOSPITAL RESOURCES FOR THE BURN PATIENT

It is important during this time to determine the seriousness of the patient's injury in relation to his or her need for hospitalization. The American Burn Association has developed the following specific optimal criteria for hospital resources for care of patients with burn injury. Patients with a partial-thickness injury of less than 15 percent of the TBSA or a full-thickness injury of 2 percent of the TBSA may be treated on an outpatient basis but must be seen every 48 hours. Those who have sustained a partial-thickness injury of less than 25 percent of the TBSA or a full-thickness injury of 10 percent TBSA can be treated in the average hospital. All patients with full-thickness injuries of more than 10 percent TBSA; partial-thickness injuries of more than 25 percent TBSA; partial-thickness or full-thickness burns of the face, eyes, ears, hands, feet, or perineum; electrical injury, respiratory tract injury, associated fracture, or major soft-tissue injury; and all poor-risk patients should be treated in a burn unit or center.

PAIN

Assessment of pain in the burn patient is difficult. Thermally injured victims with partial-thickness injury have a great deal of pain because the nerve endings are exposed. Even the slightest air current across the sensitive tissue will cause extreme discomfort. On the other hand, some patients with massive injury have little discomfort, since the nerve endings are destroyed in full-thickness injury. In addition, patients in the shock phase are not so likely to complain or they complain inappropriately. Once a satisfactory response has been obtained from the resuscitation fluids, the patients' complaints are lucid.

The importance of the correct interpretation of the patient's symptoms cannot be overemphasized. The patient in pain may be restless, but restlessness is also a sign of hypoxia that can easily be misinterpreted as pain. An example of a clinical picture of hypoxia is one in which the patient thrashes about complaining vehemently of discomfort. Assessment of shock and hypoxemia, including monitoring of arterial blood gases, is critical.

To relieve the pain of patients in shock, analgesics are given in small doses intravenously because of the irregular absorption of medication administered intramuscularly. Soft-tissue perfusion is decreased as a result of edema formation and the low flow state.

Fluid and Electrolyte Balance

The thermally injured patient has all the problems of the acutely ill trauma patient compounded by the ramifications of the most severe form of stress known to man. The major problems of the first 4 to 5 days are related to alterations in fluid and electrolyte status.

FLUID VOLUME, CONCENTRATION, AND COMPOSITION

The most prominent alteration following thermal injury is sequestration of fluid into the injured area. The ability of the wound to swell is enormous. This sequestration or shift in body fluids results in a transfer of fluid volume from a functional space to a nonfunctional one. Soon after injury, large quantities of the isotonic fluid are translocated into this nonfunctional or third space, and this fluid must be replaced to offset the problems of the low flow or burn shock state.

Clinically, burn shock seems to be helped by all the fluid resuscitation regimens. Prompt institution of therapy is crucial [47]. In general, parenteral treatment is necessary for all patients with an injury involving more than 20 percent of the TBSA, except for elderly patients and children with injuries involving less than 20 percent of the TBSA. The particular formula used for fluid resuscitation does not make a significant difference in the survival of patients with an injury of less than 40 percent of the TBSA; however, if it exceeds 40 percent, survival will depend on the careful selection of and response to fluid therapy [10].

The primary goal of initial resuscitation is a rapid and complete restoration of cardiac output. Moncrief [46] states that the rapid drop in cardiac output (approximately 50 percent) precedes any measurable change in blood or plasma volume, and cardiac output continues to decrease after the plasma and blood volume begin to decline. Animal studies using a burn model have shown that the cardiac output usually approaches 20 percent of resting normal values [46]. Although the significant decreases in cardiac output suggest depressed cardiac efficiency that is directly attributable to the injury, the decrease is also attributable to a circulating myocardial depressant factor (MDF) (Chap. 16). The cause or source of this factor is unknown, although the pancreas and fibrinogen breakdown products have been suggested as sources, and the effects of MDF are particularly detrimental in patients with injuries involving more than 65 percent of the TBSA and in the elderly [8, 10].

Volume deficit is of extreme importance. One may think of the injury as three-dimensional: volume, surface area extent, and depth. The deficit in blood volume is approximately proportional to the extent and depth of injury. The plasma deficit is more significant, since the erythrocyte loss is less than 10 percent. Measurements of plasma and extracellular fluid volume deficits with ^{125}iodine and ^{35}sulfur respectively show that the decrease in extracellular volume is even larger than the decrease in plasma volume [8]. This volume decrease or translocation is highest during the initial 12 hours after injury, lasts for a total of 18 to 24 hours, and is the rationale for the rapid administration of resuscitation fluid [59].

Plasma proteins are lost into the interstitial spaces all over the body but primarily into the burned area. It is generally accepted that capillary and venular walls are permeable only to electrolytes and water, but after thermal injury, the capillaries are also permeable to proteins. This capillary injury is not sealed off for approximately 24 hours although the time is variable and may range from 18 to 36 hours. Colloid cannot remain in the intravascular space until the capillary injury seals [6]. The findings of one study [32] have supported an alternative explanation for the loss of fluid in the burn wound: that osmotic alterations in burn tissue and the negation of Starling's law are the primary factors rather than increased capillary permeability; however, the latter concept is generally accepted. In any case, the loss of fluid into the wound reflects the magnitude of injury, and the vascular changes account for the presence of plasma protein. A further finding is fibrinogen in the interstitial spaces in concentrations up to 3 gm per 100 ml [21]. This forms a gel-like edema that blocks drainage of the lymphatics and venules supplying the area, resulting in edema extending laterally and in-depth beyond the injured area.

An additional response is the release of aldosterone from the adrenal cortex with maximal sodium reabsorption. The result is oliguria with increased urine concentration and decreased sodium concentration. As volume is replaced, renal blood flow improves and urine volume increases. Complications in renal function are usually the result of inadequate fluid and electrolyte replacement. Baxter [8] states that low urinary sodium concentrations (below 20 mg per liter) imply inadequate volume replacement.

Alterations in water balance or concentrations of body fluids are also a problem. A physiologic response to all trauma is the release of antidiuretic hormone from the posterior pituitary, which results in water reabsorption from the distal renal tubules. This response to stress continues for an indefinite period of time, and high urine concentration persists. In instances where a severe imbalance is not properly treated, the urine will contain only the amount of water necessary to excrete a normal solute load. Increasing the water intake will not change the urine concentration but will lead to water intoxication.

Water balance should be monitored until the wound is covered. The **stratum corneum,** a condensed fibrous membrane that is tough and resilient and closely resembles a fine sheet of semitransparent plastic, constitutes the vapor barrier of the skin. When this barrier is removed by burn, evaporative water loss increases from 4 to 15 times normal [9]. Jelenko et al. [30] found that burned human and rabbit skin contained approximately 0.25 percent of the normal amount of water-holding lipid. Increased loss of water from second-degree burns is as significant as that from deeper burns and is proportional to the total burned area. If the burn wound is covered with a piece of plastic, drops of condensed water vapor will show on the patient side of the plastic in a few minutes. Losses as high as 3.5 ml/kg/percent TBSA burned can occur every 24 hours. The average loss is estimated at 1.5 ml/kg/percent TBSA burned, and loss continues until the wound is covered with a physiologic dressing or reepithelialization occurs.

The amount of water lost is also determined by the amount of burn surface exposed to the air, by air currents, and by wound care. For example, in patients burned on the abdomen and back and who lie on their backs, more water will evaporate from the abdomen than from the back. On the other hand, hydrotherapy may result in the loss of sodium and in the absorption of significant amounts of water. Thus, the exact quantity of water required by the individual burn patient cannot be calculated precisely. Generally, patients with burns of 40 to 70 percent of the TBSA require between 3 to 5 liters per day for replacement [9]. The following formula can be used to approximate water needs [69]:

$$(25 + \%\text{TBSA burned}) \times (\text{body surface area in meters}^2) = \text{ml H}_2\text{O/hour (evaporate water loss)}$$

Example:

$$[25 + 50 (\% \text{ TBSA burned})] \times 2 (\text{body surface area in meters}^2) = 150 \text{ ml H}_2\text{O/hour}$$

Mobilization of burn wound edema begins within 48 hours and continues gradually until the body weight reaches preburn levels between the tenth and fourteenth postburn day. Assessment remains difficult since weight loss to preburn level is not entirely indicative of mobilization of burn wound edema. Since the patient is in a hypermetabolic state during this period, he or she also loses body weight in an amount proportional to the extent of the injury. Indeed, the complex systemic ramifications of injury are compounded by alterations in fluid volume and concentration, so that both clinical signs and laboratory values are difficult to evaluate during this period [10].

Alterations in fluid composition can be a significant problem. All the compensatory hemodynamics occur at the expense of adequate perfusion. To maintain arterial pressure and venous return, the splanchnic bed constricts, and blood flow to the kidneys, liver, and intestines decreases. Decreased blood flow causes decreased cellular oxygenation, and cellular hypoxia results in cellular alterations and metabolic acidosis. The magnitude of this response is proportional to the severity of the injury and the physiologic status of the patient at the time of injury.

Intracellular potassium deficits are large. Potassium is excreted in large amounts in the urine because of the presence of respiratory alkalosis, high urine output, and high aldosterone levels, and later is needed for cell synthesis as the major intracellular cation. Large amounts of potassium (80 to 200 mEq) are administered to offset the intracellular deficit. *Digitalis is ordered only for the person with specific cardiovascular problems, and if it is ordered, the patient must be closely observed and monitored by ECG* [10, 13]. Hyperkalemia does not tend to be a problem in patients with adequately functioning kidneys.

Although serum magnesium levels may remain within low normal limits, total body magnesium may be decreased. One of the most common signs of the problem is a total body tremor that is particularly noticeable in the extremities. As a preventive measure, parenteral magnesium sulfate is usually administered daily, and magnesium-containing antacids are used. Additionally, serum calcium values tend to be slightly below normal and are related to the decreased total serum protein values. Replacement medication is usually not ordered unless significantly low levels or infection supervenes. Vitamin and mineral supplements are necessary. [10].

Hematologic alterations are noted in many of the formed elements of the blood. For the first 5 days following injury, platelet destruction is rapid, and the patient exhibits a progressive thrombocytopenia as low as 30,000 to 100,000 per ml. Then platelet levels rise rapidly to 300,000 per ml and above by 10 days after injury. Hypercoagulation is a problem, but the administration of heparin is not recommended [10, 13, 58].

The patient also suffers from anemia. Initial erythrocyte destruction is caused by the thermal insult and is followed by a progressive anemia. Previously, mobilization of burn wound edema was thought to expand blood volume so that hemoglobin concentrations only appeared to be low; however, it has been established that a profound anemia is actually present. The severity of the anemia correlates directly with the extent and severity of the injury. Loebl and colleagues [33] postulated that the anemia is caused by a microangiopathic condition probably produced by an unidentified plasma factor. In their study, erythrocytes from burn patients transfused into normal persons had a normal half-life, but erythrocytes from normal persons transfused into burn patients showed a significantly reduced half-life. Thus, a circulating factor probably causes anemia; wound debridement, monitoring samples, and surgical therapy also contribute. The patient needs frequent transfusions of packed red cells to correct the anemia and maintain the hematocrit between 35 and 40 percent.

Since thermally injured patients receive so many blood transfusions, reactions are a significant potential problem. The incidence of transfusion reactions increases in proportion to the number of transfusions administered (Chap. 5). Major transfusion reactions may be hemolytic or nonhemolytic, and early recognition is of crucial importance. Symptoms may occur any time after transfusion is begun; close to the end of the transfusion, or 1 to 2 hours after completion. Any one or more of several particularly significant symptoms may be observed: (1) inappropriate severe aching pain, commonly in the back, shoulders, and hamstrings; (2) very tense or anxious feeling; (3) an increase in pulse and respirations; (4) nausea; and (5) sweating. If the reaction is hemolytic the urine has a red color, hemoglobin is found in the urine, and the temperature rises (rarely higher than 38°C [101°F]).

Immediate treatment for blood transfusion reactions consists in stopping the transfusion and administering salt-containing solutions. In response to the transfusion reaction a tremendous vascular shift occurs; the vascular tree dilates so that the intravascular fluid is not sufficient to fill the intravascular space, and the patient becomes hypotensive. The usual fluid volume therapy is 2 to 3 liters of 6 M lactate or Ringer's lactate and sodium bicarbonate to alkalinize the urine and prevent precipitation in the tubules. Later, an osmotic diuretic is used to maintain urinary outflow (if necessary) and is continued until the urine becomes clear.

FLUID RESUSCITATION

Replacement of fluid sequestered as a result of a burn injury is the most important component of initial therapy. An optimal physiologic response is ultimately dependent on the ability of various solutions to restore the intravascular and extracellular fluid volume and to effect a complete and rapid cardiovascular response. Fluid replacement is dependent on the rate of fluid lost, the total quantity of fluid sequestered, and the composition of burn edema fluid [6]. Authorities differ on the quality, quantity, and rate of the fluid to be administered to replace that sequestered into the wound, to minimize systemic changes, and to reduce the systemic dysfunction due to products from the injured tissues. The crystalloid resuscitation formula is the formula most commonly used and is the one approved for use in emergency rooms by the Committee on Trauma of the American College of Surgeons. However, many different formulas are described in the literature.

Brooke Resuscitation Formula

In the Brooke resuscitation formula developed at the Brooke Army Medical Center, San Antonio, Texas, the patient receives a crystalloid solution, Ringer's lactate, and colloid. The amount of electrolyte solution is calculated as 1.5 ml/kg/percent TBSA burned for the first 24 hours. Colloid-containing solutions, usually plasma protein fraction (Plasmanate), are given, using the formula calculated as 0.5 ml/kg/percent TBSA burned (the traditional maximum of 50% has been altered in current medical practice). In addition, the adult is given 2,000 ml of 5% dextrose in water. Half the total calculated fluid is administered in the first 8 hours and the second half in the remaining 16 hours of the first postburn day.

In the second 24 hours, one-half to three-fourths of the amount of crystalloid and colloid fluids given in the first 24 hours is administered, plus 2,000 ml of 5% dextrose in water. Frequent observation is necessary to determine the patient's response to therapy. Vital signs (blood pressure, pulse, respirations) and general mental status are noted. A urinary output of 30 to 50 ml per hour in adults (1.0 to 1.5 ml/kg/hour in children) is considered adequate.

Moore's Burn Budget Formula

In the Moore burn budget formula, 75 ml of plasma and 75 ml of electrolyte-containing fluid are given for every 1 percent of the TBSA burned. In addition, 2,000 ml of 5% dextrose in water is given. One-half the total amount of fluid calculated is administered in the first 8 hours. The remainder of the fluid is administered over the next 16 hours.

Evans Formula

In the Evans formula, 1 ml of colloid and 1 ml of electrolyte solution per kilogram of body weight per percent of the TBSA burned are administered in the first 24 hours; 2,000 ml of 5% dextrose in water is also administered. One-half the total fluid calculated is administered in the first 8 hours and the second half in the remaining 16 hours. In the second 24 hours, one-half to three-fourths of the electrolyte and colloid solution given in the first 24 hours is administered, together with 2,000 ml of 5% dextrose in water.

Hypertonic Resuscitation Formula

In the hypertonic resuscitation formula, a hypertonic salt solution containing 300 mEq of sodium, 100 mEq of chloride, and 200 mEq of lactate is administered. The rate of administration is adjusted to maintain a urinary output of 30 to 40 ml per hour. The formula is used for resuscitation, but deficits in cardiac output and plasma volume of about 40 percent below normal are found [46]. By 24 hours after burn injury, both plasma and cardiac output are within normal limits. In addition to the intravenous salt solution, fluids are usually given by mouth [44].

The decreased cardiac output and plasma volume are reasons the formula is used in some institutions for the elderly or for patients with preexisting cardiopulmonary disease in whom the amount of fluid load is thought best kept to a minimum. The thesis proposed by the authors is that these patients in particular would have an increased left atrial pressure, which would tend to compound the increased pulmonary vascular resistance and blood volume [47].

Crystalloid Resuscitation Formula

In the crystalloid resuscitation formula (also called the Baxter formula or Parkland formula) Ringer's lactate is administered during the first 24 hours according to the following formula:

4 ml × weight in kilograms
× %TBSA burned

(Fig. 15-4), with one-half given in the first 8 hours, one-fourth in the second 8 hours, and one-fourth in the third 8 hours [9]. In essence, fluid is given as rapidly as possible and continued until the signs of shock are abated. Alternatively, in several institutions, crystalloid therapy is administered according to pulmonary artery pressures. One significant factor is that, even in the presence of bright red urine (hemoglobinuria), an osmotic diuretic is not necessary since the urine clears in the first 300 to 400 ml. Criteria for adequate resuscitation are the following:

1. Urine volume 50 to 100 ml per hour
2. A lucid patient
3. A pulmonary wedge pressure in normal range
4. Pulse below 120 beats a minute
5. Disappearance of nausea and paralytic ileus
6. Improvement in the acidosis of burn shock usually corrected in 18 to 24 hours

At the end of the 24-hour period and during the fourth 8 hours after the burn injury, plasma is administered according to the extent of body surface area burned. The amount of plasma administered is normally within the range of 0.3 to 0.5 ml/kg/percent TBSA. At this time, it is thought that the capillary leak is sealed and the plasma ad-

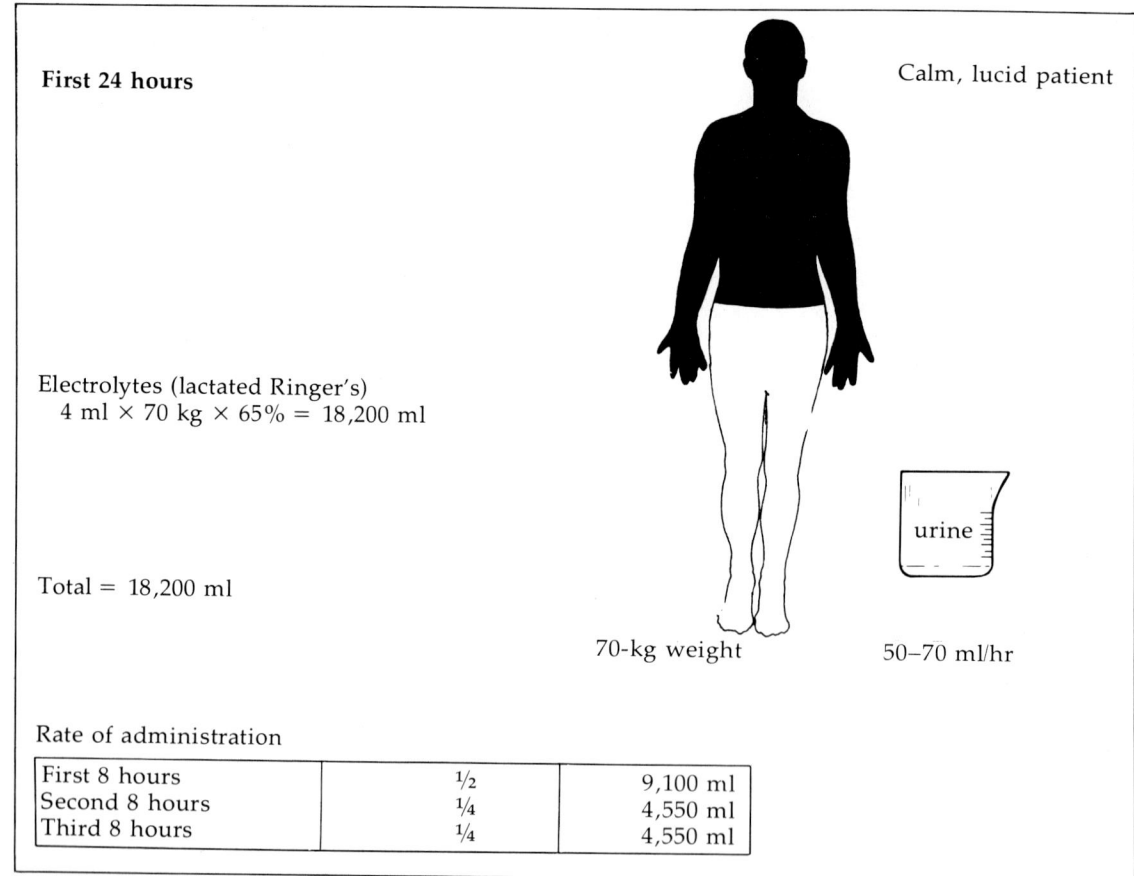

Figure 15-4
Fluid administration for the first 24 hours following thermal injury according to the crystalloid resuscitation formula.

ministered will remain in the intravascular space. The hematocrit is used to assess plasma restoration at this time, but it is not an accurate assessment tool for blood volume after 48 hours. In some instances, the patient's capillaries may not seal until after 24 hours, and a second or even third administration of colloid is ordered by the physician. The fluid administered in the second 24 hours is 5% dextrose in water in amounts from 2,000 to 6,000 ml. The amount of water administered is guided and evaluated by the serum sodium level (Fig. 15-5).

This formula is systematically derived from studies of serial changes in plasma and extracellular fluid volumes, cardiac output, and acid-base equilibrium. Fluid translocation occurs by 18 hours post burn, so the intravenous replacement of fluid is planned at a rapid rate. Due to the late phase of the development of burn edema, the amounts of fluid administered are even greater than anticipated [59].

It is important to note that the formula for fluid replacement is calculated from the time the patient is burned, not from the time he or she arrives in the emergency room. For example, a person arriving in the emergency room 3 hours after injury frequently will not have received any intravenous therapy; 5 hours remain to infuse half the total amount of fluid calculated for the first 24 hours.

Ringer's lactate solution is a balanced salt solution with a composition close to that of the extracellular fluid, except for a slight difference in the amounts of sodium; in extracellular fluid it is at 140 mEq per liter and Ringer's lactate, at 130 mEq per liter. The ratio of lactate to chloride is 27:103, hence the term **balanced.** The lactate is rapidly converted in the body to bicarbonate, and the acidosis of burn shock disappears within 12 to 24 hours after injury despite the large amounts of lactate administered [8, 9, 10, 11].

The most common reason burn patients have decreased urinary output is that the calculated amount of fluid is behind schedule. The second most common reason is that the

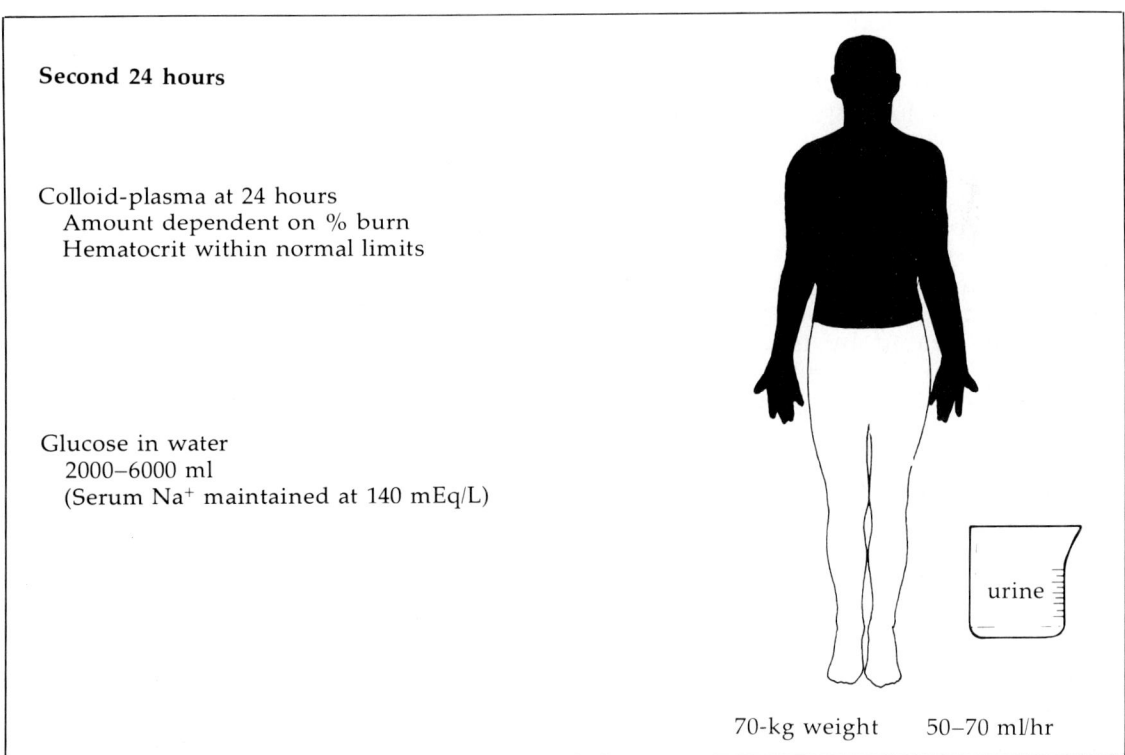

Figure 15-5
Fluid administration for the second 24 hours following thermal injury according to the crystalloid resuscitation formula.

extent of the burn has been underestimated, especially in children. A method to avoid this error is to recalculate the extent of injury after initial care is completed. Other reasons for decreased urine output include associated injuries, respiratory injury, disseminated intravascular coagulation, and myocardial depression.

Studies have shown that the functional extracellular fluid is maintained near the normal 20 percent during the administration of Ringer's lactate. Cardiac output usually returns to a near normal rate of 3.12 liters per minute per square meter within 12 to 24 hours. Tachycardia and postural hypotension are physical signs indicating the decreased plasma volume that remains until colloid is administered [10, 46].

In patients treated with the crystalloid resuscitation formula, no additional fluid therapy with Ringer's lactate is needed after the first 24 hours, although clinically the burn edema continues to increase. First, cell integrity is restored. Excess fluid simply accumulates around the cells and is available as needed for translocation into the damaged tissue. The difference between the measured rates of fluid volume losses and the rate of edema formation is explained by this phenomenon. The mechanism differs in the second phase of edema formation, in which tissues that have not been damaged contain most of the edema. The resulting denaturation of collagen causes an increased uptake of sodium and water, and the area is much like a sponge. Edema in surrounding tissues probably is caused by the effects of histamine, bradykinin, and other biogenic amines released from the damaged tissue [10].

Problems in Respiratory Status

Changes occur in the lungs after injury. The initial stable pulmonary blood volume is followed by a change in the venous pulmonary vasculature, resulting in pulmonary engorgement with increased pulmonary blood volume and vascular resistance, a possible reason for the tachypnea that is observed [7]. Respiratory alkalosis commonly follows initial acidosis in severe cases.

Decreased arterial oxygenation is often present early. The reason for this decrease is not known, but restoration of cardiac output improves the oxygenation. One must be careful to attribute this decreased oxygenation to poor tissue perfusion and shock rather than to airway obstruction. A falling arterial Po_2 is indicative either of airway obstruction or a declining left heart output [10, 47].

The problems in respiratory status that will be discussed include carbon monoxide poisoning, airway obstruction, oxygen delivery, and pneumonia.

CARBON MONOXIDE POISONING

Carbon monoxide poisoning is frequently overlooked. Often the patient has crawled out of a burning building, inhaling a significant amount of carbon monoxide on the way, and arrives at the hospital disoriented and possibly even deranged. Significant carbon monoxide poisoning is indicated by carboxyhemoglobin levels greater than 10 percent 4 hours after injury, and careful observation of the unburned and burned skin will often reveal a cherry red color. Carbon monoxide poisoning should always be suspected in a patient who is hypoxic, restless, and confused several hours after the accident. The treatment is administration of 100% oxygen. Careful observation for cerebral dysfunction following the disappearance of carbon monoxide from the body is mandatory, since the incidence of cerebral damage is high.

AIRWAY OBSTRUCTION

Early recognition of upper airway obstruction is particularly important. Here, the history is invaluable. Physical examination may reveal singed nasal hairs, dry, red mucosa, and soot in the sputum. The immediate causes of respiratory distress are often laryngeal edema or spasm and accumulation of mucus. Suctioning and indirect laryngoscopy help to clear the mucus and aid the evaluation of the extent of involvement.

Actual signs of obstruction do not become apparent for several hours. The patient is observed for any drooling or inability to handle secretions and, most important, for increasing hoarseness. The latter can be observed by asking the patient the same question every 15 minutes and evaluating the tone of the response. The upper airway may be compared to a hollow tube that does not produce a significantly changed tone until it is almost occluded. Thus, by the time hoarseness occurs, the diameter of the airway has been significantly diminished. Once noted, the hoarseness is monitored closely, so that steps can be taken to keep the airway patent.

Development of edema may continue for 72 hours, and endotracheal intubation or a tracheostomy is often needed. Tracheotomies are no longer performed as prophylactic measures and sufficient need must be established before surgery is indicated. A tracheostomy is frequently necessary because of airway obstruction that prevents adequate oxygenation of the blood or interferes with the patient's ability to handle respiratory secretions or to expel vomitus. Supportive measures required during this period include frequent suctioning, analgesics to reduce pain and hyperventilation, and humidified oxygen to avoid mucosal dehydration and drying of secretions.

Lower airway obstruction arising from a respiratory burn or inhalation injury impairs pulmonary function by increasing the resistance to breathing, lowering the distribution of inspired air, and decreasing the diffusion of gases across the alveolar membrane [23]. Usually, the lower respiratory injury is not directly attributable to the burn, since rapid vaporization results in cooling that protects the pulmonary tree. Moritz et al. [50] showed that 260°C (500°F) air introduced by a blowtorch into an endotracheal tube caused minimal damage beyond the carina. Only inhalation of steam results in true burning of the lower respiratory tract.

Most commonly, especially in closed-space injuries, inhalation of the products of incomplete combustion leads to chemical pneumonitis. First, the pulmonary tree is irritated, then it becomes edematous, and this is followed by a pneumonitis. Inflammatory changes occur during the first 24 hours following injury but are often not noticeable until the second 24 hours. Pulmonary edema may occur any time from the first few hours to 7 days after injury.

Early diagnosis of lower airway obstruction can be difficult. In many patients with lower airway obstruction, the findings on physical examination and the chest x-rays on admission are negative. Subsequent critical evaluation is essential. The history is the first clue. Patients who have sustained burn injury in a closed space or who have inhaled significant amounts of smoke should be closely watched. Although the most reliable sign is carbonaceous sputum, the patient may also exhibit hoarseness, cough, increased secretions, and wheezing [3, 28, 61]. Burns of the face and neck are neither necessary nor sufficient criteria for diagnosis of inhalation injury, but respiratory problems occur more frequently in patients with these injuries. Even though symptoms are clinically insignificant, the patient may be hypoxic. Similarly, the early chest x-rays may be clear, but later ones may show patchy or peribronchial infiltrates [28]. Bronchoscopy may be performed, and the ^{133}xenon lung scan may show positive findings. According to Moylan et al. [52], a positive scan shows delayed clearance (greater than 90 seconds) and unequal scintillation density.

The signs and symptoms usually described for airway obstruction, such as cyanosis, severe respiratory distress, and severe cerebral hypoxia, are not early signs of respiratory injury but are much later signs of impending disaster. One needs to observe signs and symptoms before the patient becomes this debilitated.

Management includes, first, vigorous pulmonary toilet. The patient may need nasotracheal suction or bronchoscopy to clear the bronchial tree of debris. Second, humidified oxygen and intravenous bronchodilators are given. Third, the administration of steroids is helpful if the patient is undergoing severe bronchospasm. Arterial blood gases are closely monitored. Antibiotics are used only for pneumonia. Tracheostomy and mechanical ventilation are utilized when indicated.

OXYGENATION

Movements of the thorax may be decreased by circumferential full-thickness burns of the chest. The patient will show increasing symptoms of respiratory distress, since the tight eschar prevents adequate movement of the chest and proper oxygenation. An escharotomy will allow for expansion of the underlying tissue and alleviation of the symptoms.

Another problem is maintaining oxygen delivery to the tissues. Normal oxygen-carrying capacity is dependent on the amount of hemoglobin in the blood; as seen in the following formula, 15 gm of hemoglobin per

100 ml of blood is sufficient to attain the necessary 20 ml of O_2 per 100 ml of blood, since each gram carries 1.39 ml of oxygen.

$$\frac{15 \text{ gm hemoglobin}}{100 \text{ ml blood}}$$

$$\times \frac{1.39 \text{ ml oxygen}}{1 \text{ gm hemoglobin}}$$

$$= \frac{20.85 \text{ ml oxygen}}{100 \text{ ml blood}}$$

If the hemoglobin is decreased, the amount of inspired oxygen must be increased tremendously for tissue oxygen to be maintained at adequate levels. Even if oxygen toxicity is ignored, it is difficult, if not impossible, to attain adequate levels of oxygenation by relying solely on high concentrations of inspired oxygen [25]. It is much more satisfactory to ensure delivery of oxygen by maintaining an adequate amount of hemoglobin.

Tissue oxygenation levels also become decreased if the oxygen dissociation curve is shifted to the left, since, in this event, oxygen is not released at the same arterial tensions (Chap. 3). The shift is caused by hypothermia, respiratory alkalosis, administration of cold parenteral fluids, and administration of old blood or blood stored in acid-citrate-dextrose rather than in citrate-phosphate-dextrose solution [41, 54].

PNEUMONIA

Bronchopneumonia may be superimposed on other problems at any time and may be either hematogenous or airborne in origin. Hematogenous pneumonia (miliary pneumonia) begins as a bacterial abscess secondary to another septic source, usually the burn wound. However, it may be secondary to another source, such as suppurative thrombophlebitis (septic phlebitis in veins used for intravenous fluid administration). The onset is usually more than 2 weeks after injury. Airborne pneumonia (bronchopneumonia) is more common (65 percent) and is contracted from an external source. The onset tends to be soon after the injury and often is associated with lower airway injury or aspiration.

SUMMARY

Management of patients with respiratory complications involves attention to detail. Ongoing assessment of pulmonary status, including a chest examination, is important. Changes in the rate and pattern of breathing are monitored by inspection. Palpation and percussion are used, but auscultation is of primary importance. Rales or wheezes must be reported to the physician. Arterial blood gases are monitored. Patients must be encouraged to cough, breathe deeply, and change position frequently.

A thorough understanding of the suctioning technique is essential for the care of patients maintained on mechanical ventilators. Sterile suctioning technique has been well described in the literature; however, several misconceptions about the technique must be clarified. First, adequate suctioning is extremely difficult when an endotracheal tube is in place unless an extra-long suction catheter is used. Length is also important if a tracheostomy tube is in place, but here the converse is true, and the entire length of catheter need not be inserted. Anatomy and the person's size should be taken into account, so that the catheter is inserted appropriately and coughing is stimulated. Second, two or three deep sighs on the ventilator after suctioning are beneficial. However, if the patient sighs before suctioning, the mucus will only be driven further into the tracheobronchial tree. Last, contrary to popular opinion, patients on pulmonary positive end-expiratory pressure should be suctioned as needed, and airway pressure will return to preset levels in a very few minutes [63].

Problems in Metabolism and Nutrition

In the absence of supplemental nutritional support, the burned patient slips into a cachectic state. The exceptionally large caloric intake necessary for maintenance is based on an altered metabolic response.

PATHOPHYSIOLOGY

The metabolic response to thermal injury as described by Wilmore [69] consists in hypermetabolism, severe protein wasting, and weight loss.

Apparently mediated by the secretion of catecholamines, the metabolic rate is characterized by a rapid increase from its normal value to a peak (hypermetabolic) rate and then a gradual rate decrease as the wound is closed. The peak rate is reached between the sixth and tenth postinjury day. The amplitude of the response is proportional to the size of the injury, with a maximum reached with wounds involving 40 to 50 percent of the TBSA. Oxygen consumption returns to normal when the wound is closed.

The amount of protein in the body decreases; in particular, skeletal muscle is depleted. If left untreated, respiratory muscles will eventually decrease in size and strength, so that adequate expansion and ventilation are difficult, and the stage is set for pneumonia. The severe protein wasting is thought to be mainly from the catabolism of skeletal muscle. Amino acids are converted to glucose and nitrogen as well as other intracellular constituents are lost [24].

A weight loss greater than 20 percent of the preinjury weight may be expected in patients with an injury of more than 40 percent of the TBSA unless attention is given to caloric support. The amount of weight loss is also related to sex, body build, preinjury nutritional status, severity of injury, and complicating factors [28]. A loss in body weight greater than 10 percent of preburn weight and decreased body water then result. Death is likely to ensue if one-fourth to one-third of the protein mass or 40 to 50 percent of body weight is lost. An increase in body protein and weight gain do not usually occur until wound closure.

Protein and caloric intake to support basic energy levels is crucial early in the postinjury period. Caloric support must be continued until the wound is closed, and approximately 2000 calories per square meter of total body surface per day for patients with injuries involving more than 40 percent of the TBSA is frequently needed. Curreri et al. [17] showed that an intake of 6000 calories per day in thermally injured patients stabilizes red blood cells so that a normal concentration of intracellular sodium is maintained. He suggested that thermal injury either inhibits active transport of red blood cells or produces a defect in the red blood cell membrane, and that the problem may be reversed by maintenance of a positive energy balance. Red blood cells may serve as an example of the functioning of other body cells, and intracellular sodium concentrations thus reflect the effectiveness of nutritional support. In addition, nitrogen requirements must be met and approximately 15 gm per square meter of total body surface per day for patients with an injury involving more than 40 percent of the TBSA is frequently needed.

Underlying the metabolic response following thermal injury is the response to stress [69]. Physiologically, sympathetic stimulation, adrenergic activity, and energy needs are increased, so that body fuels are utilized rather than stored. Many different mechanisms may result in the stress phenomenon, but the same response seems to result: The greater the stress, the greater the response. In the thermally injured patient, it is theorized that stimuli (nervous or hormonal) first alter central nervous system function. Next, a reset phenomenon occurs in the hypothalamus, causing increased adrenergic stimulation. The result in turn is increased catecholamine and glucagon levels and decreased insulin levels.

$$\begin{array}{c}\text{afferent}\\\uparrow\\\text{stimuli}\end{array}\to\begin{array}{c}\text{alter}\\\text{CNS}\\\text{function}\end{array}\to\begin{array}{c}\text{reset}\\\\\text{hypothalamus}\end{array}\to\begin{array}{c}\uparrow\\\text{catecholamines}\end{array}\begin{array}{c}\uparrow\\\text{glucagon}\end{array}\begin{array}{c}\downarrow\\\text{insulin}\end{array}$$

The change in the normal glucagon-insulin ratio directly affects the cells, altering substrate flow. Increased levels of glucagon are consistent with catabolism—glycogenolysis, gluconeogenesis, and ureagenesis—rather than the synthesis of protein. Once protein and calorie support levels are attained, insulin flow increases and reverses the glucagon-insulin ratio. Protein synthesis (anabolism) is then possible. Substrate flow is increased, and the negative nitrogen balance and weight loss are decreased. Hypermetabolism continues until closure of the wound [69, 72].

Previously, it was accepted that the hypermetabolic response was due to the increased caloric expenditure necessary to provide for the evaporation of water [22]. Further definitive work has identified other salient features. First, Zawacki et al. [73] proved the raised metabolic rate in burn patients was not the direct result of the evaporation of water. They showed that prevention of this evaporative water loss by covering the injured area with an impermeable piece of plastic film for periods up to 12 hours did not significantly reduce oxygen consumption. Additional studies by Wilmore and colleagues [68–72] demonstrated that the evaporative water loss is not primary in the metabolic response but that the increased energy production is related to the reset of metabolic activity. The thermally injured person produces great quantities of heat as a consequence of injury and is internally warm, not externally cold. Increased water loss is a means of transferring the heat generated.

NUTRITIONAL SUPPORT

In the first week following injury, nutritional support does not have the highest priority. Other situations must first be alleviated. The gastrointestinal system must begin to function, and the body must restabilize in order to handle the protein and glucose load. Patients receive glucose-containing solutions until oral support can be started. Then, liquid protein supplements are used extensively to provide protein and calories [18, 68, 69].

To encourage the intake of food, a dietary history is obtained, since it is important to find out what the patient likes and to serve those foods in an appealing, appetizing manner. If necessary, meals may be brought in from home. It is of utmost importance that meal plans and total daily caloric allotments be individualized, since patients cannot eat more after injury than they could before; and, in fact, they eat 10 percent less on the average [70]. Young athletic patients are often used to eating 5000 calories per day and find the task easy; others have difficulty taking in 2500 calories.

In the first weeks after injury, high-calorie protein supplements (1 cal per gram) continue to be the mainstay of nutritional support. A high-carbohydrate, tasteless liquid such as Polycose may be added to all beverages to increase calories. As the patient's appetite improves, the need for supplements may decrease. It is important to calculate dietary needs and make certain that ancillary personnel are aware of the patient's requirements. All staff members must be cognizant of what the patient has already eaten and what remains to be taken, so that efforts are made to provide for the total caloric requirement for that day. Protein requirements are generally 2 to 3 gm/kg body weight/day. The total caloric requirements may be calculated by the following formula [18].

25 kcal/kg of body weight
$\quad$ + 40 kcal × % burn = kcal/day

Example:

25 kcal × 70 kg
$\quad$ + 40 kcal × 50% = 3750 kcal/day

Every opportunity is taken to encourage the patient to eat or drink. Sips of fluid are offered every 5 minutes during bathing. Medications are given with high-calorie drinks rather than with water. A rule of thumb is always to give a beverage with calories. Mouth care is essential to promote the appetite. Procedures, particularly painful ones, should not interfere with meals or other nourishment.

In some patients, additional calories are given through a small nasogastric feeding tube. If constant nasogastric tube feedings are administered, the stomach contents are withdrawn every 4 hours to ascertain the amount remaining. Potential catastrophe lurks: ileus, distention, emesis, aspiration, pneumonia, and death.

Attention must also be paid to increasing the concentration of fluids slowly. If diarrhea begins, the concentration is decreased, maintained at the decreased level for 2 days, and then it is increased slowly each day. Small increments will increase tolerance and enhance absorption. In some instances, the physician orders Kaopectate or paregoric to treat the diarrhea. Every effort is made to utilize the gastrointestinal system for nutrition; however, most patients are unable to take in more than 3000 calories per day, even with the combination of eating and nasogastric feedings. Total parenteral nutrition is often necessary for adequate caloric support [68, 69], but problems can occur (Chap. 2).

Problems of Environmental Support

PREVENTION OF INFECTION

Of particular importance in the burn patient's environment are measures to prevent infection. Attention to detail can keep the infection rate relatively low. The high glucose levels make the hyperalimentation solution an excellent culture medium for microorganisms.

Aseptic technique during total parenteral nutrition is essential. Daily catheter care must be exacting. Solutions are prepared using strict technique, preferably under a laminar air hood. An in-line micron filter is used, and no bottle of solution is infused for more than 8 hours.

The central entry site is changed every 3 days. In the event of burns over the entry site, iodine-soaked gauze sponge pads are kept over the site and changed a minimum of every 8 hours.

All tubing, down to the needle, is changed each time a new bottle of hyperalimentation solution is added, making certain that no excess tubing is used. The lines are never violated by piggy-back medications, blood or other fluids, stopcocks, or central venous pressure measuring devices or by withdrawal of blood specimens.

DECREASING ANXIETY AND DISCOMFORT

It is important to help dissipate the patient's anxiety and relieve discomfort. An accepted principle is that knowledge decreases anxiety. It is important that the patient understand the rudiments of his care plan and that his cooperation be elicited. Patient education is kept simple, and information is repeated as frequently as necessary. Analgesics complemented by nursing techniques to decrease pain are beneficial. Tranquilizers tend to blunt responses, making a physiologic assessment inaccurate, and are thus used as little as possible.

McCaffery [40] has described several methods of altering pain perceptions. One is that of administering the medication intravenously immediately before bathing or debridement. An alternative method is helping the patient focus on pleasant thoughts during debridement and administering the medication afterward, when true relief and rest are possible. Many people can tolerate significant amounts of pain for short periods if they then have relief and time to recuperate.

Sleep and planned rest periods throughout the day are extremely important. If the patient has a good night's sleep, he or she will be better able to cope with the pain and frustration of therapy. Sleep habits and patterns are assessed, and fundamental principles to induce sleep are followed. Procedures and care are planned so that periods of uninterrupted sleep are allowed.

External sources of heat increase comfort. Burn patients are internally warm, but their skin feels cool, and they even shiver because of the heat transfer required by the heat of evaporation. This coolness is easier to understand if one remembers that on a hot July afternoon even healthy persons feel cool while standing near a lawn sprinkler evaporating large quantities of water. First, the room should be warm. Patients who have been allowed to maintain and regulate their room temperature have adjusted it to 33 to 35°C (92 to 95°F) [68]. Second, heat lamps are used; no sheets or blankets are placed between the patient and the heat lamp. Third, in some instances, heat is provided by placing blankets over a bed cradle.

Problems Associated with the Gastrointestinal System

The burn patient is truly one of the most critically ill patients encountered in nursing. Every system within the body is likely to go awry. Gastrointestinal problems that start silently and sometimes erupt violently are among the most dramatic and potentially lethal of those encountered.

Gastric dilatation and paralytic ileus develop in almost everyone who has sustained an injury of more than 20 percent of the TBSA. The danger of vomiting and subsequent aspiration is significant. A nasogastric tube is inserted on admission and remains in place until bowel sounds return (usually from 24 to 72 hours).

Sepsis is also frequently accompanied by gastric distention and paralytic ileus. Slight distention, mild abdominal pain, and a subtle increase in respiratory rate herald gastric distention. The danger of vomiting and aspiration is great because the gastrointestinal tract is used as much as possible for alimentation. In the case of supplementation by nasogastric tube, periodic quantitation of gastric contents prior to tube feeding is necessary. If distention occurs, oral and nasogastric feedings are withheld, and a nasogastric tube is connected to intermittent suction until an accurate patient assessment can be performed.

Since potassium is the major intracellular cation, large amounts are necessary for cell synthesis. Thus, hypokalemia also is suspected whenever gastric distention or an intestinal ileus develops.

Painless upper abdominal distention associated with vomiting can be accompanied by partial and at times complete intestinal obstruction resulting from compression of the duodenum by the superior mesenteric artery. The superior mesenteric artery syndrome, found particularly in tall, slender people, is compounded by a rapid accentuated weight loss. Dilatation in the first and second parts of the duodenum leads to gastric reflux, which in turn leads to gastric dilatation. Vomiting characteristically occurs after meals. Therapy is conservative or surgical. Conservative therapy entails initial gastric decompression, metabolic support via intravenous hyperalimentation, and liquid alimentation enhanced by proper patient positioning. Positioning encompasses eating in an upright position and then turning to a prone or left lateral position after meals. Upper gastrointestinal fluoroscopy is invaluable in determining the most advantageous patient position for gastric drainage. As the liquid diet is increased and weight is gained, more and more solid food is added. If conservative therapy is not successful or if ulceration and perforation occur, surgical intervention is mandatory.

HEMATEMESIS

Another sign of gastrointestinal dysfunction is **hematemesis.** Two important causes of bright red or coffee-ground hematemesis are hemorrhagic gastritis and Curling's ulcer. Other uncommon causes include peptic ulcer, disseminated intravascular coagulation, and gastric erosion from a nasogastric tube.

Hematemesis of small amounts of coffee-ground material in the first 48 hours after injury is characteristic of **hemorrhagic gastritis.** Congested gastric capillaries rupture and produce the emesis. The congestion and irritation may possibly set the stage for further acute gastroduodenal disease. A nasogastric tube is inserted and connected to intermittent suction, and antacids are administered [19].

Curling's ulcer remains the enigma of the burn patient. The incidence has been greatly reduced by the introduction of prophylactic antacid therapy. The diagnosis can be made at autopsy in approximately 25 percent of all burn patients who die [47]. Its presence may be heralded by a massive hematemesis of bright red blood or the passage of tarry stools. However, its presence may also be identified on investigation of mild abdominal discomfort or even as an incidental finding in an asymptomatic patient. Perforation is the initial symptom in 10 percent of patients. Typically, bleeding occurs near the end of the first week but may occur at any time [38, 46].

The etiology of Curling's ulcer is unknown, but early ischemia and adrenal hormone secretion appear to play a significant role. Hyperacidity and preexisting ulcer diseases do not seem to be causative factors in this particular syndrome. According to Moncrief and Pruitt [49], the influence of sepsis is still incompletely delineated, but the presence of sepsis acts as an additive stress. In a 2-year period 77 percent of the patients they studied had sepsis at the time the ulcer was diagnosed. Other possible etiologic factors are (1) elevated steroid levels, (2) decreased gastroduodenal blood flow (hemoconcentration, elevated catecholamines, hypovolemia), (3) the lytic effect of regurgitated chyme, and (4) a quantitative or qualitative change in mucus.

The most plausible explanation comes from evaluation of the initial gastric congestion. In an effort to determine the incidence and natural history of acute gastroduodenal disease, Czaja et al. [19] performed early and serial gastroduodenoscopies in 32 patients following thermal injury. In areas of intense superficial mucosal injury after the first 72 hours post burn, 22 percent of patients had a gastric ulcer and 28 percent had a duodenal ulcer. Moncrief [47] has postulated that the lesions are associated with intense congestion of capillaries in the gastroduodenal region that is localized to discrete areas of the gastric or duodenal mucosa. The resulting tissue slough, combined with changes in the character of gastric mucus, results in mucosal susceptibility to normal quantities of acid. When the localized area lies over a major artery, hemorrhage occurs.

If bleeding occurs, therapy is antacids with pH monitoring, gastric decompression, iced saline lavage, and blood administration. Surgical intervention is indicated if hemorrhage continues and the patient needs more than 2,500 ml of blood in 12 hours, or if the ulcer perforates. If possible, vagotomy with partial gastric resection is performed. Most patients with large burns progress well following surgery; however, statistics show an increased incidence of associated complications later in the hospitalization of these patients [55].

Sepsis

Sepsis is the most formidable complication facing the thermally injured patient. The seeding source may be any part of the body, but it is likely to be wound-related.

The presence of sepsis must be identified as early as possible. Early clinical signs are (1) a change in mental orientation; (2) increased respiratory rate and depth; (3) glucose intolerance, hyperglycemia, and glycosuria; and (4) decreasing platelet count.

Systemically, early sepsis induces a hyperdynamic state. High cardiac output develops over a period of days, and the patient is prone to arrhythmias. The stress is extremely significant, since these patients are already in a hypermetabolic state with increased oxygen consumption from the altered metabolic response to injury. Some have already responded maximally and are unable to meet the increased demands. Management is difficult and is likely to change hour by hour.

If the infection continues unabated, the patient decompensates. It is now generally known that gram-positive and gram-negative organisms produce a similar clinical syndrome. The infectious process is on a continuum and ends in decompensation and death. The vascular tree dilates, and hypovolemia is a problem. Then the low flow state results in decreased perfusion all over the body. Decreased cardiac output is particularly significant and results in decreased myocardial, cerebral, renal, and intestinal perfusion. Large amounts of fluid must be infused. An early respiratory alkalosis gives way to metabolic acidosis from the low flow state. Renal function may be greatly impaired from the toxic products of sepsis, drug toxicity, and/or low flow state. Treatment requires surgical drainage of the seeding source (if possible), administration of antibiotics specific for the organism(s), fluid replacement, and administration of glucocorticosteroids and a vasodilator such as dopamine.

SEEDING SOURCES

Sepsis can have multiple seeding sites: a Foley or an intravenous catheter, suppurative thrombophlebitis, chondritis, pneumonia, and the burn wound itself. Any invasive procedure or monitoring device increases the likelihood of infection. Thus, all catheters are removed from the patient as soon as possible.

Suppurative thrombophlebitis is an infectious complication following intravenous catherization in which the vein that contained the cannula is infected. It may occur in all patients, not only in burn patients, and must be considered as a possible source of sepsis any time the primary site of infection cannot be identified. If suppurative thrombophlebitis is suspected, all veins into which a catheter has been inserted are explored by the physician and are gently compressed or "milked" toward the catheter site in an effort to express suppurative material. Frequently, the area above the entry site that approximates the catheter tip is also explored. If any suppuration is found, the entire vein is removed.

Chrondritis is an infection of the ear, usually bacterial, and follows direct burn injury. The ear is extremely tender and swollen, and the infection is difficult to treat, since cartilage has a poor blood supply. If local antibiotic therapy is unsuccessful, the ear is bivalved and the cartilage removed (partial or total chondrectomy).

BURN WOUND

Fundamental to any discussion of sepsis in the thermally injured patient is the burn wound itself. The skin, which is the first line of defense from microorganisms in the environment, is lost. The area of destruction is deeper than one would anticipate [53]. Thermal injury is characterized by coagulation necrosis of blood vessels in the skin and the adjacent subcutaneous tissue. Immediately after a full-thickness injury, the vascular supply is interrupted, and the area of destruction remains without a vascular supply until granulation tissue develops at the interface between burned and unburned tissue. Granulation tissue (including fibroblasts and new blood vessels) begins to form at approximately 14 days after injury and is completed at approximately 21 days [53]. In partial-thickness injury, the underlying blood vessels begin to form new canals approximately 2 days after injury, and the process is completed in approximately 7 days [47].

Infection plays a significant role and can

alter the normal processes. Bacteria on the surface of the burn wound proliferate because the necrotic tissue is an excellent culture medium. Delivery of humoral and cellular defense mechanisms is impaired. If infection is not controlled in areas of partial-thickness injury, a progressive tissue necrosis converts the wound to a full-thickness injury. Following bacterial colonization of the wound, the adjacent subcutaneous tissues are invaded. **Burn wound sepsis** is now defined as the proliferation and active invasion of the burn wound by microorganisms in the quantity of 100,000 (10^5) or more per gram of tissue.

ASSESSMENT OF PRESENCE AND TYPE OF INFECTION

Early in the patient's course, the external appearance of the burn wound gives little hint to what might be transpiring in and under the eschar (the subeschar space). It is absolutely crucial to be able to monitor the infectious process before sepsis becomes clinically apparent and invasive. Therefore, bacteriologic methods have been developed to sample the area and determine the presence and nature of bacterial growth.

Full-thickness wound biopsies [34] are used to quantitate bacterial colonization and to determine the predominating organism(s) and antibiotic sensitivities. A small piece of the entire thickness of eschar and underlying tissue (1 to 2 cm × 0.5 cm × depth, which contains a portion of unburned fat) is excised from selected sites three times a week and the number of organisms per gram of tissue determined. Burn wound sepsis is considered to be present when bacterial counts reach 10^5 per gram of tissue [48, 65]. Since the laboratory determinations require 24 hours, patients with biopsy cultures of 10^4 per gram of tissue are often treated for sepsis based on the assumption that bacteria have continued to proliferate and are at invasive concentrations. Utilizing this technique, the staff can evaluate the effectiveness of therapy and monitor the progression or regression of bacterial growth.

Monitoring by surface culture techniques has not proved satisfactory, since the correlation between surface and deep tissue colonization is poor [12, 34]. Contact plates (Rodac plates) are helpful in predicting what organism is likely to cause sepsis, but their use has a number of disadvantages. The contact plate is likely to identify a variety of organisms. Great variability in surface cultures results from the surface therapy used. Bathing changes surface cultures and increases the bacterial count. Any mechanical agitation during bathing will break up the colonies so it appears that a greater number of bacteria are present.

The blood cultures may be positive only a small portion of the time the patient is septic, but in blood drawn from a patient close to death, a high percentage of cultures will be positive. Thus, blood cultures have limited usefulness in the early diagnosis of sepsis. One investigation demonstrated positive blood cultures in only 4 percent of the patients studied, although 13 percent died with sepsis, 19 percent demonstrated clinical signs, and 27 percent had burn wound biopsy cultures showing more than 10^4 organisms per gram of tissue [37].

It is important to realize that sepsis is related to the total quantity of bacteria present. Fewer bacteria will be present in a patient with an injury affecting 15 percent of the TBSA whose biopsy counts are 10^5 of bacteria per gram of tissue than in a patient with an injury involving 80 percent of the TBSA and counts of 10^3 of bacteria per gram of tissue. Survival is usually not possible if bacterial concentrations remain greater than 10^6 or 10^7 of bacteria per gram of tissue for more than 12 days, or if more than one type of organism is present with a combined concentration greater than 10^{10} of bacteria per gram of tissue. On the other hand, if the base is healthy granulation tissue, bacterial concentrations of 10^7 per gram of tissue can be withstood [1, 12].

Infection in the wound can be caused by a variety of organisms. Early after the injury, the organisms are likely to be gram positive; later, often in the first week, the organisms are likely to be gram negative (*Pseudomonas, Klebsiella, Enterobacter, Escherichia coli, Serratia*). Other opportunistic organisms such as *Candida, Phycomycetes, Aspergillus,* and viruses may cause significant problems.

TREATMENT OF BURN WOUNDS

Topical Agents

One of the most important advances in burn wound care has been the development of topical therapy to control the bacterial population of the burn wound. Topical agents such as mafenide acetate (Sulfamylon) and silver sulfadiazine (Silvadene) diffuse through the eschar and help retard bacterial growth. Since no systemic antibiotics enter the avascular eschar, it is imperative to have an active agent present at the site of infection [45, 48].

Antimicrobial agents control but do not prevent sepsis. However, sufficient time is gained for the areas of partial-thickness injury to heal rather than convert to full-thickness injury and for the development of granulation tissue that is resistant to bacterial invasion. This has significantly decreased the mortality rate of thermally injured patients with burns involving 40 to 60 percent of the TBSA [5]. Various schedules of topical agents are used across the country: (1) one primary agent is used; (2) several agents are used and therapy is rotated (for example, every 3 days); or (3) therapy is changed as necessary according to its effectiveness against bacterial growth.

Silver sulfadiazine 1% is a combination of a sulfonamide and a heavy metal, silver. This agent is effective against a wide range of gram-positive and gram-negative organisms, as well as against *Candida albicans*. Unfortunately, several disadvantages are associated with its use: (1) Resistant strains of *Pseudomonas* often appear; (2) a few cases of leukopenia have been reported; and (3) occasionally a patient will exhibit hypersensitivity. However, it also has many advantages. Dressings are not necessary (although a thin, dry dressing may be used), and this "open" method of treatment, combined with a softened eschar, allows increased joint mobility. Since the agent is poorly absorbed, no systemic metabolic derangements occur, and wounds are kept white with cream for comfort as well as antimicrobial action. The method of application is shown in Figure 15-6. Sensitive areas are thus protected from air currents, and the patient feels more comfortable.

Mafenide acetate (Sulfamylon) 11% is in a water-soluble base and diffuses through the entire avascular eschar. It is thus the agent of choice in patients with electrical injuries. Called "burn butter," it was developed specifically to combat *Pseudomonas* organisms, but it is effective against a wide spectrum of gram-positive and gram-negative organisms. It is not effective against fungi and some strains of gram-negative rods. In institutions where it has been the sole topical agent used, resistant organisms such as *Providencia stuartii* have emerged.

Mafenide acetate is an excellent agent, and, as with silver sulfadiazine, the open method of therapy can be used. Bulky dressings are not necessary, and the patient has greater mobility. Unfortunately, its use may result in metabolic acidosis from two causes. First, the end product of breakdown is an acid salt that increases the hydrogen ions in the body's buffer system. Second, an alkaline urine is produced by the inhibition of car-

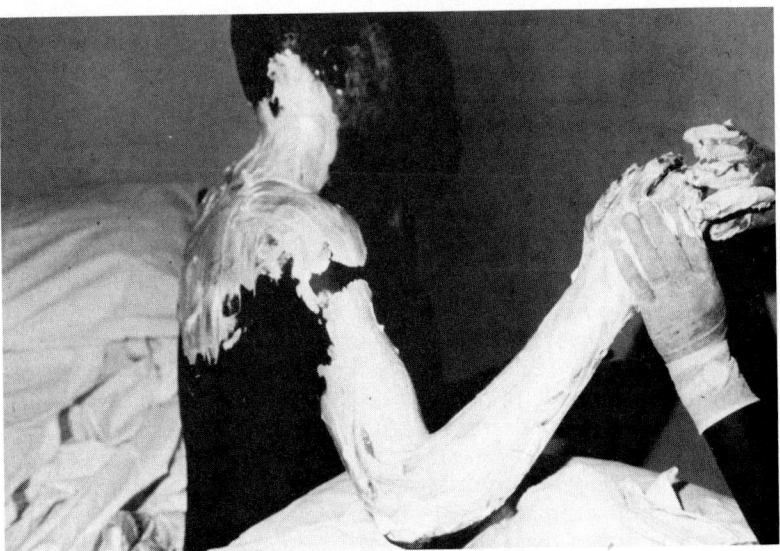

Figure 15-6
Application of silver sulfadiazine.

bonic anhydrase. Tachypnea is the body's means of compensation. If pulmonary complications arise, compensatory mechanisms are altered, and the physician will temporarily withdraw the agent. Application is limited to a thin layer (3 mm) every 12 hours. A great deal of discomfort, specifically in areas of partial-thickness injury, is associated with its application, and pain relief is frequently necessary. Hypersensitivity also occurs in 5 percent of patients. The reaction is characterized by a maculopapular rash, but therapy is discontinued only if the rash is severe.

Povidone-iodine (Betadine) ointment is a new agent in burn therapy that is currently being evaluated. Iodine has been long known for its germicidal properties, but actual guidelines for its use cannot be given until the investigation is completed. The question of iodine toxicity is unanswered. At body temperature, the ointment changes from a semisolid to a liquid, so that a light wrap must be used. The dressing, combined with a hardened eschar, makes decreased mobility a potential problem. Quantitative burn wound biopsies for monitoring of bacterial growth are not entirely accurate while this agent is being used. The tissue specimen may contain iodine concentrations that will inhibit bacterial growth during the laboratory test in a patient whose infection may be increasing. Besides its antibacterial activity, povidone-iodine ointment has two major advantages: The wound becomes translucent, and depth of injury can therefore be more easily identified; and preoperative application hardens the eschar and aids surgical removal.

Silver nitrate solution 0.5% is applied as a continuous wet soak in large bulky dressings. It is effective against staphylococci, streptococci, and *Pseudomonas* but is ineffective against *Enterobacter, Klebsiella,* and *Serratia*. Dressings must be placed on the patient's wound 3 to 5 days prior to bacterial colonization, since silver nitrate does not penetrate the eschar and is not effective after colonization; active debridement to remove the crust must accompany therapy in order for any infection to be reached. The silver ion is inactivated and precipitated, once combined with tissue fluid. A crust results under which bacteria proliferate, so that the crust must be frequently removed by debridement. The dressing should be at least 14 layers thick (5 cm) and kept totally saturated with a warm solution. Dressings are saturated every 2 to 4 hours and are changed completely every 12 hours; if the dressing is allowed to dry, the concentration of silver becomes so high that it is toxic to the tissues. Then the whole body is covered with a dry, light blanket to retain heat and decrease evaporation.

Several major disadvantages limit the use of silver nitrate solution. First, it is a hypotonic agent, and significant electrolyte losses of sodium, potassium, calcium, and chloride occur. The burn wound acts as a semipermeable membrane, and all four electrolytes diffuse quickly into the dressings. Methemoglobinemia is a potential complication, since nitrate is oxidized to nitrite in the wound and absorbed. An occlusive dressing must be used, and the bulky dressings limit mobility, thus increasing the possibility of contractures. Last, but certainly not least, silver nitrate stains everything black with which it comes in contact.

Other agents such as gentamicin and nitrofurazone (Furacin) have been studied but have not been successful for use as primary topical agents. The ideal topical agent has not yet been developed, and the laboratory search continues.

Subeschar Antibiotic Therapy

An alternative method of combating the bacterial population in the burn wound is subeschar clysis. A specific antibiotic for the bacteria present in the burn wound is delivered by a hypodermoclysis technique directly to the subeschar space. Preliminary studies indicate that the antibiotic is absorbed systemically. Subeschar antibiotic therapy may be used as an adjunct to topical therapy in burn patients admitted late with infections, as well as in clinical burn wound sepsis, as prophylaxis for bacterial colonization of 10^4 per gram of tissue, and in patients with severe allergies or toxicity to topical therapy. Normal saline or half normal saline is the vehicle used, since the calcium in Ringer's lactate is likely to precipitate in the alkaline medium and is incompatible with many antibiotics. The quantity of antibiotic solution ordered is divided into 100 ml aliquots and administered 25 ml at a time by injection or by gravity drip from a chamber infusion set. The needle is inserted at a 45° angle; 25 ml of solution covers an area 7.5 cm in diameter, or approximately the size of a softball (Fig. 15-7). The needle is then withdrawn and changed, and the process is re-

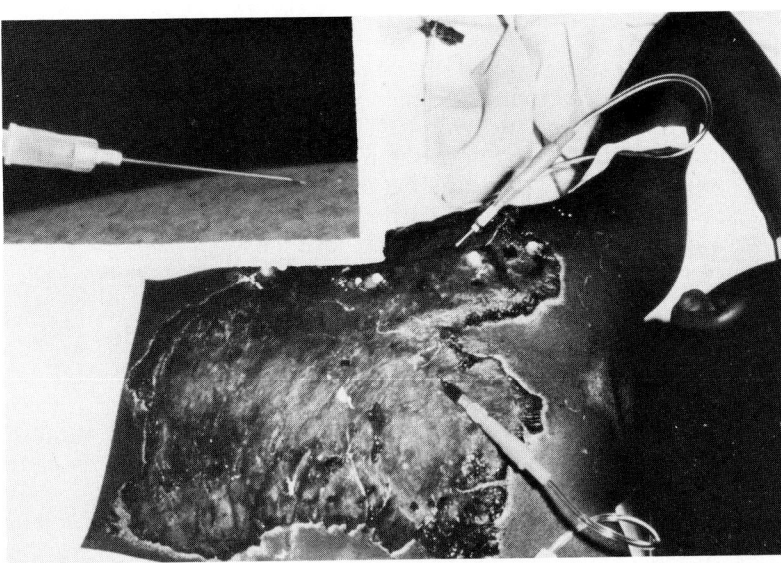

Figure 15-7
Administration of antibiotic by subeschar clysis technique.

peated. Another 25 ml is administered at a distance of approximately 15 cm. An ordered progression of injection ensures coverage of the entire wound.

Evolving Methods of Treatment

Methods of treatment have evolved in the laboratory. Gamma globulin has been administered when levels are depressed, but, unfortunately, such administration has not affected the overall survival rate. What is known at this time is that catabolism and synthesis of the immunoglobulin are both increased initially, and measured levels are depressed. Unless sepsis and accentuated catabolism intervene, normal levels are regained by the end of the second week [62]. In some institutions, a great deal of success has resulted from the use of a *Pseudomonas* vaccine. Many strains of *P. aeruginosa* have been combined as a polyvalent antigen vaccine to stimulate antibody production and resistance in the patient [1]. Unfortunately, in other institutions, growth from strains of *Pseudomonas* not included in the vaccine has been overwhelming. The infusion of white blood cells when levels are subnormal offers a great deal of promise [26, 35].

Other methodologies evolved from the laboratory have met with varying degrees of success. The nitroblue tetrazolium (NBT) dye test measures the ability of neutrophils to kill ingested bacteria [2]. The cyclic variation in neutrophil function that exists in normal man is accentuated and negatively affected after burn injury. Burn wound sepsis occurs when the ability of phagocytic cells to kill ingested bacteria is depressed. Preliminary studies have shown that a reduction in phagocytic function precedes and accompanies burn wound sepsis [16].

Still in the investigational stages is the chemotactic index that measures the attraction of leukocytes [66]. Transfer of R factors from resistant bacteria to previously susceptible bacteria has been identified as a significant factor in antibiotic resistance [43]. Complement levels are depressed, but no relation has as yet been found between sepsis and total levels or complement component levels [20].

Wound Care

Wound care is initiated on admission and directed toward prevention of infection. Attention must be paid to all details of asepsis, since the patient is extremely susceptible to infection. Emergency care of the wound at the site of injury entails application of shaving cream and coverage with a sterile sheet for transfer to the burn facility. The treatment of the wound can be delayed until the patient has shown a satisfactory response from fluid therapy, but it must be initiated early, since bacteria readily begin to proliferate. Tetanus prophylaxis and penicillin (if ordered) are given for beta-hemolytic streptococcus prophylaxis.

INITIAL CLEANING AND DEBRIDEMENT

The initial cleaning and debridement must take place in a clean room, and personnel must wear gowns, masks, and gloves. The wound is gently washed, and loose epidermis is removed with a gauze pad using slight pressure. Scissors are used for gentle trimming away of the devitalized tissue; scrub brushes are not used. Blisters are excised, except for those on the palms and soles. Hair is shaved from the burned area and adjacent surrounding unburned skin surface (Fig. 15-8). The wound is then covered with an appropriate topical agent.

BATHING

Topical agents are removed at least once a day and reapplied. A bed bath, shower, or hydrotherapy is used, depending on the results of a daily physiologic assessment. In many institutions, hydrotherapy is called either tubbing or tanking.

The type of tub used varies from a regular bathtub to a small tub for arms or legs, to a large stainless steel tub (Fig. 15-9). The type of tub used depends on the specific purpose of hydrotherapy. The large stainless steel tub (Hubbard tank) is of no particular benefit in the early postburn period when the injury involves more than 50 percent of the TBSA, and another type of tub will suffice during this time. On the other hand, it is most beneficial later in the burn course, when the patient can be submerged in water as an adjunct to physical therapy.

Tubbing allows for easy removal of the topical agent, softens the eschar (and so helps with daily removal of the eschar), and allows increased range of motion. However, its disadvantages are significant and include heat loss, increased stress and pain, sodium loss, and the danger of cross-contamination.

Assessment prior to tubbing includes cardiopulmonary status, fluid therapy, bacterial count, and location of infection. The nurse must appropriately plan care. Intramuscular injection of medication for pain is given 15 to 30 minutes before tubbing or intravenous injections are given immediately before tubbing. An explanation of the procedure is followed by the removal of dressings or cream (hastened by the use of a tongue blade), perineal care, and preparation of the Foley catheter. This is the ideal time to obtain a daily weight on the metabolic scales. Physiologic and psychological assessment is continuous throughout the procedure.

Time in the tub is limited to 20 minutes, since sodium losses are increased because water is hypotonic and therefore hypothermia may result. Stress must be kept to a minimum. The environment is kept warm with heat shields, and the water temperature should be comfortable. The patient is helped on and off any movable devices used for the transfer. This is a painful procedure, and nar-

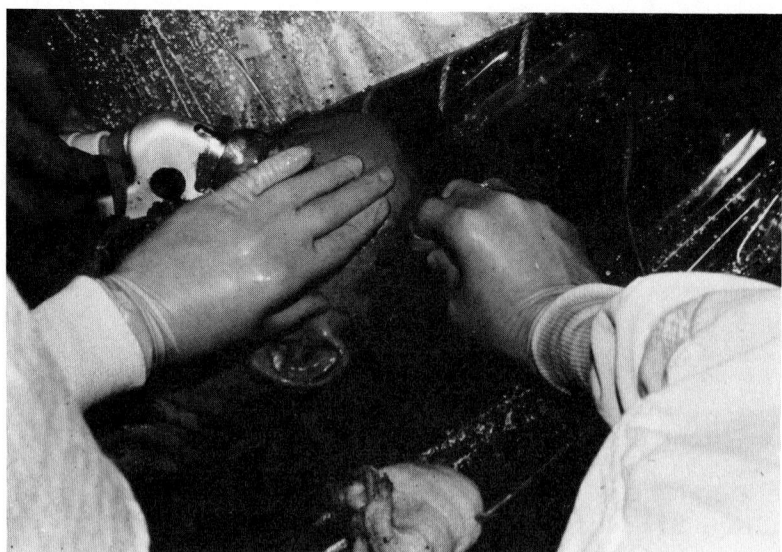

Figure 15-8
Initial cleaning and debridement. Shaving of hair in and surrounding injured area.

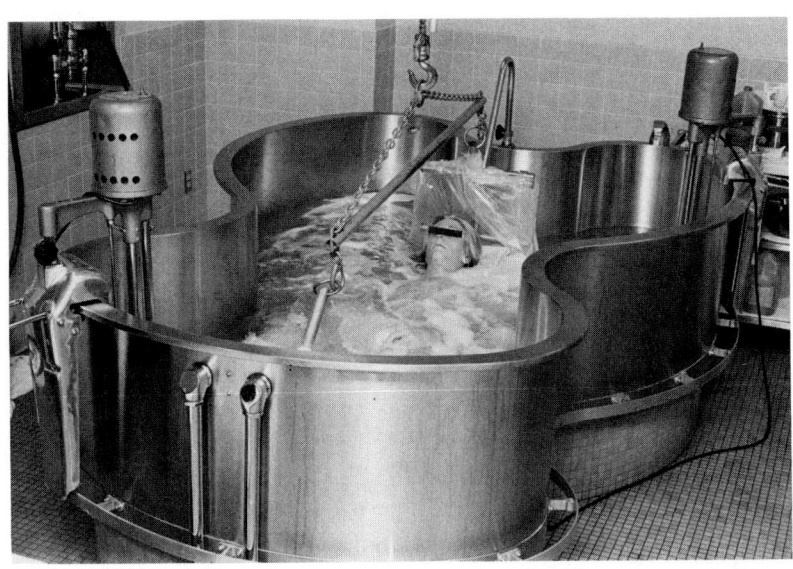

Figure 15-9
Hydrotherapy in Hubbard tank.

cotics as well as nursing techniques are necessary to diminish pain as much as possible.

In implementation of care, rigid adherence to the principles of asepsis is important. The patient with open wounds should not be submerged in the water but should lie on a plinth over the tub and be gently sprayed with water (Fig. 15-10). Submersion in water allows organisms (particularly perineal organisms) to spread quickly all over the body. The environment must be clean; sterile gloves are changed as needed; water is prevented from pooling in areas of contact with the body; and a fresh cleaning sponge (such as a povidone-iodine sponge) is used for each area of the body burned. Scrupulous cleaning of the tub and environment after the bath (even if plastic tub liners are used) will decrease the incidence of cross-contamination. Patient evaluation continues after the patient is returned to bed, including assessment of cardiopulmonary status, temperature, condition of the wounds, and comfort.

The same principles are followed in the bathing of the critically ill patient washed by the bed-bath procedure (Fig. 15-11).

Figure 15-10
Equipment model for use in hydrotherapy without submersion.

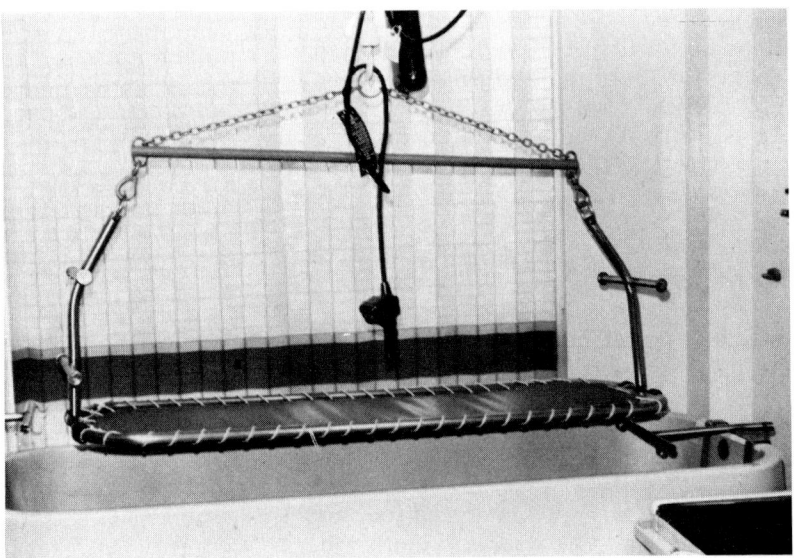

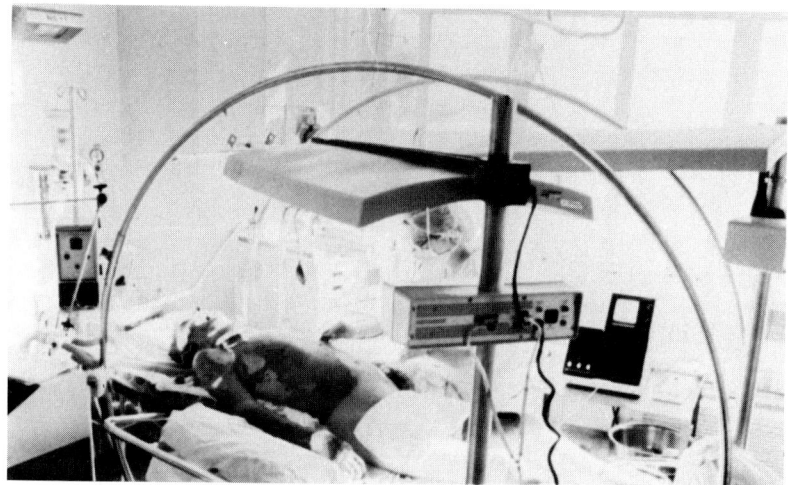

Figure 15-11
Bed-bath procedure utilized for washing a critically ill patient. Principles of asepsis and environmental support are followed.

PREVENTION OF CROSS-CONTAMINATION

Isolation may be required to prevent cross-contamination. The decision about the appropriate type of isolation to prevent the transfer of infection depends on the unique qualities of each burn unit environment. Considerations in developing a system of isolation are (1) physical facilities available, (2) type of personnel and the numbers available, (3) types of burn patients to be treated, (4) cost, and (5) psychological effect on patient, family, and staff. Total isolation does not seem to be the answer, since adults isolated in "life islands" have colonized their wounds with their own endogenous organisms at the same rate as those not in total isolation. The small space makes the administration of patient care difficult. An additional problem is the difficulty of maintaining adequate social interaction and prevention of serious psychological disturbances. Laminar airflow equipment is currently under investigation in many units across the country and seems to offer many advantages. In any situation, the principles of reverse isolation and medical asepsis must be followed to prevent cross-contamination.

The environment does not have to be sterile but must be immaculate. All equipment used must be thoroughly cleaned. Nonsterilized linen may be used as long as laundry procedures are thorough and the linen is directed from the dryer to the ward in closed carts with no chance for contamination. In some settings, sterile disposable linen is the best choice. Tap water can be used in most areas but should be monitored for quantities and types of bacterial flora. However, water should not be allowed to stand in any area—in the nebulizer, bathtub, water hose, or drain.

Cross-contamination is a significant problem in most units. Each patient procedure must be carefully analyzed to determine where contamination might occur and the necessary safeguards implemented. Careful, thorough hand washing before administering care to the patient is essential.

Another prime offender in cross-contamination is the uniform. As the nurse or physician leans across the bed of patient A to help the patient, any organisms on the bed are transferred to the uniform. Then, at patient B's bedside, the nurse or physician leans across the bed to help the patient, and the organisms are transferred from the uniform to the bed. Patient B now has patient A's organisms. The problem is a complex one to solve. Gowns or plastic aprons worn over the uniform are part of the answer. Infection control personnel are an invaluable aid; they do not currently recommend routine, simple environmental cultures (Chap. 1). Probably the most important preventive measure of all is an alert staff.

Adjustment to Stress

The burned patient undergoes many severe physiologic and psychological stresses. The injury itself produces fear and pain, and the victim still must face numerous anxieties. Powerlessness, depersonalization, fear of the unknown, pain, dependency, change in body image, disfigurement, loss of function, and even death are all problems the patient faces daily. The literature is filled with research studies that describe these problems, but definitive criteria on which to base care are sparse.

Initially the nurse must be aware that the patient is concerned primarily with survival and the most rudimentary facets of life. Simple explanations, kindness, attention to details of comfort, and skillful, knowledgeable care will do more to allay the patient's anxiety and apprehension than any outpouring of feelings. Even patients with potentially massive disfiguring injuries are more concerned initially with survival than with an alteration in body image.

During this initial phase, the family must also be included in explanations and kept informed of the patient's status and progress. The nurse is able to answer questions and explain the appearance of their loved one and the necessary care. Appropriate explanations accompanied by pictures of burn patients may prepare the family for seeing the patient.

The family may be considered as a redundantly coupled system so that alterations in one part of the system will affect other parts. Thus, the family members are affected by the patient's injury, and the patient is affected by the response of the family. Sometimes the patient is able to cope with the stresses of the illness, but another family member, another part of the system, breaks down. That breakdown will then add increased stress to the system and may seriously affect the patient. Families are different in style and in the manner in which they function, and these differences are correlated with syndromes found in their children [14]. Therefore, assessments of the family will be helpful to plan patient care objectives. If there is an extended family, friends, and/or community support on which to rely, the family members are more likely to be able to cope with the stress of the illness and hospitalization. The nurse must be cognizant of their responses, family structure, and body language during an early interview and use the data to help predict whether or not the family is likely to have overwhelming problems. Weekly educational classes will help increase the level of knowledge so that family members' active participation in care can be elicited. These classes provide a setting in which anxieties can be shared and alleviated.

Evaluation of the patient's psychological problems and coping mechanisms may be incorrect at any time. Indeed, problems that are considered to be psychological are often actually problems of electrolyte imbalance or sepsis. Any change in orientation and any increase in respiratory rate indicate sepsis until proved otherwise. An accurate physiologic appraisal is therefore imperative.

Probably the best people on the team to help the burned person adjust to stress and loss are the nurses. Psychologists, social workers, and chaplains have a great deal of expertise, but their numbers are small, and often they are not in the right place at the right time. Nurses are present at all hours of the day and night and are totally involved in the patient's care. They are present to listen, provide understanding, and act as a buffer. However, nurses tend to become part of the patient's system and are affected by all the stimuli surrounding the patient. Thus, some nurses begin to wonder about their perspective on the total patient situation and their ability to intervene appropriately. Group sessions are therefore extremely important to keep the nurses' stress at a tolerable level, to help them learn interpersonal skills, and to provide guidance for nurse-patient interactions [39]. Perhaps the most important role of the psychologist in the burn unit is to help the nurses help the patients [57].

The long, weary road to recovery is filled with ups and downs, and few patients recover without some complications. Patients respond in their individual ways, and it is difficult to generalize about the personality characteristics of burn patients. In general, however, basic personality patterns are not changed by the experience. People who were well adjusted and flexible before injury tend to be well adjusted and flexible after injury. If they were unstable before injury, they are unstable after injury.

Often, during the period of hospitalization, the pain and stress will alter the patient's defenses for an indefinite period [4]. Regression and denial are often present and seem to be protective mechanisms. The stages of grief are frequently seen, and denial tends to be prolonged: it is commonplace for the patient not to seem to realize the actual extent of the injury. Denial can be viewed as an adaptive mechanism, indicating that the person is not yet ready to cope with his problems. The burn unit is not the place to force or even encourage people to look at these problems and come up with a solution. Patients should have the freedom to deal with problems at their own pace. Once they are ready to begin to work, the clues will be given by their behavior. Supportive mechanisms and assistance may then be offered.

What can nurses really do to help patients in their struggles? First, the nurse must be clinically competent, knowing what should be done and why it should be done, and being able to do it. Life-endangering problems take priority. The nurse must understand that each patient is a unique individual and must be accepted and treated as such. The first obligation is to understand what is going on from the patient's point of view. The nurse must examine motivations for behavior. It is helpful to remember that emotions have basis in thoughts and beliefs, which may be the crux of the problem.

How can patients be motivated to participate in their exercise regimens? A helping person with skills can assist others to modify their attitudes and become more rational about the goals they can attain. The first step is to define the patient's motivation. What is the objective? What is the probability of attainment of the objective? If the objective is to attain full range of motion in a burned extremity, what does the patient see as his or her chances for successfully achieving that goal? Next, what is the usefulness of the objective? What does it personally mean to the patient? If, for example, the patient is a working man with a family he wants to support, must he be able to use his hands? Or is he uninterested in returning to work? Finally, what is the cost to the patient in terms of his values and desires? The dependence of motivation on objective, probability of a successful outcome, usefulness of the goal, and cost may be summarized as follows [42]:

$$\text{Motivation} = \frac{\text{probability of outcome} + \text{objective} + \text{usefulness}}{\text{cost}}$$

Since numerical application would require the definition of subjective scales, this formula is used only for conceptualizing and evaluating the impact of the independent variables in terms of what each means to the individual patient.

Problems in Wound Coverage

The most important factor in the recovery of the thermally injured patient is closure of the burn wound. Not until the eschar is removed and the wound is covered by an autograft, or deep dermal burns are reepithelialized, are the severe derangements resulting from the open wound reversed.

An autograft is skin taken from an unburned area and transferred to a burned area of the body. Since donor sites are often limited in patients with widespread thermal injuries, new techniques for temporary coverage have evolved. Skin from another human being (homograft, usually from a cadaver donor) or another species (heterograft) can be used. Successful temporary coverage has also been reported with amniotic membrane, but synthetic skin substitutes have been unsuccessful to date.

BIOLOGIC DRESSINGS

Homografts [60] are now available from the skin bank in Dallas and can be shipped by air to hospitals all over the country. It is now possible to arrange for the postmortem donation of one's skin as well as for the donation of kidneys or eyes. Homograft procurement is done under sterile conditions, and homografts are stored in a nitrogen freezer until needed. The skin of the pig is ordinarily used for heterografts [56]. Pigskin can be readily obtained in large quantities from one of the commercial skin banks in 24 hours and can be ordered fresh, frozen, or lyophilized. A heterograft is an acceptable alternate for a homograft but certainly does not offer as many clinical advantages.

Biologic dressings offer the following benefits: They (1) restore the water vapor barrier, (2) decrease exudative protein loss, (3) protect from infection, (4) relieve pain and allow active joint function, (5) help in the debridement of dermal debris, and (6) stimulate the growth of epithelium and granulation tissue. Heterografts are so readily available from the skin banks that it is difficult to list procurement as a disadvantage. On the other hand, the supply of homograft is limited for obvious reasons. Storage can be a problem for both types of grafts. One potential problem is the trapping of infection. Subgraft suppuration and the early coverage of full-thickness injury lead to burn wound sepsis.

Several uses of biologic dressing are of particular importance. In general, the patient is remarkably more comfortable with a biologic dressing. He or she feels better, eats better, and is able to participate actively in physical therapy. Coverage of the wound is probably the best available tool for pain control. The immediate coverage of partial-thickness burns (but not of full-thickness burns) alleviates pain, and the wounds also seem to heal faster. On the second day after heterografting, small, raised areas of serous drainage may be gently pierced with a sterile needle to remove the serum, and the graft will then adhere. Occasionally, the amount of serous drainage is sufficient to require that the biologic dressing be removed and a fresh dressing (new graft) reapplied. Healing occurs under the biologic dressing.

Biologic dressings can also be used after the eschar has separated, when the wound is still not ready for grafting because of the presence of dermal debris. These spotty wounds can be prepared for an autograft by the application of biologic dressings. Normally, for the first few days, the graft becomes "soupy" with accumulation of debris, does not adhere, and must be removed daily. The patient is then bathed, and the dressing is reapplied to the wound. The process is repeated, since the biologic dressing is considered a test material prior to autografting, and once a heterograft or homograft remains on the wound bed, an autograft "take" is highly probable.

If a homograft is used on a full-thickness injury, the graft may be left in place until it becomes vascularized, thus protecting the wound until it is covered by an autograft. At this time, skin from any donor is used on any recipient, and tissue typing is not done. Probably due to the use of multiple donors, tissue rejection occurs relatively infrequently and in limited areas. Clinically, the patient with a rejection phenomenon exhibits any of the following: increased temperature and pulse, irritability, anxiety, gastrointestinal malfunction, edema in and surrounding the area, and a spotty, raised, irritated, reddened granulation tissue.

Biologic dressings are applied to the cleaned wound as a ward procedure using aseptic techniques (Fig. 15-12). The dressing is applied with the shiny side next to the burned area, and the gauze backing is removed. All the air pockets are removed by smoothing the skin with forceps or a gloved hand. With scissors, the skin is trimmed so that it covers only the wound and there is no overlapping. The biologic dressing is then covered with a layer of fine mesh gauze or gauze impregnated with an antibiotic ointment and covered with a light, dry sterile dressing. Following the procedure, the temperature often rises slightly; this is considered a normal occurrence. Occasionally after heterograft application, the patient's temperature suddenly rises to a high level, necessitating removal of the skin.

DEBRIDEMENT

The goal of burn care is to close the wound, but this cannot be accomplished until the eschar is removed. Daily debridement removes the eschar as it separates. Debridement is defined as the removal of eschar at the interface of the living and dead tissue. Preparation of the wound for grafting is initiated. The success of the open method of burn therapy depends on active debridement. The procedure is tedious and relatively painful but allows for consistent removal as areas become ready for debridement. The result is a decreased number of operative procedures.

Debridement is performed as follows: Loose pieces of tissue are gently removed with forceps and scissors; scalpels are not used (see color insert Figure 14 on page 1078D). Gentle pressure with a gloved hand is applied to the wound to identify areas of subeschar suppuration. The areas that have been lysed by bacterial growth are then unroofed and removed. Bleeding should be minimal and can be controlled with direct pressure. The patient's wounds are debrided during hydrotherapy, but if areas to be debrided remain and the 20-minute hydrotherapy time allotment has been used, the procedure is completed while the patient is on the

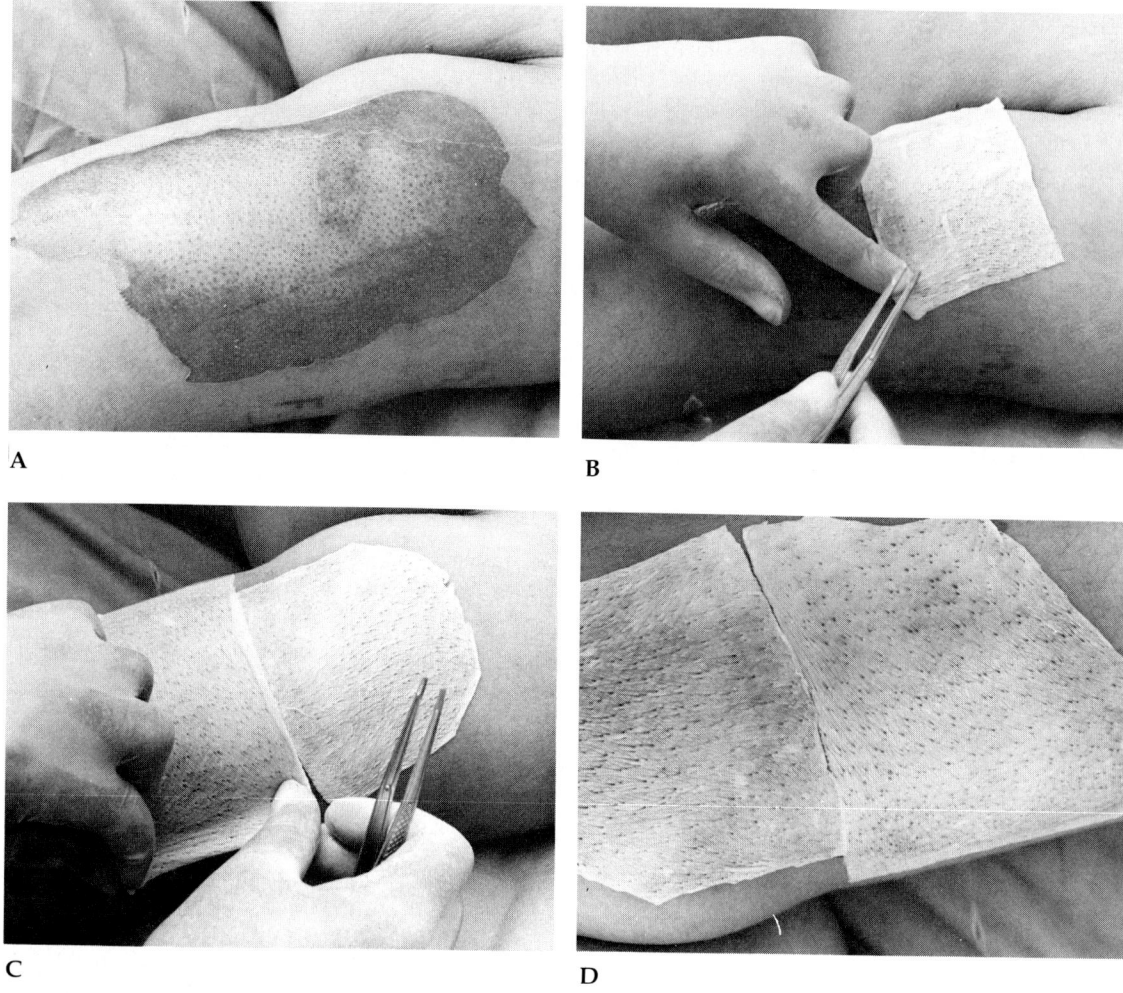

Figure 15-12
Application of biologic dressing. **A.** Partial-thickness wound after cleaning. **B.** Application of biologic dressing and removal of air pockets using aseptic technique. **C.** Placement and trimming of biologic dressing to avoid overlapping. **D.** Completed application. **E.** Biologic dressing secured by fine-mesh gauze and an expandable net-like material.

stretcher before he is returned to bed. After the debridement is completed, a topical agent is applied to the wounds.

Alternative methods of debridement are used. Enzymatic debridement is still under investigation but continues to be problematic. The major problem has been the increased incidence of infection following the application of enzymes [27].

Both heterograft application and wet-to-dry dressings are effective later in the hospital course for the mechanical removal of remaining debris. Dressings wet with saline are applied to the wounds, allowed to dry, and then removed. Although it is painful, the method is extremely effective.

EXCISIONAL THERAPY

The surgical approach to the removal of eschar is excisional therapy. Traditionally, excisional therapy has been limited to patients with burn injury involving less than 15 percent of the TBSA. Today, staged excisions are being performed on patients with large injuries in an attempt to decrease the extent of the burn. The availability of homograft is essential for success.

The procedure is first performed on or before 5 days postinjury and before significant bacterial colonization has occurred. Specific criteria for selection and further evaluation of patients undergoing excision are under investigation. Currently, candidates for excision are evaluated by weighing the following categories: age; extent, depth, and location of the injury; associated injuries and illnesses; cardiopulmonary status; bacterial colonization; ability to fight infection (white blood cell count and other laboratory procedures); clotting factors; and the patient's general physiologic status.

Primary excisional therapy entails removal of the full-thickness injury by means of the scalpel, electrosurgical cautery, carbon dioxide laser, or dermatome. The area is then covered with a biologic dressing or autograft [36]. Tangential excision (Fig. 15-13) is another form of excisional therapy. Debridement is done to the point of capillary bleeding. The eschar is shaved away layer by layer until a good bleeding bed is established and viable tissue is reached. In this procedure, shaving does not usually go deep enough to remove all skin elements, and thus regenera-

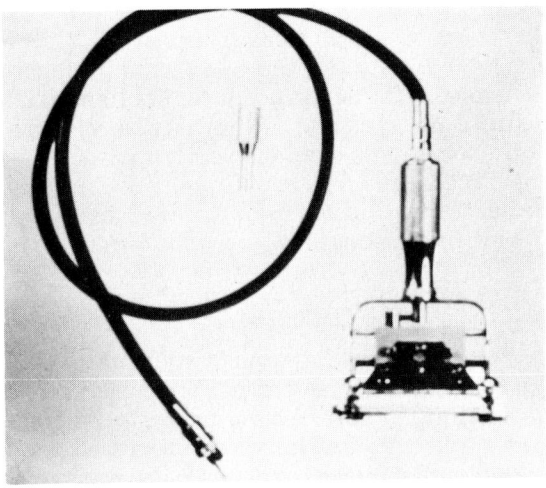

A

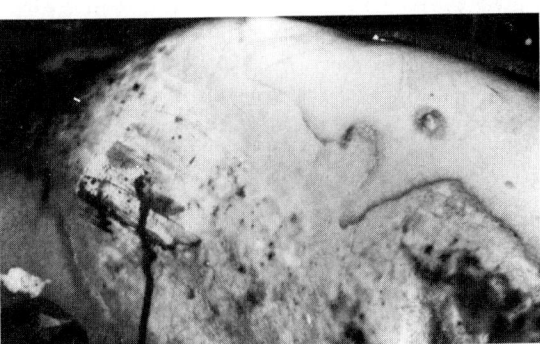

B

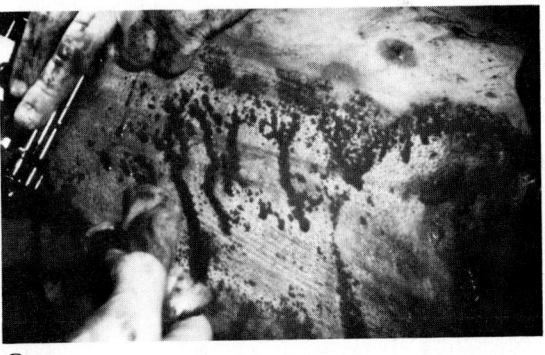

C

Figure 15-13
Tangential excision. **A.** Brown dermatome. **B.** Eschar is shaved away layer by layer. **C.** Debridement is to the point of capillary bleeding.

tion of epithelium can occur [29]. A biologic dressing is then used to protect the wound from infection until it heals or is covered by an autograft. Since the technique is relatively painless, the procedure can also be done in the ward on small areas of the wound. For elderly patients in particular, small, staged excisions as limited procedures are beneficial because the inelastic cardiovascular systems of these patients cannot tolerate more extensive procedures. The technique is also used to decrease morbidity from contractures and hypertrophic scarring.

AUTOGRAFTS

Areas of full-thickness injury require the use of an autograft for coverage. Skin grafts can be taken from any area of the body not burned and applied to the clean, red vascular bed.

Revascularization of the graft is dependent on several processes. The skin is carefully applied, usually without sutures, but Steri-strips may be used. For 3 to 5 days, the graft site is immobilized and either covered with large bulky dressings or left open, and physical therapy is temporarily discontinued. Next, a blood supply for the graft is established. Circulation is restored both by vascular anastomoses and by new vascular ingrowth from the graft bed into the graft. During the first day following grafting, a fibrin layer is produced and provides contact but not fixation between graft and graft bed. During the second day, the fibrin reticulum organizes and advances, and the granulation tissue contains immature fibroblasts and a few open spaces with erythrocytes. Then, 3 days following grafting, granulation is so organized that it is difficult to differentiate graft from graft bed on microscopic study. The percentage of graft take is high if the wound has been carefully prepared, infection does not intervene, and pressure does not disrupt the graft.

Different types of skin grafts are used. The care of each patient must be individualized since skin coverage is dependent on the site of the injury and on what areas remain to be used as donor sites for autografting. If the injury is extensive, the first consideration is the closure of as large an area as possible. Then priority is given to coverage of burns on the (1) face, (2) hands, (3) feet, (4) neck and other joint areas, (5) genitalia and perineum, and then (6) other areas such as the back [28].

Various depths of skin are used. A **full-thickness graft** uses the entire depth of skin and is applied to specific areas such as eyelids, tip of the nose, or hands. **Split-thickness grafts** (Fig. 15-14) are most commonly used and are transferred to the wound bed in a continuous sheet if enough donor sites are available. If this is not the case, the **mesh skin graft** is used [64].

Utilizing the Tanner-Vandeput mesh dermatome, multiple slits are cut so that the skin expands to an area three to nine times the size of the donor site. Unless very large areas must be covered, the skin is not expanded to a size greater than three times that of the donor site. The meshed skin is applied to the clean wound (see color insert Figure 16 on p. 1078D) and covered with a moist dressing. Tissue

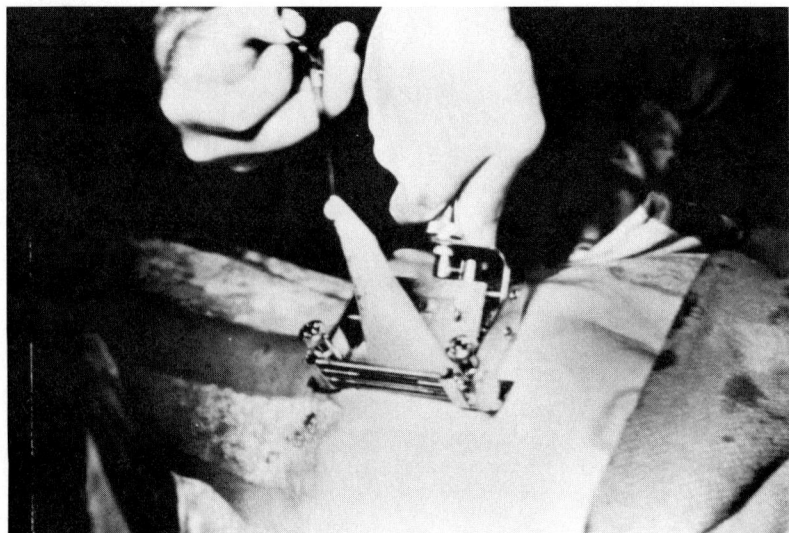

Figure 15-14
Taking of autograft from donor site.

fluid can drain from the wound, eliminating the problem of fluid collecting under the graft. However, multiple potential portals of entry for infection are open. Skin then grows outward from the outline or rows of graft and closes the interstices. Unfortunately, the healed meshed area has more scarring than a sheet graft and is not as cosmetically attractive. If possible, its use should be limited to areas where appearance is less important, such as the back, abdomen, and thighs.

Care of the donor site is important. Donor sites are covered with a single layer of fine mesh gauze, left open to the air, and exposed to a heat lamp for 24 hours. The areas tend to be relatively uncomfortable, and the patient often requires medication to relieve the discomfort. The gauze separates in 10 to 14 days as the area heals, but the gauze is not removed until the donor site heals. As healing occurs, the gauze separates from the donor site and dries. These raised and dry areas of gauze are then gently trimmed away, exposing the new tissue. Donor sites can also be covered with other dressings such as wet antibiotic dressings, Adaptic, and heterograft. Fresh porcine heterograft was used at one time but many patients incorporated some of the cells of the biologic dressing into their own skin. Currently, alternate forms of heterograft, such as lyophilized products, are being evaluated for this purpose.

After a successful autograft, the patient is ready for discharge. Patients with extensive burn injuries will face many subsequent admissions and operative procedures for reconstructive surgery. Physical functioning may be impaired from the injury—from contractures or from bands of scar tissue that form after discharge. The patient's cosmetic appearance may need to be revised by softening of scar lines and other techniques utilized by the skillful reconstructive burn surgeon. Cosmetic devices may have to be constructed for missing body parts, most commonly for the ear, since reconstructive techniques are not as normal looking as prosthetic reconstruction. Actually, the prosthetic ear looks normal, particularly with the longer hair styles, and is preferred by most patients.

Problems with Decreased Range of Motion and Contractures

Rehabilitation of the thermally injured patient starts with admission. Prevention of decreased range of motion and contractures is always better than treatment. Function must be maintained and active range of motion encouraged. It behooves everyone on the health team to pay heed to the physical medicine regimen. On the other hand, not all contractures and disabilities are caused by inadequate physical therapy. Frequently, injuries are deep and vital structures are destroyed. Infection may supervene and cause additional damage.

POSITIONING AND SPLINTING

The contracture is caused by the scar, or cicatrix. Scarring of the skin and deeper structures follows most injuries. The surrounding normal tissue is drawn toward the scar, and blood flow to distal areas is hampered. The scar is very deep and dense, and the surface tends to be avascular and thus injures easily. Blood vessels cannot get to the top, so ulcerations and blisters form. The skin may be so thin that healing is slow and difficult even after a minor trauma.

Flexion contractures are common and primarily involve the skin, although deeper structures are also involved. Positions of flexion tend to be positions of comfort. Infections also contribute to flexion contractures, since they delay healing; and when healing is delayed, the amount of red, moist, vascular granulation tissue increases, which in turn results in greater contracture. In addition, the shortening of muscles and fibrosis of joint capsules lead to contracture.

Current therapy is based on the findings of studies of granulation tissue in burn wounds [67]. It has been noted on tissue biopsy that if whirlpools of collagen are present, these whirlpools continue to grow and evolve into swirls of nodular collagen. These swirls appearing on the skin surface are called hypertrophic scarring. If the fibers of collagen develop parallel to the direction of stress, the nodular swirls are not as likely to form. Thus, current therapy attempts to maintain extension and parallel fibers of collagen by proper positioning, splinting, and traction.

Early positioning maintains functional range of motion and proper body alignment, decreases edema, and prevents deformities and decubiti by avoiding positions of flexion and pressure areas. Potential problems include maceration of tissue, refractory edema, and soft-tissue calcification, which results in ankylosis of the joints. Positions for all burned and unburned areas of the body must be considered in a systematic manner.

For the first 2 to 3 days following injury, any burned extremities are elevated above the level of the heart. The arms are covered with a flexible net-like material and it is then suspended from IV poles (Fig. 15-15). Every hour, the suspension is temporarily discontinued, and active exercise for 5 minutes is encouraged. If the legs are burned, the foot of the bed is also elevated (Fig. 15-16). Moylan et al. [51] have suggested that for patients admitted with adequate arterial blood flow, elevation combined with active motion appears to maintain arterial blood flow by relieving venous obstruction.

An injury covering the anterior surface of the patient's neck requires hyperextension after the first 48 to 72 hours. A small pillow roll is used under the neck to provide minimal hyperextension if the patient has respiratory problems, is very edematous, or is elderly; greater hyperextension is attained by placing the patient on a double mattress. A short or pediatric mattress is placed on the top of a

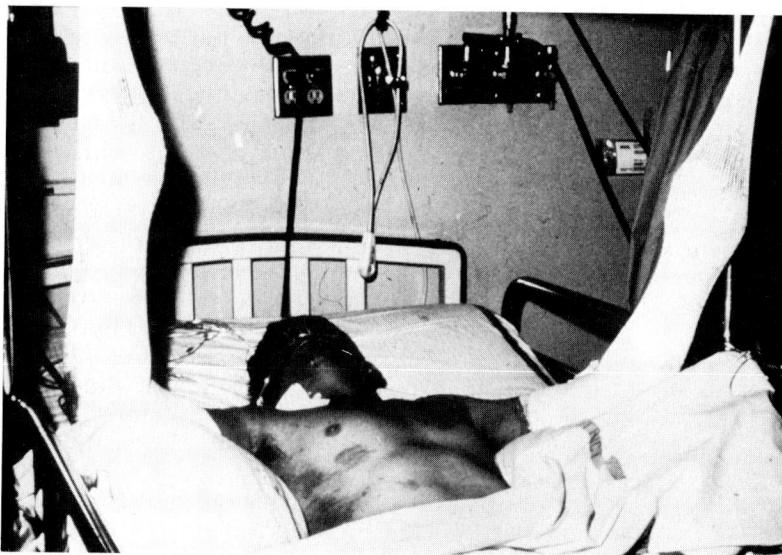

Figure 15-15
Technique for elevation of upper extremities.

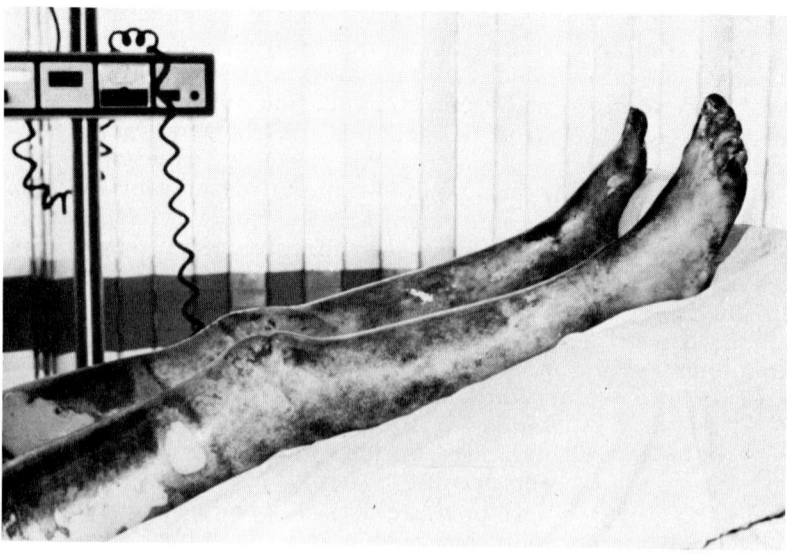

Figure 15-16
Elevation of lower extremities.

regular hospital bed mattress. The patient lies on the pediatric mattress with the shoulders close to its top and the head over the edge and resting on the regular mattress. For comfort, a small roll is used under the head, and the patient's position is slightly altered hourly.

Shoulder boards are attached to the head of the bed, and the patient's shoulders and arms are abducted. The elbows are extended on the boards in a spread-eagle fashion. The forearm and palms are supinated, with the hands and wrist extended (neutral to 35°). Pillows are used to elevate the hands and arms above the level of the heart. Each distal part is elevated higher than the proximal part to decrease edema. The position is difficult for the patient to maintain, but frequent minor changes in position help. Occasionally, a light restraint is necessary to help remind the patient to maintain the abduction.

Attention must be given to the trunk area. A small roll placed lengthwise against the spine will give enough support to allow the shoulders to fall backward in proper alignment. Later, the roll will also help keep the patient's back straight and prevent lateral pulling.

Hips are kept straight, knees are extended, and legs are maintained in very slight abduction (15°). A trochanter roll is usually sufficient, and additional pillow support is not necessary. It is important to prevent the patient's knees from falling outward into a frog-leg position. Several problems may arise. Pressure on the peroneal nerve may cause a palsy, or the stretch may cause a foot drop. The inversion of the foot may also cause a stretch on the lateral side of the foot. Tissue breakdown is common on the bottom or sides of the feet, and pressure sores frequently form around the heel. Feet should be flat against a footboard (90°) and foam placed to relieve pressure between feet and board. If possible, the leg should be slightly elevated so the heel does not touch the end of the bed.

Various types of beds (for example, Circ-Olectric, Stryker, alternating-pressure, air flow, and oscillating beds) are available to assist with positioning and turning. Frequently, the patient is in one type of bed for several days and is then transferred to another for several more. Each bed has advantages and disadvantages, depending on the patient's situation at any given time. For example, a CircOlectric bed is most helpful in turning the patient from back to abdomen or assisting him or her to stand. However, such a bed is harmful to a patient who cannot be turned to a prone position because the bed is relatively uncomfortable and so narrow that side-to-side positioning is difficult.

Splinting is often necessary to help hold basic positions, maintain functional position, and prevent deformities. Occasionally, swelling may be reduced early with the appropriate use of splints. In general, the ideal position does not entail the use of splints unless a problem has arisen. Frequently, the patient is too ill to participate in an active exercise regimen, and splints are required.

Therapy for the hands is an area of considerable controversy, but most authorities agree on the benefits of excisional therapy. Hand care must be highly individualized and frequently altered according to the patient's progress [15]. A static splint is constructed from thermoplastic material with the wrist in 30° extension, MP joints in 65° flexion, and the proximal and distal interphalangeal joints in full extension (Fig. 15-17). Problems are likely to arise when the wrist becomes flexed, the metacarpophalangeal joints become hyperextended, the interphalangeal joints are flexed, the fingers are abducted, and the thumb is adducted. A dynamic splint or a splint molded from Isoprene will permit acute flexion of the hand, abduction of the thumb, and extension of the wrist. Finger-thumb opposition (prehensile position) is important to maintain because 50 percent of hand function is in the thumb. Well-functioning hands are essential if patients are to return to work and to their preinjury life-styles.

If the patient has a full-thickness dorsal injury, the physiatrist initially performs a careful assessment and is likely to immobilize the hand because of the danger of loss of the extensor mechanism. Full range of motion is not a primary goal in these patients. Hand function is maintained by keeping movements minimal and the hand "loose." Then, when possible, the wound is covered by an autograft, and the hand is internally splinted or pinned. If the patient has a partial-thickness injury, his hand is covered with a biologic dressing and exercise is encouraged. Full range of motion is maintained during healing.

Traction devices are used in many burn units. Limbs may be kept off the bed so that

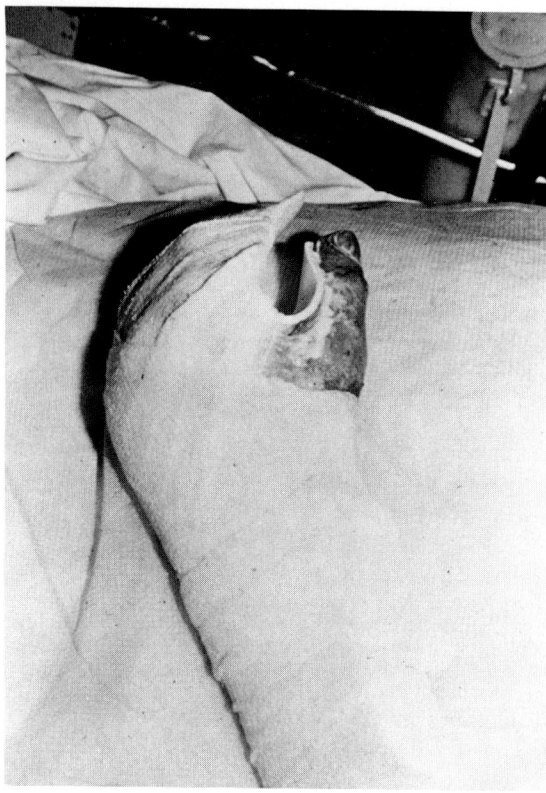

Figure 15-17
Hand splint to maintain extension.

grafts may heal without undue pressure. Weights should be altered and exercise encouraged between procedures.

EXERCISE

Gentle active and passive exercise is started early. Active exercise and "self-exercise" regimens are encouraged. Active motion minimizes edema and prevents the adherence of flexor and extensor tendons to surrounding tissues and shortening of capsular structures. The best type of program includes carrying out the activities of daily living. Hand exercises are encouraged in every possible way. If patients have problems feeding themselves, a self-help device to hold the fork is used. The program is adjusted to the tolerance of the individual patient.

Several short exercise sessions are preferred to one long session. Commonly, the patient starts early in the day and participates in a sustained active exercise program three to five times a day. At night, he maintains the position by wearing splints. Active exercise can be unlimited, but passive exercise must be done gently, since too vigorous a regimen will be harmful.

Exposed tendons are a significant problem. If the patient is allowed to exercise the area actively or if passive exercise is pursued, the tendon may snap, causing a flexion deformity. Thus, the shiny viable tendon should be covered with moist gauze or pigskin and immobilized. Patients are not allowed to feed themselves or do anything by themselves until an extension splint is ready. When the danger of tendon rupture is detected, internal fixation or pinning is usually indicated. Thus, the joint is internally splinted in 15° to 20° of flexion with a Kirschner wire for a period of 6 to 8 weeks [15, 31].

Bed exercises such as gluteal tightening and range of motion are encouraged. Muscle strengthening is started when the patient's condition has stabilized. It is important to have the patient out of bed for short periods, as his condition permits. Walking is encouraged. When the patient has burns below the knees, the lower extremities should be wrapped with Ace bandages.

Rehabilitation

As the patient's condition improves, the focus of therapy changes: Range of motion and strengthening become most important. The entire body must be built up because of the muscle wasting and atrophy. If available, electromyelography is a useful tool to determine muscle status. Areas of scarring require sustained stretching. If certain body areas are tight, opposing muscle groups need strengthening. Posture is reattained and mobility of the trunk assured. If neuropathies are present, muscle groups require reeducation. Ulnar nerve palsies with the presenting symptoms of numbness in the fourth and fifth finger are caused by pressure on the ulnar nerve at the olecranon. A change in resting position usually relieves the pressure, and the numbness disappears.

The patient should walk as much as possible. Patients whose feet have been burned may need sheepskin-lined shoes to prevent skin breakdown. Any abnormalities in gait are assessed and corrected. Occasionally, devices such as canes, braces, or drop-foot supports are needed.

Splints and wraps are devised to provide stretch and pressure to areas of hypertrophic scarring. Finger, hand, axillary area, or other body area splints are provided to help with the particular problem the patient has or is about to develop. Isoprene neck splints are molded and are worn 24 hours a day for many months to prevent the contracture bands that previously developed without such splints.

If needed, pressure wraps such as Ace bandages, Elastinette, or Jobst garments are worn 24 hours a day for approximately 6 months to maintain pressure and decrease hypertrophic scarring. As soon as the grafted area has healed, pressure wraps may be applied to scars to soften, smooth, and splint the skin [67]. Additionally, creams with a vegetable or mineral oil base are applied to lubricate and soften the reepithelialized or grafted skin. Itching becomes a significant problem, helped to a slight degree by medications such as diphenhydramine hydrochloride (Benedryl) and baths with sodium bicarbonate added to the water.

Discharge planning and patient education are vital to ensure adherence to a therapy program. Initially, patients may return to the hospital daily for therapy, followed by visits three times a week and then weekly. The time intervals and length of the follow-up depend on the patient's status. It is important that patients understand the regimen, so that they can participate actively in the program. Exercise must be continued for many months. Frequent short sessions will increase strength and range of motion more than a few long sessions.

Patient problems during rehabilitation change dramatically from those in the acute phase. No longer is the situation concerned with life or death, but the problems are just as vital and meaningful to the patient. Hospitalizations are long and costly. Often, the patient has to adapt by changing his or her life-style. Formation of scar tissue and contracture bands require extensive physical therapy and, if this fails, release of contracture. Patients are often unrealistically optimistic about the possibilities of plastic surgery. Progress is tedious, and miracles cannot be performed. Many questions will arise: "Can I return to work? Can I return to the same job? My family has been O.K. since I've been gone. Do they still need me? Does it matter that I look different? Is my wife or husband still interested in me as a sex partner? Will my new boss understand that I have to take time off periodically to go to the hospital? Will I be able to meet new friends?" All these questions and many, many more must be answered. Helping is really a team effort. All members of the health team are needed to provide input and assistance for patients in their quest to readjust to their life situations.

References

1. Alexander, J. W. Immunologic Consideration and the Role of Vaccination in Burn Injury. In Polk, H., and Stone, H. H. (eds.), *Contemporary Burn Management*. Boston: Little, Brown, 1971. Pp. 265–280.
2. Alexander, J. W. Periodic variation in the antibacterial function of human neutrophils and its relationship to sepsis. *Ann. Surg.* 173:206, 1971.
3. Ambiavagar, M. B., Chalon, J., and Zargham, I. Tracheobronchial cytologic changes following lower airway thermal injury. *J. Trauma* 14:280, 1974.
4. Andreasen, N. J. C., Noyes, R., Hartford, C. E., Brodland, G., and Proctor, S. Management of emotional reactions in seriously burned adults. *N. Engl. J. Med.* 286:65, 1972.
5. Artz, C. P., and Moncrief, J. A. *The Treatment of Burns*. Philadelphia: Saunders, 1969.
6. Baxter, C. R. Burns. In Shires, G. T. (ed.), *Care of the Trauma Patient*. New York: McGraw-Hill, 1966. Pp. 197–222.
7. Baxter, C. R. Evaluation of the Burned Patient. In H. F. Conn and R. B. Conn, Jr. (eds.), *Current Diagnosis*. Philadelphia: Saunders, 1968. Pp. 915–919.
8. Baxter, C. R. Crystalloid Resuscitation of Burn Shock. In Polk, H., and Stone, H. H. (eds.), *Contemporary Burn Management*. Boston: Little, Brown, 1971. Pp. 7–32.
9. Baxter, C. R. Response to Initial Fluid and Electrolyte Therapy of Burn Shock. In Lynch, J. B., and Lewis, S. R. (eds.), *Symposium on the Treatment of Burns*. St. Louis: Mosby, 1973. Vol. 5, pp. 42–48.
10. Baxter, C. R. Fluid volume and electrolyte changes of the early postburn period. *Clin. Plast. Surg.* 1:673, 1974.
11. Baxter, C. R., Curreri, P. W., and Marvin, J. A. Fluid and electrolyte therapy of burn shock. *Heart Lung* 2:707, 1973.
12. Baxter, C., Curreri, P. W., and Marvin,

J. The control of burn wound sepsis by the use of quantitative bacteriologic studies and subeschar clysis with antibiotics. *Surg. Clin. North Am.* 53:1509, 1973.
13. Baxter, C. R., Curreri, P. W., and Marvin, J. A. Early management of thermal burns. *Postgrad. Med.* 55:131, 1974.
14. Bell, H. W. Extended Family Relations of Disturbed and Well Families. In Ackerman, N. W. (ed.), *Family Process.* New York: Basic Books, 1970.
15. Boswick, J. The management of fresh burns of the hand and deformities resulting from burn injuries. *Clin. Plast. Surg.* 1:621, 1974.
16. Curreri, P. W., Heck, E., Browne, L., and Baxter, C. Stimulated nitroblue tetrazolium test to assess neutrophil antibacterial function: Prediction of wound sepsis in burned patients. *Surgery* 74:6, 1973.
17. Curreri, P. W., Wilmore, D., Mason, A., Newsome, T. W., Asch, M. J., and Pruitt, B. A. Intracellular cation alterations following major trauma: Effect of supranormal caloric intake. *J. Trauma* 11:390, 1971.
18. Curreri, P. W., Richmond, D., Marvin, J., and Baxter, C. Dietary requirements of patients with major burns. *J. Am. Diet. Assoc.* 65:415, 1974.
19. Czaja, A., McAlbany, J. C., and Pruitt, C. A. Acute gastroduodenal disease after thermal injury. *N. Engl. J. Med.* 291:925, 1974.
20. Daniels, J., Larson, D., Aleston, A., and Ritzmann, E. Serum protein profiles in thermal burns. II: Protease inhibitors, complement factors, and C-reactive protein. *J. Trauma* 14:153, 1974.
21. Davies, J. W. L. The Metabolism of Fibrinogen in Burn Patients. In Wallace, A. B., and Wilkinson, A. W. (eds.), *Research in Burns.* Edinburgh: Livingstone, 1966.
22. Davies, J. W. L., and Liljedahl, S. O. Metabolic Consequences of an Extensive Burn. In Polk, H., and Stone, H. H. (eds.), *Contemporary Burn Management.* Boston: Little, Brown, 1971. Pp. 151–169.
23. DiVincenti, F. C., Pruitt, B. A., and Reckler, J. M. Inhalation injuries. *J. Trauma* 11:109, 1971.
24. Gump, F., Martin, P., and Kinney, J. Oxygen consumption and caloric expenditure in surgical patients. *Surg. Gynecol. Obstet.* 137:499, 1973.
25. Guyton, A. C. *Textbook of Medical Physiology.* Philadelphia: Saunders, 1971.
26. Howard, R. J., and Simmons, R. L. Acquired immunologic deficiencies after trauma and surgical procedures. *Surg. Gynecol. Obstet.* 139:771, 1974.
27. Hummel, R. P., Kautz, P. D., MacMillan, B. G., and Altemeier, W. A. The continuing problem of sepsis following enzymatic debridement of burns. *J. Trauma* 14:572, 1974.
28. Hunt, J. L., and Pruitt, B. A. *Management of Thermal Injury.* In press.
29. Janzekovic, Z. The burn wound from the surgical point of view. *J. Trauma* 15:42, 1975.
30. Jelenko, C., Jennings, W., O'Kelly, W., and Byrd, H. Threshold burning effects in distant microcirculation. *Arch. Surg.* 102:617, 1971.
31. Koepke, G. H. The role of physical medicine in the treatment of burns. *Surg. Clin. North Am.* 50:1385, 1970.
32. Leape, L. Initial changes in burn tissue in burned and unburned skin of rhesus monkeys. *J. Trauma* 10:450, 1970.
33. Loebl, E. C., Baxter, C. R., and Curreri, P. W. The mechanism of erythrocyte destruction in the early post burn period. *Ann. Surg.* 178:681, 1973.
34. Loebl, E. C., Marvin, J. A., Heck, E. L., Curreri, P. W., and Baxter, C. R. The use of quantitative biopsy cultures in bacteriologic monitoring of burn patients. *J. Surg. Res.* 16:1, 1974.
35. Lowenthal, R. M., Goldman, J. M., Buskard, N. A., Murphy, B. C., Grossman, L., Storring, R. A., Parks, D. S., Spiers, A. S. D., and Galton, D. A. G. Granulocyte transfusions in treatment of infections in patients with acute leukemia and aplastic anemia. *Lancet* 1:353, 1975.
36. MacMillan, B. G. Deep Excision and Early Grafting. In Polk, H., and Stone, H. H. (eds.), *Contemporary Burn Management.* Boston: Little, Brown, 1971. Pp. 357–365.
37. Marvin, J. A., Heck, E. L., Loebl, E. C., Curreri, P. W., and Baxter, C. R. Usefulness of blood cultures in confirming septic complications in burn patients: Evaluation of a new culture method. *J. Trauma* 15:657, 1975.
38. Mason, A. D., and Pruitt, B. Curling's Ulcer. In Lynch, J. B., and Lewis, S. R. (eds.), *Symposium on the Treatment of Burns.* St. Louis: Mosby, 1973. Vol. 5, pp. 79–81.
39. Mattsson, E. I. Psychological aspects of severe physical injury and its treatment. *J. Trauma* 15:217, 1975.
40. McCaffery, M. *Nursing Management of the Patient in Pain.* Philadelphia: Lippincott, 1972.
41. McCann, R. The oxyhemoglobin dissociation curve in acute disease. *Surg. Clin. North Am.* 55:627, 1975.
42. McDaniel, J. W. *Physical Disability and Human Behavior.* New York: Pergamon, 1969. P. 138.
43. Minshew, B., Holmes, R., Sanford, J., and Baxter, C. Transferrable resistance to tobramycin in *Klebsiella pneumoniae* and *Enterobacter cloacae* associated with enzymatic acetylation of tobramycin. *Antimicrob. Agents Chemother.* 6:492, 1974.

44. Monafo, W. W. The treatment of burn shock by the intravenous and oral administration of hypertonic lactated saline solution. *J. Trauma* 10:575, 1970.
45. Moncrief, J. A. Topical therapy. *Surg. Clin. North Am.* 50:1301, 1970.
46. Moncrief, J. A. Medical progress. *N. Engl. J. Med.* 288:444, 1973.
47. Moncrief, J. A. Burns. In Schwartz, S. T. (ed.), *Principles of Surgery.* New York: McGraw-Hill, 1974. Pp. 253–274.
48. Moncrief, J. A., Lindberg, R. B., Switzer, W. E., and Pruitt, B. A. Use of topical antibacterial therapy in the treatment of the burn wound. *Arch. Surg.* 92:558, 1966.
49. Moncrief, J. A., and Pruitt, B. A. The Massive Burn with Sepsis and Curling's Ulcer. In Hardy, J. P. (ed.), *Critical Surgical Illness.* Philadelphia: Saunders, 1971. Pp. 207–226.
50. Moritz, A. R., Henriques, F. C., and McLean, R. The effects of inhaled heat on the air passages and lungs: An experimental investigation. *Am. J. Pathol.* 21:311, 1945.
51. Moylan, J. A., Wellford, W. I., and Pruitt, B. A. Circulatory changes following circumferential extremity burns evaluated by the ultrasonic flowmeter: An analysis of 60 thermally injured limbs. *J. Trauma* 11:763, 1971.
52. Moylan, J., Wilmore, D., Mouton, D., and Pruitt, B. Early diagnosis of inhalation injury using ^{133}xenon long scan. *Ann. Surg.* 176:477, 1972.
53. Order, S. E., and Moncrief, J. A. *The Burn Wound.* Springfield, Ill.: Thomas, 1965.
54. Proctor, H. J., Fry, J., and Lennon, D. Pharmacologic increases in erythrocyte 2, 3-diphosphoglycerate for therapeutic benefit. *J. Trauma* 14:127, 1974.
55. Pruitt, B. A., Foley, F. D., and Moncrief, J. A. Curling's ulcer: A clinical pathology study of 323 cases. *Ann. Surg.* 172:523, 1970.
56. Pruitt, B. A., and Curreri, P. W. The Use of Homograft and Heterograft Skin. In Polk, H., and Stone, H. H. (eds.), *Contemporary Burn Management.* Boston: Little, Brown, 1971. Pp. 397–418.
57. Quinby, S., and Bernstein, N. Identity problems and the adaptation of nurses to severely burned children. *Am. J. Psychiatry* 128:58, 1971.
58. Saliba, J. J., Jr., Dempsey, W. C., and Krugyel, J. L. Large burns in humans: Treatment with heparin. *J.A.M.A.* 225:261, 1973.
59. Shires, C. T., Carrico, C. J., Baxter, C. R., Giesecker, A. H., Jr., and Jenkins, M. T. Early Resuscitation of Patients with Burns. In Welch, C. (ed.), *Advances in Surgery.* Chicago: Year Book, 1970. Vol. 4, pp. 308–324.
60. Shuck, J., Pruitt, B. A., and Moncrief, J. A. Homograft skin in wound coverage. *Arch. Surg.* 98:472, 1969.
61. Stone, H. H. Management of Respiratory Injury According to Clinical Phase. In Polk, H., and Stone, H. H. (eds.), *Contemporary Burn Management.* Boston: Little, Brown, 1971. Pp. 111–123.
62. Stone, H. H., Graber, C. D., and Martin, J. D. Evaluation of gamma globulin for prophylaxis against burn sepsis. *Surgery* 58:810, 1965.
63. Suter, P. M., Fairly, H. B., and Isenburg, M. D. Optimum end-expiratory airway pressure in patients with acute pulmonary failure. *N. Engl. J. Med.* 292:284, 1975.
64. Tanner, J. C., Vandeput, J., and Olley, J. F. The mesh skin graft. *Plast. Reconstruct. Surg.* 34:287, 1964.
65. Teplitz, C., Davis, D., Mason, A. D., Walker, H. L., Raulston, G. L., Mason, A. D., and Moncrief, J. A. Pseudomonas burn wound sepsis. I: Pathogenesis of experimental Pseudomonas burn wound sepsis. *J. Surg. Res.* 4:200, 1964.
66. Warden, G., Mason, A., and Pruitt, B. Evaluation of leukocyte chemotaxis in vitro in thermally injured patients. *J. Clin. Invest.* 54:1001, 1974.
67. Willis, B., Larson, D., and Abston, A. Positioning and splinting the burned patient. *Heart Lung* 2:696, 1973.
68. Wilmore, D. Energy Requirements of Seriously Burned Patients and the Influence of Caloric Intake on Their Metabolic Rate. In Cowan, G., and Scheetz, W. (eds.), *Intravenous Hyperalimentation.* Philadelphia: Lea & Febiger, 1972. Pp. 97–108.
69. Wilmore, D. W. Nutrition and metabolism following thermal injury. *Clin. Plast. Surg.* 1:603, 1974.
70. Wilmore, D. W., Curreti, P. W., Spitzer, K. W., Spitzer, M. E., and Pruitt, B. A. Supranormal dietary intake in thermally injured hypermetabolic patients. *Surg. Gynecol. Obstet.* 132:881, 1971.
71. Wilmore, D. W., Lindsey, C. A., and Moylan, J. A. Hyperglucagonemia following thermal injury: Insulin and glucagon in the posttraumatic catabolic state. *Lancet* 1:73, 1974.
72. Wilmore, D. W., Long, J. M., Mason, A. D., Skreen, B. S., and Pruitt, B. A. Catecholamines: Mediator of the hypermetabolic response to thermal injury. *Ann. Surg.* 180:653, 1974.
73. Zawacki, B. E., Spitzer, K. W., Mason, A. P., and Johns, L. A. Does increased evaporative water loss cause hypermetabolism in burn patients? *Ann. Surg.* 171:236, 1970.

chapter 16 Patients in Shock

Mary Ann Krol

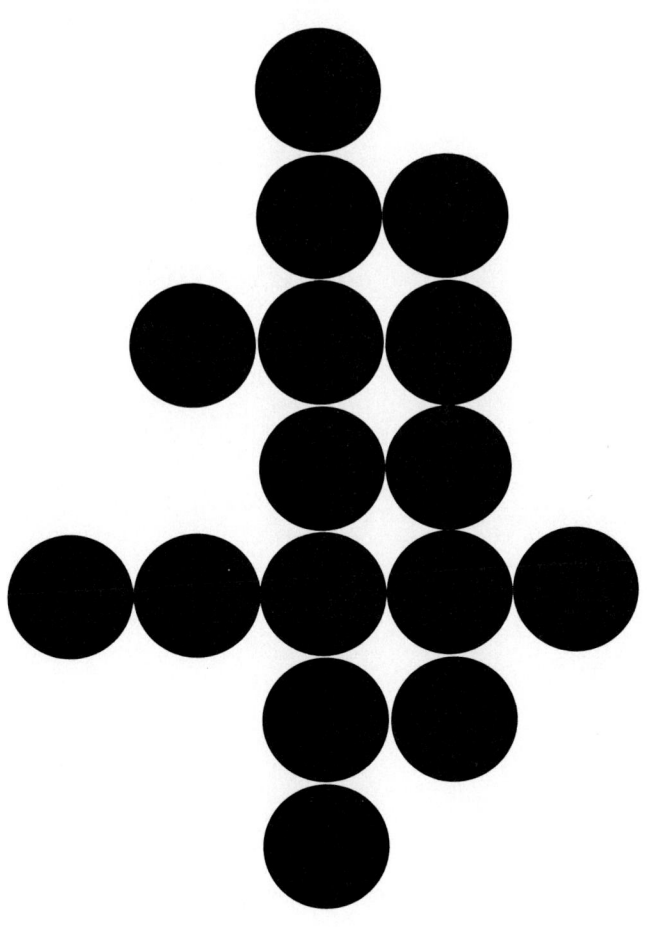

Shock is a state in which the lack of effective circulating blood volume results in reduced tissue perfusion and cellular hypoxia. The relative simplicity of this definition underestimates the complexity of the subject as well as the controversy that surrounds it.

A historical review of shock research illustrates some of the complexities of the subject. Shock has been described in the medical literature for two hundred years, but little systematic investigation of this entity was done until the beginning of the twentieth century. Until that time the treatment of shock utilized alcohol, strychnine, digitalis, and phlebotomy.

Studies at the turn of the century demonstrated that diminished venous return is a component of the shock state. By the end of World War I, physiologists and surgeons working at the battlefields attempted to relate hypotension to cardiac failure and decreased blood volume. Metabolic acidosis during shock was investigated. The use of vasopressors or vasodilator therapy was questioned [67]. Work in the field of shock advanced sporadically in the following years. Every subsequent war or new technologic development added momentum. Today, shock research is conducted internationally both in animal laboratories and in clinical research settings. Despite the exhaustive investigations, knowledge of the precise mechanism of shock has yet to be determined.

Many problems exist in shock research and in the clinical management of shock patients. The use of experimental animal models is not uniform, and it is not always clear which data from animal experiments can be transferred to human subjects. Clinical research experiments, similarly, are not uniform and have many uncontrollable variables. The sobering fact is that, despite treatment, many patients with prolonged hypotension will not survive. The survival rates for patients in shock secondary to sepsis or myocardial infarction have not improved in the past decade [39].

Since the cause of shock is not clearly understood, treatment remains controversial and variable. For example, after fifty years, the use of vasopressors or vasodilators is still debated. More recently the use of massive doses of steroids has been argued in the literature. These events illustrate that (1) controversy in the subject is the rule, (2) many knowledge gaps exist, and (3) clinically one can expect to see many variable forms of treatment for the same type of problem.

The nursing care of the patient in shock is managed in intensive care units in most institutions. The role of the nurse in other settings is not diminished, however; shock can occur in any setting and can be an acute complication of almost any disease. The nurse should be aware of the potential for shock in particularly vulnerable patients, such as the patient with a myocardial infarction, dehydration, infection, multiple injuries, trauma, or burns, and the postsurgical patient. Through astute observations the nurse can detect early or impending shock and thereby improve the patient's chance of survival, because the duration of shock is an important variable in survival. This vital role of all nurses in early detection, as well as the possibility of shock occurring to patients in all clinical situations, mandates that all nurses have a working knowledge of the pathophysiologic processes involved and of the signs and symptoms of shock and their significance in order to be able to initiate prompt and appropriate action.

Related Concepts of Anatomy and Physiology

The following paragraphs are a review of normal circulatory physiology. These concepts are basic to the understanding of the pathophysiology of shock and the compensatory mechanisms that take place during shock.

The circulatory system functions as the distributor of essential nutrients and oxygen to all body cells and as the remover of toxic waste products. This function is admirably achieved through a closed system of vessels in which no body cell is more than 20 to 30 microns away from the system. A liquid medium (blood) transports the materials and a pump (the heart) serves as the driving force. Thus the three essential components of the circulatory system: (1) the heart, (2) the blood, and (3) blood vessels are established. They function interdependently, each component affecting the function of the others.

CIRCULATORY SYSTEM COMPONENTS

The blood volume of the average 70-kg person is 5 liters. Blood cells compose 45 percent of this volume and plasma accounts for 55 percent. The blood volume is maintained at a relatively steady state. Any increase in blood volume increases the venous return to the heart, which increases the cardiac output and arterial pressure. Increased arterial pressure results in increased blood flow to the kidney with greater water excretion and a return of the blood volume to normal. The red blood cells comprise the greatest portion of the blood cell composition. An increase in the number of red blood cells increases the viscosity of the blood. The hematocrit value reflects the percentage of blood cells in whole blood. The plasma is similar to interstitial fluid, with the exception that plasma contains the plasma proteins albumin, globulin, and fibrinogen. These proteins remain in the vascular compartment and exert the colloid osmotic pressure that maintains capillary equilibrium.

The **heart** is a four-chambered hollow muscular organ that is capable of its own intrinsic beat. In addition, the heart is supplied by fibers from the sympathetic nervous system, which accelerate the heart rate and increase the strength of contraction, and parasympathetic fibers (vagus nerve), which decelerate the heart rate. The normal cardiac output is 5,000 ml per minute and is a measurement of the amount of blood pumped by the left ventricle per minute. It is the product of the stroke volume (amount of blood ejected with each contraction) times the heart rate. Cardiac output may vary from 3,000 ml per minute at rest to 35,000 ml per minute in a well-trained athlete during strenuous activity. The stroke volume is determined by the amount of venous return to the heart (Frank-Starling principle). The heart rate can be altered by sympathetic and parasympathetic stimulation. Cardiac output can be affected by many factors. For example, an increase in blood volume increases the venous return to the heart and results in increased cardiac output.

The cardiac index is a measurement of cardiac output per square meter of body surface and allows for comparative measurements between individuals of varying body sizes. Figure 16-1 depicts the normal cardiac index at varying ages.

The myocardium itself is supplied with blood via the coronary circulation. Approximately 4 to 5 percent of the cardiac output is coronary blood flow. The coronary vessels fill during diastole since blood flow through the myocardium is obstructed during systolic contraction. Sympathetic stimulation has a vasodilator effect on the coronary arteries.

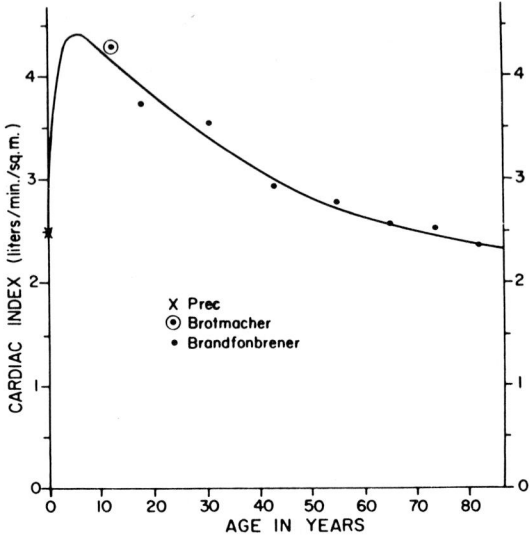

Figure 16-1
Cardiac index at different ages. [From A. C. Guyton, *Textbook of Medical Physiology* (4th ed.). Philadelphia: W. B. Saunders Company, 1971. Reproduced with permission.]

Blood flow through the coronary arteries is regulated by the nutrient demands of the myocardium [28].

The blood vessels subdivide the circulatory system into two segments: the **pulmonary circulation,** which circuits blood through the lungs; and the **systemic circulation,** which circuits blood through the remainder of the body. The circulation in the arteries and veins is the **macrocirculation** while that of the arterioles, capillaries, and venules is the **microcirculation.** The amount of blood in each segment of the circulatory vasculature is seen in Figure 16-2 [28].

The arteries are composed of three layers, consisting of an endothelial lining and a thick muscular layer interwoven with fibrous tissue. The thick musculature allows blood to flow through the vessel under pressure. Arterioles are 8 to 50 microns thick and have an endothelial lining; the musculature layer is much thinner. It is the contraction of the smooth muscle layer of the arteriole that provides a great part of the peripheral vascular resistance required to maintain blood pressure. Arterioles further subdivide into metarterioles, which give rise to capillaries. Each arteriole supplies 10 to 100 capillaries with blood [28].

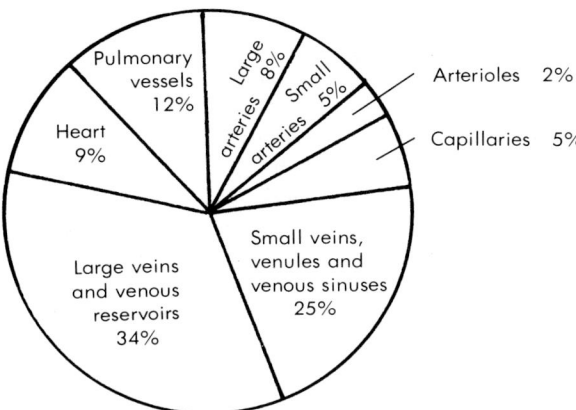

Figure 16-2
Percentage of total blood volume in each portion of the circulatory system. [From A. C. Guyton, *Textbook of Medical Physiology* (4th ed.). Philadelphia: W. B. Saunders Company, 1971. Reproduced with permission.]

The capillary wall is a single layer of endothelial cells. Capillaries usually are subdivided into preferential channels and true capillaries. The preferential channels are larger; the true capillaries are smaller. A smooth muscle fiber, the precapillary sphincter, encircles the capillary at the entrance to the true capillary. Some capillary beds, especially in the skin, ears, and hands, have arteriovenous channels that allow blood to be circulated to an area to exchange heat without going through nutritive channels. The functions of the circulatory system are accomplished at the capillary level, for it is here that exchange between the blood and the cells occurs. No exchange occurs at any other level. Blood flow is slowest through the capillaries since the capillaries, taken collectively, are the largest in diameter of all blood vessels [28]. This flow pattern is analogous to the flow in a river that suddenly widens. The capillaries comprise one of the largest organs in the body; their total length is estimated at 60,000 miles [76]. Blood flow through the capillaries is not continuous, but occurs in spurts; this action is called vasomotion. Not all capillary beds are open at any given time, but rather they close and open in response to the nutritional demands of the cells that surround them [28].

The venules are composed of a lining of endothelial cells and fibrous tissue, but they are still capable of contracting. Finally, the veins are composed of an inner layer of endothelial cells, covered by a fine muscle layer sheathed in fibrous tissue. All blood vessels are distensible; however, the veins are 6 to 10 times as distensible as arteries. With any rise in blood pressure veins are 24 times as compliant and can store large quantities of blood. Consequently, they are often referred to as capacitance vessels. As seen in Figure 16-2, the veins hold more than 50 percent of the blood in the circulatory system [28].

CIRCULATORY HEMODYNAMICS

Blood pressure (B.P.) is the force exerted by the blood against any unit area of vessel wall. It is the product of cardiac output times peripheral resistance. The latter, as mentioned before, is governed largely by the constriction of the arterioles.

Regulation of blood pressure is achieved by several mechanisms. Short-term regulation is accomplished by the baroreceptors located in the aortic arch and the carotid sinus. These detect changes in pressure, with stimulation of the vasomotor center in the medulla and a correction of the pressure toward normal. It is a negative feedback system in which a rise in pressure is corrected to lower the pressure and vice versa. The baroreceptors operate in the range of 60 to 200 mm Hg pressure. Chemoreceptors in the carotid and aortic bodies respond to reduced oxygen concentrations; however, they do not exert much control until the arterial pressure is in the 40 to 80 mm Hg range. The central nervous system ischemic response is powerful when the B.P. drops to 20 to 50 mm Hg. Long-term regulation of blood pressure is maintained primarily by kidney function [28].

Blood pressure decreases as the blood flows from the arterial to the venous side. As seen in Figure 16-3, blood pressure is greatly reduced as blood returns to the heart and the normal central venous pressure in the right atrium is 0 mm Hg [28].

Blood flow is the amount of blood that passes through any point in the circulation within any given unit of time. The amount of blood flow is regulated by the resistance in the vessels and the pressure gradient between both ends of the vessel. The amount of blood flow to any organ depends on its metabolic activity, not on its size. The brain,

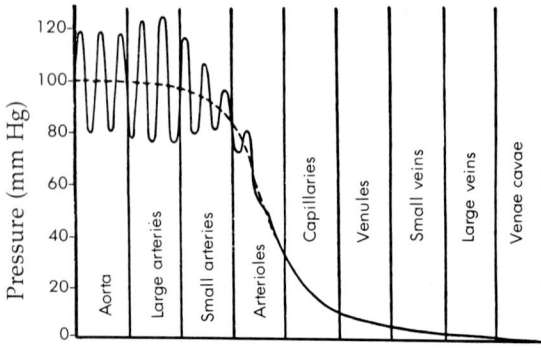

Figure 16-3
Blood pressures in the different portions of the systemic circulatory system. [From A. C. Guyton, *Textbook of Medical Physiology* (4th ed.). Philadelphia: W. B. Saunders Company, 1971. Reproduced with permission.]

which comprises less than 2 percent of the body weight, for example, requires 15 percent of the resting cardiac output (i.e., 750 ml per minute) [28].

In normal capillary function the quantity of fluid that leaves the capillary at the arterial end is equal to the quantity that returns at the venous end or through the lymphatics (Starling's law). Four forces that operate at this level to determine movement across the capillary membrane are

1. **Capillary pressure,** which is the force of the blood against the capillary wall, tends to drive fluid out of the capillary.
2. **Interstitial fluid pressure,** which is the pressure of the interstitial fluid between cell spaces, exerts a force that would tend to keep fluid in the capillary. For many reasons, however, it actually is a negative pressure and therefore tends to draw fluid out of the capillary.
3. **Interstitial fluid colloid osmotic pressure,** which is the osmotic force exerted by plasma proteins that escape from the capillary and tends to draw fluid out of the capillary.
4. **Plasma colloid osmotic pressure,** which is the osmotic force exerted by the plasma proteins albumin, globulin, and fibrinogen. It is the force which draws fluid into the capillaries at the venous end [28].

At the arterial end of the capillary, therefore, several forces work in a combined effort to push fluid out of the capillary. These various forces are the capillary pressure, the negative interstitial fluid pressure, and the interstitial fluid colloid osmotic pressure. The sum total of their combined force is 36.5 mm Hg.

A summary of the forces that operate at the capillary level is depicted in Table 16-1.

The force that tends to hold fluid in the capillary is the plasma colloid osmotic pressure, which is measured at 28 mm Hg. Therefore a pressure gradient of 8.5 mm Hg exists at the arterial end to push fluid out of the capillary.

The reverse occurs at the venous end of the capillary. The plasma colloid osmotic pressure remains the same at 28 mm Hg. The capillary pressure is reduced to 9 mm Hg since fluid was removed from the capillary as it traversed from the arterial to the venous side. The interstitial fluid pressure and the interstitial fluid colloid osmotic pressure remain the same. The net result is a pressure gradient of 7.5 mm Hg to draw fluid back into the capillary (Table 16-1). The 1 mm Hg pressure difference in gradients is accounted for by the accidental loss of plasma proteins through the capillary pores. These proteins are returned to the circulation via lymphatic drainage. This function of the lymphatics is so important that without the lymphatic system circulation would collapse within 24 hours. It can be appreciated from Table 16-1 that any change in the pressures operating at

Table 16-1
Summary of capillary forces*

Movement	Arterial end (mm Hg)	Venous end (mm Hg)
Out of capillary:		
Capillary pressure	25	9
Negative interstitial fluid pressure	7	7
Interstitial fluid colloid osmotic pressure	4.5	4.5
Total	36.5	20.5
Into capillary:		
Plasma colloid osmotic pressure	28	28
Exit gradient	8.5	
Reentry gradient		7.5

*Adapted from A. Guyton, *Textbook of Medical Physiology* (4th ed.). Philadelphia: Saunders, 1971.

the capillary level will alter the fluid exchange equilibrium. These alterations will be pointed out when various mechanisms that initiate shock are discussed.

Concept of Shock

Shock is not a disease entity or a syndrome of related symptoms. It is sometimes referred to as a clinical state, but this can imply a static condition, which is inaccurate. Shock is a dynamic body response to a life-threatening injury [67]. The life-threatening injury which may result in shock can occur at any age and which most often involves some insult to the circulatory system, whether it be loss of blood, failure of the heart, or vasodilatation of the blood vessels.

Whatever the injury, the body response follows the same pattern of sympathoadrenal stimulation. This response serves the initial function of maintaining blood flow to the vital organs (the heart and the brain) by causing extensive vasoconstriction of all the other vascular beds. If the injury is minor, this response corrects the situation. For example, withdrawal of blood for donation is essentially an injury to the circulatory system. The removal causes a sympathetic response which constricts the blood vessels, elevates the blood pressure, and maintains normal circulation [39]. If the injury is major, however, maintaining the sympathetic response becomes detrimental to the body. The intense vasoconstriction causes decreased tissue perfusion; the cells are not adequately oxygenated and must produce energy anaerobically, which in turn produces a metabolic acidosis. Essentially, the feedback systems become positive, that is, a decrease in blood flow causes a response to decrease it further. Eventually the cellular conditions become incompatible with life and the patient expires.

The severity of the injury is an important factor in the survival of shock patients. A rapid loss of blood gives the body little time to respond. The survival of patients with shock resulting from myocardial infarction is directly related to the extent of myocardial damage [12]. Time is another variable that affects survival in shock patients. Experimentally, dogs that are bled and then retransfused within 2 hours have a 10 percent mortality rate whereas dogs that are bled and retransfused after 4 hours have a 90 percent mortality rate [29]. The underlying disease process and the physical condition of the patient are also variables in shock. The patient who has latent coronary disease will be less capable of withstanding any myocardial hypoxia during the shock state, no matter what the original cause of the shock. The elderly patient with arteriosclerotic vessels will have a lesser response than young persons who have no vascular pathology [67].

Shock therefore is a dynamic body response to a life-threatening injury in which there is a lack of effective circulating blood volume, causing decreased tissue perfusion and cellular hypoxia. Variables that affect this response are severity of injury, duration of shock, and the original state of health. The shock state ensues when the body cannot sufficiently correct any hemodynamic derangements. Shock is a progressive state, as positive feedback mechanisms per se cause continuing deterioration.

Initiating Events Resulting in Shock

The number and variety of events and injuries that can result in shock is so large that a classification is required for clarification. The simplest classification used by many investigators is based on the circulatory component, which is affected by the initial defect or injury. Such a classification is seen in Table 16-2. Septic shock is added as a fourth category since its mechanism is so poorly understood that it would be misleading to classify it otherwise.

It should be reemphasized that eventually the same pathophysiologic process occurs in all types of shock. Labeling shock as cardiogenic, hypovolemic, neurogenic, or septic

Table 16-2
Classification of initiating events in shock

I. Hypovolemic	Marked loss of blood volume
II. Cardiogenic	Failure of the heart as a pump
III. Neurogenic	Vasodilatation and pooling of blood
IV. Septic	Possible vasodilatation, AV shunting, or primary cellular defect

HYPOVOLEMIC SHOCK

Hypovolemic shock is produced in conditions in which there is a marked decrease of the blood volume. As Table 16-3 indicates, more than 10 percent of the blood volume (assuming an original normal volume) is lost before symptoms of shock appear. The pathophysiologic mechanism is that blood volume loss results in decreased venous return to the heart and decreased cardiac output and tissue perfusion. Blood volume can be diminished by loss of whole blood through hemorrhage or loss of plasma from the vascular compartment. The latter situation occurs in burns and peritonitis.

Whole blood loss occurs frequently as a result of traumatic injury with severance of blood vessels or injury to the liver or spleen. Other common causes of hemorrhage are postpartal bleeding, carcinomas, and bleeding into a third space, such as the peritoneal or pelvic cavity. It should be clarified that intracranial bleeding does not produce enough hypovolemia to cause shock, because the amount required to do so is much greater than the amount that would cause increased intracranial pressure, brain displacement, and death. This fact has implications for the nurse who is observing and caring for a patient with apparent head injury. If there is decreased blood volume in such a patient, another source of internal hemorrhage must be investigated as a cause of hypovolemic shock.

Loss of plasma occurs in a variety of conditions that are not as obvious as gross hemorrhage. Plasma loss occurs in all burns or thermal injuries. The capillaries in the burned area are either damaged or become more permeable, allowing plasma to ooze into the area. The increased permeability results in greater loss of plasma proteins into the interstitial spaces. With the loss of plasma proteins the colloid osmotic force is decreased, resulting in less fluid return across the capillary membrane. The capillary equilibrium is disturbed with a net increase in fluid loss and

Table 16-3
Correlation of clinical findings and the magnitude of volume deficit in hemorrhagic shock[a]

Severity of shock	Clinical findings	% Reduction in blood volume
None	None; normal blood donation	Up to 10% (500 ml)[b]
Mild	Minimal tachycardia Slight decrease in blood pressure Mild evidence of peripheral vasoconstriction with cool hands and feet	15–25% (750–1,250 ml)
Moderate	Tachycardia 100–120 Decrease in pulse pressure Systolic blood pressure 90–100 mm Hg Restlessness Increased sweating Pallor Oliguria	25–35% (1,250–1,750 ml)
Severe	Tachycardia, over 120 Blood pressure below 60 per mm Hg systolic and frequently unobtainable by cuff Mental stupor Extreme pallor, cold extremities Anuria	Up to 50% (2,500 ml)

[a]Blood volume changes based on the clinical observations of Beecher et al.
[b]Based on a blood volume of 7 percent in a 70-kg male of medium build.
Source: M. Weil and H. Shubin, *Diagnosis and Treatment of Shock.* Baltimore: Williams & Wilkins Company, 1967.

subsequent decrease in blood volume. A similar loss of plasma proteins can occur as a result of nephrosis and acute kidney disease.

Any disease or pathologic condition that results in a depletion of body water can lead to hypovolemia. Prolonged vomiting and diarrhea (especially in infants or the elderly), heat exhaustion, diabetic acidosis, and adrenal insufficiency deplete body fluids to the extent that plasma fluid is drawn from the vascular compartment to the interstitial spaces with subsequent hypovolemia.

Certain types of venous obstruction lead to either a decreased venous return to the heart or a relative hypovolemia. For example, an enlarged uterus during pregnancy can obstruct the vena cava when the patient is in a supine position and produce shock. The symptoms fortunately can be relieved immediately by having the patient turn on her side, thus reestablishing circulation. Pulmonary embolism, if massive enough, will initially cause a decreased venous return to the left side of the heart in a similar manner.

Intestinal obstruction can lead to decreased blood volume because distention of the intestine results in a large amount of fluid loss through the capillary walls. This fluid loss may be the result of damage to the capillaries or increased resistance caused by collapsed venules, which produces an increase in hydrostatic pressure and net fluid loss [12]. Peritonitis also can cause a large amount of fluid loss and hypovolemia [16]. (Peritonitis is discussed on page 547.)

Crushing injuries frequently cause hypovolemia. One frequently hears of accident victims who were alert for many hours while pinned under objects but went into profound shock after obstructing objects were removed. The mechanism that produces shock in these instances is similar to that occurring in burns. The crushed capillaries are damaged but retain blood while pressure is exerted by the obstructing object. Once the object is removed, whole blood or plasma leaks into the interstitial spaces. The amount of blood loss is often difficult to determine. For example, the amount of blood that can be lost in a fractured hip can range from 800 to 2,000 ml. A case has been reported of an elderly man with crushing injuries of both legs who required 8,000 ml of blood before adequate blood volume was restored [42].

Hypovolemic shock is also called traumatic, hemorrhagic, or surgical shock, which delineates the cause further. In all initiating events, the loss of blood volume reduces the venous return to the heart, which in turn diminishes cardiac output and tissue perfusion.

Hypovolemic shock is relatively common in the United States because of the high accident rate. Treatment results in a good prognosis if the variables of duration, severity, and previous diseases are within realistic limitations. The experiences in the Korean and Vietnam conflicts demonstrated that survival could be improved significantly in traumatic shock when prompt and adequate treatment was instituted. This principle of prompt and adequate treatment also applies in civilian situations. When first-aid measures to control bleeding and maintain patent airways are instituted immediately and there is rapid transfer to emergency room settings for appropriate and intensive treatment, survival is facilitated.

Hypovolemia frequently becomes a complication of other types of shock. Hypovolemia occurs in approximately 20 percent of patients in cardiogenic shock as a result of diuretic therapy and inadequate fluid intake [69]. The patient in septic shock also has alterations in capillary dynamics which result in hypovolemia.

CARDIOGENIC SHOCK

Cardiogenic shock occurs in any disease or situation in which the heart fails to pump sufficient blood to maintain tissue perfusion and oxygenation. Approximately 20 percent of the individuals who suffer myocardial infarction develop cardiogenic shock. The ischemic damage to the myocardium decreases the stroke volume and cardiac output. The extent of the myocardial damage correlates positively with the incidence of cardiogenic shock, which usually occurs when 40 percent of the myocardium is damaged [12, 52]. Congestive heart failure can develop into cardiogenic shock. Uncorrected arrhythmias may also severely damage the heart's pumping ability.

Cardiogenic shock is a significant complication of open heart surgery and is referred to as the **low output syndrome.** Among the causes of this syndrome are (1) prolonged extracorporeal circulation, (2) ventricular fibrillation, (3) myocardial hypoxia due to cross clamping of the aorta, (4) coronary microemboli, (5) prosthetic valve failure, and (6) associated coronary disease [12].

Cardiogenic shock is encountered frequently today due to both the rising incidence of myocardial infarcts and the improved treatment of previously fatal arrhythmias. The mortality rate for patients in cardiogenic shock is approximately 80 percent and has not changed in the past decade despite the improvement in treatment modalities [39]. Cardiogenic shock may at times be superimposed upon other types of shock. A patient with initial profound hypovolemia or sepsis eventually will have insufficient coronary blood flow and resultant myocardial damage.

NEUROGENIC SHOCK

Neurogenic shock occurs in conditions in which insufficient vasomotor tone results in widespread vasodilatation. Vasodilatation produces an increased capacity of the vascular bed with decreased systemic pressure and causes inadequate venous return to the heart, decreased cardiac output, and inadequate tissue perfusion. Therefore the shock in this instance may be normovolemic, in that "normal" amounts of blood are available, but are incapable of filling the increased vascular capacity.

The term **neurogenic** refers to a loss of vasomotor tone caused by decreased activity of the vasomotor center in the medulla. **Vasogenic** refers to vasodilatation caused by factors operating on the blood vessels locally. Neurogenic shock can result from high cervical injury. The vasomotor tone mediated through the sympathetic nerves is lost at the level of injury. High spinal anesthesia can produce neurogenic shock on the same basis. Severe brain damage with loss of the medullary vasomotor center produces neurogenic shock also.

Insulin shock operates basically on the same mechanism. Inadequate blood glucose affects the function of the vasomotor center, and the typical signs of shock appear. Fainting is another form of neurogenic shock resulting from vasodilatation [28]. Severe pain can produce shock by inhibition of the vasomotor center, again resulting in massive vasodilatation. Barbiturate, narcotic, and tranquilizer overdoses also produce vasodilatation, although the mechanism is not clearly understood [60].

Although not central in origin, shock can be produced on the basis of vasodilatation by rapid removal of fluid from the peritoneal cavity of a patient with ascites or rapid removal of urine from a greatly distended bladder. The abdominal veins, having been compressed by the additional fluid, enlarge with rapid change in pressure and the available blood volume is inadequate to fill the system; shock ensues [28].

Neurogenic shock occurs less frequently than the other forms of shock. Treating the primary cause is the goal of therapy in neurogenic shock. For example, insulin shock is treated by the administration of glucose. Neurogenic shock resulting from severe pain is treated by the use of analgesics to relieve the pain. Little can be done for shock resulting from brain damage. **Vasogenic shock** is similar to neurogenic shock, and differs only insofar as the cause of vasodilatation occurs at the blood vessel level and not the vasomotor center. The most significant form of vasogenic shock is anaphylactic shock, which is the end result of a violent antigen-antibody response in a sensitized individual. It is produced by the release of four substances: (1) **histamine,** which causes arteriolar dilatation and increased capillary permeability, (2) **serotonin,** which causes venular constriction and increased capillary permeability, (3) **slow-reacting substance** (SRS), which causes bronchiolar constriction, and (4) **bradykinin,** which causes vasodilatation and increased capillary permeability. The massive vasodilatation and increased capillary permeability cause a decreased venous return to the heart, decreased cardiac output, and decreased tissue perfusion. The onset of the reaction is often only minutes after exposure to the antigen. Penicillin, foreign sera, pollen extracts, vaccines, iodides, and local anesthetics are some common antigens that cause anaphylactic shock. The course of anaphylactic shock is often too rapid to produce any cellular changes. If the victim is fortunate enough to receive immediate medical treatment, rapid infusion of epinephrine, antihistamines, bronchodilators, and anti-inflammatory drugs can be life-saving [6]. Prevention is a more substantial approach. Patients should always be informed of what medication they are to receive prior to administration; allergic tendencies should be determined prior to any treatment. Similarly, depending on the substances to be injected, test doses may be indicated. Individuals with a history of allergic responses should wear Medic-Alert bracelets or medallions or carry Medic-Alert cards.

SEPTIC SHOCK

Septic shock most often occurs as a result of bacteremia caused by gram-negative bacteria. It can be caused by gram-positive bacteria, but the incidence of this type of septic shock is much lower [42]. The incidence of gram-negative sepsis has increased 5 to 8 times in the past twenty years [15] and almost equals trauma and myocardial infarction as a cause of shock [39]. It was not described clinically until 1951 [42, 39]. Some investigators attributed its increased frequency to the promiscuous use of antibiotics that are more effective against gram-positive bacteria and therefore have allowed gram-negative bacteria to proliferate.

In some studies, 25 to 30 percent of the patients with bacteremia develop septic shock [42, 74]. The patient is usually over 45 years of age and has one of the following predisposing conditions: (1) indwelling urinary catheter, (2) previous gastrointestinal or genitourinary surgery, (3) peritonitis, (4) urinary tract infection, or (5) chronic or acute debilitating disease such as neoplasms or diabetes [15, 42, 74]. Intravenous infusions, piggyback intravenous administration, and indwelling venous catheters have also been implicated with increasing frequency as a cause of hospital-acquired bacteremia [30]. Women with septic abortions or postpartal infections are also particularly susceptible. The mortality rate of patients in septic shock is approximately 60 percent.

The pathophysiologic mechanisms that initiate septic shock are elusive and the most formidable challenge in shock research. Two factors predominate: (1) the physiologic changes resulting from the release of endotoxin, and (2) the effects of living bacteria [39].

These factors will be explained later in this chapter. Ultimately they lead to the same cellular problems that are present in cardiogenic or hypovolemic shock.

Septic shock resulting from gram-positive bacteria is produced by the effect of an exotoxin. The circulatory result is similar to that in gram-negative shock. As is true with other types of shock, septic shock can occur in the progression of hypovolemic or cardiogenic shock. With decreased tissue perfusion and inadequate cellular oxygenation, the reticuloendothelial system fails. Bacteria are released from the intestine into the bloodstream, resulting in sepsis, because the reticuloendothelial system is unable to detoxify endotoxins released by the gram-negative organisms.

In summary, many singular or multiple events and diseases may initiate the dynamic response of shock. Hypovolemic, cardiogenic, neurogenic, and septic are terms that indicate the component of the vascular system in which the primary defect occurred. As shock progresses and multiple organs begin to fail, these terms lose their significance since all circulatory components will be affected.

The Pathophysiology of Shock

The observation of a Harvard surgeon in 1895 accurately illustrates the classic symptoms of the patient in shock [42]:

A patient is brought into the hospital with a compound comminuted fracture . . . , where the bleeding has been slight. As the litter is gently deposited on the floor he makes no effort to move or look about him. He lies staring at the surgeon with an expression of complete indifference as to his condition. There is no movement of the muscles of the face; the eyes, which are deeply sunken in their sockets, have a weird, uncanny look. The features are pinched and the face shrunken. A cold, clammy sweat exudes from the pores of the skin, which has an appearance of profound anaemia. The lips are bloodless and the fingers and nails are blue. The pulse is almost imperceptible; a weak, thread-like stream may, however, be detected in the radial artery. The thermometer, placed in the rectum, registers 96° or 97° F. The muscles are not paralyzed anywhere, but the patient seems disinclined to make any muscular effort. Even respiratory movements seem for the time to be reduced to a minimum. Occasionally the patient may feebly throw about one of his limbs and give vent to a hoarse, weak groan. There is no insensibility . . . , but he is strangely apathetic, and seems to realize but imperfectly the full meaning of the questions put to him. It is of no use to attempt an operation until appropriate remedies have brought about a reaction. The pulse, however, does not respond; it grows feebler and finally disappears, and "this momentary pause in the act of death" is soon followed by the grim reality. A post-mortem examination reveals no visible changes in the internal organs.

The description above points out some of the classic symptoms of patients in shock: apprehension or apathy, tachycardia, cold clammy skin, and muscular weakness. Other common symptoms not specifically described are decreased urine output and hypotension. These symptoms occur from the initial sympathoadrenal response to injury and can be easily understood. What is not clearly understood is why the patient died and why the postmortem examination revealed no visible changes. These two questions have consumed the energies of shock researchers for the past half century.

Some of the pathophysiologic mechanisms that occur in shock have been elucidated to some degree. The body's initial response to injury is one of sympathoadrenal stimulation with negative feedback systems maintaining homeostasis. The continued sympathetic stimulation, however, becomes detrimental and results in positive feedback systems operating on two levels: (1) the microcirculation and (2) the cell. These body responses will now be explained in greater detail.

SYMPATHOADRENAL RESPONSE

The initiating event in hypovolemic, cardiogenic, or neurogenic shock results in a decreased venous return to the heart and a subsequent decrease in cardiac output. The decrease in cardiac output triggers a response by the baroreceptors in the aortic arch and carotid sinus that initiates the sympathoadrenal response. In this body response to stress, catecholamines (epinephrine and norepinephrine) are released from the adrenal medulla, while additional norepinephrine is released from the postganglionic fibers of the sympathetic nervous system. The epinephrine primarily stimulates the beta receptors of the sympathetic nervous system, causing an increase in the myocardial contractility (inotropic effect) and in the heart rate (chronotropic effect). Alpha receptors in the periphery are located primarily in the precapillary sphincters; when stimulated, they increase the arterial blood pressure. Such an effect occurs from the stimulation of norepinephrine, which causes intense vasoconstriction in almost all vascular beds, except the cerebral and coronary beds. The net effect of the sympathoadrenal response is to increase peripheral resistance and the effectiveness of the heart.

Venous vasoconstriction also occurs as a result of norepinephrine stimulation. The capacitance vessels, which normally store large amounts of blood, now release the blood into the circulation and concomitantly augment the blood volume.

The sympathoadrenal response also increases the blood volume by transcapillary filling. Arteriolar and venous vasoconstriction lowers intracapillary pressure, causing a net influx of fluid into the vascular compartment since the other factors that influence fluid movement across the capillary membrane remain unchanged. A common example of the compensatory mechanism of transcapillary filling is the restoration of normal blood volume following blood donation [39]. The sympathoadrenal response thus causes an increase in peripheral resistance, in the heart rate and contractile force, and also in blood volume by the addition of stored blood from the venous reservoir and transcapillary influx of interstitial fluid.

The hemodynamic adjustments resulting from the shock episode stimulate the production of four hormones: angiotensin II, aldosterone, antidiuretic hormone, and cortisol. The decreased blood flow to the kidney causes a stimulation of the juxtaglomerular apparatus releasing renin. Renin catalyzes the conversion of angiotensinogen to angiotensin I, which is then converted to angiotensin II. The latter effects an increase in vasoconstriction and stimulation of the hormone aldosterone. Aldosterone secretion by the adrenal cortex results in retention of sodium ions and water and is a mechanism to increase blood volume.

Antidiuretic hormone production is stimulated by changes in the plasma osmolarity (detected by osmoreceptors in the hypothalamus), decreased left atrial filling, and increased baroreceptor firing [42, 67]. This hormone increases reabsorption of water by the distal tubules of the kidney and thereby increases intravascular volume. ACTH secretion, which occurs within seconds of the onset of circulatory failure, stimulates cortisol production. In addition to the carbohydrate metabolism stabilizing effect and anti-inflammatory properties, cortisol also exerts a positive inotropic effect to augment cardiac output [46].

The total body response to this point reflects negative-feedback functioning in which homeostasis is maintained. These responses are depicted graphically in Figure 16-4. For example, a decrease in arterial pressure produces a response to increase arterial pressure. A decrease in blood volume stimulates responses to increase blood volume.

The initial response of sympathoadrenal stimulation is beneficial to the organism only in the early stages of shock. There is practically universal agreement that continued sympathetic stimulation is detrimental to the patient, causing shock to be progressive and irreversible with time. **Irreversible** indicates that the state of shock has progressed to a point at which death is inevitable despite all treatment and even if circulatory homeostasis is restored. The body response becomes one of positive feedback, which consistently increases the circulatory defect [67]. Experimentally it is possible to produce shock in animals simply by injecting large doses of epinephrine and norepinephrine [39]. This fact is the basis for understanding the poten-

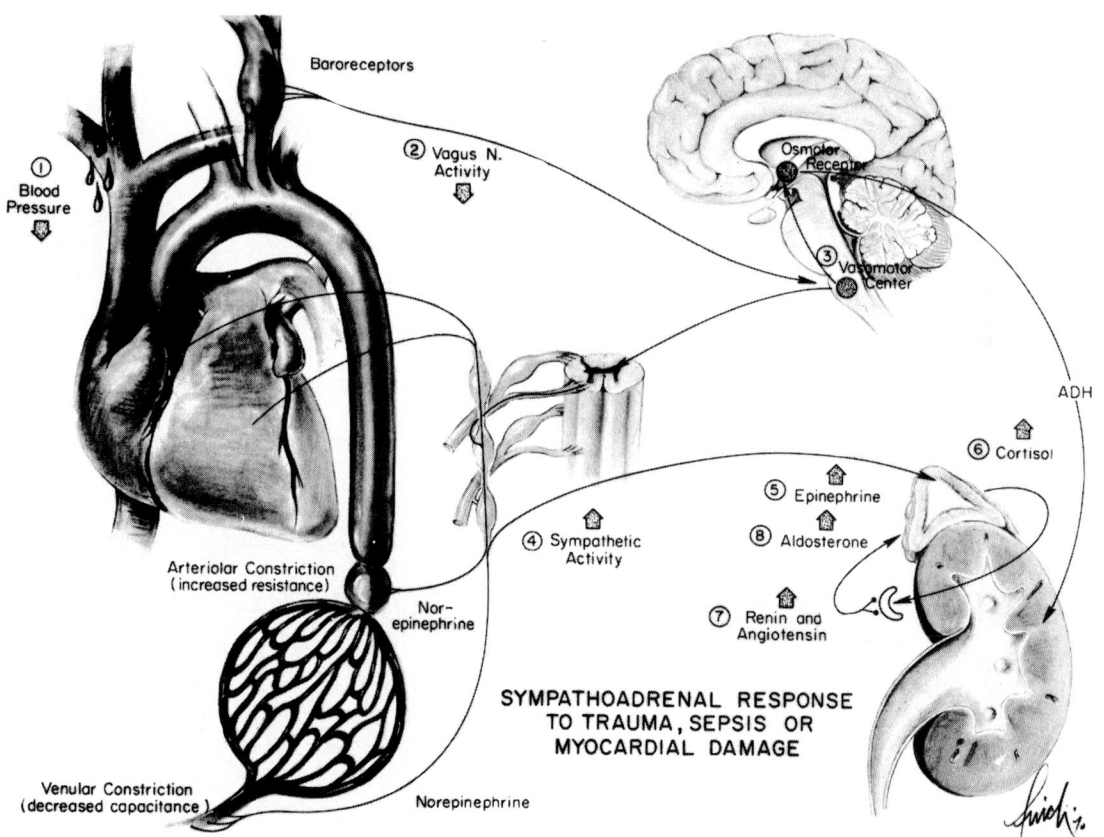

Figure 16-4
Sympathoadrenal response to trauma, sepsis, or myocardial damage. [From S. I. Schwartz (ed.), *Principles of Surgery* (2nd ed.). Copyright © 1974 by McGraw-Hill Book Company. Used with permission of McGraw-Hill Book Company.]

tial dangers of the prolonged use of vasopressor drugs in the treatment of shock, particularly in the absence of an adequate blood volume.

CHANGES IN MICROCIRCULATION

The constant vasoconstriction of the arterioles and venules resulting from the increased catecholamines decreases blood flow in the microcirculation. Consequently the cells do not receive sufficient oxygen or nutrients, which results in a state of ischemic anoxia [39]. The energy metabolism of the cells becomes predominantly anaerobic with an increase in lactic acid production. The pH environment surrounding the cells becomes acidotic and causes the arterioles to dilate. The venules, however, remain constricted. The blood is able to enter the microcirculation but is unable to exit, and a state of stagnant anoxia ensues. There is no complete explanation as to why the venules remain constricted after the arterioles dilate. It has been postulated that the venules fail to respond to the lower pH because they have adapted to these conditions normally, since venous blood has a higher lactic acid content and lower pH [39].

Stagnant anoxia mediates other changes. The hemodynamic pressure is increased and plasma fluid escapes into the interstitial spaces with edema formation. The capillary wall itself is damaged by anoxia, allowing plasma proteins to be lost into the interstitial spaces with an additional loss of plasma. The states of ischemic and stagnant anoxia are depicted in Figure 16-5.

Tissue acidosis and slow blood flow provide the basis for the development of disseminated intravascular clotting (DIC). This syndrome, which may also complicate a variety

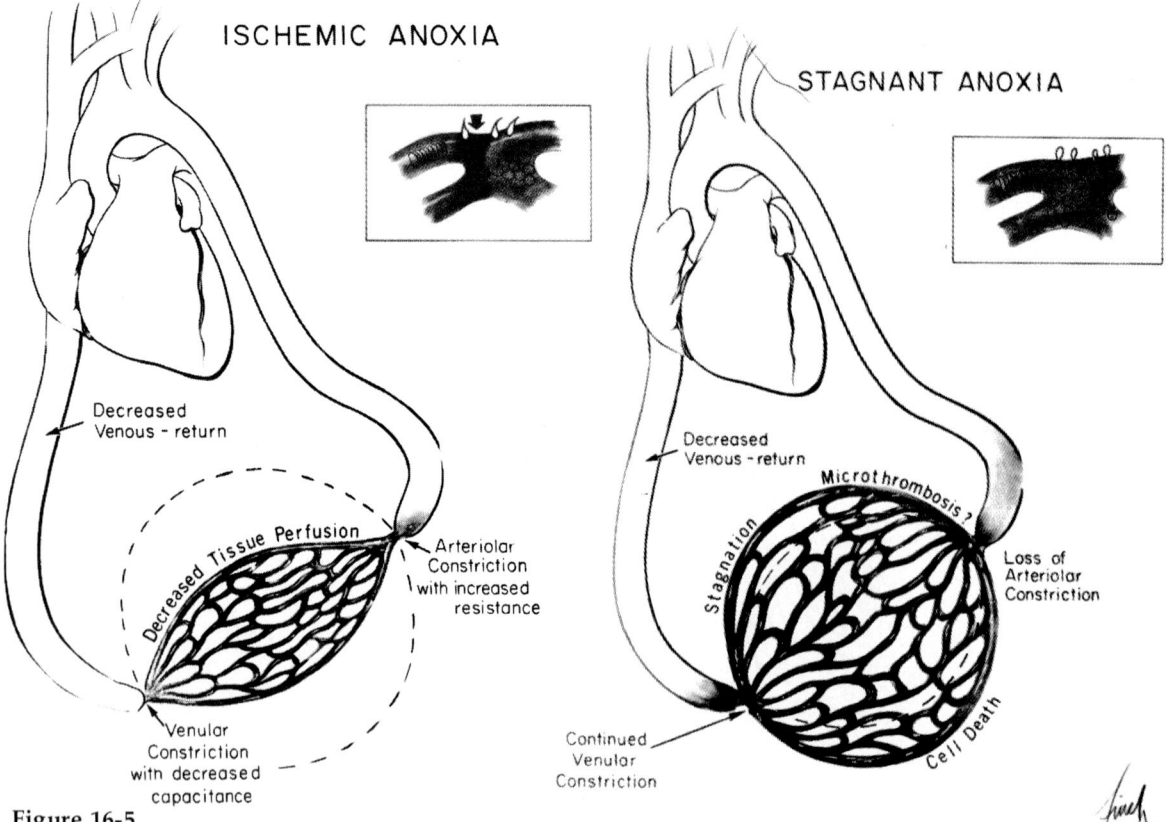

Figure 16-5
States of ischemic and stagnant anoxia. [From S. I. Schwartz (ed.), *Principles of Surgery* (2nd ed.). Copyright © 1974 by McGraw-Hill Book Company. Used with permission of McGraw-Hill Book Company.]

of other clinical disorders, is characterized by the inappropriate initiation of the clotting process in large segments of the capillary bed.

There are two major initiating factors, capillary stasis and hypercoagulability. Disseminated intravascular coagulation occurs more frequently in septic and traumatic shock than in other types of shock. Depending on other factors operant in the individual situation, the patient may have a minor episode and recover. If excessive clotting occurs, the clotting factors in the blood are consumed and the patient begins to hemorrhage. Bleeding occurs from the mucous membranes, gastrointestinal tract, or from any recent surgical wound [18, 30, 67]. The onset of DIC indicates a poor prognosis for the patient in shock. (DIC is also discussed on page 463.)

CELLULAR RESPONSE

The normal cell produces energy in the form of adenosine triphosphate (ATP) primarily from the metabolism of glucose. Fatty acids and amino acids can also be metabolized for energy production. ATP maintains the functions required for cellular life such as energy transport systems, protein synthesis, and enzyme production.

The breakdown of nutrients for energy occurs along two pathways. The first pathway is anaerobic (glycolytic) and does not require oxygen. Approximately 10 percent of the cell's energy requirements are produced in this sequence. The glycolytic process occurs in the cytoplasm of the cell and ends in the formation of pyruvate from the breakdown of glucose. Pyruvate enters the second energy pathway, the citric acid cycle (Krebs cycle), which occurs in the mitochondria. Here the pyruvate is converted into acetyl coenzyme A, and through a long series of breakdown reactions releases energy with carbon dioxide and water remaining. The citric acid cycle is aerobic and produces approximately 90 percent of the cell's energy requirements [39, 57].

In inadequate oxygenation, pyruvate cannot be degraded in the Krebs cycle and the energy supply of the cells must be maintained by the anaerobic pathway. The pyruvate is combined with hydrogen ions, which are released in the glycolytic process to form lactic acid, which diffuses out of the cell and into the surrounding interstitial fluid. The lactic acid gains access to the circulatory system and produces metabolic acidosis. The respiratory center in the medulla is stimulated by the acid environment, causing increased respirations and a compensatory respiratory alkalosis. Eventually all the body buffer systems are exhausted and acidosis ensues.

The release of catecholamines and cortisol during shock also stimulates the release of fatty acids for energy production. The degradation of the fatty acids produces substantial quantities of ketones, which are normally oxidized in the liver. In hypoperfusion, the liver is not able to fulfill this function adequately and the metabolic acidosis is increased [57].

Without sufficient energy production, normal cellular function cannot be maintained. The cell membrane transport systems begin to falter with the consequent release of potassium ions out of the cell and influx of sodium and water into the cell. Protein synthesis diminishes, being affected by both the decreased energy supply and the low intracellular potassium. Immunoprotein production is decreased and the immune system also begins to fail. Lastly, it is believed that vasoactive substances are released into the circulation from damaged cells. The substances generally considered to be released are histamine, serotonin, and bradykinin.

Histamine, which is present in all body tissue, exerts a vasodilator effect on arterioles and venules and increases tissue permeability. **Serotonin** is found chiefly in platelets, gastrointestinal tissue, and brain cells. It also can exert a vasodilator or vasoconstrictor effect. **Bradykinin** belongs to a group of body substances known as kinins. The kinins are polypeptides that are released from the alpha globulin molecules by the action of a proteolytic enzyme. In the case of bradykinin, the enzyme is kallikrein. Bradykinin is one of the most potent vasodilator substances known. Recent research indicates that it may be excreted through the lungs while angiotensin II is formed in the pulmonary tissue.

It is generally agreed that these substances are released during septic and anaphylactic shock as a result of the antigen-antibody reaction that occurs. Their release in other types of shock is more controversial. Some investigators believe that the lysosome membrane integrity is disturbed as a result of prolonged anoxia and acidosis, so that enzymes are released and give rise to vasoactive substances. Others postulate that prolonged ischemia depresses the reticuloendothelial system. Gram-negative bacteria are liberated from the intestines into the general circulation and the reaction becomes identical to septic shock. According to this theory, all prolonged shock would eventually be septic.

Experimentally a myocardial depressant factor, which is released from the pancreas during ischemia, has been isolated. It is believed to be a factor in the cause of myocardial failure in irreversible shock [38].

Decreasing cellular function is reflected in the multiple organ failure that occurs in the progression of shock. The multiple organ failure compounds the existing problems. Renal ischemia and diminished function of the kidneys increase the acidosis. Decreased hepatic function diminishes protein, fat, and glucose metabolism as well as the integrity of the reticuloendothelial system. Intestinal ischemia allows release of bacteria into the bloodstream. Pulmonary function is reduced by edema formation, resulting in arteriovenous shunting. Acidosis and cellular hypoxia eventually depress myocardial functioning and death ensues. Some of the sequences described in the pathophysiologic progression remain to be validated sufficiently in clinical research. The theories, however, provide a model on which to base therapy [30, 39, 42, 57, 67, 68, 72].

DYNAMICS OF SEPTIC SHOCK

While it is clear that the initiating events of cardiogenic, hypovolemic, and neurogenic shock lead to either reduced venous return or impaired myocardial function, the precise mechanism that leads to septic shock is unclear. Some of the confusion exists because septic shock (endotoxic) as produced experimentally in animals does not correlate with septic shock in man [39]. Generally two types of septic shock have been described in humans. In the hyperdynamic type, the patient has a high cardiac output, high central venous pressure, and low peripheral resistance with warm, dry extremities. Urine output remains good, and the patient's sensorium remains clear. The hypodynamic type of septic shock presents a picture similar to hypovolemic shock with low cardiac output, high peripheral resistance, and decreased kidney output [15, 42, 67]. Experiments with animals produced only the hypodynamic syndrome. The missing factor apparently was the effect of the living bacteria on circulation. When this was added to the experimental model, which had used endotoxin from dead bacteria, the circulatory dynamics between humans and experimental animals were more uniform [39].

As is presently conceived by most authorities, two factors operate in septic shock. The **first factor** is the effect of endotoxin liberated from dead bacteria. This endotoxin combines with the serum globulins or antibodies and activates the complement system, which in turn releases epinephrine, norepinephrine, histamine, and serotonin. The release of epinephrine and norepinephrine causes the sympathoadrenal response similar to that in other forms of shock with consequent microcirculatory changes [39]. The **second factor** postulated is the effect of living bacteria on the circulation. Bacteria in the infected area react with the damaged tissue with the release of kinin. Kinin causes widespread vasodilatation in the area. As a result a large amount of fluid may be sequestered in the area, causing hypovolemia [57]. It also appears that the blood flow through the area does not follow the course of nutritive channels but of arteriovenous shunts [39]. It is now known that serotonin may cause some primary cellular disturbance in which normal oxidative reactions in the mitochondria cannot take place [57]. The increased blood flow through the inflamed areas in addition to low peripheral resistance from vasodilatation may account for the phenomenon of increased cardiac output [31, 67].

It is not known why some patients in septic shock exhibit the hyperdynamic state for several days before becoming hypodynamic, or why others remain in the hyperdynamic state until death [39]. It is also unclear what causes the conversion from bacteremia to septic shock.

The progression of septic shock is similar to the mechanisms of the other types of shock in terms of the microcirculatory changes and cellular metabolic derangements. There is considerable controversy, however, about the mechanism of the initiating sequence and the high cardiac output syndrome. Finally, the initial pathophysiologic response in shock is sympathoadrenal stimulation, which augments blood volume, improves cardiac function, and produces vasoconstriction. If the basic cause is not corrected, however, this response becomes detrimental and leads to cellular hypoxia, acidosis, and multiple organ failure.

Assessment of the Patient

Shock is a clinically dynamic state in which the patient's condition is constantly changing either in the direction of progressive deterioration or of improvement. The very nature of the disorder dictates that the observations and assessments of the patient must be made continuously and must encompass a wide range of physiologic measurements, since the entire organism is affected. Constant monitoring of the patient is necessary to detect these changes and to determine the need for alterations in interventions and treatments. The nurse often functions in the role of primary observer of the patient. Accurate observations are based on an understanding of the pathophysiology involved, that is, one must know what to look for. Similarly, monitoring data that are essential for adequate assessment of the patient has value only if the data are accurate and properly evaluated. The nurse's role in assessment of the patient is discussed in greater detail later in this chapter.

In general, assessment of the patient's status can be divided into two general areas: (1) noninvasive assessments made by observation of the patient or with simple monitoring equipment and (2) invasive assessments made after withdrawal of blood or entrance into the circulatory system via catheters or other instruments.

NONINVASIVE ASSESSMENTS

Respirations

Initially the patient in shock will have an increased respiratory rate as a result of sympathoadrenal stimulation with its subsequent increased metabolic rate. Pain and anxiety may also cause hyperventilation. As the patient develops metabolic acidosis, a compensating respiratory alkalosis is produced. In advanced shock, the patient may have a respiratory acidosis with diminished respiratory work. The general muscular weakness associated with shock often makes respiratory excursion ineffective. It should be remembered that tachypnea is an early sign in septic shock and a direct effect of endotoxin on the respiratory center [15]. The respiratory rate and the quality of the respirations should be measured continuously. Changes in the quality or rate of respirations will dictate the need for further evaluation (e.g., the measurement of arterial blood gases), as well as the need for intubation, oxygenation, or other interventions.

Pulse

An increased pulse rate is often an early sign of shock and is an effect of increased circulating epinephrine. Generally the pulse rate in shock is increased, but a bradycardia can also occur as a reflex secondary to increased cardiac output. In addition, medications used in the treatment of shock may alter the heart rate in either direction. Beta-adrenergic drugs such as isoproterenol can increase the heart rate, even over the rate of 160 beats per minute. A persistent tachycardia is a poor prognostic sign [26].

The quality of the pulse also reflects the circulatory status. A thready pulse in the peripheral vessels indicates vasoconstriction and reflects decreased cardiac output. If vasoconstriction is intense, the peripheral pulses may be absent. On the other hand, a bounding pulse can indicate overload during fluid administration. The pulse rate may be measured via monitor oscilloscopes; however, the quality of the pulse must be assessed also, by direct palpation, and evaluated at other sites, such as in the carotid, femoral, and radial arteries. A comparative apical-radial rate is measured at intervals to determine whether there is a pulse deficit.

Arterial Blood Pressure

Use of blood pressure as an assessment measurement is controversial and often misunderstood. In the first place, hypotension is a late sign of shock and indicates lack of compensation in the circulatory system. The effects of norepinephrine initially keep the arterial blood pressure elevated. Second, a drop in blood pressure must be considered in relation to the patient's normal pressure. A patient whose normal pressure, for example, is 190/120 may well be in shock with a pressure of 130/90. Similarly, individuals who normally have a lower range of blood pressure may tolerate blood pressures below 90 systolic. Generally, a systolic pressure of 70 mm Hg is considered minimal, and most adults would be considered hypotensive with a systolic reading below 90 mm Hg [33]. Third, an adequate arterial pressure does not guarantee tissue perfusion. The blood pressure can be normal; however, if the microcirculation is in a state of stagnant anoxia or if multiple capillary beds are clotted, the cells will not receive nutrients or oxygen, and the state of shock will progress despite normal blood pressure. The use of a sphygmomanometer to evaluate blood pressure in shock patients is not reliable. The peripheral vasoconstriction makes it difficult to obtain accurate readings. Studies have demonstrated wide discrepancies between pressure measurements made with a sphygmomanometer and an intra-arterial line [69]. Measurements of arterial pressure may be made as frequently as every 2 to 15 minutes, especially when vasopressor drugs are being initiated or discontinued.

Emphasis has been placed on the systolic blood pressure in the past, but it is also important to note the pulse pressure when evaluating blood pressure measurements. As cardiac output decreases, there is generally a corresponding fall in the pulse pressure.

Electrocardiogram

An ECG tracing is not ordinarily used to initially diagnose shock; however, ECG readings are important in the continued monitoring of the patient. Patients in cardiogenic shock following myocardial infarction are vulnerable to a wide range of arrhythmias. In other types of shock, patients can develop arrhythmias as a result of acidosis, hyperkalemia, or hypokalemia, which occur with cellular metabolic derangements. Arrhythmias must be diagnosed promptly since they can be rapidly fatal.

Urine Output

One of the earliest signs of shock is a decrease in urine output below 30 ml per hour. The vasoconstrictor effect of norepinephrine decreases blood flow to the kidneys which in turn decreases the glomerular filtration rate and the output of urine. If vasoconstriction is intense and prolonged, renal damage occurs (see Complications of Shock). The decreased urine output also can be a reflection of hypovolemia. Patients in shock require the insertion of a Foley catheter for accurate measurement of hourly urine output. Specific gravity is also measured to determine the concentration or osmolarity of the urine. The inability of the patient to concentrate urine may indicate renal damage. An increase in urine output is a good indication of improved tissue perfusion.

Skin Changes

The skin reflects the amount of peripheral vasoconstriction. The patient in shock typically has cold and clammy skin, although in the hyperdynamic type of septic shock the skin may be warm and dry. The pallor of the skin is determined by the intensity of vasoconstriction. Slow blood flow produces coldness; clamminess is produced by increased sympathetic stimulation of sweat glands. The state of capillary blood flow can be evaluated by applying pressure on the nail beds. Normally, color returns almost instantaneously when the pressure is relieved; the return will be slow in shock. Cyanosis indicates deoxygenated blood and is best noted in the nail beds, lips, mucous membranes, and the tip of the nose. Cyanosis appears earlier in septic shock than in the other forms [15]. Skin changes toward normal indicate improved tissue perfusion.

Sensorium

The restlessness and anxiety seen in shock patients in the early stages of shock is attributed to diminished cerebral blood flow [67]. Patients often complain of "feeling funny" but cannot pinpoint any specific problem. The cerebral circulation is usually well protected; as blood flow is reduced, the brain compensates by extracting more oxygen. Anoxia does not become a problem until the systolic pressure is reduced to below 50 mm Hg [51]. Fortunately, brain damage does not occur often in shock patients who survive. The patient's level of consciousness must be assessed frequently. As shock progresses, the patient becomes apathetic and possibly comatose. Frequently the patient is more aware of the environment than his general appearance indicates. Communication with the patient must be based on accurate evaluation of his level of consciousness. Conversations concerning his condition are never appropriate at the bedside.

Muscular Function

Muscle weakness predominates in all forms of shock, most probably as a result of decreased energy supply. This consideration is particularly pertinent in assessing the patient's ventilation status. Muscular weakness can compromise respiratory function.

Temperature

Usually the temperature of shock patients decreases as the metabolic activity in the cells decreases. In septic shock, however, the temperature may remain elevated. Temperature is measured by rectal probe. The temperature of the great toe has been used as an indicator of tissue perfusion. An increase in toe temperature indicates improvement in the patient's status, with 67 percent predictability in one study [35]. The use of the predictor requires some calculation in order to account for room temperature changes.

Weight

Measurement of weight may be required to determine fluid retention. Since the patient in shock should not be moved, a bed scale is required and comparative measurement of weight change can be made. Weight measurements, however, are not commonly made on shock patients, except in research units.

Chest X-ray

Initial and frequent chest x-rays may be required to assess the pulmonary status of the patient.

INVASIVE ASSESSMENTS

Invasive monitoring techniques involve the withdrawal of blood for analysis or the cannulation of arteries or veins to obtain hemodynamic measurements.

Arterial Blood Gases

The pH, Po_2 and Pco_2 are used to determine the state of acidosis or alkalosis and the adequacy of ventilation. The time intervals for these measurements vary, depending on the observed changes in the patient's symptoms. It is of paramount importance that an accurate account of blood withdrawn for these tests be recorded and included as blood loss.

Arterial Pressure

The intra-arterial pressure measurements are more accurate than those measured with a sphygmomanometer. Indirect (via sphygmomanometer) pressures are usually reported as lower than direct intra-arterial pressures in low-flow states. Catheters may be inserted percutaneously or through a cutdown into the radial, brachial, axillary, or femoral artery. Most intra-arterial catheters are attached to transducers, which display continuous arterial pressure readings on an oscilloscope. The dangers of intra-arterial catheterization are introduction of air emboli, infection, and loss of blood supply to the distal portion of the limb. Complication rates generally remain low when proper techniques by skilled practitioners are utilized. Intra-arterial lines can be used for the withdrawal of blood samples for blood gas analysis.

Pulmonary Artery Pressure

The measurement of the pulmonary artery pressure has become clinically feasible with the introduction in 1970 of the Swan-Ganz catheter. This multilumen catheter has a flow-directed, balloon-tipped end. It can be inserted via a cutdown into the antecubital vein. The balloon is filled with carbon dioxide after entrance into the thorax to avert an air embolus if the balloon should rupture. With the balloon inflated, the catheter flows through the right atrium and ventricle into the branches of the pulmonary artery. An advantage of the catheter is that it can be inserted without fluoroscopy with relative safety and accuracy. The placement of the balloon in the pulmonary artery provides the means for continuous monitoring of the pulmonary artery pressure, which reflects the functioning of the right heart.

Pulmonary Wedge Pressure

Probably more important than the pulmonary artery pressure is the measurement of the pulmonary wedge pressure (PWP), which reflects the functioning of the left heart. The PWP is obtained by inflating the balloon of the Swan-Ganz catheter. The tip is then sealed off from the right side of the heart and measures the pressure reflected backward from the left atrium. The balloon can be inflated only momentarily as it blocks blood flow through the parts of the lung distal to the branch of the pulmonary artery in which it lies [66]. The PWP may not accurately reflect left atrial pressure in patients who develop pulmonary resistance. Complications with the use of the Swan-Ganz catheter are infrequent, although perforation of the pulmonary artery and knotting have been reported. Arrhythmias may occur during insertion of the catheter [69].

Central Venous Pressure

Measurement of the central venous pressure (CVP) is obtained by inserting a catheter into the superior vena cava via the median cubital vein. The normal CVP measures under 2 mm Hg, or 5 to 10 cm of water pressure. The CVP measures the filling pressure of the right atrium, which is a combination of three separate factors: (1) the blood volume, (2) the venous tone, and (3) the compliance of the right ventricle. The CVP, however, is altered by changes in intrathoracic pressure [69].

The value of CVP measurement is not in its absolute numerical value, but in the changes that occur over a period of time. A low CVP reading can indicate hypovolemia, but if the venous tone is increased the CVP reading will remain normal. Similarly, a high CVP reading may indicate volume overload, but it may also indicate right ventricular failure. Respirators must be temporarily disconnected in order to obtain accurate CVP readings. Some common sources of errors in CVP readings are (1) incorrect placement of the catheter, (2) poor patency in the catheter, and (3) failure to maintain a consistent zero level. A chest x-ray should be taken following insertion of the catheter to determine accurate placement. The intravenous fluids should run freely through the catheter before measuring, and the baseline zero mark should be marked on the patient's chest.

Coagulation Studies

Studies to evaluate blood coagulation factors provide information about the potential development of DIC. Disseminated intravascular clotting occurs more frequently in septic shock but may be a problem in prolonged hypotension of any cause. Fibrinogen titer, platelet estimation, thrombin, prothrombin, fibrin split products, plasminogen, and fibrinogen levels, as well as platelet adhesiveness, are studies that can provide a composite picture of the coagulation status of the patient. (These factors are discussed in Chapter 5).

Hematocrit

The hematocrit reflects the percentage of red blood cells in whole blood. It is a useful index in determining the type of fluid that should be administered to the patient.

Blood Lactate Levels

Blood lactate is generally the best prognostic indicator in all types of shock [2, 59, 67, 75]. It reflects the status of cellular anaerobic metabolism.

Complete Blood Count

A complete blood count may be obtained at intervals to determine the presence of anemia or leukocytosis or both.

Blood Urea Nitrogen (BUN)

A BUN is obtained when presumptive evidence of renal damage exists.

Blood Cultures

Blood cultures are required in septic shock to determine appropriate antibiotic treatment.

Other Studies

Depending on the institution and on its capabilities, many other measurements can be made to determine more accurately the clinical state of the patient and his response to therapy. These studies include

1. Cardiac output studies
2. Blood volume
3. Mean transit time
4. Oxygen consumption
5. Left ventricular end diastolic pressure
6. Left ventricular ejection time
7. Blood flow measurements
8. Systemic vascular resistance
9. Stroke work index

Treatment

The treatment plan for the patient in shock is determined by the medical staff. Because the majority of these interventions are implemented by the nurse, a thorough understanding of the rationale, physiologic responses, and expected outcomes of therapy is essential for safe and therapeutic care.

Two basic principles of shock treatment are universally agreed on: (1) treat the underlying cause, and (2) restore tissue perfusion. The specific treatment modalities, however, vary greatly among practitioners and often are directly opposed. The treatment of shock is difficult for many reasons. First, the etiology and pathophysiology are often unclear; second, the state of shock is a dynamic one in which the patient's condition is constantly changing, necessitating continuous assessment and reevaluation. Third, shock is a cellular problem and assessment tools measure function of cellular activity indirectly. Finally, the patient usually has multiple problems that must all be considered in assessment and treatment.

TREATING THE UNDERLYING CAUSE

The causes of shock are so multiple and varied that each situation must be evaluated individually and specific causes must be treated with the same degree of specificity. Some forms of shock are resolved simply by treating the underlying cause. In hemorrhagic shock, hemostasis and blood replacement will usually restore circulatory homeostasis if the duration of shock has not been too long. The administration of glucose in insulin shock will restore circulation. Placing the patient in a supine position will correct vasomotor failure in shock related to fainting.

INCREASING TISSUE PERFUSION

Treatment to restore tissue perfusion directly revolves around efforts to improve circulation (restore the blood volume, assist the heart, and alter peripheral resistance by vasoconstricting or vasodilating the blood vessels). Other interventions are aimed directly at treatment of problems on the cellular level. These generally consist in (1) oxygenation, (2) correction of acid-base imbalance, (3) administration of steroids and antibiotics, (4) correction of clotting disorders, and (5) provision of renal support. General interventions that support tissue perfusion will be discussed at the end of this section.

Restoring Blood Volume

Hypovolemia is a problem not only in hypovolemic shock but also in septic shock and in some cases of cardiogenic shock. Patients in cardiogenic shock lose fluids from diuretic therapy, inadequate fluid intake, and fluid shifts across capillary membranes. Approximately 20 percent of patients in cardiogenic shock have hypovolemia [40]. Fluid loss in septic shock can occur when fluid is sequestered in infected tissues or as a result of dehydration from fever or from fluid shifts to the intracellular and third space compartments.

The amount of fluid to be replaced can be determined by fluid challenge. While the procedure is institutionally specific, generally fluid in amounts ranging from 200 to 1,000 ml are given over a 20-minute period [5, 67]. A rapidly rising CVP indicates that the heart is overloaded. An increase in arterial pressure without a significant increase in CVP indicates that hypovolemia exists. Continuous CVP measurement during fluid administration is required to prevent heart overload. A favorable response to volume replacement can also be assessed by increased urine output and improved skin circulation. The volume of fluid needed to adequately replace blood volume and fluid loss is specific to each patient.

The type of fluid selected for replacement is determined by the amount and type of body fluid lost. Fluid replacement will be either colloidal, which remains in the vascular space, or crystalloid, which moves into the interstitial fluid spaces.

Colloid Whole blood is replaced when the hematocrit drops below 35 percent. The heart during hypotension functions best at a hematocrit level of 35 to 40 percent [69]. Plasma expanders such as plasma, albumin, and dextran provide vascular volume expansion. These colloidal solutions decrease the viscosity of the blood by hemodilution and prevent blood cell aggregation. Plasma is required when plasma proteins are lost from the vascular space as in burns and peritonitis. Albumin solutions prepared from fractionating human blood may also be used. Dextran is a glucose polymer which is available in molecular weights of 70,000 and 40,000. It is used as a plasma expander. Low-molecular dextran is thought to specifically prevent red blood cell aggregation, but experimental evidence has not confirmed this [67].

Crystalloid Crystalloid solutions provide extravascular space expansion and electrolyte replacement. Ringers lactate resembles the electrolyte content of extracellular fluid. Its use in shock must be evaluated when liver function is diminished since the liver must metabolize the lactate to bicarbonate. Normal saline is indicated in many cases in which there is excessive fluid loss. Glucose solutions without electrolytes are not commonly used.

Assisting the Heart

Cardiac output is diminished in most forms of shock. In cardiogenic shock, the myocardium itself is damaged and its effectiveness is reduced. In hypovolemic and septic shock the decreased coronary perfusion, acidosis, and hyperkalemia also provide an insult to the myocardium and alter its function. Cardiac support can be provided by drugs or by mechanical devices. The aim of therapy is to improve cardiac output. Drug therapy improves the contractility, controls the rate, and corrects arrhythmias. Mechanical assistance devices reduce the workload of the heart.

Drugs Digitalis has a direct inotropic effect, improving cardiac contractility without increasing the oxygen demands of the myocardium. A suitable intravenous form of digitalis is administered; however, dosage must be controlled when renal failure, hypokalemia, or hyperkalemia exists. Experimental evidence shows that digitalis may protect the myocardium from damage in endotoxic shock [39].

Isoproterenol (Isuprel) is a pure beta stimulator which has inotropic and chronotropic effects, increasing cardiac output and rate. It also causes vasodilatation in the muscles innervated by beta receptors, thereby decreasing peripheral resistance. The major disadvantage of the use of isoproterenol is that it increases the oxygen demand of the myocardium and may aggravate myocardial damage [52]. Isoproterenol also causes tachycardia with arrhythmia development. Tachycardia may also decrease diastolic filling time and reduce the cardiac output.

Glucagon, which is produced by the alpha cells of the pancreas, also possesses positive inotropic properties. Its use has been advocated recently in mild hypotensive states. It is a relatively safe drug, with nausea and vomiting as the chief side effects [69].

The use of drugs to treat arrhythmias is discussed on page 366.

Mechanical assistance The mechanical assistance devices reduce the workload of the heart, providing time to determine whether surgical procedures are warranted to save the patient's life. These devices are most often used in cardiogenic shock but have application in other forms of shock as well.

The **intra-aortic balloon pump** was first used clinically in 1967. It provides internal **counterpulsation** to improve coronary perfusion and decrease the workload of the left ventricle. The balloon is inserted retrograde into the thoracic aorta via the femoral artery. The pump, synchronized with the ECG, inflates the balloon with helium during diastole and deflates it during systole. Counterpulsation is beneficial in two ways: it creates a diastolic pressure wave which benefits the perfusion of all organs but especially the myocardium. Coronary perfusion is greatest during diastole, and the sudden systolic collapse of the balloon lowers the peripheral resistance, thereby reducing the work of the contracting left ventricle. Complications of intra-aortic balloon pumping include femoral artery embolism, thrombosis, aortic wall damage, infection, and foot drop [20, 43, 71]. Most clinical studies indicate that use of the intra-aortic balloon improves the survival rate for patients in cardiogenic shock by approximately 20 percent [58]. Increased skill in using the technique can be anticipated to decrease the rate of complications in cardiogenic shock.

External counterpulsation is accomplished by the use of a water-filled bag to surround the patient's lower extremities. Water is pumped in and out of the bag in synchronization with the ECG. During diastole, positive pressure is exerted through the water pumped into the bag. This pressure propels blood retrograde through the arteries, thereby increasing coronary perfusion. Venous blood is also propelled toward the heart, augmenting venous return and right atrial filling. During systole, the water is pumped out of the bag so that the pressure becomes negative. This negative pressure during systole pulls blood from the heart and decreases the workload of the heart. The retrograde flow in the veins is prevented by the venous valves. When the counterpulsation is functioning properly the blood pressure reading is reversed, with the systolic reading falling below the diastolic reading. Because the heart does not have to pump the blood against increased peripheral resistance, the work of the heart is decreased. Another benefit of counterpulsation is improved perfusion of the heart during diastole so that the increased oxygen supply that results augments the healing process. Clinical use of external counterpulsation is limited; however, one study indicates a 45 percent survival rate when counterpulsation is used with patients in cardiogenic shock [8].

Altering Peripheral Resistance
Peripheral resistance can be altered in two directions, by either increasing or decreasing it. There is a great deal of controversy over which approach to use. Medical practitioners who advocate increasing peripheral resistance believe that arterial pressure must be maintained to ensure adequate tissue perfusion. Vasopressor drugs are used to increase peripheral resistance and maintain arterial pressure. The opposite view is held by those who advocate the use of vasodilating drugs.

The rationale for the use of vasodilator therapy is based on the conclusion that decreased arterial pressure is not the cause, but a symptom of shock, and that raising arterial pressure does not guarantee organ perfusion. Hence the vascular beds are dilated with simultaneous fluid therapy to increase blood flow and improve tissue perfusion. Vasodilator therapy is achieved through use of adrenergic alpha-blocking drugs.

The sympathetic nervous system receptors have been divided into two basic types, alpha receptors and beta receptors. Alpha receptors cause vasoconstriction; beta receptors act primarily in the heart. The effects of alpha and beta stimulation are summarized in Table 16-4. Dopamine receptors, which cause renal and mesenteric vasodilatation, have recently been described [23].

Vasopressor drugs are adrenergic drugs. The following represent the drugs most commonly used in shock treatment. Norepinephrine (Levophed) acts on both alpha and beta receptors. It increases myocardial contractility through its beta effects, but causes intense vasoconstriction by its alpha effects. If used in low concentrations, its beta effects predominate. Levophed can be useful in certain instances in cardiogenic and neurogenic shock or as an initial emergency measure to maintain vital organ blood flow in traumatic shock.

Epinephrine (adrenalin) also has alpha- and beta-stimulating properties. Its beta effects operate at low doses, having an inotropic and chronotropic effect and increasing cardiac output. A decreased peripheral resistance occurs at low doses [67]. Epinephrine is the drug of choice in the treatment of anaphylactic shock since it antagonizes the most adverse effects of histamine [23]. Metaraminol (Aramine) is almost identical to norepinephrine and acts by displacing norepinephrine at receptor sites. In small doses, it has a positive inotropic effect. Prolonged treatment with metaraminol leads to a state of refractoriness and hypotension. It does not have any effect on patients who are taking reserpine or any norepinephrine-depleting drugs. Methoxamine (Vasoxyl) is a pure alpha-stimulating drug. It causes intense vasoconstriction but decreases cardiac output and causes reflex bradycardia [67]. Dopamine (Intropin) is an intermediate in the formation of norepinephrine and epinephrine. It has properties similar to norepinephrine. However, it is not as powerful a vasoconstrictor. It also has a vasodilating effect on the renal and mesenteric vessels.

All the vasopressor drugs are extremely potent and they are used for their vascular and

Table 16-4
Receptors acted on by sympathomimetic amines and their antagonists

Receptor	Results of receptor activation	Antagonists
Beta$_1$	Myocardial contractility heart rate AV conduction	Propranolol Practolol
Beta$_2$	Vasodilation (especially skeletal muscle vascular bed); bronchodilation	Propranolol
Alpha	Vasoconstriction (less prominent in coronary and cerebral vascular beds)	Phenoxybenzamine Phentolamine
Dopamine	Vasodilation—renal, mesenteric (coronary, intracerebral)	Haloperidol Chlorpromazine

Source: L. Goldberg, Use of sympathomimetic amines in shock. *American Family Physician* 10:80, 1974.

Table 16-5
Actions of sympathomimetic amines on receptors

	Isoproterenol	Dopamine	Epinephrine	Norepinephrine	Methoxamine
Beta$_1$	+++	++	+++	+	0
Beta$_2$	+++	0	+	0	0
Alpha	0	+[a]	+[b]	+++	++
Dopamine	0	++	0	0	0

[a]Small doses, little or no alpha-adrenergic action; large doses, alpha-adrenergic action predominates.
[b]Small doses, beta-adrenergic response predominates; large doses, alpha-adrenergic receptors predominate.
Source: L. Goldberg, Use of sympathomimetic amines in shock. *American Family Physician* 10:80, 1974.

cardiac effects. The alpha and beta effects of these drugs are summarized in Table 16-5. Intravenous administration of these drugs must be precisely monitored and requires pressure measurements every 2 to 5 minutes when therapy is initiated and every 15 minutes when the patient's condition has been stabilized with the drug. The nurse must observe for extravasation of the drug into the patient's subcutaneous tissue. If this should occur, intense vasoconstriction produced in the local tissue will cause necrosis and sloughing. Phentolamine (Regitine) is usually injected into the site to counteract this effect.

Vasodilating drugs have alpha adrenergic-blocking properties. Fluid replacement must be done simultaneously to avoid profound hypotension. Alpha-blocking agents can be used with some sympathomimetic drugs; blocking the alpha effect of the drug, the desired inotropic beta effects can be produced.

Phenoxybenzamine (Dibenzyline) is an alpha adrenergic-blocking agent with no effect on beta receptors. The drug action begins in 3 to 4 hours following intravenous administration and lasts 48 hours. The drug has some antihistaminic and antiserotonin effects. Phenoxybenzamine is not widely used since the FDA approval has been granted for limited use only. Phentolamine (Regitine) is an alpha adrenergic-blocking agent with properties similar to those of phenoxybenzamine but with a faster onset and shorter duration of action. Chlorpromazine (Thorazine) has alpha adrenergic-blocking properties in addition to central nervous system effects; it was used in 1950 in the first trials of vasodilator therapy by drug action. Its results are unpredictable, and it is not used extensively by those advocating vasodilator therapy [58].

CORRECTION OF CELLULAR PROBLEMS

Oxygenation

Arterial oxygen tension must be kept at normal levels if maximum hemoglobin saturation and tissue oxygenation are to occur. The patient who is in shock is vulnerable to many respiratory problems. General muscular weakness can cause inadequate respiratory excursion with retention of secretions and development of atelectasis. Sedation and hypoxia can cause additional respiratory depression; fluid overload or heart failure may develop into pulmonary edema. Arteriovenous shunting may decrease effective ventilation. Generally, intubation and placement on a volume-cycled respirator are required for most patients in prolonged shock. Continuous adjustments are required to maintain normal oxygen tension.

Acid-Base Balance

The development of anaerobic metabolism leads to metabolic acidosis, which may be initially compensated for by respiratory alkalosis. Eventually, as the body buffer stores are utilized, respiratory acidosis ensues [58]. The correction of acidosis is dependent on correction of the hemodynamic equilibrium. Use of bicarbonate or THAM as buffers is indicated in some situations.

Steroids

The administration of massive doses of steroids is advocated by some practitioners. Results of animal experiments demonstrate an increased survival rate for animals pretreated with steroids [39]. Steroids in large doses have an inotropic effect, decrease peripheral resistance, and stabilize lysosomal membranes. Adrenal function is usually accelerated in shock. Patients receiving massive doses of steroids do not need to be weaned from the drugs since the duration of administration is short [39].

Antibiotics

Antibiotics are required in septic shock as primary treatment. Since gram-negative bacteria are most often the causative agent, an antibiotic to cover a wide range of gram-negative bacteria is chosen. Specific treatment must await blood culture and sensitivity studies. Dosages must be adjusted in the presence of oliguria or anuria. The nephrotoxicity of many antibiotics also presents problems [69]. The use of antibiotics as a prophylactic measure in other types of shock is controversial, but based on the rationale that hypovolemia reduces the patient's resistance to infection [72].

Correction of DIC

Disseminated intravascular clotting is a problem in progressive shock. It is treated by administration of whole blood less than 24 hours old and still containing platelets and coagulation factors. Heparin is also administered to prevent coagulation and to allow clotting factors to return to normal levels [42].

Providing Renal Support

Oliguria during hypotension may be caused by hypovolemia, decreased renal blood flow, or acute renal failure. Renal function is evaluated by the response to rapid infusion of a large amount of fluid. Mannitol, an osmotic diuretic, is administered rapidly during oliguria to determine whether renal damage has occurred. A 25-gram dose of mannitol is infused over a 10- to 30-minute period. If urine output does not improve, renal damage is assumed and fluid administration is restricted. Furosemide (Lasix) may also be administered for the same reason.

General Measures

Position   The supine position is the best one for the patient in shock. Various studies have proved that the Trendelenberg position is detrimental to the patient. Originally used in the 1890s to provide better surgical exposure during pelvic surgery, it became the traditional position for the shock patient. The rationale for using this position was that placing the head down would provide better cerebral circulation and venous return to the heart [27]. Studies on animals have shown that the Trendelenberg position causes a decrease in arterial pressure due to the stimulation of baroreceptors. In addition, effective lung volume is decreased by pressure of the abdominal contents against the diaphragm. The vital capacity falls 15 to 20 percent [73]. This position also increases the risk of cerebral edema. The supine position with the patient's legs elevated at a 45-degree angle is advocated by some. This position may be initially helpful, but the supine position is preferred in prolonged shock [27].

Temperature   Hypothermia has been used for patients in shock to reduce the metabolic rate and oxygen demands. No data have indicated that hypothermia has been effective. Below 90°F, the potential for arrhythmias is increased [72]. Patients with fever should have their temperatures lowered to normal. Providing warmth by external covering is not advised, since it would promote vasodilatation and counteract the body's vasoconstricting effect. On the other hand, shivering must be avoided since it increases the oxygen demands by as much as 100 percent.

Pain control   Pain can aggravate or cause shock and therefore must be treated. Pain control must be accomplished by intravenous medications for the patient in shock since inadequate circulation makes absorption from other routes unpredictable. Morphine is the most effective analgesic and has the added value of reducing the cerebral metabolic demands by as much as 50 percent [51]. However, the benefits of morphine sulfate and other narcotics must be weighed against their adverse effect on respiratory function, that is, respiratory depression.

Treatment is based on the broad principles of (1) treating the underlying cause and (2) increasing tissue perfusion. Despite improved technology and better understanding of the pathophysiologic process, the survival rate often is discouraging.

Nursing Care

The nursing care for the patient in shock can be best described through analysis of each component of the nursing process: assessment, planning, intervention, and evaluation.

ASSESSMENT

The most valuable assessments made by the nurse are those that detect impending shock. Observations of the signs of early shock, for example, apprehension, tachycardia, and decreased urine output, should be made in any patient who has suffered some circulatory insult. The increasing incidence of septic shock should alert nurses to carefully observe debilitated, elderly patients who have undergone gastrointestinal or genitourinary tract surgery or who are on continuous intravenous therapy. It must be emphasized that the duration of shock is an important variable that affects the survival of the patient. Prompt recognition and treatment improve the prognosis for the patient.

Assessment of the physiologic status of the patient consumes a great portion of the nurse's time with the patient. The nature of the assessments and their interpretation have been outlined previously. Observations must be made continuously. The volume of data mandates some systematic approach to provide for accuracy and continuity. Generally some type of flow sheet is required to keep assessment data in perspective and to determine patterns of response.

The use of invasive monitoring equipment provides valuable data but demands additional attention. Most invasive monitoring catheters require radiologic confirmation of correct placement. All monitoring equipment requires periodic calibration to guarantee accuracy. Data obtained from sophisticated monitoring equipment have value only insofar as they are accurately and properly interpreted. Complications that occur secondary to invasive monitoring procedures are outweighed by the advantages of monitoring equipment.

Patients who are admitted in shock to the hospital require additional assessment regarding their previous illnesses and current drug therapy. Especially significant data are previous pulmonary and cardiovascular disease, a history of diabetes, and antihypertensive or anticoagulant therapy.

PLANNING

On an institutional level, providing for the nursing care of the patient in shock must be pre-planned since equipment and qualified personnel must be available on short notice.

For the individual patient a nursing care plan can be projected only in general goals since each patient is unique and changes constantly. The major goals of care are to (1) correct underlying causes of shock, (2) maintain maximum oxygenation, and (3) increase tissue perfusion. These goals provide a simple but valid priority. Any nursing intervention that does not promote these goals is not therapeutic for the patient. Common comfort measures such as bathing, frequent position changes, and oral hygiene require an energy expenditure by the patient and increase his oxygen demands. Although these energy expenditures are normally minimal, they become extraordinary for the individual who is having difficulty with perfusion of vital organs and must be delayed until the patient's hemodynamic status is stabilized. The multiplicity of procedures and interventions that must be done for the patient often necessitates more than a 1:1 patient-to-nurse ratio. The nurse cannot leave the bedside of the patient in shock, and additional personnel are required to secure supplies and to provide psychological support to the family or friends of the patient.

INTERVENTIONS

The nurse's role in intervention supports that of the physician. The primary interventions are directed toward treatment of the underlying cause of shock. Often the situation is reversed and circulation is stabilized with these measures. If the patient does not recover with the initial treatment, efforts must then be directed toward improving tissue perfusion and oxygenation. Specific measures have been discussed in the section on treatment. In addition, some general methods to provide safe care should be considered: (1) The patient's energy must be conserved; unnecessary care and moving of the patient are not indicated and can be detrimental; and (2) The patient's immune response is impaired during shock. Aseptic techniques must be meticulous. This is often difficult when emergency cutdowns and arterial catheters are being inserted.

Maintaining precise records is difficult in most cases. The multiplicity of orders, frequent changes, and general confusion present a formidable challenge in record keeping. The use of tape recorders has been introduced at some institutions to alleviate this problem.

The patient's psychological needs must be considered throughout the crisis and require conscious effort by the nursing staff. The most natural impulses lead one to be carried with the momentum of activities to save the patient's physical body. Patients often do remain aware during the entire period of shock. The patient feels helpless, powerless, and frightened as well as feeling physiologic apprehension. Simple explanations of procedures are sufficient; nonverbal communication is equally important. Appearing confident and performing efficiently will assure the patient. Use of touch as a therapeutic intervention has its place in this type of situation. The fascinating study of Lynch et al. demonstrated that human contact and touch elicited a beneficial effect on heart rate in patients who were given curare and were artificially ventilated [41]. General conclusions cannot be made because the study group was too small. However, the study supports empiric assumptions of the inseparability of mind and body.

The family and friends of the patient need assistance and emotional support. Clinical specialists in crisis intervention can be most therapeutic in these situations.

EVALUATION

Evaluation is continuous in the nursing care of the patient in shock and provides the basis for reassessment. The most valuable indicator of improved tissue perfusion is adequacy of urine output. Skin changes toward normalcy, stability of the blood pressure, and pulse are also good indicators of improving tissue perfusion.

Complications of Shock

Three major complications can occur in successfully resuscitated shock patients. The complications are extremely serious and are frequently fatal. Renal failure and stress ulceration result from the particular vulnerability of the renal tubules and gastric mucosa to ischemia. The shock lung syndrome is of more recent discovery and its etiology remains unclear.

Acute renal insufficiency most often develops following shock caused by sepsis, trauma, or burns. The precise mechanism by which renal failure is produced is not clearly understood. The previous acceptance of renal ischemia as being the sole cause of tubular necrosis has not been substantiated by microscopic data or research evidence. Other causes that have been considered are (1) plugging of the nephrons with cellular casts, (2) renal vasospasm, (3) intravascular clotting, and (4) high interstitial hydrostatic pressure [67]. Nephrotoxic antibiotics used in shock resuscitation may aggravate the problem.

The clinical picture presented by the patient is one of persistent oliguria (below 400 ml per 24 hours) or anuria (urinary output of less than 20 ml per 24 hours), with increasing blood urea nitrogen levels following restoration of arterial blood pressure and volume. Some patients with acute renal failure may have a high urine output with an increasing blood urea nitrogen. The oliguric phase of acute renal failure may last from 5 to 15 days before diuresis begins. Adequate renal function may return in several weeks, but it may be 6 months before normal renal function is restored. The use of peritoneal dialysis or hemodialysis to prevent uremia while allowing the nephrons time to heal has increased the survival rate of patients.

Gastric ulceration, or stress ulcers, can occur after any episode of shock, trauma, or neurologic injury. They are most common after episodes of septic shock. The patient may appear deceptively well when acute bleeding suddenly occurs. The bleeding episode may occur several days after the shock period. The cause of stress ulcers is unknown. Gastric hyperacidity, abnormal permeability of the gastric mucosa to hydrogen ions, altered gastric secretion of mucus, and gastric mucosal necrosis have been suggested as possible causes. Nasogastric tubes and the tendency to bleed during shock are aggravating factors. The gastric lesions are superficial in depth and most frequently appear on the lesser curvature of the stomach. They are treated by a variety of modes, which include iced saline lavage, blood replacement, gastric resection with vagotomy, hyperalimentation, antacids, and anticholinergic medications. Often the treatment is institutionally specific. Stress ulcers appear to be increasing in frequency as more patients survive shock. Some hospitals report the largest cause of gastrointestinal bleeding to be stress ulceration [13].

Shock lung is pulmonary insufficiency following successful resuscitation from hypotension. The development of shock lung as a complication is increasing in frequency, quite possibly because more patients survive the original hypotensive episode and therefore develop the shock lung as a consequence of shock [39]. There is a positive correlation between the severity of hypotension and the development of shock lung [45].

Typically the syndrome manifests itself insidiously anywhere from 1 to 6 days following the original shock period. The patient looks deceptively well, but begins to hyperventilate and becomes progressively dyspneic with rapid shallow breathing and a productive cough. The minute volume is increased, the compliance of the lung decreases, and the Pco_2 becomes elevated [61]. Extensive and diffuse interstitial and alveolar edema and hemorrhage have occurred, resulting in the development of arterial venous shunting in the lung with reduced gas exchange across the alveolar membranes [21]. As much as 42 percent of the cardiac output can traverse the pulmonary capillary beds without any gas exchange in this condition.

There is a high mortality rate with shock lung [45]. Current treatment includes ventilatory support with the use of positive end-expiratory pressure (PEEP), oxygen therapy, diuretics, heparin, and steroids. On an experimental basis, selected institutions have maintained patients on continuous extracorporeal membrane oxygenators for up to 12 days with limited success [22]. The cause of shock lung is unknown. Agents that have been postulated as causes include toxins, microemboli, neurogenic stimuli, and vasoactive substances. The possibility of overhydration during initial resuscitation and oxygen toxicity as causative mechanisms is debated [45].

The histologic response produced in shock lung is similar to that produced in a wide variety of other conditions, such as fat embolism, aspiration pneumonia, and inhalant injuries. These similar syndromes have been grouped by various authors into a broader syndrome, the **adult respiratory distress syndrome** [45].

Nursing the patient in shock is a challenging experience that commands all the skills of the nurse. When the patient recovers, it is also a very satisfying experience. Unfortunately, certain types of shock patients have a high mortality rate despite the best nursing care and medical treatment. Nurses in intensive care settings often need psychological support themselves to help them cope with valid feelings of frustration and helplessness. Fortunately this need has been recognized, and many institutions provide support through group work with nursing consultants or psychiatric staff members.

References

1. Abernathy, R. S. Shock Due to Hypersensitivity and Anaphylaxis. In M. Weil and H. Shubin (eds.), *Diagnosis and Treatment of Shock*. Baltimore: Williams & Wilkins, 1967.
2. Adler, D. C., and Brown, C. B. Use of axillary artery for intravascular monitoring. *Crit. Care Med.* 1:148, 1973.
3. Afifi, A., et al. Prognostic indexes in acute myocardial infarction. *Am. J. Cardiol.* 33:826, 1974.
4. Allardyce, B. D. Parenteral fluid therapy in septic shock: An evaluation of crystalloid and colloid. *Am. Surg.* 40:542, 1974.
5. Armstrong, P. W., and Parker, J. D. The complications of brachial arteriotomy. *J. Thorac. Cardiovasc. Surg.* 61:424, 1971.
6. Ayres, S., and Mueller, H. The overall approach to the patient with hypotension. *Heart Lung* 3:463, 1974.
7. Baird, J. N., et al. Shock lung. *Am. J. Obstet. Gynecol.* 115:583, 1974.
8. Begley, L. A. External counterpulsation for cardiogenic shock. *Am. J. Nurs.* 75:967, 1975.
9. Bentley, D. W., and Lepper, M. H. Septicemia related to indwelling venous catheters. *J.A.M.A.* 206:1729, 1969.
10. Berman, L. Renal Failure in Shock. In M. Weil and H. Shubin (eds.), *Diagnosis and Treatment of Shock*. Baltimore: Williams & Wilkins, 1967.
11. Bilodeau, C. The nurse and her reactions to critical care nursing. *Heart Lung* 2:358, 1973.
12. Buja, L. M., and Roberts, W. C. The Coronary Arteries and Myocardium in Acute Myocardial Infarction and Shock. In R. M. Gunnar et al. (eds.), *Shock in Myocardial Infarction*. New York: Grune & Stratton, 1974.
13. Butterfield, W. C. Experimental Stress Ulcers: A Review. *Surgery Annual 1975*, vol. 7. New York: Appleton-Century-Crofts, 1975.
14. Cassem, N. H., and Hackett, T. P. Stress on the nurse and therapist in the intensive care unit and coronary care unit. *Heart Lung* 4:252, 1975.
15. Christy, J. H. Pathophysiology of gram-negative shock. *Am. Heart J.* 81:694, 1971.

16. Cohn, J. N. Monitoring technique in shock. *Am. J. Cardiol.* 26:565, 1970.
17. Cohn, J. N. Blood pressure measurement in shock: Mechanism of inaccuracy in auscultatory and palpatory methods. *J.A.M.A.* 199:972, 1967.
18. Coleman, R. W. Disseminated intravascular coagulation: A problem in critical care medicine. *Heart Lung* 3:789, 1974.
19. DaLuz, P. L., et al. Effectiveness of phentolamine for reversal of circulatory failure (shock). *Crit. Care Med.* 1:135, 1973.
20. Dorr, K. S. The intra-aortic balloon pump. *Am. J. Nurs.* 75:52, 1975.
21. Fishman, A. P. Shock lung—A distinctive nonentity. *Circulation* 47:921, 1973.
22. Follat, R. J. Treatment of acute respiratory failure with prolonged extracorporeal oxygenation. *Chest* (supplement) 66:385, 1975.
23. Goldberg, L. Use of sympathomimetic amines in shock. *Am. Fam. Physician* 10:80, 1974.
24. Gunnar, R. M., et al. Hemodynamic measurements in coronary care units. *Proc. Cardiovasc. Dis.* 11:29, 1968.
25. Gunnar, R. M., et al. Hemodynamic Studies in Shock with Myocardial Infarction. *Shock in Myocardial Infarction.* New York: Grune & Stratton, 1974.
26. Gunnar, R. M., et al. *Shock in Myocardial Infarction.* New York: Grune & Stratton, 1974.
27. Guntheroth, W. G., et al. The effect of Trendelenberg's position on blood pressure and carotid flow. *Surg. Gynecol. Obstet.* 119:345, 1964.
28. Guyton, A. *Textbook of Medical Physiology* (4th ed.). Philadelphia: Saunders, 1971.
29. Hardaway, R. Disseminated intravascular coagulation as a possible cause of acute respiratory failure. *Surg. Gynecol. Obstet.* 137:419, 1973.
30. Herman, C. M. Advances and Newer Concepts in Shock. *Surgery Annual 1972,* vol. 4. New York: Appleton-Century-Crofts, 1972.
31. Hopkins, R. W., and Damewood, C. A. Septic shock: Hemodynamics of endotoxin and inflammation. *Am. J. Surg.* 127:477, 1974.
32. Horovitz, J. H., and Luterman, A. Postoperative monitoring following critical trauma. *Heart Lung* 4:269, 1975.
33. Jahre, J. A., et al. Medical approach to the hypotensive patient and the patient in shock. *Heart Lung* 4:577, 1975.
34. Johnston, A. O. B., and Clark, R. G. Malpositioning of central venous catheters. *Lancet* 2:1395, 1972.
35. Joly, H. R., and Weil, M. H. Temperature of the great toe as an indication of the severity of shock. *Circulation* 39:131, 1969.
36. Kelly, W. F. Psychiatric aspects of critical care. *Crit. Care Med.* 2:139, 1974.
37. Kones, R. J. Cardiogenic shock. *Angiology* 25:317, 1974.
38. Lefer, A. M., and Spath, J. A. Pancreatic hypoperfusion and the production of a myocardial depressant factor in hemorrhagic shock. *Ann. Surg.* 179:868, 1974.
39. Lillehei, R. C., and Dietzman, R. H. Circulatory Collapse and Shock. In S. I. Schwartz (ed.), *Principles of Surgery* (2nd ed.). New York: McGraw-Hill, 1974.
40. Loeb, H. S., et al. Hypovolemia in shock due to acute myocardial infarction. *Circulation* 40:653, 1969.
41. Lynch, J. J., et al. Effects of human contact on the heart activity of curarized patients in a shock-trauma unit. *Am. Heart J.* 88:160, 1974.
42. MacLean, L. D. Shock: Causes and Management of Circulatory Collapse. In D. C. Sabiston (ed.), *Textbook of Surgery.* Philadelphia: Saunders, 1972.
43. Malinin, T. F., et al. *Acute Fluid Replacement in the Therapy of Shock.* New York: Stratton Intercontinental, 1974.
44. McCann, W. J., and Soares, D. M. The use of intraaortic balloon counterpulsation in the management of cardiogenic shock. *Heart Lung* 4:211, 1975.
45. McCorkle, R. Effects of touch on seriously ill patients. *Nurs. Res.* 23:125, 1974.
46. Melby, J. C. Hormonal Factors. In M. Weil and H. Shubin (eds.), *Diagnosis and Treatment of Shock.* Baltimore: Williams & Wilkins, 1967.
47. Menguy, R., and Masters, Y. F. Gastric mucosal energy metabolism and stress ulceration. *Ann. Surg.* 180:538, 1974.
48. Moore, F. D., et al. *Post-Traumatic Pulmonary Insufficiency.* Philadelphia: Saunders, 1969.
49. Moran, J. M., et al. A clinical and bacteriological study of infections associated with venous cutdown. *N. Engl. J. Med.* 272:554, 1965.
50. Morgan, B., et al. Effect of position on leg volume. *J.A.M.A.* 187:1024, 1964.
51. Moyer, J. H., and Mills, L. C. Vasopressor agents in shock. *Am. J. Nurs.* 74:48, 1974.
52. Mueller, H., et al. Principal defects which account for shock following myocardial infarction in man. *Crit. Care Med.* 1:27, 1973.
53. Nielsen, M. A. Intra-arterial monitoring of blood pressure. *Am. J. Nurs.* 74:48, 1974.
54. Norden, C. W. Application of antibiotic ointment to the site of venous catheterization: A controlled trial. *J. Infect. Dis.* 120:611, 1969.
55. O'Rourke, M. Cardiogenic shock following myocardial infarction. *Heart Lung* 4:3, 1975.
56. Rodriquez, T., et al. Use of non-invasive monitoring in hemorrhagic shock. *Crit. Care Med.* 1:141, 1973.
57. Schumer, W. Metabolic Aspects of Shock. *Surgery Annual 1974,* vol. 6. New York: Appleton-Century-Crofts, 1974.

58. Schumer, W., and Nyhus, L. M. *Treatment of Shock: Principles and Practice.* Philadelphia: Lea & Febiger, 1974.
59. Shubin, H., et al. Selection of hemodynamic, respiratory and metabolic variables for evaluation of patients in shock. *Crit. Care Med.* 2:326, 1974.
60. Shubin, H., and Weil, M. H. Shock Following Suicidal Doses of Barbiturate, Narcotic and Tranquilizer Drugs. In M. H. Weil and H. Shubin (eds.), *Diagnosis and Treatment of Shock.* Baltimore: Williams & Wilkins, 1967.
61. Shoemaker, W. C. *Shock: Chemistry, Physiology and Therapy.* Springfield, Ill.: Thomas, 1967.
62. Shoemaker, W. C., et al. Early prediction of death and survival in post-operative patients with circulatory shock by nonparametric analysis of cardiorespiratory variables. *Crit. Care Med.* 2:317, 1974.
63. Simeone, F. A. Shock, trauma and the surgeon. *Ann. Surg.* 158:759, 1963.
64. Simeone, F. A. Hemorrhagic shock. *Am. J. Cardiol.* 12:589, 1963.
65. Sutton, F. D., et al. Recognition and management of adult respiratory distress syndrome. *Chest* (supplement) 66:345, 1975.
66. Swan, H. J. C., et al. Catheterization of the heart in man with use of a flow-directed balloon-tipped catheter. *N. Engl. J. Med.* 283:447, 1970.
67. Thal, A. P. *Shock: A Physiological Basis for Treatment.* Chicago: Year Book, 1971.
68. Tharp, G. D. Shock: The overall mechanisms. *Am. J. Nurs.* 74:2208, 1974.
69. Towne, W. O. Physiologic Monitoring of Patients in Shock. In R. M. Gunnar et al. (eds.), *Shock in Myocardial Infarction.* New York: Grune & Stratton, 1974.
70. Vaisrub, S. Myocardial depressant factor in cardiogenic shock. *J.A.M.A.* 228:500, 1974.
71. Weber, J. T., and Jancki, J. S. Intraaortic balloon counterpulsation. *Ann. Thorac. Surg.* 17:603, 1974.
72. Weil, M., and Shubin, H. *Diagnosis and Treatment of Shock.* Baltimore: Williams & Wilkins, 1967.
73. Weil, M. H., et al. The head down position in treatment of shock. *Surg. Gynecol. Obstet.* 116:669, 1963.
74. Weil, M. H., and Shubin, H. Shock Associated with Infection—Bacterial Shock. In M. Weil and H. Shubin (eds.), *Diagnosis and Treatment of Shock.* Baltimore: Williams & Wilkins, 1967.
75. Weil, M. H., and Shubin, H. Monitoring and Measurement in Shock. In M. Schumer and L. M. Nyhus (eds.), *Treatment of Shock: Principles and Practice.* Philadelphia: Lea & Febiger, 1974.
76. Zwiebach, B. W. The microcirculation of the blood. *Sci. Am.* January, 1959.

Index

Abdomen
 distention of
  in ascites, 695–697
  in burns, 1154
 examination of, 530–531
 muscles of, 818
 palpation of, 531
Abdominal-perineal resection, 574
Abdominal reflexes, 911
Abducens nerve, 898
 assessment of, 908
Ablative surgery, indications for, 635–636
ABO blood groups, 423–424
 in erythroblastosis fetalis, 442
 and matching blood transfusions, 33
Abortion
 induction of, 796–798
  prostaglandins in, 797
  saline in, 797
 septic, 798
 spontaneous, 796
Abrasions, 21
Abscess, 20
 of brain, 936
 of liver, 592
 of lung, 292–293
 in mastoid bone, 1054
 perinephric, 489
 perirectal, 582
 peritonsillar, 1073
 in spine, 936
 in urinary tract, 486
Absorption of nutrients, intestinal, 527, 566–567
 disorders of, 535–536, 566–569. See also Malabsorption
Accessory nerve, 899
 assessment of, 909
Accoucheur's position, in hypoparathyroidism, 670
Accretion of bone, 813–814
Acetabulum, prosthetic, in total hip replacement, 844–846
Acetazolamine
 as diuretic, 380
 in glaucoma, 1011, 1022
Acetylcholine, 30
 activity in myasthenia gravis, 962
 and hydrochloric acid secretion, 543
 as neurotransmitter, 319, 904
 vascular effects of, 394
Acetylcysteine as mucolytic agent, 226
Acetylsalicylic acid (aspirin)
 anticoagulant effects, 353
 and dehydration in salicylate poisoning, 165
 in osteoarthritis, 860
 in rheumatoid arthritis, 864
 as ulcerogenic, 544
Achalasia, 527, 561–562
 motility test in diagnosis of, 562
Achilles reflex, in thyroid disease, 647, 911
Achlorhydria, 434, 532, 534
Acid, definition of, 161, 162
Acid-base balance, 161. See also Fluids
 regulation of, 504–505
 in respiratory failure, 244
Acidosis, 14
 diabetic, 699, 723–726
 lactic acid, 14, 185
  in diabetes, 721, 727–728
 metabolic, 184–186
  in cardiac arrest, 370–371
  diagnosis of, 185
  disorders with, 185
  from extracorporeal circulation, 388
  nursing care in, 186
  in shock, 1191, 1193, 1200
 in renal failure
  acute, 506–507
  chronic, 510
 respiratory, 181–184
  in acute respiratory failure, 230
  diagnosis of, 183
  disorders with, 182
  from hyperventilation, 203
  nursing care in, 183–184
  symptoms and signs of, 182
 tubular, 506

Acne, 1096, 1108–1110
 in Cushing's disease, 681
 rosacea, 1110
 treatment of, 1109–1110
 vulgaris, 1108–1110
Acoustic nerve, 1041, 1044
 neuroma, 946
Acrocyanosis, 404
Acromegaly, 628–629, 815, 820
ACTH, 631
 affecting learning, 16
 hypersecretion of, 680
 hyposecretion of, 680
 releasing factor, 674
 secretion by pituitary, 674
  in Addison's disease, 678
  diurnal rhythm of, 674
  in shock, 1189
  stress affecting, 674
 serum levels of
  adrenal tumors affecting, 683
  in Cushing's disease, 683
 tests with, 675
Actin, 315, 817
Action potential, of cardiac cells, 316
Acupuncture, for pain relief, 47–48
Acute illness, 63
Adam's apple, 1076
Adams-Stokes syndrome, 360
Adaptive responses, 7, 17–50, 151. See also Psychological aspects
 in dying patients, 136–139
 immune response as, 22–39
 inflammatory response as, 18–22
 nursing implications in, 50–64
 pain response, 39–50
 in terminal illness, 132–136
Addiction, to narcotics, 46
Addison's disease, 676–680
 and calcifications in ear, 1037
 causes of, 676–677
 crisis in, 677, 678
 hyperkalemia in, 177
 signs and symptoms of, 677–678
 treatment of, 679–680
 water intoxication in, 169
Adductor muscles, 818
Adenine, as purine base, 8
Adenitis, cervical, acute, 408
Adenocarcinoma, 107
 of breast, 786
 of lung, 305–306
 of prostate, 778
Adenohypophysis, 625, 628
Adenoid tissue, enlarged, 1072
Adenoidectomy, 1072
Adenoma, 107
 bronchial, 306
 of ear, 1052
 parathyroid, location of, 667–668
 of pharynx, 1074
 pituitary, 632, 946
 thyroid, toxic, 658
Adenomyosis, 771
Adenosine diphosphate, 9
Adenosine triphosphate, 8–9, 1191
 muscular production of, 817
Adenosis, of breast, 785
ADH. See Antidiuretic hormone
Adhesions
 in endometriosis, 771
 intestinal, 573
 in pelvic inflammatory disease, 757–758
 of wounds, in postoperative care, 101–105
Adipose layer of skin, 1095
Adolescence
 acne in, 1109
 spinal cord injuries in, 979
Adrenal glands, 672–692
 aldosteronism, 685–692
 anatomy of, 672
 cortex of, 673
  zones in, 672
 corticosteroid hormones. See Corticosteroids
 Cushing's disease, 680–685
 dysfunction of, 675–692
 enzymatic deficiencies of, 688
 function of, 672–675

function tests, 675–676
 ganglioneuroma of, 690
 insufficiency of. See Addison's disease
 medulla of, 672
  insufficiency of, 688–690
  neuroblastoma of, 690
  shock affecting, 1188–1189
 surgery of, 684–685, 690
 tumors of, 682–683
Adrenalectomy, 684–685
 in breast cancer, 788
 in palliative treatment for cancer, 115
Adrenergic blocking agents
 in hypertension, 340
 in shock, 1200
Adrenergic drugs
 as bronchodilators, 225–226
 as mydriatics, 1010
Aerosol therapy
 bronchodilators in, 218–219, 226
 oxygen in, 234
Agammaglobulinemia, 38
Agencies for help
 in blindness, 994–1030
 in cancer, 114
 in convulsive disorders, 929
 in diabetes, 706
 in hearing loss, 1059
 in Huntington's chorea, 961–962
 in laryngectomy, 1089–1090
 in multiple sclerosis, 958
 in myasthenia gravis, 964
 in ostomy care, 560
 in paraplegia, 982
Agglutination, in transfusion reactions, 425
Agglutinins, in blood groups, 423, 424
Agglutinogens, in blood groups, 423, 424
Aging
 and body function, 12
 and cataract formation, 1019
 dehydration in, 164
 integumentary system in, 1099
 and menopause, 799–801
 and osteoporosis, 861
Agnosia, 907
Agranulocytosis, 444–445
 from antithyroid drugs, 653
 in aplastic anemia, 436
 drug-induced, 36, 653
 symptoms of, 653
Air embolism, in transfusion therapy, 426
Air flow unit, laminar, 128–129
Airway maintenance
 airway tubes in, 238
 in anesthesia recovery, 97
 in cardiopulmonary resuscitation, 368
 in coma, 920
 complications of, 243–244
 endotracheal intubation in, 238–239
 in laryngeal foreign bodies, 1078
 in respiratory failure, 238–243
 in stroke patients, 952
 in thoracic trauma, 300
 tracheostomy in, 239–243
Airway obstruction, chronic, 216, 217–227
Albumin
 cortisol bound to, 674
 serum, 415
  levels in liver disease, 586
  therapeutic uses of, 428
 solutions in shock, 1197
Alcohol use
 in diabetes, 708
  hypoglycemia from, 721
 liver damage from, 592
 and Mallory-Weiss syndrome, 542
 and spermatogenesis, 751
 therapeutic
  for pain relief, 49

polyvinyl alcohol as eye lubricant, 1011
Alcoholism, 600–601
 cirrhosis in, 592
 and folic acid deficiency, 435–436
 and pancreatitis, 612
 polyneuritis in, 967
 and withdrawal symptoms, 600
Aldosterone, 159, 504, 672, 673
 release in burns, 1143
 secretion of, 673
  in cardiogenic shock, 384
  hyposecretion, 677
  in shock, 1188
  in water intoxication, 169
Aldosteronism, 676, 685–692
 hypokalemia in, 175
 primary, 685–687
  signs and symptoms of, 685–686
  treatment of, 686
 pseudoaldosteronism, 687
 secondary, 685, 687–692
  causes of, 686–687
  diagnosis of, 687
  treatment of, 687
 secretion rates, evaluation of, 686
Alimentary canal, 525
Alimentation. See Nutrition, parenteral total
Alkali, alkalosis from, metabolic, 187
Alkaline phosphatase levels
 in hyperparathyroidism, 667
 in liver disease, 586
 in pancreatic disease, 609
 in thyroid disease, 647
Alkaloids, chemotherapy with, 123, 125
Alkalosis
 from antacids, 546
 metabolic, 186–188
  diagnosis of, 187
  disorders with, 187
  in hypokalemia, 176
  nursing care in, 187–188
 respiratory, 184
  disorders with, 184
  from hyperventilation, 203
  nursing care in, 184
  in shock, 1191, 1193, 1200
Alkylating agents, 123, 124
Alleles, 16
Allergens, 32
Allergic reactions, 22, 29, 30–31. See also Hypersensitivity and allergic reactions
Allotypes, immunoglobulin, 23
Allport's syndrome, 1058
Alopecia, 1096
 from chemotherapy, 128, 446, 453
Alpha receptors, agents affecting, 1199
Alveolar ventilation, and carbon dioxide in blood, 163
Alveoli, pulmonary, 197–198
 fluid accumulation in, 201
Ambenonium, in myasthenia gravis, 963
Ambu bag, 235
 in cardiopulmonary resuscitation, 370
 in narcotic overdose, 230
Ambulation. See also Musculoskeletal system
 postoperative, 100
  after cardiopulmonary bypass, 392
  after laminectomy, 984
 in spinal cord injuries, 978
 for stroke patients, 954–955
Amelia, 819
Amenorrhea, 765, 766–768
 in gonadotropin deficiency, 631
 primary, 766
 secondary, 766
 treatment of, 767–768
American Cancer Society, 114
Amino acids, 11
γ-Aminobutyric acid deficiency, in Huntington's disease, 961

1207

By Betty Herr Hallinger

1208 Index

ε-Aminocaproic acid
  as antifibrinolytic agent, 956
  in disseminated intravascular coagulation, 464
Aminophylline
  in asthma, 266
  as bronchodilator, 226
Ammonia
  conversion into urea, 584
  production of, 505
    in hepatic coma, 598
Ammonium chloride, acidosis from, metabolic, 185
Amniocentesis, in abortion induction, 797
Amphotericin B, in fungus infections of lung, 287–288
Ampulla of Vater, 602
Amputations, 868–881
  above-elbow, 874
  above-knee, 871, 872–873
  at ankle, 871
  below-elbow, 873–874
  below-knee, 871–872
  closed, 870
  complications from, 876
  contractures from, 876
  exercises after, 876–877
  of hand or digits, 873
  and immediate postsurgical prosthesis, 878
  indications for, 868–869. See also Diabetes mellitus, neuropathy in; Peripheral vascular system, diseases of
  in lower extremity, 871–873
  major, 870
  minor, 869–870
  open, 870
  operative procedures in, 870–871
  phantom limb sensations and pain in, 43, 878–879
  postamputation care in, 876–878
  prostheses for, 874–876
  psychologic factors in, 869
  and rehabilitation, 881
  at shoulder, 874
  site of, factors affecting, 871
  stumps in
    dressings for, 871, 876, 877–878
    wrapping or banding of, 879–880
  Syme's, 871
  traumatic or accidental, 869
  types of, 869–874
  in upper extremity, 873–874
  and wheelchair use, 881
  at wrist, 873
Amygdaloid nucleus, 896
Amyl nitrite, in angina pectoris, 346
Amylase
  intestinal, 567
  pancreatic, 567
  serum levels, 609
    in pancreatic disease, 609
  urinary, 609
    in pancreatic disease, 609
Amyloidosis, 455
  liver in, 601
Anabolism, 11
Anal canal, 525
Analgesic drug therapy, 45–47
  dependency on, 46
  in osteoarthritis, 860
  postoperative, 99–100
  in rheumatoid arthritis, 864
  in terminal illness, 134
Anamnestic response, 27
Anaphylactic reactions, 29, 30, 36–37
  shock in, 30, 1186
Anasarca, 376
Androgens. See also Erythropoiesis
  adrenal secretion of, 672, 674, 736
    excessive, 687–688
  and bone growth, 815, 820
  as therapy in cancer, 126
Anemia, 428–443

aplastic, 436–437
  in burn patients, 443, 1144
  in cancer, 128
  in chemotherapy, 128, 436
  in folic acid deficiency, 435–436
  glossitis in, 419
  in glucose 6-phosphate dehydrogenase deficiency, 441
  hemolytic, 437–438
    autoimmune, 36, 443
    crises in, 443
    extracorpuscular factors in, 442
  from hemorrhage, 443
  hypoplastic, 436
  iron deficiency, 430–433
    from hemorrhage, 443
    pica in, 432
  in lead poisoning, 442
  macrocytic normochromic, 430
  in malaria, 442
  megaloblastic, 435–436
  microcytic hypochromic, 430
  in myeloma, multiple, 454
  nail changes in, 419
  normocytic normochromic, 430
  nursing care in, 429–430
  in panhypopituitarism, 635
  in paroxysmal nocturnal hemoglobinuria, 441
  pernicious, 433–435
    nursing care in, 435
    Schilling test in, 434
  pure red cell, congenital aplastic, 436
  refractory, primary, 436
  in renal failure, 512, 516
  sickle cell, 438–441
  and spherocytosis, hereditary, 438
  stomatitis in, 419
  in surgical patients, 83
  thalassemia, 441
  in thyroid disease, 642
  in vitamin B_{12} deficiency, 433–435
Anesthesia, 90–97
  caudal, 95–96
  complications from, 95, 97
  for eye surgery, 1002, 1010
  general, 90
    neuromuscular blocking agents with, 93–94
  hyperthermia from, malignant, 96–97
  hypothermia in, 96
    in cardiac surgery, 387
  inhalation, 90–94
    agents in, 92
    stages in, 91
  intravenous, 94
    agents in, 92–93
  recovery from, 98
  rectal, 94
  regional, 90, 94–96
    agents in, 93
  respiratory acidosis from, 182
  saddle block, 95
  spinal, 95
  topical, 94
Anesthesiologist, 86–87
Aneurysms
  arterial, 399–400
  cerebral, rupture of, 955
  dissecting, 399
  fusiform, 399
  saccular, 399
  surgical repair of, 400
  ventricular
    excision of, 386
    in myocardial infarction, 353–354, 386
Angina
  abdominal, 566
  cerebral, 950
  Ludwig's, 1073
  pectoris, 345–346
    and myocardial infarction, 347
  Vincent's, 542, 1073
Angiofibroma, of pharynx, 1073

Angiography
  celiac, 610
  cerebral, 915–916
  cholangiography, 603–604
  coronary
    cinearteriography, 386
    selective, 334
  fluorescent, of retinal vessels, 1002
  hepatic and portal, 588
  in peripheral vascular disease, 396
  pulmonary, 212
    in thromboembolism, 294
  renal, 478
Angioma, spider, in liver disease, 585
Angiotensin, 159, 504, 673–674
  and aldosterone secretion, 685
  secretion in shock, 1188
Anisocytosis, 415
Anisometropia, 1004
Ankle
  amputations in, 871
  sprains of, 821
Ankylosis, in rheumatoid arthritis, 862
Anomalies
  of ear, 1051–1052
  of musculoskeletal system, 819
  of nervous system, 932–934
  of urinary tract, 503
Anorectal disorders, 582–583
Anorexia, 527, 538–540
  in cancer, 117
  nervosa, 538–539
Anorexiants, 540
Anosmia, 908, 1061
Anoxia, in shock, 1190, 1194, 1200
Antabuse, in alcoholism, 601
Antacids, in peptic ulcer, 545–546
Antibiotics
  in acne, 1109
  chemotherapy with, 123, 125
  in emphysema, 260
  before intestinal surgery, 573
  in lung disease, chronic, 225, 227
  organisms resistant to, 73–74
  in pneumonia, 278
  in shock, 1201
  subeschar, in burns, 1158–1159
  in urinary tract infections, 487
Antibodies, 23. See also Immune response
  antiantibodies, 27
  antinuclear, 35
  antireceptor, 27
  control of responses in, 27
  formation in response to antigens, 22, 23
  heterophil, in mononucleosis, 454
  to insulin, 720
  reaginic, 30
  to sperm, in cervical mucus, 752
  to thyroid, 647
Anticholinergic drugs
  as mydriatics, 1010
  in pancreatitis, 611
  in Parkinson's disease, 960
  in peptic ulcer, 545, 546
  in prostatic hypertrophy, 763
Anticoagulant therapy, 397–399. See also Heparin
  adrenal hemorrhage from, 677
  drugs affecting, 398–399
  excessive, 462–463
  hypoprothrombinemia from, 460
  in thrombophlebitis, 407
Anticonvulsants, 927–928
  side effects of, 928
Antidiuretic hormone, 158–159, 504, 626
  affecting learning, 16
  in bleeding esophageal varices, 595
  deficiency of, 626–627
  release in burns, 1143
  secretion of
    in shock, 1189
    in water intoxication, 169
  in test for diabetes insipidus, 627

therapy with, after hypophysectomy, 634
  vascular effects of, 394
Antiemetic drugs, 562
Antigen(s), 23
  hepatitis-associated, 588
  histocompatible, 32
  HL-A system of, 33
  isoantigens, 33
Antigenic determinants, 26
Antigenicity, 23
Antihemophilic factor, concentrates of, 428, 461
Antihistamines, as cough suppressants, 227
Antilymphocytic serum, 33
Antimetabolites, chemotherapy with, 123, 124
Antistreptolysin O titer, 327
Antitoxin
  in diphtheria, 273
  tetanus, 939
α_1-Antitrypsin deficiency, and emphysema, 253, 254
Antrectomy, 548
Antrostomy, intranasal, 1062
Anulus fibrosis, 892, 983
Anuria, 471
  in renal failure, 506
  in shock, 1201
Anxiety. See Psychological aspects
Aorta, 313, 320
  balloon pump in, in shock, 1198
  coarctation of, hypertension in, 342
  diseases of, 399
Aortic bodies
  receptors in, 1181
  and respiration control, 204
Aortic valve, 313
  insufficiency of, stenosis of, 372
Aortitis, 399
Aphakia, 1020
  and retinal detachment, 1024
Aphasia, 907, 930–932
  expressive, 930
  global, 930
  jargon, 930
  nursing care in, 931–932
  receptive, 930
Aphonia, 1076
  functional, 1077
Apneustic breathing, 924
Apocrine glands, 1096
Aponeurosis, 817
Appendicitis, 581
Appendix, 525
Appetite reduction, drugs for, 540
Apraxia, 907, 930
Aqueous humor, 995
  drainage in glaucoma, 1021
  venous shunt of, in glaucoma management, 1022
Arachnoid, 892
Areola, of mammary gland, 784
  in mammaplasty, 791, 792
Arm
  amputations in, 873–874
  examination of, 808
  muscles of, 818, 819
Arrest
  cardiac, 368
  sinus, 357
Arrhenoblastoma, 780
Arrhythmias, cardiac, 328, 354–360. See also Hyperkalemia; Hypokalemia
  in aldosteronism, 685
  atrial, 357–358
    fibrillation, 358
    flutter, 357
    paroxysmal tachycardia, 357
    premature contractions, 357
  atrioventricular node in, 358–360
  bradycardia, 360
  bundle-branch block, 360
  cardiac arrest, 368

Index

after cardiopulmonary bypass, 390–391
cardiopulmonary resuscitation in, 368–371
from digitalis, 378
drugs in, 365–368
electrocardiogram in, 355–356
extrasystoles, 357
heart block, 359
from hypoxemia, 237–238
in myocardial infarction, 350, 353
premature contractions
  atrial, 357
  nodal, 359
  ventricular, 364
sinus, 356–357
  arrest, 357
  sick sinus syndrome, 356–357
supraventricular, 357
in thyrotoxicosis, 640
ventricular, 364–368
  asystole, 368
  fibrillation, 365
  tachycardia, 364–365
Wolff-Parkinson-White syndrome, 357
Arteries, 1180
  anatomic layers of, 320
  coronary. See Coronary arteries
  peripheral vascular disease, 313–314, 320–321, 393–409
Arteriography. See Angiography
Arterioles, 320–321, 1180
  of eye, 1001
Arteriosclerosis, 342
Arthritis
  in acromegaly, 629
  infectious, 867
  osteoarthritis, 858–860
  rheumatoid, 35, 861–866
    fibrous tissue changes in, 862–863
    immunologic factors in, 861–862
    infectious theory of, 862
    knee in, 847
    nursing care in, 865
    pannus formation in, 862
    personality factors in, 862
    pleural effusion in, 297
    synovitis in, 862
    treatment of, 863–865
Arthrography, 810
Arthroplasty
  of hip, 843–846
  of knee, 846–848
Arthropods, 65
Arthroscopy, 810
Arthus reaction, 34–35
Articular cartilage, 812, 815, 816
Arytenoid cartilage, 1074
Arytenoid muscle, 1074
Arytenoidectomy, 1078
Asbestosis, 290–291
Aschoff bodies, in rheumatic fever, 372
Ascites, 596–597
  dehydration in, 165
  in liver disease, 585
  paracentesis in, 597
  sodium loss in, 172
Asepsis, surgical, 88–90
L-Asparaginase, 123, 126
  toxic effects of, 129
Aspergillosis, pulmonary, 287
Aspiration
  of foreign bodies, 1077–1078
  pneumonia from, 279
  in respiratory failure, 243–244
Aspiration procedures
  bone marrow, 423
  cul-de-sac, 747–748
Assessment of patient, 53–55. See also Examination
  in biliary tract disorders, 602–604
  in bronchitis, 263
  in burns, 1137–1138
  and cancer detection, 111

cardiovascular data in, 321–335
in cerebral injuries, 942–943
in dehydration, 165–166
ear function tests in, 1036–1041
in emphysema, 256–258
eye examinations in, 996–1003
in gastrointestinal disorders, 527–535
in hematopoietic disorders, 418–423
in laryngeal disorders, 1076
in musculoskeletal disorders, 807–810
in nervous system dysfunction, 905–917
in peripheral vascular disease, 394–396
in respiratory system dysfunction, 206–216
in shock, 1193–1196, 1202
in thyroid disorders, 638–642
in urinary system disorders, 471–481, 486–487
Asterixis
  in carbon dioxide narcosis, 205
  in emphysema, 256
  in hepatic coma, 598
  in liver disease, 585
Asthma, 263–268
  adaptation to, 267–268
  allergic, 264–267
  attacks in, 265
  causative factors in, 264
  idiopathic, 264
  status asthmaticus, 265–266
  treatment of, 266–267
Astigmatism, 1004
Astrocytoma, 946
Ataxic breathing, 924
Atelectasis, postoperative, 97, 99
  after extracorporeal circulation, 388, 391
  respiratory failure in, 232
  after splenectomy, 456
Atherosclerosis, 342–343
  and aneurysm formation, 399
  cerebral, 951
  cholesterol levels in, 326
  in diabetes, 700
  of mesenteric arteries, 566
  and myocardial infarction, 347
  myocardial revascularization in, 385–387
Atopy, 29
Atrioventricular node, 317, 318
  in arrhythmias, 358–360
Atrium, cardiac, 313
  in arrhythmias, 357–358
Atrophy, muscular, 818
Atropine
  affecting autonomic nervous system, 319
  in arrhythmias, 367
  as mydriatic, 1010
Audiometry, 1042–1043
Auricle, 1037
Auricular lymph nodes, 420
Auscultation
  of the abdomen, 531
  of cardiovascular system, 323–325
  in chest examination, 209–210
  in peripheral vascular disease, 395
Australia antigen, 588
Autochthonous relation, between tumor and host, 37
Autografts, 32
  in burns, 1168–1169
Autoimmune diseases, 22. See also Collagen diseases; Lupus erythematosus; Rheumatoid arthritis; Ulcerative colitis
Automatic speech, 930
Automaticity, in cardiac cells, 317, 318
Autonomic nervous system, 318–319, 904–905
  assessment of, 910–911
  and hyperreflexia, 970–971
  in spinal cord injuries, 967

Autosplenectomy, 439
Avidity, of antigen-antibody bond, 26
Axillary lymph nodes, 420
Axon, 891
Azotemia, 506
Azulfidine
  in enteritis, regional, 568
  in ulcerative colitis, 552

B cells, lymphocyte, 24, 26, 418
Babinski reflex, 911
Bacteremia and septic shock, 1187
Bacteriostatic agents, 89
Bacteriuria, 473, 486, 487
  and stone formation, 503
Balance, maintenance of, 1035
Balanitis, 777
Ballistocardiogram, 329
Balloon pump, intra-aortic, 1198
  in cardiogenic shock, 385
Ballottement of nail base, in carcinoma of lung, 306
Bárány test, of vestibular function, 1043
Barium x-rays
  enema in, 534
  of stomach, 533
Baroreceptors
  and blood pressure regulation, 1181
  and control of respiration, 204
Barron food pump, 539
Bartholin's cyst, 754
Bartter's syndrome, 687
Basal cells, 1095
Basal ganglia, 896
Base
  definition of, 161
  strong, 162
  weak, 162
Basilar artery, 899
Basilar membrane, of cochlear duct, 1041
Basophils, 417, 418
  in allergic reactions, 29
Bathing
  in burns, 1160–1161
  in skin diseases, 1148
Baxter formula, in burns, 1146
BCG vaccine, in malignant melanoma, 132, 1125
BCNU, in cancer, 126
Bearded areas
  sycosis barbae, 1114
  tinea barbae, 1117
Beau's lines, in nails, 1098
Bed sores, 1129. See also Decubitus ulcers
Behavior changes. See also Psychological aspects
  in alcohol withdrawal, 600
  in brain tumors, 945
  in Cushing's disease, 682
  factors affecting, 57–58
  in thyroid disease, 639, 641, 654
Behavior modification
  in anorexia nervosa, 539
  for pain relief, 45
Belching, 527
Bell's palsy, 966, 1058
Bence Jones proteinuria, in multiple myeloma, 454–455
Beriberi, heart in, 375
Bernstein test, for acid reflux, 562
Berylliosis, 291
Beta receptors, agents affecting, 1199
Bezold's mastoiditis, 1054
Bicarbonate
  ratio to carbonic acid, 162, 201
  renal tubular reabsorption of, 163, 505
Biceps, 818
Biceps reflex, 910
Bigeminal rhythm, 323
  in digitalis toxicity, 378
Biguanides
  as hypoglycemic agents, 709
  side effects of, 710
Bile, 567, 583

characteristics of, 536
passage into duodenum, 602
pigments of, 583
salts of, 583
Biliary tract, 602–608
  assessment of, 602–604
  cholecystitis, 605
  cholelithiasis, 604–605
  in cirrhosis, 592
  drainage with T tube, 606–608
  fistulas in
    acidosis from, 185
    sodium loss in, 172
  surgery of, 606–608
Bilirubin, 422, 583
  direct, 422
  indirect, 422
  in jaundice, 584
  serum levels of
    in hemolytic anemia, 438
    measurements of, 586
  in urine, 587, 604
Biliverdin, 583
Billroth procedures, 548
Biopsy, 80–81
  of bone marrow, 423
  of cervix uteri, 748
  excisional, 81
  frozen-section technique in, 80–81
  of liver, 587–588
  of lung tissue, 214
  punch, 81
  renal, 479–480
  of reproductive tract tissue, 747
  of skin, 1104
  of small intestine, 568
  of thyroid tissue, 647
Birth control, 792–796
  and basal body temperature, 746
  condoms in, 795
  diaphragms in, 793
  intrauterine devices in, 793–794
    pelvic inflammatory disease from, 757
  oral contraceptives in, 794–795
    amenorrhea from, 767
    complications from, 794–795
    and folic acid deficiency, 436
    hypertension from, 338
    and pulmonary infarction, 294
    and thrombophlebitis, 407
  rhythm method of, 793
Birthmarks, 1128
Bishydroxycoumarin, 398
  overdosage of, 460, 463
Black eye, 1019
Black light, use of, 1108
Blackheads, 1108–1109
Bladder, 469–470
  automatic, 470
  autonomous, 470
  care of
    in autonomic hyperreflexia, 970
    in comatose patients, 921
    in multiple sclerosis, 958
    in spinal cord injuries, 974–976
    in stroke patients, 953
  cystocele, 773, 774
  cystometry of, 480
  cystoscopy of, 478–479
  decompression of, in prostatic hypertrophy, 763
  distention of, 475
    postoperative, 99
  drugs affecting function of, 470
  ectopic, 503
  electronic stimulation of, 976
  in micturition, 469–470
  neurogenic, 483, 974–976
  obstruction in, 489
  palpation of, 475
  pressure in, 469
  spasms after prostatectomy, 765
  in spinal cord injury, 470, 483, 974–976

Bladder *Continued*
  suprapubic drainage of, 483
  training program for, 483
  trauma of, 501
  tumors of, 491
    chemotherapy in, 494
    cystectomy in, 494
    radiation therapy in, 493–494
    urinary diversion in, 494–500
Blakemore-Sengstaken tube, 537
Blastomycosis, pulmonary, 287
Blebs, emphysematous, 254
Bleeding. *See* Hemorrhage
Bleeding time, 457
Blenderized foods, use of, 539
Bleomycin, 125
  toxic effects of, 129
Blepharitis, 998
Blind spot, physiologic, 995
Blindness
  agencies for help with, 994, 1030
  from cranial nerve lesions, 908
  in diabetes, 729
  from glaucoma, 1021
  legal, definition of, 997
  and nursing care in hospital, 1012–1014
  prevention of, 993–994
  and rehabilitation, 1028–1030
Blinking reflex, 998
  loss of, in Bell's palsy, 966
Blister formation, 1128
Blood. *See also* Hematopoietic and lymphatic system
  in cerebrospinal fluid, 913
  clotting factors in, 459
  erythrocytes in, 415–417
  function of, 415
  leukocytes in, 417–418
  platelets in, 418
  transfusions of. *See* Transfusion therapy
  in urine, 472
  in prostatic hypertrophy, 763
Blood-brain barrier, 900
Blood flow. *See* Circulation
Blood groups
  in erythroblastosis fetalis, 442
  and matching blood transfusions, 33
  and transfusion reactions, 36
Blood pressure, 320–321
  arterial, 330–331
  in cardiogenic shock, 383
  in coma, 920
  diastolic, 330, 336
  hypertension, 336–342
  intra-arterial measurement of, 331, 1195
  normal values for, 336
  pulmonary arterial, 198, 333
  readings by patients, 338
  regulation of, 1181
  in shock
    direct measurements, 1195
    indirect measurements, 1193–1194
  systolic, 330, 336
  venous, 331–333
    central, 331
Blood vessels. *See also* Arteries; Capillaries; Veins
  of adrenal glands, 672
  anatomy and physiology of, 1180–1181
  of brain and spinal cord, 899–900
  of breast, 784
  of gastrointestinal system, 525–526
  of liver, 583
  of myocardium, 313, 1180
  of parathyroid glands, 669
  peripheral vascular system, 313–314, 320–321, 393–409
  of pituitary gland, 626
  renal, anomalies of, 503
  of reproductive tract, 777
  of thyroid gland, 638
Blood volume, 1179–1180

expanders in cardiogenic shock, 384–385
  in hypovolemic shock, 1184
  restoration of, 1197
Bock knee, 873, 875
Body function
  assessment of, 12–13
  and homeostasis, 50–51
  optimum, 50
Body mechanics, 882
Boils, 1114
Bone(s), 810–815
  accretion of, 813–814
  in acromegaly, 629
  cells of, 813
  in Cushing's disease, 681–682
  flat, 810
  in hypoparathyroidism, 666–667
  infection of, 820
  irregular, 810
  long, 810
  marrow of, 814
    aspiration and biopsy of, 423
    chemotherapy affecting, 128
    in hemolytic anemia, 438
    in myeloma, multiple, 454
  matrix of, 813
  muscle attachment to, 817
  and osteogenesis, 814–815
  parathyroid hormone affecting, 665
  in pseudohypoparathyroidism, 671
  resorption of, 813–814
  scanning of, 810
  short, 810
  in skeletal traction, 853–856
  in thyroid disease, 642, 659–660
  tumors of, 820
    amputations in, 868
Bonney test, in stress incontinence, 775
Borborygmi, 527
Botulin toxin, 940
Botulism, 940
Bowel management
  in autonomic hyperreflexia, 970
  in comatose patients, 921
  in Parkinson's disease, 961
  in spinal cord injuries, 976–977
  in stroke patients, 953
Bowel sounds, 531
Bowen's disease, 1123
Bowman's capsule, 504
Braces, care of, 978
Brachioradialis reflex, 910–911
Bradycardia, 316
  and Stokes-Adams syndrome, 360
Bradykinin, 1191
  anaphylactic shock from, 1186
  vascular effects of, 394
Braille, use of, 1029
Brain. *See also* Central nervous system; Cerebrum
  abscess of, 936
  cerebral injuries, 941–944
  electroencephalography of, 914
  scanning of, 915
  stereotaxic surgery of, for pain relief, 50
  tumors of, 944–947
    diagnosis of, 945
    hypernatremia in, 173
    symptoms of, 944–945
    treatment of, 946–947
    types of, 945–946
Brainstem, 896
Breast(s), 784–792
  anatomy of, 784
  cancer of, 786–792
    chemotherapy in, 788
    factors related to, 786–787
    mastectomy in, 787–788
    metastasis of, 787, 790–791
    nursing care in, 789–791
    risk factors in, 785
    staging of, 787
    treatment of, 787–789
  cystic disease of, 743, 786

diagnostic tests of, 785
  epitheliosis of, 786
  examination of, 112, 742–744
    in females, 742–744
    in males, 744
    self-examination, 744
  fibrocystic disease of, 785–786
  function of, 784
  mammaplasty of, 791–792
  nodules in, 743
  Paget's disease of nipple, 786
  papilloma of, 786
  prosthesis for, 790
Breath sounds, 209–210
  bronchial, 209
  bronchovesicular, 209
  cavernous, 209
  in emphysema, 258
  tubular, 209
  vesicular, 209
Breathing exercises, 222, 223–224
Breathlessness. *See* Dyspnea
Brenner tumors, ovarian, 779
British anti-Lewisite (BAL), in lead poisoning, 442
Bromides, acne from, 1109
Bromsulphalein test, of liver function, 586–587
Bronchi
  adenoma of, 306
  injuries of, 303
Bronchial hygiene, 218–222, 226
  effectiveness of, 222
Bronchial washings, 213
Bronchiectasis, 268–270
  diagnosis of, 269
  treatment and nursing care, 270
Bronchitis, chronic, 261–263
  and assessment of patient, 263
  progression of, 262–263
  reversible, 263
Bronchodilators, 225–227
  aerosol, 218–219, 226
  in asthma, 266
  in emphysema, 260
Bronchogram, 213
  in bronchiectasis, 269
Bronchopneumonia, 276
Bronchoscopy, 212–213
Bronchospasm, in bronchitis, 262
Brooke resuscitation formula, 1145
Brown-Sequard syndrome, 970
Brudzinski's sign, in meningitis, 934
Buck's extension, in traction for fractures, 837, 850, 852–853
Budd-Chiari syndrome, 593
Buerger-Allen exercises, 396
Buerger's disease, 403
Buffers, definition of, 162
Buffy coat, between erythrocytes and plasma, 427
Bullae, 1099
  emphysematous, 254
Bundle branch, 317
Bundle-branch block, 360
Bunions, 866
Burkitt's lymphoma, 453
Burns, 21, 1137–1173
  anemia from, 443
  antibiotics in, subeschar, 1158–1159
  anxiety and discomfort in, 1153
  assessment of depth, 1138–1140
  autografts in, 1168–1169
  bathing in, 1160–1161
  biologic dressings for, 1164–1165
  carbon monoxide poisoning in, 1148
  chemical, of esophagus, 570
  contractures from, 1169
  cross-contamination in, prevention of, 1161–1162
  debridement of, 1160, 1165–1167
  dehydration in, 165
  emergency care in, 1137
  eschartomy in, 1140
  estimate of total body surface area burned, 1138

excisional therapy in, 1167–1168
  exercise in, 1172
  of eyes, 1018
  fasciotomy in, 1140
  first degree, 1138
  fluid and electrolyte balance in, 1142–1144
  fluid resuscitation in, 1138
    formulas for, 1145–1148
  gamma globulin in, 1159
  gastrointestinal disorders in, 1153–1154
  hand care in, 1171
  hematemesis in, 1154
  hematologic changes in, 1144
  and hospital resources for care, 1141
  hypernatremia in, 173
  infections in, 1156
    prevention of, 1152–1153
  magnesium levels in, 1144
  metabolic response to, 1150–1152
  nutrition in, 1151–1152
  oxygen therapy in, 1149–1150
  pain in, 1141–1142
  phagocytosis in, 1159
  pneumonia in, 1150
  and positioning of patient, 1169–1171
  potassium deficit in, 1144
  pressure wraps in, 1173
  Pseudomonas vaccine in, 1159
  psychological problems in, 1162–1164
  rehabilitation in, 1172–1173
  respiratory problems in, 1137, 1118–1150
    management of, 1150
  Ringer's lactate solution in, 1147–1148
  second degree, 1138
  sepsis in, 1153, 1155
  shock from, 1184
  smoke inhalation in, 1137, 1149
  sodium loss in, 171
  splinting in, 1171
  third degree, 1140
  topical agents in, 1156–1158
  transfusion reactions in, 1144
  treatment of, 1156–1172
  urinary output in, 1143, 1147–1148
  water loss in, 1143
Burow's solution, in atopic dermatitis, 1112
Bursitis, 866
Busulfan, 124
Byssinosis, 291

Cachexia, 527
  in terminal illness, 132
Calcifications in ear, in Addison's disease, 1037
Calcitonin, 638
  and bone resorption, 815
Calcium
  absorption of, 665
  in bone, 813
  as coagulation factor, 457, 459
  dietary, recommended amounts of, 155
  function in body, 154, 664
  hypercalcemia, 178–179
    in cancer patients, 133–134
    diseases causing, 668–669
  hypocalcemia, 178
  and insulin release, 694
  levels in plasma, 664
    in hyperparathyroidism, 667
    in hypoparathyroidism, 669
    metastatic carcinoma affecting, 668–669
    in pancreatic disease, 609
    and parathyroid hormone release, 664
    in renal failure, 511
  metabolism of, thyrocalcitonin affecting, 636, 642
  and osteogenesis, 814
  parathyroid hormone affecting, 179

tolerance test in hypoparathyroidism, 670
urinary, 161, 665
Calcium gluconate
 in cardiopulmonary resuscitation, 371
 in hypocalcemia, 178
 in hypoparathyroidism, 671
 in test of parathyroid function, 667
Calcium oxalate stones, 502
Calculi
 choledocholithiasis, 606
 cholelithiasis, 604–605
 otoliths, 1043
 in pancreatic duct, 613
 urinary, 501–503
  calcium oxalate, 502
  causes of, 502
  cystine, 502
  phosphate, 502
  prevention of, 503
  types of, 502
  uric acid, 502
Callus formation, 826, 1101
Caloric intake, for burn patients, 1151, 1152
Caloric stimulation tests, 1039, 1043–1044
Calorie, 10
Canaliculi, biliary, 583
Cancer, 105–136. See also Tumors and anatomic sites of cancer
 of breast, 786–792
 and carcinoembryonic antigen, 37, 535, 614
 and carcinogenesis, 109–111
 of cervix uteri, 781
  Schiller test in, 747
 chemotherapy in, 122–131
 of colon
  and polyposis, 572
  surgery in, 574
  and ulcerative colitis, 553
 danger signals of, 113
 detection and diagnosis of, 111–114
  exfoliative cytology in, 113
  laboratory tests in, 113
  mammography in, 112, 785
  Papanicolaou smear test in, 112–113, 740, 747
  radionuclides in, 120–122
  thermography in, 112, 785
  xerography in, 112, 785
 of ear, 1052
 of esophagus, 569–570
 of fallopian tubes, 781
 of gallbladder, 605–606
 from immunosuppressive therapy, 37–38
 immunotherapy in, 131–132
 of kidney, 490
 of larynx, 1079–1090
 of lung, 304–309
 metastasis of, 108–109. See also Metastasis
 nature of, 107–108
 oral, detection of, 529
 of ovary, 779–780
 of pancreas, 613–614
 of prostate, 492
 radiation therapy in, 116–122
 of skin, 1123–1124
 staging of, 109
 of stomach, and peptic ulcer, 547–548
 surgery in, 114–116
  cryosurgery, 115
  radiation with, 116–117
  rehabilitation after, 115
  resection, 115
 and terminal illness, 132–136
 terminology of, 105–107
 of thyroid, 663
 of tonsil, 1074
 treatment of, 114–132
 and tumor growth fraction, 123
 of vagina, 782
 of vulva, 782–783

Candidiasis, 1115
 oral, 542
 of reproductive tract, 756
Canes, use of, 882–883
Cantor tube, 536–537
Capillaries, 313, 321, 1181
 diabetes affecting, 700
 fragility of
  in infections, 458
  test of, 458
 injuries in burns, 1142
 movement across membranes of, 1182–1183
 pressure in, increase in, 180
 pulmonary, 313
  blood flow in, 199
 in shock, 1188, 1190
Caput medusae, 585, 593
Carbohydrate
 dietary, in diabetes, 706, 707
 malabsorption of, 568
 metabolism of, 10
Carbon dioxide
 and chronic hypercapnia, 227–228
 diffusion of, 201
 narcosis from, 205
  in emphysema, 256
  in myxedema coma, 662
 partial pressure of, 199, 201
 removal from body, 197
 serum levels of
  renal regulation of, 163–164
  in respiratory acidosis, 181
  respiratory rate affecting, 163
 transport of, 201
Carbon monoxide poisoning, in burn patients, 1148
Carbon tetrachloride, liver damage from, 591
Carbonic acid, ratio to bicarbonate, 162, 201
Carbonic anhydrase
 and bicarbonate reabsorption, 505
 inhibitors of
  acidosis from, metabolic, 185
  as diuretics, 380
  in glaucoma, 1011
  hypokalemia from, 175
 in red cells, 201
Carbuncles, 1114–1115
Carcinoembryonic antigen, 37
 in pancreatic cancer, 614
 radioimmunoassay for, 535
Carcinogenesis, 109–111
Carcinoid tumors, 564
Carcinoma, 107. See also Cancer
Cardiac index, 1180
Cardiac output, 1180
 in burns, 1142
Cardiac surgery, 385–393
Cardinal ligaments, 772
Cardiogenic shock. See Shock, Cardiogenic
Cardiomyopathy, 375
Cardiopulmonary bypass, 387–393
 ambulation after, 392
 delirium after, 391
 extracorporeal circulation in, 387–388
 postoperative care, 390–393
 preoperative care, 389–390
 sleep patterns after, 392
Cardiopulmonary resuscitation, 368–371
Cardiospasm, 561
Cardiovascular system, 313–409
 in acidosis
  metabolic, 185
  respiratory, 182
 in alkalosis, metabolic, 187
 anatomy and physiology of, 313–321
 angina pectoris, 345–346
 arrhythmias, 354–360
 assessment of, 321–335
 atherosclerosis, 342–343
 cardiomyopathy, 375
 cardiopulmonary bypass, 387–393

complications from immobilization, prevention of, 841
 in dehydration, 165
 in diabetes, 700–701
 diagnostic tests of, 325–330
 disorders of, 336–371
  epidemiology and prevention of, 335–336
  risk factors in, 336
  in specific structures, 371–385
 endocarditis, bacterial, 373–374
 heart, 313, 314–320
 heart failure, congestive, 375–381
 in hyperkalemia, 177
 in hyperlipoproteinemia, 326, 343–345
 in hypermagnesemia, 180
 hypertension, 336–342
 in hypokalemia, 175
 in hypomagnesemia, 179
 in hyponatremia, 172
 myocardial infarction, 347–354
 myocarditis, 375
 pacemakers, cardiac, 360–364
 pericarditis, 374–375
 peripheral vascular system, 313–314, 320–321, 393–409
 pulmonary edema, 381–383
 resuscitation, cardiopulmonary, 368–371
 revascularization procedures, myocardial, 385–387
 rheumatic fever, 372
 shock, cardiogenic, 383–385, 1185–1186
 surgery of, 385–393
 tamponade, cardiac, 374
 in thyroid disease, 640
 transplantation of heart, 393
 tumors of heart, 375
 valvular lesions, 372–373
Cardioversion
 in atrial fibrillation, 358
 in atrial flutter, 357
 in atrial tachycardia, paroxysmal, 357
 procedures in, 358
 in ventricular tachycardia, 365
Carotid arteries, 899, 1044
Carotid bodies, receptors in, 1181
 and respiration control, 204
Carpal tunnel syndrome
 in acromegaly, 629
 in myxedema, 642
Carpopedal spasm, 178
Carriers of disease, 64
Cartilage
 articular, 812, 815, 816
  in osteoarthritis, 859
 grafts for ear, 1051
 laryngeal, 1074
Caruncle, urethral, 491
Casts
 for fractures, 828–834
 urinary, 473
Catabolism, 11
Cataracts, 1000, 1019–1021
 bilateral, 1021
 congenital, 1019
 in diabetes, 701
 immature, 1019
 intraocular lenses in, 1020
 mature, 1019
 phacoemulsification in, 1020
 senile, 1019
 surgery of, 1019–1021
Catecholamine levels, in pheochromocytoma, 688, 689
Cathartics, 565
Catheterization
 cardiac, 333–335
  left-heart, 334
  nursing care after, 334–335
  right-heart, 334
 for cardiac pacemakers, 360
 in cystoscopy, 479

and dialysis tubing placement, 514–515
 for intra-arterial blood pressure measurements, 331
 nasal, for oxygen therapy, 232–233
 for pulmonary artery pressure, 333
 of subclavian vein, in total parenteral nutrition, 189
 urinary, 476–478
  Foley catheter in, 482
  infections from, 76–77
  intermittent, 976
  male catheter taped to abdomen, 921, 974–975
  nursing care with, 482–483
 for venous pressure measurements, 332, 333
Cauda equina, 902
Caudal anesthesia, 95–96
Caudate nucleus, 896
Cauliflower ear, 1051
Causative agents, for disease, 65
Cauterization
 in cervicitis, 781
 in epistaxis, 1063
 for sterilization of females, 749
Cecostomy, 574
Cecum, 525
Celiac arteriography, 610
Celiac disease, 568
Cell(s), 7–9
 in blood, 415–418
 and blood volume, 1179
 in bone, 813
 in bone marrow, 814
 in cerebrospinal fluid, 913
 cytotoxic or cytolytic reactions, 35–36
 in inflammatory response, 19
 membrane permeability of, 155–156
 in muscle, 817
 neurons, 891
 in pancreas, 692
 in parathyroid glands, 664
 in pituitary gland, 625
 proliferation in cancer, 107–108
 shock affecting, 1191–1192
 in skin, 1095
 in thyroid gland, 638
Cell-mediated immune response, 22, 26, 29
 and delayed hypersensitivity, 32
Cellulitis, 1115
 orbital, in ethmoid sinusitis, 1062
Cement
 in arthroplasty procedures, 845
 in ostomy appliances, 556
Central nervous system, 891–904
 in acidosis
  metabolic, 185
  respiratory, 182
 in alkalosis
  metabolic, 187
  respiratory, 184
 in anemia, 429, 434
 assessment of, 907–910
 blood-brain barrier, 900
 brainstem, 896
 cerebellum, 896
 cerebrospinal fluid, 900–902
 cerebrum, 892–896
 cranial nerves, 896–899
 dehydration affecting, 165
 in hypernatremia, 174
 in hypokalemia, 175
 in hyponatremia, 172
 nerve tracts in, 903–904
 in pheochromocytoma, 689
 reflex arc in, 902–903
 in renal failure, 511
 spinal cord, 902
 in thyroid disease, 641
 vascular system of, 899–900
 in water intoxication, 169
Centrioles, cellular, 9
Centrisomes, cellular, 9
Cephalin flocculation test, 586

Cerebellum, 896
  assessment of, 909–910
Cerebral arteries, 899
  angiography of, 915–916
Cerebral palsy, 934
Cerebrospinal fluid, 892, 900–902
  analysis of, 912–913
  in cerebral injuries, 942
  drainage of, 925
  in encephalitis, 935
  in hydrocephalus, 933
  in meningitis, 935
  otorrhea of, 1050
  pH changes in, chemoreceptor responses to, 204, 256
  rhinorrhea of, 1066, 1068
Cerebrovascular disease, 950–955
  ambulation in, 954–955
  causes of, 951
  and discharge planning for patients, 955
  lacunar strokes, 951
  and nursing care of stroke patients, 951–955
  from oral contraceptives, 794
  psychological aspects of, 953–954
  and subarachnoid hemorrhage, 955–956
  symptoms of, 950–951
  and transient ischemic attacks, 950–951
Cerebrum, 892–896
  cortex of, 891
    evaluation of function, 907
  dominant hemisphere in, 892
  injuries of, 941–944
    assessment of, 942–943
    dehydration in, 165
    emergency care of, 942
    nursing care in, 943–944
    treatment of, 943
  tumors of. See Brain, tumors of
Cerumen, 1037–1039
  accumulation of, 1049
Ceruminoma, 1052
Cervical lymph nodes, 420
  adenitis of, acute, 408
  in laryngeal carcinoma, 1081
  palpation of, 1071
Cervical rib, 404
Cervical spine
  cordotomy for pain relief, 49
  fractures of
    casts for, 831
    traction in, 851, 854
  herniation of intervertebral disks, 983, 984
  injuries of, 968
  function in, 971–972
Cervicitis, chronic, 781
Cervix uteri
  biopsy of, cone, 748
  carcinoma of, 781
    Schiller test in, 747, 781
    staging of, 781
    treatment of, 782
  mucus of
    affecting sperm, 752
    evaluation of, 752
    ferning of, 747, 752
  polyps of, 781
Chalazion, 999
Chancre, 756
Charcot's triad, in multiple sclerosis, 957
Cheilitis, 1116
Chemicals
  agranulocytosis from, 444
  aplastic anemia from, 436
  as carcinogens, 110
  esophageal burns from, 570
  eye injuries from, 1018
  hemolytic anemia from, 442
  leukemia from, 445
  pneumonia from, 278
Chemonucleolysis, in intervertebral disk herniation, 984–985

Chemoreceptors
  and blood pressure regulation, 1181
  and control of respiration, 204
  responses to pH changes in cerebrospinal fluid, 204, 256
Chemosurgery in skin lesions, 1125–1126
Chemotaxis, 19, 418
  in burns, 1159
Chemotherapy, cancer, 122–131
  in adrenal hyperplasia or tumors, 684, 685
  agents in, 124–127
  alopecia from, 128, 446, 453
  aplastic anemia from, 436
  in bladder tumors, 494
  in brain tumors, 947
  in breast cancer, 788
  combinations of drugs in, 129
  folic acid deficiency from, 436
  in Hodgkin's disease, 452
  intra-arterial infusion in, 130
  investigational therapy in, 130–131
  in leukemia, 446–447
  in myeloma, multiple, 455
  in ovarian carcinoma, 780
  in pancreatic cancer, 614
  Pneumocystis carinii pneumonia from, 453
  in prostatic tumors, 778
  regional perfusion in, 129–130
  stomatitis from, 127–128
  toxic effects of, 123, 127–129, 446–447
Chenodeoxycholic acid, in cholelithiasis, 604
Chest examination, 207–210
  auscultation in, 209–210
  breath sounds in, 209–210
  inspection and palpation in, 208
  movements in, 207–208
  percussion in, types of sounds in, 208–209
  x-rays in, 212
Chest surgery, 246–252
Chest tubes, 250–252
  clamping of, tension pneumothorax from, 252
  milking of, 252
  one-bottle system with, 250
  pleur-Evac with, 250–251
  removal of, 252
  three-bottle system with, 250
  two-bottle system with, 250
  water seal system with, 250
Cheyne-Stokes respiration, 228, 923
Chickenpox, 1120
Chloride
  in cerebrospinal fluid, 913
  dietary, recommended amounts of, 155
  serum levels in Cushing's disease, 682
  urinary, 161
Chocolate cysts of ovary, 771
Cholangiography, 603–604
  endoscopic, 604
  transhepatic, percutaneous, 603, 610
Cholecystectomy, 605
  complications of, 608
Cholecystitis, 605
  acute, 605
  chronic, 605
Cholecystography, 602–603
Cholecystokinin, 602
Cholecystokinin-pancreozymin, 609
Choledochitis, 606
Choledochoduodenostomy, 606
Choledochojejunostomy, 606
Choledocholithiasis, 606
Choledochostomy, 606
Cholelithiasis, 604–605
Cholesteatoma, of ear, 1052–1053
Cholesterol, 343–345
  adrenal synthesis of, 672
  dietary, effects of, 344
  serum levels of, 326

  in liver disease, 586
  in thyroid disease, 640, 647
Cholinergic drugs
  as miotics, 1010
  in myasthenia gravis, 963
Cholinesterase, 30
Chorda tympani nerve injury, from stapedectomy, 1057
Chorea, Huntington's, 961–962
Choriocarcinoma, thyroid hormone levels in, 643
Chorionepithelioma, 784
Chorionic gonadotropin, human, 631
Choroid, 995
Choroid plexus, 901
Christmas disease, 460
Chromosomes, 8
  and sex-linked diseases, 17
Chronic illness, 63
Chronic obstructive pulmonary disease (COPD). See Respiratory system
Chronotropic effect, of autonomic nervous system stimulation, 319
Chvostek sign, in tetany, 178, 670
Chylothorax, 297
Chyme, 561, 567
Chymopapain in chemonucleolysis, 984–985
Cigarette smoking. See Smoking
Cilia, in bronchitis, 262
Ciliary body, 995
Cinearteriography, coronary, 386
Cinefluorography in musculoskeletal disorders, 810
Circadian rhythms, 15. See also Rhythms
Circle of Willis, 899
CircOlectric bed, 854, 972–973, 1171
Circulating nurse, 87
Circulation
  of blood, 313, 1181–1182
  of cerebrospinal fluid, 900–901
  extracorporeal, 387–388
  hemodynamics of, 1181–1183
  impairment from casts, in fractures, 832
  lymphatic, 408
  macrocirculation, 1180
  microcirculation, 1180
  peripheral, 393
  pulmonary, 198–199, 1180
  systemic, 1180
  in venous system, 404–405
Circumcision
  and appearance of penis, 739
  and carcinoma of penis, 777
  and cervical carcinoma, 781
Cirrhosis, 592–593
  biliary, 592
  congestive, 592
  dehydration in, 165
  Laennec's, 592
  nursing care in, 593
  and portal hypertension, 593
  postnecrotic, 592
  thyroid function in, 648
Cisterna magna, 892
Cisternal puncture, 912
Cistron, 33
Citrate intoxication, from blood transfusions, 426–427
Citric acid cycle, shock affecting, 1191
Claudication, intermittent, 400–401
Clavus, 1101
Climacteric, 766
Clinistix, 696
Clinitest tablets, 696
Clot retraction, 457, 458
Clotting time, 457–458
  in cardiovascular disorders, 327
Clubbing of fingers or nails, 1098
  in respiratory system dysfunction, 206
  in thyroid disease, 651
Cluster headache, 918
Coagulation, 456–458
  anticoagulant therapy affecting, 462–463

  blood clotting factors in, 459
  and clot retraction, 457, 458
  disorders of, 457, 459–462
    disseminated intravascular, 463–464
      in shock, 1190–1191, 1201
    extrinsic system in, 456–457
    in hemophilia, 460–461
    in hypoprothrombinemia, 459–460
    intrinsic system in, 457
    in liver disease, 585
    in shock, 1196
  tests of, 457–458
  in thrombocytopenia, 462
  and vascular abnormalities, 458
  in von Willebrand's disease, 461–462
Coagulopathy, consumption, 463
Coal miner's pneumoconiosis, 291
Coarctation of aorta, hypertension in, 342
Coccidioidomycosis, pulmonary, 287
Cochlea, 1040, 1041, 1045
  electronic, 1048
Codominance, of genes, 17
Coitus, painful, 776
Cold applications. See also Cryosurgery
  compresses for eyes, 1009
  gastric freezing in peptic ulcer, 546
  for pain relief, 46–47
  in rheumatoid arthritis, 863
Cold exposure, effects of
  in asthma, 264, 268
  in bronchitis, 262
  in emphysema, 253, 257
  in hypothyroidism, 659
  and paroxysmal hemoglobinuria, 442
  and Raynaud's disease, 403–404
Cold sore, 542
Colds, common, 272
Colectomy, total, with ileostomy, 553
Colic, 528
  biliary, 602
  relief of, 605
Colitis
  granulomatous, 567
  ulcerative, 551–553
    and cancer of colon, 553
    dehydration in, 165
    disorders with, 552
    ileostomy in, 553–561. See also Ileostomy
    medical treatment of, 552–553
    psychologic factors in, 552, 559
    symptoms of, 552
Collagen, 813
Collagen diseases, 34–35. See also specific diseases
Collagen fibers, dermal, 1095
  in burn wounds, 1169
Colloidal gold test, of cerebrospinal fluid, 913
Colloidal osmotic pressure, plasma, 321, 1182
Colon, 525
  cancer of
    and polyposis, 572
    surgery in, 574
    and ulcerative colitis, 553
  for esophageal replacement, 570
  polyps of, 572
  spastic, 564
Colonoscopy, 534
Colostomy, 574–580
  abdominal-perineal resection, 574
  adaptation to, 577
  appliances with, 577, 578
  ascending, 574
  compared to ileostomy, 557
  descending or sigmoid, 574
  double barrel, 574
  irrigation of, 578–579
  loop, 574
  Mikulicz procedure in, 574
  nutrition in, 579
  perineal wound in, 576
  postoperative care in, 576–577
  preoperative preparation for, 573

and sexual activity, 580
transverse, 574
wet, 495
Colpocleisis, in prolapse of uterus, 774
Colporrhaphy, anterior, in prolapse of uterus, 774
Colposcopy, 749
in cervical carcinoma, 781–782
Colpostomy, 747
Coma, 919
in drug overdose, 229–230
hepatic, 597–598
hyperosmolar, in diabetes, 726–727
hypoglycemic, 722
myxedema, 661–662
nursing care in, 920–922
in renal failure, 511
Comedones, 1108–1109
in mammary ducts, 786
Commando procedure, 542, 569
Commissurotomy, mitral, 373, 385
Communicable diseases and infections, 64–80
community implications of, 79–80
control methods, 66–79
APHA recommendations for, 67
hand washing in, 74, 78
immunizations in, 66
international quarantine in, 67
isolation measures in, 77–79
nurse's role in, 71–72
public education programs in, 68–71
and public safety, 72–74
surveillance in, 67–68
hospital-acquired infections, 74, 75–77
transmission of, 65–66
Communicating arteries, 899
Communication
and aphasia, 930–932
and blindness, 1029
and deafness, 1046–1047
laryngectomy affecting, 1081–1082
in neurologic abnormalities, 907
noise affecting, 1050
in respiratory failure, 245–246
with retarded persons, 933
Complement system, 36
in burns, 1159
Compliance, pulmonary, 197, 205
in restrictive diseases, 227
Compresses, for eyes, 1009
Computerized transverse axial tomography, of brain, 915
Conchae, nasal, 1060
Concussion, cerebral, 941
Condoms, use of, 795
Conduction deafness, 1045
Conductive system, cardiac, 317
Condylomata acuminata, 1118
Cones and rods, in eye, 995
Congenital anomalies. See Anomalies
Congestive heart failure. See Cardiovascular system
Conjunctiva
bulbar, 999
examination of, 999
palpebral, 999
Conjunctivitis, 999, 1016–1017
Connective tissue, 813
diseases of, 861
Consciousness
changes in levels of, 918–922
in intracranial pressure increase, 922
loss of, 919–922
Consensual reaction, pupillary, 908
Consent for treatment, obtaining of, 84, 130–131
Constipation, 528, 565–566
Contact with infected persons, 64
direct, 65
indirect, 65
Contact lenses, 1006
for cataract patients, 1020

corneal, 1005
hydrophilic, 1006
removal of, 1005–1006
scleral, 1005
soft, 1006
Contamination, 64
of transfused blood, 426
of wounds, 104
Contraception. See Birth control
Contractility, myocardial, 315
force-velocity relationship in, 320
Frank-Starling principle in, 319–320
Contraction of muscle, 817
and headache, 917
isometric, 882
Contractures
from amputations, 876
from burns, 1169
from immobilization, 952
Contusion, 21
cerebral, 941
Convergence of eyes, 997
Convulsive disorders, 925–929
agencies for help with, 929
anticonvulsants in, 927–928
in brain tumors, 944–945
focal motor or sensory seizures in, 926
grand mal seizures in, 926
in hypocalcemia, 178
in hypoglycemic coma, 722
in hypomagnesemia, 179
in intracranial pressure increase, 924
nursing care in, 927
patient education in, 928–929
petit mal seizures in, 926
postresuscitation, 371
psychologic aspects of, 929
psychomotor epilepsy, 926
status epilepticus, 926–927
surgery in, 928
treatment of, 927–928
Coombs tests, 422
in erythroblastosis fetalis, 442
in hemolytic anemia, 438
Coping mechanisms in behavior, 51
Copper metabolism, in Wilson's disease, 601
Cor pulmonale, 199, 376
in emphysema, 256
in pickwickian syndrome, 228
Cordotomy, cervical, for pain relief, 49
Cornea, 995
diseases of, 1026
examination of, 999
transplantation of, 1026
Corneal reflex, 909
loss of, 920
Corns, 1101
Coronary arteries, 313, 1180
arteriography of, selective, 334
atherosclerosis of, 342–343
cinearteriography of, 386
in myocardial revascularization procedures, 385–387
perfusion of, factors affecting, 319
Coronary Care Units, 348
Corpus callosum, 892
Corpus luteum, 736, 745
cysts of, 779
involution of, 745
in pregnancy, 745
Corpus striatum, 896
Corpuscular indices, 421–422
mean corpuscular hemoglobin, 422
mean corpuscular hemoglobin concentration, 422
mean corpuscular volume, 421
Corti organ, 1041
Corticospinal tract, 903–904
Corticosteroid therapy, 690–692
in Addison's disease, 679–680
before adrenalectomy, 684–685
affecting wound healing, 103
in asthma, 266
in breast cancer, 788
in cancer, 126

in cerebral injuries, 944
Cushing's disease from, 680, 681
in emphysema, 261
hypernatremia from, 173
hypokalemia from, 175
after hypophysectomy, 633, 634
for immunosuppression, 33
indications for, 691
injections in osteoarthritis, 860
in intracranial pressure increase, 924
in lupus erythematosus, 1127
in myasthenia gravis, 963
in psoriasis, 1111
in shock, 1200
side effects of, 691
in ulcerative colitis, 552
Corticosterone, 673
Corticotropin, 631. See also ACTH
Cortisol, 673
affecting fluid and electrolyte regulation, 159
binding of, 674–675
hyposecretion of, 677
release in shock, 1189, 1191
serum levels of
in Cushing's disease, 682
in panhypopituitarism, 635
as therapy after hypophysectomy, 634
urinary levels of, 675
Cortisone, 675
in test of parathyroid function, 667
as therapy in rheumatoid arthritis, 864
Coryza, 272
Costen's syndrome, 1049
"Cotton wool" patches, in eyes, 1001
Cough
in bronchiectasis, 269
in bronchitis, 262
chronic, 211
dry, 211
from ear irritation, 1059
induction of, 221–222
after cardiopulmonary bypass, 391
in respiratory acidosis, 183
paroxysmal, 211
in pneumonia, 274, 277
postoperative need for, 99
productive, 211
in respiratory system dysfunction, 210–211
suppressants of, 227
Coumarin derivatives, 398
Counseling of patients, 61–62
Counterpulsation techniques
in cardiogenic shock, 385
external, 1198–1199
internal, 1198
Coxsackie virus, pharyngitis from, 273
Cranial nerves, 896–899
function tests of, 907–909
Craniectomy, 947
Cranioplasty, 947–948
Craniosacral division, of autonomic nervous system, 904
Craniotomy, 947
complications of, 633
Creams, for skin care, 1105
Creatine, urinary, in thyroid disease, 642
Creatinine clearance tests, 480, 481, 667
Creatinine phosphokinase, 326
levels in myocardial infarction, 349
Credé method, for manual expression of urine, 483, 975–976
Cremasteric reflex, 911
Crepitus, in fractures, 822
in nasal fractures, 1066
Cretinism, 640, 659
Cricoarytenoid muscles, 1074
Cricoid cartilage, 1074
anterior prominence of, 1076
carcinoma of, 1081
trauma of, 1078
Crisis
adrenal, 677, 678
myasthenic, 964

sickle cell, 439, 440
thyroid, 657–658
Crista ampullaris, 1043
Crohn's disease, 567
Cromolyn sodium, in asthma, 268
Crushing injuries, hypovolemia from, 1185
Crusting of skin, 1099
at laryngectomy stoma, 1084
Crutches, use of, 882–883
Cryopexy, transconjunctival, in retinal holes, 1025
Cryosurgery
in acne, 1109
in cancer, 115
in glaucoma, 1022
for hypophysectomy, 633
in skin lesions, 1108
Cryptococcosis, pulmonary, 287
Crystalloid resuscitation formula, 1146–1147
Crystals, in synovial fluid, in gout, 866
Cubic centimeter, 152
Culdocentesis, 747–748
Culdoscopy, 749
Cullen's sign, in pancreatitis, 611
Cultural factors
in behavior patterns, 58
in health care, 7
Curling's ulcer, in burns, 1154
Cushing's disease, 676, 680–685
alkalosis, metabolic, 187
and diabetes, 677
diagnosis of, 682–683
hypokalemia in, 175
lung cancer in, 683–684
nursing care in, 684–685
pituitary tumors in, 683
signs and symptoms of, 681–682
treatment of, 683–685
Cutaneous sensations, 1096–1097. See also Skin
Cyanosis, 201, 1098
acrocyanosis, 404
in blood disorders, 419
in bronchiectasis, 269
in bronchitis, 262
in Raynaud's disease, 404
in shock, 1194
Cyclic body processes. See Rhythms
Cyclodialysis, in glaucoma, 1022
Cyclodiathermy, in glaucoma, 1022
Cycloplegic agents, 1003
Cyst(s)
Bartholin, 754
of breast, 743, 786
cutaneous, 1099
of ear, sebaceous, 1037
of kidney, 503
polycystic disease, 503
ovarian, 778–779
chocolate, 771
of pancreas, 613
pilonidal, 581–582
testicular, 759
thyroglossal duct, 1073
Cystadenoma, ovarian, 779
Cystectomy, 494
Cystic duct, 583, 602
Cystine stones, 502
Cystitis, 486
cystica, 488
honeymoon, 482
interstitial, 488
Cystometry, 480
Cystoscopy, 478–479
Cystostomy, 495
Cystourethrocele, 773, 774
Cytology, exfoliative, 113
Cytosine, as pyrimidine base, 8
Cytosine arabinoside, 125
Cytotoxic or cytolytic reactions, 35–36

D and C, uterine. See Dilatation and curettage, uterine

D and E. *See* Dilatation and evacuation, for abortions
Dacarbazine, 127
Dacryocystitis, 999, 1017
Dacryocystorhinostomy, 1017
Dead space, 198
 anatomical, 198
 in emphysema, 256
 physiological, 198
Deafness. *See* Hearing, loss of
Death and dying, reactions to, 135, 136–139
 and definition of death, 139
 and life-sustaining techniques, 139
Debridement
 in burns, 1160, 1165–1167
 enzymatic agents for, 1132
 surgical, in decubitus ulcers, 1133
Deceleration injuries, 303
 flail chest from, 302–303
Decibels, 1043
Decongestants, nasal, 1061
Decubitus ulcers, 920, 1129–1133
 predisposing factors in, 1130
 prevention of, 170, 977, 1130–1131
 sites of, 1130
 treatment of, 1132–1133
Defecation, stimulus for, 561
Defibrillation, in ventricular fibrillation, 365
Defibrination syndrome, 463
Degenerative disease
 of central nervous system, 956–964
 of joints, 858–868
Dehiscence, wound, 104
Dehydration, 164–168
 in aged persons, 164
 diagnosis of, 166
 disorders with, 165
 and mechanisms in thirst, 158
 nursing care in, 166–167
 skin in, 1098
 symptoms and signs of, 165–166
 in total parenteral nutrition, 191
Dehydroepiandrosterone, 675
Delirium
 after cardiac surgery, 391
 tremens, 600
Deltoid muscle, 819
Demecarium bromide, as miotic, 1010
Dementia paralytica, 938
Dendrites, 891
Denial of illness, 137
 in burns, 1163–1164
11-Deoxycorticosterone, 673
Depolarization, 316
 in ear, 1041
Depression
 from immobilization, prevention of, 842
 in spinal cord injuries, 978–979
 in stroke patients, 954
DeQuervain's thyroiditis, 663
Dermabrasion, for keloids, 1110
Dermatitis
 atopic, 1112
 in blood disorders, 419
 seborrheic, 1111
 of eyelids, 998
Dermatophytosis, 1117
Dermis, 1095
Desensitization, in allergies, 37, 268
Detachment of retina, 1023–1025
Developmental defects. *See* Anomalies
Dexamethasone, 673
 in cancer, 126
 tests with
  for adrenal function, 676
  in Cushing's disease, 682–683
 topical, in eye conditions, 1010
Dextran solutions, in shock, 1197
Dextrostix, use of, 722, 726
Diabetes insipidus, 626–627
 dehydration in, 165
 diagnosis of, 627

hypernatremia in, 173
 treatment of, 627
Diabetes mellitus, 692, 693–729
 adult-onset, 695, 696
 and atherosclerosis, 700
 blood sugar tests in
  fasting, 697
  postprandial, 698–699
 cardiovascular changes in, 700–701
 chemical, 695
 in Cushing's disease, 677
 dehydration in, 165
 diet in, 704–709
  and alcohol consumption, 708
  calorie distribution in, 707
  carbohydrate in, 706, 707
  dietetic foods in, 708
  exchange diet method, 706
  fat in, 706, 707
  liquids in, 708
  protein in, 706, 707
  weighed diet method, 706
  and weight reduction, 705
 emotional disorders in, 728
 encephalopathy in, 728
 glucose tolerance tests in, 697–698
 health practices in, 729
 hypernatremia in, 173
 hyperosmolar coma in, 726–727
 hypoglycemia in, 715, 717, 721–723
 infections in, 728
 insulin in, 710–717
 ketoacidosis in, 723–726
  treatment of, 725–726
 kidney in, 701
 lactic acidosis in, 727–728
 neuropathy in, 702–703
 oral hypoglycemic agents in, 703, 709–710
 overt, 695
 and panhypopituitarism, 634–635
 peripheral vascular disease in, 702
 prediabetes, 695
 retinopathy in, 700–701, 1001–1002
  hypophysectomy in, 636
  treatment of, 1025
 suspected, 695
 symptoms of, 699
 and teaching plan for patients, 704
 theories of, 693–694
 and thyroid disease, 640
 urine tests in, 696–697
 vision loss in, 729
 xanthomas in, 1128
 youth-onset or juvenile, 695–696, 703
Diagnex Blue test, 532
Diagnosis of illness, responses to, 56, 135, 137
Dialysis
 hemodialysis, 514–516
 home programs for, 516
 nursing care in, 517–518
 peritoneal, 516–517
  in diabetic hyperosmolar coma, 727
 in renal failure, 506, 509, 514–518
 tubing placement in, 514–515
 uses of, 517
Diapedesis, 19, 418
Diaphoresis, sodium loss in, 172
Diaphragm
 contraceptive, 793
 hiatus hernia of, 563
 injuries of, 303–304
Diaphysis, 810
Diarrhea, 528, 564–565
 acidosis from, metabolic, 185
 alkalosis from, metabolic, 187
 from chemotherapy, 127
 in diabetes, 728
 functional, in irritable colon, 564
 hypocalcemia from, 178
 hypokalemia from, 175
 hypomagnesemia from, 179
 from radiation therapy, 134
 in regional enteritis, 567

sodium loss in, 172
 in ulcerative colitis, 552
Diarthroses, 815–816
Diascope, 1104
Diastix, use of, 696
Diastole, 313
Diastolic pressure, 330, 336
Diathermy, in glaucoma, 1022
Diethylstilbestrol
 for abortion induction, 796
 in cancer, 126
 in pregnancy, affecting daughters, 782
Diffusion, 156
 of carbon dioxide and oxygen, 201
 facilitated, 156
 lung dysfunction affecting, 199
 and osmosis, 156–157
 simple, 156
Di George syndrome, 38, 669
Digestion, mechanisms in, 525–527, 561
Digitalis
 arrhythmias from, 378
 in atrial fibrillation, 358
 in atrial flutter, 357
 in atrial tachycardia, paroxysmal, 357
 calcium affecting action of, 178
 in cardiogenic shock, 384
 in heart failure, congestive, 378–379
 preparations of, 379
 in pulmonary edema, 382
 in shock, 1198
 toxicity of, 378
Digitalization, 378
Digitoxin, 379
Dilatation and curettage, uterine, 748
 in abnormal uterine bleeding, 769, 770
 in endometrial carcinoma diagnosis, 783
Dilatation and evacuation, for abortions, 796–797
2,3-Diphosphoglycerate, in red cells, 202
Diphtheria, 273
Diplopia, 908, 997
Disarticulation, 868
Discharge from hospital, planning for, 59–60, 105
 for amputees, 869, 881
 for blind patients, 1028
 in burns, 1173
 for eye patients, 1016
 in spinal cord injuries, 981
 for stroke patients, 955
Discography, 810
Discrimination, two-point, 894, 910
Disease, 63–64
 acute, 63
 basic concepts in, 5–139
 chronic, 63
 communicable, 64–80
 and definition of illness, 6
 denial of, 137
  in burns, 1163–1164
 epidemiology of, 63
 exacerbation of, 63
 incidence of, 63
 individual reactions to, 56, 57–58
 morbidity rates in, 63
 and mortality rates, 63
 and population at risk, 64
 prevalence of, 63
 remission of, 63
 response to diagnosis of, 135, 137
Disinfectants, 89
Dislocation, 821
Dissociation curve, oxygen-hemoglobin, 200, 201–202
 in hypoxia, 232
Distention
 abdominal
  in ascites, 695–697
  in burns, 1154
 of bladder, 475
 postoperative, 99
Diuretics
 alkalosis from, metabolic, 187

in ascites, 597
 in cerebral injuries, 943, 944
 in diabetes insipidus, 627
 dosage of, 380
 in heart failure, congestive, 379
 hyperkalemia from, 177
 in hypertension, 339
 hypokalemia from, 175
 hypomagnesemia from, 179
 in intracranial pressure increase, 924
 potassium loss from, 339
 potassium-sparing, 339, 340, 380
 in pulmonary edema, 382
 side effects of, 380
 sodium loss from, 172
Diurnal rhythms. *See* Rhythms
Diverticulitis, 573
Diverticulosis, 573
Diverticulum
 esophageal, 570
 ureteral, 491
Dizziness, 906, 918
DNA, 8
Dominant gene traits, 16
 autosomal, 16
Donor sites in burns, 1164–1165
Dopamine
 in cardiogenic shock, 384
 in cardiopulmonary resuscitation, 371
 deficiency in Parkinson's disease, 959
 receptors for, 1199
 in shock, 1199
Down's syndrome, 933
Drainage
 biliary, with T tube, 606–608
 of cerebral ventricles, 925
 chest, postoperative, 249–252
 and complications from drains, 103
 from Hemovac, after mastectomy, 789
 of mastoid abscess, 1054
 Penrose drains in, 102
 postural, 219–220
  in acidosis, respiratory, 183
 urinary, appliances used for, 497–498
Dressings
 for amputation stumps, 871, 876, 877–878
 biologic, for burns, 1164–1165
 for ear, 1054
 for skin care, 1105–1106
  dry, 1106
  wet, 1105
Dressler's syndrome, 354
Dribbling, urinary, 472
Dromotropic effect of autonomic nervous system stimulation, 319
Drowning accidents, 304
Drugs
 acidosis from, respiratory, 182
 affecting autonomic nervous system, 319
 affecting bladder function, 470
 affecting thyroid uptake, 644
 agranulocytosis from, 36, 444
 anticoagulants, 397–399
 anticonvulsants, 927–928
 aplastic anemia from, 436
 for appetite reduction, 540
 in arrhythmias, 365–368
 contraceptive agents, oral, 794–795
 as haptens, 29
 hemolytic anemia from, autoimmune, 443
 hypoglycemic agents, oral, 703, 709–710
 interactions with anticoagulants, 463
 liver damage from, 592
 narcotic overdose, 229–230
 ototoxicity of, 1056
 patent medications, 272
 preoperative medication, 85, 86
 side effects and toxicity of. *See* Toxicity
 ulcerogenic agents, 544
Dumping syndrome, postoperative, 551

Duodenoscopy, 610
  in pancreatic cancer, 614
Duodenum, 525
  bile duct anastomosis to, 606
  intubation of, 603–604
  pancreaticoduodenal surgery, 614
Dura mater, 892
Dust inhalation and pneumoconiosis, 288
Dwarfism, 630, 815, 820
Dysarthria, 931
Dysgammaglobulinemia, 38
Dysgerminoma, ovarian, 780
Dysgraphia, 932
Dyslexia, 932
Dysmenorrhea, 766, 768
Dyspareunia, in retroversion of uterus, 776
Dyspepsia, 528
Dysphagia, 528, 561
  in laryngeal disorders, 1076, 1077
  in myasthenia gravis, 964
  in renal failure, 511
Dyspnea
  in anemia, 429
  in asthma, 265
  breathing technique in, 223–224
  in bronchitis, 262
  in emphysema, 257
  paroxysmal nocturnal, 237, 376
Dysuria, 472

Ear, 1035–1059
  absence of, 1051
  assessment of function, 1036–1041
  atticoantral disease of, 1054
  caloric stimulation tests of, 1039, 1043–1044
  cerumen accumulation in, 1049
  cleaning of, 1048
  congenital deformities of, 1051–1052
  dressings for, 1054
  drops for, 1039, 1048
  examination of, 1037
  foreign bodies in, 1049
  functions of, 1035
    tests of, 1041–1044
  infections of, 1053–1056
  irrigation of, 1039
  itching of, 1049
  keratosis obturans of, 1049–1050
  labyrinthitis, 1055–1056
  mastoiditis, 1054
  ointment application, 1049
  otitis media, 1053–1054
  otosclerosis, 1056–1057
  physiology of, 1041–1045
  piercing of, 1048
  protrusion of, 1052
  reconstructive surgery of, 1051
  rupture of drum, 1039, 1040, 1050
  trauma of, 1050–1051
  tubotympanic disease of, 1054
  tumors in, 1052–1053
  tympanoplasty, 1054
  vestibular dysfunction, 1057–1059
Earache, 1049
Eardrum, 1039
Eating behavior
  excessive intake in, 535, 540–541
  inadequate intake in, 535, 538–540
Ecchymoses, 419
  in fractures, 822
Eccrine sweat glands, 1096
Echocardiography, 329
Echoencephalography, 915
  in brain tumors, 945
Echography
  in biliary tract disease, 604
  of breast, 785
Ecthyma, 1113, 1114
Ectopia
  of kidneys, 503
  of testis, 758
Ectropion, 999

Eczema
  atopic, 1112
  hand, 1112
  nummular, 1112
Edema, 180–181
  in burns, 1143
  cerebral, 922
  dehydration in, 165
  of epiglottis, 1077
  of eyelids, 998
  in glomerulonephritis, 508
  in hypothyroidism, 660
  in inflammation, 19
  lymphedema, 409
  in nephrotic syndrome, 508–509
  orbital
    in ethmoid sinusitis, 1062
    in exophthalmos, 650
  papilledema, 898, 995
  periocular, postoperative, 949
  pitting, 181
  pulmonary, 180, 381–383
    after chest surgery, 249
    in fractures, 827
    in narcotic overdose, 230
    respiratory failure in, 232
    in transfusion reactions, 426
  scrotal, after herniorrhaphy, 581
  in spinal cord injuries, 969
  in surgery, 82
  venous pressure in, 405
Edrophonium test, in myasthenia gravis, 962
EDTA, in lead poisoning, 442
Education programs for disease control, 68–71
  and cancer detection, 113
  and eye health, 993
  for hypertensive patients, 338
Effusions, pleural, 296–298
Ejaculatory ducts, 761
Elastic stockings, use of, 406
Elasticity
  of articular cartilage, 816
  pulmonary, 197
    in emphysema, 254
    in restrictive lung diseases, 216, 227
Elastin fibers, dermal, 1095
Elbow
  disarticulation of, 874
  prosthesis for, 874
Electrical potentials of cardiac cells, 316
Electrical shock, direct-current synchronized. See Cardioversion
Electrical stimulation
  of bladder, 976
  of peripheral nerves, for pain relief, 48–49
Electrocardiogram, 317, 328
  in arrhythmias, 355–356
  artifacts in, 355
  after pacemaker insertion, 363
  in dialysis procedures, 506
  in hypoparathyroidism, 670
  in myocardial infarction, 349
  P wave in, 317
  in pericardiocentesis, 374
  QRS wave in, 317
  in shock, 1194
  T wave in, 317
Electrocoagulation, 1108
Electrodesiccation, 1108
Electroencephalography, 914
  provocative tests in, 914
Electrolytes, 152
  absorption of, 567
  active transport of, 157–158
  balance of, 151–191. See also Fluids, and electrolyte balance
  problems in, 171–180
  diffusion of, 156
  in extracellular fluid, 154
  and hydrogen ion balance, 161–164
  levels in cardiac assessment, 325–326
  loss in gastrointestinal suction, 572
  metabolism regulation by hormones, 12

  postoperative balance of, 99
  renal tubular absorption of, 160
  and total parenteral nutrition, 188–191
Electromyography, 914–915
Electronystagmography, 1044
Electrophoresis of serum proteins, 586
Electrosurgery, in skin lesions, 1108
Elephantiasis, 409
Ellsworth-Howard test
  in hypoparathyroidism, 670
  in pseudohypoparathyroidism, 671
Embden-Meyerhof pathway, for glucose metabolism, 10
Embolectomy, 403
Embolism, 397
  air, in transfusion therapy, 426
  cerebral, 951
  fat, in fractures, 827
  mesenteric, 403
  pulmonary, 293–295, 408
    nursing care in, 295
    and thrombophlebitis, 407
    treatment of, 294–295
Emergency care. See also Trauma
  in burns, 1137
  in cerebral injuries, 942
  in fractures, 822–824
  in spinal cord injuries, 968
  in surgery, 82
Emiocytosis, 693
Emmetropia, 1004
Emotions. See Psychological aspects
Emphysema, 253–261
  aging, 254
  and α_1-antitrypsin deficiency, 253, 254
  and assessment of patient, 256–258
  centrilobular, 254
  classifications of, 253–254
  destructive, 254
  diagnostic tests in, 258–259
  familial, 254
  focal, 254
  hospitalization in, 260
  mediastinal, 303
  overdistention, 254
  panacinar dilatation, 254
  panlobular, 254
  pneumothorax in, 261
  polycythemia in, 256, 261
  progression of, 254–256
  senile, 254
  smoking affecting, 257, 259
  subcutaneous, 303
  symptoms of, 256
  treatment of, 259–261
  ventilation and perfusion in, 198
Empyema, 298–299
Emulsions, for skin care, 1105
Encephalitis, 935–936
  lethargica, 935
  St. Louis, 935
  treatment of, 936
Encephalomyelitis, 936
Encephalopathy
  diabetic, 728
  hepatic, 597
  hypertensive, 341
Endarterectomy
  in chronic arterial insufficiency, 402
  mortality from, 385
Endemic disease, 64–65
Endocarditis, bacterial, 373–374
Endocardium, 315
Endocrine system, 623–729
  adrenal glands, 672–692
  hormone activity. See Hormones
  pancreas, 692–729
  parathyroid glands, 664–672
  pineal gland, 672
  pituitary gland, 624–636
  and reproductive tract function, 736–738
  thyroid gland, 636–664
Endolymph, 1041
  hydrops of, 1057

Endometriosis, 770–771
  treatment of, 771
Endometrium
  carcinoma of, 783
  changes in menstrual cycle, 745
  evaluation of, 752–753
Endoplasmic reticulum, 9
Endoscopy
  and cholangiography, 604
  gastric, 533–534
Endosteum, 813
Endotoxin, and septic shock, 1192
Endotracheal intubation, 97, 238–239
Enema, preoperative, 84–85
Energy expenditure, 10
  and heat production, 14–15
  and mechanical efficiency, 13
  and oxygen consumption, 13–14
Enteritis, regional, 567–568
Enterocele, 773
Enterogastric reflex, 561
Enterogastrone, 525, 561
Enterokinase, 567
Entropion, 998–999
Enucleation of eyeball, 1026–1028
Environmental factors
  pollutants in. See Pollutants
  and skin changes, 1098
  temperature affecting thyroid function, 648, 659
Enzymes, 8
  activity in myocardial infarction, 349
  in cardiac cells, 326
Eosinophilia, 418
Eosinophils, 417, 418
  in inflammation, 19
Ependymoma, 946
Ephedrine, as bronchodilator, 226
Epidemic disease, 65
  contact, 80
  point, 80
Epidemiology of disease, 63
Epidermis, 1095
Epiglottis, 1074
  carcinoma of, 1081
  edema of, 1077
Epilepsy, 925. See also Convulsive disorders
Epinephrine
  in arrhythmias, 367
  as bronchodilator, 225–226
  in cardiopulmonary resuscitation, 371
  in hypoglycemia, 723
  as mydriatic, 1010
  racemic, as aerosol agent, 226
  in shock, 1199
  vascular effects of, 394
Epiphora, 999
Epiphysis, 810–812
  closure of, 812
Epistaxis, 1063
Epithelioma, 1124
Epitheliosis, of breast, 786
Epitrochlear lymph nodes, 420
Epstein-Barr virus, and infectious mononucleosis, 454
Equilibrium, 1035
  and body maintenance, 152
  disequilibrium, 152
  dynamic, 152
  and vertigo, 1036–1037
Equivalent, definition of, 152
Erb's point, 325
Erection, penile, mechanisms in, 761
Erosions of skin, 1099, 1128–1129
Eructation, 528
Erysipelas, 1115
Erythema, 1101
  in heat injuries, 21
  marginatum, in rheumatic fever, 372
  nodosum, 1102
  palmar, in liver disease, 585
Erythroblastosis fetalis, 36, 424, 442–443
Erythrocytes, 415–417
  in anemia. See Anemia
  count of, 325, 421

1216 Index

Erythrocytes *Continued*
  disorders of, 428–444
  fragility of, 422
  freezing of, for transfusions, 427
  life span determinations, 422
  mean corpuscular volume of, 421
  packed cell preparations, transfusions of, 427
  phagocytosis of, 417
  in polycythemia, 444
  sedimentation rate, 326
  in urine, 473
Erythropoiesis, 417
Erythropoietin, 417
  formation in renal failure, 512
Eschar, 1102, 1129
  in burns, 1140
Escharotomy, in burns, 1140
Esophageal speech, 1085–1086
Esophagitis
  in hiatal hernia, 563
  reflux, 563
Esophagomyotomy, 570
Esophagus
  achalasia of, 561–562
  acid perfusion test, 562
  cancer of, 569–570
  caustic burns of, 570
  colonic replacement of, 570
  diverticulum of, 570
  in dysphagia, 561
  motility test of, 562–563
  obstruction of, 569–570
  strictures of, 570
  varices of, 593–595
    portasystemic shunting procedures in, 595–596
17β-Estradiol, 736
Estrogen
  for abortion induction, 796
  adrenal secretion of, 674
  and bone growth, 815, 820
  and breast development, 784
  function of, 736
  and lactation inhibition, 784
  in oral contraceptives, 794
  ovarian secretion of, 736, 745
  therapy with
    in breast cancer, 788
    in cancer, 126
    in menopause, 800
Ethmoid sinus, 1060
  sinusitis, 1062
Eustachian tube, 1040
  blockage in, 1040
  intubation of, 1053, 1056
Euthanasia, 139
Evans formula, in burns, 1145
Evisceration, wound, 104
Ewald tube, 536
Exacerbation of disease, 63
Examination. *See also* Assessment of patient
  abdominovaginal, bimanual, 741–742
  of breast, 112, 742–744
    in females, 742–744
    in males, 744
    self-examination, 744
  of chest, 207–210
  of ear, 1037
  of eye, 996–1003
  of gastrointestinal system, 529–532
  of integument, 1103–1104
  of larynx, 1076
  of lymph nodes, 419–420
  in musculoskeletal disorders, 807–809
  of neck, 1071
  of nose, 1059–1061
  in peripheral vascular disease, 394
  of pharynx, 1071
  physical, 55
    and cancer detection, 111
  rectal, 532, 740
    in cancer detection, 113
  of reproductive system, 739–742
  of skin, 419
  of sputum, 224–225
  of thyroid gland, 638
  of urinary tract, 475
  of urine, 472–473
Excisional therapy, in burns, 1167–1168
Exenteration, pelvic, 495
Exercises
  after amputations, 876–877
  breathing, 222, 223–224
    in emphysema, 259
  Buerger-Allen, 396
  in burns, 1172
  circulatory effects of, 14
  and energy requirements during work, 10
  of facial muscles, in Bell's palsy, 966
  heat production in, 14
  and insulin dosage, 716–717
  isometric, 882
  after mastectomy, 789–790
  metabolic effects of, 13
  in osteoarthritis, 860
  in prolapse of uterus, 774
  respiratory alkalosis from, 184
  in respiratory failure, 244–245
  in retroversion of uterus, 776
  in rheumatoid arthritis, 863
  in spinal cord injuries, 977–978
  in stress tests, 224
  testing of cardiac patients, 329–330
Exophthalmometer, 650–651
Exophthalmos
  in thyroid disorders, 650–651
  unilateral, 998
Expectorants, 227
  in asthma, 266
Expiration
  in emphysema, 258, 259
  ratio to inspiration, 207
Expiratory flow rate, 215
Expiratory reserve volume, 215
Expiratory time, forced, 215
Expiratory volume, forced, 215
Expressivity, concept of, 16
Extensor muscles, 818, 819
Extracorporeal circulation, 387–388
Extracorporeal hemodialysis, 514–516
Extrapyramidal motor tract, 904
  in Huntington's disease, 961
  in Parkinson's disease, 959
Extrasystoles
  atrial, 357
  ventricular, 364
Exudates, 20
  in pleural effusion, 296
Eye(s), 993–1030. *See also* Blindness
  anatomy and physiology of, 994–996
  anesthetics for, 1002, 1010
  assessment of, 996–1003
  black eyes, 1019
  in blood disorders, 419
  burns of, 1018
  cataracts, 1019–1021
  chemical injuries of, 1018
  compresses for, 1009
  corneal diseases, 1026
  in diabetes, 700–701
  drops for
    administration of, 1007–1008
    in glaucoma, 1010, 1022, 1023
    preoperative, 1015
    systems for controlled release of, 1011–1012
  enucleation of, 1026–1028
  in exophthalmos, 650–651
  external, 998–999
  foreign bodies in, 1017–1018
  glaucoma, 1021–1023
  in hypertension, 337
  in hypoparathyroidism, 666
  infections of, 1016–1017
  internal, 1001–1002
  intraocular pressure in
    in glaucoma, 1021
    measurements of, 1002–1003
  prevention of increase in, 1015–1016, 1023
  irrigation of, 1009
  measurement of visual acuity, 996–997
  measurement of visual field, 997–998
  movements of, 997
    rapid, in sleep, 15
  ointments for, administration of, 1008
  patches for, application of, 1008–1009
  perforating wounds of, 1017
  periocular edema, postoperative, 949
  promotion of eye health, 993, 1006–1007
  prosthesis for, 1027–1028
  refractive errors of, 1003–1006
  retinal disorders, 1023–1026
  surgery of
    in cataract, 1019–1021
    in corneal diseases, 1026
    enucleation, 1026–1028
    postoperative care, 1015–1016
    preparation for, 1014–1015
    in retinal detachment, 1024–1025
  sympathetic ophthalmia, 1019
  topical medications for, 1009–1012
  trauma of, 1017–1019
Eyeglasses, 1004, 1005
  for cataract patients, 1020
  sunglasses, 1007
Eyelashes, examination of, 998–999
Eyelids,
  examination of, 998
  laceration of, 1018–1019
  lag in hypothyroidism, 660
  ptosis in Cushing's disease, 681
  retraction in exophthalmos, 650

Face, injuries of, 1067–1071
Facial muscles, 818
Facial nerve, 898, 1044
  assessment of, 909
  Bell's palsy of, 966, 1058
  paralysis after stapedectomy, 1057
Facies
  in acromegaly, 629
  adenoid, 1072
  in Cushing's disease, 681
  in hypothyroidism, 660
  in Parkinson's disease, 959
Factors, clotting, 457, 459, 460, 461
Fallopian tubes, 736
  carcinoma of, 781
  ligation for sterilization, 795–796
  patency of, diagnosis of, 749, 752
  Rubin test for patency, 749
Falx cerebri, 892
Families of patients, contact with, 58, 61
Farmer's lung, 291–292
Farsightedness, 1004
Fasciotomy, in burns, 1140
Fasting, weight loss in, 540–541
Fat
  dietary, in diabetes, 706, 707
  emboli from, in fractures, 827
  metabolism of, 10–11
Fatigue
  in anemia, 429
  in thyroid disease, 641
Favism, 441
Fecal impaction. *See* Impaction, fecal
Feces. *See* Stools
Feedback mechanisms, 152
  and ACTH secretion, 674
  and aldosterone secretion, 673
  and hormone regulation, 623
  and sex hormone secretion, 736, 744
  in shock, 1189
Femoral head prothesis, 834–844
  after methotrexate therapy with citrovorum factor, 868
  in total hip replacement, 844–846
Femoral hernia, 580
Femoral lymph nodes, 420
Fenestration surgery, of ear, 1057
Ferning, of cervical mucus, 747, 752

α-Fetoprotein, 37
Fetor hepaticus, 585
Fever, 929–930
  blister, 542
  dehydration from, 165
  after extracorporeal circulation, 388
  in intracranial pressure increase, 923
  in malignant hyperthermia, 96–97
  postoperative, 101
  reduction of, 930
  in total parenteral nutrition, 191
Fibrillation
  atrial, 323, 358
  ventricular, 368
Fibrin, 457
  intravascular deposits in DIC, 463
Fibrinogen, 415, 459
  transfusions of, 428
Fibrinolysis, 457
Fibroblasts, in wound healing, 102
Fibrocystic disease, of breast, 785–786
Fibroma, 107
  ovarian, 779
  of uterus, 783
Fibroplasia, retrolental, 1025
Fibrositis, in rheumatoid arthritis, 862
Filum terminale, 902
Fimbrioplasty, 752
Fingers
  amputation of, 873
  clubbing of. *See* Clubbing
Fissures
  cerebral, 892
  cutaneous, 1101
  rectal, 582
Fistula, 20
  acidosis from, 185
  anal, 582
  arteriovenous, 404
  biliary tract, postoperative, 608
  gastrointestinal
    in cancer of esophagus, 570
    from ileostomy, 557
  pancreatic, postoperative, 614
  perirectal, 582
  rectovaginal, 775
  in reproductive tract, female, 775
  sodium loss in, 172
Flail chest, 302–303
Flare, at inflammation site, 19
Flatulence, 528
Flatus, 528
Flexor muscles, 818, 819
Fluids
  absorption of, 567
  administration of, 167–168
    in acidosis, metabolic, 186
    in burns, 1138
    calculation of flow rates in, 167–168
    postoperative, 99
    preoperative, 85
    in shock, 1197–1198
    in spinal cord injuries, 974
    in total parenteral nutrition, 188–191
  in body
    active transport of, 157–158
    alterations in, 164
    composition of, 153–154
    in dehydration, 164–168
    diffusion of, 156
    distribution of, 153
    in edema, 180–181
    function of, 154–155
    movement of, 155–158
    normal balance of, 155
    osmosis of, 156–157
    regulation of, 158–160
    and electrolyte balance, 151–191
      in burns, 1142–1144
      concepts in, 151–152
      after hypophysectomy, 634
      after ileostomy, 557
      normal state of, 152–164
      problems in, 171–180
    in thyroid storm, 657

Index

excretion from renal system, 158–159
extracellular, 153
and hydrogen ion balance, 161–164
intake in dehydration, 166–167
interstitial, 153
intracellular, 153
loss of
  measurement of, 477
  in renal failure, 506
  in pulmonary alveoli, 201
  restriction of, in heart failure, congestive, 381
  retention of, measurement of, 477. See also Edema
volume of, 153
  deficit in burns, 1142
  and water intoxication, 169–171
Fluorescence, of skin lesions, 1104
Fluoroscopy of chest, 212
Flutter, atrial, 357
Foley catheters, care of, 482
Folic acid, 416
  deficiency of, 435–436
Follicle(s), ovarian
  maturation of, 745
  rupture of, 745
Follicle-stimulating hormone, 631, 736, 744
Folliculitis, 1114
Food
  botulism from, 940
  and nutrition. See Nutrition
Foot
  care of, 396–397, 401–402, 406–407
  prosthetic, 871, 873
  tinea pedis, 1118
  verruca plantaris, 1118
Foramen magnum, 892
Forbes-Albright syndrome, 630, 632
Forearm, amputations through, 873
Foreign bodies
  in ear, 1049
  in eyes, 1017–1018
  in larynx, 1077–1078
Fovea centralis, 995
Fox shield, for eyes, 1017
Fractures, 819, 821–843
  and callus formation, 826
  casts for, 828–834
    circulatory impairment from, 832
    Lightcast II in, 828–829
    for lower extremity, 830–831
    Minerva jacket, 831
    nerve impairment from, 832
    nursing care with, 831–833
    odor from, 832–833
    pain from, 832
    Plaster of Paris in, 829–830
    removal of, 833–834
    skin care in, 833
    spica, 831
    for spine, 831
    types of, 830–831
    for upper extremity, 830
  of cervical spine, 968
  classification of, 824–825
  closed, 824
  closed reduction of, with external fixation, 828–834
  comminuted, 825
  complications of, 826–828
    prevention of, 841–843
  compressed, 825
  delayed union of, 826
  depressed, 825
  displaced, 825
  ear damage in, 1050
  emergency care in, 822–824
  of facial bones, 1068
  fat embolism from, 827
  greenstick, 825
  healing of, 825–826
  of hip, 836–841
    arthroplasty in, 843–846
    impacted techniques in, 838

and position changes for patient, 840–841
  postoperative nursing care in, 840
  preoperative nursing care in, 839–840
  skin traction in, 837
  immobilization in, and prevention of complications, 841–843, 857
impacted, 825
of larynx, 1078
of mandible, 1068–1069
of maxilla, 1068–1069
non-union of, 826–827
of nose, 1065–1066, 1068, 1069–1070
oblique, 825
open, 824
open reduction of, with internal fixation, 834–836
  nursing care in, 835–836
of orbit, 1068
pathologic, 821–822
and photographs of patients, 836, 856
of ribs, 301
signs and symptoms of, 822
of skull, 825, 940–941
spiral, 825
splinting of, 823
traction in, 848–858
  Buck's extension in, 837, 850, 852–853
  cervical, 851, 853
  countertraction with, 848
  manual, 849
  nursing care in, 856–858
  pelvic, 852–853
  pin insertion in, 855–856
  pulleys in, 849
  Russell, 837, 850
  skeletal, 853–856
  skin, 837, 849–851
  Thomas splint with, 854–855
  Varco, 852
  Williams position in, 852
transverse, 825
treatment of, 828–831
of zygoma, 1069
Frank-Starling principle, 319–320, 1180
Freckles, 1101
Freezing procedures. See Cold applications
Frequency, of sound, 1041
  in phonation, 1076
Friction rubs, 325
  pericardial, 374
  pleural, 210
Friedländer's pneumonia, 275, 277
Frontal lobe, 895
Frontal sinus, 1060
  sinusitis, 1062
Fructose, in seminal fluid, 747
Fundoscopy, 1001
Fundus oculi, examination of, 1001
Fungus infections
  of lung, 287–288
    treatment of, 287–288
  of skin, 1115–1118
Furuncles, 1114

Gag reflex, 909, 1071
  and endotracheal intubation, 238
Gait, in Parkinson's disease, 959
Galactose tolerance test, 587
Gallbladder, 602
  cancer of, 605–606
  cholecystitis, 605
Gallop
  atrial, 324
  ventricular, 324
Gallstones, 604–605
Gamma globulins
  in cerebrospinal fluid, 913
  deficiency disorders of, 38–39
  in serum, 415
  therapeutic uses of, 428
  in burns, 1159

Ganglia, 891
  of autonomic nervous system, 904
  basal, 896
Ganglioneuroma, of adrenal medulla, 690
Gangrene, 403
  in diabetes, 702
  dry, 702
  wet, 702
Gardner's syndrome, 572
Gas exchange, 197–198
Gases, blood
  in cardiovascular disorders, 327
  oxygen therapy affecting, 233
  in shock, 1195
Gasserian ganglion, 898
Gastrectomy
  partial, 548
  total, 550, 570
  in Zollinger-Ellison syndrome, 614
Gastric juice, 525
  characteristics of, 536
Gastrin, 525, 543
Gastritis, 542–543
  hemorrhagic, in burns, 1154
Gastrocnemius muscle, 819
Gastroduodenostomy, 548
Gastroenterostomy, 548
Gastrointestinal system, 525–615
  absorption problems, 566–569
  in acidosis, metabolic, 185
  adhesions of, 573
  in alkalosis, metabolic, 187
  anorectal conditions, 582–583
  appendicitis, 581
  assessment of, 527–535
  biliary tract, 602–608
  colostomy, 574–580
  complications from immobilization, prevention of, 841–842
  constipation, 565–566
  in dehydration, 165–166
  diabetes affecting, 728
  diagnostic tests of, 532–535
  diarrhea, 564–565
  disorders of, 535–615
  diverticulosis and diverticulitis, 573
  fistulas of
    acidosis from, 185
    sodium loss in, 172
  functional disorders of, 563–564
  gastric analysis, 532–533
  hemorrhoids, 582–583
  hernias, 580–581
  hyperfunction of, 564–565
  in hyperkalemia, 177
  hypofunction of, 565–566
  in hyponatremia, 172
  ileostomy, 553–561
  intubation of, 536–538
  large intestine, 525
  lesions in lining of, 535, 541–561
    in large intestine, 551–561
    in oral cavity and esophagus, 541–542
    in stomach and small intestine, 542–551
  liver, 582–602
  motility disorders, 535, 561–566
  nutrient intake. See Nutrition
  obstruction of, 535, 569–580. See also Ileus
  oral cavity. See Mouth
  peptic ulcer, 543–551
  physical examination of, 529–532
  pilonidal cyst, 581–582
  polyps of, 572–573
  radiology of, 533–535
  shock affecting, 1192
  small intestine, 525
    absorption activity in, 527, 566–567
    biopsy of, 568
    characteristics of secretions in, 536
    lesions in lining of, 542–551
    obstruction of, 571–572

  peptic ulcer of, 543–551
  regional enteritis of, 567–568
stomach, 525
surgery of, 573–580
  postoperative care in, 576–579
  preoperative preparation for, 573
  in thyroid disease, 641
  ulcerative colitis, 551–553
  volvulus, 573
Gastrojejunostomy, 548
Gastroscopy, 533–534
Gastrostomy, permanent, 570
Gate control theory, of pain response, 40–41
Gavage feedings, 539
Gellhorn pessary, 774
Genes, 8, 16–17
Genetics, 16–17
Geniculate body, 897
Genitalia, external, examination of, 739–740
Genotype, 16
Germicidal agents, 89
Germicidal lamps, 1108
Giant cells, 20
Gigantism, 628, 815, 820
Gingivae, examination of, 529
Giordano-Giovannetti diet, 513
Glasses. See Eyeglasses
Glaucoma, 1021–1023
  angle-closure, 1022
  miotics in, 1010, 1022, 1023
  nursing care in, 1022–1023
  open-angle, 1021–1022
  surgery in, 1022
  tonometry in, 1002
  water provocative test in, 1002–1003
Glia, 891
Glioblastoma multiforme, 946
Gliomas, 945–946
Globulin
  serum, 415
    levels in liver disease, 586
  thyroxine-binding, 643
Globus hystericus, 561
Glomerulonephritis
  acute, 508
  and Arthus reaction, 34
  chronic, 508
  in ecthyma, 1113
  renal failure in, 507–508
Glomerulus, 159, 469, 504
  filtration rate, 160
    measurement of, 480
Glomus tumors of ear, 1052
Glossitis, in anemia, 419, 434
Glossopharyngeal nerve, 898–899
  assessment of, 909
Glottis, 1074, 1076
  carcinoma of, 1081
Glucagon, 692, 694
  in cardiogenic shock, 384
  in hypoglycemia, 723
  secretion of, 694–695
  in shock, 1198
Glucocorticoids, 672, 673. See also Corticosteroids
  and bone growth, 815, 820
  therapy with, 690–692
Gluconeogenesis, insulin affecting, 711
Glucose
  blood levels of, 697
    in cardiovascular disorders, 327
    in hyperosmolar coma, 727
    in hypoglycemia, 722
    in ketoacidosis, 725
    liver function affecting, 584
  cellular, insulin affecting, 695
  in cerebrospinal fluid, 913
  hyperglycemia, 692
    from insulin, 720
  hypoglycemia, 692. See also Hypoglycemia

Glucose   *Continued*
  metabolism of, 10
    in glucose 6-phosphate dehydrogenase deficiency, 441
    in shock, 1191
  as therapy
    in hypoglycemia, 723
    in narcotic overdose, 230
  tolerance tests, 697–698
    in Addison's disease, 677
    in Cushing's disease, 681
    factors affecting, 698
    in pseudohypoparathyroidism, 671
    variations of, 698
  in urine, 473, 699
  and insulin action, 715
  tests for, 696–697
Glucose 6-phosphate, 10
Glucose 6-phosphate dehydrogenase, deficiency of, 441
Glue ear, 1056
Glutamic oxaloacetic transaminase, serum, 326
  in liver disease, 586
  in myocardial infarction, 349
Gluteal muscles, 819
Gluteal reflex, 911
Gluten, sensitivity to, in celiac disease, 568
Glycerin, oral, in glaucoma, 1011, 1022
Glycosuria. *See* Glucose, in urine
Goblet cells, in bronchitis, 262
Goeckerman technique, in psoriasis, 1111
Goiter, 638
  diffuse toxic, 649–650
  factors in formation of, 639
  nontoxic, 662–663
  toxic nodular, 657
  treatment of, 662–663
Goitrogens, 648
Gold
  colloidal, in test of crebrospinal fluid, 913
  compounds in rheumatoid arthritis, 865
  radioactive, 122
    in bladder tumors, 493–494
Golgi apparatus, 9
Gomco suction machine, 537
Gonad(s), 9
Gonadotropin
  human chorionic, 631
    for ovulation induction, 753
  human menopausal, for ovulation induction, 753, 767
  hypersecretion of, 631
  hyposecretion of, 631
  releasing hormone, 736, 744
  secretion of, 736
Gonioscopy, 1002
Gonorrhea, 755
Gordon reflex, 911
Gout, 866–867
  tophi in, 866, 1037
Gradenigo syndrome, 1054
Grafts and transplants, 32–34
  ABO blood group affecting, 33
  autografts, 32
  in burns, 1168–1169
  for cardiac valve replacement, 385
  of cornea, 1026
  of heart, 393
  heterografts, 385
  in burns, 1164
  HL-A system affecting, 33
  homografts, 32, 385
    in burns, 1164–1165
  kidney, 34, 509, 518–519
  of liver, 600
  rejection of, 32–34
  skin. *See* Skin, grafts
Granulation, and wound healing, 21
Granulocytes, 415, 417
Granulocytopenia. *See* Agranulocytosis

Granulomatous reaction, 34
  in immune response, 29
Graphesthesia, testing of, 910
Graves' disease
  diagnosis of, 652
  treatment of, 652–655
Gravity, specific
  of cerebrospinal fluid, 913
  of urine, 473, 480
Gravlee jet wash, in endometrial carcinoma diagnosis, 783
Gray matter, 891
Grey-Turner's sign, in pancreatitis, 611
Grief, anticipatory, in dying patients, 138
Groin
  intertrigo of, 1115
  ringworm of, 1117
Ground substance, intracellular, 9
Growth hormone, 626, 628
  and bone growth, 815, 820
  hypersecretion of, 628–629
  hyposecretion of, 629–630
  levels in panhypopituitarism, 635
  supply from human cadaver pituitary glands, 630
Guanine, as purine base, 8
Guarding, in abdominal musculature, 528
Guillain-Barré syndrome, 937
Gyri of brain, 892
  precentral, 894

Hair, 1095–1096
  alopecia, 1096
    from chemotherapy, 128, 446, 453
  folliculitis, 1114
  growth of, 1096
  loss of, 1096
    in metabolic disorders, 1098
  sycosis barbae, 1114
  terminal, 1095
  vellus, 1095
Haldane effect, 201
Halothane, 92
  liver damage from, 591
Halstead radical mastectomy, 787
Hamstring muscles, 819
Hand
  amputations in, 873
  burned, care of, 1171
  clubbing of fingers. *See* Clubbing
  eczema of, 1112
  pain in, paraffin baths for, 860, 863
  prosthesis for, 873–874
  washing of, and infection control, 74, 78
Hand-Schüller-Christian disease, 632
Haptens, 23, 32
  drugs as, 29
Harris tube, 537
Hashimoto's thyroiditis, 663–664
Haversian system, 814
Hay fever, 1062
Head injuries, 940–944
Headache, 917–918
  in brain tumors, 945
  cluster, 918
  from lumbar puncture, 912
  migraine, 917–918
  muscle contraction, 917
Healing of wounds. *See* Wound healing
Health care
  fragmentation of services in, 69, 80
  teaching of, 71–72
  variability in, 52–53
Health and disease, 5–139
  adaptive responses in, 7, 17–50
  body rhythms in, 15–16
  cellular activity in, 7–9
  and concept of wellness, 59
  and definition of health, 6
  genetic factors in, 16–17
  metabolism in, 9–15
Hearing, 1041

aids for, 1047
loss of
  adaptation to, 1045–1046
  adventitious, 1045
  agencies for help with, 1059
  central, 1045, 1048
  conduction deafness, 1045
  congenital, 1045
  indications of, 1036
  in Ménière's disease, 1057
  from noise, 1050–1051
  nursing care in, 1045–1049
  in otosclerosis, 1056
  sensorineural, 1045, 1047–1048
  after stapedectomy, 1057
  transient, 1045, 1046
tests of, 1041–1043
Heart, 1180. *See also* Cardiovascular system
  anatomy and physiology of, 313, 314–320
  arrest, cardiac, 368
  assessment of, 323–335
  block in
    first-degree, 359
    Mobitz types, 359
    pacemaker in, 360
    second-degree, 359
    third-degree, 359
    Wenckebach, 359
  cardiac index, 1180
  cardiac output, 313, 316, 1180
  catheterization of, 333–335
  failure, congestive, 375–381
    in anemia, 429
    digitalis in, 378–379
    diuretics in, 379
    hypokalemia in, 175
    left-sided, 376
    nursing care in, 377–378
    nutrition in, 377, 379–381
    refractory, 381
    right-sided, 376
    signs and symptoms of, 376–377
    sodium loss in, 171
    in thyroid disease, 640
    water intoxication in, 169
  force-velocity relationship in, 320
  Frank-Starling law of, 319–320, 1180
  injury of, 303
  length-tension relationship in, 319–320
  rate, 316–319
  in shock, assistance for, 1198–1199
  sounds, 324–325
    first, 324
    fourth, 324
    murmurs, 324
    paradoxical splitting of, 324
    second, 324
    third, 324
Heartburn, 528
Heart-lung machines, 387. *See also* Cardiopulmonary bypass
Heat
  application of,
    in burns, 1153
    compresses for eyes, 1009
    for pain relief, 46
  exposure to, effects of
    in Addison's disease, 677
    in thyrotoxicosis, 648
  injuries from, 21, 1137–1173. *See also* Burns
  mechanisms in production of, 14–15
Heat rash, 1110
Heberden's nodes, 859
Hemangioblastoma, 946
Hemangioma, 1128
  intracranial, 946
  racemose, 1128
Hemarthrosis, in sprains, 820
Hematemesis, 528
  in burns, 1154
  in Mallory-Weiss syndrome, 542
Hematocele, 759

Hematocrit, 325, 421, 1180
  in shock, 1196
Hematoma
  affecting wound healing, 103
  cerebral, 941–942
  epidural, 941–942
  nasal, 1066
  subdural, 941
Hematopoietic and lymphatic system, 415–464
  in acidosis
    metabolic, 185
    respiratory, 182
  in alkalosis
    metabolic, 187
    respiratory, 184
  anemia, 428–443
  assessment of, 418–423
  blood content and function, 415–418
  blood tests, 420–423
  bone marrow aspiration and biopsy, 423
  coagulation disorders, 457, 459–462
  in dehydration, 166
  erythrocyte disorders, 428–444
  hemostasis disorders, 456–458
  Hodgkin's disease, 449–453
  in hyponatremia, 172
  leukocyte disorders, 444–455
  lymphomas, 453–454
  mononucleosis, infectious, 454
  myeloma, multiple, 454–455
  polycythemia, 444
  spleen disorders, 455–456
  thrombocytopenia, 462
  transfusion therapy, 423–428
  vascular disorders, 458
  in water intoxication, 169
Hematuria, 472
  in prostatic hypertrophy, 763
Heme, 416
Hemianopia
  bitemporal, 898
  homonymous, 898, 908
Hemimelia, 819
Hemipelvectomy, prosthesis in, 873
Hemochromatosis, 601
Hemodialysis, 514–516
Hemodynamics, circulatory, 1181–1183
Hemoglobin
  adult, 417
  as buffer of carbonic acid, 163
  fetal, 417
  mean corpuscular, 422
  mean corpuscular concentration, 422
  normal values for 325, 416, 421
  oxygen-hemoglobin dissociation curve, 201–202
  and oxygen perfusion, 232
  and oxygen transport, 198, 416
  and oxyhemoglobin formation, 200, 201
  in sickle cell disease, 438–439
Hemoglobinuria, paroxysmal nocturnal, 441–442
Hemolysis
  from extracorporeal circulation, 388
  in glucose 6-phosphate dehydrogenase deficiency, 441
  immune, 442–443
  in sickle cell disease, 439
  from transfusion therapy, 425
Hemolytic anemia, 437–438
  autoimmune, 36, 443
  extracorpuscular factors in, 442
Hemophilia, 460–461
  AHF concentrates in, 428, 461
  nursing care in, 461
  type A, 460–461
  type B, 460
  type C, 460
Hemoptysis, 211
  in bronchiectasis, 269
Hemorrhage
  adrenal, from anticoagulants, 677
  anemia from, 443

Index **1219**

cerebral, 951
and cerebral hematomas, 941–942
after chest surgery, 249
dehydration from, 165
and epistaxis, 1063
in esophageal varices, 593–594
in eye, 1001
in facial injuries, 1068
in laryngectomy, 1083
in orthopedic injuries, 823, 824
in pancreatitis, 612
in peptic ulcer, 546
pituitary, in Sheehan's syndrome, 632
postoperative, 98
shock from, 1184
sodium loss in, 172
in spinal cord injuries, 967
splinter, in nails, 1098
subarachnoid, 955–956
uterine, 769
Hemorrhoidectomy, 582
Hemorrhoids, 582–583
Hemosiderosis, 601
Hemostasis, 456–458. *See also* Coagulation
 tests for, 457–458
Hemothorax, 297
Hemovac drainage, 103
 after laryngectomy, 1081
 after mastectomy, 789
Henderson-Hasselbalch equation, 161, 201
Henoch-Schönlein disease, 458
Heparin, 30, 398
 antidote for, 398
 in disseminated intravascular coagulation, 464
 in extracorporeal circulation, 387
 in myocardial infarction, 349, 354
 overdosage of, 462–463
 in pulmonary embolism, 295
 in thrombophlebitis, 407
Hepatic duct, 602
Hepatitis, 588–592
 hospital-acquired, 77
 infectious or epidemic, 588
 serum, 588
 thyroid function in, 648
 toxic, 591–592
 type A, 588, 589
 type B, 588, 589
  carriers of, 589
 viral, 588–591
  chronic active, 591
  chronic persistent, 591
  fulminating, 591
  placental transmission of, 590
  prevention of spread of, 590
  from transfusions, 591
Hepatoma, 107, 599
Hepatomegaly, 585
Hepatorenal syndrome, 593
Heredity, 16–17
Hering-Breuer reflexes, 204
Hernia, 580–581
 abdominal, 580
 direct, 580
 femoral, 580
 hiatus, 563
 at ileostomy stoma site, 557
 incisional, 581
 inguinal
  in emphysema, 257
  indirect, 580
 of intervertebral disk, 983–985
 irreducible or incarcerated, 580
 of pelvic structures, in females, 773
 reducible, 580
 strangulated, 580
 umbilical, 580–581
Herniorrhapy, 581
Heroin, overdose of, 229–230
Herpes infections, 1119–1120
 in Ramsey Hunt syndrome, 1058
 simplex, 1119

and keratitis, 1017
of lips, 542
zoster, 938, 1119–1120
Heterografts, 385
 in burns, 1164
Heterotopic grafts, 32
Heterozygous genes, 16
Hiccups, 528
 postoperative, 101
Hip
 arthroplasty of, 843–846
  cup arthroplasty, 844
  for total hip replacement, 844–846
 dislocation of, 821
 fractures of, 836–841
 prosthesis for, 873
Hippuric acid test, of liver function, 587
Hirschsprung's disease, 566
His, bundle of, 317
 and bundle-branch block, 360
Histamine, 30, 1191
 anaphylactic shock from, 1186
 release in inflammatory response, 19
 in tests
  for gastric acid, 532
  in pheochromocytoma, 689–690
 vascular effects of, 394
Histamine headaches, 918
Histiocytes, 19
Histocompatibility, 32–34
Histoplasmosis, pulmonary, 287
Hives, 1099
HL-A system of antigens, 33
Hoarseness, 1076
 in airway obstruction from burns, 1148–1149
 in laryngeal cancer, 1079
Hodgkin's disease, 449–453
 chemotherapy in, 452
 diagnosis of, 450–451
 prognosis of, 452
 Reed-Sternberg cells in, 450
 staging of, 450
 treatment of, 452–453
Hollander test, of gastric secretion, 533
Homan's sign, 395, 407
Homatropine methylbromide, as mydriatic, 1010
Home care, and contact with families, 58
Homeostasis, 50–51, 151
 adrenal role in, 676, 690
 blood role in, 415
 of body fluids, 155
 cardiovascular system, role in, 394
 hypothalamus role in, 905
 pituitary role in, 628, 633
 shock affecting, 1189
 thyroid role in, 636
Homografts, 32, 385
 in burns, 1164–1165
Homosexuality, 735, 738
Homozygous genes, 16
Hordeolum, 999
Hormones. *See also* Endocrine system; Reproductive system
 adrenal, 672–675
 classes of, 623
 hypothalamus, 625
 interdependency of, 624
 metabolic effects of, 11–12
 of pancreas, 692
 parathyroid, 664–665
 of pineal gland, 672
 pituitary. *See* Pituitary gland
 regulation of, 623
 therapy with
  in Addison's disease, 679
  in cancer, 126
  after hypophysectomy, 634
 thyroid. *See* Thyroid hormones
Horner's syndrome, in carcinoma of lung, 307
Hospital-acquired infections, 74, 75–77
Hospitalization
 of burn patients, 1141

and discharge planning, 59–60, 105
 See also Discharge from hospital
 effects of, 58–59
Host, of infectious agents, 65
Humidification procedures, 219
 in asthma, 266
 in emphysema, 260
 for laryngectomy patients, 1084
 in oxygen therapy, 234
Hunger
 recognition of, hypothalamus in, 11
 temperature related to, 11
Huntington's disease, 961–962
 nursing care in, 961–962
 symptoms of, 961
 treatment of, 961
Hyaluronic acid, 9
Hydatidiform mole, 783
Hydration
 dehydration, 164–168
 overhydration, 169–171
 and skin fluid content, 1098
Hydrocele, 758–759
 infected, 759
Hydrocephalus, 901, 933
Hydrochloric acid, in gastric juice, 525
 control of secretion, 543
 tests for, 532–533
Hydrogen ion balance, 161–164
 in acidosis
  metabolic, 184–186
  respiratory, 181–184
 in alkalosis
  metabolic, 186–188
  respiratory, 184
 alterations in, 181–188
 chemical buffering system in, 162–163
 renal regulation of, 163–164
 respiratory regulation of, 163
 and secretion of hydrogen ion, 504–505
Hydrogen peroxide, as mouthwash, 538
Hydronephrosis, 490
Hydrophobia, 939
Hydrops
 fetal, 443
 labyrinthine, 1057
Hydrostatic pressure, 157, 321
Hydrotherapy
 in burns, 1160–1161
 in rheumatoid arthritis, 863
 in skin diseases, 1148
Hydrothorax, 297
Hydroureter, 489
α-Hydroxybutyrate dehydrogenase, serum, 326
17-Hydroxycorticosteroids, urinary, 675, 676
 in Cushing's disease, 683
17α-Hydroxylase deficiency, 688
20-Hydroxylase deficiency, 688
21-Hydroxylase deficiency, 688
Hydroxyprogesterone caproate, in cancer, 126
Hydroxypropyl methylcellulose, as eye lubricant, 1011
18-Hydroxysteroid deficiency, 688
3β-Hydroxysteroid dehydrogenase deficiency, 688
Hydroxyurea, in cancer, 126
Hyperalimentation. *See* Nutrition, parenteral total
Hypercalcemia, 178–179. *See also* Calcium
Hypercapnia
 chronic, 227–228
 in respiratory failure, 230, 237, 244
Hyperglycemia, 692
 from insulin, 720
Hyperkalemia, 176–178. *See also* Potassium
Hyperkeratosis, 1101
Hyperlipoproteinemia, 326, 343–345
Hypermagnesemia, 180
Hypermenorrhea, 765, 769
Hypernatremia, 173–174

Hyperopia, 1004
Hyperparathyroidism, 666, 667–669
 secondary, 668–669
 surgery in, 668
Hyperpyrexia, 929–930
Hyperreflexia, autonomic, 970–971
Hypersensitivity and allergic reactions, 22, 29, 30–31
 and anaphylactic shock, 1186–1187
 Arthus type, 34–35
 and asthma, 264, 267
 classification of, 36–38
 cytotoxic or cytolytic, 35–36
 delayed, 29, 31–32, 37
 desensitization in, 37, 268
 and eczema, 1112
 granulomatous, 34
 from insulin, 716
 and Ménière's disease, 1057
 and nasal allergies, 1062
 patch test in, 1104
 purpura in, 458
 and sarcoidosis, 285
 from transfusion therapy, 426
 treatment of, 31
Hypertension, 336–342
 in aldosteronism, 685
 and blood pressure readings by patients, 338
 and cerebrovascular disease, 951
 drugs in, 339–341
  combinations of, 338
  compliance with, 337
  side effects of, 339
 encephalopathy from, 341
 eye changes in, 337
 malignant, 341
 in nephrotic syndrome, 508
 nursing care in, 337–339
 in pheochromocytoma, 689
 portal, 593
 pulmonary
  in hypoxemia, 237
  in thromboembolism, 293
 secondary, 342
Hyperthermia, malignant, 96–97. *See also* Fever
Hyperthyroidism, 636, 648–659
 cardiovascular effects of, 640
 metabolic disorders in, 640
 symptoms of, 639–642
Hypertonic resuscitation formula, 1145
Hyperventilation, 202–203
 central neurogenic, 924
 in emphysema, 255–256
Hyphema, 1017, 1019
Hypnosis, for pain relief, 47
Hypnotics, with analgesic drugs, 46
Hypocalcemia, 178
 nursing care in, 178
Hypodermoclysis, for subeschar antibiotic therapy, 1158
Hypogammaglobulinemia, transient, 38
Hypoglossal nerve, 899
 assessment of, 909
Hypoglycemia, 692
 in Addison's disease, 677
 coma in, 722
 in diabetes, 721–723
 from insulin, 715, 717, 721
 in narcotic overdose, 230
 postgastrectomy, 551
 from sulfonylureas, 721–722
 treatment of, 723
Hypoglycemic agents, oral, 703, 709–710
 hypoglycemia from, 721–722
Hypokalemia, 174–176, *See also* Potassium
Hypomagnesemia, 179–180
 nursing care in, 179–180
Hypomenorrhea, 765
Hyponatremia, 171–173
Hypoparathyroidism, 666–667, 669–672, 815
 diseases causing, 669
 idiopathic, 669

Hypoparathyroidism *Continued*
  symptoms and signs of, 669
  treatment of, 670–671
Hypopharynx, 1071
Hypophysectomy, 633–634
  as ablative measure, 635–636, 947
  in Cushing's disease, 683, 684
Hypoprothrombinemia, 459–460
Hypostatic pneumonia, 279
Hypotension
  postural, in pheochromocytoma, 689
  in transfusion reactions, 425
Hypothalamus, 625, 895
  and breast development, 784
  corticotropin-releasing factor in, 674
  cyclic center in, 744
  and gonadal hormone secretion, 744–745
  and homeostasis, 905
  hormones secreted in, 626
  and hunger recognition, 11
  and reproductive function, 744
  symptoms of dysfunction, 633
  tonic center in, 744
Hypothermia
  from blood transfusions, 427
  induced, 96
    in cardiac surgery, 387
    in intracranial pressure increase, 925
Hypothyroidism, 636, 659–662
  in adults, 660
  cardiovascular effects of, 640
  juvenile, 659–660
    symptoms of, 659–660
  metabolic disorders in, 640
  in panhypopituitarism, 635
  symptoms of, 639–642
  thyroprival, 646
  treatment of, 660–661
  trophoprival, 646
Hypoventilation, 203
  alveolar, 227–228
  causes of, 228–229
  from narcotics during anesthesia, 96
  in pneumonia, 277
Hypoxemia, 203, 205
  in emphysema, 256
  in pulmonary thromboembolism, 293
  in respiratory failure, 230, 237–238
Hypoxia, 205
  postoperative, 97
  and respiratory alkalosis, 184
Hysterectomy, 779, 782, 800–801
  in cervical carcinoma, 782
  complications from, 800–801
  in ovarian tumors, 779, 780
  psychological reactions to, 801
Hysterosalpingography, 749

Icterus index, 586. *See also* Jaundice
Idoxuridine, topical, in eye conditions, 1011
Ileal conduit, for urinary diversion, 494, 499
Ileostomy, 553–561
  appliances with, 554
    adhesives for, 556
    changing of, 556
    discs with, 554–555
    leakage of, 556
    odor control with, 555–556
  compared to colostomy, 557
  complications from, 553
  continent, 560–561
  dietary management in, 559
  dysfunction of, 557
  fluid and electrolyte imbalance with, 557
  and hernias at stoma site, 557
  lavage of, 557
  pregnancy after, 560
  prolapse of stoma in, 557
  retraction of stoma in, 557

  and sexuality, 560
  and skin barriers for peristomal care, 558
  stoma site in, 553
Ileum, 525
Ileus, 528
  hyponatremia in, 171
  paralytic (adynamic), 566
    in burns, 1153
    from gastric surgery, 551
Iliac crest puncture, for bone marrow aspiration, 423
Illness. *See* Disease
Illumination, of breast tissue, 785
Immobilization
  and assistance in mobility, 881–884
  complications from, prevention of, 841–843, 857, 952–953
  contractures from, 952
  and position changes for patient, 952, 953. *See also* Position changes
  in stroke patients, 952–953
Immune response, 22–39. *See also* Antibodies; Antigens
  allergic reactions in, 29, 30–31
  alterations in, 29
  anaphylactic reactions in, 29
  antibodies and antigens in, 23
  Arthus reaction in, 34–35
  and blood compatibility for transfusions, 423–424
  cell-mediated, 22, 26, 29
    in delayed hypersensitivity, 32
  chemical mediators in, 29–30
  and control of antibody responses, 27
  cytotoxic or cytolytic reactions in, 35–36
  in erythroblastosis fetalis, 442
  in grafts and transplants, 32–34
  granulomatous reaction in, 34
  humoral, 22, 24
  hypersensitivity in, 29
    delayed, 29, 31–32
  laboratory tests for, 28
  lymphocytes in, 24, 26
  primary, 26
  secondary, 26–27
  specificity in, 26
  tolerance in, 27
  in tumors, 37–38
Immunity
  active, 27
  passive, 27
Immunizations, 27–28
  combination vaccines in, 70
  declining rates of, 69
  and disease control, 66
  effectiveness of, 28
  in hepatitis A, 589
  influenza vaccines, 274
  for poliomyelitis, 70, 936–937
  priorities in, 70
  Pseudomonas vaccine in burns, 1159
  in rabies, 939
  records of, 70
  routes of administration in, 28
  for rubella, 70
  Sabin vaccine in, 936
  Salk vaccine in, 936
  substances used in, 28
  in tetanus, 939
Immunodeficiency disorders, 22, 38–39
  agammaglobulinemia, 38
  dysgammaglobulinemia, 38
  hypogammaglobulinemia, transient, 38
  Swiss type, 39
  United States type, 39
Immunofluorescence, 28
Immunogenicity, 23
Immunoglobulins, 23
  deficiency of, 38
  IgA, 23
  IgD, 23
  IgE, 23
    in allergic reactions, 30

IgG, 23
IgM, 23
Immunosuppression therapy
  agents in, 33–34
  carcinoma from, 37–38, 131
Immunotherapy, in cancer, 131–132
Impaction, fecal, 565–566
Impetigo, 1113
Incontinence, urinary
  nursing care in, 477
  in prostatic hypertrophy, 763
  in spinal cord injuries, 975
  from stress, 775
Incudostapedal junction, 1039
Incus, 1040
Infarction
  cerebral. *See* Cerebrovascular disease
  myocardial, 347–354
  pulmonary, 293–294
Infections
  and arthritis, 862, 867
  in burns, 1156
    prevention of, 1152–1153
  communicable. *See* Communicable diseases
  definition of, 64
  in diabetics, 728
  of ear, 1053–1056
  of eye, 1016–1017
  of nervous system, 934–940
  of reproductive system, 754–758
  in respiratory tract, 270–279
  of skin, 1113–1120
  in urinary tract, 481–489
Infertility, 750–754
  and artificial insemination, 753–754
  in females, 751–753
  in males, 750–751
  treatment of
    in females, 753
    in males, 751
Inflammatory response, 18–22
Influenza, 273–274
  vaccines in, 274
Informed consent, obtaining of, 84, 130–131
Inguinal hernia, 580
Inguinal lymph nodes, 420
Inhalation injury, in burns, 1149
Insemination, artificial, 753–754
Inspection
  of cardiac patients, 323
  of chest, 208
  of musculoskeletal system, 807
  of neck, in thyroid disease, 639
  in peripheral vascular disease, 394–395
Inspiration, ratio to expiration, 207
Inspiratory reserve volume, 215
Insufficiency
  arterial, chronic, 400–402
  renal, 509
  valvular, cardiac, 372
  venous, chronic, 405
Insulin, 692, 694
  allergy to, 716
  antibodies to, 720
  automatic injectors of, 718–719
  combinations of, 713
  concentrations or units of, 718
  dosage of, 713–717
    exercise affecting, 716–717
  function of, 711
  globin zinc, 713, 717
  hyperglycemia from, 720
  hypoglycemia from, 715, 717, 721
  intravenous injection of, 719
  lente, 713, 717
  metabolism of, 695
  NPH, 713, 717
  preparations of, 713
  protamine zinc, 713, 717
  regular, 713, 717
    acid, 713
    neutral, 713
  resistance to, 716

secretion and release of, 694
  shock from, 1186
  sites for injection of, 719–720
  syringes for, 718
  in test for growth hormone levels, 630
  as therapy
    in diabetes, 710–717
    in ketoacidosis, 725–726
Integumentary system, 1095–1133. *See also* Skin
  aging affecting, 1099
  anatomy of, 1095–1097
  disorders of, 1108–1133
    nursing care in, 1102–1103
    surgery in, 1108
    treatment of, 1104–1108
  examination of, 1103–1104
  factors affecting, 1098–1099
  infections of, 1113–1120
  parasitic infestations of, 1120–1122
Intensity of sound, 1041
Intercostal muscles, 818
Internal capsule, 896
Interstitial-cell-stimulating hormone, 631
Interstitial cells, 631, 736
Interstitial fluid, 153
Intertrigo, 1115–1116
Intervertebral disks, 893
  herniated, 983–985
Intervertebral foramen, 892
Intestinal juice, 567
Intestines. *See* Gastrointestinal system
Intracranial pressure increase, 922–925
  in brain tumors, 945
  in cerebral injuries, 943
  and measurements of pressure, 924–925
  signs and symptoms of, 922–924
  treatment and nursing care in, 924–925
Intrinsic factor, 433
  replacement therapy, 435
Intubation
  airway tubes in, 238
  chest tubes in, 250–252
  dehydration from, 165
  duodenal, 603–604
  endotracheal, 97, 238–239
    complications of, 238
    tracheostomy with, 238, 239–243
  for esophageal tamponade, 594
  of eustachian tube, 1053, 1056
  gastrointestinal, 536–538
    and gavage feedings, 539
  laryngectomy tubes in, 1082, 1083
  for emergencies, 1089
  tracheostomy tubes in, 240
Intussusception, 573
Inulin clearance test, 480
Iodine
  affecting thyroid uptake, 644
  butanol-extractable, test with, 644
  deficiency of, 646
  as mucolytic agent, 226–227
  protein-bound, test with, 644
  radioactive, 121–122
    in thyroid disease, 655
    in thyroid function tests, 644, 645, 646
    as therapy in Graves' disease, 652
  and thyroid function, 637
Ion, definition of, 152
Iridectomy, in glaucoma, 1022
Iridencleisis, in glaucoma, 1022
Iris, 995
  examination of, 999–1000
Iritis, 1000
Iron
  daily requirements for, 416, 431
  deficiency anemia, 430–433
    from hemorrhage, 443
  metabolism in hemochromatosis, 601
  parenteral administration of, Z track technique in, 432
  therapy with, 432–433

Irrigation
 of colostomy, 578–579
 of ear, 1039
 of eye, 1009
 of ileostomy, 557
 of maxillary sinus, 1062
 of orbit, after enucleation, 1027
Irritable bowel syndrome, 564
Ischemia
 in acute arterial occlusion, 402
 cerebral. *See* Cerebrovascular disease
 digital, in Raynaud's disease, 403
 in mesenteric occlusion, 566
 muscular, from casts in fractures, 832
 myocardial, 347
 and skin ulcers, 1129
Islet cells, pancreatic, 692
Isoantigens, 33
Isolation measures, in infections, 77–79
 laminar air flow unit in, 128–129
 life island in, 128
 reverse isolation in, 78, 128
Isometric exercises, 882
Isoproterenol
 affecting autonomic nervous system, 319
 in arrhythmias, 367
 as bronchodilator, 218, 226
 in cardiogenic shock, 384
 in cardiopulmonary resuscitation, 371
 in shock, 1198
Isotypes, immunoglobulin, 23
Itching. *See* Pruritus

Jaeger chart, 997
Jaundice, 584–585
 in biliary tract obstruction, 606
 in erythroblastosis fetalis, 443
 in hematopoietic disorders, 419
 in hemolytic anemia, 438
 icterus index in, 586
Jaw
 fractures of, 1068–1069
 wiring of, for weight loss, 541
Jaw jerk, 909
Jejunoileal bypass, in obesity, 541
Jejunum, 525
 bile duct anastomosis to, 606
Jock itch, 1117
Joints, 815–816
 capsule of, 816
 degenerative disease of, 858–868
 disarticulation of, 868
 prostheses for, 875
Jugular vein, 1044
 in central venous pressure measurements, 331

Kartagener's syndrome, 268
Karyopyknotic index, 747
Kayexalate
 affecting potassium levels, 506–507
 in hyperkalemia, 177
Kayser-Fleischer ring, in Wilson's disease, 601
Keloid, 1102
 dermabrasion of, 1110
Keratin, 1095
Keratinization, 1095
Keratinocytes, 1095
Keratitis, 1017, 1026
 herpes simplex, 1017
Keratolytic agents
 in acne, 1109
 in psoriasis, 1111
 for wart removal, 1119
Keratoplasty, 1026
Keratosis
 actinic, 1122
 obturans, of ear, 1049–1050
 seborrheic, 1122
 of vocal cords, 1079
Kerion, 1117
Kernicterus, in erythroblastosis fetalis, 443

Kernig's sign, in meningitis, 934
Ketamine hydrochloride, 93
Ketoacidosis, in diabetes, 699, 723–726
 treatment of, 725–726
Ketone bodies, in diabetes, 699
17-Ketosteroids, urinary, 675
Ketostix, 696
Kidneys, 159–160, 469, 503–519
 acute failure of, 505
  dialysis in, 506
  diuretic phase of, 507
  hyperkalemia in, 177
  management of, 505–507
  nutrition in, 507
  oliguric phase of, 507
  potassium levels in, 506
  water intoxication in, 169
 anomalies of, 503
 biopsy of, 479–480
 calculi of, 501–503
 chronic failure of, 505
  dialysis in, 509, 514–518
  dietary management of, 512–514
  management of, 509–519
  progression of, 510
  symptoms of, 510–512
  transplantation in, 509, 518–519
  treatment plans in, 512
  vitamin D activity in, 510, 511
 clearance tests of, 480–481
 cysts of, 503
 in diabetes, 701
 dialysis of, 506, 509, 514–518
 diseases of. *See also* Glomerulonephritis
  acidosis in, metabolic, 185
  hypokalemia in, 175
 ectopic, 503
 erythropoietic factor in, 417
 excretion of fluids from, 158–159
 failure of, 505–519
  acute, 505
  causes of, 505, 507–509
  chronic, 505
  in glomerulonephritis, 507–508
  management of, 505–507, 509–519
  in nephrotic syndrome, 508–509
  in prostatic hypertrophy, 763
  symptoms of, 505
  wound healing in, 506
 function tests, 479, 480–481
 horseshoe, 503
 in hydrogen ion regulation, 163–164
 in hydronephrosis, 490
 insufficiency of, 509
  hypermagnesemia in, 180
 nephrectomy, 492
 nephron, 159, 469, 504
 nephrosclerosis, 505, 509
 nephrosis, thyroid uptake in, 644
 nephrotic syndrome, 508–509
 obstruction of, 490
 palpation of, 475
 parathyroid hormone affecting, 666
 physical examination of, 475
 polycystic disease of, 503
 and renin-angiotensin system, 673
 shock affecting, 1192, 1201, 1203
 spinal cord injuries affecting, 974
 sponge, 503
 structure and function of, 504–505
 transplantation of, 34, 509, 518–519
 trauma of, 500–501
 tubules of
  acidosis in, 506
  reabsorption in, 504
 tumors of, 490–491
  nephrectomy in, 492–493
  renin-secreting, 687
Kimmelstiel-Wilson syndrome, 701
Kinins, 1191
Kirschner wires, use of, 855
Klinefelter's syndrome, 750
Knee
 prosthesis for, 873, 875
 total replacement of, 846–848

Knee jerk, 903
Koilonychia, 419, 1098
Korotkoff sounds, 330, 331
Krause's end bulbs, 1097
Krebiozen, 114
Krebs cycle, 10
 shock affecting, 1191
Kupffer cells, 583
Kussmaul breathing
 in acidosis, 185
 in renal failure, 512
Kveim test, in sarcoidosis, 286
Kyphosis, 808
 in Cushing's disease, 681

L-Dopa, 959–960
Labyrinth, 1037, 1040
 hydrops of, 1057
Labyrinthitis, 1055–1056
Lacerations, 21
 of eyelids, 1018–1019
 facial, 1068
 of scalp, 940
Lacrimal system, 995
 examination of, 999
Lactate
 levels in shock, 1196
 ratio to pyruvate, 727
Lactation, 784
 prolactin secretion in, 632
Lactic acid acidosis, 14, 185
 in diabetes, 721, 727–728
Lactic dehydrogenase
 in cardiac cells, 326
 serum levels
  in liver disease, 586
  in myocardial infarction, 349
Lactulose, in hepatic coma, 598
Laennec's cirrhosis, 592
Laetrile, 114
Laminar air flow unit, 128–129
Laminectomy
 in intervertebral disk herniation, 984
 for pain relief, 49
Language. *See* Speech
Laparoscopy, 749
 in liver disease, 588
Laparotomy, staging, in Hodgkin's disease, 451
Laryngeal nerve, recurrent, damage to, 639, 656
Laryngectomy
 adjustment to, 1089–1090
 agencies for help with, 1089–1090
 hemorrhage from, 1083
 neck breathing in, 1084
 partial, supraglottic, 1078
 postoperative care in, 1082–1085
 preoperative care in, 1080–1082
 and recurrence of carcinoma, 1089
 respiratory distress from, 1082, 1088
 speech training in, 1085–1086
 stoma care in, 1083–1084, 1087–1088
 total, 1080–1090
 tubes used with, 1082, 1083
  for emergencies, 1089
 vertical hemilaryngectomy, 1080
 and VoiceBak prosthesis, 1086–1087
Laryngitis, 1076–1077
Laryngocele, 1078–1079
Laryngoscopy, 1076
 direct, 1076
 indirect, 1076
Larynx, 1074–1090
 anatomy of, 1074
 assessment of function, 1076
 carcinoma of, 1079–1090
  glottic, 1081
  laryngectomy in, 1080–1090
  metastasis of, 1081
  recurrence after surgery, 1089
  sites of, 1081
  subglottic, 1081
  supraglottic, 1081

dysfunction of, 1076–1090
 foreign bodies in, 1077–1078
 fractures of, 1078
 paralysis of, 1077
 polyps of, 1079
 spasm of, 97
  from foreign bodies, 1077
 trauma of, 1077–1078
 ulcers of, 1079
Lasers
 in canes for blind persons, 1029
 in treatment of eye lesions, 1025
Lashes, examination of, 998–999
Lavage. *See* Irrigation
Laxatives, 565
LE cells, 35, 1126
Lead poisoning, 442
Learning, ACTH and vasopressin affecting, 16
Le Fort procedure, in prolapse of uterus, 774
Leg
 amputations of, 871–873
 examination of, 808–809
 muscles of, 818, 819
 raising test in herniation of intervertebral disk, 983
 ulcers of, 1129
Legal aspects
 and definition of blindness, 997
 and informed consent, 84, 130–131
Lens of eye, 995
 loss of, 1020
 and retinal detachment, 1024
 opacities of, 1000, 1001, 1019
Lenses
 contact, 1006
  for cataract patients, 1020
  corneal, 1005
  hydrophilic, 1006
  removal of, 1005–1006
  scleral, 1005
  soft, 1006
 intraocular, for cataract patients, 1020
Leptomeningitis, 934
Leukapheresis, 428
Leukemia, 445–449
 acute, 445
  lymphocytic, 447–448
  myelogenous, 448
 chemotherapy in, 446–447
 chronic, 445
  lymphocytic, 449
  myelogenous, 448–449
 induction therapy in, 447
 lymphocytic, 446
  acute, 447–448
  chronic, 449
 myelogenous, 445–446
  acute, 448
  chronic, 448–449
  and polycythemia vera, 444
 stem cell, 447
Leukocytes, 417–418
 count of, 325, 422
  chemotherapy affecting, 128
  in pharyngitis or tonsillitis, 272
  preoperative, 83
  subleukemic, 446
 disorders of, 444–455
 in inflammation, 19
 transfusions of, 445
 in urine, 473
Leukocytosis, 417
Leukopenia, 417, 444
Leukoplakia
 oral, 529, 1122–1123
 in reproductive tract, 777
 of vocal cords, 1079
 and vulvar carcinoma, 782
Leukopoiesis, 417
Leukorrhea, 741
Levin tube, 536
Leydig cells, testicular, 631, 736
Lice, 1120–1122
Lichen planus, 1110

Lichenification, 1101
Lid of eye. See Eyelids
Lidocaine, 93
 in anesthesia, 94
 in arrhythmias, 367
 for pain relief, 49
Life island, as isolation system, 128
Life patterns of patients, variables in, 57–58
Life-sustaining techniques, resuscitative, 139
Ligaments, 816
 in female pelvis, 772
Ligation of veins, 406
Ligatures, 89
Lightcast II, use of, 828–829
Linens, affecting skin lesions, 1107
Lip(s), examination of, 529
Lip reading, 1046
Lipase
 pancreatic, 567
 serum levels of, 609
 in pancreatic disease, 609
Lipids, 343
 metabolism of, 10–11
 serum, 326
Lipodystrophy, 711
Lipogenesis, 11
Lipoid pneumonia, 278–279
Lipophages, 20
Lipoprotein levels, 326
Liter, definition of, 153
Lithiasis. See Calculi
Little's area, epistaxis in, 1063
Livedo reticularis, 404
Liver, 583–602
 abscess of, 592
 alcoholism affecting, 600–601
 amyloidosis of, 601
 anatomy of, 583
 angiography of, 588
 biopsy of, 587–588
 cirrhosis of, 592–593
 detoxifying functions of, 584
 disorders of
  ascites in, 596–597
  bleeding tendencies in, 585
  coma in, 597–598
  and esophageal varices, 593–595
  hypernatremia in, 173
  jaundice in, 584–585
  portal hypertension in, 593
  symptoms of, 585
  thyroid function in, 648
 function tests, 585–588
 gluconeogenesis in, 711
 in glucose metabolism, 584
 in hemochromatosis, 601
 in hepatitis. See Hepatitis
 hepatomegaly, 585
 Hodgkin's disease of, 451
 palpation of, 531
 scanning of, 587
 secretory function of, 583
 shock affecting, 1192
 surgery of, 599–600
 transplantation of, 600
 tumors of, 598–600
  from oral contraceptives, 795
 in Wilson's disease, 601
Lobectomy
 hepatic, 599
 pulmonary, in carcinoma, 307
Lobotomy
 frontal, for pain relief, 49
 psychological, hypnosis as, 47
Lockjaw, 938
Lomotil, in ulcerative colitis, 552
Lordosis, 808
Lotions, 1105
Louis Bar syndrome, 38–39
Lower extremity. See Leg
Lubricants
 for eyes, 1011
 intestinal, 565
Ludwig's angina, 1073

Lumbar spine
 herniation of intervertebral disks, 983, 984
 puncture of, 912
  in brain tumors, 945
 sympathetic block of, as test in peripheral vascular disease, 396
Lung. See also Respiratory system
 carcinoma of
  adenocarcinoma, 305–306
  alveolar, 305
  bronchial cell, 305
  cell types in, 305–306
  and Cushing's disease, 683–684
  diagnosis of, 306
  epidermoid, 305
  metastasis of, 308
  oat cell types, 306
  radiation in, 308
  squamous cell, 305
  surgery in, 307
  symptoms and signs of, 306–307
  treatment and nursing care in, 307–309
  undifferentiated cell, 305
 edema of, 180
 fat embolism in fractures, 827
 function tests, 214–216
 scans of, in burns, 1149
 segmental resection of, 246
  in carcinoma, 307
 shock affecting, 1192, 1204
 volume studies, 215–216
Lupus erythematosus, 35, 443, 866, 1126–1127
 treatment of, 1126–1127
Lupus pernio, 286
Luschka foramen, 901
Luteal conditions. See Corpus luteum
Luteinizing hormone, 631, 736, 744
 surge in secretion of, 745
Lymph nodes
 axillary
  examination of, 744
  removal with mastectomy, 788, 790
 cervical, palpation of, 1071
 examination of, 419–420
 location of, 420
Lymphangiography, in Hodgkin's disease, 451
Lymphangitis, 408
Lymphatic system, 321
 of breast, 784
 disorders of, 408–409
 in edema, 180
 of reproductive tract, 777
 role in circulation, 1182
Lymphedema, 409
 after mastectomy, 790
 in pneumonia, 276
Lymphocytes, 24, 26, 415, 417, 418
 antilymphocytic serum, 33
 B cells, 24, 26, 418
 in cerebrospinal fluid, 913
 T cells, 24–26, 418
Lymphoid tissue, 24
Lymphoma, 107, 453–454
 Burkitt's, 453
 Hodgkin's. See Hodgkin's disease
Lymphosarcoma, 453
Lysosomes, 9
 in inflammatory response, 19

Mackenrodt ligaments, 772
Macroglobulinemia, Waldenstrom's, 455
Macrophages, 19, 20, 418
Macula
 retinal, 995
 of saccule, 1043
 of utricle, 1043
Macules, 1099
Magnesium
 deficiency in burns, 1144
 dietary, recommended amounts of, 155

function in body, 154–155
 hypermagnesemia, 180
 hypomagnesemia, 179–180
Malabsorption of nutrients, 535–536, 566–569
 in celiac disease, 568
 hypomagnesemia in, 179
 nursing care in, 568–569
 in Peutz-Jeghers syndrome, 569
 in regional enteritis, 567–568
 and vitamin B_{12} deficiency, 433
 in Whipple's disease, 569
Malacoplakia, 488
Malaria, hemolytic anemia in, 442
Malformations. See Anomalies
Malignancies, 106. See also Tumors
Malleus, 1039
Mallory-Weiss syndrome, 542
Mammaplasty, 791–792
Mammary artery implantation, for myocardial revascularization, 385
Mammary glands. See Breast
Mammography, 112, 785
Manchester procedure, in prolapse of uterus, 774
Mandible, fractures of, 1068–1069
Mandibular nerve, 898
Mantoux test, 282
Marchetti test, in stress incontinence, 775
Marrow, bone, 814
Marshall-Marchetti procedure, in stress incontinence, 775
Mast cells, in allergic reactions, 29
Mastectomy, 787–788
 and axillary lymph node resection, 788, 790
 nursing care in, 789–791
 subcutaneous, 791–792
Master's exercise test, 330
Mastoid bone, examination of, 1044
Mastoiditis, 1054
Maturity, sexual, 736
Maxilla, fractures of, 1068–1069
Maxillary nerve, 898
Maxillary reflex, 909
Maxillary sinus, 1060
 sinusitis, 1062
McBurney's point, in appendicitis, 581
Mechanics, body, 882
Mechanoreceptors, cutaneous, 1097
Mecholyl test, for esophageal motility, 562
Mediastinal emphysema, 303
Mediastinoscopy, 213–214
Medulla oblongata, 896
Medulloblastoma, 946
Megacolon
 constipation in, 566
 toxic, in ulcerative colitis, 552
Megakaryocytes, 415
Meibomian glands, infection of, 998
Meigs' syndrome, 779
Meissner's corpuscles, 1097
Melanin, 1098
 and hyperpigmentation, 1101
Melanin-stimulating hormone, 626, 632
 secretion in Addison's disease, 678
Melanoma, malignant, 107, 1125
 BCG vaccine in, 132
Melanotropin, 631
Melatonin, 672
Melena, 528
Membranes
 alveolar, 198
 capillary, movement across, 1182–1183
 cellular
  and electrolyte transport, 316
  permeability of, 155–156
  potential in, 8
 synovial, 816
Menarche, 736
Ménière's disease, 1036, 1057–1058
 treatment of, 1057–1058
Meningeal arteries, 909

Meninges, 892
Meningioma, 946
Meningitis, 934–935
 from craniotomy, 633
 diagnosis of, 935
 Hemophilus influenzae, 934, 935
 meningococcal, 934, 935
 symptoms of, 934
 treatment and nursing care in, 935
 tubercular, 935
 viral, 935
Meningocele, 932
Meniscus, 816
Menopause, 736, 766, 799–801
 and postmenopausal bleeding in carcinoma, 781, 784
 premature, 768
Menorrhagia, 765–766
Menstrual cycle, 745
 and abnormal uterine bleeding, 768–770
 in carcinoma, 784
 and amenorrhea, 765, 766–768
 cessation at menopause, 736
 disorders in, 765–768
 and dysmenorrhea, 766, 768
 follicular phase in, 745
 luteal phase in, 745
 onset of, 736
 ovulation phase in, 745
 postmenopausal bleeding in carcinoma, 781, 784
 and premenstrual syndrome, 766, 768
Mental retardation, in Down's syndrome, 933
Mental status, evaluation of, 907
 in brain tumors, 945
Mercurial diuretics, 380
Merkel's disks, 1097
Mesenteric arteries
 embolism of, 403
 occlusion of, 566
 syndrome in burns, 1154
Mesentery, 527
Metabolism, 9–15. See also Endocrine system
 anabolism in, 11
 and assessment of body function, 12–13
 basal rate of, 10, 647
 in burns, 1150–1152
 carbohydrate, 10
 catabolism in, 11
 in diabetes, 711–712
 and energy expenditure, 10, 13
 exercise affecting, 13
 fat, 10–11
 hormones affecting, 11–12
 oxygen consumption in, 13–14
 protein, 11
 regulatory controls of, 11–12
 shock affecting, 1191
Metaphysis, 812
Metastasis, 108–109
 affecting calcium levels, 668–669
 to brain, 946
 of breast cancer, 787, 790–791
 of laryngeal carcinoma, 1081
 of lung carcinoma, 308
 of reproductive tract tumors, 776–777
 to spine, 982
Metrorrhagia, 766
Metyrapone test, 675–676
 in Cushing's disease, 683
Microangiopathy, in diabetes, 700
Microcirculation, 313, 321, 1180
 in shock, 1190–1191
Micturition, 469–470
 anuria, 471
 dribbling in, 472
 dysuria, 472
 frequency of, 471
 hesitancy in, 472
 and incontinence, 472
 intermittent, 472
 nocturia, 471

oliguria, 471
  in prostatic hypertrophy, 762
  reflex control of, 469, 470, 975
    in neurogenic bladder, 483
  urgency in, 471–472
  and voiding patterns, 469
  voluntary inhibition of, 470
Midbrain, 896
Migraine, 917–918
  in Ménière's disease, 1057
Mikulicz procedure, in intestinal surgery, 574
Miliaria, 1110
  crystallina, 1110
  profunda, 1110
  pustulosa, 1110
  rubra, 1110
Milk production, mechanisms in, 784
Miller-Abbott tube, 536
Milliequivalent, definition of, 152
Milligrams percent, 153
Milliliter, 152
Millimole, 153
Milliosmol, 153
Mineralocorticoids, 672, 673
  as therapy in Addison's disease, 679
Minerva jacket, 831
Miotic drugs, 1010
  in glaucoma, 1010, 1022, 1023
Mitosis, 8
Mitral valve, 313
  commissurotomy of, 373, 385
  insufficiency of, 372
  stenosis of, 372
Mittelschmerz, 768
Mobility of patient
  assistance in, 881–884
  lack of. See Immobilization
Mobitz types of heart block, 359
Mole
  cutaneous, 1101
  hydatidiform, 783
Mole (M), 153
Molecule, 152
Molluscum sebaceum, 1123
Moniliasis, 1115
  oral, 542
  of reproductive tract, 756
Monocytes, 19–20, 417
Monoiodotyrosine, 644–645
Mononucleosis, infectious, 454
  respiratory tract in, 279–280
Monro foramen, 901
Montgomery glands, 784
Moore's burn budget formula, 1145
Morbidity rates, 63
Mortality rates, 63
Motility disorders, gastrointestinal, 535, 561–566
Motion sickness, 1037, 1043
Motor area of brain, 894
Motor end plate, 816
Motor function
  assessment of, 910
  in intracranial pressure increase, 922–923
Motor seizures, focal, 926
Motor tract
  extrapyramidal, 904
  pyramidal, 903
Mouth
  blood supply of, 525
  infections of, 541–542, 1073
  lesions in lining of, 541–542
  leukoplakia of, 1122–1123
  malignant lesions in, 542
  oral hygiene
    agents as mouthwashes in, 538
    in anemia, 430
    in chemotherapy, 128, 446
    in comatose patients, 921
    after gastric surgery, 550
    in laryngectomy patients, 1088
    with nasogastric intubation, 538
    in radiation therapy, 117–118
    in renal failure, 511

physical examination of, 529–530
  ulcerations in, 1073
Mouth-to-mouth resuscitation, 368–370
Mouthwashes, 538
Mucolytic agents, 226–227
Mucormycosis, pulmonary, 287
Mucosa
  nasal, 1060
  oral, examination of, 530
Mucous cells, gastric, 525
Mucus, cervical
  evaluation of, 752
  ferning of, 747, 752
Mumps
  immunization in, 70
  and orchitis, 756
Murmurs, cardiac, 324
Murphy Pattee test, of thyroid function, 643
Muscle(s), 816–818
  atrophy of, 818
  attachment to bone, 817
  contraction of, 817
    and headache, 917
  electromyography of, 914–915
  of eye, 996, 997
  hypoventilation in neuromuscular disorders, 228
  insulin affecting, 711
  laryngeal, 1074
  myoneural junction, 817
  neuromuscular blocking agents, with general anesthesia, 93–94
  relaxants of
    with analgesic drugs, 46
    in osteoarthritis, 860
    spasms in spinal cord injuries, 969
    in thyroid disease, 641–642
Musculoskeletal system, 807–884
  amputations, 868–881
  arthritis. See Arthritis
  assessment of, 807–810
  bones, 810–815
  bursitis, 866
  complications from immobilization, prevention of, 842
  conditions affecting, 818–820
  congenital anomalies of, 819
  gout, 866–867
  hip arthroplasty, 843–846
  in hypercalcemia, 179
  in hyperkalemia, 177
  in hypermagnesemia, 180
  in hypernatremia, 174
  in hypokalemia, 175
  in hypomagnesemia, 179
  in hyponatremia, 172
  joints, 815–816
  knee replacement, total, 846–848
  mobility assistance, 881–884
  muscles, 816–818
  osteomalacia, 867
  osteomyelitis, 867–868
  osteoporosis, 860–861
  rheumatic diseases, 858–868
  trauma of, 819, 820–843
Myasthenia gravis, 962–964
  agencies for help with, 964
  crisis state in, 964
  diagnosis of, 962–963
  nursing care in, 963–964
  symptoms of, 962
  and thyroid dysfunction, 642
  treatment of, 963
Mycosis fungoides, 1126
Mycotic infections. See Fungus infections
Mydriatics
  adrenergic, 1010
  anticholinergic, 1010
Myelin, 891
Myelinated nerve fibers, 40
Myelitis, 936–937
  transverse, 936
Myelography, 810, 913
Myeloma, multiple, 454–455

Myelomeningocele, 932
Myocarditis, 375
Myocardium, 315
  blood supply of, 313, 1180
  cardiomyopathy, 375
  contraction mechanisms in, 315
    force-velocity relationship in, 320
    Frank-Starling principle in, 319–320, 1180
  depressant factor release from pancreas, 1192
  infarction of, 347–354
    arrhythmias in, 350, 353
    and cardiogenic shock, 383, 1185
    complications of, 353–354
    and coronary care units, 348
    diagnosis of, 349
    enzyme levels in, 326, 349
    hyperkalemia in, 177
    nursing care in, 349–353
    pericarditis in, 354
    postinfarction syndrome, 354
    psychological state in, 351–352
    and shoulder-hand syndrome, 354
    thromboembolic disease with, 354
    ventricular aneurysm in, 353–354, 386
    ventricular rupture in, 353
  revascularization procedures, 385–387
Myofibrils, 817
Myofilaments, 817
Myomas, uterine, 783
Myopia, 1004
Myosin, 315, 817
Myringoplasty, 1054
Myringotomy, in otitis media, 1053
Myxedema, 640, 659
  coma in, 661–662
  mucinous deposits in, 642
  pretibial, 651
Myxoma, cardiac, 375

Nails, 1097
  aging affecting, 1099
  clubbing of, 1098
  examination of, 419
  koilonychia, 419, 1098
  in metabolic disorders, 1098
  onychomycosis, 1116–1117
  paronychia, 1115
  splinter hemorrhages of, 1098
Naloxone, in narcotic overdose, 230
Narcosis, carbon dioxide, 205
  in emphysema, 256
Narcotics
  addiction to, 46
  as cough suppressants, 227
  hypoventilation from, 96
  overdose of, 229–230
  for pain relief, 46
  postoperative use of, 99–100
  in terminal illness, 134
Nasogastric tubes, 536–538
  feeding by, 539
  after gastric surgery, 550
  for laryngectomy patients, 1083
Nasolacrimal duct, 1060
Nasopharynx, 1071
National Cancer Institute, 114
National Eye Institute, 993, 1030
National Society for the Prevention of Blindness, 994, 1030
Nearsightedness, 1004
Nebulizers, 218–219, 226
  in asthma, 266
  infections from, 243
  in oxygen therapy, 234
Neck
  dissection of, radical, 542
    in laryngeal carcinoma, 1080
    in parathyroid disorders, 668
  examination of, 1071
  inspection of, in thyroid disease, 639
Negri bodies, in rabies, 939

Nelson's syndrome, 631
Neoplasia, 106. See also Tumors
Nephrectomy, 492–493
Nephroblastoma, 490
Nephron, 159, 469, 504
Nephropathy, tubular, 506
Nephrosclerosis, 505, 509
Nephrosis, thyroid uptake in, 644
Nephrotic syndrome, 508–509
Nerves and nervous system, 891–895
  anatomy and physiology of, 891–906
  in aphasia, 930–932
  assessment of, 905–917
  autonomic, 318–319, 904–905. See also Autonomic nervous system
    of bladder, 469
  central, 891–904. See also Central nervous system
  cerebrovascular disease, 950–955
  convulsive disorders, 925–929
  cranial nerves. See Cranial nerves
  degenerative disease of, 956–964
  developmental defects of, 932–934
  diabetic neuropathy, 702–703
  diagnostic tests of, 911–917
  disorders of, 932–947
    manifestations of, 917–932
  of eye, 995
  headache, 917–918
  hyperpyrexia, 929–930
  impairment from casts, in fractures, 832
  infections of, 934–940
  intracranial pressure increase, 922–925
  laryngeal, 1074
  motor nerves, 817, 903–904
  myelinated fibers in, 40
  myoneural junction, 817
  neuropathies, 964–967
  nonmyelinated fibers in, 40
  optic nerve, 897–898, 995
  parasympathetic system, 318–319, 904–905
    and bladder control, 469
  pathways from ear to brain, 1041, 1045
  peripheral nerves
    neuritis of, 966–967
    stimulation for pain relief, 48–49
    tumors of, 964–965
  of pituitary gland, 626
  regional blocks of, 94–96
    for pain relief, 49
  of reproductive tract, 776
  sensory nerves, 40, 817, 904
  surgery, intracranial, 947–950
    postoperative care in, 949–950
    preoperative preparation for, 948–949
  sympathetic system, 318–319, 904–905
    receptors in, 1199
    of thyroid gland, 638
  trauma of, 940–944
  tumors of
    brain, 944–947
    spinal, 982–983
  unconsciousness, 918–922
  vertigo, 918
Neuralgia
  in herpes zoster, 1120
  trigeminal, 965–966
Neurectomy, for pain relief, 49
Neurilemmoma, 964
Neuritis, 937–938, 966–967
Neuroblastoma, of adrenal medulla, 690
Neurofibroma, 964
Neurogenic bladder, 483
Neuroglia, 891
Neurohypophysis, 625
Neurology, 891
Neuroma, acoustic, 946
Neuron, 891
  afferent, 903
  efferent, 903
Neuronitis, vestibular, 1058

Neuropathies, 964–967
  diabetic, 702–703
Neurophysin, 626
Neurosurgery, for pain relief, 49–50
Neurosyphilis, 938
Neurotransmitters, 891
  acetylcholine, 904
Neutropenia, 444
Neutrophils, 417, 418
  burns affecting, 1159
Nevus, 1124–1125
  in choroid layer of eye, 1001
  flammeus, 1128
Nickerson-Kveim test, in sarcoidosis, 286
Nicotine acid tartrate test, in diabetes insipidus, 627
Nipples
  anatomy of, 784
  examination of, 742–743
  in mammaplasty, 792
  Paget's disease of, 786
Nitroblue tetrazolium dye test, in burns, 1159
Nocardiosis, pulmonary, 287
Nocturia, 471
  in prostatic hypertrophy, 762
Nodules, 1099
  Heberden's, 859
  vocal, 1079
Noise
  hearing loss from, 1050–1051
  startle effect of, 1050
  tolerance for, 1050
Norepinephrine
  as neurotransmitter, 319
  in shock, 1199
  vascular effects of, 394
Nose, 1059–1067
  assessment of, 1059–1061
  cauterization of, 1063
  decongestants for, 1061
  drops for, 1062
    overuse of, 1067
  dysfunction of, 1061–1067
  foreign bodies in, 1064–1065
  fractures of, 1065–1066, 1068, 1069–1070
  functions of, 1059
  hematomas of, 1066
  lypressin spray for, in diabetes insipidus, 627
  packing of, 1063–1064
  perforations of septum, 1065
  polyps in, 1063
  rhinitis, 1061
  rhinophyma, 1110
  rhinoplasty, 1065
  septal deviation in, 1065
  sinusitis, 1061–1062
  tumors of, 1066–1067
Nosocomial infections, 75–77
Nucleolus, cellular, 9
Nucleotides, bases of, 8
Nucleus
  of cells, 8
    and antinuclear antibodies, 35
  pulposus, 892, 983
Numbness, 906
Nurse's role
  circulating nurse, 87
  in communicable disease control, 71–72
  occupational health (industrial) nurse, 289
  school nurse, 335–336
  scrub nurse, 87
Nursing care
  and assessment of patient, 53–55
  basic concepts in, 5–139
  for cancer patients, 105–136
  in communicable diseases, 64–80
  counseling in, 61–62
  and discharge planning, 59–60
  evaluation of, 62–63
  patient variables affecting, 56–59

  planning of, 55–62
  for surgical patients, 80–105
  and teaching of patients, 60–61
  in terminal illness, 132–136
Nutrition
  and acne, 1109
  in alcoholism, 600
  in anemia, 429
  in ascites, 597
  assessment of, 418
  Barron food pump in, 539
  blenderized foods in, 539
  in burns, 1151, 1152
  in cancer, 133
  in chemotherapy in leukemia, 446
  and cholesterol in diet, 344
  in cirrhosis, 593
  for colostomy patients, 579
  in comatose state, 920–921
  in constipation, 565
  in diabetes, 704–709
  in diarrhea, 564
  and digestive process, 525
  in emphysema, 260
  in enteritis, regional, 568
  and excessive intake, 535, 540–541
  and eye health, 1006
  Giordano-Giovannetti diet, 513
  in glomerulonephritis, 508
  and goitrogens in food, 648
  in Graves' disease, 654
  in heart failure, congestive, 377, 379–381
  in hepatic coma, 598
  in hepatitis, 589
  in hyperkalemia, 177
  in hyperlipoproteinemia, 344–345
  in hyponatremia, 173
  in hypothyroidism, 661
  for ileostomates, 559
  and inadequate intake, 535, 538–540
  in laryngectomy patients, 1083
  low carbohydrate diet, effects of, 528
  in malabsorption, 568, 569
  malnutrition with sodium loss, 171
  in myocardial infarction, 350
  and needs of hospitalized patients, 528, 529
  in nephrotic syndrome, 509
  parenteral, total, 188–191, 539
    and insertion of subclavian line, 189
    nursing care in, 189–191
  in peptic ulcer, 545
  phenolic acid in foods, 689
  postoperative, 100
  in radiation therapy, 117–118
  in renal failure
    acute, 507
    chronic, 512–514
  in respiratory failure, 244
  in rheumatoid arthritis, 863, 865
  sodium restriction in, 379–381
  in spinal cord injuries, 969
  for stroke patients, 953
  in terminal illness, 133
  in thyroid disease, 640–641
  tube feedings in, 539
  Vivonex in, 539
  and wound healing, 103
Nystagmus, 908, 918, 1043–1044
  from caloric stimulation, 1039
  in multiple sclerosis, 957

Oatmeal baths, in skin diseases, 1148
Obesity
  in diabetes, 705
  and excessive intake of nutrients, 540–541
  fasting in, 540–541
  jejunoileal bypass in, 541
  medications in, 540
  in pickwickian syndrome, 228
  psychotherapy in, 540
  in surgical patients, 83
  and surgical wiring of jaws, 541

Obstipation, 528
Obstruction
  of airway, chronic, 216, 217–227
  of bile ducts, 606
  of esophagus, 569–570
  gastrointestinal, 535, 569–580
  of pylorus, 571
  of salivary glands, 1073
  of small intestine, 571–572
  of stomach, 570–571
  of urinary tract, 489–503
Obstructive lung disease, chronic, 252, 253
Occipital lobe, 895
  blindness from lesions of, 908
Occipital lymph nodes, 420
Occlusion, arterial
  acute, 402–403
  chronic, 403
  coronary arteries, 347
  mesenteric, 566
Occupational health (industrial) nurse, role of, 289
Ochronosis, 1037
Oculist, 993
Oculomotor nerves, 898
  assessment of, 908
  in pituitary tumors, 633
Ocusert Pilocarpine Delivery System, 1012
Oddi sphincter, 526, 602
Odor
  from casts, in fractures, 832–833
  control in ostomy care, 555
  detection of, 1059, 1061
Ointments, for skin, 1105
Olfaction, 1059, 1061
Olfactory nerve, 896–897, 1060–1061
  assessment of, 907–908
Olfactory receptors, 1060, 1061
Oligodendroglioma, 946
Oligomenorrhea, 765
Oliguria, 471
  in burns, 1143, 1147–1148
  in renal failure, 506
  in shock, 1194, 1201, 1203
  in transfusion reactions, 425
Omentum, great, 527
Oncology, 105–106
Oncotic pressure, 157
Onycholysis, in thyroid disease, 651
Onychomycosis, 1116–1117
Oophorectomy
  in breast cancer, 788
  and menopause induction, 800, 801
  in ovarian malignancies, 780
  psychological reactions to, 801
Opacities, ocular, 1000, 1001, 1019–1021
Operant conditioning. See Behavior modification
Ophthalmia, sympathetic, 1019
Ophthalmic nerve, 898
Ophthalmologist, 993
Ophthalmoscope, 1001
Opiates, for pain relief, 46
Opisthotonos, in tetanus, 939
Opsonins, 19
Opsonization, 28
Optacon, use of, 1029
Optic chiasm, 897
Optic disc, 1001
Optic nerve, 897–898, 995
  assessment of, 908
  damage from pituitary enlargement, 633
Optician, 993
Oral cavity. See Mouth
Orbit of eye, 995
  cellulitis of, in ethmoid sinusitis, 1062
  edema of, in ethmoid sinusitis, 1062
  fractures of, 1068
  irrigation of, after enucleation, 1027
Orchidopexy, 758
Orchitis, mumps, 756
Oropharynx, 1071
Orthopnea, 376

Oscillometry, in peripheral vascular disease, 395
Osmol, 153, 156
Osmolality, 157
Osmolarity, 157
  of urine, 161
Osmosis, 152, 156–157
Osmotic pressure, 152, 156, 321
  colloidal, 157, 1182
Ossicles, auditory, 1040, 1041, 1045
Osteoarthritis, 858–860
  signs and symptoms of, 859
  treatment of, 860
Osteoblasts, 813
Osteoclasts, 813
Osteocytes, 813
Osteogenesis, 814–815
  imperfecta, 819
Osteoid substance of bone, 813
Osteoma, of ear, 1052
Osteomalacia, 815, 867
Osteomyelitis, 820, 867–868
Osteoporosis, 860–861
  postmenopausal or senile, 800, 861
Ostomy care. See Colostomy; Ileostomy
Otitis media, 1053–1054
  complications of, 1055
  secretory, 1056
  after stapedectomy, 1057
Otoliths, 1043
  movements of, 1043
Otorrhea, cerebrospinal fluid, 1050
Otosclerosis, 1056–1057
Otoscope, 1037
Ototoxic drugs, 1056
Ouabain, 379
Ova, 736
Oval window, of ear, 1040, 1041
Ovariopexy, in Hodgkin's disease, 451–452
Ovary, 736
  arrhenoblastoma of, 780
  Brenner tumors of, 779
  carcinoma of, 779–780
    with endometrial tumors, 783
    staging of, 780
    treatment of, 780
  cystadenoma of, 779
    mucinous, 779
    serous, 779
  cysts of, 778–779
    chocolate, 771
    dermoid, 779
    follicular, 778
    luteal, 779
  dysgerminoma of, 780
  endometriosis of, 771
  fibroid tumors of, 779
  follicular maturation in, 745
  granulosa-theca cell tumors of, 780
  teratomas of, 779
Overhydration, 169–171
Ovulation, 736, 745
  and basal body temperature, 746
  failure of, 753
    and abnormal uterine bleeding, 769
  induction of, 634, 753, 767
Oxygen
  anoxia in shock, 1190, 1194, 1200
  consumption of, 13–14
  diffusion of, 201
  dissociation curve, 200, 201–202
  hypoxia, 204
    postoperative, 97
    and respiratory alkalosis, 184
  partial pressure of, 199–200
  perfusion of, 197, 232
  saturation of, 200, 201
  therapy with, 232–237
    in acidosis, respiratory, 183
    in asthma, 266
    blood gas levels in, 233
    in burns, 1149–1150
    concentrations of oxygen in, 233–234
    in emphysema, 260

in heart failure, congestive, 377
humidification in, 234
importance of flow rate and concentration in, 234–235
intermittent positive pressure breathing with, 234
and mechanically assisted ventilation, 235–237
in myocardial infarction, 350
in narcotic overdose, 230
nasal cannulas and catheters in, 232–233
in pulmonary embolism, 295
in respiratory failure, acute, 230, 231, 232–237
results of, 237
and retrolental fibroplasia, 1025
toxicity of, 235
transport by hemoglobin, 198, 201, 416
uneven distribution of, 200–201
Oxygenator, in heart-lung machine, 387
Oxyhemoglobin, 200, 201, 417
dissociation curve in hypoxia, 232
Oxytocin, 626, 628

Pacemakers
for bladder stimulation, 976
cardiac, 360–364
battery life of, 362
battery replacement for, 363–364
demand, 361–362
emergency use of, 361, 362
fixed-rate, 361
in heart block, 360
nursing care with, 362–364
precautions with, 363
signs of failure in, 363
in Stokes-Adams syndrome, 360
synchronous, 361
temporary, 360, 362
transthoracic insertion of, 361
transvenous insertion of, 360
Pachymeningitis, 934
Pacinian corpuscles, 1097
Packing, intranasal, 1063–1064
Paget's disease of bone, 814
Pain, 39–50
acupuncture in, 47–48
acute, 42–43
analgesics in, 45–47
in angina pectoris, 345
assessment of, 43–45
in Bell's palsy, 966
in biliary colic, 602
relief of, 605
in breast, 787
in burns, 1141–1142, 1153
after cardiopulmonary bypass, 390–391
from casts, in fractures, 832
causes of, 20
chronic, 43
colic, in urinary calculi, 501
deep, 42
in dysmenorrhea, 768
in dyspareunia, 776
in earache, 1049
gate control theory of, 40–41
in hands, paraffin baths for, 860, 863
in headache, 917
in herniation of intervertebral disk, 983
in herpes zoster, 1120
hypnosis in, 47
intercostal, 210
intractable, 43
management of, 45–50
mechanisms in, 40–41
in musculoskeletal disorders, 808
in myeloma, multiple, 454
neurosurgery in, 49–50
in orthopedic injuries, 824
in osteoarthritis, relief of, 860

in pancreatitis, 610–611
in peptic ulcer, 544
perception of, 41–42
in pericarditis, 374
peripheral nerve stimulation in, 48–49
in peripheral vascular disease, 394, 395
phantom limb, 43, 878–879
placebos in, 47
pleuritic, 210, 296
postoperative, 98
narcotics in, 99–100
as protective influence, 39–40
psychogenic, 43
psychological gains from, 50
in pulmonary embolism, 295
reactions to, 42
receptors for, 1097
referred, 42
in reproductive tract infections, 754
in respiratory system dysfunction, 210
in rheumatoid arthritis, 863
in shock, 1201
in sickle cell disease, 439
in spinal cord injuries, 969
superficial, 42
in terminal illness, 134
thoracic, generalized, 210
in trigeminal neuralgia, 965
types of, 42–43
in urination, 472
Palatal reflex, 909
Palate, examination of, 529
Pallor, 419
in anemia, 429
in orthopedic injuries, 824
in shock, 1194
Palpation
of abdomen, 531
of bladder, 475
of breasts, 742
of cervical lymph nodes, 1071
of chest, 208
of heart, 325
of kidneys, 475
of liver, 531
of musculoskeletal system, 807
of paranasal sinuses, 1060
of pelvic organs, 739
bimanual, 741–742
of peripheral pulses, 395
of thyroid gland, 638
Palpitations, cardiac, 320, 364
Palsy
Bell's, 966
cerebral, 934
Pancoast syndrome, 305–306, 307
Pancreas, 608–615, 692–729
acinar cells of, 608
anatomy and function of, 608–609
cancer of, 613, 614
cystadenoma of, 614
cysts of, 613
in diabetes mellitus, 692
function of, 692
function tests of, 609–610
in hyperglycemia, 692
in hypoglycemia, 692
islet cells of, 608
tumors of, 613, 614
myocardial depressant factor released from, 1192
pancreatitis, 610–613
pseudocysts of, 613
scanning of, 610
surgery of, 614
tumors of, 613–615
in Zollinger-Ellison syndrome, 548, 613, 614
Pancreatectomy, total, 614
Pancreatic duct, 602, 608
Pancreatic juice, 567, 608
characteristics of, 536
Pancreatitis, 610–613
acute, 610–612
diagnostic tests in, 611

hyponatremia in, 171
nursing care in, 612
treatment of, 611
chronic, 612–613
hemorrhagic, 612
in hyperparathyroidism, 666
Pancreozymin-secretin test, 609–610
Pancytopenia, in aplastic anemia, 436, 437
Panhypopituitarism, 628, 631, 634–635
and adrenal insufficiency, 680
Pannus formation, in rheumatoid arthritis, 862
Papanicolaou smear test, 112–113, 740, 747
Papilledema, 898, 995, 1001
in hypertension, malignant, 341
Papilloma
of breast, 786
of vocal cords, 1079
Papules, 1099
Paracentesis, in ascites, 594, 597
Paraffin baths, for pain in hands, 860, 863
Paralysis
agitans, 959
facial, 909, 966
flaccid, in spinal shock, 968
in hypokalemia, 175
laryngeal, 1077
in spinal cord injuries. See Spine, injuries of
in stroke patients. See Cerebrovascular disease
of vocal cords, 1077
Paraplegia
exercises in, 977–978
in spinal tumors, 983
and tilt table use, 974
Parasitic infestations of skin, 1120–1122
Parasympathetic nervous system, 318–319, 904–905
and bladder control, 469
Parathyroid glands, 664–672
anatomy of, 664
dysfunction of, 665–667
treatment of, 668–672
function of, 665
function tests, 667–668
in hypercalcemia, 179
hyperparathyroidism, 666, 667–669. See also Hyperparathyroidism
in hypocalcemia, 178
hypoparathyroidism, 666–667, 669–672. See also Hypoparathyroidism
surgery of, 668
in thyroid surgery, 656
Parathyroid hormone, 664–665
activity in renal failure, 511
affecting fluid and electrolyte regulation, 159
and bone growth, 815, 820
feedback relationship with calcium, 179
forms of, 666
function of, 665
in hypermagnesemia, 180
in hypomagnesemia, 179
in venous samples, radioimmunoassay of, 667–668
vitamin D affecting, 665
Parathyroidectomy, 668
Paresis, general, 938
Paresthesia, 906
in herpes zoster, 1120
in orthopedic injuries, 824
Pargyline hydrochloride, in hypertension, 340
Parietal cells, gastric, 525
Parietal lobe, 894
blindness from lesions of, 908
Parieto-occipital fissure, 894
Parkinson's disease, 959–961
medical treatment of, 959–960
nursing care in, 960–961

postencephalitic, 935
surgery in, 960
Parkland formula, in burns, 1146
Paronychia, 1115
Parotid glands, 525, 1071
tumors of, 569
Parotitis
acute, postoperative, 101
from nasogastric intubation, 538
Pastes, for skin disorders, 1105
Patch tests, in allergies, 1104
Patellar reflex, 911
Patent medications, 272
Patients
assessment of, 53–55
counseling of, 61–62
families of, 58
physical examination of, 55
responses to diagnosis, 56
teaching of, 60–61
variables in, 56–59
Paul-Bunnell heterophil agglutination test, in infectious mononucleosis, 454
Pearson attachment, with Thomas splint, 855
Peau d'orange, of breast, 743, 787
Pectoral muscles, 818
Pediculosis, 1120–1121
Pelvic exenteration, 495, 780–781
Pelvic inflammatory disease, 754, 757–758
Pelvic organs
palpation of, 739
bimanual, 741–742
relaxation of, 771–775
Pelvic traction, 852–853
Pemberton's sign, in thyroid disease, 639
Pemphigus, 1114, 1128
Penetrance, concept of, 16
Penis
disorders of, 760–761
erection of, mechanisms in, 761
examination of, 739
Penrose drain, 102
Pentolinium, in hypertension, 340
Pentose phosphate pathway, for glucose metabolism, 10
Pepsin, 525, 543
Pepsinogen secretion, 525
Peptic ulcer, 535, 543–551
antacids in, 545–546
anticholinergic drugs in, 545, 546
and cancer of stomach, 547–548
duodenal, 543
in emphysema, 257
esophageal, 543
gastric, 543
gastric freezing in, 546
hemorrhage in, 546
in hypoparathyroidism, 666
intractable, 547
jejunal, 543
nursing care in, 544–546
pain in, 544
perforation of, 547
plication procedure in, 547
postoperative care in, 550–551
psychologic factors in, 544
in shock, 1203
surgery in, 547, 548–550
and Zollinger-Ellison syndrome, 548, 613
Percussion
of abdomen, 531
in cardiac assessment, 325
of chest, 208–209
with postural drainage, 220–221
Perforation, of peptic ulcer, 547
Perfusion of gases, 197–202
ratio to ventilation, 198
Pericardiocentesis, 374
Pericarditis, 374–375
acute, 374

Pericarditis *Continued*
  chronic, 375
  in myocardial infarction, 354
Pericardium, 314
Perichondritis, of pinna, 1053
Perilymph, 1041, 1043
Perimeter, for visual field testing, 998
Perineum, in colostomy, 576
Periosteum, 813
Peripheral nerves
  neuritis of, 966–967
  stimulation for pain relief, 48–49
  tumors of, 964–965
Peripheral vascular system, 313–314, 320–321, 393–409
  acute arterial occlusion, 402–403
  aneurysms, 399–400
  aortic diseases, 399
  arterial disorders, 399–404
  assessment of, 394–396
  chronic arterial insufficiency, 400–402
  in diabetes, 702
  diagnostic tests of, 395–396
  diseases of
    amputations in, 868
    anticoagulant therapy in, 397–399
    bone disorders in, 820
    nursing care in, 396
    preventive measures in, 396–397
  fistulas, arteriovenous, 404
  foot care, 396–397, 401–402, 406–407
  hemorrhagic disorders, 458
  Raynaud's disease, 403–404
  thoracic outlet syndrome, 404
  thromboangiitis obliterans, 403
  thrombophlebitis, 407–408
  varicose veins, 405–406
  venous disorders, 404–408
Peristalsis
  gastrointestinal, 561
    bowel sounds in, 531
    in intestinal obstruction, 571
    and motility disorders, 561–566
  ureteral, 469
Peritoneal cavity, 527
Peritoneal dialysis, 516–517
Peritoneoscopy, in liver disease, 588
Peritoneum, 527
  parietal, 527
  visceral, 527
Peritonitis, 527
  hyponatremia in, 171
  in pelvic inflammatory disease, 757
Perlèche, 1116
Permeability, membrane, 155–156
Peroneal sign, in hypoparathyroidism, 670
Personality changes. *See* Behavior changes
Pessaries
  in prolapse of uterus, 774–775
  in retroversion of uterus, 776
Petechiae, 419
Peutz-Jeghers syndrome, 569, 572
Peyronie's disease, 760
pH, 161. *See also* Hydrogen ion balance
  of blood, 202, 415
    in acidosis, 182, 185
    in alkalosis, 184, 186
  of cerebrospinal fluid, chemoreceptor responses to, 204, 256
  of gastrointestinal secretions, 536
  of synovial fluid, 816
  urinary, 161, 473
    and stone formation, 503
  of vaginal secretions, 736
Phacoemulsification, in cataract, 1020
Phagocytosis, 19, 20, 417
  in burns, 1159
Phagosomes, 19
Phantom limb sensations and pain, 43, 878–879
Pharyngitis, 272–273, 1071–1072
  from coxsackievirus, 273
  streptococcal, 273

Pharynx, 1071–1074
  blood supply of, 525
  infections of, 1073
  tonsillectomy and adenoidectomy, 1072–1073
  tumors of, 1073–1074
Phenolic acid, foods containing, 689
Phenolsulfonphthalein excretion test, 480, 481
Phenotype, 16
Pheochromocytoma, 688–690
  diagnosis of, 689–690
Phimosis, 739
Phlebitis, 407
Phlebothrombosis, 408
Phlebotomy, in pulmonary edema, 382
Phonation, 1074, 1076
Phonocardiography, 329
Phosphate
  buffering system, 162
  deprivation test, for parathyroid function, 667
  excretion test, for parathyroid function, 667
  stones, 502
Phospholipids, 343
Phosphorus
  absorption of, 665
  functions in body, 664–665
  levels in plasma, 664
    in hyperparathyroidism, 667
    in hypoparathyroidism, 669
    in renal failure, 511
  radioactive, 122
Photocoagulation, of retinal holes, 1025
Photographs of patient, in fracture cases, 836, 856
Photophobia, 999
Physical examination, 55. *See also* Examination
Physical therapy
  in osteoarthritis, 860
  in rheumatoid arthritis, 863
Physis, 812
Pia mater, 892
Pica, and iron deficiency, 432
Pickwickian syndrome, 228
Pigmentation
  of ear, in ochronosis, 1037
  of fundus oculi, 1001
  in retinitis pigmentosa, 1025
  of skin, 1098
    in Addison's disease, 678
    hyperpigmentation, 1101
    hypopigmentation, 1101
Pilonidal cyst, 581–582
Pineal gland, 672
  displacement of, in brain tumors, 945
  function of, 672
  and reproductive function, 744
  tumors of, 672, 946
Pinealoma, 946
Pinna, 1037
  large, surgical repair of, 1052
  perichondritis of, 1053
  trauma of, 1051
Pitch, of sound, 1041–1042
Pitressin. *See* Antidiuretic hormone
Pituitary gland, 624–636
  ACTH secretion in, 674
  adenoma of, 946
  blood supply of, 626
  dysfunction of, 628–633
    adrenal dysfunction in, 677
    treatment and nursing care in, 633–636
  function of, 626–628
  function tests, 675–676
  gonadotropin secretion in, 736, 744
  hormone replacement therapy, 634
  hypophysectomy, 633–634. *See also* Hypophysectomy
  nerve supply of, 626
  panhypopituitarism, 628, 631, 634–635
  radiation of, in Cushing's disease, 684

  surgery of, in Cushing's disease, 683, 684
  tumors of, 632–633, 946
    and Cushing's disease, 683
    treatment of, 633
Pityriasis rosea, 1110
Placebos, for pain relief, 47
Planigraphy, of chest, 212
Plantar reflex, 911
Plaques, 1099
Plasma, 153
  and blood volume, 1179
  constituents of, 415
  expanders of, 1197
  transfusions of, 428
Plasmablasts, 418
Plasma cells, 418
  in multiple myeloma, 454
Plasmapheresis, 427
Plasminogen, 457
Plaster of Paris, for casts, 829–830
Plastic material, for joint prostheses, 844
Platelets, 418
  aggregation of, 456
  count of, 422, 458
  factor 3 in, 457
  in hemostasis, 456
  thrombocytopenia, 462
  transfusions of, 427–428
Pleocytosis, 913
Plethora, in Cushing's disease, 681
Pleural friction rub, 210
Pleur-Evac system, 250–251
Pleurisy, 296
  dry, 296
  fibrinous, 296
  nursing care in, 298
  in pneumonia, 277
  wet, 296–298
Pleuritic pain, 210, 296
Plication, in peptic ulcer, 547
Plumbism, 442
Plummer's nails, in thyroid disorders, 651
Plummer-Vinson syndrome, postcricoid carcinoma in, 1081
Pneumoconiosis, 254, 288–292
  asbestosis, 290–291
  benign, 289
  berylliosis, 291
  byssinosis, 291
  coal miner's, 291
  disease process in, 288
  farmer's lung, 291–292
  and role of industrial nurse, 289
  siderosis, 290
  silicosis, 289–290
  types of, 289–292
Pneumocystis carinii pneumonia, from chemotherapy, 453
Pneumoencephalography, 916
Pneumonectomy, 246
  in carcinoma of lung, 307
  postoperative care in, 248–249
Pneumonia, 274–279
  aspiration, 279
    in narcotic overdose, 230
    prevention of, 244
  atypical, 279
  bacterial, 276
  bronchopneumonia, 276
  in burns, 1150
  chemical, 278
  Friedländer, 275, 277
  hypostatic, 279
  lipoid, 278–279
  lobar, 276
  nursing care in, 278
  postoperative, 99
  progression of, 276–277
  pulmonary function in, 277–278
  radiation-induced, 279
  respiratory failure in, 231–232
  segmental, 276
  after splenectomy, 456
  staphylococcal, 277

  symptoms and signs of, 277
  viral, 274–275
Pneumonitis
  chemical, 1149
  after extracorporeal circulation, 388, 391
Pneumothorax
  in emphysema, 261
  spontaneous, 299
  tension, 301–302
    from clamping of chest tubes, 252
Poikilocytosis, 415
Polarizing therapy, in myocardial infarction, 350
Poliomyelitis, 70, 936–937
Pollutants
  atmospheric
    and bronchitis, 261
    and emphysema, 253
    and laryngitis, 1077
    and nasal cancer, 1077
  noise, 1050
  smoke. *See* Smoking
Polycythemia, 444
  in emphysema, 256, 261
  vera, 419, 444
Polydactyly, 819
Polydipsia
  in aldosteronism, 685
  in diabetes insipidus, 626
  in diabetes mellitus, 699
  in hypoparathyroidism, 666
  psychogenic, water intoxication in, 169
Polymenorrhea, 766, 769
Polyneuritis, 937, 966–967
Polyp(s)
  of cervix uteri, 781
  of ear, 1054
  intestinal, 572–573
    familial, 572
    in Gardner's syndrome, 572
    pedunculated, 572
    in Peutz-Jeghers syndrome, 572–573
    sessile, 572
    villous, 572
  laryngeal, 1079
  nasal, 1063
  of uterus, 783
Polyphagia, in diabetes, 699
Polyuria, 471
  in aldosteronism, 685
  in diabetes insipidus, 626
  in diabetes mellitus, 699
  in hypoparathyroidism, 666
  in thyrotoxicosis, 642
Pompholyx, 1112
Pons, 896
Port wine stain, 1128
Portacaval shunt, 595
Portal hypertension, 593
Porter-Silber chromagen method, for plasma cortisols, 675
Position changes for patient
  in decubitus ulcer prevention, 1130
  in heart failure, congestive, 377
  in hip fractures, 840–841
  after laminectomy, 984
  in myocardial infarction, 351
  in spinal cord injuries, 972–974
  in stroke patients, 952, 953
Positioning of patient
  in burns, 1169–1171
  in coma, 920
  in intervertebral disk herniation, 984
  in shock, 1201
  in spinal cord injuries, 968, 969
Positive airway pressure, continuous, in adult respiratory distress syndrome, 229
Positive end-expiratory pressure technique, 229
Positive pressure breathing, intermittent, 234

in acidosis, respiratory, 183
in emphysema, 259
Postoperative care, 97–105
Postural drainage, 219–220
in acidosis, respiratory, 183
Posture, 808
affecting renin secretion, 686
decerebrate, 923
decorticate, 923
Potassium
active transport of, 157
dietary, recommended amounts of, 155
function in body, 154
hyperkalemia, 176–178
in Addison's disease, 677
diagnosis of, 177
disorders with, 177
nursing care in, 177–178
symptoms and signs of, 177
hypokalemia, 174–176
in aldosteronism, 685
in burns, 1144
in Cushing's disease, 682
diagnosis of, 175
disorders with, 175
from diuretics, 339
nursing care in, 176
symptoms and signs of, 175
intoxication from blood transfusions, 426
replacement therapy, 176
in digitalization, 378
in myocardial infarction, 350
serum levels
in cardiac assessment, 325–326
Kayexalate affecting, 506–507
in renal failure, 506
tubular reabsorption of, 504
urinary, 161
Potential
in cardiac cells, 316
in cellular membrane, 8
Povidone-iodine, in burns, 1158
Powders, for skin care, 1105
Prausnitz-Küstner reaction, 30
Prealbumin, thyroxine-binding, 643
Preauricular lymph nodes, 420
Precentral gyrus, 894
Precocious puberty, 631
Pregnancy
abortion for termination of, 796–798
antithyroid drugs in, affecting fetus, 653
and breast cancer, 788
corpus luteum in, 745
diethylstilbestrol in, affecting daughters, 782
ectopic
bleeding from rupture of, 769
culdocentesis in, 748
and erythroblastosis fetalis, 442
folic acid deficiency in, 436
in ileostomy patients, 560
molar, 783
and placental transmission of hepatitis, 590
progesterone role in, 738
Sheehan's syndrome in, 632
and spinal cord injuries, 981
thyroid hormone levels in, 643
urinary tract infections in, 488
Premenstrual syndrome, 766, 768
Preoperative care, 82–86
Presbycusis, 1047, 1058
Presbyopia, 997, 1003
Pressure
blood, 320–321, 1181
capillary, increase in, 180
of cerebrospinal fluid, 912, 913
hydrostatic, 157
intracranial
increased, 922–925
measurement of, 924–925
intraocular, 1002–1003
in glaucoma, 1021

prevention of increase in, 1015–1016, 1023
intravesical, 469
oncotic, 157
osmotic, 152, 156
colloidal, 157, 1182
partial, of oxygen and carbon dioxide, 199–200
receptors for, 1097
sores from, 1129
wraps for burn patients, 1173
Prevalence of disease, 63
Priapism, 761
Prickle cells, 1095
Primidone, as anticonvulsant, 927
Probenecid, in gout, 867
Procainamide, in arrhythmias, 358, 366
Procaine, 93
Procarbazine, in cancer, 126
Proctoscopy, 534
Progesterone, 673
and basal body temperature, 746
deficiency of, 752–753
function of, 738
and lactation inhibition, 784
ovarian secretion of, 736, 745
Progestins
in oral contraceptives, 794
as therapy in cancer, 126
Prognathism, 629
Prolactin, 632
levels in panhypopituitarism, 635
and milk production, 784
Prolapse, of uterus, 772–775
Prophylactic surgery, 82
Proprioception, 894
Prostaglandins, for abortion induction, 797
Prostate
anatomy of, 761
carcinoma of, 492
hypertrophy of, 491–492, 761–765
diagnosis of, 763
prostatectomy in, 763–765
treatment of, 763
tumors of, staging, 778
Prostatectomy, 763–765
nursing care in, 764–765
perineal, 764
retropubic, 764
suprapubic, 764
transurethral, 764
Prostatitis, 757
in hypertrophy of prostate, 762
Prostheses, 874–876
in above-knee amputations, 873
in ankle disarticulation, 871
in below-knee amputations, 871–872
for breast, 790
complications from, 880
for ears, 1051
for elbow, 874
electrolarynx, 1085
electronic cochlea, 1048
femoral head, 843–844
for hand, 873–874
for heart valves, 373, 385
for hip replacement, 844–845, 873
immediate postsurgical fitting of, 878
for knee replacement, 847, 873, 875
ocular, 1027–1028
patellar-tendon-bearing, 872
solid-ankle cushion-heel, 871, 873
in stapedectomy, 1056
VoiceBak, 1086–1087
Protease, and thyroid hormone release, 645
Protein
as buffer, 162–163
in cerebrospinal fluid, 913
dietary
in diabetes, 706, 707
recommended amounts of, 155
electrophoresis of, 586
function in body, 155

high protein feedings, hypernatremia from, 173
malabsorption of, 568
metabolism of, 11
insulin affecting, 699–700
plasma, 415, 1180
decrease in, 180
loss in burns, 1142
osmotic force of, 1182
synthesis in shock, 1191
in urine. See Proteinuria
Proteinuria, 161, 473
in aldosteronism, 685
Bence Jones, in multiple myeloma, 454–455
in glomerulonephritis, 508
in nephrotic syndrome, 509
Prothrombin, 415, 457, 459
activator of, 456
extrinsic, 457
intrinsic, 457
conversion to thrombin, 457
hypoprothrombinemia, 459–460
levels in liver disease, 586
Prothrombin time, 458
in cardiovascular disorders, 327
Pruritus, 1101
in atopic eczema, 1112
in biliary tract obstruction, 606
in blood disorders, 419
cholestyramine in, 606
of ear, 1049
in hepatitis, 590
in Hodgkin's disease, 450
in jaundice, 584
mechanisms in itching, 1097
in pediculosis, 1121
in renal failure, 510
in scabies, 1121
in vulvar carcinoma, 782
Pseudoaldosteronism, 687
Pseudocysts, pancreatic, 613
Pseudoephedrine, as bronchodilator, 226
Pseudogout, 867
Pseudohermaphroditism, female, 688
Pseudohypoparathyroidism, 671, 815
Pseudomonas vaccine, in burns, 1159
Pseudoparkinsonism syndrome, 959
Pseudopseudohypoparathyroidism, 671–672
Pseudotumor cerebri, 946
Psoriasis, 1111–1112
Psychogenic conditions
pain, 43
polydipsia, water intoxication in, 169
and respiratory alkalosis, 184
Psychological aspects
in ACTH secretion, 674
in adaptation, 51
in alcoholism, 601
in amputations, 869
in anorexia nervosa, 538–539
in asthma, 264
in burns, 1162–1164
in cardiac arrest and resuscitation, 371
in cardiac surgery, 391–392
in colostomy, 577
in Cushing's disease, 682, 684
in dependence on analgesics, 46
in diabetes management, 728
in epilepsy, 929
in functional disorders of gastrointestinal tract, 564–565
in Graves' disease, 649, 654
in Huntington's disease, 961
in laryngectomy, 1081–1082
in lung cancer, 308
in menopause, 799
in myocardial infarction, 351–352
in noise tolerance, 1050
in obesity, 540
in ovulation failure, 753
in pain, 50
in panhypopituitarism, 635
in Parkinson's disease, 959, 961

in peptic ulcer, 544
preoperative, in cardiopulmonary bypass, 389–390
in rape victims, 799
in rheumatoid arthritis, 862, 865
in shock, 1203
in skin lesions, 1102–1103, 1106
in spinal cord injuries, 969–970, 978–980
in stroke patients, 953–954
in thyroid disease, 641
in thyroid function, 638
in ulcerative colitis, 552, 559
Psychomotor epilepsy, 926
Pterygium, 999
Ptosis, of eyelids, 998
Ptyalin, 525
Puberty, 736
and acne, 1108
precocious, 631
Public education
and cancer detection, 113
and disease control, 68–71
Public safety, and communicable disease control, 72–74
Pubocervical ligament, 772
Pulmonary artery pressure, 333
in shock, 1195
Pulmonary edema. See Cardiovascular system
Pulmonary valve, 313
Pulse
bigeminal, 323
in digitalis toxicity, 378
in chronic arterial insufficiency, 401
deficit detection, 323
in orthopedic injuries, 824
paradoxical, 323
peripheral, palpation of, 395
ratio to respiration, 207
in shock, 1193
in thyrotoxicosis, 640
Pulsus alternans, 323
Puncture
cisternal, 912
lumbar, 912
Pupil of eye
in cerebral injuries, 943
consensual reaction of, 908
cycloplegic agents for, 1003
dilatation of, unilateral, 908
examination of, 1000
in intracranial pressure increase, 923
reactions of, 908, 1000
Purgatives, 565
Purine
bases of nucleotides, 8
metabolism in gout, 866
Purkinje fibers, 317
Purpura, 419, 1102
allergic, 458
idiopathic, 458, 462
senile, 458
thrombocytopenic, 462
idiopathic, 462
secondary, 462
Pus formation, 20
in urine, 472
Pustules, 1099
Putamen, 896
Pyelogram
intravenous, 477–478
retrograde, 478
Pyelonephritis, 486
chronic, 488
Pyloromyotomy, 570
Pyloroplasty, 548, 571
in obstruction from peptic ulcer, 547
Pylorus, obstruction of, 571
Pyoderma gangrenosum, in ulcerative colitis, 552
Pyorrhea, 528
Pyramidal cells, 894
Pyramidal motor tract, 903
Pyrimidine bases, of nucleotides, 8
Pyrosis, 528

Pyruvate, ratio to lactate, 727
Pyuria, 472

Quadriplegia
　devices for aids in, 978
　wheelchair use in, 971
Quarantine, international, 67
Queckenstedt's sign, 912
Quinsy, 1073

Rabies, 939–940
Radiation therapy, 116–122
　in bladder tumors, 493–494
　in breast cancer, 789
　in cervical carcinoma, 782
　in Cushing's disease, 684
　external, 117–118
　in Hodgkin's disease, 452
　internal sealed, 116, 118–120
　in laryngeal carcinoma, 1080
　in lung cancer, 308
　in myeloma, multiple, 455
　nutrition during, 117–118
　in ovarian carcinoma, 780
　in pituitary tumors, 633
　pneumonia from, 279
　radionuclides in, 120–122
　radium in, 118–120
　skin reactions from, 118
　surgery with, 116–117
　in thyroid disease, 655
　toxic effects of, 117
　unsealed, 116
Radiculitis, 937
Radioallergosorbent test (RAST), 30
Radioimmunoassay, 28
　of carcinoembryonic antigen, 535
　of gonadal hormones, 744, 746, 753
　of parathyroid hormone in venous samples, 667–668
Radioimmunosorbent test (RIST), 30
Radioiodine
　therapy with, in thyroid disease, 655
　in thyroid function tests, 644, 645, 646
Radiology
　angiography in. See Angiography
　chest x-rays, 212
　　in cardiac disease, 327–328
　　in emphysema, 258
　　in pneumonia, 275
　　in sarcoidosis, 286
　　in shock, 1195
　　in silicosis, 290
　cholecystography, 602–603
　of gastrointestinal tract, 533–535
　of musculoskeletal system, 810
　myelography, 913
　in pancreatic disease, 610
　in peptic ulcer, 547
　pneumoencephalography, 916
　of reproductive tract, 748–749
　in rheumatoid arthritis, 863
　urinary tract studies, 477–478
　ventriculography, 917
Radionuclides, 120–122
Radium therapy, 118–120
　in bladder tumors, 493
　in cervical carcinoma, 782
Rales, 210, 324
Ramsey Hunt syndrome, 1058
Rape, 798–799
Rauwolfia compounds, in hypertension, 339
Raynaud's disease, 403–404
Raynaud's phenomenon, 403
Reactose, in hypoglycemia, 717
Receptors
　cutaneous, 1096–1097
　in immune response, 26, 28
　　alpha and beta adrenergic receptors, 31
　　and antireceptor antibody, 27
　mechanoreceptors, 1097
　olfactory, 1060, 1061

for pain, 1097
　in parasympathetic nervous system, 319
　for pressure, 1097
　in reflex arc, 903
　in sympathetic nervous system, 319, 1200
　for temperature, 1097
　touch, 1097
Recessive gene traits, 16–17
　autosomal, 16, 17
Recklinghausen's disease, 964–965
Recognition, in immune response, 26
　and antireceptor antibodies, 27
Reconstructive surgery, 81–82
　of ear, 1051
　in facial injuries, 1070
　of nose, 1065
Recruitment, in hearing, 1047
Rectal anesthesia, 94
Rectal examination, 532, 740
　in cancer detection, 113
Rectocele, 773, 774
Rectum, 525
　anorectal disorders, 582–583
　bleeding from, in intestinal obstruction, 571
　fissures in, 582
Reed-Sternberg cells, in Hodgkin's disease, 450
Reflex
　abdominal, 911
　Achilles, in thyroid disease, 647
　autonomic hyperreflexia, 970–971
　Babinski, 911
　biceps, 910
　blinking, 998
　　loss of, in Bell's palsy, 966
　brachioradialis, 910–911
　corneal, 909
　　loss of, 920
　cremasteric, 911
　enterogastric, 561
　gag, 909, 1071
　gluteal, 911
　Gordon, 911
　maxillary, 909
　and micturition, 469, 470, 975
　　in neurogenic bladder, 483
　palatal, 909
　patellar, 911
　plantar, 911
　pupillary, 908, 1000
　spinal, 903
　swallowing, in stroke patients, 953
　triceps, 910
　vestibulo-ocular, 1043
　vomiting, 562
Reflex arc, 902–903
Reflex center, 903
Reflux of urine, 484–486
Refractive errors in eyes, 1003–1006
　correction of, 1004–1006
Regitine test, in pheochromocytoma, 690
Rehabilitation
　of amputees, 881
　of aphasic patients, 931
　and assistance in mobility, 881–884
　of blind patients, 1028–1030
　in burns, 1172–1173
　after cancer surgery, 115
　of cardiac patients, 353
　in cerebral injuries, 944
　after colostomy, 579–580
　of the deaf, 1045–1048
　of laryngectomees, 1085–1090
　in spinal cord injuries, 981–982
Reiter's syndrome, 756
Relaxation, of pelvic structures, 771–775
Remission of disease, 63
Renin, 159, 504, 673
　and aldosterone secretion, 685
　measurement of production, 686
　secretion of
　　affected by position of body, 686

by kidney tumors, 687
　in shock, 1188
Rennin, in gastric juice, 525
Renogram, 478
Repolarization, 316
Reproductive system, 735–801
　abortion, 796–798
　amenorrhea, 765, 766–768
　assessment of, 738–749
　biopsy of, 747
　birth control, 792–796
　blood and lymph supply of, 777
　breast conditions, 784–792
　diagnostic tests of, 744–749
　endometriosis, 770–771
　female disorders, 765–776
　fistulas in, 775
　hormonal factors affecting, 736–738
　infections of, 754–758
　　secondary, 756–758
　infertility, 750–754
　male disorders, 758–765
　menopause, 799–801
　nerve supply of, 776
　pelvic inflammatory disease, 754, 757–758
　prostatitis, 757
　rape victims, 798–799
　relaxation of pelvic structures, 771–775
　retroversion of uterus, 776
　trauma of, 756
　tumors and cysts of, 776–784
　　in females, 778–784
　　in males, 777–778
　　metastasis of, 776–777
　uterine bleeding, abnormal, 768–770
Reservoir, of disease agents, 65
Residual volume, 215
Resistance
　to disease, 64, 65–66. See also Susceptibility
　of organisms to antibiotics, 73–74
Resorption of bone, 813–814
Respiration
　apneustic, 924
　ataxic, 924
　central neurogenic hyperventilation, 924
　Cheyne-Stokes, 228, 923
　in coma, 920
　control of, 203–206
　　receptors in, 204
　　reflexes in, 204
　in emphysema, 258
　in intracranial pressure increase, 923–924
　Kussmaul, 185, 512
　neck breathing after laryngectomy, 1084
　nose in, 1059
　in pulmonary edema, 382
　rate of, 207
　　and carbon dioxide in blood, 163
　　ratio to pulse, 207
　in renal failure, 512
　in shock, 1193
　and work of breathing, 205–206
Respiratory acidosis, 181–184
Respiratory alkalosis, 184
Respiratory centers, depression of, hypoventilation in, 228
Respiratory distress
　adult syndrome of, 229–230
　in burns, 1137, 1148–1150
　in laryngectomy patients, 1082, 1088
　in myasthenia gravis, 964
Respiratory system
　abscess of lung, 292–293
　in acidosis
　　metabolic, 185
　　respiratory, 182
　acute respiratory failure, 230–246
　　acid-base imbalance in, 244
　　airway maintenance in, 238–243
　　aspiration from, 243–244

causes of, 231–232
　　and communication with patient, 245–246
　　compared to respiratory insufficiency, 231
　　goals of therapy in, 230–231
　　hypoxemia in, 237–238
　　nursing care in, 244–246
　　nutrition in, 244
　　oxygen therapy in, 230, 231, 232–237
　　rest and exercise in, 244–245
　adult respiratory distress syndrome, 229–230
　in alkalosis, respiratory, 184
　asthma, 263–268
　bronchiectasis, 268–270
　bronchitis, chronic, 261–263
　bronchospasm, 222–223
　carcinoma of lung, 304–309
　cardiopulmonary bypass, 387–393
　cardiopulmonary resuscitation, 368–371
　chronic obstructive lung disease, 252 253
　colds, common, 272
　compliance in, 197, 205
　complications from immobilization, prevention of, 841
　and control of respiration, 203–206
　dead space in, 198
　diffusion of carbon dioxide and oxygen, 201
　diphtheria, 273
　in drowning accidents, 304
　dysfunction of, 206–309
　　aerosol bronchodilators in, 218–219, 226
　　angiography in, pulmonary, 212
　　antibiotics in, 225, 227
　　assessment techniques in, 206–207
　　biopsy in, 214
　　breathing exercises in, 222, 223–224
　　bronchial hygiene in, 218–222, 226
　　bronchoscopy in, 212–213
　　chest drainage in, postoperative, 249–252
　　chest examination in, 207–210
　　chest x-rays in, 212
　　classification of, 216–217
　　cough in, 210–211
　　cough induction in, 221–222
　　diagnostic testing in, 211–216
　　endotracheal intubation in, 238–239
　　exercise stress tests in, 224
　　fluoroscopy in, 212
　　humidification in, 219
　　mediastinoscopy in, 213–214
　　medication in, 225–227
　　nebulizers in, 218–219, 226
　　nursing care in, 216–309
　　pain in, 210
　　percussion in, 220–221
　　postural drainage in, 219–220
　　scanning of lungs in, 212
　　signs and symptoms of, 210–211
　　skin tests in, 211
　　smoking withdrawal in, 217–218
　　sputum in, 211
　　surgery in, 246–252
　　tracheostomy in, 239–243
　　vibration in, 221
　dyspnea, 223–224
　edema, pulmonary, 381–383
　and elasticity of lung, 197
　emphysema, 253–261
　empyema, 298–299
　function of, 197–206
　function tests of, 214–216
　fungus infections of, 287–288
　　treatment of, 287–288
　in hyperventilation, 202–203
　in hypoventilation, 203
　infarction, pulmonary, 293–294
　infections of, 270–279
　　hospital-acquired, 77

microorganisms in, 271
susceptibility to, 270–271
influenza, 273–274
lung volume, 214–216
reduced, 228–229
in mononucleosis, infectious, 279–280
nursing care in dysfunction of, 216–309
in obstructive disease, 217–227
in restrictive disease, 227–246
in specific diseases, 252–309
for surgical patients, 246–252
obstructive dysfunction of, 216, 217–227
postoperative, 97
after thyroid surgery, 656
oxygen distribution in, uneven, 200–201
and partial pressure of oxygen and carbon dioxide, 199–200
pharyngitis, 272–273
pleural disorders, 296–298
pneumoconiosis, 288–292
pneumonia, 274–279
pneumothorax, spontaneous, 299
and pulmonary circulation, 198–199
respiratory insufficiency compared to acute respiratory failure, 231
restrictive diseases of, 216, 227–246
in sarcoidosis, 285–287
sputum examination, 224–225
surfactant in, 197
surgery of, 246–252
cardiac tamponade from, 249
chest drainage after, 249–252
hemorrhage from, 249
pneumonectomy, 246, 248–249
postoperative care, 247–252
preoperative care, 247
pulmonary edema from, 249
segmental resection of lung, 246
thoracotomy, 246, 248
thromboembolism, pulmonary, 293–295
tonsillitis, 272–273
transport of oxygen and carbon dioxide, 201
and trauma, thoracic, 299–304
in tuberculosis, 280–285
ventilation and perfusion in, 197–202
Rest
as essential need, 14
hazards of
in cardiovascular system, 336, 351
in musculoskeletal system, 807, 881
in heart failure, congestive, 377
in myocardial infarction, 350–351
in pneumonia, 278
in respiratory failure, 244–245
in rheumatoid arthritis, 863
Resting potential, of cardiac cells, 316
Resuscitation, cardiopulmonary, 368–371
drug therapy in, 371
external massage in, 370
mouth-to-mouth procedures in, 368–370
and postarrest nursing care, 371
reactions of patient to, 371
Resuscitative techniques, life-sustaining, 139
Retardation, mental, in Down's syndrome, 933
Reticular formation, 896
Reticulocyte count, 422
Reticulocytosis, in hemolytic anemia, 438
Reticuloendothelial system, 20–21
Reticulospinal tract, 904
Reticulum, endoplasmic, 9
Reticulum fibers, dermal, 1095
Retina, 995
degeneration of, 1025
detachment of, 1023–1025
nonrhegmatogenous, 1024

rhegmatogenous, 1024
treatment of, 1024–1025
disorders of, 1023–1026
holes in, repair of, 1025
Retinal vessels
examination of, 1001
fluorescent angiography of, 1002
occlusion of vein, 1001
in retrolental fibroplasia, 1025
Retinitis pigmentosa, 1025
Retinoblastoma, 1025–1026
Retinopathy, diabetic, 700–701, 1001–1002
hypophysectomy in, 636
treatment of, 1025
Retroversion of uterus, 776
Revascularization
myocardial, procedures for, 385–387
of skin grafts, 1168
Rh blood groups, 424
in erythroblastosis fetalis, 442
Rheumatic diseases, 858–868
Rheumatic fever, 372, 865
Rheumatoid arthritis, 35, 861–866
Rheumatoid factor, 35, 861–862
Rhinitis, 1061
medicamentosa, 1067
Rhinophyma, 1110
Rhinoplasty, 1065
Rhinorrhea
of cerebrospinal fluid, 1066, 1068
from craniotomy, 633
Rhizotomy
for pain relief, 49
retrogasserian, 965
radio-frequency, 965
Rhonchi, 210
Rhythms of body, 15–16
and ACTH secretion, 631, 674
and melatonin secretion, 672
temperature cycle in, 14
Rib
cervical, 404
fractures of, 301
Ribosomes, 8
Rickets, 815
Riedel's thyroiditis, 663
Rigidity, in Parkinson's disease, 959
Ringer's lactate solution
in burns, 1147–1148
in shock, 1197–1198
Ringworm, 1117–1118
Rinne hearing test, 1042
Risk groups for diseases, 64
in rubella, 69
RNA, 8
vitamin B_{12} affecting production of, 416, 434
Rods and cones, in eye, 995
Rolando fissure, 892
Romberg's sign, 703
Round window, of ear, 1040, 1041
Rubella
immunization in, 70
risk groups in, 69
Rubin test, for tubal patency, 749
Rubor, in blood disorders, 419
Ruffini's endings, 1097
Rupture
of eardrum, 1039, 1050
of spleen, 456
Russell's skin traction, in fractures, 837, 850

Sabin vaccine, 936
Saccule, 1037, 1043
Saddle block anesthesia, 95
St. Louis encephalitis, 935
Salem sump tube, 536
Salicylate poisoning, dehydration in, 165
Saliva, 525
characteristics of, 536
Salivary glands, 525
obstruction of, 1073
tumors of, 569

Salk vaccine, 936
Salpingectomy, 800
Salpingitis, gonorrheal, 755
Salpingolysis, 752
Salpingo-oophorectomy, 779
Saphenous vein
bypass graft, 386
stripping of, 406
Sarcoidosis, 285–287, 1126
Sarcolemma, 817
Sarcoma, 107
of breast, 786
osteogenic, 820
of uterus, 783
Sarcomeres, 315
Sarcoplasm, 817
Sarcoplasmic reticulum, 817
Sartorius muscle, 818
Scab formation, 1099
Scabies, 1121–1122
Scalenus anticus syndrome, 404
Scaling, of skin, 1099
Scalp
folliculitis of, 1114
lacerations of, 940
ringworm of, 1117
Scanning, scintillation, 120–122
of biliary tract, 604
of bone, 810
of brain, 915
of kidney, 478
of liver, 587
of lungs, 212
in burns, 1149
in thromboembolism, 294
of pancreas, 610
of thyroid gland, 648, 662
Scar formation, 1102
from burns, 1169
hypertrophic, 1169
Schiller test, in cervical carcinoma, 747, 781
Schilling test, 434
in malabsorption syndromes, 568
Schiøtz's tonometer, 1002
Schlemm's canal, 1021
Schönlein-Henoch disease, 458
School nurse, role of, 335–336
Schrapnell's membrane, 1039
Schultz-Dale test, 30
Schwabach hearing test, 1042
Sciatica, 983
Scintillation scanner, 120
Sclera, 995
buckling procedure in retinal detachment, 1024–1025
Scleroderma, 1127
Sclerosis
amyotrophic lateral, 958
multiple, 956–958
agencies for help with, 958
management of, 957–958
symptoms and course of, 957
Scoliosis, 808
Scotoma, 908
Scrotum
cancer of, 777
examination of, 740
Scrub nurse, 87
Scurvy
bleeding tendency in, 458
bone pain in, 815
Sebaceous cysts, of ear, 1037
Sebaceous glands, 1096
Seborrheic dermatitis, 1111
of eyelids, 998
Seborrheic keratosis, 1122
Sebum, 1096
inflammation from, 1109
Secretin, 609
Sedatives, with analgesics, 46
Sedimentation rate, erythrocyte, 326
Seizures, 925. See also Convulsive disorders
Self-awareness, development of, 12

Sella turcica, 625
pituitary tumors affecting, 683
Semicircular canals, 1037, 1040, 1043
vestibular impulses in, 1043
Seminal fluid
collection of, 747
evaluation of, 747
fructose in, 747
Sengstaken-Blakemore tube, for esophageal tamponade, 594–595
Sensorium, in shock, 1194
Sensory area of brain, 894
Sensory field, 1096
Sensory nerve fibers, 40
Sensory seizures, focal, 926
Sensory tests, 910
Sensory tracts, 904
Sepsis
from abortion, 798
in burns, 1153, 1155
shock in, 1187, 1192–1193
Serotonin, 30, 1191
anaphylactic shock from, 1186
vascular effects of, 394
Serum sickness, 34
Sex of child, determination of, 688
Sex hormones, 736
function of, 736–738
Sex-linked diseases, 17
Sexual arousal, male, factors in, 761
Sexuality, 735
in adrenal dysfunction, 687
and behavior patterns, 57–58
biologic factors in, 738
in colostomy patients, 580
in ileostomy patients, 560
in panhypopituitarism, 634
in spinal cord injuries, 980–981
in thyroid disease, 642
Sharpey's fibers, 813
Sheehan's syndrome, 632
Shingles, 938, 1119–1120
Shock, 1179–1201
acid-base balance in, 1191, 1193, 1200
anaphylactic, 30, 1186
assessment of patient in, 1193–1196, 1202
blood gases in, 1195
blood pressure in
direct measurements of, 1195
indirect measurements of, 1193–1194
in burns, 1142, 1184
cardiac assistance in, 1198–1199
cardiogenic, 383–385, 1185–1186
counterpulsation in, 385
drug therapy in, 384
volume expanders in, 384–385
cellular problems in, 1191–1192
correction of, 1200–1201
central venous pressure in, 1196
coagulation studies in, 1196
complications of, 1203–1204
concept of, 1183
counterpulsation in, 385, 1198–1199
disseminated intravascular coagulation in, 1190–1191, 1201
drugs in, 1198
electrocardiogram in, 1194
fluid replacement in, 1197–1198
colloidal solutions in, 1197
crystalloid solutions in, 1197–1198
gastric ulceration in, 1203
hematocrit in, 1196
hypovolemic, 1184–1185
in cerebral injuries, 942
in dehydration, 166
hyperkalemia in, 177
in thoracic trauma, 300–301
initiating events in, 1183–1187
insulin, 721, 722, 1186
kidneys in, 1192, 1201, 1203
lactate levels in, 1196
lung disorders in, 229, 1204
microcirculation in, 1190–1191
neurogenic, 1186–1187

Index

Shock *Continued*
  nursing care in, 1201–1203
  in orthopedic injuries, 824
  pathophysiology of, 1187–1192
  postoperative, 98
  psychological needs in, 1203
  pulmonary artery pressure in, 1195
  pulmonary wedge pressure in, 1195–1196
  pulse in, 1193
  and related concepts of anatomy and physiology, 1179–1183
  respiration in, 1193
  sensorium in, 1194
  septic, 1187, 1192–1193
  skin changes in, 1194
  in spinal cord injuries, 968–969
  sympathoadrenal response in, 1188–1190
  in transfusion reactions, 425
  treatment of, 1196–1201
  urine output in, 1194, 1201, 1203
  vasogenic, 1186
  vasopressors in, 1199–1200
Shoulder
  bursitis in, 866
  disarticulation of, 874
Shoulder-hand syndrome, in myocardial infarction, 354
Shunts
  anatomical, 198
  arteriovenous, for hemodialysis, 514–515
  for hydrocephalus, 933
  physiologic, in thoracic trauma, 300
  portasystemic procedures for, 595–596
Sickle cell disease, 438–441
  crisis states in, 439, 440
  genetic transmission of, 440
  nursing care in, 439–440
  screening programs for, 440
  signs and symptoms of, 439
Sickle cell trait, 439, 440
Siderophages, 20
Siderosis, 290
Sigmoidoscopy, 534
Sign language, 1046
Silicosis, 289–290
Sims-Huhner test, 752
Singer's nodes, 1079
Singultus, 528
  postoperative, 101
Sinoatrial node, 317, 318, 354
  in arrhythmias, 356–357
Sinuses, paranasal, 1060
  infections of, 1062, 1071
  tumors of, 1066
Sinusitis, 1061–1062, 1071
  and bronchiectasis, 268
  complications of, 1062
Sinusoids, hepatic, 583
Sitosterols, as antilipemic agents, 345
Skeleton, 810. *See also* Bone; Musculoskeletal system
Skin, 1095–1133
  acne, 1108–1110
  in acromegaly, 629
  in Addison's disease, 678
  aging affecting, 1099
  anatomy of, 1095
  biopsy of, 1104
  blister formation, 1128
  Bowen's disease, 1123
  cancer of, 1123–1124
    chemosurgery in, 1125–1126
    staging of, 1125
  care of
    in casts for fractures, 833
    preoperative, 85, 89
    in spinal cord injuries, 977
  color of, 1098
  complications from immobilization, prevention of, 842
  in Cushing's disease, 681
  dehydration affecting, 165

dermatitis, 1111, 1112
disorders of, 1108–1133
  bacterial, 1113–1115
  fungal, 1115–1118
  treatment of, 1104–1108
  viral, 1118–1120
dressings for, 1105–1106
  dry, 1106
  wet, 1105
eczema, 1112
of eyelids, examination of, 998
flaps, in amputations, 870
functions of, 1096–1097
grafts
  in burns, 1164–1165, 1168–1169
  for ear, 1051
  revascularization of, 1168
in hematopoietic disorders, 419
hydration affecting, 1098
in hyponatremia, 172
in hypoparathyroidism, 670
keratosis, 1122
leukoplakia, 1122–1123
lichen planus, 1110
melanoma, malignant, 1125
miliaria, 1110
molluscum sebaceum, 1123
nevus of, 1124–1125
pallor of, 419
pityriasis rosea, 1110
psoriasis, 1111–1112
reactions to radiation therapy, 118
receptors in, 1096–1097
in sarcoidosis, 286, 1126
in scleroderma, 1127
in shock, 1194
temperature changes in peripheral vascular disease, 395–396
tests
  in respiratory system dysfunction, 211
  in tuberculosis, 282
  in thyroid disease, 641, 660
topical medications for, 1105
traction in fractures, 837, 849–851
ulcers of, 1128–1133
vascular disorders of, 1127–1128
in venous insufficiency, 405
in water intoxication, 169
Skull, 891–892. *See also* Tongs, for cervical traction
  fractures of, 825, 940–941
Sleep, 919
  circadian pattern of, 15–16
  desynchronized, 15
  noise affecting, 1050
  patterns after cardiopulmonary bypass, 392
  problems in laryngectomy patients, 1088
  REM periods in, 15
  slow wave, 15
  temperature changes in, 14
Sleeping sickness, 935
Slow-reacting substance, 30
  anaphylactic shock from, 1186
Smegma, 739
Smell, sense of, 1059, 1061
Smith-Hodge pessary, 775
Smoke inhalation, in burns, 1137, 1149
Smoking
  and cerebrovascular disease, 951
  and coronary artery disease, 343
  and emphysema, 257, 259
  and lung cancer, 110, 304–305
  and thromboangiitis obliterans, 403
  vasoconstriction from, 396, 402
  withdrawal from, 217–218
Snellen chart, 996
Soap, abrasive, in acne, 1109
Sodium
  dietary
    recommended amounts of, 155
    restriction of, in congestive heart failure, 379–381
  function in body, 154

hypernatremia, 173–174
  disorders with, 173
  nursing care in, 174
  symptoms and signs of, 174
hyponatremia, 171–173
  diagnosis of, 172
  disorders with, 171–172
  nursing care in, 172–173
  symptoms and signs of, 172
loss of, in Addison's disease, 677
retention of
  edema from, 180
  in glomerulonephritis, 508
  in nephrotic syndrome, 509
serum levels
  in cardiac assessment, 326
  in Cushing's disease, 682
  dehydration affecting, 166
transport of, 157, 316
tubular reabsorption of, 504
urinary, 161
  in burns, 1143
Solute, definition of, 152
Solutions
  definition of, 152
  for skin care, 1105
Solvent, definition of, 152
Somatomedin, 628, 630
Somatotropin. *See* Growth hormone
Sound waves, transmission of, 1041
Sounds
  bowel, 531
  breath, 209–210
  chest, 208–209
  heart, 324–325
  voice, 210, 1074, 1076
Spasm
  laryngeal, 97, 1077
  in spinal cord injuries, 969
Spastic colon, 564
Specific gravity
  of cerebrospinal fluid, 913
  of urine, 473, 480
Specificity, in immune response, 26
Speculums
  aural, 1037
  nasal, 1060
  vaginal, 740
Speech. *See also* Voice
  and aphasia, 930–932
  discrimination testing, 1043
  esophageal, after laryngectomy, 1085–1086
  hearing loss affecting, 1046
  in multiple sclerosis, 957
  production of, 1074, 1076
  reception threshold, 1043
  and VoiceBak prosthesis, 1086–1087
Speech therapy, in aphasia, 931
Sperm, 736
  antibodies to, in cervical mucus, 752
  cervical mucus affecting, 752
  evaluation of, 747
  fertilization of, 752
Spermatic vein, varicocele of, 759
Spermatogenesis, factors affecting, 751
Spermicidal creams, 795
Sphenoid sinus, 1060
Spherocytosis, hereditary, 438
Sphincters
  of bladder, 469
  cardiac, 526
  gastrointestinal, motility disorders of, 561
  of Oddi, 526, 602
  pyloric, 526
Spica casts, 831
Spina bifida, 932
  aperta, 932
  occulta, 932
Spinal arteries, 900
Spine and spinal cord, 892, 902
  abscess in, 936
  anesthesia of, 95
  examination of, 808
  fractures of, casts for, 831

herniated intervertebral disk, 983–985
  chemonucleolysis in, 984–985
  medical treatment of, 983–984
  surgery in, 984
injuries of, 967–982
  bladder care in, 974–976
  bladder function in, 470, 483
  bowel management in, 976–977
  discharge planning in, 981
  edema in, 969
  emergency care in, 968
  exercise and ambulation in, 977–978
  and factors in rehabilitation, 978, 981–982
  level of injury affecting function, 971–972
  nursing care in, 972–978
  nutrition in, 969
  pain and muscle spasms in, 969
  positioning of patient in, 968, 969
  psychological aspects of, 969–970, 978–980
  sexual aspects of, 980–981
  shock in, 968–969
  skin care in, 977
intervertebral disks, 892
  herniated, 983–985
tumors of, 982–983
Spinnbarkeit, 747
Spinothalamic tract, 891
Spiral arteries, endometrial, 745
Spironolactone, 380
  in aldosteronism, 686
  hyperkalemia from, 177
  in hypertension, 339, 340
  suppression test in aldosteronism, 686
Spleen
  autosplenectomy, 439
  disorders of, 455–456
  rupture of, 456
Splenectomy, 456
Splenorenal shunt, 595
Splinting
  for burn patients, 1171
  of fractures, 823
  for stroke patients, 953
Spongiosis, 1102
Sporadic diseases, 65
Sprain, 820–821
Sprue, tropical, 568
Sputum
  blood-tinged, 211
  in bronchiectasis, 269
  in bronchitis, 262
  examination of, 211, 224–225
  mucoid, 211
  mucopurulent, 211
  in pneumonia, 277
  in pulmonary edema, 382
  purulent, 211
  rusty, 211
Stab wounds, 21
Staging procedures, in cancer, 109
Standstill, cardiac, 368
Stapedectomy, 1056–1057
  complications of, 1057
Stapes, 1040, 1041
Staphylococcal infections
  and impetigo, 1113
  and osteomyelitis, 867
  and pneumonia, 277
Starr-Edwards valve, 373
Startle effect of noise, 1050
Starvation, sodium loss in, 171
Status asthmaticus, 265–266
Status epilepticus, 926–927
Steatorrhea, in malabsorption syndrome, 568
Stein-Leventhal syndrome, 779
Steinmann pins, use of, 955
Stenosis
  of laryngectomy stoma, 1083
  valvular, 372
Stereognosis, 894
  testing of, 910

Stereotaxic brain surgery, for pain relief, 50
Sterility. *See* Infertility
Sterilization
 of females, 795–796
  cauterization in, 749
 of males, 796
 of materials and instruments, 88
Sternum
 injuries of, 303
 puncture for bone marrow aspiration, 423
Steroids, adrenocortical. *See* Corticosteroids
Stethoscope, 323
Stiff lung, 229
Stimulators, transcutaneous, for pain relief, 48–49
Stockings, elastic, 406
Stokes-Adams syndrome, 360
 pacemaker in, 360
Stoma. *See also* Colostomy; Ileal conduit; ileostomy
 care of, in laryngectomy, 1083–1084, 1087–1088
 site of, in ileostomy, 553
 skin care in, 558
 in urinary diversion, 497
  drainage appliances with, 497–498
Stomach, 525
 analysis of contents, 532–533
 barium x-rays of, 533
 blood supply of, 525–526
 cancer of, and peptic ulcer, 547–548
 freezing techniques in peptic ulcer, 546
 gastritis, 542–543
 intrinsic factor in, 433
 lesions in lining of, 542–551
 obstruction of, 570–571
 surgery of, 548–550
  complications from, 551
  dumping syndrome after, 551
  hypoglycemia from, 551
  postoperative care in, 550–551
 ulcers of, 543–551. *See also* Peptic ulcer
Stomatitis, 541–542
 in anemia, 419
 angular, 1116
 from chemotherapy, 127–128
 in renal failure, 511
Stone formation. *See* Calculi
Stools
 analysis of specimens, 532
 in biliary tract obstruction, 604
 in hepatitis, 588
 impaction of, 565–566
 in jaundice, 585
 in pancreatic disease, 609
 urobilinogen in, 422
Strabismus, 997, 1006
 nonparalytic, 1006
 paralytic, 1006
Straight-leg-raising test, 983
Strain(s), 820
Stratum
 corneum, 1095
  burns of, 1143
 germinativum, 1095
 granulosum, 1095
 spinosum, 1095
Strawberry mark, 1128
Streptococcal infections
 in abortions, 798
 and endocarditis, 373
 and glomerulonephritis, 508
 and impetigo, 1113
 and pharyngitis, 273
 and rheumatic fever, 372
Stress incontinence, urinary, 775
Striae, 1102
Strictures
 esophageal, 570
 ureteral, 501
 urethral, 501
Stridor, 210

Stroke patients. *See* Cerebrovascular disease
Stryker frame, 854, 973, 1171
Stumps, amputation
 dressings for, 871, 876, 877–878
 wrapping or bandaging of, 879–880
Stupor, 919
Sty, 999
Subarachnoid space, 892
Subclavian arteries, 899
Subclavian vein catheterization, in total parenteral nutrition, 189
Subcutaneous tissue, 1095
Subdural space, 892
Sublingual glands, 525
Subluxation, 821
Submaxillary glands, 525
Submaxillary lymph nodes, 420
Submental lymph nodes, 420
Suctioning
 closed, in surgical wounds, 103
 gastrointestinal, 537
  alkalosis from, metabolic, 187
  electrolyte loss in, 572
  hypokalemia from, 175
  hypomagnesemia from, 179
  hyponatremia from, 172
  and irrigation of apparatus with normal saline, 173
 nasotracheal, 242
 for patients on mechanical ventilators, 1150
 of tracheostomy tube, 240–243
Sulci of brain, 892
Sulfonylureas
 hypoglycemia from, 721–722
 as hypoglycemic agents, 709
 side effects of, 710
Sump tube, use of, 103
Sunglasses, use of, 1007
Sunlamps, excessive exposure to, 1007, 1018
Sunlight, exposure to
 and actinic keratosis, 1123
 and skin cancer, 1123–1124
Suppuration, in inflammatory response, 20
Supraclavicular lymph nodes, 420
Surfactant, pulmonary, 197
Surgery, 80–105
 ablative, in tumors, 635–636
 adenoidectomy, 1072
 adrenal, 684–685, 690
 anesthesia in, 90–97
 asepsis in, 88–90
 of biliary tract, 606–608
 biopsy procedures in, 80–81
 in brain tumors, 946
 in cancer, 114–116
 cardiac, 385–393
  psychological reactions to, 391–392
 in cervical carcinoma, 782
 cholecystectomy, 605
 complications from, 97–99
 in convulsive disorders, 928
 curative, 81
 cystectomy, 494
 and discharge planning, 105
 ear reconstruction, 1051
 elective, 82
 emergency, 82
 exploratory, 81
 of eyes
  in cataract, 1019–1021
  in corneal diseases, 1026
  enucleation, 1026–1028
  postoperative care, 1015–1016
  preparation for, 1014–1015
  in retinal detachment, 1024–1025
 gastric, 548–550
  complications from, 551
  dumping syndrome after, 551
  hypoglycemia from, 551
  postoperative care in, 550–551
 hemorrhoidectomy, 582
 herniorrhaphy, 581

 hip arthroplasty, 843–846
 informed consent for, 84
 intracranial, 947–950
 intraoperative care in, 86–97
 knee arthroplasty, 846–848
 laminectomy, 984
 laryngectomy, 1080–1090
 of liver, 599–600
 in lung cancer, 307
 mammaplasty, 791–792
 mastectomy, 787–788
 myringoplasty, 1054
 myringotomy, 1054
 nephrectomy, 492–493
 optional, 82
 for pain relief, 49
 palliative, 81, 115–116
 of pancreas, 614
 of parathyroid glands, 668
 in Parkinson's disease, 960
 in peptic ulcer, 547, 548–550
 pituitary, 633–636
  in Cushing's disease, 683, 684
 portasystemic shunting procedures, 595–596
 postoperative care in, 97–105
 preoperative care in, 82–86
 prophylactic, 82
 prostatectomy, 763–765
 reconstructive, 81–82
 in respiratory disease, nursing care in, 246–252
 rhinoplasty, 1065
 rhizotomy, retrogasserian, 965
 stapedectomy, 1056–1057
 thymectomy, 963
 of thyroid gland, 655–657
 tonsillectomy, 1072–1073
 transplantations. *See* Grafts
 tympanoplasty, 1054
 urgent, 82
 urinary diversion procedures, 494–500
 in uterine prolapse, 774
 vulvectomy, 782–783
 wounds in
  clean, 104
  clean-contaminated, 104
  closed suction of, 103
  contaminated, 104
  dehiscence of, 104
  dirty, 104
  evisceration through, 104
  healing of, 101–105
  open exposure of, 103
Surgical team, 86–87
Surveillance, and disease control, 67–68
Susceptibility to disease, 64, 65–66
 to respiratory tract infections, 270–271
 to tuberculosis, 280
 to urinary tract infections, 488
Sutures, 89–90
 absorbable, 89
 nonabsorbable, 89
 removal of, 102
 retention, 90
Swallowing reflex, in stroke patients, 953
Swan-Ganz catheter, 333
 complications from, 1196
Sweat glands, 1096
Sweating, and miliaria, 1110
Sycosis barbae, 1114
Sylvian aqueduct, 901
Sylvian fissure, 892
Syme's amputation, 871
Sympathectomy
 in hypertension, 341
 lumbar, in chronic arterial insufficiency, 402
Sympathetic nervous system, 318–319, 904–905
 and bladder control, 469
 lumbar block as test in peripheral vascular disease, 396
 receptors in, 1199

Sympathomimetic drugs, as bronchodilators, 226
Synapse, 891
Synarthroid joints, 815
Synovial fluid, 816
Synovial membrane, 816
Synovitis
 in gout, 866
 in rheumatoid arthritis, 862
Syphilis, 756, 938
Syringes, for insulin, 718
Syringomyelia, 958–959
Syringomyelocele, 932
Systole, 313
Systolic blood pressure, 330, 336

T cells, lymphocyte, 24–26, 418
T tube, for biliary drainage, 606–608
Tabes dorsalis, 938
Tachycardia, 316, 319
 in anemia, 429
 atrial paroxysmal, 357
 nodal, 359
 in thyrotoxicosis, 640
 ventricular, 364–365
Tamponade
 cardiac, 374
  after cardiopulmonary bypass, 391
  from chest surgery, 249
 esophageal, with Sengstaken-Blakemore tube, 594–595
Taste sensation, testing of, 909
Teaching
 of health care, 71–72
 of patients, and nursing care, 60–61, 84
 and public education programs, 68–71
Tears
 formation and drainage of, 995–996
 substitutes for, 1009, 1011
Teeth
 examination of, 529
 in hypoparathyroidism, 670
Telangiectases, 1128
Telangiectasia, hereditary hemorrhagic, 458
Telemetry monitoring, cardiac, 352
Temperature
 affecting ventilation, 204
 basal body, 746
 environmental, affecting thyroid function, 648, 659
 fever, 929–930. *See also* Fever
 hunger related to, 11
 hypothermia. *See* Hypothermia
 and mechanisms in heat production, 14–15
 natural cycle of, 14–15
 receptors for, 1097
 in shock, 1195, 1201
 of skin, in peripheral vascular disease, 395–396
 in sleep, 14
 and spermatogenesis, 751
 and sweat gland function, 1096
Temporal bone, 1040
 examination of, 1044
 in otosclerosis, 1056
Temporal lobe, 895
 blindness from lesions of, 908
 epilepsy, 926
Tendons, 816, 817
 exposed, in burns, 1172
Tentorium cerebelli, 892, 896
Teratoma, ovarian, 779
Terminal illness, 132–136
 and reactions to death and dying, 135, 136–139
Tes-Tape, 696
Testes, 736
 cysts in, 759
 disorders of, 758–760
 ectopic, 758
 examination of, 740
 imperfect descent of, 758
 torsion of, 758

1232 Index

Testes *Continued*
 tumors of, 777–778
 staging of, 777
Testosterone, 736
 function of, 738
 as therapy
  in cancer, 126
  in endometriosis, 771
  and spermatogenesis, 751
Tetanus, 938–939
Tetany, 178
 diagnostic signs in, 669–670
 diseases causing, 671
 in hypoparathyroidism, 669–670
 latent, 669
 overt, 669
 after parathyroid surgery, 668
 treatment of, 670–671
Texture discrimination, 910
Thalamus, 895
Thalassemia, 441
 alpha type, 441
 beta type, 441
 major, 441
 minor, 441
 sickle cell, 438
Thanatology, 136
Theophyllines, as bronchodilators, 225–226
Thermal injuries. *See* Burns
Thermography, 112
 of breast, 785
Thiazide diuretics, 380
 in hypertension, 339
Thionamide drugs, in thyroid disease, 652–653
Thirst, mechanisms in, 158
Thomas splint, 854–855
 Pearson attachment with, 855
Thoracic outlet syndrome, 404
Thoracic surgery, 246–252
Thoracocentesis, for biopsy of lung, 214
Thoracolumbar division, of autonomic nervous system, 904
Thoracoplasty, 246
Thoracotomy, 246
 for biopsy of lung, 214
 postoperative care in, 248
Throat. *See* Pharynx
Thrombin, 456, 457
Thrombin time, 458
Thromboangiitis obliterans, 403
Thrombocytes. *See* Platelets
Thrombocytopenia, 462
 in aplastic anemia, 436
 in burns, 1144
Thromboembolic disorders, 397. *See also* Embolism; Thrombosis
 and acute arterial occlusion, 402–403
 in myocardial infarction, 354
Thrombolytic agents, in pulmonary embolism, 295
Thrombophlebitis, 407–408
 postoperative, 101
Thromboplastin, 456–457
Thromboplastin time, partial, 458
Thrombosis, 397
 cerebral, 951
 venous, 407
Thrush
 oral, 542, 1073, 1116
 vaginal, 1116
Thymectomy, in myasthenia gravis, 963
Thymine, as pyrimidine base, 8
Thymol turbidity test, 586
Thymomas, immunodeficiency from, 39
Thymus
 alymphoplasia of, 39
 tumors of, in myasthenia gravis, 962
Thyrocalcitonin, 636
 and calcium metabolism, 636
 in hyperthyroidism, 642
 and parathyroid hormone activity, 665
Thyroglobulin, 645
Thyroglossal duct cysts, 1073

Thyroid cartilage, 1074
Thyroid extract, 660
Thyroid gland, 636–664. *See also* Goiter
 anatomy of, 638
 antibodies to, 647
 assessment of, 638–642
 biopsy of, 647
 carcinoma of, 663
  anaplastic, 663
  follicular, 663
  medullary, 663
  papillary, 663
 disorders of, 648–664
  antithyroid drugs in, 652–653
  behavior changes in, 639, 641, 654
  cardiomyopathy in, 375
  crisis or storm in, 657–658
  diagnosis of, 652
  exophthalmos in, 650–651
  signs of, 651
  treatment of, 652–656
 function of, 636–638
  tests of, 642–648, 652
 Graves' disease, 649–650
 hyperthyroidism, 648–659. *See also* Hyperthyroidism
 hypothyroidism, 659–662. *See also* Hypothyroidism
 involution of, 656
 myxedema, 659
 scanning of, 648, 662
 surgery of, 655–657
 thyrotoxicosis, 648–659
Thyroid hormones
 affecting fluid and electrolyte regulation, 159
 binding proteins for, 643
 biosynthesis of, 644–645
 therapy with, 660
  affecting iodine uptake, 644
  after hypophysectomy, 634
  weight loss from, 661
Thyroid stimulator, long-acting, 647
Thyroid tissue, lingual, 659, 1073
Thyroidectomy, hypoparathyroidism from, 669
Thyroiditis, 663–664
 acute pyogenic, 663
 de Quervain's, 663
 Hashimoto's, 663–664
 Riedel's, 663
Thyrotoxicosis. *See also* Hyperthyroidism
 factitia, 658–659
 treatment of, 652–653
Thyrotropin, 632, 636
 releasing hormone, 626, 636
 stimulation test, 646–647
Thyroxine, 636
 half-life of, 643
Thyroxine-binding globulin, 643
Thyroxine-binding prealbumin, 643
Tic douloureux, 965
Tickle sensation, 1097
Tidal volume, 214
Tilt table, use of, 974
Tinea
 barbae, 1117
 capitis, 1117
 corporis, 1117
 cruris, 1117
 manuum, 1118
 pedis, 1118
 versicolor, 1117
Tinnitus, 1036, 1058
 in otosclerosis, 1056
Tobacco use. *See* Smoking
Tolerance, immunologic, 27
 acquired, 27
 natural, 27
 reversal of, 27
Tolerogen, 27
Tomography
 of chest, 212
 of kidney, 477
 in musculoskeletal disorders, 810

transverse axial, computerized, of brain, 915
Tongs, for cervical traction, 854
Tongue
 in anemia, 419, 434
 blood supply of, 525
 examination of, 530
 lingual thyroid, 659, 1073
 malignant lesions of, 542
Tonometry, 1002–1003
Tonsil(s), 1071
 carcinoma of, 1074
 peritonsillar abscess, 1073
Tonsillar lymph nodes, 420
Tonsillectomy, 1072–1073
Tonsillitis, 272–273, 1072
Tophi, in gout, 866
 in ear, 1037
Torsion, of testis, 758
Touch receptors, 1097
Tourniquets, rotating, in pulmonary edema, 382
Toxicity and side effects
 of anticonvulsants, 928
 of antihypertensive agents, 339
 of chemicals. *See* Chemicals
 of chemotherapeutic agents, 127–129, 446–447
 of digitalis, 378
 of diuretics, 380
 of L-dopa, 960
 of glucocorticoid therapy, 691
 of hypoglycemic agents, oral, 710
 of lead, 442
 of oxygen, 235
 of radiation, 117
Trachea, intubation of, 238–239
Tracheostomy, 239–243
 in acidosis, respiratory, 183
 in burn patients, 1149
 and button insertion in stoma, 243
 care of equipment in, 240
 and communication with patient, 240, 245–246
 complications of, 239–240
 cuff deflation in, 242
 emergency, in thoracic trauma, 300
 nursing care in, 240
 removal of tubes in, 243
 suctioning techniques in, 240–243
 in vocal cord paralysis, 1077
 weaning from, 243
Trachoma, 993
Tract(s), nerve
 motor, 903–904
 sensory, 904
Traction
 for burn patients, 1171–1172
 in fractures, 848–858
 in intervertebral disk herniation, 984
Tractotomy, for pain relief, 49
Tragus, 1037
Tranquilizers, with analgesics, 46
Transcortin, cortisol bound to, 674
Transfusion therapy, 423–428
 ABO blood groups in, 423–424
 agglutination from, 425
 air embolism from, 426
 allergic reactions to, 426
 antihemophilic factor concentrates in, 428, 461
 circulatory overload from, 426
 citrate intoxication from, 426–427
 contaminated blood in, 426
 crossmatching of blood for, 424
 in disseminated intravascular coagulation, 464
 fibrinogen in, 428
 freezing of erythrocytes for, 427
 hemolytic reactions to, 425
 in hemophilia, 461
 hepatitis from, 591
 hypothermia from, 427
 leukocytes in, 428, 445
 packed red cells in, 427
 plasma in, 428

 and plasmapheresis, 427
 platelets in, 427–428
 potassium intoxication from, 426
 precautions in, 424
 procedures in, 425
 reactions to, 36, 425–427
  in burns, 1144
 in renal failure, 512, 516
 Rh blood groups in, 424
 in shock, 1197
 typing of blood for, 423–424
 in ulcerative colitis, 553
 whole blood in, 427
Transmission of communicable diseases, 65–66
Transplantation of heart, 393
Transplantations. *See* Grafts
Transudates, in pleural effusion, 296
Trapezius muscle, 819
Trauma
 amputations from, 869
 of bladder, 501
 burns in. *See* Burns
 cerebral, 941–944
  water intoxication in, 169
 of ear, 1050–1051
 emergency care in, 21
 of eyes, 1017–1019
 facial, 1067–1071
 flail chest in, 302–303
 and healing of wounds. *See* Wound healing
 of heart, 303
 of kidney, 500–501
 of larynx, 1077–1078
 musculoskeletal, 819, 820–843. *See also* Fractures
 in rape victims, 798
 of reproductive tract, 756
 scalp lacerations, 940
 shock in. *See* Shock
 sodium loss in, 172
 of spinal cord, 967–982
 of sternum, 303
 and tension pneumothorax, 301–302
 thoracic, 299–304
 types of wounds in, 21
 of urinary tract, 500–501
Treadmill exercise test, 330
Tremor
 intention, in multiple sclerosis, 957
 in Parkinson's disease, 959
Trench mouth, 1073
Trendelenburg test
 in peripheral vascular disease, 396
 in venous valvular incompetence, 406
Trephination, scleral, in glaucoma, 1022
Triceps, 819
Triceps reflex, 910
Trichomonas, 755–756
Tricuspid valve, 313
Trigeminal nerve, 898
 assessment of, 908–909
 neuralgia, 965–966
Triglycerides, 343
Triiodothyronine, 636
 half-life of, 643
Trismus, in quinsy, 1073
Trochlear nerve, 898
 assessment of, 908
Trousseau's sign, in tetany, 178, 670
Trypsin, pancreatic, 567
Tubercle bacillus, action of, 281
Tuberculin test, 32, 282
Tuberculosis, 280–285
 and bronchiectasis, 269
 causative factors in, 280
 classification of, 282
 follow-up care in, 285
 incidence of, 280–281
 isolation measures in, 78–79
 and meningitis, 935
 nursing care in, 284–285
 preventive therapy in, 282–283
 of reproductive tract, 756
 and silicosis, 290

skin tests in, 282
treatment of, 283–284
tubercle bacillus in, 281
Tubules, renal, 504
Tumors. *See also* Cancer
ablative surgery in, 635–636
of adrenal gland, 682–683
affecting adrenal hormone secretion, 681
autochthonous relation to host, 37
of bladder, 491
of bone, 820
amputations in, 868
of brain, 944–947
of breast, 786–792
of cervix uteri, 781–782
definition of, 106
of ear, 1052–1053
of fallopian tubes, 781
ganglioneuroma, 690
of heart, 375
immune response in, 37–38
intracranial, 944–947
of kidney, 490–491
renin-secreting, 687
of larynx, 1079–1090
of liver, 598–600
neuroblastoma, 690
of nose, 1066–1067
of pancreas, 613–615
in Zollinger-Ellison syndrome, 548
of peripheral nerves, 964–965
of pharynx, 1073–1074
pheochromocytoma, 688–690
of pineal gland, 672, 946
pituitary, 632–633, 946
and Cushing's disease, 683
treatment of, 633
of prostate, 492, 778
of reproductive tract, 776–784
in females, 778–784
in males, 777–778
metastasis of, 776–777
retinoblastoma, 1025–1026
of salivary glands, 569
of scrotum, 777
of skin, 1123–1126
of spine, 982–983
of testis, 777–778
of thymus, in myasthenia gravis, 962
of urinary tract, 490–500
of uterus, 783–784
of vagina, 782
Tunica vaginalis
hematocele in, 759
hydrocele in, 758
Tuning fork, 910
in hearing tests, 1042
sound produced by, 1041
Turbinates, nasal, 1060
Two-point discrimination, 894, 910
Tympanic membrane, 1039, 1040
Tympanoplasty, 1054
Tympanostomy tube, 1056

Ulcer, 20
Curling's, in burns, 1154
cutaneous, 1099, 1128–1133
decubitus, 920, 1129–1133
prevention of, 170, 977, 1130–1131
of larynx, 1079
in oral cavity, 1073
peptic, 535, 543–551. *See also* Peptic ulcer
venous, 406–407, 1129
Ulcerative colitis, 551–553
Ultrasound
in diagnosis of biliary tract disease, 604
and echoencephalography, 915
Ultraviolet light therapy
in acne, 1109
in psoriasis, 1111
in skin lesions, 1108
Umbilical hernia, 580–581

Umbo, 1039
Unconsciousness, 919–922
in cerebral injuries, 942
nursing care in, 920–922
Unna's paste, 407
Upper extremity. *See* Arm
Urate crystals, in gout, 866
Urea clearance tests, 480–481
Urea nitrogen, blood, 480
in cardiovascular disorders, 326
in hypernatremia, 174
Uremia, 509
Ureter(s), 469
diverticula of, 491
ectopic, 503
obstruction in, 489–490
strictures of, 501
Ureteritis, 486
Ureterocele, 503, 773
Ureterosigmoidostomy, for urinary diversion, 494, 499
Ureterostomy, cutaneous, for urinary diversion, 494, 499
Urethra
caruncle of, 491
in prostatic hypertrophy, 761, 762
strictures of, 501
Urethritis, 486
Urethrovesical reflux, 484
Uric acid levels
in gout, 866
in leukemia, after chemotherapy, 446
Uric acid stones, 502
Urinary tract, 469–519
anomalies of, 503
assessment of, 471–481
calculi of, 501–503
catheterization of, 482–483
complications from immobilization, prevention of, 842
diagnostic tests of, 475–481
disorders of, 481–503
dilatation of, 469–471
infections in, 481–489
assessment of patient in, 486–487
causative organisms in, 486
hospital-acquired, 76–77
long-term consequences of, 488–489
prevention of, 488–489
treatment of, 487–488
intake and output measurements, 477
kidney disorders, 503–519. *See also* Kidney
neurogenic bladder, 483. *See also* Bladder
obstruction of, 489–503
in anomalies, 503
in calculi, 501–503
in trauma, 500–501
in tumors, 490–500
physical examination of, 475
radiographic studies of, 477–478
reflux of urine, 484–486
trauma of, 500–501
tumors of, 490–500
urine tests, 476–477
and voiding patterns, 469
Urination. *See* Micturition
Urine
in acidosis, metabolic, 185
bilirubin in, 604
in cardiac disease, 327
casts in, 473
collection of specimens, 473, 476
concentration tests, 480
constituents of, 161
in dehydration, 165
dilution tests, 480
diversion procedures, 494–500
drainage appliances in, 497–498
follow-up care in, 500
ileal conduit in, 494, 499
long-term management of, 498–500
postoperative care in, 495–497
preoperative preparation for, 495

stoma placement in, 497
ureterosigmoidostomy in, 494, 499
ureterostomy in, cutaneous, 494, 499
drainage appliances for, 497–498
examination of, 472–473
flow of, 469
hematuria, 472
in hypokalemia, 175
in hyponatremia, 172
in liver disease, 587
manual expression with Credé method, 975–976
output measurements, 477
pH of, 473
and stone formation, 503
pyuria, 472
reflux of, 484–486
prevention of, 469, 470
urethrovesical, 484
vesicoureteral, 484–486
in renal failure, 506
retention of
in obstruction of urinary tract, 489
in prostatic hypertrophy, 762–763
specific gravity of, 473, 480
tests of, 476–477
for diabetes, 696–697
urobilinogen in, 422, 587, 604
in water intoxication, 169
Urobilin, 583
Urobilinogen, 422
fecal, 422
urinary, 422, 587, 604
Urticaria, 1101
Uterosacral ligaments, 772
Uterus
adenomyosis of, 771
bleeding from, abnormal, 768–770
in carcinoma, 784
cervical conditions. *See* Cervix uteri
dilatation and curettage of, 748
in abnormal uterine bleeding, 769, 770
in endometrial carcinoma diagnosis, 783
dilatation and evacuation of, for abortion, 796–797
endometrial conditions. *See* Endometrium
estrogen affecting, 736
intrauterine contraceptive devices, 793–794
myomas of, 783
polyps of, 783
prolapse of, 772–775
pessaries in, 774–775
surgical repair of, 774
retroversion of, 776
sarcoma of, 783
tumors of, 783–784
Utricle, 1037, 1043
Uveal tract, 995
Uveitis, 1017
and sympathetic ophthalmia, 1019
Uvula, 1071

Vaccine administration. *See* Immunization
Vacuoles, cellular, 9
as phagosomes, 19
Vagina
cancer of, 782
estrogen affecting, 736
examination of, 740
pH of secretions, 736
pyknotic cells in smears from, 747
thrush in, 1116
vulvovaginitis, 1116
Vagotomy, 548–550
in peptic ulcer, 547
selective, 550
Vagus nerve, 899, 904
assessment of, 909
and hydrochloric acid secretion, 543

Valley fever, 287
Valsalva maneuver, 333
affecting intracranial pressure, 924
glottis closure in, 1076
hazards in, 351, 392
Valves, venous, 405
testing of competence, 406
Valvular heart disease, 372–373
prostheses in, 373, 385
surgical repair of, 373, 385
Van den Bergh test, 586
Vanillylmandelic acid excretion, in pheochromocytoma, 689
Varco's traction, 852
Varicella, 1120
Varicocele, 750, 759–760
repair of, 751
Varicose veins, 405–406
esophageal, 593–595
portasystemic shunting procedures in, 595–596
and hemorrhoids, 582
Vasculature. *See* Blood vessels
Vasectomy, 796
Vasoconstriction, 320
pulmonary, mechanisms in, 199, 201
Vasoconstrictors, in cardiogenic shock, 384
Vasodilatation, 320
in neurogenic shock, 1186
pulmonary, agents causing, 199
Vasodilators
in cardiogenic shock, 384
in chronic arterial insufficiency, 402
in peripheral vascular disease, 396
Vasopressin. *See* Antidiuretic hormone
Vasopressor agents, in shock, 1199–1200
Vater ampulla, 602
Vectorcardiogram, 328–329
Vehicles, for transmission of disease, 65
Veins, 321, 1181
disorders of, 404–408
of eye, 1001
thrombophlebitis, 407–408
ulcers of, 406–407, 1129
valves of, 405
testing of competence, 406
varicose, 405–406
ligation of, 406
Vellus hairs, 1095
Venacavagraphy, in Hodgkin's disease, 451
Venipunctures, repeated, discomfort from, 430
Venous pressure, central, in shock, 1196
Ventilation, 197–202
acute ventilatory failure, 230–246
alveolar, and carbon dioxide in blood, 163
control of, 203–206
hyperventilation, 202–203
dehydration from, 165
hypoventilation, 203
maximum voluntary, 215
ratio to perfusion, 198
Ventilatory assistance methods, 235–237
in acidosis, respiratory, 183
Ambu bag in, 235
for burn patients, 1150
in carcinoma of lung, 307
continuous positive airway pressure in, 229
intermittent positive pressure breathing with, 234
and mouth-to-mouth resuscitation, 368–370
nursing care with, 236–237
positive end-expiratory pressure in, 229
types of ventilators in, 235–236
weaning from, 237
Ventricles
cardiac
fibrillation in, 368
left, 313
right, 313

1234 Index

Ventricles, cardiac *Continued*
  rupture in myocardial infarction, 353
  cerebral, 900
    drainage of, 925
Ventriculography, 917
Ventriculostomy, in hydrocephalus, 933
Venules, 321, 1181
  in shock, 1190
Verbalization. *See* Speech
Vermis cerebelli, 896
Verruca
  filiformis, 1118
  plana, 1118
  plantaris, 1118
  vulgaris, 1118
Vertebra. *See* Spine and spinal cord
Vertebral arteries, 899
Vertigo, 906, 918, 1036–1037
  from caloric stimulation, 1039
  in Ménière's disease, 1057
  nystagmus with, 1043
  in otosclerosis, 1056
  after stapedectomy, 1057
Vesicles, 1099
Vesicotomy, 495
Vesicoureteral reflux, 484–486
Vestibular apparatus, 1037, 1040, 1043
  dysfunction of, 1057–1059
Vestibular functions of ear, 1035
  assessment of, 1036–1037
  caloric stimulation tests of, 1039, 1043–1044
Vestibule, of nose, 1060
Vestibulocochlear nerve, 898
  in acoustic neuroma, 946
Vestibulo-ocular reflexes, 1043
Vibration
  and ear function, 1040, 1041, 1045
  in phonation, 1076
  techniques in respiratory system dysfunction, 221
Vincent's angina, 542, 1073
Virilization, female, 688
Viruses
  and carcinogenesis, 110
  and common cold, 272
  in hepatitis, 588–591
  in influenza, 273–274
  in meningitis, 935
  in mononucleosis, infectious, 454
  pharyngitis from coxsackievirus, 273
  pneumonia from, 274–275
  in skin infections, 1118–1120
Vision, 993
  acuity measurements, 996–997
  fields of, testing of, 908, 997–998
  loss of. *See* Blindness
  physiology of, 994–995
  and prevention of blindness, 993–994
  substitution devices for, 1029
Vital capacity, 214
Vitamin A
  deficiency of, eyes in, 1006
  therapy in acne, 1109

Vitamin B deficiency, eyes in, 1006
Vitamin B_{12}, 415–416
  daily requirements for, 416
  deficiency of, 416, 433–435
  and RNA production, 416, 434
Vitamin C
  and bone growth, 815
  deficiency of, bleeding tendency in, 458
Vitamin D
  activity in renal failure, 510, 511
  and calcium metabolism, 665
  deficiency of
    hypocalcemia in, 178
    osteomalacia in, 867
  intoxication from, hypercalcemia in, 669
  malabsorption of, 568
  and osteogenesis, 814–815
  and parathyroid hormone activity, 665
  therapy with
    in hypocalcemia, 178
    in hypoparathyroidism, 671
Vitamin K
  deficiency of
    and hypoprothrombinemia, 459–460
    in liver disease, 586
  malabsorption of, 568
  as therapy in hemorrhage, 398
Vitiligo, 1101
Vitreous humor, 996
Vocal cords, 1074
  corectomy, 1080
  leukoplakia of, 1079
  nodules of, 1079
  papilloma of, 1079
  paralysis of, 1077
  removal of, 542
Voice
  in laryngeal dysfunction, 1076
  in thyroid disease, 639, 660
  thyroid surgery affecting, 656
Voice sounds, 210
  production of, 1074, 1076
VoiceBak prosthesis, 1086–1087
Voiding of urine. *See* Micturition
Volkmann's canals, 814
Volume
  blood. *See* Blood volume
  pulmonary, 214–216
    expiratory reserve, 215
    forced expiratory, 215
    inspiratory reserve, 215
    reduction of, diseases with, 228–229
    residual, 215
    tidal, 214
Volvulus, 573
Vomiting, 528, 562
  alkalosis from, metabolic, 187
  antiemetic drugs in, 562
  dehydration from, 165
  hematemesis in burns, 1154
  hypokalemia from, 175

reflex mechanisms in, 562
sodium loss in, 171
Vomitus, in intestinal obstruction, 571
Von Willebrand's disease, 461–462
Vulva, carcinoma of, 782–783
Vulvectomy, 782–783
Vulvovaginitis, 1116

Waldenstrom's macroglobulinemia, 455
Waldeyer's tonsillar ring, 1071
Walkers, use of, 882–883
Wangensteen suction machine, 537
Warfarin sodium, 398
  overdosage of, 460, 463
Warts, 1118–1119
  removal of, 1119
Washing of hands, and infection control, 74, 78
Watch test, for hearing acuity, 1042
Water
  intoxication, 169–171
    diagnosis of, 169–170
    disorders with, 169
    gradual onset of, 169
    nursing care in, 170–171
    rapid onset of, 169
  metabolism regulation by hormones, 12
  provocative test in glaucoma, 1002–1003
  restriction test in diabetes insipidus, 627
Waterhouse-Friderichsen syndrome, 678
Wax in ear. *See* Cerumen
Weakness
  in Cushing's disease, 681
  in myasthenia gravis, 962
  in renal failure, 511
  in shock, 1195
Weaning
  from mechanically assisted ventilation, 237
  from tracheostomy tube, 243
Weber hearing test, 1042
Wedge TM turning frame, 973
Weight
  control with low carbohydrate diet, 528
  gain in water intoxication, 169
  loss of
    in Addison's disease, 678
    in burns, 1151
    from thyroid hormone therapy, 661
  measurements in shock, 1195
  reduction of, 540–541
    in diabetes, 705
  thyroid disease affecting, 640–641
Wellness, definition of, 59
Wenckebach phenomenon, 359
Wertheim operation, in cervical carcinoma, 782
Wheal, 19, 1099
Wheelchairs, use of, 881, 883–884
  and care of, 978

in quadriplegia, 971
and skin care, 977
Wheezing, 210
  in asthma, 265
  in bronchitis, 262
Whipple's disease, 569
Whipple's procedure, in pancreatic cancer, 614
Whispered voice test, for hearing acuity, 1042
White cell count. *See* Leukocytes, count of
Whiteheads, 1108–1109
White matter, 891
Williams position, in traction, 852
Wilms' tumor, 490
Wilson's disease, 601
Wiring of jaws
  in fractures, 1068–1069
  in obesity, for weight reduction, 541
Wirsung duct, 608
Wiskott-Aldrich syndrome, 39
Withdrawal
  from alcohol, symptoms from, 600
  from cigarette smoking, 217–218
Wolff law, of bone growth, 814
Wolff-Parkinson-White syndrome, 357
Wood's light, 1104, 1117
Word-finding problems, in aphasia, 930
Work, and energy requirements, 10
Wound healing, 21, 101–105
  in amputations, 876
  in burns, 1155
  delayed, 103
  disease affecting, 22
  in fractures, 825–826
  healing phase in, 102
  lag phase in, 102
  in laryngectomy, 1083
  maturation phase in, 102
  primary union in, 101–102
  in renal failure, 506
  secondary union in, 102
  of surgical wounds, 101–105
Wrist, disarticulation of, 873

Xanthochromic cerebrospinal fluid, 913
Xanthomas, 1127–1128
Xenografts, 32
Xenon arc photocoagulation, for retinal holes, 1025
Xerography, 112
  of breast, 785
X-ray studies. *See* Radiology
Xylose tolerance tests, 568
  in pancreatic disease, 610

Z track technique, for parenteral iron administration, 432
Zollinger-Ellison syndrome, 548, 613, 614
Zygoma, fractures of, 1069
Zymogen granules, in chief cells, 525